This book is due for return on or before the last date shown below.

19/7/21		

Caffey's **Pediatric Diagnostic Imaging**

EDITOR-IN-CHIEF

Brian D. Coley, MD

Professor
Departments of Radiology and Pediatrics
University of Cincinnati College of Medicine
Radiologist-in-Chief
Department of Radiology
Cincinnati Children's Hospital Medical Center
Cincinnati, Ohio

Caffey's **Pediatric Diagnostic Imaging**

Twelfth Edition

VOLUME I

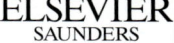

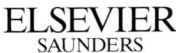
SAUNDERS

1600 John F. Kennedy Blvd.
Ste 1800
Philadelphia, PA 19103-2899

Senior Content Strategist: Don Scholz
Content Development Manager: Maureen Iannuzzi
Publishing Services Manager: Patricia Tannian
Project Manager: Carrie Stetz
Design Direction: Ellen Zanolle

Printed in China

Last digit is the print number: 9   8   7   6   5   4   3   2   1

To my family:
Elizabeth, Ian, Connor, and Kate;

To my teachers:
Gordon, Rosengard, Halasz, Mattrey, Olson,
Talner, Leopold, Forrest, Shultz, Patterson, Johnson,
Babcock, Siegel, Slovis, and others;

To my students, residents, and fellows
whom I have been privileged to teach;

To my many brilliant colleagues
who have taught and guided me;

And to the children whom I hope
to have played some role in helping:

Thank you all.

Tribute to Drs. John P. Caffey, Frederic N. Silverman, and Thomas L. Slovis

Caffey's Pediatric Diagnostic Imaging (titled *Caffey's Pediatric X-Ray Diagnosis* for the first nine editions) is the oldest continuous comprehensive textbook in this subspecialty. First published in 1945, it was the first English language text on the subject since Thomas Morgan Rotch's 1910 *The Roentgen Ray in Pediatrics*.

This book began as a labor of love for John Caffey in an era without computers, digital images, or internet bibliographic searches. Each chapter was meticulously dictated, typed, corrected, and typed again. Each radiograph was carefully selected from Dr. Caffey's own teaching file at Babies Hospital in New York City. Dr. Caffey, initially trained as a pediatrician, was an astute clinician who stressed that the radiographic findings were only one part of the diagnostic evaluation; proper patient care required the integration of the history, physical examination, laboratory data, and imaging. Despite the great effort involved, he was the sole author of the first four editions.

With the 1967 fifth edition, former Caffey fellow Dr. Frederic N. Silverman of Children's Hospital Cincinnati participated in preparation of the text, and continued as a co-editor of the sixth and seventh editions. With the death of Dr. Caffey in 1978, Dr. Silverman became sole editor of the eighth edition in 1985. Also trained as a pediatrician, he, too, stressed the importance of the physical examination and the need for accurate clinical information to properly interpret imaging studies.

Over time, Dr. Silverman added authors and expanded sections. Due to the increasing amount of information, he edited a one-volume *Essentials of Caffey's Pediatric X-Ray Diagnosis* in 1989 aimed at trainees, which was my first exposure to this text. Dr. Jerald P. Kuhn joined Silverman as co-editor with the 1993 ninth edition, and then succeeded him as editor. For the 2003 tenth edition, Dr. Kuhn added Drs. Jack O. Haller and Thomas L. Slovis as co-editors, two important figures in pediatric radiology education. Dr. Slovis (also originally trained as a pediatrician) lead the production of the eleventh edition, which was a significant modernization of the text and figures. This addition had eight associate editors overseeing subsections of the text, reflecting the growing complexity and expertise required in delivering pediatric imaging care.

In an era when information is so readily obtainable, it is easy to forget the importance books such as Caffey's have played in education and training. For decades, this was the definitive source of pediatric imaging information, crafted by experts in the field who brought their understanding of the literature and practical experience to the interested reader. Caffey and Silverman devoted more than half of their lives to creating the best book possible in an era when the work was done with typewriters, carbon paper, film, and darkrooms. That this book has survived is testimony to the quality of their work. Dr. Slovis continued that care and attention to detail to reflect the modernization of pediatric imaging, while at the same time continuing to stress the importance of the physical examination and keeping the child at the center of our focus. The impact of Caffey, Silverman, and Slovis on the education of prior generations of pediatric imagers cannot be underestimated and is certain to continue far into the future.

Brian D. Coley
Editor, twelfth edition
2013

Contributors

Sami Abedin, MD Department of Radiology, University of Missouri–Kansas City, Kansas City, Missouri

Brent Adler, MD Associate Clinical Professor, Department of Radiology, The Ohio State University, Nationwide Children's Hospital, Columbus, Ohio

Prachi P. Agarwal, MD Clinical Associate Professor, Department of Radiology, Division of Cardiothoracic Radiology, University of Michigan, Ann Arbor, Michigan

Kimberly E. Applegate, MD Professor of Radiology and Pediatrics, Director of Practice Quality Improvement, Department of Radiology and Imaging Sciences, Emory University School of Medicine, Atlanta, Georgia

E. Michel Azouz, MD Pediatric Radiologist, Medical Imaging, Montreal Children's Hospital; Pediatric Radiologist, Shriners Hospital for Children, Montreal, QC, Canada

Paul Babyn, MDCM Radiologist-in-Chief, Hospital for Sick Children, Toronto, ON, Canada; Head of University of Saskatchewan and Saskatoon, Health Region, Royal University Hospital; Professor of Medical Imaging, University of Saskatchewan, Canada

D. Gregory Bates, MD Clinical Associate Professor of Radiology, Ohio State University College of Medicine and Public Health; Assistant Chief, Clinical Operations and Section Chief Fluoroscopy, Nationwide Children's Hospital, Columbus, Ohio

Mary P. Bedard, MD Associate Neonatologist, Neonatal-Perinatal Medicine, Children's Hospital of Michigan, Detroit, Michigan

Gerald G. Behr, MD Department of Radiology, Morgan Stanley Children's Hospital of New York-Presbyterian and Columbia University, New York, New York

Sadaf T. Bhutta, MBBS Associate Professor, Department of Radiology, University of Arkansas for Medical Sciences, Little Rock, Arkansas

Larry A. Binkovitz, MD Associate Professor, Department of Diagnostic Radiology, Mayo Clinic, Rochester, Minnesota

Susan Blaser, MD Department of Diagnostic Imaging, The Hospital for Sick Children, Toronto, ON, Canada

Stefan Bluml, MD Associate Professor of Research Radiology; Director, New Imaging Technologies; Departments of Radiology and Pediatrics, Children's Hospital, Keck School of Medicine, University of Southern California, Los Angeles, California

Danielle K.B. Boal, MD Professor of Radiology and Pediatrics, Department of Radiology, Pennsylvania State University College of Medicine; Professor of Radiology and Pediatrics, Department of Radiology, Milton S. Hershey Medical Center, Hershey, Pennsylvania

Phillip M. Boiselle, MD Department of Radiology, Beth Israel Deaconess Medical Center and Harvard Medical School, Boston, Massachusetts

Timothy N. Booth, MD Professor, Department of Radiology, Children's Medical Center, University of Texas Southwestern Medical Center, Dallas, Texas

Emma E. Boylan, BA Department of Medical Imaging, Ann and Robert H. Lurie Children's Hospital of Chicago, Chicago, Illinois

Dorothy Bulas, MD Professor of Pediatrics and Radiology, Department of Diagnostic Imaging and Radiology, Children's National Medical Center, Washington, DC

Angela Byrne, MD Department of Radiology, Children's Hospital of British Columbia, Vancouver, BC, Canada

Alicia M. Casey, MD Department of Medicine, Division of Respiratory Diseases, Boston Children's Hospital and Harvard Medical School, Boston, Massachusetts

Christopher I. Cassady, MD Clinical Associate Professor, Department of Radiology, Baylor College of Medicine; Chief of Fetal Imaging, Pediatric Radiology, Texas Children's Hospital, Houston, Texas

Kim M. Cecil, PhD Departments of Radiology, Pediatrics, Neuroscience and Environmental Health, Cincinnati Children's Hospital Medical Center, University of Cincinnati College of Medicine, Cincinnati, Ohio

Rafael C. Ceschin, MD Department of Radiology, Children's Hospital of Pittsburgh of UPMC; Department of Biomedical Informatics, University of Pittsburgh, Pittsburgh, Pennsylvania

Frandics P. Chan, MD, PhD Associate Professor, Department of Radiology, Stanford University Medical Center, Stanford, California

Teresa Chapman, MD Staff Radiologist, Seattle Children's Hospital; Assistant Professor, Department of Radiology, University of Washington, Seattle, Washington

Grace R. Choi, MD Assistant Professor, Department of Pediatrics, Northwestern University Feinberg School of Medicine; Attending Physician, Pediatrics, Division of Cardiology, Ann and Robert H. Lurie Children's Hospital of Chicago, Chicago, Illinois

Winnie C.W. Chu, MB ChB Department of Imaging and Interventional Radiology, Prince of Wales Hospital and The Chinese Univerisity of Hong Kong, Hong Kong SAR, China

Harris L. Cohen, MD Professor and Chairman, Department of Radiology; Professor, Pediatrics and Obstetrics & Gynecology, University of Tennessee Health Science Center; Medical Director, Radiology, LeBonheur Children's Hospital, Memphis, Tennessee

Brian D. Coley, MD Professor, Departments of Radiology and Pediatrics, University of Cincinnati College of Medicine; Radiologist-in-Chief, Department of Radiology, Cincinnati Children's Hospital Medical Center, Cincinnati, Ohio

Moira L. Cooper, MD Associate Clinical Professor, University of Victoria, Victoria, BC, Canada

Hannah Crowley, MD Department of Radiology, Children's Hospital of Pittsburgh of UPMC, Pittsburgh, Pennsylvania

J.A. Gordon Culham, MD Professor, Department of Radiology, University of British Columbia; Pediatric Radiologist, Department of Radiology, British Columbia's Children's Hospital, Vancouver, BC, Canada

Pedro Daltro, MD Clinica de DiagnOstico Por Imagem, Rio de Janeiro, Brazil

Amy R. Danehy, MD Division of Pediatric Neuroradiology, Boston Children's Hospital; Instructor in Radiology, Harvard Medical School, Boston, Massachusetts

Alan Daneman, MB BCh Radiologist, Department of Diagnostic Imaging; Division Head of General Radiology and Body Imaging, The Hospital for Sick Children; Professor, Medical Imaging, University of Toronto, Toronto, ON, Canada

Karunamoy Das, MD King Fahad Hospital, Dammam, Saudi Arabia

Andrew deFreitas, MD Assistant Professor of Pediatrics, Northwestern University Feinberg School of Medicine; Director, Adult Congenital Heart Disease, Ann and Robert H. Lurie Children's Hospital of Chicago, Chicago, Illinois

Katyucia de Macedo Rodrigues, MD Research Fellow, Radiology, Boston Children's Hospital; Research Fellow, Radiology, A.A. Martinos Center/Massachusetts General Hospital, Boston, Massachusetts

Jonathan R. Dillman, MD Assistant Professor, Department of Radiology, Section of Pediatric Radiology, University of Michigan Health System, Ann Arbor, Michigan

Lincoln O. Diniz, MD Department of Radiology, Cincinnati Children's Hospital Medical Center, Cincinnati, Ohio

Mary T. Donofrio, MD Associate Professor of Pediatrics, George Washington University; Director of the Fetal Heart Program, Children's National Heart Institute, Children's National Medical Center, Washington, DC

Andrea Schwarz Doria, MD, PhD, MSc Staff Radiologist/Clinician-Scientist, Department of Diagnostic Imaging; Scientist, Research Institute, The Hospital for Sick Children; Associate Professor, Faculty of Medicine, University of Toronto, Toronto, ON, Canada

Adam L. Dorfman, MD Clinical Associate Professor, Departments of Pediatrics and Radiology, University of Michigan, Ann Arbor, Michigan

Laura A. Drubach, MD Department of Radiology, Division of Nuclear Medicine, Boston Children's Hospital and Harvard Medical School, Boston, Massachusetts

Josée Dubois, MD, MSc Professor, Department of Radiology, Radio-Oncology, and Nuclear Medicine, University of Montreal; Chief, Department of Medical Imaging, CHU Sainte-Justine, Montreal, QC, Canada

Jerry Dwek, MD Clinical Adjunct Assistant Professor of Radiology, University of California at San Diego; Department of Radiology, Rady Children's Hospital and Health Center, San Diego Imaging, San Diego, California

Eric L. Effmann, MD Professor of Radiology, Department of Radiology, University of Washington; Division Chief, General Diagnosis, Department of Radiology, Seattle Children's Hospital, Seattle, Washington

Wendy D. Ellis, MD Assistant Professor, Department of Radiology, Vanderbilt University, Nashville, Tennessee

Monica Epelman, MD Department of Radiology, The Children's Hospital of Philadelphia, Philadelphia, Pennsylvania

Eric N. Faerber, MD Professor of Radiology and Pediatrics, Drexel University College of Medicine; Director, Department of Radiology, St. Christopher's Hospital for Children, Philadelphia, Pennsylvania

Nancy R. Fefferman, MD Assistant Professor of Radiology, Department of Radiology; Section Chief, Pediatric Radiology, NYU School of Medicine, New York, New York

Kate A. Feinstein, MD Professor of Radiology and Surgery; Section Chief, Pediatric Radiology, Comer Children's Hospital at University of Chicago, Chicago, Illinois

Celia M. Ferrari, MD Department of Radiology, Hospital de Ninos Sor Maria Ludovic, La Plata, Argentina

Tamara Feygin, MD Assistant Professor of Radiology, University of Pennsylvania School of Medicine, Neuroradiology, The Children's Hospital of Philadelphia, Philadelphia, Pennsylvania

Kristin Fickenscher, MD Assistant Professor and Fellowship Program Director, Radiology and Pediatrics, University of Missouri-Kansas City; Pediatric Radiologist, Children's Mercy Hospital and Clinics, Kansas City, Missouri

A. Michelle Fink, MD Department of Medical Imaging, The Royal Children's Hospital, Melbourne, Australia

Martha P. Fishman, MD Department of Medicine, Division of Respiratory Diseases, Boston Children's Hospital and Harvard Medical School, Boston, Massachusetts

Donald P. Frush, MD Chief of Pediatric Radiology, Duke University, Durham, North Carolina

Andre D. Furtado, MD Department of Pediatric Radiology, Department of Pediatrics, Division of Neurology, Children's Hospital of Pittsburgh of UPMC, Pittsburgh, Pennsylvania

Ana Maria Gaca, MD Assistant Professor, Department of Radiology, Duke University Medical Center, Durham, North Carolina

Asvin M. Ganapathi, MD Department of Surgery, Duke University Medical Center, Durham, North Carolina

Seth Gibson, DO Department of Radiology, University of Missouri-Kansas City; Radiology Fellow, Children's Mercy Hospitals and Clinics, Kansas City, Missouri

Hyun Woo Goo, MD Department of Radiology and Research Institute of Radiology, Asan Medical Center, University of Ulsan College of Medicine, Seoul, Korea

P. Ellen Grant, MD Associate Professor, Department of Radiology; Director, Fetal-Neonatal Neuroimaging and Developmental Science Center, Boston Children's Hospital, Boston, Massachusetts

J. Damien Grattan-Smith, MBBS Department of Radiology, Children's Healthcare of Atlanta, Atlanta, Georgia

S. Bruce Greenberg, MD Professor of Radiology and Pediatrics, Department of Radiology, University of Arkansas for Medical Sciences, Little Rock, Arkansas

John P. Grimm, MD Assistant Professor, Children's Hospital Los Angeles, Keck School of Medicine, University of Southern California, Los Angeles, California

R. Paul Guillerman, MD Associate Professor of Radiology, Baylor College of Medicine, Edward B. Singelton Department of Pediatric Radiology, Texas Children's Hospital, Baylor College of Medicine, Houston, Texas

Stephen M. Henesch, DO Director of Pediatric Radiology, Radiology Consulting of Long Island; Imaging Services Department, Good Samaritan Hospital Medical Center, West Islip, New York

James René Herlong, MD Associate Clinical Professor of Pediatrics, University of North Carolina School of Medicine; Division Chief, Pediatric Cardiology, Sanger Heart and Vascular Institute, Charlotte, North Carolina

Marta Hernanz-Schulman, MD Professor of Radiology and Pediatrics, Vanderbilt University Medical Center; Medical Director, Diagnostic Imaging, Monroe Carell, Jr. Children's Hospital at Vanderbilt, Nashville, Tennessee

Melissa A. Hilmes, MD Assistant Professor, Department of Radiology & Radiological Sciences, Vanderbilt University School of Medicine, Nashville, Tennessee

Hollie A. Jackson, MD Associate Professor, Department of Radiology, Children's Hospital Los Angeles, Keck School of Medicine University of Southern California, Los Angeles, California

J. Herman Kan, MD Associate Professor, Baylor College of Medicine; Section Chief, Musculoskeletal Imaging, E.B. Singleton Pediatric Radiology, Texas Children's Hospital, Houston, Texas

Ronald J. Kanter, MD Professor, Departments of Pediatrics & Medicine; Director, Pediatric Electrophysiology, Duke University Medical Center, Durham, North Carolina

Sue Creviston Kaste, DO Professor of Radiology, University of Tennessee Health Science Center; Member, Radiological Sciences, St. Jude Children's Research Hospital, Memphis, Tennessee

Paritosh C. Khanna, MD Department of Radiology, Seattle Children's Hospital, Seattle, Washington

Stanley T. Kim, MD Assistant Professor, Department of Radiology, Northwestern University Feinberg School of Medicine, Chicago, Illinois

Sunhee Kim, MD Assistant Professor, Department of Diagnostic Radiology, University of Pittsburgh, Children's Hospital of Pittsburgh of UPMC, Pittsburgh, Pennsylvania

Joshua Q. Knowlton, MD, MPH Pediatric Radiologist, Department of Radiology, Children's Mercy Hospital, Kansas City, Missouri

Amy B. Kolbe, MD Pediatric Radiology Fellow, Department of Radiology, Mayo Clinic, Rochester, Minnesota

Korgün Koral, MD Associate Professor, Department of Radiology, University of Texas Southwestern Medical Center; Department of Radiology, Children's Medical Center, Dallas, Texas

Rajesh Krishnamurthy, MD Director of Cardiovascular Imaging, EB Singleton Department of Pediatric Radiology, Texas Children's Hospital; Associate Professor of Radiology and Pediatrics, Baylor College of Medicine, Houston, Texas

Anita Krishnan, MD Pediatric Cardiologist, Children's National Medical Center, Washington, DC

Ralph Lachman, MD Emeritus Professor, Radiology & Pediatrics, UCLA School of Medicine; International Skeletal Dysplasia Registry, Medical Genetics Institute, Cedars-Sinai Medical Center, Los Angeles, California; Consulting Clinical Professor, Stanford University, Stanford, California

Tal Laor, MD Professor of Radiology and Pediatrics, University of Cincinnati College of Medicine; Co-Section Chief, Musculoskeletal Imaging, Department of Radiology, Cincinnati Children's Hospital Medical Center, Cincinnati, Ohio

Bernard F. Laya, MD, DO Associate Professor of Radiology; Director, Institute of Radiology, St. Luke's Medical Center, Global City, Taguig City, The Philippines

James Leach, MD Associate Professor, Department of Radiology, Cincinnati Children's Hospital Medical Center; Associate Professor, Department of Radiology, University of Cincinnati College of Medicine, Cincinnati, Ohio

Henrique M. Lederman, MD Professor of Radiology, Department of Diagnostic Imaging, Federal University of Sao Paulo; Chief, Center of Diagnostic Imaging, Pediatric Oncology Institute, Sao Paulo, Brazil

Edward Y. Lee, MD, MPH Associate Professor of Radiology and Chief, Division of Thoracic Imaging; Director, Magnetic Resonance Imaging, Departments of Radiology and Medicine, Pulmonary Division, Boston Children's Hospital and Harvard Medical School, Boston, Massachusetts

Craig W. Lillehei, MD Department of Surgery, Boston Children's Hospital and Harvard Medical School, Boston, Massachusetts

Andrew J. Lodge, MD Assistant Professor, Department of Surgery; Assistant Professor, Department of Pediatrics, Duke University Medical Center, Durham, North Carolina

Lisa H. Lowe, MD Professor, Department of Pediatrics, Children's Mercy Hospitals and Clinics; Professor, Academic Chair and Residency Program Director, Department of Radiology, University of Missouri-Kansas City, Kansas City, Missouri

Jimmy C. Lu, MD Clinical Assistant Professor, Departments of Pediatrics and Radiology, University of Michigan, Ann Arbor, Michigan

Cathy MacDonald, MD Assistant Professor, Department of Medical Imaging, University of Toronto; Staff Radiologist, Department of Diagnostic Imaging, The Hospital for Sick Children, Toronto, ON, Canada

Maryam Ghadimi Mahani, MD Clinical Assistant Professor, Department of Radiology, University of Michigan, Ann Arbor, Michigan

Diana V. Marin, MD Pediatric Radiologist, Department of Radiology, Miami Children's Hospital, Miami, Florida

John B. Mawson, MB, CHB (NZ) Assistant Professor, Department of Radiology, University of British Columbia; Pediatric Radiologist, Department of Radiology, British Columbia's Children's Hospital, Vancouver, BC, Canada

Charles M. Maxfield, MD Associate Professor of Radiology and Pediatrics, Duke University Medical Center, Durham, North Carolina

William H. McAlister, MD Professor of Radiology and Pediatrics, Department of Pediatric Radiology, Washington University Medical School, St. Louis, Missouri

M. Beth McCarville, MD Associate Member, Department of Radiological Sciences, St. Jude Children's Research Hospital, Memphis, Tennessee

James S. Meyer, MD Associate Professor of Radiology, University of Pennsylvania School of Medicine; Associate Radiologist-in-Chief, Department of Radiology, Children's Hospital of Philadelphia, Philadelphia, Pennsylvania

Sarah S. Milla, MD Assistant Professor, Department of Radiology, New York University Langone Medical Center, New York, New York

Elka Miller, MD Chief/Medical Director and Research Director, Diagnostic Imaging Department, Children's Hospital of Eastern Ontario; Assistant Professor, Department of Radiology, University of Ottawa, ON, Canada

David M. Mirsky, MD Pediatric Neuroradiology Fellow, The Children's Hospital of Philadelphia, Philadelphia, Pennsylvania

David A. Mong, MD Department of Radiology, The Children's Hospital of Philadelphia, Philadelphia, Pennsylvania

Kevin R. Moore, MD Vice Chair of Radiology; Director of MR Imaging, Department of Medical Imaging, Primary Children's Medical Center; Adjunct Associate, Professor of Radiology, Department of Radiology, University of Utah, Salt Lake City, Utah

Oscar Navarro, MD Assistant Professor, Department of Medical Imaging, University of Toronto; Staff Radiologist, Department of Diagnostic Imaging, The Hospital for Sick Children, Toronto, ON, Canada

Marvin D. Nelson Jr, MD, MBA Chairman, Department of Radiology, Children's Hospital Los Angeles; Professor, Department of Radiology, Keck School of Medicine, University of Southern California, Los Angeles, California

Beverley Newman, BSc, MB BCh Associate Professor, Department of Radiology, Lucile Packard Children's Hospital at Stanford University, Stanford, California

Julie Currie O'Donovan, MD Pediatric Radiologist, Department of Radiology, Nationwide Children's Hospital; Clinical Assistant Professor of Radiology, The Ohio State University Medical Center, Columbus, Ohio

Robert C. Orth, MD, PhD Assistant Professor of Radiology, Baylor College of Medicine, Edward B. Singleton Department of Pediatric Radiology, Texas Children's Hospital, Houston, Texas

Deepa R. Pai, MHSA, MD Assistant Clinical Professor, Department of Radiology, Section of Pediatric Radiology, University of Michigan, Ann Arbor, Michigan

Michael J. Painter, MD Department of Pediatric Radiology, Department of Pediatrics, Division of Neurology, Children's Hospital of Pittsburgh of UPMC, Pittsburgh, Pennsylvania

Harriet J. Paltiel, MD Radiologist, Boston Children's Hospital; Associate Professor of Radiology, Harvard Medical School, Boston, Massachusetts

Ajaya R. Pande, MD Department of Radiology, Children's Hospital of Pittsburgh of UPMC, Pittsburgh, Pennsylvania

Ashok Panigrahy, MD Radiologist-in-Chief, Associate Professor of Radiology, Children's Hospital of Pittsburgh of UPMC, Pittsburgh, Pennsylvania

Angira Patel, MD, MPH Assistant Professor of Pediatrics, Department of Pediatric Cardiology, Northwestern University Feinberg School of Medicine; Attending Physician, Pediatric Cardiology, Ann and Robert H. Lurie Children's Hospital of Chicago, Chicago, Illinois

Grace S. Phillips, MD Assistant Professor, Department of Radiology, University of Washington School of Medicine; Division Chief, Computed Tomography, Department of Radiology, Seattle Children's Hospital, Seattle, Washington

Avrum N. Pollock, MD Associate Professor of Radiology, Department of Radiology, Division of Neuroradiology, The Children's Hospital of Philadelphia, Philadelphia, Pennsylvania

Andrada R. Popescu, MD Radiology Fellow, Ann and Robert H. Lurie Children's Hospital of Chicago, Chicago, Illinois

Tina Young Poussaint, MD Professor of Radiology, Harvard Medical School; Attending Neuroradiologist, Department of Radiology, Boston Children's Hospital, Boston, Massachusetts

Sanjay P. Prabhu, MBBS Instructor in Radiology, Harvard Medical School; Attending Neuroradiologist, Department of Radiology, Boston Children's Hospital, Boston, Massachusetts

Sumit Pruthi, MD Assistant Professor, Department of Radiology & Radiological Sciences, Vanderbilt University, Memphis, Tennessee

Anand Dorai Raju, MD Department of Radiology, LeBonheur Children's Hospital, Memphis, Tennessee

Brenton D. Reading, MD Assistant Professor of Radiology, Department of Pediatric Radiology, University of Missouri-Kansas City, Kansas City, Missouri

Brian Reilly, RT(R) 3D Imaging Specialist, Department of Medical Imaging, Ann and Robert H. Lurie Children's Hospital of Chicago, Chicago, Illinois

Ricardo Restrepo, MD Department of Radiology, Miami Children's Hospital, Miami, Florida

John F. Rhodes, MD Associate Professor, Departments of Pediatrics & Medicine; Chief, Duke Children's Heart Center; Director, Pediatric & Adult Congenital Cardiac Catheterization Laboratory, Duke University Medical Center, Durham, North Carolina

Michael Riccabona, MD University Professor, Department of Radiology, Division of Pediatric Radiology, Universitätsklinikum-LKH Graz, Auenbruggenplatz, Graz, Australia

Cynthia K. Rigsby, MD Professor of Radiology and Pediatrics, Northwestern University Feinberg School of Medicine; Division Head, Body Imaging and Vice Chair, Medical Imaging, Ann and Robert H. Lurie Children's Hospital of Chicago, Chicago, Illinois

Douglas C. Rivard, DO Assistant Professor, Department of Radiology, Children's Mercy Hospital and Clinics, Kansas City, Missouri

Richard L. Robertson, MD Radiologist-in-Chief, Division of Pediatric Neuroradiology, Boston Children's Hospital; Associate Professor of Radiology, Harvard Medical School, Boston, Massachusetts

Ashley J. Robinson, MD Department of Radiology, Children's Hospital of British Columbia, Vancouver, BC; Department of Diagnostic Imaging, The Hospital for Sick Children, Toronto, ON, Canada

Joshua D. Robinson, MD Division of Cardiology, Children's Memorial Hospital, Department of Pediatrics, Northwestern University Feinberg School of Medicine, Chicago, Illinois

Caroline D. Robson, MB ChB Operations Vice Chair and Division Chief of Neuroradiology, Department of Radiology, Boston Children's Hospital; Associate Professor, Department of Radiology, Harvard Medical School, Boston, Massachusetts

Diana P. Rodriguez, MD Radiologist, Boston Children's Hospital, Boston, Massachusetts

Nancy Rollins, MD Medical Director, Department of Radiology, Children's Medical Center; Professor, Department of Radiology, University Texas Southwestern Medical Center, Dallas, Texas

Lucy B. Rorke-Adams, MD Senior Neuropathologist, Division of Neuropathology; Clinical Professor, Pathology and Laboratory Medicine, Perelman School of Medicine at the University of Pennsylvania, Philadelphia, Pennsylvania

Arlene A. Rozzelle, MD Associate Professor, Department of Surgery, Wayne State University School of Medicine; Chief, Plastic & Reconstructive Surgery, Children's Hospital of Michigan; Director, CHM Cleft/Craniofacial Anomalies Program Director, CHM Vascular Anomalies Team, Children's Hospital of Michigan, Detroit, Michigan

Gauravi Sabharwal, MBBS Section Head, Pediatric Radiology, Henry Ford Hospital and Health Network; Clinical Assistant Professor of Radiology, Wayne State University School of Medicine, Detroit, Michigan

Vincent J. Schmithorst, PhD Department of Radiology, Children's Hospital of Pittsburgh of UPMC, Pittsburgh, Pennsylvania

Erin Simon Schwartz, MD Associate Professor of Radiology, Perelman School of Medicine at the University of Pennsylvania; Clinical Director, The Lurie Family Foundation's Magnetoencephalography Imaging Center, Department of Radiology, Division of Neuroradiology, The Children's Hospital of Philadelphia, Philadelphia, Pennsylvania

Jayne M. Seekins, DO Instructor, Department of Radiology and Radiological Sciences, Vanderbilt University, Nashville, Tennessee

Sabah Servaes, MD Assistant Professor, Department of Radiology, The Children's Hospital of Philadelphia, Philadelphia, Pennsylvania

Virendersingh K. Sheorain, MD Radiology Fellow, University of Tennessee Health Science Center, Memphis, Tennessee

Richard M. Shore, MD Divison Head, General Radiology and Nuclear Medicine, Medical Imaging, Ann & Robert H. Lurie Children's Hospital of Chicago; Professor, Radiology, Northwestern University Feinberg School of Medicine, Chicago, Illinois

Sudha P. Singh, MBBS, MD Assistant Professor, Department of Radiology and Radiological Sciences, Vanderbilt University, Nashville, Tennessee

Carlos J. Sivit, MD Professor of Radiology and Pediatrics, Case Western Reserve School of Medicine; Vice Chairman, Clinical Operations, University Hospitals Case Medical Center, Cleveland, Ohio

Thomas L. Slovis, MD Professor, Department of Pediatric Imaging, Wayne State University School of Medicine; Emeritus Chief, Pediatric Imaging, Children's Hospital of Michigan, Detroit, Michigan

Christopher J. Smith, MD University of Missouri-Kansas City School of Medicine, Kansas City, Missouri

Gloria Soto, MD Department of Radiology, Clinica Alemana de Santiago, Santiago, Chile

Vera R. Sperling, MD Assistant Clinical Professor, Department of Radiology, Children's Hospital of Pittsburgh of UPMC, Pittsburgh, Pennsylvania

Stephanie E. Spottswood, MD, MSPH Associate Professor of Radiology, Department of Diagnostic Imaging, Monroe Carell, Jr. Children's Hospital at Vanderbilt University, Nashville, Tennessee

Gayathri Sreedher, MD Department of Pediatric Radiology, Children's Hospital of Pittsburgh of UPMC, Pittsburgh, Pennsylvania

Jan Stauss, MD Medical X-Ray Consultants, Eau Claire, Wisconsin

Peter J. Strouse, MD Professor and Director, Section of Pediatric Radiology, Department of Radiology, University of Michigan Health System, Ann Arbor, Michigan

George A. Taylor, MD Radiologist-in-Chief Emeritus, Department of Radiology, Boston Children's Hospital; John A. Kirkpatrick Professor of Radiology (Pediatrics), Department of Radiology, Harvard Medical School, Boston, Massachusetts

Paul Thacker, MD Instructor, Pediatric Radiology, Children's Mercy Hospitals and Clinics, Kansas City, Missouri

Darshit Thakrar, MD Advanced Pediatric Radiology Fellow, Department of Medical Imaging, Children's Memorial Hospital, Northwestern University Feinberg School of Medicine, Chicago, Illinois

Mahesh M. Thapa, MD Program Director, Radiology Medical Education, Seattle Children's Hospital; Associate Professor, Department of Radiology, UW Medicine, Seattle, Washington

Jean A. Tkach, PhD Associate Professor, Department of Radiology, Imaging Research Center, Cincinnati Children's Hospital Medical Center, Cincinnati, Ohio

Alexander J. Towbin, MD Assistant Professor of Radiology, Department of Radiology, Cincinnati Children's Hospital Medical Center, Cincinnati, Ohio

Donald A. Tracy, MD Assistant Professor of Radiology, Tufts University School of Medicine; Chief of Pediatric Radiology, Tufts Medical Center and Floating Hospital for Children, Boston, Massachusetts

Jeffrey Traubici, MD Assistant Professor, Medical Imaging, University of Toronto; Radiologist, The Hospital for Sick Children, Toronto, ON, Canada

S. Ted Treves, MD Chief, Division of Nuclear Medicine and Molecular Imaging, Radiology, Boston Children's Hospital; Professor of Radiology and Director of the Joint Program in Nuclear Medicine Radiology, Harvard Medical School, Boston, Massachusetts

Shreyas S. Vasanawala, MD, PhD Assistant Professor, Department of Radiology, Stanford University, Stanford, California

Arastoo Vossough, PhD, MD Assistant Professor of Radiology, University of Pennsylvania; Department of Radiology, Children's Hospital of Philadelphia, Philadelphia, Pennsylvania

Robert G. Wells, MD Associate Professor of Radiology and Pediatrics, Medical College of Wisconsin; Pediatric Radiologist, Pediatric Diagnostic Imaging, Milwaukee, Wisconsin; Director, Pediatric Radiology, Northwestern Lake Forest Hospital, Lake Forest, Illinois

Sjirk J. Westra, MD Associate Professor of Radiology, Department of Radiology, Massachusetts General Hospital and Harvard Medical School, Boston, Massachusetts

Elysa Widjaja, MBBS, MRCP, MD, MPH Neuroradiologist, Department of Diagnostic Imaging, The Hospital for Sick Children; Associate Professor, Medical Imaging, University of Toronto, Toronto, ON, Canada

Sally Wildman, DO Pediatric Radiologist, Department of Radiology, Nationwide Children's Hospital; Assistant Professor, Department of Radiology, The Ohio State University Medical Center, Columbus, Ohio

Peter Winningham, MD Department of Radiology, University of Missouri–Kansas City, Kansas City, Missouri

Jessica L. Wisnowski, PhD Department of Pediatric Radiology, Department of Pediatrics, Division of Neurology, Children's Hospital of Pittsburgh of UPMC, Pittsburgh, Pennsylvania; Department of Radiology, Children's Hospital Los Angeles; Brain and Creativity Institute, University of Southern California, Los Angeles, California

Ali Yikilmaz, MD Associate Professor of Radiology, Department of Pediatric Radiology, Erciyes University Medical Center, Erciyes University; Department of Pediatric Radiology, Children's Hospital, Kayseri, Turkey

Adam Zarchan, MD Assistant Clinical Professor, Department of Diagnostic Radiology, University of Kansas-Wichita; Pediatric Radiologist, Wesley Medical Center, Wichita, Kansas

Giulio Zuccoli, MD Radiology Department, Children's Hospital of Pittsburgh of UPMC, Pittsburgh, Pennsylvania

Evan J. Zucker, MD Radiology Resident, Tufts Medical Center and Floating Hospital for Children; Clinical Associate in Radiology, Tufts University School of Medicine, Boston, Massachusetts

Foreword

The twelfth edition of *Caffey's Pediatric Diagnostic Imaging* reflects the evolution of a powerful educational tool. It is shorter as a book but infinitely longer when one includes the many online images, videos, and supplemental text.

Since the 1945 first edition, the organization of topics and their placement in "The Book" has varied from purely anatomic to organ system and disease. In 1972, the sixth edition, the neonatal section first appeared and continued through the most recent edition. Modality chapters were specifically noted in the table of contents when Dr. Frederic Silverman became the editor of the eighth edition in 1985. The incorporation in 2003, when Drs. Jerald Kuhn, Thomas Slovis, and Jack Haller shared the editorship, of an initial section on the "Effects of Radiation" followed by "Neonatal Imaging" emphasized the importance of these topics in our practice. Chapters on prenatal imaging first formally appear with this edition.

Through the years the authorship has grown from Dr. John Caffey alone to Drs. Caffey and Silverman to literally more than 100 hundred experts. This is important because the authors are not only pediatric radiologists, but also superb pediatric subspecialists and scientists in the technical aspects of multimodality imaging. This mix has brought us back to our clinical roots.

Caffey's Pediatric Diagnostic Imaging is more than an imaging text. The twelfth edition reflects the evolution of pediatric radiology and pediatric medicine. The initial section, "Radiation Effects and Safety," expresses our concern for the safety of our patients in the broad context of radiation, use of magnetic resonance imaging, and contrast effects.

Neonatal and perinatal imaging has been incorporated into organ system chapters to emphasize the continuum of an abnormality throughout the patient's life. The concept of "the best test" has allowed elimination of the modality approach, and each test is discussed when appropriate in the disease state. Interventional radiology has been incorporated into those chapters when it is useful.

Dr. Brian Coley and his team have a done a superb job of making our educational experience more efficient. The continual change we see with each edition not only reflects the need for us to "keep up" with the science, but also emphasizes what is best for our patients.

Congratulations, Brian.

Thomas L. Slovis, MD
Professor Emeritus
Department of Radiology
Wayne State School of Medicine
Emeritus Chairman
Department of Imaging
Children's Hospital of Michigan
Detroit, Michigan

How and where we seek information differ today from 1945, when the first edition of *Caffey's Pediatric X-Ray Diagnosis* was published. There was no Internet, Google, or PubMed; you could make a Photostat of an article, but no Xerox machines existed yet. Journals of the day contained the latest research, but the synthesis of that knowledge with practical experience came in the form of the textbook. Historically, the landmark textbooks were written by the most influential leaders in their fields and were usually solo efforts (one can speculate whether ego or difficulties of collaboration played the greater part). A small number of valuable and influential texts have outlived their creators, evolving over years through the efforts of new authors and editors. Sir William Osler's *The Principles and Practice of Medicine* was published from 1892 to 2001; Sir Vincent Zachary Cope's *Early Diagnosis of the Acute Abdomen,* currently in its twenty-second edition, first appeared in 1921. Other such venerable texts still being published include Harrison's *Principles of Internal Medicine* (1950), Nelson's *Textbook of Pediatrics* (1945), and Goodman & Gilman's *The Pharmacological Basis of Therapeutics* (1941). *Caffey's Pediatric Diagnostic Imaging* has also proven its lasting value and importance over almost six decades.

But how we collect, store, and access information has changed. Even the most technophobic among us obtains information regularly via electronic means. For those of us fond of our computers and mobile devices, we can indulge in a deluge of data at any time or location. The ability to find information and answers to specific questions is a tremendous benefit to medical care and education. The quality of the information retrieved online, however, is sometimes unclear. Further, freely available Internet content is often truncated and condensed to suit a culture of shortened attention span. How well are subtleties or syntheses conveyed by a single screen page summary or bullet point list? As we learn more about the science of education, what is the best method of presenting information to learners both young and old?

Are books such as this one still relevant? Clearly, I have a somewhat biased viewpoint. I believe that well-constructed prose from an author with expert knowledge and practical real-world experience, coupled with illustrative images and diagrams, is a powerful and efficient way to transmit information and facilitate learning. Lists of facts and bullet point paragraphs cannot convey more complex concepts and syntheses. No matter what the medium, content counts. And books such as this one have tremendously valuable content.

That said, there is ongoing debate as to the best medium in which to disseminate complex and comprehensive content. Books are simple to use. They are familiar. It is easy to flip from section to section, to go back a few pages without losing your place. You can take notes in the margins. Books can also be heavy and cumbersome. They are costly to manufacture. Electronic formats have their pros and cons as well. A light, portable laptop or tablet may contain thousands of books' worth of information. Images can be manipulated as in actual practice. Video and animations can augment the learning experience. Online texts can be accessed anywhere with an Internet connection. Content length need not be dictated by physical page limitations. However, the device screen size dictates and somewhat limits the amount and method of information display. Moving back and forth between content sections can be awkward.

The twelfth edition of this text reflects the conflict and state of flux in publishing. There is a physical book. There are more explanatory diagrams and illustrations with better use of color, and I have tried to continue the work of Dr. Slovis in updating and improving the images. This edition adds a significant online and electronic presence. Additional images, animations, and videos are available online to supplement the print volume and to allow those who prefer electronic media to take advantage of the material in an alternate way.

The authors and section editors have contributed significant updates regarding newer imaging modalities, the understanding of disease processes, imaging appropriateness, and the importance of minimizing radiation exposure. As with the last edition, there has been input from many clinical specialists, providing perspective on the important role of imaging in the care of children. The authors and section editors have my thanks.

I would like to thank the team at Elsevier. Rebecca Gaertner and Kristina Oberle helped to get this edition started. Maureen Iannuzzi and Don Scholz were my main partners in this project. I especially appreciate Maureen's hard work in keeping us on task and her sense of humor. Carrie Stetz oversaw the layout and proof part of the production, helping to give the book its updated look.

I hope that this twelfth edition of Caffey is helpful to you and to the patients you serve.

Brian D. Coley, MD

Preface to First Edition

*Shadows are but dark holes in radiant streams, twisted rifts
beyond the substance, meaningless in themselves.*

*He who would comprehend Röntgen's pallid shades need always
to know well the solid matrix whence they spring. The physician
needs to know intimately each living patient through whom the
racing black light darts, and flashing the hidden depths reveals
them in a glowing mirage of thin images, each cast delicately in
its own halo, but all veiled and blended endlessly.*

*Man — warm, lively, fleshy man — and his story are both root
and key to his shadows; shadows cold, silent and empty. —*
JOHN CAFFEY

Within a few weeks after Röntgen announced his now
renowned discovery to the world in December 1895, the
x-ray method of examination was applied to infants and
children. The Vienna letter of February 29 (M. Rec. 49:312,
1896) contained a roentgen print of the arm of an infant
made of Kreidl in Vienna: this is the second reproduction of
a roentgen image in the American literature. Credit for the
first recorded roentgen examination of an infant in the United
States undoubtedly belongs to Dr. E.P. Davis of New York
City, who described the roentgen shadows cast by the trunk
of a living infant and the skull of a dead fetus in March 1896.
In his remarkable article (The study of the infant body and
the pregnant womb by the roentgen ray, Am. J. M. Sc.
111:263, 1896), Dr. Davis also included three drawings of
shadows visualized by means of a skiascope—shadows of the
feet, elbows, and orbit of a living infant. Feilchenfeld's discussion of spina ventosa in May 1896 is probably the first roentgen description of morbid anatomy in children (Berlin. Klin.
Wchnschr. 33:403, 1896). There were only two roentgen
pediatric publications in 1896; the number increased to 14
in 1897.

In 1898, Escherich of Graz had had sufficient experience
with pediatric roentgen examinations to write a general
exposition on the merits and weaknesses of the method (La
valeur diagnostique de la radiographie chez les enfants, Rev.
d. mal. de l'enf. 16:233, May 1898). This is a highly interesting and illuminating discussion in which Escherich points out
the roentgen examination was already not being used as commonly in young patients as in adults. He states that a roentgen
laboratory was established especially for children at Graz in
1897, and it seems probable that this was the first of its kind.
A single film is reproduced—a print of an infantile hand and
forearm which shows rachitic changes. The uncertainties of
the mediastinal shadows, which still bedevil us, were fully
appreciated by Escherich, and he was quite unhappy about
this baffling structure "in which so many important infantile
lesions lie concealed." He was enthusiastic in regard to the
possible estimation of the state of hydration of soft tissues in
infantile diarrhea from their roentgen densities.

Reyher's German monograph in 1908 is the earliest
review of the world literature of pediatric roentgenology
which I have found (Reyher, P.: Die roentgenologische
Diagnostik in der Kinderheilkunde, Ergebn. d. inn. Med. U.
Kinderh. 2:613, 1908). In it there are 276 references to
articles published during the first 12 years following Röntgen's discovery, and these furnish a good key for the study
of the early writings in this field. The appendix contains 40
small but clear roentgen prints.

Rotch's *The Roentgen Ray in Pediatrics* appeared in 1910—
the first book in any language devoted exclusively to pediatric
x-ray diagnosis and still, I believe, the only one in English.
Dr. Thomas Morgan Rotch was Professor of Pediatrics,
Harvard University, and an outstanding podiatrist of his
time.★ In this pioneer treatise he stresses the importance of
mastering the shadows of normal structure before attempting
the recognition and interpretation of the abnormal, and he
carefully correlates the clinical findings with the roentgen
findings in the cases illustrated; 42 of 264 figures depict the
"normal living anatomy of infants and children." This material was taken largely from the files of the Boston Children's
Hospital, and the author's statement that more than 2,300
cases were available for study demonstrates that roentgen
examination had long been a commonplace in his clinic. Dr.
Rotch's early fostering of roentgen examination of infants
and children, his appreciation of the special problems in
applying this method to the young, his careful anatomic
roentgen studies and his text, monumental for this time, all
mark him as the father of pediatric roentgenology in America.

Two years later—1912—the first German book, Reyher's
Das Roentgenverfahren in der Kinderheilkunde, was published.
Later and more familiar texts are Gralka's *Roentgendiagnostik
im Kindesalter* (1927), Becker's *Roentgendiagnostik und Strahlen-
therapie in der Kinderheilkunde* (1931), and the *Handbuch der
Roentgendiagnostik und Therapie im Kindesalter* by Engel and
Schall (1933). As far as I have been able to determine, no
book on pediatric roentgen diagnosis has been published in
English during the 35 years which have passed since Rotch's
unique publication in 1910. The absence of pediatric roentgenology in the flood of medical texts which has streamed
from the American and English presses during the last three
decades constitutes a dereliction unmatched in other equally
important fields of medical diagnosis—a literary developmental hypoplasia which it is hoped *Pediatric X-Ray Diagnosis* will
remedy.

This book stems from the roentgen conferences held
semimonthly at the Babies Hospital during the last 20 years.
The films reproduced herein were all selected from our
own roentgen files save those for which credit to others is

★Jacobi, A.: In memoriam Thomas Morgan Rotch, Am. J. Dis. Child. 8:245,
1914.

indicated in the legends. The purpose of the author is two-fold: description of shadows cast by normal and morbid tissues, and clinical appraisal of roentgen findings in pediatric diagnosis. Roentgen physics, technique, and therapy have been omitted intentionally. As references and acknowledgments testify, the writer has borrowed freely from the literature and is indebted to many contributors for subject matter and illustrations. To all of them I am sincerely grateful. In the broad and deep field of pediatric diagnosis, selection of the most appropriate material has posed many dilemmas. In the main, data have been chosen which have proved the most useful and instructive in solving the common and important diagnostic problems which have arisen during two decades in a large and busy pediatric hospital and out-patient clinic.

The limitations of space do not permit adequate recognition here of all those to whom credit is due for the making of this book. The roentgen examinations which are its foundation could not have been made without the cooperation of thousands of patients—many weak and pain weary; to all of these I am profoundly thankful. Intimate clinical contacts have been maintained and essential collateral examinations have been made possible through the sustained collaboration of my colleagues—attending physicians and surgeons, resident physicians and nurses. I am under deep and solid obligation to Dr. Rustin McIntosh who read the entire manuscript; his discerning criticism and valuable suggestions are responsible for numerous corrections and improvements in the text. The sympathetic reception given to our early endeavors by Dr. Ross Golden will always be remembered gratefully, as well as his continuing wise and friendly counsel. We have benefited much and often from the discipline of the necropsy table—from the instructive dissections of Dr. Martha Wollstein, Dr. Beryl Paige, and Dr. Dorothy Anderson.

To none, however do I owe more than to my loyal coworkers in the roentgen department of the Babies Hospital—Edgar Watts, Cecelia Peck, Moira Shannon, Mary Fennell, and Mary Jean Cadman—for their gentle handling of patients, unfailing industry, and superlative technical skill. Mrs. Cadman typed the manuscript; I am grateful to her for the speedy completion of a thorny chore. The drawings are the work of Alfred Feinberg, and they reflect his rich experience in medical illustration.

The final phase in the preparation of the manuscript was saddened by the death of Mr. H.A. Simons, President of the Year Book Publishers. His stimulating enthusiasm and generosity were indispensable to the completion of the book during these unsettled war years. His passing was a grievous loss. The task of publication has fallen to the capable and patient hands of Mr. Paul Perles and Mrs. Anabel Ireland Janssen.

John Caffey
Babies Hospital
New York 32
June 10, 1945

Contents

SECTION 4
Respiratory System

SECTION 5

Heart and Great Vessels

VOLUME II

SECTION 6
Gastrointestinal System

SECTION 7
Genitourinary System

SECTION 8
Musculoskeletal System

Video Contents

Videos are available at the *Caffey's Pediatric Diagnostic Imaging* collection online at www.expertconsult.com.

SECTION 1

Radiation Effects and Safety

Radiation Bioeffects, Risks, and Radiation Protection in Medical Imaging in Children

DONALD P. FRUSH and THOMAS L. SLOVIS

Diagnostic imaging has evolved from the single technique of radiography discussed in the first edition of *Caffey's Pediatric X-Ray Diagnosis* in 1945 to a specialty with a choice of many modalities and techniques. Many of these modalities use ionizing radiation, and some entail relatively high doses of radiation, such as computed tomography (CT) and nuclear imaging, including positron emission tomography.[1] For this reason, the imaging community (and our medical colleagues) must jointly adhere to two of the principles of radiation protection for our patients: justification (i.e., the examination is appropriate) and optimization (i.e., the appropriate technique is used). For example, we can substantially influence the radiation dose range within the radiographic arena depending on how we perform computed or direct digital radiographic examinations. Image processing for this digital technology can accommodate overexposures; that is, from a contrast and brightness standpoint, the image can be adjusted to appear as if it was obtained using standard techniques, whereas with screen film technology, the film image would be recognized as overexposed (dark) (Fig. 1-1). In addition, without accountability for displaying dose metrics (such as the exposure index available with digital radiography), it is difficult or impossible to account for patient exposures in clinical practice.[2] In addition, uninformed and potentially irresponsible justification of medical imaging occurs when persons are unfamiliar with the methods of estimating an effective radiation dose during CT examinations in children.[3,4] Increasing accountability is expected from the medical community with regard to the use of imaging modalities that expose children (as well as adults) to ionizing radiation, especially for the risk part of the risk/benefit ratio. Because of the need for such accountability, a basic understanding of radiation biology, including bioeffects, radiation doses of various types of imaging examinations, and risks of radiation, is essential for the pediatric imager. A glossary of terms and dose descriptors is found in the addendum at the end of this chapter.

Trends in Medical Radiation Exposure to Children

Approximately 4 billion imaging examinations using ionizing radiation (i.e., radiography, fluoroscopy/angiography, CT, and nuclear imaging) are performed annually worldwide.[5] In the United States, medical imaging currently accounts for a significant percentage of the annual radiation exposure to

the population (Fig. 1-2),[6] and most sources demonstrate continued increased use during the past decade. For example, one study showed a fivefold increase in CT examinations in the pediatric acute care setting from 1995 to 2008.[7] Natural or background sources account for about 50% of the annual radiation exposure in the United States, and diagnostic medical radiation accounts for most of the remainder, an approximately sixfold increase during the past 30 years. CT alone accounts for nearly 25% of all radiation exposure to the U.S. population.[6] Many reasons exist for the increased use of diagnostic medical radiation, and much use of such radiation is based on sound medical decision making. However, other factors determine use as well, including defensive medicine.

Pathophysiology of Radiation Effects

Hall[8] has written an excellent review of radiobiology for the radiologist. The biologic effects of radiation result primarily from damage to deoxyribonucleic acid (DNA)—the critical target. The first step in the absorption of x-rays is that the x-ray particle, the photon, gives up its energy to produce a fast recoil electron. The electron may damage DNA directly, but the electron also can interact with a molecule of water to produce a free radical (Fig. 1-3). A free radical is a highly reactive atom or molecule with an unpaired electron in the outer shell:

$$H_2O \rightarrow H_2O^+ + e^-$$
$$H_2O^- + H_2O \rightarrow H_3O^+ + OH^*$$

where the asterisk indicates a free radical.

The hydroxyl radical (OH) can diffuse a short distance to cause DNA damage. The fact that two thirds of x-ray damage occurs via OH suggests that someday this component of radiation damage might be reduced through the use of chemical radioprotectants. The topic of radioprotectants was recently well reviewed.[9]

The biologic effects of radiation result primarily from damage to double-stranded DNA as opposed to single-strand injury (see Fig. 1-3). Single-strand breaks of DNA are readily repaired and are presumed to have a negligible effect. Breaks in both DNA strands that are opposite or separated by a few base pairs are much more difficult to repair. These double-strand breaks can cause important biologic effects, including genetic mutations, carcinogenesis, and cell death. Dicentric

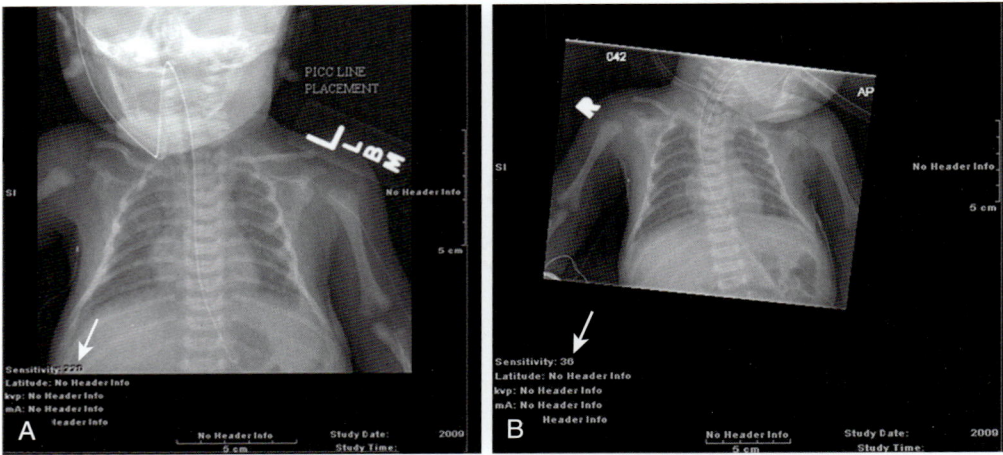

Figure 1-1 A, The initial neonatal chest radiograph has an exposure index ("S" value 39) (*arrow*) that was very low, indicating a relatively high radiation exposure. which would have rendered this image dark with film screen technology. This radiograph was processed to yield appropriate contrast and brightness. **B,** After adjustment to a more appropriate exposure index ("S" value 220) (*arrow*). The image quality is very similar. The left arm was included because assessment was for percutaneous indwelling central catheter placement. (From Frush DP. Radiation protection in children undergoing medical imaging. In Daldrup-Link HE, Gooding CA, editors: *Essentials of pediatric radiology*, Cambridge: Cambridge University Press; 2010. Used with permission.)

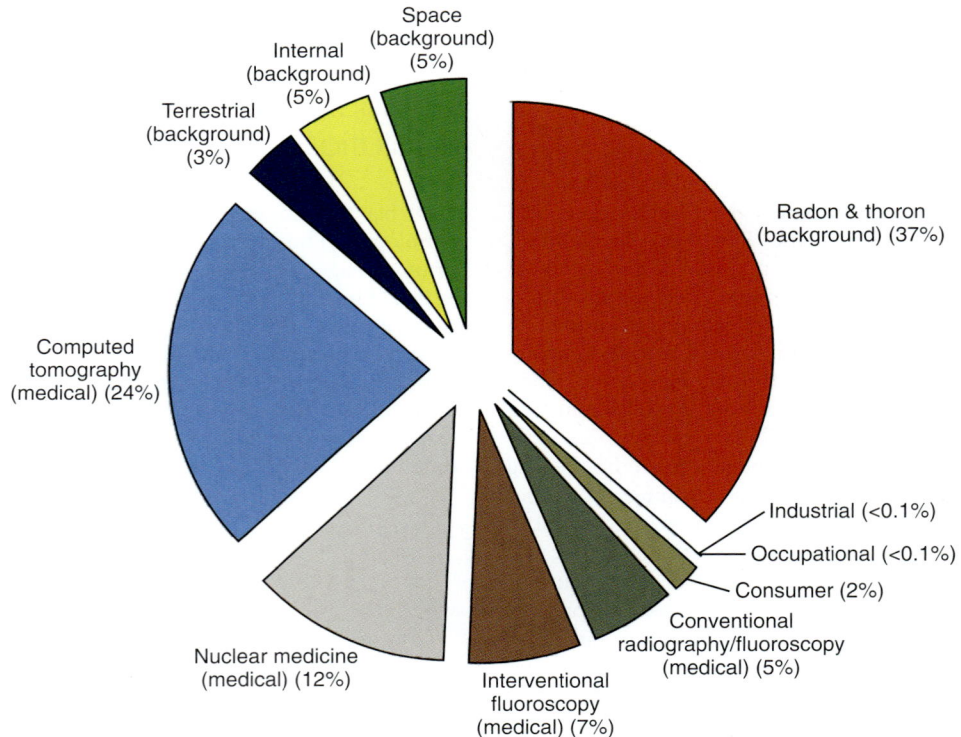

Figure 1-2   All exposure categories for the collective effective dose (%), 2006. (From National Council on Radiation Protection & Measurements. *Ionizing radiation exposure of the population of the United States (NCRP report No. 160)*, Bethesda, Md: National Council on Radiation Protection & Measurements; 2009. Used with permission.)

and fragmented breaks typically result in cell death, whereas nonlethal translocation repairs may cause impaired cellular function, including development of an oncogene.[8]

The biochemical and physiologic damage produced by radiation generally occurs within hours or days, but the impact of these changes, such as the induction of cancer, can take decades to manifest. This carcinogenesis process has several steps. Aberrations in chromosomes (e.g., deletions, translocations, or aneuploidy) are produced by DNA damage. Because these impaired cells survive, they become "stable

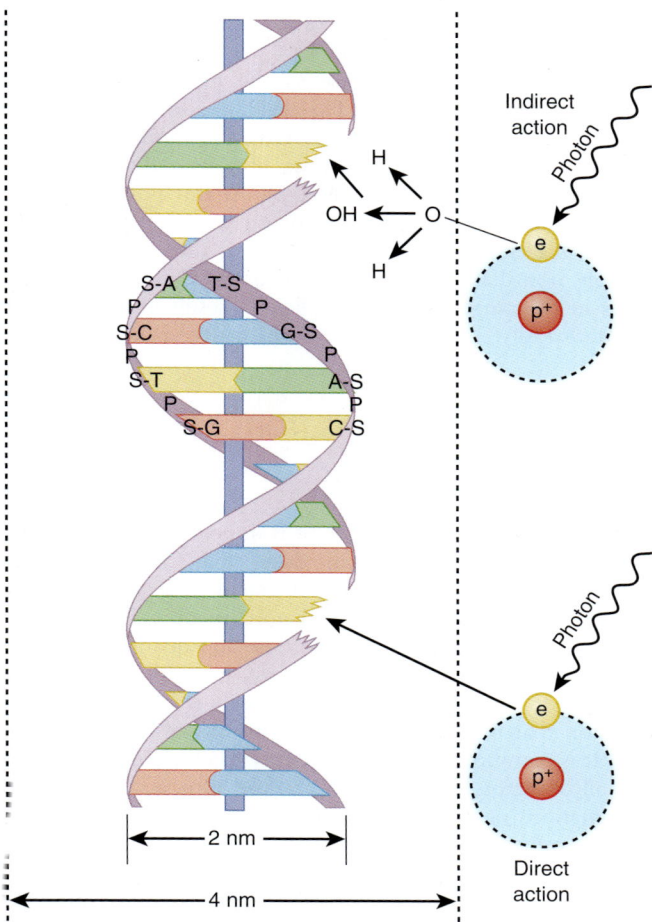

Figure 1-3 *Direct and indirect action.* Indirect action (top part of figure), an electron damages the deoxyribonucleic acid (DNA). In indirect action, the secondary electron interacts with a water molecule to produce a hydroxyl radical that then damages DNA, in this case affecting a single strand. (From Hall EJ. Radiation biology for pediatric radiologists, *Pediatr Radiol* 39(1):S57-S64, 2009. Used with permission.)

Table 1-1

Deterministic Dose Rates	
Skin Injury	**Approximate Threshold**
Skin	
Transient erythema	200 rad (2 Gy)
Dry desquamation	1000 rad (10 Gy)
Moist desquamation	1500 rad (15 Gy)
Temporary epilation	200 rad (2 Gy)
Permanent epilation	700 rad (7 Gy)
Late effects on tissue	**More variable**

Modified from Hall EJ. *Radiobiology for the radiologist*, ed 5, Philadelphia: Lippincott Williams & Wilkins; 2000.

Types of Radiation Bioeffects

The two types of biologic effects from radiation are deterministic and stochastic (random). Deterministic bioeffects are characterized by a threshold dose, and the severity of the effect is dose dependent. For example, cataracts traditionally are reported not to occur with less than a 2.0 Gy exposure, although recent data suggest that this threshold is below 1.0 Gy.[11] Table 1-1 shows some of the doses for deterministic effect. In general, deterministic effects from the doses used in diagnostic imaging are extremely rare. Recent exceptions with head perfusion CT scanning in adults have been reported.[12] Deterministic effects such as skin ulcers and burns should never occur from diagnostic imaging, but they are seen with relatively lengthy interventional procedures.

Stochastic effects are more of a concern because they have the potential to occur at any dose, and the severity of the effect is independent of the dose. No threshold exists with stochastic effects, but the probability of an effect (e.g., cancer) increases with increasing doses.

Fetuses and Children Have Greater Radiation Risks

From a public health perspective, all ionizing radiation from medical imaging is considered to be potentially harmful because we assume that no threshold exists below which radiation is safe (i.e., no harmful effects will occur). This

aberrations" (some with neoplastic transformation), a morphologic change that is the first step of a multistep process to radiation-induced carcinogenesis. The second step of the process is cellular immortality. That is, most cancer cells are descendents of a single cell that originally underwent neoplastic transformation. The third step is tumorgenicity. The radiation exposure induces a cellular genomic instability that is transmitted to progeny, which Little[10] described as "a persistent enhancement in the rate of which genetic changes arise in the descendents of the irradiated cells after many generations of replication … [this process] has been termed a nontargeted effect of radiation as genomic damage occurs in the cells that in themselves receive no direct radiation exposure."

Most childhood tumors (about 85%) occur sporadically, but in 15% of the cases, a strong family association and genetic basis for radiation sensitivity are present. Persons with certain diseases are uniquely sensitive to radiation-induced cancers, although the exact mechanism is unclear (Box 1-1).

"linear no threshold" model is applied to low-level radiation exposure.[13,14]

The effects of radiation are greatest on rapidly developing organisms—that is, fetuses, infants, and young children. In pregnancy, the major biologic effects of fetal demise, growth restriction, organ malformations, and cognitive deficits are seen only with doses far in excess of routine diagnostic imaging.[15] The risk of developing cancer from exposure of a fetus to radiation is uncertain, as it is with exposure of a child to radiation; potential effects could be seen with uterine doses that occur as a result of relatively high direct exposures (e.g., a pelvis CT scan for possible appendicitis). No data in humans indicate that genetic effects result from diagnostic levels of radiation.

Compared with middle-aged adults, children have been reported to be from 2 to 15 times more sensitive to radiation-induced carcinogenesis.[16,17] However, Shuryak et al[18] recently noted that the cancer induction risk (greater at younger ages) must be balanced with the radiation-induced promotion of premalignant damage (greater in middle age), which may differ for certain types of cancer. Thus cancer risks may be higher in the adult population than traditionally believed.[18]

Low-dose effects have been described by Pierce and Preston,[19] who studied the data from atomic bomb survivors reported by the Radiation Effects Research Foundation. Among persons who had received dosages of 0.005 to 0.2 sievert (500 mrad to 20 rad), 35,000 people survived, and 5000 cases of cancer developed. The authors made the following conclusions: first, the solid cancer risk persists for more than 50 years. Second, there is a 10% increase over the expected cancer rate.[19] Low-dose relative risk factors are shown in Figure 1-4.

The overall risk of cancer for the entire population suggested by the International Commission on Radiological Protection is 5% per sievert for low doses and low-dose rate. However, this value is an average value. For adults in late middle age, the risk decreases to only 1% per sievert, whereas

for children in the first decade of life, the risk may be as high as 16% per sievert for girls and 12% per sievert for boys. The female dose is higher because of the greater incidence of breast and thyroid cancers (Fig. 1-5). Radiation risks from diagnostic imaging low-level radiation were reviewed recently.[20] Two excellent reviews also recently were published by Linet et al[21,22] (Table 1-2). At this point, we have cautious uncertainty regarding cancer risk and low-level radiation. As Hricak et al[23] state, "In brief, there is reasonable, though not definitive, epidemiologic evidence that organ doses in the range from 5 to 125 mSv result in a very small but statistically significant increase in cancer risk."

Radiation Exposures from Various Imaging Modalities

When discussing radiation dose, it is important to state clearly whether entrance dose, skin dose, exit dose, or organ (absorbed) dose is considered. For example, a vast difference can exist between skin dose and gonadal dose for the same incident radiation. (The terms for dose and quantitative comparisons are provided in the glossary, and dose metrics are provided in Box 1-2.) "Effective dose" is one measure of radiation that is widely used in discussions of medical radiation. It is commonly used because it is relatively easily derived and allows gross comparisons of dose estimations between examinations of different regions as well as different modalities. However, the application of effective dose in medical imaging is problematic.[24,25]

Published estimates for radiation doses in adults and children include those by Fahey et al.[26] and Mettler et al.[27] In summary, radiographic dose ranges from a fraction of a millisievert (for extremity evaluation) to somewhat larger doses of more than 1.0 mSv for more extensive examinations, such as a lumbar spine series. Fluoroscopic doses depend on

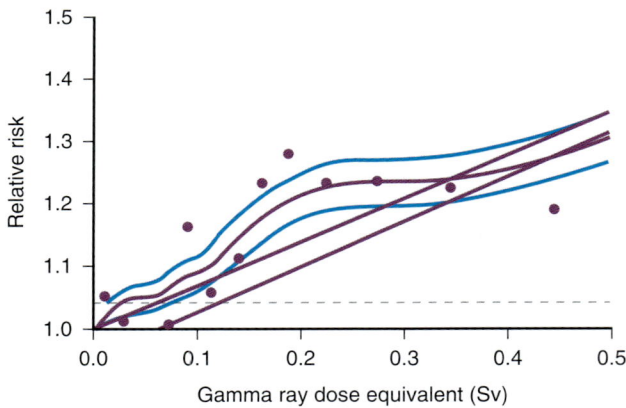

Figure 1-4 Estimated low-dose risks. Age-specific cancer rates over the 1958 through 1994 follow-up period relative to the rates for unexposed people averaged over the follow-up for sex and for age at exposure. The dashed line represents ±1 standard deviation error for the smooth purple curve. The upper straight line is the linear risk estimate computed from the range 0 to 2 Sv. The second straight line beginning at 0.06 Sv is the upper 95% confidence limit for such a quantity. (From Pierce DA, Preston DL. Radiation-related cancer risks at low doses among atomic bomb survivors. *Radiat Res.* 154:178-186, 2000.)

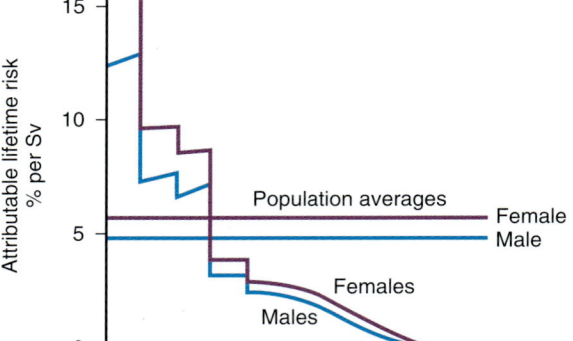

Figure 1-5 Lifetime risk of excess cancer per sievert as a function of age at the time of exposure. Data from atomic bomb survivors. Although the average risk for a population is about 5% per sievert, the risk varies considerably with age; children are much more sensitive than adults. At early ages, girls are more sensitive than boys. (From Hall EJ: Introduction to session I. helical CT and cancer risk, *Pediatr Radiol.* 32:225-227, 2002.)

Table 1-2

Risk of Specific and Total Childhood Cancers Associated with Early Life Postnatal Medical Radiation Exposure

Study	Upper Age Limit (y)	Type/No. of Cases	Type/No. of Controls	Method of Exposure to Assessment	Type of Exposure	Exposure Prevalence in Controls	Estimated Relative Risk
Leukemia							
Stewart et al, U.K. (1953–1955)	10	Deceased (619)	Population (619)	Interview, medical records	Diagnostic	12.9	1.2
					Therapeutic	0.2	5.0
Polhemus & Koch, U.S. (1950–1957)	NS	Incident (251)	Hospital (251)	Questionnaire	Diagnostic	41.4	2.1*
					Fluoroscopic	3.2	3.5*
					Therapeutic	3.6	3.7*
Ager et al, U.S. (1965)	4	Deceased (109)	Siblings (102)	Interview, medical records	Any	16.7	1.3
			Neighborhood (110)			18.2	1.1
Graham et al, U.S. (1966)	14	Incident (319)	Population (884)	Medical records	Any	36.0	1.2
					>1 site	7.6	2.1
Shu e al, China (1974–1986)	14	Incident, prevalent (309)	Population (618)	Interview	Any	27.3	0.9
Fajardo-Gutierrez et al, Mexico (1993)	14	Incident, prevalent (79)	Population, hospital (148)	Interview	Any	27.0	1.1
Acute Lymphocytic Leukemia							
Shu, China (1974–1986)	14	Incident, prevalent (172)	Population (618)	Interview	Any	27.3	0.9
Magnani et al, Italy (1981–1984)	NS	Incident, prevalent (142)	Hospital (307)	Interview	Diagnostic	45.9	0.7
Shu et al, China (1986–1991)	14	Incident (166)	Population (166)	Interview	Any	—	1.6
Shu, U.S. (1989–1993)	15	Incident (1842)	Population (1986)	Interview	Diagnostic	39	1.1
Infante-Rivard, Canada (1980–1998)	14	Incident (701)	Population (701)	Interview	Diagnostic, 1	19.1	1.1
					Diagnostic, ≥2	18.8	1.5*
Acute Myeloid Leukemia							
Shu et al, China (1974–1986)	14	Incident, prevalent (92)	Population (618)	Interview	Any	27.3	1.0
Lymphoma							
Shu et al, China (1981–1991)	14	Incident (87)	Population (166)	Interview	Any	—	1.6*
Brain Tumors							
Howe et al, Canada (1977–1983)	19	Incident (74)	Population (138)	Interview	Chest diagnostic	8.0	2.1
					Skull diagnostic	4.3	6.7*
McCredie et al, Australia (1985–1989)	14	Incident (82)	Population (164)	Interview	Dental	9.1	0.4
					Skull diagnostic	2.4	2.3
Shu et al, China (1981–1991)	14	Incident (107)	Population (107)	Interview	Any	—	1.5
Schuz et al, Germany (1993–1997)	15	Incident (466)	Population (2458)	Interview	Any	4.3	0.8
Astrocytoma							
Kuijten et al, U.S. (1980–1986)	14	Incident (163)	RDD (163)	Interview	Head or neck	NS	1.0
					Dental	NS	0.9
Bunin et al, U.S./Canada (1986–1989)	5	Incident (155)	RDD (155)	Interview	Head, neck, or dental	13.5	1.2
					Dental	9.0	1.0
					Head	3.2	1.1

Continued

Table 1-2

Risk of Specific and Total Childhood Cancers Associated with Early Life Postnatal Medical Radiation Exposure—cont'd

Study	Upper Age Limit (y)	Type/No. of Cases	Type/No. of Controls	Method of Exposure to Assessment	Type of Exposure	Exposure Prevalence in Controls	Estimated Relative Risk
Peripheral Neuroepithelioma							
Bunin et cl, U.S./Canada (1986–1989)	5	Incident (166)	RDD (166)	Interview	Head, neck, or dental	12.0	1.1
					Dental	8.4	0.5
					Head	4.2	0.9
Neuroblastoma							
Greenberg et al, U.S. (1972–1981)	14	Incident (104)	Hospital (208)	Medical records	Chest	33.2	0.3*
			Wilm's (105)			11.7	2.0
					Cranial	6.2	0.3
						1.3	1.6
					Abdominal	6.7	0.4
						3.9	0.8
Osteosarcoma							
Gelberg et al, U.S. (1997)	24	Incident (130)	Population (130)	Interview	Medical	NS	1.0
Ewing Sarcoma							
Daigle et al, U.S. (1975–1981)	20	Incident, prevalent (98)	RDD (98)	Interview	Any	NS	1.0
		Incident, prevalent (95)	Siblings (95)			NS	1.0
Winn et al, U.S. (1983–1985)	22	Incident (204)	RDD (204)	Interview	Diagnostic	37.7	1.6*
					Dental	50.0	1.2
All Sites							
Stewart et al, U.K. (1953–1955)	10	Deceased (1299)	Populaton (1299)	Interview, medical records	Diagnostic	13.6	1.0
					Therapeutic	0.2	2.7
Hartley et al, U.K. (1980–1983)	14	Incident (535)	General practitioner (1068)	Interview, medical records	Neonatal	0.3	2.0
		Incident (465)	Hospital (928)		Diagnostic	1.0	1.1
Shu et al, China (1994)	14	Incident (642)	Population (642)	Interview	Any	—	1.3*

RDD, random-digit dialing.
*Statistically significant.
From Linet MS, Slovis TL, Miller DL, et al. Cancer risks associated with external radiation from diagnostic imaging procedures. *CA Cancer J Clin* 2012 (epub ahead of print).

technical parameters, especially fluoroscopy time and frame rate, and can vary widely from very low dose cystography to doses in tens of millisieverts for complex interventional procedures. CT is a modality that can deliver a relatively large dose of ionizing radiation. The number of these examinations has been increasing at a rapid rate, with children (birth to 15 years old) undergoing approximately 11% of all CT examinations.[28] More recent information has shown that the dose (the CTDI; see glossary) from CT (conventional and spiral examinations) in adults is less than 1.0 mSv to as much as 40 mSv.[26,27] Typical pediatric CT doses should be less than 10 mSv,[26,29] and with new iterative reconstruction technologies, an increasing fraction of body examinations are approaching or being performed in the sub-millisievert range. Data on radiation doses from select pediatric imaging examinations are found in Table 1–3.

Strategies for Optimizing Radiation Doses for Children

The fundamental principles for protecting children from radiation during imaging include justification and optimization. Justification for a study can be difficult to define, although summary recommendations and appropriateness criteria for medical imaging are available.[30] The use of imaging modalities that do not depend on ionizing radiation, especially magnetic resonance imaging and sonography, is fundamental in justification considerations.

When an examination is considered justified, the imaging technique should be optimized. Radiation reduction is not always appropriate because some examinations require multiple and additional projections, greater fluoroscopy time or

---

Box 1-2   Radiation Metrics

A. Absorbed Dose—Radiation Absorbed Dose (rad), Gray (Gy)

1 Gy = 100 rad

1 cGy = 1 rad = 1000 mrad

1 mGy = 100 mrad

B. Use of Absorbed Dose Equivalent—Radiation-Equivalent—Man (rem), Sievert (Sv)

1 Sv = 100 rem

10 mSv = 1 rem = 1000 mrem

1 mSv = 100 mrem

Rem = rad × quality factor

Rem = rad × 1

Because the quality factor for x-ray and γ-rays = 1, rad = rem

C. Nuclear Medicine

1. Unit of radioactivity—becquerel (Bq)
   Bq = 1 disintegration/sec
2. Unit of radioactivity—curie (Ci)
   1 Ci = 3.7×10^{10} Bq (disintegration/sec)
   1 Ci = 2.2×10^{12} disintegration/min
   10 mCi = 370 mBq

Table 1-3

Radiation Dose to Children by Age at Diagnostic Examination

Examination*	Dose (mSv) (by Age at Exposure (y))					
	0	1	5	10	15	Adult
Radiography††						
Skull AP	—	0.037	0.058	—	—	0.084
Skull LAT	—	0.025	0.031	—	—	0.041
Chest PA	0.023	0.024	0.037	0.025	0.026	0.051
Abdomen AP	0.077	0.197	0.355	0.509	0.897	2.295
Pelvis AP	0.085	0.121	0.230	0.309	0.556	1.783
Dental Radigraphy†						
Intraoral		0.008				0.011
Panoramic		0.015				0.015
Diagnostic Fluoroscopy Procedures†						
MCU	0.807	0.763	0.688	0.640	0.677	2.789
Barium swallow	0.645	0.589	0.303	0.760	0.581	1.632
Barium meal	2.205	2.226	1.427	2.137	2.386	5.158
Cardiac ASD occlusion				3.88		5.158
Cardiac PDA occlusion				.021		
Cardiac VSD occlusion				12.1		
Computed Tomography§						
Brain	2.3	2.2	1.9	20.	2.2	1.9
Facial bone/sinuses	1.4	0.5	0.5	0.5	0.6	0.9
Chest	1.9	2.2	2.5	3.0	3.3	5.9
Entire abdomen	3.6	4.8	5.4	5.8	6.7	10.4
Spine	4.4	11.4	8	7.6	6.9	10.1

AP, anteroposterior; ASD atrial septal defect; LAT, lateral; MCU, micturating cystourethrography; PA, posterolateral; PDA, patent ductus arteriosus; VSD, ventricular septal defect.

*Dosimetric quantities are all effective doses in millisieverts (mSv).

†From Hart D, Hillier MC. *Dose to patients from medical x-ray examinations in the UK–2000 review.* Chilton, UK: National Radiological Protection Board; 2007.

‡From Hart D, Hillier MC. *Dose to patients from medical x-ray examinations in the UK—2002 review.* Chilton, UK: National Radiological Protection Board; 2002.

§From Galanski M, Nagel HD, Stamm G. *Paediatric CT exposure practice in the Federal Republic of Germany—results of a nation-wide survey in 2005/2006.* Hannover, Germany, 2006, Hannover Medical School. Radiation doses are based on a German nationwide survey on multislice CT. The radiation dose in each age group category is the dose administered to pediatric patients who are newborn (the 0-year category), those ages >0-1 year (the 1-year category), those ages 2- 5 years (the 5-year category), those ages 6-10 years (the 10-year category), and those ages 11-15 years (the 15-year category).

---

magnification, or lower image noise (requiring a higher dose) to answer specific clinical questions. Implicit here is the "as low as reasonable achievable" principle, which entails using the amount of radiation necessary for diagnosis.

Patient preparation and examination planning are paramount for any examination. Planning includes communicating with the ordering clinician when necessary to clarify examination indications.[31] Communication also is important both before and during fluoroscopic and angiographic examinations to minimize potentially nonuseful fluoroscopy. Use of appropriately trained staff and involvement with qualified medical physicists, along with licensing, certification, and accreditation considerations and routine reviews of equipment function and protocols as part of quality control and assessment, are becoming expected components of radiation protection in medicine.[32]

Strategies for computed radiography and direct radiography dose management in pediatric imaging include appropriate collimation, evaluation of the number of projections required, consideration of the source to film and patient to film distances, shielding, use of grids, filtering, consideration of exposure factors, and use of postprocessing techniques. General strategies for protecting patients from radiation during radiography can be found in International Atomic Energy Agency educational material.[33]

A number of radiation protection management strategies exist for fluoroscopy and interventional radiology, including those by the International Atomic Energy Agency and Alliance for Radiation Safety in Pediatric Imaging (Image Gently Campaign).[34-36] These strategies include avoiding field overlap among different projection series, avoiding electronic magnification, placement of the image intensifier before fluoroscopic activation, use of appropriate grids and positioning (i.e., source to patient and patient to intensifier distances), collimation, and use of pediatric-specific filters. In addition, image hold, pulsed fluoroscopy, image store, video capture, and alerts are part of examination optimization for children.

Video recording during studies can provide review without use of additional fluoroscopy.

Contemporary strategies and examination optimization for radiation dose management in pediatric CT, including protocol optimization (especially related to clinical indication), are available.[37-40] Adjustment in the parameters that are primarily responsible for the dose delivered—tube current (milliamperes), gantry cycle time in seconds, peak kilovoltage, and pitch—should be based on the size of the child, examination indication, prior examinations, and region examined.

Additional efforts should include minimizing multiphase examinations, excessive scan length, and overlapping regions of examination. Tube current modulation, organ-based dose modulation (in which the tube current is reduced in an arc to reduce the surface dose to anterior structures such as the breasts when the patient is supine), iterative reconstructive technologies, and dual-source/dual-energy technology also have provided real or potential opportunities for dose reduction, improved examination quality, or a combination of both. The use of shielding in the region of scanning, which usually is discussed for breast tissue, is debated.[41,42] A more in-depth discussion of radiation protection in children undergoing diagnostic imaging is available.[43]

Educational efforts are extremely important, particularly given increased scrutiny and concern regarding medical radiation and the risk of cancer. To these ends, the Alliance for Radiation Safety in Pediatric Imaging, through the Image Gently campaigns,[44,45] has been a successful education and awareness organization for pediatric imaging involving ionizing radiation.

Continued needs include more evidence-based research and decision support to improve utilization,[46] better dose estimations,[3,4] development of diagnostic reference levels for pediatric imaging, alerts and notifications on imaging equipment,[47] and cumulative dose estimation reporting for all modalities as well as dose tracking.[48]

Key Points

Radiation can have a direct action on DNA or operate indirectly through free radicals.

In medicine, biologic effects from radiation are primarily a result of double-strand DNA breaks.

In diagnostic imaging, radiation effects are stochastic effects, primarily cancer induction (vs. deterministic effects such as skin burns seen at much higher doses).

Fetal and childhood tissues are more susceptible to the stochastic effects of radiation.

Key principles of protecting persons from radiation that apply to medicine are justification (only perform indicated examinations) and optimization (use appropriate techniques when examinations are warranted).

Dose metrics (i.e., exposure or dose estimations) should be part of the examination information for every modality that uses ionizing radiation.

Suggested Readings

Fahey FH, Treves ST, Adelstein SJ. Minimizing and communicating radiation risk in pediatric nuclear medicine. *J Nucl Med.* 2011;52:1240-1251.

Frush DP. CT dose and risk estimates in children. *Pediatr Radiol.* 2011;41:483-487.

Hall EJ. Radiation biology for pediatric radiologists. *Pediatr Radiol.* 2009;39(1):S57-S64.

Hricak H, Brenner DJ, Adelstein SJ, et al. Managing radiation use in medical imaging: multifaceted challenge. *Radiology.* 2011;258:889-905.

Linet MS, Slovis TL, Miller DL, et al. Cancer risks associated with external radiation from diagnostic imaging procedures. *CA Cancer J Clin.* 2012 [epub ahead of print].

McCollough CH, Schueler BA, Atwell TD, et al. Radiation exposure and pregnancy: when should we be concerned? *Radiographics.* 2007;27:909-917.

References

Full references for this chapter can be found on www.expertconsult.com.

Addendum

GLOSSARY AND DOSE DESCRIPTORS

As we probe more deeply into the effects of radiation, it is important to use precise definitions. Some of the most pertinent terms are provided in this glossary.*

Absolute risk: The risk of an adverse effect that is independent of other causes of that same health effect.

Absorbed dose (D): The energy imparted to matter per unit of mass by ionizing radiation at a specific point. The Systeme Internationale (SI) unit of absorbed dose is joules per kilogram (J/kg). The special name for this unit is the gray (Gy). The previously used special unit of absorbed dose, the rad, was defined as being an energy absorption dose of 100 erg/g; 1 Gy = 100 rad.

ALARA (as low as reasonably achievable): The principle of limiting the radiation dose administered to exposed individuals to levels as low as are reasonably achievable, taking into account economic and social factors.

Background radiation: The radiation in the natural environment, including cosmic rays and radiation from the naturally radioactive elements, found outside and inside the bodies of humans and animals. Background radiation also is called natural radiation. The term also may mean radiation that is unrelated to a specific experiment.

CTDI (computed tomography dose index): A measure of radiation dose obtained using dosimeters in a standard phantom (e.g., 32- or 16-cm acrylic cylinder).

Deterministic effect: An effect with a threshold, the severity of which increases as the dose increases.

Effective dose: The radiation dose, allowing for the fact that some types of radiation are more damaging than are others and some parts of the body are more sensitive to radiation than are others. It is defined as the sum, over specified tissues, of the products of the equivalent doses in the tissues and the weighting factors for the tissues.

Exposure: Exposure is used more often in its more general sense and not as the specially defined radiation quantity. It is a measure of the quantity of x-radiation or gamma radiation based on its ability to ionize air through which it passes. The previously used special unit of exposure, the roentgen (R), has been replaced with the SI unit of exposure, coulombs per kilogram (C/kg); 1 R = 2.58 × 10^{-4} C/kg (exactly). The physical quantity exposure may be replaced by the quantity air kerma in air, especially for calibration of monitoring instruments: 1 R = 10 mGy air kerma.

---

*Modified from Hall EJ: *Radiobiology for the radiologist*, ed 5, Philadelphia, 2000, Lippincott Williams & Wilkins.

Free radical: A fragment of an atom or molecule that contains an unpaired electron in the outer shell and is very reactive.

Gamma rays: High-energy, short-wavelength electromagnetic radiation (γ). Gamma radiation frequently accompanies α and β emissions and always accompanies fission. Gamma rays are very penetrating and are best stopped or shielded against by dense materials, such as lead or depleted uranium. Gamma rays are indistinguishable from x-rays except for their source: gamma rays originate inside the nucleus, and x-rays originate from outside.

Gray (Gy): The special name for the SI unit of absorbed dose (kerma) and specific energy imparted equal to 1 J/kg. The previous unit of absorbed dose, the rad, has been replaced by the gray: 1 Gy = 100 rad.

Hereditary effects of radiation: Radiation effects that can be transferred from parent to offspring; any changes in the genetic material of sex cells caused by radiation.

Kerma (kinetic energy released per unit mass): The sum of the initial kinetic energies of all the charged ionizing particles liberated by uncharged ionizing particles per unit mass of a specified material. Kerma is measured in the same unit as absorbed dose. The SI unit of kerma is joules per kilogram (J/kg), and its special name is the gray (Gy). Kerma can be quoted for any specified material at a point in free space or in an absorbing medium.

Lifetime risk: The risk of dying of some particular cause over the entire course of a person's life.

Linear no threshold (LNT): The theory that no level of radiation exposure can be assumed to be absolutely safe.

Rad: The old unit of absorbed dose, equivalent to an energy absorption of 100 erg/g. Superseded by the gray (see absorbed dose).

Relative risk: The situation in which the risk of a disease resulting from some injury is expressed as some percentage increase of the spontaneous rate of occurrence of that disease. Relative risk is in contrast to an absolute risk, in which the risk of a disease resulting from an injury does not depend on the normal rate of occurrence of that disease.

Rem: Old unit of equivalent or effective dose. It is the product of absorbed dose (in rads), the radiation weighting factor, and the tissue weighting factor; 1 rem = 0.01 Sv.

Roentgen (R): A unit of exposure to ionizing radiation named after Wilhelm Röntgen, the German scientist who discovered x-rays in 1895. It is that amount of γ rays or x-rays required to produce ions carrying one electrostatic unit of electric charge (either positive or negative) in 1 cm^3 of dry air under standard conditions.

Sievert (Sv): Unit of equivalent dose or effective dose: 1 Sv = 100 rem.

Stochastic effect: The effect, the probability of which, rather than its severity, is a function of radiation dose without threshold. (More generally, stochastic means random in nature.)

Chapter 2

Complications of Contrast Media

GAURAVI K. SABHARWAL

Allergic-Like Reactions

INTRODUCTION

Contrast media are an essential aid in diagnostic medical imaging. A multitude of radiologic examinations are performed daily using these agents. They are used primarily to enhance the visibility of blood vessels, organs, and pathology in the body. Contrast media are considered pharmacologic agents, and, like any other medication, they are not without adverse effects.

INCIDENCE

Scant data are available regarding the incidence of contrast reactions in children for at least three reasons: (1) few clinical trials with children as subjects have been performed to obtain federal approval of an agent,[1] (2) assessing symptoms, particularly mild ones in very young children, is difficult, and (3) differentiating true contrast reactions from symptoms is difficult because of sedation, synchronous medications, anxiety, and other preexisting diseases.[2]

In the pediatric population, use of nonionic contrast media is discriminative and exclusive when administered intravenously.[3] Administration of nonionic contrast is associated with a much lower incidence of contrast media–related adverse effects.[2] Dillman et al[4] reported a 0.18% incidence of acute allergic-like reactions to intravenous (IV) administration of nonionic iodinated contrast material in children. This finding is very similar to an incidence of 0.23% in the adult population reported by Cochran et al.[5] Most of the contrast reactions are mild in both children[4] and adults.[2,5-7] Of all the reported allergic reactions in children, 15% (<0.03% overall) were severe in degree.[4] Fatal reactions to contrast media have occurred, but they are very rare. A large Japanese study did not blame any fatalities on contrast media in more than 170,000 injections.[6] The very low or negligible reported fatalities likely suggest aggressive preventive measures and advancement in management of these reactions.[2] Delayed reactions have been described in adults and may occur between 1 hour and 2 days after contrast administration. These reactions are predominantly cutaneous and usually resolve within 7 days.[8-10]

RISK FACTORS

As with adults, children need to be appropriately screened before contrast media are administered. Screening includes a complete and specific history from the accompanying parents/responsible adults. Attempts should be made to identify any variables that may preclude the use of the contrast media or potentially increase the eventuality of an adverse reaction to this agent. The following list outlines a few of these factors.

1. Known prior reaction to contrast media, which markedly increases the risk of subsequent reactions.[6,11-13]
2. Known allergies to food products or medications; minor allergies do not pose a significant risk, but a prior anaphylactic reaction to any substance should heighten awareness of the possibility of a similar reaction to contrast media administration.
3. A history of asthma may increase the incidence of contrast reaction.[6,13]
4. Known renal disease; renal function in such patients can worsen after administration of contrast media.
5. Known heart disease, sickle cell disease, or diabetes mellitus; patients with these diseases may be at increased risk for contrast reactions.

Other disease entities, such as pheochromocytoma, dehydration, heart failure, severe hyperthyroidism, and β-blocker therapy, that are known risk factors in adults have not been studied in the pediatric population (Box 2-1).

PATHOGENESIS

The exact pathogenesis of untoward events after the administration of contrast media remains obscure and poorly understood. Most of the symptoms resemble an allergic or anaphylactoid reaction to a medication or allergen. However, definitive evidence is lacking that these reactions are truly allergic reactions because antibodies and the typical allergic cascade to these agents have not been identified.[13]

CLASSIFICATION OF ALLERGIC-LIKE CONTRAST REACTIONS

Based on severity, contrast reactions can be classified as mild, moderate, or severe. Flushing and a sensation of warmth are considered physiologic responses (Box 2-2).

Mild reactions are usually of short duration and resolve without the need for any treatment. However, patients should be carefully observed until the symptoms resolve because the symptoms could progress to more severe reactions.

Moderate reactions require some form of treatment. More importantly, close observation is essential until the symptoms resolve. Vital signs should be monitored and IV access should be secured.

> **Box 2-1 Risk Factors for Allergic-Like Contrast Reactions**
>
> Prior reaction to contrast media
> Prior anaphylactic reaction
> Moderate to severe allergies to food products or medications
> History of asthma
> Preexisting renal or heart disease
> Diabetes mellitus or sickle cell disease
> Concomitant use of certain medications

> **Box 2-2 Classification of Allergic-Like Contrast Reaction**
>
> **Mild**
> Nausea/vomiting
> Mild urticaria
> Pallor
>
> **Moderate**
> Severe vomiting
> Significant urticaria
> Mild vasovagal reaction
> Mild bronchospasm
> Dyspnea
> Tachycardia and hypotension
>
> **Severe**
> Laryngeal edema
> Pulmonary edema
> Moderate to severe bronchospasm
> Cardiovascular collapse
> Bradycardia and hypotension
> Seizures

Severe reactions, which are rare, can be life threatening. They could present a worsening of mild or moderate reactions. Prompt and aggressive treatment may be required. The assistance of a rapid response or code team often may be necessary.

MANAGEMENT

In the event of any adverse reaction to contrast media, the IV contrast injection should be discontinued. All reactions and management of the reactions should be documented in the patient care notes, and notation of a contrast allergy should become part of the patient's permanent medical record. The following protocols closely follow the American College of Radiology (ACR) guidelines for management of acute reactions in children.[2] The specific agents used in the management of an adverse reaction are determined by individual institutional pharmacy formulary and policy. Some institutions require the radiology personnel to call for assistance (e.g., a rapid response team) if they administer IV epinephrine for the management of these adverse reactions (given the rare incidence of these events and hence the lack of uniformity in preparedness for these reactions).[14,15] To be prepared for such reactions, weight-based dosages of the medications used for management should be posted in clearly visible areas where contrast media are administered to children. Regular review of treatment protocols and practice of contrast reaction scenarios should be performed by radiologists and staff. If at any time a patient does not respond to treatment or the situation seems troublesome, it is appropriate to seek additional medical support immediately. This support may be sought from another radiologist in the department or through activation of an institutional rapid response or code team.

URTICARIA

Urticaria, which is the most common reaction to contrast media, is limited to skin and subcutaneous tissue. Worsening of symptoms can be caused by the accompanying pruritus. Findings on physical examination include:
- Red raised wheals that blanch with pressure
- Patchy, symmetric involvement
- Itching, which is often intense
- Stable vital signs

Mild urticaria is usually self-limiting and does not require treatment.

Close observation for 30 to 60 minutes, or until resolution, is recommended because urticaria may progress to a moderate reaction. Medications may include H1-receptor blockers (such as diphenhydramine) or α-agonists (such as epinephrine). The accompanying parents/responsible adults should be cautioned about the possibility of drowsiness when diphenhydramine is administered. If urticaria is extensive, pay close attention to the patient's blood pressure and watch for signs and symptoms of hypotension, especially orthostatic hypotension.

BRONCHOSPASM

The patient may present with varying degrees of cough, wheezing, and/or difficulty breathing. It is most important to ensure the presence of an adequate airway. Six to 10 L/min of oxygen should be administered via a face mask. Vital signs should be monitored. Medications may include β-agonists (i.e., bronchodilators), subcutaneous epinephrine for mild symptoms, and IV epinephrine for more acute and severe symptoms.

FACIAL OR LARYNGEAL EDEMA

Swelling of the face may be mild without any significant progression. At this time, only observation may be required. An adequate airway and IV access should be secured. However, if the patient presents with other symptoms such as varying degrees of cough, hoarseness, dysphagia, and/or difficulty breathing, more aggressive measures need to be taken. Medications include subcutaneous, intramuscular, or IV epinephrine. The patient should be closely monitored.

PULMONARY EDEMA

The patient may present with tachypnea, tachycardia, shortness of breath, diaphoresis, agitation, and/or bibasilar rales. Blood-tinged sputum is a late-presenting sign. The airway must be secured and supplemental oxygen should be administered. Medications may include diuretics. Pulmonary edema is a severe response that usually should involve a rapid response or code team.

Box 2-3 Management of Acute Reactions in Children

Urticaria

- No treatment is needed in most cases.
- For moderate itching, consider an H1-receptor blocker such as diphenhydramine (Benadryl), PO/IM or via a slow IV push, 1 to 2 mg/kg, up to 50 mg.
- If severe itching is present or the urticaria is widely disseminated, consider an α-agonist such as epinephrine (1:10,000), 0.1 mL/kg via a slow IV push over 2 to 5 minutes, up to 3 mL.

Facial Edema

- Secure the airway and administer O_2, 6 to 10 L/min (via mask, face tent, or blow-by stream). Monitor electrocardiogram, O_2 saturation (pulse oximeter), and blood pressure.
- Administer an α-agonist such as epinephrine (1:10,000), 0.1 mL/kg via a slow IV push over 2 to 5 minutes, up to 3 mL/dose. Repeat in 5 to 30 minutes as needed.
- Consider administering an H1-receptor blocker such as diphenhydramine (Benadryl) IM or via a slow IV push, 1 to 2 mg/kg, up to 50 mg.
- Note: If facial edema is mild and no reaction progression occurs, observation alone may be appropriate. If the patient is not responsive to therapy, call for assistance.

Bronchospasm

- Secure the airway and administer O_2, 6 to 10 L/min (via mask, face tent, or blow-by stream). Monitor electrocardiogram, O_2 saturation (pulse oximeter), and blood pressure.
- Administer an inhaled β-agonist (e.g., a bronchiolar dilator such as albuterol (Proventil or Ventolin), 2 to 3 puffs from a metered dose inhaler. Repeat as necessary.
- If bronchospasm progresses, administer epinephrine (1:10,000), 0.1 mL/kg via a slow IV push over 2 to 5 minutes, maximum 3 mL/dose. Repeat in 5 to 30 minutes as needed. If the patient is not responsive to therapy, call for assistance for severe bronchospasm or if O_2 saturation <88% persists.

Laryngeal Edema

- Secure the airway and administer O_2, 6 to 10 L/min (via mask, face tent, or blow-by stream). Monitor electrocardiogram, O_2 saturation (pulse oximeter), and blood pressure.
- Administer epinephrine (1:10,000), 0.1 mL/kg via a slow IV push over 2 to 5 minutes, maximum 3 mL/dose. Repeat in 5 to 30 minutes as needed.

Pulmonary Edema

- Secure the airway and administer O_2, 6 to 10 L/min (via mask, face tent, or blow-by stream). Monitor electrocardiogram, O_2 saturation (pulse oximeter), and blood pressure.
- Administer a diuretic: IV furosemide (Lasix), 1 to 2 mg/kg.

Hypotension with Tachycardia (Anaphylactic Shock)

- Secure the airway and administer O_2, 6 to 10 L/min (via mask). Monitor electrocardiogram, O_2 saturation (pulse oximeter), and blood pressure.
- Elevate the legs 60° or more (preferred) or use the Trendelenburg position.
- Keep the patient warm.
- Administer a rapid infusion of IV or IO normal saline solution or Ringer's lactate.
- If severe, administer an α-agonist such as epinephrine (1:10,000), 0.1 mL/kg via a slow IV push over 2 to 5 minutes, up to 3 mL/dose. Repeat in 5 to 30 minutes as needed. If the patient is not responsive to therapy, call for assistance (e.g., cardiopulmonary arrest response team or 911).

Hypotension with Bradycardia (Vagal Reaction)

- Secure the airway and give O_2, 6 to 10 L/min (via mask). Monitor electrocardiogram, O_2 saturation (pulse oximeter), and blood pressure.
- Elevate the legs 60° or more (preferred) or use the Trendelenburg position.
- Keep the patient warm.
- Administer a rapid infusion of IV or IO normal saline solution or Ringer's lactate. Caution should be used to avoid hypervolemia in children with myocardial dysfunction.
- Administer atropine IV, 0.02 mg/kg if the patient does not respond quickly to steps 2, 3, and 4. Use a minimum initial dose of 0.1 mg. The maximum initial dose is 0.5 mg (for an infant/child) or 1.0 mg (for an adolescent). May repeat every 3 to 5 minutes up to maximum dose up to 1.0 mg (for an infant/child) or 2.0 mg (for an adolescent). If the patient is not responsive to therapy, call for assistance.

IO, Intraosseous; *IM*, intramuscular; *IV*, intravenous; *PO*, by mouth.
From American College of Radiology Committee on Drugs and Contrast Media. *ACR manual on contrast media*, 7th ed. 2010. Available at http://www.acr.org/~/media/ACR/Documents/PDF/QualitySafety/Resources/Contrast%20Manual/FullManual.pdf. Accessed June 26, 2012.

HYPOTENSION WITH TACHYCARDIA (ANAPHYLAXIS)

Anaphylaxis can be a life-threatening response to contrast media. Symptoms may include difficulty breathing, chest tightness, a thready pulse, a rapid or irregular heart rate, dizziness, hoarseness, and/or loss of consciousness. The rapid response or code team should be called the moment this adverse effect is suspected. Meanwhile, management should be initiated with Trendelenburg positioning, securing of the airway, rapid fluid resuscitation, and administration of IV epinephrine.

HYPOTENSION WITH BRADYCARDIA (VASOVAGAL REACTION)

Patients may present with pallor, a decreased level of consciousness, diaphoresis, and a decreased heart rate. Management should be initiated with Trendelenburg positioning, securing of the airway, hydration, and administration of atropine if bradycardia persists (Box 2-3).

DELAYED REACTIONS

Delayed reactions appear to occur more frequently than acute/immediate reactions to administration of contrast media. The incidence ranges from 2% to 12%.[8,9] No definite data are available on the incidence and symptoms of delayed reactions in children. In adults, rash, itching and other cutaneous manifestations predominate.[9] Other symptoms include fevers, chills, nausea, vomiting, headaches, abdominal pain, drowsiness, and dizziness.[9] These symptoms can manifest any time from 1 hour to 2 days after administration of the contrast agent and usually resolve spontaneously by 7 days.[8-10]

Table 2-1

Pediatric Premedication Regimen for Prevention of Contrast Reaction		
Medication	Dosage	Timing
Prednisone	0.5-0.7 mg/kg PO (up to 50 mg)	13, 7, and 1 hour before contrast injection
Diphenhydramine	1.25 mg/kg PO (up to 50 mg)	1 hour before contrast injection

PO, by mouth.
From American College of Radiology Committee on Drugs and Contrast Media. *ACR manual on contrast media*, 7th ed. 2010. Available at http://www.acr.org/~/media/ACR/Documents/PDF/QualitySafety/Resources/Contrast%20Manual/FullManual.pdf. Accessed June 26, 2012.

PREVENTION

Before any study requiring administration of IV contrast media is begun, it is imperative to identify patients who would be at high risk for adverse reactions. If risk factors are identified, the need for the examination should be reassessed with the ordering clinician. Other modalities that may offer the same level of diagnosis but do not require administration of contrast agents should be considered. The possibility of performing the same test without the use of contrast media also should be entertained.

Ultimately, if the examination is considered absolutely necessary, the patient with known risk factors for adverse reactions should be premedicated with a combination of an antihistamine and corticosteroids. The regimen suggested by the ACR[2] is described in Table 2-1.

EXTRAVASATION

Extravasation is a well-recognized complication of contrast-enhanced imaging that occurs in approximately 0.7% of all injections.[16-19]

Risk Factors

Extravasation is more prone to occur in patients who are unable to verbalize their symptoms, such as infants, younger children, and severely ill and unconscious patients.[20,21] Increased rates also are noted in patients receiving chemotherapy, likely because of increased friability of the vein wall.[21,22,23]

Other risk factors include the site of injection, IV access type, and the method of injection.[21] Wang et al[16] noted that although the antecubital fossa was the single most common extravasation site, most of these events occurred in patients with venous access elsewhere. Increased incidents have been noted with injections at the dorsum of the hand.[24] Other risk factors also include venous thrombosis, extremity edema, multiple venous access attempts, and use of a tourniquet.[2,20,21] Extravasations are more frequent where preexisting catheters are used as access sites for administration of the contrast media.[22] At least two studies did not note any significant difference in the incidence of extravasation with the use of power injectors (Box 2-4).[24,25]

Box 2-4 Risk Factors for Intravenous Contrast Extravasation

Infants, young children, severely ill patients, and unconscious patients
Patients with friable veins
Presence of venous thrombosis or extremity edema
Injection sites other than antecubital fossa
Large volume of contrast medium
Injection through indwelling catheters
Multiple venous access attempts
Use of a tourniquet

Box 2-5 Signs and Symptoms of Contrast Extravasation

Pain, erythema, burning and/or tingling, tightness, swelling at the affected extremity
Blisters, skin ulceration, soft tissue necrosis
Compartment syndrome
Altered tissue perfusion
Paresthesia
Diminished arterial pulses

Presentation

The immediate symptoms of extravasation can be quite variable. Some patients present with a burning sensation, whereas others remain asymptomatic. Close attention should be paid to young children and unconscious patients because they may not be able to express these sensations. On physical examination, the extravasation site may be red, swollen, and tender.[2]

Most incidents are self-limiting and resolve spontaneously within 1 to 2 days. These incidents usually are restricted to the skin and subcutaneous tissue.[2] The injuries can range from transient tightness of the skin to tissue ulceration and necrosis to acute compartment syndromes. Severe reactions have been observed with both small and large volumes of extravasated contrast. However, the majority of severe reactions have been observed with larger volumes (Box 2-5).[26]

Management

A definite treatment approach has not been accepted because of a lack of consensus on the appropriate management of extravasation.[20,27,28] Minor symptoms can be treated with elevation of the affected extremity above the level of the heart to help reduce edema by promoting resorption of the fluid.[2,21] Sufficient data are lacking to support either warm or cold compresses over the affected limb.[2] Hyaluronidase injected subcutaneously may help speed resorption, but insufficient evidence exists to suggest routine use. Regardless, close monitoring of the patient is warranted. These events should be documented in the patient's medical records and appropriate directions should be provided to seek medical attention in the event of worsening symptoms.

Severe extravasation injuries require a surgical consultation. Such injuries may present as worsening of pain or swelling, skin blistering, decreased capillary refill, diminished pulses, and a change in sensation of the affected extremity.[2,20] Wang et al[16] noted in their observations that compartment

---

Box 2-6 Management of Contrast Extravasation

Elevation of extremity
Cold/warm compresses
Frequent monitoring of capillary refill, arterial pulses
Frequent questioning for progression of symptoms
Surgical consult

---

syndrome can develop even with less than 100 mL of extravasated fluid. Thus it is prudent to conclude that signs and symptoms, rather than the volume extravasated, should be used as a scale for seeking surgical consultation (Box 2-6).

CONTRAST-INDUCED NEPHROPATHY

Limited data are available on the nephrotoxic effects of iodinated contrast media in children. The ACR recommends following the principles used for adults in the prevention and management of contrast-induced nephropathy (CIN).[2] Risk factors for the development of CIN include preexisting renal insufficiency, diabetes mellitus, and multiple contrast media administrations during the same day.

CIN has been described as either an absolute increase in serum creatinine by at least 0.5 mg/dL within 48 hours of contrast injection[29] or an increase of more than 25% within 72 hours of contrast administration.[30] However, serum creatinine cannot be reliably used as a measure of renal function in this setting in the pediatric population.[2] The estimated glomerular filtration rate (GFR) is used widely for this purpose. The National Kidney Disease Education Program has provided information regarding the measurement of GFR at its website (http://www.nkdep.nih.gov/lab-evaluation/gfr-calculators.shtml) and advocates use of the bedside isotope dilution mass spectrometry–traceable Schwartz GFR calculator for children equation[31]:

$$GFR \ (mL/min/1.73 \ m^2) = (0.41 \times Height \ [cm])/ Creatinine \ [mg/dL]$$

A GFR of less than 30 mL/min is associated with an increased risk of CIN. Cystatin C, a protein that is produced by all nucleated cells and is exclusively eliminated by glomerular filtration, has been suggested as a better indicator of GFR than serum creatinine.

No significant studies have been conducted to understand the nephrotoxic effects, risk factors, or prevention of CIN in children. Hence when CIN is a concern for a pediatric patient, the clinician ordering the test and the radiologist must carefully consider the need for the study and the potential use of other modalities or unenhanced imaging.

NEPHROGENIC SYSTEMIC FIBROSIS

Nephrogenic systemic fibrosis is a disease characterized primarily by skin fibrosis, but it may involve multiple organs. Its association with gadolinium-based contrast agents has been realized and was first documented in 2006.[32] Nine pediatric cases have been reported as of 2008, with the patients ranging in age from 8 to 19 years.[33] Not enough data exist in the pediatric population to provide guidelines for the prevention of nephrogenic systemic fibrosis in children. The ACR[2] recommends following adult guidelines for identifying patients at risk and the use of gadolinium-based contrast media. The suggested risk factors are acute renal failure, decreased renal function with GFR less than 30 mL/min, high doses of administered gadolinium, and postsurgical status.[32,34,35] Only a limited number of gadolinium-based contrast agents have been studied and approved by the Food and Drug Administration for use in children younger than 2 years.[33] Gadolinium agents should be used with caution in infants and preterm babies because their renal function is immature.[33]

Key Points

Although allergic-like reactions are rare, they sometimes happen after injection of iodinated contrast media; thus screening for risk factors is important.

A guide describing management and weight-based doses of the medications should be within reach of every radiologist and should be posted in every room where a contrast injection occurs.

All reactions and the management provided should be documented in the medical record.

Patients with extravasation (any volume) should be closely monitored for worsening of pain and development of other symptoms suggesting compartment syndrome or tissue necrosis.

The GFR should be calculated for all children before the injection of iodinated contrast material.

Gadolinium should be used with caution in infants because of the immaturity of their renal function.

Suggested Reading

American College of Radiology Committee on Drugs and Contrast Media. *ACR manual on contrast media.* 7th ed. 2010. Available at http://www.acr.org/~/media/ACR/Documents/PDF/QualitySafety/Resources/Contrast%20Manual/FullManual.pdf. Accessed June 26, 2012.

Brockow K. Immediate and delayed reactions to radiocontrast media: is there an allergic mechanism? *Immunol Allergy Clin North Am.* 2009;29(3):453-468.

Mendichovszky IA, Marks SD, Simcock CM, et al. Gadolinium and nephrogenic systemic fibrosis: time to tighten practice. *Pediatr Radiol.* 2008;38:489-496.

Namasivayam S, Kalra MK, Torres WE, et al. Adverse reactions to intravenous iodinated contrast media: a primer for radiologists. *Emerg Radiol.* 2006;12:210-215.

Rudnick MR, Keselheim A, Goldfarb S. Contrast-induced nephropathy: how it develops, how to prevent it. *Cleve Clin J Med.* 2006;73:75-80.

Schaverein MV, Evison D, McCulley SJ. Management of large volume CT contrast medium extravasation injury: technical refinement and literature review. *J Plast Reconstr Aesthet Surg.* 2008;61(5):562-565.

References

Full references for this chapter can be found on www.expertconsult.com.

Chapter 3

Magnetic Resonance Safety

JEAN A. TKACH

Magnetic resonance imaging (MRI) has proved to be a powerful diagnostic imaging tool in children and adults. MRI uses low-energy nonionizing radio waves, and as such it is particularly well suited for pediatric and longitudinal imaging studies. MRI exploits a wide variety of intrinsic tissue-specific properties to generate a wide spectrum of tissue contrast, thus providing detailed information about anatomy, physiology, and function. For clinical MR exams, the acquisition techniques used and the specific acquisition parameters selected are manipulated to generate the type of image contrast most relevant to the underlying medical question. Unlike MRI, ultrasound is limited by the restriction of bone anatomy, and radiography uses ionizing radiation. Compared with other diagnostic imaging modalities, MRI has proved to be superior at imaging soft tissues. In addition, MRI enables images to be obtained in numerous planes and/or it enables true volumetric data acquisition without the need to reposition the patient. Once collected, the imaging data can be reformatted to any arbitrary plane and/or rendered to provide a three-dimensional representation of anatomy and/or physiologic and functional parameters.

The MR environment is the term used to describe the area immediately surrounding and including the MR scanner.[1] It is characterized by the three types of electromagnetic fields used to generate images: (1) the strong static magnetic field and associated spatial gradients (fringe field), (2) the smaller time-varying magnetic gradient fields (imaging gradients, measured in kilohertz), and (3) the radiofrequency (RF) magnetic fields (RF pulses, megahertz FM radio band). When performed under the appropriate conditions, no safety risks are inherent to MRI, and millions of MRI examinations are performed each year without incident. However, when not appropriately managed, safety concerns exist for each of the three electromagnetic fields used for MRI (Table 3-1) as well as the associated acoustic noise. Notably, most MR-related injuries and the few fatalities that have occurred primarily were a result of the failure to adhere to MR safety guidelines for the MRI environment, or they occurred because inaccurate or outdated MR safety-related information for biomedical implants and devices was used.[2,3] To prevent similar adverse MR safety-related incidents from occurring, it is imperative that the potential safety risks intrinsic to the MR environment be understood and respected by users of this powerful imaging technology (Boxes 3-1 and 3-2).

Safety Considerations of the Magnetic Resonance Environment

MAIN STATIC MAGNETIC FIELD

Biologic Effects of Static Magnetic Fields

The majority of MR units in clinical use today operate at main or static magnetic field strengths of 0.2 to 3.0 tesla (T). For comparison, the static field of a 1.5-T scanner is approximately 30,000 times stronger than Earth's magnetic field (roughly 0.00005 T). The most recent United States Food and Drug Administration (FDA) guidelines state that for adults, children, and infants older than 1 month, diagnostic MRI systems that operate at or below 8 T are considered to be a nonsignificant risk. For neonates, the limit is 4 T.[4] In practice, 3 T is the highest field strength in common clinical use. Initially, some concern was expressed that the strong magnetic fields might have irreversible detrimental biologic/health effects in humans, including alterations in cell growth and morphology, cell reproduction and teratogenicity, DNA structure and gene expression, prenatal and postnatal reproduction and development, blood-brain barrier permeability, nerve activity, cognitive function and behavior, cardiovascular dynamics, hematologic indexes, temperature regulation, circadian rhythms, immune responsiveness, and other biologic processes.[5-23] However, a comprehensive review of the literature indicates that short-term exposures (of a duration comparable to an MR examination) to high-static magnetic fields produce no appreciable detrimental biologic effects.[24,25]

Although no lasting adverse effects of short-term exposures to high magnetic field strengths have been reported, several relatively transient reversible biologic effects are known to occur, including electrocardiographic changes and benign sensory effects. These effects have been reported primarily at field strengths greater than 2 T and the sensory effects appear to occur most often when a person's head is moved rapidly within the static magnetic field. The elevation in electrocardiographic T waves is believed to be due to magnetohydrodynamic phenomena. When an electrically conductive fluid, such as blood, flows within a magnetic field, an electric current is produced, as is a mechanical force opposing the flow. Hence the movement of blood in the magnetic field of the MRI causes a magnetohydrodynamic

Table 3-1

Principal Mechanisms of Interaction of the Three Main MRI Energy Fields with Tissues and Some Related Effects		
Magnetic Resonance–Related Electromagnetic Field	Mechanism of Interaction	Potential Effects
Static magnetic field (T)	Polarization/ magnetization	Elevated electrocardiographic T wave and/or transient sensory effects (e.g., vertigo, nausea, phosphenes, and metallic taste)
Transient gradient magnetic field (dB/dt)	Induced currents Acoustic noise	Peripheral nerve stimulation Physiologic stress, anxiety, temporary hearing loss
Radio frequency field (specific absorption rate)	Thermal heating	Local burns

From Bushong SC. Biologic effects of magnetic resonance imaging. In: *MR safety, magnetic resonance imaging: physical and biological principles.* 3rd ed. St Louis: Mosby; 2003.

Box 3-1 Magnetic Resonance Safety Organizations

International Electrotechnical Commission (IEC)
Food and Drug Administration (FDA)
National Electrical Equipment Manufacturer's Association (NEMA)
American Society for Testing and Materials (ASTM)
American College of Radiology (ACR)

From Center for Devices and Radiological Health, Food and Drug Administration. *FDA guidelines for magnetic resonance equipment safety.* Available at http://www.aapm.org/meetings/02AM/pdf/8356-48054.pdf. Accessed July 25, 2012.

Box 3-2 Magnetic Resonance Imaging Safety Standards

International Electrotechnical Commission
  60601-2-33—Requirements for the Safety of MR Equipment for Medical Diagnosis
Food and Drug Administration—Guidelines for Premarket Notifications for MR Diagnostic Devices
National Electrical Equipment Manufacturer's Association MS 1 through 12—Safety and Performance Standards
American Society for Testing and Materials—Test Methods for MR Safety of Implanted Medical Devices
American College of Radiology—Site Safety Guidelines

From Center for Devices and Radiological Health, Food and Drug Administration. *FDA guidelines for magnetic resonance equipment safety.* Available at http://www.aapm.org/meetings/02AM/pdf/8356-48054.pdf. Accessed July 25, 2012.

---

effect that produces a voltage across the vessel. Typically, the voltage is negligible except in large arteries such as the aorta (on the order of 5 mV/T) and for high blood velocities. Because the peak flow rate occurs during the repolarization phase of the cardiac cycle, the added voltage from the flowing blood manifests as an artifactual elevation of the T wave.[26,27] The voltage associated with the magnetohydrodynamic effect is not considered hazardous at the magnetic field strengths that are approved for clinical use. However, at higher field strengths, the possibility exists that the induced potential might exceed 40 mV, which is the threshold for depolarization of cardiac muscle.[28]

Several short-term, relatively benign sensory effects have been reported at higher field strengths, including vertigo, nausea, headaches, flashing lights (also known as *magnetophosphenes*), a metallic taste, and/or sensation in dental fillings.[29] The magnetophosphenes are believed to be a result of torque upon the rods or cones in the retina imposed by the magnetodynamic resistive forces during quick movements of the head and/or eyes within the magnetic field. Similarly, the vertigo, nausea, and/or headache have been posited to be associated with torque on the hair cells in the semicircular canals (causing disequilibrium). Electrical currents induced in saliva or metallic fillings are believed to account for the incidences of a metallic taste and/or sensations that have been reported.

Interaction of the Main Magnetic Field with Ferromagnetic Objects

5 Gauss Line

Although exposure to high magnetic fields may not inherently be unsafe, failure to adhere to safe practices within the MR environment have led to most of the MR–related accidents and fatalities that have occurred. These incidents have involved the inappropriate and/or inadvertent introduction of metallic objects and or implanted medical devices into the scan room. The term *fringe field* typically is used to refer to the full spatial extent of the magnetic field gradient associated with an MR magnet. Five gauss (G) (0.0005 T) and below are considered "safe" levels of static magnetic field exposure for the general public.[1] The 5 G line identifies the perimeter around an MR scanner within which the static magnetic fields are higher than 5 G; it is the most commonly recognized MR safety policy.[26] Safety considerations require that this distance from the magnet be determined and that potentially unsafe areas be identified with appropriate and conspicuous signage. Importantly, the 5G line extends in three dimensions; thus when the MR area is sited, the extent of the fringe field to the floors above and below the magnet must be considered. Notably, the term *MR environment* also is often used synonymously to refer to the area within the 5 G line. Because of the potential hazards, access to this area must be rigorously controlled and supervised.

Magnetic Field Interactions: Torque and Attractive Forces

The field associated with an MR scanner can be separated into two spatial regions defined by the types of interaction with ferromagnetic objects that predominate in each region. The first region surrounds the magnet isocenter and is contained within the bore of the MRI scanner. The magnetic field in this region essentially is temporally constant and homogeneous in strength. A magnetic object introduced into this region of the static field is subjected to a torque that acts to align it with the magnetic field, just as magnetic material aligns itself with the poles of a permanent bar magnet or a compass needle aligns itself with the earth's magnetic field.[1] Hence any nonspherical metallic object that enters the spatially homogenous static region of the field will be subjected to a rotational force or torque such that its long axis will be aligned with that of the main magnetic field. If metallic implants are not sufficiently anchored by the surrounding tissue (e.g., bone in the case of an orthopedic implant), this rotational motion of metallic implants will cause trauma to the surrounding tissue. The magnitude of these effects depends on the geometry and mass of the object, as well as the characteristics of the MR system's magnetic field.

In the second region (the fringe field), the strong magnetic field strength drops off rapidly as the distance from the magnet increases, producing a large spatial gradient that typically is greatest in regions immediately adjacent to the magnet. Metallic objects introduced into this magnetic field gradient experience a translational (attractive) and rotational force. The translation will be in the direction of the higher field strength. The strength of the attractive/translational force will depend on the size of the object and its location within the gradient field and will increase rapidly as the object approaches the magnet. As such, the metallic object will be accelerated along the direction of the spatial gradients in the static field and quickly can become a dangerous projectile. Depending on the size and composition of the metallic object, these attractive/translational effects may begin as soon as the object is introduced into the scan room. Once the object enters the uniform field within the bore of the magnet, acceleration will cease and the object will come to a stop.[26]

The potential hazards associated with the spatial gradients are greatest for high magnetic field strengths and large fringe fields. In general, the forces increase approximately as the square of the field strength but will vary depending on the composition of the object.[30] For example, at 3 T compared with 1.5 T, the force on a paramagnetic material (e.g., a stainless steel scalpel) is five times greater, whereas the force on a ferromagnetic object (e.g., a steel wrench) is 2.5 times greater.[30] Finally, but importantly, even for a given field strength, the magnitude and footprint of the spatial gradients can vary between magnet configurations. For example, it has been reported that short-bore MR systems have significantly higher spatial gradients than do long-bore scanners, particularly those operating at 3 T.[31,32] This finding highlights the multiple nuances and factors that must be considered when evaluating and establishing MR safety guidelines and operating procedures for any object before it may be introduced into a specific MRI environment. The potential risks associated with the introduction of metallic objects into regions of high and or rapidly spatially varying magnetic field strengths cannot be underestimated. It is a common misconception that the magnet is only "on" when the images are being acquired. However, the magnet is *always* on, and signage to indicate the "Magnet is ON" should be displayed conspicuously on the door to the MR scan room.

Missile/Projectile Effect

The projectile/missile effect, wherein a ferromagnetic object is accelerated toward the isocenter of the magnet, is the most widely recognized and publicized safety hazard associated with MRI. Objects constructed partially or entirely of ferromagnetic materials (e.g., iron, nickel, cobalt, and the rare earth metals chromium, gadolinium, and dysprosium) are strongly attracted to the magnet bore. Steel objects also are highly ferromagnetic, as are some medical grades of stainless steel.

Notably, working a metal by machining, molding, and/or bending it, for example, can alter its magnetic properties and, as a result, some forms of nonmagnetic stainless steel can be made magnetic. For this reason, the MR safety of a given metallic object must be evaluated in its final form.[33] Although metals such as aluminum, tin, titanium, gold, and lead are not ferromagnetic, objects are rarely made of a single metal (e.g., the ferromagnetic screws used to secure the wheels to the frame of an aluminum cart).[33] Consequently, carefully inspecting all objects before introducing them into the MR environment is necessary. If any doubt remains regarding the presence of ferromagnetic material, the object should be checked with a permanent magnet and/or a ferromagnetic wand as a final precautionary measure before it enters the scan room.

As noted previously, within the MR environment, a ferromagnetic object will experience a magnetic pull that increases greatly as it approaches the magnet bore. Depending on the size of the object, the magnetic field strength, and the proximity of the object to the magnet, the attractive force may be so great that it becomes impossible for an individual to continue to hold onto the object. Any individual—whether a patient or a staff member—who is in the path between the object and the center of the magnet (e.g., the patient lying in the magnet bore) can be seriously injured or killed.[34] Numerous instances of MR-related accidents involving objects such as scalpels, scissors, oxygen tanks, intravenous line poles, wheelchairs, transport carts, floor buffers, mop buckets, vacuum cleaners, other medical devices, and even firearms have been documented. Any injuries related to ferromagnetic projectiles must be documented; the necessary forms can be accessed on the FDA website.[35,36] More comprehensive information regarding these online resources is provided in a later section of this chapter.

To prevent potentially devastating MR-related accidents from occurring, it is essential that access to areas that exceed the 5 G line must be rigorously restricted and vigilantly supervised at all times. All patients, accompanying family members, and hospital personnel with a demonstrated need to enter the MR environment must be appropriately educated to the potential hazards and rigorously screened for contraindications.

TIME-VARYING GRADIENT MAGNETIC FIELDS

During imaging acquisition, gradient magnetic fields are transiently imposed along the main magnetic field to spatially localize and encode the spins. These gradient magnetic fields are much weaker than the static magnetic field and are generated by gradient coils located inside the magnet bore. Each orthogonal axis (i.e., x, y, and z) has a pair of gradient coils. For a given direction, a linear gradient magnetic field is generated within the main magnetic field by applying electrical current in opposite directions to the coil pair over a short time interval.[28] When this gradient magnetic field is applied, the magnetic field intensity changes rapidly, giving rise to a time-varying magnetic field. The rate of change in magnetic field (dB) occurs over time (dt) and usually is measured and reported in units of dB/dt expressed in milliteslas per meter per millisecond (mT/m/msec) or in gauss per centimeter per second (G/cm/sec). During the rise time of the magnetic field, an electrical current can be induced in any electrical conductor (e.g., implanted medical device, wire, human body). Notably, the magnitude of the time-varying magnetic field along each of the three spatial directions (i.e., x, y, and z) is zero at the center of the magnet and increases linearly with increasing distance from the isocenter.

Because the human body is a conductor, the rapidly switching magnetic fields can induce electrical fields and current in a patient (as described by Faraday's law of induction) that may lead to the stimulation of muscle and nerve tissues.[28] The mean threshold levels (measured in tesla per second) for various stimulations are 3600 T/sec for the heart, 900 T/sec for the respiratory system, 90 T/sec for pain, and 60 T/sec for the peripheral nerves. However, the exact values differ significantly among individuals.[26] Experience has shown that sufficient dB/dt levels can produce brief muscle twitches and peripheral nerve stimulation (PNS) that is perceptible as a "tingling" or "tapping" sensation. This sensation can become uncomfortable and/or painful as the gradient magnetic field increases to 50% to 100% above perception thresholds.[37] For these reasons, threshold sensations, when reported, should not be ignored, because they may readily escalate to uncomfortable levels. Although cardiac stimulation is a concern, studies conducted in dogs have shown that the cardiac stimulation threshold for the most sensitive 1% of the population is 20 times, and the mean defibrillation threshold is 500 times, the energy required for PNS.[33] The exceedingly strong and/or rapidly switching gradient magnetic fields necessary to achieve cardiac stimulation threshold levels are more than an order of magnitude greater than those used in commercially available MR systems.[37-39]

In addition to varying from person to person, stimulation thresholds also depend on gradient direction. Assuming equal dB/dt for each of the three gradient axes, the associated gradient-induced electric fields are highest for the largest perpendicular body cross section. Accordingly, the y gradient has the lowest dB/dt PNS threshold since the x-z cross section of the human body is usually larger than the other cross sections.[40,41,41a] In addition, the mean PNS threshold for the y gradient was further reduced (by approximately 32%) when the patient's hands were clasped; the x and z gradient PNS thresholds were not similarly affected.[40,41,41a] In practice, the potential for PNS is greatest for fast imaging (e.g., echo planar imaging [EPI]) acquisitions, particularly when oblique imaging planes are obtained where the combined contributions of gradients from more than one axis result in a higher effective slew and/or when the readout (i.e., frequency encode) lies along the craniocaudal direction.[26]

When the threshold for PNS is exceeded, the anatomic site of the stimulation depends on the direction along which the magnetic field gradient is applied. Anatomic sites stimulated by the activation of the x gradients include the bridge of the nose, left side of the thorax, iliac crest, left thigh, buttocks, and lower back. Stimulation sites associated with the application of the y gradient include the scapula, upper arms, shoulder, right side of the thorax, iliac crest, hip, hands, and upper back. For the z gradient, stimulation sites are the scapula, thorax, xiphoid, abdomen, iliac crest, and upper and lower back.[37] In addition, it has been noted that the PNS sites typically correspond to bony prominences. Because bone is less conductive than the surrounding tissue, it is believed that current densities are increased in narrow regions of tissue between bone and skin, resulting in lower than expected nerve stimulation thresholds.[37]

Normal imaging sequences (e.g., conventional spin echo and gradient echo) induce currents of a few tens of milliamperes per square meter, a level that is far below that present in the normal brain and heart tissue. However, as noted previously, PNS is quite possible for the rapid imaging techniques such as EPI and for high-performance gradients. These effects can be controlled by limiting the maximum rate of change in the magnetic field gradients. Early limits imposed by the FDA to prevent PNS were 1 dB/dt at 20 T/sec for pulse durations greater than 120 microseconds.[33] However, the increasingly apparent diagnostic benefits and widespread use of EPI, single-shot fast-spin echo, and other fast imaging techniques for routine clinical MR imaging caused the FDA to reevaluate and revise these limits. It is now recognized that although these rapid imaging techniques have the potential to cause PNS, the sensation in itself is not harmful. However, painful stimulation still should be avoided. Thus the current FDA standard is based on the threshold for sensation, rather than a specific numerical value of dB/dt. Specifically, "current FDA guidance limits the time rate of change of magnetic field (dB/dt) to levels which do not result in painful peripheral nerve stimulation." This policy reflects in part the complexity of modeling and calculating the current distribution in the body associated with the pulsed gradient fields. Correspondingly, dB/dt levels below that resulting in painful stimulation are considered a nonsignificant risk by the FDA. It is important to note that dB/dt is a function of the gradient strength and rise time and not of the static field strength. Thus dB/dt is of equal concern for both lower and higher field scanners.

Clinically, two operating modes for the RF and gradient field levels used for imaging are permissible, normal and first level controlled (Table 3-2). In normal mode, the system output levels are below those that will cause physiologic stress and therefore are appropriate for all subjects. Alternatively, in first level conditional mode, one of the MR system outputs (e.g., dB/dt) may reach a value that may cause physiological stress and thus may not be appropriate for the most medically compromised patients. Operation in this mode requires authorization by appropriate clinical staff and vigilant medical supervision during the examination. Institutional Review Board approval is required for operation above these levels (second level controlled). In practice, the commercial MR

Table 3-2

International Electrotechnical Commission/Food and Drug Administration Operating Modes for Magnetic Resonance Imaging Diagnostic Equipment	
Operating Mode	**Conditions/Qualifications**
Normal mode	Will not cause stress; suitable for all patients
First level controlled mode	May cause stress; requires medical supervision and positive action by operator to enter
Second level controlled mode	Institutional Review Board approval required

From Center for Devices and Radiological Health, Food and Drug Administration. *FDA guidelines for magnetic resonance equipment safety* (website): http://www.aapm.org/meetings/02AM/pdf/8356-48054.pdf. Accessed July 25, 2012.

systems monitor dB/dt throughout the examination and generate a warning for the specific protocols for which PNS is likely. The PNS limits are derived from the empirical results obtained from clinical trials. For normal operating mode, the dB/dt threshold level is set at 80% of the mean threshold value for PNS stimulation, and it is set at 100% for the first level.[3C] In addition, the MR operator should remain in constant verbal contact with the patient and instruct him or her to report any tingling, muscle twitching, or painful sensations that occur during scanning. This contact is not possible for infants and for sedated, noncommunicative, or otherwise compromised patients. Operationally, dB/dt can be reduced by increasing the field of view and/or slice thickness, reducing the matrix size, and decreasing receiver bandwidth. In addition, because the y gradient has the lowest stimulation threshold, whenever possible, the most rapidly changing gradient waveform (e.g., read out; i.e., frequency encode in EPI) should be placed along a direction other than y.

RADIOFREQUENCY FIELDS

Biologic Effects

One of the primary safety concerns in MRI is tissue heating. The conductivity of tissue allows the absorption of RF energy, which is transformed into heat as a result of resistive losses.[42,43] The heating is greatest at the periphery of the body, and thus the skin is the most prone to this effect.[30] When thermally challenged, the body responds by thermoregulatory mechanisms and attempts to dissipate the heat by means of convection, conduction, radiation, and evaporation. If these attempts are not completely successful, the heat accumulates and is stored, resulting in a rise in local tissue and/or systemic core temperatures,[42-44] which has the potential to produce physiological changes.[28] For humans, the typical skin temperatures are about 33° C, whereas core temperatures are about 37° C. Experience has shown that when the body is subjected to significant RF power levels, it immediately attempts to dissipate the heat load through vasodilatation of the blood vessels of the skin, with the skin approaching core temperature. This response mechanism allows the body to reduce heat fairly rapidly and typically is evidenced by flushing of the skin, which in itself is not harmful and usually subsides within several hours.

The dose measure used to describe this energy absorption or heat dose is the specific absorption rate (SAR). SAR is defined in the International Electrotechnical Commission standard as the amount of RF power (measured in watts) absorbed per patient mass in kilograms (W/kg). The MR system software calculates an SAR for each acquisition and enforces the limits established by the FDA. Because SAR depends on patient weight, it is important that an accurate value be entered during the patient registration procedure. The amount of RF energy that is absorbed is dependent on the frequency (as determined by the static magnetic field strength), the RF coil used, the volume (size), composition (conductivity), and configuration of the exposed tissue and the duty cycle and type of RF pulses applied, as well as other factors.[42-46] Notably, SAR increases with the square of the frequency (and hence magnetic field strength) and patient size.[30] Consequently, for a given pulse sequence, doubling the field strength (e.g., 1.5 vs. 3 T) results in a factor of four increase in SAR. SAR can be minimized by decreasing the power and/or duty cycle of the RF pulses. In practice, this minimization can be accomplished by increasing the repetition time, reducing the number of slices, and, when feasible, reducing the RF flip angle (because SAR is proportional to the square of the flip angle). In addition, for fast-spin echo and EPI acquisitions, SAR also can be reduced by increasing the interecho spacing and/or reducing the echo train length (for a fixed repetition time).

A person's ability to respond to the thermal challenge and effectively dissipate the heat is influenced by the rate at which the energy is deposited and the duration of the exposure. Underlying health conditions such as cardiovascular disease, hypertension, diabetes, fever, old age, obesity, or a compromised ability to perspire can impair a person's ability to tolerate the thermal challenge.[47-51] In addition, certain medications such as diuretics, β-blockers, calcium channel blockers, amphetamines, muscle relaxants, and sedatives can alter the body's thermoregulatory responses significantly, with some medications actually having a synergistic effect with respect to tissue heating caused by RF exposure.[3] Finally, the ability of the subject to dissipate heat also is affected by the ambient temperature, relative humidity, and airflow in the MR scan room.

To prevent excessive heat stress and/or local tissue damage, the FDA has established guidelines to limit allowable whole-body SAR levels to those that produce no more than a 1° C increase in tissue and/or core temperature beyond the normal 37° C.[28] As with dB/dt, two levels of clinical operation are possible for SAR. Note, however, that only the whole-body SAR limit is increased, from 2 W/kg to 4 W/kg, in the advancement from normal to first level controlled operation. The SAR limit for normal and first level controlled operating modes for the head is 3.2 W/kg (1°C maximum temperature increase) averaged over head mass and 10 W/kg temperature over any 10 g of tissue for the torso and extremities.[52] These SAR limits correspond to time-averaged values over a 6-minute interval. Exceptions to the specified FDA guidelines include infants and pregnant women, for whom the FDA recommends that the limits be reduced by a factor of two. Similarly, for patients with thermoregulatory compromise (e.g., cardiovascular impairment, cerebral vascular impairment, and diabetes), the FDA recommends a whole-body SAR limit of 1.5 W/kg.[33] In addition, the SAR limits are reduced when the ambient temperature rises above 24° C (75° F) or if the humidity exceeds 60%.

Interaction with Other Devices

Additional safety concerns associated with RF irradiation exist when objects made from conductive materials that have an elongated shape or are looped, such as electrodes, monitor leads, guidewires, and certain types of catheters (e.g., catheters with thermistors or other conducting components), are present in the magnet bore.[38,53-58] The rapidly changing magnetic field associated with the RF can induce an electromotive force in the conductor and, hence, current flow, which, because of electrical resistance, will lead to heating of the conductor. If the conductor is in contact with the skin, burns can result. Incidents of first-, second- and third-degree burns have been reported.[3,26] Notably, maximum current induction occurs when the plane of the conducting loop is perpendicular to that of the changing magnetic field. Inductive heating also can occur when the active-decoupling circuitry associates with a receive-only coil fails. In addition, because the body is a conductor, inadvertent conductive loops can arise in the absence of any external conductors, when, for example, the patient's hands or calves are in contact to form a closed loop. In such cases, heating can occur at the high-resistance skin-to-skin contact point, which can result in local redness and blistering. To minimize the possibility of RF burns, all conductors (e.g., leads and coils) that are not being used should be removed from the magnet bore. In addition, the integrity of all conductors that must remain in the magnet bore should be verified before the MR examination, and these cables, leads, and/or wires should be kept as straight as possible and run down the center of the bore. In addition, the patient should be thermally and/or electrically isolated (e.g., using pads and/or sheets or blankets) from direct contact with all conductors and all RF body transmitters, as well as surface coils, and skin to skin contact should be avoided. The MR operator must be extra vigilant to mitigate the potential heating risks for infants and sedated or other noncommunicative patients. Any metallic object in or on the patient may absorb RF energy, resulting in excessive heating that may lead to thermal damage of surrounding tissue; the potential for this effect is greatest at higher field strengths.[28,33]

ACOUSTIC NOISE

The predominant and most widely recognized source of MRI-related acoustic noise is the time-varying gradient magnetic field applied during MR imaging. The rapid pulsed currents within the gradient coils in the presence of the static magnetic field create strong Lorentz forces that produce a torque on the coil itself, causing it to move and/or vibrate against its mounting. This movement, analogous to that of the diaphragm of a loudspeaker, creates the loud chirping, tapping, knocking, and banging noises heard by the subject during MR imaging.[3,28] Sound levels for MRI are measured in A-weighted decibels (dBA), which takes the frequency response of the human auditory system into account. As a reference, normal conversation is approximately 60 dBA (www.osha.gov), and a difference of 6 dBA represents a doubling of sound intensity. Sound pressure levels (SPL) of 81 to 117 dBA are common for standard 1.5 T MRI examinations[59] and can be as high as 130 dBA for high-speed acquisitions such as EPI and techniques that use nontraditional (i.e., non-Cartesian) k-space trajectories, such as propeller, radial, and spiral sequences. Although many factors influence the intensity of the MR-related acoustic noise (e.g., gradient coil design, gradient amplitude and slew rate, size of patient, location of patient in magnet bore), higher field strength systems tend to be louder.

MRI-related acoustic noise may lead to simple annoyance, difficulties in verbal communication, heightened anxiety, and temporary or potentially permanent hearing loss for both the patient and other persons in or near the MR scan room.[60-72] In addition, the noise may cause confusion and or extreme anxiety in more vulnerable patients such as children and elderly persons and in persons with psychiatric disorders.[60,62,73] MRI-related noise also has been reported to produce alterations in physiologic parameters in neonates, which may be problematic in light of their immature cardiac physiology and cerebrovascular regulation.[64] Furthermore, the acoustic noise

levels may cause discomfort to sedated patients, and certain drugs are known to increase hearing sensitivity.[63] Because exposure duration is one of the most influential factors in determining the effect of noise on hearing, it is unlikely that the noise levels experienced during the relatively short MR examinations will have a long-term negative effect on hearing.[74,75] It is the short-term effects of MR-related acoustic noise that are the primary concern.

The FDA indicates that MR-related acoustic noise levels must be below the level of concern established by pertinent federal regulatory or other recognized standard-setting organizations.[76] Guidelines for acceptable acoustic noise levels associated with MRI are based on Occupational Safety and Health Administration (OSHA) guidelines for industrial workers, which recognize that the risk is a function of its intensity and the duration of exposure.[26] OSHA standards stipulate that to avoid hearing damage, the peak unweighted SPL cannot exceed 140 dB[28] and the A-weighted root mean square SPL cannot exceed 99 dBA, with hearing protection in place. Because the acoustic noise level for many sequences can exceed 99 dBA, the MR manufacturer must recommend that it is necessary for the MR system operator to provide the patient with hearing protection.[3] Hearing protection should also be given to all other persons who will be present in the scan room during the MR exam.

The Noise Reduction Rating (NRR) is the standard for hearing protection devices established by the Environmental Protection Agency. For a given noise attenuator, the NRR value is the mean attenuation value (in dB) for the device minus two standard deviations, corresponding to the minimum noise reduction achieved by 98% of the population. For MR examinations, adequate hearing protection can be most easily and effectively accomplished with earplugs (≈29 to 32 dBA NRR) and/or headphones (≈29 to 49 dBA for adults and 7 to 12 dBA mini muffs for infants). Notably, the NRR reported for earplugs will not be realized if they are improperly inserted or do not fit snugly, as often may be the case for young pediatric patients. Although the combined use of earplugs and headphones do not produce additive effects in hearing protection per se, they can increase the NRR by 5 to 6 dB (equivalent to approximately half the sound intensity) for frequencies ≤2000 Hz (http://www.biac.duke.edu/research/safety/tutorial.asp). At frequencies higher than 2000 Hz, hearing protection is limited by bone conduction, and the combined use of headphones and earplugs is less beneficial. Nevertheless, the harmonic response of MR systems for a wide spectrum of imaging protocols contains a significant amount of energy at or below 2000 Hz so that combined use is still advisable (Fig. 3-1). MR manufacturers are actively working to further decrease noise levels by using methods such as quieter MR sequences, active noise cancellation filters, acoustic hoods,[59] and vacuum packing.[73]

CLAUSTROPHOBIA

Many persons find the confinement of the MRI bore at least somewhat disconcerting, particularly when a head coil is used. For some persons, this discomfort is extreme and can result in anxiety that may escalate into panic. In these cases, sedation is required to perform the MR examination. Claustrophobic reactions in the scanner typically are characterized

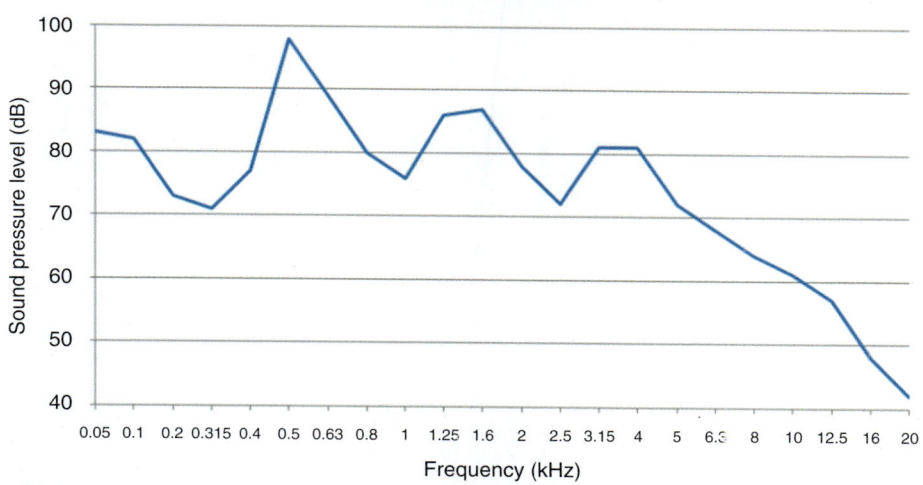

Figure 3-1 Harmonic response of a conventional 1.5 T magnetic resonance scanner for a standard spin echo acquisition demonstrating significant energy below 2 kHz. The human auditory range is 20 Hz to 20 kHz.

Table 3-3

Magnetic Resonance Environment Medical Device Concerns		
Component of Magnetic Resonance Environment	**Medical Device Concern**	**Potential Adverse Effect**
Static magnetic field (always on)	Rotational force (torque) on object Translational force on object	Trauma to tissue as object rotates to align with main field Tissue damage as object accelerates toward magnet bore (projectile/missile effect)
Gradient magnetic field (pulsed during imaging)	Induced currents due to dB/dt	Device malfunction or failure
Radio frequency field (pulsed during imaging)	Radio frequency–induced currents resulting in heating Electromagnetic interference—active	Patient burns (thermal and electrical) Device malfunction, induced noise (monitoring devices)

From Food and Drug Administration. *Primer on medical device interactions with magnetic resonance imaging, US Food and Drug Administration (FDA) Systems.* Available at http://www.fda.gov/MedicalDevices/DeviceRegulationandGuidance/GuidanceDocuments/ucm107721.htm. Accessed July 25, 2012.

by a fear of suffocation and/or a fear that something will happen while they are confined.[77] Operationally, experience suggests that this reaction can be minimized by maintaining frequent verbal contact with the individual throughout the examination and sufficient airflow (e.g., a bore fan) to reduce heat and mitigate the fear of suffocation. In addition, the individual also should be provided with an emergency panic notification device (e.g., a pneumatic squeeze bulb) to allow him or her to summon help at any time throughout the examination. In fact, such a device should be provided to all nonsedated communicative patients as a means of notifying the MR operator immediately upon any sign of discomfort, including local heating or tugging of ferromagnetic objects (e.g., a belt or shoes).

MEDICAL IMPLANTS, DEVICES, AND OTHER METALLIC POTENTIAL HAZARDS

Passive and Electrically Active Medical Devices

The MR environment may be unsafe for persons with certain medical implants or devices that are made out of ferromagnetic materials. For passive implants (i.e., any medical device that serves its function without the supply of power, such as aneurysm clips, shunts, or stents) made of ferromagnetic materials, the primary concern is movement and/or dislodgement,[31,32,35,36,54,78-87] although excessive heating of the implant is also possible (Table 3-3). Several incidents have occurred in which metallic implants were mistakenly introduced into the MR environment and were dislodged within or from the body, resulting in blindness or death.[26] For electrically active implants such as deep brain or vagal nerve stimulators and drug pumps, excessive heating at the lead tips and associated tissue damage is the primary safety concern.[56,88-90] Device malfunction, device heating, induced currents, and movement and/or dislodgement also are potential hazards (Table 3-3).

When it is known that a patient has an implant (passive or active), the implant should be considered a contraindication for MRI until documented proof of its MR compatibility and safety is verified. The information must correspond to the exact model and serial number of the device, which should be recorded in the patient's medical record. If such

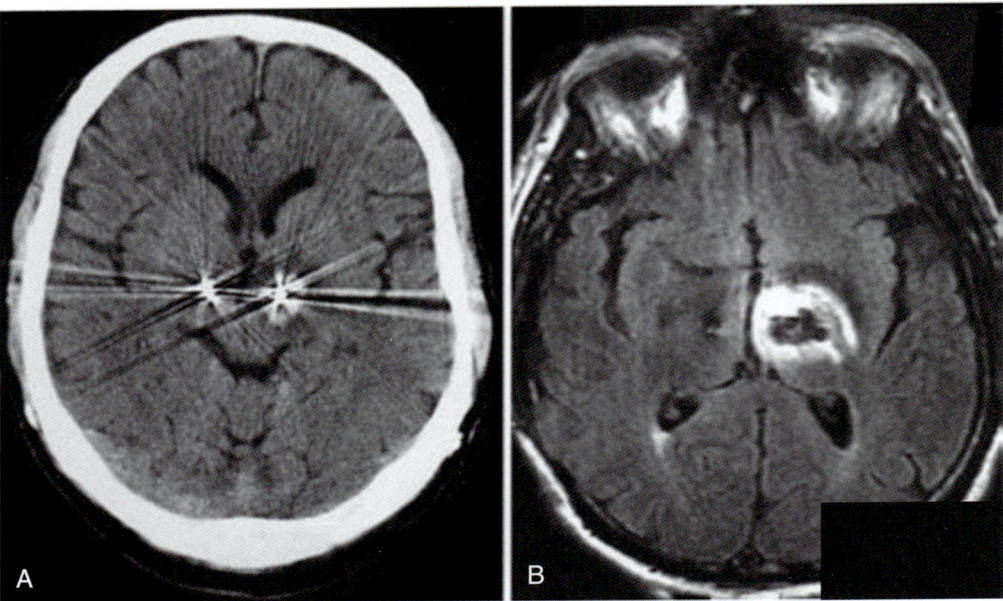

Figure 3-2   Adverse event due to failure to adhere to medical device product guidelines. Tissue damage (hemorrhage on computerized tomography (CT) (**A**) and edema on magnetic resonance imaging (MRI)) as a result of radiofrequency heating at the deep brain stimulator (DBS) lead tip that occurred during a routine MR examination of the lumbar spine. The CT and MRI images of the brain were acquired immediately after a lumbar spine MR scan performed on a 1.0 T MR scanner using the body coil to transmit and a surface coil to receive, and a relatively specific absorption rate (SAR) aggressive imaging protocol. Alternatively, the DBS device manufacturers specified the MR conditions under which MR imaging can be accomplished safely for patients implanted with this device as a 1.5 T scanner using a Transmit receive head coil and head SAR levels at or below 0.1 W/kg. (From Henderson JM, Tkach JA, Phillips M, et al. Permanent neurological deficit related to magnetic resonance imaging in a patient with implanted deep brain stimulation electrodes for Parkinson's disease: case report. *Neurosurgery.* 2005;57:1063.)

information is not available, the radiologist or MR technologist should consult the implanting or monitoring physician. Once the device is identified, the associated device documentation typically is available online, posted on the device manufacturer's website. The device labeling should be carefully reviewed for information regarding behavior in the MR environment specific to the exact MR scanner and set of imaging conditions to be used to perform the examination. Salient MR-related information present in the labeling includes system parameters such as field strength(s), magnet types and manufacturers, RF transmit coils, system software versions and imaging conditions (e.g., RF power levels and gradient slew rates [dB/dt]). In addition, when appropriate, information regarding the configuration of the device itself, such as lead length and routing, that were evaluated and reported in the device labeling must also be considered. Note that the safety information for any implantable medical devices (passive or active) and medical equipment applies only to the magnetic field strengths, MR system configurations, RF coils, and/or imaging conditions evaluated. Safety at 1.5 T does not necessarily imply safety at 3 T, and vice versa. The consequences of failing to strictly adhere to the product information regarding MR safety can be catastrophic to the patient (Fig. 3-2).[88,91]

Several comprehensive reviews of the topic of MR safety and implants have been published,[3,78,92-96] and more than 1200 objects have been tested for MR safety, with more than 200 evaluated at 3 T or higher.[97] This MR safety information is readily available to the public as published reports, compiled lists online (www.MRIsafety.com), and in the *Reference Manual for Magnetic Resonance Safety, Implants and Devices*, a publication that is compiled and updated annually.[98]

Other Metallic Potential Hazards

In addition to implantable devices, it must be documented that the patient has no other form of metal in his or her body, including metal filings, shrapnel, and abandoned leads (e.g., a pacemaker). If the patient indicates that such materials may be present, a radiograph must be obtained, and if the presence of such materials is confirmed, the MR examination should not be performed. All of the precautions and considerations previously outlined apply not only to patients but also to any hospital personnel and/or patient family members who may accompany the patient to the MR environment.

Some body piercing jewelry is ferromagnetic, and certain tattoos and permanent cosmetics may contain irregularly shaped iron oxide or other metal-based pigments and therefore may be of concern. In these instances, mild to moderate movement or displacement in the MR environment may occur that, in the case of the tattoos and/or permanent cosmetics, may result in localized swelling and/or irritation. In addition, when the jewelry or pigments are contained within the transmit RF coil, a risk of localized heating also exists. For these reasons, patients and/or individuals should be informed of the potential risks. Body jewelry should be removed before entering the MR environment. If removal is not possible and the individual chooses to proceed, the jewelry should be stabilized (e.g., with application of adhesive tape or a bandage) and, if it is contained within the transmit RF coil, it should be wrapped with gauze or tape to insulate it from underlying skin.[97] Similarly, for tattoos and permanent cosmetics, if any concern exists that heating may occur, an ice pack or cold compress can be applied to the site as a precautionary measure. Adverse events associated with tattoos and/or permanent cosmetics are relatively infrequent, and when they do occur, they are relatively minor and transient.[35,36,97,99] In the opinion of the FDA, "The risks of avoiding an MRI when your doctor has recommended one are likely to be much greater than the risks of complications from an interaction between the MRI and tattoo or permanent makeup. Instead of avoiding an MRI, individuals who have tattoos or permanent makeup should inform the radiologist or technician of this fact in order to take appropriate precautions, avoid complications, and assure the best results."[3,100]

A comprehensive and updated list of reported adverse MR safety-related incidents can be accessed online from the Manufacturer and User Facility Device Experience Database (MAUDE; available at www.fda.gov/cdrh/maude.html)[36] and the Medical Device Report (available at www.fda.gov/CDRH/mdrfile.html),[35] both of which are compiled and maintained by the FDA Center for Devices and Radiological Health.[97]

MAGNETIC RESONANCE "SAFETY" LABELING

In response to the severity of the potential hazards of the presence of ferromagnetic objects in the MR environment, the FDA has developed and implemented a well-defined and stringent evaluation and labeling convention. Medical equipment, devices, and/or implants are now classified as "MR safe," "MR unsafe," and "MR conditional."[101,102] These terms replace the previous MR-related evaluation and labeling convention of "MR safe" and "MR compatible." In the prior labeling convention, "MR safe" was applied to devices and implants that, when present and/or used in the MR environment, presented no additional risk to the patient or any other individual but may, however, have affected the diagnostic quality of the images. "MR compatible" implied that in addition to being "MR safe," the device had no significant effect on the diagnostic quality of the images, nor was its operation affected by the MR system.

The replacement of these previous designations and definitions by "MR safe," "MR unsafe," and "MR conditional" was deemed necessary because the earlier designations were confusing and the terms often were used inappropriately. To clarify and prevent misuse, the new set of terms and associated icons was developed (Fig. 3-3).[101-103] "MR safe" and/or "MR unsafe" designates an item (e.g., a medical device, equipment, or implant) as unequivocally safe or unsafe in any or all MRI environments (e.g., field strength, magnet type, and RF coils) and imaging conditions (e.g., RF power levels and gradient slew/switching rates [dB/dt]) and for all configurations of device/object use. "MR safe" objects include nonconducting, nonmetallic, and/or nonmagnetic items such as plastic or gauze tape. "MR unsafe" items include any magnetic object such as a pair of ferromagnetic/metal scissors, scalpel, wrench, or cleaning bucket.[97]

Alternatively, "MR conditional" indicates an item that has no known hazards for very specific combination(s) of MR environment and imaging conditions. When appropriate, additional conditions of use of the item (e.g., routing of leads associated with a neurostimulation system) also are specified. For MR conditional items, the testing must include the assessment of the magnetically induced displacement force and torque, RF heating, and other potential hazards such as thermal injury, induced currents and voltages,

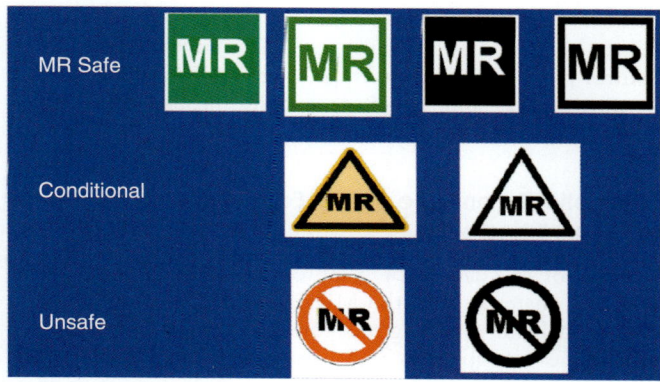

Figure 3-3 *International magnetic resonance safety labeling icons.* U.S. Food and Drug Administration (FDA) labeling criteria (developed by American Society for Testing and Materials International) for portable objects (e.g., medical devices, implants, medical equipment, oxygen tanks, housekeeping equipment, and tools) that may or may not enter the magnetic resonance (MR) environment. Square/green "MR safe" labels correspond to objects that are totally nonreactive, triangular/yellow labels correspond to objects with "MR conditional" status, and round/red labels identify an object as being "MR unsafe." The use of the new labeling convention has been adopted by the FDA and applied to items prospectively (but not retrospectively), beginning approximately in August 2005. (From ASTM International. *Standard practice for marking medical devices and other items for safety in the magnetic resonance environment* (designation F2035), West Conshohocken, PA: ASTM International; 2005.

electromagnetic compatibility, and neurostimulation. In addition, the function and operational status of the item during and after exposure to the MR environment must be evaluated, along with its impact on the MR system itself (e.g., image artifact). The salient results of this testing should be documented in the product's labeling, and any parameters that affect or alter the safety of the item should be noted and the potential influence described.[97] The original and complete definition of the new terms and testing conditions are provided in the American Society for Testing and Materials International document.[97,101,103] Notably, the use of the new labeling convention has only been applied to items prospectively, beginning approximately as of August 2005.[97] Because it has not been applied by the FDA retrospectively, the labeling for many currently used items may still adhere to the prior definitions of and labeling as "MR safe" and "MR compatible."

MAGNETIC RESONANCE SAFETY, FACILITY OPERATION, AND PATIENT CARE GUIDELINES

Magnetic Resonance Safety Risks and Considerations

In light of the extreme severity of the potential hazards associated with the improper management of the MR environment, all hospital personnel who may have reason to be in the MR department, patients, and patient family members must be appropriately educated and screened for metallic objects and/or electrically active devices on or within their person well before entering the scan room. The education must include information about the behavior of metallic objects in static magnetic fields and the associated hazards.[97] The importance and necessity of these measures are highlighted by the fact that the majority of adverse MR safety incidents have been due either to deficiencies in and/or failure to enforce screening or MR environment access control procedures and practices, resulting in contraindicated personal items and other potentially problematic objects entering the MR scan room.[35,36]

Magnetic Resonance Safety Education and Screening

Because of the danger of inappropriately introducing ferromagnetic materials into the MR environment, the following educational and screening procedures have been implemented for facilities and apply to both patient and nonpatient populations. Access to areas that exceed the 5 G line must be vigilantly restricted and supervised at all times.[26] It is important to remind all persons entering the MR facility that the magnet is always "on," even when no examinations are being performed. Screening involves both written documentation and a verbal review. The written screening questionnaire is designed to elicit information about the presence of a medical device, implant, or other ferromagnetic object within or on the individual and/or of the existence of an underlying condition (e.g., pregnancy or disability) that may require special consideration. Once completed, an oral interview is conducted to verify the information reported, and the individual is given the opportunity to express concerns and have any remaining questions about the examination answered before entrance into the MR environment is finally allowed.

The education and screening must be performed by a health care worker specially trained in MR safety who has a comprehensive appreciation and understanding of the potential hazards of the MR environment and procedures and is familiar with the information and implications of the contents of the screening forms for patients and other individuals. Because some of the questions included on the patient screening form may not be relevant for nonpatients, separate screening forms for the patient and nonpatient groups have been compiled. Template screening forms for patients (English and Spanish versions) and a screening form for nonpatient individuals can be downloaded for use at www.MRI safety.com.[93,94]

The fact that a patient has had a previous MR examination without incident does not ensure the safety of current or future studies. For example, the patient may have undergone a surgical procedure and/or experienced an accident involving a metallic foreign body in the interim that now makes him or her ineligible to enter the MR environment. The exact conditions (e.g., static magnetic field strength of the MR system, RF coil used, orientation of the patient, body part evaluated, or orientation of a metallic implant or object) also can alter the safety profile substantially.[96,104,105] Therefore comprehensive screening must be conducted each time any person prepares to enter the MR environment.

With respect to pregnancy, in 1991, the Safety Committee of the Society for Magnetic Resonance Imaging issued a document entitled "Policies, Guidelines, and Recommendations for MR Imaging Safety and Patient Management,"[3,106] which stated that "MR imaging may be used in pregnant women if other non-ionizing forms of diagnostic imaging are inadequate or if the examination provides important information that would otherwise require exposure to ionizing radiation (e.g., fluoroscopy, computed tomography).

Pregnant patients should be informed that, to date, there has been no indication that the use of clinical MR imaging during pregnancy has produced deleterious effects." This policy was adopted by the American College of Radiology (ACR) and remains the current "standard of care"; it is applicable to MR systems operating at static magnetic field strengths up to and including 3 T.[3] Because no deleterious effects of MR imaging exposure on the fetus have been documented during any stage of development, pregnant women can undergo MRI examinations at any point during their pregnancy.

Magnetic Resonance Facility Operating Procedure Guidelines

In recognition and acknowledgement of the appreciable potential hazards and severe consequences of failure to adhere to safety precautions associated with the MR environment, the ACR formed the Blue Ribbon Panel on MR Safety. First convened in 2001, the panel reviewed and refined the current MR safety practices and guidelines and established new ones when appropriate. The results of this first review were published in 2002[106] and became the de facto industry standards for safe and responsible practice in both clinical and research MR environments. These guidelines were reviewed and updated in May 2004[107] and again in 2006-2007, incorporating recommendations and feedback from the MR community.[95] The results of the 2006–2007 review were published as the "ACR Guidance Document for Safe MR Practices: 2007."[95]

The ACR outlines well-defined methodologies and procedures to ensure and enforce safe and restricted exposure and access to the MR environment most appropriate to the existing state of the MR technology, recognizing that this is continuously evolving. Specifically, in their 2007 publication, the ACR stated that the ACR MR Safe Practice Guidelines document was intended to be used as a template for MR facilities to follow in the development of their own individualized MR safety program.[95] In addition, the ACR recommended that once established, each site should regularly review, reevaluate, and update its safety program as the field of MR, and MR safety, continues to evolve. The ACR also recommended that each site name an MR medical director whose responsibilities include ensuring that MR safe practice guidelines are established and maintained as current and appropriate for the site.[95]

One of the recommendations is the separation of the general MR facility into four zones of increasing potential MR-related danger.[95] Zone One is to include all areas that are freely accessible to the general public, such as outside areas surrounding a freestanding MRI facility or the corridor in an imaging department. Zone Two is defined as the area controlled and supervised by the MR personnel, such as the reception area and patient preparation area. Zone Three is the area where there is potential for injury from ferromagnetic objects and equipment. Access to this zone must be vigilantly and strictly controlled and limited by MR personnel. These areas include the operator control room, computer room, and/or any areas immediately adjacent to the MR scan room. Finally, Zone Four is the MR scan room itself. This zone must be clearly marked with warning signs and notification of high magnetic field strengths within this area, including a sign that the magnet is always on. Access to Zone Four is strictly limited to persons with a demonstrated need to be there (i.e., patients and medical personnel), and then only after comprehensive education about the MR environment and a rigorous screening.

CONCLUSION

The potential health hazards associated with MR are directly attributable to the three main components that make up the MR environment: (1) a strong static magnetic field, including its associated spatial gradient; (2) pulsed gradient magnetic fields; and (3) pulsed RF fields. For a properly operating system, the hazards associated with direct interactions of these fields and the body is negligible. However, it is the interactions of these fields with medical devices and/or ferromagnetic objects inadvertently introduced within the fields that create potential concerns for human safety. To prevent adverse MR safety–related incidents and allow the full benefit of this powerful imaging modality to be realized, it is imperative that the potential safety risks intrinsic to the MR environment be understood and respected by all persons exposed to the MR environment. Comprehensive education and screening to rule out contraindications of both patient and nonpatient groups who enter the MR environment is imperative.

Suggested Readings

MR safety *(Journal of Magnetic Resonance Imaging special edition),* J Magn Reson Imaging 12(1), 2000.

Hornak JP. The basics of MRI. Available at http://www.cis.rit.edu/htbooks/mri/. Accessed July 25, 2012.

Shellock FG, ed. *Magnetic resonance procedures: health effects and safety.* Boca Raton, FL: CRC Press; 2001.

Stafford RJ. *Physics of MRI safety.* Available at http://www.aapm.org/meetings/amos2/pdf/59-17207-59975-979.pdf. Accessed July 25, 2012.

Bushong SC. *Magnetic resonance imaging: physical and biological principles.* 3rd ed. St Louis: Mosby; 2003.

MR Safety Websites

Danger! Flying objects! is an illustrative gallery from the educative "Simply Physics" site, an MRI portal created by Dr Moriel NessAiver, PhD. The gallery, which is available at http://simplyphysics.com/flying_objects.html (accessed July 27, 2012), depicts the dangers resulting from common hospital-based ferromagnetic medical equipment.

ECRI Institute is an independent, nonprofit organization that researches the best approaches to improving the safety, quality, and cost-effectiveness of patient care. ECRI is designated an Evidence-Based Practice Center by the U.S. Agency for Healthcare Research and Quality and is listed as a federal Patient Safety Organization by the U.S. Department of Health and Human Services. The organization has a Website at https://www.ecri.org (accessed July 27, 2012).

MRIsafety.com is available at http://www.mrisafety.com/ (accessed July 27, 2012). This site, developed and maintained by Dr. F.G. Shellock, provides up-to-date information on MRI safety-related topics. Impressively, the latest information regarding screening patients with implants, materials, and medical devices is provided. A key feature of the site is The List, a searchable database that contains more than 1200 implants and devices, including more than 200 objects tested at 3 T for MRI safety. Moreover, the site includes a summary section that is a presentation of more than 100 peer-reviewed articles on MRI bioeffects and safety. Other features include a downloadable Pre-MRI Screening form and safety information.

ReviseMRI.com is designed principally as a revision aid but also may be used as an educational resource. Contents include a detailed question and answer section, Web-based animated tutorials, interactive learning tools, and links to resources for further reading in common textbooks and online for nearly every question and answer posed. The site can be accessed at http://www.revisemri.com/questions/safety (accessed July 27, 2012).

The Institute for Magnetic Resonance Safety, Education and Research is a multidisciplinary professional organization headed by Director Dr. Frank Shellock. It focuses on information and research on magnetic resonance (MR) safety, while "promoting awareness, understanding, and communication of MR safety issues through education and research." The Web site is available at http://www.imrser.org/ (accessed July 27, 2012) and has useful sections, including MRI Safety Guidelines and MR Safety Papers.

The U.S. Food and Drug Administration has a **Center for Devices and Radiological Health,** which is an integral part of the Department of Health & Human Services. Online documents available include "A Primer on Medical Device Interactions with Magnetic Resonance Imaging Systems" at http://www.fda.gov/MedicalDevices/DeviceRegulationandGuidance/GuidanceDocuments/ucm107721.htm (accessed July 27, 2012) and "MRI Safety" at http://www.fda.gov/MedicalDevices/Safety/AlertsandNotices/ucm135362.htm (accessed July 27, 2012).

Two important **MRI accident databases** derived from the Database of Medical Device Related Accidents and Events are available from Maude Accidents Database (http://www.accessdata.fda.gov/scripts/cdrh/cfdocs/cfMAUDE/search.cfm; accessed July 27, 2012) and the UK Medical Devices Agency (http://www.mhra.gov.uk/index.htm#page=DynamicListMedicines; accessed July 27, 2012).

medicalphysicsweb, which was launched in 2006, is a unique site for the medical physics community. It provides in-depth analysis and incisive commentary on the fundamental research, emerging technologies, and clinical applications that underpin the dynamic disciplines of medical physics and biomedical engineering. It can be accessed at http://medicalphysicsweb.org (accessed July 27, 2012).

References

Full references for this chapter can be found on www.expertconsult.com.

SECTION 2

Head and Neck

Chapter 4

Embryology, Anatomy, Normal Findings, and Imaging Techniques

ERIC N. FAERBER

Embryology of the Eye

Development of the eye originates from neuroectoderm, surface ectoderm, and neural crest cells.[1-3] The neuroectodermal layer gives rise to the retina, iris, and optic nerve, the surface ectoderm gives rise to the lens, and the neural crest cells are responsible for vascular structures, sclera, choroid, and mesenchymal tissue from which the adnexal structures, bony orbit, fat, and nerve sheaths arise.[4,5]

The prime regulatory gene for human eye development is *PAX6*, a member of the PAX (paired box) family of transcription factors. This gene initially is expressed in a band contained in the anterior neural ridge of the neural plate before the process of neurulation.[6] A single eye field is present at this stage, which then separates into two primordial optic structures under the direction of sonic hedgehog (*SHH*), which belongs to a family of vertebrate genes involved with encoding inductive signals during embryogenesis and is part of a vast signaling network that affects development of many tissues and organs.[6]

The earliest sign of eye development is the appearance in a 22-day-old embryo of a pair of shallow grooves evaginating on either side of the prosencephalon or forebrain.[6] The grooves form the optic vesicles in contact with surface ectoderm. Invagination of the optic vesicle leads to formation of a double-walled optic cup. This cup has two layers that become the retina, separated by the intraretinal space. The outer layer contains pigment granules that appear during the fifth week of development. The inner layer has two parts. The pars optica retinae occupies the posterior four fifths and contains cells that ultimately differentiate into the rod and cone cells responsible for light reception. The pars ceca retinae, within the anterior fifth of the inner layer, divides into the pars iridica retinae, which will form the inner layer of the iris, and the pars ciliaris retinae, which will be involved with formation of the ciliary body. The central retinal artery results from the residuum of the embryonic hyaloid artery, which regresses by 4 months of gestation. The lips of the choroid fissure fuse during the seventh week; the mouth of the optic cup becomes the future pupil.

Elongation of surface ectoderm cells in contact with the optic vesicle results in formation of the lens placode, which develops into the lens vesicle. The lens vesicle becomes located in the mouth of the optic cup (Fig. 4-1). Cells located in the posterior wall of the vesicle elongate, forming long fibers that fill the lumen of the vesicle, reaching the anterior wall of the lens vesicle by the seventh week of development. The vascular capsule is a mesenchymal condensation that covers the lens. The hyaloid artery supplies the lens, forming a plexus on its posterior surface.[7]

The primary vitreous develops from mesenchyme within the optic cup, which has an embryonic fissure, known as the canal of Cloquet. The hyaloid artery reaches the globe through this canal.

The hyaloid artery and its branches are a transient vascular system that nourishes structures of the eye, subsequently involuting by the 35th week of gestation.[5]

The choroid and sclera are formed from mesenchyme surrounding the optic cup. The ciliary body and ciliary processes are formed from the anterior portion of the choroid.[7]

The optic cup and brain are connected by the optic stalk. The choroid fissure is a groove on the ventral surface of the optic stalk, wherein lie the hyaloid vessels. The fissure closes at 7 weeks' gestation, during which time a narrow tunnel is formed inside the optic stalk. The inner and outer walls of the stalk fuse, becoming the optic nerve. The center contains a portion of the hyaloid artery, the central artery of the retina. The exterior of the optic nerve is covered by a continuation of the choroid and sclera, along with the pia, arachnoid, and dura.[6]

Development of the eye continues into postnatal life. The fovea centralis of the retina becomes differentiated by 4 months after birth. The cones remain poorly developed until 4 months after birth.[8] The infant globe and orbit reach 80% of adult size during the first few years of life, with full size reached by approximately 13 years of age.

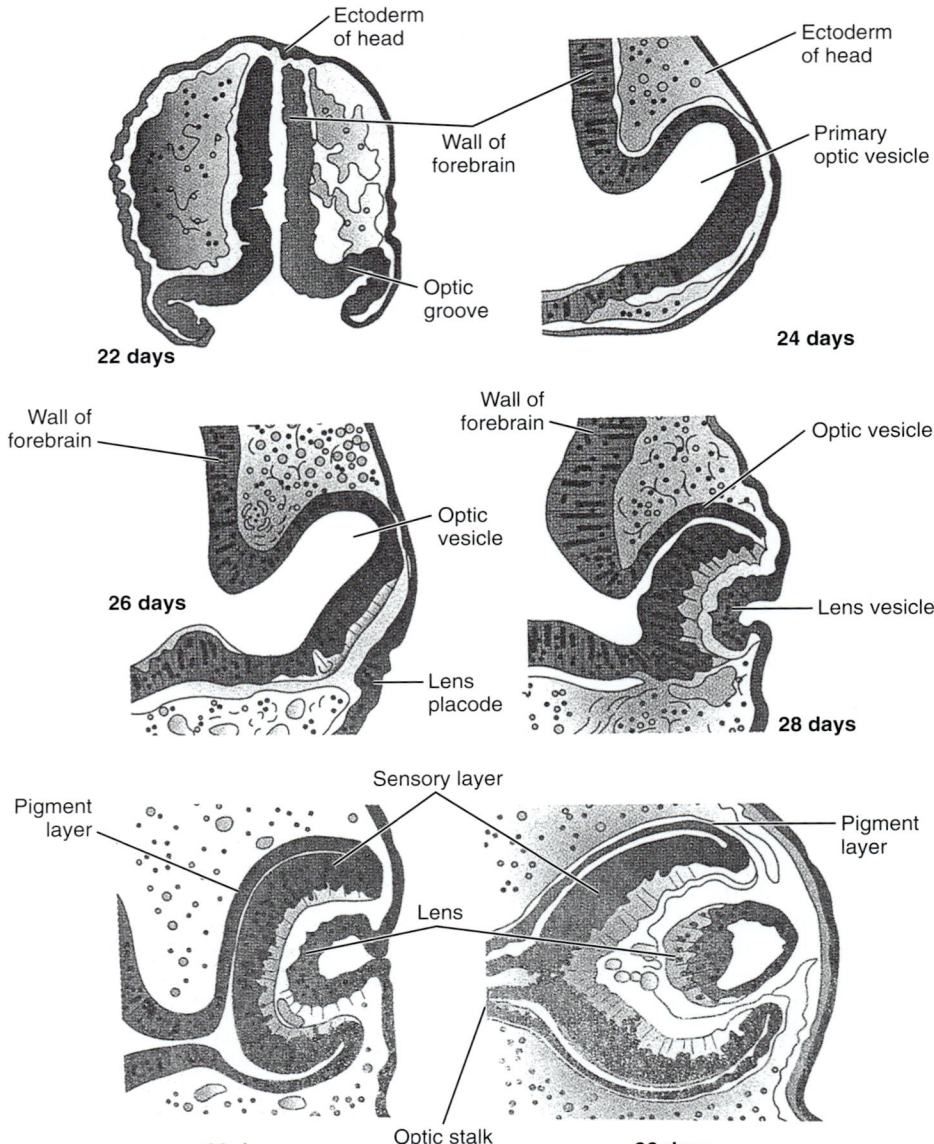

Figure 4-1   Early development of the human eye. (From Carlson BM: *Human embryology and developmental biology*, ed 2, St Louis, 1999, Mosby.)

Normal Anatomy of the Orbit and Eye

The orbits are cone-shaped cavities containing the globes, extraocular muscles, blood vessels, nerves, retrobulbar fat, and lacrimal glands. Each orbit is bounded by the floor of the anterior cranial fossa superiorly, the maxillary sinus inferiorly, the ethmoid sinus medially, and the temporal bone and middle cranial fossae anterolaterally and posterolaterally (Figs. 4-2 and 4-3).

The orbital septum is a thin connective tissue membrane that arises from the peripheral periosteum of the anterior osseous orbit and attaches to the tarsal plates of the eyelids. The septum divides the orbit into an anterior preseptal space and a deeper postseptal space. The postseptal space is divided by the extraocular muscle cone (consisting of the four rectus muscles) into intraconal, conal, and extraconal compartments. The lacrimal gland lies in the superolateral quadrant of the orbit.

The globe occupies about 20% of the orbital cavity. It is divided by the lens into an anterior chamber filled with aqueous humor and a posterior chamber containing vitreous humor found between the lens and retina. The globe contains the retina, uveal layer, and sclera. The sclera is covered anteriorly by the conjunctiva, continuous with the mucous membrane of the eyelid (Fig. 4-4). Tenon fascia separates the globe and extraocular muscle insertions from the orbital fat.

The retrobulbar space extends from the orbital septum anteriorly to the orbital apex posteriorly. The space contains six extraocular muscles (the superior, inferior, lateral, and medial rectus muscles and the inferior and superior oblique muscles), vascular structures, and the optic nerve, surrounded by fat.

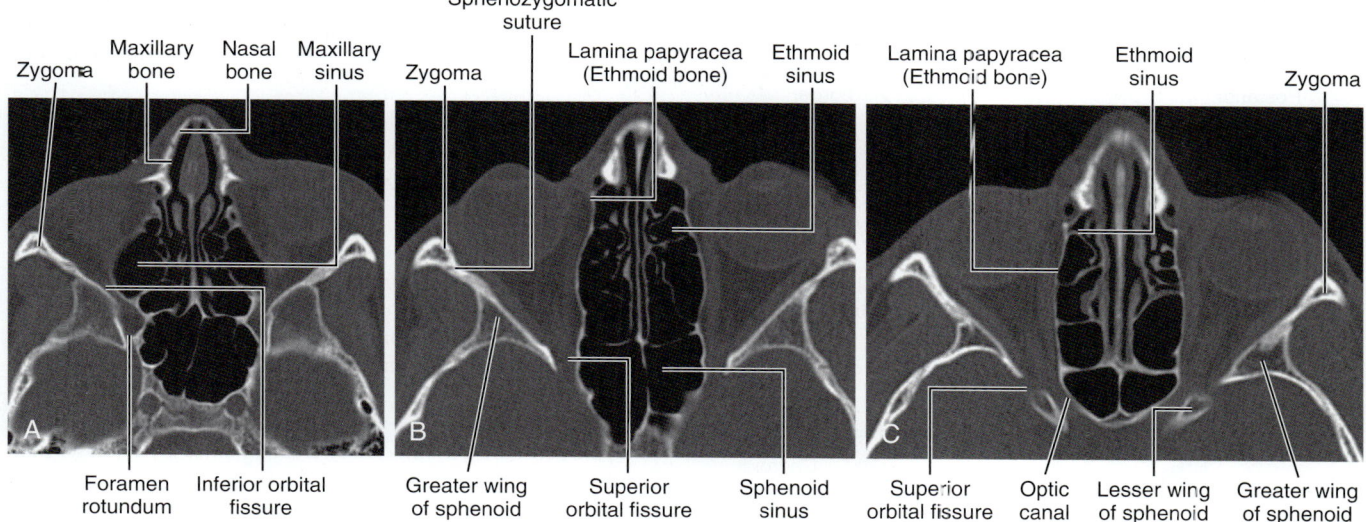

Figure 4-2 **Bony orbit.** Axial noncontrast computed tomography images from inferior to superior location.

The optic nerve is divided into four segments: (1) an intraocular segment penetrating the sclera, (2) an intraorbital segment in the intraconal space, (3) an intracanalicular segment in the optic canal, and (4) an intracranial segment extending from the optic canal to the optic chiasm. It is fully myelinated by 7 months of age. It continues to increase in thickness for the first 8 years of life.

Optic nerve sheath diameter in children as measured on magnetic resonance imaging (MRI) is 3.1 mm in the 0- to 3-year age group, 3.41 mm between 3 and 6 years, 3.55 mm between 6 and 12 years, and 3.56 mm in the 12- to 18-year age group.[9]

Imaging Techniques

Computed tomography (CT) and MRI are the main imaging modalities for the orbit and visual pathways. Ultrasonography may be useful for specific indications.

ULTRASOUND

Ultrasound is extremely beneficial in infants and children because it does not use ionizing radiation, it is widely available, and the need for sedation is rare. The primary indications are disease or conditions of the anterior chamber preventing funduscopic examination of the remainder of the eye, such as hyphema and trauma, non-neoplastic leukokoria, assessment of vascular integrity of the retina or an underlying lesion, and follow-up of neoplastic causes of leukokoria after treatment.[10] Secondary indications include further elucidation of intraconal and extraconal lesions and assessment of lacrimal masses.[7] Ultrasound is less helpful in showing osseous abnormalities of the orbit.

The procedure is performed with the patient supine. Initially a small amount of gel is placed over the upper eyelid. Images are obtained using a high-resolution (7.0 to 10.0 MHz) linear-array transducer with color Doppler capability.[10] Power output must be decreased to avoid mechanical or thermal

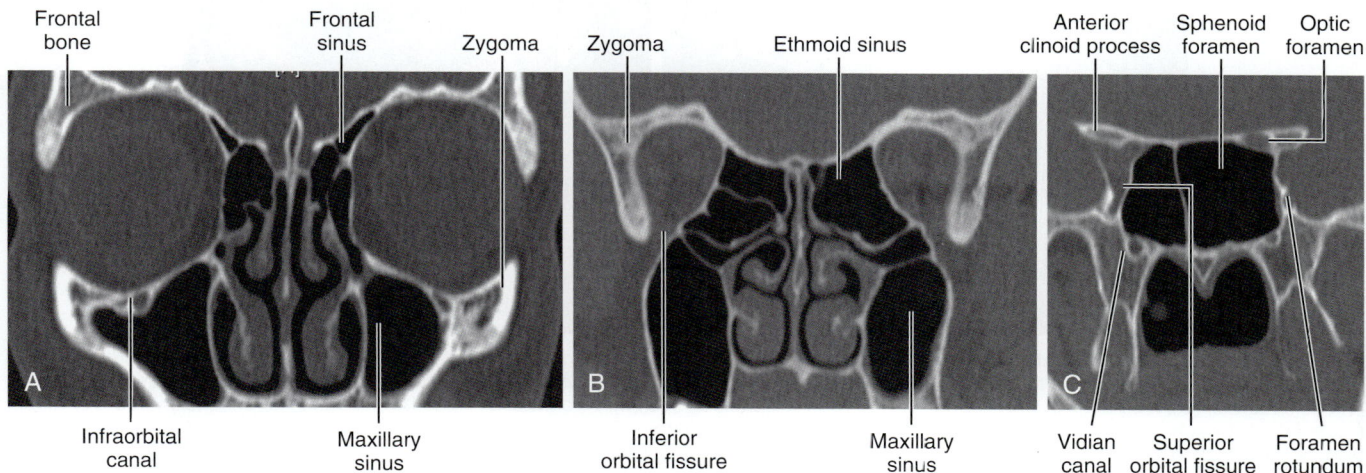

Figure 4-3 **Bony orbit.** Coronal noncontrast computed tomography images from anterior to posterior location.

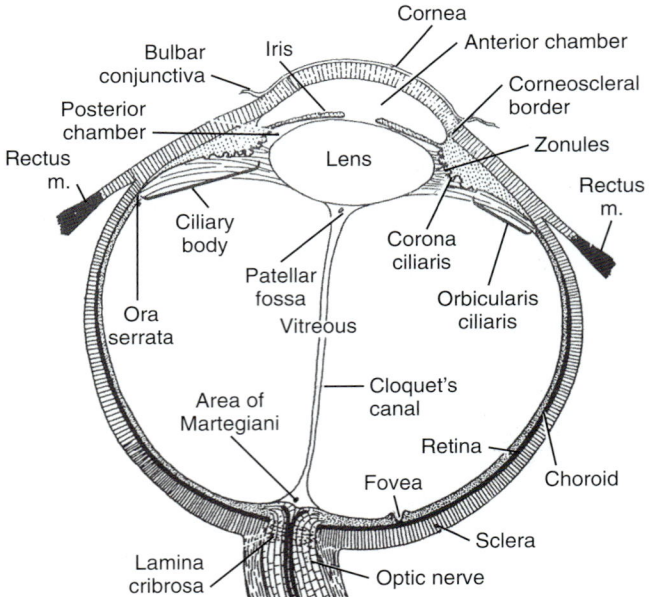

Figure 4-4   Normal anatomy of the eye. *(From Jakobiec FA, Ozanics V: General topographic anatomy of the eye. In Jakobiec FA, editor: Ocular anatomy, embryology and teratology, New York, 1982, Harper & Row.)*

injury. Scanning is usually performed in the axial plane; however, other planes also may be used to evaluate the entire globe[10] (Fig. 4-5, *A*).

Color Doppler imaging is an important component of the ultrasound examination because it permits demonstration of the ophthalmic artery and vein, the central artery of the retina, the retinal vein, ciliary and lacrimal arteries and accompanying veins, and the superior ophthalmic vein (Fig. 4-5, *B*).[10]

COMPUTED TOMOGRAPHY SCAN

CT is ideal for showing osseous abnormalities, calcification, and foreign bodies. Excellent anatomic detail is obtained rapidly, with high contrast of orbital tissues. Rapid scan times also decrease the need for sedation in many patients. Disadvantages of CT include use of ionizing radiation, limited imaging planes compared with MRI, beam-hardening artifact, and the potential risk from iodinated contrast media.

High-resolution, thin-section scans with a slice thickness of 2 to 3 mm are obtained in the axial planes with subsequent coronal and sagittal reformatted images, which eliminate further radiation to the patient (Fig. 4-6, *A*, *B*, and *C*). The axial plane is usually parallel to the canthomeatal line. Thinner images, especially in the coronal plane, may be obtained when indicated, such as visualization of the orbital floor for a blow-out fracture. Direct coronal images may be obtained in either the supine or the prone position.

MAGNETIC RESONANCE IMAGING

MRI is of great value for showing soft tissue abnormalities of the orbit. Although the lack of ionizing radiation is appealing in infants and children, MRI requires a longer scan time than other modalities, and it is not helpful in detecting

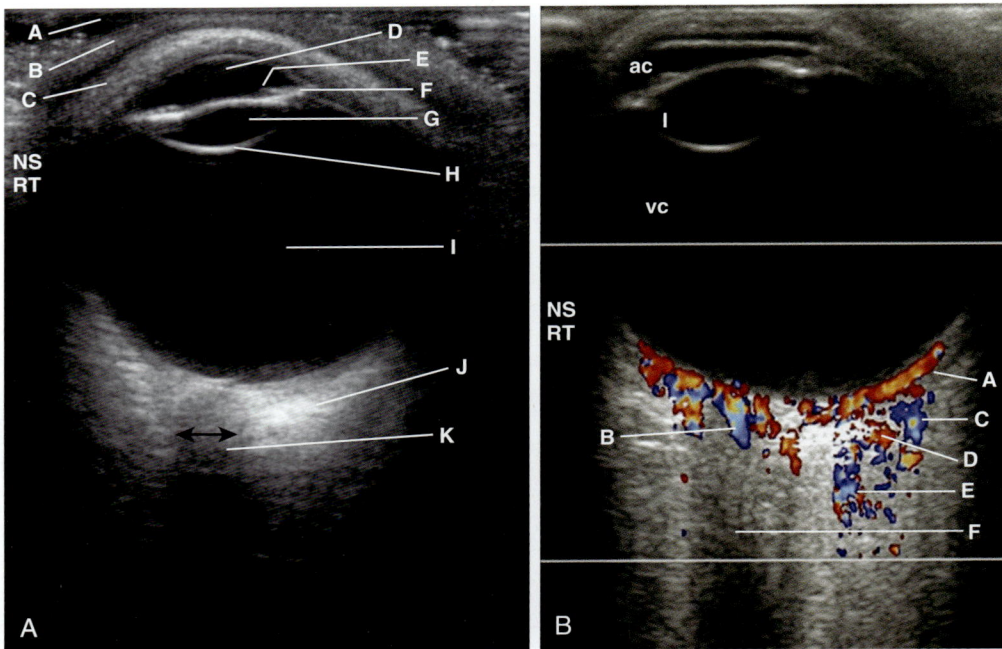

Figure 4-5   Normal ophthalmic axial ultrasound of a teenager. **A,** Using a broadband, high-resolution linear array transducer (5-17 MHz extended-frequency range), sterile gel (*A*) is placed on the skin (*B*) over the upper eyelid (*C*), which remains shut throughout the examination. The anechoic anterior chamber (*D*), the iris (*E*), the ciliary apparatus (*F*), the anechoic lens (*G*) with the posterior reflective echo (*H*), the anechoic vitreous chamber (*I*), and the hypoechoic optic nerve (*J*) are demonstrated and the optic nerve width (*double-ended black arrow*) can be measured. **B,** Normal color Doppler examination of the eye in the same patient. Color Doppler imaging shows very good flow in the choroidal vessels (*A*), central retinal artery (*B*), lacrimal vein (*C*) and artery (*D*), as well as in the ophthalmic artery (*E*). The anterior chamber (*ac*), lens (*I*), and vitreous chambers (*vc*) are again noted. Different parts of the eye can be examined by having the patient move the eye as instructed. *(Courtesy Faridali Ramji, MD.)*

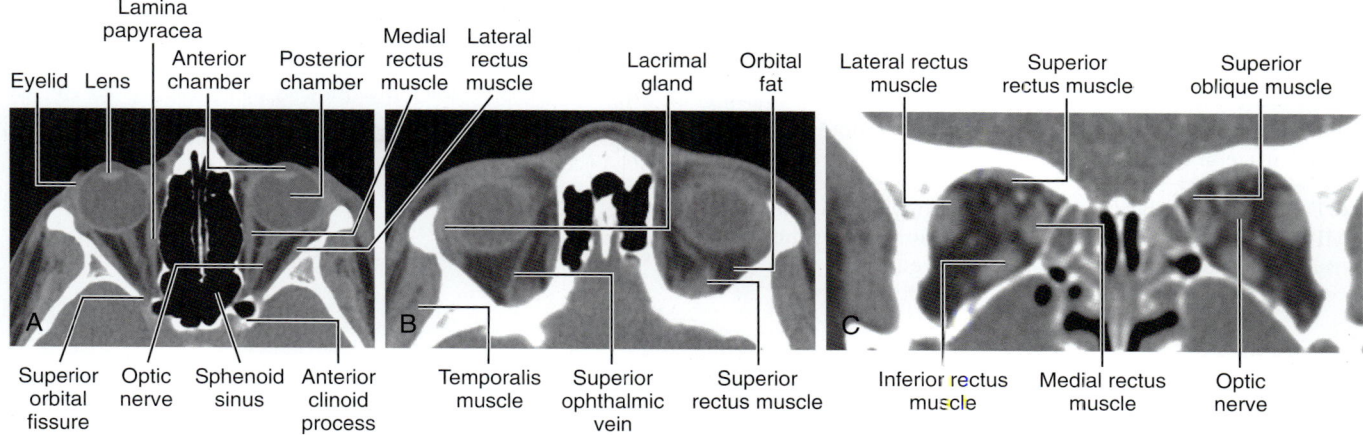

Figure 4-6 Computed tomography of the orbit. **A,** Axial. **B,** Coronal. **C,** Axial (after administration of contrast material).

calcifications. Orbital MRI requires high-resolution imaging with thin sections (Fig. 4-7). MRI of the brain often is performed concomitantly.

For purely orbital pathology, T1-weighted and fast spin echo (FSE) T2-weighted images with fat saturation or short tau inversion recovery images that suppress the orbital fat are used. Axial and coronal T1-weighted images usually are obtained in an oblique plane parallel to the optic nerve with thin sections with a small field of view (e.g., 20 cm) and a high-resolution matrix (512 × 192). Axial and coronal FSE inversion recovery images are performed through the orbit and chiasm.

Contrast material is administered intravenously for ocular and orbital disease, such as neoplasms, inflammatory and infectious processes, and vascular malformations, with T1-weighted imaging performed with fat saturation in the axial and coronal planes. In some centers, small surface coils are used, which may provide better spatial resolution but are not useful for imaging apical lesions or intracranial disease extension.

Contrast-enhanced MRI of the orbit and brain, using a head coil, is recommended for the evaluation of suspected retinoblastoma, possible subarachnoid seeding of retinoblastoma, and bilateral retinoblastoma. Early detection is made possible for optic nerve involvement, orbital spread, and asymptomatic pineoblastoma and suprasellar tumors.[11]

Chiasmatic lesions, such as gliomas, are studied in a manner similar to that of other supratentorial brain tumors. The fast three-point Dixon technique, which combines with FSE acquisition, has been used to look at the retrobulbar space within the orbit.[12] However, the Dixon method is rarely used because it requires a minimum of two data acquisitions and is as susceptible to static field inhomogeneities as is fat saturation.[15]

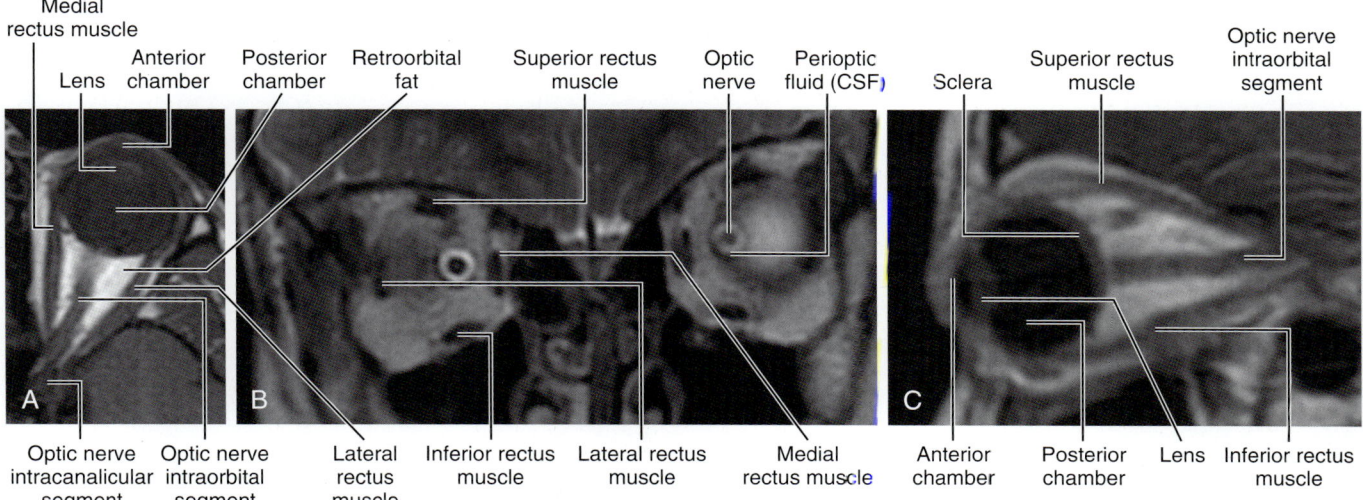

Figure 4-7 Magnetic resonance imaging of the orbit. **A,** Axial T1-weighted image. **B,** Coronal T2-weighted image. **C,** Sagittal oblique T1-weighted image. CSF, Cerebrospinal fluid.

Key Points

The globe reaches its full size by 13 years.

The orbital septum divides the orbit into an anterior pre-septal space and a deeper postseptal space.

CT provides the best images of the bony orbit, whereas MRI is the modality of choice for demonstrating the soft tissues and adjacent intracranial structures.

Suggested Reading

Bilaniuk LT, Farber M. Imaging of developmental anomalies of the eye and the orbit. *Am J Neuroradiol.* 1992;13:793-803.
Mafee MF, Karimi A, Shah J, et al. Anatomy and pathology of the eye: role of MR imaging and CT. *Neuroimaging Clin N Am.* 2005;15:23–47.
Ramji FG, Slovis TJ, Baker JD. Orbital sonography in children. *Pediatr Radiol.* 1996;26:245-258.

References

Full references for this chapter can be found on www.expertconsult.com.

Chapter 5

Prenatal, Congenital, and Neonatal Abnormalities

ASHLEY J. ROBINSON, ANGELA BYRNE, and SUSAN BLASER

Assessment of the orbits is part of a detailed fetal sonographic or magnetic resonance imaging (MRI) scan, particularly in the setting of suspected central nervous system malformation. When further assessment is performed by fetal MRI, quite obvious ocular pathologies can be missed, particularly if they are bilateral and symmetrical. Diagnoses can be further honed or even altered completely when a coexisting ocular pathology is found.

Ocular evaluation comprises assessment for the presence or absence of eyes, the morphology of the lens and vitreous, and ocular biometry.[1]

Presence or Absence of the Eyes

ANOPHTHALMIA AND MICROPHTHALMIA

The only way that anophthalmia and microphthalmia truly can be differentiated is pathologically, with anophthalmia being complete absence of the globe but the presence of the ocular adnexa (i.e., eyelids, conjunctiva, and lacrimal apparatus).

Primary Anophthalmia

With primary anophthalmia, ocular tissue in the orbit is completely absent because no development of the eyes has occurred. Primary anophthalmia usually is associated with chromosomal abnormalities such as trisomy 13 or genetic syndromes such as CHARGE syndrome, incontinentia pigmenti, Norrie disease, *SOX2*-related eye disorders, Walker-Warburg syndrome, and oculo-auriculo-vertebral spectrum.[2-7]

Secondary Anophthalmia

Loss of ocular tissue caused by an insult during development results in secondary anophthalmia. Etiologies include infection (e.g., rubella), a vascular event (e.g., Goldenhar syndrome), or a toxic or metabolic event (e.g., low or high vitamin A levels). The ocular diameter is below the fifth percentile.[8]

Matthew-Wood syndrome (also known as *Spear syndrome, PMD,* or *PDAC syndrome*) is composed of pulmonary hypoplasia/agenesis, diaphragmatic hernia/eventration, anophthalmia/microphthalmia, and cardiac defect.[9] In a case of congenital diaphragmatic hernia, associated abnormal orbital morphology and biometry and cardiac anomalies can allow this diagnosis to be made antenatally (Fig. 5-1).

Walker-Warburg syndrome, a type of congenital muscular dystrophy, also can be diagnosed antenatally through the association of Dandy-Walker spectrum, along with a Z-shaped brainstem on midline sagittal MRI views, an occipital cephalocele, and ocular asymmetry (Fig. 5-2 and e-Fig. 5-3).

Aicardi syndrome is a rare genetic malformation syndrome that can be diagnosed antenatally by the association of partial or complete absence of the corpus callosum, ocular abnormalities, and a posterior fossa cyst. Aicardi syndrome is thought to be caused by a defect on the X chromosome because it has only been seen in girls and in boys with Klinefelter syndrome (Fig. 5-4 and e-Fig. 5-5).

Morphology of the Lens and Vitreous

On ultrasound examination, the lens and vitreous are equally hypoechoic; however, the outline of the lens can be seen as a thin hyperechoic ovoid anteriorly within the globe. Typically, however, the only reflection from the lens is from the surfaces perpendicular to the insonating beam, and it can be difficult to see (Fig. 5-6).

On MRI, the entire lens has a low signal compared with the high signal of the vitreous (Fig. 5-7). By endovaginal ultrasound, the lens is visible by 14 weeks as a thin echogenic rim with an anechoic center. The hyaloid artery can be seen as an echogenic line bisecting the vitreous, which, during conversion of the primary vitreous to mature secondary vitreous, gradually becomes beaded as it involutes, a process that should be completed by 30 weeks menstrual age.[10,11] The remnant channel through the vitreous is known as the *Cloquet canal.*

PERSISTENT HYPERPLASTIC PRIMARY VITREOUS

Failure of involution of the hyaloid artery results in a spectrum of abnormalities known as persistent hyperplastic primary vitreous, which is seen frequently with trisomy syndromes and other forms of abnormal brain development.[12,13] It is usually unilateral. Clinically the presentation is variable

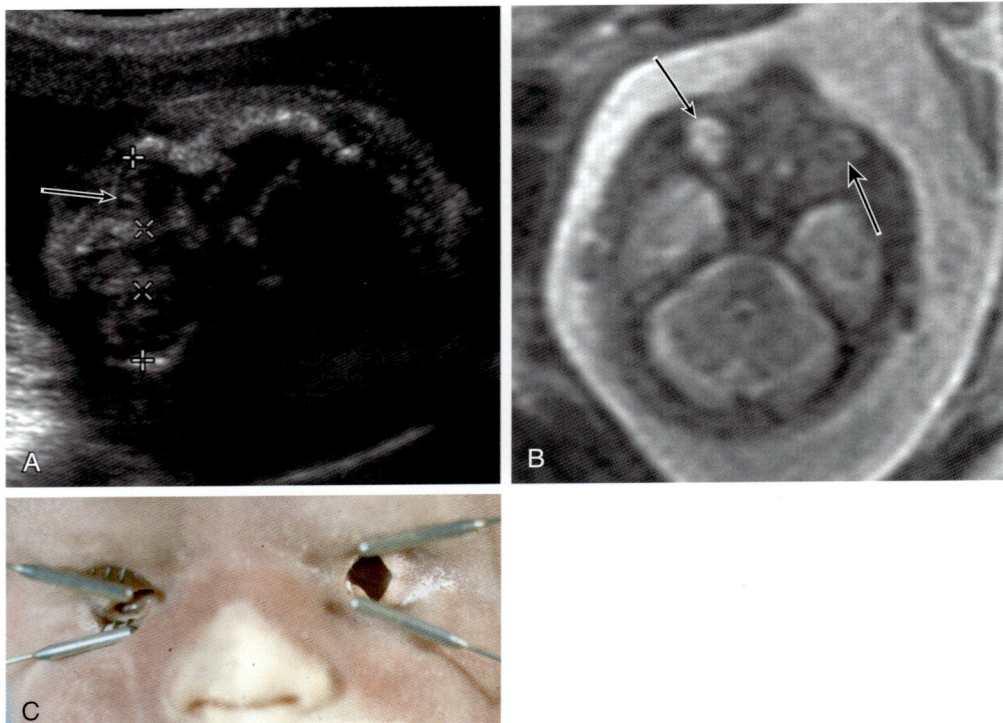

Figure 5-1 Matthew-Wood syndrome. **A,** Fetal ultrasonography shows that biometry was delayed and the lens and globe have an abnormal appearance, appearing echogenic (*arrow*). **B,** Fetal magnetic resonance imaging shows apparent anophthalmia (*large arrow*) and microphthalmia (*small arrow*). **C,** A postmortem examination reveals that the globes are absent. (From Robinson AJ, Blaser S, Toi A, et al. Magnetic resonance imaging of the fetal eyes—morphologic and biometric assessment for abnormal development with ultrasonographic and clinicopathologic correlation. *Pediatr Radiol.* 2008;38:971-981.)

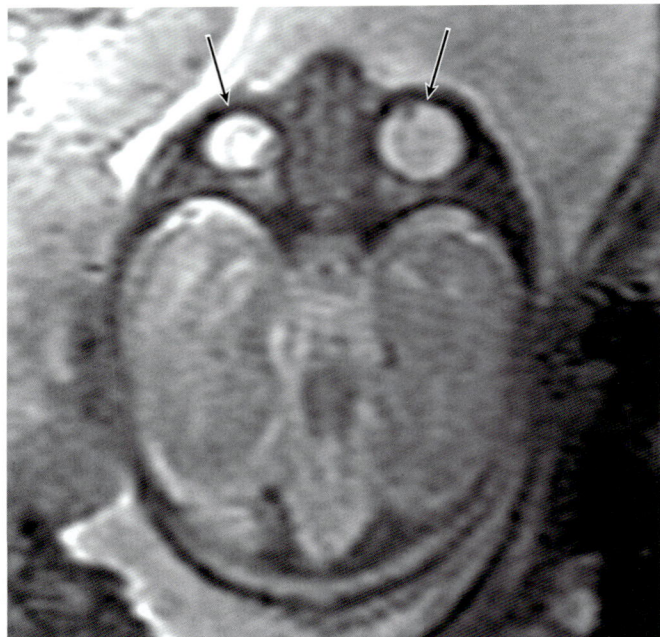

Figure 5-2 Walker-Warburg syndrome. A fetal magnetic resonance image shows symmetric globes (*arrows*). (From Robinson AJ, Blaser S, Toi A, et al. Magnetic resonance imaging of the fetal eyes—morphologic and biometric assessment for abnormal development with ultrasonographic and clinicopathologic correlation. *Pediatr Radiol.* 2008;38:971-981.)

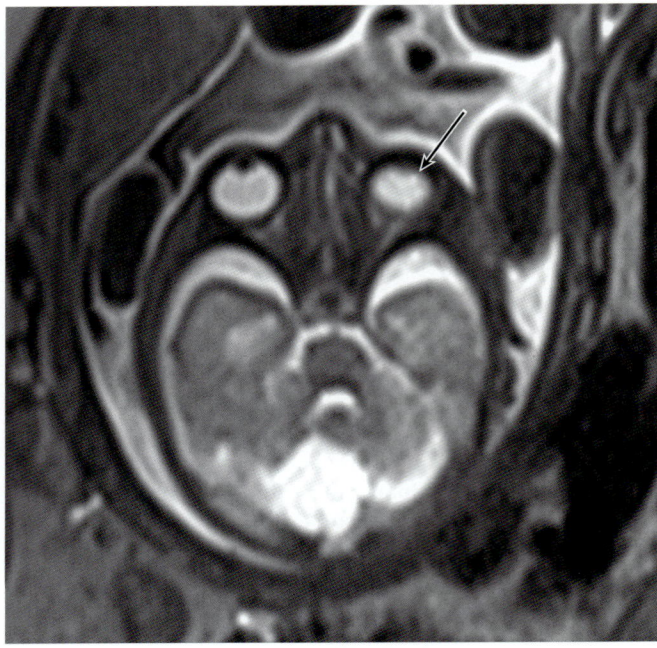

Figure 5-4 Aicardi syndrome. Fetal magnetic resonance imaging demonstrates unilateral microphthalmia (*arrow*).

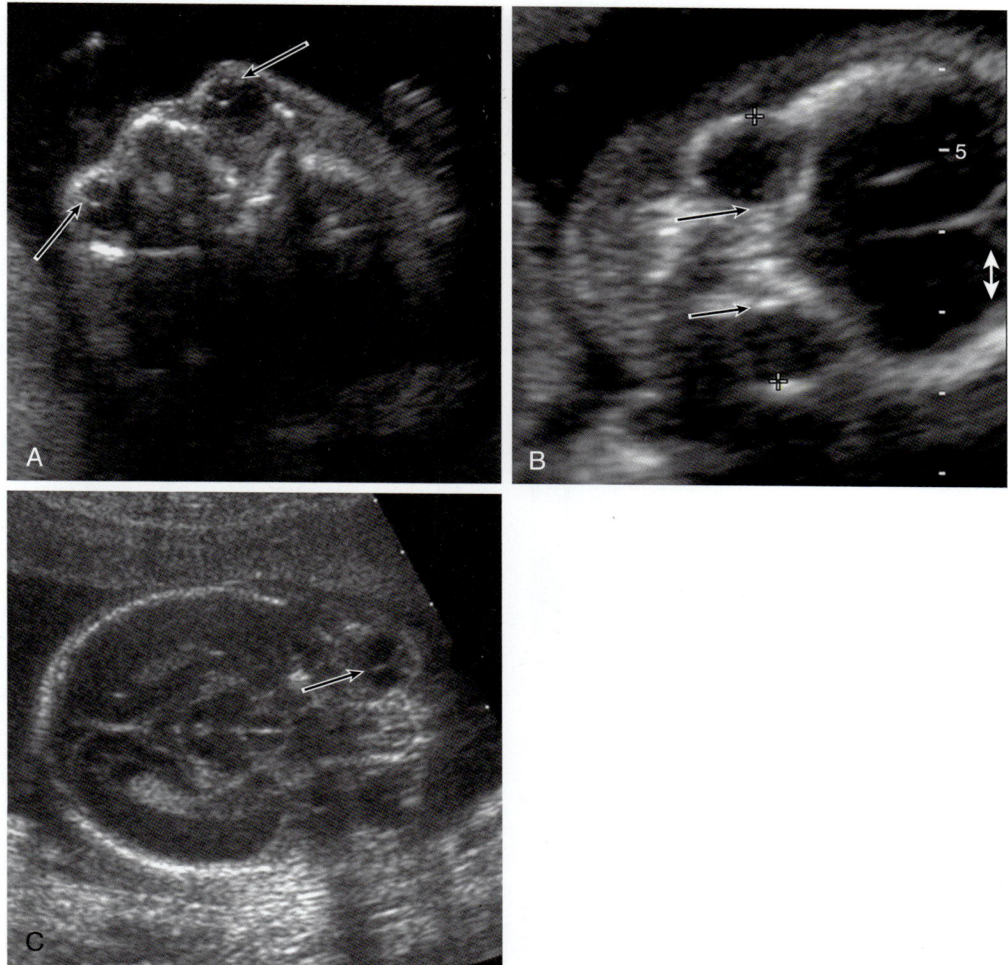

Figure 5-6 Sonographic appearances. **A,** Lens and vitreous. The surfaces of the lenses are seen as faint curvilinear echoes in the anterior globe (*arrows*). **B,** A transorbital view of the fetal face shows the measurement of the binocular distance with the calipers on the malar margins of the orbit. The interocular distance is measured between the two ethmoidal margins (*arrows*). **C,** An ultrasound image shows the appearance of the hyaloid artery (*arrow*). (From Robinson AJ, Blaser S, Toi A, et al. Magnetic resonance imaging of the fetal eyes—morphologic and biometric assessment for abnormal development with ultrasonographic and clinicopathologic correlation. *Pediatr Radiol.* 2003;38:971-981.)

and includes leukokoria, vitreous hemorrhage, retinal detachment, microphthalmos, and lens opacification.

The diagnosis can be made antenatally or by ultrasound, computed tomography (CT), or MRI postnatally. Ultrasound can detect the hyaloid vessel. A cone-shaped retrolental density is the characteristic finding on CT and MRI. Findings described on CT include a small irregular lens with a shallow anterior chamber; intravitreal densities of variable shape, suggesting the persistence of fetal tissue in the Cloquet canal; and enhancement of abnormal intravitreal tissue after intravenous administration of contrast media. On MRI the appearance is that of low-signal intensity linear plaques extending from the posterior part of the lens to the optic nerve head. Calcification is unusual (Fig. 5-8 and e-Fig. 5-9).

CATARACTS

Cataracts are seen in a variety of metabolic, infectious, genetic, and chromosomal abnormalities that affect the fetus,

including toxoplasmosis; X-irradiation; in-vitro fertilization; persistent hyperplastic primary vitreous; Nance-Horan, Adams-Oliver, Walker-Warburg, and Neu-Laxova syndromes; rhizomelic chondrodysplasia punctata; trisomy 17 mosaicism; and trisomy 21 (Fig. 5-10).[5,14-23]

OPTIC NERVE HYPOPLASIA

Optic nerve hypoplasia is usually sporadic and difficult to detect prenatally; however, it has a number of associations that potentially can be diagnosed prenatally because of associated structural abnormalities, several of which are discussed in this chapter (Box 5-1 and Fig. 5-11).

Septo-optic dysplasia can be extremely difficult to diagnose antenatally and is usually suspected because of the absence of the cavum septi pellucidi. Associated optic nerve hypoplasia potentially can be detected by measurement of the transverse diameter of the optic chiasm, normal growth of which has been described by ultrasound[24-26] and can, with some difficulty, be assessed by MRI.[27]

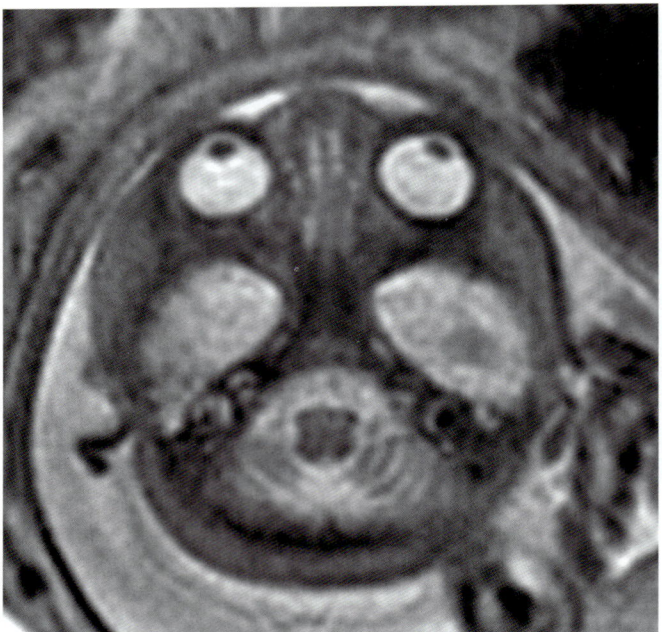

Figure 5-7 Fetal magnetic resonance imaging orbital appearance. The entire lens has a low signal compared with the high signal of the vitreous. (From Robinson AJ, Blaser S, Toi A, et al. Magnetic resonance imaging of the fetal eyes—morphologic and biometric assessment for abnormal development with ultrasonographic and clinicopathologic correlation. *Pediatr Radiol.* 2008;38:971-981.)

COLOBOMA, MORNING GLORY DISC, AND PERIPAPILLARY STAPHYLOMA

Coloboma, morning glory syndrome, and peripapillary staphyloma are all congenital anomalies that are excavations of the optic disc and can significantly impair visual function.[28]

Coloboma is a unilateral or bilateral congenital condition caused by incomplete closure of the embryonic fissure. Clinical features include visual field defects. On examination, coloboma appears as an enlarged, sharply circumscribed, deeply excavated optic disc, usually occurring inferiorly with increased risk of macular detachment. Other associated ocular findings include microphthalmos with an orbital cyst, a persistent hyaloid artery, and retinal dysplasia. Coloboma also may be part of the CHARGE syndrome (i.e., coloboma, heart defects, choanal atresia, growth retardation, and genital and ear abnormalities), and it may be associated with numerous other syndromes. Coloboma can be detected by fetal MRI (Fig. 5-12).[29]

Morning glory syndrome is a congenital anomaly of the optic disc in which there is a funnel-shaped excavation of the posterior fundus incorporating the optic nerve, surrounded by an elevated annulus of chorioretinal pigment. It is named for the ophthalmoscopic resemblance to the morning glory flower. Morning glory syndrome occurs more frequently in females and presents with poor vision, amblyopia, and strabismus with leukokoria. In the first months of life there is an increased risk of retinal detachment and associated cerebral abnormalities, including moyamoya disease (e-Fig. 5-13).

Staphyloma occurs as a result of weakening of the outer layer of the eye (cornea or sclera) by an inflammatory or degenerative condition and is an abnormal protrusion of uveal tissue caused by sclero-uveal ectasia. It is most commonly unilateral and nonhereditary.

COATS DISEASE

Coats disease is a rare, congenital, nonhereditary disorder characterized by retinal telangiectasia resulting in massive intraretinal and subretinal lipid accumulation, exudative retinal detachment, and blindness. It is usually isolated, unilateral, and occurs predominantly in young males, with the onset of symptoms occurring in the first decade of life. It appears as a hyperechoic mass on ultrasound without posterior acoustic shadowing. Vitreous and subretinal hemorrhage may be present. On CT, the globe is hyperdense and enhancement of the subretinal exudate is seen. This exudate is hyperintense on T1- and T2-weighted MRI sequences. It is important to differentiate this entity from retinoblastoma, which usually presents as a calcified mass and may require enucleation of the globe (Fig. 5-14).

NORRIE DISEASE

Norrie disease is an X-linked recessive disorder leading to congenital blindness in male infants. It is caused by mutations in the *NDP* gene. The ocular findings are characterized by retinal dysplasia and the development of a white, vascularized, retrolental mass that may lead to phthisis bulbi. Cataracts and leukocoria also may be present. Norrie disease is associated with progressive hearing loss in one third of patients, whereas up to 50% of patients have developmental delay, movement

---

Box 5-1 Associations with Optic Nerve Hypoplasia

Aicardi syndrome

Anticonvulsants

CHARGE association

Congenital muscular dystrophy

Distal 5q deletion syndrome

Dominant inheritance

Duane retraction syndrome

Partial deletion of chromosome 6p

Chromosome 7(q22-q34) and 7(q32-34) interstitial duplication

Chromosome 17 interstitial deletion

Ethanol toxicity

Frontonasal dysplasia

Goldenhar–Gorlin syndrome

Idiopathic growth hormone deficiency

Isotretinoin toxicity

Jadassohn sebaceous nevus

Maternal diabetes mellitus

Orbital hemangioma

Periventricular leukomalacia

Septo-optic dysplasia

Suprasellar teratoma

Valproic acid toxicity

Modified from Dutton GN. Congenital disorders of the optic nerve: excavations and hypoplasia. *Eye (Lond).* 2004;18:1038-1048.

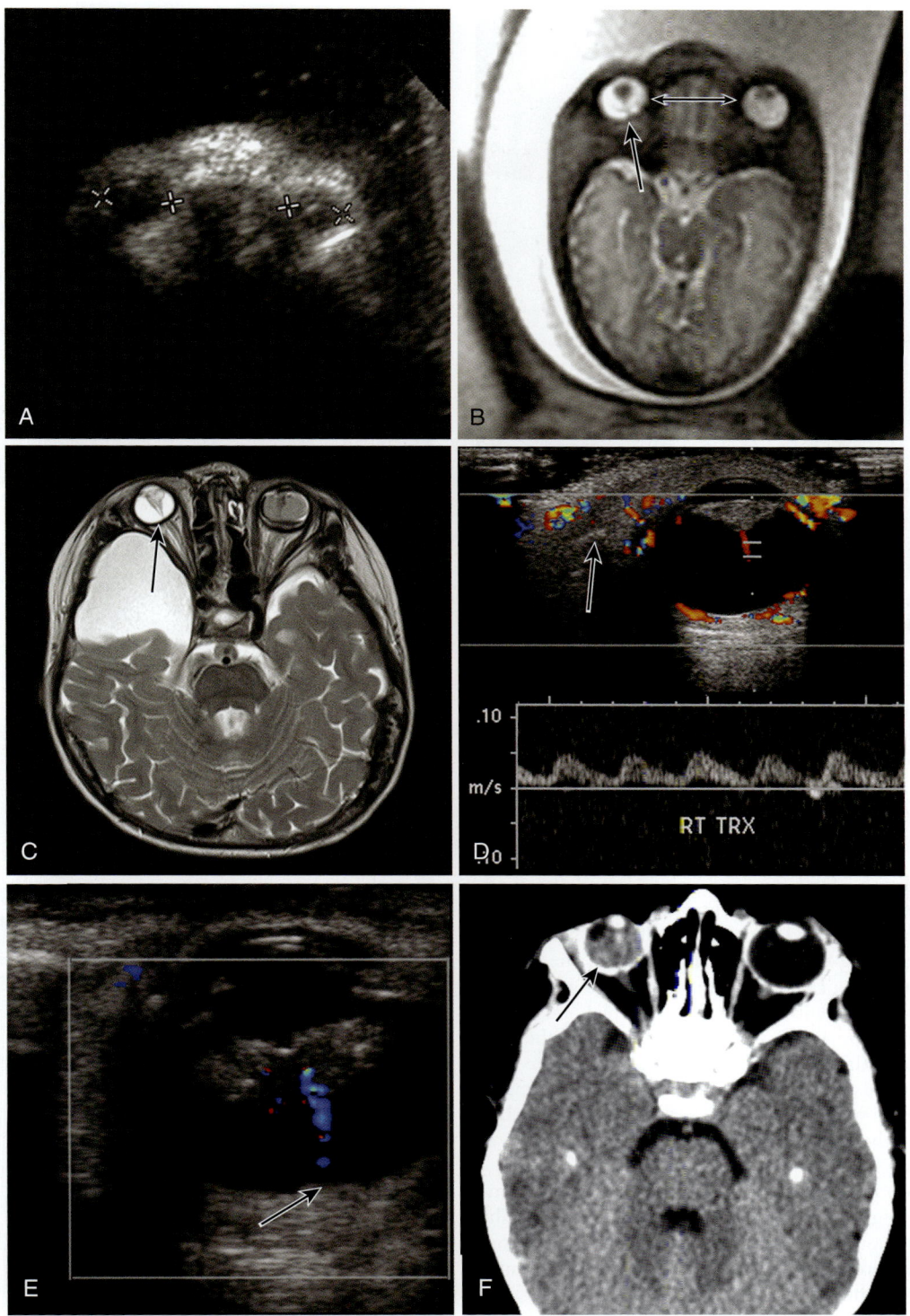

Figure 5-8 Persistent hyperplastic primary vitreous. **A,** Fetal ultrasonography shows the absence of normal anatomy and ocular hyperechogenicity. **B,** Fetal magnetic resonance imaging (MRI) shows hypertelorism (*double-headed arrow*) plus a persistent hyaloid artery (*large arrow*) and a triangular-shaped lens. **C,** An axial T2-weighted MRI demonstrates a low funnel-like signal extending from the right posterior lens to the optic nerve head (*arrow*). A similar low signal is noted on the left with associated vitreous hemorrhage. Note the incidental right middle cranial fossa arachnoid cyst. **D,** Doppler ultrasound reveals an arterial waveform within the hyaloid artery (*arrow*). **E,** Ultrasound shows thickening of the soft tissues posterior to the lens and a hyaloid vessel (*arrow*). **F,** An axial noncontrast computed tomography image shows increased attenuation in the right posterior chamber in keeping with vitreous hemorrhage (*arrow*) with linear high density centrally in persistent hyperplastic primary vitreous.

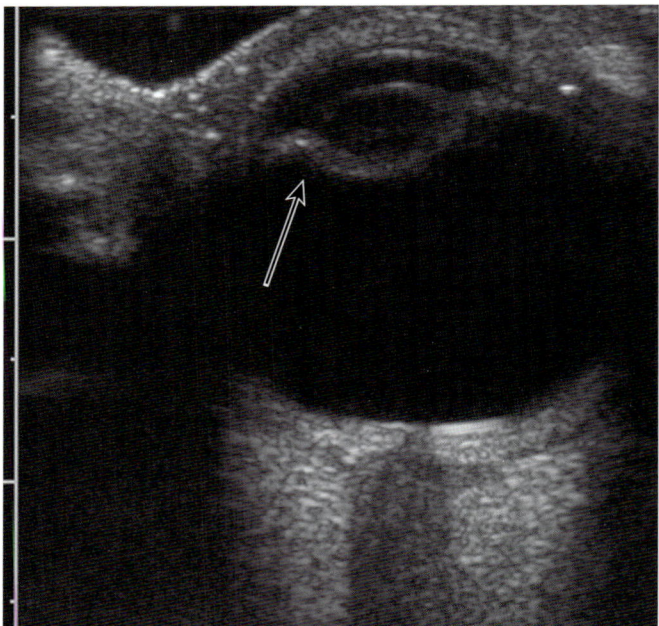

Figure 5-10 Cataract. Transverse ultrasound of the left eye shows increased echogenicity of the lens (*arrow*) in keeping with a cataract.

disorders, psychotic features, or behavioral problems. CT demonstrates dense vitreous chambers as a result of vitreous or subretinal hemorrhage, microphthalmia, optic nerve atrophy, a retrolental mass, and retinal detachment.

Biometry

Growth charts for the fetal lens and orbit[30,31] and the measurements of binocular and interocular distances (BOD and IOD) have been determined sonographically.[32-34] The orbits are measured according to the bony landmarks of the medial and lateral orbital walls. The orbital measurements ideally are made in the axial plane, with both orbits of equal and largest possible diameter.[8] The BOD is measured between the two malar margins, and the IOD is measured between the two ethmoidal margins of the bony orbits. These bony landmarks are difficult to see with fetal MRI and therefore standard sonographic growth charts cannot accurately be applied to fetal MR studies.

On MRI, the entire lens is of low-signal intensity compared with the high signal intensity of the vitreous. The BOD and IOD measurements can be made in any plane from true axial to true coronal, provided both eyes can be seen in the same image and have the most equal and largest possible transverse diameters. The BOD and IOD are respectively measured between the two malar or ethmoidal margins of each vitreous (Fig. 5-15). These measurements can be plotted against gestational age (Table 5-1).[1] Other available nomograms also include measurements of the anteroposterior globe diameter[37] and the diameter of the lens.[38]

HYPOTELORISM

Hypotelorism is defined as an IOD below the fifth percentile.[8]

Primary

During normal embryologic development, the opening for the eye forms during development of the face, when the paired nasal swellings on either side migrate medially and inferiorly and fuse with the midline frontal swelling to form the nose. Overmigration results in primary hypotelorism; the two halves of the face (and more often than not the underlying halves of the brain) lie too close together ("the face predicts the brain"),[39] and both the BOD and IOD therefore are decreased. This scenario most commonly results in an anomaly within the spectrum of holoprosencephaly,[35,40] which in around 55% of cases is associated with a variety of

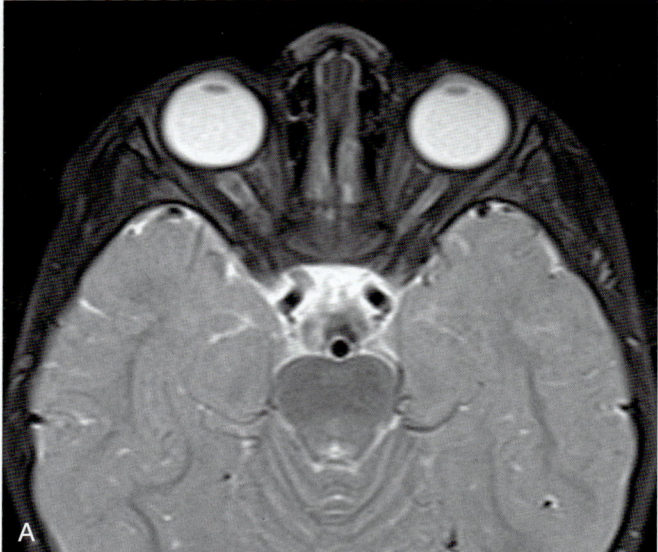

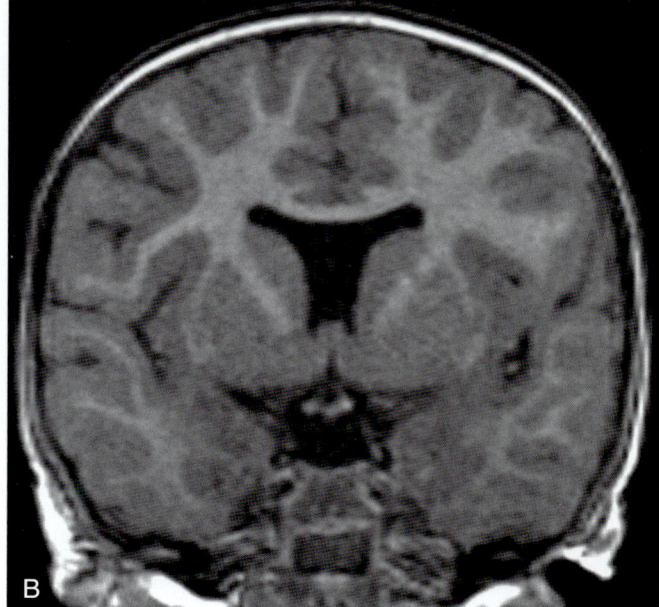

Figure 5-11 Optic nerve hypoplasia/septo-optic dysplasia. **A,** An axial T2-weighted fat saturation magnetic resonance image (MRI) of the orbits shows bilateral optic nerve hypoplasia. **B,** A coronal T1-weighted MRI demonstrates an associated small chiasm and absent cavum septi pellucidi.

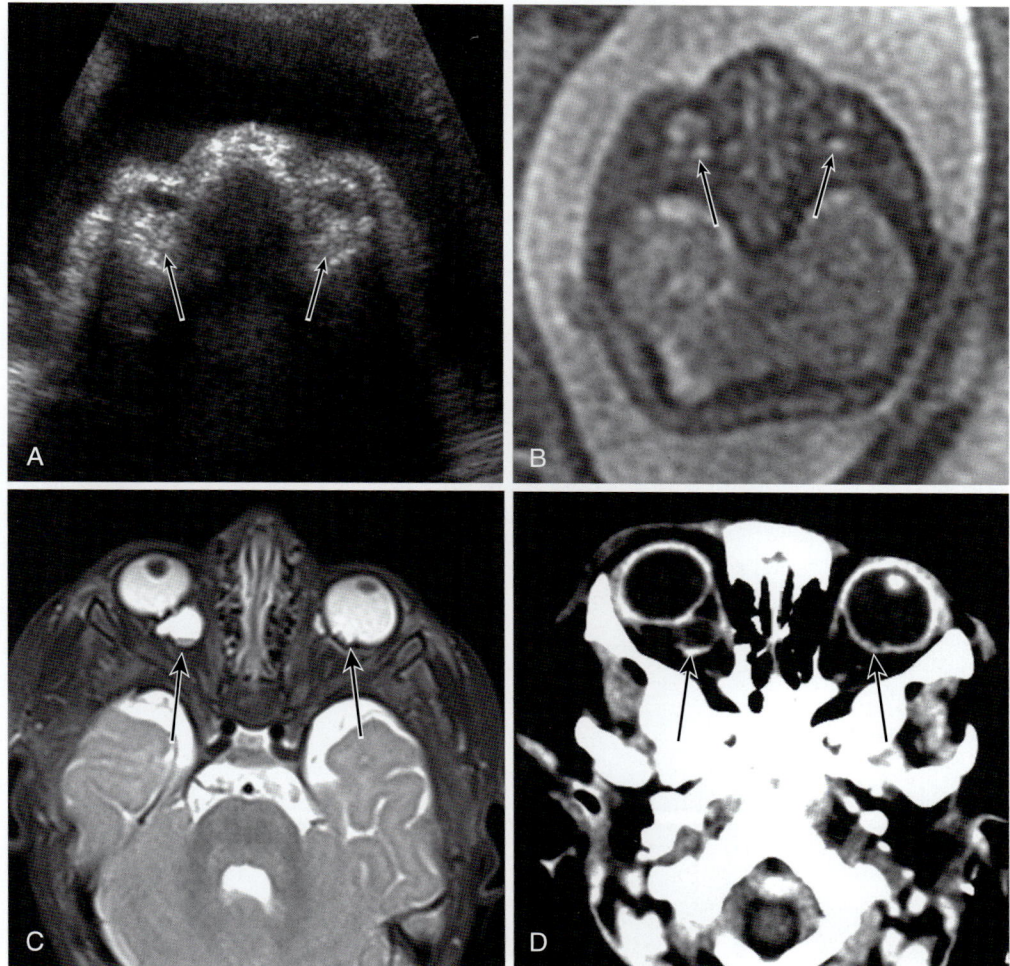

Figure 5-12 Coloboma. **A,** A prenatal ultrasound image demonstrates an abnormal echogenicity of the globes (*arrows*), but the lenses appear relatively normal. **B,** An axial fetal magnetic resonance image (MRI) shows bilateral, symmetrical, abnormal globes with mixed low- and high-signal vitreous (*arrows*) and no definite lens structures. **C,** A postnatal axial T2-weighted MRI of the orbits showing bilateral cystic colobomata (*arrows*). **D,** A noncontrast computed tomography image showing cystic coloboma of the posterior right orbit (*arrows*). (**B,** From Robinson AJ, Blaser S, Toi A, et al. Magnetic resonance imaging of the fetal eyes—morphologic and biometric assessment for abnormal development with ultrasonographic and clinicopathologic correlation. *Pediatr Radiol.* 2008;38:971-981.)

chromosomal abnormalities, most commonly trisomy 13 (Fig. 5-16 and e-Fig. 5-17).[8,32]

Secondary

Secondary hypotelorism is usually the result of abnormalities of the bony skull, such as microcephaly, plagiocephaly, and metopic synostosis (Fig. 5-18).[8]

HYPERTELORISM

Hypertelorism is defined as an IOD above the 95th percentile.[8]

Primary

During fetal development, if the nasal swellings do not migrate medially and inferiorly far enough that they fuse with the midline frontal swelling, the result is primary hypertelorism, in which the two halves of the face (and often the underlying halves of the brain) lie too far apart. Primary hypertelorism can result from many chromosomal anomalies and syndromes,[2] including median facial cleft syndrome, also known as *frontonasal dysplasia* (Fig. 5-19 and e-Fig. 5-20). This median facial cleft syndrome is composed of hypertelorism, facial clefting, and as a result of the two cerebral hemispheres "being too far apart," callosal agenesis. IOD may be the most reliable means of making the diagnosis of hypertelorism, because by ultrasound this measurement is usually more than two standard deviations from the mean, whereas the BOD remains at the upper limit of normal.[8]

Secondary

Secondary hypertelorism typically results from abnormalities of the skull, the most common being anterior cephalocele and craniosynostoses (e-Figs. 5-21 and 5-22).[2,40,41]

Text continued on page 48.

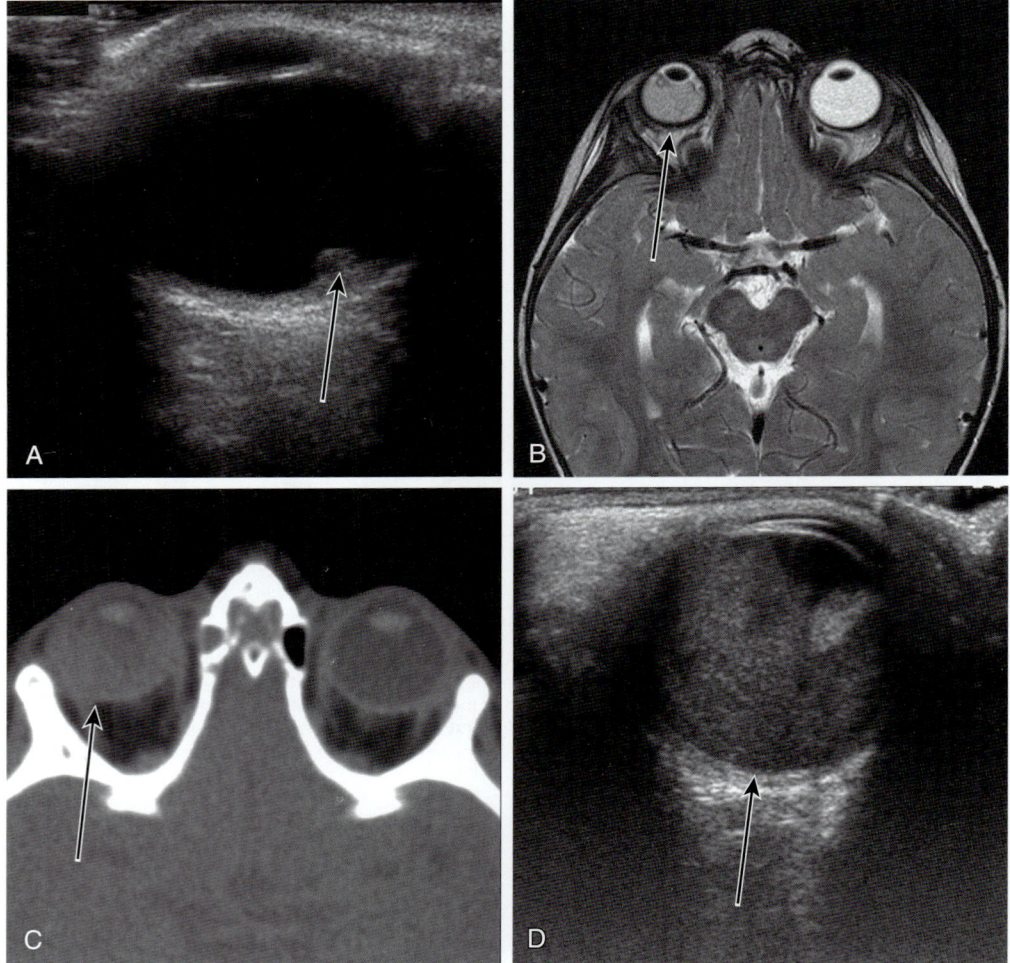

Figure 5-14 Coats disease. **A,** Ultrasound shows a hyperechoic mass in the posterior vitreous (*arrow*) without posterior acoustic shadowing. **B,** An axial T2-weighted magnetic resonance image shows intermediate signal within the right vitreous (*arrow*) in keeping with proteinaceous exudate. **C,** An unenhanced computed tomography scan of the orbits demonstrates homogenous hyperattenuation of the right globe (*arrow*) and a normal left globe. **D,** Ultrasound of the right eye shows hyperechogenicity within the posterior chamber (*arrow*) and a more focal area of increased echogenicity anteriorly.

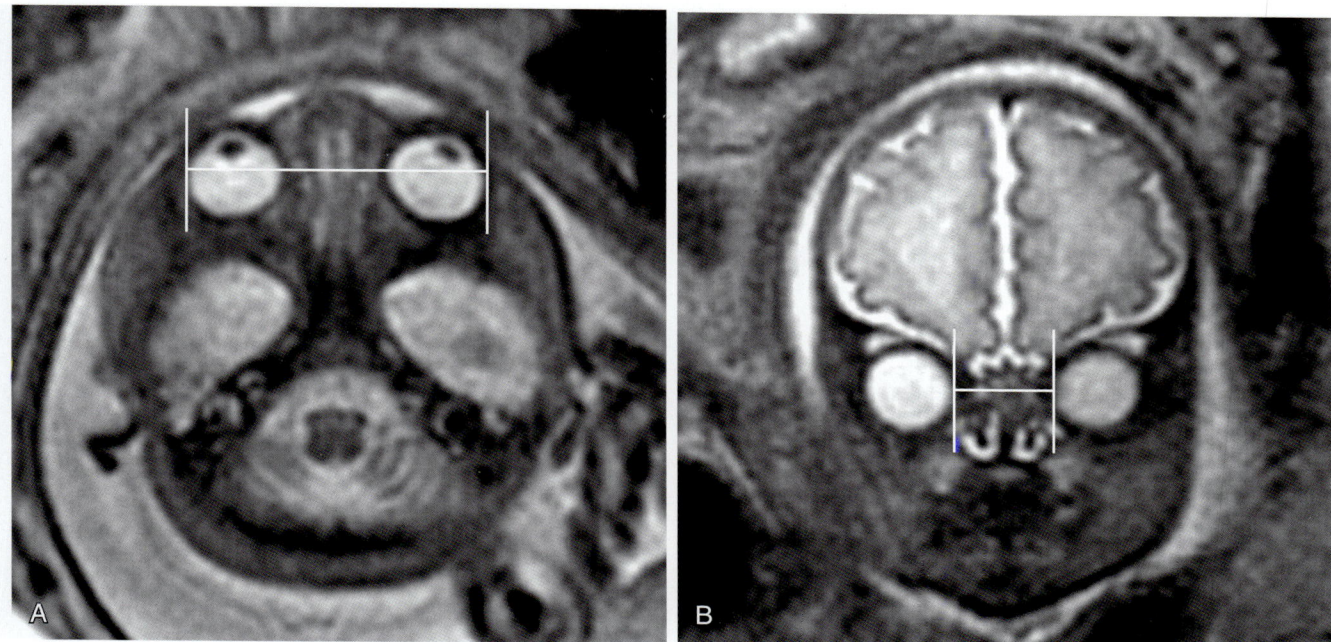

Figure 5-15   Ocular biometry measurements by magnetic resonance imaging. **A,** The binocular distance is measured between the two malar margins of each high-signal vitreous. The measurements can be made in any plane orthogonal to the sagittal plane. **B,** The interocular distance is measured in the coronal plane between the two orbital margins of each high-signal vitreous. (From Robinson AJ, Blaser S, Toi A, et al. Magnetic resonance imaging of the fetal eyes—morphologic and biometric assessment for abnormal development with ultrasonographic and clinicopathologic correlation. *Pediatr Radiol.* 2008;38:971-981.)

Table 5-1

Fetal Magnetic Resonance Imaging Measurements of Binocular Distance, Interocular Distance, and Ocular Diameter in Relation to Gestational Age									
	BOD			**IOD**			**OD**		
GA	**5% CI**	**50% CI**	**95% CI**	**5% CI**	**50% CI**	**95% CI**	**5% CI**	**50% CI**	**95% CI**
15	16.6	20.8	21.4	7.4	9.8	12.3	3.4	5.5	6.4
16	19.0	22.8	24.0	8.2	10.6	13.3	4.2	6.1	7.1
17	21.3	24.8	26.5	9.0	11.4	14.3	5.0	6.7	7.9
18	23.4	26.8	28.9	9.7	12.1	15.2	5.7	7.3	8.5
19	25.4	28.7	31.1	10.4	12.9	16.1	6.4	7.9	9.2
20	27.3	30.5	33.2	11.1	13.6	15.9	7.0	8.5	9.8
21	29.1	32.3	35.2	11.7	14.3	17.6	7.6	9.0	10.4
22	30.8	34.1	37.1	12.3	14.9	18.4	8.2	9.6	10.9
23	32.4	35.8	38.9	12.8	15.6	19.1	8.8	10.1	11.4
24	34.0	37.4	40.7	13.4	16.2	19.8	9.3	10.6	11.9
25	35.5	39.0	42.4	13.9	16.8	20.4	9.8	11.1	12.4
26	37.0	40.6	44.0	14.4	17.4	21.0	10.3	11.6	12.9
27	38.4	42.1	45.5	14.9	17.9	21.6	10.8	12.0	13.3
28	39.7	43.5	47.0	15.3	18.5	22.2	11.3	12.5	13.8
29	41.0	44.9	48.5	15.8	19.0	22.8	11.7	12.9	14.2
30	42.3	46.3	49.9	16.2	19.5	23.3	12.1	13.4	14.6
31	43.5	47.6	51.2	16.6	19.9	23.8	12.5	13.8	15.0
32	44.6	48.8	52.5	17.0	20.4	24.3	12.9	14.2	15.4
33	45.8	50.0	53.8	17.4	20.8	24.8	13.3	14.6	15.7
34	46.9	51.2	55.0	17.8	21.2	25.3	13.7	15.0	16.1
35	48.0	52.3	56.2	18.2	21.5	25.7	14.1	15.3	16.4
36	49.0	53.3	57.3	18.5	21.9	26.2	14.4	15.7	16.7
37	50.0	54.4	58.5	18.9	22.2	26.6	14.8	16.0	17.1
38	51.0	55.3	59.6	19.2	22.5	27.0	15.1	16.3	17.4
39	52.0	56.2	60.6	19.5	22.7	27.4	15.4	16.6	17.7
40	52.9	57.1	61.7	19.9	23.0	27.8	15.8	16.9	18.0

BOD, Binocular distance; *CI,* confidence interval; *GA,* gestational age; *IOD,* interocular distance; *OD,* ocular diameter.

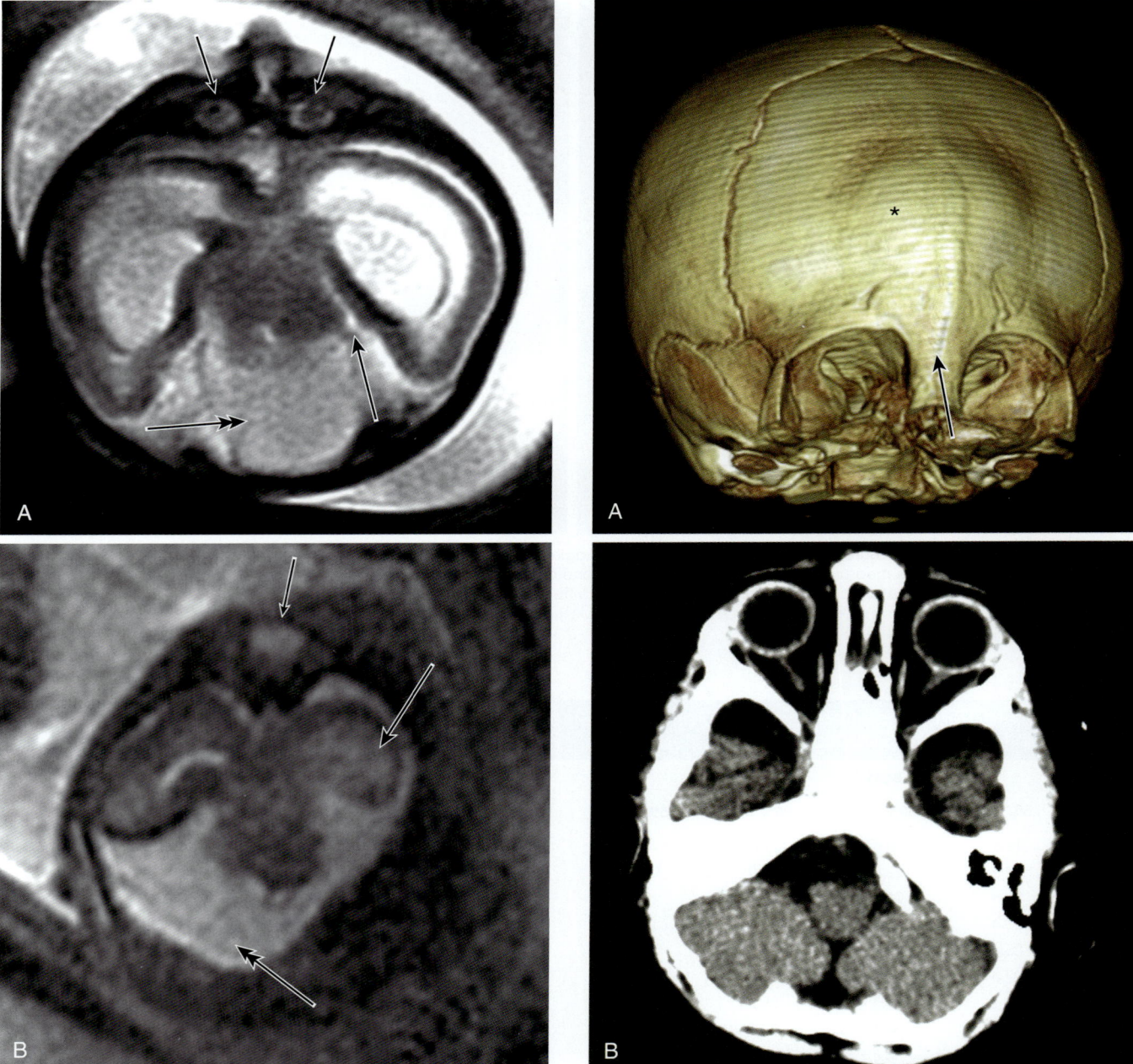

Figure 5-16 Holoprosencephaly. **A,** An axial magnetic resonance (MR) image shows severe hypotelorism and microphthalmia (*small arrows*). A dorsal interhemispheric cyst is present (*double arrow*), and the hippocampus touches the brainstem at the ambient cistern (*long arrow*) in keeping with lobar holoprosencephaly. **B,** An axial MR image shows a single small midline globe (*small arrow*). The hippocampus is not touching the brainstem (*long arrow*), and wide communication of the ambient cistern with the dorsal interhemispheric cyst is present (*double arrow*) in keeping with alobar holoprosencephaly. (From Robinson AJ, Blaser S, Toi A, et al. Magnetic resonance imaging of the fetal eyes—morphologic and biometric assessment for abnormal development with ultrasonographic and clinicopathologic correlation. *Pediatr Radiol.* 2008;38:971-981.)

Figure 5-18 Metopic synostosis. **A,** A three-dimensional computed tomography (CT) reconstruction of the skull showing metopic synostosis (*arrow*) and associated bowing of the adjacent frontal bone (*asterisk*) **B,** An axial CT scan in the same patient shows hypotelorism.

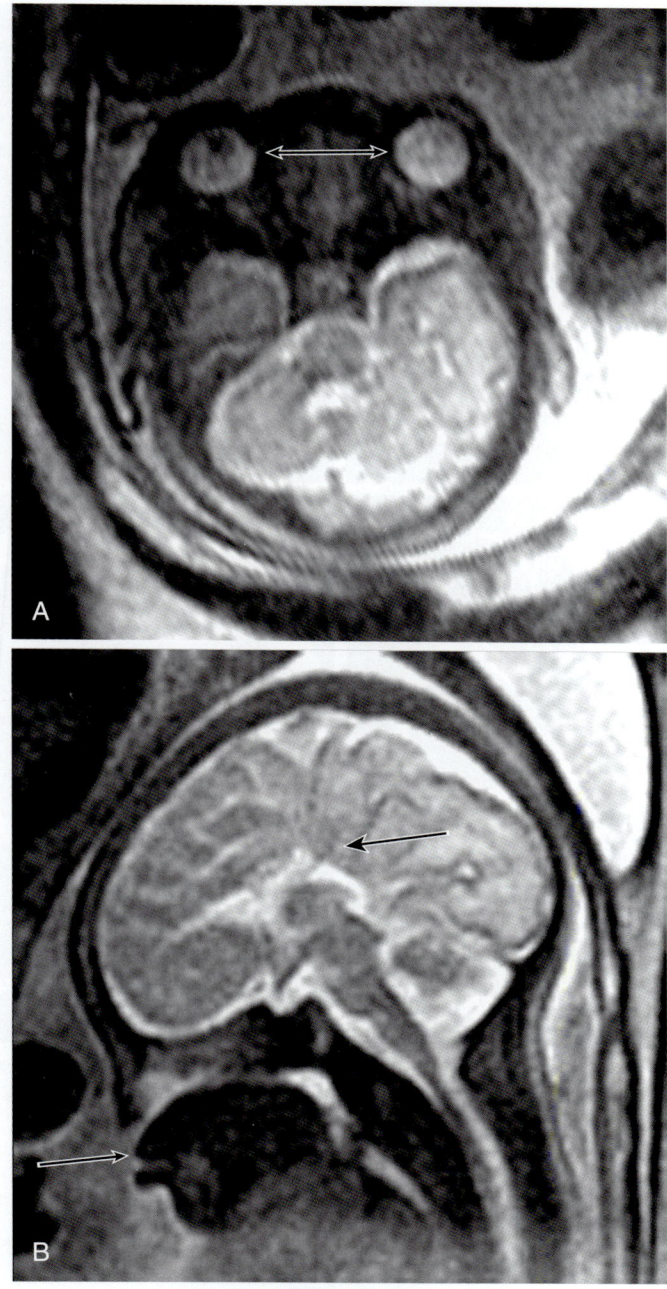

Figure 5-19 Frontonasal dysplasia. **A,** An axial magnetic resonance image shows hypertelorism (*double-headed arrow*). The binocular distance and interocular distance were both greater than the 95th percentile for gestational age. **B,** Absence of the corpus callosum (*large arrow*) and a facial defect with absence of the hard palate separating the nasal and oral cavities, with the tongue protruding through the defect (*small arrow*). (**A,** From Robinson AJ, Blaser S, Toi A, et al. Magnetic resonance imaging of the fetal eyes—morphologic and biometric assessment for abnormal development with ultrasonographic and clinicopathologic correlation. *Pediatr Radiol.* 2008.38:971-981.)

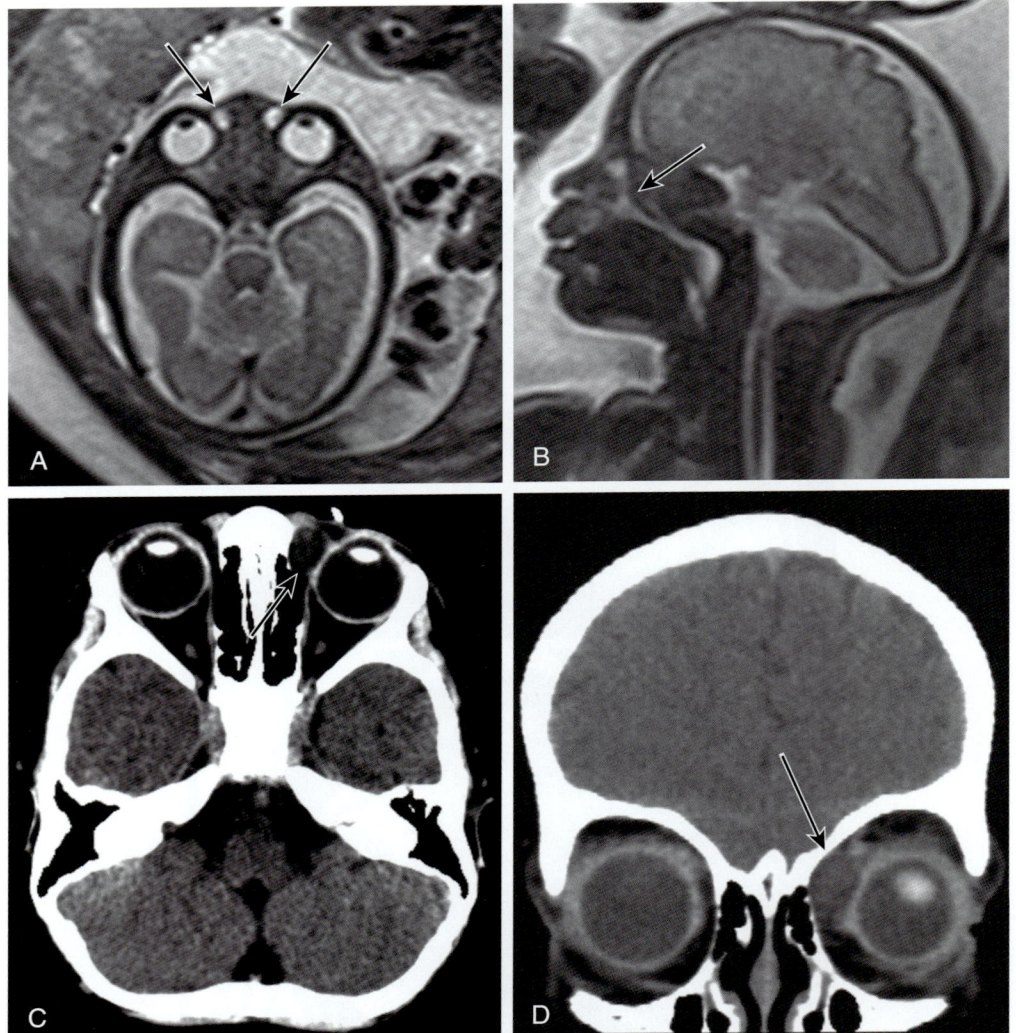

Figure 5-23 Dacryocystocele. **A,** Fetal magnetic resonance imaging (MRI) showing bilateral cysts in the medial canthi (*arrows*). **B,** Fetal MRI showing a dilated nasolacrimal duct (*arrow*). **C,** An axial noncontrast computed tomography (CT) scan shows a well-circumscribed low attenuation in the region of the left nasolacrimal duct (*arrow*). **D,** A coronal CT scan shows a left dacryocystocele (*arrow*).

Orbital Abnormalities (Nonneoplastic)

DACRYOCYSTOCELE

Congenital dacryocystocele is a distension of the nasolacrimal duct, usually as a result of obstruction at its distal end at the valve of Hasner. Prenatal ultrasound and MRI can be used to make the diagnosis (Fig. 5-23).[42,43] The incidence on prenatal MRI studies has been reported to be between 0.7% and 2.7%, depending on the definition, and only 50% of affected eyes were symptomatic postnatally. Congenital dacryocystocele is not expected to be seen before 24 weeks' gestation because nasolacrimal duct canalization is incomplete, and even normal fluid-filled nasolacrimal ducts can only be seen by MRI after 24 weeks' gestation. Dacryocystoceles also can resolve spontaneously before delivery as a result of rupture of the valve of Hasner.[44,45]

Key Points

Routine assessment of the orbit should include the presence or absence of the eyes, morphology of the lens and vitreous, and ocular biometry.

Detection of orbital abnormalities often can be a critical step in diagnosing fetal dysmorphology.

The existing sonographic growth charts for ocular biometry cannot be directly applied to fetal MRI; dedicated MRI nomograms should be used.

Suggested Readings

Babcook C. The fetal face and neck. In: Callen P, ed. *Ultrasonography in obstetrics and gynecology*. Philadelphia: W.B. Saunders; 2000.

Bardakjian T, Weiss A, Schneider A. Anophthalmia/microphthalmia overview. Available at http://www.ncbi.nlm.nih.gov/books/NBK1378/; Accessed October 19, 2012.

Dutton GN. Congenital disorders of the optic nerve: excavations and hypoplasia. *Eye (Lond).* 2004;18:1038-1048.

Paquette LB, Jackson HA, Tavare CJ, et al. In utero eye development documented by fetal MR imaging. *Am J Neuroradiol.* 2009;30:1787-1791.

Li XB, Kasprian G, Hodge JC, et al. Fetal ocular measurements by MRI. *Prenat Diagn.* 2010;30:1064-1071.

Ramji FG, Slovis TL, Baker JD. Orbital sonography in children. *Pediatr Radiol.* 1996;26:245-258.

Robinson AJ, Blaser S, Toi A, et al. Magnetic resonance imaging of the fetal eyes—morphologic and biometric assessment for abnormal development with ultrasonographic and clinicopathologic correlation. *Pediatr Radiol.* 2008;38:971-981.

References

Full references for this chapter can be found on www.expertconsult.com.

Chapter 6

Orbit Infection and Inflammation

JOHN P. GRIMM

A wide variety of disease processes can cause inflammatory changes in the orbit, including infection, idiopathic inflammation, granulomatous disease, thyroid-related disease, optic neuritis, and sickle cell disease. Even metabolic diseases can affect the optic nerves, leading to vision loss. Although many of these conditions also occur in adults, they behave differently in children. Furthermore, many of these disease processes can share a similar imaging appearance. As a result, a good understanding of their pathophysiology and clinical presentation is needed to formulate a useful differential diagnosis.

Periorbital and Orbital Cellulitis

Etiologies, Pathophysiology, and Clinical Presentation The orbital septum, the anterior reflection of the periosteum of the orbital wall onto the tarsal plate of the eyelid, divides the orbit into preseptal and postseptal compartments.

Periorbital cellulitis refers to infection anterior to the orbital septum involving the eyelid and adnexa. Orbital cellulitis refers to infection posterior to the orbital septum. This distinction is important because orbital cellulitis carries the risks of abscess, blindness, venous thrombosis, intracranial extension, and death. Defects in the orbital septum, direct extension from sinus infection, and valveless veins provide infection with access to the postseptal orbit. Sinusitis is the most common cause (60% to 85%), with stye, dacryoadenitis/cystitis, dental abscess, skin breaks, and hematogenous seeding being less common.[1,2] *Staphylococcus aureus*, *S. epidermidis*, and *S. pyogenes* account for ~75% of infections; rates of *Hemophilus influenzae* and streptococcal pneumonia are declining as a result of immunization.[1] Patients present with erythema, swelling, warmth, and tenderness of the eyelid. Although ophthalmoplegia and proptosis predict postseptal involvement and abscess, approximately 50% of patients with an abscess do not have these symptoms. As a result, the guidelines for imaging are unclear and vary: edema preventing a complete examination, signs of central nervous system involvement, deteriorating vision, proptosis, ophthalmoplegia, and/or deterioration after 24 to 48 hours of treatment.[3-5]

Imaging Periorbital cellulitis presents with eyelid swelling and thickening of the preseptal soft tissues on computed tomography (CT), with T2 hyperintensity on magnetic resonance imaging (MRI) (Fig. 6-1, *A*).[2,6,7] In orbital cellulitis, similar inflammatory changes of the extraconal and/or intraconal orbital fat are present. The most common complication of orbital cellulitis is subperiosteal abscess, frequently involving the lamina papyracea, and directly extending from ethmoid sinus disease. A subperiosteal abscess presents as a broad-based, peripherally enhancing fluid collection along the medial wall of the orbit that displaces the medial rectus muscle laterally (Fig. 6-2, *A*). Less commonly, an abscess can form in the extraconal or intraconal orbit separate from the bone, which also is seen as a peripherally enhancing fluid collection. MRI can be helpful in identifying an abscess by demonstrating restricted diffusion.[8]

Treatment Treatment consists of oral antibiotics covering staphylococcus and streptococcus for periorbital cellulitis and admission to the hospital with administration of intravenous (IV) antibiotics for orbital cellulitis. Surgical intervention for drainage of an abscess is required in only 12% of admitted patients,[3] and an orbital abscess can be treated with IV antibiotics if it is small or appears in a young child.[9,10]

Dacryocystitis

Dacryocystitis is the result of bacterial overgrowth of stagnant fluid in the nasolacrimal sac presenting with epiphora, erythema, and edema at the medial canthus. In neonates, dacryocystitis can complicate 33% to 65% of cases of congenital dacryocystocele caused by incomplete canalization of the distal nasolacrimal duct.[11,12] In older children, dacryocystitis can result from other causes of nasolacrimal duct obstruction, including rhinitis/sinusitis, tumor, or trauma and fracture. CT or MRI demonstrates a cystic medial canthus mass with adjacent inflammatory changes (Fig. 6-1, *B*).[13-15] Although infection is most commonly associated with periorbital cellulitis, it rarely can extend into the postseptal orbit with abscess formation.[16] Treatment typically consists of antibiotics and dacryocystorhinostomy.

Superior Ophthalmic Vein Thrombosis

Superior ophthalmic vein (SOV) thrombosis is a complication of orbital cellulitis that results from inflammatory thrombophlebitis or direct venous invasion by infection; 33% to 75% of isolated SOV thrombosis leads to cavernous sinus

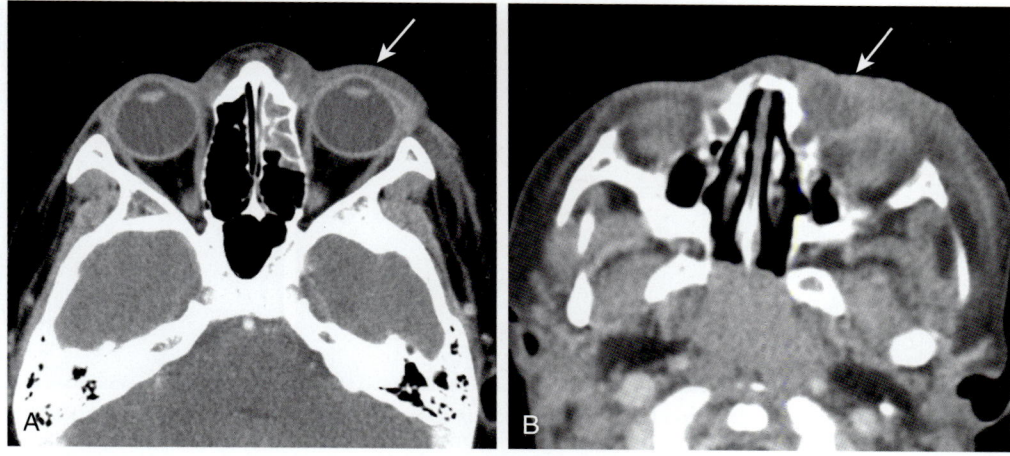

Figure 6-1 Periorbital cellulitis. **A,** A computed tomography (CT) image of periorbital cellulitis from adjacent sinusitis demonstrates preseptal soft tissue swelling (*arrow*). **B,** A CT image of dacryocystitis causing periorbital cellulitis demonstrates a cystic medial canthus mass (*arrow*) with adjacent inflammatory changes.

thrombosis, which carries a mortality rate of 20%.[17,18] Imaging with CT or MRI demonstrates an enlarged S-shaped SOV below the superior rectus muscle with a filling defect and peripherally enhancing vasa vasorum on postcontrast images (Fig. 6-2, *B*).[19] Restricted diffusion of the SOV also has been reported, facilitating identification.[20] Treatment consists of aggressive use of antibiotics with or without corticosteroids and anticoagulation, which are not proven therapies.[17,18]

Ocular Toxocariasis

Ocular toxocariasis refers to infection of the globe by the nematodes *Toxocara canis* or *Toxocara cati*. It is one of several ocular infections caused by parasitic worms, including onchocerciasis (*Onchocerca volvulus*), cysticercosis (*Taenia solium*), and diffuse unilateral subacute neuroretinitis. Ocular toxocariasis is most common in the southeastern United States in children 6 to 12 years of age as a result of ingestion of food or soil contaminated by the feces of dogs or cats. It presents with painless unilateral vision loss, strabismus, and leukocoria.[21]

CT and MRI demonstrate an intravitreal enhancing mass with or without adjacent uveoscleral thickening and retinal detachment. A normal-sized globe containing a mass without calcification differentiates toxocariasis from other common causes of leukocoria (e.g., retinoblastoma, persistent hyperplastic primary vitreous, Coats disease, and retinopathy of prematurity).[22,23]

Orbital Pseudotumor (Idiopathic Orbital Inflammation)

Etiologies, Pathophysiology, and Clinical Presentation Orbital pseudotumor (OP) is a noninfectious inflammatory condition of the orbit of unclear etiology. In adults it is the most common painful orbital mass, accounting for ~10% of orbital masses, and is the third most common orbital disease. Pediatric OP is rare, with only 68 cases reported in the medical literature as of 2008, accounting for only 7% to 16% of cases of OP.[24,25] Children present similarly to adults with pain,

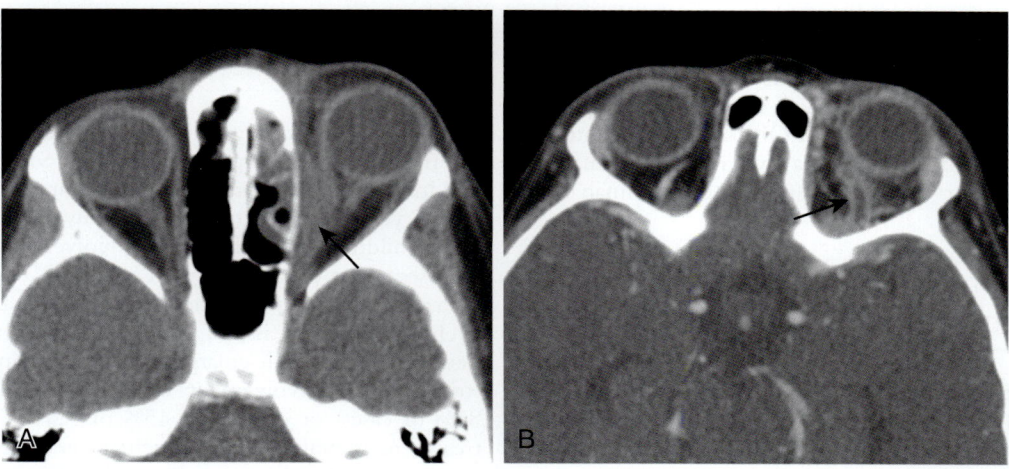

Figure 6-2 Orbital cellulitis. **A,** A computed tomography (CT) scan of orbital cellulitis with a subperiosteal abscess demonstrates inflammatory changes of the fat of the postseptal orbit with a broad-based, peripherally enhancing fluid collection adjacent to the lamina papyracea (*arrow*). **B,** A CT scan of superior ophthalmic vein (SOV) thrombosis demonstrates an enlarged S-shaped SOV with a filling defect and peripheral enhancement (*arrow*).

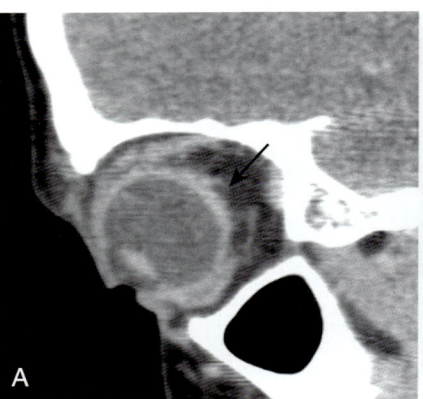 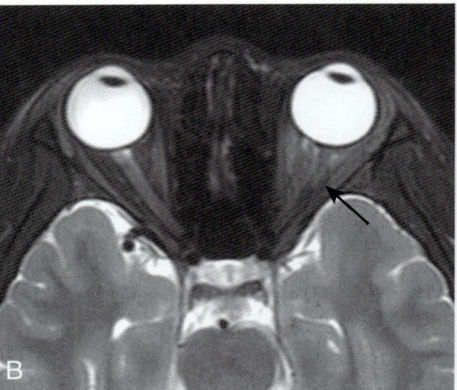 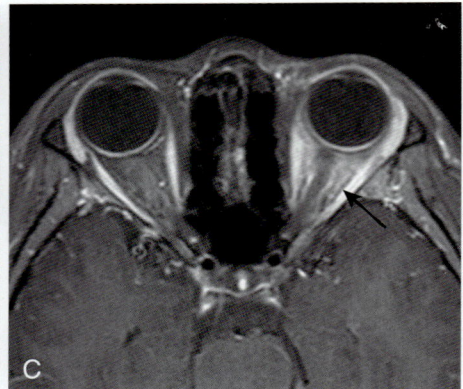

Figure 6-3   Orbital pseudotumor. **A,** A sagittal computed tomography image of scleral involvement by a pseudotumor causing posterior scleritis with subtle thickening of the posterior sclera (*arrow*). **B,** A T2-weighted fat-saturated magnetic resonance image in a different patient with a pseudotumor demonstrating ill-defined T2 hyperintensity of the intraconal fat (*arrow*). **C,** A T1-weighted fat-saturated postcontrast image demonstrating corresponding "tramline" enhancement of the optic nerve sheath and ill-defined enhancement of the intraconal fat (*arrow*).

proptosis, a mass, swelling, and motility restriction; however, children more frequently demonstrate ptosis and bilateral or intraocular involvement.

Imaging   Both CT and MRI are useful in evaluating OP.[26-28] Lacrimal gland involvement is most common, with enlargement and adjacent inflammatory change. Myositis also occurs frequently, typically with unilateral tubular thickening of extraocular muscles and tendons (compared with Graves orbitopathy, which tends to be bilateral with tendon sparing). OP may involve the uvea and sclera with thickening and enhancement (Fig. 6-3, *A*). Perineuritis, which involves the optic nerve sheath, demonstrates "tramline" inflammatory changes and enhancement surrounding the optic nerve (Fig. 6-3, *B-D*). Inflammation can extend through the orbital fissures and optic canal into the cavernous sinus and middle cranial fossa. The differential diagnosis includes infection, lymphoma, Wegener granulomatosis, sarcoidosis, and Graves orbitopathy. Diffusion-weighted imaging may be helpful in the diagnosis with the intensity of lymphoid lesions > OP > cellulitis on b–value = 1000 images.[29]

Treatment   Administration of oral corticosteroids often results in a rapid response (within 1 to 2 days); radiation is used in refractory cases.[25,30] Recurrence after withdrawal of steroids occurs frequently in adults (~50%) but has been reported in only one child.[24,31] Biopsy is reserved for atypical symptoms or poor response. Recently, cases of OP have been identified as part of IgG4-related disease, a systemic inflammatory disease demonstrating excellent response to rituximab and corticosteroids.[32,33]

Graves Orbitopathy (Thyroid Orbitopathy)

Etiologies, Pathophysiology, and Clinical Presentation   Graves orbitopathy is an orbital inflammatory process seen in persons with Graves disease, which is an autoimmune thyroid disease from thyroid-stimulating hormone receptor autoantibodies. Pediatric Graves disease is uncommon, yet children who have the disease experience Graves orbitopathy at similar rates as

do adults, in one third to two thirds of cases.[34-36] Graves orbitopathy is milder in children than in adults, with mild proptosis and mild eyelid retraction or lag. In children, no cases of compressive optic neuropathy have been reported, and strabismus is rare.

Imaging   Imaging demonstrates fusiform enlargement of extraocular muscles (involving muscle bellies and sparing tendons), which is bilateral in 90% of cases and frequently involves the inferior and medial recti. Increased volume of orbital fat and lacrimal gland enlargement also can be seen.[37] Active disease can be differentiated from fibrotic disease by evaluating the T2 signal intensity and dynamic contrast enhancement of the muscles (T2 hyperintensity, shorter time to peak, and greater enhancement and washout ratios are found in persons with active disease). This distinction is important, because medical therapy is not effective in persons with fibrotic disease.[38-40]

Treatment   Most pediatric cases can be controlled with antithyroid medication alone; steroids, radiation therapy, or surgery are not required, as is often the case with adults.[34-36]

Sarcoidosis

Sarcoidosis is a multisystem disease of unclear etiology characterized by noncaseating granulomas. Sarcoidosis is rare in children; however, a unique form appears in children younger than 5 years and presents with rash, uveitis, and arthritis.[41] In older children and adults, ocular involvement is seen in ~25% of cases, most commonly with uveitis.[41-44] Additional orbital structures involved can include the lacrimal gland and sac, eyelid, orbital soft tissues, optic nerve and sheath, and extraocular muscles, with enlargement and enhancement of these structures.[45,46] Involvement can be well circumscribed (in 85% of cases) or diffuse (in 15% of cases). The mainstay of treatment is oral steroids, which generally results in a good response; methotrexate or surgery is used for refractory cases. In patients with isolated orbital involvement (63%), systemic disease develops in 8% within 5 years.[47]

Wegener Granulomatosis

Wegener granulomatosis is a necrotizing granulomatous vasculitis of small and medium-sized vessels associated with antineutrophil cytoplasmic antibodies. Pediatric Wegener granulomatosis is rare; it presents in adolescence with a female predominance.[48,49] Orbital involvement occurs in approximately 50% of adults (and is the presenting feature in 15%), but it is less common in children.[50,51] Orbital disease may be primary or extend from the sinuses with osseous erosion. The globe (conjunctivitis and scleritis), lacrimal gland, retrobulbar space, optic nerve, and extraocular muscles all can be involved. Imaging demonstrates granulomatous masses with variable enhancement and characteristic T2-weighted hypointensity on MRI, presumably related to fibrocollagenous tissue (Fig. 6-4).[52,53] Visual impairment related to optic nerve compression or vasculitis is seen in up to 20% to 50% of adults. Nasolacrimal duct obstruction from sinus disease can result in dacryocystitis. Treatment in children can vary but typically consists of administration of steroids and cyclophosphamide.

Optic Neuritis

Etiologies, Pathophysiology, and Clinical Presentation Optic neuritis (ON) is an inflammatory disease of the optic nerve with acute onset of vision loss and periocular pain (in >90% of adults). ON may be idiopathic or related to multiple sclerosis (MS), neuromyelitis optica, or acute disseminated encephalomyelitis. ON behaves differently in children than in adults, likely reflecting different etiologies, with parainfectious ON being common in children (in one third to two thirds of cases).[54-58] Compared with adults, ON in children is more often bilateral (in 37% to 66% of cases), less often painful (in 37% of cases), and more often demonstrates disk swelling (in 46% to 85% of cases) and profound vision loss. In children it tends to have better visual recovery and is less often associated with MS.

Imaging MRI demonstrates contrast enhancement (>90%), T2-weighted hyperintensity, and mild enlargement of the optic nerves acutely, with mild volume loss developing chronically (Fig. 6-5).[59,60] If frank enlargement of the optic

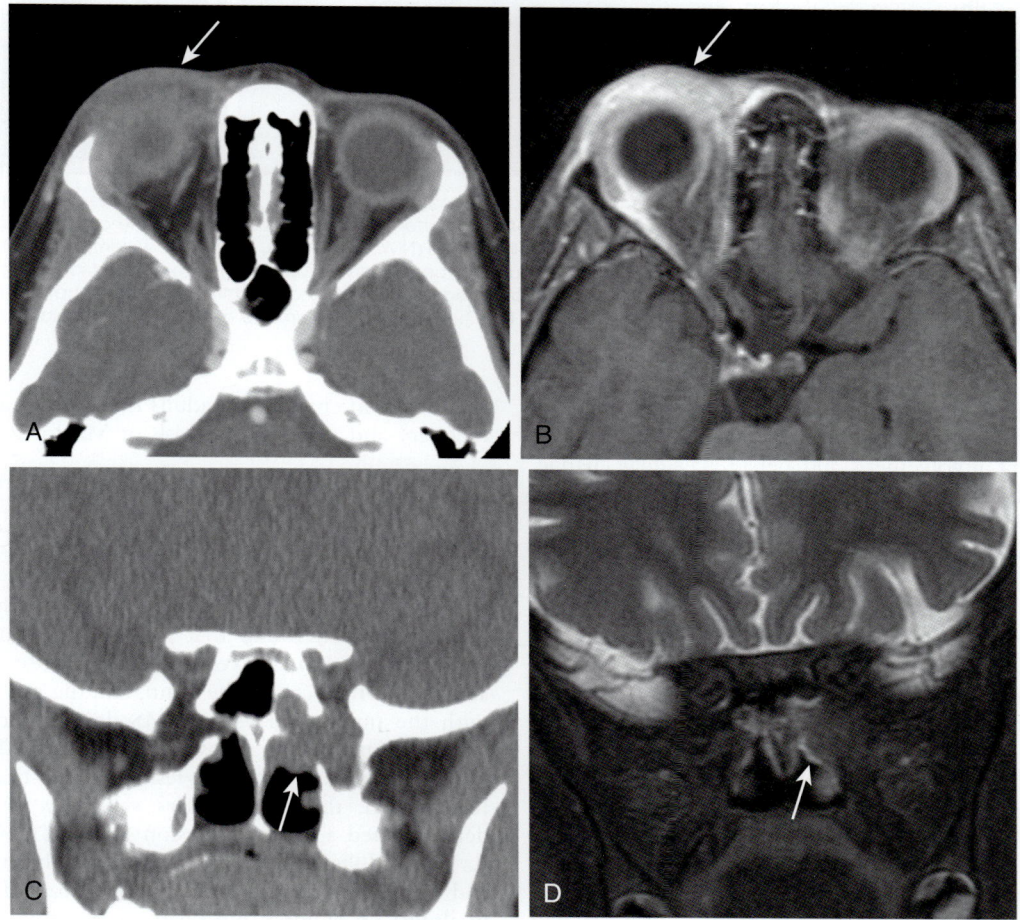

Figure 6-4 Wegener granulomatosis. **A** and **B,** Computed tomography (CT) and T1-weighted fat-saturated postcontrast magnetic resonance (MR) images of the orbit demonstrating inflammatory changes and enhancement adjacent to the lacrimal gland in the preseptal orbit, similar in appearance to periorbital cellulitis (*arrow*). **C** and **D,** Coronal CT and T2-weighted fat-saturated MR images demonstrating a mass centered on the sphenopalatine foramen with osseous erosion and extension to the orbital apex with characteristic T2 hypointensity, making it difficult to visualize on MR imaging (*arrows*).

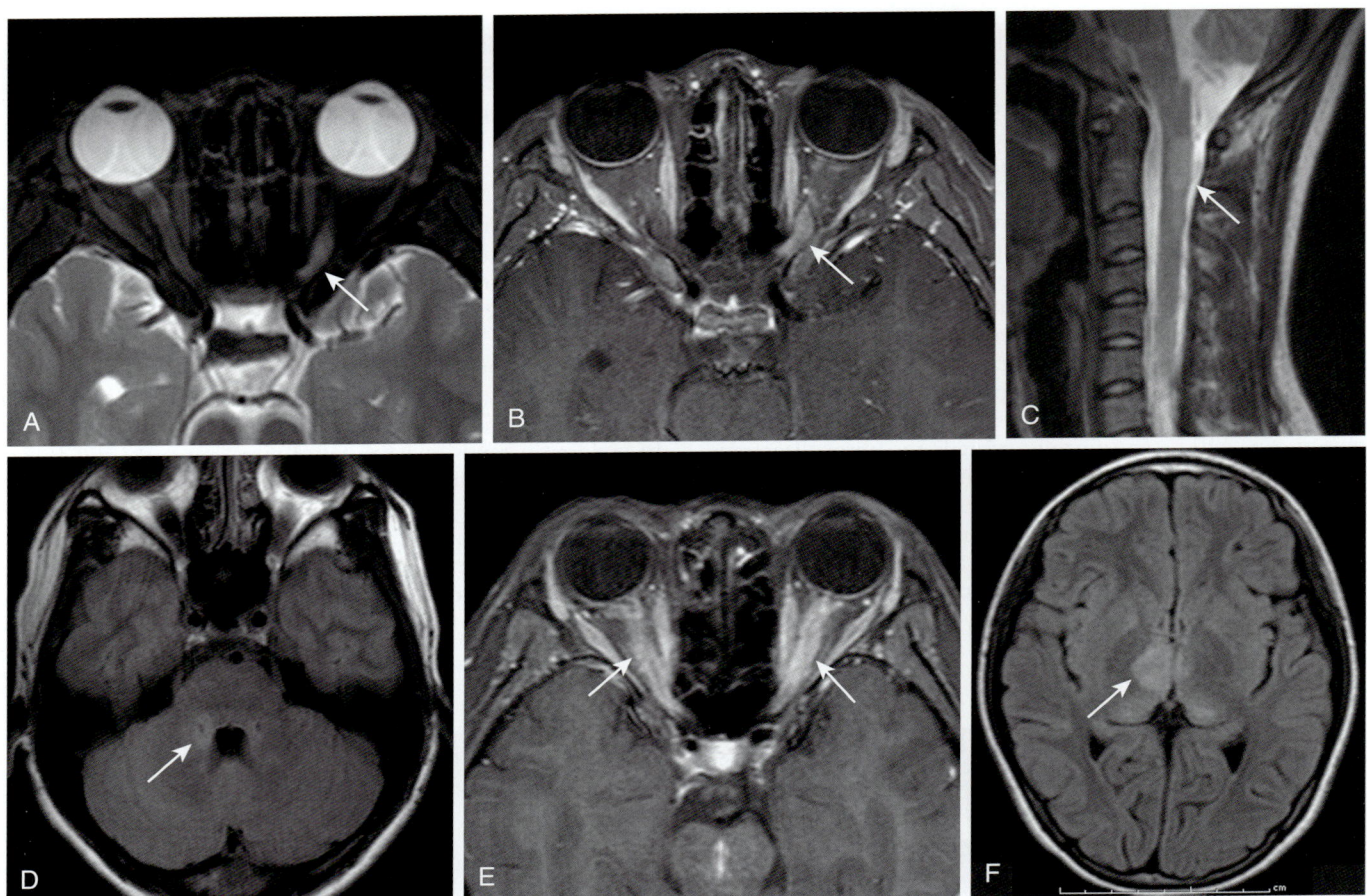

Figure 6-5   Optic neuritis. T2- (**A**) and T1-weighted fat-saturated postcontrast (**B**) magnetic resonance (MR) images of the orbits demonstrating abnormal T2 hyperintensity and enhancement of the left optic nerve (*arrows*). **C,** A sagittal T2-weighted MR image of the cervical spine demonstrates a characteristic central long segment cord lesion in a patient with neuromyelitis optica (NMO) (*arrow*). **D,** An axial T2-weighted fluid attenuated inversion recovery (FLAIR) MR image in the same patient with NMO demonstrating subtle hyperintensity adjacent to the fourth ventricle in regions of high aquaporin 4 concentration (*arrow*). **E,** A T1-weighted fat-saturated postcontrast image of the orbits demonstrating bilateral optic nerve enhancement (*arrows*) in a patient with acute disseminated encephalomyelitis (ADEM). **F,** A T2-weighted FLAIR image of the brain in the same patient with ADEM showing lesions in the thalami (*arrow*).

nerve is seen, an optic pathway glioma should be considered. Intraorbital involvement is most common. Intracanalicular and long segment involvement and persistent signal change over time correlate to worse visual outcomes. Retinal nerve fiber layer thinning on optical coherence tomography also correlates to vision loss.[61,62] Diffusion tensor imaging of optic nerves is difficult perform clinically, yet demonstrates decreased axial diffusivity acutely and increasing radial diffusivity and apparent diffusion coefficient values during recovery, correlating to changes in visual acuity and retinal nerve fiber layer thinning.[63-65] Decreased fractional anisotropy values also can be seen in the optic tracts and radiations, possibly as a result of Wallerian and transsynaptic degeneration.[66-68] Magnetization transfer ratios (MTRs), which are thought to decrease with demyelination, are more sensitive than T2 spin echo imaging. They progressively decrease in the optic nerve, with a nadir at 240 days, and then mildly increase (possibly from remyelination), also correlating to changes in visual acuity.[69,70]

Treatment   ON in children is usually treated with IV methylprednisolone followed by an oral prednisolone taper.[71] Although no large randomized controlled trials have been performed in children, in adults this therapy accelerates visual recovery and decreases the risk of MS for 2 years.[72]

Optic Neuritis and Multiple Sclerosis

Most ON research has been conducted with adult subjects, and it has been found that MS develops in 50% of adults with ON within 15 years.[72] The greatest predictor is an abnormal MRI scan of the brain, and the risk of MS increases with the number of lesions: MS develops in 25% of adults with a normal MRI at baseline, whereas it develops in 75% of adults with one or more lesions in the brain at baseline.[73] In children, the largest series with the longest follow-up demonstrated a 19% conversion to MS (13% in 10 years).[57] As with adults, almost all children in whom MS developed had an abnormal MRI scan at baseline, and MS developed in almost no children who had a normal MRI scan.[54,55] Furthermore, optic disk swelling is associated with a decreased risk of MS in adults and is a common feature of pediatric ON, likely reflecting the often parainfectious nature of ON in children.[54-58]

Optic Neuritis and Neuromyelitis Optica (Devic Disease)

Etiologies, Pathophysiology, and Clinical Presentation Neuromyelitis optica (NMO) is an inflammatory demyelinating disease of the optic nerves and spinal cord related to NMO–immunoglobulin G (IgG), a serum autoantibody targeting aquaporin 4, a water channel on astrocytes at the blood–brain barrier.[74,75] The distinction of NMO from MS is important because NMO has a worse prognosis and requires different treatment. Diagnostic criteria for children are similar to those for adults: clinical diagnosis of ON and transverse myelitis with either a cord lesion on MRI or NMO-IgG seropositivity.[76,77] The prognosis is poor: >50% of patients have vision loss or lose the ability to ambulate within 5 years. Death as a result of respiratory failure also is seen.[78] NMO-IgG seropositivity may indicate a worse prognosis with a relapsing course.[79-81] Parainfectious NMO is common in children and typically is NMO-IgG negative and monophasic.[82,83] Accordingly, pediatric NMO has a better prognosis and a longer time before the onset of disability.[84,85]

Imaging Characteristic cord lesions are centrally located and extend three or more segments in length (Fig. 6-5, C). Up to 60% of patients also demonstrate brain lesions, which are part of the new diagnostic criteria.[86] Findings include nonspecific signal changes, MS-like lesions (10%), and T2-weighted hyperintensity in areas of high aquaporin 4 concentration adjacent to the third and fourth ventricles (Fig. 6-5, D). Signal changes in the distribution of aquaporin 4 may be specific for NMO and are seen more frequently in children.[86,87]

Treatment Treatment of persons with NMO consists of immunosuppression (IV methylprednisolone ± plasmapheresis acutely, with oral prednisone and azathioprine for maintenance), compared with immunomodulation for persons with MS.[74,84] NMO-IgG positivity in persons with isolated ON or transverse myelitis may represent a limited form of NMO, requiring more aggressive treatment.[81] Similarly, NMO-IgG negativity in children may predict a parainfectious etiology with a monophasic course not requiring immunosuppressive therapy.[79,80]

Optic Neuritis and Acute Disseminated Encephalomyelitis

Acute disseminated encephalomyelitis (ADEM) is an autoimmune inflammatory and typically monophasic demyelinating disease of the central nervous system that occurs days to weeks after a viral illness or vaccination. Visual loss is seen in up to one fourth of patients with ADEM, and ON in persons with ADEM tends to be bilateral with swollen optic disks (Fig. 6-5).[88-90] Although no clear guidelines exist, treatment usually consists of IV steroids with favorable outcomes.[91] The high frequency of parainfectious ON in children (in one third to two thirds of cases) likely contributes to the different presentation and more favorable prognosis of ON in children compared with adults.

Papilledema

Papilledema is another cause of optic disk swelling in children. It is the result of elevated intracranial pressure as a result of intracranial masses/inflammation, hydrocephalus, venous sinus thrombosis, or pseudotumor cerebri. Visual loss may result.[92] MRI demonstrates optic disc elevation, dilated perioptic subarachnoid spaces, and optic nerve tortuosity.[93,94] Enhancement and restricted diffusion of the optic disk have been described, perhaps as a result of venous congestion and ischemia (e-Fig. 6-6).[95,96]

Sickle Cell Disease

Etiologies, Pathophysiology, and Clinical Presentation Sickle cell disease (SCD) is an inherited autosomal-recessive disease of the sickle beta globin gene that results in chronic hemolytic anemia and recurrent vaso-occlusive crises and infection. A vaso-occlusive crisis can affect any bone with active bone marrow. Orbital wall involvement is seen almost exclusively in children because of a greater volume of marrow space in this location during childhood. Patients present with acute periorbital pain, swelling, proptosis, and restricted extraocular movements. Subperiosteal hemorrhage can be a complication in 36% of cases. Resultant orbital compression syndrome can cause optic nerve compression and vision loss.[97-100]

Imaging MRI demonstrates bone marrow edema (T2-weighted hyperintensity) and hemorrhage with or without subperiosteal hemorrhage (Fig. 6-7, A). It is important to differentiate bone marrow infarction from osteomyelitis given that both can occur in persons with SCD. On MRI, infarction demonstrates thin peripheral contrast enhancement, whereas infection demonstrates thick peripheral, geographic, or irregular contrast enhancement with or without cortical defects.[101] Areas of high signal intensity on T1-weighted fat-saturated noncontrast images due to sequestration of red blood cells also has been found to be helpful in detecting areas of infarction and distinguishing them from infection (Fig. 6-7, B).[102]

Treatment Treatment consists of conservative management for SCD crises. In cases of optic nerve compression and vision change, IV steroids and/or surgical drainage of hematomas may be required.

Leber Hereditary Optic Neuropathy

Etiologies, Pathophysiology, and Clinical Presentation Leber hereditary optic neuropathy (LHON) is the most common genetic mitochondrial disease, affecting 1 in 25,000 persons.[103] Deficient adenosine triphosphate production leads to degeneration of retinal ganglion cells. Three mitochondrial deoxyribonucleic acid mutations (G3460A, G11778A, and T14484C) account for >90% of cases with incomplete penetrance: 50% in males and 10% in females. Accordingly, LHON is most common in young males, with a median age of 24 years. Painless bilateral clouding of vision, centrocecal scotoma, and impairment of color vision progresses to vision

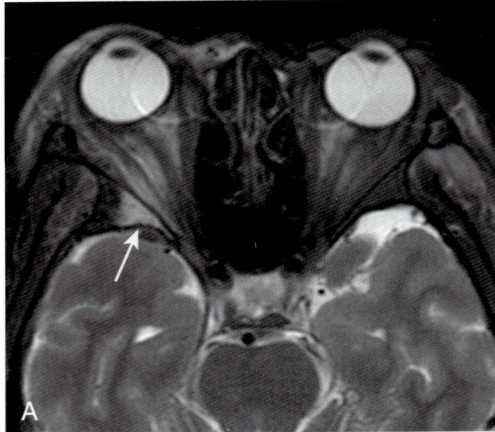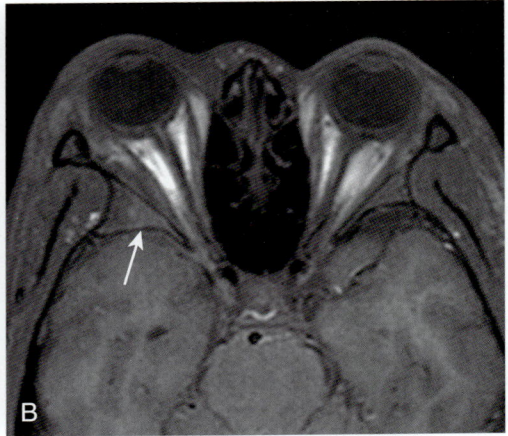

Figure 6-7 **Sickle cell disease. A,** A T2-weighted fat-saturated magnetic resonance (MR) image of the orbits demonstrating bone marrow infarction in a patient with sickle cell disease, with T2 hyperintensity of the bone marrow of the lateral wall of the right orbit and adjacent inflammatory changes of the extraconal fat (*arrow*). **B,** A T1-weighted fat-saturated noncontrast MR image of the orbit in the same patient demonstrating subtle T1 hyperintensity of the bone marrow from sequestration of red blood cells (*arrow*).

loss and optic nerve atrophy in 6 months. Most patients show no functional improvement, remaining legally blind.

Imaging Most patients demonstrate no imaging findings, yet acutely, T2 hyperintensity, enlargement, and enhancement of the optic nerves, chiasm, and tracts can be seen. Chronically, T2 hyperintensity, volume loss, and decreased MTR values of these structures have been described.[104-109] A small portion of patients, particularly females, demonstrate MS-like lesions in the brain preceding or more commonly following optic nerve involvement after an average of 4.3 years.[110,111] These MS-like lesions may progress with a relapsing course; difficulties with ambulation develop in 75% of patients. Even brain that appears normal in patients with LHON demonstrates abnormal MTR and mean diffusivity values, suggesting more extensive subclinical neurologic disease.[105]

Treatment No treatment is available that significantly improves visual outcome, but recent trials have focused on Idebenone.[112,113] Patients with LHON and MS-like lesions may need immunosuppressive therapy.

Autosomal-Dominant Optic Atrophy

Autosomal-dominant optic atrophy (ADOA) is the most common hereditary optic neuropathy related to mutations in the optic atrophy 1 (*OPA1*) gene (encoding a mitochondrial guanosine triphosphatase).[114] Selective retinal ganglion cell loss results in isolated, progressive, and permanent vision loss, typically in the first two decades of life. Extraocular neurologic involvement is seen in up to one sixth of patients, with sensorineural hearing loss being the most common manifestation, likely as a result of *OPA1* expression in the inner ear.[115] Few studies describe the imaging appearance of ADOA, although a decrease in the size of the optic nerves throughout their length can be seen.[116]

Krabbe Disease (Globoid Cell Leukodystrophy)

Krabbe disease is an autosomal-recessive neurodegenerative disorder with a deficiency in galactosylceramide β-galactosidase, a lysosomal enzyme responsible for myelin breakdown and turnover. This deficiency leads to accumulation of neurotoxic psychosine and galactosylceramide, which form globoid cells. Early, late, and adult-onset forms are described. Presentation is most common at 3 to 6 months of age, with death by 2 to 3 years of age. Optic nerve enlargement is an uncommon manifestation, perhaps as a result of globoid cell accumulation in optic nerves, as described at autopsy (e-Fig. 6-8).[117-120] The major differential considerations in children with enlarged optic nerves and signal changes in both the white matter and deep grey nuclei are Krabbe disease and neurofibromatosis type 1 with optic pathway gliomas.

Key Points

Infection involving the postseptal orbit carries the risks of abscess formation, vision loss, venous thrombosis, intracranial extension, and death, requiring admission for monitoring and IV antibiotics.

Many disease processes in the orbit can look similar on imaging, with presentation as an ill-defined inflammatory mass: infection, orbital pseudotumor, Wegener granulomatosis, sarcoidosis, and lymphoma.

Causes of ON in children include an idiopathic cause, MS, NMO, and ADEM.

ON behaves differently in children, which likely is related to its frequent parainfectious nature: it is painless, bilateral, presents with disk edema and profound vision loss, generally results in a good recovery, and infrequently progresses to MS.

Although uncommon, metabolic disease also should be considered in a child with vision loss and changes to the optic nerves upon imaging.

Suggested Readings

Gorospe L, Royo A, Berrocal T, et al. Imaging of orbital disorders in pediatric patients. *Eur Radiol.* 2003;13:2012-2026.

Hopper KD, Sherman JL, Boal DK, et al. CT and MR imaging of the pediatric orbit. *Radiographics.* 1992;12:485-503.

Narla LD, Newman B, Spottswood SS, et al. Inflammatory pseudotumor. *Radiographics.* 2003;23:719-729.

Saito N, Nadgir RN, Flower EN, et al. Clinical and radiologic manifestations of sickle cell disease in the head and neck. *Radiographics.* 2010;30:1021-1035.

Smirniotopoulos JG, Bargallo N, Mafee MF. Differential diagnosis of leukokoria: radiologic-pathologic correlation. *Radiographics.* 1994;14:1059-1079.

References

Full references for this chapter can be found on www.expertconsult.com.

Chapter 7

Orbital Neoplasia

TAMARA FEYGIN and AVRUM N. POLLOCK

A wide variety of primary and secondary neoplasms may affect the orbit. Most orbital masses are benign and slow growing; however, approximately 20% are malignant. As is often the case in pediatrics, obtaining a precise history and conducting a physical examination may be challenging. Presenting symptoms of different entities may overlap considerably; for example, leukocoria, a worrisome sign of retinoblastoma, also can be a manifestation of infectious/inflammatory or developmental conditions masquerading as retinoblastoma. Imaging findings also may overlap; for example, some forms of orbital rhabdomyosarcoma (RMS) initially may present as inflammatory cellulitis or may closely resemble a hemangioma based on imaging features. Some non-neoplastic orbital masses may present quite dramatically with visual loss and destructive changes of the orbit (e.g., Wegener granulomatosis and Langerhans cell histiocytosis [LCH]) and must be differentiated from a malignancy. Pertinent clinical information, such as patient age and duration of symptoms, may be of added value when trying to narrow the diagnostic possibilities. The location of the lesion within the orbit may be a clue to its underlying nature because different lesions have the propensity to originate from specific compartments of the orbit. Knowledge of the rate of growth of the mass also may help narrow the differential diagnosis. Rapid progression is suggestive of more aggressive lesions such as RMS, acute leukemic infiltration, or LCH (one of the great mimickers of malignant bone diseases in children). A more indolent course, with little to no progression in visible growth, can be observed in lesions such as dermoid cysts, optic nerve gliomas, or meningiomas.

A precise and timely diagnosis of an orbital mass may be crucial for successful treatment of many disorders and may lead to improved quality of life, preserved vision, or prevention of blindness. Imaging plays an important role in the accurate diagnosis of orbital masses, and at times more than one imaging modality may be required. The primary imaging modalities used to evaluate orbital masses are ultrasonography, computed tomography (CT), and magnetic resonance imaging (MRI). Ultrasound eye examination is performed with use of a linear, or three-dimensional high-frequency transducer with a small footprint, which is placed over the closed eyelids. It is an effective imaging tool for the evaluation of the globe, papilledema, retinal detachment, and the proximal optic nerve. Color Doppler allows evaluation of the vascularity of intraocular lesions. Orbital ultrasound may be used as a primary imaging tool in the evaluation of young children with leukocoria and for confirmation of papilledema and retinal detachment. However, it is suboptimal for the assessment of extraocular lesions.

CT is excellent at depicting ocular calcifications and evaluating potential orbital bony involvement. It is an easily accessible test and may be used in the primary evaluation of acute proptosis. Modern CT equipment allows for the acquisition of high-resolution images in the axial plane with additional computed reconstruction images in the coronal and/or sagittal planes, thus avoiding the need for direct acquisition of images in orthogonal planes and thereby preventing additional radiation exposure. The speed of current CT scanners may allow the imaging team to avoid patient sedation in many cases.

Orbital masses are optimally imaged with MRI. The use of high-resolution, 2- to 3-mm thick T1-weighted and T2-weighted sequences, as well as thin-slice postgadolinium multiplanar sequences, are mandatory for precision imaging of orbital structures. Fat suppression often is essential in orbital imaging to allow for tissue differentiation and distinction from intraorbital fat, as well as in the assessment of the marrow within the bony orbit and of pathologically enhancing tissues. Diffusion-weighted imaging (DWI) plays an important role in further characterizing the tissues within and around tumors. Apparent diffusion coefficient mapping may help in the differentiation of benign and malignant lesions and occasionally may allow for assessment of treatment response. Half-Fourier acquisition single-shot turbo or fast spin-echo imaging is helpful for depiction of cystic components of orbital mass and for better visualization of sinus tracts.

Use of a high-resolution matrix, a small field of view, and routine use of fat-saturation techniques, as well as the administration of intravenous (IV) contrast (gadolinium), are all necessary components in successfully imaging orbital pathology. When analyzing images, particular attention should be given to the presence of bone erosion, the avidity of contrast uptake, and lesion vascularity, as well as the presence of intracranial extension. Tumor extension through the orbital fissures is better delineated on MRI, whereas erosive bony changes are better depicted on CT. CT and MR are complimentary imaging techniques in the evaluation of orbital tumors, and in some cases, both may be indicated for proper and complete evaluation of complex orbital masses, both before treatment and when assessing for potential residual or recurrent disease. Most protocols for imaging of orbital tumors include brain imaging for the evaluation of potential intracranial extension.

Certain orbital tumors may be a manifestation of more complex or systemic conditions or syndromes and may thus require further evaluation of extraorbital regions for involvement of other organ systems. Examples of known associations of orbital lesions potentially involving other organ systems are

(1) hemangiomata associated with PHACES syndrome (**p**osterior fossa abnormalities, **h**emangiomas of the cervical facial region, **a**rterial anomalies, **c**ardiac defects, **e**ye anomalies, and **s**ternal defects) and (2) kaposiform hemangioendotheliomas and their association with Kasabach-Merritt syndrome, a severe, life-threatening consumptive coagulopathy.

Although analysis of imaging findings along with clinical signs and symptoms may lead to a narrowed differential diagnosis, the definitive diagnosis almost always is based on histopathologic findings.

The following discussion of imaging of orbital pathology is divided into four categories: ocular lesions, optic nerve sheath lesions, primary orbital lesions, and lesions that secondarily involve the orbit.

Ocular Lesions

RETINOBLASTOMA

Retinoblastoma, which is the most common intraocular pediatric tumor, typically affects children younger than 4 years. Even though retinoblastoma is considered a congenital type of malignant tumor, it is rarely recognized neonatally. Two forms of retinoblastoma—hereditary and sporadic—are described. These forms differ in their clinical presentation and prognosis.

Hereditary retinoblastoma is usually bilateral and multifocal and clinically presents at an earlier age (mean, 6 months). It is associated with a germline mutation in the tumor suppression *RB1* gene, located on chromosome 13q14. In a small percentage of patients with heritable retinoblastoma (3% to 7%), intracranial neuroectodermal pineal or suprasellar tumors, termed trilateral retinoblastoma, will develop. Trilateral tumors usually present months after the initial discovery of the ocular lesions and have an associated dismal prognosis. Patients with hereditary *RB1* mutations have increased risk (progressive throughout their lifetime) of the development of other malignancies; such malignancies especially develop in patients who have undergone radiation therapy. Secondary tumors that develop most often include osteogenic and other soft tissue sarcomas, leukemia, and malignant melanoma. Secondary nonocular tumors are the leading cause of death in these patients, rather than the primary retinoblastoma itself.

Sporadic retinoblastoma is usually solitary and unilateral and is associated with spontaneous somatic mutations of the *RB1* gene. The average age at presentation varies from 13 to 18 months. Patients with sporadic noninvasive intraocular tumors have an excellent prognosis, with a survival rate approaching 90%.

Approximately two thirds of all retinoblastoma cases are unilateral, and one third are bilateral. Several classification systems have been developed for intraocular retinoblastoma, all of which are based on expected results of therapy and predicted salvage of the globe. The rapid evolution of newer retinoblastoma treatment has resulted in the replacement of the previously widely accepted Reese-Ellsworth classification, which is based on intraocular tumor staging and is used in tumor management after external beam radiation. A new International Classification of Retinoblastoma is based mainly on the natural history of retinoblastoma (early disease [group A] to late disease [group E]) and upon the extent of tumor seeding within the vitreous and subretinal space (Box 7-1).

Box 7-1 International Classification of Retinoblastoma

The International Classification of Retinoblastoma is a new classification system for retinoblastoma that is based on tumor size, location, and associated seeding. This new classification system is designed to simplify grouping and assist in predicting treatment outcomes.

Group A = Retinoblastoma ≤3 mm

Group B = Retinoblastoma >3 mm, macular location, or minor subretinal fluid

Group C = Retinoblastoma with localized seeds

Group D = Retinoblastoma with diffuse seeds

Group E = Massive retinoblastoma necessitating enucleation

This classification is more applicable for patients treated with chemotherapy.

For purposes of disease prognostication, it is important to assess tumor growth pattern, which is described according to the retinal spread of tumor. Endophytic tumors grow anteriorly into the vitreous, whereas exophytic tumors grow into subretinal space and tend to have earlier choroidal involvement and increased risk of metastatic spread. Optic nerve involvement is a marker for aggressive and advanced tumors and is associated with a high risk of metastatic disease and consequent increased mortality rates. The most uncommon pattern of spread is that of diffuse infiltrative tumor growth within the retina, which is not characterized by the presence of a nodular mass or by intralesional calcifications. This type of retinoblastoma presents at a later age, with the clinical symptoms sometimes mimicking an inflammatory process.

Leukocoria (or white pupillary reflex) is the most common presenting sign of retinoblastoma. For tumors located in the posterior globe, leukocoria may indicate advanced disease because a lesion in the posterior retina must be sufficiently large to produce leukocoria. Strabismus is the second major presenting sign of retinoblastoma. In contrast to leukocoria, tumors presenting with strabismus as their initial sign are associated with a higher survival rate and a higher chance of salvage of the globe. Patients with exophytic tumor growth may present with retinal detachment surrounding the tumor, indicating tumor extension into the subretinal space.

Leukocoria in a young child that is confirmed by an ophthalmoscopic examination requires further evaluation. Imaging may reliably distinguish retinoblastoma from a host of other conditions that also may present with leukocoria (e.g., persistent hyperplastic primary vitreous, Toxascaris infection, Coats disease, and medulloepithelioma). In many retinoblastoma centers, eye ultrasonography has replaced orbital CT for initial disease assessment. Three-dimensional high-frequency ultrasound is sufficient for assessment of tumor and calcifications but is less suitable for the evaluation of extraocular spread. Retinoblastoma is readily visible on ultrasound as an echogenic irregular retinal mass with focal acoustic shadows. CT is an excellent tool for depicting ocular calcifications (Fig. 7-1, *A*), but its use in retinoblastoma evaluation has markedly decreased because of the associated radiation risks. MRI has become a relatively quick and convenient modality for the evaluation of retinoblastoma. A variety of tailored MR sequences are beneficial in illustrating the different features of these masses. Specifically, intraocular hemorrhages and calcifications are depicted best on gradient

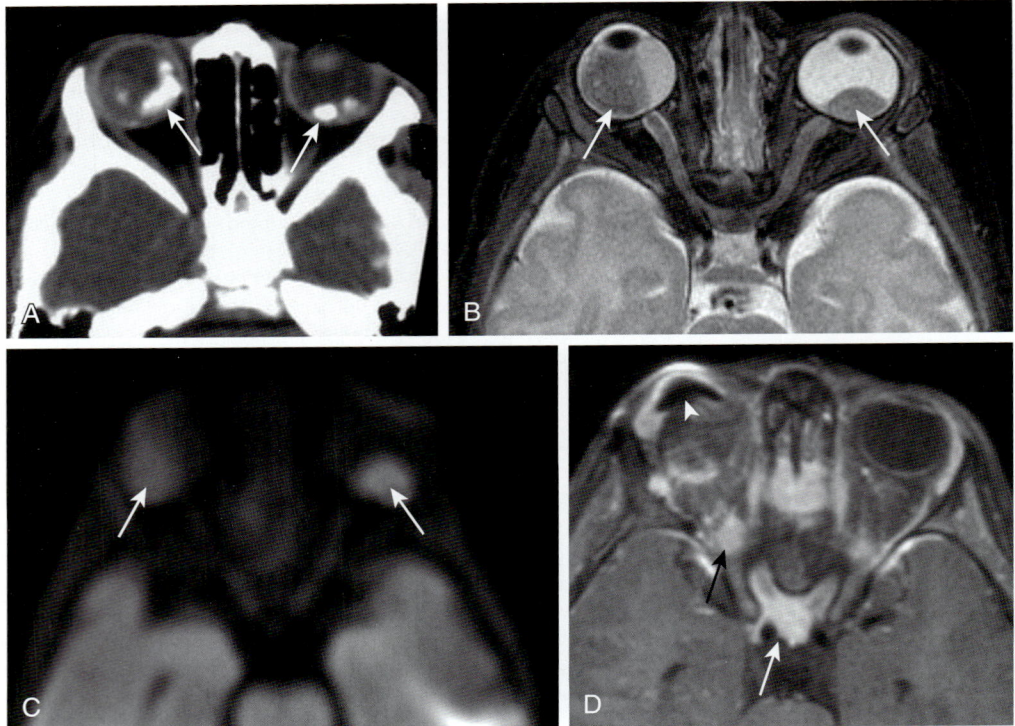

Figure 7-1   Retinoblastoma of the orbits in three different patients. **A,** An orbital computed tomography scan demonstrates bilateral, markedly calcified orbital masses (*arrows*). Orbital magnetic resonance images (MRI), including an axial fat-saturated T2-weighted image (**B**) and a diffusion-weighted image (**C**), demonstrate bilateral, lobulated, T2-hypointense, retinal-based masses that exhibit diffusion restriction (*arrows*). **D,** In another patient with known recurrent retinoblastoma who has had right enucleation and prosthesis insertion (*arrowhead*), postcontrast T1-weighted fat-saturated MRI demonstrates fusiform enlargement and enhancement of the stump of the optic nerve sheath throughout its intraorbital (*black arrow*) and intracanalicular components, with associated posterior extension to the optic chiasm (*white arrow*).

sequences, whereas the malignant, markedly cellular nature of these tumors (composed of immature retinoblasts) is confirmed on T2-weighted and DWI sequences (Fig. 7-1, *B* and *C*). Contrast-enhanced sequences provide important information that may affect prognosis and treatment options with respect to tumor spread into the optic nerve (Fig. 7-1, *D*), anterior chamber, or other adjacent orbital structures. In addition, MRI serves as a surveillance examination of the brain when monitoring for possible leptomeningeal spread of tumor or for the presence of retinoblastoma in more remote locations.

Standard treatment for retinoblastoma has evolved in the past several decades from prior methods of surgical enucleation or external radiation. Most retinoblastoma referral centers are now using alternative therapies that are aimed at eye salvage and avoiding the risks inherent with radiation. These methods include systemic chemotherapy (chemoreduction) along with focal treatments (eye-sparing radiotherapy [local plaque radiation], laser photocoagulation, and cryotherapy) as the primary treatment modality, especially when tumors are small. Orbital imaging is therefore an essential step in deciding the appropriate treatment.

MEDULLOEPITHELIOMA

A medulloepithelioma is another pediatric malignant intraocular tumor that may present with leukocoria. This tumor is a rare embryonal type of neoplasm arising from the nonpigmented epithelial lining of the ciliary body. Patients usually are diagnosed in the first decade of life (at a mean age of 6 years); only rarely is medulloepithelioma seen in adults. Many imaging features of medulloepithelioma may closely resemble those of a retinoblastoma, such as presentation with a nodular enhancing intraocular mass, which occasionally will have calcifications (Fig. 7-2). A medulloepithelioma differs from a retinoblastoma mainly by its anterior

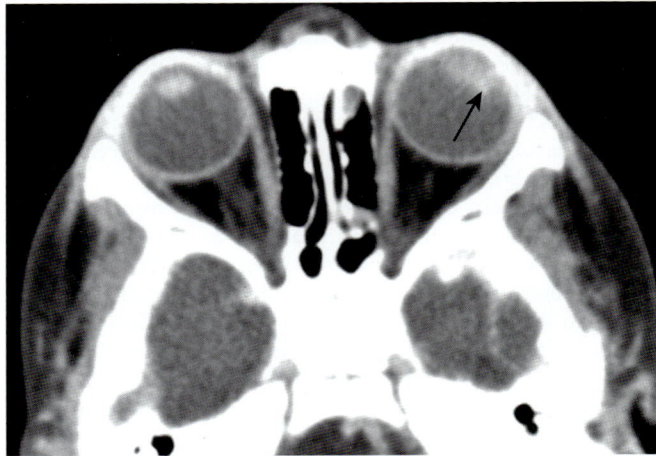

Figure 7-2   Medulloepithelioma. Contrast-enhanced computed tomography of the orbit in a patient with a known medulloepithelioma shows an amorphous lesion in the anterior chamber of the left eye with associated punctate calcification in the region of the ciliary body (*arrow*).

location, but it may appear identical to a retinoblastoma when it is located in the vicinity of the optic nerve. Medulloepitheliomas have been divided into two types, teratoid and nonteratoid (diktyoma), based on their histologies. More complex teratoid medulloepitheliomas are composed of heteroplastic elements, including cartilage, which may have associated calcifications, whereas the nonteratoid diktyoma presents as a well-defined, noncalcified mass with associated diffuse contrast enhancement.

HEREDITARY ORBITAL HAMARTOMATOSIS

Many neurocutaneous disorders (phakomatoses) may have typical ocular masses that may or may not be visible with modern imaging techniques. These lesions represent hereditary hamartomas, which are composed of tissues with limited capacity for proliferation. Examples of these entities may be seen in the settings of tuberous sclerosis, neurofibromatosis (NF), and von Hippel-Lindau disease.

Ocular manifestations of tuberous sclerosis include astrocytic hamartomas of the retina and optic disk. These lesions have a typical appearance on ophthalmologic examination; however, they may calcify as the patient ages and may in fact resemble drusen when located on the optic disk. On thin-section high-resolution T2-weighted imaging, hamartomas of tuberous sclerosis are visible as small hypointense nodules within the posterior globe (e-Fig. 7-3).

Ocular stigmata of NF may present as neuronal hamartomas of the iris, called Lisch nodules, which only occur with NF type 1. Lisch nodules can only rarely be visualized with imaging.

Persons with Sturge-Weber syndrome and von Hippel-Lindau disease may have ocular vascular lesions. Choroidal vascular lesions in persons with Sturge-Weber syndrome may be diffuse or localized and can simulate melanoma on ophthalmoscopic examination, but they may be differentiated from one another on MRI examination. Choroidal vascular lesions demonstrate a typical hyperintense signal on T1-weighted and T2-weighted sequences, which is opposite to the signal characteristics expected with melanoma (a bright T1-weighted signal and a hypointense T2-weighted signal). Ocular manifestations of von Hippel-Lindau disease consist of retinal angiomatosis, which may cause severe complications, including retinal detachment and ocular destruction, and usually present later in childhood or in early adulthood (in the second and third decades of life).

DRUSEN

Disc drusen are nonhamartomatous subretinal lesions without astrocytic hyperplasia that are associated with the presence of intrapapillary, partially calcified hyaline bodies that form concretions of unknown nature. Drusen likely are the most common etiology for congenital bilateral elevation of the optic nerve discs. Drusen may be detected on funduscopic evaluation or may be seen as an incidental finding on imaging. In both scenarios, it is important to establish the benign nature of disk elevation so as not to confuse drusen (which cause pseudopapilledema) with true papilledema. Equivocal results of ophthalmoscopic examination may lead to orbital imaging, which will either confirm the presence of disc drusen or detect the source of the increased intracranial

pressure. Drusen may be diagnosed with use of ultrasound, appearing as foci of increased echogenicity, or drusen can be seen on noncontrast CT most often as bilateral punctuate calcifications within the optic nerve heads (e-Fig. 7-4). MRI demonstrates isolated mild protrusion of the optic discs into the vitreous without perioptic cerebrospinal fluid space enlargement or other imaging features of papilledema. Clinically, drusen are usually asymptomatic and only rarely may be associated with slowly progressive visual loss.

Optic Nerve-Sheath Complex Tumors

Optic nerve-sheath complex lesions include neoplasms of the optic nerves (gliomata), optic nerve sheaths (meningiomas), or rare cases of intraconal peripheral primitive neuroectodermal tumors (PNETs).

OPTIC NERVE GLIOMA

Optic nerve glioma (ONG) is the most common primary neoplasm of the optic nerve in children. ONG may be seen in the setting of NF type 1 (Fig. 7-5, *A*) or may present as an isolated tumor (nonsyndromic) (Fig. 7-5, *B*). ONGs, which are associated with NF, most often are bilateral lesions that may involve the nerve and surrounding subarachnoid space and are remarkable for their low-grade nature and favorable prognosis. Nonsyndromic ONGs are usually unilateral and histologically are either pilocytic or fibrillary astrocytomas. The mortality rate for these tumors is approximately 5% when the tumor involves only the optic nerve, but hypothalamic involvement portends a more ominous prognosis; despite their benign histology, some series report mortality rates approaching 50%.

ORBITAL MENINGIOMA

Orbital meningioma is not a common pediatric tumor but has been reported in patients in the first decade of life. Meningiomas of the orbits may be perioptic (e-Fig. 7-6, *A-C*), arising from the optic nerve sheath, or may extend through the optic canal from an intracranial origin, that is, arising from the area of anterior clinoid process of the sphenoid bone or from the tuberculum sella, with extension anteriorly into the orbit (e-Fig. 7-6, *D*).

Perineural meningioma is the most common form seen in children, possibly because of early presentation with visual symptoms. Pediatric meningiomas are much more aggressive than the adult form. These tumors may occur as isolated neoplasms or in the setting of NF type 2.

In general, CT is useful in the detection of the orbital portion of some meningiomas but not in differentiating whether the tumor originates from the optic nerve itself or from the optic nerve sheath. These tumors are usually hyperattenuating on CT, often with calcifications (but not in the early stages), seen as the so-called "rail road track sign," which implies that the surrounding tumor of the nerve sheath is enhancing, not the optic nerve itself. Meningiomas ideally should be imaged with MRI. They most often appear hypointense on T1-weighted and T2-weighted sequences and

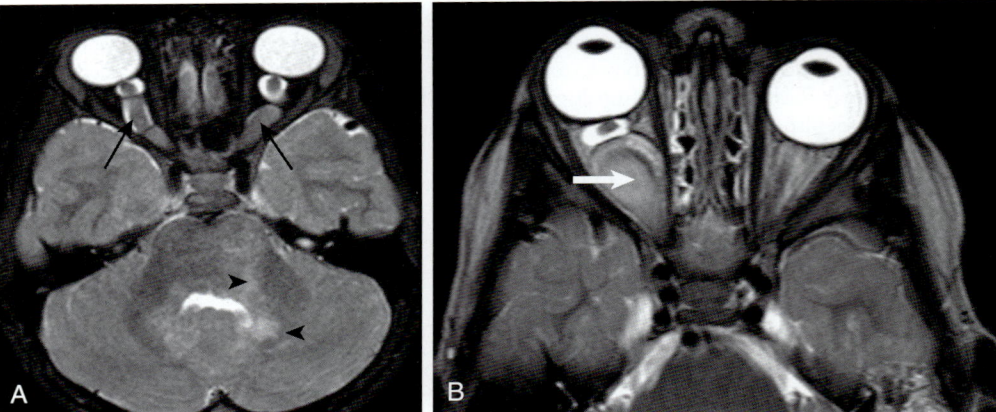

Figure 7-5   Optic glioma. **A,** An optic glioma in a patient with neurofibromatosis (NF) type 1. An axial fat-saturated T2-weighted image of the orbits shows bilaterally symmetrically enlarged intracanalicular portions of the optic nerves associated with marked tortuosity (*arrows*), which commonly is seen in patients with NF type 1. An additional clue to the diagnosis is the areas of signal abnormality within the cerebellar white matter, in keeping with spongiform changes of NF type 1 (*arrowheads*). **B,** An isolated right optic nerve glioma in a different patient. Magnetic resonance imaging shows an optic nerve glioma with similar expansion and tortuosity of the optic nerve (*arrow*) but with unilateral involvement of the right optic nerve and without additional imaging findings of NF type 1.

exhibit avid gadolinium enhancement and restricted diffusion on DWI because of their high cellularity (e-Fig. 7-6, *A-C*).

Primary optic nerve tumors are not the only cause of optic nerve enlargement. Other causes include non–neoplastic conditions such as inflammatory pseudotumor, optic neuritis, and sarcoid granulomata. Enlargement of the optic nerve–sheath complexes may be caused by true papilledema (related to increased intracranial pressure), perineural hematoma, or granulomatous disease, or it may represent a normal variant.

PRIMITIVE NEUROECTODERMAL TUMOR

A PNET is a small, round, blue cell malignant tumor of neuroectodermal origin. PNETs that present outside of the central nervous system are referred to as peripheral PNET. It appears that PNET is the least aggressive subtype of tumor among other similar small cell tumors, with a favorable prognosis seen after complete tumor resection. This tumor, similar to Ewing sarcoma, expresses the *MIC-2* gene (CD99) on cell membranes, which allows for their differentiation from other tumors. This rare tumor of the orbit presents as an enhancing, heterogeneous, T2-hypointense, intraconal lesion with

associated restricted diffusion on DWI (Fig. 7-7, *A-C*). DWI characteristics are important imaging features that favor a highly cellular lesion, which includes PNET within the limited differential diagnosis. Treatment usually includes globe enucleation, high-dose chemotherapy, and stem cell transplantation.

Orbital Lesions

VASCULAR LESIONS

Vascular orbital mass lesions constitute a heterogeneous group of both true neoplasms and non–neoplastic vascular malformations. Orbital vascular masses occur on a spectrum, ranging from benign lesions such as the common infantile hemangioma (true neoplasm), congenital lesions such as venolymphatic malformations, orbital varices, and arterial-venous malformations, to the rarer locally aggressive lesion known as kaposiform hemangioendothelioma. Mulliken and Glowacki have classified this spectrum of vascular masses based on differing therapeutic approaches for different lesions. Much

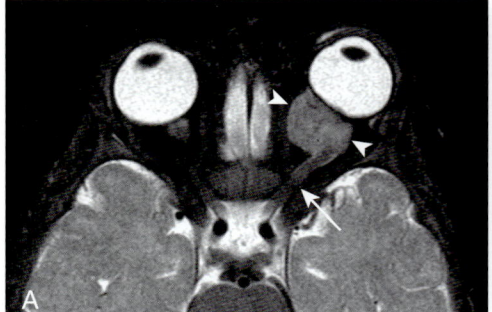
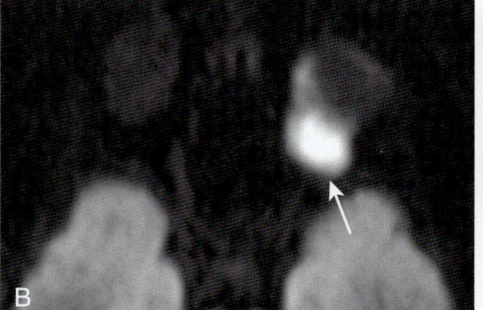
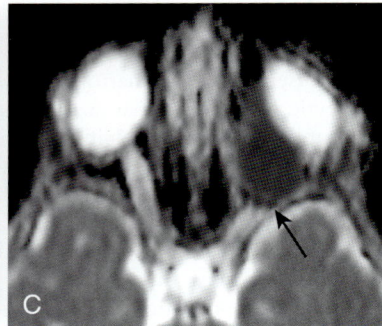

Figure 7-7   Primitive neuroectodermal tumor. An axial fat-saturated T2-weighted image (**A**), an axial diffusion-weighted image (**B**), and an axial apparent diffusion coefficient image (**C**) of a patient with a left orbital primitive neuroectodermal tumor (PNET). Note the left-sided posteriorly located intraconal T2-hypointense lesion with associated marked restricted diffusion (*arrows*). The restricted diffusion suggests a densely cellular tumor, a finding almost invariably seen with PNETs.

controversy still exists regarding the nomenclature and classification of these entities. The most common accepted view is that they belong to a spectrum of vascular lesions. Vascular malformations are congenital lesions but usually are clinically occult at birth and tend to present later in life, at times after an upper respiratory tract infection or as a result of spontaneous hemorrhage. In contradistinction, infantile hemangiomas become clinically apparent shortly after birth, and some of the rarer orbital vascular tumors may even be diagnosed prenatally. Imaging protocols also should include evaluation of the brain because of the association of orbital vascular lesions with intracranial vascular anomalies.

Orbital Hemangioma

Orbital hemangiomas are not uncommon lesions and are classified as benign infantile hemangiomas. Orbital hemangiomas usually appear shortly after birth, although up to 40% may be visible at birth only as a faint cutaneous (birth) mark. During the proliferative phase of growth they will become raised, bulky, and compressible. In rare instances, the proliferative phase may be biphasic. The most variable attribute of these lesions is the stage of involution, which may occur over a period of years and results in involution and fatty replacement, without the presence of calcifications. Even after resolution, some persistent fibrofatty mass or abnormal cutaneous pigmentation may remain, mainly leading to cosmetic and aesthetic concerns rather than functional issues.

Only a small percentage of hemangiomas lead to complications, such as ulcerations and bleeding. However, because of their location, early age at presentation, and potential for very rapid growth, orbital hemangiomas may lead to devastating visual impairment as a result of obscuration of light delivery to the eye, especially if the eyelids are involved. Lack of visual input early in life prevents the formation of neural pathways necessary for proper vision later in life and will lead to amblyopia and blindness.

These lobulated lesions often appear bright on T2-weighted imaging, avidly take up gadolinium, and may have multiple flow voids and increased vascularity seen on perfusion imaging (Fig. 7-8, *A-C*). Although usually nonsyndromic, some hemangiomas are known to occur in conjunction with other systemic abnormalities, such as PHACES (*p*osterior fossa abnormalities, *h*emangiomas of the cervical facial region,

arterial anomalies, *c*ardiac defects, *e*ye anomalies, and *s*ternal defects) (e-Fig. 7-9).

The imaging differential diagnosis for hemangioma includes RMS, vascular malformation, infantile fibromatosis, and infantile fibrosarcoma. The vascular features of hemangioma, particularly the flow voids on MR images, help to distinguish hemangiomas from these other lesions. RMS may be very vascular and contain flow voids but typically occurs in an older age group and often will demonstrate restricted diffusion on DWI. Most hemangiomas are managed conservatively because they tend to resolve on their own. However, tumors that can or do compromise vision are aggressively treated. Therapeutic options include propranolol, systemic or intralesional corticosteroids, α-2a or α-2b interferon, and laser therapy or surgery.

Venolymphatic Malformation

Venolymphatic malformations encompass a group of vascular lesions consisting of vascular channels of varying sizes and histologic types. Most lesions are composed of a combination of anomalous lymphatic and venous vessels. Some lesions consist primarily of lymphatic vessels and are called lymphangiomas or lymphatic malformations, whereas others are composed mainly of venous channels and thus are called venous malformations (formerly known as cavernous hemangiomas). However, most lesions contain both types of vessels, and their clinical presentation and imaging appearances depend on the prevalence of lymphatic or venous components within the individual lesion.

Rootman et al classified combined orbital venolymphatic malformations on the basis of anatomic location into three groups: superficial, deep, or combined lesions. The superficial lesions (and the superficial components of combined lesions) contain lymphatic components at pathologic evaluation. In contrast, deep lesions, as well as the deep component of combined lesions, are predominantly or completely venous in nature, reflecting the distribution of vessels within the normal orbit. When these lesions are superficial, they will involve the eyelid and/or conjunctiva, and they tend to manifest clinically at an early age. Deep lesions in the retrobulbar orbit, although present from birth, may present later in life and even into young adulthood. Unlike hemangiomas, venolymphatic malformations grow with the patient, and

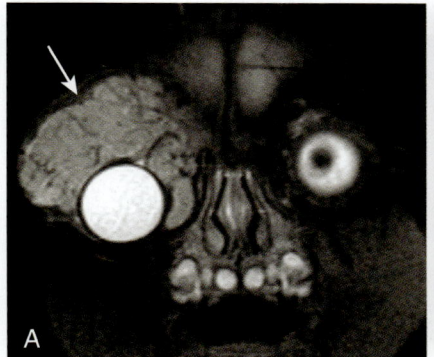 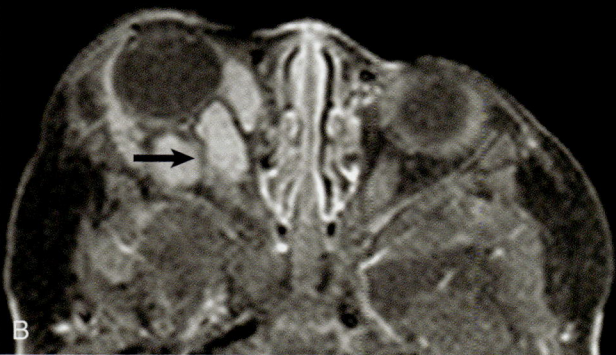 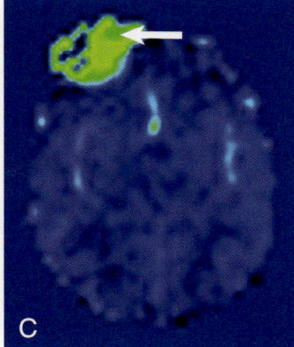

Figure 7-8 **Hemangioma.** A coronal fat-saturated T2-weighted image (**A**), an axial postcontrast fat-saturated T1-weighted image (**B**), and an axial arterial spin labeling perfusion color map (**C**) from a patient with a right orbital region hemangioma. Note the fleshy mass surrounding the right globe in the supraorbital region (*arrow* in **A**) with associated flow voids, avid contrast enhancement (*arrow* in **B**), and increased blood flow (*arrow* in **C**).

they never involute spontaneously. Clinically, these lesions usually present with progressive or acute painless proptosis, but they may present with restricted movement of the extraocular muscles. Intermittent change in size may occur as a result of recurrent hemorrhage, secondary to fragile vessels within the intervening connective tissue septations.

Imaging features may reflect the dual nature of these vascular malformations, with multicystic lymphatic components often containing blood–fluid levels and enhancing solid venous components, which may contain phleboliths. Uncomplicated lymphatic malformations usually do not demonstrate contrast enhancement, or at most may show some peripheral enhancement of the septations. On ultrasound, lymphangiomas exhibit no Doppler flow and demonstrate cystic spaces filled with blood and fluid. On CT their appearance may be inconclusive, not fully reflecting the internal complexity of the lesion (Fig. 7-10, *A*), but they can appear as a soft tissue mass with associated proptosis. MRI is capable of fully evaluating their true nature and distinguishing them from masses such as RMS lesions (Fig. 7-10, *B*).

Treatment of orbital vascular lesions remains challenging. In the past it consisted of conservative management if the patient's vision was not jeopardized. Surgical excision often is difficult and associated with numerous complications, as well as with a high rate of recurrence. Intralesional sclerosing therapy appears to be an effective method for debulking low-flow malformations and is not associated with vision-threatening complications, and thus it is an attractive alternative to surgical resection.

Orbital Varix

Primary congenital venous varices (uncommonly affecting children) represent distensible venous malformations in the retrobulbar compartment of the orbit (e-Fig. 7-11), which may enlarge with dependent posture. The varix may consist of marked enlargement of a single orbital vein or may present as a tangled multivascular mass. Clinically these lesions may present with globe displacement that may augment and increase in conspicuity when the Valsalva maneuver is performed, but at times the lesions are collapsed and may be undetectable. Occasionally these lesions may lead to spontaneous orbital hemorrhage. Secondary varices may occur in the setting of intracranial dural venous thrombosis or arteriovenous shunting.

Nonvascular Lesions

Orbital Tumors

Congenital orbital tumors mostly consist of benign tumors such as teratomas or the more aggressive kaposiform hemangioendotheliomas; however, more aggressive malignant tumors such as angiosarcomas and rhabdoid tumors also occur. The most common malignant orbital tumor in children is rhabdomyosarcoma.

Orbital Teratoma

Orbital teratoma is a very rare congenital tumor that often is diagnosed prenatally with ultrasound and fetal MRI (Fig. 7-12). These tumors usually present as a large heterogeneous mass containing multiple tissue types, including fat, calcium, and bone. Teratomas of the orbit are most often benign and well differentiated; however, they may lead to significant proptosis when located at the orbital apex. The imaging appearance of a teratoma is quite distinctive, with the presence of a very large multicystic mass that includes a solid component and calcification. The solid components may exhibit enhancement after administration of a contrast agent. The enhancement pattern may help to distinguish a teratoma from a dermoid cyst, which, when present, tends to have peripheral enhancement.

A kaposiform hemangioendothelioma may be very large and may sequester platelets, thereby leading to a consumptive coagulopathy as a result of the Kasabach-Merritt phenomenon. This phenomenon is not known to occur with hemangiomas.

Rhabdoid tumors of the orbital region occur in young children (with a mean age of 15 months at presentation) and can be highly vascular and mimic more benign lesions such as hemangiomas. These rare malignant tumors are highly aggressive and lethal (death occurs within 12 months of presentation). Their dense cellularity can produce restricted diffusion on DWI (e-Fig. 7-13, *A* and *B*).

Rhabdomyosarcoma

RMS is the most common malignant soft tissue tumor in childhood. The orbits and paranasal sinuses are the second most common location. The embryonal type is the most

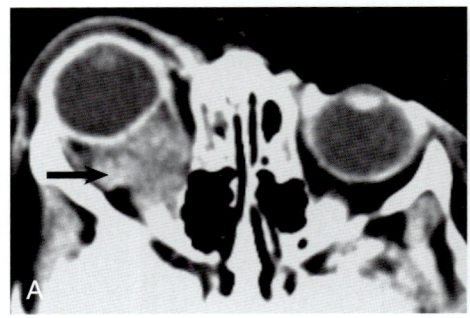 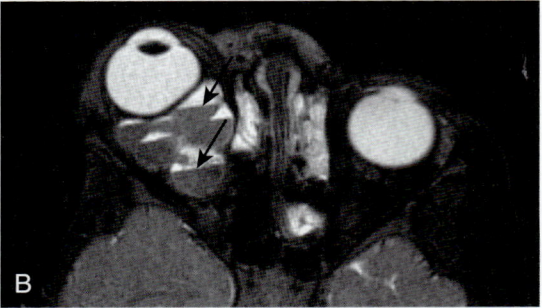

Figure 7-10   Venolymphatic malformation. An axial contrast-enhanced computed tomography (CT) scan (**A**) and an axial fat-saturated T2-weighted magnetic resonance image (MRI) of the orbit (**B**) show a soft tissue intraconal mass posterior to the right globe (*arrow* in **A**), which is associated with anterior displacement of the globe. Although the finding on CT is nonspecific, the multiple fluid-fluid levels on MRI (*arrows* in **B**) are highly suggestive of the diagnosis.

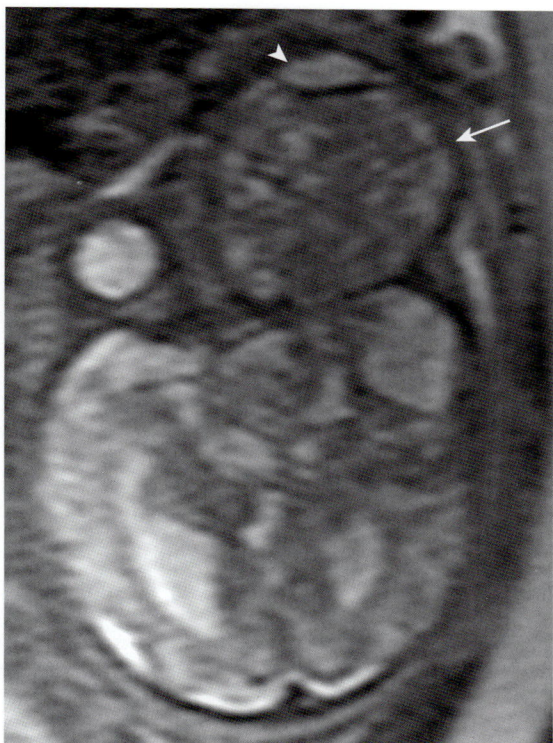

Figure 7-12 Fetal teratoma. An axial half-Fourier acquisition single-shot turbo spin-echo magnetic resonance image of the orbital region shows a very large, slightly T2-hypointense lesion in the region of the left orbit (*arrow*), with associated marked anterior/ventral displacement of the globe (*arrowhead*) representing a teratoma.

common variety of orbital RMS; the alveolar and pleomorphic varieties occur rarely. The mean age at presentation is 6 years.

RMS previously was thought to arise from skeletal muscle but now is generally believed to originate from pluripotential mesenchymal cells that have the capacity to differentiate into skeletal muscle. RMS is an aggressive, fast-growing tumor that most often manifests with rapidly progressive proptosis or globe displacement and should be considered in any child

with that clinical presentation. Other common signs and symptoms include conjunctival and palpebral swelling, which may erroneously suggest the clinical diagnosis of orbital cellulitis and may lead to confusion with respect to presentation and imaging appearance.

Most tumors are extraconal in location, but intraconal components also may be present. The most typical location for the common embryonal form is in the superonasal quadrant. The less prevalent alveolar form more often affects the inferior orbit. RMS grows rapidly and behaves aggressively, frequently invading the adjacent bones and soft tissues. However, advanced disease is less often encountered today because of greater awareness of the diagnosis.

Both CT and MR imaging play important roles in the preoperative evaluation, staging, and follow-up of orbital RMS tumors. On T2-weighted imaging, these lesions may appear as hypointense, isointense, and even hyperintense with respect to both extraocular muscles and orbital fat (Fig. 7-14, *A* and *B*). Because of the high degree of RMS cellularity, the lesions may be predominantly hypointense on T2-weighted imaging, hyperattenuating on CT, and exhibit restricted diffusion on DWI. On T1-weighted contrast-enhanced images, RMS will have moderate to marked enhancement, and in some cases a component of highly vascular internal tissue may mimic the appearance of a hemangioma. Meticulous attention is required in the assessment of local invasion because RMS may invade the paranasal sinuses, as well as for more remote invasion because RMS can spread to the intracranial space via the orbital fissures and then into cavernous sinuses and even the middle cranial fossa. Favorable prognostic factors include lack of distant metastases, a primary site in the orbit, disease confined to the orbit, gross total surgical resection, a patient age of younger than 10 years, an embryonal histologic type, hyperdiploid deoxyribonucleic acid content, and a tumor size of 5 cm or less. The most important prognostic factor is response to therapy, which is assessed with follow-up imaging.

Advances in chemotherapy and radiotherapy have improved survival rates of patients with orbital RMS. This improved survival rate has allowed observation of the late effects of radiotherapy on both facial growth (e.g., bony hypoplasia of the orbit and facial asymmetry) and visual function (e.g., cataract, keratopathy, and retinopathy).

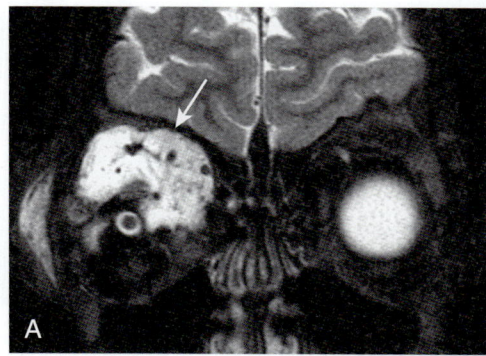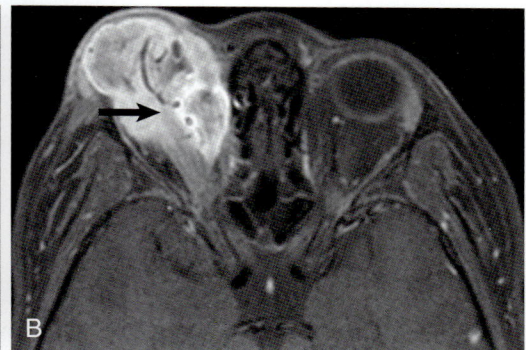

Figure 7-14 Rhabdomyosarcoma. A coronal fat-saturated T2-weighted image (**A**) and an axial fat-saturated postcontrast T1-weighted image (**B**) in a patient with a right orbital rhabdomyosarcoma show a large, mainly extraconal lesion with flow voids seen on the T2-weighted image (*white arrow*) and with associated enhancement within the superior aspect of the right orbit (*black arrow*) indicative of the highly vascular nature of this tumor.

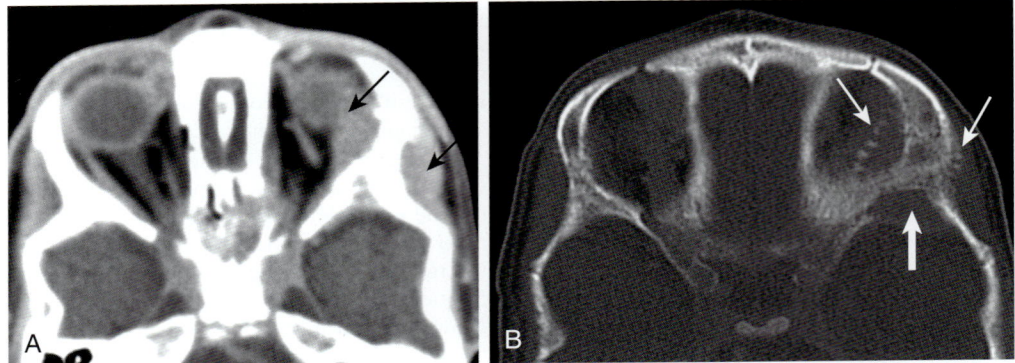

Figure 7-15 Neuroblastoma metastases. Axial contrast-enhanced computed tomography scans of the orbits with soft tissue (**A**) and bone windows (**B**) in a patient with known metastatic neuroblastoma show enhancing soft tissue masses on either side of the lateral orbital wall (*arrows* in **A**). In addition, the bone surrounding the orbit has a moth-eaten appearance, which is a typical appearance of neuroblastoma that has metastasized to the orbits/skull base (*arrows* in **B**).

Lesions that Secondarily Involve the Orbit

METASTATIC LESIONS INVOLVING THE ORBITS

Orbital metastases are less common in children than in adults. Primary tumors that can metastasize to the bony orbit are neuroblastoma, lymphoma and leukemia, and very rarely Wilms tumor and Ewing sarcoma. Ocular choroid metastases, which are quite common in adults, are exceedingly rare in children.

Neuroblastoma

Neuroblastoma is the most common metastatic tumor of young pediatric patients (Figs. 7-15 and 7-16). In 8% of cases, neuroblastoma first presents with acute orbital symptoms related to tumoral hemorrhage, sudden proptosis, and ecchymosis (raccoon eyes). Neuroblastoma metastases to the head and neck favors the bony skull base and the cranial sutures, at times leading to sutural diastasis on conventional radiographs, with the additional extraaxial soft tissue masses only discernable on cross-sectional CT and MR imaging.

Leukemia and Lymphoma

The marrow malignancies lymphoma and leukemia account for 10% to 15% of orbital masses. The two forms of these marrow diseases that most frequently involve the orbit are granulocytic sarcoma (also called chloroma or extramedullary myeloid tumor), which is associated with acute myelogenous leukemia (AML) in younger children, and non-Hodgkin lymphoma (NHL) in older children. In patients with AML, the metastatic focus is referred to as chloroma (derived from the Greek word chloros [green]), because of their green tint. Rarely, this finding is the initial presenting sign of AML, although it more commonly occurs with recurrent disease. A

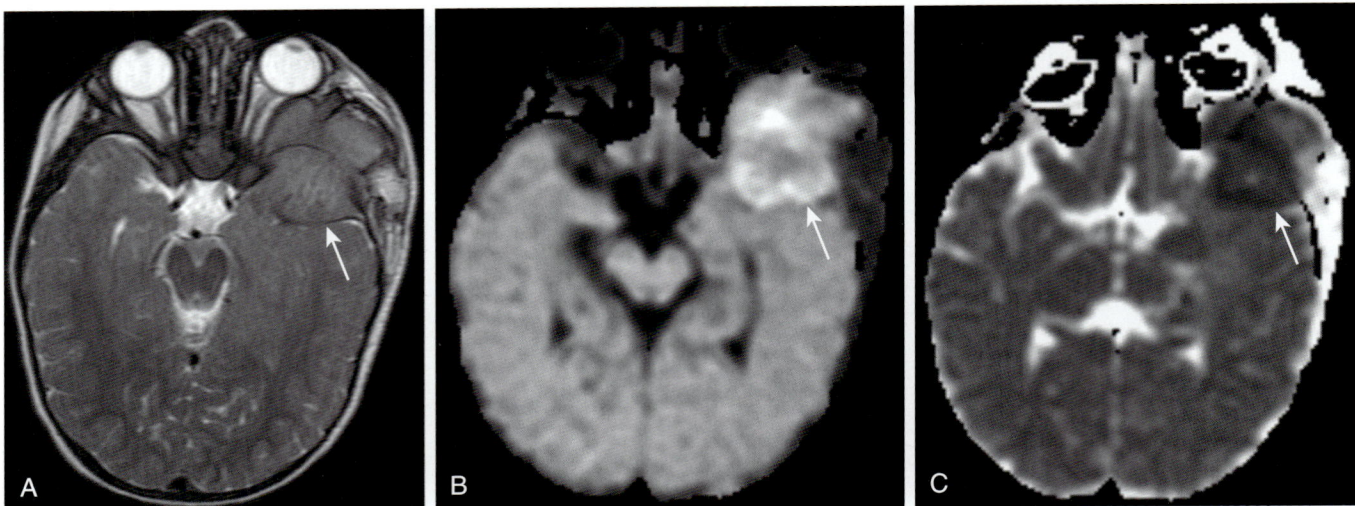

Figure 7-16 Neuroblastoma metastases. Axial T2-weighted magnetic resonance imaging (**A**), axial diffusion-weighted imaging (DWI) (**B**), and axial apparent diffusion coefficient (ADC) imaging (**C**) of the orbit in a patient with known metastatic neuroblastoma. A large, nearly isointense mass is seen on the T2-weighted image at the level of the mid orbit; it is extraaxial in location and produces posterior displacement of the ipsilateral temporal lobe (*arrow* in **A**). Corresponding restricted diffusion (*arrows*) is identified on DWI (**B**) and ADC (**C**) images at the same level, indicating marked cellularity of the tumor.

predilection exists for involvement of the subperiosteal space, and on imaging they resemble the bony metastases of a neuroblastoma.

NHL (a tumor composed of B cells) often presents with extranodal disease. Most patients with orbital lymphoma also have systemic disease. The locations involved may include the lacrimal glands, anterior orbit, retrobulbar region, and the superior orbital compartment. CT may demonstrate a hyperattenuating mass with sharply defined margins. MRI findings include hypointense masses on T2-weighted imaging, with associated restricted diffusion on DWI (e-Fig. 7-17, A and B).

DERMOID AND EPIDERMOID CYSTS

Dermoid and epidermoid cysts are congenital developmental ectodermal inclusion cysts, and they constitute up to 5% of all orbital masses. Both dermoids and epidermoids arise from entrapped embryonic epithelium, often within the orbital sutures, but they also may be intraorbital or even corneal in location. Epidermoid cysts contain epithelial elements and cholesterol crystals and may be bounded by a thin capsule, whereas dermoid cysts may contain dermal appendages, including hair and sebaceous glands, and are surrounded by a fibrous capsule. Dermoid cysts usually appear as a painless subcutaneous nodule, and they mainly cause cosmetic deformity, but later in life they may grow, partially rupture, and become inflamed and symptomatic. Imaging sometimes is indicated when deep extension of the lesion is suspected and cannot be ruled out clinically.

Dermoid and epidermoid cysts may occur anywhere within the orbit, but most reside in the superolateral aspect of the orbit, at the frontozygomatic suture, or in a superonasal position at the frontolacrimal suture. Osseous remodeling may occur but without associated periosteal reaction. These lesions are well-demarcated, cystic-appearing extraconal masses with differing degrees of fatty content. Uncomplicated superficial dermoid cysts are well depicted on orbital CT without the need for IV contrast because these lesions should not enhance (Fig. 7-18, A). MRI is superior for more detailed depiction of possible intracranial connection and the presence of a potential sinus tract. These lesions are hyperintense on T1-weighted imaging because of their fatty content. Mild rim enhancement occasionally may be seen and is considered normal, whereas the appearance of a more irregular type of enhancement is suggestive of prior rupture with a secondary inflammatory reaction. Epidermoid cysts are hyperintense on fluid attenuated inversion recovery sequences and exhibit restricted diffusion on DWI (Fig. 7-18, B and C).

LANGERHANS CELL HISTIOCYTOSIS

LCH is a granulomatous disease resulting from proliferation and infiltration of abnormal histiocytes within various tissues. Orbital lesions occur mainly in young children ages 1 to 4 years. Orbital disease may accompany widespread disease, but occasionally it may be the first manifestation of LCH. The lesions arise from the orbital bone or bone marrow and spread directly to the orbit. Orbital disease may present clinically with proptosis and rapidly enlarging periorbital masses. CT demonstrates expansile soft tissue masses associated with smoothly marginated ("punched out") areas of osseous destruction in the posterolateral orbits, with a predilection for the frontosphenoid sutures (e-Fig. 7-19, A). MR imaging demonstrates periorbital heterogeneous lesions that may demonstrate blood-fluid levels and restricted diffusion (e-Fig. 7-19, B). The masses exhibit diffuse enhancement on CT and MRI. Evaluation for intracranial extension is imperative on postcontrast sequences (e-Fig 7-19, C). Discovery of a solitary orbital LCH lesion necessitates additional examination for other possible sites of involvement. Multiple soft tissue masses may resemble neuroblastoma metastases by certain imaging features; that is, both lesions may demonstrate restricted diffusion, diffuse enhancement, and intraosseous and extraosseous components. The type of osseous involvement may help to distinguish the "clear-cut" margins of LCH from the permeative pattern and aggressive periosteal reaction of a neuroblastoma. Orbital LCH also can simulate the imaging appearance of an RMS tumor with bone invasion, although bone destruction with LCH typically is more pronounced.

ORBITAL PSEUDOTUMOR (IDIOPATHIC ORBITAL INFLAMMATION)

An orbital pseudotumor, which is a condition of unknown etiology, represents a noninfectious infiltration of the orbital structures by lymphocytes and plasma cells, usually without associated osseous involvement. The disease may present as unilateral, isolated involvement of the extraocular muscles but also may manifest with a more diffuse pattern that involves multiple orbital sites. It also can present with neuritis or an extrabulbar mass. CT and MRI are equally effective in depicting the extent of disease (Fig. 7-20).

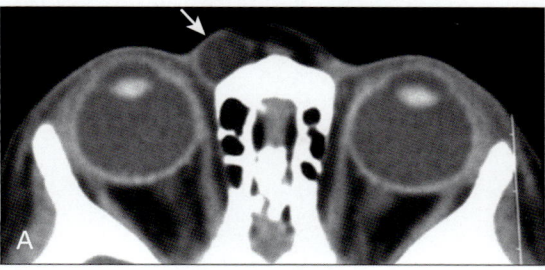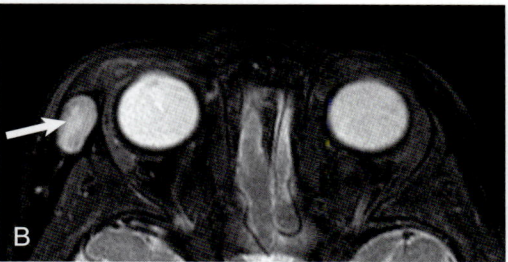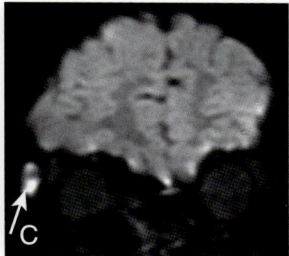

Figure 7-18 Epidermoid. **A,** An axial noncontrast computed tomography scan shows an ovoid area of low-attenuation (fat) within the anterior soft tissues medial to the right globe (*arrow*). In another patient, an axial fat-saturated T2-weighted image (**B**) and coronal diffusion-weighted image (**C**) show a similar lesion along the right lateral orbital soft tissues, which is bright on the T2-weighted fat-saturated axial image (*arrow* in **B**) but exhibits restricted diffusion on the coronal diffusion-weighted image (*arrow* in **C**), as typically is seen with epidermoid cysts.

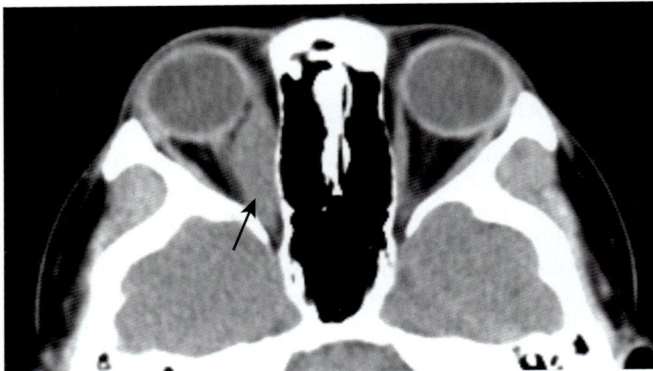

Figure 7-20 **Inflammatory orbital pseudotumor.** A contrast-enhanced computed tomography scan of the orbit in a patient with a known right-sided inflammatory orbital pseudotumor. Note the fusiform enhancement and enlargement of the right medial rectus muscle (*arrow*) with extension to the myotendinous junction.

In children, orbital pseudotumor presents with an acute onset of painful proptosis and painful eye movement. The clinical presentation of orbital pseudotumor may be the best discriminator between this disease process and Graves disease (formerly known as Graves ophthalmopathy and now referred to as thyroid-associated orbitopathy). Orbital myositis usually appears as enlargement of the extraocular muscles with mild surrounding inflammatory changes and anterior extension into the tendinous insertion. The imaging features of orbital myositis may be fairly similar to the early stage of thyroid-associated orbitopathy, although the tendinous portion/insertion of the extraocular muscles is spared in patients with thyroid-associated orbitopathy. Excellent response to steroid treatment with cessation of pain is typical for persons with orbital pseudotumor. In rare cases, a biopsy is necessary to exclude malignancy.

OSTEOMA

Osteomas are benign, slow-growing, bone-forming tumors. Although osteomas of the facial region are not common, they sometimes occur within the region of the paranasal sinuses. If a lesion is of a large enough size and occurs within either the frontal or ethmoid sinus, an adjacent bony break through into the orbit can occur, mimicking an orbital lesion.

Osteomas within the orbits demonstrate typical imaging features of a broad-based expansile osseous mass, sometimes with an inner ground-glass lucent area, surrounded by dense compact bone. Osteomas usually do not cause bony destruction, even when the lesions are large in size. CT is the best imaging modality to delineate the lesion's characteristics and extension (e-Fig. 7-21). MRI findings may be confusing, because the mature dense bone of the osteoma (and its absence of protons), composing most of the lesion's volume, may not be distinguishable from the air in the paranasal sinuses.

Suggested Readings

Bilaniuk LT. Vascular lesions of the orbit in children. *Neuroimaging Clin North Am.* 2005;15:107-120.

Brennan RC, Wilson MW, Kaste S, et al. US and MRI of pediatric ocular masses with histopathological correlation. *Pediatr Radiol.* 2012;42:738-749.

Chung EM, Smirniotopoulos JC, Specht CS, et al. Pediatric orbit tumors and tumor like lesions: nonosseous lesions of the extraocular orbit. *Radio-Graphics.* 2007;27:1777-1799.

Razek A, Elkhamary S, Mousa A. Differentiation between benign and malignant orbital tumors at 3T diffusion MR imaging. *Neuroradiology.* 2011;53:517-522.

Rootman J. Distribution and differential diagnosis of orbital disease. *In Diseases of the orbit: a multidisciplinary approach.* 2nd ed. Philadelphia: Lippincott Williams & Wilkins; 2003:52-84.

Chapter 8

Nose and Sinonasal Cavities

DIANA P. RODRIGUEZ

Development and Anatomy of the Sinonasal Cavities

NASAL CAVITY

The nasal cavity is triangular and is separated in the midline by the nasal septum. The nasal cavity is composed of a cartilaginous portion anteriorly and an osseous portion posteriorly, which is formed by the perpendicular plate of the ethmoid posterosuperiorly and the vomer posteroinferiorly. The opening to each nasal cavity is known as the vestibule, which is bounded medially by the columella and nasal septum and laterally by the nasal alae. The cribriform plate is the roof of the nasal cavity, and the floor is the hard and soft palate. Posteriorly, the nasal cavity communicates with the nasopharynx via the choanae, after rupture of the oronasal membrane during the fetal period. From the lateral wall of the nasal cavity, three pairs of turbinates (superior, middle, and inferior) project into the nasal cavity, each with a corresponding meatus below them. The middle turbinate is attached to the cribriform plate via the vertical lamella and to the lamina papyracea via the basal lamella (Fig. 8-1).

PARANASAL SINUSES

The paranasal sinuses form as diverticula from the walls of the nasal cavities and become air-filled extensions in the adjacent bones—maxilla, ethmoid, frontal, and sphenoid. The original openings of the diverticula persist as the ostia of the sinuses that communicate with the nasal cavity (Fig. 8-2, *A* and *B*).

The mucosal lining of the nasal cavities is contiguous with the paranasal sinuses and consists of pseudostratified, columnar, ciliated epithelium containing mucinous and serous glands,[1] whereas the nasal septum is lined by squamous mucosa.[2] In the human embryo, ethmoidal and maxillary sinus budding can be detected at 11 to 12 gestational weeks and at 14 to 15 gestational weeks, respectively.[3] In general, only rudimentary maxillary and ethmoid sinuses, which continue to expand until puberty or early adulthood, are present at birth.[4] The sinuses also are linked to facial growth and dentition and have been studied extensively by different anatomic and imaging methods (Fig. 8-3, *A-C*).[4-11]

ETHMOID SINUSES

At birth the ethmoid sinuses are already developed in number and pneumatized, but they continue to expand, reaching adult proportions at about 12 years of age.[12] The ethmoid sinuses consist of a paired group of a variable number of cells (3 to 18) within the lateral masses of the ethmoid bone, also known as labyrinths. In addition to the lateral masses, the ethmoid bone consists of the cribriform plate superiorly and the perpendicular plate, which is part of the nasal septum (see Fig. 8-3, *A*). The ethmoid sinus is bordered medially by the nasal cavity and laterally by the lamina papyracea; its roof is formed by the cribriform plate and fovea ethmoidalis (see Fig. 8-1). The anterior and posterior ethmoid air cells are separated by the basal lamella (see Fig. 8-3, *C*), which is the lateral attachment of the middle turbinate to the lamina papyracea. Drainage of the anterior ethmoid air cells occurs via the ethmoid bulla into the hiatus semilunaris and middle meatus. The posterior ethmoid air cells drain into the superior meatus and then into the sphenoethmoid recess (see Fig. 8-2, *A*).

The anterior ethmoidal artery arises from the ophthalmic artery in the orbit, pierces the lamina papyracea, and exits via its respective foramina by passing through the ethmoid roof in the superomedial wall of the orbit, 2 to 3 mm behind the anterior wall of the bulla ethmoidalis. Occasionally the anterior ethmoidal artery passes within bony septae of the ethmoid sinuses and is suspended in a mesentery without bony cover (e-Fig. 8-4).[13]

Anatomic Variants

The roof of the anterior ethmoid sinus is formed by the cribriform bone medially and the fovea ethmoidalis laterally (see Fig. 8-1). Any asymmetry in the height of the ethmoid roof should be documented by the radiologist because a higher incidence of surgical penetration occurs during endoscopic surgery on the side where the position of the roof is lower.[14,15] An increased risk of inadvertent intracranial penetration may occur if the fovea ethmoidalis plane passes through the midorbital plane or below.

Concha bullosa refers to the pneumatization of the middle turbinate as a result of intramural extension of posterior ethmoid air cells (Fig. 8-5, *B*). A large concha bullosa eventually can cause obstruction of the airway.

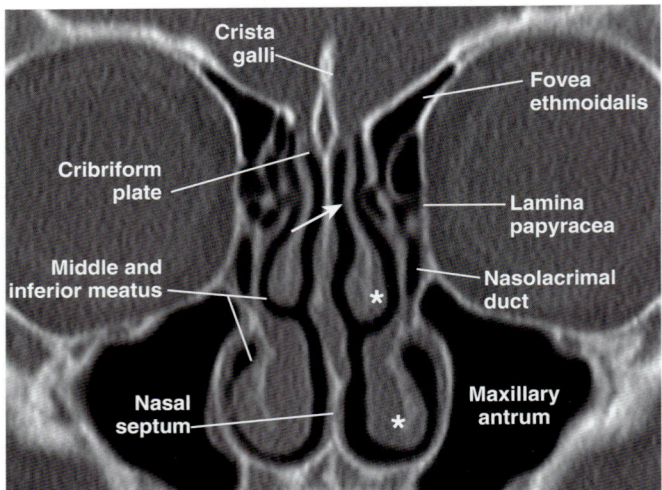

Figure 8-1 Anatomy of the nasal cavity demonstrated in a 13-year-old child. A coronal computed tomography scan shows middle and inferior turbinates (*asterisks*) and vertical lamella of the middle turbinate attached to the cribriform plate (*arrow*).

Extramural expansion of ethmoid air cells can result in anatomic variants, including the following: Agger nasi cells (Fig. 8-5, *A*), which are the most anterior and inferior cells involving the lacrimal bone or maxilla; Haller cells, which are middle ethmoid air cells extending into the inferomedial floor of the orbit (Fig. 8-5, *C*); and Onodi cells, which are posterior sphenoethmoid air cells with prominent superolateral pneumatization in close relationship to the optic nerve canal.[13]

MAXILLARY SINUSES

The maxillary sinuses are very small and pneumatized at birth, measuring an ellipsoid volume (sinus volume index) of approximately 0.24 ± 0.36 cm^3.[4] During the first years of life, the maxillary sinuses undergo rapid inferolateral expansion, reaching full size between 15 to 18 years of age. The floor of the maxillary sinus usually is seen at the level of the middle meatus during infancy; it reaches the level of the nasal floor by 8 to 9 years of age, and by age 12 years, it is located at the level of the hard palate.[6] However, variation exists in the final descent of the floor, which lies below the level of the nasal floor in 65% of adults (e-Fig. 8-6, *A-D*).[16]

The maxillary sinus is the largest of the sinuses. Its roof is formed by the orbital floor, which carries the bony canal for the infraorbital nerve; the medial wall is formed by the lateral nasal wall. The posterior wall of the maxillary sinus forms the pterygopalatine fossa (Fig. 8-7, *A*). The maxillary sinus drains via the maxillary ostium located superomedially into the infundibulum, the hiatus semilunaris, and the middle meatus (Fig. 8-2, *A*).

Developmental variations of the maxillary sinus include an accessory ostium, isolated unilateral hypoplasia, and prominent septa that appear to compartmentalize the sinus cavity. Occasionally the roots of the maxillary molars impinge on the walls of the sinuses.

SPHENOID SINUS

The sphenoid sinus begins to pneumatize in a ventrodorsal direction from 7 months to 2 years of age. A significant acceleration in sinus expansion occurs between 3 and 8 years of age, with complete pneumatization usually present by age 10 years (e-Fig. 8-8, *A-E*).[9] Its border is formed superiorly by the sella turcica, posteriorly by the clivus, anteriorly by the ethmoid sinus, and inferiorly by the nasopharynx (see Fig. 8-2, *A* and *B*). This sinus drains anteriorly via the sphenoethmoid recess. Lateral recesses of the sphenoid sinus are formed from pneumatization of the pterygoid process in 44% of people (see Fig. 8-7, *A*). Benign sphenoid marrow variants, which sometimes are mistaken for lesions, can be seen adjacent to the pneumatized sphenoid sinus (e-Fig. 8-9, *A-C*).

Important anatomic relationships of the sphenoid sinus include the optic canal and nerve located superolaterally; the foramen rotundum with the maxillary nerve that courses along the inferolateral margin of the sphenoid sinus; the vidian canal, which usually runs along the floor of the sphenoid sinus; and the cavernous portion of the internal carotid artery, which protrudes laterally into the sinus (see Fig. 8-7, *B*).

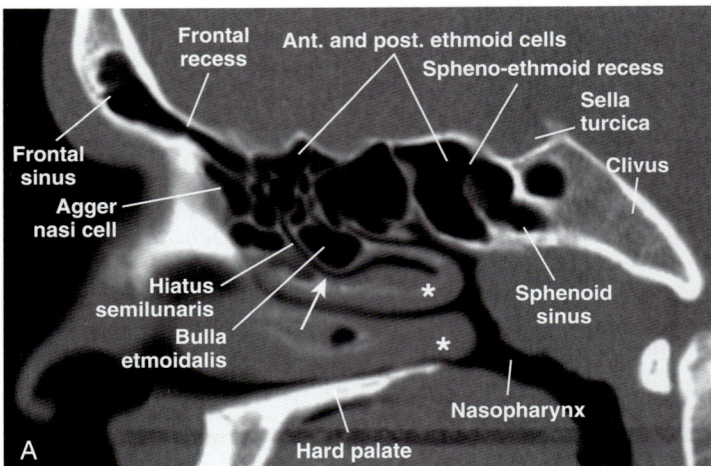

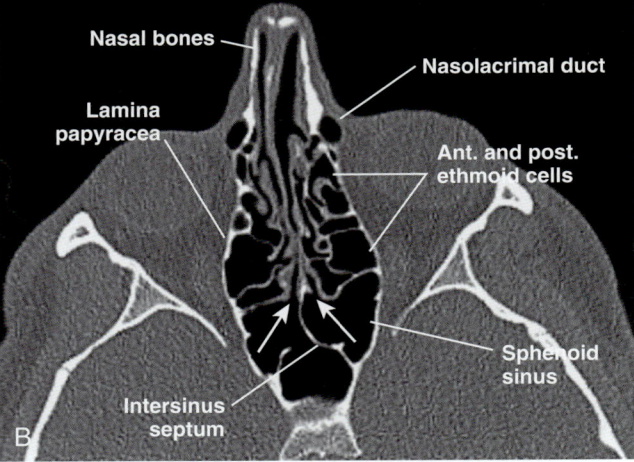

Figure 8-2 Normal sinus openings. **A,** A sagittal computed tomography (CT) scan shows frontal recess of the frontal sinus, hiatus semilunaris, middle meatus (*arrow*), sphenoethmoid recess, and middle and inferior turbinates (*asterisks*). **B,** An axial CT view shows sphenoethmoid recesses (*arrows*).

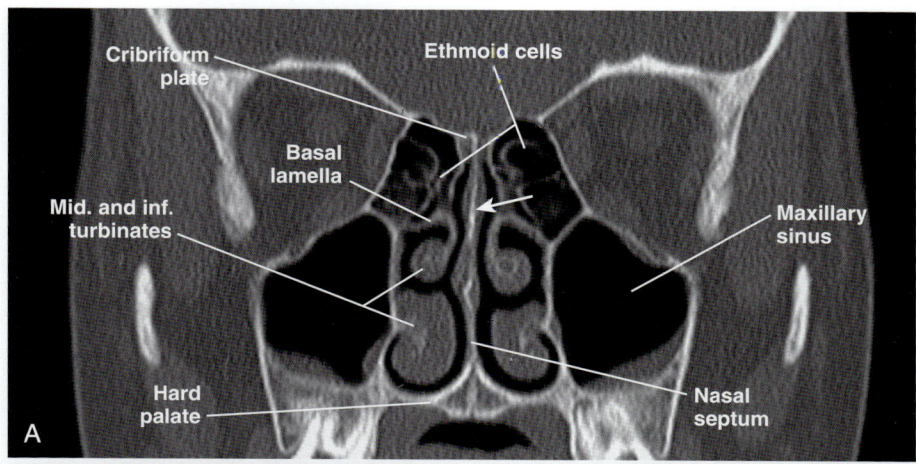

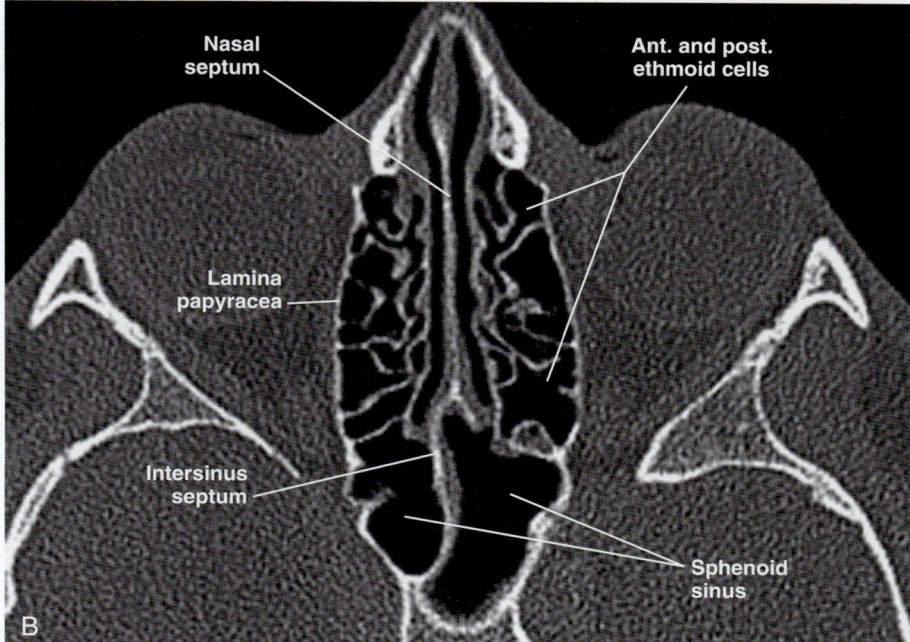

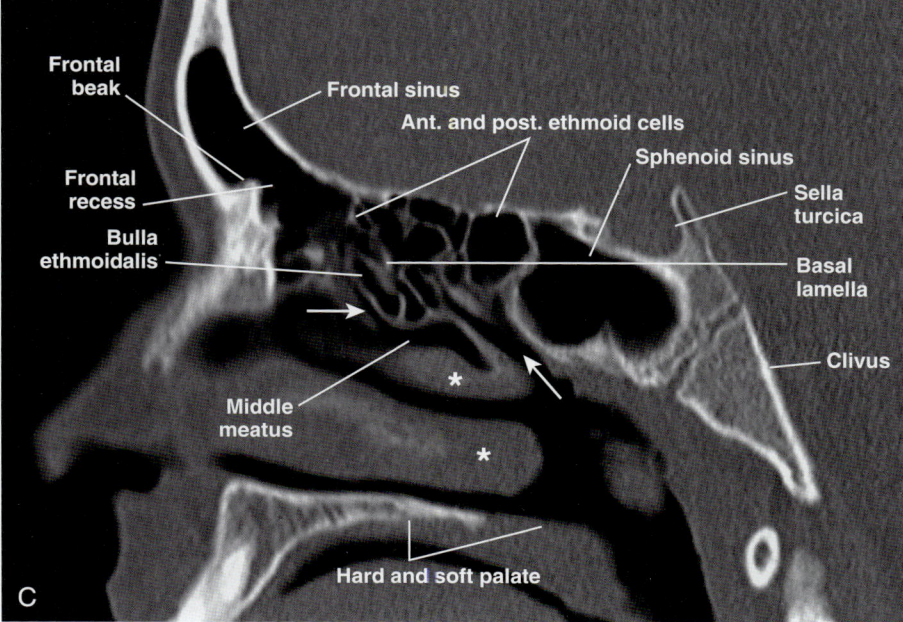

Figure 8-3 Normal anatomy of the sinuses demonstrated by fully developed sinuses in a 13-year-old boy. **A,** A coronal computed tomography (CT) scan shows the perpendicular plate of the ethmoid bone (*arrow*). **B,** An axial CT image. **C,** A sagittal CT image shows hiatus semilunaris (*arrow at left*), drainage passage of posterior ethmoid cells (*arrow at right*), and middle and inferior turbinates (*asterisks*).

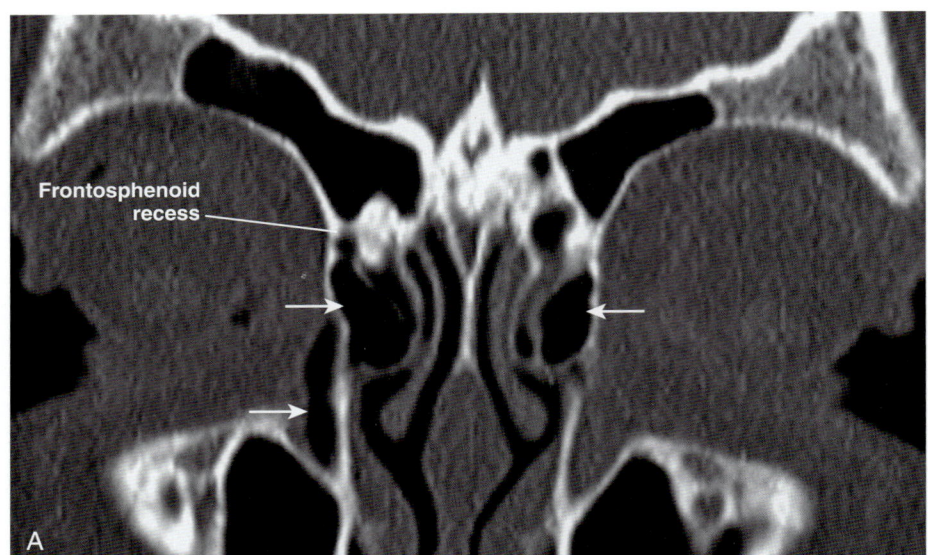

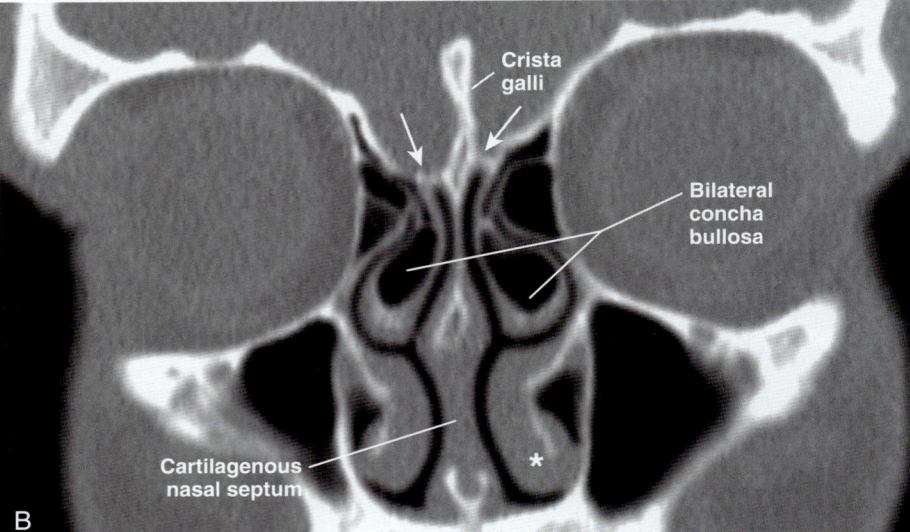

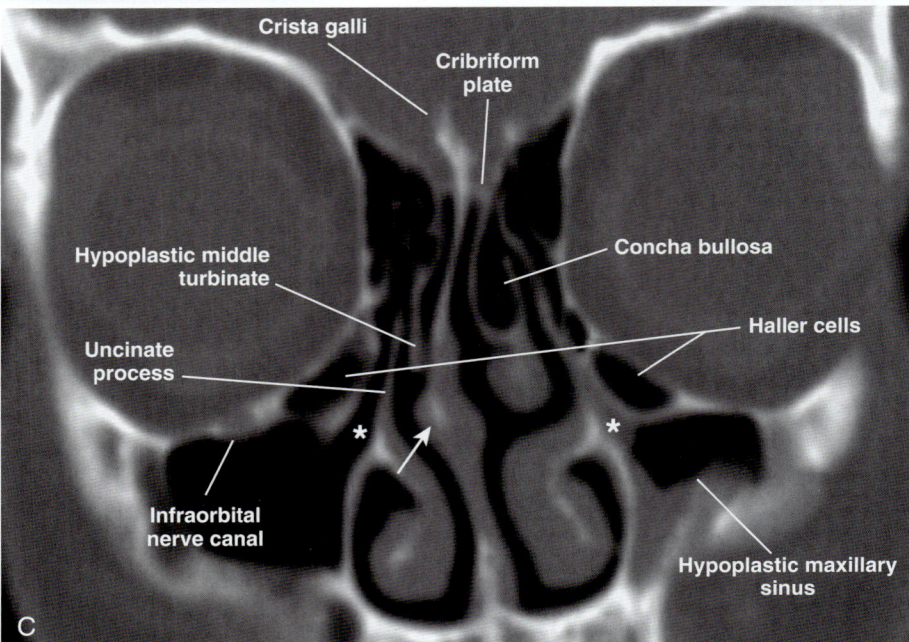

Figure 8-5 Anatomic variants. **A,** A coronal computed tomography scan shows bilateral agger nasi cells (*top arrows*), the nasolacrimal canal (*bottom arrow*), and the right fronto-ethmoidal recess. **B,** Bilateral concha bullosa, asymmetric height of the ethmoid roofs (*arrows*), and the inferior turbinate (*asterisk*) are shown. **C,** A hypoplastic right middle turbinate, rightward nasal septal deviation, Haller cells, and infundibulum (*asterisks*) are shown.

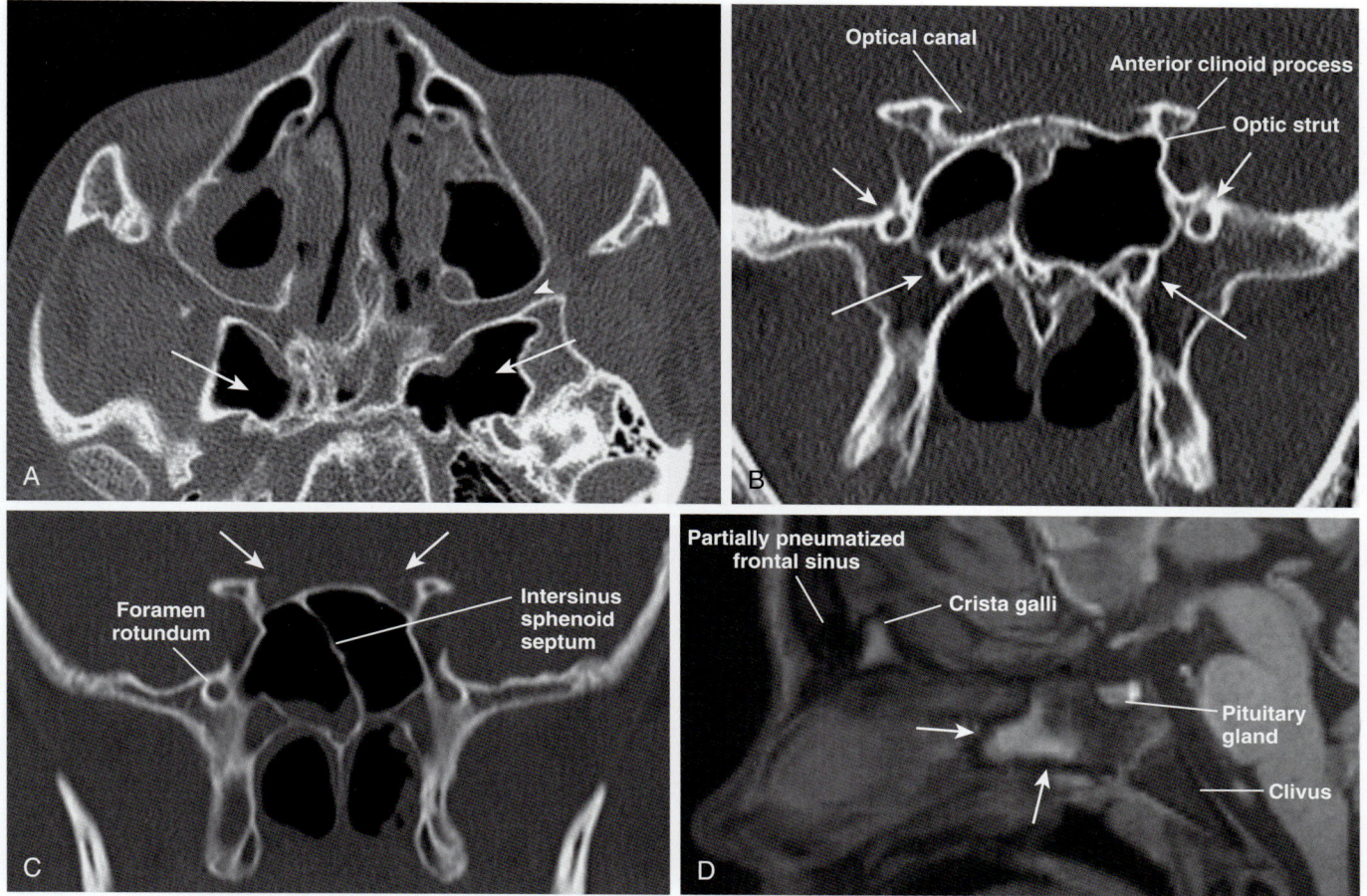

Figure 8-7 Sphenoid sinus anatomy and variants. **A,** An axial computed tomography (CT) image shows hyperpneumatization of the sphenoid sinus involving the pterygoid plates bilaterally (*arrows*); the pterygopalatine fossa (*arrowhead*) also is shown. **B,** A CT image shows foramen rotundum (*short arrows*) and the vidian canal (*long arrows*) bilaterally. **C,** A coronal CT image shows insertion of the intersinus septum into the right optic canal (*arrows*). **D,** A sagittal T1-weighted magnetic resonance image demonstrates a nonpneumatized sphenoid sinus in an 11-year-old boy with fatty transformation of its anteroinferior portion (*arrows*).

The sphenoid sinus septum usually is aligned anteriorly with the nasal septum, but the sinus septum can deviate posteriorly, forming unequal sphenoid cavities (see Fig. 8-7, *C*). Absent pneumatization in a child older than 9 years is usually abnormal and warrants clinical investigation (see Fig. 8-7, *D*).

FRONTAL SINUSES

The frontal sinuses are absent at birth and are the last to develop once bone marrow conversion has occurred. The frontal sinus is considered an extension of the anterior ethmoid air cells and pneumatizes between 2 to 8 years, with the most significant growth taking place between ages 1 to 5 years. The frontal sinuses can continue to expand up until the second decade of life.[6,11] The frontal sinuses consist of paired, often asymmetric cells. The anterior wall corresponds to the outer cortical table of the frontal bone, and the posterior wall of the sinus separates it from the anterior cranial fossa. Drainage of this sinus occurs via the frontal recess, which is an hourglass-like narrowing between the frontal sinus and the anterior middle meatus (see Fig. 8-2, *A*). Hypoplasia and aplasia of the frontal sinus can be seen in 4% and 5% of the population, respectively.

Imaging of the Paranasal Sinuses

RADIOGRAPHY

Although plain radiography is less costly and more widely available than computed tomography (CT), it has significant limitations in evaluating the paranasal sinuses. Specifically, plain radiography often overestimates or underestimates findings, it does not localize pathology well, and it does not provide important anatomic detail.[17] Traditionally, the paranasal sinus series has consisted of four views (Caldwell, Waters, posteroanterior, and lateral) that are technically difficult to perform in children. The Waters view is obtained by angulating the beam in 5-degree increments per year (up to age 6 years) to compensate for the progressive enlargement of the maxillary antra throughout childhood (Fig. 8-10, *A* and *B*). Although this approach improves visualization of the maxillary sinuses by projecting them over the petrous pyramids, it also creates double contours that can simulate mucosal thickening. Radiographic density also is critical because overpenetration of the films can completely obscure density differences created by disease, whereas underpenetration can simulate disease. Air fluid levels also can be obscured as a

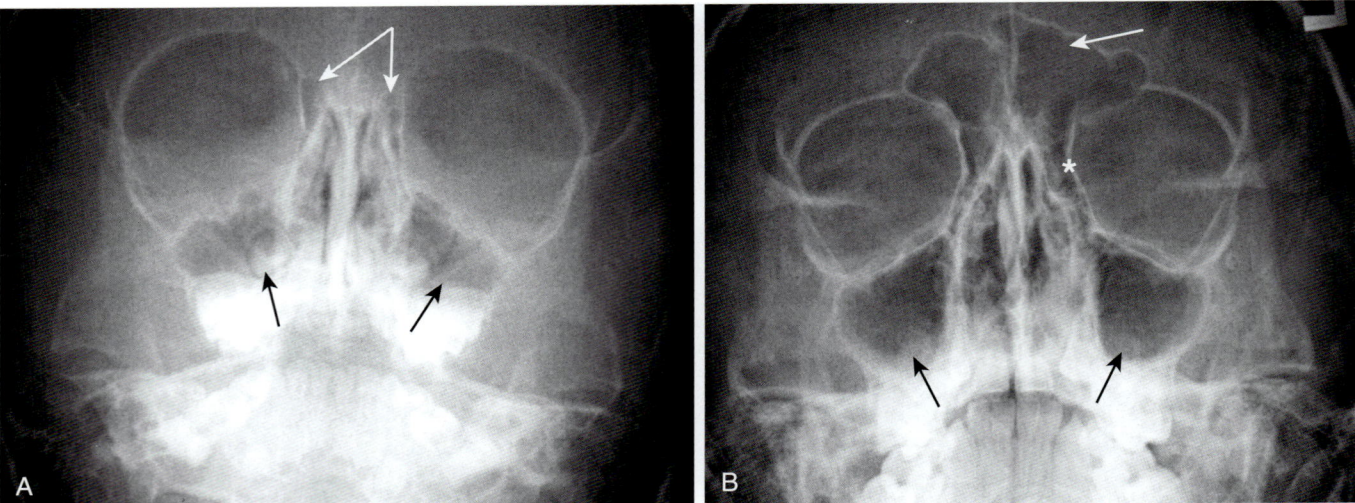

Figure 8-10 Plain radiograph—Waters view. **A,** Maxillary sinuses (*single arrows*) and ethmoid air cells (*attached arrows*) in a 3-year-old child. **B,** Maxillary sinuses (*bottom arrows*), frontal sinus (*top arrow*), and ethmoid air cells (*asterisk*) in an 11-year-old child.

result of beam angulation. Although some have suggested using only the Waters view radiograph, this modality has been shown to have 32% false-negative results and 49.2% false-positive results when compared with CT. Moreover, most of the abnormalities in the ethmoid and sphenoid sinus are not detected in the Waters radiograph.[18] Ethmoid disease on the Caldwell projection can be overdiagnosed or underdiagnosed because of technical and anatomic factors. The lateral view for evaluating the sphenoid sinus is of very little value in children younger than 4 years.[17,19]

The American College of Radiology does not recommend the use of plain radiography in diagnosing sinusitis in children. Sinusitis is considered a clinical diagnosis that should not be made on the basis of imaging findings alone.[20] Similarly, American Academy of Pediatrics (AAP) guidelines state that plain radiographs are unnecessary for diagnosing sinonasal disease in children younger than 6 years.[21] Further, plain films do not play a role in evaluating sinonasal masses or complications of sinusitis.

COMPUTED TOMOGRAPHY

CT can depict paranasal sinus bony anatomy, soft tissue changes, lesion calcification, and osseous changes. Coronal CT images best demonstrate the anatomy of the ostiomeatal unit, as well as important anatomic landmarks and variants of the sinuses, effectively providing a road map for functional endoscopic sinus surgery. For these reasons, CT is considered the imaging modality of choice for evaluating inflammatory disease of the paranasal sinuses (i.e., recurrent and chronic sinusitis). CT also plays an important role in detecting orbital and intracranial complications of acute or chronic sinusitis. Along with magnetic resonance imaging (MRI), CT is an excellent tool for evaluating sinonasal masses.

When using nonhelical CT, images of the paranasal sinuses are obtained in a direct coronal plane with the patient in a prone position with the head hyperextended. Multidetector CT with volume isometric imaging allows axial image acquisition perpendicular to the table with the patient in a neutral supine position; images subsequently are reconstructed in

coronal and sagittal planes. Slice thickness is usually 2.5 mm, and anatomic coverage extends from the upper teeth to 2 cm above the frontal sinus. If orbital or intracranial complications of sinusitis are suspected clinically, the study should be performed after the intravenous (IV) administration of contrast material, and imaging also should include the brain. Images are reconstructed in both soft tissue and bone algorithms.

In recent years, there has been heightened awareness of and concern about the potentially harmful side effects associated with radiation exposure, particularly in the pediatric population.[22,23] For this reason, the practice of the "as low as is reasonably achievable" principle among the radiologic community is critical, with special attention given to CT protocols and parameters.[22,24] In evaluating paranasal sinuses, it is possible to reduce radiation techniques for maxillofacial CT imaging, even to a level comparable to that used for standard radiographic images, *without* sacrificing diagnostic image quality.[25]

MAGNETIC RESONANCE IMAGING

The role of sinus MRI in imaging inflammatory disease is limited, but it is valuable in evaluating complications of sinusitis (e.g., intracranial extension), as well as inflammatory disease associated with sinus or parasinal neoplasm. However, MRI does not depict bony detail and is less sensitive for bony erosions. Other limitations include its availability, higher costs, and the frequent need for sedation in young children.

The normal nasal cycle of vasodilation and mucosal edema followed by vasoconstriction and mucosal shrinkage can produce signal changes that can create significant variability in findings and thus differing interpretations. This cycle varies from 50 minutes to 6 hours, and the signal intensity during the edematous phase is indistinguishable from that of inflammatory change. As with CT and plain radiographs, sinus MRI typically shows a high incidence of findings in asymptomatic persons (13% to 37%) and mucosal thickening of <3 mm that is likely insignificant.[2] MRI can differentiate mucosal thickening from sinus secretions (Fig. 8-11, *A–E*).

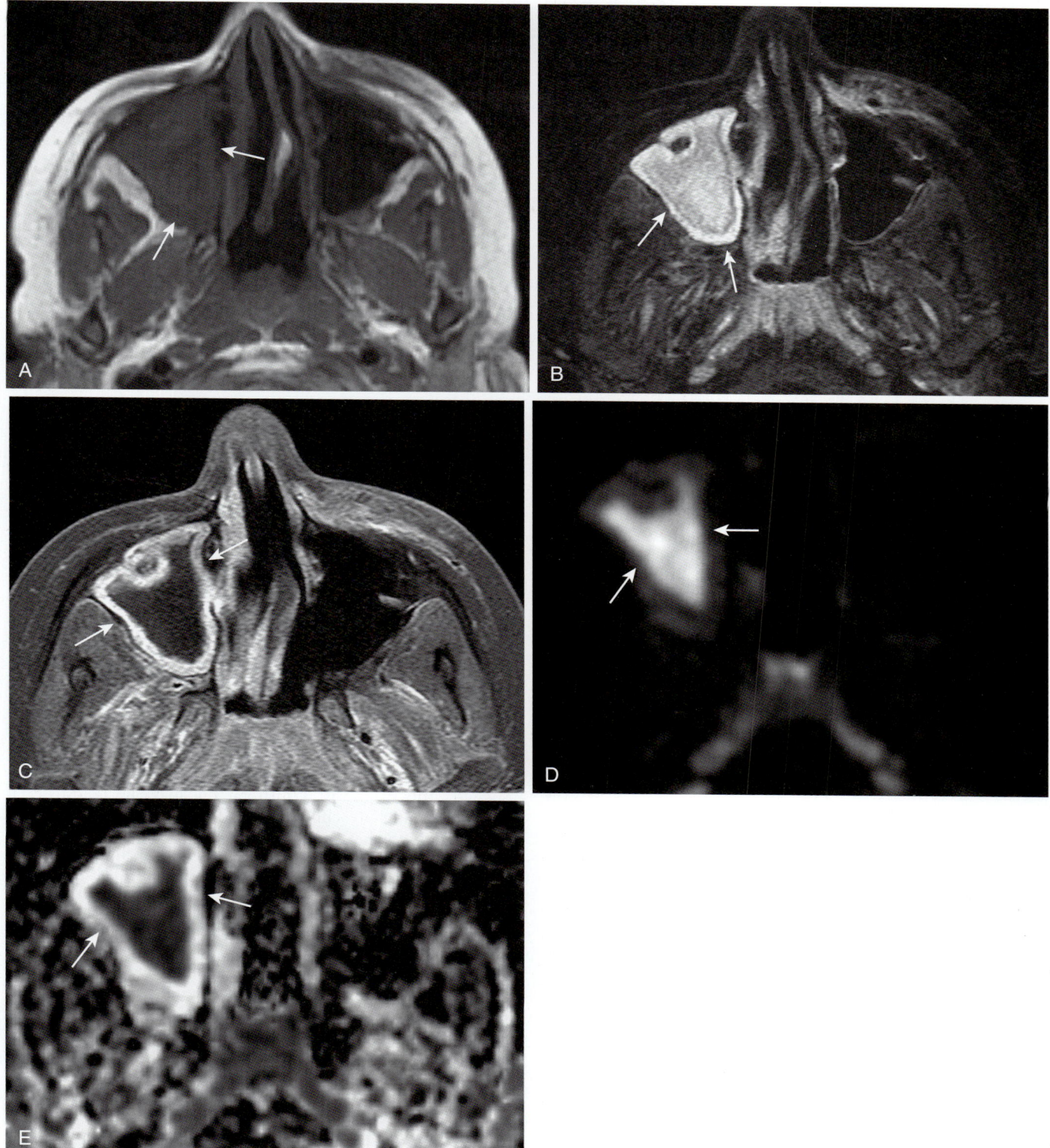

Figure 8-11 Acute bacterial sinusitis in a 10-year-old boy. **A,** An axial T1-weighted magnetic resonance (MR) image shows hypointense material in the right maxillary sinus (*arrows*). **B,** An axial T2-weighted MR image shows corresponding T2-hyperintense material (*arrows*). **C,** An axial T1-weighted MR image with fat saturation and contrast shows circumferential mucosal enhancement. **D** and **E,** Corresponding decreased diffusivity in the right maxillary sinus is shown on diffusion-weighted imaging and apparent diffusion coefficient maps consistent with purulent material.

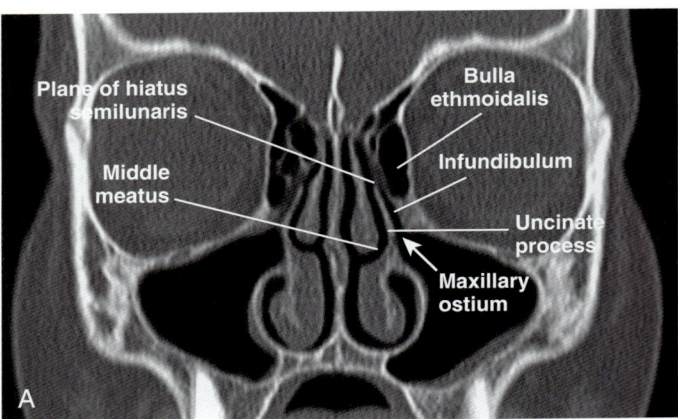
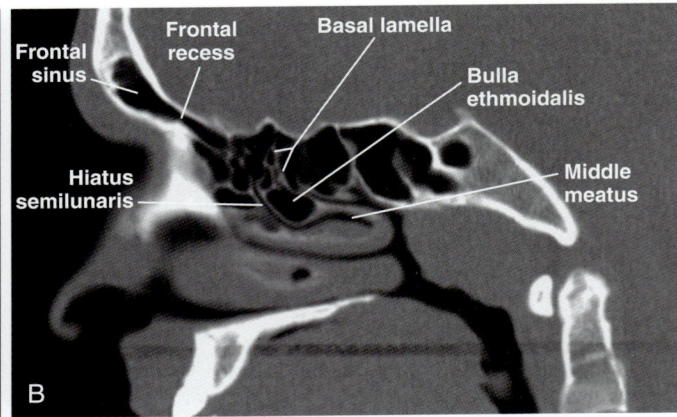

Figure 8-12 Ostiomeatal unit (OMU). **A,** A coronal computed tomography (CT) image shows the OMU components: middle meatus, uncinate process, infundibulum, bulla ethmoidalis, maxillary ostium, and plane of the hiatus semilunaris. **B,** A sagittal CT image demonstrates the hiatus semilunaris.

Along with CT, MRI is very useful in evaluating neoplasms. An estimated 90% to 95% of tumors in the sinuses or nasal cavity exhibit moderately lower signal intensities on T2-weighted images (from hypercellularity) compared with most acute inflammatory diseases (including polyps, mucoceles, and retention cysts), which produce a bright signal on T2-weighted images. However, more mature granulation tissue and fibrosis also have a lower T2 signal, making it difficult to distinguish from tumor. Certain fungal infections, in contrast to other types of acute inflammatory disease, also have a lower T2 signal.

Imaging Anatomy of the Sinonasal Cavities

OSTIOMEATAL UNIT

Regarded as an important anatomic region for potential surgical intervention, the ostiomeatal unit is a complex anatomic structure at the crossroads of mucociliary drainage from the frontal, anterior ethmoid, and maxillary sinuses.[26] It includes the uncinate process, infundibulum, ethmoid bulla, hiatus semilunaris, and middle meatus (Fig. 8-12, A and B).[13]

The uncinate process arises from the upper medial maxillary wall and defines the wall of the infundibulum.[27] The infundibulum is the channel defined laterally by orbit or Haller cells and medially by the uncinate process. The ethmoid bulla is a dominant middle ethmoid air cell that protrudes inferomedially into the infundibulum and hiatus semilunaris. The hiatus semilunaris is a semilunar region between the tip of the uncinate process and ethmoid bulla (see Fig. 8-12, A and B).

Congenital Lesions of the Nose

CHOANAL ATRESIA

Choanal atresia, the most common congenital abnormality of the nasal cavity, is thought to result from failure of rupture of the oronasal membrane during the sixth week of fetal life. It consists of obstruction of the posterior opening of the nasal cavity, which is mixed bony-membranous in approximately 70% of cases and pure bony atresia in 30% of cases. The existence of a purely membranous atresia has been questioned, and evaluation with high-resolution CT often has failed to demonstrate a membranous atresia without a bony component.[28] Choanal atresia can be unilateral (in 50% to 60% of cases) or bilateral, and it is more common in girls (the female:male ratio is 2:1).

Clinical Presentation Bilateral choanal atresia presents with severe immediate onset of respiratory distress in the newborn, because infants are obligate nasal breathers. Symptoms are aggravated by feeding and relieved by crying. The inability to pass a nasogastric tube in a neonate with well-aerated lungs suggests the diagnosis. Unilateral choanal atresia usually is diagnosed later in childhood and presents with unilateral purulent rhinorrhea.

Imaging Noncontrast CT is the imaging modality of choice. Nasal secretions should be suctioned before imaging is performed; administration of a nasal topical vasoconstrictor spray helps in reducing mucosal thickening. High-resolution imaging in bone algorithm will aid in delineating the bone margins. Findings consist of narrowing of the posterior choana (<0.34 cm in children <2 years of age) and enlargement and thickening of the vomer (>0.23 cm), which sometimes is fused to the maxilla.[29] Medial bowing and thickening of the posterior aspect of the lateral wall of the nasal cavity also is seen. The nasal cavity often is filled with air, soft tissue, and fluid (Fig. 8-13, A and B). CT will identify other causes of bilateral nasal obstruction such as pyriform aperture stenosis and bilateral nasolacrimal duct cysts. Bilateral choanal atresia can be associated with other congenital abnormalities in 75% of cases, such as in persons with CHARGE syndrome.

Treatment The oral airway should be secured and surgical correction of bilateral atresia should be performed as soon as possible after diagnosis. Transpalatal or transnasal endoscopic surgical techniques may be used.

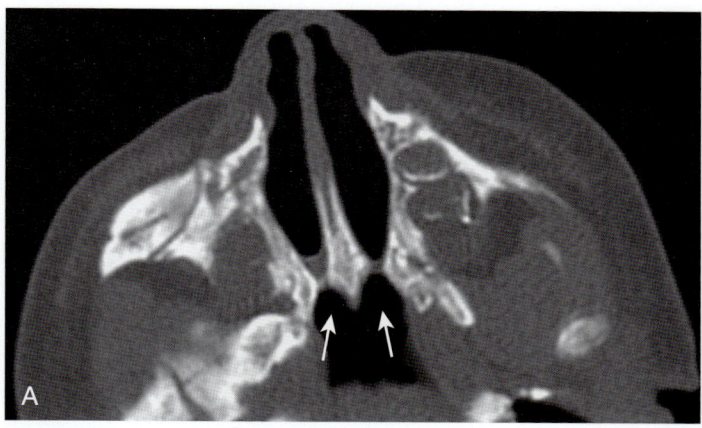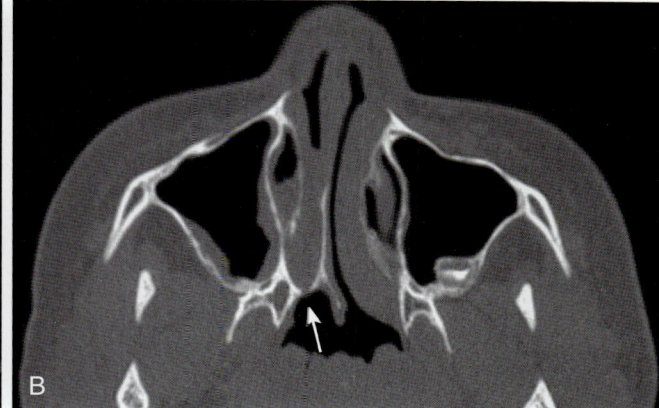

Figure 8-13 A, Choanal atresia in a 1-day-old neonate with severe respiratory distress. An axial computed tomography (CT) image shows bilateral bony choanal atresia with retained fluid in the right nasal cavity, medial bowing of the lateral nasal wall, and a thickened vomer. **B,** A 12-year-old child with chronic nasal obstruction and purulent rhinorrhea. An axial CT image shows unilateral (right) bony atresia with fluid in the nasal cavity.

CONGENITAL NASAL PYRIFORM APERTURE STENOSIS

Congenital nasal pyriform aperture stenosis is a rare form of nasal obstruction that consists of narrowing of the nasal pyriform aperture as a result of bony overgrowth of the nasal process of the maxilla.[30] It should be suspected in any neonate with upper respiratory obstruction and needs to be differentiated from choanal atresia and other congenital nasal masses.

Clinical Presentation Symptoms depend on the severity of the stenosis and are similar to those in patients with choanal atresia, including cyanosis in the neonatal period that is exacerbated with feeding and relieved by crying. Congenital nasal pyriform aperture stenosis can present in association with other congenital anomalies such as holoprosencephaly, hypopituitarism, a single mega-incisor, hypotelorism, cleft palate, clinodactyly, or absent olfactory bulbs.[31,32] A central mega-incisor often is associated with intracranial abnormalities, and thus further evaluation with MRI of the brain is indicated in these cases.

Imaging Congenital nasal pyriform aperture stenosis is confirmed with CT and is characterized by overgrowth of the medial nasal process of the maxilla, resulting in narrowing of the anterior bony nasal cavity, and is usually bilateral. A pyriform aperture of less than 11 mm in a term infant is diagnostic.[30] The choanae are usually normal in caliber, but choanal atresia may coexist.[31] The hard palate is usually hypoplastic and in the shape of a triangle with the presence of a median maxillary single incisor tooth (mega-incisor) (Fig. 8-14, *A-C*).

Treatment Treatment consists of securing the airway, with surgical intervention required in severe cases.

CONGENITAL NASOLACRIMAL DUCT DACROCYSTOCELES

Congenital nasolacrimal duct dacryocystoceles consist of a cystic dilatation of the nasolacrimal apparatus as a result of proximal and or distal obstruction of the nasolacrimal duct, which is thought to result from failure of duct canalization. Dacryocystoceles can be unilateral or bilateral. Ductal dilatation can occur at any level from the lacrimal sac (a proximal lesion at the medial canthus) to the opening of the duct in the inferior meatus (a distal lesion in the inferior meatus underturbinate), with enlargement of the bony duct.

Clinical Presentation A proximal lesion, a dacryocystocele, presents clinically as a round, bluish, medial, canthal mass usually identified at birth; it may vary in size from 5 to 10 mm. A distal lesion, a nasolacrimal duct cyst, usually presents in the neonatal period as an intranasal mass causing airway obstruction if it is bilateral. Neonates also can present with difficulty breathing while feeding.

Imaging CT findings include a well-circumscribed, rounded, unilateral or bilateral hypodense "cystic" lesion in the medial canthus and/or anteroinferior nasal cavity. The cyst can communicate with an enlarged nasolacrimal duct (Fig. 8-15, *A*). Large cysts may cause nasal septal deviation. Association with choanal atresia has been described. Contrast-enhanced CT will show no enhancement or minimal wall enhancement. Infected dacryocystoceles present with thick rim enhancement.

MR findings include a T1-weighted hypointense and T2-weighted hyperintense well-circumscribed mass at the medial canthus and/or nasal cavity with no enhancement or minimal wall enhancement (Fig. 8-15, *B* and *C*). Dacryocystoceles can be diagnosed prenatally with fetal ultrasound or MRI.[33]

Treatment Congenital dacryocystoceles may resolve with conservative treatment, but many become infected and require systemic antibiotic treatment; most need surgical intervention. Early referral to an ophthalmologist can help in timely intervention.[33]

Other Nasal Masses

Other frontonasal or intranasal masses that can present similarly include naso-orbital cephaloceles, hemangiomas, dermoid

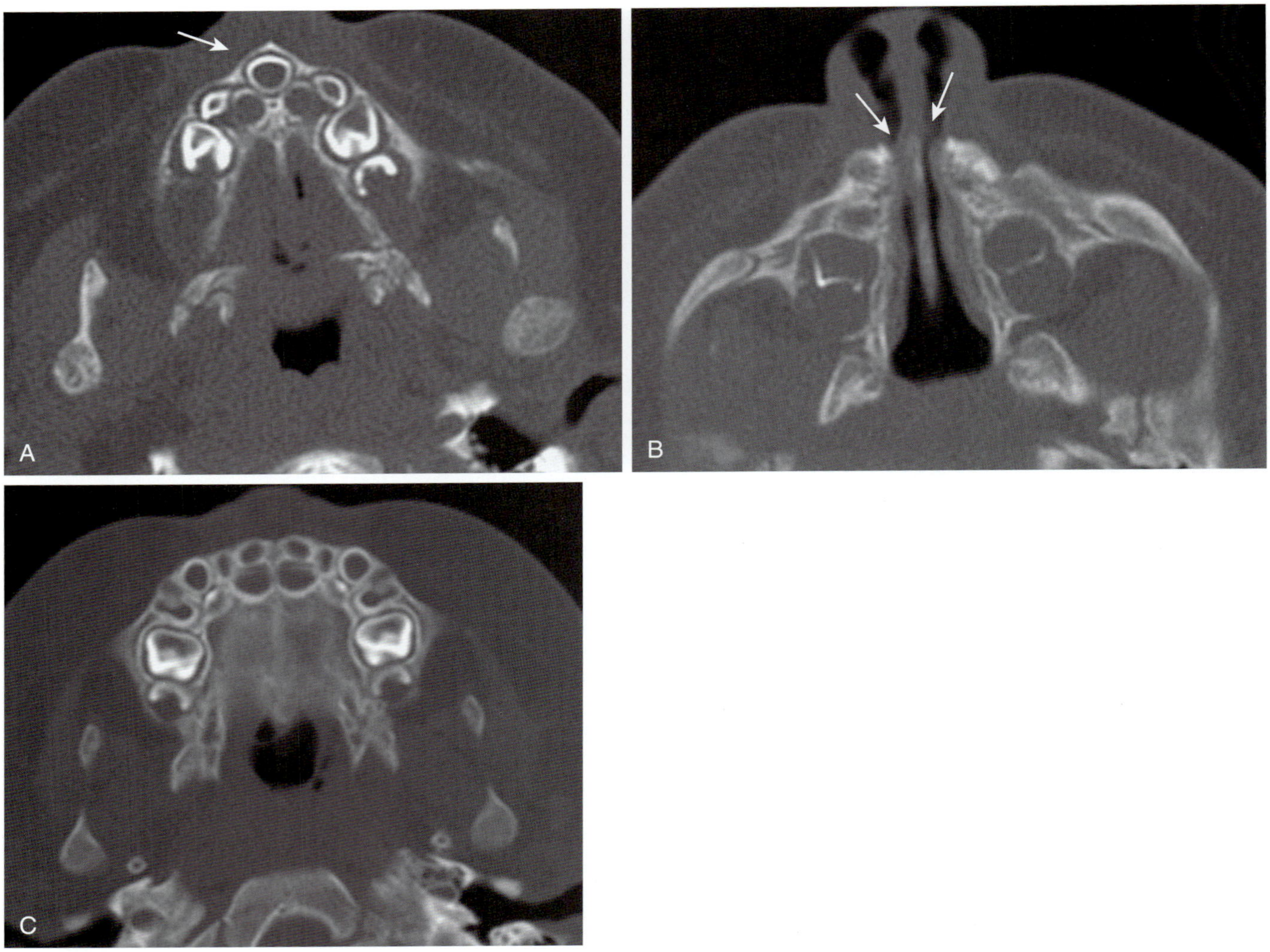

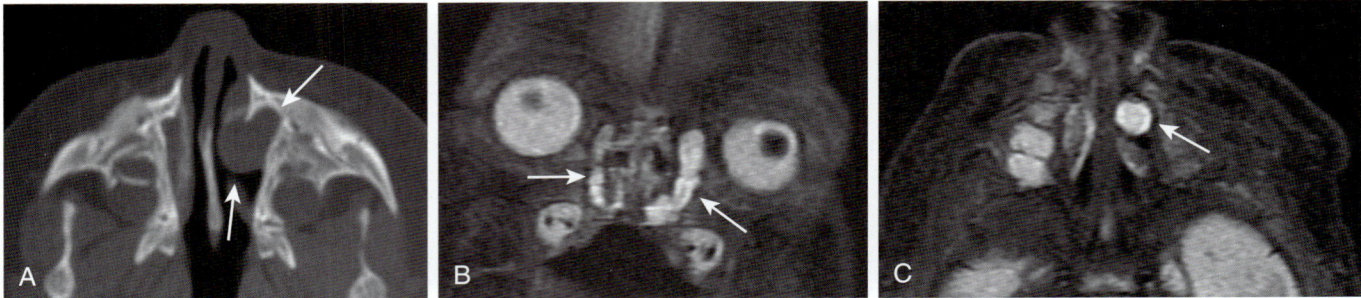

Figure 8-14 Congenital nasal pyriform aperture stenosis in a 1½-month-old infant with episodes of respiratory distress during breastfeeding. **A,** An axial computed tomography (CT) image shows a triangular hard palate and solitary central maxillary mega-incisor (*arrow*). **B,** An axial CT image shows narrowing of the anterior and inferior nasal passages. **C,** A normal infant maxilla for comparison.

cysts, and nasal gliomas and should be included in the differential diagnosis.

Naso-orbital cephaloceles present as frontal, nasal, or medial orbital nonenhancing soft tissue masses contiguous with the intracranial brain, which extends through a bony defect. The adjacent meninges may enhance (e-Fig. 8-16, *A*).

A hemangioma of infancy is a well-defined, lobular mass that enhances diffusely and intensely.

A nasal glioma (nasal glial heterotopia) is a nonenhancing extranasal (along the nasal dorsum) or intranasal solid soft tissue mass without connection between the mass and intracranial contents (e-Fig. 8-16, *B* and *C*).

Figure 8-15 Congenital nasolacrimal duct dacryocystoceles in a 1-day-old neonate. **A,** An axial computed tomography image shows a left nasal round soft tissue mass with enlargement of the ipsilateral nasolacrimal duct and canal (*arrows*). **B** and **C,** Coronal and axial magnetic resonance fast spin-echo inversion recovery images show bilateral cystic enlargement of the nasolacrimal sacs and ducts (*arrows*).

A nasal dermal sinus with or without a cyst presents as an enhancing tract from the tip of the nose to the foramen cecum (intracranially) just anterior to the crista galli with or without a dermoid/epidermoid cyst along its tract (e-Fig. 8-16, *D*). On diffusion-weighted imaging, the cyst will demonstrate high signal restricted diffusion.

Imaging of Specific Sinonasal Disease Entities

SINUSITIS

Rhinosinusitis is characterized by inflammation of the sinonasal mucosa, usually after an upper respiratory infection (URI). Children contract an average of three to eight viral URIs per year that are generally self-limited, with no antimicrobial therapy required.[34] However, acute bacterial sinusitis (ABS) can complicate viral rhinosinusitis in up to 13% of affected children.[21] Other predisposing conditions for sinusitis are allergic rhinitis, immunoglobulin deficiency, immotile cilia syndrome, cystic fibrosis (CF), and anatomic abnormalities causing obstruction of the drainage pathways. The AAP has defined five categories of bacterial rhinosinusitis: acute, subacute, recurrent acute, ABS superimposed on chronic disease, and chronic sinusitis.[21]

Bacterial sinusitis remains a challenging clinical diagnosis because the signs and symptoms of sinusitis typically seen in adults are noted less frequently in children. Because specific clinical signs in children are generally few, it often is difficult to differentiate ABS from viral rhinosinusitis. Signs and symptoms in children vary and may include cough, purulent nasal discharge, facial pain, fever, headache, and malodorous breath. A frequent cough and the urge to clear the throat usually is due to posterior nasopharyngeal drainage. Nasal congestion is frequent and leads particularly to nocturnal mouth breathing, which results in a sore throat upon awakening in the morning. Constitutional complaints are frequent, including malaise, poor appetite, easy fatigability, and irritability.[34]

The gold standard for diagnosis of acute or chronic sinusitis remains aspiration from the sinus cavities with the recovery of bacteria in a high density (>10 colony-forming units/mL).[21] However, this method is impractical, invasive, and time-consuming and is rarely performed. For this reason, the diagnosis of sinusitis usually is based on clinical criteria; it is the duration rather than the severity of symptoms that raises suspicion for ABS. This diagnosis is considered when a URI with purulent discharge lasts for >10 days.

ACUTE SINUSITIS

The AAP defines ABS as sinusitis in which symptoms resolve completely and that lasts <30 days. Common causative microorganisms are *Streptococcus pneumoniae*, *Haemophilus influenzae*, and *Moraxella catarrhalis*.

Imaging Imaging of the paranasal sinuses in children with uncomplicated ABS is unnecessary and generally is not recommended because the results will not affect treatment decisions. Imaging cannot differentiate between viral and bacterial sinusitis. Mucosal abnormalities are reported routinely on radiographs, CT, and MRI in asymptomatic patients who undergo imaging for other indications. The incidence of abnormal findings is very high in infants and young children. For example, in a study of infants who had a cold in the 2 weeks preceding a head CT performed for reasons other than sinusitis, mucosal abnormalities were detected in the sinuses of 97% of the babies examined. Soft tissue changes can persist for months on MRI after an acute infection.[20] For these reasons, clinical correlation is vital when evaluating imaging findings in children.

Treatment A course of antibiotics is recommended to speed resolution of symptoms and to prevent possible complications. Amoxicillin for 10 to 14 days is the usual treatment, although other antibiotics may be used.

CHRONIC SINUSITIS

The AAP defines chronic sinusitis as episodes of inflammation of the paranasal sinuses lasting >90 days. Patients have persistent residual respiratory symptoms such as cough, rhinorrhea, and/or nasal obstruction. Children who experience chronic sinusitis usually are older (at least 4 to 7 years of age) and often have a history of recurrent ABS. Other associated factors are recurrent viral URIs, allergic and nonallergic rhinitis, CF, immunodeficiency, ciliary dyskinesia, sinus and facial anatomic abnormalities, and gastroesophageal reflux.[35]

Clinical findings are similar to those of acute infection but are characterized mostly by a continuous nasal discharge and congestion with a persistent nighttime cough. Other symptoms include chronic headache, chronic halitosis, intermittent fever, sleep deprivation, and general malaise. In persons with chronic sinusitis, *Staphylococcus aureus*, coagulation negative *Staphylococcus*, anaerobic organisms, gram-negative bacteria, and fungi are the most commonly encountered colonizing organisms.[35]

Imaging Radiography can show mucosal thickening or sinus opacification and, occasionally, sclerotic, thickened walls. CT findings include peripheral mucosal thickening in a hypodistended or contracted sinus with sclerotic thickened walls, although these findings are uncommon in children. Calcifications may be seen occasionally, and sinonasal polyposis also may be present. Secretions can be dense depending on their content. MR findings include mucosal thickening that enhances with administration of contrast material. Retained secretions will vary in signal intensity depending on content (see Fig. 8-11, *A-E*). Desiccated secretions are hypointense on T2-weighted imaging.

Treatment Initial trial therapy includes environmental control, allergic therapy if indicated, antibiotics for 21 days directed to resistant organisms, saline solution irrigation, and topical nasal corticosteroids. Second-line therapy includes oral decongestants and oral corticosteroids. Endoscopic sinus surgery remains the most definitive therapy.[35]

COMPLICATIONS OF RHINOSINUSITIS

Orbital and intracranial complications of rhinosinusitis can result from delayed diagnosis and treatment, antibiotic-resistant or aggressive organisms, or incomplete treatment.

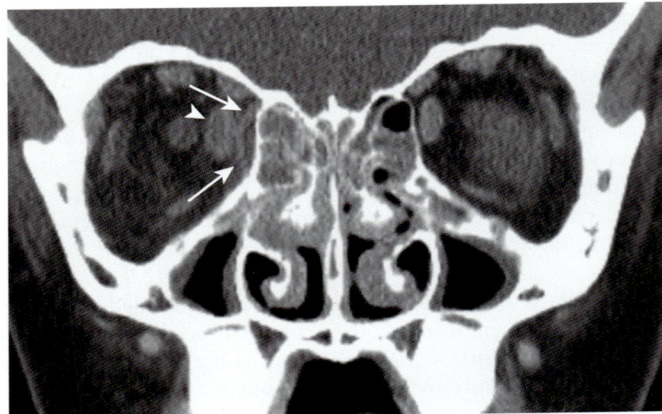

Figure 8-17 An orbital subperiosteal abscess in a 9-year-old girl. A coronal contrast-enhanced computed tomography image shows a small, low-attenuation, rim-enhancing fluid collection consistent with an abscess (*arrows*) in the medial aspect of the orbit with mass effect on the medial rectus muscle (*arrowhead*), which is thickened. Bilateral ethmoid sinus disease with infiltration of the right retro-orbital fat is demonstrated.

Signs and symptoms of orbital complications include periorbital edema, proptosis, chemosis, decreased visual acuity, and/or limited ocular motility. Potential intracranial complications should be suspected when a patient has a history of acute sinusitis combined with severe intractable headache, an altered level of consciousness, focal neurologic deficits, or signs of meningitis.[36]

Orbital complications usually result from the spread of ethmoid infection that occurs via valveless ethmoid veins that traverse the lamina papyracea. Extension of disease also can arise from the sphenoid, frontal, and maxillary sinuses in order of frequency. Complications include orbital cellulitis with inflammatory edema, preseptal cellulitis, postseptal cellulitis, subperiosteal abscess (Fig. 8-17) (see Chapter 6), orbital abscess (e-Fig. 8-18), optic neuritis, and cavernous sinus thrombosis.

Intracranial complications include epidural empyema, subdural empyema, meningitis, cerebritis, and parenchymal abscess (e-Fig. 8-19, *A-G*). Subgaleal involvement such as

with Pott puffy tumor and osteomyelitis also can occur (Fig. 8-20, *A* and *B*). Vascular complications are infrequent and include mycotic aneurysm, stenosis of the cavernous segment of the internal carotid artery (which, in very rare instances, can result in brain infarction[37]), and venous sinus thrombosis. Superior sagittal thrombosis usually results from frontal sinusitis, whereas sigmoid sinus thrombosis and cavernous sinus thrombosis are associated more often with sphenoid sinusitis (Fig. 8-21, *C*).

Imaging Imaging enables diagnosis and accurate presurgical planning when necessary. For the initial evaluation, contrast-enhanced CT is the imaging modality of choice and should include both the paranasal sinuses and brain. Noncontrast CT should not be performed because it increases the radiation dose without providing any additional diagnostic information. CT can demonstrate fluid collections with rim enhancement consistent with subperiosteal abscesses (see Fig. 8-17) and bone erosion of osteomyelitis as seen with Pott puffy tumor (extracranial subperiosteal abscess from frontal sinusitis) (Fig. 8-20, *A* and *B*).[38,39]

MRI is indicated to further assess known or suspected intracranial extension of disease and should include imaging of the brain, sinuses, and orbits. MRI protocols for the brain should include diffusion and contrast-enhanced sequences and should evaluate for venous thromboses. MRI protocols for the paranasal sinuses and orbits should include high-resolution axial and coronal images before and after administration of gadolinium. MRI is more sensitive than CT in the assessment of leptomeningeal enhancement, small extraaxial fluid collections, and parenchymal abnormalities such as cerebritis and cerebral abscess (see e-Fig. 8-19, *E-G*). MRI also can detect early stages of osteomyelitis by demonstrating bone marrow edema with associated contrast enhancement. Diffusion-weighted imaging will show restricted diffusion of fluid collections with purulent contents (see Fig. 8-11, *A-E*).

Subperiosteal abscesses will appear hypointense on T1-weighted imaging and hyperintense on T2-weighted imaging with peripheral contrast enhancement. Signs of cavernous sinus thrombosis include enlargement or heterogeneous enhancement of the cavernous sinus with associated enlargement or thrombosis of the superior ophthalmic vein

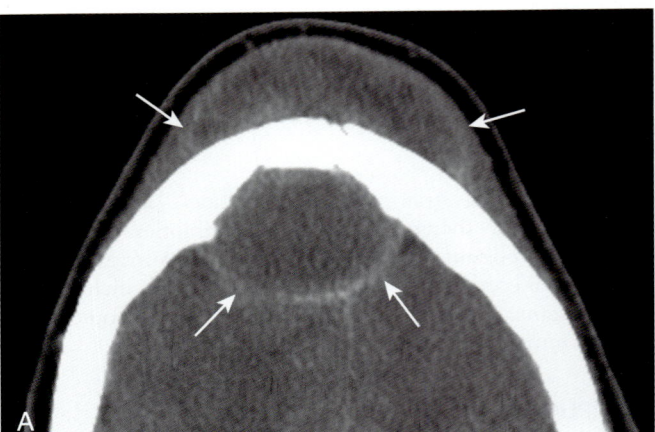

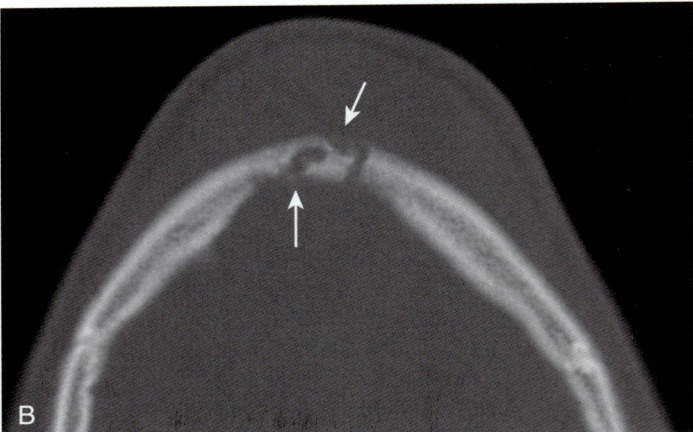

Figure 8-20 Pott puffy tumor and epidural abscess in a 16-year-old boy. **A,** A contrast-enhanced computed tomography image in a soft tissue window shows a large subperiosteal abscess (*top arrows*) and a large epidural abscess (*bottom arrows*). **B,** An axial image in a bone window shows erosion of the frontal bone consistent with osteomyelitis (*arrows*).

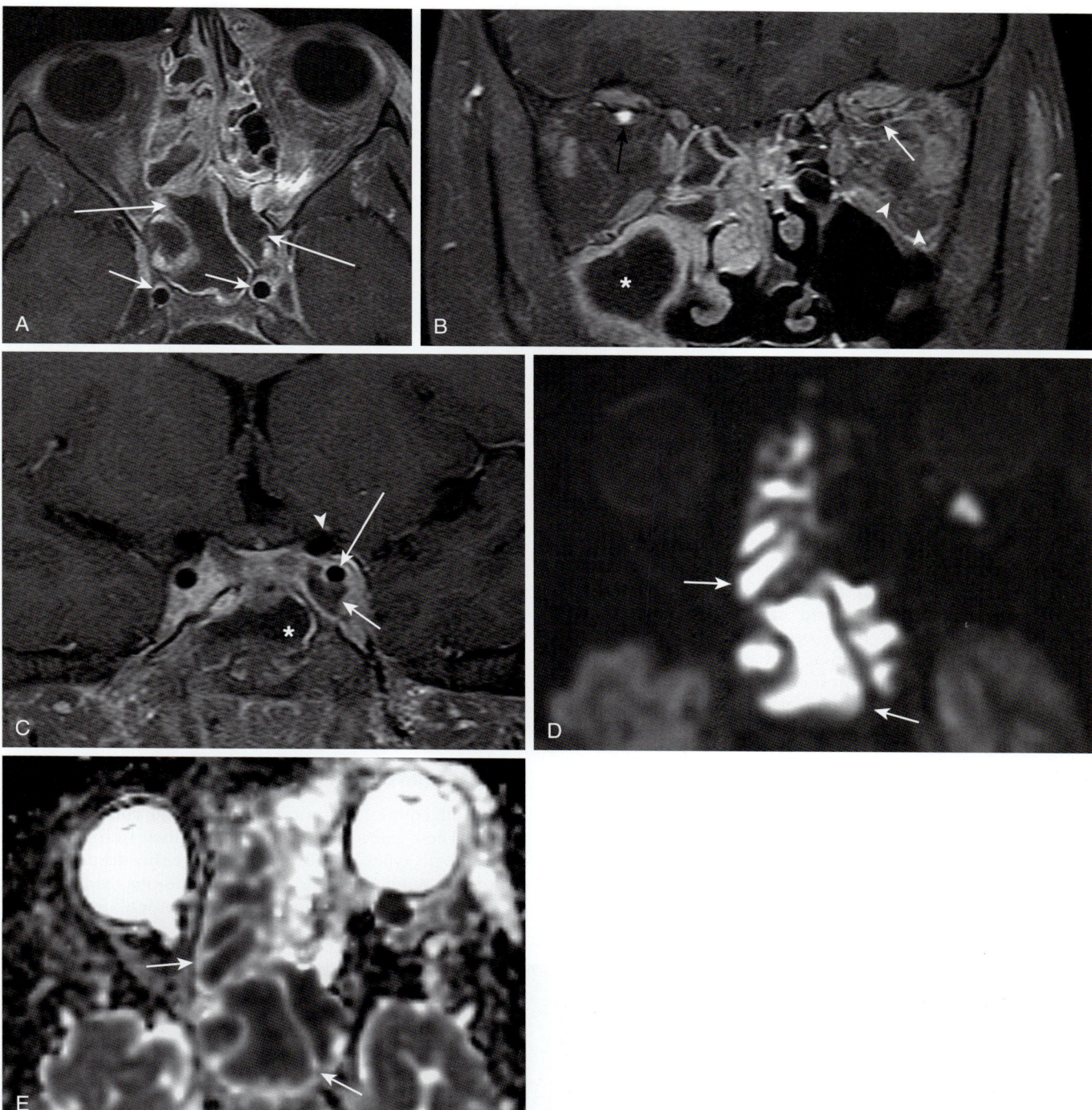

Figure 8-21 Sinusitis with a left periorbital abscess and cavernous sinus thrombosis in a 10-year-old boy. **A,** A postcontrast axial T1-weighted magnetic resonance image with fat saturation shows hypointense fluid within the ethmoid and sphenoid sinuses with circumferential mucosal enhancement (*long arrows*) and normal flow voids of the cavernous internal carotid artery (ICA) segments (*short arrows*). **B,** A coronal T1-weighted image with fat saturation shows a thrombus in the left superior ophthalmic vein (*white arrow*), normal enhancement of the right superior ophthalmic vein (*black arrow*), and inflammatory changes in the retro-orbital fat (*arrowheads*). **C,** A coronal T1-weighted image with fat saturation shows a thrombus in the left cavernous sinus (*bottom arrow*) and normal flow void of the left ICA cavernous segment (*long arrow*) and left ICA supraclinoid segment (*arrowhead*). A fluid-filled sphenoid sinus is shown (*asterisk*). Corresponding restricted diffusion on diffusion-weighted imaging (**D**) and apparent diffusion coefficient maps (**E**) consistent with purulent material.

(Fig. 8-21, *A-E*). Subdural and epidural empyemas appear as T1-hypointense and T2-hyperintense fluid collections with adjacent dural enhancement and central decreased diffusivity as a result of the presence of purulent material (see e-Fig. 8-19, *B-D*). Cerebritis appears as a poorly defined area of T2 prolongation without ring enhancement, whereas a cerebral abscess will present as a ring-enhancing lesion with central decreased diffusivity and perilesional edema (see e-Fig. 8-19, *E* and *F*).

Treatment Treatment includes combinations of systemic intravenous antibiotics and surgical interventions such as drainage of the sinuses, functional endoscopic sinus surgery, and craniotomy. Because of the high incidence of seizures associated with intracranial abscess, anticonvulsant therapy is recommended as prophylaxis in patients with intracranial complications.[36]

SINONASAL DISEASE IN PERSONS WITH CYSTIC FIBROSIS

CF is caused by a genetic defect in the long arm of chromosome 7, which affects the protein that regulates transmembrane passage of chlorine ion and causes dysfunction of multiple organs and systems.[40] High concentrations of chlorine, mucus thickness, and reduction of mucociliary clearance predisposes to inflammation and chronic infection of the respiratory tract. Nearly 100% of persons with CF present clinically with nasal obstruction and chronic rhinosinusitis (Fig. 8-22, *A* and *B*).[41] The most common organisms colonizing the sinonasal mucosa in order of frequency are *Pseudomonas aeruginosa*, *S. aureus*, and *Streptococcus viridans*.[42]

Imaging CT is the imaging modality of choice for evaluating sinus disease in patients with CF and will show abnormalities in nearly all of these persons. Findings include mucosal thickening and sinonasal polyposis. The incidence of nasal polyposis in children with CF varies between 10% and 86%.[43-45] High–attenuation material often is present in the sinus cavities, consistent with inspissated secretions (see

Fig. 8-22, *A*). However, superimposed fungal infection has a similar appearance and cannot be excluded on the basis of imaging. Bony sclerosis and thickening of the sinuses can be seen in older patients. Frontal sinus hypoplasia or aplasia is a common finding and may be a result of poor aeration from chronic obstruction. The severity of the imaging findings does not necessarily correlate with the severity of symptoms.[41]

Treatment Medical and surgical treatment depends on symptoms and the overall condition of the patient, including pulmonary status and infection frequency. Not all patients will require surgery.[46] Imaging findings of CF cannot be differentiated from other causes of chronic sinusitis such as allergic sinusitis with polyposis or fungal allergic sinusitis.

ALLERGIC SINUSITIS

It is estimated that allergic rhinosinusitis affects about 10% of the population. In the United States, the most common form is seasonal pollinosis, resulting from an immunoglobulin E reagin–antibody reaction (type I immunologic disorder), which manifests clinically with sneezing, nasal obstruction, and rhinorrhea. This condition can result in hypertrophic, thickened, and redundant mucosa, known as hypertrophic polypoid mucosa, which is prone to bacterial infection. Allergic sinusitis often coexists with chronic asthma, and 30% of patients will present with polyps (e-Fig. 8-23, *A* and *B*). Conversely, up to 80% of patients with polyps have asthma.[47,48] The association of allergic asthma, allergy to aspirin, and aggressive polyposis is known as the Samter triad (e-Fig. 8-23, *A* and *B*). Polyps in this condition can be destructive and invade the anterior cranial fossa.[2]

FUNGAL RHINOSINUSITIS DISORDERS

Fungal infections can cause both acute and chronic rhinosinusitis. These infections have been classified into four clinicopathologic types that can present as either tissue-invasive disorders (acute invasive fulminant disease and chronic invasive infection) or noninvasive disorders (noninvasive

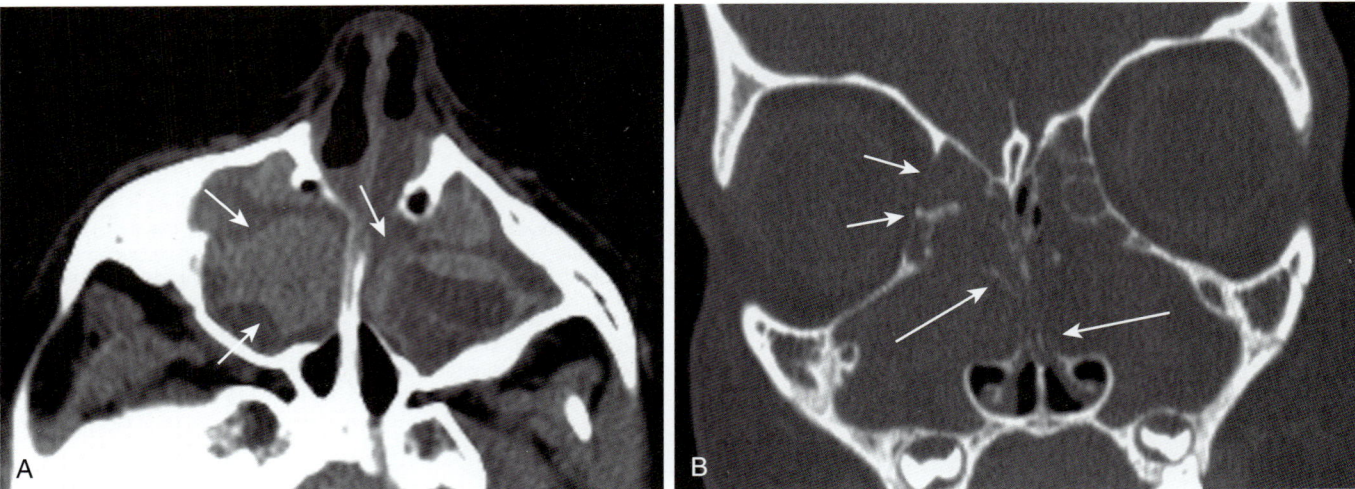

Figure 8-22 Cystic fibrosis in an 8-year-old child. **A,** High attenuation secretions in the maxillary sinuses shown on axial computed tomography (CT) (*arrows*). **B,** Polyps causing expansion of the sinuses (*short arrows*) and nasal cavity with demineralization of septations shown on a coronal CT image (*long arrows*).

mycotic colonization ["fungus ball" or mycetoma] and allergic fungal [mycotic] sinusitis).[49] All of these entities are rare in children.

Acute invasive fulminant disease occurs in persons who are immunosuppressed and clinically presents as pale mucosa that can progress to gangrene. Spread through neuronal routes can cause vascular invasion with intracranial spread and parenchymal infarcts. Mucormycosis is a disease caused by several types of fungi and can have an acute and fulminant course. In persons with diabetes, mucormycosis can present more as a chronic tissue-invasive infection and frequently causes periorbital invasion (orbital apex syndrome).[49]

A fungal ball or "mycetoma" consists of fungal hyphae compressed into a thick exudate within a sinus lumen.[49] It is a benign fungal colonization and may occur in patients with previous sinus surgery, oral-sinus fistula, a history of chemotherapy or radiotherapy for cancer, or in those without any known predisposing factor.

Allergic fungal rhinosinusitis should be considered in all adults with chronic sinusitis, but it is rarely seen in young children. Clinical presentation may include a history of allergic sinusitis, chronic rhinosinusitis, nasal polyps, allergic asthma, and immunosuppression, and it can present with proptosis from an inflammatory mass.[35,50] The diagnosis is primarily histopathologic. At surgery a characteristic inspissated sinonasal inflammatory exudate called allergic mucin is encountered and must be positive for fungal hyphae on fungal staining or cultures. No evidence for mucosal fungal invasion should be present.[50]

Imaging Radiographically, fungal disease is difficult, if not impossible, to distinguish from bacterial infection. Radiographic signs include sinonasal polyposis with a heterogenous soft tissue inflammatory mass with remodeling or destruction of bone and increased densities in the sinuses, which can represent calcifications. Allergic mucin is largely responsible for the sinus CT hyperattenuation.[50] MRI findings can suggest fungal infection because, in contrast to the high signal intensity on T2-weighted images seen with acute bacterial disease, the presence of calcium, air, or ferromagnetic elements in the fungus causes decreased signal intensity on T1-weighted and T2-weighted images. However, inspissated secretions as seen in patients with CF can have a similar appearance.

Benign Masses in the Sinuses

CYSTS, POLYPS, AND MUCOCELES

Cysts and polyps are frequent complications of inflammatory rhinosinusitis. A mucous retention cyst results from the obstruction of a submucosal mucinous gland, and the cyst wall is the duct epithelium. These cysts can occur in any sinus but are more frequently found in the inferior aspect of the maxillary sinus. A serous retention cyst results from the accumulation of serous fluid in the submucosal layer of the sinus mucosal lining.[2] These cysts are not inflammatory lesions and appear as dome-shaped, well-defined, homogeneous, nonenhancing structures on CT; they are hypointense on T1-weighted MR images and hyperintense on T2-weighted images (Fig. 8-24, A). Cysts also can be found incidentally in 10% to 30% of patients.[51]

Polyps, in contrast, are a manifestation of an allergic or inflammatory process, or both. When they are associated with an allergy, polyps tend to be multiple. These lesions can become large and cause bony distortion with expansion and erosion. Polyps can be difficult to distinguish from mucous retention cysts in some cases and malignancies in others. Polyps have a high T2-weighted MR signal, in contrast to most neoplasms, which helps in the diagnosis.

An antrochoanal polyp (sinonasal solitary polyp) is a maxillary sinus polyp that fills the sinus, expands the sinus ostium, and prolapses through it into the posterior choana, presenting as a nasal or nasopharyngeal polyp (Fig. 8-24, B and C). Although they are rare, sphenochoanal and ethmochoanal polyps also can occur. In the general population these polyps represent 4% to 6% of all nasal polyps; however, in children the incidence increases to 28% to 33%.[52] Antrochoanal polyps differ from inflammatory polyps; they tend to be fibrotic with minimal inflammation and are composed of a cystic portion filling the maxillary sinus and a solid dumbbell-shaped portion that emerges into the nasal cavity through the maxillary infundibulum or through an accessory ostium of the maxillary sinus. These polyps are usually unilateral solitary lesions; however, bilateral antrochoanal polyps can be seen in 20% to 25% of cases. The clinical presentation is nasal obstruction and discharge, mouth breathing, snoring, and sleep apnea.

On CT, most antrochoanal polyps have mucoid attenuation. When contrast material is administered, mucosal surface enhancement can occur, but without central enhancement. Antrochoanal polyps can appear denser when inspissated secretions are present. On MRI, antrochoanal polyps usually appear hyperintense on T2-weighted images because of their high water content.

Mucoceles, which are most common in the frontal (60%) and ethmoid (30%) sinuses and result from obstruction or sequestration of a portion of the sinus, are cystic lesions lined with respiratory epithelium and filled with mucoid secretions.[53] Mucoceles are rare in the sphenoid[54] and maxillary sinuses. The association of mucoceles and CF is frequent.[55] Clinical symptoms result from the mass effect of the lesion and depend on location; these symptoms may include proptosis, headache, cranial nerve impingement, or nasal obstruction (e-Fig. 8-25, A-D).

On CT, mucoceles are low-density, nonenhancing masses that can expand the sinus. Thin rim enhancement can occur; however, if enhancement is thick or nodular, infection should be considered. Calcification in the wall suggests remote infection. The signal varies on MRI, depending on the relative concentrations of water, protein, and mucus.

If the bony wall of the portion of the sinus bordering the brain is disrupted and the rim of the sinus enhances, it is likely that the mucocele is adherent to thickened dura that may lead to complications such as empyema, meningitis, and abscess. A mucocele within the sphenoid sinus before enhancement may mimic the appearance of a pituitary adenoma or chordoma. After administration of IV contrast material, however, these entities should be differentiated easily.

NEOPLASMS OF THE SINONASAL CAVITY

Benign neoplasms and tumorlike conditions of the sinonasal cavity in children include fibro-osseous lesions and tumors

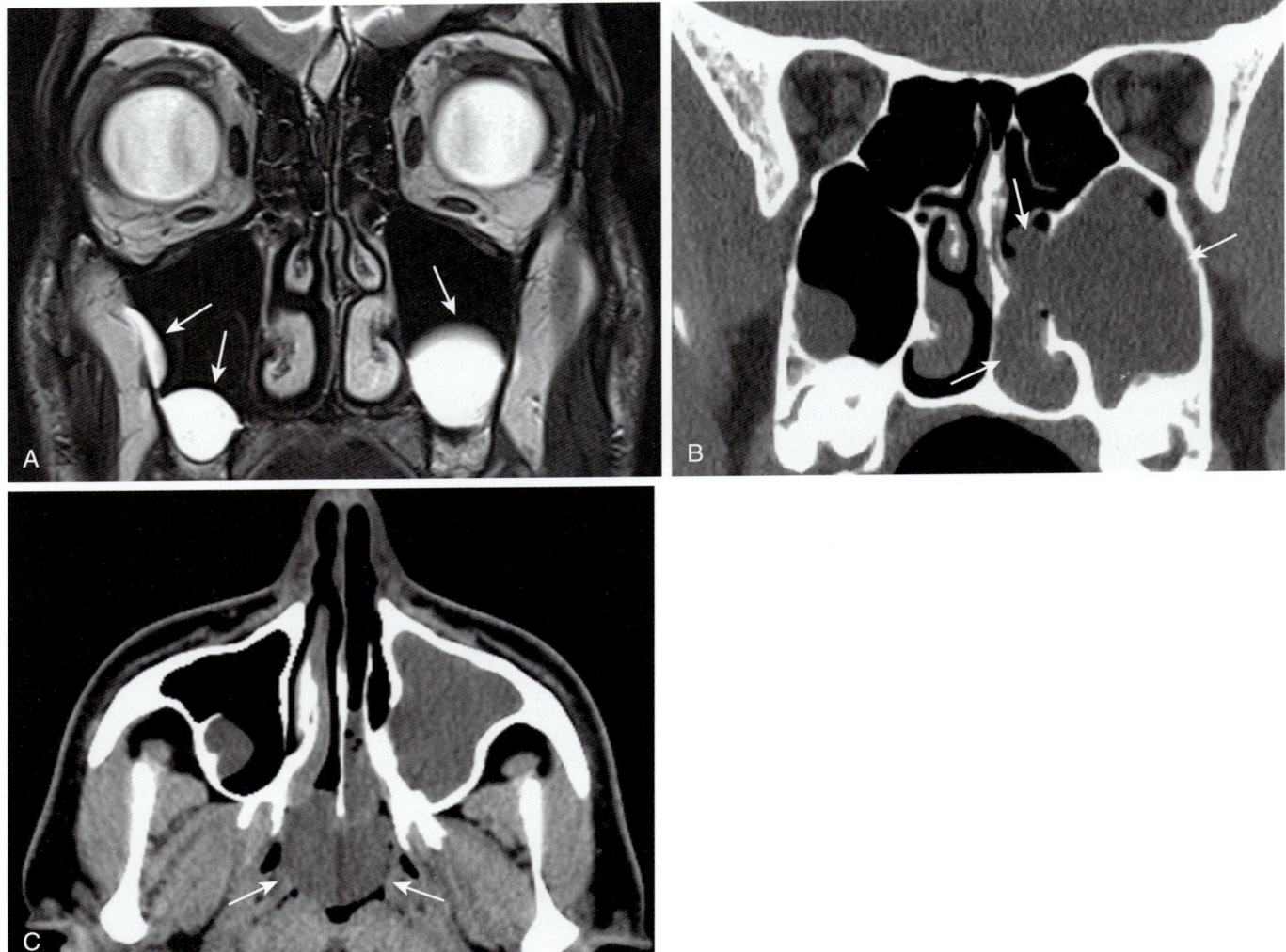

Figure 8-24 A, Retention cysts in a 17-year-old boy. Maxillary retention cysts are hyperintense on a T2-weighted magnetic resonance image (*arrows*). **B,** An antrochoanal polyp in a 16-year-old boy. An axial computed tomography (CT) image shows a large polyp that fills in the left maxillary antrum extending through the ostium to the nasal cavity (*arrows*). **C,** A coronal CT image shows posterior extension of the polyp to the nasal choana, crossing the midline to the right (*arrows*).

(e.g., fibrous dysplasia and ossifying fibroma), extramedullary hematopoiesis in anemias (e.g., sickle cell anemia and thalassemia), bony tumors (e.g., giant cell tumor and aneurysmal bone cyst) (e-Fig. 8-26), juvenile nasopharyngeal angiofibroma (Fig. 8-27, *A-E*) and odontogenic cysts or tumors.

Malignant neoplasms of the sinonasal cavity in children include rhabdomyosarcoma (e-Fig. 8-28, *A-C*), lymphoma/leukemia (e-Fig. 8-29, *A* and *B*), esthesioneuroblastoma, nasopharyngeal adenocarcinoma, and metastatic disease (neuroblastoma). These neoplasms will be discussed in greater detail in Chapter 16.

Fractures of Facial Bones

Nasal fractures, which typically result from direct frontal impact, occur most often in the lower third of the nasal bone.

Lateral blows cause more complex fractures and often are associated with other facial fractures. Associated dislocation of the septal cartilage and fracture of the nasal spine also can be seen.

Plain radiographs may evaluate simple fractures, but CT is the preferred method to evaluate more complex fractures and often is used in preoperative planning.[56] High-resolution ultrasonography also has proven to be a reliable diagnostic tool for the evaluation of nasal fractures, especially in low-grade nasal fractures.[57,58]

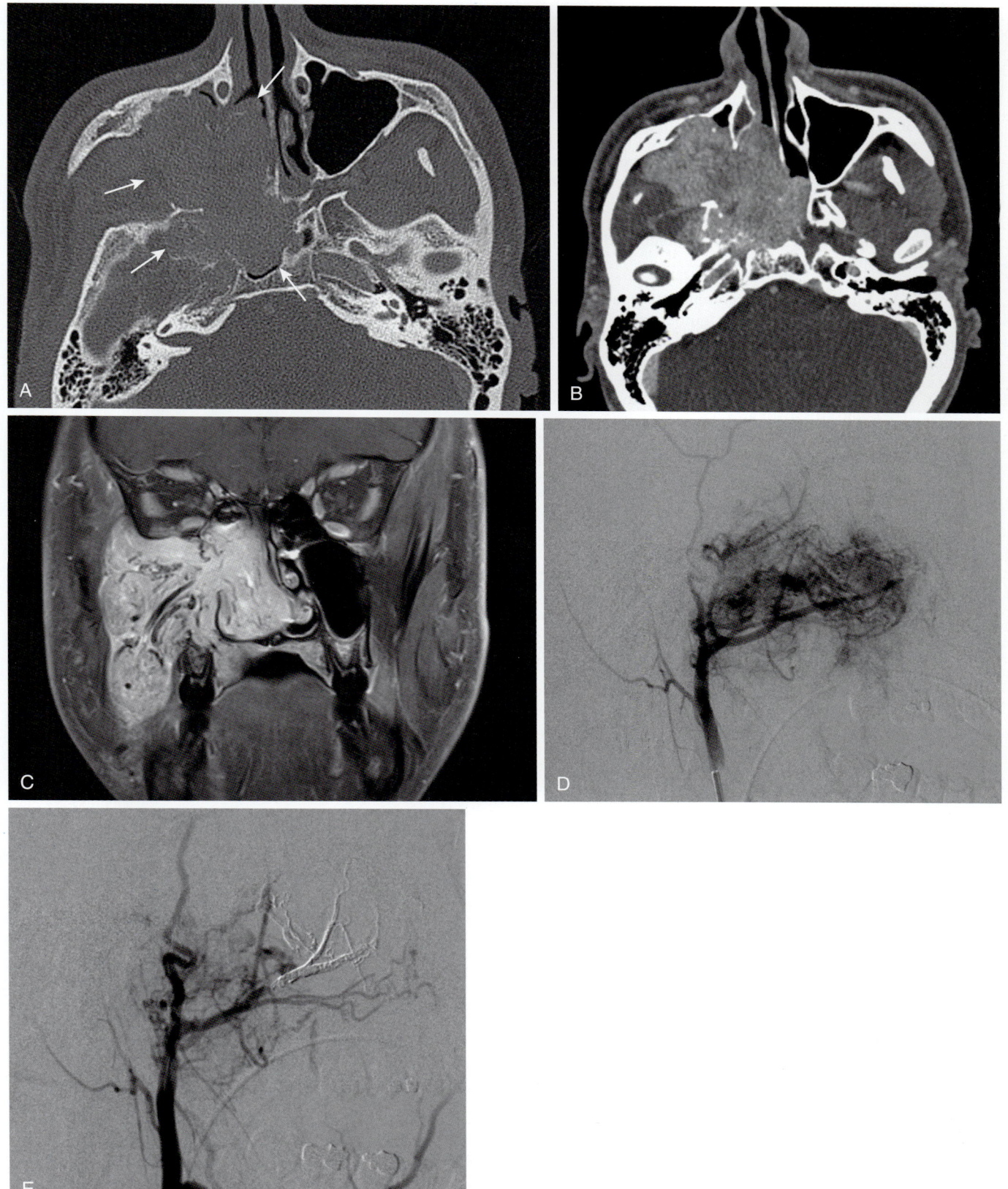

Figure 8-27 Juvenile nasopharyngeal angiofibroma in a 15-year-old boy. **A,** An axial contrast-enhanced computed tomography (CT) image in a bone window shows a large nasopharyngeal soft tissue mass with extension through the pterygopalatine fossa and extensive bony destruction. **B,** An axial contrast-enhanced CT image in a soft tissue window shows a large, enhancing, lobulated mass. **C,** A coronal T1-weighted postcontrast magnetic resonance image shows an avidly enhancing mass with intrinsic prominent flow voids. **D,** Conventional angiography shows intense capillary blush fed by large feeding external carotid artery vessels. **E,** Preoperative, postembolization angiography.

Key Points

Maxillary and ethmoid sinuses are present at birth. Sphenoid sinuses develop after fatty marrow transformation of the sphenoid bone. Frontal sinuses appear between 6 and 12 years of age.

Plain radiographs are extremely limited in the evaluation of the paranasal sinuses and are not indicated in children younger than 2 years.

With all imaging, a high incidence of mucosal thickening is seen in asymptomatic individuals.

CT is indicated in persons with complicated acute sinusitis and is the gold standard study that guides management of recurrent or chronic sinusitis and serves as a road map for functional endoscopic sinus surgery.

MRI is the imaging modality of choice in evaluating intracranial complications of sinusitis.

CT and MRI are complementary in assessing and mapping neoplasms.

Suggested Readings

Karmazyn B, Coley BD, Robertson ME, et al. Sinusitis—child. American College of Radiology (ACR) appropriatness criteria, 2012. Available at http://www.acr.org/~/media/485AEEC108E941C6B5551A8D21017 EED.pdf.

Mafee MF, Tran BH, Chapa AR. Imaging of rhinosinusitis and its complications: plain film, CT, and MRI. *Clin Rev Allergy Immunol.* 2006;30(3):165-186.

Steele RW. Chronic sinusitis in children. *Clin Pediatr (Phila).* 2005; 44(6):465-471.

Steele RW. Rhinosinusitis in children. *Curr Allergy Asthma Rep.* 2006; 6(6):508-512.

Ummat S, Riding M, Kirkpatrick D. Development of the ostiomeatal unit in childhood: a radiological study. *J Otolaryngol.* 1992;21(5):307-314.

References

Full references for this chapter can be found on www.expertconsult.com.

Embryology, Anatomy, Normal Findings, and Imaging Techniques

KORGÜN KORAL

Embryology

A detailed study of the development of the ear is beyond the scope of this chapter; thus only the key embryologic events and their timing are discussed. It is important to appreciate that the inner ear is derived from neuroectoderm, whereas the middle ear and the external ear develop from the branchial apparatus, which explains why the abnormalities of the inner ear generally are isolated from the abnormalities of the middle and external ear and vice versa. It also is important to remember that the pharyngeal clefts give rise to the ectodermal structures, pouches give rise to the endodermal structures, and the intervening arches give rise to the mesodermal structures.

EXTERNAL EAR

The external auditory meatus (canal) is derived from the first pharyngeal cleft. At the beginning of the third month, the epithelial cells at the bottom of the meatus proliferate and form the meatal plug. The meatal plug dissolves in the seventh month, and the epithelial lining of the floor of the meatus participates in the formation of the definitive tympanic membrane. The lateral part of the tympanic membrane arises from ectoderm, and the medial part of it arises from endoderm. Located in between is an intermediate layer of connective tissue, the fibrous stratum, which is derived from mesoderm.

The pinna (auricle) develops from six mesenchymal proliferations, called hillocks, which are located at the dorsal ends of the first and second pharyngeal arches. They surround the first pharyngeal cleft (the future external auditory meatus). These hillocks gradually fuse and form the definitive auricle.[1]

MIDDLE EAR

The tympanic cavity is derived from endoderm and develops from the first pharyngeal pouch. This pouch grows laterally until it comes in contact with the floor of the first pharyngeal cleft. The lateral part of the pouch gives rise to the primitive tympanic cavity. The medial part of the pouch is smaller and forms the eustachian tube. The malleus and incus are derived from the cartilage of the first pharyngeal arch, whereas the stapes is derived from the second pharyngeal arch. The ossicles remain embedded in the mesenchyme until the eighth month, when the surrounding tissue dissolves. The tympanic cavity expands dorsally to form the mastoid antrum late during fetal life. Pneumatization of the mastoid process continues after birth.[1]

INNER EAR

The otic placodes become visible on each side of rhombencephalon on day 22 of gestation; they are the first indications of developing ears. The otic placodes invaginate rapidly and form the otic (auditory) vesicles. From the ventral component of the otic placode, the cochlea and the saccule develop. From the dorsal components, the utricle, the semicircular canals, and the endolymphatic duct arise. These epithelial structures are collectively named the membranous labyrinth.

Between the sixth and eighth weeks of gestation, the cochlear duct, arising from the saccule, penetrates the surrounding mesenchyme and completes the two and a half turns. The thin residual connection between the cochlea and saccule is the ductus reuniens. At the tenth week, the cartilage that differentiated from the mesenchyme surrounding the cochlear duct undergoes vacuolization and two perilymphatic spaces are formed: the scala tympani and the scala vestibuli. The cochlear duct (scala media) is separated from the scala vestibuli by the vestibular membrane and from the scala tympani by the basilar membrane. The lateral wall of the cochlear duct remains attached to the surrounding cartilage by the spiral ligament. Medially, the cochlear duct is attached to the modiolus, which is the axis of the bony cochlea. At 6 weeks gestation, semicircular canals appear as outpouchings of the utricular (posterior) component of the otic vesicle.[1]

Anatomy and Normal Findings

The normal imaging anatomy of the temporal bone is exquisitely displayed on computed tomography (CT) and magnetic resonance imaging (MRI). An exhaustive review of the temporal bone anatomy is beyond the scope of this chapter.

The temporal bone consists of tympanic, squamous, petrous, and mastoid parts and a styloid process.[2] The temporal bone may be divided into compartments when studying its anatomy or reviewing imaging studies. These compartments are described from lateral to medial.

PINNA AND EXTERNAL AUDITORY CANAL

Detecting subtle abnormalities of the pinna with imaging may be difficult, but in general it is possible to identify gross malformations or absence of pinna on CT. Ossicular abnormalities are present in 98% of the temporal bones with microtia and external auditory canal (EAC) abnormality.[3]

In cross section, the EAC is oval in shape. Its walls (anterior and posterior; superior and inferior) run parallel to each other throughout the course of the EAC. The EAC consists of two segments: a membranous (fibrocartilaginous) segment that makes up the lateral third of the EAC, and a medial bony segment that forms the remainder of it.[4]

The tympanic membrane separates the EAC from the middle ear cavity and is attached to the tympanic annulus, which is a circumferential bony prominence at the medial-most aspect of the bony EAC. Superiorly, the tympanic membrane attaches to the scutum (e-Fig. 9-1), which is an important bony landmark in the diagnosis and evaluation of cholesteatoma. If the tympanic membrane is not thickened, wide window settings on CT are required to visualize it.

MIDDLE EAR CAVITY (CLEFT)

The tympanic cavity is an aerated space medial to the tympanic membrane. Air reaches the middle ear cavity from the nasopharynx via the eustachian tube. The middle ear cavity is arbitrarily divided into three compartments: epitympanum (attic), mesotympanum, and hypotympanum. With lines drawn parallel to the superior and inferior walls of the bony segment of the EAC on the coronal plane, the part of the middle ear cavity above the upper line is the epitympanum (attic), which is the largest portion and houses the bulk of the ossicular chain. The mesotympanum lies between the two lines. The hypotympanum is below the lower line and normally is non-existent or very small in children (Fig. 9-2).

Ossicles

The malleus, incus, and stapes form the ossicular chain, which is responsible for amplification (~30%) and transmission of sound waves from the tympanic membrane to the oval window on the vestibule.[5]

The manubrium (handle) and the lateral process of the malleus are embedded in the tympanic membrane. The tympanic membrane has two parts, divided by the lateral process of the malleus: a smaller pars flaccida superiorly, and a larger pars tensa inferiorly.[6] Cranial to the manubrium is the neck of the malleus, to which the tendon of the tensor tympani muscle attaches. The tensor tympani muscle is derived from the first branchial arch and is innervated by the only branch of the trigeminal nerve that has motor fibers: V3 (mandibular branch). The head of the malleus forms the "ice cream" of the familiar "ice cream and cone" appearance and articulates with the body of the incus (Fig. 9-3). The malleoincudal joint is a diarthrodial (synovial) articulation, as is the incudostapedial joint (Figs. 9-3 and 9-4).

The incus is the largest of the three middle ear ossicles. Its body articulates with the head of the malleus and forms

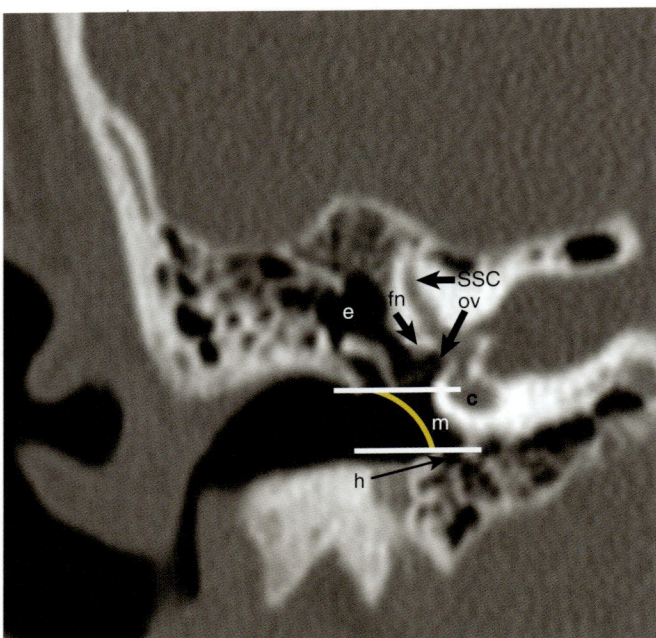

Figure 9-2 A reconstructed coronal computed tomography image shows the lines drawn to define epitympanum (*e*), mesotympanum (*m*), and hypotympanum (*h*). The tympanic membrane is outlined by a yellow curvilinear line. *c*, Cochlea; *fn*, facial nerve; *ov*, oval window; *SSC*, Superior semicircular canal.

the "cone." The short process of the incus (which is better appreciated on the axial images) extends from the body dorsally and resides in the fossa incudis, to which it is secured by ligaments that are invisible on CT. The long process of the incus extends inferiorly from the body. The lenticular process of the incus joins the long process, forming a nearly 90° angle. The long and lenticular processes of the incus are very delicate and are more prone to erosion as a result of infection and/or inflammation than are other parts of the ossicular chain. The lenticular process is cup shaped medially and articulates with the head (capitulum) of the stapes. The head of the stapes is connected to the crura (anterior and

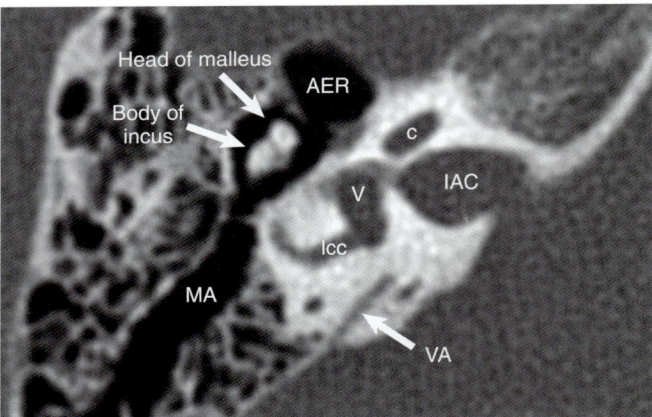

Figure 9-3 An axial computed tomography image demonstrates the "ice cream cone" appearance of the head of the malleus and incus. *AER*, Anterior epitympanic recess; *c*, cochlea; *IAC*, internal auditory canal; *lcc*, lateral semicircular canal; *MA*, mastoid antrum; *V*, vestibule; *VA*, vestibular aqueduct.

posterior), which subsequently join the footplate of the stapes. The opening between the crura of the stapes is the obturator foramen, where the stapedial artery is located in fetal life. The stapes footplate articulates with the oval window, forming the syndesmotic (fibrous) stapediovestibular joint.[5]

Recesses and Ridges of the Middle Ear Cavity

The sinus tympani is the medial and posterior recess of the middle ear cavity. Sinus tympani may be deep, making the visualization of lesions within it difficult at surgery. Lateral to the sinus tympani is the pyramidal eminence, which is a triangular bony prominence. The stapedius muscle (innervated by the facial nerve) occasionally may be imaged on CT arising from the pyramidal eminence and extending to the stapes. Lateral to the pyramidal eminence is the facial recess.

The Prussak space is medial to the scutum and lateral to the malleolar head. This space is important because soft tissue lesions within it, such as cholesteatomas, may be inaccessible upon clinical examination. The superior malleolar ligament (which is not seen on CT) forms the cranial border of the Prussak space.

The anterior epitympanic recess (Figs. 9–3 and 9–4) is contiguous with the middle ear cavity through an incomplete septum, named "cog," the integrity of which may be lost because of infection or inflammation.[5]

Mastoid Air Cells

The interconnected, air-filled mastoid air cells open into the mastoid antrum, which in turn communicates with the middle ear cavity (Figs. 9–3 and 9–4). The connection between the middle ear cavity and mastoid antrum is the aditus ad antrum (opening to antrum). The mastoid air cells are separated by innumerable thin septa. The Körner septum is the bony thickening that runs obliquely through the mastoid air cells; it is an important surgical landmark.

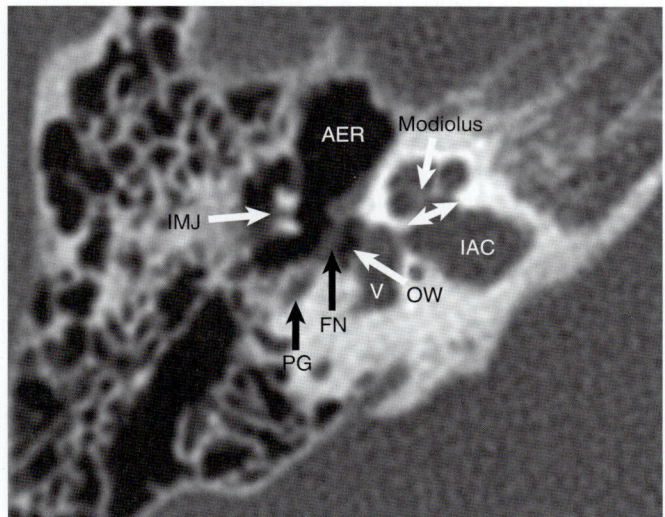

Figure 9-4 An axial computed tomography image shows the cochlear aperture (*double arrow*) and modiolus. *AER,* Anterior epitympanic recess; *FN,* facial nerve; *IAC,* internal auditory canal; *IMJ,* incudomalleolar joint; *OW,* oval window; *PG,* posterior genu of the facial nerve; *V,* vestibule.

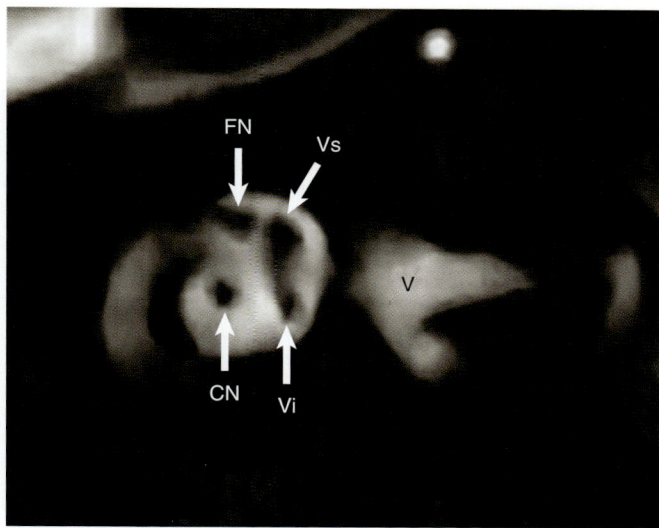

Figure 9-6 An oblique sagittal balanced fast field echo image through the fundus of the internal auditory canal shows the facial nerve (*FN*), cochlear nerve (*CN*), and superior (*Vs*) and inferior (*Vi*) branches of the vestibular nerves. *V,* vestibule.

The roof of the middle ear cavity is the tegmen tympani (e-Fig. 9-1).

Facial and Vestibulocochlear Nerves and Internal Auditory Canal

The facial nerve has motor, parasympathetic, and special sensory (taste) fibers. Its nucleus lies in the dorsal pons. It is important to remember that the facial nerve has a rather long intraaxial segment extending from the nucleus through the nerve exit zone at the surface of the lateral pons. The cisternal and canalicular segments of the facial nerve are evaluated on high-resolution T2-weighted images of the temporal bone. The cisternal segment, the longest segment of the facial nerve, can be identified routinely on high-resolution MRI. The facial nerve enters the internal auditory canal (IAC) through the porus acusticus and is named the canalicular segment thereafter. In the IAC, the facial nerve lies in the anterior-superior quadrant. The lateral-most aspect of the IAC is the fundus, which is divided by the crista falciformis (e-Fig. 9-1) into superior and inferior compartments. The superior compartment is further divided into anterior and posterior parts by vertical, variably ossified arachnoid tissue, known as the Bill bar. The cochlear nerve occupies the anterior-inferior quadrant, and the vestibular nerve (superior and inferior branches) is seen in the posterior quadrants[7] (e-Figs. 9-5 and 9-6).

The facial nerve enters the labyrinthine canal and fills approximately 95% of this canal. The labyrinthine segment of the facial nerve is particularly susceptible to ischemia because its bony confines do not permit swelling during inflammation. The labyrinthine segment synapses at the geniculate ganglion, from which the parasympathetic greater superficial petrosal nerve arises. The greater superficial petrosal nerve recruits some sympathetic fibers and become the vidian nerve, providing the parasympathetic innervation of the lacrimal gland. Distal to the geniculate ganglion, the facial nerve makes a dorsal turn and becomes the tympanic segment. The distal labyrinthine segment, geniculate ganglion, and proximal tympanic segment make up the anterior genu. The tympanic segment of the facial nerve lies at the medial wall of the tympanic cavity and below the lateral semicircular canal. The tympanic segment has a thin, inconsistent bony covering. The tympanic segment lies in close proximity but lateral to the oval window. The posterior genu is a nearly 90° bend where the tympanic segment meets the mastoid (or descending) segment (Fig. 9-4). The mastoid segment exits the temporal bone through the stylomastoid foramen. Just proximal to the stylomastoid foramen, the chorda tympani arises from the mastoid segment, extends into the middle ear cavity in its own canal, and traverses the middle ear cavity within the tympanic membrane, between the manubrium of the malleus and incus. The chorda tympani contains the taste sensation fibers from the anterior two thirds of the tongue, as well as the parasympathetic fibers to the submandibular and sublingual glands.[2] After exiting the temporal bone, the facial nerve traverses the parotid gland (but does not innervate it) and innervates the facial musculature. The parotid gland is divided by the facial nerve into deep and superficial lobes.

The cochlear nerve is equal in size or slightly larger than the facial nerve, as seen on oblique-sagittal T2-weighted images. It enters the cochlea through the cochlear aperture, which can be appreciated on both CT and MRI. Stenosis or atresia of the cochlear aperture usually is associated with deficiency or absence of the cochlear nerve.

Oval Window/Round Window

The stapes footplate rests on the oval window (Fig. 9-4). It can be appreciated easily on both axial and coronal CT images. The abnormalities of the oval window include atresia and stenosis, which usually are associated with abnormalities of the ossicles and external ear. The round window is easier to appreciate on coronal images because of the fluid–air interface at the inferior aspect of the vestibule.

Jugular Bulb/Carotid Canal

The right jugular bulb is generally the dominant jugular bulb. The term "high-riding" is used when the jugular bulb and basal turn of the cochlea are seen on the same axial image. Without bony dehiscence or protrusion of the internal jugular vein into the posterior tympanic cavity, a high-riding jugular bulb is insignificant. The carotid canal should be identified in all temporal bone examinations. An aberrant internal carotid artery running in the tympanic cavity is a very rare but important anomaly.

Vestibular Aqueduct/Cochlear Aqueduct

The vestibular aqueduct (seen on CT) is the bony housing of the endolymphatic duct and sac. It is seen on MRI when enlarged (Fig. 9-3). The vestibular aqueduct is considered enlarged when it measures greater than 1.0 mm at its midpoint.[8] Although its enlargement is commonly associated with sensorineural hearing loss, this observation does not alter the management if the patient is otherwise a good candidate for cochlear implantation.

Foramen Ovale/Foramen Spinosum

The foramen spinosum is positioned posterolateral to the foramen ovale. Identifying the foramen spinosum is important because when it is absent, in about one third of cases it is associated with a persistent stapedial artery. The obturator foramen of the stapes should be inspected thoroughly for a soft tissue density when the foramen spinosum is not visualized.

Temporomandibular Joint and Mandibular Head/Condyle

Evaluation of the temporomandibular joint is important because dysplasia often is associated with abnormalities of the auricle (particularly aural atresia) and ossicles.

INNER EAR

The inner ear consists of bony and membranous labyrinths. The bony labyrinth contains the vestibule, cochlea, and semicircular canals. The membranous labyrinth is a system of epithelial spaces and tubes filled with endolymph. The main components are the utricle, saccule, endolymphatic sac and duct, three semicircular ducts and their ampullae, and the cochlear duct.

MRI is the modality of choice in the assessment of the inner ear; however, many inner ear abnormalities also may be appreciated by examining the bony labyrinth with CT. The cochlea lies anterior to the IAC and is made up of basal, middle, and apical turns. The basal and middle turns are complete 360-degree turns, whereas the apical turn covers 180 degrees, hence the normal two and a half turns. The modiolus is the bony axis of the cochlea; it has a "star" or "crown" shape and can be seen atop the cochlear aperture (Fig. 9-4 and e-Fig. 9-5). The vestibule has a delicate, nearly cylindrical shape (Fig. 9-3 and e-Fig. 9-5). The semicircular canals (superior, posterior, and lateral) are at right angles to each other and connect to the vestibule. Although six openings in the inner surface of the vestibule (two for each semicircular canal) are expected, five openings exist because the posterior limb of the superior semicircular canal and the superior limb of the posterior semicircular canal unite to form the common crus, which has its own opening to the vestibule. The lateral semicircular canal is slightly larger than the other two semicircular canals.

Petromastoid (Subarcuate) Canal

The petromastoid canal is almost always visualized on CT. It lies underneath the arch of the superior semicircular canal and is closer to its posterior limb. Its size decreases with age. When fluid is present in the petromastoid canal (due to cerebrospinal fluid in the dural sleeve about the subarcuate artery that travels in the canal to reach the mastoid air cells and middle ear cavity), the petromastoid canal occasionally can be identified on MRI examinations of young children (e-Fig. 9-7). It is a normal structure and should not be confused with a pathologic lesion.

Imaging Techniques

CT is reserved for conductive hearing loss, whereas MRI is used in the evaluation of sensorineural hearing loss.[9] A low-dose technique is used in volumetric CT acquisition; the imaging parameters include a kVp of 90 and an mA of 80, resulting in a dose length product of approximately 90 mGy/cm. Attention is required to keep the lenses outside the field of the primary beam. Coronal and, if necessary, oblique-sagittal reformations are generated.

For high-resolution MRI, three-dimensional acquisition (e.g., balanced fast field echo, fast imaging steady state acquisition, and constrictive interference in steady state) of the membranous labyrinth is performed in the axial plane. The reconstructed images yield an effective slice thickness of 0.75 mm. Oblique-sagittal images of the cerebellopontine angles and IACs are acquired. It is prudent to complement the MRI of the temporal bones with a brain MRI, including sagittal T1-weighted, diffusion-weighted axial fluid attenuated inversion recovery and T1-weighted images, to exclude central causes of hearing loss.

Key Points

Developmental abnormalities of the external ear and middle ear generally coexist and are separate from the abnormalities of the inner ear, because the external ear and middle ear are derived from the pharyngeal apparatus, whereas the inner ear arises from neuroectoderm.

In general, CT is reserved for the evaluation of conductive hearing loss (e.g., aural atresia, cholesteatoma, and ossicular disruption), whereas MRI is used in the workup of sensorineural hearing loss (primarily in the evaluation of candidates for cochlear implantation).

The lenses should be kept outside the primary beam during CT acquisition. The low-dose technique allows for dose reduction without significant loss in the image quality.

Suggested Readings

Fatterpekar GM, Doshi AH, Dugar M, et al. Role of 3D CT in the evaluation of the temporal bone. *Radiographics.* 2006;26(suppl 1):S117-S132.

Lane JI, Lindell EP, Witte RJ, et al. Middle and inner ear: improved depiction with multiplanar reconstruction of volumetric CT data. *Radiographics.* 2006;26(1):115-124.

Niu Y, Wang Z, Liu Y, et al. Radiation dose to the lens using different temporal bone CT scanning protocols. *AJNR Am J Neuroradiol.* 2010;31(2):226-229.

Shah LM, Wiggins 3rd RH. Imaging of hearing loss. *Neuroimaging Clin N Am.* 2009;19:287-306.

References

Full references for this chapter can be found on www.expertconsult.com.

Chapter 10

Congenital and Neonatal Abnormalities

TIMOTHY N. BOOTH

The discussion of congenital and neonatal temporal bone abnormalities in this chapter is approached from lateral to medial. External canal atresia and associated middle and inner ear anomalies are discussed first. Isolated middle ear anomalies with associated branchial arch malformations are then addressed, along with associated anomalous development of the oval window. A classification and description of inner ear malformations is discussed along with potential surgical outcomes. Finally, vascular anomalies involving the temporal bone is briefly discussed.

External Auditory Canal Atresia

Clinical Presentation and Etiologies The external and middle ear both are derived from the branchial apparatus, in contrast to the inner ear, which is of neuroectodermal origin. As a result, dysplasia of the external auditory canal (EAC) is commonly associated with a malformed auricle and anomalies of the middle ear and the mandible. These children usually present with a malformed pinna and conductive hearing loss. Inner ear anomalies occur in 20% of children with aural atresia and are more likely to involve the vestibular apparatus. A profound sensorineural component of hearing loss usually is not present.[1] In general, anomalies of the external and middle ear are more common than those of the inner ear. The incidence of EAC atresia is one in 10,000 to 20,000 at birth and is bilateral in one third of cases, but it appears to be more common in the United States than elsewhere.[2]

Imaging A spectrum of involvement is seen, with only mild bony stenosis of the EAC present in some children. When the canal is atretic, the atresia may be membranous or bony. The severity of middle ear anomalies correlates with the extent of external malformation. Preoperative high-resolution computed tomography (CT) plays an integral role in determining potential candidates for hearing restorative surgery and should be performed shortly before intended surgery.[3] If a sensorineural component to the hearing loss is present, magnetic resonance imaging (MRI) may offer additional information that may affect treatment.

Ossicular anomalies often are found in association with EAC atresia. The handle of the malleus may be fused to the atretic plate (e-Fig. 10-1). Less commonly, the malleus may be fused to the incus, with severe dysplasia usually present. The incudostapedial joint can be involved as well and can be well demonstrated on axial and coronal images. Patent oval and round windows are essential in achieving a good surgical outcome. Atresia of the oval window often is seen with syndromic EAC atresia (Fig. 10-2). The stapes can be dysplastic, malpositioned, or absent. Significant abnormalities of the stapes often necessitate removal and placement of a prosthesis. The size of the middle ear cavity is significant, because small hypoplastic cavities are associated with a poor surgical outcome. The degree of mastoid pneumatization also may affect the surgical approach.[3-5]

The course of the facial nerve is critical to the evaluation of children with EAC atresia. The most common anomaly involves anterior displacement of the descending segment of the facial nerve, with the stylomastoid foramen lying just posterior to the temporal mandibular joint. The posterior genu usually is more anteriorly positioned immediately posterior to the level of the oval window[6] (Fig. 10-3). Less commonly, the tympanic segment may be malpositioned into the oval window niche or even more inferiorly over the cochlear promontory. The anomalous position of the tympanic segment of the facial nerve usually is associated with atresia or stenosis of the oval window. The facial nerve can be hypoplastic and difficult to visualize, but other labyrinthine segment anomalies are uncommon.[7]

Syndromic EAC atresia usually is associated with more severe middle ear anomalies and a higher incidence of inner ear anomalies; these patients are poorer surgical candidates. Syndromes associated with EAC atresia include Goldenhar syndrome, Treacher Collins syndrome, and Pierre Robin sequence[8,9] (Tables 10-1 to 10-4; e-Fig. 10-4).

Treatment Grading systems have been developed to assess the probability of surgical success. These systems take into account such findings as middle ear volume, ossicular anomalies, and the status of the oval window.[2] Transmastoid and anterior surgical approaches are used, with formation of a new tympanic membrane, mobilization of the ossicles, and possibly placement of a stapes prosthesis. The presence of a cholesteatoma also is a potential issue in both the imaging evaluation and surgical management of these patients.

Isolated Middle Ear Anomalies

Clinical Presentation and Etiologies Minor ear anomalies are associated with a normal external ear canal and are much less common than EAC atresia. Children with minor ear anomalies usually present with a nonprogressive conductive hearing

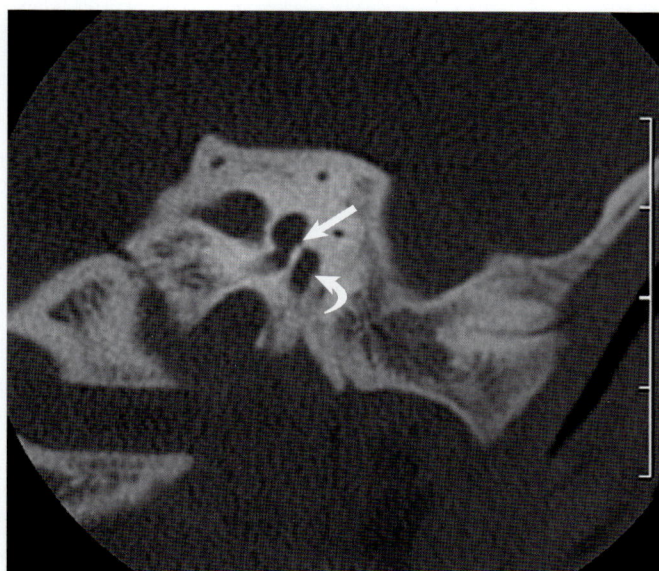

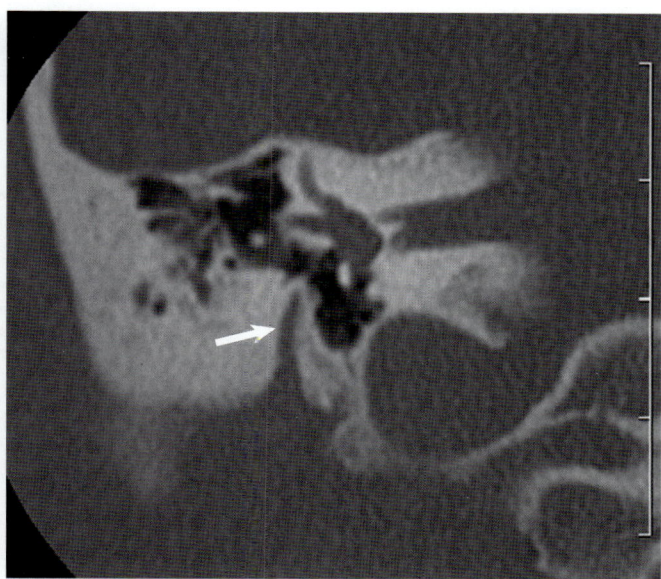

Figure 10-2 A 5-year-old with bilateral microtia and conductive hearing loss. A coronal high-resolution computed tomography image at the expected level of the oval window demonstrates that the middle ear cavity is markedly hypoplastic and opacified (*curved arrow*). The oval window is atretic and the facial nerve is not well demonstrated (*straight arrow*). This patient would be a poor surgical candidate for middle ear reconstructive surgery.

Figure 10-3 External auditory canal atresia. A coronal high-resolution computed tomography image shows anterior displacement of the descending facial nerve (*arrow*) with the posterior genu at the level of the oval window.

Table 10-1

Otocraniofacial Syndromes with Congenital Abnormalities of the Ear			
Syndromes	Outer Ear	Middle Ear	Inner Ear
Treacher Collins syndrome (mandibulofacial dysostosis)	Deformed, low-set auricles	Deformed/absent ossicles	Occasional abnormal vestibule
	Stenosis/atresia of EAC	Decreased size of middle ear cavity Abnormal facial nerve (anterior displacement)	Short LSCC
Crouzon disease (craniofacial dysostosis)	Stenosis/atresia of EAC	Narrow tympanic cavity Ossicular chain fixation	
Apert syndrome (acrocephalosyndactyly)		Fixation of stapes footplate	
Hemifacial microsomia	Microtia Atresia/stenosis Vertically oriented EAC Ossicles deformed/absent	Descent of tegmen	

EAC, External auditory canal; *LSCC*, lateral semicircular canal.
From Hasso AN, Casselman JW, Broadwell RA. Temporal bone congenital anomalies. In Som PM, Carter HD, editors: *Head and neck imaging.* 3rd ed. St Louis: Mosby; 1996:1352-1355.

Table 10-2

Otocervical Syndromes with Congenital Abnormalities of the Ear			
Syndrome	Outer Ear	Middle Ear	Inner Ear
Goldenhar syndrome (oculoauricular vertebral dysplasia)	Preauricular appendage	Severe dysplasia	Hypoplastic cochlea and petrous ridge
	Deformed auricle Atresia of EAC	Narrow cavity Absent ossicles	Short IAC with acute upward inclination
Klippell-Feil syndrome	Microtia	Thickening and fixation of stapes	Range from cochlear hypoplasia and semicircular canals to simple otocyst
	Atresia/vertical orientation of EAC	Bony obliteration of tympanic cavity	Stenotic IAC
Wildervanck syndrome (cervico-oculoacoustic syndrome)			Aplasia/hypoplasia of various structures
Cleidocranial dysostosis	Narrowed EAC	Marked sclerosis of mastoid	Marked sclerosis of petrous bone

EAC, External auditory canal; *IAC*, internal auditory canal.
From Hasso AN, Casselman JW, Broadwell RA. Temporal bone congenital anomalies. In Som PM, Carter HD, editors: *Head and neck imaging.* 3rd ed. St Louis: Mosby; 1996:1352-1355.

Table 10-3

Otoskeletal Syndromes with Congenital Abnormalities of the Ear			
Syndrome	Outer Ear	Middle Ear	Inner Ear
Pyle disease (craniometaphyseal dysplasia)	Sclerosis of EAC	Osseous proliferation in tympanic cavity Constriction of facial canal Obliterans of mastoids	Sclerosis of IAC
Hart syndrome (frontometaphyseal dysplasia)		Deformed ossicles	Osseous infiltration around cochlea
van der Hoeve syndrome		Stapes abnormalities	Loss of otic capsule
Alber-Schönberg disease (osteopetrosis)	Narrowed EAC	Sclerotic bone that narrows facial canal and tympanic cavity, covering oval and round windows Obliterates mastoid sinuses	IAC narrowed

EAC, External auditory canal; *IAC,* internal auditory canal.
From Hasso AN, Casselman JW, Broadwell RA. Temporal bone congenital anomalies. In Som PM, Carter HD, editors: *Head and neck imaging.*
3rd ed. St Louis: Mosby; 1996:1352-1355.

loss. Ossicular abnormalities may be unilateral or bilateral. Unilateral ossicular abnormalities are usually sporadic and isolated. Bilateral anomalies may be associated with autosomal-dominant inheritance, and syndromic associations include Goldenhar and Treacher Collins syndrome. Round window atresia is caused by a deficiency in the development of cartilage during ossification of the otic capsule and typically is associated with conductive hearing loss. Oval window atresia is likely caused by anomalous development of the second branchial arch (innervated by the seventh cranial nerve) and often is associated with a mixed sensorineural conductive hearing loss. Oval window atresia can be seen with the CHARGE association (*C*oloboma of the eye, *H*eart defect, *A*tresia of choanae, *R*etarded growth and development, *G*enital anomalies, and *E*ar defect with deafness).

Imaging High-resolution CT using both axial and reconstructed coronal planes is the imaging modality of choice in evaluating patients with isolated middle ear anomalies. Anomalies of the stapes include aplasia, partial absence, columnar deformity, fusion of the head to the promontory, and footplate fixation. The incus can be aplastic, it can be fused to the lateral semicircular canal or scutum, it can have a malformed long process, it may be absent, or it may be fixed to an incudostapedial joint (e-Fig. 10-5). Similar anomalies involve the malleus; rarely, a bony bar fixes the malleus to the anterior lateral epitympanic wall[9,10] (Fig. 10-6). These anomalies have been classified into five classes on the basis of their surgical success rate and include (from better to worse):
Class 1: Normal stapes with abnormal incus or malleus
Class 2: Mobile stapes footplate
Class 3: Stapes footplate fixation only
Class 4: Stapes footplate fixation with other anomaly
Class 5: No stapes footplate[11,12]

Congenital stapes deformity or fixation may be associated with a perilymphatic fistula.[13]

Round window atresia is not associated with malposition of the facial nerve or ossicular abnormalities, but it has been reported in association with oval window atresia.[14,15] Atresia of the oval window can occur in the absence of EAC atresia or stenosis. The absent oval window often is associated with malposition of the tympanic segment of the facial nerve into or inferior to the atretic oval window. The stapes typically is deformed or hypoplastic and appears oriented toward a segment of facial nerve rather than the oval window. The long and lenticular portions of the incus also are malformed.

Table 10-4

Miscellaneous Syndromes with Congenital Abnormalities of the Ear			
Syndrome	Outer Ear	Middle Ear	Inner Ear
Pendred syndrome			Incompletely developed cochlea with hypoplasia, flattening of promotory
Waardenburg syndrome			Posterior semicircular absence LSCC slightly dilated Vestibule irregular in shape
Möbius syndrome	Auricular malformation	Facial canal absent with no enlargement at geniculate ganglion	Semicircular canals and vestibule dilated Hypoplastic cochlea (may be a cystic cavity)
Chromosome 18 deletion syndrome	Low-set auricles Stenosis/atresia of EAC	Ossicular abnormalities	
DiGeorge syndrome		Ossicular deformities Small tympanic cavity	Varying degrees of aplasia/dysplasia of cochlea

EAC, External auditory canal; *LSCC,* lateral semicircular canal.
From Hasso AN, Casselman JW, Broadwell RA. Temporal bone congenital anomalies. In Som PM, Carter HD, editors: *Head and neck imaging.*
3rd ed. St Louis: Mosby; 1996: 1352-1355.

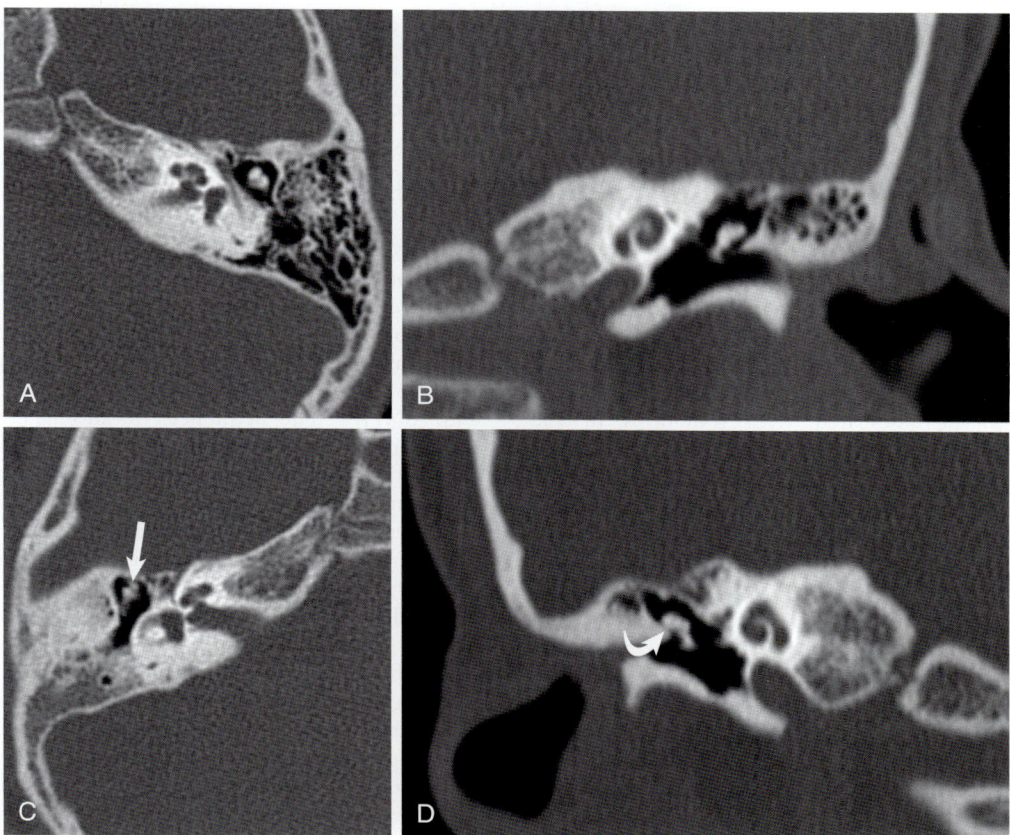

Figure 10-6 A 10-year-old boy with right-sided conductive hearing loss. **A** and **B,** Axial and coronal high-resolution computed tomography through the normal left middle ear. **C** and **D,** Corresponding axial and coronal computed tomography images of the right middle ear shows incomplete separation of the malleolar head from the tegmen (*straight arrow*) and narrowing of Prussak space (*curved arrow*). Ossicular fixation was confirmed surgically.

Anomalous development of the second branchial arch is likely the cause, with the facial nerve, incus, and a portion of the stapes arising from this structure.[16,17] (Fig. 10-7).

The CHARGE association has typical features on high-resolution CT of the temporal bone, and oval window atresia is present in nearly all cases (e-Fig. 10-8). Anomalies of the incus and stapes are found along with fixation of the malleus to the anterior tympanic wall. The inner ear is malformed in all cases, with the cochlea and vestibular system involved. The typical vestibular findings are a small vestibule and absent semicircular canals. The facial nerve often is difficult to identify in these patients and may be hypoplastic or malpositioned.[18,19]

Treatment Ossicular chain reconstruction is the mainstay of treatment. Accurate preoperative assessment is essential to plan the appropriate procedure. The status of the oval window is important because atresia imparts a poor surgical prognosis. Determining the position of the facial nerve is essential in these patients.

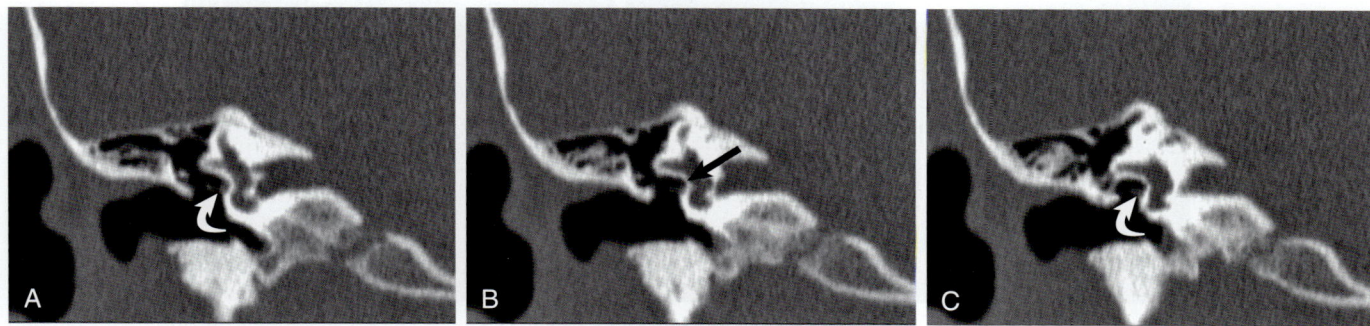

Figure 10-7 A 7-year-old with mixed hearing loss and a 60-dB threshold. **A, B,** and **C,** Coronal high-resolution computed tomography images from anterior to posterior. The oval window is atretic (*arrow*), with displacement of the facial nerve within and slightly below the structure (*curved arrows*). The stapes was not visualized, and the lenticular process of the incus appears adherent to the displaced facial nerve.

Inner Ear Anomalies

Clinical Presentation and Etiologies Study of the genetic defects associated with congenital sensorineural hearing loss (SNHL) is increasing. Nonsyndromic congenital hearing loss is not associated with additional medical anomalies and constitutes 70% of the cases. Genetic mutations are found in persons with nonsyndromic congenital hearing loss, with approximately 50% of nonsyndromic recessive hearing loss caused by a mutation in the *GJB2* gene.[20] Children with enlarged endolymphatic ducts have mutations of the *SLC26A4 (PDS)* gene in up to 82% of the hereditary cases and 30% of the sporadic cases.[21] Auditory neuropathy/dyssynchrony may be associated with mutations in the *OTOF* gene, as well as suggested by the associated brain anomalies. These patients typically have a poor response to hearing aids and may benefit from earlier cochlear implantation.[22,23] The future classification of congenital hearing loss is likely to be based on a combined genetic and morphologic evaluation.

Syndromic congenital hearing loss accounts for 30% of cases. A wide spectrum of syndromes is associated with congenital anomalies of the ear, which include inner ear malformations (Tables 10-1 through 10-4).[9] Toriello et al.[24] also have produced a definitive text on syndromic associations and congenital hearing loss.

It is important to understand that diagnosing congenital SNHL can be difficult in sporadic cases, and perinatal insults can be responsible. Congenital cytomegalovirus infection, hypoxia, ototoxic drugs, kernicterus, and, rarely, tumors are additional etiologies that should be considered and are at times suggested by imaging[25] (Fig. 10-9).

Imaging Congenital SNHL is a common indication for inner ear imaging evaluation and may be accomplished with high-resolution CT and/or MRI. Cochlear and vestibular anomalies, intracranial abnormalities, and deficiency of the cochlear nerve often are found in children with congenital SNHL.[26] MRI is preferred because it provides improved evaluation of the membranous labyrinth and endolymphatic sac and direct visualization of the cochlear nerve; it also permits a better evaluation of intracranial structures compared with other imaging modalities.

The wide spectrum of congenital inner ear anomalies previously were all grouped together as "Mondini dysplasia." These anomalies were reclassified by Jackler and colleagues into five types, based on the stage of arrested development and appearance of the cochlea.[27] More recently, a revised classification by Sennaroglu has been proposed to better describe the anomalies of the cochlea found in children with SNHL. The sequence of anomalies corresponds to the timing of the potential insult to the developing inner ear, with the more severe anomalies occurring earlier in gestation[28]:

1. Complete labyrinthine aplasia (Michel malformation): Labyrinthine structures are completely absent (Fig. 10-10).
2. Cochlear aplasia: The cochlea is completely absent and the cochlear promontory is absent on coronal high resolution CT. A normal or malformed vestibule and semicircular canals may be present (e-Fig. 10-11).
3. Common cavity: A single cystic cavity represents the cochlea and vestibule without further differentiation (e-Fig. 10-12). Formed semicircular canals may be present.
4. Incomplete partition type I: The modiolus and cribriform area are absent, resulting in a cystic appearance. The vestibule is abnormally enlarged and cystic but remains a separate structure.
5. Cochlear hypoplasia: The cochlea shows further differentiation with the presence of a small cochlea, with a height less than 4 mm and fewer than two and a half turns (e-Fig. 10-13). A spectrum of severity is present, ranging from a small cochlear bud to a well-formed basal turn and small apical and middle turns.

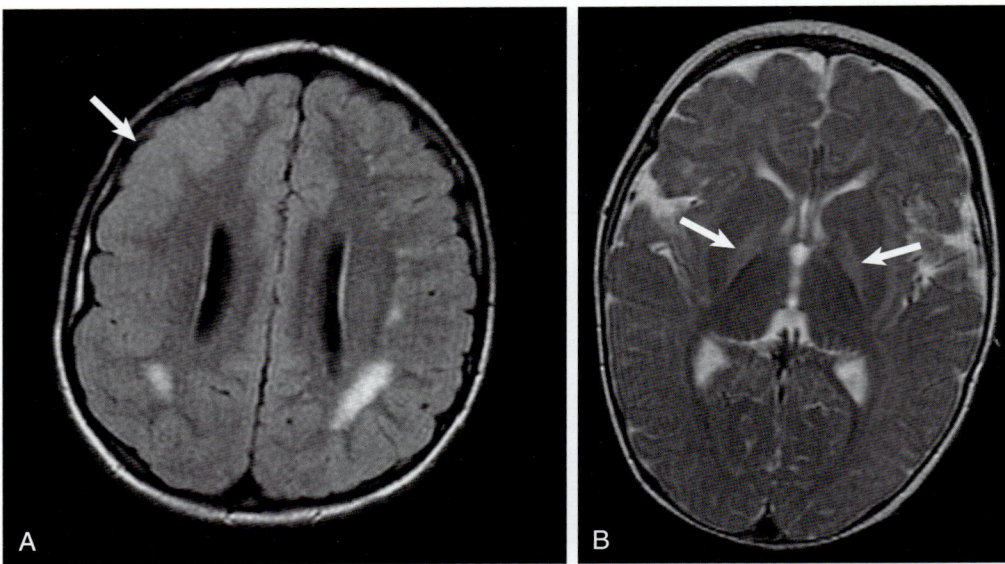

Figure 10-9   Congenital sensorineural hearing loss. **A,** An axial fluid attenuated inversion recovery image shows that an abnormal increased T2-weighted signal is present within the supratentorial white matter. Cortical dysplasia is present within the right frontal region (*arrow*). The findings are consistent with congenital cytomegalovirus infection. **B,** An axial T2-weighted image through the basal ganglia in a young child with sensorineural hearing loss and a history of prematurity shows an increased T2-weighted signal in the bilateral globus pallidus (*arrows*), consistent with kernicterus.

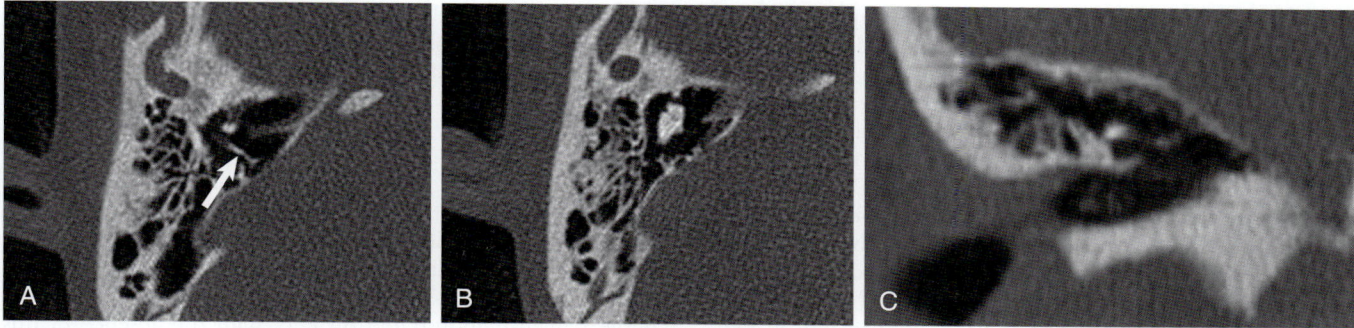

Figure 10-10 A child with profound hearing loss. Axial high-resolution computed tomography images (**A** and **B**) and a coronal reformatted image (**C**) show complete absence of the membranous labyrinth. Imaging findings are consistent with an early embryologic insult and resultant aplasia (Michel deformity). The ossicles are abnormally oriented (*arrow*). (Images courtesy of Nafi Aygun, MD, Johns Hopkins, Baltimore, MD.)

6. Incomplete partition type II (classic Mondini deformity): A normal basal turn of the cochlea is present. The middle and apical structures become a single cystic structure with an incomplete or absent interscalar septum and scalar asymmetry. A dilated vestibule and enlarged vestibular aqueduct/endolymphatic duct often are associated (Fig. 10-14). Numerous syndromes may have an associated Mondini defect, including DiGeorge, Waardenburg, Alagille, Klippel-Feil, Wildervanck, and Pendred syndromes and chromosomal trisomies.[29]

It has been suggested that cochlear hypoplasia may be further subcategorized into cochlear bud, basal turn cochlea, and hypoplastic cochlea.[30] Measuring the cochlea, including the height and width of the second turn, may allow for increased sensitivity in evaluating patients with SNHL for cochlear hypoplasia, and it might be useful in assessing the success of implantation.[31,32] MRI has allowed for improved visualization and categorization of the milder forms of cochlear malformation. Modiolar deficiency often is found in children undergoing evaluation for SNHL, with the cochlear modiolus appearing flattened and with a diminished number of bony projections extending into the cochlea (e-Fig. 10-15).

In normal ears, the scala vestibuli (anterior) is approximately equal in size to the scala tympani (posterior). Scalar asymmetry is present when the anterior chamber is larger and can be present in children with SNHL (see Fig. 10-14).[33]

Anomalies of the vestibule usually are associated with other inner ear abnormalities and are seldom isolated. The semicircular canals may be partially or completely assimilated into the vestibule. The diameter of the vestibule should be equal to the diameter of the bony plug between the vestibule and lateral semicircular canal.[33] The small bony island should be 3 mm or larger; if it is small, abnormal dilation of the lateral semicircular canal or vestibule is indicated[34] (e-Fig. 10-16). Although the abnormal vestibule is usually dilated, it can be small. If the vestibule is small, the oval window is frequently stenotic or atretic and the facial nerve is often malpositioned. These constellation of findings are found in the CHARGE association, along with absent semicircular canals.[18]

Enlargement of the vestibular aqueduct often is reported as the most common inner ear anomaly to be demonstrated by imaging, but with high-resolution CT and three-dimensional T2-weighted MRI, milder forms of cochlear

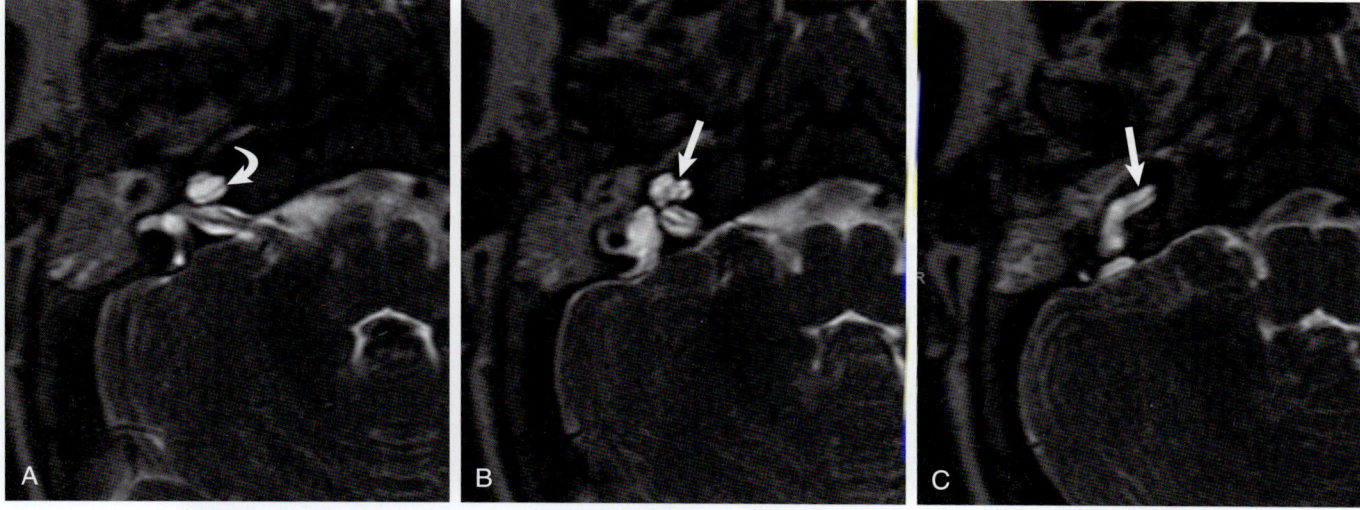

Figure 10-14 A 9-month-old with bilateral sensorineural hearing loss. **A, B,** and **C,** Axial three-dimensional T2-weighted images show a mildly dysplastic basal turn with coalescent apical and middle turns (*straight arrows*). The intrascalar septum is deficient and scalar asymmetry is present (*curved arrow*). A dilated endolymphatic duct and enlarged vestibule also are noted. The constellation of findings is typical for incomplete partition type II (Mondini deformity).

dysplasia may be more common.[26] An enlarged vestibular aqueduct is considered to result from arrested development of the endolymphatic duct and sac and is associated with progressive hearing loss, as well as complete hearing loss after trauma. The aqueduct is enlarged when the anteroposterior diameter or lateral-medial dimension is 1.5 mm or greater; this enlargement is best demonstrated on axial CT. It has been suggested that the upper limit of normal of the aqueduct on CT may be smaller than 1.5 mm, and possibly as small as 1.0 mm.[34] MR fast spin echo T2-weighted images can directly demonstrate a dilated endolymphatic duct and sac. The finding may be seen as an isolated abnormality in children with SNHL or in association with a dilated endolymphatic duct. MRI has demonstrated that a large percentage of these cases have associated anomalies of the membranous labyrinth (84%), which include modiolar deficiencies, scalar asymmetry, an enlarged vestibule, and an enlarged lateral semicircular canal[33] (e-Fig. 10-17). CT has also been shown to demonstrate a high association of superior and posterior semicircular canal dehiscence.[35]

Embryologically, the endolymphatic duct and sac form at the same time as partitioning of the cochlea occurs, which may explain the common association of cochlear dysplasia. Most cases of large vestibular aqueduct are sporadic, but it also has been reported in persons with Pendred syndrome, distal renal tubular acidosis, CHARGE association, and branchio-oto-renal syndrome.[36,37] The presence of heterogeneous signal within the sac on steady-state T2-weighted images may correlate with high protein levels and indicate the presence of Pendred syndrome and possibly the development of goiter.[38]

The size and contents of the internal auditory canal (IAC) should be evaluated on MRI in all patients. The IACs are usually symmetric; however, considerable variability is found in shape, size, and orientation. The IAC may be absent or hypoplastic. Aplasia or severe narrowing of the IAC is present in children with SNHL, which is commonly associated with deficiency or absence of the cochlear nerve. Two small channels may be present in place of the single canal, which is termed a duplicated IAC. One channel represents the facial nerve canal and the other a hypoplastic IAC with the presence of a deficient or absent cochlear nerve.[39] A duplicated IAC has been reported to be associated with Pontine tegmental cap dysplasia and other entities[40] (e-Fig. 10-18).

It is important to note that the size of the IAC correlates with the presence or absence of the cochlear nerve; however, a normal sized cochlear nerve can be associated with a small IAC, and a deficient or absent cochlear nerve can be seen with a normal IAC.[32] The osseous channel for the cochlear nerve is well demonstrated on CT, with the absence of this structure representing an indirect sign of cochlear nerve deficiency or absence[41] (e-Fig. 10-19). The cutoff value of 1.5 mm has been suggested for the size of the cochlear nerve canal, with a value of equal or lower suggesting deficiency of the cochlear nerve.[42]

The size and presence of the cochlear nerve is best assessed on MRI using oblique sagittal images through the IAC. The cochlear nerve should be greater or equal in size to the adjacent facial nerve (Fig. 10-20). If the IAC is stenotic and the cochlear nerve is not well seen, the vestibulocochlear nerve complex can be found in the cerebellopontine cistern. The vestibulocochlear nerve complex is usually greater than two times the size of the adjacent facial nerve.[43,44] The IAC may be enlarged in persons with neurofibromatosis as a result of dural ectasia or in association of translabyrinthine fistulae in children who have severe malformations of the inner ear.[45]

Treatment   Hearing aids and cochlear implantation are the most common interventions in a child with SNHL. CT and MRI are able to classify the severity of inner ear malformations encountered. MRI is better able to evaluate the intracranial contents and directly visualize the cochlear nerve, which allows the otolaryngologist to better assess the potential success of implantation and potentially directs the side to be implanted. After implantation, CT becomes the mainstay in the evaluation of complications and implant position.

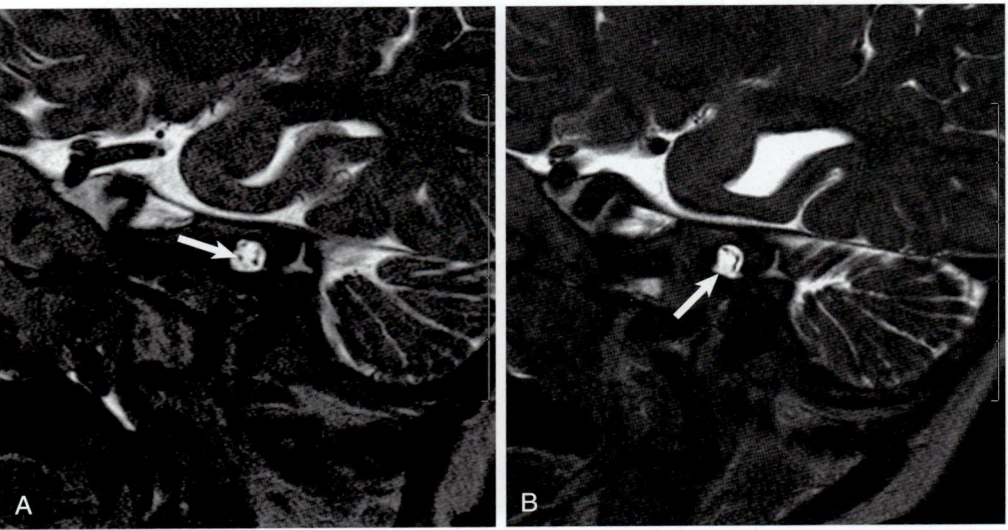

Figure 10-20   A 1-year-old with profound right sensorineural hearing loss. **A** (left) and **B** (right) oblique sagittal three-dimensional T2-weighted images show absence of the right cochlear nerve and a normal left cochlear nerve (*arrows*).

Cerebrospinal Fluid Fistula and Recurrent Meningitis

Clinical Presentation and Etiologies Recurrent meningitis may result from the association of severe inner ear anomalies and abnormal communication between the subarachnoid space and middle ear. Congenital perilymphatic fistula is a cause of unexplained asymmetric SNHL in children, and recurrent meningitis and vertigo may result. The most common site of a fistula is in the region of the stapes footplate, resulting from malformation of the stapes. Fistulas may occur via a dilated cochlear aqueduct or more commonly via a deficient lamina cribrosa. Leakage of perilymph usually occurs through the oval window.

Imaging CT findings include deficient lamina cribrosa and demonstration of fluid or soft tissue protruding though the oval window. This bulging oval window is well demonstrated on MRI as well (e-Fig. 10-21). Less commonly, the labyrinthine facial nerve canal may be enlarged and the IAC has an undulating contour.[46]

Treatment Knowledge of the potential perilymphatic fistula is important preoperatively and can obviate the need for a second surgery. A preemptive packing procedure can prevent the development of a significant leak during manipulation of the oval window.

Vascular Abnormalities

Clinical Presentation and Etiologies Vascular abnormalities often are encountered in the temporal bone. The anomalies can be asymptomatic but may alter potential surgery. Vascular abnormalities are associated with conductive hearing loss as a result of contact with the ossicular chain. A child with a glomus tumor or hemangioma may present with a vascular, bluish mass within the middle ear cavity.

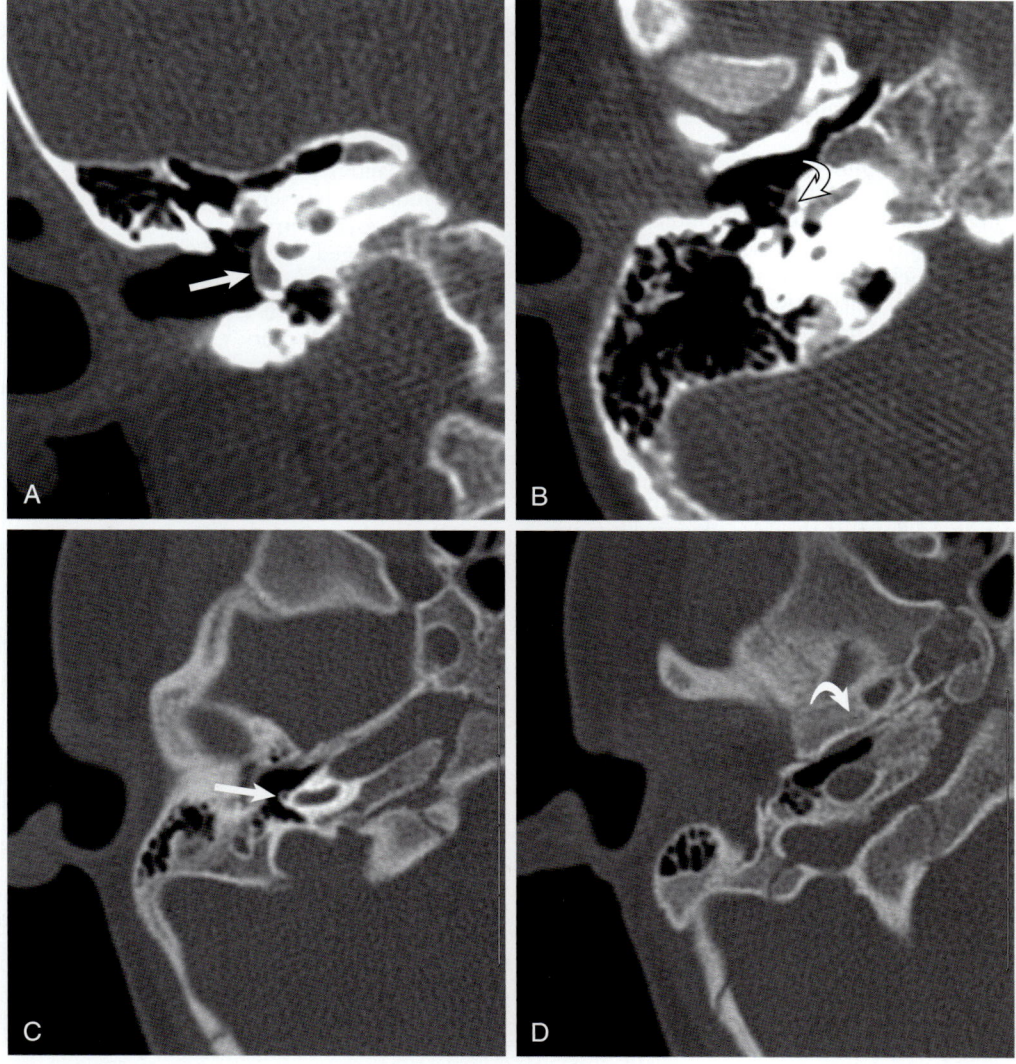

Figure 10-23 A persistent stapedial artery. **A** and **B,** Coronal and axial high-resolution computed tomography (CT) images show a vascular structure ascending vertically along the cochlear promontory (*straight arrow*) through the stapedial crura (*curved arrow*). **C** and **D,** Axial CT images in a different patient demonstrating a bony covered vessel on the cochlear promontory (*straight arrow*) and absence of the foramen spinosum (*curved arrow*).

Imaging   Arterial: The internal carotid artery (ICA) may be congenitally absent on either one or both sides. The entity can be confirmed by documenting absence of the associated carotid canal on CT.

With an aberrant ICA, the cervical portion of the ICA may regress during embryogenesis and is replaced by an anastomosis of the enlarged inferior tympanic and carotico-tympanic arteries. The aberrant ICA enters the tympanic cavity, posterior to the course of the normal ICA, through an enlarged tympanic canaliculus. It joins the horizontal carotid canal through a dehiscence in the carotid plate. This abnormality may be unilateral or bilateral. Clinical presentations include tinnitus, vertigo, hearing loss, and ear pain. The CT findings are characteristic, but an aberrant ICA also can be associated with a persistent stapedial artery (e-Fig. 10-22).

The stapedial artery usually regresses during the third month of gestation. The persistent stapedial artery is a rare anomaly that may be unilateral or bilateral and may occur with or without an aberrant ICA. The anomalous artery originates at the genu of the ICA. The artery courses superiorly over the cochlear promontory and through the crura of the stapes into the tympanic segment of the facial nerve canal. The CT appearance includes enlargement of the tympanic segment of the facial nerve and absence of foramen spinosum[47,48] (Fig. 10-23). It is important to know that the foramen spinosum can be absent in 3% of the normal population.[49]

Venous: Variants of the jugular bulb include agenesis, atresia, stenosis, diverticulum, protrusion, and high location. Agenesis of the jugular bulb is extremely rare. Associated agenesis of the sigmoid bulb may be present, with redirection of flow via transmastoid channels into regional scalp veins. Associated dilated venous collaterals should be described because they may affect potential surgery. Jugular atresia and stenosis may be isolated or associated with other disorders such as achondroplasia or Crouzon syndrome. MR or CT venography may be used to assess for venous obstruction in these patients[50] (e-Fig. 10-24).

A high jugular bulb is the most common variant, characterized by elevation of the roof of the jugular bulb above the inferior tympanic ring or floor of the IAC. It usually is unilateral but may be bilateral in up to 12% of cases. It is well demonstrated by CT or jugular venography.

Protrusion of the jugular bulb through a dehiscence of the floor of the middle ear into the hypotympanum is a common vascular anomaly of the temporal bone (e-Fig. 10-25). Clinically, the bluish mass behind the tympanic membrane may be mistaken for a vascular mass in the middle ear. Symptoms include hearing loss (usually conductive), pulsatile tinnitus, and headaches. The enhancing soft tissue mass in the middle ear and the bony defect above the jugular bulb in the floor of the hypotympanum are demonstrated on CT.[51]

A jugular diverticulum emanates from a jugular bulb that rises superomedially in the petrous pyramid. In contrast to a protruding bulb, it is more medially and posteriorly located in the petrous bone and does not invade the middle ear. The diagnosis is made only by imaging because it is not visible clinically.

Treatment   These lesion abnormalities need to be recognized and qualify them as "don't touch" lesions, with surgery usually being avoided in these children. The presence of a jugular diverticulum may affect surgery involving the IAC and should be commented on in the imaging report.[47]

Key Points

Preoperative imaging evaluation of EAC atresia should include the following:
- Ossicular chain (presence, position, fixation)
- Middle ear size
- Status of oval and round window
- Position of facial nerve
- Coexisting inner ear malformations

Round window atresia usually is associated with conductive hearing loss.

Isolated oval window atresia is a second branchial arch anomaly associated with mixed hearing loss. A malformed incus and stapes often is associated with mixed hearing loss, along with a malpositioned facial nerve.

Imaging findings in persons with CHARGE association include ossicular fixation, a small vestibule, absent semicircular canals, and oval window atresia.

An enlarged endolymphatic duct is associated with other abnormalities:
- Modiolar deficiency
- Scalar asymmetry
- An enlarged vestibule and lateral semicircular canal
- Dehiscent semicircular canals
- *SLC26A4* (*PDS*) gene
- Mondini deformity

The cochlear nerve canal should be greater or equal to 1.5 mm.
   Vascular abnormalities of the middle ear include:
- Agenesis ICA
- Aberrant ICA
- Persistent stapedial artery
- Dehiscent-protruding jugular bulb
- Jugular bulb diverticulum
- Venous agenesis—obstruction

Suggested Readings

Glastonbury CM, Davidson HC, Harnsberger HR, et al. Imaging findings of cochlear nerve deficiency. *AJNR Am J Neuroradiol.* 2002;23:635-643.

Jahrsdoerfer RA, Yeakley JW, Aguilar EA, et al. Grading system for the selection of patients with congenital aural atresia. *Am J Otol.* 1992;13:6-12.

Koesling S, Kunkel P, Schul T. Vascular anomalies, sutures and small canals of the temporal bone on axial CT. *Eur J Radiol.* 2005;54:335-343.

McClay JE, Booth TN, Parry DA, et al. Evaluation of pediatric sensorineural hearing loss with magnetic resonance imaging. *Arch Otolaryngol Head Neck Surg.* 2008;134;945-952.

Park K, Choung YH. Isolated congenital ossicular anomalies. *Acta Oto Laryngol.* 2009;129:419-422.

References

Full references for this chapter can be found on www.expertconsult.com.

Chapter 11

Infection and Inflammation

TIMOTHY N. BOOTH

Infectious and inflammatory disorders commonly involving the temporal bone; external, middle, and inner ear; and the facial nerve are discussed in this chapter.

The auricle, the cartilaginous canal, and the bony external canal comprise the external ear, with the tympanic membrane representing the division between the external and middle ear.

The middle ear is predominately composed of the tympanic cavity and its contents. The eustachian tube connects the middle ear to the nasopharynx and can be a path for the spread of infection. All air spaces are lined with mucosa, which makes them susceptible to the spread of infection and inflammation. The membranous and bony labyrinths make up the inner ear, with potential communications present within the subarachnoid space.

External Ear

EXTERNAL OTITIS

Clinical Presentation and Etiologies Children present with variable degrees of pain, as well as secretions that can be serous early and progress to frank purulence. External otitis is associated with swimming and can be caused by a number of pathogens, including fungi. Otomycosis is more common in the postsurgical ear and presents in a similar fashion to a bacterial infection.[1]

Imaging The diagnosis of otitis externa should be made clinically; however, the diagnosis can be made in the evaluation for possible mastoiditis. Soft tissue swelling and inflammation of the external canal in isolation, without evidence of involvement of the parotid or mastoids, may be demonstrated on computed tomography (CT) (e-Fig. 11-1). The acute inflammatory stage can be classified from mild to severe, and when infection spreads to surrounding tissues, the condition is then termed *malignant* or *necrotizing otitis externa*.[2] Langerhans cell histiocytosis can infiltrate the soft tissue of the external canal but is more often associated with bony involvement (Box 11-1).

Treatment Usual treatment comprises appropriate antibiotics and antifungal treatment in the postoperative ear. Surgical intervention is typically not necessary.

Malignant (Necrotizing) Otitis Externa

Clinical Presentation and Etiologies Usually, the presentation is acute, with associated systemic symptoms of fever and leukocytosis. *Pseudomonas aeruginosa* is the most common cause of this severe infection of the external canal. Diabetes is a common predisposing condition; however, any condition resulting in immunodeficiency can be associated with malignant otitis externa.[3-5] Children are reported to have better outcomes compared with adults.

Imaging CT shows more extensive inflammation within the external canal and can demonstrate bony destruction. Magnetic resonance imaging (MRI) with gadolinium demonstrates osteomyelitis, with increased signal on fat-suppressed T2-weighted images and abnormal enhancement, within bone. MRI is useful in confirming central skull base involvement, especially in the presence of multiple cranial nerve palsies, and in evaluating for intracranial complications. Facial nerve paralysis, intracranial extension, and additional cranial nerve involvement may result.[5]

Single photon emission CT (SPECT) technetium-99m bone scan is an effective way to confirm or exclude bone involvement in a patient whose condition evokes high clinical suspicion, and bone scan can be positive in the absence of osseous destruction on CT.[6]

Treatment Several weeks of intravenous antibiotics are required for adequate treatment. High-resolution CT helps assess the extent of inflammation and surrounding bony involvement and is used to stratify patients into nonsevere and severe groups, with the latter offered early surgical intervention and debridement.[7]

Other Lesions Encountered Within the External Auditory Canal

Acquired cholesteatoma may present as debris or a mass within the external auditory canal (e-Fig. 11-2), as can keratosis obturans.[8] Exostoses of the external canal may result from chronic inflammation caused by prolonged exposure to water. These lesions tend to be bilateral, broad based, and of bony density.

Foreign bodies and osteomas can also occur in the external canal, with osteomas appearing pedunculated and very dense (e-Fig. 11-3).[9]

Mastoid and Middle Ear

ACUTE INFECTIONS

Otitis Media

Clinical Presentation and Etiologies Otitis media is the most common childhood infection that is treated with antibiotics. The otoscopic findings are critical to the diagnosis. Acute otitis media typically presents with fever, ear pain, and a red tympanic membrane.[10] The initial cause of the infection is likely viral, but it may be bacterial or represent a secondary bacterial infection. Antibiotic therapy does appear to be moderately more effective than no treatment. Complications may occur in up to 10%, and this rate may be increasing; this could be associated with more conservative treatment.[11]

Imaging CT and MRI have little place in the evaluation of uncomplicated acute otitis media, with studies showing fluid in the middle ear and an associated mastoid effusion. It is important to realize that fluid in the middle ear and mastoid is also often found in asymptomatic individuals.

Mastoiditis

Clinical Presentation and Etiologies Acute mastoiditis is the most common complication of acute otitis media and usually presents with high fever and elevated systemic inflammatory markers. Bacterial infections are most commonly caused by *Streptococcus pneumoniae* and group A beta-hemolytic streptococci. Nonbacterial causes include tuberculosis and fungal infections. Disease in the very young or infections that are not responsive to antibiotic therapy should raise the suspicion of an atypical infection or possible Langerhans cell histiocytosis.[12] Facial nerve paralysis is uncommon in bacterial mastoiditis and usually is temporary, which may suggest atypical etiologies. Complications of acute mastoiditis are common, reported in up to 25% of cases.[13-15]

Imaging Mastoid air fluid levels can be seen in uncomplicated acute mastoiditis; however, the diagnosis remains a clinical diagnosis. Imaging becomes useful in evaluating for possible complications of acute mastoiditis, with CT being the primary acute imaging modality. CT facilitates the diagnosis of complications of mastoiditis with a high sensitivity and positive predictive value.[16] MRI and magnetic resonance venography (MRV) are valuable in assessing intracranial involvement and associated dural sinus thrombosis.

The initial CT finding is decreased definition of the mastoid trabeculae caused by inflammatory hyperemia. As the trabeculae are absorbed and periostitis develops, coalescent mastoiditis develops with infected fluid within the mastoid.[17] The subsequent development of a subperiosteal abscess is, by far, the most common complication and typically occurs in the postauricular region where bone is thin, termed the *Macewen triangle*. CT demonstrates a rim-enhancing fluid collection that is adhering close to bone; underlying bone is usually intact but may show focal destruction (Fig. 11-4). The abscess rarely may arise from the zygomatic root and present with an abscess anterior to the ear. The infection may also

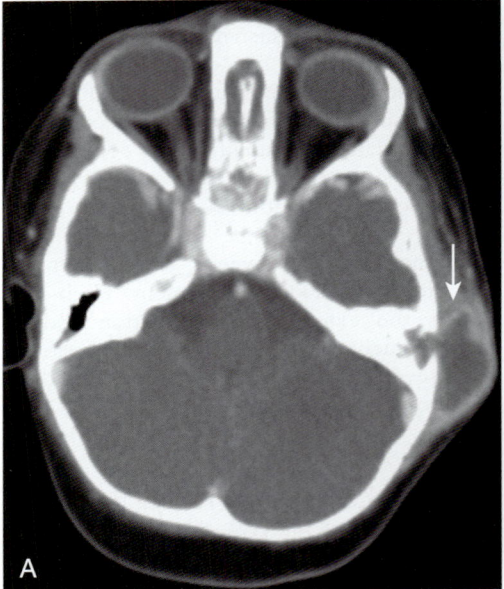 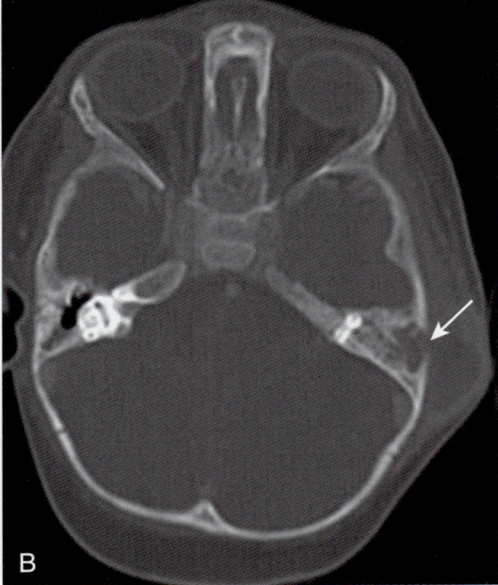

Figure 11-4 Mastoiditis in a 2-year-old with post auricular swelling. **A,** Axial computed tomography image through the mastoids shows a large subperiosteal abscess (*arrow*). **B,** Axial computed tomography with bone windows demonstrates destruction of the lateral mastoid wall (*arrow*). No intracranial extension is present with a normally enhancing sigmoid sinus.

progress inferiorly through the mastoid tip, resulting in a Bezold abscess (e-Fig. 11-5). The eustachian tube allows infection to spread into the retropharyngeal space, and children with mastoiditis may present with a retropharyngeal abscess.

Mastoid infection may extend to the petrous apex and central skull base though the continuous mucosal spaces, resulting in petrous apicitis and osteomyelitis, respectively. Petrous apicitis classically presents as the clinical Gradenigo triad of purulent otorrhea, pain in the distribution of the fifth cranial nerve, and ipsilateral sixth cranial nerve palsy.[18] CT demonstrates bony destruction and associated epidural empyema, but normal asymmetric pneumatization may make evaluation difficult. MRI demonstrates a peripherally enhancing fluid collection within the apex, and diffusion-weighted images show restricted diffusion with associated empyema or, less commonly, brain abscess (Fig. 11-6).

The major pathways that allow infectious intracranial extension include bone erosion, thrombophlebitis, and preformed pathways. The oval and round windows, cochlear and vestibular aqueducts, internal auditory canal, dehiscent tegmen, and patent petrosquamosal suture are preformed pathways that allow early or late intracranial extension. These pathways may lead to the development of suppurative labyrinthitis, as shown by abnormal enhancement of the internal auditory canal and membranous labyrinth (e-Fig. 11-7). Meningitis can occur via these pathways by spread to the subarachnoid space.[17]

Meningitis, epidural empyema, dural sinus thrombosis, and cerebellar or cerebral abscesses are the most common intracranial complications. Bony erosion commonly involves the relatively thin sigmoid plate (Trautmann triangle) and may result in an epidural empyema or anterior lateral cerebellar abscess. Usually, significant compression of the adjacent sigmoid sinus occurs, and it may be difficult to distinguish between extrinsic mass effect and thrombosis of the sinus. Erosion through the tegmen results in a middle cranial fossa epidural empyema and or temporal lobe abscess (Fig. 11-8). Veins allow organisms to readily traverse both bone and dura, resulting in thrombophlebitis and spread of infection. The sigmoid sinus is the most common to become thrombosed; however, the lateral, petrosal, and cavernous sinuses may be involved, especially with infection of the petrous apex.[17,19,20] Venous sinus thrombosis may lead to venous infarctions or otitic hydrocephalus caused by impaired venous drainage.[21] MRI and gadolinium-enhanced MRV can be helpful in diagnosing dural sinus thrombosis (e-Fig. 11-9). Diffusion-weighted images show purulent material to have increased signal, which may be especially helpful in postoperative imaging (Fig. 11-10 and Box 11-2).[19]

Box 11-2 Complications of Mastoiditis

Subperiosteal abscess

Central skull base osteomyelitis

Venous thrombosis

Meningitis

Epidural or subdural empyema

Intraparenchymal abscess

Treatment Subperiosteal abscess and other complications have traditionally been treated with drainage, cortical mastoidectomy, and ventilation tube.[13,14] However, more conservative surgical management has been recently reported. Antibiotic therapy, followed by retroauricular puncture and grommet insertion, has been proven to be an effective alternative to surgical management of complicated mastoiditis.[22,23] Intracranial involvement is treated more aggressively with neurosurgical consultation and drainage of extraaxial empyemas and intraparenchymal abscesses.

CHRONIC INFECTIONS

Chronic Otomastoiditis

Clinical Presentation and Etiologies Persistent retraction of the tympanic membrane and fluid within the middle ear cavity may be associated with chronic otitis media (COM). Tympanic membrane perforations from chronic middle ear infections typically involve the pars tensa. In contrast, retraction and perforation involving the pars flaccida portion of the tympanic membrane are usually caused by eustachian tube dysfunction. Children often present for imaging because of development of conductive hearing loss. Hearing loss may have been from ossicular erosions caused by chronic suppurative otomastoiditis or may be related to ossicular fixation, tympanosclerosis, or both.

Imaging Ossicular erosions associated with COM frequently involve the distal portion of the long process of the incus and are associated with retraction rather than bulging of the tympanic membrane.[24] Tympanosclerosis is caused by the deposition of hyalinized, often calcific, granulation tissue in the middle ear cavity. On CT, tympanosclerosis may appear as multiple middle ear masses with regions of increased density. Isolated involvement of the tympanic membrane may occur or be seen in conjunction with middle ear involvement (Fig. 11-11). Increased thickness of the ossicles may be present on imaging studies, suggesting osteitis, and CT classically demonstrates the ossicle that is not visualized too well.[20,25]

Treatment Imaging is helpful in determining the extent of ossicular erosion and disease prior to surgical intervention in COM. High-resolution CT should be used selectively and only if complications are suspected.[26] Surgical outcome is generally poor for tympanosclerosis but appears to depend on the extent of disease.[27]

Acquired Cholesteatoma

Clinical Presentation and Etiologies Cholesteatoma is composed of squamous epithelium and keratin debris, most commonly introduced into the middle ear and mastoid via retractions or perforations in the tympanic membrane. A careful otoscopic examination of the ear is essential in the initial diagnosis of cholesteatoma, and CT is typically used to diagnose the extent of the lesion or associated complications.[28] These can be subdivided into pars flaccida and pars tensa cholesteatoma. Pars flaccida lesions are caused by eustachian tube dysfunction and begin in the Prussak space before spreading into the epitympanum. Pars tensa lesions are the result of COM and perforations within the more inferior

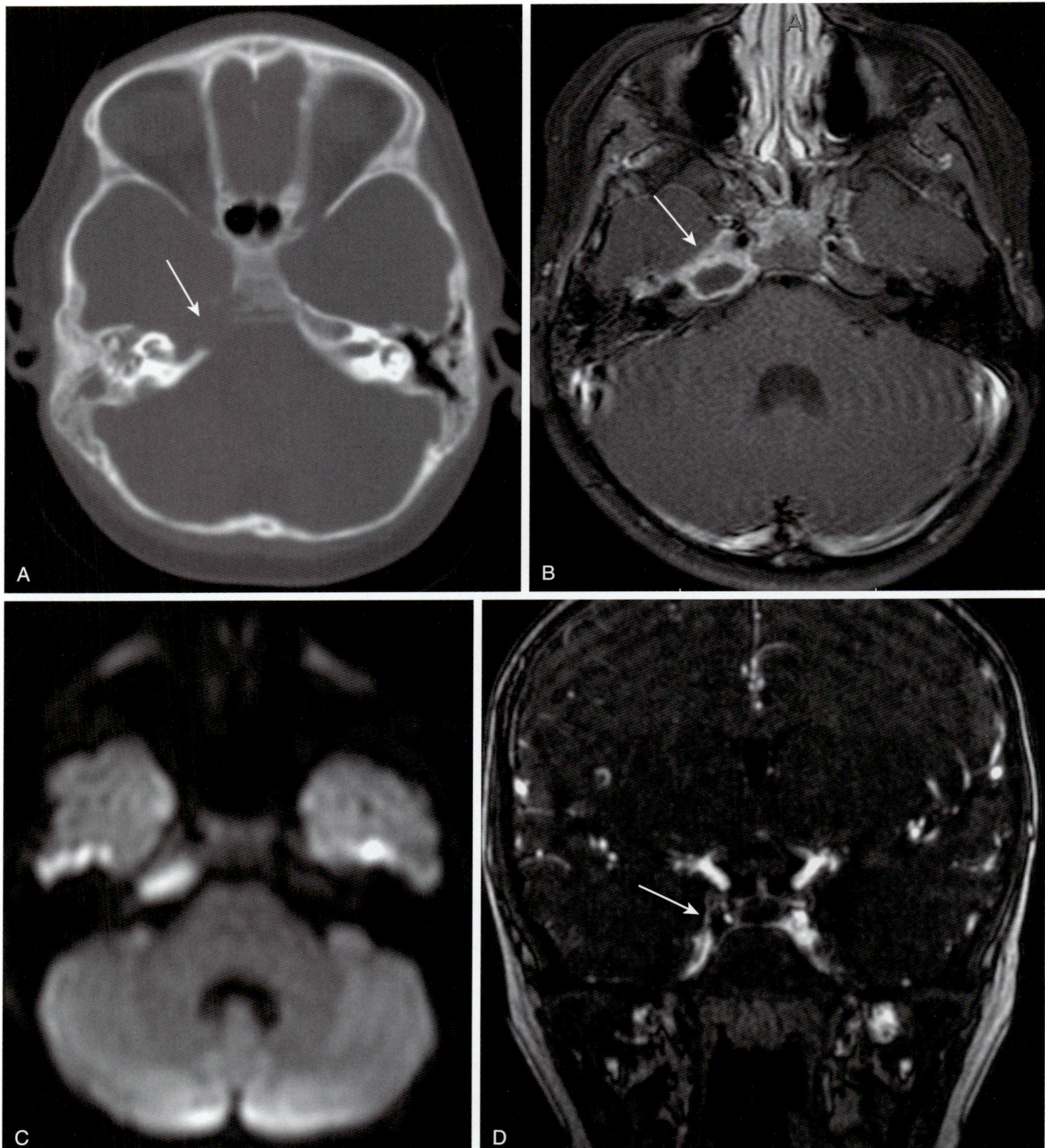

Figure 11-6 Petrous apicitis. A 6-year-old with headache and right sixth nerve palsy. **A,** Axial computed tomography shows absence of the right petrous apex (*arrow*). **B,** Axial post-gadolinium T1-weighted images show a rim-enhancing fluid collection in the right petrous apex with associated dural enhancement. The left internal carotid artery is narrowed, likely relating to inflammation within the cavernous sinus (*arrow*). **C,** Restricted diffusion is present on the axial diffusion-weighted image. **D,** Gadolinium-enhanced magnetic resonance venography shows a filling defect in the right cavernous sinus consistent with thrombosis (*arrow*).

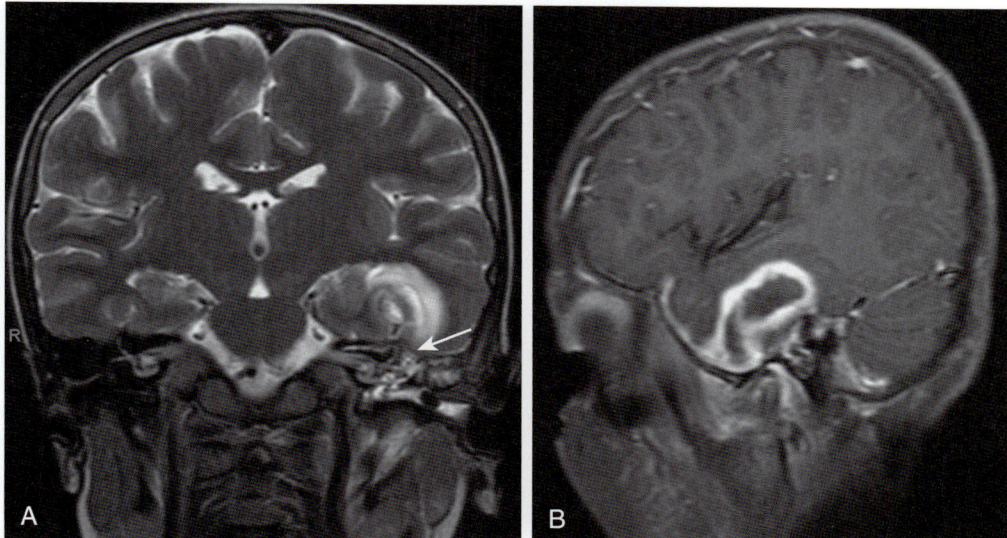

Figure 11-8 Brian abscess. An 8-year-old with complicated mastoiditis. **A,** Coronal T2-weighted image shows fluid in the left mastoid and middle ear. A defect is present within the tegmen (*arrow*) associated with a large temporal intraaxial lesion. **B,** Left parasagittal post-gadolinium T1-weighted image demonstrates rim enhancement of the temporal mass, consistent with abscess.

tympanic membrane, with extension of disease medial to the ossicles and into the oval window.

Imaging High-resolution CT is the primary imaging modality in children. The differentiation of chronic otomastoiditis without cholesteatoma from COM with cholesteatoma may be difficult with CT. Cholesteatoma usually is associated with more extensive bony erosions, including short process of the incus, lateral wall of the attic, facial nerve canal, tegmen tympani, and superior margin of the external canal or scutum (e-Fig. 11-12). Mass effect is also a significant suggestive finding, with ossicular displacement and bulging of the tympanic membrane noted on CT.[24] The ossicular chain typically lies an equal distance from the medial and lateral walls of the middle ear cavity. The position of the ossicles should be evaluated on all imaging studies, with the structures displaced medially with a pars flaccida and laterally with a pars tensa cholesteatoma (Fig. 11-13). Associated erosion of Korner septum in the mastoid antrum may also be seen. Erosion may also involve the bony separation of the middle ear cavity and the lateral semicircular canal, resulting in a fistula and sensorineural hearing loss. Cholesteatomas are histologically benign but may be locally aggressive and extend outside the confines of the temporal bone (Box 11-3).[29,30]

MRI is usually not necessary in the initial evaluation of a suspected cholesteatoma, unless intracranial involvement or labyrinthine fistula is suspected. CT evaluation of the postoperative ear is quite difficult, and differentiation of fluid from granulation tissue and recurrent cholesteatoma is nearly impossible. Echoplanar diffusion-weighted imaging was performed in the past, but small recurrent cholesteatomas were missed. Newer spin echo–based sequences have demonstrated cholesteatomas that are less than 5 mm in diameter.[31] Increased signal compared with the brain on diffusion-weighted images is considered consistent with cholesteatoma. Increased signal on T2-weighted images and peripheral enhancement on postgadolinium T1-weighted images are present (Fig. 11-14).[32] Delayed imaging can be helpful as well, but not as useful in the pediatric population because of sedation issues.

Treatment High-resolution CT allows for improved operative management in patients with COM and suspected cholesteatoma. MRI, specifically diffusion-weighted imaging, has shown promise in evaluation of postoperative patients and may eventually replace the standard second-look surgery for residual cholesteatoma.[32]

Inner Ear and Petrous Temporal Bone

LABYRINTHITIS

Clinical Presentation and Etiologies Bacterial labyrinthitis usually is caused by extension from an acute otomastoiditis or petrous apicitis. Other causes of labyrinthitis include viral, syphilitic, posttraumatic with labyrinthine hemorrhage, and autoimmune disorders.[29] Cholesteatoma with resultant translabyrinthine fistula may also result in labyrinthitis.[30] In the pediatric population, congenital infections, classically cytomegalovirus, may lead to labyrinthitis and hearing loss, but evaluation of the inner ear in the nonacute setting is most often normal.

Box 11-3 Important Structures to Evaluate in the Assessment of Cholesteatoma

Tegmen tympani and tegmen mastoidinium

Facial canal

Bony margin of lateral semicircular canal

Ossicles

Extratemporal extension

Labyrinthine involvement

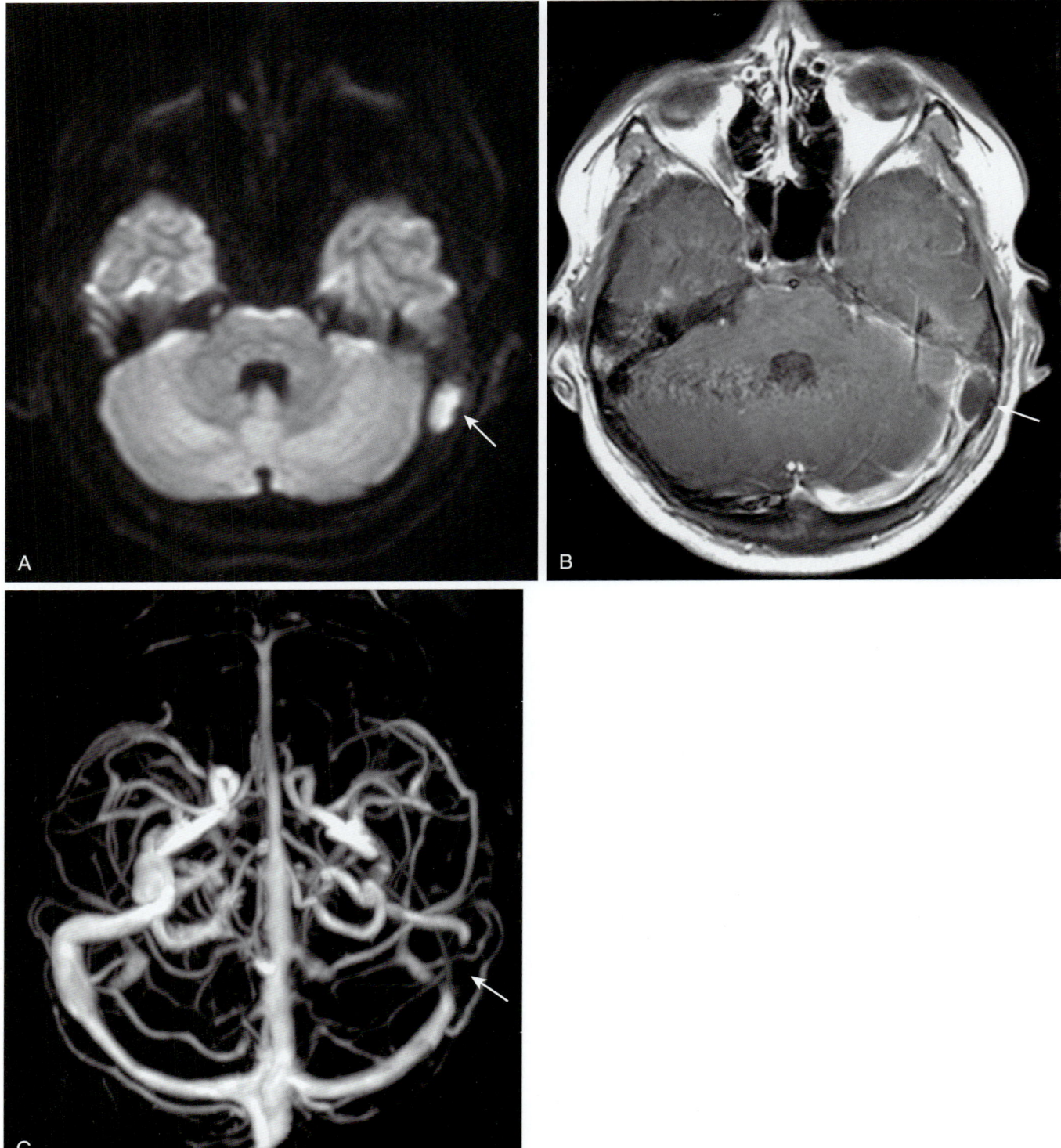

Figure 11-10 Epidural abscess. An 11-year-old with mastoiditis. **A** and **B,** Axial diffusion-weighted and post-gadolinium T1-weighted image shows restricted diffusion in a rim-enhancing fluid collection (*arrows*). **C,** Axial maximum-intensity projection image from a gadolinium enhanced magnetic resonance venogram shows extrinsic mass effect on the sigmoid sinus, with no intrinsic filling defect (*arrow*). No thrombus was demonstrated after surgical drainage of the epidural abscess.

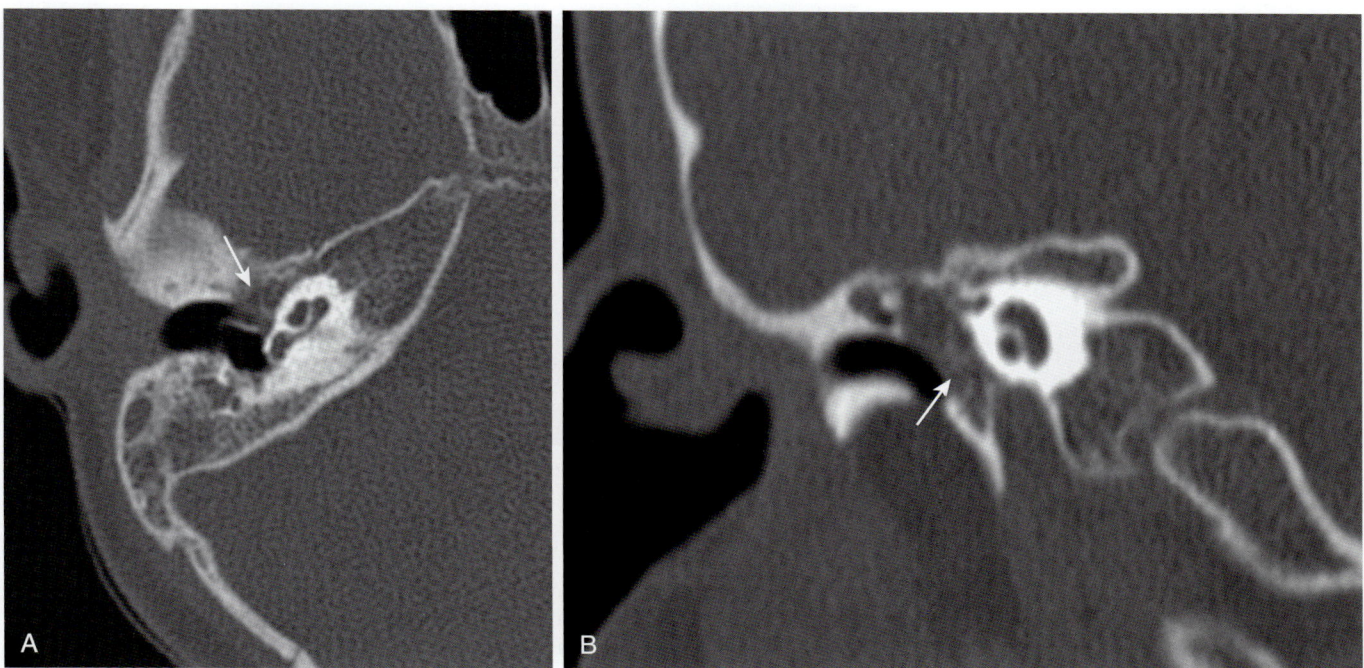

Figure 11-11   A 9-year-old with chronic otitis media and tympanosclerosis. **A** and **B,** Axial and coronal high-resolution computed tomography images though the middle ear. Abnormal soft tissue is present throughout the anterior middle ear cavity with lacelike increased density (*arrows*).

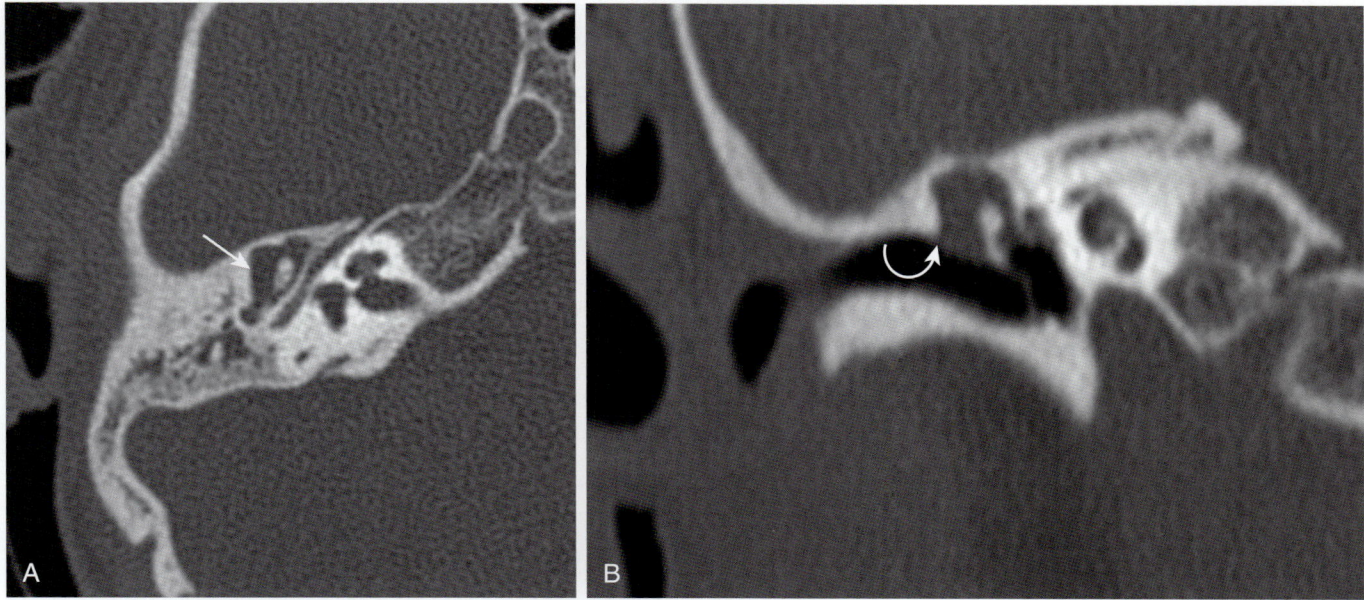

Figure 11-13   Cholesteatoma. A 5-year-old with chronic ear infections. **A** and **B,** Axial and coronal high-resolution computed tomography images through the middle ear. The ossicles are displaced medially with abnormal soft tissue in Prussak space and epitympanum (*arrow*). The scutum is eroded (*curved arrow*). At surgery, a pars flaccida cholesteatoma was removed.

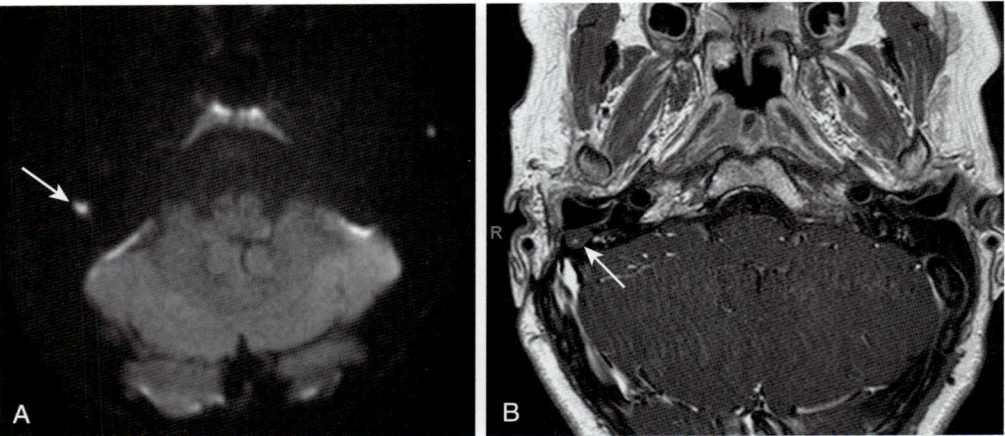

Figure 11-14 Recurrent cholesteatoma. A 9-year-old after mastoidectomy for cholesteatoma. **A,** Axial diffusion-weighted image demonstrates a focus of increased signal within the right mastoid (*arrow*). **B,** Axial post gadolinium T1-weighted image shows the lesion to be fluid intensity without enhancement (*arrow*). Surgery confirmed a 5-mm cholesteatoma.

Sickle cell disease has a known association with sensorineural hearing loss and labyrinthine hemorrhage.[33]

Imaging Labyrinthine hemorrhage manifests as increased T1-weighted signal on precontrast T1-weighted images. Enhancement within the membranous labyrinth can be demonstrated on post-gadolinium T1-weighted and fluid-attenuated inversion-recovery (FLAIR) images (see e-Fig. 11-7).[34]

LABYRINTHITIS OSSIFICANS

Clinical Presentation and Etiologies Labyrinthitis ossificans is the end result of a labyrinthine infection, hemorrhage, or toxic insult to the membranous labyrinth. Bacterial meningitis is the most common cause. A significant inflammatory process occurs and results in profound sensorineural hearing loss, which may occur as early as 2 weeks after the initial infection. Fibrous tissue is initially deposited within the membranous labyrinth, followed eventually by ossification.

Imaging Acutely, MRI may demonstrate findings of labyrinthitis; however, the normal high T2-weighted signal within the cochlea and vestibular system is preserved. In the subacute fibrous phase of the inflammatory response, MRI shows loss of the normal high T2-weighted signal in the membranous labyrinth. Ossification occurs in the latter stages of labyrinthitis and is well demonstrated on CT (e-Fig. 11-15). Both scalar chambers of the cochlea that are visualized should be evaluated in these children, as the scala tympani may be involved in isolation (e-Fig. 11-16 and Fig. 11-17).[35] CT shows increased density within the labyrinth late in the course of disease, but at this stage, cochlear implantation is more difficult. Complete ossification of the cochlea must be differentiated from cochlear aplasia, which is done by examining the cochlear promontory. The structure is absent in aplasia and normal in labyrinthitis ossificans.

Treatment The only treatment available for children with labyrinthitis ossificans is cochlear implantation. The early diagnosis of cochlear obstruction caused by labyrinthitis is

important because as the process continues, cochlear implantation may become more difficult and possibly unsuccessful.

CHOLESTEROL GRANULOMA

Clinical Presentation and Etiologies Cholesterol granuloma is the result of inflammation and obstruction that initiates repetitive hemorrhage and subsequent formation of granulation tissue. Sites of involvement include the middle ear cavity and petrous apex. Petrous apex cholesterol granuloma may be found incidentally or present with headaches and deficits in cranial nerves VI, VII, IX, X, XI, and XII.[36]

Imaging The CT appearance is that of an expansile nonenhancing soft tissue mass with sharply marginated bone destruction. The mass is of high signal intensity on both T1- and

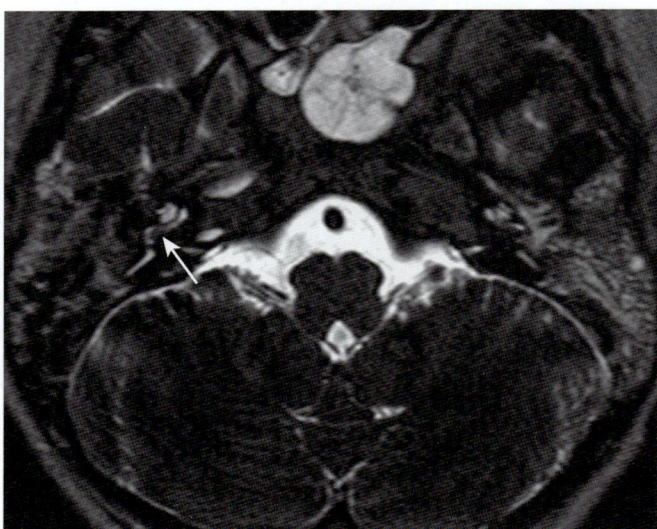

Figure 11-17 A 5-year-old with sensorineural hearing loss and meningitis. Axial three-dimensional T2-weighted image through the right cochlea shows a T2-weighted hypointense plug at the junction of the scala tympani and vestibule (*arrow*), which was confirmed at cochlear implantation. Sphenoid sinus disease is also present.

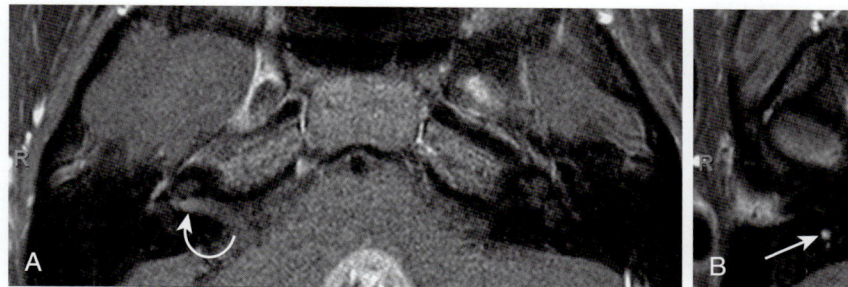
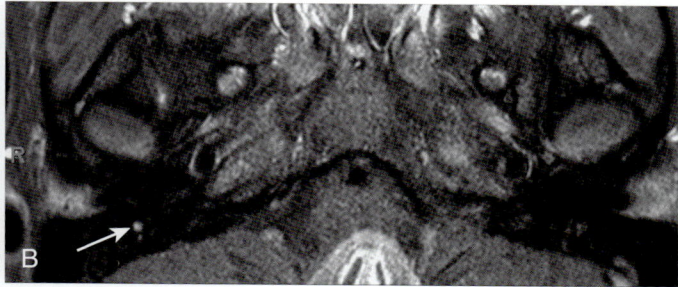

Figure 11-21 A 16-year-old female with recurrent left facial paralysis and likely Bell palsy. **A** and **B,** Axial post-gadolinium T1-weighted fat-suppressed images. Abnormal enhancement of the right intracanalicular facial nerve (*curved arrow*) and asymmetric enhancement of the tympanic and descending facial nerve on the right (*arrow*) are seen. No mass is demonstrated and the right facial palsy eventually resolved.

T2-weighted MRI scans and low signal on diffusion-weighted images, which differentiates the lesion from a congenital or acquired cholesteatoma (e-Fig. 11-18).[37]

Treatment Asymptomatic lesions are usually monitored. If cranial nerve palsies are present or symptoms are progressive, surgical drainage may be performed with fenestration or tube placement.

Facial Nerve

LYME DISEASE

Clinical Presentation and Etiologies Lyme disease is multisystemic and is caused by an infection by the tick-borne spirochete *Borrelia burgdorferi*. Three stages with influenza-like symptoms exist, with a classic rash occurring in stage 1. In stage 2, cardiac and neurologic symptoms occur. Stage 3 manifests with arthritic and chronic neurologic symptoms, sometimes years later. Clinical central nervous system involvement has been reported to occur in up to 15% of patients. Neurologic symptoms include myelopathies, encephalitis, pain syndromes, cerebellar dysfunction, movement disorders, and cranial nerve palsies.[38,39] Bilateral facial nerve palsy is a common neurologic manifestation of Lyme disease and should suggest the diagnosis.

Imaging Involvement of the brain may manifest with foci of increased T2-weighted signal, but MRI abnormalities in Lyme disease are rare. Small foci of increased T2-weighted signal are quite common, thus making the finding nonspecific.[40,41] Post-gadolinium studies may show enhancement within these lesions, increasing the specificity. Meningeal enhancement may occur, but more commonly, abnormal enhancement of the involved cranial nerves is present. The facial and trigeminal nerves are most often involved, with bilateral facial nerve involvement being a classic presentation. (e-Fig. 11-19).[42,43] Hearing loss has also been reported, possibly caused by cochlear nerve involvement. The differential diagnosis would include bilateral Lyme disease, autoimmune disease, demyelinating neuropathy (Miller–Fisher syndrome), and neoplastic etiologies (e-Fig. 11-20).

Treatment Oral antibiotics are the standard treatment for early-stage Lyme disease, usually doxycycline for adults and children older than 8 years. With central neurologic involvement, intravenous antibiotics are required.

BELL PALSY

Clinical Presentation and Etiologies Bell palsy is the most common cause of acute lower motor neuron unilateral facial nerve palsy. A viral etiology has been postulated; however, ischemic and possibly autoimmune contributions are likely contributing factors.[44] Bell palsy is a diagnosis of exclusion, and other potential etiologies of facial nerve paralysis in childhood include trauma, infection, neoplasm, and congenital anomalies. Virologic tests have suggested herpes simplex type 1 and varicella-zoster as possible etiologies.

Imaging With typical Bell palsy, complete recovery usually occurs within 6 to 8 weeks, and imaging is not necessary in the acute phase. If prolonged paralysis or other neurologic signs are present, MRI evaluation is suggested.[45] Imaging of Bell palsy demonstrates abnormal, asymmetric enhancement and mild enlargement of the facial nerve. It is important to realize that the normal facial nerve segments can enhance (geniculate ganglion, tympanic, and mastoid segments). The labyrinthine segment can show some mild enhancement. Any enhancement of the facial nerve within the internal auditory canal and strong enhancement of the labyrinthine segment is considered pathologic (Fig. 11-21).[46,47] Mild enhancement of the normal canalicular facial nerve may be noted at 3-Tesla MRI.[48]

Varicella zoster virus infection can also result in the more severe Ramsay Hunt syndrome, manifesting clinically with facial nerve palsy, sensorineural hearing loss, tinnitus, vertigo, ataxia, and a painful vesicular eruption within the region of the auricle.[49] MRI demonstrates not only abnormal enhancement of the facial nerve but also the vestibulocochlear nerve and membranous labyrinth (e-Fig. 11-22).[50]

Treatment The intensity of enhancement has been correlated with the outcome for these patients, using quantitative analysis.[51] Antiviral agents and corticosteroids are the preferred treatment in the acute phase. Surgery to decompress the facial nerve is controversial when performed in patients with complete Bell palsy that has not responded to medical therapy. Imaging can potentially direct the surgeon to the more affected portion of the nerve.[52]

Key Points

Carefully inspect the images in patients with mastoiditis for intracranial and venous complications.
A cholesteatoma demonstrates mass effect and bony erosion.
MRI is more sensitive in demonstrating cochlear obstruction in labyrinthitis ossificans.
Lyme disease should not be in the differential diagnosis on foci of increased T2-weighted signal in the cerebral white matter, unless clinically suspected.

Suggested Readings

Dobben GD, Raofi B, Mafee MF, et al. Otogenic intracranial inflammation: role of magnetic resonance imaging. *Topics Magnetic Res Imaging.* 2000;11:76-86.

Fernandez RE, Rothberg M, Ferencz G, et al. Lyme disease of the CNS: MR imaging findings in 14 cases. *AJNR Am J Neuroradiol.* 1990;11: 428-431.

Lemmerling MM, De Foer B, Verbist BM, et al. Imaging of inflammatory and infectious diseases of the temporal bone. *Neuroimag Clin North Am.* 2009;19:321-337.

Oestreicher-Kedem Y, Raveh E, Kornreich L. Complications of mastoiditis in children at the onset of the new millennium. *Ann Otol Rhinol Laryngol.* 2005;114:147-152.

Schwartz KM, Lane JI, Bolster BD, et al. The utility of diffusion weighted imaging for cholesteatoma evaluation, *AJNR Am J Neuroradiol.* 2011; 32:430-436.

References

Full references for this chapter can be found on www.expertconsult.com.

Chapter 12

Neoplasia

KORGÜN KORAL

Overview

Pediatric neoplasms of the temporal bone are relatively infrequent. The imaging specialist must be familiar with the common malignancies and their imaging appearances. Defining the extent of the lesion, both within the temporal bone and in the presence of intracranial extension, is an important task of the radiologist. Reports of temporal bone tumors should include discussion of the tumor location (external ear, middle ear and mastoid air cells, inner ear, cerebellopontine angle cistern, or internal auditory canal), facial nerve and vascular involvement, and the presence or absence of intracranial extension.

Rhabdomyosarcoma

Rhabdomyosarcoma (RMS) is the most common soft tissue sarcoma of childhood, accounting for approximately 60% of all soft tissue sarcomas and 5% to 8% of all childhood cancers.[1] Approximately 40% of all RMSs occur in the head and neck region. Temporal bone RMS is relatively rare. In a study of 39 pediatric head and neck RMS cases, 6 patients (15%) had temporal bone involvement.[2]

Most patients present before age 12 years, and 40% are younger than 5 years at presentation. An equal gender incidence is observed. The embryonal form is the most common type to involve the middle ear.[3] The onset may be insidious, with presentations of serosanguineous otorrhea or nonsuppurative granulation tissue simulating otitis externa or otitis media. The most common presentation of temporal bone RMS is chronic otitis media that is not responsive to therapy.[2] Many patients present with swelling or facial nerve palsy.[3]

The role of computed tomography (CT) is to demonstrate bone erosion and a soft tissue mass. Magnetic resonance imaging (MRI) is indicated for evaluation of intracranial extension and involvement of vascular structures (internal carotid artery, jugular vein, and dural venous sinuses). MRI appearance is usually a nonspecific, enhancing, destructive mass (Fig. 12-1, *A* and *1B*). Partial or total sparing of the otic capsule leaves the bony cochlea, vestibule, and semicircular canals isolated, creating an appearance referred to as *skeletonization*.

Treatment regimens combining chemotherapy and radiotherapy, with or without surgery, have improved the once-dismal outcomes of patients with temporal bone RMS. In a study of 14 patients, 82% of 5-year disease-free survival rate was reported.[3]

Langerhans Cell Histiocytosis

Langerhans cell histiocytosis (LCH) is a histiocytic proliferation of unknown etiology occurring primarily in infants and children. The diagnosis of LCH is made histologically by demonstration of the characteristic electron microscopic features of CD1a positivity in the involved tissue.[4] In children younger than 15 years, the annual incidence of LCH is estimated to be 0.5 in 100,000.[5] The mean age at presentation is 12 years, and no sex predilection is observed. The most common form of LCH is a solitary osteolytic lesion of the skull and spine.[6] The temporal bone may be involved in isolation or as part of polyostotic or systemic disease.[7] Temporal bone involvement may be unilateral or bilateral (30% of cases).

Although ear and temporal bone involvement is relatively rare, otologic signs and symptoms may be the only manifestations of LCH, including ear infection, otorrhea, postauricular swelling, or aural polyp. The ossicles may be eroded. Conductive hearing loss is occasionally seen in temporal bone LCH.[8] Sensorineural hearing loss and vertigo may result from destruction of the bony labyrinth. The lesion is characterized on CT as a nonspecific, lytic soft tissue mass. As in calvarial LCH, no periosteal reaction of the residual bone, which has sharp, well-defined margins, is seen (Fig. 12-2). The role of MRI is to demonstrate the soft tissue mass and the associated intracranial involvement and evaluate the hypothalamic-pituitary axis, which may be concomitantly involved in systemic LCH. Chemotherapy is generally the treatment of choice for temporal bone LCH.

Lymphoma

Primary lymphoma of the temporal bone is rare.[9] The lesions are generally lytic and may be associated with epidural components (Fig. 12-3).

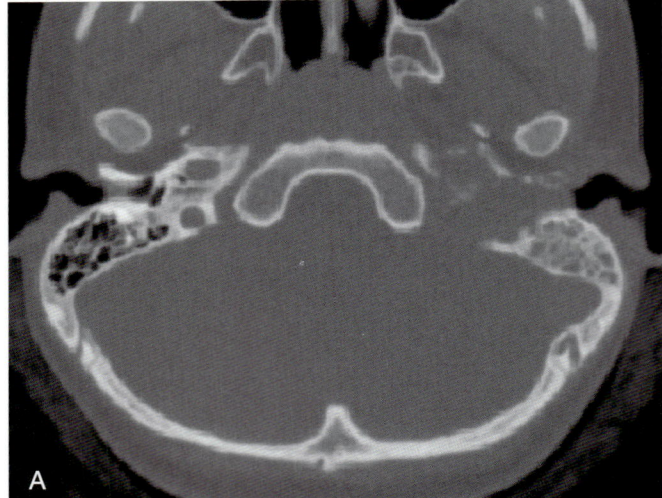

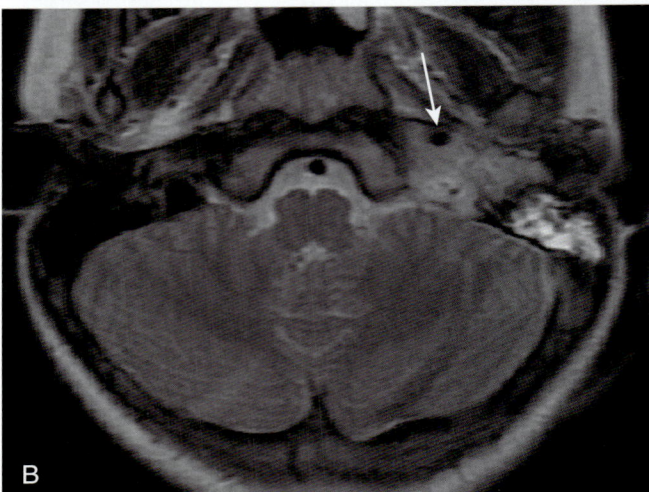

Figure 12-1   Rhabdomyosarcoma in a 12-year-old girl with hearing loss. **A,** Axial noncontrast computed tomography image shows a destructive soft tissue mass involving the petrous and tympanic segments of the left temporal bone. The mastoid air cells are opacified. **B,** Axial T2-weighted magnetic resonance image displays that the mass is less hyperintense than the fluid in the mastoid air cells. The signal void of the petrous segment of the left internal carotid artery (*arrow*) is displaced anteriorly. (Courtesy Arzu Kovanlikaya, MD, New York.)

Endolymphatic Sac Tumor

Endolymphatic sac tumor (ELST) is a rare neoplasm arising from the epithelium of the endolymphatic sac. This adenomatous neoplasm is typically located at the posterior aspect of the temporal bone. ELST is rare in adults and even rarer in children. Patients with von Hippel–Lindau disease have an increased risk of developing ELST, particularly bilaterally.[10] The characteristic imaging finding is a retrolabyrinthine mass resulting in bone erosion (Fig. 12-4). The lesions show intense enhancement with intravenous gadolinium administration. Signal voids are rarely seen on MRI despite the increased vascularity of the tumor.[11] The treatment is wide surgical resection.

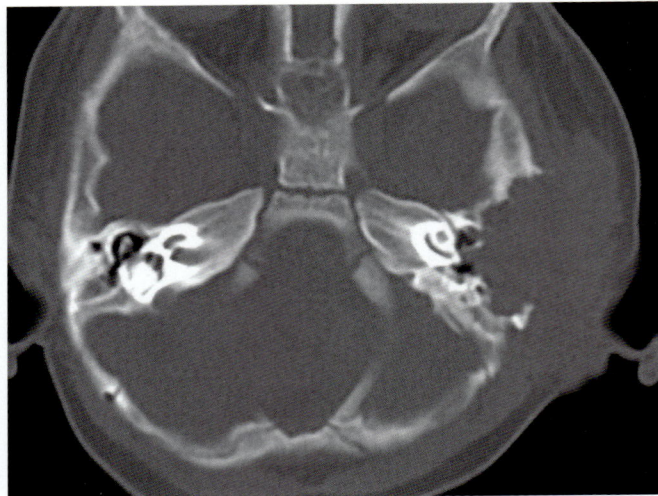

Figure 12-2   Langerhans cell histiocytosis in a 2-year-old boy with scalp and neck swelling. Axial computed tomography shows a large, destructive soft tissue mass of the left temporal bone. Note the sharp margins of the bone–mass interface.

Osteosarcoma

Primary osteosarcoma of the temporal bone is exceedingly rare.[12] The lesions can be osteoblastic, lytic, or mixed (Fig. 12-5).

Exostosis and Osteoma

Exostoses and osteomas are benign bony tumors of the external auditory canal.[11] These tumors are rarely encountered in children. Exostoses generally result from prolonged exposure

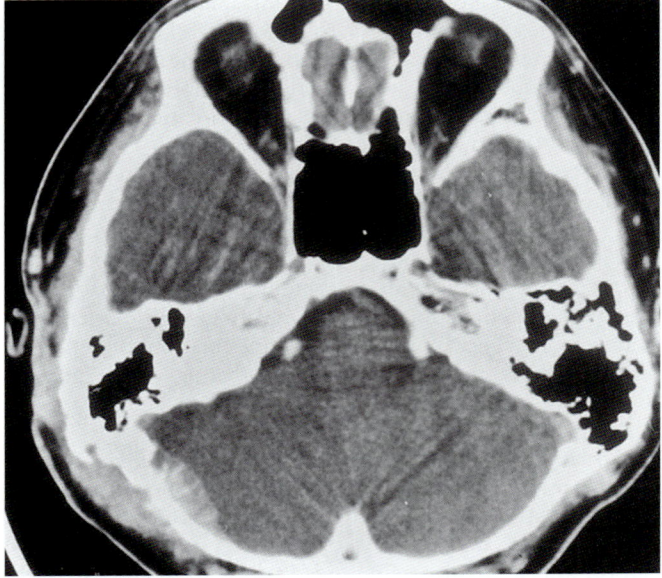

Figure 12-3   Lymphoma in a 15-year-old boy with retroauricular mass. Contrast-enhanced computed tomography shows a lytic, enhancing mass arising from the mastoid segment of the right temporal bone and involving the occipital bone. (From Koral K, Curran JG, Thompson A. Primary non-Hodgkin's lymphoma of the temporal bone. CT findings. Clin Imaging 27:386-388.)

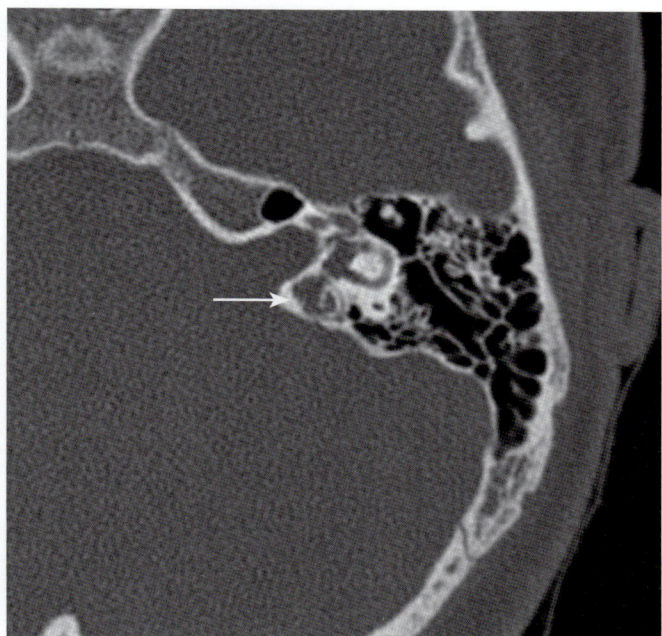

Figure 12-4 Endolymphatic sac tumor in a 14-year-old boy with sensorineural hearing loss. Axial, noncontrast computed tomography shows a lytic, expansile lesion (*arrow*) posterior to the vestibule, in the expected location of the vestibular aqueduct.

to cold water and are referred to as the "surfer's ear" or "swimmer's ear." Osteomas are rarer than exostoses and may also arise in the middle ear, mastoid, or petrous segments of the temporal bone.

Acoustic Schwannoma (Vestibular Schwannoma)

Schwannomas are rare in children, but they are encountered in children with neurofibromatosis type 2 (NF2). They arise from the acoustic nerve (cranial nerve VIII) more commonly than any other cranial nerve, and the vestibular division is more commonly involved than the cochlear division. Bilateral enhancing cerebellopontine angle or internal auditory canal masses are pathognomonic for NF2 (Fig. 12-6), although unilateral involvement should also be suggestive for NF2. Both the vestibular nerve and facial nerve may be involved in the cerebellopontine angle or internal auditory canal. Most lesions arise within the internal auditory canal, although a labyrinthine lesion may occur in the modiolus, cochlea, and vestibule or expand into the middle ear through the oval window. Treatment is resection, the goal being preservation of hearing.

Schwannomas may be seen in other cranial nerves, including the trigeminal, facial, and chorda tympani nerves, as well as cranial nerves IX, X, and XI in the jugular foramen. Intracranial and spinal meningiomas and ependymomas may be seen in patients with NF2.[13]

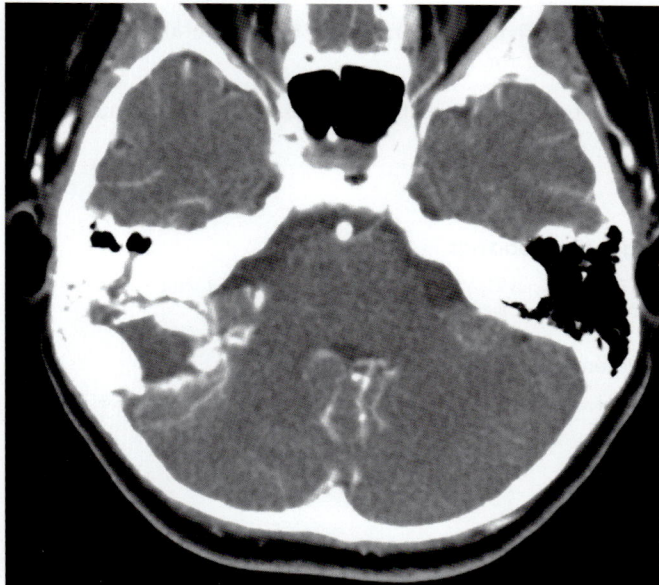

Figure 12-5 Osteosarcoma in a 9-year-old female with right facial nerve palsy who underwent heart transplantation 4 years earlier. Contrast-enhanced axial computed tomography image shows a lytic, vascular mass arising from the mastoid segment of the temporal bone with intracranial extension.

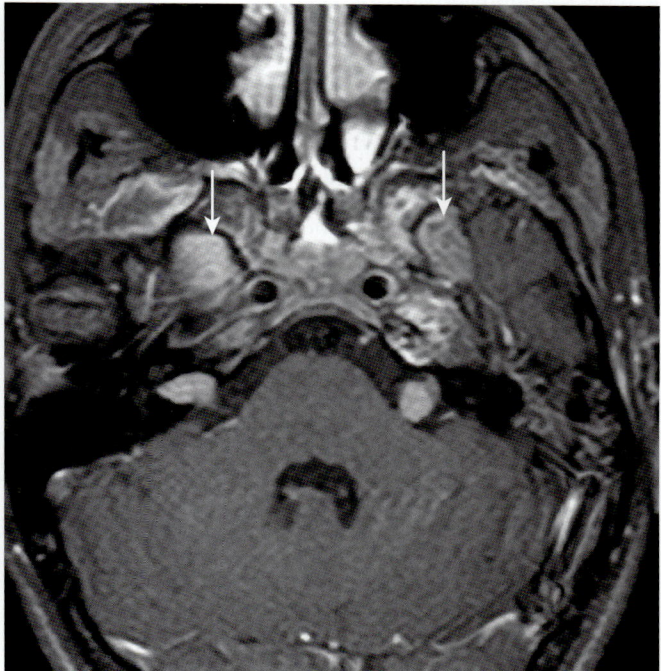

Figure 12-6 Acoustic schwannomas in a 15-year-old male with neurofibromatosis type 2. Bilateral internal auditory canal masses are present. There are enhancing masses in the enlarged bilateral foramina ovale (*arrows*).

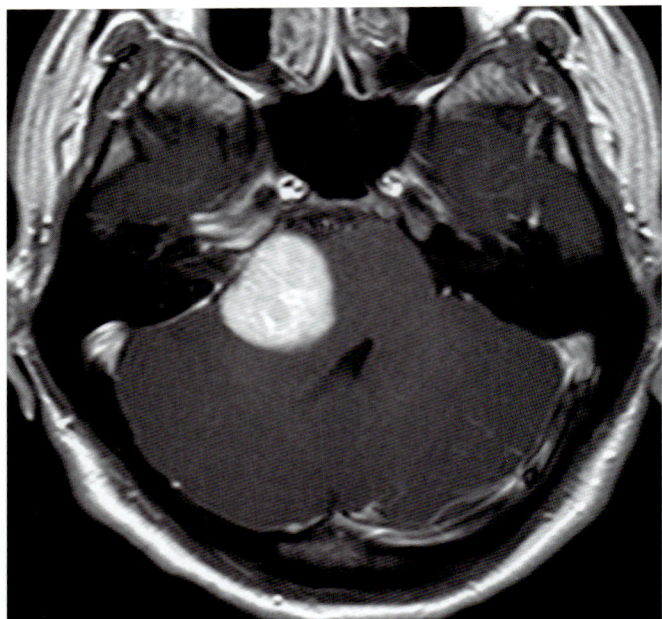

Figure 12-7 Hemangiopericytoma in a 15-year-old male with an intensely enhancing right cerebellopontine angle mass. The mass does not extend into the internal auditory canal. The primary differential diagnosis is meningioma.

Hemangiopericytoma

Hemangiopericytoma is a highly vascular tumor rarely seen in children.[14] In the cerebellopontine angle, the main differential consideration is meningioma (Fig. 12-7). Treatment is with resection, usually followed by radiotherapy.

Paraganglioma

Paragangliomas of the temporal bone arise from the jugulotympanic paraganglia of neural crest origin. Tumors arising from the middle ear nerves are termed *tympanic paragangliomas* or *glomus tympanicum*, and tumors arising from the jugular bulb are termed *glomus jugulare*. These tumors are rare in childhood but may present with symptoms of recurrent otitis media, unilateral pulsatile tinnitus, and aural fullness from conductive hearing loss. Bleeding, vertigo, sensorineural hearing loss, and cranial nerve palsies indicate advanced disease.

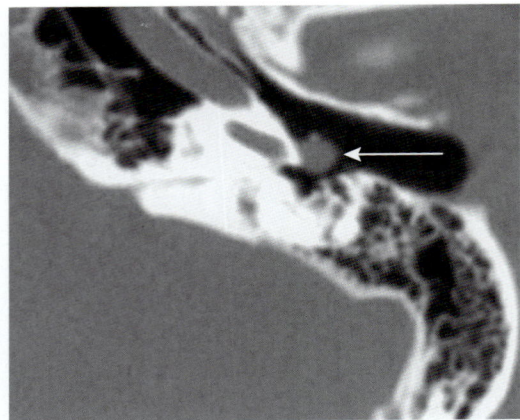

Figure 12-8 Paraganglioma. Axial computed tomography of the left ear shows a soft tissue mass (*arrow*) adjacent to the promontory consistent with a paraganglioma (glomus tympanicum).

CT and MRI scans show a mass in the mesotympanum or jugular foramen (Fig. 12-8). These are highly vascular tumors that enhanced intensely with intravenous contrast. In larger lesions, MRI may show arborizing vessels and a typical "salt and pepper" pattern of hyperintense TI-weighted signal and hypointense T2-weighted signal. The preferred treatment is surgical excision.

Key Points

- Temporal bone tumors are rare in children.
- LCH and RMS are the most common neoplasms.
- Bilateral lytic temporal bone masses are almost pathognomonic for LCH.
- Bilateral acoustic schwannomas are pathognomonic for NF2.

Suggested Readings

De Foer B, Kenis C, Vercruysse JP, et al. Imaging of temporal bone tumors. *Neuroimaging Clin N Am.* 2009;19(3):339-366.

References

Full references for this chapter can be found on www.expertconsult.com.

Embryology, Anatomy, Normal Findings, and Imaging Techniques

VERA R. SPERLING

Embryology of the Neck

Accurate diagnosis and successful treatment of congenital anomalies and masses of the neck are dependent on an understanding of the complex embryologic development of this region and the anomalies that result from abnormal development.

This chapter will focus on the embryology of the neck and the oral cavity. The embryology of the orbit, face and sinuses, temporal bone, and ear are addressed in Chapters 4, 8, 9, and 18.

Many of the structures of the head and neck form from an interaction between somitomeres, somites, the mesenchyme, and the branchial apparatus.

DEVELOPMENT OF THE MESENCHYME

The mesenchyme is derived from three main sources:
1. The lateral plate mesoderm, which forms the laryngeal cartilages and regional connective tissue
2. The neural crest cells, whose migration initiates the formation of the pharyngeal arch skeletal structures and regional bone, cartilage, tendons, and glandular stroma
3. The ectodermal placodes, from which originate the fifth, seventh, ninth, and tenth cranial nerves (CNs)

DEVELOPMENT OF THE MESODERM, SOMITOMERES, AND SOMITES

After neurulation occurs, the mesoderm subdivides into the lateral, intermediate, and paraxial mesoderm. The lateral mesoderm forms most of the throat and larynx. The intermediate mesoderm does not form any part of the head and neck. The paraxial mesoderm forms the seven somitomeres and 42 to 44 paired somites. The five most rostral somites are involved in the formation of head and neck musculature (Fig. 13-1). The somitomeres and somites form before the development of the branchial apparatus.

The branchial apparatus, that is, the branchial arches, clefts, pouches, and membrane, begin to form late in the third week of gestation. The buccopharyngeal membrane breaks down and the mesodermal branchial bars begin to form six pairs of branchial arches. The fifth arch is rudimentary and disappears.

The fourth somitomere invades the first branchial arch and generates the formation of the muscles of mastication, that is, the masseter, pterygoid, and temporalis muscles. These muscles are innervated by the trigeminal nerve (CN V).

The seventh somitomere interacts with the third branchial arch to form the stylopharyngeus muscle, which is innervated by the glossopharyngeal nerve (CN IX).

The first four occipital somites invade the fourth and sixth branchial arches and thus stimulate the formation of the extrinsic and intrinsic laryngeal muscles innervated by the vagus nerve (CN X) and the cranial segment of the spinal accessory nerve (CN XI).

The third through seventh somites form the sternocleidomastoid muscle and trapezius and are innervated by the spinal accessory nerve (CN XI).

The intrinsic and extrinsic tongue muscles are likely derived from the second through fourth occipital somites and are innervated by the hypoglossal nerve (CN XII).

The contribution of the somitomeres and somites to the formation of muscles and their distinct innervation is unchanged throughout growth and development. Thus although many muscles migrate in location, their nerve supply is maintained and hence their branchial arch origin can always be identified (see Fig. 13-1).

DEVELOPMENT OF THE BRANCHIAL APPARATUS

Formation of the branchial apparatus occurs between the fourth through seventh weeks of development. The pharynx constitutes much of the foregut during the first few weeks of development. Formation of the five branchial arches (I, II, III, IV, and VI) results from the breakdown of the buccopharyngeal membrane and segmentation of the mesoderm. Migration of neural crest cells to this location stimulates growth and development. Each arch has its own outer epithelial lining of ectoderm separated by five clefts and an inner epithelial lining of endoderm with five corresponding pouches and a central cartilaginous core, which is a mesenchymal derivative that participates in the formation of the characteristic skeletal, muscular, ligamentous, vascular, and neural components of each arch.

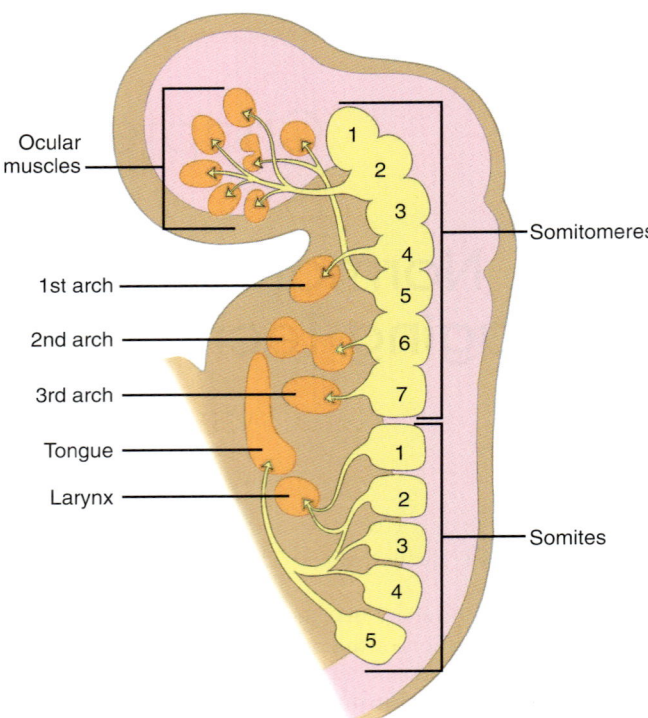

Ocular muscles

1st arch

2nd arch

3rd arch

Tongue

Larynx

Somitomeres

Somites

Figure 13-1 Embryology. A sagittal section shows the relationship of somitomeres and somites and their corresponding derivatives. (From Som P, Curtin H. *Head and neck imaging.* 4th ed. Philadelphia: Mosby; 2003.)

Shortly after formation of the branchial arches, the first and second arches undergo mesodermal proliferation, thus creating the epicardial ridge, which contains the mesodermal precursor of the sternocleidomastoid, the trapezius, and the infrahyoid and lingual muscles. The nerves of the epicardial ridge are the hypoglossal (CN XII) and spinal accessory (CN XI) nerves. The proliferation of mesenchyme overgrows branchial arches II, III, and IV and narrows branchial clefts II, III, and IV. Subsequently, an ectodermal pit is formed— the cervical sinus of His—which obliterates with further development; failure of obliteration results in formation of branchial sinus, clefts, or cysts of types II, III, or IV.

Branchial Apparatus and its Contribution to the Structures of the Neck

Branchial Arches

The first branchial arch (Fig. 13-2) is composed of a dorsal segment known as the maxillary process and a ventral segment known as Meckel cartilage or the mandibular process; both involute. The ossification around Meckel cartilage is the precursor of the mandible and the sphenomandibular cartilage in the neck. The muscle derivatives of the first arch are the muscles of mastication (the masseter, pterygoid, and temporalis muscles), the tensor tympani and tensor veli palatine muscles, the anterior belly of the digastric muscle, and the mylohyoid muscle. The trigeminal nerve (CN V) provides motor and sensory innervation to the first branchial arch.

The second branchial arch is also known as Reichert cartilage. It gives rise to the upper body and lesser cornu of the

hyoid bone, the styloid process, and stylohyoid ligament. The muscle derivatives include the platysma, the posterior belly of the digastric, and the stylohyoid. The nerve of the second brachial arch is the facial nerve (CN VII), which is primarily motor. The main sensory component is the chorda tympani branch that is carried with a branch of the trigeminal nerve (CN V3) to supply taste to the anterior two thirds of the tongue. The artery of the second brachial arch is the stapedial artery, which normally regresses aside from some contributions to the internal and external carotid arteries.

The third branchial arch cartilage derivatives include the greater cornu and inferior body of the hyoid. The muscle derivatives include the stylopharyngeus and superior and middle pharyngeal constrictors. The nerve of the third brachial arch is the glossopharyngeal nerve (CN IX). The neural crest cells of the third branchial arch also form the carotid bodies. The artery of the third branchial arch contributes to the common carotid artery and the internal and external carotid arteries.

The fourth and sixth branchial arch cartilage derivatives fuse to form the larynx and the laryngeal cartilages (the thyroid, cricoid, arytenoid, corniculate, and cuneiform). Muscle derivatives include the cricothyroid muscle, the levator veli palatini, and the inferior pharyngeal constrictors. The muscle derivatives of the sixth arch are the remaining intrinsic muscles of the larynx. The nerve of the fourth arch is the superior laryngeal nerve, and the nerve of the sixth arch is the recurrent laryngeal nerve. Both are branches of the vagus nerve (CN X). The artery of the fourth branchial arch contributes to the aortic arch on the left and the subclavian artery on the right. The artery of the sixth branchial arch becomes the ductus arteriosus and the pulmonary artery. Between the branchial arches lie the paired branchial pouches and clefts.

Branchial Pouches

The first branchial pouch does not contribute to the structures of the neck. The second branchial pouch gives rise to the palatine tonsils and tonsillar fossa. The third branchial pouch gives rise to the inferior parathyroids and thymus. The early embryologic connections to the pharynx normally are obliterated. The fourth branchial pouch gives rise to the superior parathyroid glands and the ultimobranchial body, which contains the parafollicular cells (C cells) of the thyroid gland. The fifth branchial pouch degenerates. The branchial clefts do not contribute to any neck structures and are obliterated as development occurs (Tables 13-1 and 13-2).

Embryology of the Tongue

The tongue forms from the first four branchial arches. Two lateral and one central swelling, the tuberculum impar, form from the first branchial arch. A second central swelling, the copula/hypobranchial eminence, forms from the second, third, and fourth branchial arches. A third central swelling from the fourth branchial arch forms the epiglottis. Thus the anterior two thirds or body of the tongue forms from the first branchial arch, whereas the root of the tongue forms from the second, third, and fourth branchial arches. The groove that is formed where the anterior and posterior portions of the tongue fuse is called the terminal sulcus.

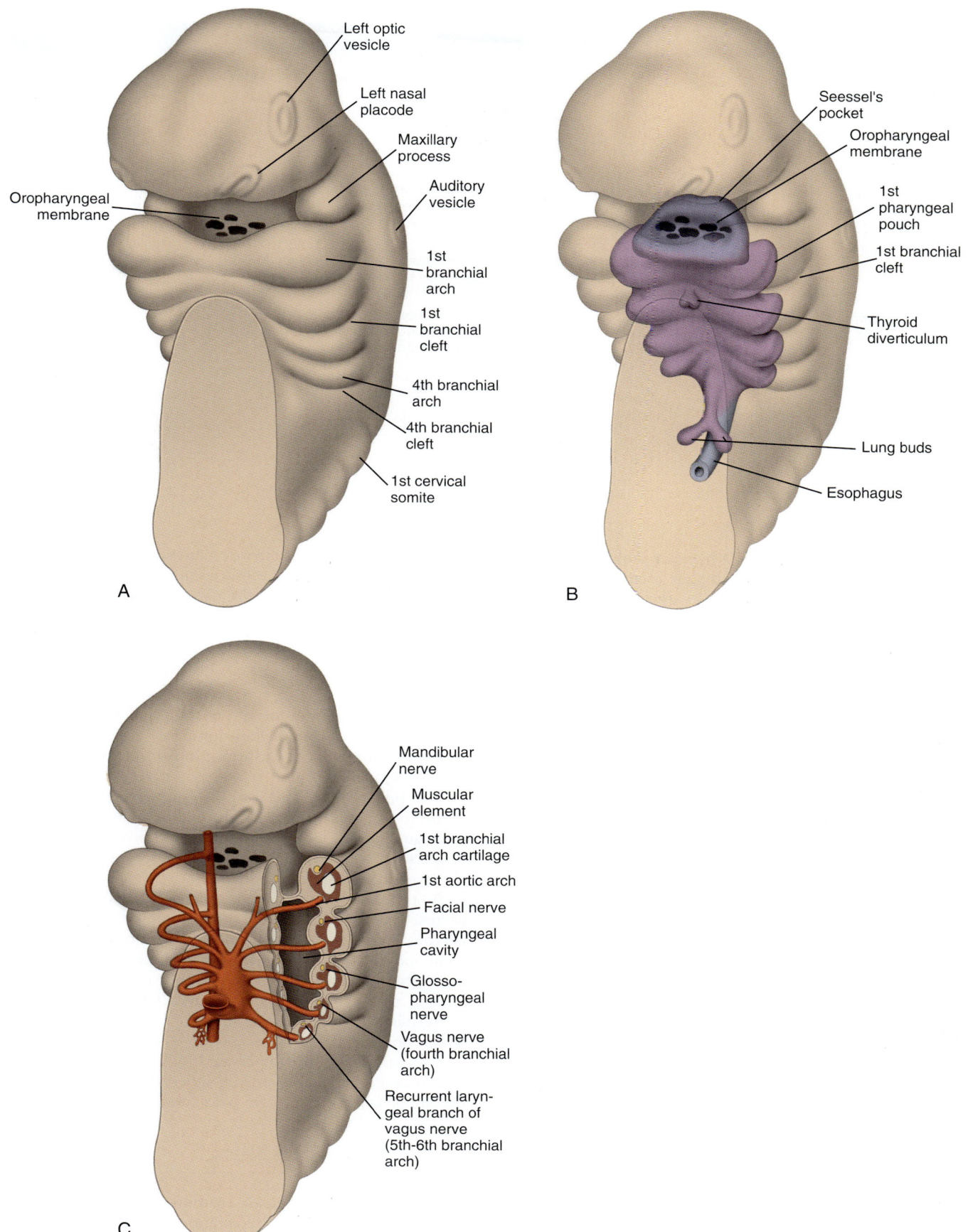

Figure 13-2 Embryology. Relationship of branchial arches and clefts and subsequent derivative structures. (From Som P, Curtin H. *Head and neck imaging.* 4th ed. Philadelphia: Mosby; 2003.)

Table 13-1

Derivatives of the Branchial Arches					
Arch	**Nerve**	**Muscles**	**Skeletal Structures**	**Ligaments**	**Artery**
First (mandibular)	Trigeminal nerve (CN V) (maxillary and mandibular branches only)	Muscles of mastication, mylohyoid,; anterior belly of digastric, tensor tympani, tensor veli palatine	Malleus incus	Anterior ligament of malleus, sphenomandibular ligament	Maxillary artery
Second (hyoid)	Facial nerve (CN VII)	Muscles of facial expression, stapedius, stylohyoid, posterior belly of digastric	Stapes, styloid process, lesser cornu and upper body of the hyoid bone	Stylohyoid ligament	Stapedial artery (rarely)
Third	Glossopharyngeal nerve (CN IX)	Stylopharyngeus, superior and middle pharyngeal constrictors	Greater cornu and lower part of body of the hyoid bone		Contributions to the carotid arteries
Fourth and sixth	Superior laryngeal branch of vagus nerve (CN X)—fourth arch; recurrent laryngeal branch of vagus nerve (CN X)—sixth arch	Cricothyroid, levator veli palatine, inferior pharyngeal constrictors, intrinsic muscles of larynx, striated muscles of the esophagus	Thyroid, cricoid, arytenoid, corniculate, cuneiform cartilages		The artery of the fourth arch contributes to the subclavian artery on the right and the aortic arch on the left; the artery of the sixth arch forms the ductus arteriosus and the pulmonary artery

CN, Cranial nerve.
Adapted from Moore KL, Persaud MG, Torchia MG. *Before we are born*. Philadelphia: Saunders/Elsevier; 2008.

The hypoglossal nerve (CN XII) innervates all the intrinsic tongue muscles and all extrinsic tongue muscles but the palatoglossus. Sensory innervation is by the lingual branch of CN V3, the chorda tympani branch of CN VII, the lingual branch of CN IX, and the recurrent laryngeal branch of CN X.

Embryology of the Thyroid Gland

The thyroid gland originates from a median endodermal thickening in the floor of the primitive pharynx in the third to fourth week of development. The thyroid primordium develops between the tuberculum impar and the copula of the first and second pouches. The foramen cecum is the remnant of the thyroid promordium in this location, between the anterior two thirds and the posterior one third of the tongue. The thyroid gland passes anterior to the hyoid and laryngeal cartilages and descends anterior to the thyrohyoid membrane and the strap muscles. The thyroid gland reaches its final position by the seventh week of development. During its inferior migration, the thyroid anlage is connected to the tongue by the normally transient thyroglossal duct. Innervation of the thyroid gland is primarily by the sympathetic middle cervical ganglion.

Embryology of the Salivary Glands

The common pathway for salivary gland development is the ingrowth of surface epithelium (primarily ectoderm, but also endoderm for minor salivary gland formation) into the underlying mesenchyme.

The precursors of the parotid gland appear between the fourth to sixth weeks of gestation, and the submandibular and sublingual glands appear between the sixth to eighth weeks of gestation. The minor salivary glands do not develop until the twelfth week of gestation.

A process of proliferation, division, and canalization occurs. Interaction with and stimulation by the autonomic nervous system is essential for normal salivary gland development and function. The final process of encapsulation occurs in reverse to the order of development and growth. Encapsulation of the parotid gland occurs after formation of the lymphatic system, accounting for the presence of intraparotid lymph nodes.

The parotid gland is innervated by CN IX, the submandibular and sublingual glands are innervated by CN VII, and the minor salivary glands are innervated by CN V.

Anatomy of the Neck

Clinical evaluation and classic anatomy divides the neck into triangles. The largest are the anterior and posterior triangles, which are defined and separated by the sternocleidomastoid

Table 13-2

Derivatives of the Branchial Pouches	
Pouch	**Derivatives**
First	Eustachian tube, middle ear, portions of mastoid bone
Second	Palatine tonsils, tonsillar fossa
Third	Inferior parathyroids, thymus
Fourth and sixth	Superior parathyroids, parafollicular cells of thyroid

Adapted from Moore KL, Persaud MG, Torchia MG. *Before we are born*. Philadelphia: Saunders/Elsevier; 2008.

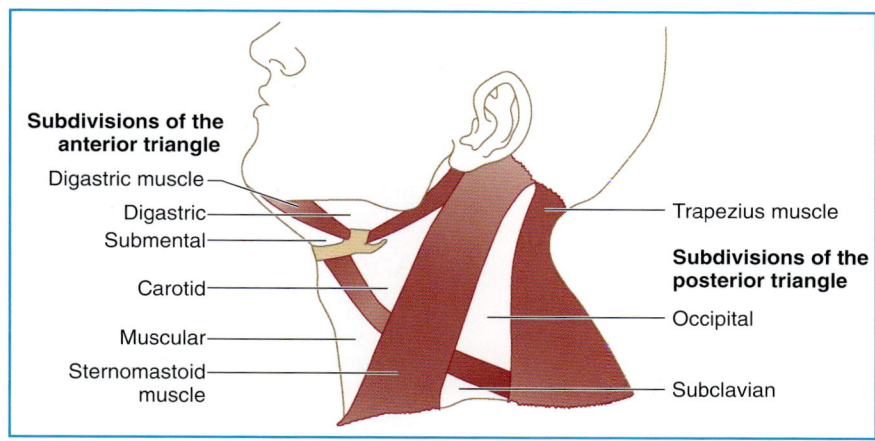

Subdivisions of the anterior triangle

Digastric muscle

Digastric

Submental

Carotid

Muscular

Sternomastoid muscle

Trapezius muscle

Subdivisions of the posterior triangle

Occipital

Subclavian

Figure 13-3 Traditional triangular division of neck spaces.

muscles. The anterior triangle is further subdivided into the paired carotid and submandibular triangles (separated by the posterior belly of the digastric muscle) and the single midline submental and infrahyoid muscular triangles. The posterior triangle consists of the paired occipital and subclavian triangles, which are separated by the inferior belly of the omohyoid muscle (Fig. 13-3). The central cavity is divided into the nasopharynx, oropharynx, hypopharynx, and oral cavity.

This approach to neck anatomy does not reflect anatomy as defined by the fascial layers, that is, the superficial and deep cervical fascia of the head and neck. The deep cervical fascia is composed of three layers:

1. The superficial layer of the deep cervical fascia (SL-DCF), also known as the investing fascia, which defines the masticator, parotid, and submandibular spaces; it also contributes to the carotid space

2. The middle layer of the deep cervical fascia (ML-DCF), also known as the visceral fascia, which primarily forms the buccopharyngeal and pharyngobasilar fascia and the fascia of the tensor veli palatine; it also contributes to the carotid space

3. The deep layer of the deep cervical fascia (DL-DCF), also known as the prevertebral fascia, which forms the perivertebral space and then is subdivided into the anterior prevertebral and posterior paraspinal compartments; the alar fascia is a small component of the DL-DCF and also contributes to the carotid sheath

The advent of cross-sectional imaging enabled a new approach to neck anatomy defined by the concept of dividing the neck into the suprahyoid and infrahyoid compartments, with further subdivision of each compartment into fascially defined spaces (Figs. 13-4 and 13-5). The resultant refined approach to differential diagnosis, combined with the use of surgically and pathologically defined common terminology and nomenclature, has improved communication between radiologists and clinicians.

The pharyngeal mucosal space, which is located in the suprahyoid neck, is the surface of pharynx. It encompasses the nasopharyngeal, oropharyngeal, and hypopharyngeal mucosa. Centrally located, it is posterior to the retropharyngeal space and lateral to the parapharyngeal space. It is not a true fascially enclosed space because only its deep margin is bound by the ML-DCF.

The parapharyngeal space is located in the suprahyoid neck; it extends from the skull base to the submandibular space. The medial fascial boundary is the visceral/buccopharyngeal fascia. The pterygomandibular raphe and masticator space is its anterior boundary. Laterally and posteriorly it is bounded by the carotid and retropharyngeal space.

The carotid space, which is located in both the suprahyoid and infrahyoid neck, extends from the skull base to the aortic arch. All three layers of deep cervical fascia form the carotid sheath. The carotid sheath is better defined in the infrahyoid neck and more loosely formed in the suprahyoid neck.

The retropharyngeal space, which is located in both the suprahyoid and infrahyoid neck, extends from the skull base to T3. The ML-DCF constitutes the anterior wall, and the DL-DCF constitutes the posterior wall. The lateral wall is the alar fascia, a small fragment of the DL-DCF. It is posterior to the pharyngeal mucosal space in the suprahyoid neck and the visceral space in the infrahyoid neck, anterior to the danger space posterior, and medial to the carotid space.

The masticator space, which is located in the suprahyoid neck, extends from the superior aspect of suprazygomatic masticator space/temporal fossa at the level of parietal bone to the inferior aspect of the infrazygomatic masticator space/undersurface of the posterior body of the mandible. It is bounded by a sling of the SL-DCF that extends from the inferior mandible to the skull base and zygomatic arch. It is anterior to the parotid space, anterolateral to the parapharyngeal space, and lateral to the pharyngeal mucosal space. Superior to it is the skull base, including the foramina ovale and spinosum.

The parotid space, which is located in the suprahyoid neck, extends superiorly from the external auditory canal and mastoid tip to below angle of mandible. It is enclosed by the SL-DCF.

The perivertebral space, which is located in both the suprahyoid and infrahyoid part of the neck, extends from the skull base to T4 and consists of a prevertebral and a paraspinal component. It is enveloped by the DL-DCF. The perivertebral space is posteromedial to the carotid space and medial to the posterior cervical space.

The visceral space, which is located in the infrahyoid neck, lies anterior to the retropharyngeal space in the midline and is enclosed by the ML-DCF.

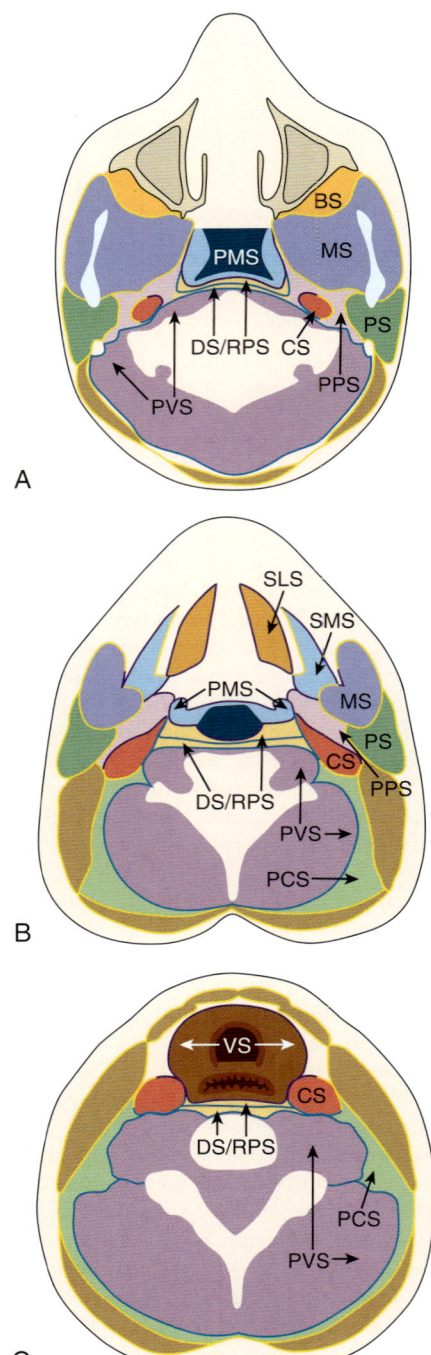

Figure 13-4 Fascial compartments of the neck. **A,** Spaces and investing fascia of the suprahyoid neck and the level of the nasopharynx. **B,** Spaces and investing fascia of the suprahyoid neck at the level of the oropharynx. **C,** Spaces and investing fascia of the infrahyoid neck. *BS,* buccal space; *CS,* carotid space; *DS,* danger space; *MS,* masticator space; *PCS,* posterior cervical space; *PMS,* pharyngeal mucosal space; *PPS,* parapharyngeal space; *PS,* parotid space; *PVS,* perivertebral space; *RPS,* retropharyngeal space; *VS,* visceral space. (Redrawn from Harnsberger HR, Hudgins P, Wiggins R, et al. *Diagnostic imaging: head and neck.* Salt Lake City, Utah: Amirsys Inc; 2004.)

The posterior cervical space extends from the mastoid tip to the level of the clavicle. Its superficial boundary is the SL-DCF, and its deep boundary is the deep cervical DL-DCF. It lies posterior to the carotid sheath, posteromedial to the sternocleidomastoid muscle, and anterolateral to the paraspinal component of the perivertebral space (Tables 13-3 and 13-4).

Anatomy of the Oral Cavity

The oral cavity is located anterior to the oropharynx. It is separated from the oropharynx by the soft palate, anterior tonsillar pillars, and circumvallate papillae. The mylohyoid muscle separates the lower oral cavity into the submandibular and sublingual spaces and forms the floor of the mouth, arising from the mandible and attaching to the hyoid.

The submandibular space, which is located inferior and lateral to the mylohyoid muscle and superior to the hyoid bone, is enveloped by the SL-DCF. Posteriorly no fascial separation is found between the submandibular space, the sublingual space, and the inferior parapharyngeal space.

The sublingual space, which is located superior and medial to mylohyoid muscle and lateral to genioglossus–geniohyoid muscle complex, is not enclosed by fascia (Table 13-5).

Table 13-3

Anatomic Spaces of the Suprahyoid Neck	
Space	**Contents**
Pharyngeal mucosal space	Mucosa, minor salivary glands and lymphoid tissue, pharyngobasilar fascia, buccopharyngeal fascia, superior and middle pharyngeal constrictor muscles, levator veli palatini muscle, cartilaginous end of eustachian tube (torus tubarius)
Parapharyngeal space (prestyloid parapharyngeal space)	Deep portion of parotid gland, minor salivary glands, pterygoid venous plexus, internal maxillary artery, ascending pharyngeal artery, branches of cranial nerve V3, cervical sympathetic chain and fat
Carotid space (retrostyloid parapharyngeal space)	Internal carotid artery, internal jugular vein, cranial nerves IX-XII, sympathetic chain, lymph nodes—deep cervical chain
Retropharyngeal space	Fat, lymph nodes—retropharyngeal (medial and lateral)
Masticator space	Ramus and posterior body of mandible, muscles of mastication—pterygoid, masseter, and temporalis; mandibular division trigeminal nerve (V3)—inferior alveolar and lingual nerves, inferior alveolar vein and artery, pterygoid venous plexus
Parotid space	Parotid gland and duct, cranial nerve VII, external carotid artery, retromandibular vein, lymph nodes—intraparotid and periparotid
Perivertebral space	Prevertebral muscles, scalene muscles, vertebral artery and vein, brachial plexus, phrenic nerve Vertebral bodies and discs

Adapted from Som PM, Curtin HD. *Head and neck imaging.* 4th ed. St Louis: Mosby; 2003.

Imaging Techniques

Cross-sectional imaging has become an integral tool in the diagnosis, characterization, and staging of neck pathology. Each modality has its strengths and drawbacks. The modalities chosen depend on the clinical question to be answered and the patient's clinical presentation and condition. In a given situation, one modality may suffice or a combination may be required to provide a diagnosis and to assist in planning treatment, as well as to provide assessment of disease progression or treatment efficacy.

Ultrasonography should always be considered because it is readily available, relatively inexpensive, and uses no ionizing radiation. High-frequency linear array transducers provide optimal spatial resolution, although sector or curved array transducers can be useful to image deeper neck structures. Ultrasound readily differentiates cystic from solid lesions, and Doppler imaging can determine vascularity. Additionally, ultrasound is valuable in guiding interventions such as aspiration or biopsy.

Computed tomography (CT) is extremely useful in evaluating neck pathology. New multidetector scanners provide rapid scan times, resulting in diminished motion artifact and little need for sedation. Volumetric thin-section acquisitions allow multiplanar and three-dimensional reconstructions, which can aid in the detection and display of abnormalities. Drawbacks include ionizing radiation and the need for iodinated contrast material. As with all CT studies, the imaging protocol and radiation dose should be tailored for patient size and desired image quality.

Magnetic resonance imaging (MRI) allows exquisite delineation of anatomy and pathology, with superior soft tissue contrast resolution relative to CT. MRI allows direct acquisition in any desired anatomic plane and does not expose patients to ionizing radiation. However, many younger patients require sedation for this procedure, and patients with implants that are not compatible with MRI may not be

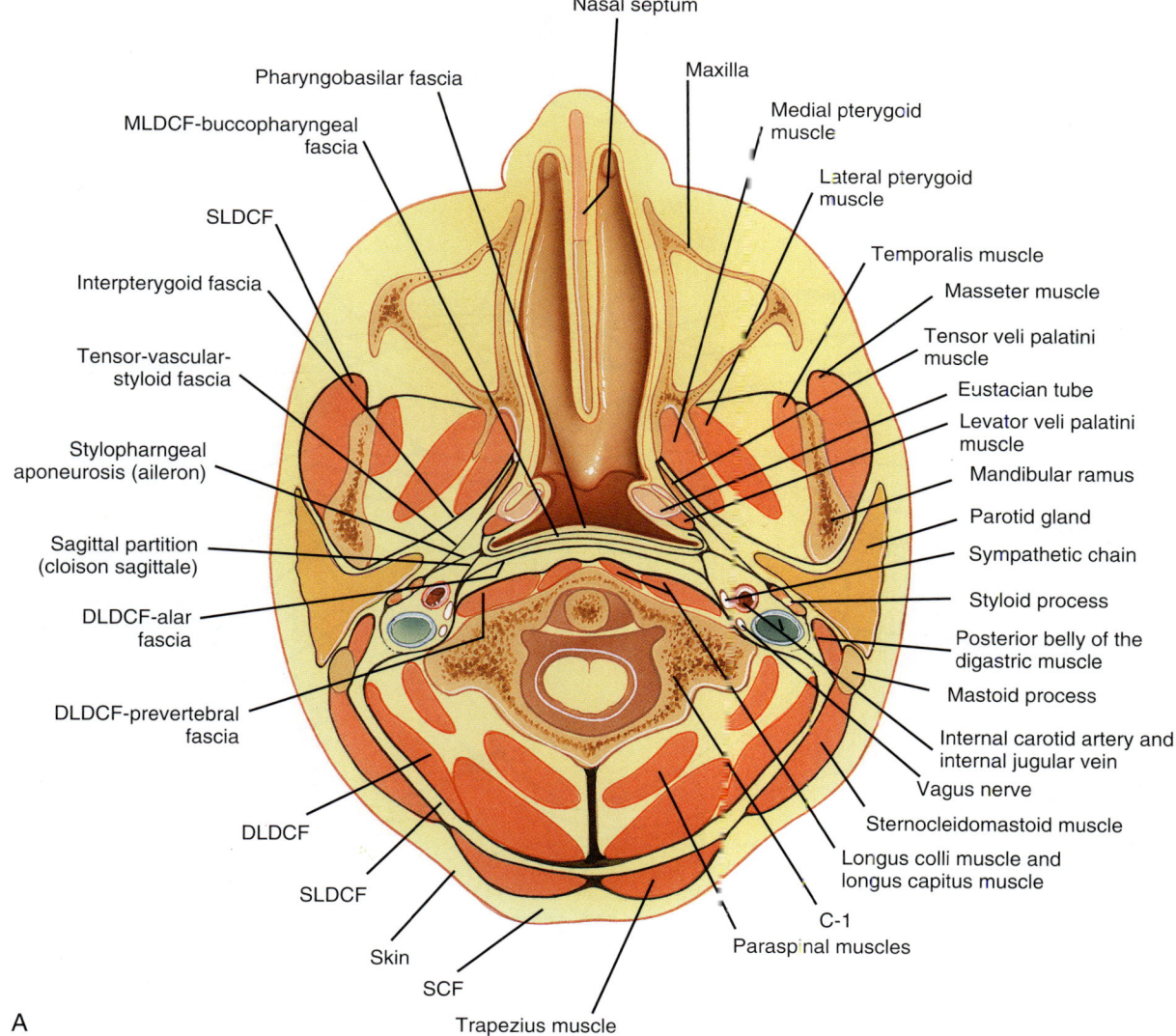

Figure 13-5 Fascial compartments of the neck. Axial sections at the level of C4 (**A**), C7 (**B**), and T1 (**C**) show the relationship of the investing fascial layers with anatomic structures. (From Som P, Curtin H. *Head and neck imaging.* 4th ed. St Louis: Mosby; 2003.)   *Continued*

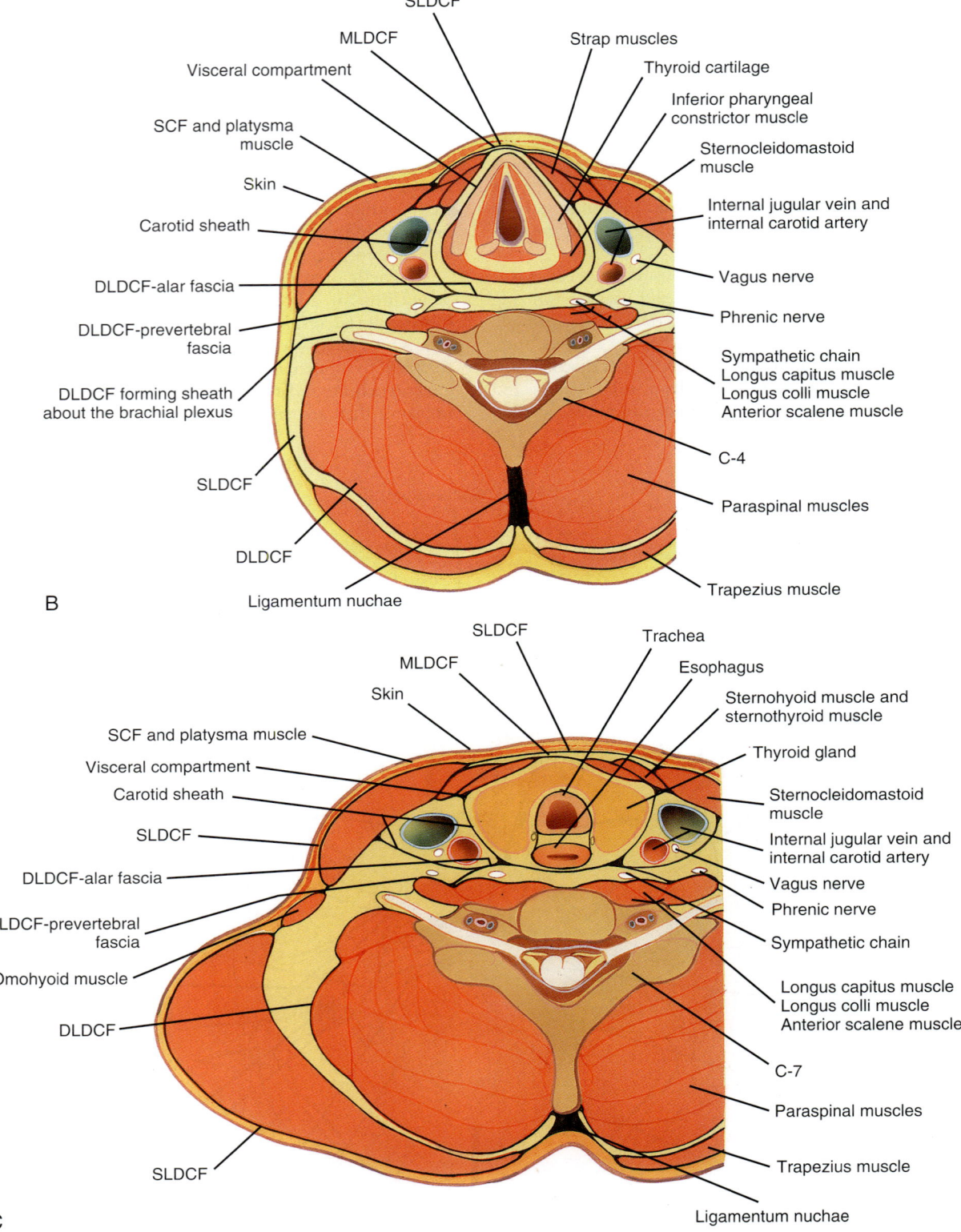

Figure 13-5, cont'd.

Table 13-4

Anatomic Spaces of the Infrahyoid Neck

Space	Contents
Visceral space	Larynx, hypopharynx and cervical esophagus, trachea, thyroid gland, parathyroid glands, lymph nodes, recurrent laryngeal nerve (branch cranial nerve X), third and fourth branchial apparatus and thyroid/parathyroid anlage remnants
Retropharyngeal space	Fat, remnants of third branchial apparatus
Carotid space	Common and internal carotid arteries, internal jugular vein, cranial nerve X, sympathetic chain, lymph nodes, carotid body, second branchial apparatus remnants
Perivertebral space	Prevertebral, scalene, and paraspinal muscles, brachial plexus, phrenic nerve, vertebral artery and vein. Vertebral bodies and discs
Anterior cervical space	Extension of submandibular space of suprahyoid neck. Composed of fat
Posterior cervical space	Cranial nerve XI, spinal accessory nodes, preaxillary brachial plexus, fat

candidates. A combination of T1-weighted, T2-weighted, inversion recovery, and other sequences can help delineate different tissue types. Angiographic techniques are useful to better delineate the vasculature.

Positron emission tomography using fluorine-18 fluorodeoxyglucose is not a first-line imaging modality, but it is valuable in the assessment of neck masses. It is sensitive for the detection of increased glucose metabolism, which often is present with malignancy. Differentiation between physiologic uptake, posttreatment uptake, and pathologic uptake is critical; standard uptake values should be used. Spatial resolution is relatively poor, but acquisition of images with concurrent CT or MRI, or fusion of positron emission tomography studies with recent CT or MRI, allows more precise anatomic localization of areas of abnormal uptake.

Table 13-5

Contents of the Submandibular and Sublingual Spaces

Space	Contents
Submandibular	Submandibular gland, submandibular and submental lymph nodes, facial artery and vein, inferior cranial nerve XII, anterior belly of digastric muscle
Sublingual	Hyoglossus muscle (anterior margin), lingual nerve (sensory branches of cranial nerve V3 and the chorda tympani branch of cranial nerve VII), distal cranial nerve IX and cranial nerve XII, lingual artery and vein, sublingual gland and duct, deep portion of the submandibular gland and duct

Key Points

Knowledge of embryology and anatomy of the neck is essential in interpreting imaging studies and formulating an effective differential diagnosis.

Choosing an appropriate imaging modality should be based on the clinical presentation and the clinical questions to be answered. More than one modality may be required.

Imaging protocols require contrast-enhanced, high-resolution, and thin-section, multiplanar images with appropriate anatomic coverage.

Cross-sectional imaging has resulted in replacement of the clinically oriented subdivision of neck structures by fascially based anatomic spaces that more closely correspond to surgical and pathologic landmarks.

Suggested Readings

Dolinskas CA. *ACR-ASNR practice guidelines for the performance of magnetic resonance imaging (MRI) of the head and neck [online publication]*. Reston, VA: American College of Radiology; 2012.

Harnsberger HR, Wiggins III RH, Hudgins PA, et al. *Diagnostic imaging head and neck, part III*. Salt Lake City, Utah: Amirys Inc; 2004.

Jinkins JR. *Atlas of neuroradiologic embryology, anatomy, and variants*. Philadelphia: Lippincott Williams & Wilkins; 2000.

Ludwig BJ, Foster BR, Saito N, et al. Diagnostic imaging in nontraumatic pediatric head and neck emergencies. *Radiographics*. 2010;30(3):781-799.

Mafee MF, Valvassori GE, Becker M, eds. *Imaging of the head and neck*. 2nd ed. New York: Thieme Stuttgart; 2004.

Moore K, Persaud TVN. *Before we are born: essentials of embryology and birth defects*. 7th ed. Philadelphia: Saunders; 2008.

Mukherji SK, Wippold FJ II, Cornelius RS, et al. *ACR Appropriateness Criteria neck mass/adenopathy [online publication]*. Reston, VA: American College of Radiology; 2009.

Siegel MJ. *Pediatric sonography*. 4th ed. Philadelphia: Lippincott Williams & Wilkins; 2010.

Som PM, Curtin HD. Fascia and spaces of the neck. In: Som PM, Curtin HD, eds. *Head and neck imaging*. 4th ed. St Louis: Mosby; 2003.

Som PM, Smoker WRK, Balboni A, et al. Embryology and anatomy of the neck. In: Som PM, Curtin HD, eds. *Head and neck imaging*. 4th ed. St Louis: Mosby; 2003.

Weiss KL, Cornelius RS, Greeley AL, et al. Hybrid convolution kernel: optimized CT of the head, neck, and spine. *AJR Am J Roentgenol*. 2011;196(2):403-406.

Wippold FJ 2nd. Head and neck imaging: the role of CT and MRI. *J Magn Reson Imaging*. 2007;25(3):453-465.

Chapter 14

Prenatal, Congenital, and Neonatal Abnormalities

TAMARA FEYGIN

Congenital lesions of the neck consist of a variety of entities, some of which become apparent at birth or shortly thereafter, whereas others present clinically later in life. This chapter will focus on congenital lesions that can be recognized in the fetus or the newborn. Currently, many congenital cervical lesions may be diagnosed prenatally, making it essential for pediatric radiologists to be familiar with general patterns of these lesions in fetal imaging.

Other congenital lesions that cause symptoms only when enlarged or infected will be discussed elsewhere in the relevant chapters.

Presence of mass lesions in the fetal neck may considerably influence other fetal organs and organ systems because of the complex anatomy of the neck and the proximity of the lesion to vascular, upper gastrointestinal, and, especially, airway structures.

Conditions that may result in tracheolaryngeal obstruction and, thus, could be life threatening include extrinsic causes such as cervical teratomas, venolymphatic malformations, and vascular rings, and intrinsic causes such as congenital high airway obstruction syndrome and upper airway hemangiomas. Giant fetal neck masses may grow to obstruct the esophagus, thereby leading to an accumulation of amniotic fluid and polyhydramnios and increasing the risk of preterm labor.

Accurate depiction and distinction of these conditions with imaging facilitate prenatal counseling and delivery planning. In addition, some congenital cervical lesions may be associated with other serious anomalies and may be the first manifestation of a systemic disease or syndrome, potentially requiring further investigation.

Fetal neck lesions occasionally present a diagnostic challenge. Giant fetal neck masses may resemble each other, sharing many imaging features including cystic and solid components, increased vascularity, and foci of mineralization. The exact origin of a midline cervical cyst may be difficult to establish. For accurate diagnosis, it may be necessary to utilize complementary imaging modalities.

Imaging Modalities

Imaging of the fetal neck is performed by ultrasonography and magnetic resonance imaging (MRI). Evaluation of the neonatal neck may be performed by ultrasonography, computed tomography (CT) with contrast, and MRI with and without contrast. Some indeterminate hypervascular lesions may rarely require evaluation with conventional angiography. Lateral radiography of the neck may still be used in emergent initial evaluation of upper airway pathology but is rarely of value in the workup of congenital lesions.

ULTRASONOGRAPHY

Ultrasonography is a noninvasive, real-time, high-resolution imaging modality that provides anatomic images supplemented by Doppler evaluation of blood flow. It is equally useful for primary obstetric imaging and for portable bedside evaluation of a neck mass in the restless child.

Prenatal ultrasonography includes routine evaluation of normal anatomic structures of the head, face, and neck, as well as upper airway patency and pattern of swallowing. Airway patency may be difficult to confirm with ultrasonography, hence ancillary signs of airway and upper gastrointestinal tract compromise, such as a small stomach or polyhydramnios, should be routinely searched for. Ultrasonography demonstrates morphologic characteristics of cervical pathology, specifically the cystic or solid nature of any lesion and the presence or absence of fat and calcifications.

Color Doppler provides valuable characterization of a lesion's vascularity and blood supply, detects possible arteriovenous shunting, and depicts the major neck vessels. Three-dimensional reconstruction clearly depicts the relationship of cervical lesions with adjacent facial and skull base structures (e-Fig. 14-1). Potential shortcomings of ultrasonography involve cases with poor acoustic windows because of an anterior position of the placenta, maternal obesity or polyhydramnios, and abnormal fetal position with unusual flexion and extension of the fetal neck.

Ultrasonography imaging of congenital neck lesions in young children is performed with high-resolution (3 or 5, up to 12 megahertz [MHz]) transducers. The examination is fast and usually requires no sedation. Reliable distinction of the cystic or solid nature of the lesion may be sufficient for diagnosis in some instances; however, assessment of surrounding tissue invasion may be suboptimal.

COMPUTED TOMOGRAPHY

CT with contrast administration is a valuable tool in the evaluation of neonatal neck masses and, in many instances, may serve as a first imaging test. Modern multidetector CT scanners allow for fast image acquisition in the axial plane and reformatted images in orthogonal planes, thereby avoiding additional radiation to the child. Additionally, the short duration of scanning may help avoid the need for sedation. CT imaging of cervical lesions is especially helpful in the depiction of calcifications, blood products, and bony involvement. However, soft tissue resolution may be suboptimal for accurate lesion characterization, and further imaging with MRI may be necessary.

MAGNETIC RESONANCE IMAGING

MRI is a superb imaging modality for the evaluation of fetal or neonatal neck lesions and may help further clarify the lesion's relationship with surrounding structures. Fetal MRI is considered safe to perform in the second and third trimesters for further assessment of a cervical mass detected by routine obstetric ultrasonography. Fetal MRI is approved by the U.S. Food and Drug Agency for magnet field strengths up to 3.0 Tesla.

Fetal imaging prior to 18 weeks of gestational age is typically of little value because of the unknown safety profile of exposure to magnetic fields during organogenesis, as well as the relatively poor image quality in a small fetus. For fast and effective performance of fetal MRI, familiarity and optimal use of imaging sequences is crucial.

Useful MRI sequences for fetal neck imaging include the following:

1. Ultrafast spin echo T2-weighted sequences are excellent for imaging of normal anatomical structures and depiction of cervical lesions.
2. Spoiled gradient echo T1-weighted imaging is helpful for imaging of the thyroid gland and blood flow within the major cervical vessels, as well as for depiction of intralesional blood products and calcifications.
3. Gradient echo planar imaging is helpful for detection of blood products, calcifications, and bony details.
4. Steady state or balanced gradient echo sequences are valuable in the prenatal assessment of preservation or impairment of swallowing in the fetus (Video 14-1). The details of fetal airway compromise secondary to the presence of a cervical mass should always be carefully examined.

MRI sequences for imaging of neonatal neck lesions include the following:

1. High resolution 2- to 3-mm T1- and T2-weighted and postcontrast imaging with fat-suppression in orthogonal planes
2. Ultrafast spin echo imaging for optimal visualization of thin fluid–filled sinus tract or fistula
3. Diffusion-weighted imaging, which is particularly useful for identification of hypercellular tumors and infected cystic lesions with viscous, purulent content
4. Magnetic resonance angiography, which may provide crucial information regarding vascular anatomy

Prenatal neck imaging sometimes may be more useful in the evaluation of lesion extension and, particularly, airway and upper gastrointestinal tract patency, rather than the establishment of a precise diagnosis. Knowledge of airway status may help facilitate prenatal counseling and management, including the decision to utilize the ex utero intrapartum treatment procedure. This procedure may be required for fetuses diagnosed with a giant neck mass to gain time to secure an airway while the neonate is still attached to the umbilical cord.

The postnatal appearance of prenatally diagnosed cervical lesions may be of additional diagnostic value, as certain lesions may have a predictable developmental pattern. For example, congenital hemangiomas may remain stable in size or become smaller, whereas teratomas are likely to increase in size; lymphatic malformations may develop blood–fluid levels caused by intralesional hemorrhage. For this reason, it is important to evaluate a cervical lesion throughout its phases of development.

Vascular Neck Lesions

The nomenclature of vascular anomalies had been a controversial topic until Mulliken and Glowacki proposed a classification that divides pediatric vascular lesions into two major categories: (1) vascular tumors and (2) vascular malformations. This classification, based on pathologic differences as well as the clinical and cellular behavior of vascular lesions, was widely accepted and adopted by the International Society for the Study of Vascular Anomalies in 1996.

Vascular tumors in young children are almost solely hemangiomas, which are true endothelial tumors with increased mitotic activity during the proliferative phase and eventual involution. Vascular malformations are congenital nonneoplastic lesions, which are further classified according to the type of abnormal vessel comprising the lesion. Vascular malformations, therefore, may consist of abnormal capillaries, veins, lymphatic vessels, or arteries, or of a combination of different types of vessels (i.e., arteriovenous malformation).

Additionally, vascular lesions are classified on the basis of hemodynamics as high–flow and low–flow types. Low–flow lesions consist of any combination of capillary, venous, and lymphatic components, whereas high–flow lesions contain arterial components. Vascular malformations grow in proportion to the patient's growth but may exhibit rapid growth or expansion following infection, trauma, or hormonal changes such as during puberty or pregnancy. Vascular malformations do not involute spontaneously.

The current classification of vascular lesions serves to distinguish neoplastic from nonneoplastic entities, as they have different treatments and prognoses. However, this classification should not be perceived as a final arrangement. A better understanding of the molecular biology and genetics of vascular anomalies may lead to further refinement of the existing system.

Vascular Tumors

HEMANGIOMA

Hemangioma is the most common vascular tumor of infancy. Two major types are recognized: (1) congenital (rare) and (2) infantile (common). The previously used categorization of hemangioma types as capillary, juvenile, or cavernous is no longer accepted. It should be noted that all types of hemangiomas have overlapping clinical, imaging, and histo-pathologic features.

INFANTILE HEMANGIOMA

Infantile hemangiomas are benign vascular neoplasms, with an increased incidence in premature children with low birth weight. These lesions have a predictable clinical course notable for early proliferation, which is often followed by spontaneous involution. Growth and involution continue with the following stages. The nascent phase may be observed in the first 2 to 4 weeks of life. A precursor lesion such as macula, multiple telangiectasias, or discoloration in a beard distribution may be seen at birth. The proliferative phase is remarkable for rapid growth of the tumor in the first year of life. At the proliferative stage, the hemangioma appears as a bulky compressible lesion of strawberry-red color and may have cutaneous as well as deep components.

On cross-sectional imaging, it appears as a lobulated mass with intense uniform enhancement, which usually demonstrates intralesional flow voids on MRI (Fig. 14-2, *A*). Proliferation may be biphasic. Careful assessment of upper airway status is important because the deep portions of a cervical hemangioma may enlarge sufficiently at this stage to impinge on the airway and cause obstruction. During the final involution phase, which may continue for up to 12 years, the rate of regression is variable. Involution is never complete, although the residual lesion may not be grossly visible; in the neck, it leaves persistent fibrofatty tissue. Infantile hemangiomas are positive for the glucose transporter 1 (GLUT-1) marker at all stages of lesion development.

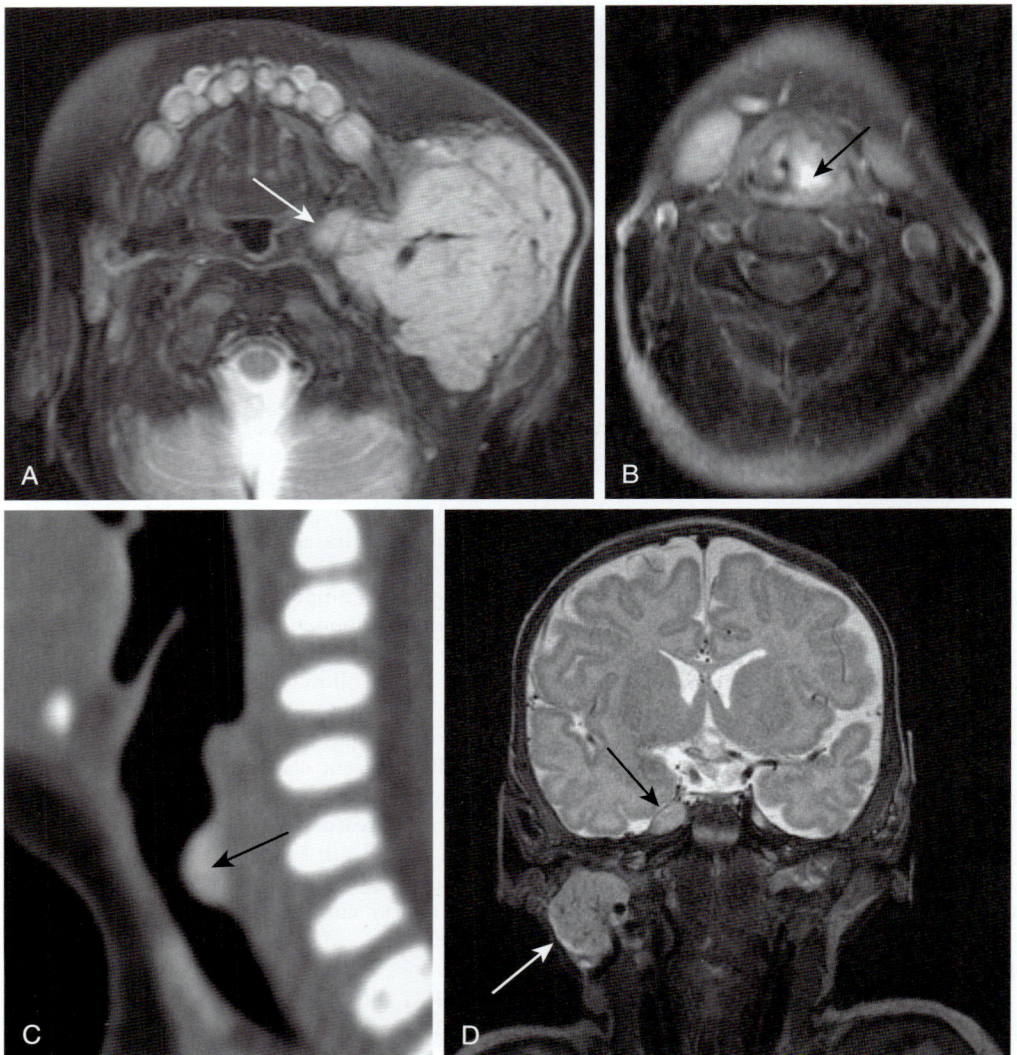

Figure 14-2 **Infantile hemangiomas. A,** Parotid infantile hemangioma. A T2-weighted axial image with fat suppression shows a well-circumscribed lobular soft tissue mass in the left parotid with intrinsic flow voids and deep extension into the ipsilateral parapharyngeal space (*arrow*). The upper airways remain patent. **B** and **C,** Upper airways infantile hemangiomas. A T2-weighted axial image with fat suppression shows a small hyperintense hemangioma in the left vocal cord (*black arrow*), causing severe airway effacement (**B**). A sagittal reconstructed computed tomography image shows a small lobulated enhancing subglottic hemangioma (*black arrow*) (**C**). **D,** Multifocal infantile hemangiomas with intracranial lesions. A T2-weighted coronal image with fat suppression shows cervical (*white arrow*) and Meckel cave (*black arrow*) hemangiomas. (**C,** Courtesy Avrum N. Pollock, MD.)

Most infantile hemangiomas do not cause any morbidity or mortality but may create cosmetic inconvenience. Nonetheless, a hemangioma of the neck is considered an alarming lesion if it assumes a beard distribution (involvement of the lower face, anterior neck, and submandibular and parotid regions) because of an increased incidence of subglottic hemangioma, high risk of airway compromise, and known association with PHACES syndrome (**P**osterior fossa malformations, **H**emangiomas, **A**rterial, **C**ardiac anomalies, **E**ye anomalies, **S**ternal cleft). The arteriopathy of PHACES syndrome commonly comprises a spectrum of congenital and progressive large arterial lesions ipsilateral to the cutaneous hemangioma. It entails careful searching (and monitoring) with imaging for potential vascular anomalies once a diagnosis of cervicofacial segmental hemangioma is established.

Upper airway hemangiomas (see Fig. 14-2, *B* and *C*) become symptomatic in the proliferative phase, causing biphasic stridor, respiratory distress, and potentially even life-threatening airway obstruction, which may require emergent intubation. These hemangiomas are often multifocal and occur above and below the vocal cords. Close monitoring with cross-sectional imaging may be indicated because laryngoscopy may not accurately depict the degree of invasion. MRI is preferred in the setting of intubation or tracheostomy.

In rare cases, cervicofacial infantile hemangioma may be associated with central nervous system hemangiomas in intracranial (see Fig. 14-2, *D*) or intraspinal locations. The reported cases of central nervous system hemangiomas indicate a specific pattern of distribution, with a predilection for the basal cisterns, ventricular system, and extradural spinal involvement.

In the past, infantile hemangiomas have been confused with other vascular neoplasms, particularly kaposiform hemangioendotheliomas (KHEs) and tufted angiomas, especially in the setting of consumptive coagulopathy, referred to as the *Kasabach-Merrit phenomenon*; it is now generally accepted that infantile hemangiomas are rarely, if ever, responsible for this phenomenon.

CONGENITAL HEMANGIOMA

Congenital hemangiomas are uncommon lesions that are fully developed at birth and do not go through the proliferative stage in postnatal life. These lesions may be diagnosed in utero, as early as at 12 weeks of gestational age. Two types of congenital hemangiomas are described: (1) rapidly involuting congenital hemangioma (RICH) and (2) noninvoluting lesions congenital hemangioma (NICH).

RICH has a predilection for scalp and neck locations. On prenatal imaging, it may appear as a large heterogeneous mass, emanating from the posterior neck (Fig. 14-3, *A*) with increased vascularity, best demonstrated on obstetric Doppler ultrasonography. Postnatal imaging features of RICH include large irregular flow voids and arterial aneurysms, direct arteriovenous shunts (seen on angiography), and calcifications. Their imaging appearance may occasionally resemble congenital infantile fibrosarcoma.

RICH may have a dramatic presentation at birth with high-output congestive heart failure, which may occur in the setting of a large hemangioma (see Fig. 14-3, *B*). Rapid involution is usually completed by 14 months of age. Usually, RICH is managed conservatively. Presence of complications may prompt surgical removal.

NICH, on the contrary, never involutes and may even grow with the child. It usually has an imaging appearance similar to infantile hemangioma, being more homogeneous with uniform parenchymal enhancement.

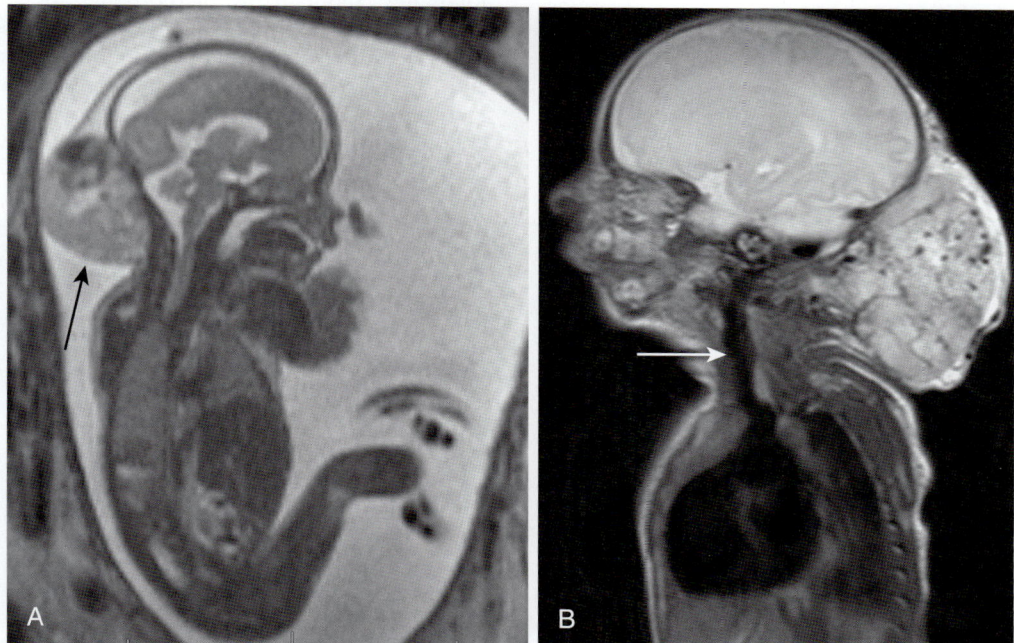

Figure 14-3 Congenital hemangiomas. **A,** A fetal magnetic resonance imaging, sagittal half Fourier acquisition single shot turbo spin echo image shows a complex soft tissue mass in the posterior neck (*black arrow*) with internal hypointensity, indicative of blood products. **B,** A sagittal magnetic resonance imaging T2-weighted image of a 1-day-old newborn's neck shows a very large heterogeneous mass with internal flow voids in the posterior neck. Enlargement of ipsilateral carotid artery (*white arrow*) and cardiomegaly indicate high-output congestive heart failure.

Most hemangiomas resolve spontaneously, however, approximately 10% to 20% require treatment, which includes pharmacologic, surgical, or laser intervention. Treatment is indicated when functional or cosmetic complications that are worse than the side effects of intervention arise. Lesion size and location, patient age, and phase of the lesion (proliferative, involuting, and mature) also influence the method and timing of intervention.

KAPOSIFORM HEMANGIOENDOTHELIOMA

KHE is a rare, aggressive vascular tumor of infancy of intermediate malignancy and differs from hemangioma by histopathology and clinical appearance. The head and neck are uncommon locations. KHE presents as an ill-defined vascular mass with stranding in the subcutaneous fat, intralesional calcifications, and prominent feeding and draining vessels (e-Fig. 14-4). It tends to cause bony destruction and may be associated with the Kasabach-Merritt phenomenon. It should be noted that thrombocytopenia occurs with the rarer KHE and not with the more commonly seen infantile hemangioma.

TUFTED ANGIOMA

Tufted angioma is another very rare vascular tumor of early childhood, typically located on the upper back and neck, and can manifest as profound thrombocytopenia. KHE and tufted angioma may represent parts of the same neoplastic spectrum. The GLUT-1 marker can be used to distinguish them from infantile hemangioma if the histologic diagnosis is uncertain. Immunopositivity for GLUT-1 may also be used to separate infantile hemangiomas from congenital hemangiomas, other vascular tumors, and vascular malformations, all of which are negative for this marker.

Venolymphatic Malformations Spectrum

Cervical venolymphatic malformations, similar to venolymphatic malformations located elsewhere in the body, represent a spectrum of entities consisting of a combination of anomalous lymphatic and venous channels. When the lymphatic vascular component is prevalent, lesions are called *lymphatic malformations*, whereas those with dominant venous components are called *venous malformations*.

Lymphatic malformations of the neck may be diagnosed prenatally or may present clinically at birth or shortly thereafter. The most pure lymphatic malformation, which seemingly consists of lymphatic channels only, is represented by a fetal posterior neck cystic hygroma. A focal nuchal translucency, perceived as a hypoechoic subcutaneous region in the posterior neck, may be identified on obstetric ultrasonography at 11 to 14 weeks' gestational age; it is considered a normal finding if it measures below a defined threshold, and eventually involutes by term.

A pathologic cystic hygroma develops in cases of failure of appropriate connections between the lymphatic jugular sac and jugular vein. Such a lesion becomes apparent as nuchal thickening at 18 to 20 weeks' gestational age. Approximately 60% of nuchal cystic hygromas result from chromosome abnormalities and are associated with aneuploidy syndromes such as Turner syndrome, trisomy 18, trisomy 21, and multiple other syndromes and conditions, including congenital diaphragmatic hernia (Fryns syndrome). Accumulation of lymph may cause lymphedema and nonimmune hydrops, a condition with a high mortality rate.

Ultrasonography demonstrates translucent nuchal thickening, with no identifiable arterial or venous flow by Doppler. MRI reveals focal edema of the posterior fetal neck (e-Fig. 14-5) and, in severe cases, depicts associated lymphedema, pleural effusions, ascites, and anasarca.

Lymphatic or venolymphatic malformations of the fetal or neonatal neck represent congenital lesions that may be apparent at birth or may "silently" grow with a child in the first few years before suddenly becoming symptomatic following spontaneous hemorrhage or infection. They usually present as large, transspatial, multicystic masses with intervening septations and fluid–fluid levels (Fig. 14-6, *A* and *B*). Ultrasonography demonstrates septated hypoechoic cystic lesions (see Fig. 14-6, *C*) without internal vascularity, although some vascular flow may be seen within the intralesional septae.

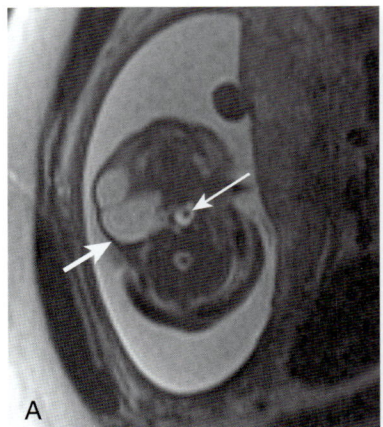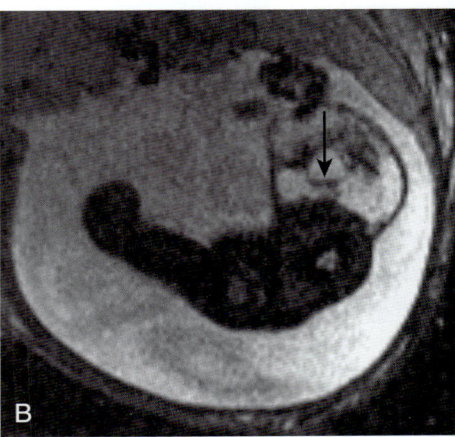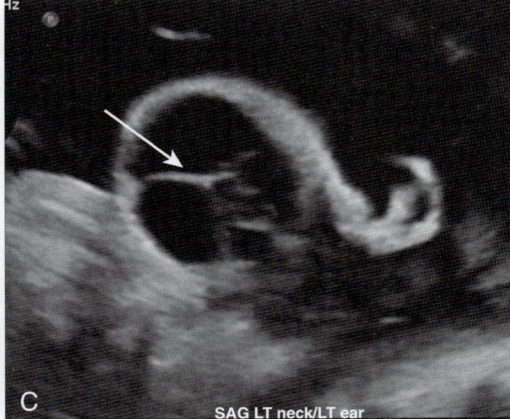

Figure 14-6 **Lymphatic malformations.** Fetal magnetic resonance imaging (**A, B**), fetal ultrasonography (**C**). Axial half Fourier acquisition single shot turbo spin echo (**A**) and gradient echo planar imaging (**B**) scans show a multicystic mass of the lateral neck (*thick white arrow*) with blood-fluid level (*black arrow*). The airways remain patent (*thin white arrow*). Fetal ultrasonography (**C**) shows hypoechoic multicystic lesion with thick intralesional septations (*arrow*). Hyperechoic debris indicates blood products.

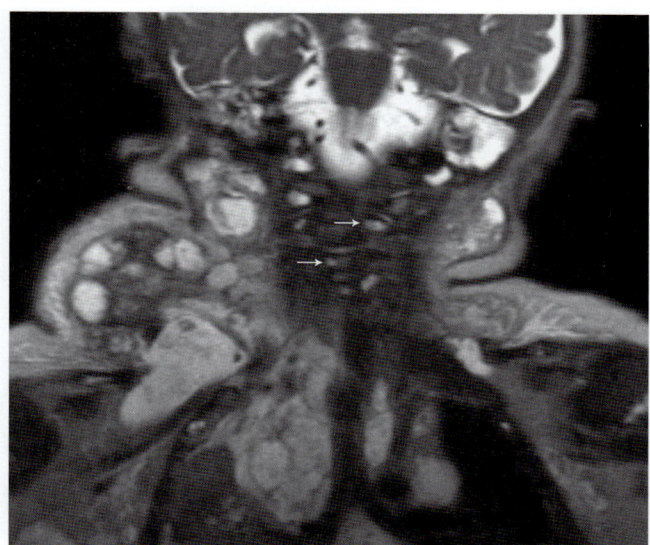

Figure 14-7 **Lymphangiomatosis.** A coronal magnetic resonance half-Fourier single-shot turbo spin echo image shows large complex cystic masses in the lateral neck, extending into the thorax, and numerous small cysts (arrows) involving the vertebra.

Lymphatic malformations may have a very complex appearance because of their multi-compartmental nature and internal hemorrhages. Relatively thick intralesional septations or foci of chronic hemorrhage may show enhancement and mimic solid portions of a cystic teratoma. Absence of calcifications and a relatively mild mass effect on surrounding structures despite the large size of the lesion lead to the correct diagnosis. Absence or presence of calcifications is easier to establish on fetal ultrasonography; blood products and calcifications may be occasionally confused on fetal MRI.

Systemic lymphatic malformations include rare conditions known as *lymphangiomatosis* and *Gorham disease (vanishing bone disease)*. These entities are poorly understood and likely represent a spectrum of congenital disorders of lymphatic development. They manifest by numerous foci of vascular and lymphatic proliferation, involving multiple organs, including bones and lungs (Fig. 14-7 and e-Fig. 14-8), and often cause serious consequences.

The current approach to treatment of venolymphatic malformations is navigation-assisted interventional sclerotherapy with doxycycline or other sclerosants, which provides excellent results for large macrocystic head and neck lesions. Therapy for microcystic and mixed lesions continues to be a challenge.

Venous Vascular Malformations

Venous malformations represent slow-growing lesions that consist of dysplastic venous channels that may have a minor lymphatic component. They are present at birth but usually manifest clinically later in life.

On imaging, they appear as well-defined, ovoid, heterogeneous lesions with strong enhancement and occasional intralesional phleboliths (Fig. 14-9). A calcified phlebolith may occasionally simulate a flow void on MRI, leading to an erroneous identification of the lesion as a hemangioma. Many lesions may be successfully treated with sclerotherapy, although larger and infiltrative lesions may be more challenging to treat.

TERATOMA

Even though teratoma is one of the most common tumors of the fetal neck, neck teratomas account for only 5% to 10% of all fetal and neonatal teratomas. Most cervical teratomas are benign, yet it is the most common mass in the fetal neck that has potential to cause fetal demise from airway obstruction. On rare occasions, large vascular teratomas may result in nonimmune fetal hydrops and subsequent fetal death. Teratomas usually originate in the anterolateral neck and may involve the face and cranial base, sometimes extending to the thorax. Interval lesion enlargement in late gestation often causes hyperextension of the neck, which is characteristic of cervical teratoma. The lesion may be intimately associated with the thyroid gland and, in addition to tracheal compression, may cause esophageal compression.

Teratomas are composed of all three germ layers with tissue differentiation that infrequently results in the presence of identifiable organs within these lesions. For instance, an oropharyngeal teratoma (epignathus) often contains

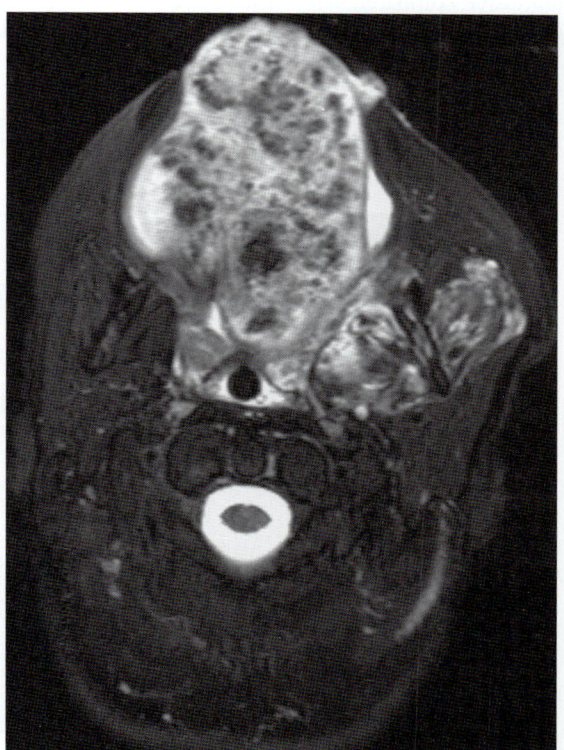

Figure 14-9 **Venovascular malformation.** A T2-weighted fat-suppressed image shows an ovoid heterogeneous lesion, almost replacing the tongue with numerous hypointense phleboliths.

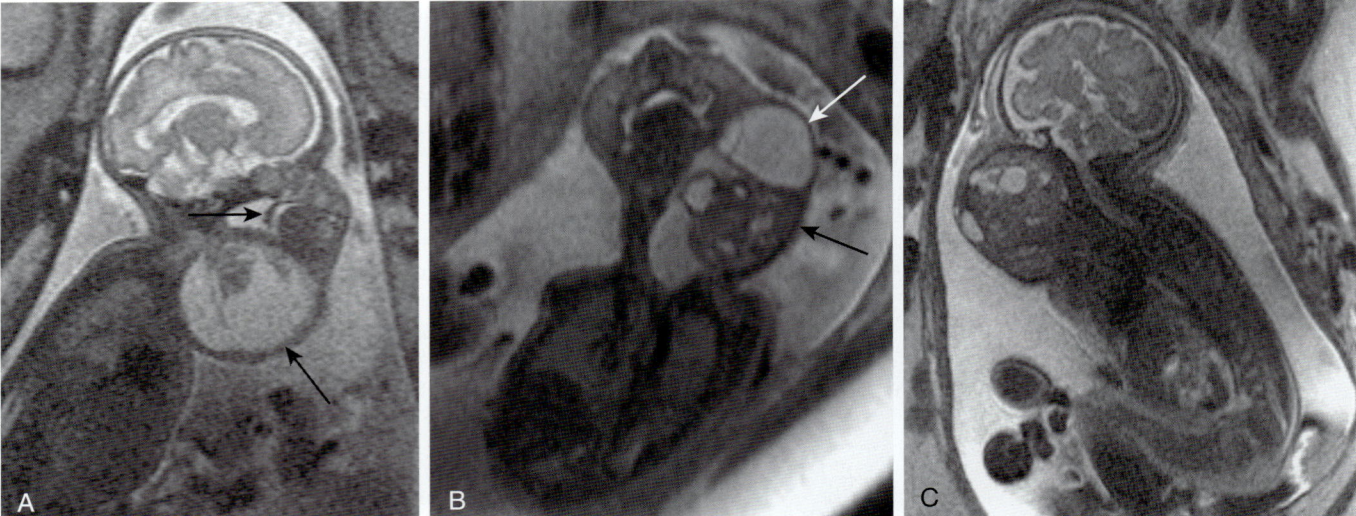

Figure 14-10   Fetal cervical teratomas. **A,** A fetal magnetic resonance imaging (MRI), sagittal half Fourier acquisition single shot turbo spin echo (HASTE) image shows predominantly cystic teratoma (*large arrow*) with small solid component in the anterolateral neck. Upper airways are distended, but motion of soft palate (*small arrow*) is preserved. **B,** A fetal MRI coronal HASTE image shows a complex cervical teratoma with mixture of cystic (*white arrow*) and solid (*black arrow*) components. **C,** A fetal MRI shows mainly solid lesion with small cystic components, extending from the skull base to the upper chest, which appears to encroach the airway. The lesion proved to be a malignant, immature teratoma.

identifiable fetal parts; this lesion is usually more aggressive and may grow more rapidly during gestation.

Teratomas are subdivided into mature, immature, and malignant types, each of which differs by histology and hence imaging appearance. Benign mature lesions are mostly cystic, whereas immature lesions tend to be more solid. Malignant teratoma types are uncommonly found in the neck and are less aggressive compared with other locations. Most teratomas demonstrate a combination of cystic and solid components (Fig. 14-10, *A* to *C*). Intratumoral foci of hemorrhage and necrosis are suggestive of malignancy. Intralesional fat and calcifications are nearly pathognomonic findings for teratoma but may not always be discernible on fetal MRI and are

better seen on ultrasonography. Cervical teratoma and congenital hemangioma share many MRI and ultrasonography features, including interval growth in utero, and establishing the correct diagnosis may be quite challenging. Both imaging modalities are often necessary for optimal assessment.

Postnatal imaging of teratomas may include CT, which is helpful for demonstration of osseous involvement. MRI, with or without contrast, is superb for precise depiction of lesion morphology and extension (Fig. 14-11, *A*). Magnetic resonance angiography may provide crucial information about the vascular supply for surgical planning (see Fig. 14-11, *B*). Surgical treatment of teratomas may be curative, although the mortality rate remains high. Persistent disfiguration of facial

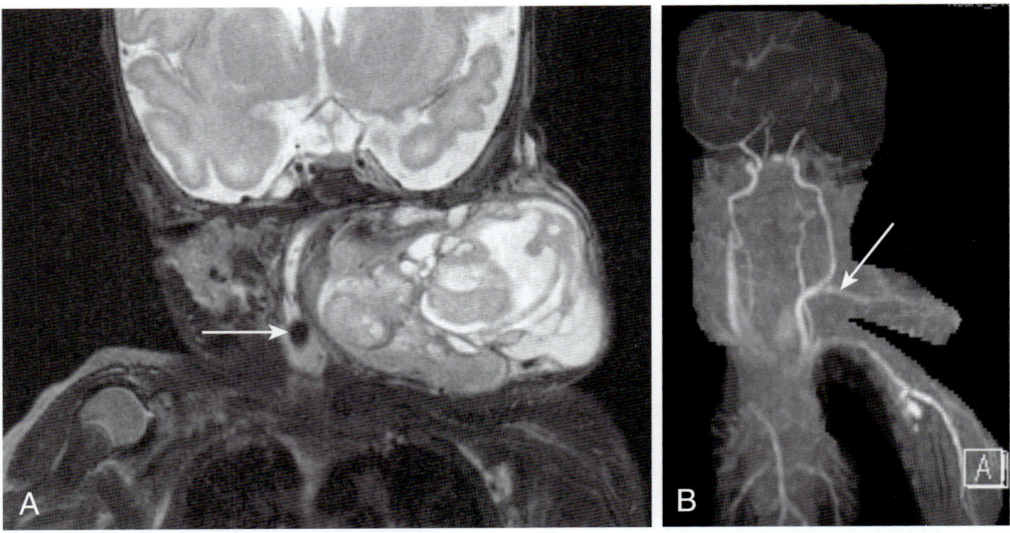

Figure 14-11   Neonatal cervical teratoma. **A,** A coronal T2-weighted image with fat suppression shows a very large complex teratoma of the lateral neck with cystic and solid components, internal flow voids, causing severe compression of airways. Endotracheal tube is evident (*arrow*). **B,** Neck magnetic resonance angiography shows a large arterial feeder (*arrow*), originating from the carotid artery, and providing blood supply to the tumor.

structure, voice issues, and hypothyroidism are among the common complications.

Cervical Cystic Lesions

A variety of unilocular cystic neck lesions may be diagnosed on prenatal imaging or may present in neonates. These lesions are uncommon; they originate from different embryonic structures, and their precise diagnosis may be challenging, especially in fetuses. Perinatal cystic neck lesions include dermoid and epidermoid cysts, laryngoceles, foregut duplication cysts, and thymic cysts.

DERMOID AND EPIDERMOID CYSTS

Dermoid cysts are congenital benign lesions that contain ectodermal elements, including hair follicles and sweat and sebaceous glands. Cervical dermoids are most commonly seen at floor of the mouth, in the submandibular or sublingual spaces, or at the suprasternal notch. They often demonstrate fatty content with imaging.

Epidermoid cysts are rare congenital unilocular lesions, which may closely resemble a thyroglossal duct cyst; however, a characteristic pattern of restricted diffusion typical for epidermoids helps distinguish these entities. Epidermoid cysts appear earlier, compared with dermoid cysts, with most lesions being evident during infancy (Fig. 14-12, *A* and *B*) or diagnosed prenatally (see Fig. 14-12, *C*). Dermoids and epidermoids have different histologies, but it is not always possible to differentiate them on imaging. It is more important to define the lesion position in relation to the oral floor muscles, as it may guide a surgical approach.

LARYNGOCELE

Most laryngoceles are acquired lesions, seen in middle-aged persons who are involved in activities that cause increased supraglottic pressure. Congenital laryngoceles are rare and likely reflect congenital enlargement of the laryngeal saccule. The three types of laryngoceles are *internal*, *external*, and *combined laryngoceles*. The internal laryngocele is found entirely within the larynx, whereas the external or mixed types protrude through the thyrohyoid membrane and may extend into the lateral neck.

Clinically, laryngoceles may manifest as fluctuating soft tissue masses causing airway obstruction in young infants, or the masses may be diagnosed prenatally (e-Fig. 14-13). Evaluation of a laryngocele with high-resolution cross-sectional imaging depicts the anatomic boundaries of the lesion and the contents of the cyst, which may be filled with air, fluid, or proteinaceous material.

FOREGUT DUPLICATION CYST

Foregut duplication cysts in the neck may be incidental findings, may present in the neonate with frank respiratory distress secondary to obstruction, or may be diagnosed prenatally as unilocular cystic masses in the anterior compartment of the fetal neck and mediastinum (e-Fig. 14-14). The cyst may or may not communicate with the esophagus; however, thorough search for this communication should be performed. Identification of abnormal canalization of the gastrointestinal tract confirms the diagnosis of foregut duplication cyst.

Preoperative imaging is recommended to differentiate these lesions from other congenital head and neck masses. Surgical excision with complete removal of the mucosal lining is curative.

THYMIC CYST

Thymic cysts may rarely present within the neck, communicating with pharyngeal structures through the thyrohyoid membrane. Thymic cysts may be found in the midline or anterior to the sternocleidomastoid muscle (e-Fig. 14-15), where they may resemble a branchial arch anomaly.

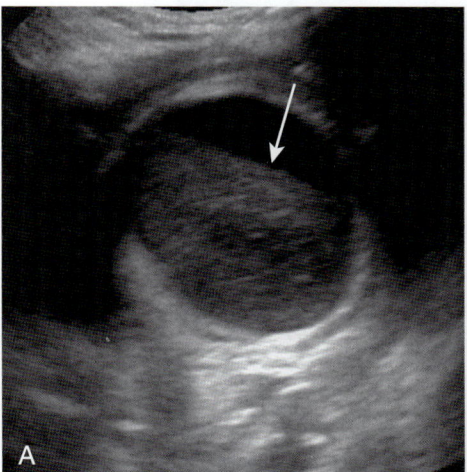 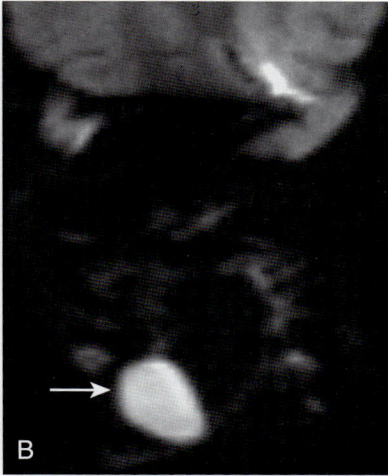 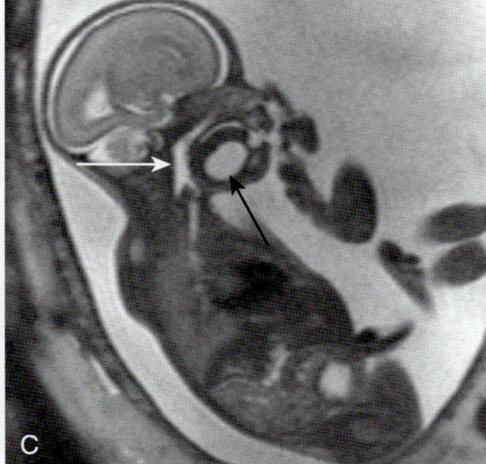

Figure 14-12   Cervical epidermoids. **A,** Submandibular unilocular cystic structure with hyperechoic content on ultrasonography and fluid level (*arrow*). **B,** Restricted diffusion pattern on magnetic resonance imaging (MRI) diffusion-weighted image. **C,** Fetal sagittal MRI shows unilocular submandibular epidermoid (*black arrow*). Airways are patent; hypopharynx is distended (*white arrow*).

Cervical Soft Tissue Masses

ECTOPIC THYMUS

Ectopic thymus is usually discovered incidentally on neck imaging performed for unrelated indications. It may be seen anywhere along the course of the primordial thymopharyngeal duct, from the mandibular angle to the thoracic inlet. It is located most often along the carotid sheath but may extend to the midline (Fig. 14-16, *A*) or may be bilateral. It may be recognized by its imaging characteristics, identical to orthotopic thymus (see Fig. 14-16, *B*). Ectopic thymus usually resolves with involution of the intrathoracic orthotopic thymus.

FETAL OR NEONATAL GOITER

Goiter is a rare cause of fetal neck mass. It may occur in the setting of maternal thyroid disorders such as Graves disease or Hashimoto thyroiditis, or as a manifestation of primary fetal hypothyroidism or hyperthyroidism. Fetal thyroid function may be assessed by ultrasound-guided umbilical cord blood sampling (cordocentesis). The fetal thyroid may be markedly enlarged, causing neck hyperextension, airway obstruction, or compression of the esophagus.

Fetal goiter may be diagnosed on ultrasonography as a bilobed echogenic mass in the anterior neck, with increased vascularity; fetal MRI demonstrates a midline symmetric cervical mass with high signal on T1-weighted imaging (Fig. 14-17). Treatment of fetal goiter includes intra-amniotic thyroxin injection, the main goal being reduction in the size of the goiter and prevention of tracheal obstruction. It may be associated with congenital deafness in the setting of Pendred syndrome (e-Fig. 14-18).

INFANTILE FIBROMATOSES

Infantile fibromatosis represents a spectrum of rare congenital disorder that involves skeletal and smooth muscles in very young children. It may manifest as a solitary form or as a multicentric form with visceral involvement. Aggressive infantile fibromatosis occurs in the first 2 years of life and may present as a nodular soft tissue mass in the head and neck, with an imaging appearance mimicking infantile fibrosarcoma or hemangioma. A desmoid type of fibromatosis may present as a nodular tumor, which often grows along the nerve sheath or vascular bundle and has a tendency to frequent hemorrhage or necrosis in the central portion, producing a target appearance on imaging (Fig. 14-19). The prognosis is good for solitary neck lesion. These lesions usually stop growing or spontaneously regress.

Fibromatosis colli is a benign condition that involves the sternocleidomastoid muscle only. It usually affects neonates and manifests as a hard unilateral soft tissue mass associated with ipsilateral torticollis caused by the muscular contraction and rotation of the chin to the opposite side. Imaging, with ultrasonography or MRI, may be performed if the clinical presentation is unusual. Both modalities reveal diffuse or focal enlargement of sternocleidomastoid muscle (Fig. 14-20) and no discrete mass or lymphadenopathy. Congenital torticollis usually spontaneously resolves in a few months. A child with cervical lymphadenitis and retropharyngeal abscess may present with a postinflammatory torticollis known as *Grisel syndrome*; this condition is caused by increased ligamentous laxity.

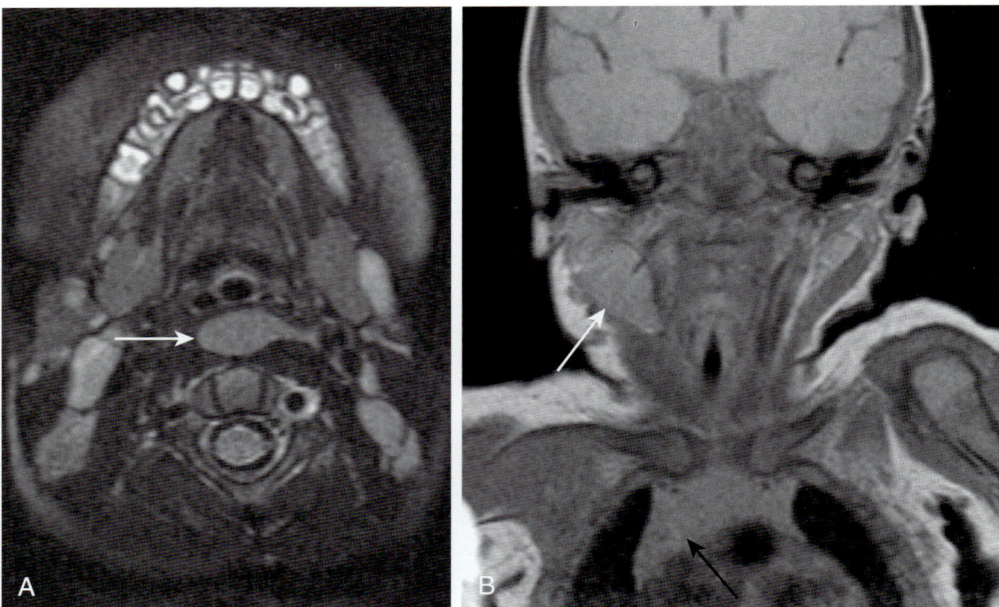

Figure 14-16 Ectopic thymus. **A,** An axial magnetic resonance imaging T2-weighted image shows unusual retropharyngeal location of ectopic thymus (*arrow*). **B,** Ectopic thymus (*white arrow*) in the right lateral neck of a 1-week-old infant has signal characteristics similar to the visualized orthotopic thymus (*black arrow*). The lesion elicits no significant mass effect. The airways are patent.

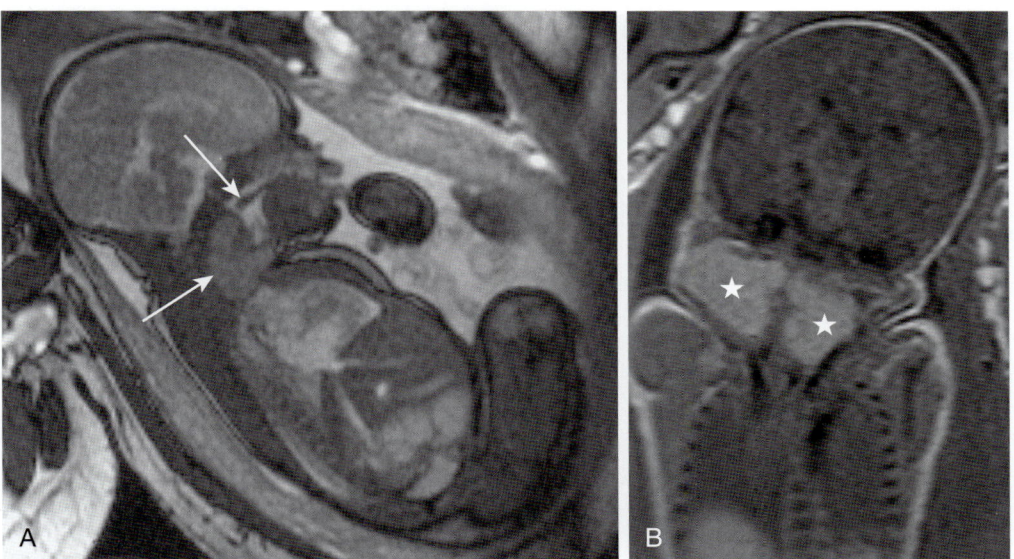

Figure 14-17 Fetal goiter. **A,** A fetal magnetic resonance imaging sagittal true fast imaging with steady precession image shows a homogeneous cervical mass (*bottom arrow*), causing mild distension of hypopharynx. Free motion of soft palate (*top arrow*) remains preserved. **B,** A coronal T1-weighted image shows the bilobed uniformly T1-hyperintense lesion (*stars*), indicative of the iodine content of thyroid gland.

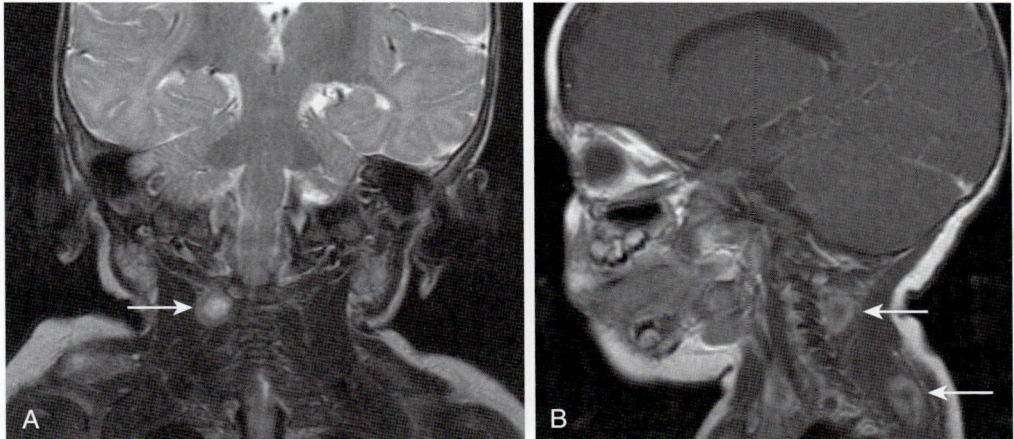

Figure 14-19 Infantile fibromatosis. Coronal T2-weighted (**A**) and sagittal postcontrast (**B**) magnetic resonance imaging scans show multiple scattered nodular masses (*arrows*) of the neonatal neck with typical "target" appearance of desmoids type of infantile fibromatosis.

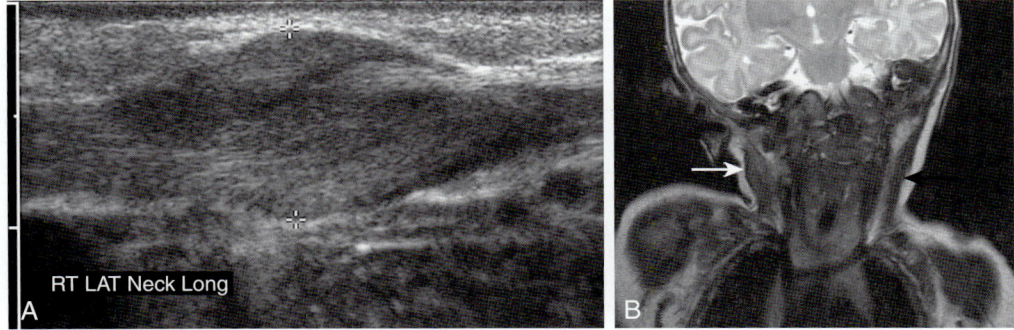

Figure 14-20 Fibromatosis colli. **A,** Ultrasonography of a 5-week-old male infant shows fusiform enlargement of the right sternocleidomastoid muscle (*cursors*). **B,** A coronal T2-weighted image in another patient shows diffuse thickening and hyperintensity of right sternocleidomastoid muscle (*white arrow*), associated with ipsilateral torticollis. The left sternocleidomastoid muscle (*black arrow*) demonstrates normal thickness and signal intensity. (**A,** Courtesy Brian D. Coley, MD.)

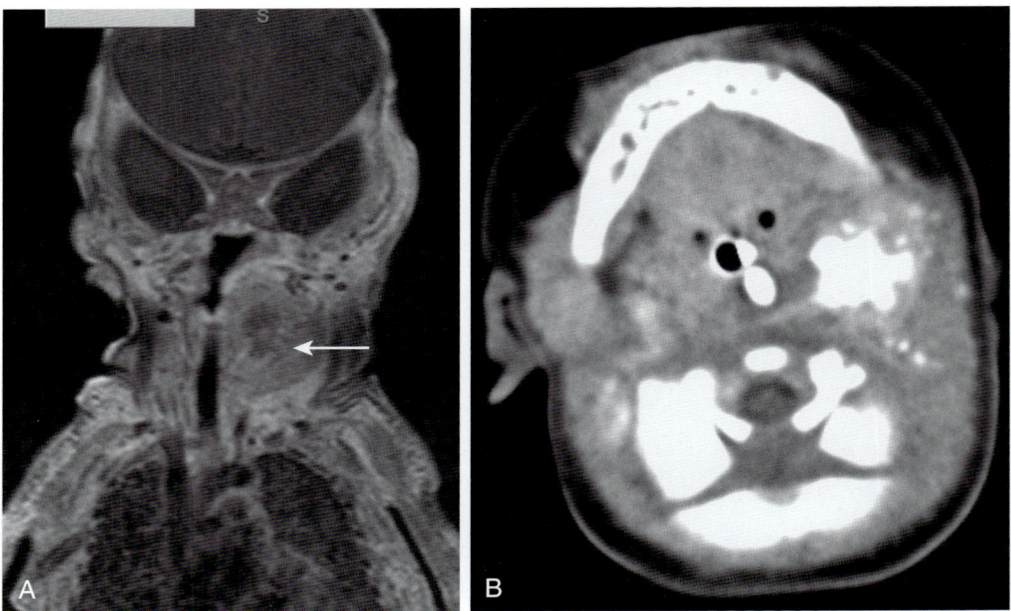

Figure 14-21 Primary cervical neuroblastoma. A coronal postcontrast T1-weighted image with fat suppression (**A**) shows a heterogeneous mass (*arrow*) within the left neck, along the presumable course of the sympathetic chain with central lack of enhancement, which prove to be chunky internal calcifications on computed tomography (**B**).

Neonatal Malignancy

NEUROBLASTOMA

Neuroblastoma is a common malignant tumor of childhood. Less than 5% occur within the neck as a primary site, arising in the sympathetic ganglia. Cervical location of neuroblastoma is more common in young infants. This tumor has known association with Horner syndrome.

The imaging of cervical neuroblastoma may be performed with CT or MRI (Fig. 14-21). Both modalities may depict tumor extension, presence of mineralization, and bony or spinal canal invasion. Restricted diffusion pattern on diffusion-weighted MRI confirms the hypercellular, malignant nature of the tumor. Intratumoral dystrophic calcifications are not uncommon and are observed in 50% of cervical neuroblastomas.

CONGENITAL INFANTILE FIBROSARCOMA

Congenital infantile fibrosarcoma, a rare tumor of infancy, has a markedly different clinical course and a more favorable prognosis compared with adult fibrosarcoma. It may present at birth or soon after or may be diagnosed in utero. Infantile fibrosarcoma has unique cytogenetic findings, which help distinguish this tumor from other infantile tumors such as embryonal rhabdomyosarcoma or from infantile fibromatosis. The tumor appears as a large solid soft tissue mass of the neck (e-Fig. 14-22), which may be rather homogeneous or have central necrosis and hemorrhage.

Key Points

The majority of congenital neck lesions are benign.

Vascular lesions are classified into vascular tumors and vascular malformations.

Lymphatic malformations of the neck may be diagnosed prenatally or present at birth or shortly thereafter.

Ectopic thymus may be found anywhere within the neck.

Suggested Readings

Berenguer B, Mulliken JB, Enjolras O, et al. Rapidly involuting congenital hemangioma: clinical and histopathologic features. *Pediatr Development Pathol.* 2003;6:495-510.

Boye E, Jinin M, Olsen BR, et al. Infantile haemangioma: challenges, new insights and therapeutic promise. *Craniofac Surg.* 2009;20(suppl 1):678-684.

Cahill AM, Nijs E, Ballah D, et al. Percutaneous sclerotherapy in neonatal and infant head and neck lymphatic malformations: a single center experience. *J Pediatr Surg.* 2011;46(11):2083-2095.

Francisca SM, Kyriaki A, Karl OK, et al. Cystic hygromas, nuchal edema, and nuchal translucency at 11-14 weeks of gestation. *Obstet Gynecol.* 2006;107(3):678-683.

Grassi R, Farina R, Floriani I, et al. Assessment of fetal swallowing with gray-scale and color doppler sonography. *AJR.* 2005;185(5):1322-1327.

Hubbard AM, Crombleholme TM, Adzick NS. Prenatal MRI evaluation of giant neck masses in preparation for the fetal exit procedure. *Am J Perinatol.* 1998;15(4):253-257.

Konez O, Burrows PE, Mulliken JB, et al. Angiographic features of rapidly involuting congenital hemangioma (RICH). *Pediatr Radiol.* 2003;33:15-19.

Laje P, Johnson MP, Howell LJ, et al. Ex utero intrapartum treatment in the management of giant cervical teratomas. *J Pediatr Surg.* 2012;47(6):1208-1216.

Murphey MD, Ruble CM, Tyszko SM, et al. Musculoskeletal fibromatosis: radiologic-pathologic correlation. *RadioGraphics.* 2009;29:2143-2183.

Nath CA, Oyelese Y, Yeo L, et al. Three-dimensional sonography in the evaluation and management of fetal goiter. *Ultrasound Obstet Gynecol.* 2005;25(3):312-314.

Restrepo R, Palani R. Hemangiomas revisited: the useful, the unusual and the new. *Pediatr Radiol.* 2011;41:895-904.

Rossler L, Rothoeft T, Teig N, et al. Ultrasound and color Doppler in infantile subglottic haemangioma. *Pediatr Radiol.* 2011;41:1421-1428.

Viswanathan V, Smith ER, Mulliken JB, et al. Infantile hemangiomas involving the neuraxis: clinical and imaging findings. *AJNR.* 2009;30:1005-1013.

Chapter 15

Infection and Inflammation

LISA H. LOWE and CHRISTOPHER J. SMITH

Primary inflammatory processes in the pediatric neck are very common. Because of their acute presentation, contrast enhanced computed tomography (CT) is the initial imaging modality of choice. Detailed characterization, including involved spaces and complicating features, is important for determining appropriate clinical management.

Pharyngotonsillitis and Peritonsillar Abscess

Overview The pharyngeal wall and tonsillar fossa are common locations of infection, particularly in children. Acute pharyngitis, which is diagnosed more than 7 million times per year, does not require imaging for diagnosis. However, when a peritonsillar abscess is suspected, imaging is indicated for diagnosis and surgical management in some cases.[1]

Etiology Most pharyngitis cases are self-limited viral infections. Accounting for up to 30% of cases, acute bacterial pharyngitis is most often secondary to group A beta-hemolytic *Streptococcus* (GAS).[1] Children with pharyngitis present with sore throat, fever, and odynophagia. Lack of improvement with antibiotics suggests the possibility of a peritonsillar abscess. The peritonsillar space is the most common abscess location in the neck.[2]

Imaging Routine pharyngitis and tonsillitis do not require imaging.[1] However, in children suspected of having complications, contrast-enhanced CT is performed.[3] Findings of uncomplicated tonsillitis include unilateral or bilateral enlarged, enhancing tonsils with inflammatory stranding of the parapharyngeal fat. Abscess formation is suggested by a central hypodense fluid collection, with peripheral enhancement within or immediately adjacent to an enlarged tonsil (Fig. 15-1).[3] Follow-up imaging is only performed in children with complications and persistent clinical symptoms.[1,2]

Treatment Viral tonsillitis is self-limiting and requires only supportive treatment, but GAS infections, confirmed by a rapid antigen test or throat culture, are initially treated with antibiotics. Children with recurrent tonsillitis are candidates for tonsillectomy.[4] Those with focal fluid collections identified by CT may require surgical aspiration and drainage. Tonsillar and peritonsillar infections have an excellent prognosis.[1,2]

Lemierre Syndrome

Overview Also known as *suppurative thrombophlebitis of the internal jugular vein*, Lemierre syndrome is an uncommon complication of oropharyngeal infection occurring most often in previously healthy teenagers.[5] Although rare, complications, including septic dissemination with abscess formation in other parts of the body (most commonly in the lungs), osteomyelitis, and arterial vasospasm or occlusion leading to infarction, may be severe.[6]

Etiology Lemierre syndrome is caused by *Fusobacterium* infection, an anaerobic gram-negative bacterium found in normal oral flora.[6] *Fusobacterium necrophorum* is the most common species, with *F. nucleatum*, *F. mortiferum*, or *F. varium* occurring less often. Recognition is important because of the high rate of morbidity and mortality associated with this syndrome.[5,7] Infection spreads from the peritonsillar space into the internal jugular vein, causing thrombus formation.[5] From the jugular vein, septic emboli may seed other organs such as the lungs and brain, leading to abscess formation.[7,8] Spread to adjacent neck spaces, including the retropharyngeal space and osseous structures, may occur, causing osteomyelitis. Patients present with a recent history of sore throat, tenderness, swelling of the lateral neck, and fever.[5] With pulmonary involvement, tachypnea, tachycardia, and hypoxia may be present. Blood cultures are positive for the causative organism.[9]

Imaging As with other head and neck infections, *Fusobacterium* infections present acutely, requiring rapid evaluation. Contrast-enhanced CT is the initial imaging modality of choice. CT findings include inflammatory changes that may involve various spaces of the neck and lack of enhancement within the jugular vein indicating thrombus.[5] Inflammatory findings range from enhancing soft tissues of cellulitis to focal fluid collections indicating an abscess (Figs. 15-2 and 15-3). Chest CT may be concurrently performed if respiratory symptoms are present, and a search for osseous involvement is part of the CT evaluation. Color Doppler ultrasonography is useful to visualize and follow thrombophlebitis but is not reliably able to visualize deep neck infection as may occur with Lemierre syndrome.[5,6] Acute neurologic symptoms may be evaluated with CT or MRI, and both may be augmented by angiographic techniques as well.[7]

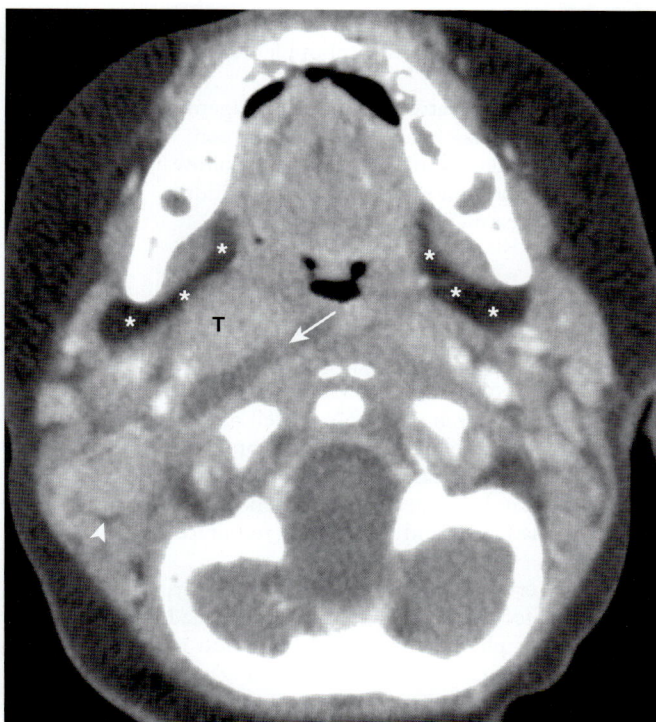

Figure 15-1 Parapharyngeal abscess in a 7-month-old male with fever and difficulty swallowing. Axial contrast enhanced computed tomography image of the suprahyoid neck just below the skull base shows a well-defined, right-sided, low-attenuation fluid collection (*arrow*) adjacent to the tonsils (*T*). The right parapharyngeal fat (*asterisks*) and carotid spaces are displaced laterally. Also, note right-sided prominent lymph nodes (*arrowhead*) and normal left parapharyngeal fat (*asterisks*).

Treatment High-dose intravenous antibiotics, including metronidazole, penicillin, and clindamycin, are the mainstay for treatment of *Fusobacterium* infection and have a high success rate. Anticoagulation therapy is used in up to 27% of patients, although its role is not completely clear.[5] Follow-up imaging is performed in patients who do not defervesce as expected and those with complications that may require closer

follow-up. Although the prognosis of *Fusobacterium* infections is good with prompt recognition and treatment, the rates of morbidity and mortality are higher than with other head and neck infections.[2,9]

Retropharyngeal Abscess

Overview Retropharyngeal abscesses in children commonly result from suppurative lymphadenitis associated with tonsillitis, as well as with sinonasal and dental infections.[10,11] Retropharyngeal abscess may rarely be caused by pharyngeal or esophageal perforation. The retropharyngeal space, the second most common location of abscess in the deep neck after the peritonsillar space, is a potential space that extends from the nasopharynx to the superior mediastinum.[10] Abscesses extending below the T4 vertebra cause concern with regard to what is termed *danger space* infections, which have a high rate of morbidity. Other uncommon conditions that cause thickening of the retropharyngeal tissues include hemorrhage (especially in hemophilia), neuroblastoma, and rarely anterior myelomeningocele.

Etiology Retropharyngeal abscesses are sequelae of GAS, but *Staphylococcus aureus* and infrequent anaerobes have also been reported as causative organisms.[2,10] The most common presenting symptoms are fever, neck pain, dysphagia, palpable neck mass, and sore throat. Cervical lymphadenopathy and torticollis are often present.[11]

Imaging Plain radiography, often ordered as the initial study to screen for large fluid collections, is otherwise limited in its ability to distinguish between cellulitis and abscess, both of which may cause convex abnormal thickening of the prevertebral soft tissues (>8 mm at C2).[4] Anterior displacement of the pharynx, esophagus, larynx, trachea, or all of these is seen from C1 to C4 (Fig. 15-4). Grisel syndrome is inflammation-induced laxity of the atlantoaxial joint, which may result in atlantoaxial rotatory subluxation or other malalignment of C1 and C2. This self-limiting sequence of

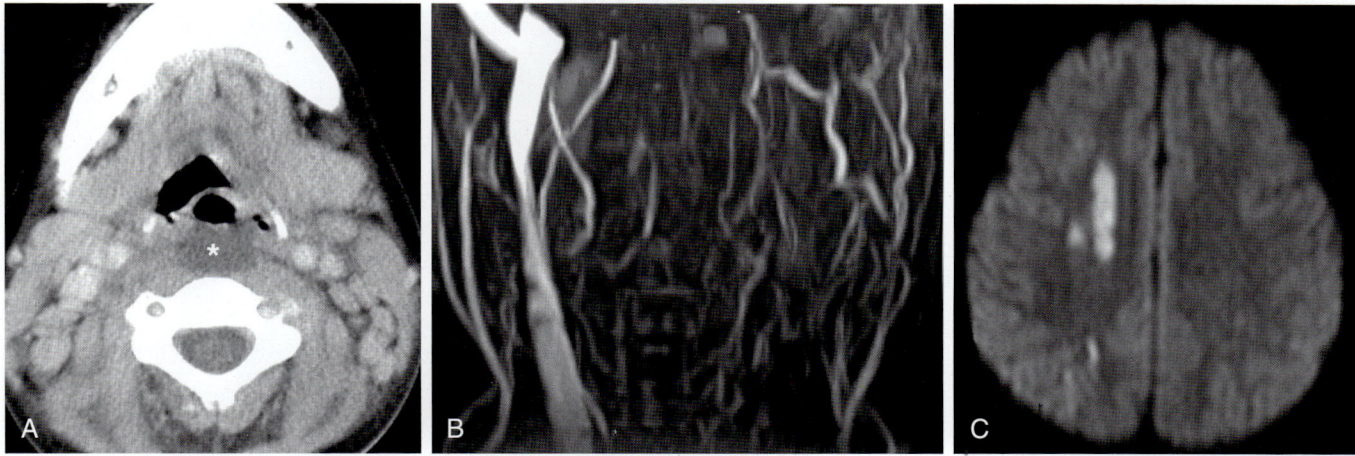

Figure 15-2 Lemierre syndrome (*Fusobacterium necrophorum* infection) complicated by stroke in a 6-year-old female presenting with fever, difficulty swallowing, and nuchal rigidity. **A,** Axial contrast enhanced computed tomography image shows low-attenuation retropharyngeal fluid (*asterisk*). **B,** Magnetic resonance imaging 2 days later, performed because of acute left arm weakness, confirms lack of left internal jugular vein patency on magnetic resonance venogram. **C,** Diffusion-weighted image of the brain reveals multiple small foci of bright signal infarction secondary to emboli from thrombophlebitis, vasospasm, or both.

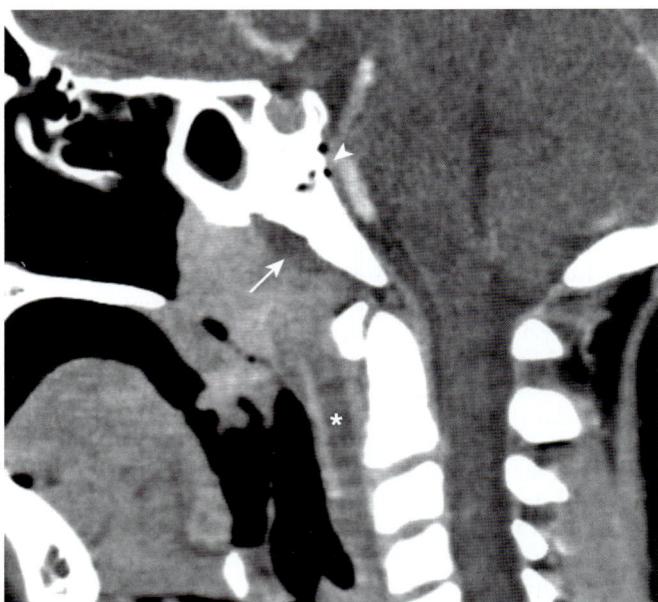

Figure 15-3 Lemierre syndrome (*Fusobacterium necrophorum* infection) complicated by osteomyelitis in a 9-year-old with fever, neck pain, and sore throat. Sagittal reconstructed contrast enhanced computed tomography image demonstrates enlarged adenoids, a low-attenuation retropharyngeal fluid collection (*asterisk*), and a subperiosteal fluid collection along the ventral clivus (*arrow*). Air within and dorsal to the clivus due to osteomyelitis (*arrowhead*) is also seen. Venous occlusion was also present (*not shown*).

symptoms and signs disappears with resolution of the inflammatory process. Contrast-enhanced CT is the study of choice to further check for hypoattenuating, rim-enhancing abscess collections and to determine the need for surgical drainage.[4,10] If an abscess is present, CT is able to define the extent of the collection, to check for mediastinal involvement, and to

detect other complications that may occur with head and neck infections such as thrombophlebitis and osteomyelitis.[4]

Treatment Conservative medical management of retropharyngeal abscess has a success rate between 18% and 57%.[10] Surgical drainage is often required. Follow-up imaging is reserved for complex cases and for children who do not respond to treatment as expected.

Cervical Lymphadenitis

Overview Cervical lymphadenitis is a common pediatric disorder. Acute cases are often caused by viral or bacterial pathogens and in general respond well to supportive care and antibiotics, respectively.[12] Imaging is only considered in subacute and chronic cases when no clinical improvement is seen with standard therapy or when distinguishing abscess from lymphadenitis and cellulitis is required.[13]

Etiology Cervical lymphadenitis is usually secondary to spread of infection from a source in the head and neck such as the tonsils, pharynx, or teeth. Common presenting symptoms include tender focal neck swelling with palpable mass and fever.[13] The most common cause of enlarged cervical lymph nodes in children is a self-limiting reactive hyperplasia as a result of viral infection.[14] However, bacterial causes, including *S. aureus* and streptococcal species, may also occur and occasionally lead to nodal suppuration. Kawasaki disease can also present with acute cervical lymphadenitis, but other organ system features such as rash and fever for at least 5 days, are also present.[13,15]

Imaging Inflamed lymph nodes are usually enlarged, measuring more than 1 cm in short axis. Necrotic or suppurative lymph nodes are characterized by a hypoechoic or hypodense

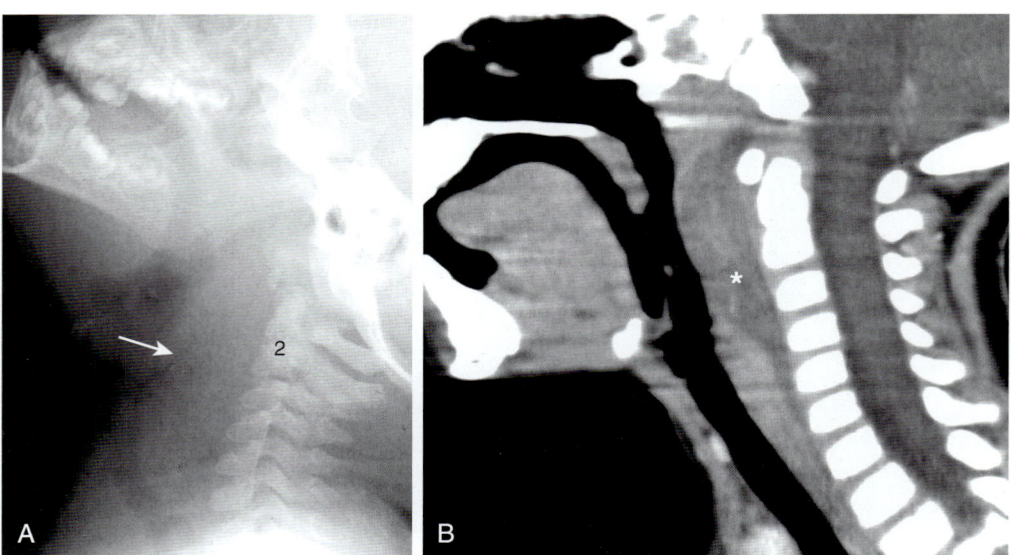

Figure 15-4 Retropharyngeal abscess in a 3-year-old female with sore throat and fever. **A,** Lateral soft tissue neck radiograph reveals extensive soft tissue swelling displacing the airway anteriorly from the skull base to C6 (*arrow*). **B,** Sagittal reconstructed contrast-enhanced computed tomography confirms thickened, enhancing retropharyngeal soft tissues indicating cellulitis. Region of hypoattenuating fluid is concerning for retropharyngeal abscess (*asterisk*).

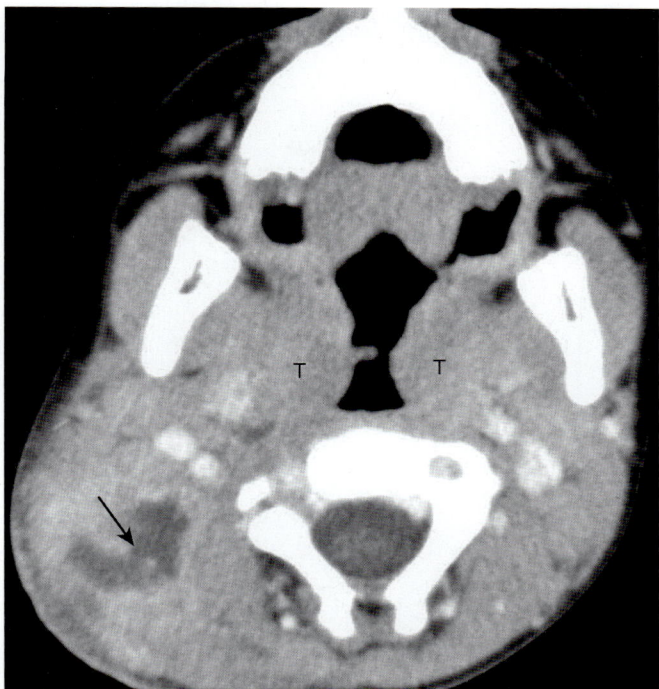

Figure 15-5 Suppurative lymphadenitis in a 5-year-old female with neck swelling and redness. Contrast enhanced computed tomography image reveals a group of enlarged nodes in the right posterior triangle with central hypoattenuating necrosis (*arrow*). Also note enlarged tonsils (*T*) in this child with recurrent tonsillitis.

NTM.[13] The term *scrofula* is used for tuberculous cervical lymphadenitis and is typically diagnosed with aspiration and culture.[17]

Imaging On CT, classic *M. tuberculosis* lymphadenitis appears as a nodal mass with a thick enhancing rim and a low–density center representing necrosis.[18] At later stages, areas of calcification may be present. Differential diagnoses include lymphoma and metastatic disease. MRI findings correlate with CT findings. The thick enhancing rim on CT appears as intermediate signal on T1-weighted images and hypointense on T2-weighted images. Central necrotic areas appear as hypointense on T1-weighted images and markedly hyperintense on T2-weighted images.[18] Chest imaging can help evaluate for pulmonary involvement. Contrast-enhanced CT imaging of NTM shows low attenuation, necrotic, ring-enhancing lesions (Fig. 15-6).[19] These lesions differ from other nodal infections in that little to no surrounding fat stranding is present. Unlike *M. tuberculosis* lymphadenitis, calcifications are uncommon in NTM infection.[19]

Treatment A 12- to 18-month course of multiple antituberculosis antibiotics such as isoniazid, ethambutol, pyrazinamide, rifampin, and streptomycin is the preferred treatment for *M. tuberculosis* lymphadenitis.[13] With this therapy, prognosis is excellent. NTM adenitis requires complete excision of the infected lymph node for optimal treatment and has a high cure rate.[16]

center (Fig. 15-5).[12] Infectious adenopathy is more common than malignant adenopathy; however, cross-sectional imaging such as ultrasonography, CT, and MRI cannot distinguish between them specifically.

Treatment Viral lymphadenitis is usually self-limiting, and acute bacterial lymphadenitis generally responds to appropriate antibiotic therapy. Lymphadenopathy unresponsive to medical therapy may require further imaging to determine if surgical intervention or biopsy is required.[2,14]

Mycobacterial Lymphadenitis

Overview Mycobacterial infection is an important cause of chronic cervical lymphadenitis. In the United States, 70% to 95% of cases of mycobacterial lymphadenitis are caused by nontuberculous mycobacteria (NTM).[13] NTM lymphadenitis commonly affects children between 1 and 5 years of age.[16] It is clinically important to differentiate tuberculous and nontuberculous causes, as they require different treatment measures.

Etiology Cervical mycobacterial lymphadenitis may be caused by various species, including *Mycobacterium tuberculosis*, *M. bovis*, and *M. avium-intracellulare*. In children, the illness is often indolent and may be self-limiting. Patients commonly present with nodal enlargement that slowly develops over several weeks. A strongly positive tuberculin skin test suggests *M. tuberculosis*, whereas a weakly positive test suggests

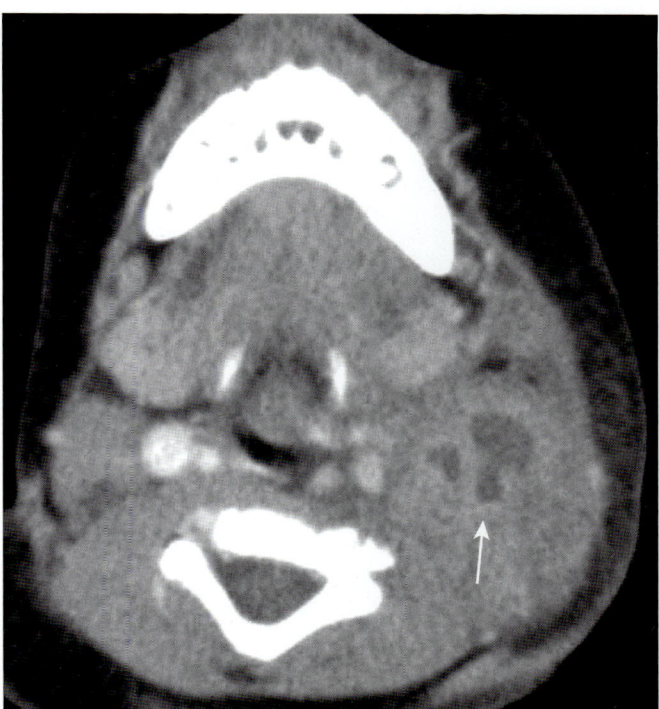

Figure 15-6 Nontuberculous mycobacterial infection in a 10-year-old male with tender left neck swelling. Axial contrast-enhanced computed tomography image shows a cluster of enlarged nodes in the left neck containing low attenuation necrotic centers (*arrow*). Other sites of infection (*not shown*) in this child included hilar nodes and a rib.

Cat Scratch Disease

Overview Cat scratch disease is a granulomatous infection that is usually self-limiting, with 87% of cases being seen in patients younger than18 years.[20] In addition to regional cervical lymphadenitis, disseminated disease can cause granulomas in the liver or spleen, osteomyelitis, discitis, encephalitis, meningitis, ophthalmitis, and cranial neuritis.

Etiology Cat scratch is caused by *Bartonella henselae*, a gram-negative bacillus. The hallmark is painful lymphadenopathy at the site of inoculation, although most patients remain afebrile and have no constitutional symptoms. Although most cases are asymptomatic, in 5% to 10% of infections, dissemination does occur, commonly affecting cervical lymph nodes.[21] The clinical diagnosis is often confirmed with serologic testing.

Imaging On ultrasonography, the affected areas show multiple enlarged and hypoechoic lymph nodes, with enhanced through transmission, as well as increased echogenicity of inflamed surrounding soft tissues.[21] Doppler ultrasonography shows hyperemia, and CT imaging reveals enlargement of lymph nodes, usually with central areas of hypodensity (Fig. 15-7).[22]

Treatment Unless severe, most cases resolve without antimicrobial therapy. Rifampin, ciprofloxacin, gentamicin, and

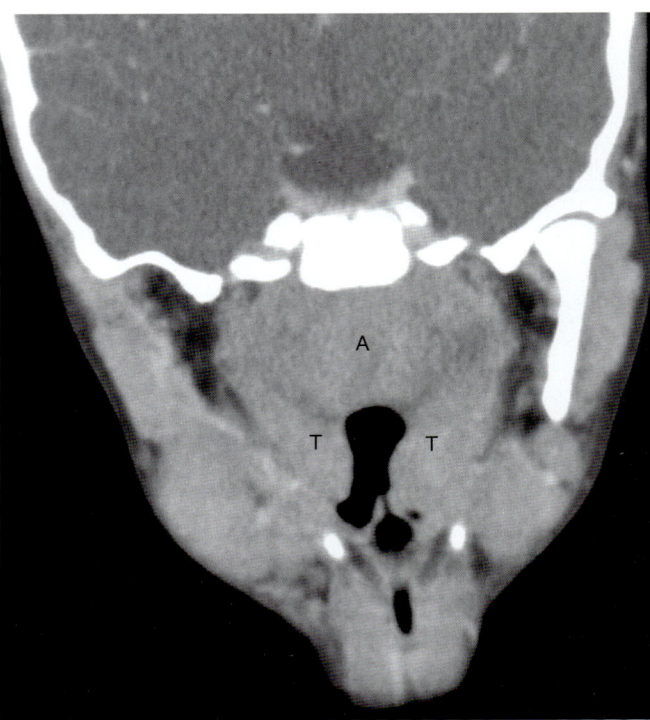

Figure 15-8 Infectious mononucleosis in a 15-year-old female with sore throat, difficulty swallowing, and fatigue. Coronal reconstructed contrast enhanced computed tomography image demonstrates nonspecific enlargement of the adenoids (*A*) and tonsils (*T*). No fluid collections were seen, and no deep neck extension was identified.

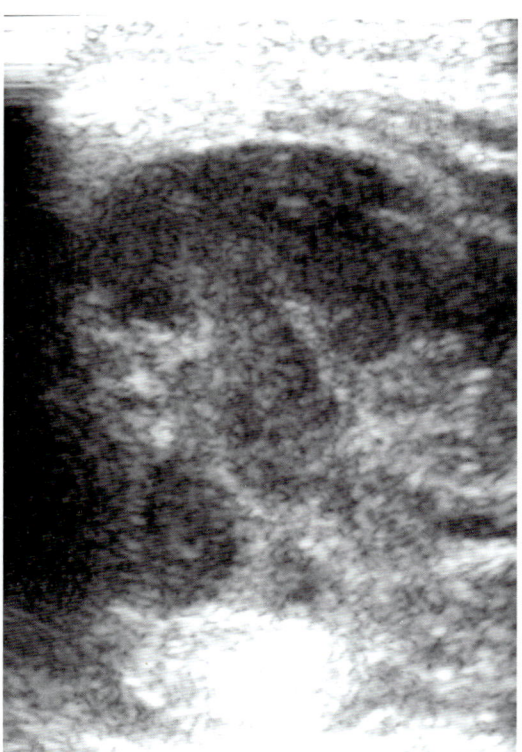

Figure 15-7 Cat scratch disease in a 4-year-old girl with right neck swelling and a new kitten. Ultrasonography demonstrates a mixed echogenicity mass suggesting a conglomeration of nodes.

trimethoprim-sulfamethoxazole have shown effectiveness and are usually reserved for disseminated disease.[23] Follow-up imaging is only necessary in patients who do not improve with antibiotic therapy.

Infectious Mononucleosis

Overview Infectious mononucleosis is a common disorder usually seen in teenagers and young adults. The annual incidence in the United States is roughly 500 cases for every 100,000 persons.[24] Diagnosis is based on clinical findings, and screening may be done with a rapid monospot test for heterophile antibodies.

Etiology Infectious mononucleosis is an acute self-limiting disorder caused by the Epstein-Barr virus. Transmission usually occurs through infected saliva. Patients commonly present with acute pharyngotonsillitis, fever, malaise, and cervical or generalized lymphadenopathy. Splenomegaly is a frequent finding.

Imaging Patients with infectious mononucleosis do not routinely require imaging. However, this disease may mimic other infectious and malignant processes, and imaging may be performed to determine the extent of involvement. Findings on CT are nonspecific but include adenoidal and tonsillar enlargement, as well as diffuse lymph node enlargement with little to no surrounding inflammatory changes (Fig. 15-8).[25]

Treatment Infectious mononucleosis is treated with supportive care. It is recommended that contact sports be avoided for at least 3 weeks following diagnosis to reduce the chances of splenic rupture.[24] The use of corticosteroids and antiviral medication such as acyclovir or valacyclovir has been suggested, but the recommendation lacks sufficient supporting data. Prognosis is excellent with the exception of possible mortality in splenic rupture cases.

Human Immunodeficiency Virus

Overview Benign cervical lymphadenopathy is one of the most common manifestations in children who are positive for the human immunodeficiency virus (HIV). HIV can also cause mediastinal and generalized lymphadenopathy. Imaging is not required for the diagnosis but should be considered along with biopsy if a neck mass persists or worsens, to rule out other causes such as malignancy.

Etiology The lymphadenopathy of HIV is usually symmetric, painless, and extensive. Although generalized lymphadenopathy in patients with HIV is considered benign, the differential diagnosis includes Kaposi sarcoma, non-Hodgkin lymphoma, metastatic disease, and multiple infections.[26] Children with HIV may present with parotid gland enlargement caused by lymphocytic infiltration and lymphoepithelial cystic and solid lesions.

Imaging Prominent adenoids are present on MRI and CT in 35% of patients who are HIV positive.[27] Numerous bilateral enlarged lymph nodes are also a common finding. Ultrasonography may show multiple parotid hypoechoic cystic and solid lesions of varying size. On CT, multiple, low attenuation, and bilateral lymphoepithelial lesions are usually seen.[26]

Treatment The frontline therapy for the treatment of HIV is multiple antiretroviral drugs, including nucleoside and non-nucleoside reverse transcriptase inhibitors, protease inhibitors, and fusion inhibitors. Although benign cervical lymphadenopathy in patients with HIV does not require specific treatment, biopsy may be necessary to rule out other etiologies.

Sialoadenitis

Overview Sialoadenitis is a relatively common condition most often affecting the parotid and submandibular glands. Inflammation is the most common etiology of parotid gland enlargement, and viral infection is the most common pathology. The diagnosis of viral infection is usually made on clinical grounds, and thus, imaging of these conditions is usually not indicated. Although many cases are caused by viruses and are self-resolving, sialolithiasis can cause recurrent episodes of inflammation.

Etiology Sialoadenitis commonly presents as a swollen, enlarged gland and fever. Sialoliths and viruses are the two most common causes. Acute bacterial (suppurative) sialoadenitis is uncommon in children, but recurrent parotitis is occasionally caused by *Streptococcus viridians*. Recurrent sialoadenitis can be caused by sialoliths, which most commonly affect the submandibular gland. Up to 85% of submandibular gland stones arise within the Wharton duct.[28] Mumps is, by far, the most common viral cause of sialoadenitis, usually affecting the parotid glands bilaterally.[29] Other viruses include HIV, influenza, and Coxsackie. Chronic salivary gland inflammation is usually caused by recurrent bacterial infections, autoimmune disorders such as Sjögren syndrome, or sarcoidosis. Lymphadenitis affecting other regions of the neck can also cause enlargement of the intraparotid lymph nodes. This is related to the fact that the parotid gland is the only salivary gland to become encapsulated after the development of the lymphatic system, resulting in the presence of intraglandular lymph nodes.

Imaging Ultrasonography has a role in detecting superficial drainable abscesses. However, it does not help visualize the deep neck to determine the full extent of disease. Nonenhanced CT is the best modality to identify salivary calculi, although contrast is needed to evaluate drainable fluid collections (Fig. 15-9).[30]

On ultrasonography, parotitis appears as an enlarged gland, with heterogeneously decreased echogenicity and irregular borders. Intraparenchymal hypoechoic foci may be found, representing small salivary fluid collections, nodes, or small abscesses.[29] Color Doppler shows hyperemia. CT shows gland enlargement with diffuse enhancement (Fig. 15-10). The presence of a low-attenuation collection with peripheral enhancement suggests an abscess.[29] Recurrent sialoadenitis on ultrasonography manifests as an enlarged gland, containing

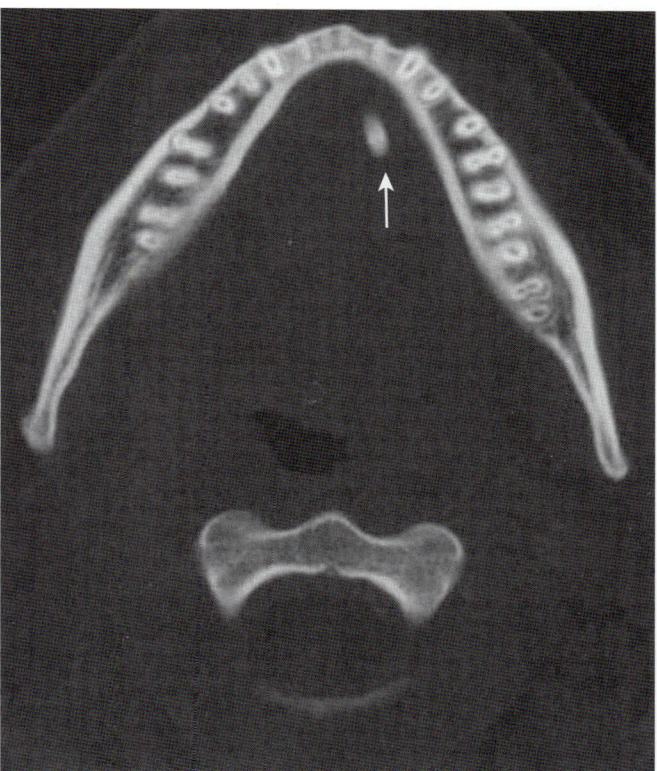

Figure 15-9 Sialoadenitis in a 17-year-old male with left jaw pain and tenderness. Axial unenhanced computed tomography image shows a large calcification in the expected location of the submandibular (Wharton) duct (*arrow*).

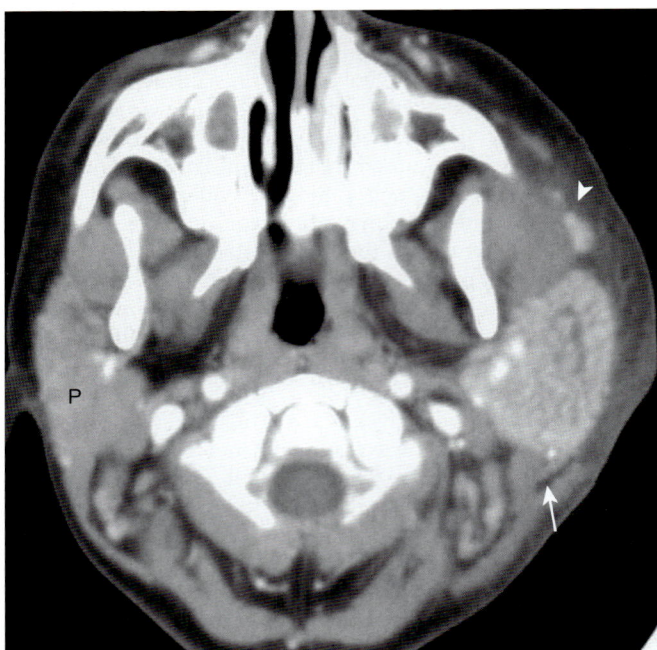

Figure 15-10 Parotitis in a 6-year-old male with painful left cheek swelling. Axial contrast enhanced computed tomography image demonstrates an enlarged, enhancing left parotid gland (*arrow*) as well as similar changes in the accessory parotid tissue (*arrowhead*) along the course of the parotid (Stensen) duct. Note inflammatory stranding in the left cheek subcutaneous fat and the normal right parotid gland (*P*).

several 2- to 4-mm hypoechoic areas that represent foci of pooled salivary secretions.

Treatment   Patients with sialoliths can be treated medically with hydration, gland massage, and sialogogues such as cevimeline or pilocarpine to increase saliva production in an attempt to flush out stones. Surgical excision may be required if symptoms do not resolve with conservative management. Total excision of the gland may also be necessary if multiple

stones are present.[28] Viral sialoadenitis usually only requires supportive treatment.

What the Clinician Needs to Know

- Extent of infection
- Need for surgical intervention
- Complications requiring additional therapy

Key Points

Although imaging features of neck infections may limit the differential possibilities, a definitive diagnosis is often not possible with imaging alone.

Imaging is important to determine extent of infection and to identify complications such as abscess, osteomyelitis, thrombophlebitis, and septic emboli, which require more aggressive treatment.

Abscess drainage is needed for symptom relief, accelerated recovery, and identification of appropriate antibiotic therapy.

Suggested Readings

Boyd ZT, Goud AR, Lowe LH, et al. Pediatric salivary gland imaging. *Pediatr Radiol.* 2009;39:710-722.

McKellop JA, Bou-Assaly W, Mukherji SK. Emergency head & neck imaging: infections and inflammatory processes. *Neuroimag Clin North Am.* 2010;20(4):651-661.

Meuwly JY, Lepori D, Theumann N, et al. Multimodality imaging evaluation of the pediatric neck: techniques and spectrum of findings. *Radiographics.* 2005;25(4):931-948.

Rana RS, Moonis G. Head and neck infection and inflammation. *Radiol Clin North Am.* 2011;49(1):165-182.

References

Full references for this chapter can be found on www.expertconsult.com.

Chapter 16

Neoplasia

CAROLINE D. ROBSON

Imaging is frequently used to evaluate neck tumors in pediatric patients. The choice of imaging modality depends on tumor location and treatment options. Ultrasound with Doppler distinguishes cystic lesions from solid lesions, detects venous or arterial vascularity, and differentiates nodal masses from nonnodal masses. Computed tomography (CT) characterizes bony changes and detects intralesional calcification. CT images are acquired as helical axial thin sections using a split-dose bolus of intravenous (IV) contrast (half of the IV bolus is administered, and images are acquired after a 3-minute pause during the administration of the second half of the bolus). Multiplanar reformatted images with bone and soft tissue reconstruction algorithms should be provided. The lowest radiation dose that produces diagnostic quality images should be used. Magnetic resonance imaging (MRI) demonstrates the soft tissue characteristics of the tumor. The MRI protocol should include multiplanar T1, fat-suppressed T2 or short-T1 inversion recovery (STIR) images, a flow-sensitive gradient echo sequence, diffusion-weighted images, and IV gadolinium-enhanced, fat-suppressed, T1-weighted sequences. Nuclear medicine studies including fluorine-18-fluorodeoxyglucose positron emission tomography (^{18}F-FDG PET) and PET CT are used for staging and follow-up of various tumor types, particularly lymphoma.

The following features are important with regard to the differential diagnosis: patient age, clinical history, physical examination, tumor location, and characteristic imaging features (e.g., mineralization, vascularity, and intensity of enhancement). The most common benign tumor is hemangioma. Lymphoma (approximately 50% of cases) and rhabdomyosarcoma (RMS) (approximately 20% of cases) account for most malignant pediatric head and neck tumors.[1,2] Thyroid, nasopharyngeal, and salivary gland carcinomas are the most frequently seen pediatric head and neck carcinomas.

Hemangioma

Overview Hemangioma is the most common vascular tumor that occurs in infants, more commonly in girls. Infantile hemangiomas proliferate during the first year of life and then involute over the next several years. Proliferating hemangiomas display prominent vascularity. With involution, progressive decrease in size and vascularity and an increase in fibrofatty matrix occur. True congenital hemangiomas are uncommon and are characterized as either rapidly involuting congenital hemangioma or noninvoluting congenital hemangioma. Approximately 20% of children have multiple hemangiomas. Hemangioma that involves skin produces a raised, knobbly, scarlet-colored mass or sometimes a macular lesion that can be confused with a port wine stain in the neonate. Complications of hemangiomas include deformity, mass effect, interference with vital functions, ulceration, and bleeding.

The acronym PHACES describes the association of *p*osterior fossa malformations, *h*emangiomas, *a*rterial anomalies, *c*oarctation of the aorta and cardiac defects, *e*ye abnormalities, *s*ternal malformations, and *s*upraumbilical raphe.[3,4] The hemangiomas are typically large plaque-like or regional cutaneous hemangiomas of the face, sometimes in the midline or appearing beard-like. The most common posterior fossa anomaly is mild unilateral cerebellar hypoplasia with prominence of the ipsilateral retrocerebellar cerebrospinal fluid space. Anomalies of the internal carotid and vertebral arteries include absence or hypoplasia, tortuosity, and ectasia or aneurysmal change, and persistence of the trigeminal artery. Progressive cerebrovascular occlusive changes with moyamoya phenomenon have also been described in patients with craniofacial hemangioma.[5]

Imaging Proliferating infantile hemangioma during the first year of life has characteristic imaging features. The tumors are solid, circumscribed, lobulated, and highly vascular by ultrasound, CT, and MRI (Fig. 16-1). Hemangiomas are isodense with muscle and enhance rapidly and intensely following the administration of contrast agent on CT. Prominent vascular signal voids on spin-echo sequences on MRI or flow-related enhancement on magnetic resonance angiography is typical. Proliferating hemangiomas are moderately hyperintense relative to muscle on T2-weighted images and enhance intensely. Involuting hemangiomas have reduced vascularity and enhancement. True intraosseous hemangioma (as opposed to osseous venous malformations, which are often erroneously referred to as "hemangioma") and small or involuting hemangiomas can be more difficult to diagnose with certainty. The differential diagnosis for hemangioma includes

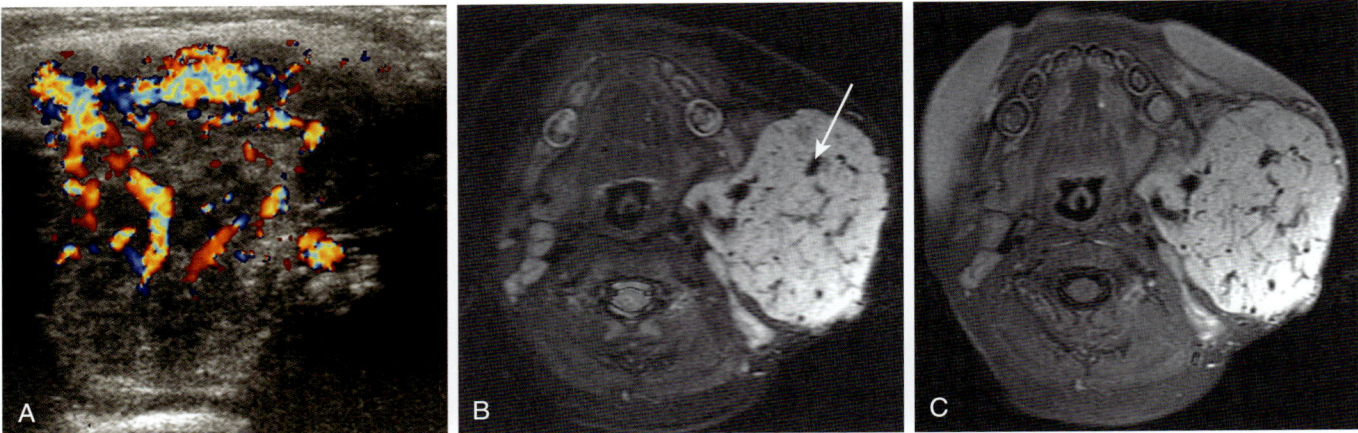

Figure 16-1 Proliferating infantile hemangioma. **A,** A 4-month-old girl with a parotid mass. Color Doppler ultrasound reveals a large, moderately echogenic hemangioma with prominent vascularity. **B,** Three-month-old baby boy with a parotid mass. Axial fast spin-echo inversion recovery magnetic resonance (MR) image shows a large, sharply circumscribed hemangioma with prominent vascular flow voids (*large arrow*). The mass is of slightly higher signal intensity than the spinal cord. **C,** Axial fat-suppressed T1-weighted MR image with intravenous contrast in the same patient demonstrates intense enhancement of the hemangioma.

pyogenic granuloma, which is usually superficial and infrequently imaged. Poorly defined or fuzzy margins are atypical for hemangioma and should prompt an alternative diagnosis such as kaposiform hemangioendothelioma. Other rare congenital tumors such as rhabdomyoma and RMS lack prominent vascularity. Infantile fibrosarcoma is sometimes somewhat vascular and hemorrhagic but usually causes more aggressive bony erosion and does not enhance as intensely as proliferating hemangioma. Hemangioma within or adjacent to bone occasionally produces bony remodeling and corticated bony erosion simulating Langerhans cell histiocytosis, but aggressive lytic bony destruction should prompt consideration of a malignant neoplasm.

Management Hemangiomas are usually treated expectantly, anticipating involution. However, if interfering with vital functions, accelerated involution is promoted by medical therapy with steroids, alpha-interferon, or, more recently, propranolol.[6] Laser therapy and embolization are therapeutic options for selected cases.

Teratoma

Overview Teratoma is the most common congenital tumor of the neck and is the second most common location of teratoma in early infancy. Histologic immaturity in congenital teratoma does not necessarily reflect an adverse outcome, as is seen in adolescents and adults.

Imaging Prenatal diagnosis of teratoma is made with fetal ultrasound or MRI. The tumor is sharply circumscribed, and heterogeneous, with solid and cystic areas. Compression of the airway by tumor may affect the timing and mode of delivery and should prompt delivery of the baby by the fetal exit procedure with elective cesarian section and securing of the airway while the neonate is receiving placental support. Midline teratoma that involves the oral cavity prevents normal development and apposition of the palatal shelves, resulting in

cleft palate. Infrahyoid teratoma frequently involves the thyroid gland and is considered by some to be of thyroid origin.[7]

On ultrasound, CT, and MRI, teratomas appear heterogeneous, with solid and cystic components (Fig. 16-2). Flecks of calcification and fat are characteristic. Other than fat, the soft tissue components typically enhance. The differential diagnosis for predominantly cystic teratoma is lymphatic malformation (LM). The presence of calcification and the apparent origin of the tumor from the thyroid gland with absence of the ipsilateral thyroid lobe or splaying of thyroid tissue around the tumor periphery are key features that distinguish teratoma from LM. Other neck tumors that contain fat include lipoma and lipoblastoma. The most common calcified tumor in the neck is pilomatrixoma, which is small, calcified, and cutaneous or subcutaneous. Less common congenital solid tumors that can be confused with teratoma include infantile myofibromatosis and kaposiform hemangioendothelioma with lymphomatoid components.

Management The treatment for teratoma is surgical resection.

Nerve Sheath Tumors

Imaging Solitary neurofibroma, plexiform neurofibroma, and malignant peripheral nerve sheath tumor (MPNST) usually occur in children with neurofibromatosis (NF) type 1. Schwannoma occurs sporadically or in patients with NF2. Solitary neurofibroma and schwannoma are well marginated and of variable signal on T1- and T2-weighted images (Fig. 16-3, *A*). Fibrous tissue in neurofibroma and Antoni A tissue in schwannoma produce T2 shortening that can simulate high-grade cellular neoplasms. These nerve sheath tumors enhance, and cystic foci can be seen in schwannoma. Plexiform neurofibromas appear multinodular or as worm-like masses extending along peripheral nerves or nerve roots, sometimes within multiple fascial compartments. Plexiform neurofibroma appears hypodense on CT and hyperintense

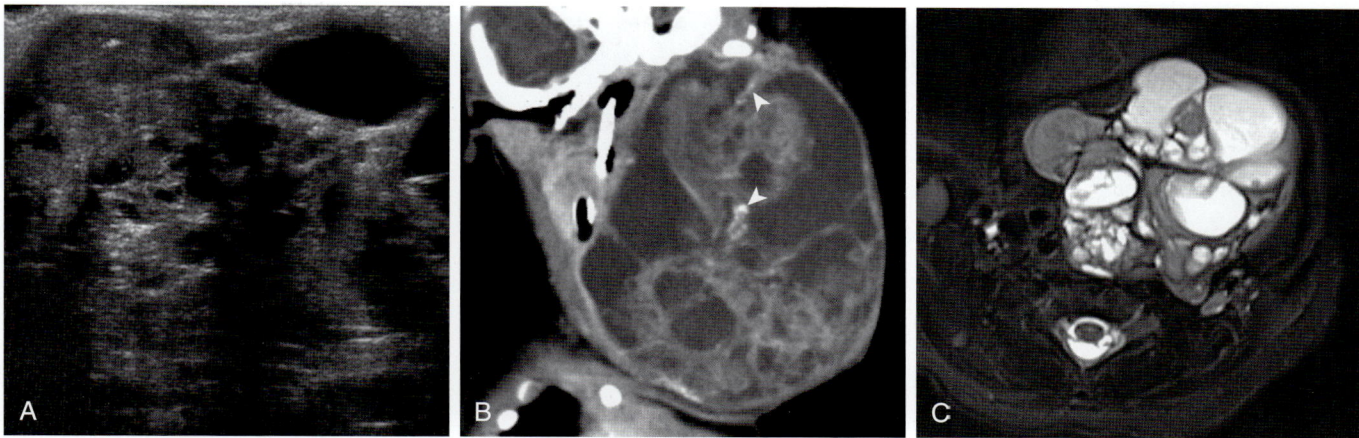

Figure 16-2 Congenital teratoma of the neck in a newborn boy. **A,** Ultrasound of the neck shows a heterogeneous cystic and solid teratoma. **B,** Reformatted coronal computed tomography image with intravenous contrast shows that the cystic and solid teratoma contains flecks of calcification (*arrowheads*). **C,** Axial fast spin-echo inversion recovery magnetic resonance (MR) image shows the cystic and solid teratoma.

relative to muscle on T2-weighted MRI and has a characteristic "target sign" on CT and central punctuate hypointensity on T2-weighted MRI (see Fig. 16-3, *B*). This feature helps distinguish this tumor from microcystic LM, which also tends to be transspatial across anatomic neck compartments. MPNST is heralded by pain, rapid increase in size of a peripheral nerve sheath tumor, change in enhancement characteristics, or the development of metastases (see Fig. 16-3, *C*). FDG PET imaging is useful for evaluation of suspected MPNST.

Management The treatment of benign nerve sheath tumors is variable, depending on symptomatology, size, location, and histology, and ranges from conservative management to complete or partial surgical resection. MPNST is an aggressive tumor for which complete surgical resection is the most effective treatment. Radiation therapy may help attain local control; the role of chemotherapy is unclear.[8,9]

Rhabdomyosarcoma

Overview RMS is the most common soft tissue sarcoma and the second most frequent head and neck malignancy after lymphoma.[1,2] About one third of cases of RMS occur in the head and neck.[10] Disease incidence is bimodal, with one peak occurring during the first decade of life and the second during adolescence. The most frequently encountered locations for RMS are the masticator space and orbit during the first decade, with an increased preponderance of paranasal sinus involvement in teenagers. RMS is typically aggressive and erodes adjacent bone. Parameningeal disease results from skull base erosion or tumor extension through the foramen ovale. Metastatic cervical adenopathy is sometimes seen. Presenting signs and symptoms include a neck mass, proptosis, airway obstruction, otalgia from eustachian tube obstruction, and cranial neuropathy.

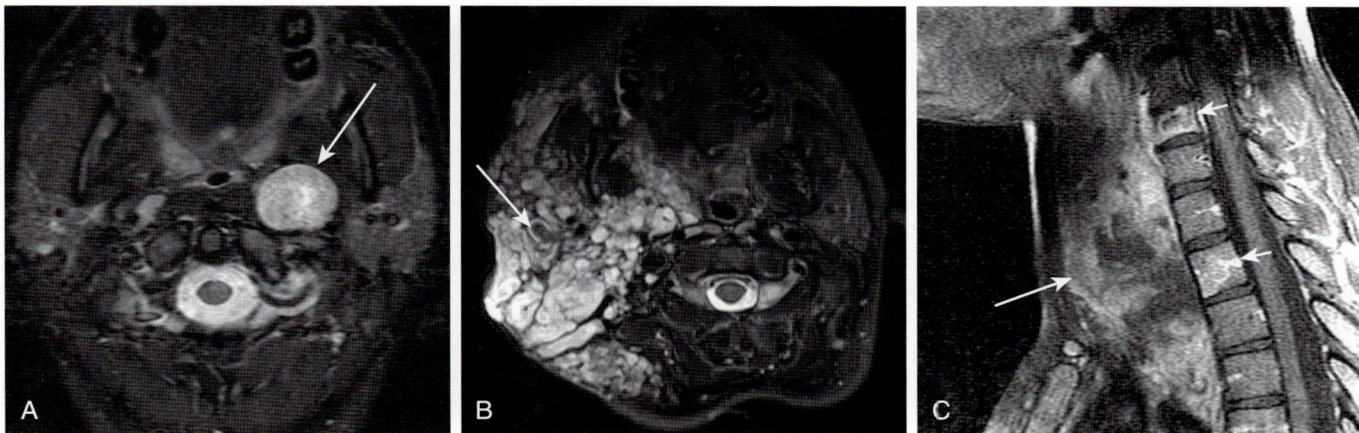

Figure 16-3 Nerve sheath tumors. **A,** Schwannoma. Axial fast spin-echo inversion recovery magnetic resonance (MR) image in a 16-year-old boy reveals an incidental sharply circumscribed, rounded tumor (*arrow*) abutting the left internal carotid artery. The tumor is of higher signal intensity than spinal cord and nodal tissue. **B,** Plexiform neurofibroma in a 19-year-old girl with neurofibromatosis type 1 (NF1). The tumor resembles a "bag of worms," with numerous tubular and rounded components located in multiple fascial compartments. The target sign is demonstrated (*arrow*). **C,** Malignant peripheral nerve sheath tumor in an 18-year-old boy with NF1, presenting with pain and a rapidly enlarging neck mass. Sagittal fat-suppressed T1-weighted magnetic resonance image shows a heterogeneously enhancing prevertebral mass (*long arrow*). Enhancement of C5 and T1 is abnormal, with loss of height of C5.

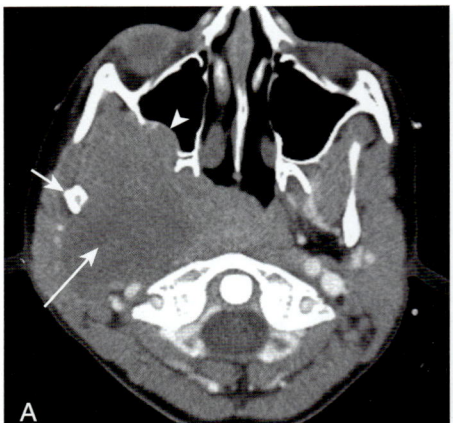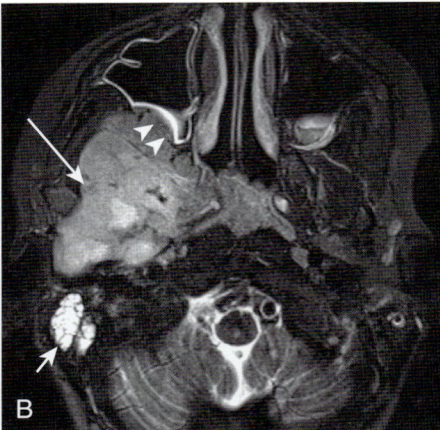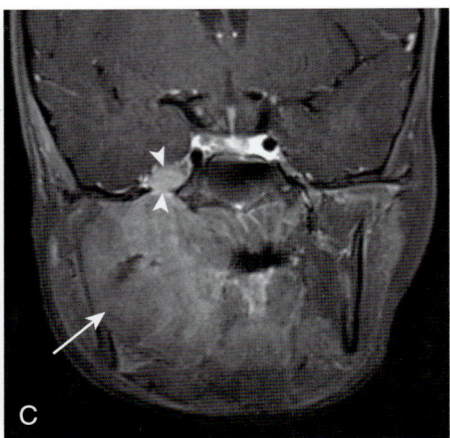

Figure 16-4   Rhabdomyosarcoma in a 7-year-old girl with a neck mass and otalgia. **A,** Contrast-enhanced computed tomography shows a tumor (*long arrow*) located in the right masticator space, involving the pterygoid muscles. Dislocation of the right temporomandibular joint (*short arrow*) and erosion of the posterolateral wall of the right maxillary antrum (*arrowhead*) are seen. **B,** Axial fast spin-echo inversion recovery magnetic resonance (MR) image shows that the tumor (*long arrow*) is of similar signal to nodal tissue. The tumor erodes through the posterior wall of the right maxillary antrum (*arrowheads*). Obstruction of the right eustachian tube results in retained secretions in right mastoid air cells (*short arrow*). **C,** Coronal fat-suppressed T1-weighted MR image reveals the enhancing tumor (*long arrow*) with parameningeal spread via the foramen ovale to the base of the right cavernous sinus (*arrowheads*).

Although most cases of RMS appear to be sporadic, some young children have identifiable constitutional mutations of the *p53* tumor suppressor gene and a possible hereditary predisposition to cancer.[11] Deletions of the *NF1* gene, a tumor suppressor and inhibitor of Ras, has also been described in some types of RMS.[12] The two most common RMS histologic types are embryonal and alveolar RMSs. Embryonal RMS is more common in younger children and is sometimes associated with loss of heterozygosity of a portion of chromosome 11. In general, the behavior, therapeutic response, and prognosis of embryonal RMS are better than for alveolar RMS, which is usually seen in teenagers. More recently, molecular criteria for RMS based on tumor genomic analysis have been described, with potential prognostic and therapeutic significance.[13] Approximately 55% to 75% of alveolar RMSs have a *FOX01* to *PAX3* or *PAX7* fusion gene. Alveolar RMS that lacks this translocation tends to behave in a fashion more like embryonal RMS.

Imaging   Imaging of RMS shows a soft tissue tumor, with lytic bone destruction and bony remodeling (Fig. 16-4, *A* and *B*). The tumor is usually heterogeneous and sometimes necrotic and has well-circumscribed borders. Tumor enhancement on CT or MRI is variable. The signal intensity of tumors on T2-weighted images is variable, but usually relatively isointense to hypointense compared with the brain because of cellularity. RMS exhibits decreased diffusion on diffusion-weighted MRI. Coronal and sagittal contrast-enhanced, fat-suppressed, T1-weighted images are used to evaluate for parameningeal spread (see Fig. 16-4, *C*). Cervical lymph nodes should be evaluated for possible metastatic adenopathy. Atypical or unusual features of RMS include marked hyperintensity on T2-weighted images and intratumoral hemorrhage. The differential diagnosis for RMS depends on tumor location and includes lymphoma, carcinoma (teenagers), other types of sarcoma, juvenile nasopharyngeal angiofibroma (e.g., adolescent boys with nosebleeds), and desmoid tumor. Desmoid tumor is typically seen along the lingual surface of the body of the mandible, is of low signal on

T2-weighted MRI, and demonstrates focal bony remodeling and a small amount of periosteal reaction on CT. Osteogenic sarcoma, or Ewing sarcoma, is suggested by a tumor that primarily involves bone and is characterized by pronounced proliferative periosteal reaction and soft tissue mass. Osteogenic sarcoma can arise primarily or secondarily as a complication of prior radiation therapy. Other sarcomas include fibrosarcoma, chondrosarcoma, and synovial sarcoma.

Management   Treatment of RMS includes surgery, radiation, and chemotherapy. Serial scans are used to detect residual or recurrent tumor. The prognosis depends on histologic and molecular subtype and is better for localized disease with complete surgical resection.

Lymphoma

Overview   Lymphoma is the most common head and neck malignancy in children. Hodgkin lymphoma (HL) occurs primarily in teenagers and is more common than non-Hodgkin lymphoma (NHL), which occurs throughout childhood.[1] HL manifests as enlarged lymph nodes that appear as firm, nontender unilateral neck masses or, less commonly, bilateral neck masses. HL typically involves contiguous lymph nodes. Constitutional symptoms usually herald systemic disease. Associated mediastinal involvement is seen in approximately 40% of patients with HL, and 80% of patients with cervical HL have disease outside of the head and neck.[1] Histologically, HL is characterized by the presence of Reed-Sternberg cells, which are giant multinucleated lymphocytes with eosinophilic nucleoli. The most common histologic subtype of HL is nodular sclerosing. Various etiologies have been implicated, including prior infection with the Epstein-Barr virus (EBV).

NHL presents as painless unilateral adenopathy or signs of airway obstruction caused by involvement of soft tissues in the region of the pharynx. Approximately 30% of patients present with extranodal disease in the head and neck, and

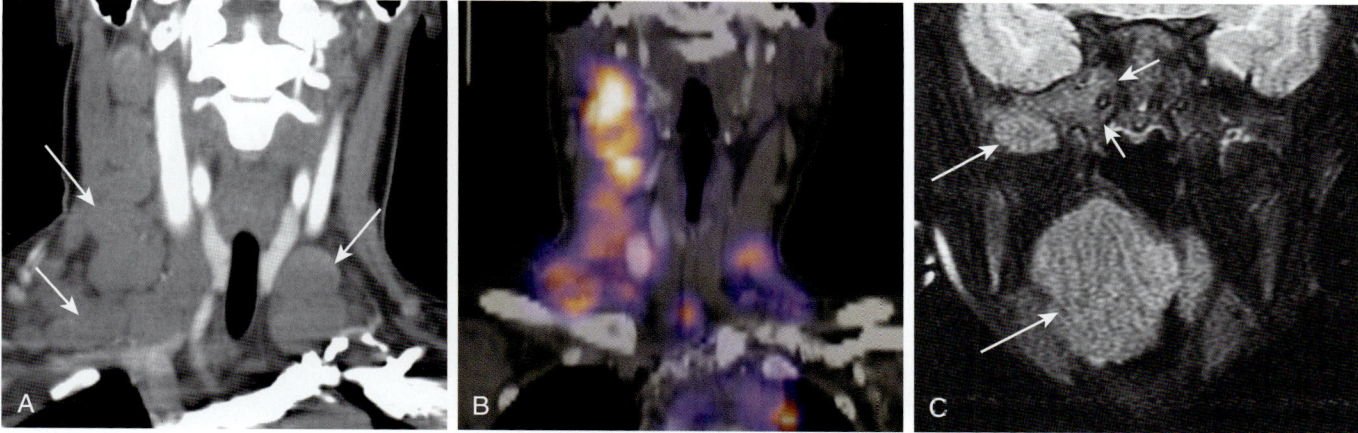

Figure 16-5 Lymphoma. **A,** A 16-year-old girl with neck masses and constitutional symptoms. Reformatted coronal computed tomography (CT) with contrast shows extensive cervical lymphadenopathy with minimally enhancing, enlarged lymph nodes. **B,** Fused fluorodeoxyglucose (FDG) positron emission tomography and CT image demonstrates FDG-avid adenopathy in the same patient, newly diagnosed with nodular sclerosing Hodgkin disease. **C,** 8-year-old boy with airway obstruction. Coronal fat-suppressed T2-weighted magnetic resonance image demonstrates homogeneous hypointense masses (*long arrows*): one involving the right palatine tonsil and the other located inferior to the right sphenoid bone. Signal abnormality and expansion of the right sphenoid bone are also present (*short arrows*). These findings are characteristic of non-Hodgkin lymphoma, in this case, it is Burkitt lymphoma.

approximately 70% of patients have disease outside of the head and neck.[1] Extranodal NHL disease involves the lymphoid tissue of the Waldeyer ring (adenoids and tonsils) or the sinonasal, thyroid, or orbital regions. Histologic subtypes of NHL in children include Burkitt's lymphoma, lymphoblastic lymphoma, diffuse large B-cell lymphoma, and anaplastic large cell lymphoma. Although the exact etiology and pathogenesis of NHL is unknown, predisposing factors include severe immunocompromise, especially when associated with certain infectious agents such as EBV, and exposure to oncogenic infections or environmental carcinogens while in an immuncompromised state.[14] In immunosuppressed children, the development of lymphoproliferative disorders, including lymphoma, is believed to be multifactorial and related to both immunosuppression and ongoing antigenic stimulation. Infectious agents associated with NHL include human immunodeficiency virus, EBV, human T-cell lymphotropic virus-1, human herpes virus 8, *Helicobacter pylori*, and *Chlamydia psittaci*.[14] EBV is also implicated in the pathogenesis of Burkitt lymphoma.

Imaging Doppler ultrasound can be helpful in distinguishing reactive from malignant adenopathy. Features of malignant nodes include displacement of vessels (which correlates with perinodal tumor spread), aberrant and subcapsular vessels, and avascular foci.[15] On CT, involved nodal tissue typically does not enhance as avidly as infectious lymphadenitis, and stranding of the surrounding fat is usually absent (Fig. 16-5, *A*). ^{18}F-FDG PET whole-body imaging is used for diagnosis, staging, and follow-up of disease (see Fig. 16-5, *B*).[16] In a study comparing FDG PET with CT, MRI, and gallium scans, FDG PET had higher sensitivity and specificity than other imaging modalities for pediatric HL and NHL.[17] The presence of a soft tissue mass, with bony involvement of the mandible and the presence of "floating teeth," is characteristic of, but not specific for, Burkitt lymphoma. On MRI, lymphomatous involvement tends to show enlargement of lymphoid tissue that is often homogeneous and of lower signal

intensity than reactive adenopathy (see Fig. 16-5, *C*), with variable but typically homogeneous enhancement that is less marked than reactive adenopathy. The differential diagnosis for lymphoma includes infection or inflammation, other lymphoproliferative disorders, and metastatic adenopathy.

Management The existing diagnostic categories of lymphoma, as exemplified by diffuse large B-cell lymphoma, consist of multiple molecularly distinct diseases that differ not only in their cells of origin and oncogenic mechanisms, but also in clinical outcome and prognosis. Tumor gene expression profiling is now being used to predict the clinical and biologic behavior of the tumor, and the genetic signature of the tumor is likely to play a crucial role in the identification of therapeutic targets and the selection of appropriate therapy.[18] Treatment regimens consist of a variety of chemotherapeutic agents with or without radiation therapy.

Carcinoma

Overview The most frequently encountered carcinomas of the head and neck are thyroid carcinoma and nasopharyngeal carcinoma (NPC). Thyroid carcinoma presents as a thyroid mass, with or without cervical adenopathy and metastatic disease. The most common histologic subtype is papillary carcinoma (Fig. 16-6, *A*). Papillary carcinoma occasionally arises in a thyroglossal duct cyst, manifesting as a calcified mural nodule.

NPC typically occurs in adolescents. Presenting symptoms and signs include a nasopharyngeal mass, cervical lymphadenopathy, unilateral otitis media, rhinorrhea, and nasal obstruction. NPC is related to prior EBV infection. On imaging, NPC manifests as a nasopharyngeal mass with cervical lymphadenopathy and aggressive characteristics such as bony destruction of the paranasal sinuses and skull base with intracranial extension. The differential diagnosis based on location is lymphoma and various types of sarcoma.

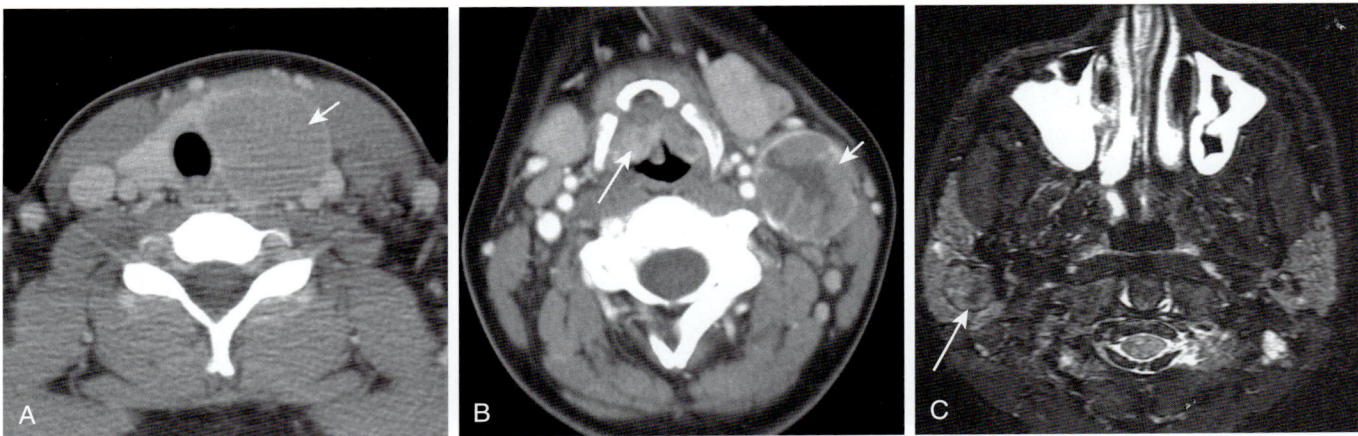

Figure 16-6 Carcinoma. **A,** Papillary carcinoma of the thyroid gland in a 15-year-old girl. Axial contrast-enhanced computed tomography (CT) image shows the mass involving the left lobe of the thyroid gland. **B,** Nuclear protein in testis midline carcinoma of the epiglottis in a 13-year-old girl presenting with hoarseness and a neck mass. The tumor exhibited the t(15,19) chromosomal translocation. Axial contrast-enhanced CT image demonstrates an irregular enhancing mass involving the epiglottis and aryepiglottic folds (*long arrow*). Necrotic adenopathy is caused by nodal metastasis (*short arrow*). **C,** Mucoepidermoid carcinoma of the parotid gland in a 19-year-old boy. Axial fast spin-echo inversion recovery magnetic resonance image shows a small, hypointense, sharply marginated tumor within the right parotid gland (*arrow*). The appearance is suggestive of, but not specific for, mucoepidermoid carcinoma.

Nuclear protein in testis (NUT) midline carcinoma is a rare, distinctive, and almost invariably highly lethal tumor characterized by a unique chromosomal rearrangement involving the *NUT* gene on chromosome 15.[19] In spite of aggressive treatment, tumors with this cytogenetic abnormality generally result in death within months due to metastatic disease. In the head and neck, these tumors involve the sinonasal region, the epiglottis, or the larynx.[20]

Imaging Relatively low signal intensity compared with lymphoid tissue on T2-weighted MRI is consistent with a cellular neoplasm. Other features include aggressive lytic destruction of bone and metastatic adenopathy (see Fig. 16-6, *B*). Imaging characteristics are indistinguishable from other high-grade neoplasms.

Carcinoma of the salivary glands is most frequently mucoepidermoid in nature.[21] Imaging does not reliably distinguish between low-grade malignant tumors and benign parotid tumors, typically pleomorphic adenoma. The signal and enhancement characteristics of mucoepidermoid carcinoma are variable, as is the histologic grade (see Fig. 16-6, *C*).

Management Treatment and prognosis of pediatric neck carcinoma depends on tumor type and cytogenetics, location, operability, and staging. For example, low-grade mucoepidermoid carcinoma can be cured by complete surgical excision alone, whereas more aggressive carcinoma types often require surgical resection, chemotherapy, and radiation therapy.

Metastatic Disease

Metastatic disease involving the neck in pediatric patients may involve bones, cervical lymph nodes, or both. During

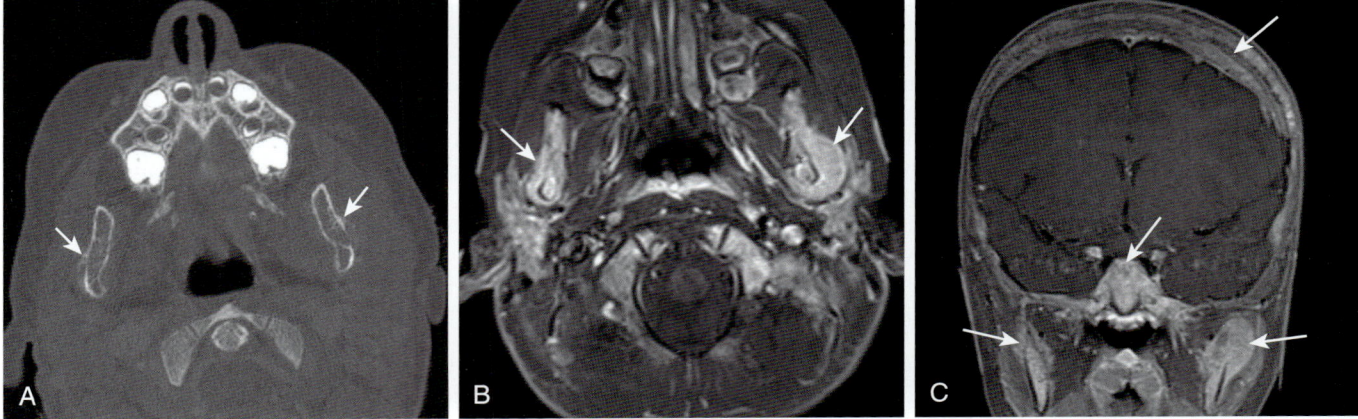

Figure 16-7 Metastatic stage 4 neuroblastoma in a 3-year-old girl. **A,** Axial contrast-enhanced computed tomography image (bone window) demonstrates poorly defined lytic destruction of the mandibular rami with ill-defined periosteal reaction (*arrows*). **B,** Axial fat-suppressed, T1-weighted magnetic resonance imaging (MRI) reveals associated enhancing soft tissue masses (*arrows*). Abnormal enhancement of the bones of the maxilla, cervical spine, and skull base is caused by metastatic neuroblastoma. **C,** Coronal fat-suppressed, T1-weighted MRI shows the enhancing metastatic deposits involving the mandible, the central skull base, and the calvarium (*arrows*).

the first decade of life, especially in children younger than 2 years, neuroblastoma is most common. Leukemic disease is also common, usually in older patients, and sometimes indistinguishable in imaging appearance. Soft tissue disease, bony metastatic disease, or a combination of both is also seen in a wide variety of other tumor types. Osseous metastases appear on CT as lytic, permeative bony destruction, spiculated periosteal reaction, and enhancing soft tissue masses (Fig. 16-7, *A*). Marrow involvement by tumor, as exemplified by neuroblastoma, produces widening of the medullary spaces that can be symmetrical, and is easily overlooked on CT. On MRI, masses are of relatively low signal on T2-weighted images, with moderate to intense enhancement (see Fig. 16-7 *B, C*).

References

Full references for this chapter can be found on www.expertconsult.com.

Chapter 17

Thyroid and Parathyroid

HOLLIE A. JACKSON

Thyroid Gland

EMBRYOLOGY

The term "thyroid" is derived from the Greek word for "shield" because of the gland's shape and relationship to the laryngeal thyroid cartilage. The thyroid gland has a dual embryonic origin.[1-3] The two thyroid cell types, thyroid follicular cells (thyrocytes) and parafollicular (C-cells), are derived from all three germ cell layers.[3]

The most abundant cells, the follicular cells, arise from the thyroid anlage. The development of the thyroid gland begins as a bud of epithelial proliferation in the floor of the primitive pharynx between the developing tuberculum impar and copula of the tongue anlage, around 24 days' gestation.[4] This thyroid anlage soon forms a ventral outgrowth known as the *thyroid diverticulum*. The progenitor follicular cells proliferate distally and then laterally, leading to the characteristic bilobed appearance of the gland connected by an isthmus.

As the embryo grows, the developing thyroid gland descends anterior to the hyoid bone and larynx, forming the thyroglossal duct. Because of the close association of the developing thyroid gland and embryonic heart, it is thought that the descent of the heart results in the thyroid gland being pulled.[3,5] The thyroid gland remains connected to the tongue by the thyroglossal duct. At approximately 7 weeks' gestation, the thyroid gland reaches its final site in front of the trachea and the thyroglossal duct disappears.[4] The original opening of the thyroglossal duct persists as a vestigial pit at the base of the tongue called the *foramen cecum*.[6,7] About 15% to 75% of people have a pyramidal lobe, which is derived from the lower part of the thyroglossal duct and extends upward from the isthmus.[8]

Around the time the thyroid gland reaches its final position, it merges with the two lateral anlagen or ultimobranchial bodies, resulting in the incorporation of the C-cells (parafollicular cells) into the thyroid gland. The ultimobranchial bodies are a pair of transient embryonic structures derived from the endoderm of the fourth pharyngeal pouch and the ectoderm of the fifth pharyngeal pouch, into which the C-cell precursors migrate from the neural crest.[9,10] The thyroid follicular cells continue to organize the thyroid follicles. As the ultimobranchial bodies merge with the thyroid, their C-cells disperse within the interfollicular space.[4]

Remnants of the ultimobranchial bodies, or solid cell nests, are seen postnatally and are usually located in the middle third of the thyroid lateral lobes.[11]

PHYSIOLOGY

The primary function of the thyroid is to produce hormones that play a vital role in regulating many cellular and physiologic activities, such as growth, development, and metabolism.

The thyroid gland synthesizes and secretes two hormones: (1) thyroxine (T4) and (2) triiodothyronine (T3). The synthesis and secretion of these hormones is closely regulated through a complex feedback mechanism known as the *hypothalamic-pituitary-thyroid axis*.

The hypothalamus synthesizes and secretes thyrotropin-releasing hormone (TRH), which is carried to the pituitary gland by the hypothalamic-pituitary portal venous system.[12-14] Once in the pituitary gland, TRH stimulates the synthesis and secretion of thyrotropin (thyroid-stimulating hormone [TSH]) from the anterior pituitary gland. TSH binds to receptors in the thyroid gland, stimulating follicular cell production and secretion of T4 and T3. Thyroid secretion and serum concentrations of T4 and T3 are maintained by a negative feedback loop involving inhibition of TSH and TRH secretion by T4 and T3.[15,16]

Iodide is actively transported into the follicular cells by the sodium-iodide symporter at the basolateral membrane.[17-21] Thyroid peroxidase (TPO) oxidizes iodide into its chemically active form. Thyroglobulin in the follicular lumen serves as a matrix for the synthesis of T4 and T3. First, TPO catalyzes the iodination of selected tyrosyl residues in thyroglobulin in a process known as *iodination and organification*. This results in the formation of monoiodotyrosine (MIT) and diiodotyrosine (DIT). TPO then catalyzes a coupling reaction in which two iodotyrosines are coupled to form T4 or T3. Iodinated thyroglobulin is stored as colloid in the follicular lumen. When needed, thyroglobulin is internalized into the follicular cell and digested in lysosomes. Subsequently, T4 (80%) and T3 (20%) are released into the bloodstream. MIT and DIT are deiodinated and released iodide is recycled for hormone synthesis.[3]

C-cells produce thyrocalcitonin, which is important in calcium homeostasis.

ANATOMY

The thyroid gland is composed of a right and left lobe usually joined by an isthmus anteriorly. The thyroid gland extends superiorly to the level of the thyroid cartilage and inferiorly to the level of the fifth or sixth tracheal ring. Occasionally, an extra midline lobe, called the *pyramidal lobe*, extends superiorly from the isthmus.

The thyroid gland is located in the visceral space of the infrahyoid neck, anterior and lateral to the trachea and posterior to the infrahyoid strap muscles. The sternocleidomastoid muscles are located anterolaterally, and the carotid space is located posterolaterally. Posteromedial to the thyroid gland are the tracheoesophageal grooves containing the recurrent laryngeal nerves, paratracheal lymph nodes, and parathyroid glands.

The middle layer of the deep cervical fascia surrounds the visceral space and ensheaths the thyroid gland. The fascia condenses to form the suspensory ligament of Berry, affixing the thyroid gland to the trachea and larynx, causing the thyroid gland to move with the larynx during deglutition. A thin fibrous capsule also covers the thyroid gland. From this true capsule, septae extend into the gland, dividing the gland into lobes and lobules. The lobules are each made up of multiple follicles. The follicles consist of an outer layer of follicular cells, which enclose a lumen that contains thyroglobulin-rich colloid. Each thyroid follicle is surrounded by a basement membrane that contains C-cells.

The thyroid gland is highly vascular being supplied by paired superior thyroidal arteries (first anterior branches of the external carotid arteries) and inferior thyroidal arteries (branches of the thyrocervical trunks that originate from the subclavian arteries). The thyroidea ima is an inconstant single vessel that has a variable origin but usually arises directly from the aortic arch or innominate artery and helps supply the inferior thyroid gland. Venous drainage is via the superior and middle thyroid veins, which drain into the internal jugular veins, and the inferior thyroid veins, which often join to form a single trunk draining to the left brachiocephalic vein. Lymphatic drainage is extensive and multidirectional. The thyroid gland is innervated by the vagus nerve and the cervical sympathetic neural plexus.[22]

NORMAL FINDINGS

Ultrasonography is usually the first choice of imaging in pediatrics because it is noninvasive, is readily available, and does not utilize radiation. A normal thyroid gland will have homogeneous echotexture, which is slightly hyperechoic relative to adjacent neck muscles.[23,24] Colloid follicles are commonly seen as small (less than 3 millimeters [mm] in diameter) anechoic cystic areas. Occasionally, the follicles contain inspissated colloid, which appear as punctate echogenic foci (Fig. 17-1).[25]

Nuclear scintigraphy provides morphologic and functional information about the thyroid gland. Thyroid scintigraphy is performed using intravenous Tc-99m pertechnetate (99mTcO4) or oral Na I-123 (I-123) (Table 17-1). Because of the large radiation dose to the thyroid gland (approximately 0.01 to 0.03 gray [Gy] per microCurie [uCi] administered), I-131 is not used for routine diagnostic imaging.[26,27] The

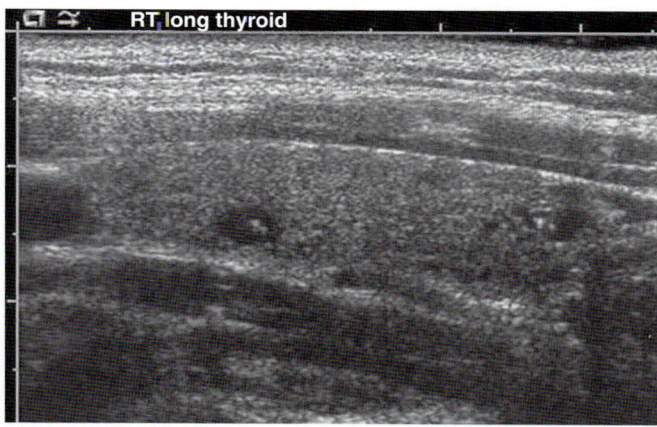

Figure 17-1 Normal thyroid ultrasound. Small anechoic foci with a central hyperechoic focus represent colloid follicles, which are a normal finding.

normal thyroid gland shows homogeneous radiopharmaceutical uptake and distribution in both lobes. The isthmus of the thyroid gland often demonstrates slightly less activity than the right and left thyroid lobes. Normal I-123 24-hour uptake ranges from 10% to 30%.

Computed tomography (CT) and magnetic resonance imaging (MRI) provide important adjunctive anatomic information to ultrasonography and thyroid scintigraphy. These modalities provide better delineation of lesions within the thyroid gland, play a critical role in the detection of lymph node metastases, and improve the detection of thyroid disease extension into adjacent neck structures. The anatomic information provided by CT and MRI is also valuable in guiding the surgical approach.

The normal thyroid gland (because of its iodide content) has a density of approximately 80 to 100 Hounsfield units on CT. A well-visualized gland usually indicates a normally functioning thyroid, whereas a poorly seen gland correlates with poor thyroid function. The injection of iodinated contrast material diffusely and homogeneously enhances the gland.[22] The use of iodinated contrast agents will alter radioactive iodine uptake, whereas gadolinium contrast material will not. The normal thyroid gland shows homogeneous signal intensity slightly greater than muscle on T1-weighted images. On T2-weighted images, the thyroid gland is relatively hyperintense to muscle. Following contrast administration, the gland enhances diffusely and homogeneously.

HYPOTHYROIDISM

Hypothyroidism is the most common disturbance of thyroid function in children. It may be congenital (Box 17-1) or may be acquired in childhood or adolescence (Box 17-2). The thyroid gland produces hormones that play a vital role in regulating many cellular and physiologic activities. Untreated congenital hypothyroidism in early infancy results in profound retardation of growth and neurocognitive development (cretinism). Untreated hypothyroidism in older children leads to growth failure as well as slowed metabolism and impaired memory.

Table 17-1

Thyroid Scintigraphy			
	Sodium Iodide (Capsule or Liquid) (1-23I)	**Tc99m-Pertechnatate (99mTcO4)**	**Perchlorate Discharge or Washout**
Advantages	Better visualization of retrosternal thyroid tissue Yields better images when uptake is low	Less expensive More readily available More rapid examination Can be performed while the patient is on thionamides	Can determine organification defects
Disadvantages	Higher cost Longer imaging times Patient must be off thionamides	Trapped, but not organified Activity in esophagus or vascular structures may be misleading Poor image quality when uptake is low	Cannot detect enzymatic defects beyond the point of organification
Dose	1.5 µCi/kg Minimum dose = 25 µCi Maximum dose = 100 µCi	0.1 mg/kg Minimum dose = 0.5 mCi Maximum dose = 1.0 mCi	Same dosing as I-123 Potassium perchlorate: Infant = 10 mg/kg Child = 400 mg Adult = 1000 mg
Route of administration	Oral	Intravenous	Oral
Time until imaging	4-6 hours 24 hours (for uptake determination)	20-30 minutes	Do I-123 thyroid uptake at 3 hours. If thyroid appears normal and uptake >10% give perchlorate Do second thyroid uptake 60-90 minutes following perchlorate administration
Radiation dosimetry (5 year old)[27] Administered activity	Assuming 25% uptake 0.1-0.3 MBq 0.003-0.01 mCi/kg	1.8-9.2 MBq/kg 0.05-0.25 mCi/kg	Same as I-123
Critical organ	Thyroid 16 mGy/MBq 59 rad/mCi	Upper large intestine 0.21 mGy/MBq 0.78 rad/mCi	
Effective dose equivalent	0.54 mSv/MBq 2.0 rem/mCi	0.04 mSv/MBq 0.15 rem/mCi	
Notes	Approximate normal uptake values (may vary greatly) 4 hours = 10%-35% 24 hours = 6%-18%		Discharge % $= 100 \times \dfrac{\text{Initial uptake} - \text{Final uptake}}{\text{Initial uptake}}$ No change = normal >10%-15% decrease (discharge) suggests an organification defect >50% discharge suggests complete organification defect 20%-50% discharge suggests partial organification defect

Congenital Hypothyroidism

Hypothyroidism in the newborn may be permanent or transient. Congenital hypothyroidism with lower than normal T4 causes retardation of growth and neurocognitive development if left untreated. The incidence of congenital hypothyroidism in the United States has dramatically increased over the last two decades, from 2.9 cases per 10,000 births in 1991 to nearly 4 cases per 10,000 births in 2000.[28,29] All states now require all newborns to be screened for hypothyroidism.

Etiologies, Pathophysiology, and Clinical Presentation The majority of cases of congenital hypothyroidism are caused by thyroid gland dysgenesis (see Box 17-1). Thyroid dysgenesis refers to a developmental defect of thyroid morphogenesis. The three types are (1) ectopia, (2) aplasia (athyrosis), and (3) hypoplasia.

Dyshormonogenesis is the second largest cause of primary congenital hypothyroidism, often inherited as an autosomal-recessive trait. Dyshormonogenesis is an abnormality of one or more of the enzymes involved in the pathway of thyroid hormone synthesis and secretion. Most inborn errors of thyroid hormone synthesis are caused by defects in iodide organification, with the most common defect being TPO deficiency. This results in a failure of oxidation of the iodide ion necessary for organification. A small percentage of infants with congenital hypothyroidism will have hypothalamic-pituitary (central) hypothyroidism, or TSH resistance, whereas the remainder will have a transient form of congenital hypothyroidism.

Congenital hypothyroidism is generally not evident clinically at birth but is usually identified by newborn screening. Less than 5% of patients are diagnosed clinically before screening.

Box 17-1 Causes of Congenital Hypothyroidism

Primary (Thyroid Gland)

Thyroid dysgenesis (80%)

- Ectopia (75%)
- Aplasia or athyrosis (25%)
- Hypoplasia (rare)

Dyshormonogenesis (15%-20%)

- Peroxidase deficiency (most common)
- Other deficiencies (less common)
- Iodide transport defect
- Iodotyrosine deiodinase defect

Secondary (Pituitary) and Tertiary (Hypothalamus)

Pituitary and hypothalamic defects (uncommon)

Miscellaneous

Thyroid-stimulating hormone resistance

Transient congenital hypothyroidism

- Functional immaturity-common in premature infants
- Transplacental transfer of maternal medication
- Transplacental transfer of maternal thyroid-blocking antibodies
- Maternal antithyroid medications
- Iodine deficiency
- Iodine excess

Newborn screening involves measuring TSH and T4 concentrations. T4 concentrations are decreased and TSH concentrations are elevated in patients with congenital hypothyroidism, except in central hypothyroidism, where the TSH is not elevated. The laboratory abnormalities tend to be more marked in cases of thyroid aplasia than in thyroid ectopia. Patients with transient hypothyroidism will also have elevated TSH concentrations and low or normal T4 concentrations, which normalize on subsequent measurements.

Imaging Imaging is not routinely used to diagnose congenital hypothyroidism. According to the most recent recommendations for congenital hypothyroidism in newborns by the American Academy of Pediatrics, the American Thyroid Association, and the Lawson Wilkins Pediatric Endocrine Society, thyroid imaging in congenital hypothyroidism is optional because of controversy regarding the risk–benefit ratio and uncertainty whether imaging findings have any bearing on patient management.[30]

Diagnostic studies for congenital hypothyroidism can include ultrasonography and thyroid scintigraphy with I-123 or 99mTcO4. Use of both ultrasonography and thyroid scintigraphy has been shown to provide a more complete depiction of congenital hypothyroidism in the newborn than either study performed alone.[31]

The role of ultrasonography is to identify the presence or absence of thyroid tissue, distinguish rudimentary glands from anatomically normal thyroid glands, and identify an enlarged gland or goiter.

99mTcO4 or I-123 can be used to help determine if thyroid dysgenesis is the cause of hypothyroidism (see Table 17-1). In patients with thyroid agenesis, the test fails to demonstrate functional thyroid tissue. It is important that the images include the oropharynx and upper neck as well as the upper portion of the chest so that an ectopic thyroid gland can be excluded.

99mTcO4 scintigraphy demonstrates a round or oval area of uptake in the midline of the upper neck in most cases of ectopia (Fig. 17-2). The ectopic gland may occupy a lingual (most common), sublingual, or prelaryngeal location. Mediastinal and lateral locations are rare. Functional thyroid tissue may be identified in more than one location, most commonly in the lingual and sublingual regions. It is unusual to identify thyroid tissue in its normal location in the presence of an ectopic gland. Patients with an ectopic thyroid gland will usually have hypothyroidism. In some unusual cases, the ectopic gland is capable of secreting sufficient thyroid hormone such that hypothyroidism is not apparent on neonatal screening. These patients often present with signs of ectopia later in life when the hyperstimulated gland enlarges and causes local symptoms.

In cases of dyshormonogenesis, 99mTcO4 scintigraphy will demonstrate a normally positioned thyroid gland that may or may not be enlarged (e-Fig. 17-3). If dyshormonogenesis is suspected, a perchlorate washout test may be performed. Perchlorate is actively transported into the thyroid gland with a greater affinity than iodide and is, therefore, a competitive inhibitor of the thyroid iodide trap. During unimpaired thyroid hormonogenesis, iodide entering the thyroid gland is rapidly oxidized and iodinates tyrosine,

Box 17-2 Causes of Hypothyroidism in Children and Adolescents

Primary (Thyroid Gland)

Chronic autoimmune (Hashimoto) thyroiditis (most common cause in the United States)

- Increased incidence in some chromosomal abnormalities and syndromes

Iodine deficiency (most common cause worldwide)

Iodine excess

External radiation therapy

Radioactive iodine therapy

Thyroidectomy

Goitrogen foods

Medications (e.g., thionamides, lithium, anticonvulsants)

Late-onset congenital hypothyroidism

- Thyroid dysgenesis
- Inborn errors of thyroid metabolism

Secondary (Pituitary) and Tertiary (Hypothalamus)

Central hypothyroidism caused by:

- Craniopharyngioma and other tumors pressing on hypothalamus or pituitary
- Septo-optic dysplasia
- Infiltrative processes
- Langerhans cell histiocytosis
- Neurosurgery
- Cranial irradiation
- Head trauma

Miscellaneous

Thyroid hormone resistance

Infection (usually not permanent)

Hemangiomas of the liver

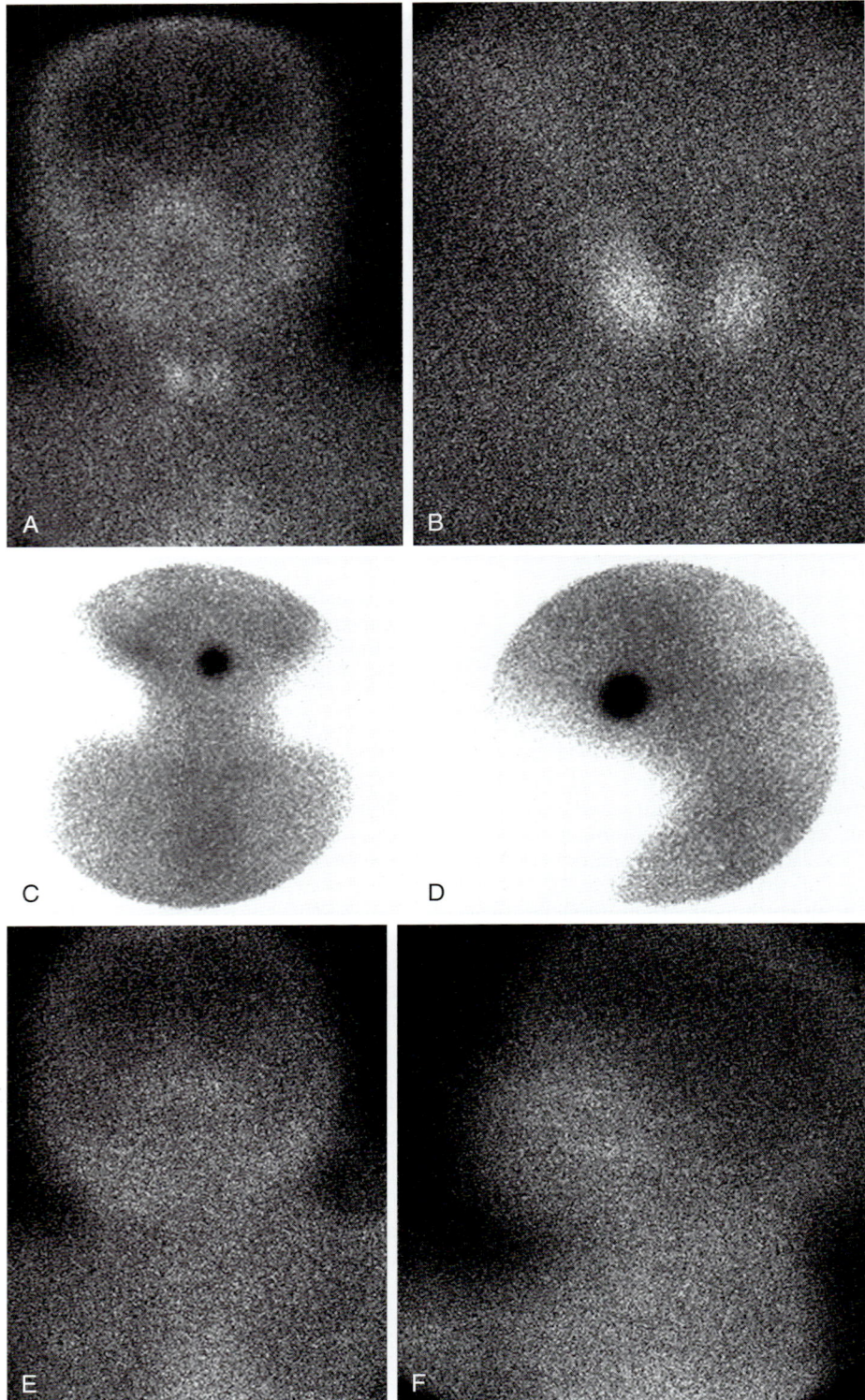

Figure 17-2   **Normal and abnormal thyroid scans. A** and **B,** Normal thyroid anatomy. Anterior and close-up (pinhole) views show normal bilobate architecture and normal position. Thyroid function cannot be meaningfully estimated from these images in an infant with known thyroid insufficiency. **C** and **D,** Thyroid ectopia. Anterior and lateral views of the neck show a solitary rounded focus of radiopharmaceutical trapping at the base of the tongue. No clinical difference exists between the terms *lingual* and *sublingual,* and they are used interchangeably. **E** and **F,** No thyroid is identified. Anterior and lateral views show no functioning thyroid tissue. Although this finding suggests thyroid agenesis, it is nonspecific because severely decreased thyroid function, particularly resulting from maternal thyrotropin receptor–blocking antibody, also may have this appearance.

forming MIT and DIT, with subsequent coupling of MIT and DIT to generate T4 and T3. Intrathyroid deiodination of the iodinated tyrosines and thyronines results in a very small pool of thyroidal inorganic iodide. Any congenital or acquired condition associated with a defect in iodide organification may yield a higher intrathyroidal inorganic iodide concentration. The perchlorate discharge or washout test is a means of estimating the size of this intrathyroidal "free" iodide pool, thereby detecting and roughly quantifying disturbances in iodide organification. The perchlorate discharge or washout test is performed by giving the patient an oral dose of I-123, followed by a dose of perchlorate and measuring the "washout" (see Table 17-1). The perchlorate test will be negative in patients who do not have an organification defect and also when enzymatic defects are present in the synthetic pathway beyond the point of organification.[32-34]

Treatment   T4 is the treatment of choice for children with hypothyroidism. The goals of the treatment are to restore normal growth and development.

Hypothyroidism in Children and Adolescents

Chronic Autoimmune (Hashimoto) Thyroiditis

Acquired hypothyroidism is caused by many factors in the pediatric population (see Box 17-1). Chronic autoimmune (Hashimoto) thyroiditis is the most common cause of acquired hypothyroidism in children and adolescents in iodine sufficient areas. It is more common in girls than in boys and increases in frequency with age during childhood and adolescence.[35-37]

Etiologies, Pathophysiology, and Clinical Presentation   Chronic autoimmune thyroiditis is a complex, thyroid-specific T-cell mediated disease with a strong genetic component.[38-40] It often coexists with other autoimmune diseases and may also be expressed as part of an autoimmune polyendocrine syndrome type 2.[41,42] The two major forms of the disorder are goitrous autoimmune thyroiditis and atrophic autoimmune thyroiditis with the common pathologic feature being lymphocytic infiltration and the common serologic feature being the presence of high serum concentrations of antibodies to TPO and thyroglobulin. Approximately 2% of all surveyed adolescents have serum TSH levels indicating hypothyroidism.[43]

The most common physical finding at presentation is a goiter, along with growth retardation and short stature.[35] The growth delay is usually insidious in onset and may be present for several years before other symptoms occur.[44] Other common symptoms include changes in school performance, sluggishness, lethargy, cold intolerance, constipation, dry skin, brittle hair, facial puffiness, and muscle aches. If the cause is from hypothalamic or pituitary disease, the patients may have headaches, visual symptoms, or pituitary disease manifestations.

Imaging   Most physicians consider the presence of serum antithyroid antibodies as sufficient evidence for chronic autoimmune thyroiditis, and thyroid ultrasonography or radionuclide scanning are rarely indicated. Children with central hypothyroidism should undergo cranial imaging, preferably MR (with contrast), and tests for other pituitary hormone deficiencies.

Ultrasound findings are nonspecific but include an enlarged relatively hypoechoic gland with coarse heterogeneous echotexture. Less commonly, the echogenicity of the gland is increased relative to adjacent muscle. Fibrotic septations in the chronic form may produce a pseudolobulated appearance of the parenchyma. Multiple discrete, hypoechoic, 1 to 6 mm micronodules may also be seen (Fig. 17-4, *A* to *C*).

In the early (preclinical) stage of Hashimoto thyroiditis, elevated I-123 uptake values with diffusely increased radionuclide activity may be seen. This happens because the initial mild decline in circulating thyroid hormone causes a compensatory rise in TSH secretion that stimulates the gland. Thyroid follicles may demonstrate a variable response to the chronic TSH stimulation, leading to patchy follicular proliferation. On the thyroid scan, this phenomenon manifests as patchy areas of increased activity (follicles that respond to TSH) and of decreased activity (those that do not respond). As more thyroid parenchyma is replaced by fibrous tissue, the radionuclide uptake becomes nonuniformly decreased (see Fig. 17-4, *D*).[45]

Treatment   T4 is the treatment of choice for children with hypothyroidism. The goals of the treatment are to restore normal growth and development.

HYPERTYHROIDISM AND THYROTOXICOSIS

Hyperthyroidism refers to overproduction of thyroid hormone by the thyroid gland. *Thyrotoxicosis* refers to the clinical and biochemical manifestations of excess thyroid hormones. Hyperthyroidism and thyrotoxicosis in children have multiple causes (Table 17-2). Most cases of thyrotoxicosis in children are associated with hyperthyroidism. Graves disease is the most common cause of hyperthyroidism in the pediatric population.

A 2008 study estimated the incidence of hyperthyroidism by using the number of new prescriptions of thionamides and data from the 2008 U.S. census and concluded that the incidence among individuals aged 0 to 11 years was 0.44 cases per 1000 population; in those aged 12 to 17 years, 0.26 cases per 1000; and in those aged 12-17 years, 0.59 cases per 1000.[46]

Graves Disease

Etiologies, Pathophysiology, and Clinical Presentation   Graves disease is the most common cause of hyperthyroidism in children and adolescents. The general cause is thyrotropin receptor-stimulating antibodies (TRS-Ab), which activate the TSH receptor.

Many of the clinical features of hyperthyroidism are similar in children, adolescents, and adults. Most children with Graves disease have a diffuse goiter.[47] Like hypothyroidism, hyperthyroidism also has an effect on growth and pubertal development. Acceleration of growth with advanced epiphyseal maturation may be seen in untreated hyperthyroidism, although changes may be subtle and the degree depends on the duration of hyperthyroidism before diagnosis. Pubertal development, in contrast, tends to be delayed or slowed in children with untreated hyperthyroidism.

Graves disease causes other unique problems not associated to the high serum thyroid hormone concentrations. They

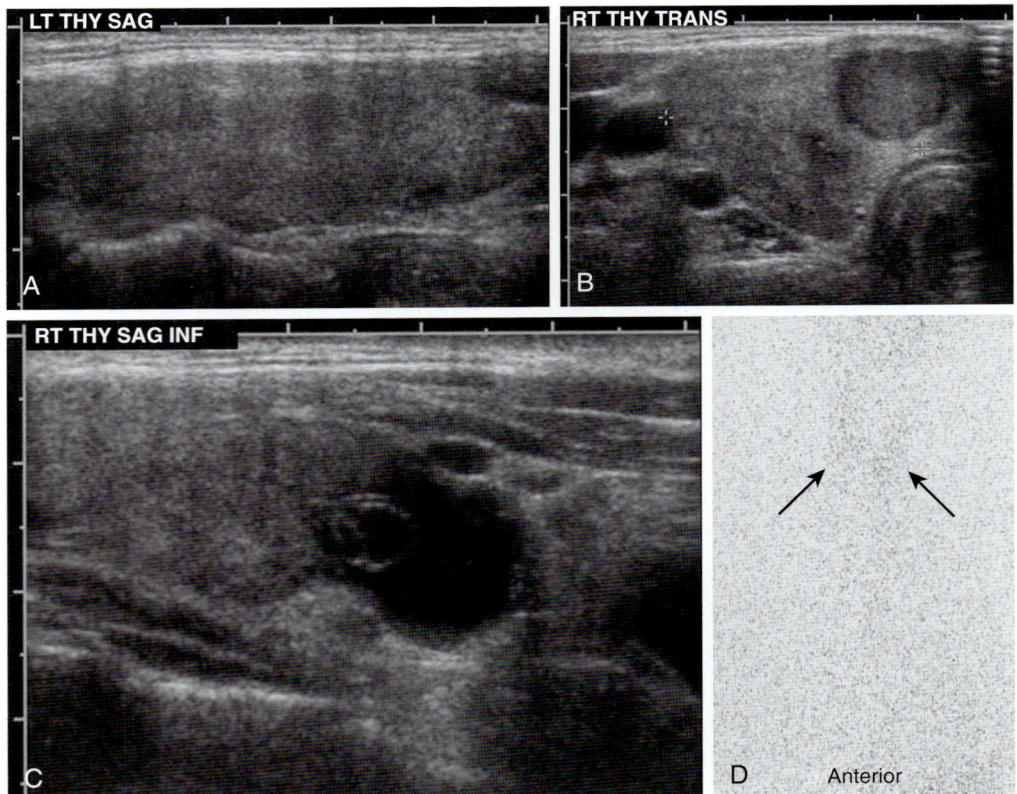

Figure 17-4 Chronic autoimmune (Hashimoto) thyroiditis. **A,** Ultrasonography demonstrates an enlarged gland that is relatively hypoechoic with heterogeneous echotexture. **B** and **C,** The right lobe of the same patient has a hypoechoic nodule and cystic changes. **D,** The I-123 scan shows diffuse decreased uptake (*arrows*). The 24-hour uptake was only 0.5%.

include Graves ophthalmopathy and pretibial myxedema. Graves ophthalmopathy is common in children but is generally less severe than in adults. The clinical manifestations of Graves ophthalmopathy stem from a combination of increased orbital fat and extraocular muscle volume. The exact etiology is unknown; however, it may result from antibodies against a TSH receptor–like protein in retro-orbital connective tissue leading to adipogenesis. Although originally thought to represent another causative agent, antibodies to extraocular muscles are now generally thought to be secondary to extraocular muscle inflammation and damage.[48,49]

Imaging In the majority of patients, no imaging is needed. The diagnosis may be made through physical examination, laboratory tests, and the onset or chronicity of symptoms. If thyrotoxicosis has been present for less than 8 weeks, transient thyrotoxicosis secondary to subacute thyroiditis or the thyrotoxic phase of autoimmune or silent thyroiditis should be considered. These conditions are self-limiting and refractory to therapy with thionamides. Thyrotoxicosis that has been present for more than 8 weeks suggests true hyperthyroidism thyrotoxicosis. However, if the diagnosis cannot be made clinically, an I-123 uptake, with or without a scan, should be performed (see Table 17-2).[50-52]

Treatment Graves disease can be treated pharmacologically, surgically, or with radioiodine ablation. The thionamide antithyroid drugs propylthiouracil and methimazole continue to be the most commonly used medications in the treatment of Graves disease in the United States.[53] Thionamides exert their antithyroid effects primarily by inhibiting thyroid hormone synthesis through interference with the oxidation and binding of iodide into thyroglobulin.[54] PTU also inhibits the peripheral conversion of T4 to T3 by type 1 deiodinase.[55,56] In resistant disease or noncompliant patients, treatment is by radioiodine ablation or thyroidectomy. Concerns over the potential long-term complications of pediatric radiation exposure have traditionally made endocrinologists hesitant about using radioiodine in the treatment of Graves disease. The use of radioactive iodine has now been detailed for more than 1000 children, with remission rates over 95% and very few complications.[57] Total-body radiation doses after I-131 therapy vary with age, and the same absolute dose of I-131 will result in more radiation exposure to a young child than to an adolescent or adult.[58-61] Thus, in addition to selecting a dose that will achieve adequate thyroid tissue destruction, the age of the patient, and the total I-131 dose need to be considered.

Infection

Acute suppurative thyroiditis is an infection of the thyroid gland that is rarely seen during childhood but is potentially life threatening.[62,63]

Etiologies, Pathophysiology, and Clinical Presentation Acute suppurative thyroiditis is usually caused by a bacterial infection. *Staphylococcus aureus, Streptococcus pyogenes, Streptococcus*

Table 17-2

Causes of Hyperthyroidism and Thyrotoxicosis in Children and Adolescents

Name	Synonyms	Mechanism of Hyperthyroidism/ Thyrotoxicosis	Laboratory Tests	RAIU Appearance on Scintigraphy	Imaging Appearance of Thyroid Gland
Hyperthyroidism, Thyroid Gland Hyperfunction (Increased Synthesis of Thyroid Hormone)					
Graves disease	Hyperthyroid goiter von Basedow disease	TRS-Ab	Low TSH Elevated free T4 Elevated T3 High thyroglobulin TSI positive TRS-Ab positive TPO-Ab positive or negative TBII positive	Elevated, often >80% Diffuse increased uptake	Ultrasonography: Enlarged gland; hypoechoic but may be normal; may be nodular; increased vascularity, "thyroid inferno"[51] CT and MRI: Nonspecific findings; enlarged gland; avid, diffuse enhancement Decreased attenuation on noncontrast CT reflecting decrease in iodine concentration
Multinodular goiter	Toxic multinodular goiter Adenomatous goiter Nodular hyperplasia Adenomatous hyperplasia	Autonomous overproduction of thyroid hormones by nodules	Low TSH Elevated free T4 Elevated T3 High thyroglobulin All thyroid antibodies negative	Normal or elevated Heterogeneous uptake; multiple foci increased uptake	Ultrasonography: Enlarged gland; multiple heterogeneous nodules; cystic changes
Autonomous nodule	Plummer disease Toxic nodule	Uncommon in children; autonomous overproduction of thyroid hormones by solitary nodule; usually produce T3	Low TSH Normal or elevated free T4 Elevated T3 High thyroglobulin All thyroid antibodies negative	Elevated Single hot focus; rest of gland suppressed	
TSH-producing pituitary adenoma		Autonomous overproduction of TSH	Normal TSH Elevated free T4 High serum TSH alpha subunit concentration All thyroid antibodies negative	High	Pituitary adenoma on MRI
Pituitary resistance to thyroid hormone		Autosomal-dominant; thyroid beta-receptor gene mutation;[52] overproduction of TSH	Normal or slightly elevated TSH Elevated free T4 Elevated T3 (less than T4) All thyroid antibodies negative	High Diffuse uptake	
Thyrotoxicosis-Excess Secretion of Preformed Thyroid Hormones					
Thyrotoxic phase of chronic lymphocytic (Hashimoto) thyroiditis	Hashitoxicosis Lymphadenoid goiter	Autoimmune; release of preformed hormones	Low TSH Elevated free T4 Elevated T3 High thyroglobulin TPO-Ab positive; Thyroglobulin positive; TRS-Ab positive or negative	Elevated Diffuse increased uptake	Ultrasonography: Findings are nonspecific; enlarged gland; hypoechoic, heterogeneous echotexture
Subacute lymphocytic thyroiditis	Painless sporadic thyroiditis Silent thyroiditis	Autoimmune; release of preformed hormones May be associated with drugs (interferon-alpha, interleukin-2, lithium)	Low TSH Elevated free T4 Elevated T3 High thyroglobulin TPO-Ab positive	Very low Diffuse decreased uptake	Ultrasonography: Findings are nonspecific; enlarged gland; hypoechoic, heterogeneous echotexture

Table 17-2

Causes of Hyperthyroidism and Thyrotoxicosis in Children and Adolescents—Cont'd					
Name	Synonyms	Mechanism of Hyperthyroidism/ Thyrotoxicosis	Laboratory Tests	RAIU Appearance on Scintigraphy	Imaging Appearance of Thyroid Gland
Thyrotoxic phase of subacute granulomatous thyroiditis	Subacute thyroiditis Painful subacute thyroiditis de Quervain thyroiditis Granulomatous giant cell thyroiditis	Viral; release of preformed hormone	Low TSH Elevated free T4 Elevated T3 High thyroglobulin TPO-Ab negative; elevated ESR	Low Diffuse decreased uptake	Ultrasonography: Findings are nonspecific; enlarged gland; hypoechoic, heterogeneous echotexture
Factitious thyroiditis	Thyrotoxicosis factitia	Intentional ingestion of too much thyroxine	Low TSH Elevated free T4 Elevated T3 Low thyroglobulin	Low	
Iodine-induced hyperthyroidism		Underlying multinodular goiter; thyroid hormone release triggered by exposure to iodine (contrast agents), amiodarone	Low TSH Elevated free T4 Elevated T3	Increased	

CT, computed tomography; *ESR*, erythrocyte sedimentation rate; *MRI*, magnetic resonance imaging; *RAIU*, radioactive iodine uptake; *T3*, triiodothyronine; *T4*, thyroxine; *TBII*, thyrotropin-binding inhibitor immunoglobulin; *TPO-Ab*, thyroid peroxidase antibodies; *TRS-Ab*, thyrotropin-receptor stimulating antibodies; *TSH*, thyroid-stimulating hormone; *TSI*, thyroid stimulating immunoglobulin.

epidermidis, and *Streptococcus pneumoniae* are the most common aerobic bacteria. The predominant anaerobic bacteria are gram-negative bacilli and *Peptostreptococcus* spp.[64]

Suppurative thyroiditis may be related to a pyriform sinus fistula or thyroglossal duct remnant, especially when recurrent infections occur.[62,65,66]

The classic clinical features of this illness include fever, neck pain, and a swollen, tender mass over the thyroid gland.

Imaging Ultrasonography, the imaging modality of choice, demonstrates unilobar or diffuse swelling and determines the presence of abscess formation.

CT or MRI is not usually necessary. On MRI, the thyroid gland will demonstrate focal or diffuse swelling with decreased signal on T1-weighted images and increased signal on T2-weighted images. MRI is superior to ultrasonography in detecting capsule rupture into adjacent soft tissue.

Treatment The primary treatment is antimicrobial therapy, directed against the likely bacterial pathogens. Surgery may be needed to drain abscesses and repair any causative developmental anomaly.

BENIGN LESIONS OR MASSES

Thyroid nodules and cysts are uncommon in children before puberty.[67-70] Most thyroid nodules are benign, although an increased incidence of malignancy exists in pediatric thyroid nodules with an overall 26.4% risk.[68]

Benign Nodules

The most common cause of benign solitary thyroid nodules is follicular adenoma (hyperplastic nodule).[71]

Etiologies, Pathophysiology, and Clinical Presentation Follicular adenomas are thought to be the result of cycles of hyperplasia and colloid involution of thyroid nodules.[24] These are encapsulated lesions, which are usually solitary and nonfunctioning. Follicular adenomas are usually asymptomatic or may present as a palpable nodule. Sudden enlargement and pain are usually related to spontaneous hemorrhage within the lesion. With the increasing number of cross-sectional studies being performed, thyroid nodules are often found incidentally.[72]

Imaging The findings of ultrasonography, CT, and MRI are nonspecific and may be seen in both benign and malignant nodules.

On ultrasonography, follicular adenomas are usually hypoechoic relative to normal thyroid tissue, although some are hyperechoic and a few are isoechoic. A thin hypoechoic "halo" or rim around the lesion may be seen. The cause of the "halo" is unknown, but the fibrous capsule, compressed thyroid parenchyma, or pericapsular inflammatory infiltration may be the cause.[24,73] Adenomas may also contain hypoechoic or anechoic areas from internal hemorrhage and necrosis. Calcifications may also be present (e-Fig. 17-5).

Thyroid scintigraphy may be used in the evaluation of a thyroid nodule. Increased uptake in a nodule almost always indicates that the nodule is benign.

Treatment   Fine-needle aspiration, biopsy, or excision may be performed to exclude malignancy.[74]

Cysts

Cysts are often thought to be caused by benign degenerative thyroid diseases.[71] However, as with thyroid nodules, a great heterogeneity exists in these disease processes in children, ranging from benign pure cysts to malignant lesions.[70]

Etiologies, Pathophysiology, and Clinical Presentation   True simple cysts lined by epithelium are rare. The majority of benign thyroid cysts are felt to be the result of cystic degeneration of a follicular adenoma.[71] Hemorrhagic cysts are usually the result of bleeding into a follicular adenoma.

Thyroglossal duct cysts (TDCs) are the result of incomplete degeneration of the thyroglossal duct. The duct remnant, which is an epithelium-lined tract, has the potential for obstruction and cyst formation because of retained secretions. These cysts can occur anywhere along the path of migration of the thyroid gland, from the foramen cecum at the tongue base to the anterior lower neck, but are most common at the level of the hyoid bone. Most TDCs are asymptomatic until they become infected. Large cysts can be clinically detected as a palpable midline or near-midline neck mass that moves with swallowing or tongue protrusion.

Imaging   Simple benign cysts are anechoic on ultrasonography and hypodense on CT. On MRI, they will follow the signal characteristics of water, demonstrating low signal on T1-weighted images and high signal on T2-weighted images. Hemorrhagic cysts will have high signal on T1-weighted images and will be hyperdense on CT.

TDCs are usually anechoic or hypoechoic on ultrasonography. The cyst may have a high protein content, which may result in some internal echoes. They may also appear complex with septations and solid-appearing areas from hemorrhage or infection.

On CT, a noninfected TDC will be well circumscribed with a thin rim of enhancement. Thick peripheral enhancement suggests infection. The attenuation of the cystic component varies on CT from hypodense (low protein content) to hyperdense (high protein content or hemorrhage).

On MRI scans, TDC usually has variably low T1-weighted signal and high T2-weighted signal intensities. Scintigraphy is not necessary in the evaluation of TDC except when a thyroid gland cannot be identified. In this case, thyroid nuclear scintigraphy may be necessary to determine if the cyst contains the patient's only functional thyroid tissue.

Treatment   Thyroid cysts and thyroglossal duct cysts may be excised for diagnosis or if they become secondarily infected, cause mass effect resulting in pain or dysphagia, or for cosmesis. The treatment of choice for TDC is the Sistrunk operation, which entails complete removal of the cyst and tract. This procedure also includes removal of the central portion of the hyoid bone.

MALIGNANT LESIONS

Thyroid malignancies are rare in children. The incidence of thyroid carcinomas is roughly 4.9 per million in children, with the peak incidence being in the 15- to 19-year-old age group (1.8 per 100,000). Papillary, follicular, and medullary carcinomas are seen in children, whereas anaplastic and poorly differentiated carcinomas are very rare.[75] Other rare thyroid neoplasms include teratomas[76] and non-Hodgkin lymphoma.[77] Most childhood thyroid malignancies are of the papillary type.

Etiologies, Pathophysiology, and Clinical Presentation   Exposure to head and neck irradiation is associated with an increased risk for the development of thyroid carcinoma.[78,79] Some thyroid cancers have a genetic predisposition and may be associated with certain syndromes. A positive family history is seen in medullary carcinoma and in 3% of papillary carcinomas (chromosome 19p13.2).[80,81] A high incidence of papillary thyroid carcinomas is seen in familial adenomatosis polyposis coli and Cowden disease.[82,83] Inherited medullary carcinoma is seen in multiple endocrine neoplasia type 2a and 2b or as part of familial medullary carcinoma.[84]

Thyroid carcinoma in children is biologically and clinically different from that seen in adults. The most common clinical presentation is a solitary thyroid nodule.[85] Other presenting manifestations such as dysphonia or dysphagia caused by local invasion of surrounding structures are rare in children. Children present with cervical node involvement (60%) and pulmonary metastases (13%) more often than adults.[86,87] Children also have more advanced disease and a higher rate of recurrence.[87] The pulmonary metastases are almost always functional and tend to be miliary.[88] Lymph nodes are the most common site of dissemination, followed by the lungs. Bone metastases are rare.[88]

Imaging   The imaging appearance of papillary carcinoma is variable. At ultrasonography, the presence of indistinct margins, hypoechogenicity, predominantly solid composition, vascularity, absence of a hypoechoic halo, and calcifications are suggestive of malignancy.[89] Ultrasonography also helps guide fine-needle aspiration, recommended for all thyroid nodules.[90] Although a solitary nodule is most common in children, multifocal nodules, diffuse infiltration with heterogeneous hypodensity, or a normal-appearing thyroid gland may be found on CT.[22] Metastatic lymph nodes are usually enlarged; may be calcified, cystic, or hemorrhagic; or contain colloid (Fig. 17-6).[91]

Cold nodules on scintigraphy are suggestive of malignancy but may also be seen in benign lesions. Some very rare thyroid carcinomas may demonstrate increased radioisotope uptake. Rare cases of a benign adenoma or carcinoma have been reported; these tumors have the ability to trap the radioisotope but do not organify the iodide, resulting in a discordant nodule that is hot on 99mTcO4 studies but cold on I-123 studies.

MRI is helpful in evaluating and delineating the extent of local invasion and lymph node metastases. Chest CT is more sensitive for pulmonary metastatic disease and detects micronodular and interstitial patterns of metastases much better than conventional chest radiography (Fig. 17-7).[92]

Treatment   A total or near-total thyroidectomy is recommended by most experts and is believed to decrease the incidence of recurrence.[86,93,94] Thyroidectomy also enables the use of thyroglobulin levels and whole body radioiodine scans for monitoring disease persistence and recurrence. Modified lateral neck dissection is recommended when lateral node

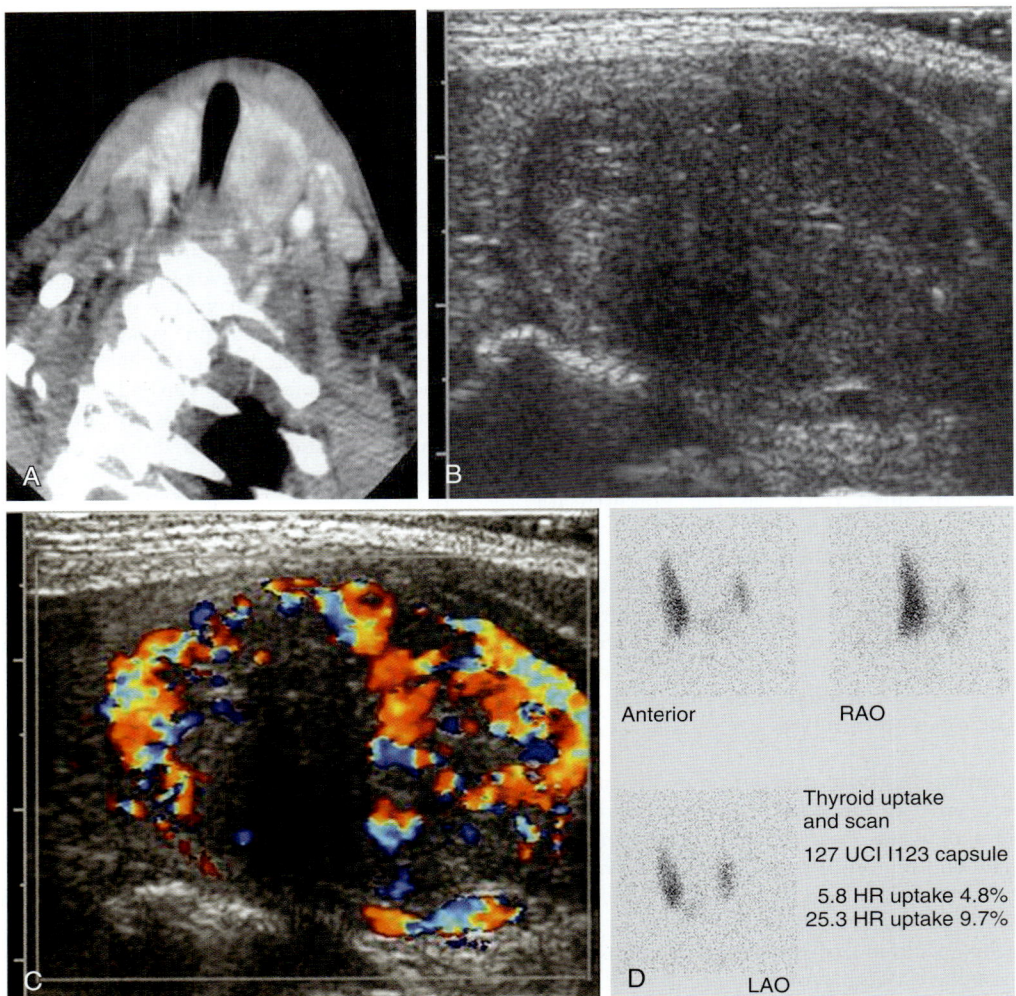

Figure 17-6   Papillary carcinoma. This patient was found to have a thyroid nodule on contrast-enhanced computed tomography being performed to assess for infection. **A,** The computed tomography scan shows a low attenuation lesion in the left lobe of the thyroid gland. **B** and **C,** Ultrasound images demonstrate a relatively heterogeneous nodule with punctate echogenicities and an eccentric round region of hypoechogenicity. Peripherally the lesion has increased vascularity. **D,** The I-123 uptake and scan demonstrates decreased uptake in the left gland and a focal "cold" lesion.

involvement is seen on clinical examination, preoperative ultrasonography, or intraoperative biopsy.[88,95]

Routine postoperative radioiodine ablation is recommended in children. Remnant thyroid tissue (greater than 0.3% uptake on radioiodine scan) is seen in most cases following thyroidectomy.[92] This tissue can interfere with the detection of residual or recurrent disease on whole body radioiodine scans or by thyroglobulin measurements. Prior to radioablation, a diagnostic whole body scan with I-123 or 0.5 to 2 milliCurie (mCi) of I-131 is obtained.[96] Images are obtained 24 to 48 hours after administration of the radioisotope. The preablation I-131 scan shows the extent of thyroid remnant as well as disease burden after thyroidectomy. Although some experts believe that preablation imaging may cause decreased I-131 uptake during ablation, no unequivocal evidence exists to suggest that this occurs when a low-dose (<2 mCi) diagnostic scan is performed.[97,98]

The uptake of radioiodine is dependent on TSH stimulation of both normal and malignant thyroid tissue. The TSH level should be greater than 30 microunits per milliliter (uU/mL) for optimal radioiodine uptake. A diagnostic scan

followed by ablation is performed 6 weeks after thyroidectomy. Thyroid hormone medications must be withheld for a sufficient time to permit an adequate rise in the TSH level. T3 has a short half-life and can be given until 2 weeks before the scan.[92] Additionally, the patient is placed on a low iodine diet for 2 weeks prior to the scan to increase the avidity of remnant tissue for iodine.[88]

The normal thyroid remnant tissue is more efficient at concentrating radioiodine than the carcinoma tissue. As a result, the first diagnostic whole body radioiodine scan following thyroidectomy might not detect residual tumor or metastases. These may show up on the scan obtained after radioablation, as much higher doses of I-131 are used for ablation.

The maximally safe radioiodine dose in children is calculated on the basis of quantitative blood and whole body dosimetry, and the minimally effective dose is calculated on the basis of lesion dosimetry.[99] Since this is complicated, most centers use a fixed dose of 30 mCi.[100] Rarely, a second treatment may be needed for complete ablation. Much higher doses of up to 200 mCi are required to ablate pulmonary

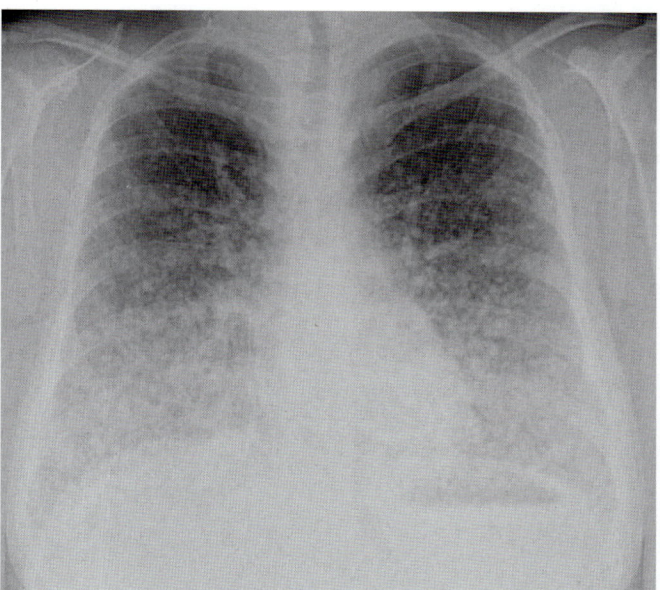

Figure 17-7 Pulmonary metastases from papillary carcinoma of the thyroid gland. The chest radiograph shows innumerable diffuse small pulmonary nodules (miliary disease).

metastases.[101] It is customary to obtain a scan 5 to 7 days after radioablation, which will demonstrate avid uptake in any thyroid remnant and may show metastases not apparent on the previous diagnostic scan.[92]

On the basis of the belief that thyroid carcinoma cells are dependent on TSH stimulation for growth, TSH suppressive therapy with thyroxine is also used to suppress tumor growth. The optimal TSH level that needs to be maintained is not known. Initially, TSH levels of less than 0.1 uU/mL are recommended, but once remission has been achieved, levels of less than 0.5 uU/mL may be acceptable.[93]

Parathyroid Glands

EMBRYOLOGY

The parathyroid glands are endodermal in origin and develop from the third and fourth pharyngeal pouches. Usually four glands (two superior and two inferior) are present; however, supernumerary or less than four glands may also occur.

The third pharyngeal pouch gives rise to the thymus and the inferior parathyroids. As both primitive inferior parathyroid glands lose their connection with the pharyngeal wall, they descend with the thymus. This migration of the inferior parathyroid glands with the thymus accounts for their lower position than the superior parathyroid glands that are derived from the fourth pharyngeal pouches.[102] The glands are usually distributed evenly between the lower pole of the thyroid gland and isthmus but may be found anywhere along their course of descent.[103]

The fourth pharyngeal pouch gives rise to the superior parathyroid glands, which attach to the posterior surface of the descending thyroid. They have a much shorter migration distance than the inferior parathyroid glands, which accounts

for their more predictable location. Generally, the superior parathyroid glands are located posterior at the level of the upper two thirds of the thyroid gland, approximately 1 centimeter above the crossing point of the recurrent laryngeal nerve and inferior thyroid artery.[104]

PHYSIOLOGY

The function of the parathyroid glands is to produce parathyroid hormone (PTH), which is one of two major hormones involved in calcium and phosphate homeostasis. PTH is produced by chief cells within the parathyroid glands. Oxyphil cells may also secret PTH, but their true function is unknown. PTH closely maintains serum ionized calcium in a narrow range through stimulation of renal tubular calcium resorption and bone resorption.[105] PTH also stimulates the conversion of calcidiol (25-hydroxyvitamin D) to calcitriol in renal tubular cells, thereby stimulating intestinal calcium absorption. PTH secretion is, in turn, regulated via a calcium-sensing receptor on the surface of parathyroid cells.[106] When the calcium-sensing receptor is activated by an increase in calcium, PTH secretion is inhibited. Conversely, deactivation of the receptor by decreases in calcium stimulates PTH secretion.

ANATOMY

The paired superior parathyroid glands are fairly constant in their position near the upper surface of the thyroid lobes. The inferior parathyroid glands are found in proximity to the lower pole of the thyroid gland. Ectopic superior parathyroid glands may be found at the level of the upper pole of the thyroid gland (2%) and above the upper pole (0.8%). Other ectopic positions of the superior parathyroid glands in the posterior neck, retropharyngeal, retroesophageal, or intrathyroid regions are even rarer (1% total).[103,104] Ectopic inferior parathyroid glands may be found anywhere along their area of descent up to the superior border of the pericardium.[103] Supernumerary glands, when present, are often found in the mediastinum associated with the thymus.

The vascular supply of the parathyroid glands is predominately the inferior thyroid artery, although the superior parathyroid glands may also be supplied by the superior thyroid artery.[104,107,108] The venous drainage is predominately to the inferior thyroid veins.[109]

The parathyroids are scantily supplied with vasomotor nerve fibers from the superior, middle, or inferior cervical sympathetic ganglia.[110,111]

NORMAL FINDINGS

Normal glands are difficult to visualize because of their small size (less than 5 mm in length). On ultrasonography, a normal parathyroid gland will have an echotexture similar to the adjacent thyroid parenchyma, which adds to the difficulty in identifying the normal glands.[24]

HYPERPARATHYROIDISM

Primary hyperparathyroidism is rare in children, with an estimated incidence of 2 to 5 in 100,000.[112,113] Primary

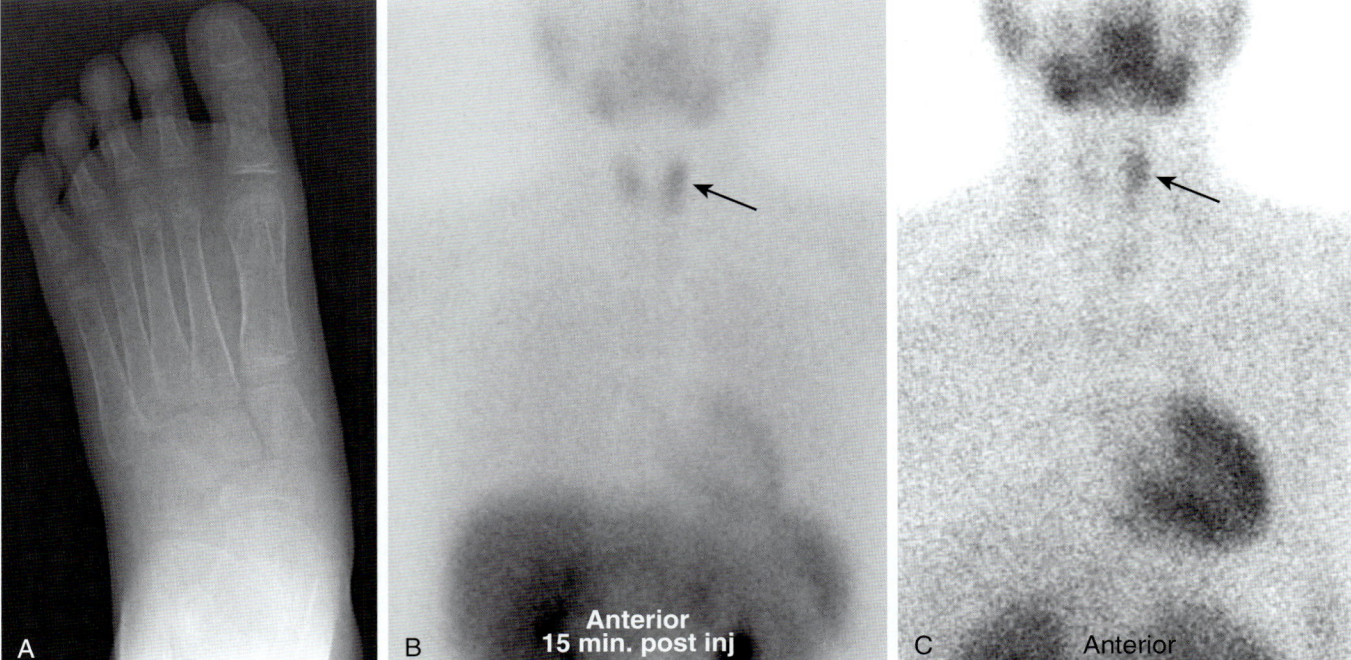

Figure 17-8 Parathyroid adenoma in a patient presenting with foot pain. **A,** Radiograph of the foot demonstrates diffuse severe osteopenia. Laboratory studies revealed marked hypercalcemia and elevated parathyroid hormone. Initial ultrasonography failed to identify an adenoma. **B,** Nuclear scintigraphy shows increased uptake is noted in the left lobe of the thyroid gland (*arrow*) on the initial 99mTc-sestamibi images. **C,** Incomplete washout of the radiopharmaceutical is seen on 2-hour delayed images (*arrow*), suggesting a parathyroid adenoma. The lesion was surgically excised, and the patient's symptoms resolved.

hyperparathyroidism is caused by overproduction of PTH by one or more parathyroid glands.

Etiologies, Pathophysiology, and Clinical Presentation Primary hyperparathyroidism is most often caused in children by a parathyroid adenoma.[112-114] Multiple endocrine neoplasia (MEN)-I or MEN-II syndromes or familial non–MEN hyperparathyroidism have also been documented and can constitute as much as 30% to 50% of pediatric hyperparathyroid disease.[115,116]

The parathyroid gland becomes overactive and secretes excess amounts of PTH, which leads to an increase in serum calcium levels. PTH stimulates calcium and phosphate mobilization through osteoclastic bone resorption. In the kidney, PTH stimulates the synthesis of calcitrol, decreases urinary calcium excretion, and increases phosphate excretion. PTH enhances the gut absorption of minerals directly and through calcitrol.

The symptoms of hyperparathyroidism may be nonspecific and include joint aches, fatigue, weakness, loss of appetite, depression, and difficulty concentrating. The commonest clinical signs in children with primary hyperparathyroidism is skeletal (bone resorption) and renal disease (hematuria, nephrocalcinosis, or nephrolithiasis).[115]

Imaging Imaging is rarely used to diagnose hyperparathyroidism. Evaluation of serum calcium and PTH levels is diagnostic. In most patients with hyperparathyroidism, both serum calcium and PTH levels are higher than normal.

Occasionally, a patient may have an elevated calcium level and a normal or minimally elevated PTH level. Since PTH should normally be low when calcium is elevated, a minimally elevated PTH is considered abnormal and indicates hyperparathyroidism.

Imaging may help in localization for surgical planning. Ultrasonography is a reliable noninvasive method for confirming parathyroid pathology in children preoperatively. A parathyroid adenoma will appear well defined and hypoechoic on ultrasonography. Adenomas are usually hyperemic on color Doppler. Differentiating an adenoma from hyperplasia or a lymph node may sometimes be difficult.

Other reliable studies include 99mTcO4 or 201Tl subtraction imaging and 99mTc-sestamibi scans, which have been reported to have a sensitivity of 67% to 80% for localizing adenomas and a sensitivity of 45% to 60% for hyperplasia in adults; however, data in children are not well established (Fig. 17-8).[117,118] Scintigraphy, occasionally along with CT and MRI, is helpful in evaluating possible mediastinal location of adenomas or hyperfunctioning parathyroid tissue.

The most specific radiographic manifestation of hyperparathyroidism is subperiosteal bone resorption. Brown tumors (osteoclastomas) are rare sequelae of hyperparathyroidism occurring in fewer than 5% of all cases.[119] The lesions localize in areas of intense bone resorption, and the bone defect becomes filled with fibroblastic tissue.

Treatment Parathyroid resection is the treatment of choice for hyperparathyroidism in children.[115,118]

Key Points

Ultrasound is the primary imaging modality for evaluating the thyroid and parathyroid glands, and for guiding aspiration and biopsy.

The majority of cases of congenital hypothyroidism are caused by thyroid gland dysgenesis.

Chronic autoimmune thyroiditis (Hashimoto thyroiditis) is the most common cause of acquired hypothyroidism in children.

Graves disease is the most common cause of hyperthyroidism in children.

Thyroid nodules are less common in children than in adults, but have a higher incidence of malignancy.

Suggested Readings

Braverman LE, Utiger RD. *Werner and Ingbar's the thyroid: a fundamental and clinical text.* 9th ed. Philadelphia, PA: Lippincott Williams & Wilkins; 2005.

Parekh C, Jackson HA. Thyroid cancer in children. In: Carroll WL, Finlay JL, eds. *Cancer in children and adolescents.* Sudbury, MA: Jones and Bartlett; 2010:459-466

Smith JR, Oates ME. Radionuclide imaging of the parathyroid glands: patterns, pearls, and pitfalls. *RadioGraphics.* 2004;24(4):1101-1115.

Sofferman RA, Ahuja AT. *Ultrasound of the thyroid and parathyroid glands.* New York, NY: Springer; 2012.

References

Full references for this chapter can be found on www.expertconsult.com.

SECTION 3

Neuroradiology

Chapter 18

Embryology, Anatomy, Normal Findings, and Imaging Techniques*

THOMAS L. SLOVIS and MOIRA L. COOPER

Anatomy of the Skull

The skull is divided into three interconnected portions: the neurocranium, the facial area, and the base. The neurocranium includes the calvarium, which is composed of the membranous portions of the occipital, parietal, frontal, and temporal bones and is bounded inferiorly by the base of the skull, which is composed of the cartilaginous portions of these bones plus the sphenoid and ethmoid bones. The facial area is the portion of the skull between the forehead and the chin.

Routine views of the skull include the frontal projection (usually posteroanterior), the Towne view of the occipital bone, and the lateral view. These views may be supplemented by submentovertical and Waters and Caldwell (posteroanterior 15 degrees) views for specific indications.

The radiation dose (with the thyroid and lens being the most sensitive structures) varies with the view obtained and the age of the patient. Best practice skin doses for a lateral vew of the skull range from 0.09 mGy in the first year of life to 0.46 mGy in a child who is 10 to 15 years old (see Huda in Suggested Readings).

Indications for plain film skull examination are listed in Box 18-1. Computed tomography (CT) and magnetic resonance imaging (MRI) generally are used for detailed evaluation of facial structures and intracranial contents.

Neonatal and Infant Skull

SIZE AND SHAPE

During infancy the neurocranium is larger relative to the face than at any other time during normal growth. Ratios of the respective areas of the neurocranium in lateral projection are roughly 3:1 to 4:1 at birth, and they decrease to 2:1 to 2.5:1 by age 6 years. The bones of the calvarium lie in their incompletely mineralized membranous capsule; they are separated by broad strips of connective tissue that form the sutures and by patches of connective tissue, the fontanelles. The six constant, or major, fontanelles are located at the four corners of the parietal bones—two in the midline of the skull and two pairs on each side (Fig. 18-1). Accessory fontanelles may occur in several parts of the cranium but usually are located in the sagittal suture. The sutures and the synchondroses in the base are prominent in newborns but diminish in width during the first 2 to 3 months. Obliteration of the sutures does not begin until the second to third decades. Figures 18-1 through 18-4 and e-Figure 18-5 illustrate sutures, fontanelles, and synchondroses.

The sphenoid bone at birth consists of a single central mass composed of the body and the lesser wings and two symmetric lateral osseous masses, each of which is made up of a greater wing and a pterygoid process. The pituitary fossa in the body of the sphenoid bone tends to be round with smooth margins; the dorsum sella is short and blunt, and the clinoid processes are rudimentary. The angle between the body of the neonatal mandible and the ascending ramus in lateral projection is about 160 degrees; the relatively large bodies are separated in the midline by a prominent cartilaginous symphysis mentalis (see Fig. 18-3). Early calcification of teeth is seen in the fifth fetal month.[1]

Components of the individual bones that are not united in infancy may lead to confusion unless they are correctly recognized. The frontal bone is divided in half laterally by the metopic suture (see Figs. 18-1 and 18-3). Apparent discontinuity of the sphenoid bone with the frontal bone superiorly and the occipital bone posteriorly indicates the sites of the sphenoid bone's synchondroses with these two bones (see Fig. 18-2). The four major components of the occipital bone (e-Fig. 18-5 and Fig. 18-2) likewise may simulate discontinuities of structure.

Growth and Development

Most of the postnatal growth and differentiation of the skull occurs during the first 2 years of life, and thus after 24 months, most of the features of the adult skull are present. During childhood, growth continues at a greatly reduced velocity but shows a slight postpubertal spurt. The thickness of the bones increases. The inner and outer tables, diploic space, vascular markings, and grooves for the dural sinuses on

---

*This chapter initially was written by Dr. John Caffey in 1945 and revised by Dr. Frederic Silverman. Although many of the tables and figures are from older references, they remain the most precise information available.

the internal surface of the calvarium all make their appearance by the end of the second year.

With increasing age, the fontanelles and sutures become smaller and narrower. The anterior fontanelle usually is reduced to fingertip size during the first half of the second year; the posterior fontanelle may be closed at birth (range of closure: birth to several months). Closure of the fontanelles occurs clinically before it is seen radiographically. The metopic suture is quite variable and may be obliterated at birth, but it usually is closed during the third year; however, it persists throughout life in about 10% of cases. In the occipital bone, the mendosal suture (see Fig. 18-4 and e-Fig. 18-5) usually disappears during the first 2 years, but it too can persist; the synchondrosis between the supraoccipital and exoccipital (supracondylar) portions usually disappears during the second or third year. The spheno–occipital synchondrosis

begins to close near the time of puberty but may persist until the twentieth year. This variation and irregularity make suture lines unreliable criteria for estimation of the developmental age of the skull. At about the twentieth year, the skull attains its definitive size.

NORMAL VARIATIONS

Intrasutural, or wormian, bones occur most frequently along the lambdoid sutures (Fig. 18-6 and e-Fig. 18-7; Box 18-2). They occur much less frequently in the fontanelles (see e-Fig. 18-7). The interparietal or Inca bone (Fig. 18-8) results from division of the supraoccipital portion of the occipital bone into two parts by the mendosal suture, with the superior part arising from membranous bone and the inferior part arising from cartilage continuous with that of the supracondylar portions and the basiocciput. A rare synchondrosis or suture line runs vertically through the squamous portion of the occipital

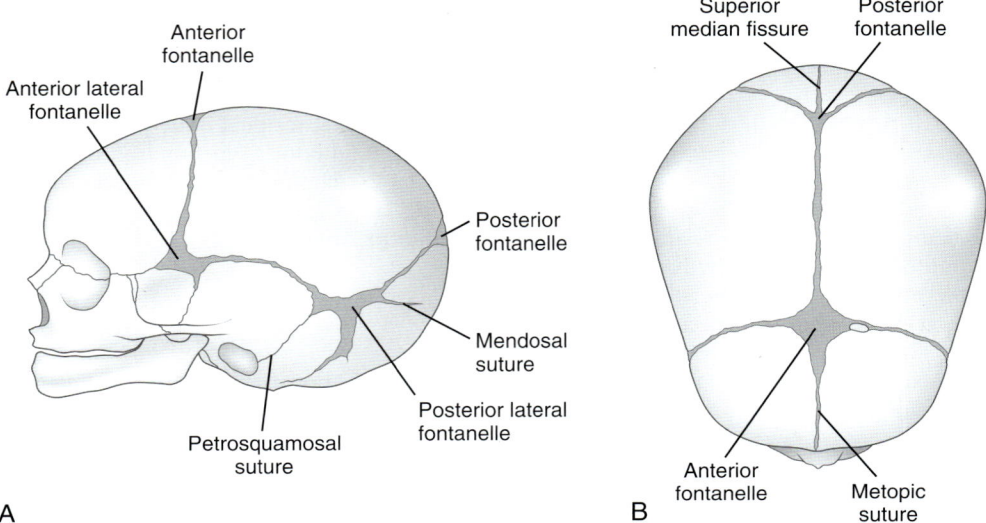

Figure 18-1 The cranium at birth showing the greater and lesser fontanelles. Lateral (**A**) and superior (**B**) views are shown.

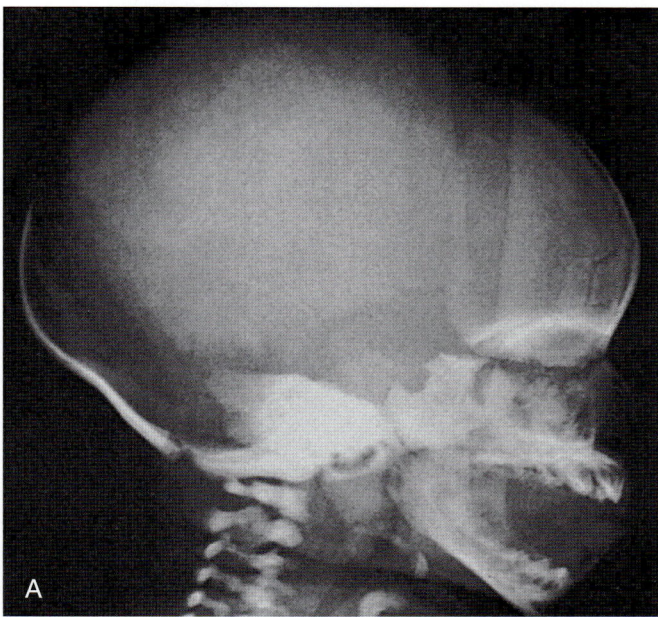

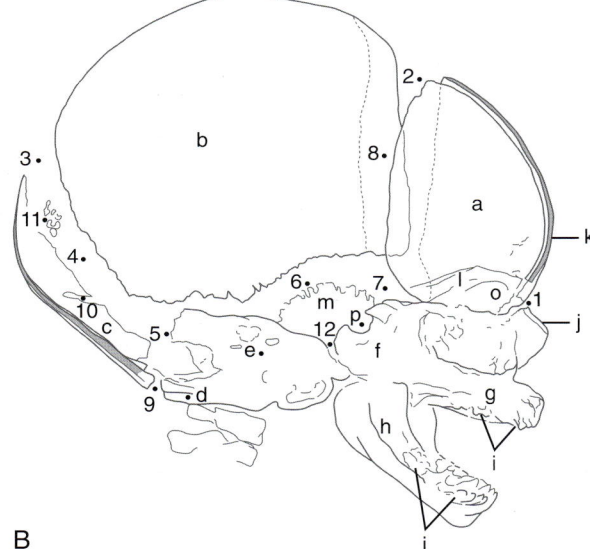

Figure 18-2 A, A radiograph of the normal neonatal skull (lateral projection). **B,** A tracing of **A**. *a,* Frontal bone; *b,* parietal bone; *c,* squamous portion of the occipital bone; *d,* exoccipital portion of the occipital bone; *e,* superimposed petrous pyramids of the temporal bone; *f,* body of the sphenoid; *g,* upper maxilla; *h,* mandible; *i,* partially mineralized deciduous teeth and dental crypts; *j,* nasal bone; *k,* squamosa of the frontal bone; *l,* horizontal plates of the frontal bone; *m,* squamosa of the temporal bone; *o,* orbit; *p,* pituitary fossa; *1,* frontonasal suture; *2,* anterior fontanelle; *3,* posterior fontanelle; *4,* lambdoid suture; *5,* posterolateral fontanelle; *6,* squamosal suture; *7,* anterolateral fontanelle; *8,* coronal suture; *9,* synchondrosis between exoccipital and supraoccipital portions of the occipital bone; *10,* mendosal suture; *11,* multiple ossification centers (wormian bones) in the lambdoid suture; *12,* occipitosphenoid synchondrosis.

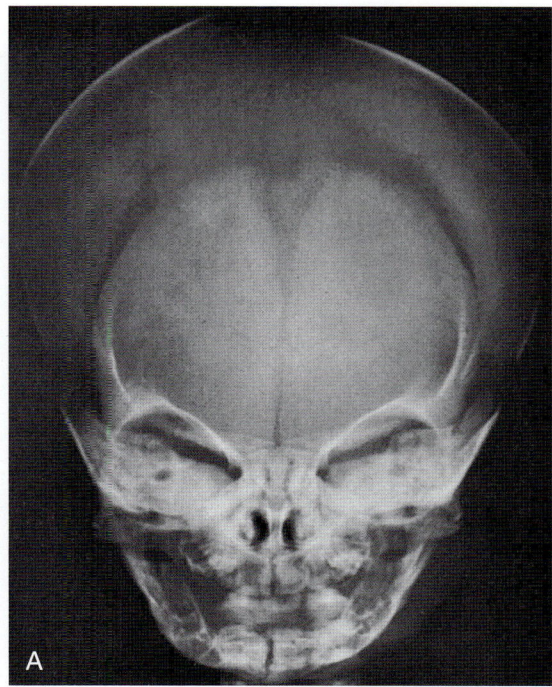

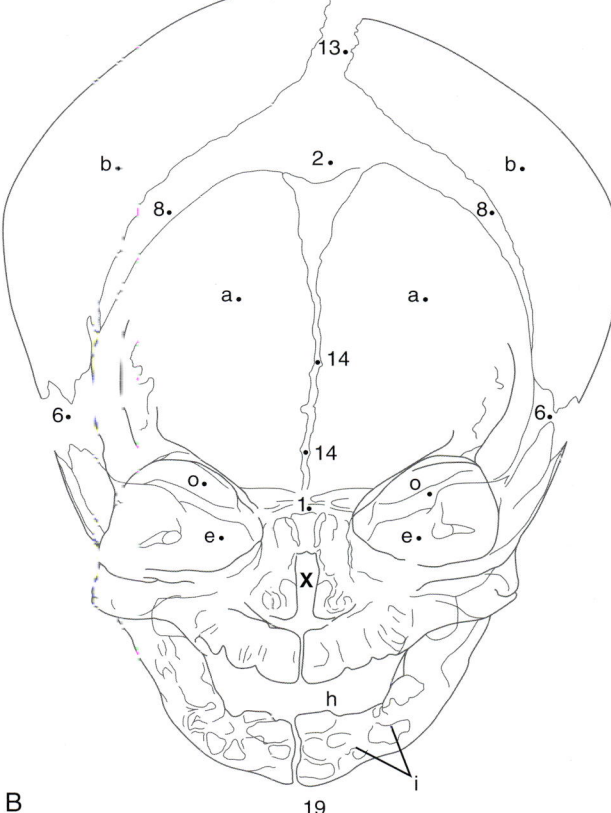

Figure 18-3 A, A radiograph of the normal skull (posteroanterior projection). **B,** Tracing of **A**. *a,* Frontal bone; *b,* parietal bone; *e,* superimposed petrous pyramids of the temporal bone; *h,* mandible; *i,* partially mineralized deciduous teeth and dental crypts; *o,* orbit; *x,* nasal septum; *1,* frontonasal suture; *2,* anterior fontanelle; *6,* squamosal suture; *8,* coronal suture; *13,* sagittal suture; *14,* metopic suture dividing the frontal bone; *19,* symphysis of the mandible.

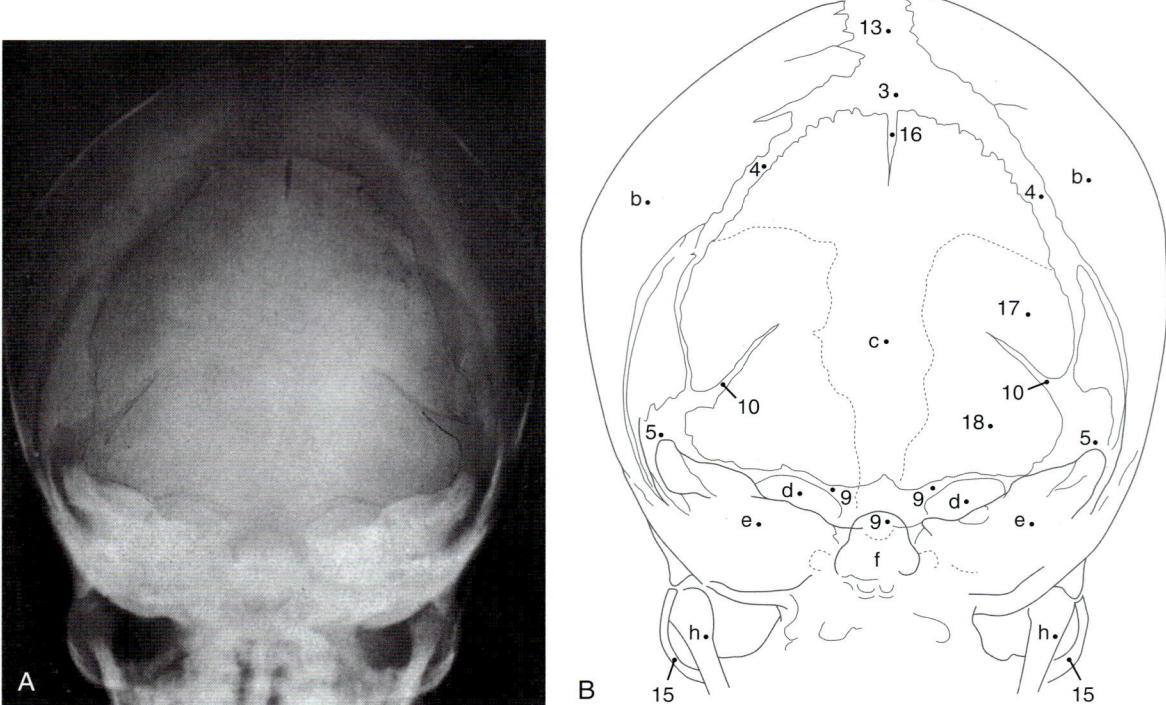

Figure 18-4   A, A radiograph of the normal neonatal skull (Towne's projection). **B,** Tracing of **A**. *b,* Parietal bone; *c,* squamous portion of the occipital bone; *d,* exoccipital portion of the occipital bone; *e,* superimposed petrous pyramids of the temporal bone; *f,* body of the sphenoid; *g,* basioccipital portion of the occipital bone; *h,* mandible; *3,* posterior fontanelle; *4,* lambdoid suture; *5,* posterolateral fontanelle; *9,* synchondrosis between exoccipital and supraoccipital portions of the occipital bone; *10,* mendosal suture; *13,* sagittal suture; *15,* zygomatic arch; *16,* superior median fissure of the occipital bone; *17,* interparietal portion of the occipital bone; *18,* supraoccipital portion of the occipital bone.

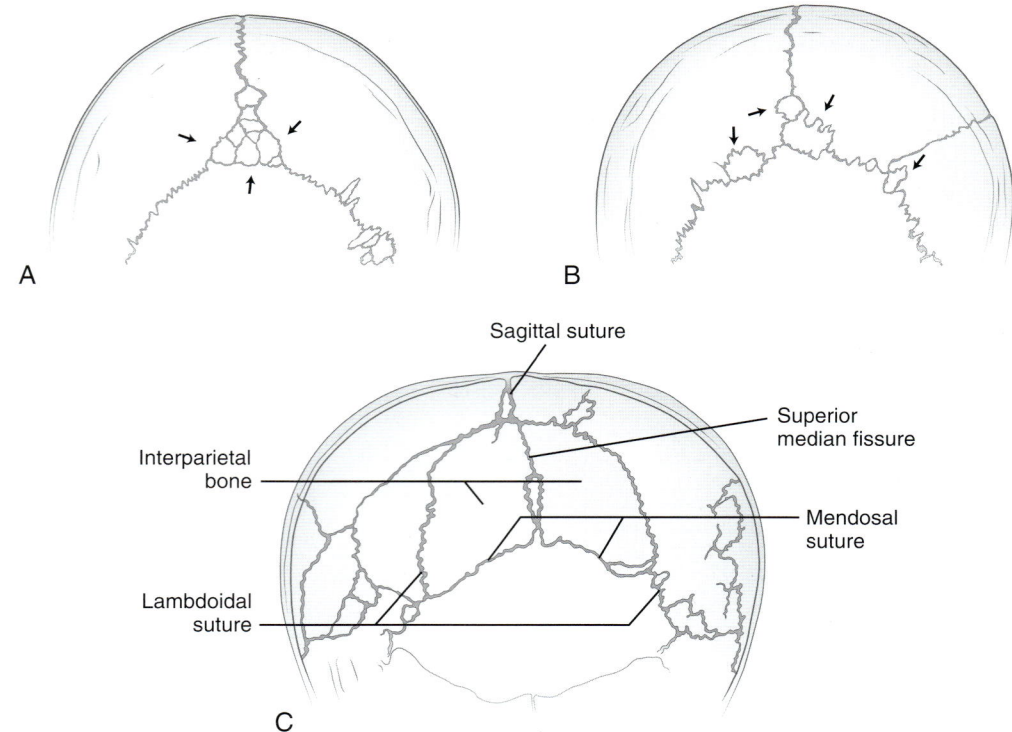

Figure 18-6   Tracings of films showing wormian bones. **A,** Multiple wormian bones (*arrows*) in the sagittal suture. **B,** Multiple wormian bones (*arrows*) in the sagittal and lambdoid sutures. **C,** Interparietal bone bounded by the lambdoid and persistent mendosal sutures. The superior median fissure also is still present and divides the interparietal bone into right and left halves.

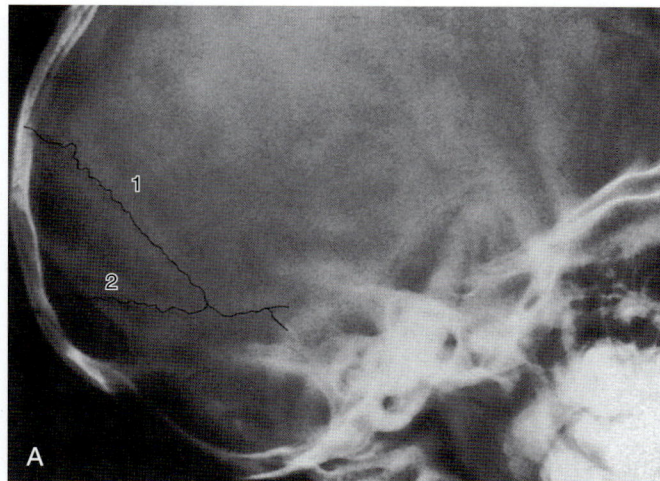

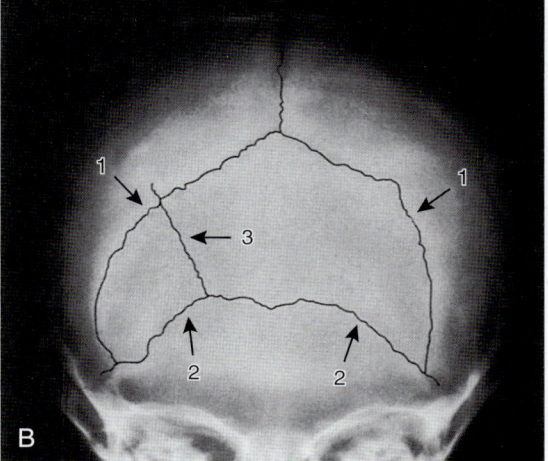

Figure 18-8 Interparietal (Inca) bone. **A,** Lateral projection. **B,** Anteroposterior Towne projection. *1,* Right and left lambdoid sutures; *2,* mendosal suture; *3,* accessory suture in interparietal bone. (Courtesy Dr. J.P. Dorst, Baltimore, MD.)

portion is practically a straight line (e-Fig. 18-15) and may be interpreted erroneously as a "fracture through a suture." Persistence of the metopic suture may simulate a vertical fracture in the occipital bone in anteroposterior, caudally angulated exposures if extension of the superimposed radiolucent line into the area of the foramen magnum is invisible

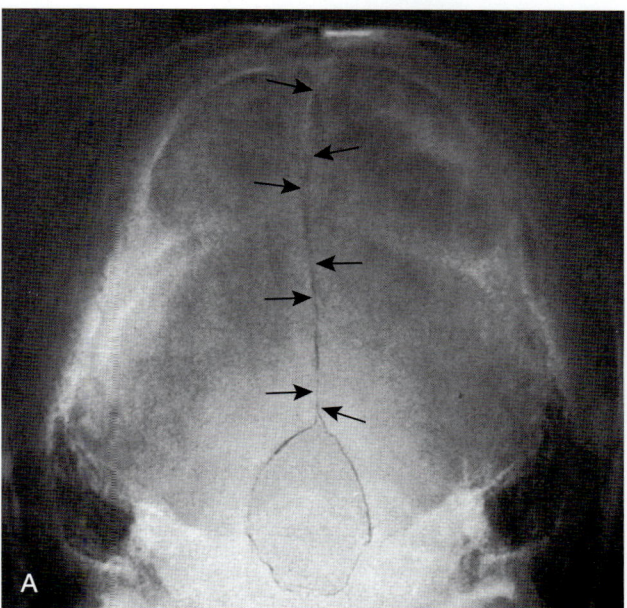

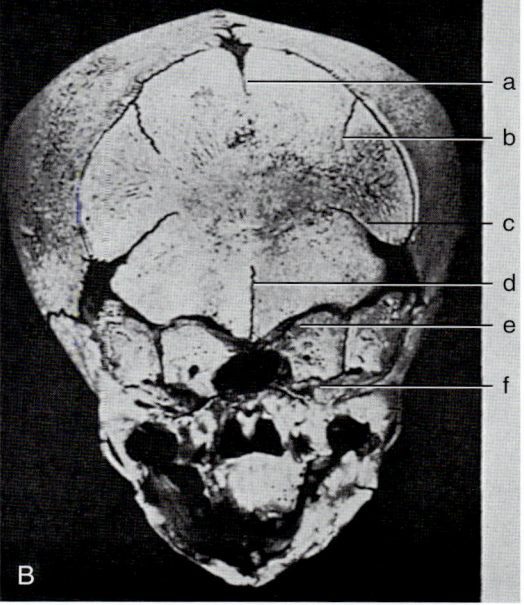

Figure 18-9 Occipital bone. **A,** A Towne projection showing radiolucent midline longitudinal or cerebellar synchondrosis (*arrows*) in the occipital squamosa of an 11-year-old girl, which resulted from failure of fusion mediad of its lateral paired ossification centers. This radiolucent strip can be mistaken for a fracture line. (Sutures were retouched with a pencil.) **B,** Persistent longitudinal or cerebellar synchondrosis (*d*) in the occipital squamosa of a skull of a newborn; only the caudal segment of the synchondrosis is still open in this case. *a,* superior median longitudinal fissure; *b,* superior lateral longitudinal fissure; *c,* mendosal suture; *e,* synchrondrosis between exoccipital and supraoccipital bones; *f,* synchrondrosis between basioccipital and exoccipital bones. (From Koehler A, Zimmer EA. *Borderlands of the normal and early pathologic in skeletal roentgenology.* 3rd ed. Philadelphia: Grune & Stratton [translated from German ed 11 by S.P. Wilk]; 1968.)

bone (Fig. 18-9); persisting superior and inferior portions of the line are known as the superior longitudinal fissure or bi-interparietal suture and the cerebellar synchondrosis or median cerebellar suture. Where the supraoccipital portion of the occipital bone forms the posterior border of the foramen magnum, accessory supraoccipital bones occasionally are found (e-Fig. 18-10). The configuration caused by an outward bulge of the occipital squamosa just above the torcular Herophili in a newborn (Fig. 18-11) is called bathrocephaly. Rarely, a horizontal interparietal suture divides the parietal bones into superior and inferior moieties (e-Fig. 18-12).

Compression of the fetal skull and its molding during passage through the maternal pelvis produce significant radiographic findings that persist after birth (Fig. 18-13).[2] During the first weeks and months of life, widths of sutures vary so much that caution is required in their evaluation for the diagnosis of increased intracranial pressure, particularly because positioning is difficult and partial superimposition of bilateral sutures can produce spurious widening (Fig. 18-14).

In children older than 2 years, the sutures extend through both tables and the diploic space. The outer table portion of the suture may be deeply serrated when the inner table

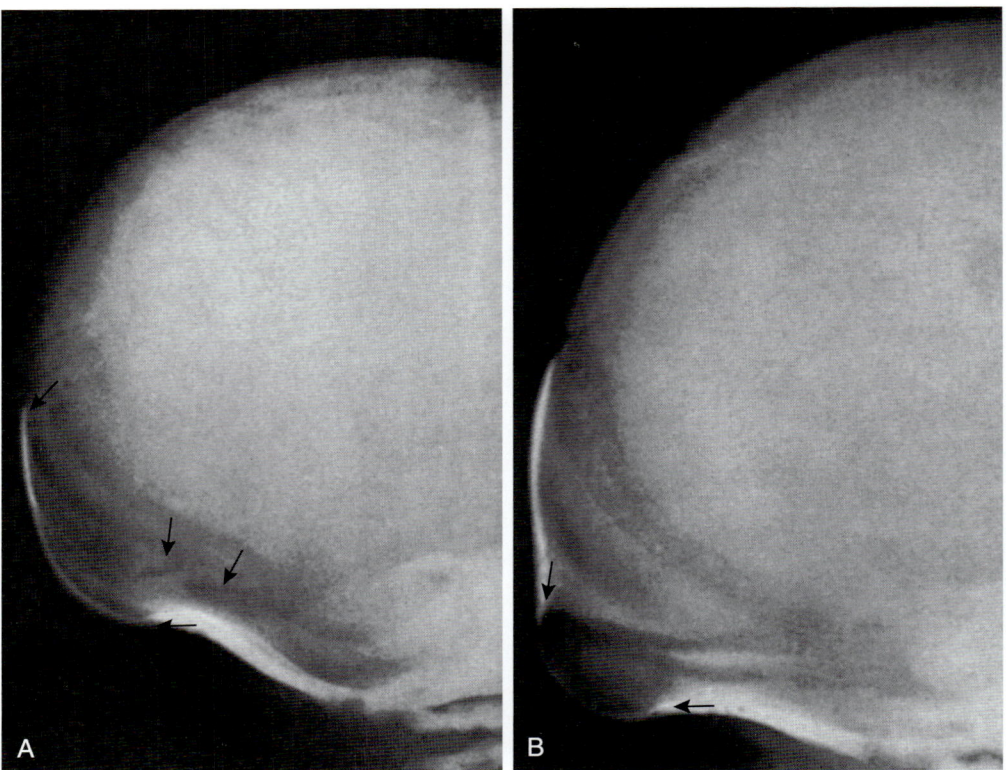

Figure 18-11 Bathrocephaly in a newborn. **A,** The external bulge (*arrows*) extends from the lambda downward to the level of the mendosal suture of a normal 3-day-old infant. **B,** The bulge (*arrows*) in this normal 5-day-old infant begins below the mendosal suture.

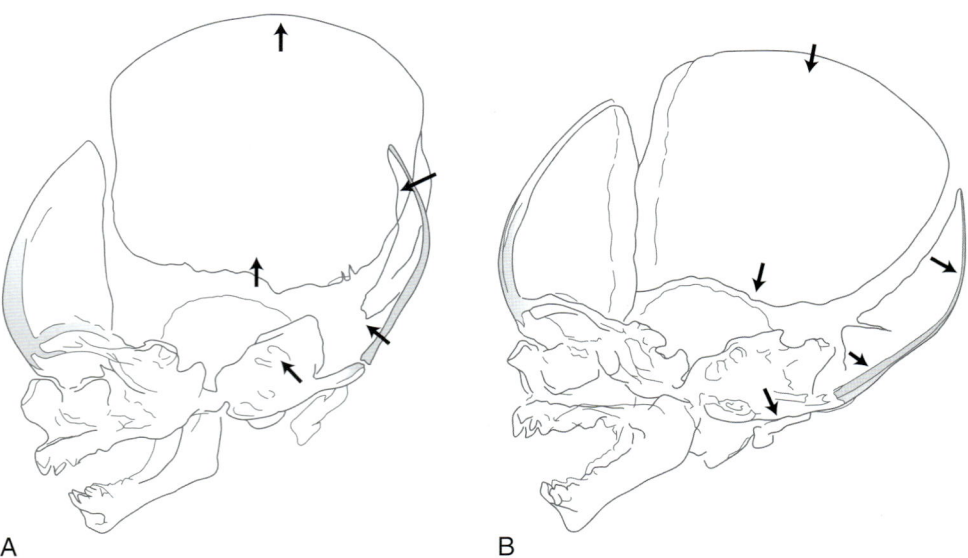

Figure 18-13 **A,** A tracing of a radiograph of the neonatal skull on the first day of life shows molding of the bones of the calvaria with overlapping of their edges and narrowing of the sutures caused by compression during passage of the head through the birth canal. The parietal bones are displaced upward, and the temporal bones and occipital bone are rotated counterclockwise (*arrows*). **B,** A tracing of a radiograph on the third day of life shows reexpansion of the cranium and widening of the sutures and fontanelles compared with **A** after the parietal, occipital, and temporal bones have returned to normal positions (*arrows*). (Courtesy Dr. H.C. Moloy.)

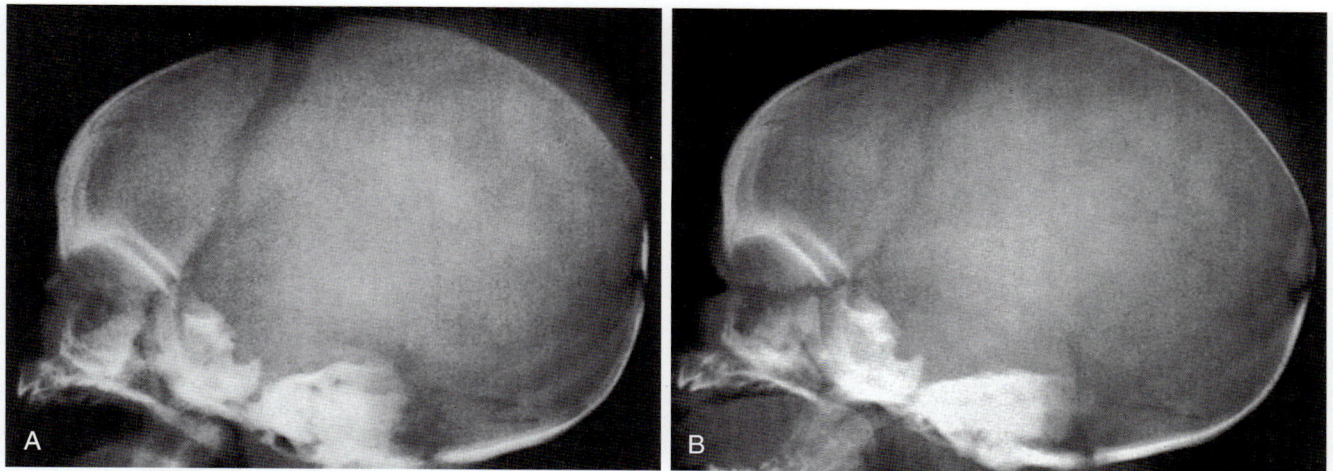

Figure 18-14 Factitious widening of the coronal suture. **A,** A slightly oblique projection in which the right and left limbs of the coronal suture overlap. **B,** A projection that is a little more oblique than **A** in which the individual, narrower, right and left limbs are seen.

or if the inferior portion of the suture has been obliterated. The frontal crest on the internal surface of the frontal squamosa in the midsagittal plane may be sufficiently prominent to simulate calcification of the falx cerebri that attaches to it (e-Fig. 18-16).

Juvenile Skull

After a child is 2 years old, the radiographic appearance of the skull is similar in most respects to that of the skull during adult life (Fig. 18-17). With advancing age, the skull gradually grows and differentiates until late in childhood, when all of the essential characteristics of the adult skull have developed (Figs. 18-18 through 18-20).

NORMAL VARIATIONS

The outstanding characteristic of the juvenile skull is its remarkable variability in size, shape, thickness and mineral content, depth of the grooves for the dural sinuses, pattern of the diploic structure and convolutional and vascular markings, degree of pneumatization of the temporal and paranasal bones, and size and shape of the pituitary fossa. These normal variants are so marked that frequently it is difficult to distinguish normal variations from early pathologic changes.

Convolutional (Digital) Markings

Convolutional (digital) markings are areas of diminished density in the calvarium that are separated by strips of normal

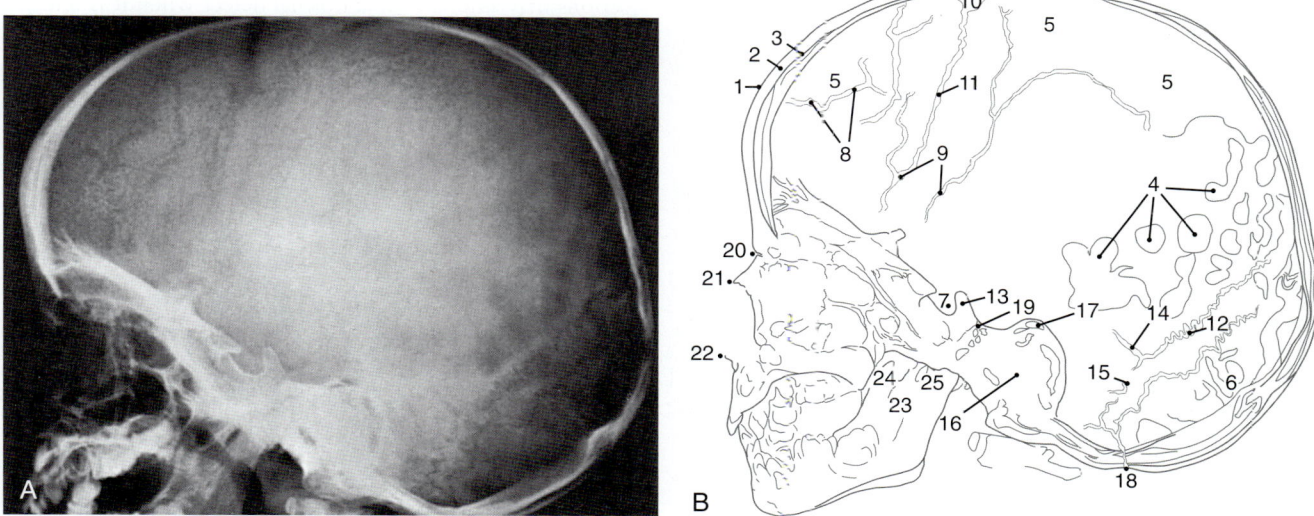

Figure 18-17 A radiograph of the normal skull at 2 years. **A,** Lateral projection. **B,** Tracing of **A**. *1,* Outer table; *2,* diploic space; *3,* inner table; *4,* convolutional markings; *5,* fine honeycomb of diploic structure; *6,* internal occipital protuberance; *7,* pituitary fossa; *8,* diploic veins; *9,* vascular grooves; *10,* anterior fontanelle; *11,* coronal suture; *12,* lambdoid suture; *13,* dorsum sellae; *14,* parietomastoid suture; *15,* occipitomastoid suture; *16,* petrous pyramids; *17,* small temporal pneumatic cell; *18,* synchondrosis between exoccipital and supraoccipital; *19,* spheno-occipital synchondrosis; *20,* nasofrontal suture; *21,* nasal bone; *22,* anterior nasal spine; *23,* mandible; *24,* coronoid process of the mandible; *25,* condyloid process of the mandible.

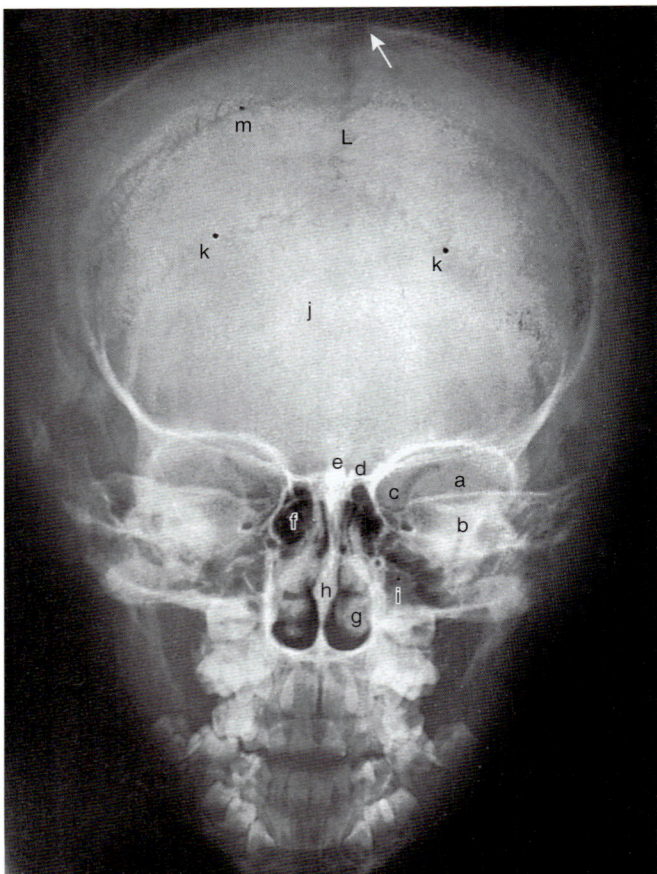

Figure 18-18 Radiographic features of a normal skull at 6 years of age—Water's projection. *a*, Orbit; *b*, petrous pyramid; *c*, superior orbital fissure; *d*, frontal sinus; *e*, crista galli; *f*, ethmoid cells; *g*, inferior turbinate; *h*, nasal septum; *i*, maxillary sinus; *j*, frontal bone; *k*, lambdoid suture; *m*, coronal suture; *L*, *arrow*, sagittal suture.

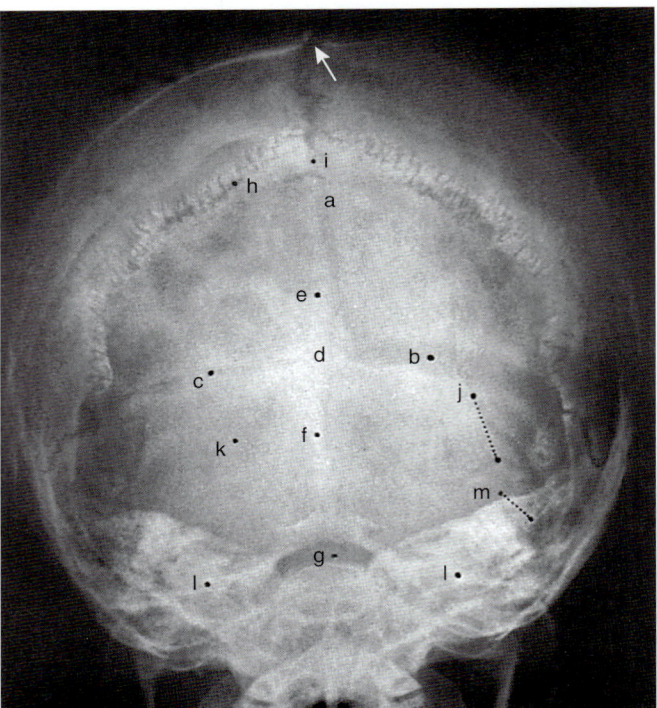

Figure 18-19 Important radiographic features of the normal skull at 3 years—Towne's projection. *a*, Groove for superior sagittal sinus; *b*, groove for right transverse sinus; *c*, groove for left transverse sinus; *d*, torcular Herophili and superimposed external and internal occipital protuberances; *e*, superior half of cruciate ridge; *f*, inferior half of cruciate ridge; *g*, foramen magnum; *h*, lambdoid suture; *i*, lambda; *j*, superimposed vascular markings in frontal bone; *k*, posterior fossa; *l*, petrous pyramid; *m*, mastoid pneumatic cells; *arrow*, sagittal sinus.

density (Fig. 18-21). These areas correspond closely to the location and configuration of cerebral convolutions.[3] They probably are formed by localized pressure of the pulsating brain on the inner table of the neurocranium.

Diploic and Vascular Markings

The diploic space between the outer and inner tables of the calvaria is filled with a cancellous bony structure that varies in volume and pattern and is responsible for the fine, honeycomb texture of the cranial vault. The diploic veins lie in large, irregular channels that appear in radiographs as irregular strips of diminished density extending through the bones of the vault in all directions (e-Fig. 18-22 and Fig. 18-23). The diploic veins vary in size, course, and visibility.

The grooves on the internal aspect of the calvarium for the arteries and veins appear in radiographs as strips of diminished density (Fig. 18-24). Compared with the venous grooves, the arterial grooves tend to taper more. The most constant of these channels is that of the middle meningeal artery, which courses upward and backward from the region of the pterion, where it may be surrounded by bone of the inner table. The largest and heaviest vascular markings are the bony thinnings over the dural venous sinuses. The superior sagittal sinus lies in a shallow groove on the internal surface

at the median plane of the vault near the attachment of the falx cerebri. At the torcular Herophili, the channels for the superior longitudinal and transverse sinuses meet; one transverse sinus may be appreciably larger and deeper than the other (see Fig. 18-18). The torcular Herophili in lateral projections may simulate an abnormal defect when it is unusually

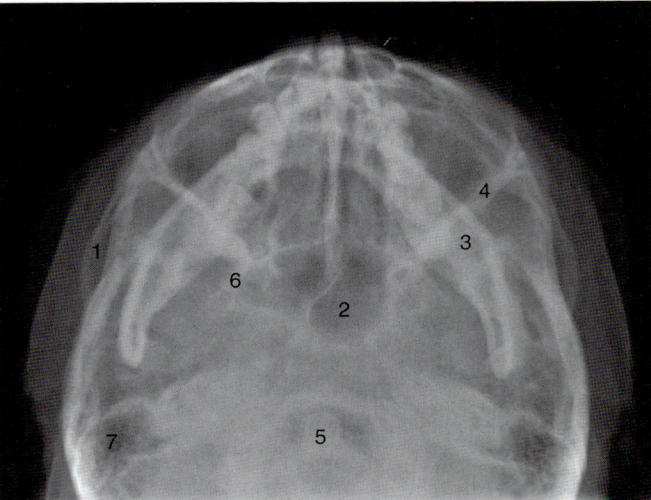

Figure 18-20 The submental vortex. The following anatomic structures are labeled: *1*, Zygomatic arch; *2*, sphenoid sinus; *3*, body of mandible; *4*, greater wing of sphenoid (orbital surface); *5*, odontoid; *6*, pterygoid plates; and *7*, mastoid air cells.

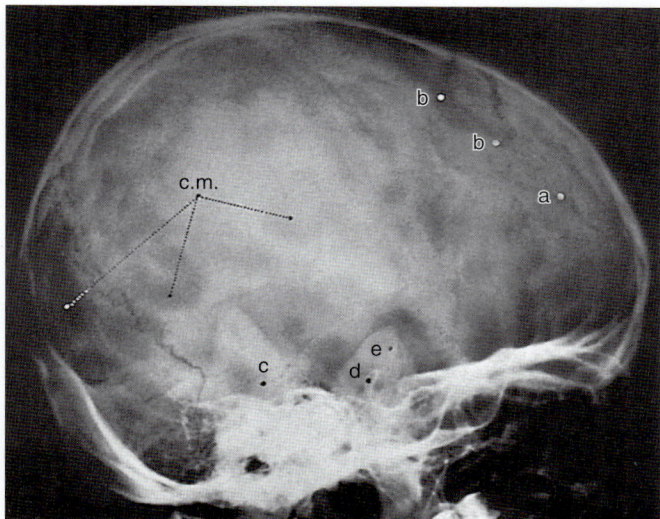

Figure 18-21 Prominent convolutional markings (c.m.) in an asymptomatic 6-year-old girl. *a,* Diploic veins; *b,* coronal suture; *c,* squamoparietal suture; *d,* dorsum sellae; *e,* shadow of external ear.

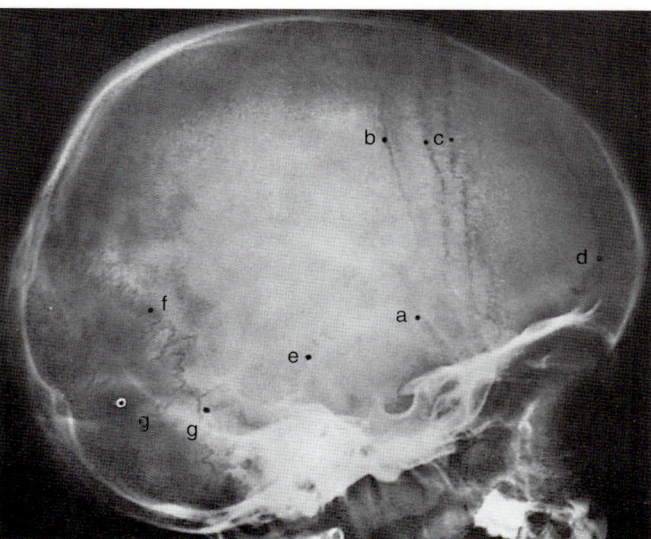

Figure 18-24 Vascular markings. *a,* Grooves for the middle meningeal artery; *b,* parietal diploic vein; *c,* coronal suture; *d,* frontal diploic veins; *e,* squamoparietal suture; *f,* lambdoid suture; *g,* large groove for the transverse dural sinus.

deep (e-Fig. 18-25). At the bend where the transverse sinus turns caudad, near the mastoid process, superimposition of the lateral end of the sulcus of the transverse sinus and the sulcus of the sigmoid sinus may produce a rounded, radiolucent patch when these sulci are unusually deep (e-Fig. 18-26). Often the groove for the bregmatic vein is seen as a conspicuous strip of diminished density on one or both lateral walls of the calvaria (e-Fig. 18-27); this groove also has been called the sphenoparietal sinus, which is a misnomer because the true sinus runs underneath the lesser wing of the sphenoid bone and does not always communicate with the bregmatic vein.

Pacchionian Bodies

The Pacchionian, or arachnoidal, granulations (e-Fig. 18-28) are attached to the undersurface of the dura. Originally they

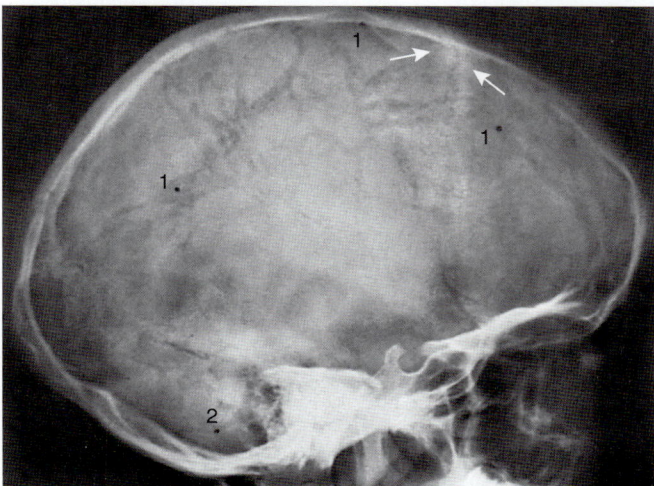

Figure 18-23 Conspicuous large diploic veins in the frontal and parietal bones in an 8-year-old girl. The veins appear as wide strips of diminished density coursing through the frontal and parietal bones. Arrows are directed at the physiologic hyperostotic ridges on either side of the coronal suture. *1,* Diploic venous lake; *2,* groove for the emissary vein of the mastoid.

were thought to be the site of absorption of cerebrospinal fluid, but this theory has been disputed.[4] These structures are irregular, sharply defined impressions with smooth edges on the inner table of skull and located in a typical parasagittal location. These normal structures appear after age 18 months.

Symmetric Parietal Foramina

About 60% of skulls show small defects (parietal foramina) in the superior posterior angles of the parietal bones through which emissary veins penetrate. The veins generally communicate with the sagittal sinus internally and with tributaries to the occipital veins externally. Occasionally, large bony defects are present in these regions; these defects have been called enlarged parietal foramina.[5] They occasionally are palpable on each side of the midline and less frequently are united to form a large, single defect (Fig. 18-29). The defects result from a failure of mineralization of the membranous bone, and thus the term "enlarged parietal foramina" is a misnomer. The defects usually are not associated with other skeletal anomalies and have no clinical significance except in the differential diagnosis of cranial defects, such as those associated with meningocele, infection, and histiocytosis.

Large parietal foramina have been recognized as an inherited trait ever since Goldsmith found them in 56 members of the Catlin family, giving rise to the term "Catlin mark."[6] Lesions may persist throughout life, although they tend to become smaller and may completely obliterate, leaving focal sclerotic residua.

Plain Radiographic Signs of Increased Intracranial Pressure

The signs of increased intracranial pressure are spread sutures, truncation of the dorsum sella, widened sella, and "beaten copper" appearance of bone (only with other changes) (Figs. 18-30 and 18-31; see Fig. 18-13). Chronic increased

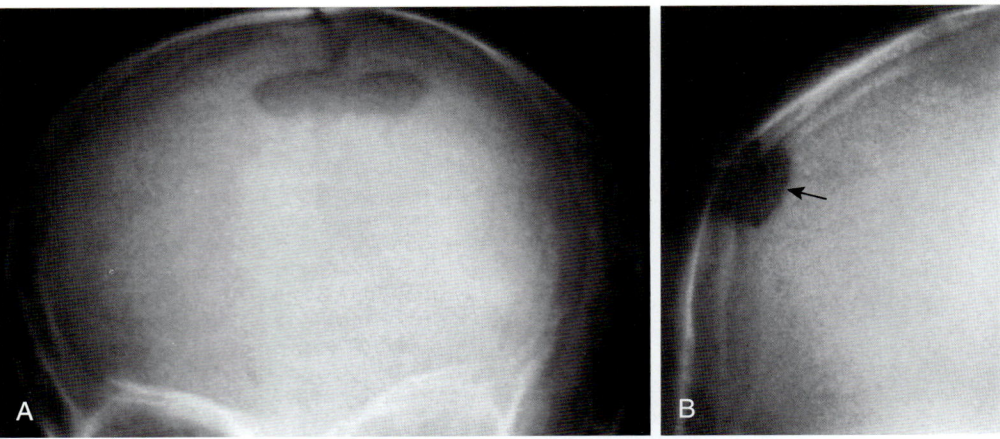

Figure 18-29 A persistent interparietal fontanelle (parietal foramen) (*arrow*) in an otherwise healthy 5-year-old boy. **A,** Frontal projection. **B,** Caldwell projection.

intracranial pressure can be revealed by increased width of sutural interdigitation.

Anatomy of the Paranasal Sinuses

NORMAL PARANASAL SINUSES

The paranasal sinuses are paired pneumatic cavities that communicate with the nasal fossae and are situated in the paranasal bones—maxilla, ethmoid, frontal, and sphenoid. Because of the continuity of their air cell mucosa with that of the nasal cavity via the eustachian tubes, the mastoid cells can be considered an additional component. The size and shape of the cavities vary in different age periods, among persons, and on the two sides of the same person.[7,8]

The sites of the openings of the sinuses into the nasal cavity are shown in Figures 18-32 and 18-33. The postnatal growth and extension of the sinuses are shown in e-Figure 18-34. The fully developed maxillary, frontal, and ethmoid sinuses are illustrated diagrammatically in e-Figures 18-35 and 18-36. Computed tomography (CT has shown extensions from adjacent sinuses into the orbital roofs and apices of the petrous temporal bone that are not easily recognized on conventional radiographs.

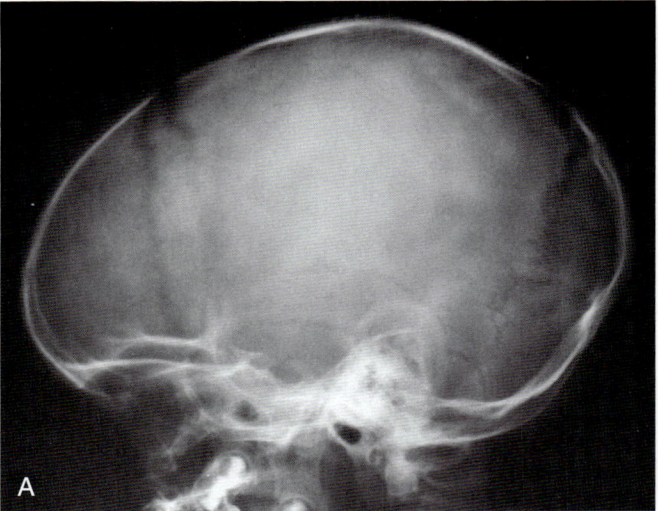

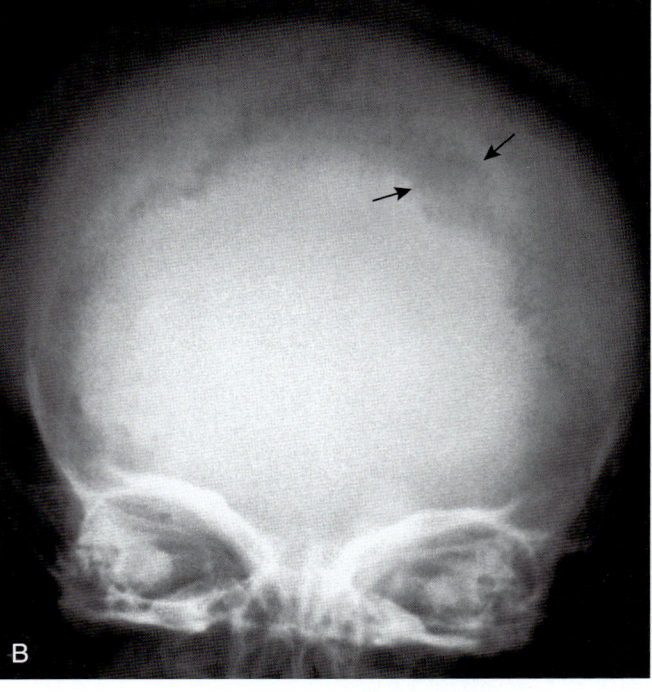

Figure 18-30 Split sutures. **A,** A lateral radiograph reveals a widened coronal suture caused by acute increased intracranial pressure. **B,** A radiograph shows the results of chronic increased intracranial pressure. The interdigitations of the lambdoid suture are widened, but the sutures are not frankly split (*arrows*). This radiograph shows an attempt of the sutures to reunite with continual increased pressure.

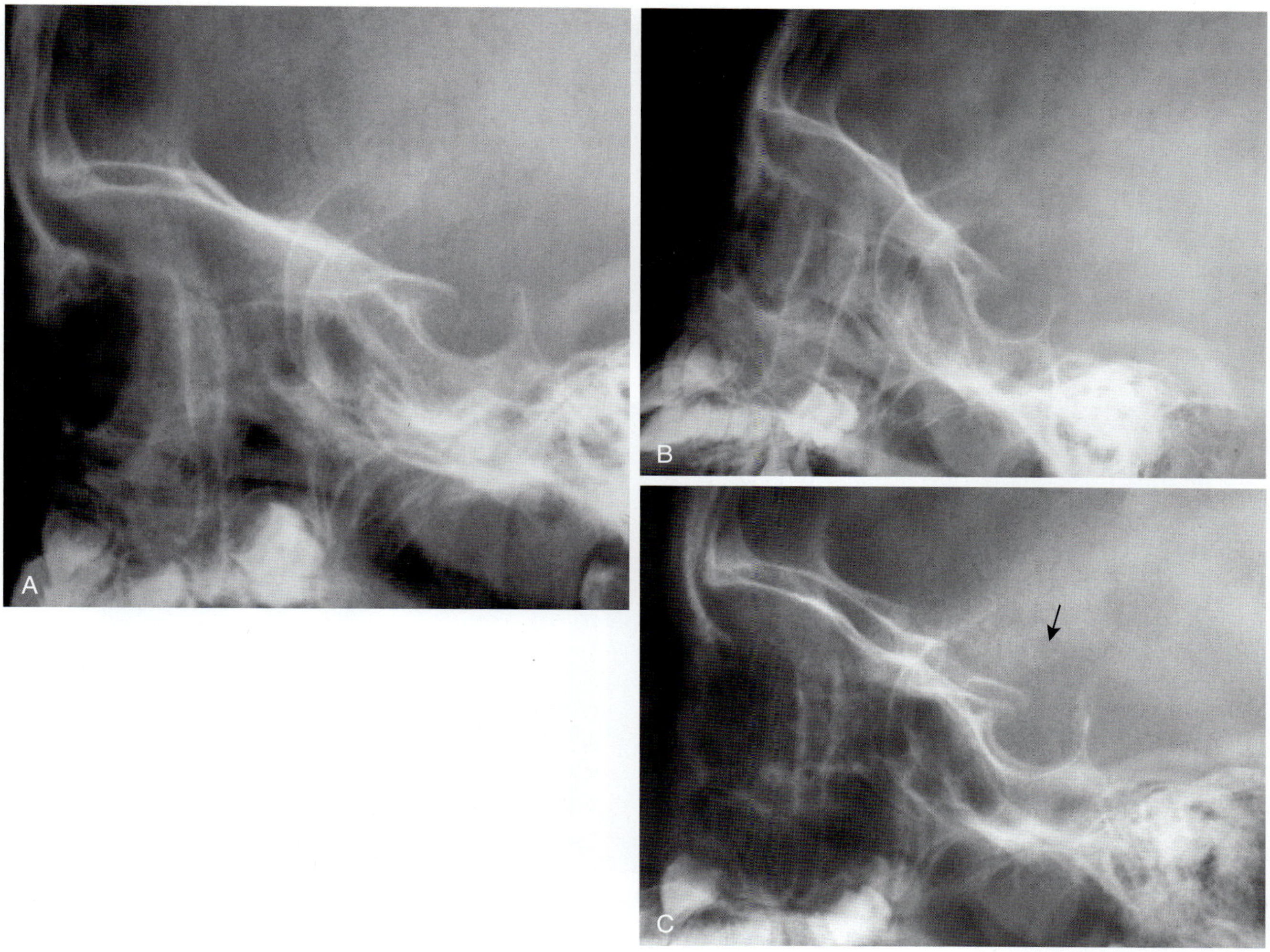

Figure 18-31   Increased intracranial pressure—sella changes. **A,** A lateral radiograph coned to the sella in an 11-year-old with headaches. **B,** The sella is wider and the dorsum is thinned 6 months later. **C,** The sella is even wider and the dorsum is truncated with flecks of calcium above (*arrow*) 1 year later. This patient had a craniopharyngioma.

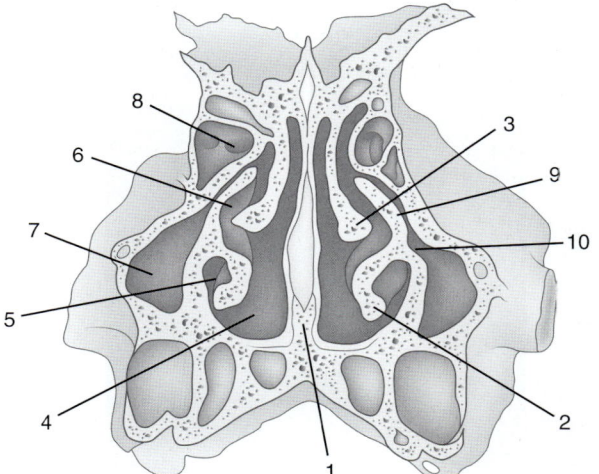

Figure 18-32   The frontal section through the nasal fossa and paranasal sinuses at the level of the ostium of the maxillary sinus in a 7-year-old child. *1,* Nasal septum; *2,* inferior turbinate; *3,* middle turbinate; *4,* nasal fossa; *5,* inferior meatus; *6,* middle meatus; *7,* maxillary sinus; *8,* ethmoid cells; *9,* infundibulum; *10,* ostium. (Modified from Schaeffer JP. *The nose, paranasal sinuses, naso-lacrimal passageways and the olfactory organ in man.* Philadelphia: P. Blakiston's Sons; 1920.)

MAXILLARY SINUSES

Changes in size and configuration of the maxillary sinuses with age are shown in e-Figure 18-36 and Figure 18-37. The maxillary sinuses are present at birth, expand steadily, and are considered mature by the time of puberty.[9] Variations in development include isolated unilateral hypoplasia and prominent septa that appear to compartmentalize the sinus cavity (Fig. 18-38). The roots of the maxillary molars occasionally impinge on the walls of the sinuses (Fig. 18-39) and sometimes produce folds in the mucous membranes. In oblique ventrodorsal projections of the skull, the roots of the teeth may be superimposed on the sinuses and artifactually appear to project into them. A molar that fails to migrate is found in its fetal position near the posterosuperomedial angle of the maxillary sinus (e-Figs. 18-40 and 18-41). Note should be made of the relative height of the antral floor and structures in the nasal cavity, which can influence surgical approaches.

FRONTAL SINUSES

Marked variation in size and shape is typical of frontal sinuses, as is asymmetry in development. The frontal sinuses are not

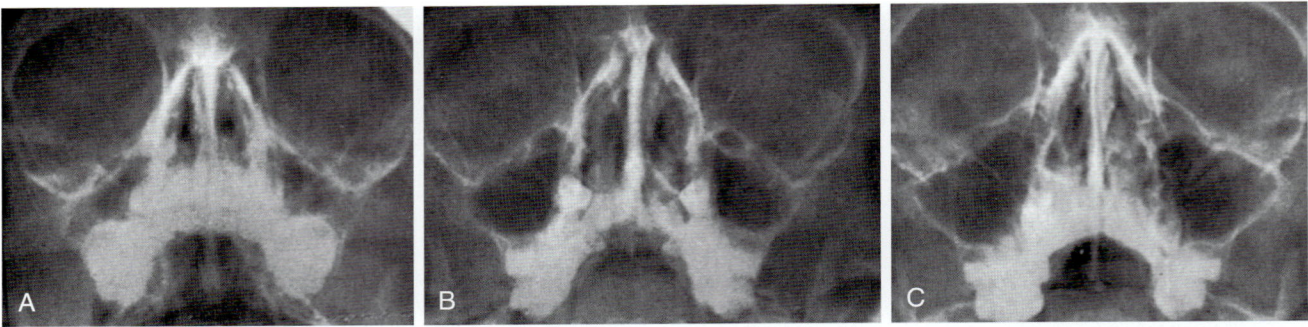

Figure 18-37 Waters projection of normal maxillary sinuses in a child at ages 4 years (**A**), 7 years (**B**), and 11 years (**C**).

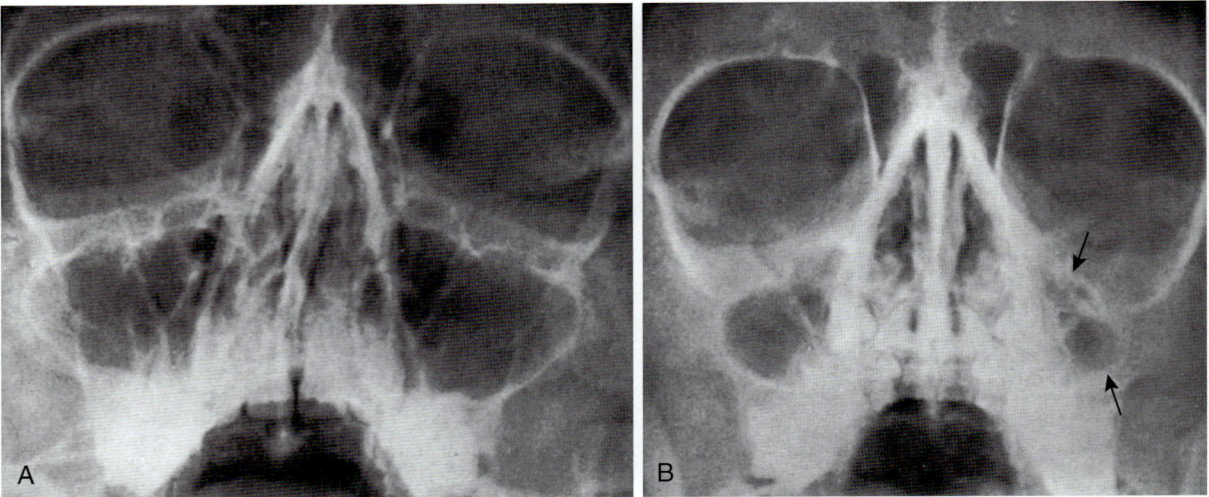

Figure 18-38 Variants of the maxillary sinus. **A,** Several septa and ridges dividing the maxillary sinus into small cavities in an 11-year-old girl. **B,** Hypoplasia of the left maxillary sinus (*arrows*) in a 7-year-old boy.

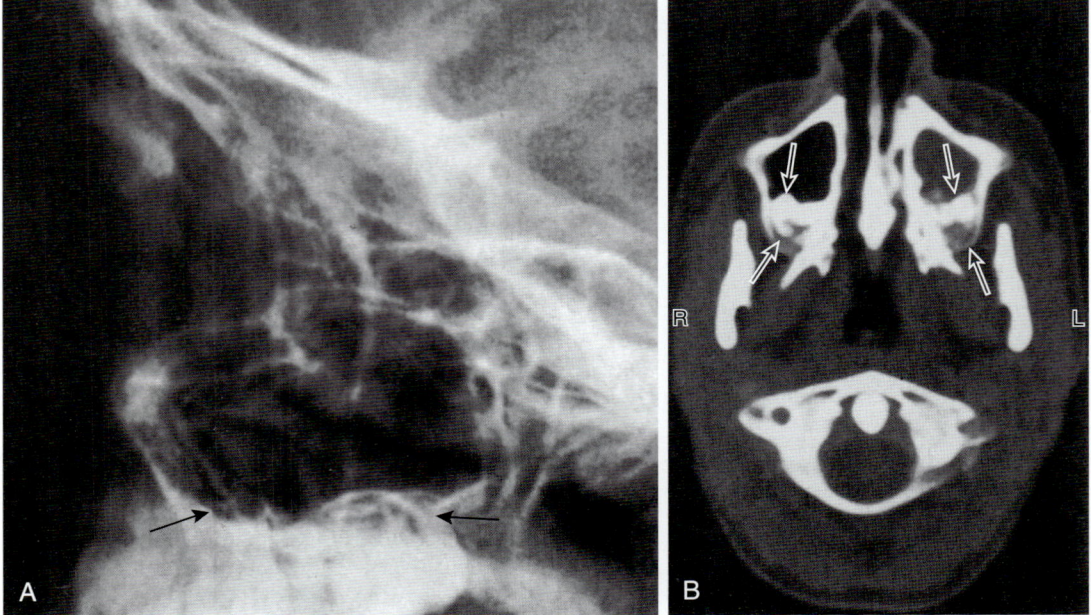

Figure 18-39 Maxillary sinuses. **A,** A lateral view of the maxillary sinus shows the roots of the molars and bicuspids in contact with the floor of the maxillary sinus (*arrows*) in an 11-year-old child. **B,** Molar-indenting maxillary sinuses in a 12-year-old child who had a computed tomography scan performed because of sinus disease. Unerupted molars indent the posterior aspects of both maxillary sinuses (*arrows*). The left sinus is opaque because of sinus disease.

sufficiently developed for radiographic identification until they extend into the base of the vertical plate of the frontal bone by 6 years of age. The rate of expansion varies; any time between 6 and 12 years they extend to the level of the orbital roofs. By puberty, most frontal sinuses have reached adult size. Some are extensions of the anterior ethmoid cells. In some cases (especially in instances of hypoplasia of the frontal lobes of the brain), exaggerated extension into the horizontal plates of the frontal bones may occur; this phenomenon is more easily recognized in lateral projections.

ETHMOID SINUSES

The ethmoid sinuses are composed of a series of cells of variable number, forming paired bony labyrinths suspended from the horizontal plate of the ethmoid bone on each side of the vertical plate, with the lateral walls forming the medial walls of the orbits. They are separated by thin osseous septa covered with mucous membrane. They all communicate with the nasal cavities either directly by independent channels or indirectly through cells of the same group. They are present at birth, expand rapidly during the first 5 years, expand less quickly until about 8 years, and usually are complete by age 12 years. They usually form three groups: anterior, middle, and posterior (see Fig. 18-33 and e-Fig. 18-36). The ethmoid cells often extend into the turbinates, crista galli, and neighboring frontal, maxillary, sphenoid, and palate bones. Three anatomic variants of ethmoid cells are found: Haller, Agger nasi, and Onodi cells. These variants are described in Chapter 8. Extension of infection from the sinus to the orbit can occur easily through the lamina papyracea (see Chapter 8).

SPHENOID SINUS

The paired cavities in the body of the sphenoid bone are separated by an osseous partition that may be displaced to one side so that the two cavities vary greatly in size and shape.[10-12] The cavities can be visualized when they are superimposed in lateral projections or side by side in submentovertical projections (e-Fig. 18-42). Ridges and septa sometimes divide each single cavity into separate compartments. The air cells are not present at birth; by age 4 years they are 4 to 8 mm in diameter, and they become adult size any time between 7 and 11 years (Fig. 18-43).

OSTEOMEATAL UNIT

The components of the osteomeatal unit (OMU) (the central sinus drainage anatomy) are present at birth, albeit crowded (see Figs. 18-32, 18-44, and 18-45). This anatomy is clearly outlined with coronal CT images obtained either directly or reconstructed from axial images.

Imaging of the Sinuses

PLAIN RADIOGRAPHS

The traditional, standard, four-view radiographic examination described next is outdated and has limited usefulness. The American Academy of Pediatrics and the American College of Radiology recommend that plain radiographic imaging be used sparingly in the diagnosis of sinusitis in children, and the American Academy of Pediatrics guidelines state that radiographs are unnecessary for diagnosing sinonasal inflammation in children younger than 6 years.[13,14] In an older child in special circumstances, radiographic imaging may prove useful, but it usually should be confined to a single Waters view.

Imaging the sinuses in children is technically demanding. The sinuses develop at varying rates, and scrupulous technique must be used when obtaining multiple views in the sometimes unhappy and moving subject. The radiation dose of a four-view examination of the sinuses is approximately 1.8 mGy to the lens and 0.12 mGy to the entire body.

A standard examination of the sinuses used to include four views (Waters, posteroanterior, Caldwell, and lateral) (see Fig. 18-43). The Waters projection is the most important and is obtained with the patient's head in just enough extension to place the shadows of the dense petrous pyramids immediately below the maxillary antral floors. It is used primarily for visualization of the maxillary sinuses.

The Caldwell (posteroanterior axial) projection, which uses a central ray angled at 15 degrees below the orbitomeatal line, provides a clear image of the ethmoid and frontal sinuses. A lateral view shows the sphenoid sinus; however, except for visualizing the tonsils and adenoids, it is of limited usefulness in a child younger than 4 years because the sphenoid sinuses are small and not well visualized, and thus they readily can appear to be partially opacified. The lateral film is important for viewing the sella and can reveal intracranial disease masquerading as sinus disease. Plain radiographs cannot adequately evaluate the anterior ethmoid air cells, the upper two thirds of the nasal cavity, the frontal recess, or the sphenoid sinuses.

Technical factors such as patient motion (even normal respiration), incorrect angulation, rotation, and underpenetration almost always overestimate the presence of disease (Box 18-3). Partial ethmoid clouding can occur in the Caldwell view because of superimposition of the ethmoid cells caused by slight rotation or nasal secretion. The normal sloping of the walls of the maxillary antra also can mimic mucosal thickening.

Although the presence of an air-fluid level appears to be evidence for acute inflammatory disease in the absence of trauma, the sensitivity of the plain radiographic finding of mucosal thickening and opacification is questionable at best. However, when radiographs are taken correctly and interpreted in view of the clinical presentation, normal findings do make a significant acute sinus infection unlikely.

Plain radiographs play no role in the investigation of a mass in the sinuses and in assessing suitability for, or complications from, sinus surgery.[15,16] Plain radiographs also are inappropriate for imaging complications of sinusitis. The

---

Box 18-3 Factors Contributing to Low Sensitivity and Specificity of Imaging Sinusitis in Pediatric Patients

Lack of clear definition of what constitutes abnormality in the sinuses

Redundant mucosa

Possible crying

Developing sinuses

High background prevalence of upper respiratory tract infections

Structural variations

Technical factors: motion, angulation, rotation, superimposition

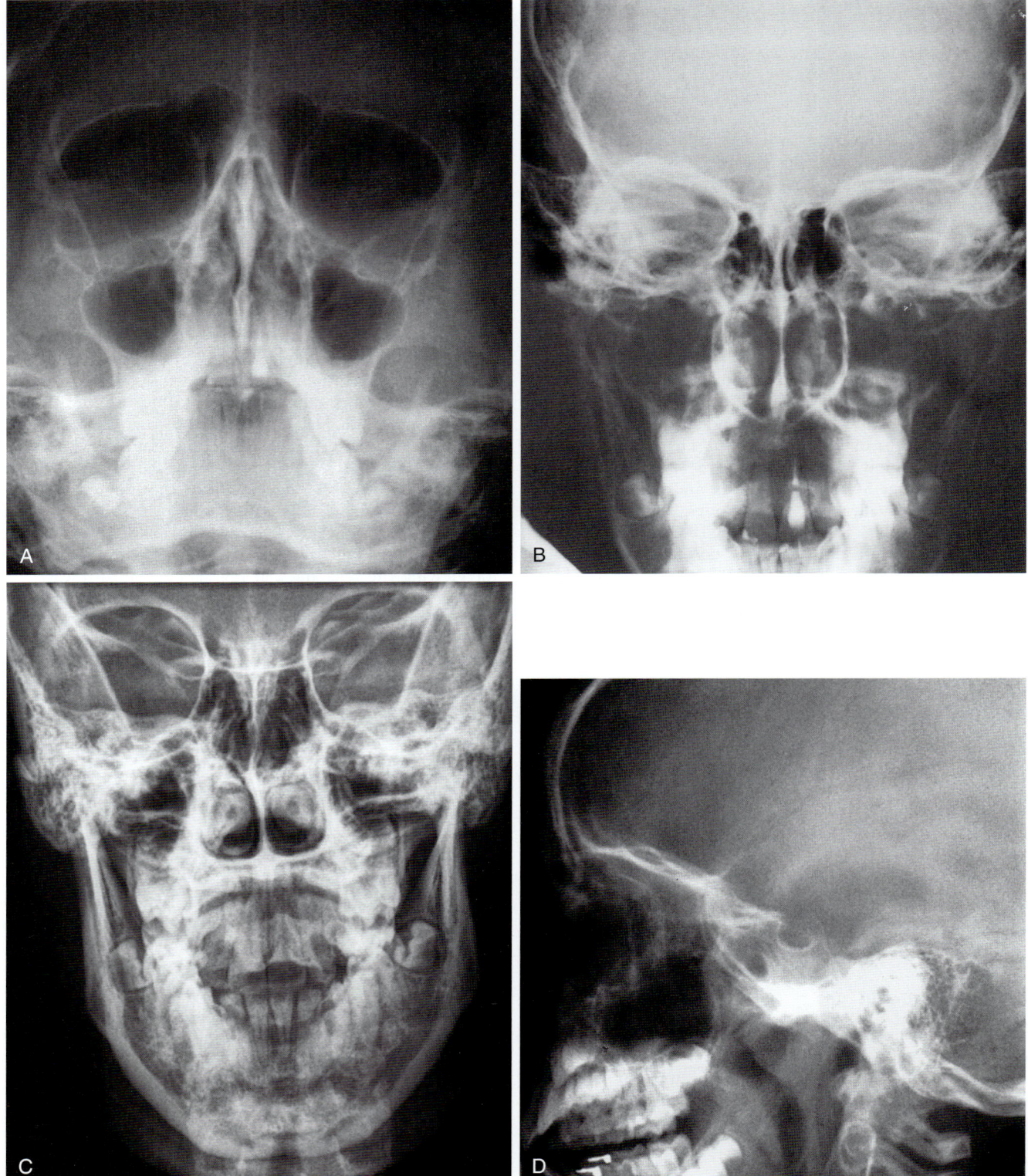

Figure 18-43 Views of the paranasal sinuses. **A,** Normal Waters (parietocanthial) axial projection. **B,** Posteroanterior axial projection. **C,** Caldwell projection. **D,** Lateral view.

capabilities of CT and magnetic resonance imaging (MRI are far superior. Plain radiographs also have little to offer in children younger than 2 years and certainly in infants younger than 1 year because such a high incidence of false-positive findings occurs.[17-21]

COMPUTED TOMOGRAPHY

Coronal CT, that is, imaging in thin sections with low milliamperage (20 to 40 mA) and kilovolts (100 to 120), provides excellent images of the sinuses and can detect changes in thin bone, surrounding soft tissue, and interposed airspaces. The CT dose index "dose" given for such an examination is approximately 6.50 mGy, which makes CT the optimal imaging modality for evaluating the paranasal sinuses and the draining pathway through the ostium and into the nasal cavity. CT is the accepted gold standard for imaging chronic inflammatory changes and their operative management. It also is the best tool for investigating complications of sinusitis and, along with MRI, for examining masses in the sinuses or surrounding soft tissue. These conditions are discussed later in this chapter.

Our current technique on a 64-slice unit is to perform axial scans (which is easier for the patient) at 5 mm reconstructed down to 0.625 mm. We scan at 100 kV with 40 mA for 0.8 seconds (32 mA). Coronal and sagittal reformatted images are obtained.

With the advent of functional endoscopic sinus surgery (FESS) for treating chronic inflammatory disease, the role of CT has expanded further.[22] Coronal imaging simulates the view through the endoscope and provides information not only about the extent of inflammation, but also regarding anatomic features that are intimately related to the pathogenesis of the disease process itself. The goal of FESS is to maintain the normal drainage pathway (the OMU) of the frontal, maxillary, and anterior ethmoid sinuses. The OMU, which is in the region of the middle meatus, consists of the ostia, infundibulum, hiatus semilunaris, and middle meatus itself. This anatomy is exquisitely shown with coronal imaging through the nose and sinuses (see Fig. 18-44). Blockage of this pathway by inflammatory tissue or exudate allows mucus and debris to accumulate in the sinus air cells and predisposes to infection. It has been suggested that anatomic variants in the OMU such as a deviated nasal septum, large concha bullosa (aerated middle turbinates), and paradoxically bent middle turbinates (concave medially, rather than the normal configuration, which is bent concave laterally) predispose to blockage of the pathway and disease. Similarly, large Haller cells (ethmoid cells located along the rim of the orbit and protruding into the maxillary antrum), ethmoid bullae (ethmoid air cells above and posterior to the infundibulum), and large Agger nasi cells (the most anterior ethmoid air cells) have been thought to compromise the drainage route and result in disease. These variants are common in asymptomatic persons, however, and have little clinical significance (see Fig. 18-5, A and C, and Fig. 18-45).[23,24]

The role of CT before endoscopic surgery also is important to assess anatomic variations that could predispose a person to have complications. The height of the cribriform plate may vary 17 mm on either side of the crista galli. It also is important to note areas of dehiscence in the cribriform plate, which are reported to be present 14% of the time.

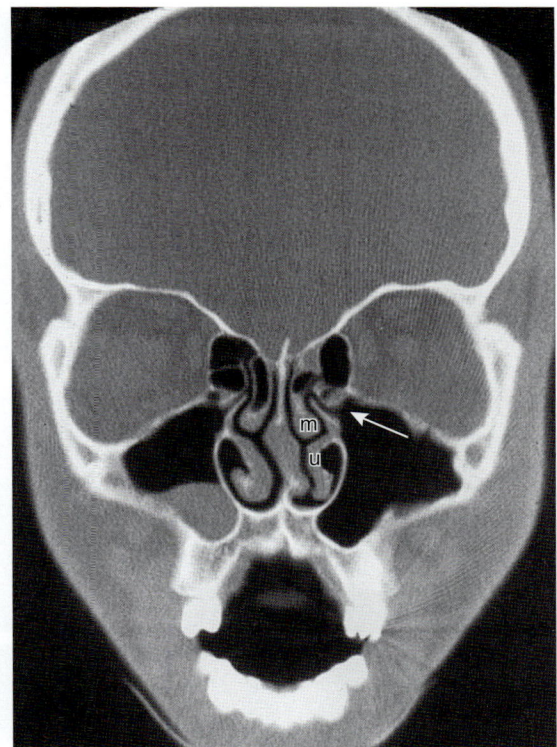

Figure 18-44 Coronal section through the midsinuses and nose showing the osteomeatal unit. Note the mucous retention cyst in the right maxillary antrum and concha bullosa in the right middle turbinate. The patient has no history or evidence of sinus disease. The ostium (opening) (*arrow*), infundibulum (airspace superior to ostia and lateral to the uncinate process of the inferior turbinate (*u*)), and middle turbinate (*m*) are shown. The circular airspace above the uncinate process is the hiatus semilunaris

No bone is found between the carotid artery and the sphenoid sinus in about 8% to 10% of the population. Also, the relationship of the optic nerve to the posterior ethmoid and sphenoid sinuses should be noted because the posterior ethmoid air cells contact the optic canal in 48% of people, and 78% to 88% of people have a very thin or no bony border between the optic nerve and the sphenoid sinus.

CT also is the study of choice for documenting complications of FESS (e-Fig. 18-46). Orbital hematomas may occur after transection of an ethmoidal artery and could potentially expand, compromising flow in the retinal artery and resulting in ischemia of the optic nerve. Postoperative cerebrospinal fluid leaks are well assessed with nuclear medicine or new cisternographic MRI techniques. CT also may provide ancillary anatomic information in these cases, and CT cisternography is a newer technique being explored. Pseudoaneurysm, is a rare complication of FESS and can be identified with CT angiography, magnetic resonance angiography, or conventional angiography.

CT is considerably more sensitive than plain radiographs in detecting rhinosinusitis. On CT scans obtained for other reasons, 100% of asymptomatic children who had a recent upper respiratory tract infection showed soft tissue changes in their sinus. Seventy percent of pediatric patients show soft tissue changes in CT scans performed for unrelated problems.[8-21] The specificity is low, and the problem

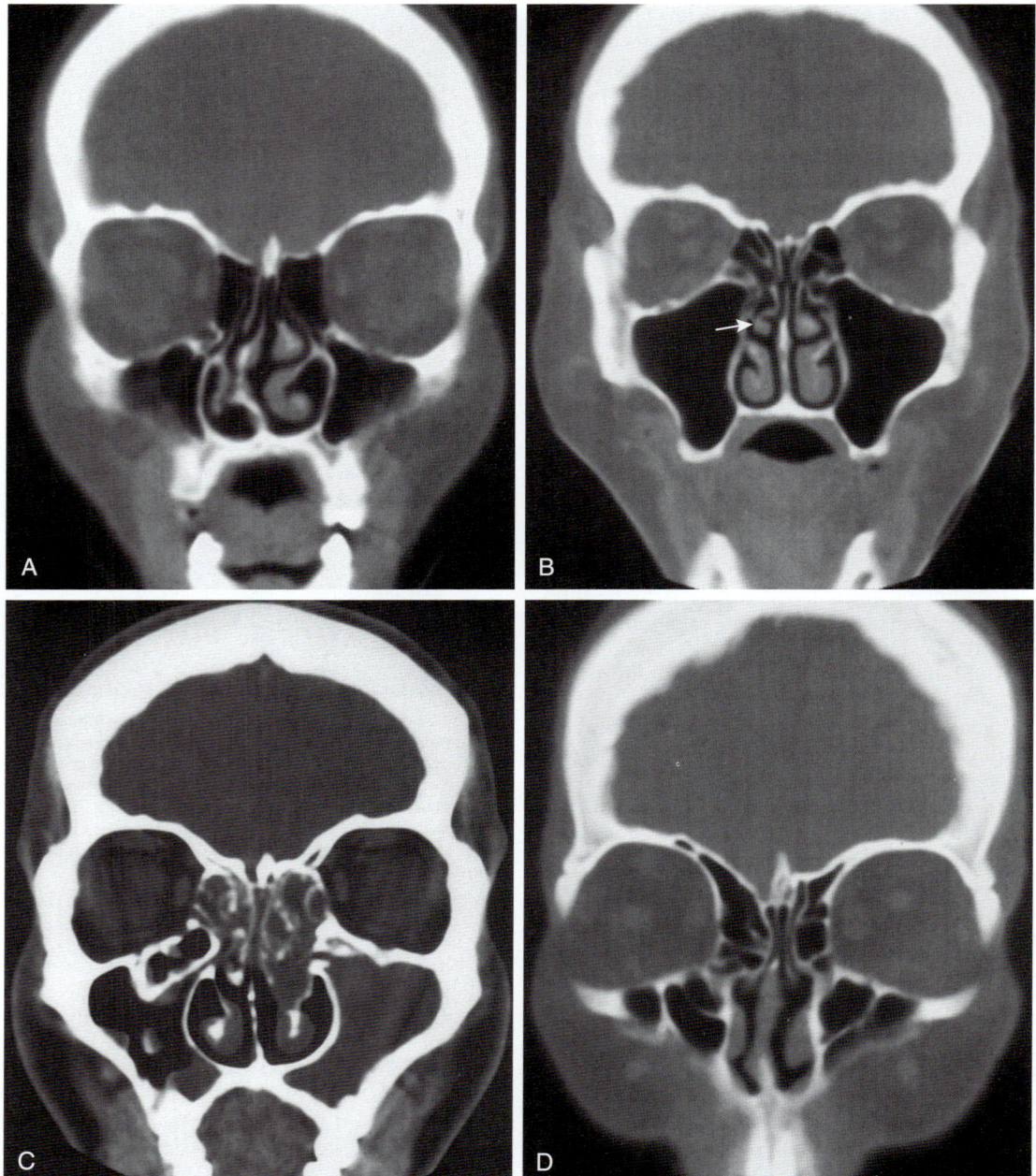

Figure 18-45   Normal variants of the nose. **A,** A deviated nasal septum. **B,** A paradoxically bent middle turbinate (*arrow*). **C,** Haller air cell (ethmoid cells located along the rim of the ostia and protruding into the maxillary antrum). **D,** Large agger nasi air cells—the most anterior air cells.

becomes an even larger issue as the use of CT for the investigation of inflammatory disease increases. Subsequently, CT should be used in cases of acute disease only when the patient is unresponsive to medical treatment, and CT should be used to assess chronic disease only when surgery is being considered.

MAGNETIC RESONANCE IMAGING

Although MRI of the paranasal sinuses is not widely advocated for assessment of inflammatory disease, it is well accepted for studying masses in this region. Limitations exist when using this modality to image the sinuses, however. Neither

bone nor air provides a signal, and thus with MRI, the bony framework and changes that are so important in the imaging of sinus disease are not visualized. It takes longer to obtain the images with MRI than with other modalities, and motion causes profound degradation of images. Most young children require sedation when MRI is performed.

The normal nasal cycle of vasodilation and mucosal edema followed by vasoconstriction and mucosal shrinkage causes signal changes that can result in problems in interpreting findings.[9,25] This cycle varies from 50 minutes to 6 hours, and the signal intensity during the edematous phase is indistinguishable from that of inflammatory change. As is the case with CT and plain radiographs, there is a high incidence of findings in asymptomatic persons (13% to 37%), and mucosal thickening less than 3 mm likely is insignificant. MRI usually is not used to image inflammatory disease, but it plays an important role in examining complex or intracranial extension of inflammatory disease or as part of the workup of a sinus or parasinal neoplasm.

Although most acute inflammatory diseases, including polyps, mucoceles, and retention cysts, produce a bright signal on T2-weighted images, 90% to 95% of tumors in the sinuses or nasal cavity exhibit moderately lower signal intensities on T2 weighting. This phenomenon largely occurs because these lesions are histologically cellular and homogeneous. More mature granulation tissue and fibrosis are difficult to distinguish from tumor because these too produce a lower T2 signal. Certain fungal infections, in contrast to other acute inflammatory disease, also exhibit a lower signal on T2 weighting.

Key Points

Maxillary air cells are present at birth.
Frontal air cells are seen between 6 and 12 years of age.
Ethmoid air cells are present at birth.
Sphenoid air cells are not present at birth.
Plain radiographic examination of the sinuses has extremely limited utility, especially in children younger than 2 years.
With all imaging modalities, a high incidence of sinus opacification or mucosal thickening occurs in asymptomatic persons

The head is larger relative to the face in neonates and infants.
Obliteration of the sutures is not complete until the second to third decade of life.
Cranial variants of normal in a child up to age 2 years include wormian bones, Inca bone, and bathrocephaly.
Cranial variants of normal children and juveniles include the paracondylar process, digital markings, and Pacchionian bodies (granulations).

Suggested Readings

Barghouth G, Prior JO, Lepori D, et al. Paranasal sinuses in children: size evaluation of maxillary, sphenoid, and frontal sinuses by magnetic resonance imaging and proposal of volume index percentile curves. *Eur Radiol.* 2002;12:1451-1458.

Belden CJ. The skull base and calvaria: adult and pediatric. *Neuroimaging Clin N Am.* 1998;8:1-20.

Bhattacharyya N, Jones DT, Hill M, et al. The diagnostic accuracy of computed tomography in pediatric chronic rhinosinusitis. *Arch Otolaryngol Head Neck Surg.* 2004;130:1029-1032.

Huda W. Assessment of the problem: pediatric doses in screen-film and digital radiography. *Pediatr Radiol.* 2004;34(suppl 3):S173-S182.

Mann SS, Naidich TP, Towbin RB, et al. Imaging of postnatal maturation of the skull base. *Neuroimaging Clin N Am.* 2000;10:1-22.

References

Full references for this chapter can be found on www.expertconsult.com.

Chapter 19

Prenatal Imaging

ASHLEY JAMES ROBINSON, SUSAN BLASER, and A. MICHELLE FINK

The fetal abnormalities described in this chapter are those most likely to be assessed by a pediatric radiologist who primarily performs fetal magnetic resonance imaging (MRI), computed tomography (CT), radiography, and ultrasound. These additional modalities are particularly useful for acquiring further characterization of fetal abnormalities, especially when a fetal autopsy will be declined but a couple needs to be counseled regarding future pregnancies.

In most of the references provided, a combination of prenatal ultrasound plus MRI and/or CT was performed. The suggested reading list includes references to several standard ultrasound texts that deal with the subject matter from the perspective of ultrasound as the primary imaging modality.

Scalp

A scalp cyst, although infrequently encountered, is likely to require further assessment by fetal MRI. The most important differential diagnosis is between an ectodermal cyst and a meningocele or encephalocele.[1-3] A fetus with an ectodermal cyst should have no underlying skull defect or transiting vessels or membranes, and the underlying brain should be normal. Because of limitations of resolution, small defects and thus the diagnosis of meningocele can be missed when MRI is used (e-Fig. 19-1).[4]

Hemangioma is another scalp abnormality that occurs infrequently but occasionally is reported (Fig. 19-2). The main differential diagnosis is encephalocele.[5,6] Further evaluation by fetal MRI can be helpful in demonstrating the absence of a skull defect or an abnormality of the underlying brain.[1,7-9]

Other lesions that should be considered in the differential diagnosis of scalp abnormalities include lymphatic malformation, edema, a sarcoma, and a teratoma perforating the skull.[1,10] Rare abnormalities that have been described on antenatal imaging include gyriform thickening of the scalp in fetuses with cutis verticis gyrata associated with Noonan syndrome[11] and hamartomata of the scalp in fetuses with encephalocraniocutaneous lipomatosis.[12]

Skull

Skull defects are a result of errors in dorsal induction, the process whereby the neural tube forms and closes (neurulation).[13,14] A spectrum of anomalies is characterized by absent flat bones of the skull.

LARGE BONY DEFECTS

Acalvaria

"Acalvaria" is the term used when the bony skull vault, meninges, and scalp muscles are absent and a normal brain is covered by skin only. "Acrania" is the term used when the skull vault, scalp muscles, and skin are absent and a dysplastic brain is covered by meninges only.[15]

Exencephaly

Exencephaly is the combination of acrania with abnormal brain tissue[15] and has been demonstrated to be the predecessor of anencephaly.[16,17] Exencephaly can be seen in association with amniotic band sequence[18-20] and limb body wall complex,[21] but can be distinguished from them because they generally form asymmetric skull defects (e-Fig. 19-3).[13]

Anencephaly

Anencephaly, which is the single most common open neural tube defect,[22] is characterized by acrania with complete absence of a normal brain above the brainstem (e-Fig. 19-3, A).[13,14] It is the end result of exencephaly with mechanical and chemical attrition of the abnormal brain tissue in utero[15]; the remaining tissue constitutes a mass of exposed vascular neural tissue. The cartilaginous skull is intact. This condition invariably is fatal. When accompanied by dysraphism of the entire spine, it is known as craniorachischisis.[13] Fetal MRI findings have been described in cases associated with omphalocele[23] and pentalogy of Cantrell.[24]

FOCAL BONY DEFECTS

Cephaloceles

Focal defects in the skull can allow internal structures to herniate. The terminology changes depending on whether the contents of the hernia include just meninges and cerebrospinal fluid (cephalocele), brain matter (encephalocele), or a ventricle (encephalocystocele). Most defects are in the midline, they generally are occipital (Fig. 19-4),[13,14] and they usually contain dysplastic brain tissue and venous sinuses.[14] They also can be part of syndromes such as Meckel-Gruber, Dandy-Walker, and Chiari III malformation.[13,14] The most common type of encephalocele in Southeast Asia is fronto-ethmoidal, particularly in children of tea garden workers in Assam, northeastern India.[25]

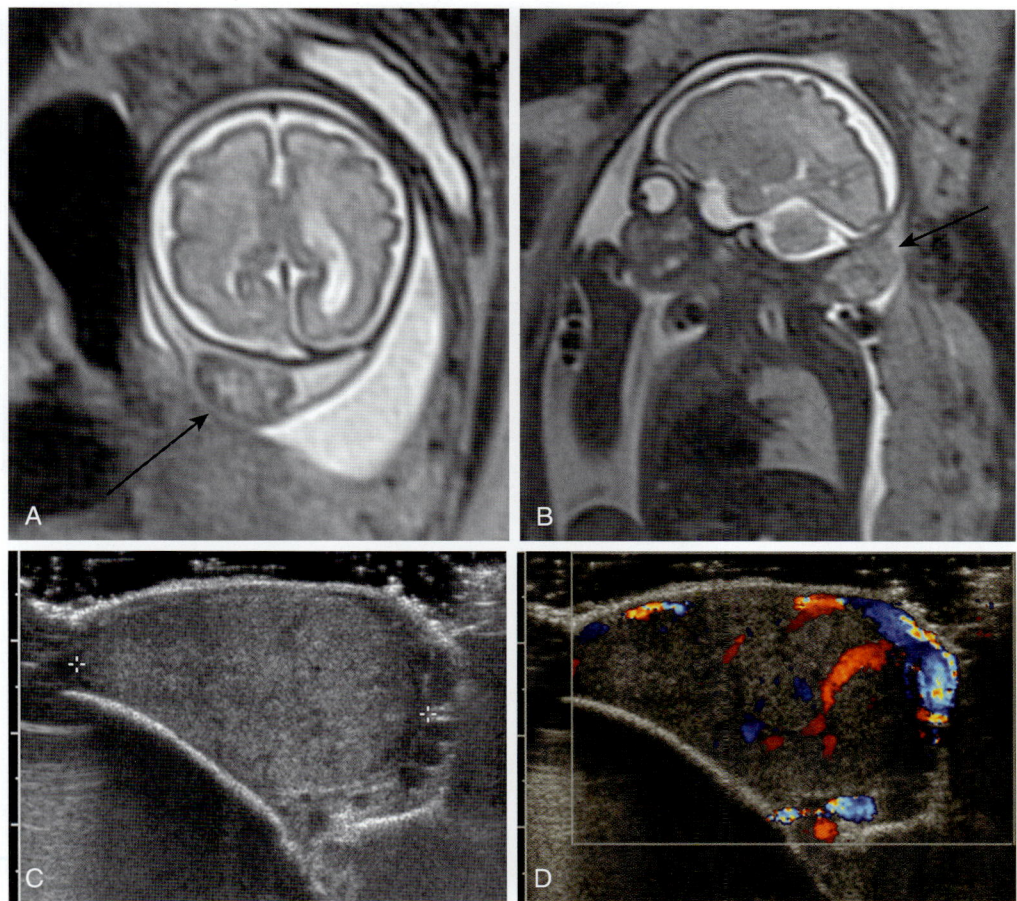

Figure 19-2 A scalp hemangioma. **A,** A fetal magnetic resonance image (MRI) shows a heterogeneous mass in the occipital scalp (*arrow*). The skull appears intact. **B,** A fetal MRI shows a sagittal view of a mass in the occipital scalp (*arrow*). **C,** A postnatal ultrasound image shows a heterogeneous mass in the scalp. The skull appears to be intact. **D,** A postnatal ultrasound image with Doppler shows vascular flow throughout.

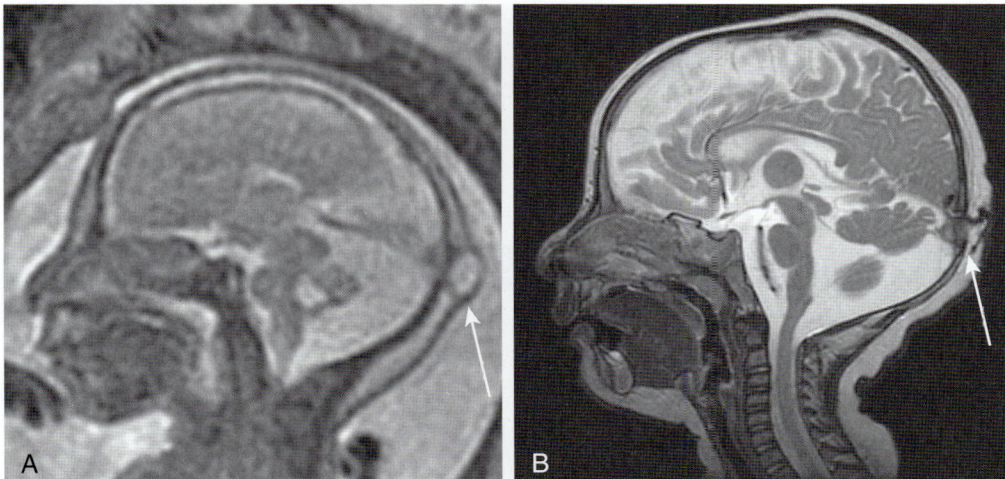

Figure 19-4 A cephalocele. **A,** A fetal magnetic resonance image (MRI) shows a small occipital cyst (*arrow*) with abnormal cerebellar vermis. **B,** A postnatal MRI shows an atretic cephalocele with a scalp abnormality (*arrow*). (From Robinson AJ, Blaser S, Toi A, et al. The fetal cerebellar vermis: assessment for abnormal development by ultrasonography and magnetic resonance imaging. *Ultrasound Q.* 2007;23(3):211-223.)

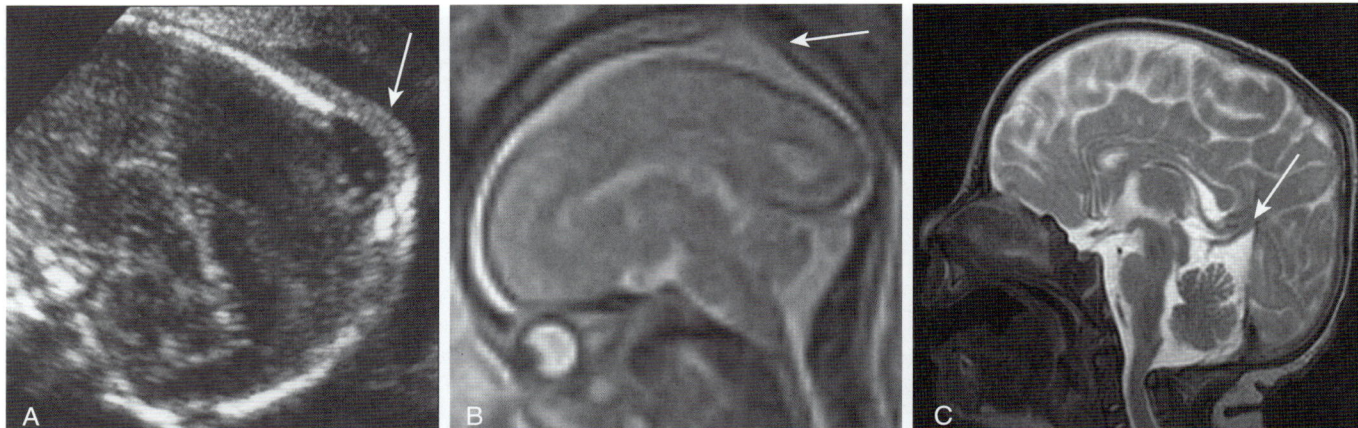

Figure 19-5 An enlarged parietal foramina. **A,** A fetal ultrasound image shows a skull defect with intact overlying scalp (*arrow*). **B,** A fetal magnetic resonance image (MRI) shows a skull defect that does not contain brain (*arrow*). **C,** A postnatal MRI shows a skull defect that now contains brain. An abnormal course of a straight sinus is present (*arrow*). (From Fink AM, Maixner W. Enlarged parietal foramina: MR imaging features in the fetus and neonate. *AJNR Am J Neuroradiol.* 2006;27:1379-1381.)

Fetal MRI can be useful to differentiate a cephalocele from a scalp cyst and to determine if it contains brain tissue.[1,26] Large encephaloceles can appear similar to anencephaly, although the calvarium typically has developed to some extent.[13] An atretic cephalocele typically presents as a midline subcutaneous nodule or cyst,[27] and underlying venous anomalies often are present that are similar to those seen with enlarged parietal foramina.[28-30]

Enlarged Parietal Foramina

Enlarged parietal foramina are thought to be the result of defective ossification of the membranous skull. During fetal life they comprise a large central defect that, because of subsequent ossification, including midline ossification (Fig. 19-5), become bilateral symmetric defects.[31] In contradistinction, encephaloceles typically are midline or unilateral. Enlarged parietal foramina can be large defects, typically closing almost completely during childhood, leaving only small bilateral foramina.[27,32] Although typically benign, they can be associated with hypoplasia or atresia of the straight sinus with a persistent falcine sinus draining to the straight sinus at the level of the anomaly, which has been demonstrated on fetal MRI.[27,31] Associated abnormalities of occipital cortical infolding can be seen postnatally.[33] Enlarged parietal foramina can be hereditary (autosomal dominant), with genes *MSX2* and *ALX4* reported to be associated with the condition.[34] Enlarged

parietal foramina also can be syndromic, as in Potocki–Shaffer syndrome.[35]

MINERALIZATION DEFECTS

A prenatal ultrasound examination reveals defective skull mineralization in fetuses with several skeletal dysplasias. Plain film radiography of the pregnant patient increasingly is being utilized, and fetal three-dimensional CT is proving to be an emerging technique in the further evaluation of fetal skeletal dysplasias[1,14,22,36-42] The main skeletal dysplasias that result in poor skull mineralization are osteogenesis imperfecta type IIa (e-Fig. 19-6), hypophosphatasia congenita, and achondrogenesis.[36] A summary of distinguishing features is provided in Table 19-1.

SIZE AND SHAPE ABNORMALITIES

Microcrania and macrocrania are defined when the head circumference differs more than three standard deviations from the mean in either direction.[22]

Microcrania

The birth incidence of microcrania is 1:1000.[37] Microcrania often is the result of an underlying small brain, that is, microcephaly[1] (e-Fig. 19-7). Causes include genetic syndromes,[37]

Table 19-1 Skull Abnormalities in Common Lethal Skeletal Dysplasias

Skull Type	Mineralization	Size	Shape	Trunk Length	Fractures
Osteogenesis imperfecta (type IIa)	Demineralized	Normal	Deformable	Short	Many
Hypophosphatasia	Demineralized	Normal	Deformable	Normal	Few
Achondrogenesis	Type I demineralized Type II normal	Large	Normal	Short	Few
Thanatophoric dysplasia	Normal	Large (megalencephaly)	Type I normal Type II cloverleaf	Normal	None

Modified from Glanc P, Chitayat D, Unger S. The fetal musculoskeletal system. In: Rumack CM, Wilson SR, Charboneau JW, eds. *Diagnostic ultrasound.* 3rd ed. St Louis: Elsevier; 2005.

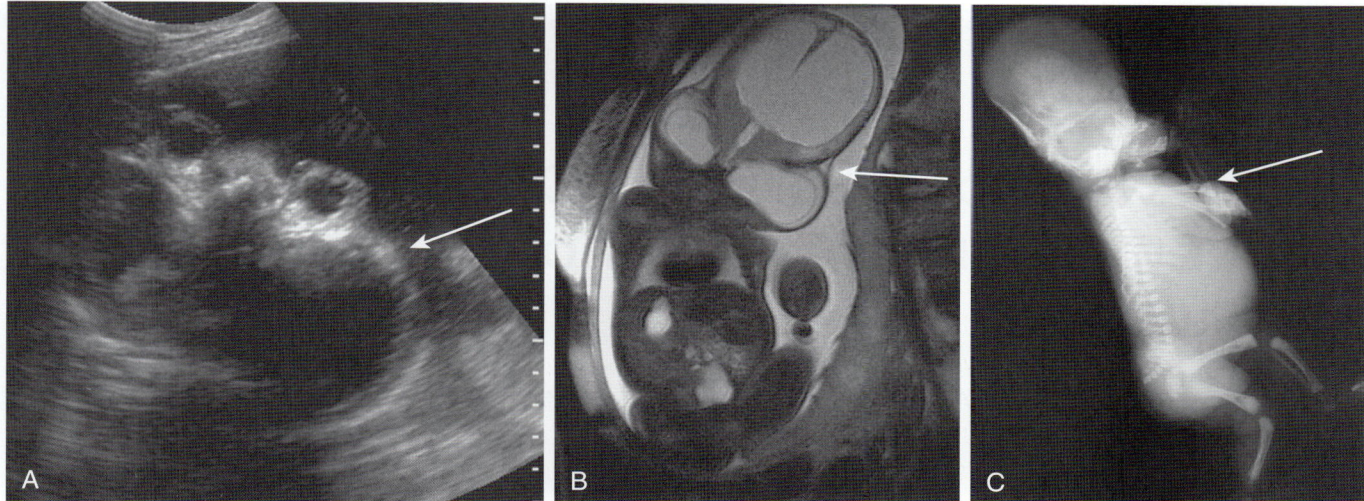

Figure 19-10 Cloverleaf skull. **A,** A fetal ultrasound shows bossing of the temporal bones (*arrow*) and bulging eyes in a case of acrocephalosyndactyly. **B,** A fetal magnetic resonance image in the coronal view shows bossing of temporal bones (*arrow*) and frontal bones. Severe ventriculomegaly is noted. **C,** A postmortem radiograph shows a severe cloverleaf skull with midface hypoplasia. Note elbow ankylosis typical of Pfeiffer syndrome. (**A** From Robinson AJ, Blaser S, Toi A, et al. Magnetic resonance imaging of the fetal eyes—morphologic and biometric assessment for abnormal development with ultrasonographic and clinicopathologic correlation. *Pediatr Radiol.* 2008;38:971-981.)

chromosomal defects (typically trisomy 13[14]), hemorrhage, teratogens, infection, radiation,[37] and encephalocele.[1,14]

Macrocrania

Macrocrania typically is seen as a result of fetal hydrocephalus. Other causes include hydrancephaly,[14,38] intracranial teratoma or astrocytoma, and, occasionally, rarer tumors.[1,39] Skeletal dysplasias that cause enlargement of the head include achondrogenesis (type 1)[36] and thanatophoric dysplasia (e-Fig. 19-8) due to an enlarged brain (megalencephaly), with preferential enlargement of the temporal lobes and coexistent cerebral malformations, in particular, abnormal premature temporal lobe sulcation, which has been demonstrated by both fetal ultrasound and MRI.[40,41] Partial callosal dysgenesis also has been reported in fetuses with this condition.[42] Table 19-1 summarizes these distinguishing features.

Dysmorphism

Lemon-Shaped Skull and Spina Bifida

A lemon-shaped skull, characterized by a concave or linear contour at the level of the coronal sutures (the "lemon sign"), is a well-known morphologic finding that is highly sensitive for open neural tube defects (see e-Fig. 19-9).[43,44] However, it has a poor positive predictive value in low-risk fetuses and is seen in fetuses with other pathologies, including encephalocele and a variety of nonneural tube structural anomalies.[22,45-47] This sign may be encountered during fetal MRI evaluation of neural tube defects.[48]

Cloverleaf Skull (Kleeblattschädel)

A cloverleaf appearance occurs as a result of bilateral coronal and lambdoid synostosis and is found in fetuses with type II thanatophoric dysplasia (see Fig. 19-10).[1,36,41] Cloverleaf skull also has been used to describe the dysmorphic appearance of the skull in fetuses with syndromic craniosynostosis,[49-51] and

which in prenatal life is often associated with abnormal karyotype, as described in Chapter 20. Several case reports have described the use of fetal MRI in its antenatal diagnosis.[49,52,53]

Strawberry Skull

A strawberry-shaped skull, characterized by flattening of the occiput and pointing of the frontal bones, is seen by ultrasound on the submentobregmatic section and is characteristic of fetuses with trisomy 18.[54] This appearance also has been described in fetal thanatophoric dwarfism.[55]

Key Points

Prenatal MRI can be used to differentiate between simple ectodermal cysts and meningoceles or encephaloceles.

Prenatal MRI can be used to differentiate between solid extracranial masses and encephaloceles or perforating intracranial tumors.

Prenatal MRI can be used to differentiate (benign) skull foramina from more serious skull defects.

Use of prenatal three-dimensional CT in the workup of skeletal dysplasias is growing.

Suggested Readings

Glanc P, Chitayat D, Unger S. The fetal musculoskeletal system. In: Rumack CM, Wilson SR, Charboneau JW, eds. *Diagnostic ultrasound*. 3rd ed. St Louis, MO: Mosby Elsevier; 2005, pp 1433-1440.

McGahan JP. Fetal head and brain. In: McGahan JP, Goldberg BB, eds. *Diagnostic ultrasound*. 2nd ed. New York: Informa Healthcare; 2008.

Toi A. The fetal head and brain. In: Rumack CM, Wilson SR, Charboneau JW, eds. *Diagnostic ultrasound*. 3rd ed. St Louis: Mosby; 2005.

References

Full references for this chapter can be found on www.expertconsult.com.

Chapter 20

Craniosynostosis, Selected Craniofacial Syndromes, and Other Abnormalities of the Skull

THOMAS L. SLOVIS, ARLENE A. ROZZELLE, and WILLIAM H. McALISTER

The basic clinical and radiologic features of craniosynostosis result either from lack of sutural formation or from premature fusion of contiguous portions of calvarial bones across the membranous sutures between them. The prevalence of premature sutural closures is displayed in e-Table 20-1.[1] Normal sutures permit growth of the skull in a direction perpendicular to their long axes. With normal endocranial stimulus to growth, cessation of growth in one suture is compensated by increased growth in others, with resulting craniofacial deformity (e-Table 20-2; Figs. 20-1 through 20-4).

The deformity of the shape of the head is present before the bony sutural changes are seen. Only a portion of the bony suture needs to be closed to have craniosynostosis (e-Fig. 20-5). The suture-associated dura mater is responsible for determining the development of the cranial suture. The dura supplies osteoinductive growth factors (e.g., transforming growth factor-β or fibroblast growth factor-2) and cellular elements. Abnormal head shape secondary to abnormal suture development can be diagnosed in utero at 13 weeks' gestational age.[2,3] Craniosynostosis is associated with genetic abnormalities (e-Box 20-1) and is a secondary finding in many systemic disorders (e-Box 20-2).[4]

Specific head shapes are associated with sutural synostoses (e-Fig. 20-6). The normal head has an egg shape, being widest in the parietal area posterior to the ears with a narrower, gently rounded forehead (Fig. 20-7).

Sagittal synosotosis is characterized by a long and narrow head (see Figs. 20-3 and 20-4). The back is usually narrower than the front, and anterior or posterior bossing may exist. *Metopic synostosis* (trigonocephaly) results in a triangular shape of the whole forehead (not just a rounded forehead with a ridge superimposed) (Fig. 20-8; see e-Fig. 20-6).

Unicoronal synostosis results in flattening of the ipsilateral forehead, flattening of the ipsilateral occipital area, the "harlequin eye" (the sphenoid is drawn up toward the closed suture and is thickened), ipsilateral temporal bulging and cheek protrusion, contralateral forehead bossing, and deviation of the nose away from the synostosed side (Fig. 20-9). Features that distinguish unicoronal synostosis from anterior deformational plagiocephaly are listed in e-Table 20-3.

Bicoronal synostosis causes a brachycephalic head (i.e., the head is wide and short). The supraorbital rims and forehead are recessed with bitemporal and upper forehead bulging (Fig. 20-10).

Lambdoid synostosis results in ipsilateral occipital flattening with compensatory bulging at the superior and inferior axes where the suture should have been (e-Fig. 20-11). The features differentiating unilateral lambdoid synostosis from posterior deformational plagiocephaly are listed in e-Table 20-4.

Synostosis of multiple sutures occurs in 14%, and the resultant head shape depends on which sutures are closed.[1] The *kleeblattschädel* ("cloverleaf skull") anomaly may result when all sutures except the squamosal are closed, resulting in severe temporal and vertex bulging with exophthalmos (Fig. 20-12). Unusual minor synostosis may exist, causing abnormal skull appearance.[5-8]

Microcrania, or a small neurocranium, may result when all sutures are closed. This usually occurs with failure of brain growth. Rarely, it may occur without failure of brain growth, and the child may develop increased intracranial pressure (Fig. 20-13).

Deformities Mimicking Craniosynostosis

Cranial deformities mimicking synostosis may result from static forces such as intrauterine crowding or prolonged recumbency. The term *plagiocephaly* refers to any flattening of the calvarium without denoting an etiology and is preceded by terms that describe the location and side (e.g., right posterior plagiocephaly). Postnatal deformational plagiocephaly may affect primarily the forehead or the occipital area. Since the 1993 recommendation by the American Academy of Pediatrics to put infants to sleep on their backs, a marked increase is seen in occipital deformational plagiocephaly (e-Fig. 20-14). The ipsilateral occipital area is flattened, with flattening of the contralateral forehead, malposition of the ipsilateral external ear, protrusion of the ipsilateral cheek, and compensatory bulging of the ipsilateral forehead and contralateral occipital area. Viewed from above, the head has a parallelogram shape (Fig. 20-15).

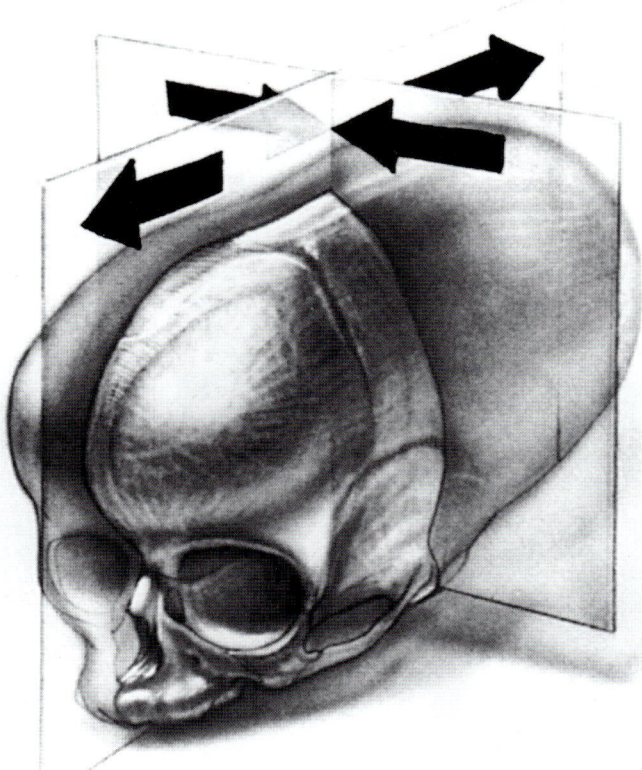

Figure 20-1　A schematic drawing of a child's skull with sagittal synosto-sis, in which growth of the skull is restricted in a plane perpendicular to the fused suture and elongated in a plane parallel to that fused suture. (From Sulica RL, Grunfast KM. Otologic manifestations of craniosynostosis syndromes. In: Cohen Jr MM, MacLean RE, eds. *Craniosynostosis.* New York: Oxford University Press; 2000:211.)

Perisutural sclerosis of the lambdoid may be seen on a plain radiograph; however, the suture is open. The concept of a "sticky lambdoid suture" is no longer considered valid.[9,10] Plagiocephaly also may occur with bony, muscular, or ocular torticollis.

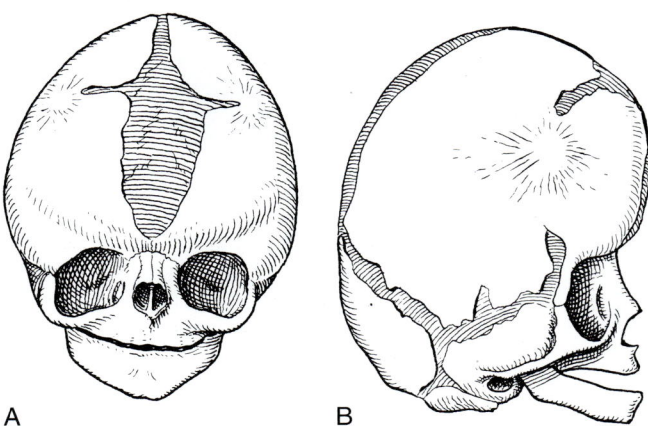

Figure 20-2　Premature synostosis of both coronal sutures. Schematic representation as seen in Apert syndrome. The suture is obliterated except for short, open terminal segments and open segments near the sagittal suture and anterior fontanel. The metopic, sagittal, lambdoid, and temporoparietal sutures all are widely open. The calvaria is short-ened in the anteroposterior direction and elongated in the craniocaudal plane. **A,** Frontal aspect. **B,** Lateral aspect.

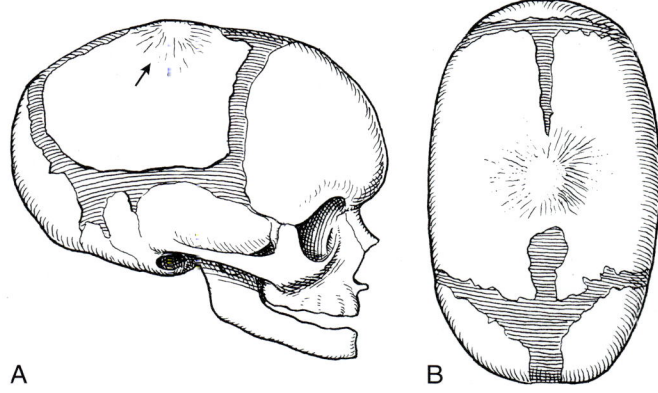

Figure 20-3　Schematic drawings of premature synostosis of the sagittal suture. **A,** Lateral aspect. **B,** Superior aspect.

In deformational plagiocephaly, the skull base (i.e., aligned from the crista galli through the foramen magnum) remains straight, with less than 7 degrees angulation, whereas in uni-lateral coronal or lambdoid synostosis, the skull base curves (Figs. 20-15 through 20-17). Pseudoscaphocephaly occurs when premature infants lie on the sides of their heads in the neonatal intensive care unit. Although the head is long and narrow, the sagittal suture is open, and the widest part of the skull is in the biparietal area.

RADIOGRAPHIC FINDINGS

Radiographic findings reflect the deformities of the cranium observed clinically. The initial examination is a skull series consisting of anteroposterior or Caldwell, Towne, and both lateral projections. The shape of the head is ascertained. The anterior fontanel should be visible at least until 7 months of age. The sagittal, coronal, and lambdoid sutures are all identi-fied. The metopic suture closes any time from before birth to after 3 months of age.[11] As many as 10% may remain open into adulthood. Closure of only a short segment of a suture is as effective in preventing separation of the opposing bones as total obliteration (see e-Fig. 20-5). The key findings to the diagnosis of craniosynostosis on skull series are (1) abnormal head shape and (2) obliteration of a portion of a suture.

According to Jane and Persing, cranial restructuring techniques have focused on (1) release of sutural synostosis, (2) remodeling of cranial bone, (3) active reduction of an abnormally long dimension of the skull, and (4) active expan-sion of abnormally narrow areas.[12]

In most instances, three-dimensional computed tomogra-phy (CT) is required in planning for cranial restructuring. It is important to keep the radiation dose as low as reasonably achievable. This is quite easy in examination for bone changes and is accomplished by lowering both the kilovolt (kV) and milliampere (mA). Exams performed at 40 mA and 100 to 120 kV at 1 second with a slice thickness of 1.25 millimeters (mm) give a CT dose index "dose" of approximately 5 mGy (500 millirads). Images are reconfigured to 0.625 mm for reformatted images and three-dimensional reconstruction (Figs. 20-16 through 20-20 and e-Fig. 20-21). In syndromic children, magnetic resonance imaging (MRI) of the brain may be performed for developmental anomalies.

Text continued on page 203.

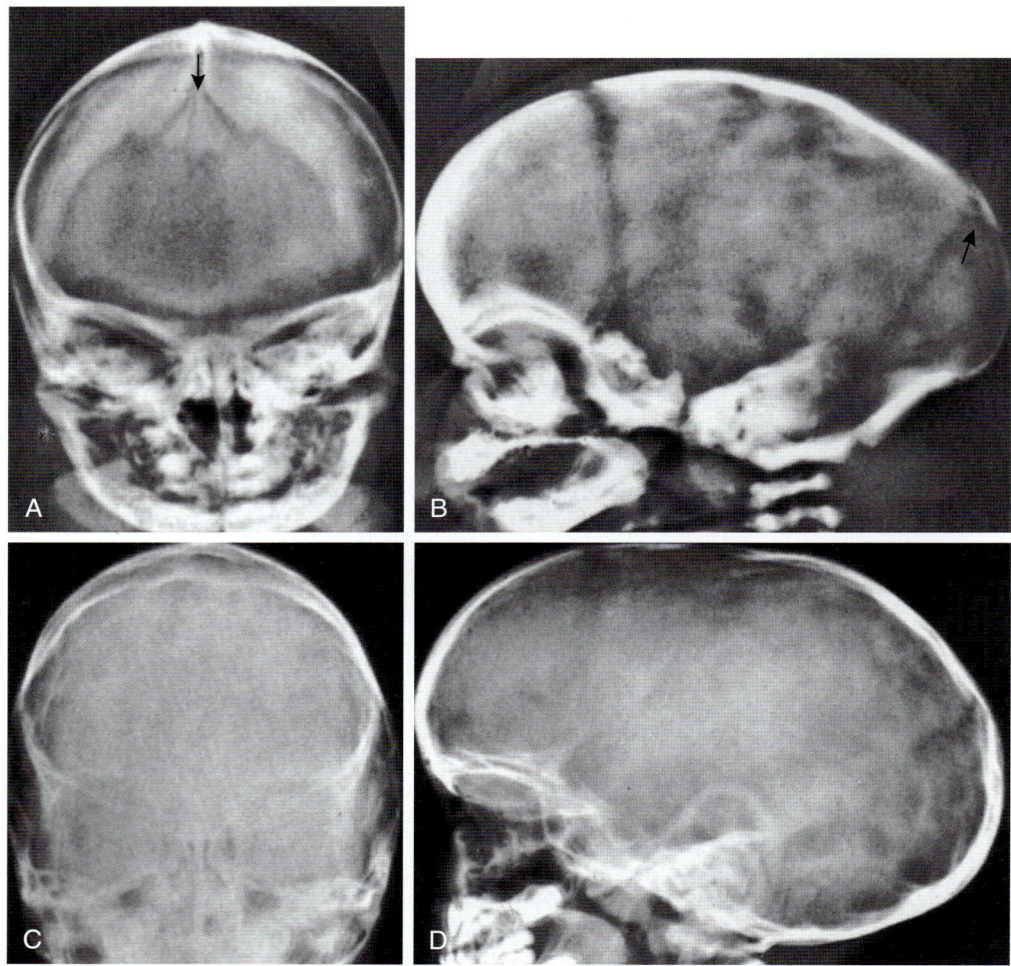

Figure 20-4 Premature synostosis of the sagittal suture with elongation of the calvaria in the occipital-frontal direction, a decrease in the transverse axis of the calvaria, and relative (to length) decrease in vertical height. The sagittal suture is ridged externally. **A** and **B,** Frontal (*A*) and lateral (*B*) projections in a 2-day-old neonate. A sutural bone is present in the region of the posterior fontanel (*arrows*). The coronal, lambdoid, and squamosal sutures are normally wide, as is the squamocondyloid synchondrosis at the base of the occipital squamosa. **C** and **D,** On frontal (*C*) and lateral (*D*) projections, similar changes are evident in the more mature skull of an 11-month-old girl.

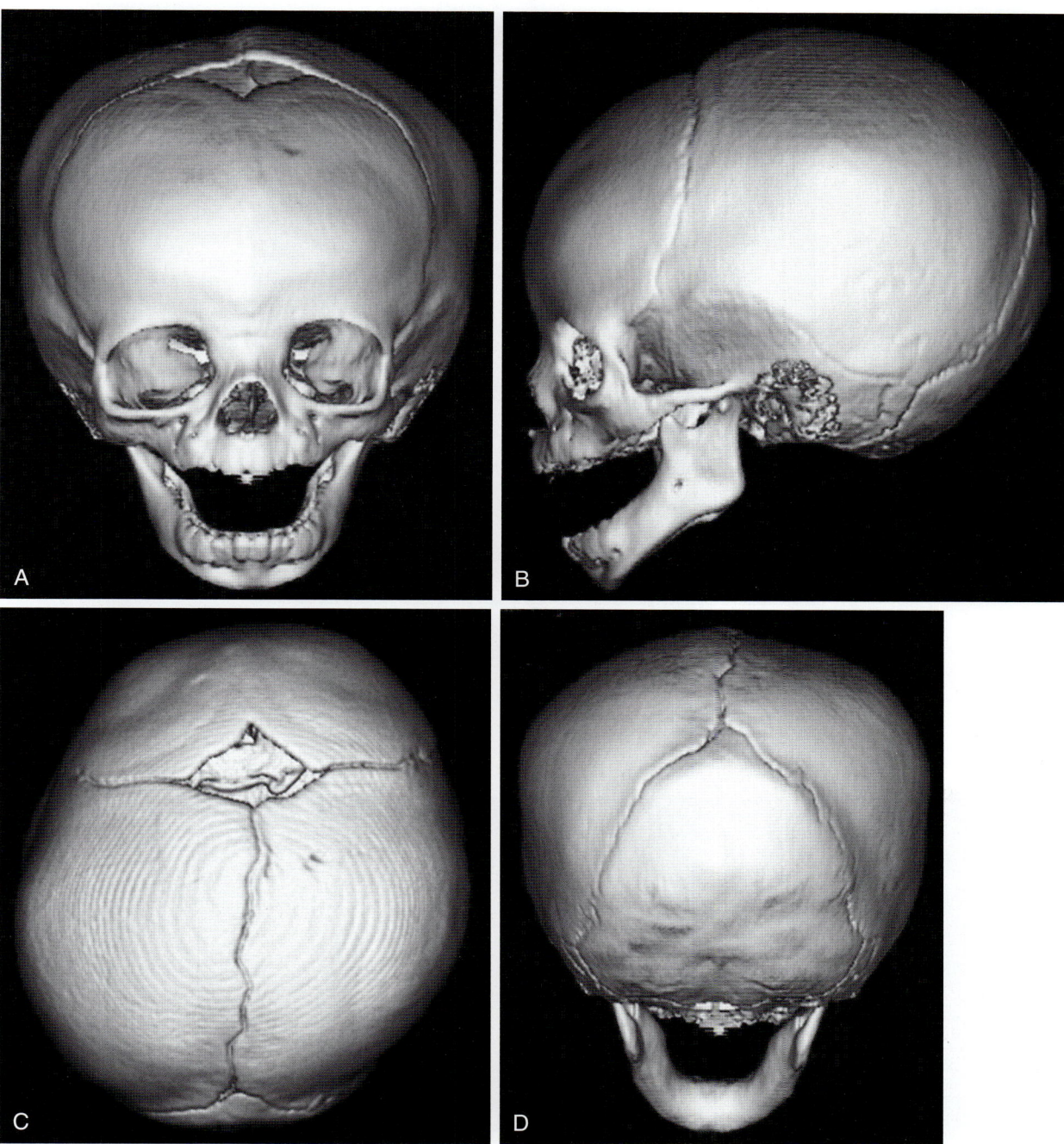

Figure 20-7   A normal three-dimensional computed tomography scan of the head in a 7-month-old infant. **A,** Frontal view clearly shows the anterior fontanel and coronal sutures. The metopic suture has closed. **B,** Lateral view shows the lambdoid and squamosal sutures and the normal coronal sutures. **C,** Bird's eye view reveals the anterior fontanel and the coronal, sagittal, and lambdoid sutures. **D,** Posterior view shows the posterior sagittal suture and the lambdoid sutures. The normal head is egg shaped, widest at the biparietal area (*C*).

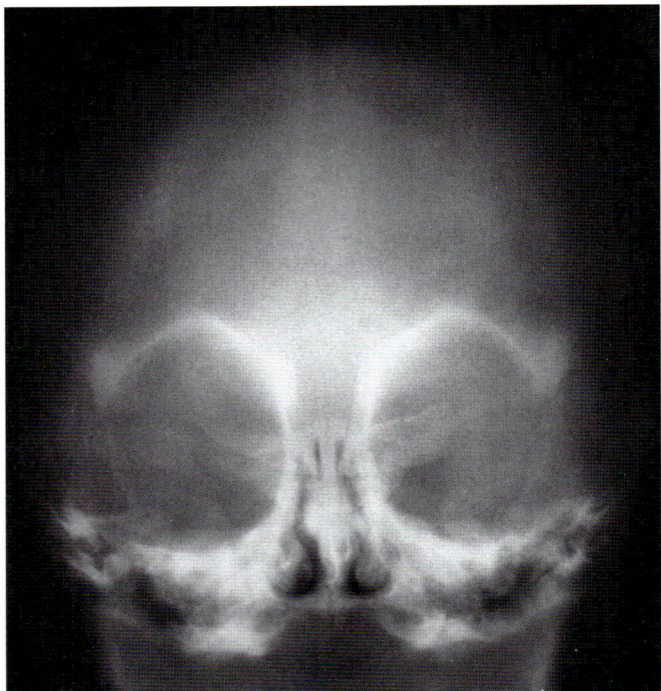

Figure 20-8 **Trigonocephaly.** Frontal projection shows the characteristic orbital hypotelorism and narrowing of the forehead. The metopic suture is invariably closed.

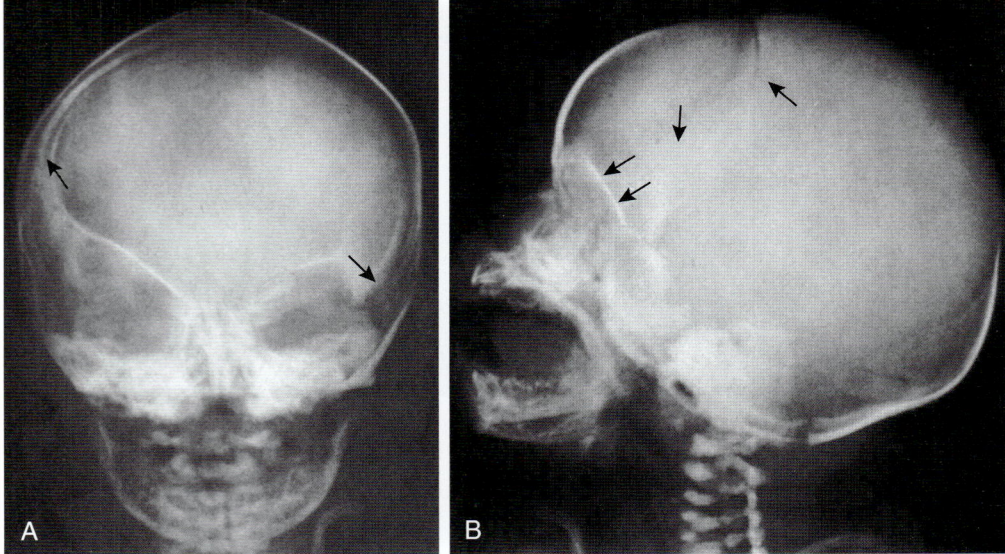

Figure 20-9 Premature synostosis of the caudal segment of the right limb of the coronal suture in a 3-week-old infant. **A,** In frontal projection, arrows are directed at the caudal ends of the right and left limbs of the coronal suture. The roof of the right orbit is lifted into a more oblique position, as is the right wing of the sphenoid. **B,** In lateral projection, the right limb of the coronal suture stops abruptly a few centimeters below the anterior fontanel. The lifting of the right orbital roof also is well seen (*two lower arrows*).

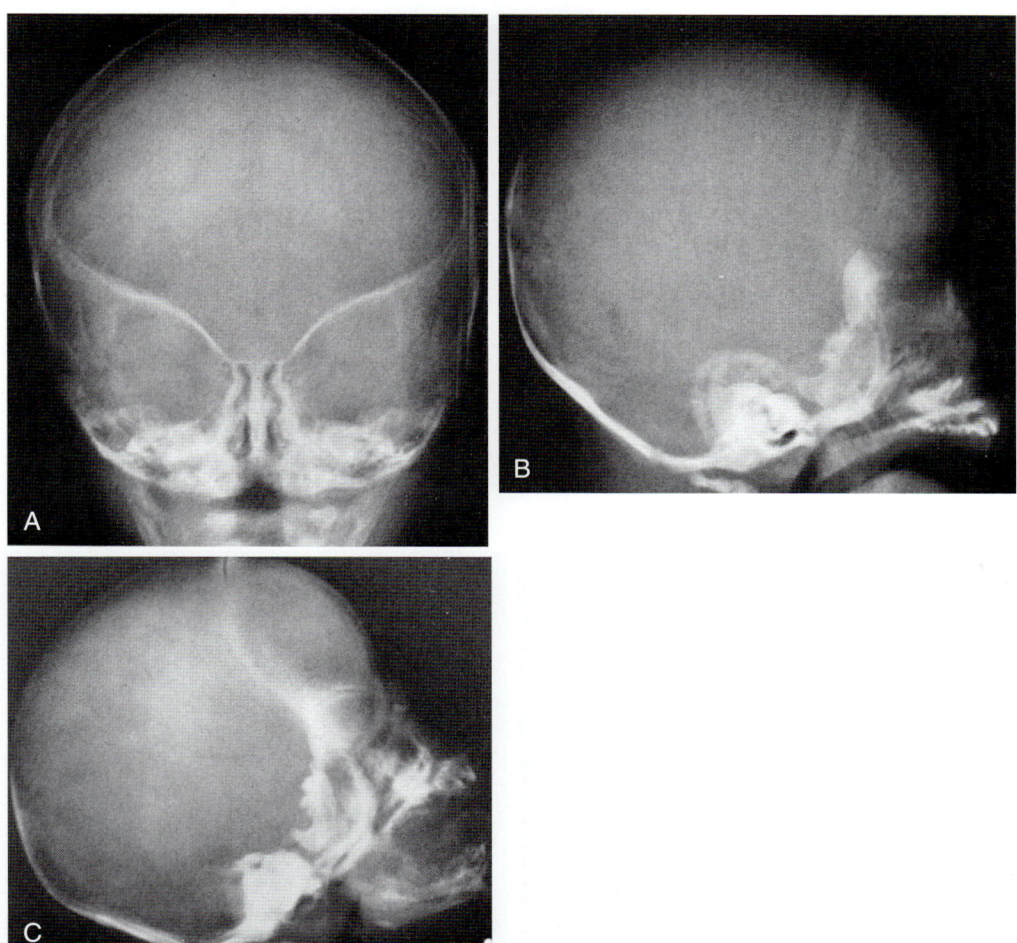

Figure 20-10 Bilateral coronal synostosis. **A,** Frontal view shows the elevated orbital roofs. **B,** The height of the skull is increased from caudad to cephalad and decreased in the anteroposterior dimension. The coronal suture is not seen. **C,** Other lateral projection showing the absence of a complete coronal suture. The head is tall (towering) and short in the anteroposterior direction.

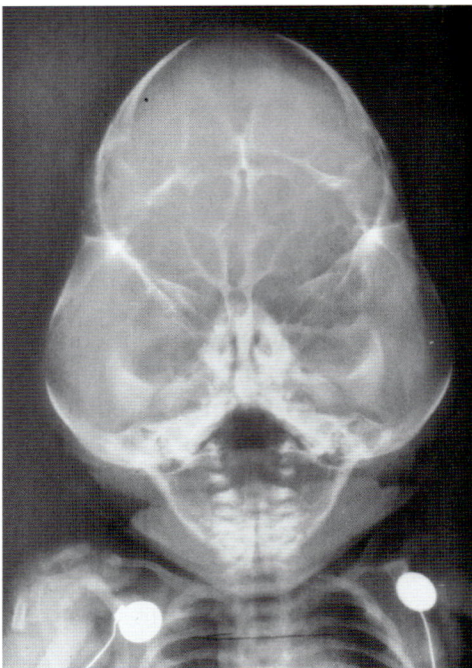

Figure 20-12   Kleeblattschädel (cloverleaf skull) anomaly. Multisuture closure has occurred, and a bizarre configuration of the face and head with bulging of the temporal region is seen.

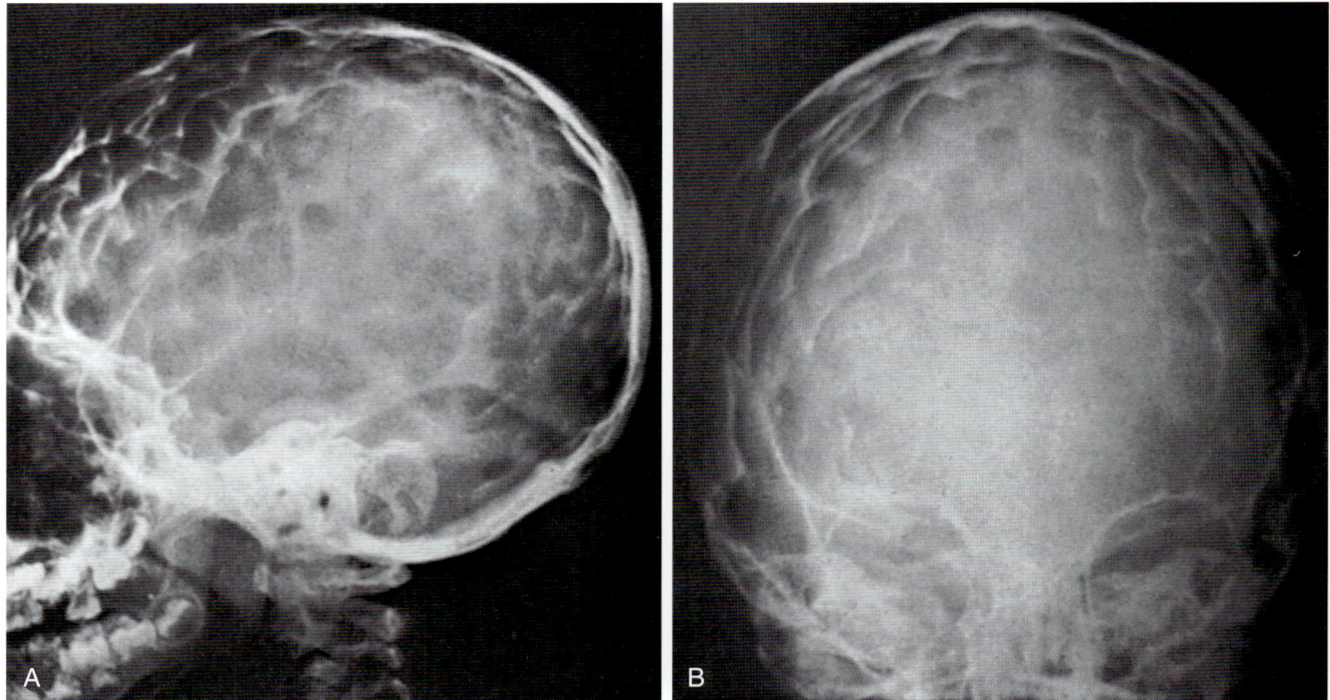

Figure 20-13   Radiographic findings in the microcephalic type of craniostenosis in a 7-year-old child. **A** and **B,** Lateral (*A*) and frontal (*B*) projections. All sutures of the cranium are obliterated, and the skull is shortened in all its diameters. The long-standing increased intracranial pressure is indicated by the heavy convolutional markings. Detailed anatomy of the sellae is not seen.

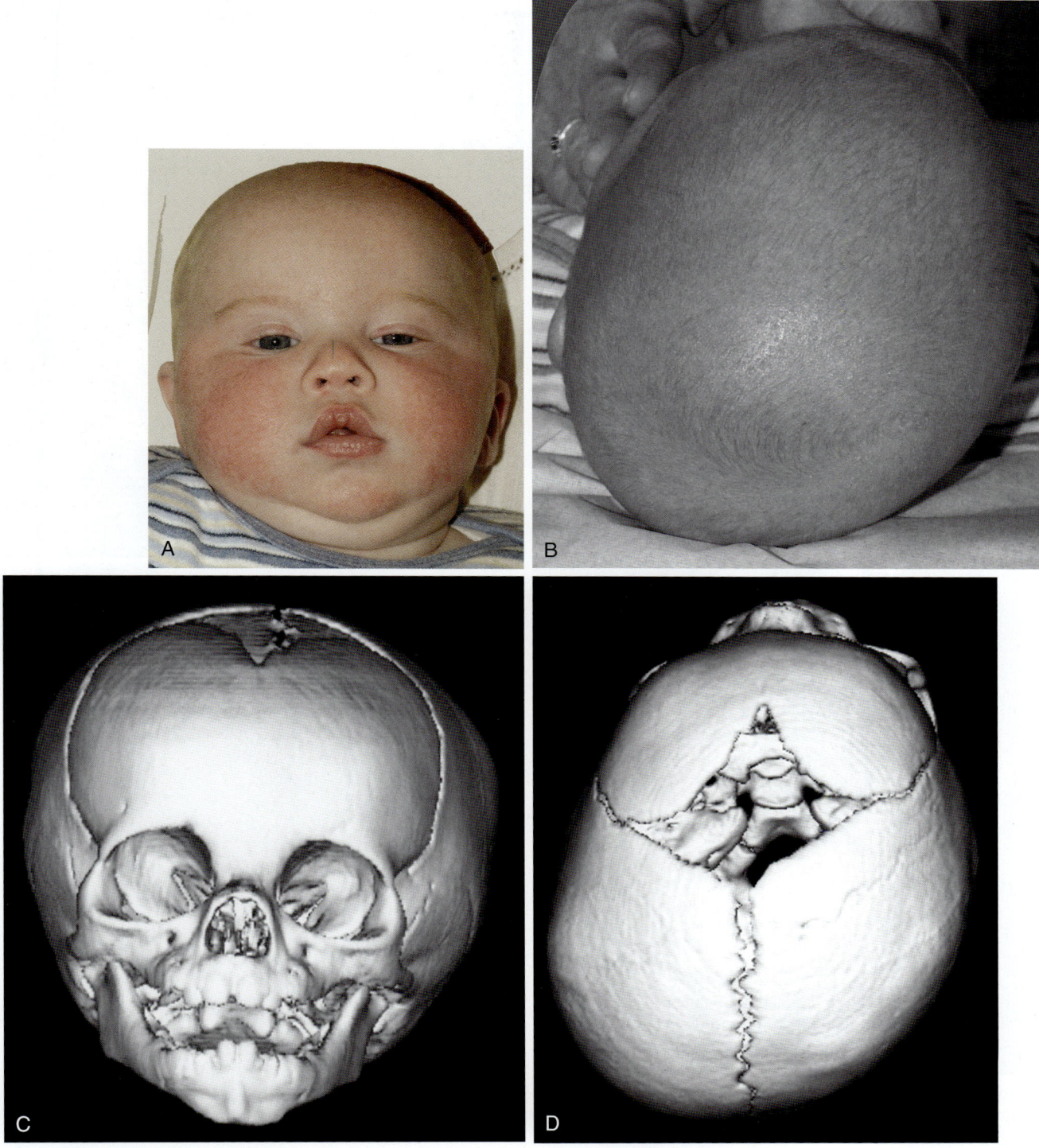

Figure 20-15 Deformational plagiocephaly. **A** and **B,** Frontal view and bird's eye view of an infant reveal the parallelogram shape of the skull and face. **C** and **D,** Frontal view and bird's eye view three-dimensional computed tomography reveals the abnormal-shaped head mimicking the clinical picture.

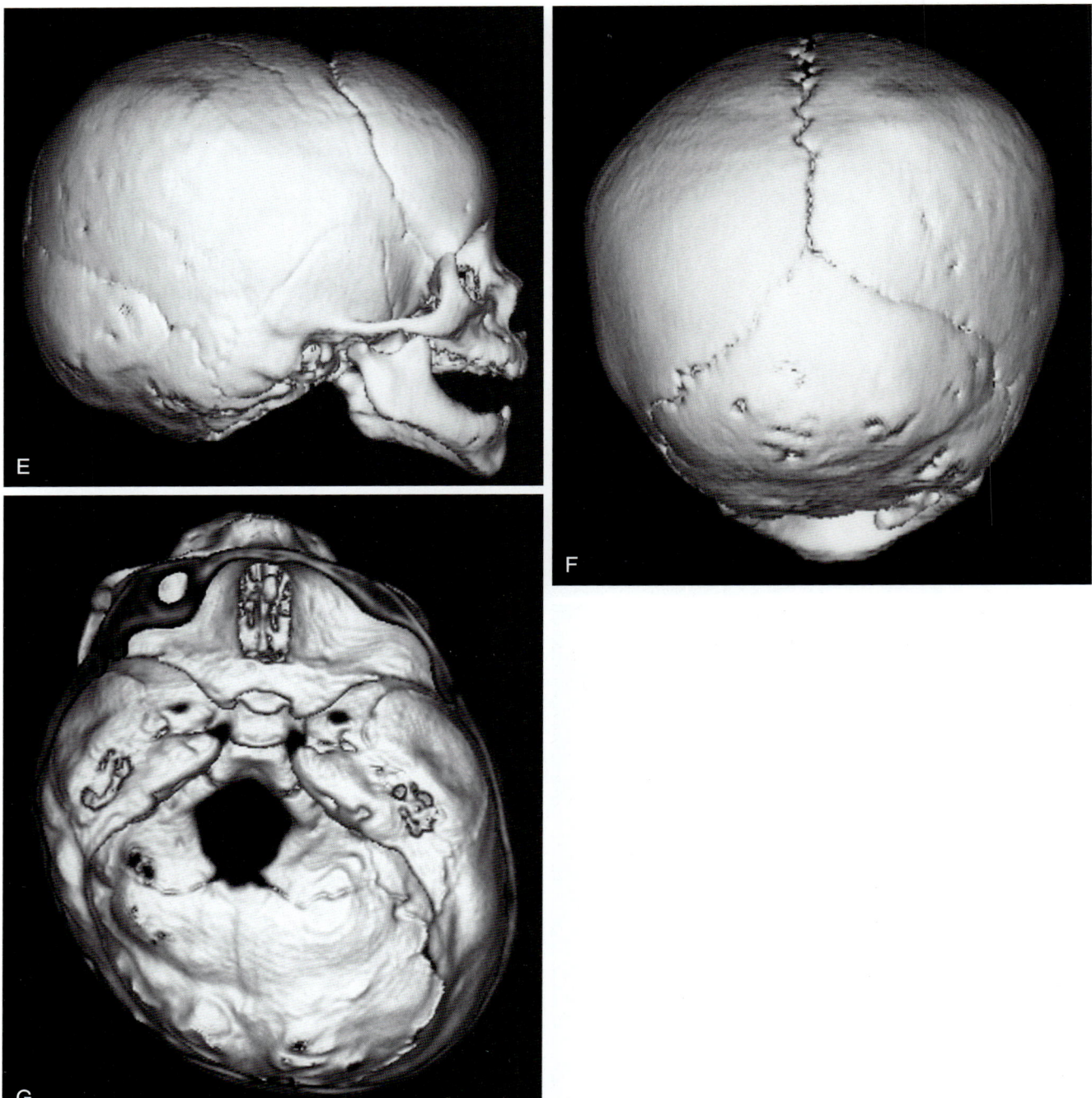

Figure 20-15, cont'd   **E** to **G,** Lateral, posterior, and basal views show all of the sutures are open despite the abnormal head shape. Right occipital flattening and left frontal flattening with compensatory right frontal and left occipital bulging are seen. This gives the parallelogram shape. No skull base angulation is evident.

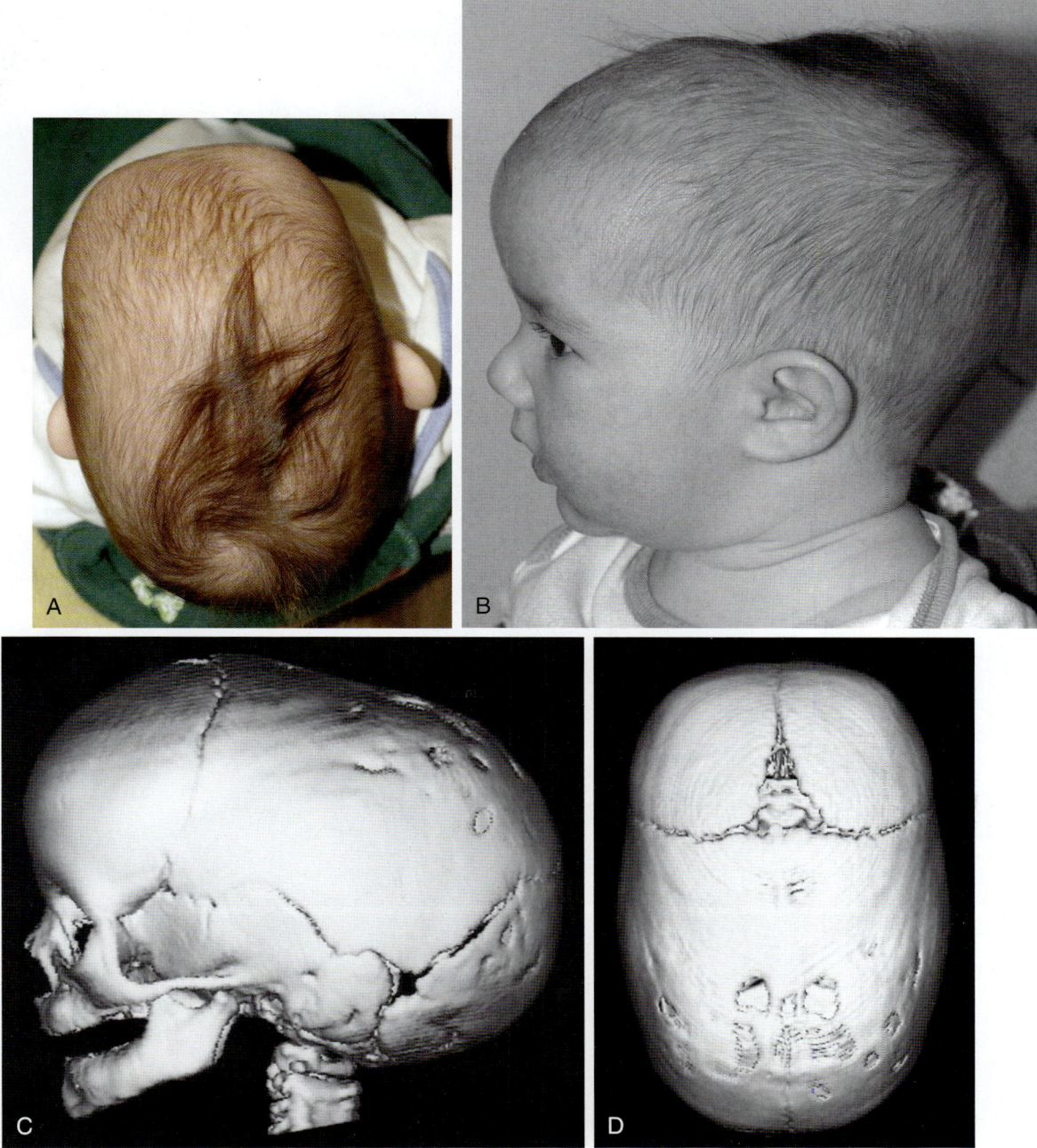

Figure 20-16   Sagittal synostosis. **A** and **B,** Bird's eye view and lateral view of an infant's head reveal a narrow, elongated calvaria from front to back. **C** and **D,** Lateral view and bird's eye view three-dimensional computed tomography shows the elongated (anteroposterior), narrow calvaria with no sagittal suture present and frontal and occipital bulging.

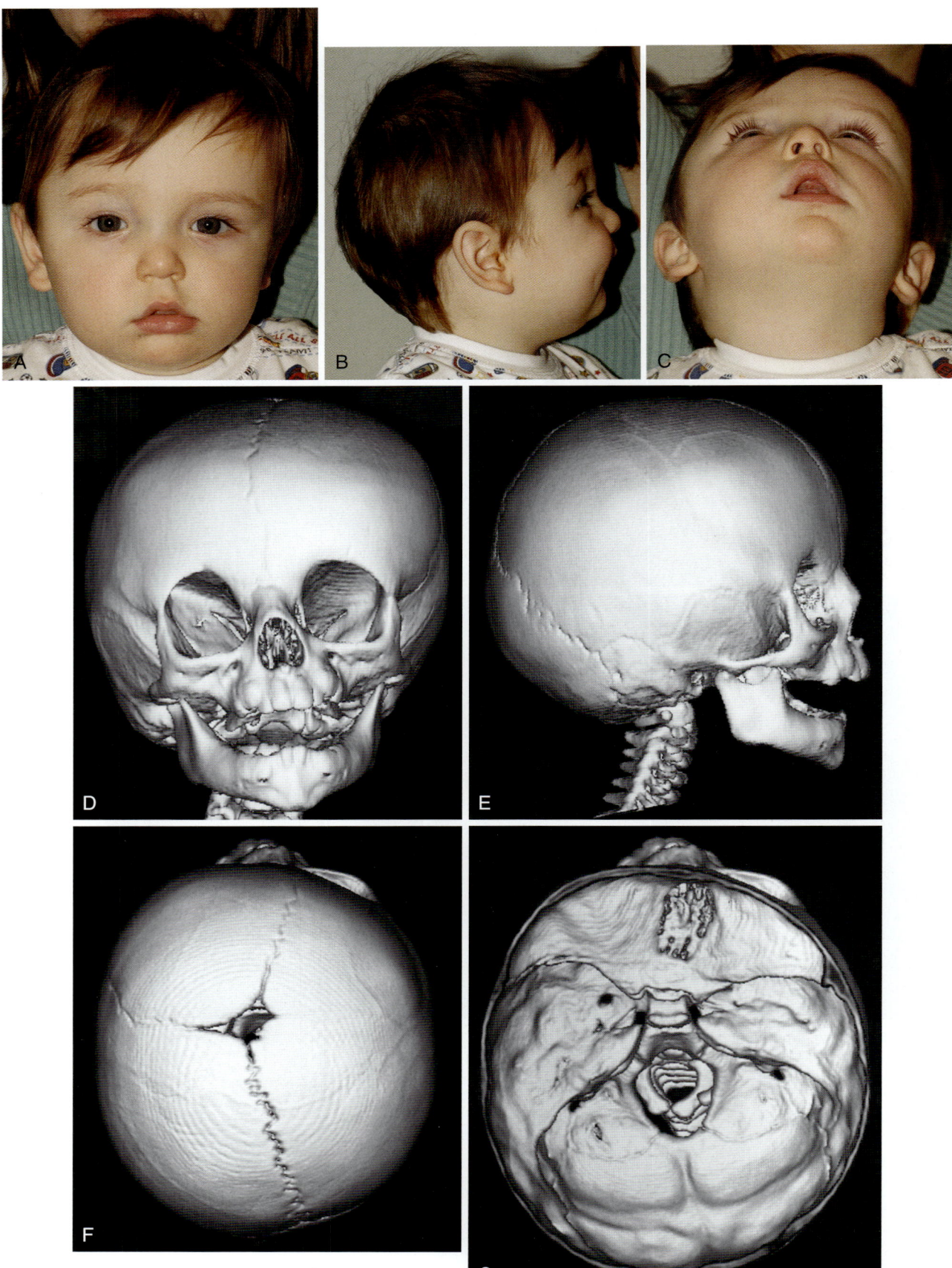

Figure 20-17 Unilateral right coronal synostosis. **A** to **C,** Three views of an infant show flattening of the right frontal and occipital regions and some recession of the right orbit. Note the elongated shape of the head from caudad to cephalad and shortening in the anteroposterior dimension. Unilateral right coronal synostosis. **D** to **G,** Three-dimensional computed tomography shows the absence of the right coronal suture, elevation of the sphenoid seen through the right orbit, right frontal and occipital flattening with a compensatory ipsilateral and temporal and contralateral frontal bulging on the left side, angulation of skull base toward side of coronal synostoses with decreased intracranial volume on affected side.

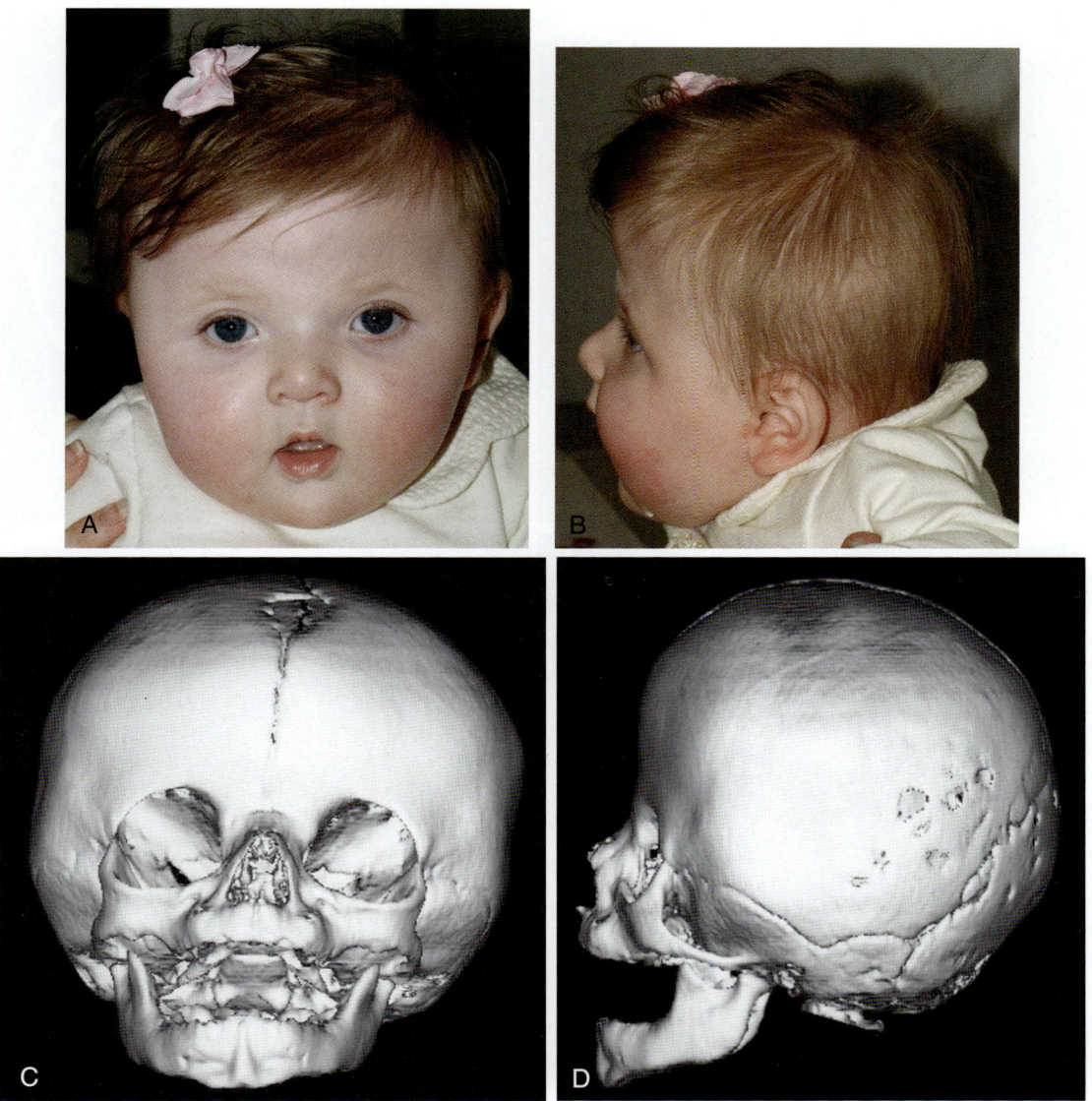

Figure 20-18 Bilateral coronal synostosis. **A** and **B,** Frontal and lateral views of a child show the towering calvaria, with some temporal bulging and orbital recession. **C** to **G,** Computed tomography and three-dimensional reconstructed images of the child reveal the absence of the coronal sutures and the increased dimension from inferior to superior of the skull (towering skull). Decreased anteroposterior dimension of the skull, temporal bulging, and orbital recession are seen.   *Continued*

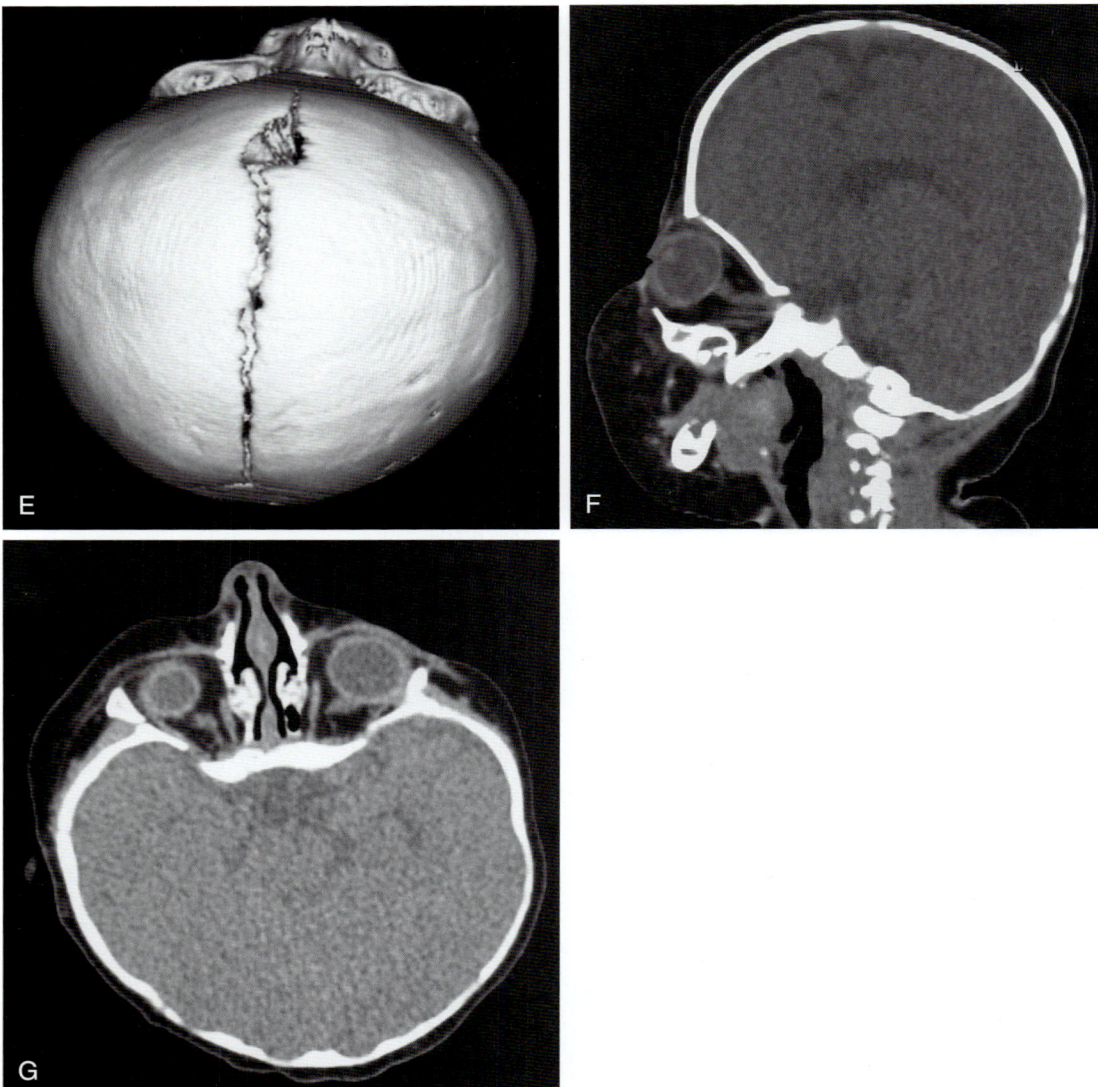

Figure 20-18, cont'd

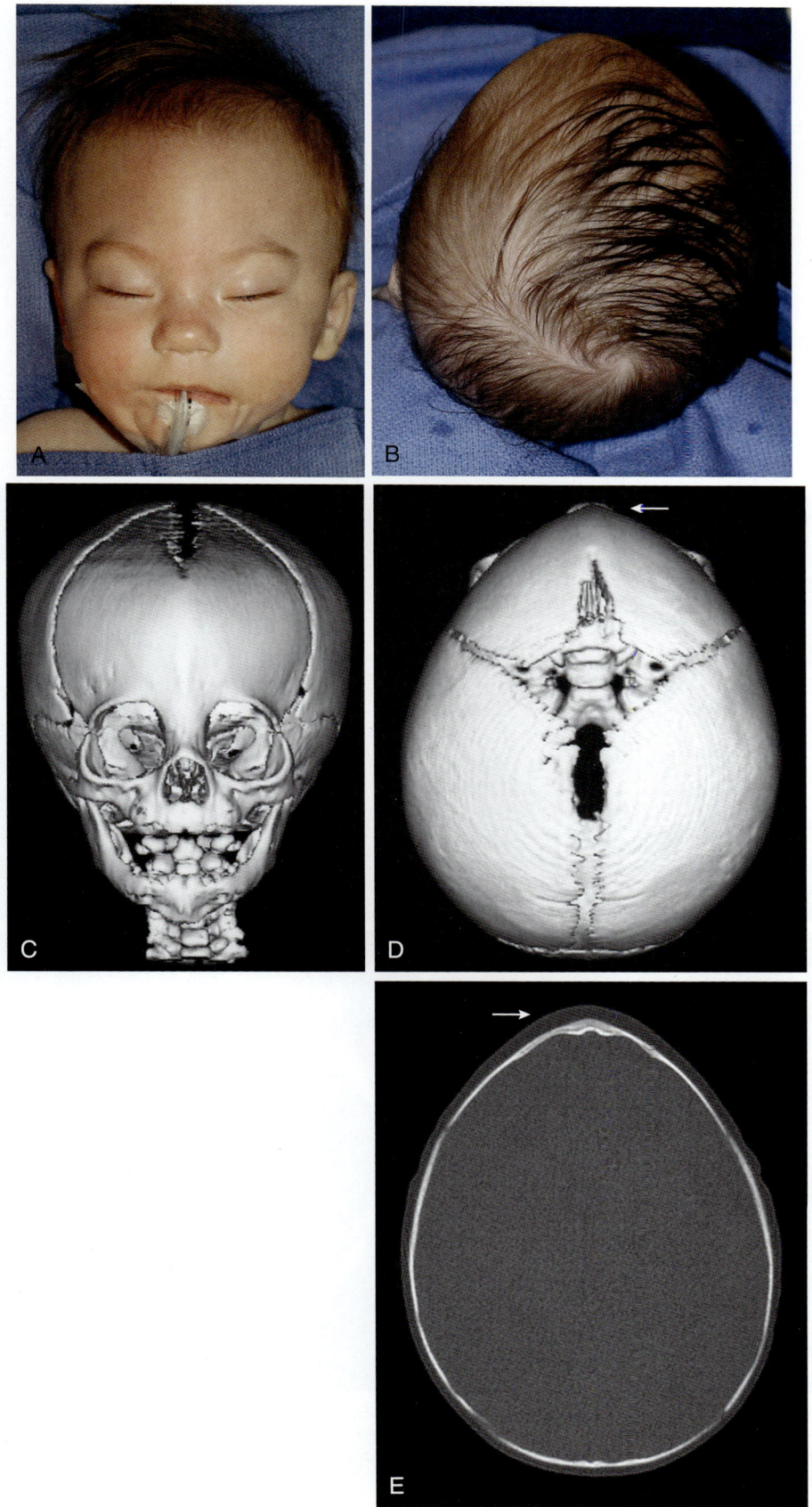

Figure 20-19 Metopic synostosis. **A** and **B,** View of a patient showing a keel-shaped forehead It is r ot round, but rather triangular, and some hypotelorism is present. **C** to **E,** Triangular or keel-shaped forehead and the closure of the metopic suture. This diagnosis cannot be made on just closure of the suture, but the patient must have the appropriate configuration of the forehead (*arrow*) (i.e., triangular shape, not rounded).

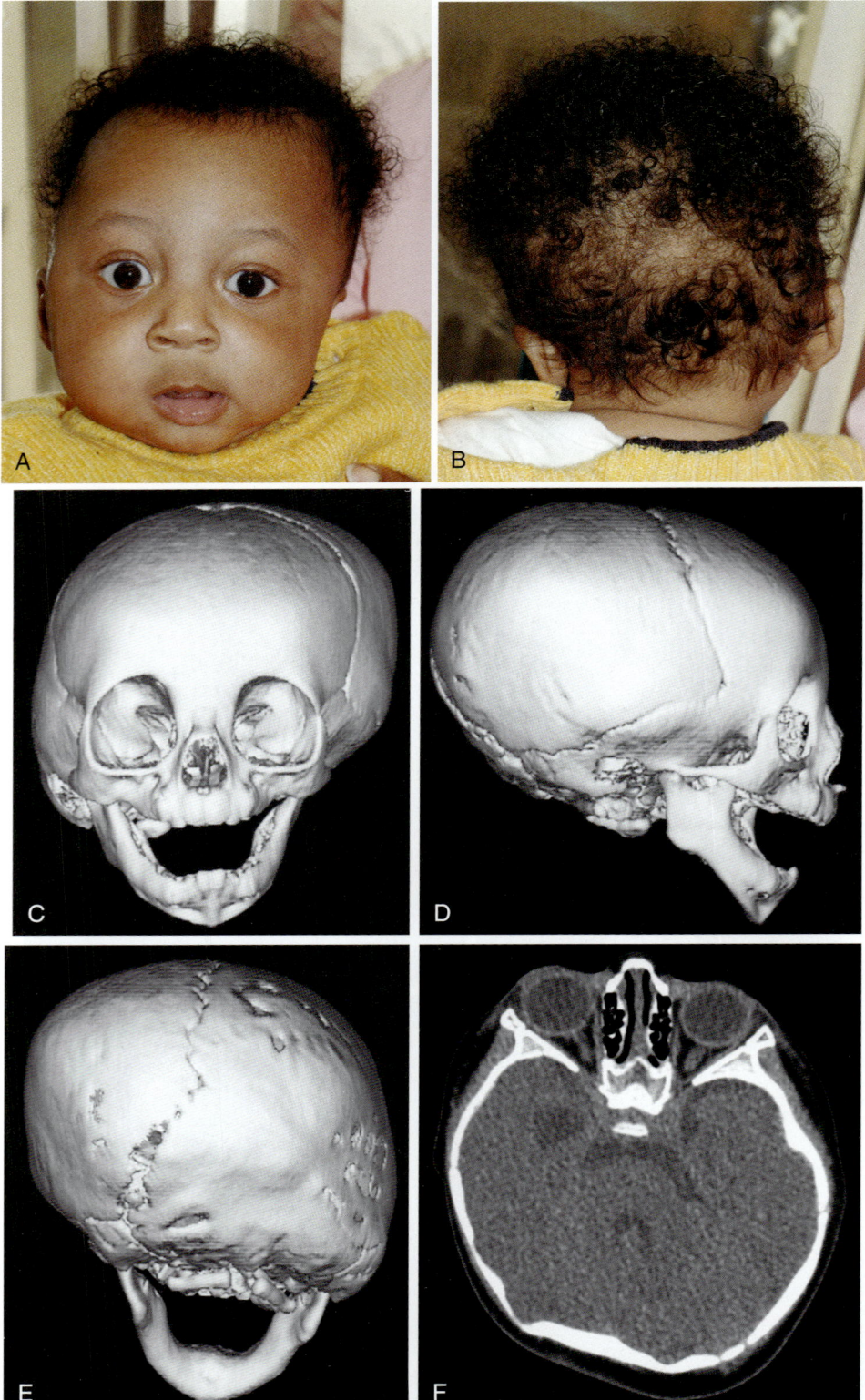

Figure 20-20   Unilateral right lambdoid synostosis. **A** and **B,** Note the asymmetry of the infant's head, with bulging of the inferior occipital region on the right. Compensatory left parietal bulging is seen superiorly. **C** to **F,** Computed tomography and reconstructed three-dimensional images show the absence of the right lambdoid suture with compensatory bulging of the superior and inferior ends of the synostosal suture (i.e., left parietal and right occipital region). Skull-base angulation is evident.

ASSOCIATED ABNORMALITIES

Limb defects are the most common feature of syndromes associated with craniosynostosis, occurring in 84%.[1] Syndactyly and polysyndactyly constitute 30% of the limb defects, and deficiencies account for 22%.

Several types of acrocephalosyndactyly and acrocephalopolysyndactyly have been described. Some are clearly defined; others are less clear and are likely to undergo reclassification as further information becomes available.

The best known acrocephalosyndactyly is *Apert syndrome* (acrocephalosyndactyly type I), in which usually bicoronal synostosis is associated with symmetric complex syndactyly of at least the second, third, and fourth digits, resulting in the "mitten-hand" and "sock-foot" appearance (e-Fig. 20-22). Mental retardation is present in varying degrees. Evaluation of craniofacial deformities may be assisted by CT (e-Fig. 20-23, Fig. 20-24, and e-Fig. 20-25).

Acrocephalosyndactyly types II, III, and IV are known as *Apert-Crouzon disease*, *Saethre-Chotzen syndrome*, and *Waardenburg syndrome*; they involve varying degrees of facial abnormality and syndactylies in patterns generally repetitive for each type. Acrocephalosyndactyly type V, *Pfeiffer syndrome*, has only soft tissue syndactyly, which is not marked, but the thumbs and great toes are deformed and broad. All forms are transmitted by dominant inheritance (Fig. 20-26).

Carpenter syndrome (acrocephalopolysyndactyly type II) is characterized by a high incidence of mental retardation and the presence of preaxial polydactyly of the feet. Types I and III are known as *Noack syndrome* and *Sakati-Nyhan syndrome*.

In *Crouzon syndrome*, the cardinal elements originally included (1) brachycephaly, (2) facial dysostosis with a hooked parrot nose and small maxilla with class III malocclusion, (3) bilateral exophthalmos, and (4) genetic transmission and familial incidence. It usually does not result in mental retardation (e-Fig. 20-27 and Fig. 20-28).

The serious complications of these syndromes include progressive exophthalmos, progressive loss of vision, progressive increase in intracranial pressure, and mental retardation. Some of these are indications for surgical therapy. In addition, the maxillary hypoplasia may cause upper airway obstruction, and affected children may have sleep apnea. Surgical procedures to move the face forward are performed to improve the airway, dental occlusion, and appearance.

Kleeblattschädel (cloverleaf skull) results from closure of all sutures except the squamosal sutures, leading to severe temporal and vertex bulging with exophthalmos (see Fig. 20-12). Hydrocephalus develops in utero, deforming the very plastic skull into a superior portion related to the position of the dilated frontal lobes and bilateral inferolateral portions corresponding to the dilated temporal lobes. Most patients do not survive infancy (see Fig. 20-12). Kleeblattschädel may be found in thanatophoric dysplasia type II.

Craniofacial Syndromes

A large number of conditions fall under the category of craniofacial syndromes; most are uncommon and beyond the scope of this book. The four syndromes that are discussed are Goldenhar syndrome, hemifacial microsomia, Treacher Collins syndrome, and Pierre Robin sequence.

GOLDENHAR SYNDROME AND HEMIFACIAL MICROSOMIA

Goldenhar syndrome is part of the oculoauricular vertebral spectrum, which includes hemifacial microsomia.[13,14] Most reported cases are sporadic. An increased incidence of Goldenhar syndrome is present in infants of mothers with diabetes. The phenotype has been reported in association with other conditions, including trisomy 18, and with maternal thalidomide, primidone, and retinoic acid use.

The hallmarks of Goldenhar syndrome are epibulbar dermoids, preauricular appendages, mandibular hypoplasia, microtia, and vertebral anomalies. Extreme variability of expression is characteristic of this anomaly. Most frequently, the orbital lesions, mandibular hypoplasia (Fig. 20-29), and microtia are unilateral and on the same side.[15] Colobomas of the upper eyelid occur in 60% of patients and may be large, requiring immediate repair to prevent corneal ulceration. Deafness is common because of associated anomalies of the middle and inner ear.[16] Vertebral anomalies occur in 60% of patients and are most often cervical; these anomalies include basilar invagination, occipitalization of the atlas, C1-2 instability, cervical synostosis, hemivertebra, butterfly vertebrae, scoliosis, kyphosis, and Sprengel deformities (e-Fig. 20-30).[17] Verterbral anomalies below the cervical spine are found in only 10% of patients. The anomalies may be severe, however, and associated with costal malformations similar to Jarcho-Levin syndrome.

Hemifacial microsomia is a variable complex malformation of asymmetric hypoplasia of the face and ear with microsomia, unilateral microtia, and ipsilateral hypoplasis of the mandibular ramus and condyle. Hemifacial microsomia implies unilateral involvement, but the structures affected are bilateral and are only affected to different degrees. Primate and rodent studies have suggested that hemifacial microsomia may be caused by a hemorrhagic event involving the stapedial artery during early stages of craniofacial development.[18] Patients with hemifacial microsomia resemble those with Goldenhar syndrome, but the presence of epibulbar dermoids, lipodermoids, auricular appendices, pretragal blind-ending fissures, and vertebral anomalies favors a diagnosis of Goldenhar syndrome.

A wide variety of additional anomalies have been described in patients with Goldenhar syndrome and hemifacial microsomia, including renal anomalies, radial anomalies, clubfoot, and congenital hip dislocation. It may be linked with VATER sequence (vertebral defects, imperforate anus, tracheoesophageal fistula, and radial and renal dysplasia). Cerebral anomalies include Chiari I malformation, lipoma, agenesis of the corpus callosum, and abnormalities in the pons. Cardiovascular anomalies, including ventricular septal defects, atrial septal defects, and pulmonic stenosis, are found. Vascular anomalies, especially portal venous anomalies (i.e., cavernous transformation) may be present. The mode of inheritance is thought to be autosomal or X-linked dominant in most cases.

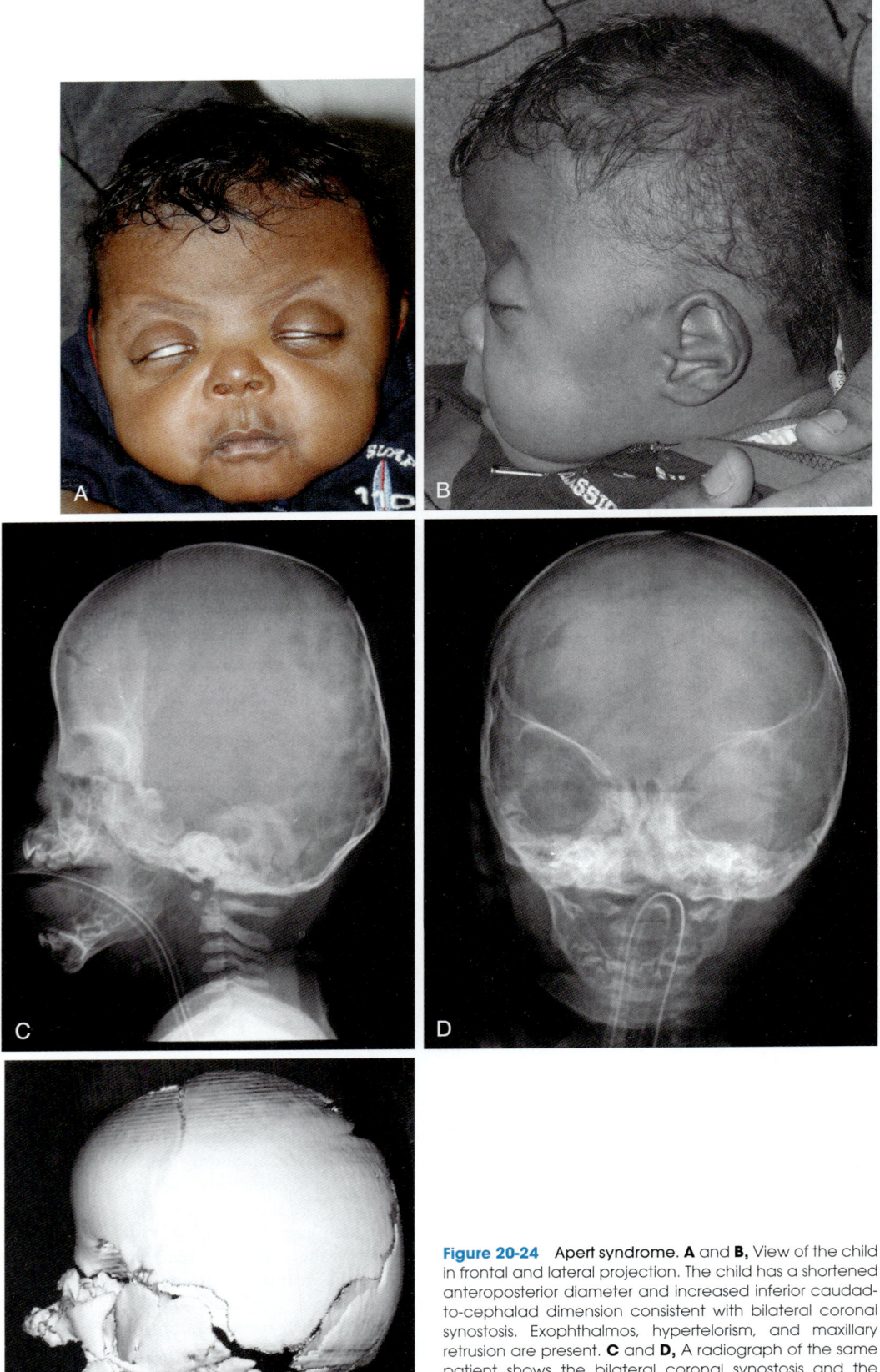

Figure 20-24 Apert syndrome. **A** and **B,** View of the child in frontal and lateral projection. The child has a shortened anteroposterior diameter and increased inferior caudad-to-cephalad dimension consistent with bilateral coronal synostosis. Exophthalmos, hypertelorism, and maxillary retrusion are present. **C** and **D,** A radiograph of the same patient shows the bilateral coronal synostosis and the expected contour of the calvaria. **E,** A three-dimensional computed tomography lateral view confirms closure of inferior coronal suture and maxillary retrusion.

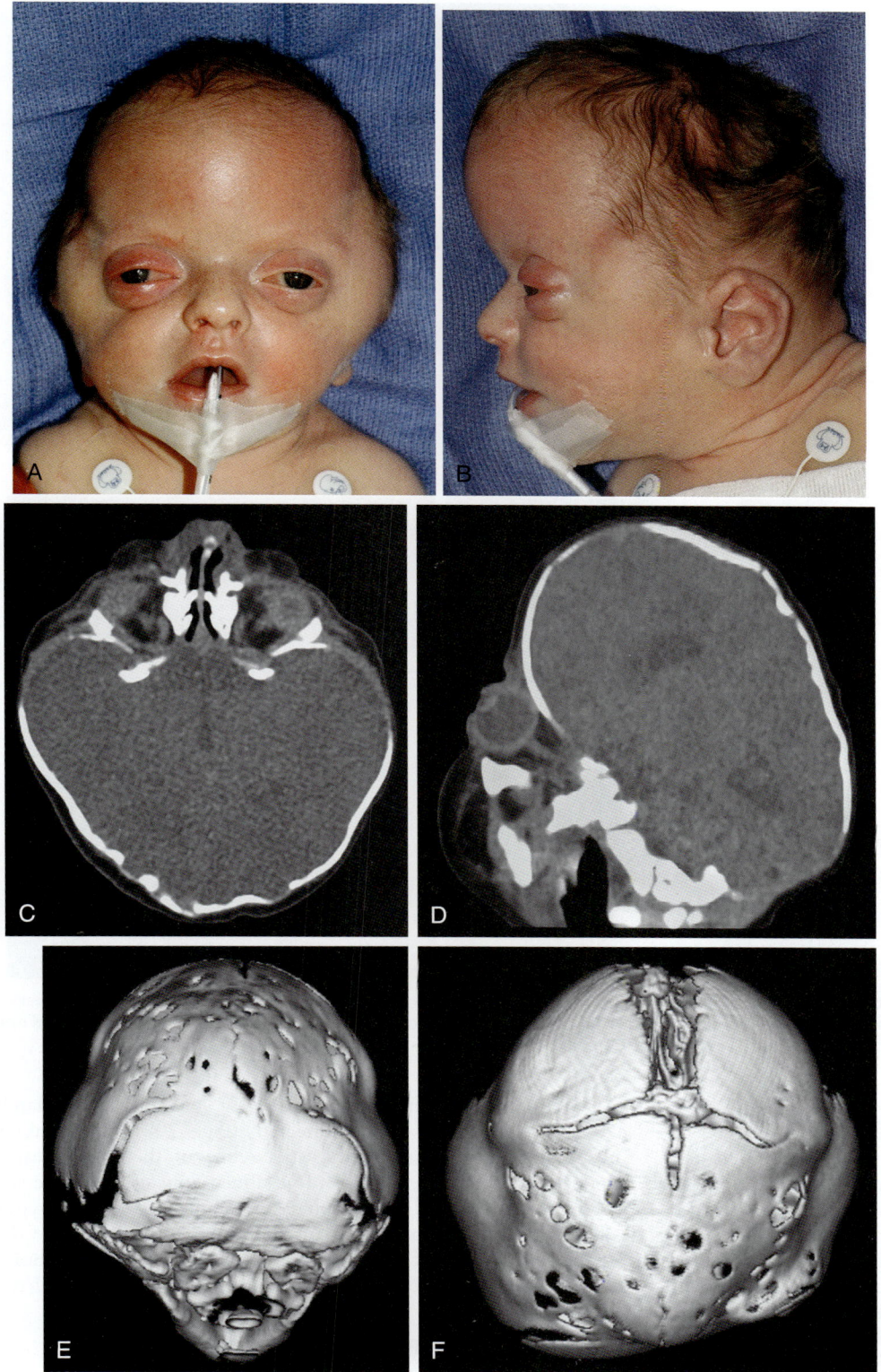

Figure 20-26 Pfeiffer syndrome. **A** and **B,** Frontal and lateral views of the child reflect the multisutural synostosis (bilateral coronal, bilateral lambdoid, and sagittal synostosis) with the resultant cloverleaf configuration. **C** and **D,** Computed tomography with bone windows shows the temporal bulging, bony fenestrations, maxillary retrusion, and exophthalmos. The characteristic deformity of the calvaria is noted. **E** and **F,** Posterior view (E) and vertex view (F), three-dimensional computed tomography shows multiple suture closures (coronal, both lambdoid and sagittal sutures).

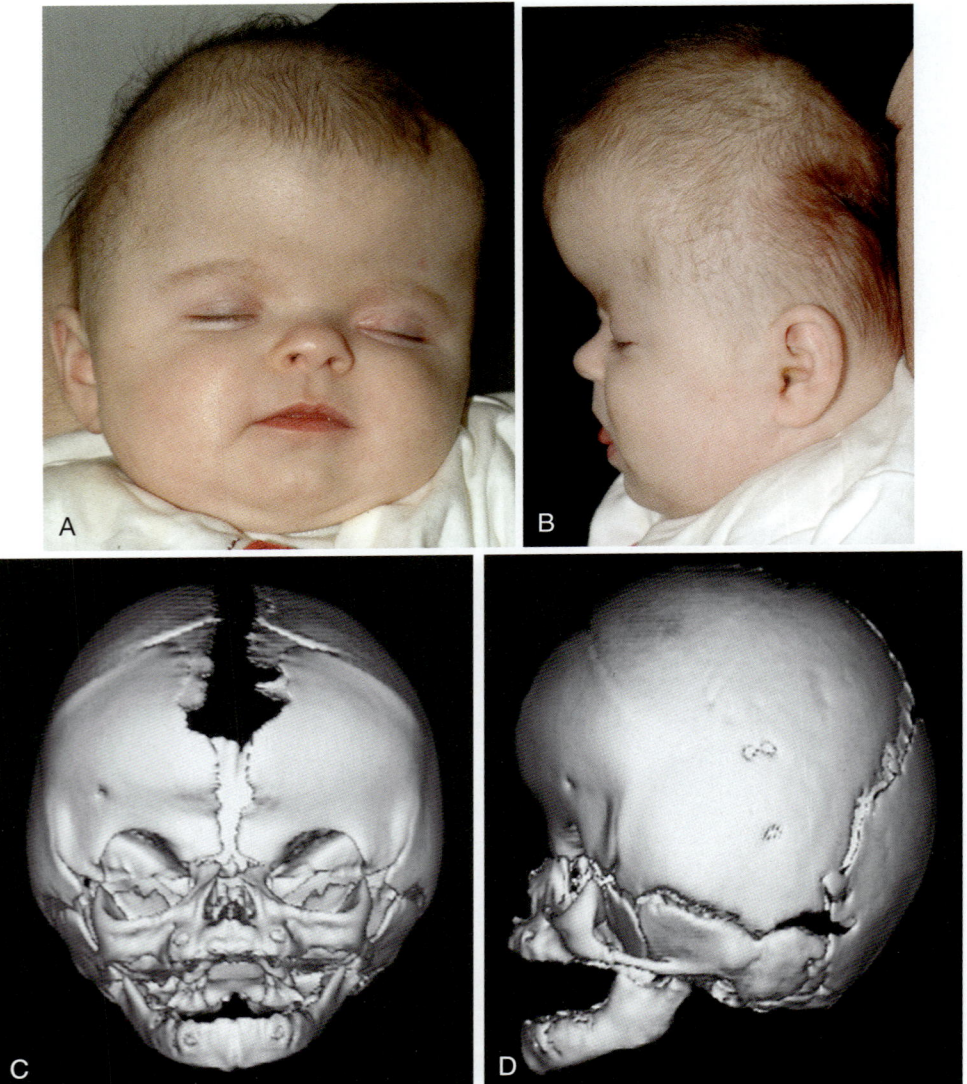

Figure 20-28 Crouzon syndrome. **A** and **B,** Frontal and lateral views of an infant reveal a head shape consistent with bilateral coronal synostosis. The dimension is increased from caudad to cranial and shortened in the anteroposterior dimension. **C** and **D,** Three-dimensional computed tomography reveals the bilateral coronal synostosis with the characteristic findings.

TREACHER COLLINS SYNDROME

The condition has been diagnosed in utero by ultrasonography and is autosomal dominant, with variable penetrance and expression. The facial features of Treacher Collins syndrome are characteristic.[19,20] Abnormalities are typically bilateral and symmetric: micrognathia, narrow face, depressed cheekbones, antimongoloid slant of eyes, malformed small ears, large downturned mouth, high-arched or cleft palate, and conductive hearing loss. The features are characterized by abnormalities in the derivatives of the first and second branchial arches.[20] Mutations in the *TCOF1* gene are associated with Treacher Collins syndrome, and numerous other associated mutations may be present.[21] The features demonstrated on imaging are primarily facial, consisting of mandibular, zygomatic, maxillary, and supraorbital hypoplasia. The orbits are described as being egg shaped. The mandibular shape of a short body and ramus is characteristic and varies with the patient's age. The mandibular condyle and coronoid process may be severely hypoplastic, flat, or even absent. Mandibular growth is severely affected (Fig. 20-31). Ear abnormalities include hypoplasia or absence of the middle ear. The ossicles and cochlea and vestibular apparatus may be severely malformed. Radiographic detection of zygomatic hypoplasia or aplasia is an important supporting finding for the diagnosis. Craniofacial three-dimensional CT for morphologic mapping has become invaluable for planning surgical treatment.[22]

PIERRE ROBIN SEQUENCE

Pierre Robin sequence, or Robin sequence, represents a nonrandom association of micrognathia, cleft palate, and glossoptosis.[23] Pierre Robin sequence is causally heterogeneous and pathogenetically and phenotypically variable.[24] Patients with Pierre Robin sequence are classified as isolated (most common), syndromic, or with associated anomalies. Numerous syndromes, including Stickler and velocardiofacial syndromes, are associated with Pierre Robin sequence.[25]

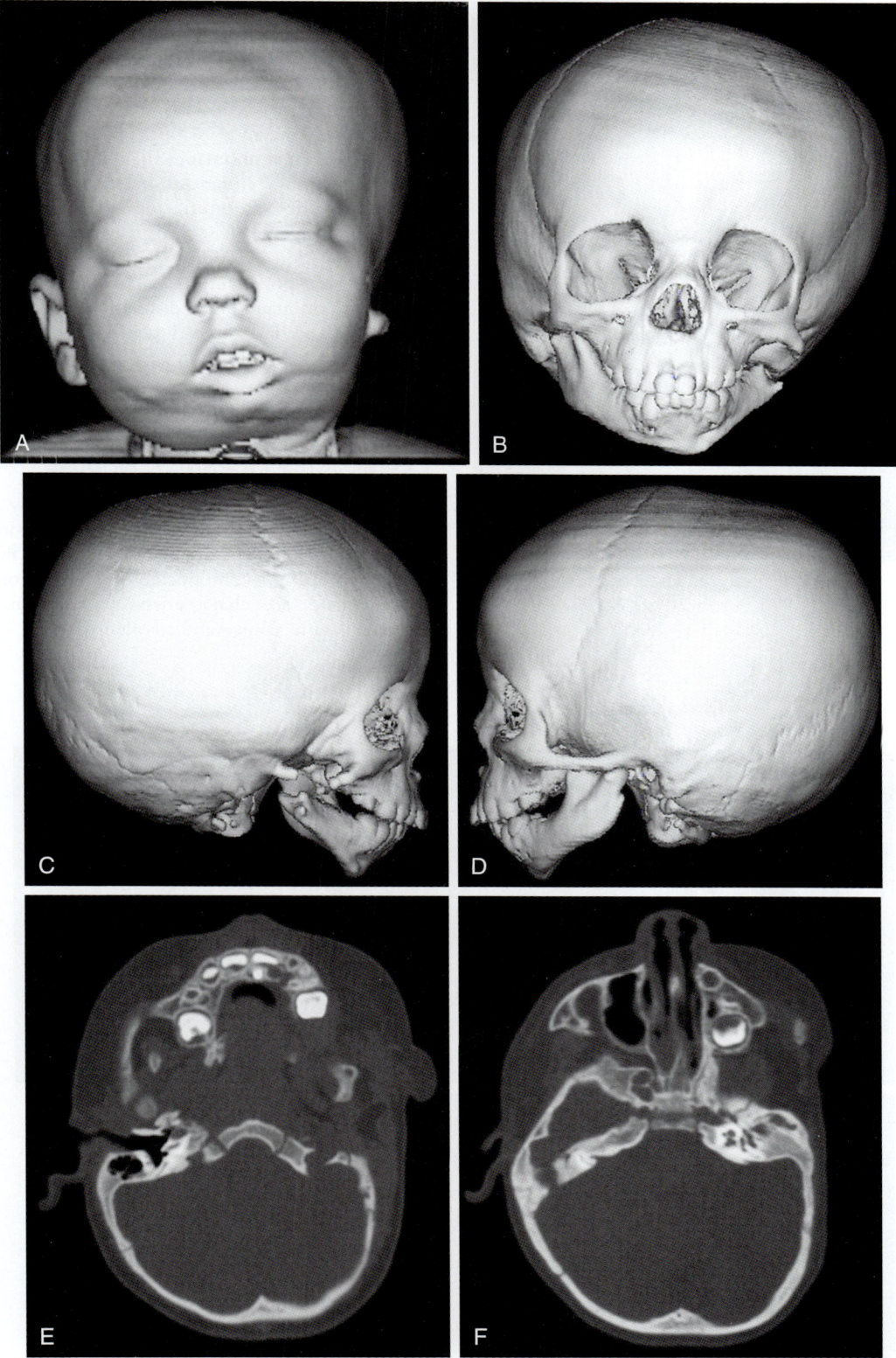

Figure 20-29 Goldenhar syndrome. **A,** Three-dimensional surface rendering image shows left hemifacial microsomia and left ear microtia. **B,** Three-dimensional computed tomography reconstruction shows hypoplastic left mandible and zygomatic arch. **C** and **D,** Lateral three-dimensional image confirms asymmetry and left microsomia. **E** and **F,** Bone window computed tomography view at skull base reveals normal right external canal and temporal bone. The left face is hypoplastic. The left external auditory canal is absent.

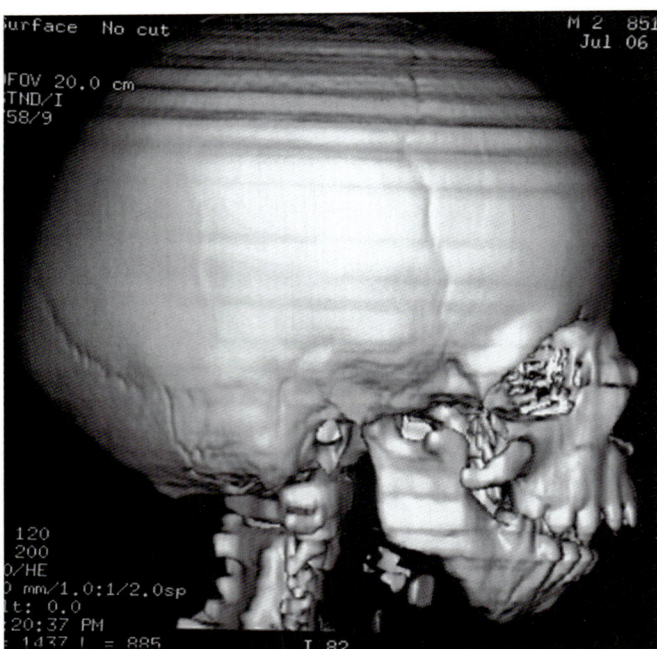

Figure 20-31 Three-dimensional imaging of Treacher Collins syndrome shows mandibular hypoplasia and absence of zygomatic arch in a 3-month-old boy.

Respiratory compromise from mechanical and central nervous system causes is common. The mandible may be small or may be normal sized and retrognathic in position as a result of a large cranial base (Fig. 20-32). Typically, a reduction in cranial base and maxillary and mandibular lengths is seen.[26] Mandibular deficiency is most pronounced in the body.

Cardiovascular anomalies include septal defects and patent ductus arteriosus. Numerous skeletal anomalies include anomalies of the ribs, sternum, and spine, and limb reductions. Airway management is similar in both nonsyndromic and syndromic Pierre Robin sequence. The infant may be managed with positioning, nasal pharyngeal airway, tie-tongue adhesions, or mandibular distraction.[27-30] Cine MRI or CT gives dynamic and three-dimensional information that may be useful in the evaluation of the airways of these patients.

Other Abnormalities of the Skull

CRANIOSCHISIS (CRANIUM BIFIDUM)

Cranioschisis, or cranium bifidum, usually occurs in the median sagittal plane, anteriorly or posteriorly (Figs. 20-32 and 20-33). Both sites are characterized by bony defects and may accompany meningocele or meningoencephalocele.[31] Meningoceles are characterized by a hernia sac, which is covered with skin and contains only meninges and

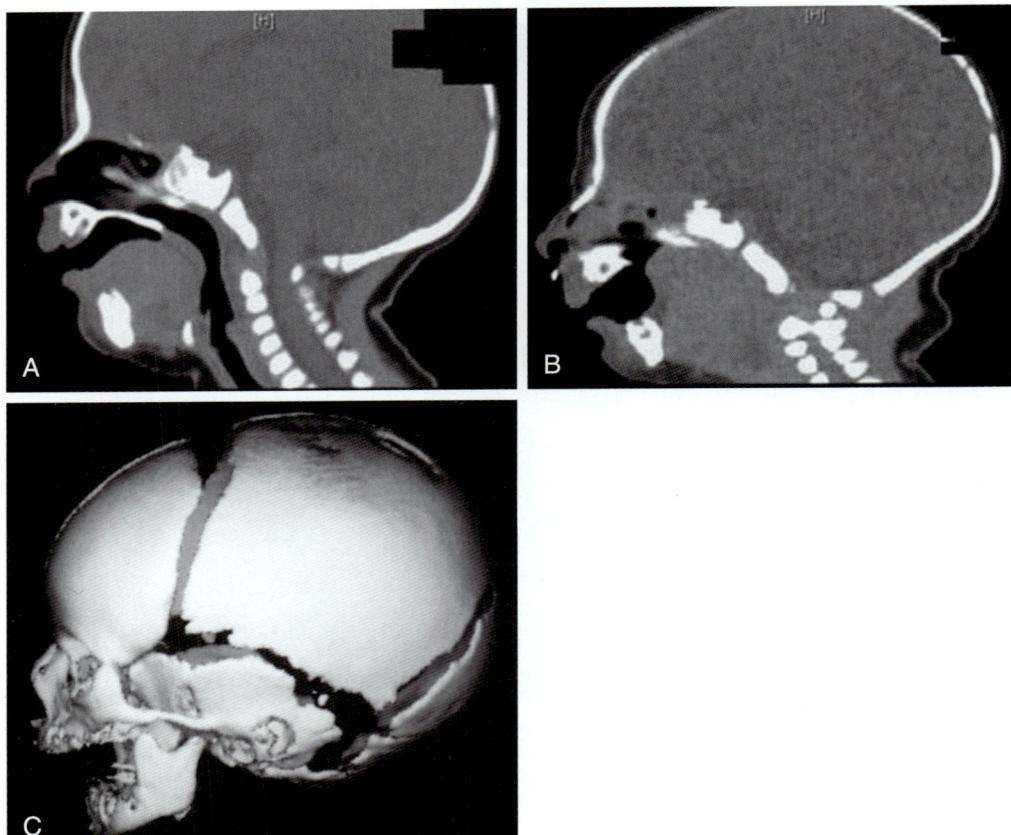

Figure 20-32 Pierre Robin sequence. **A** and **B,** Sagittal reconstructed computed tomography scans show the large tongue obstructing the oropharynx as well as the retropositioned small mandible. **C,** Three-dimensional reconstruction shows the retropositioned small mandible.

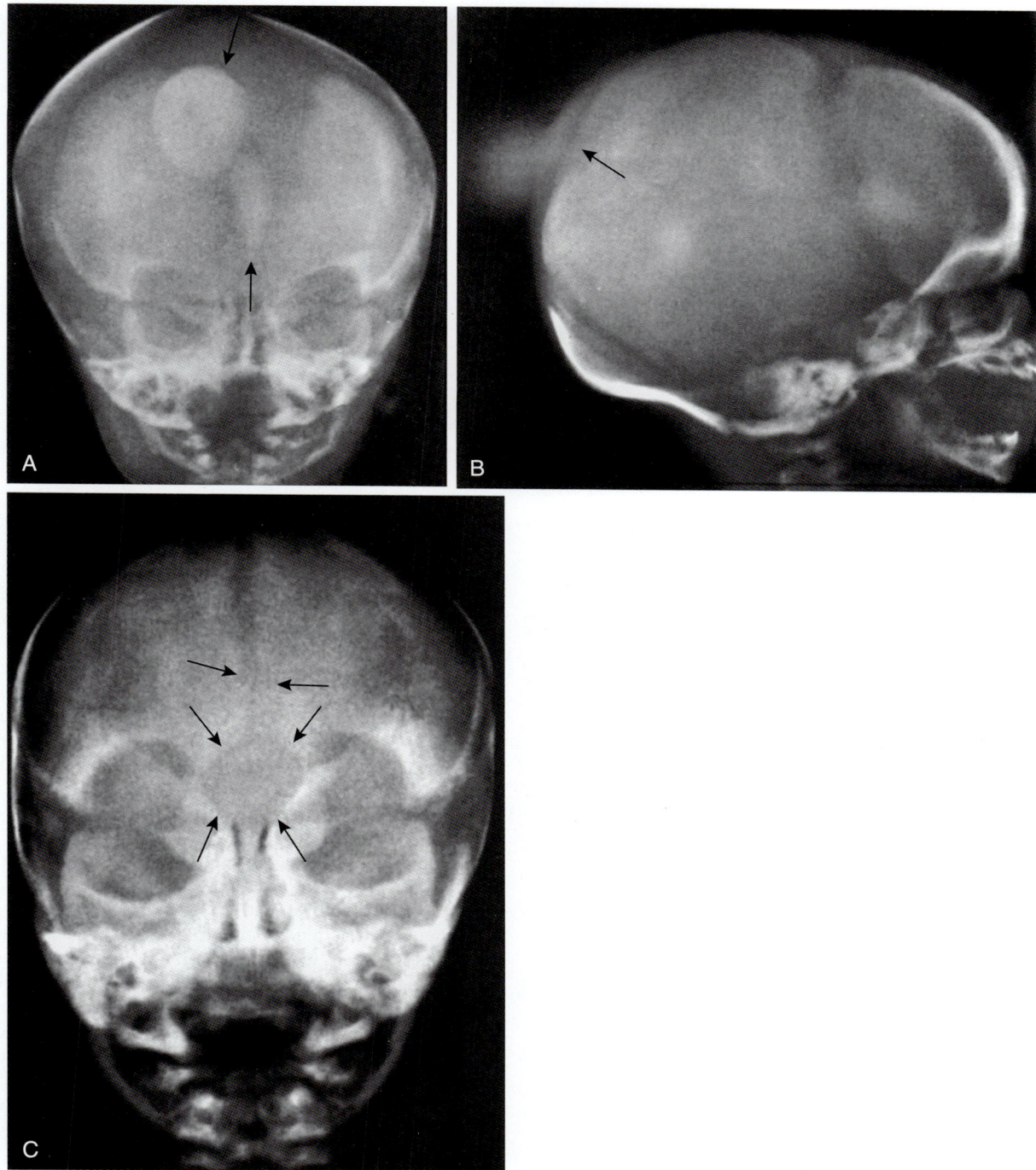

Figure 20-33　Cranium bifidum. **A** and **B,** Frontal (*A*) and lateral (*B*) projections show intrafrontal and interparietal cranium bifidum in the metopic suture and in the sagittal suture, with protrusion of a soft tissue sac (meningoencephalocele) at anterior and posterior sites, in a 2-day-old girl. The metopic suture also is widely open, and a smaller mass of soft tissue bulges externally between the two sides of the frontal squamosa. In *A,* the larger superior patch of increased density (*upper arrow*) represents the interparietal protrusion, and the lower small patch (*lower arrow*) represents the smaller and shallower intrafrontal protrusion. **C,** Large circular bone defect (cranium bifidum) at the glabella in a widely open metopic suture. A lump of soft tissue bulged externally at this site.

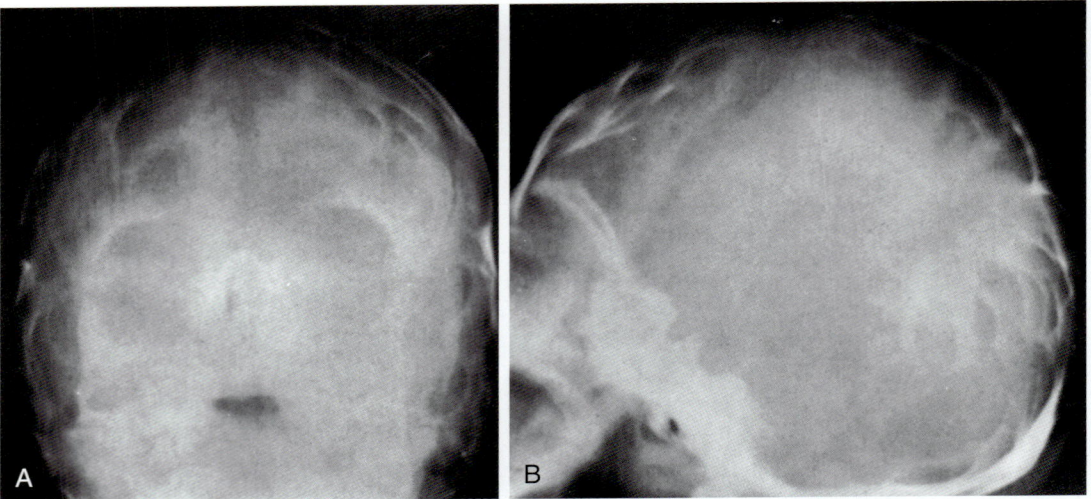

Figure 20-37   Lacunar skull on the second day of life, associated with occipital meningocele. **A** and **B,** Frontal (*A*) and lateral (*B*) projections. All bones in the calvaria show checkered rarefaction separated by bands of heavier density. The pattern resembles the mottling of beaten copper or silver.

cerebrospinal fluid (e-Fig. 20-34). Meningoencephaloceles also contain brain (e-Fig. 20-35). Rarely, cranioschisis may be associated with only a scalp nodule, with or without intracranial communication. Occasionally, small cranial defects—for example, cranium bifidum occultum—through which no herniation occurs are encountered (e-Fig. 20-36). MRI is most effective for evaluation of the sac contents.

Cranium bifidum with encephalocele often occurs in the sphenoid bone or in the cribriform plate of the ethmoid. In such cases, the protruding mass of brain and covering meninges may extend into the nasal cavity, nasopharynx, sphenoid sinus, posterior portion of one orbit, or one of the pterygoid fossae. Important clinical signs include facial deformity with increased distance between the orbits (hypertelorism) and broadened base of the nose.

LACUNAR SKULL OF THE NEWBORN (LÜCKENSCHÄDEL, CRANIOLACUNIA)

Lacunar skull develops during fetal life and is present at birth.[32] It is nearly always associated with meningomyelocele, myelocele, or encephalocele and Chiari II malformation. The cause is unknown, but it is probably a dysplasia of the calvarium and the internal periosteum (i.e., the dura). It is not caused by fetal increased intracranial pressure because it is found in infants whose skulls are normal or are small in size without evidence of hydrocephalus. The characteristic "soap bubble" rarefactions in the upper part of the calvarium are easily recognized (Fig. 20-37). These begin to fade after birth and usually disappear by 4 to 5 months of age, even in the presence of progressive hydrocephalus in some instances. Normal convolutional rarefactions differ from lacunar rarefactions in that they are not obvious until the end of the first year and tend to appear first in the posterior and lower lateral portions of the calvarium.

SINUS PERICRANII

The term *sinus pericranii* is used for a soft, fluctuant mass, often of a red-to-blue color, observed in the scalp over the region of the sagittal or transverse sinuses. It responds in size to maneuvers that tend to increase intracranial pressure and may be associated with an underlying bony defect of the calvarium. It results from an abnormal communication between the intracranial and extracranial venous systems, and its significance is cosmetic.[33-35] It must be differentiated from more serious lesions such as arteriovenous malformations, angiomas and hemangiomas, sebaceous or dermoid cysts, meningocele, encephalocele, and abscess. MRI is the best imaging modality for demonstrating the presence of an abnormal vascular communication (Fig. 20-38).

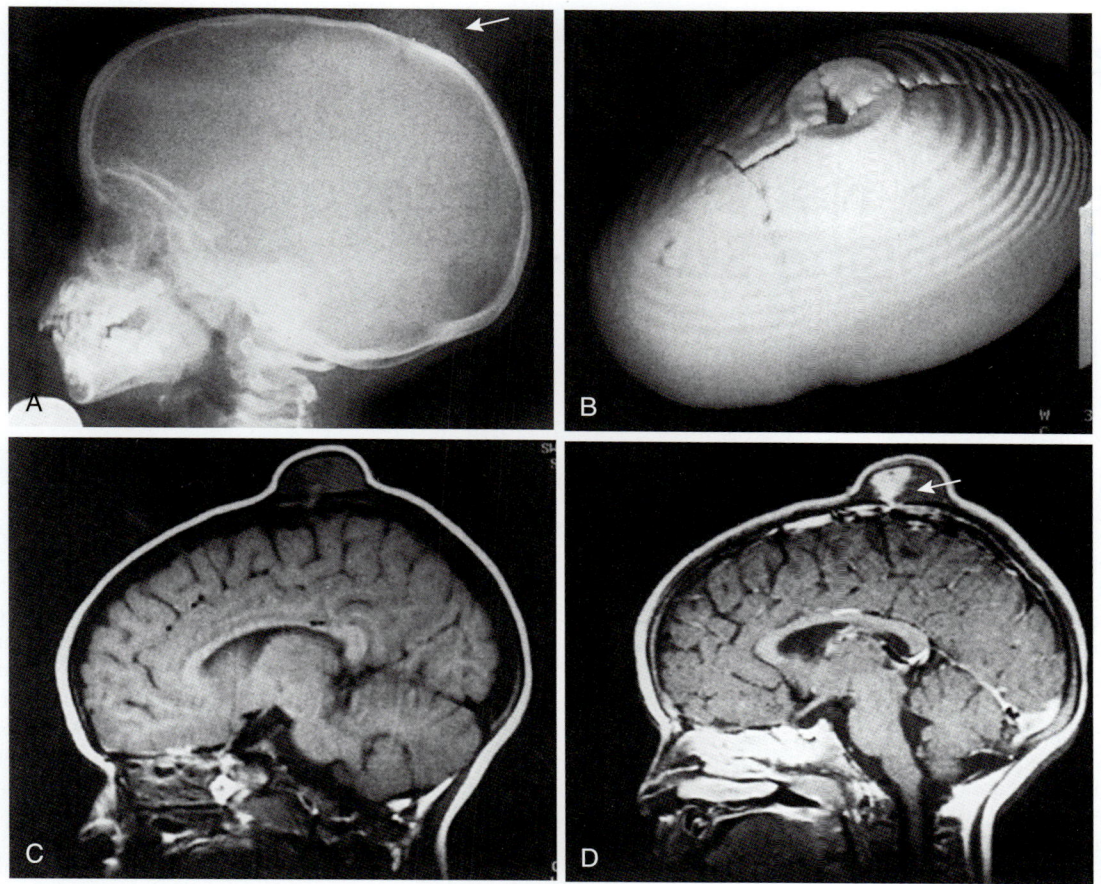

Figure 20-38 Sinus pericranii. **A,** Lateral view of the skull showing a soft tissue mass and a well-defined bone defect in the midline of the parietal region. **B,** Three-dimensional computed tomography showing erosion of both tables similar to the crater of a volcano. **C** and **D,** Magnetic resonance images (TR/TE 400/20) before (*C*) and after (*D*) gadolinium injection. **C,** The tumor shows mixed signal intensity and areas of signal void indicating flowing blood. **D,** After administration of intravenous gadolinium, heterogeneous enhancement is evident, and an emissary vein is seen extending through the parietal bone to the superior sagittal sinus (*arrow*). (From Bigot J-L, Iacona C, Lepreux A, et al. Sinus pericranii: advantages of MR imaging. *Pediatr Radiol*. 2000;30:710-712.)

Key Points

The deformities in craniosynostosis are complex, and secondary abnormalities at the base of the skull add to the structural changes.

Plagiocephaly denotes abnormal shape (usually flattening) without defining a cause.

Lacunar skull is not related to increased intracranial pressure.

Suggested Readings

Cohen Jr MM. *Perspectives on the face*. New York: Oxford University Press; 2006.

Eteson DJ, Steward RE. Craniofacial defects in the human skeletal dysplasias. *Birth Defects*. 1984;20:14-45.

Glass RB, Fernbach SK, Norton KI, et al. The infant skull: a vault of information. *Radiographics*. 2004;24:507-522.

Kirmi O, Lo SJ, Johnson D, et al. Craniosynostosis: a radiological and surgical perspective. *Semin Ultrasound CT MRI*. 2009;30:492-512.

Lachman RS, ed. *Taybi and Lachman's radiology of syndromes, metabolic disorders and skeletal dysplasias*. 5th ed, Philadelphia, PA: Elsevier; 2006.

Sood S, Rozzelle A, Shaqiri B, et al. Effect of molding helmet on head shape in nonsurgically treated sagittal craniosynostosis. *J Neurosurg Pediatr*. 2011;7:1-6.

References

Full references for this chapter can be found on www.expertconsult.com.

Chapter 21

Neoplasms, Neoplasm-like Lesions, and Infections of the Skull

THOMAS L. SLOVIS and WILLIAM H. McALISTER

Primary Neoplasms

Primary neoplasms of the skull are rare. The most commonly encountered lesions in children with a solitary nontraumatic lump on the head are dermoid tumors of the scalp (61%), cephalhematoma deformans (9%), Langerhans cell histiocytosis (LCH) (7%), and occult meningoceles and encephaloceles (4%).[1,2]

Osteochondromas may arise from the cartilaginous bones of the skull base. Osteoblastomas have been reported in the calvaria of infants, and aneurysmal bone cysts have been noted in the skull base and the calvaria (Fig. 21-1). Osteomas are small and usually limited to the outer table, although osteoid osteomas may occur in the diploë. Osteoid osteomas may present with the appearance of a button sequestrum. Malignant bone tumors are unusual, but osteogenic sarcoma and Ewing sarcoma have been reported (e-Fig. 21-2).[3-5]

Angiomas and neurofibromas of the scalp may affect the underlying skull and cause deformities, bony defects, and regional hyperostoses. Plain film findings of neurofibromatosis (NF) include lytic defect in the lambdoid suture, absence of the orbital roof and floor, elevated lesser sphenoid wing, enlarged middle cranial fossa, enlarged cranial nerve foramina, unilateral orbital enlargement, and J-shaped sella turcica (Fig. 21-3).[6,7]

Cavernous hemangiomas of the skull are characterized by rounded areas of diminished density in which there may be a honeycomb or radial pattern of greater density caused by spiculation. Calvarial hemangiomas (e-Fig. 21-4) usually thicken the outer table externally and are radially striated. They do not displace the inner table.

Lymphatic malformations of the skull are rare and may produce radiologic changes resembling cephalhematoma deformans.

Epidermoids are ectodermal rests or inclusions that may be located in the scalp, in the diploic spaces, or between the internal surface of the inner table and the dura. Epidermoids are usually benign and grow slowly. If they protrude into the cranial cavity, they may be the source of cerebral symptoms. When epidermoids grow within the bone or impinge on it, they produce local destruction of bone that appears radiographically as a sharply demarcated lucency surrounded by a smooth sclerotic margin (Fig. 21-5), which sometimes may be scalloped. The margin is due to flaring of the edge of the bone into a marginal ridge. Most cases are found in children younger than 3 years.[8] The lesions usually disappear within a few years of discovery.

Meningiomas are rare in children. Radiographic changes include hyperostosis, an increase in the caliber and number of grooves for regional blood vessels, and calcifications in the meningioma itself. The hyperostosis is composed of normal reactive bone and is a complication rather than a part of the neoplasm. Occasionally, the overlying bone is destroyed, giving rise to radiolucent patches. Rarely, interosseous meningiomas occur (e-Fig. 21-6). Multiple meningiomas sometimes occur, most commonly in association with NF. Calvarial lesions, similar to the defects in NF, can occur in persons with congenital generalized fibromatosis.[9]

Chordomas are infrequent in children; they occur predominantly in the clivus with clinical signs of diplopia, palatal or tongue weakness, and headaches.[10,11] Torticollis occasionally is present. Magnetic resonance imaging (MRI) shows the location and extent of the chordoma. The tumor is inhomogeneous on T1-weighted and T2-weighted images and shows septations (Fig. 21-7).

Melanotic neuroectodermal tumor of infancy (melanotic progonoma, retinal anlage) is a rare tumor of the skull. The tumor is believed to be of neuroectodermal origin.[12-15] More than 90% of cases involve the head and neck region; 70% occur in the maxilla, and about 13% occur in the calvarium, where the tumor has a predilection for the region of the anterior fontanelle. About 6% of cases occur in the mandible. In the calvarium, the tumor usually begins during the first year of life as a movable scalp nodule that subsequently invades the bone, becomes fixed to it (often adhering to the dura), and grows very rapidly. The bone is destroyed, but reactive spicules develop internally and externally, producing a sunburst appearance tangential to the mass on films (e-Fig. 21-8). Occasionally the mass appears as a soft tissue density. Local recurrences may occur after surgical removal. Although malignancy has been noted in extracalvarial tumors, it has not been reported for tumors in the calvarium.

"Doughnut lesions" are rounded or oval radiolucent calvarial defects with a surrounding sclerotic halo, central bone density, or both.[16] Multiple radiographic "doughnut lesions" have been described.[17] Microscopic features in the calvarial lesions included fibrous tissue with clusters of foam cells or histiocytes and surrounding sclerotic bone. Familial doughnut lesions (Fig. 21-9) of the skull have been reported, and similar radiographic changes have been found in persons with sickle

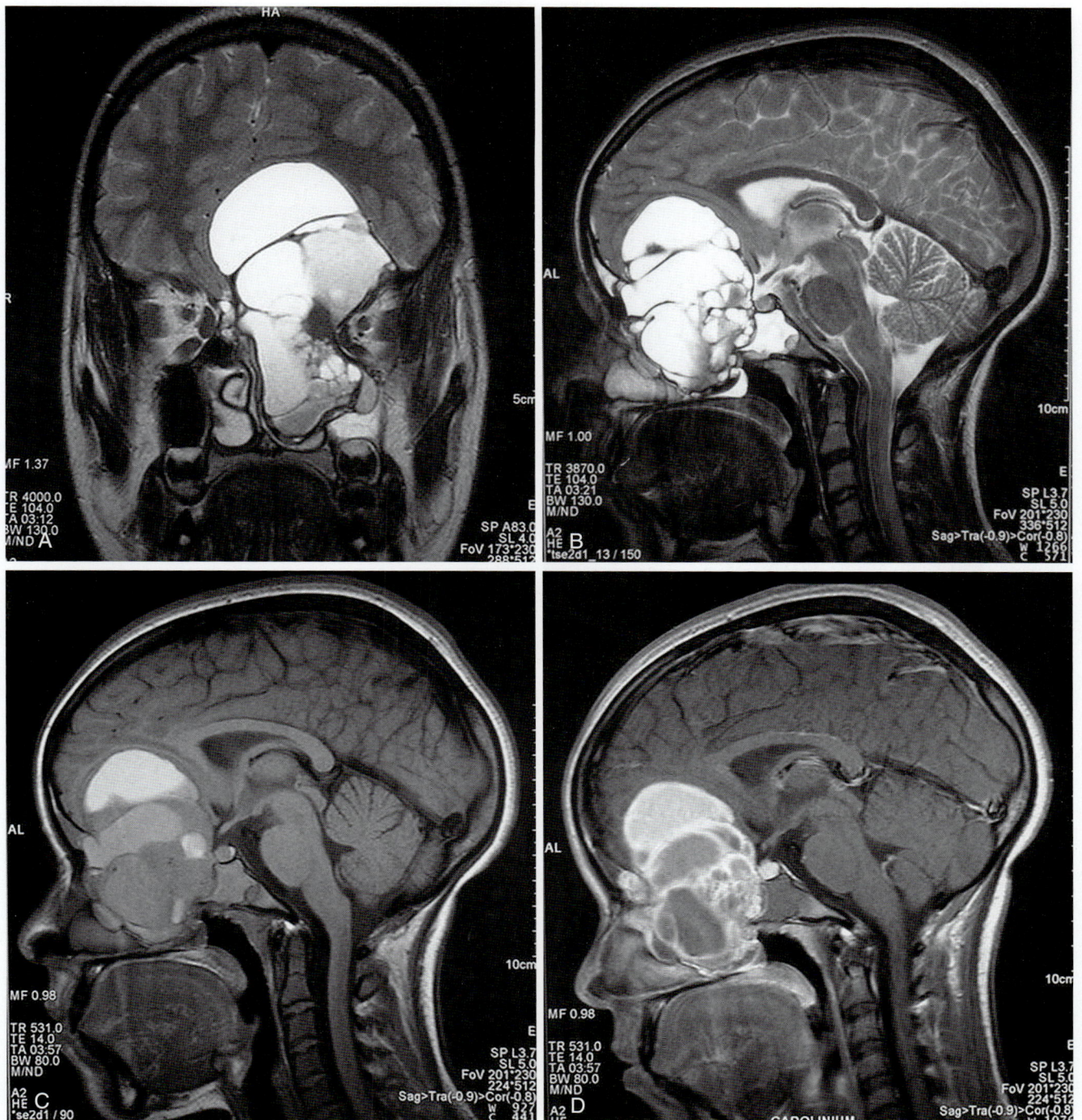

Figure 21-1 Aneurysmal bone cyst of the anterior skull base. **A,** A coronal T2-weighted magnetic resonance image shows a multicystic expansile lesion of the anterior skull base. The lesion extended into the anterior cranial fossa, left ethmoid bone, and clivus. Sagittal T2-weighted (**B**), T1-weighted (**C**), and gadolinium-enhanced (**D**) images reveal the multiple fluid levels and inhomogeneous enhancement of the central septations and periphery. Only 1% of aneurysmal bone cysts are in the skull and usually involve the cranial vault. (**A** and **B** From Theron S, Steyn F. An unusual cause of proptosis: aneurysmal bone cyst of the anterior skull base. *Pediatr Radiol.* 2006;36:997.)

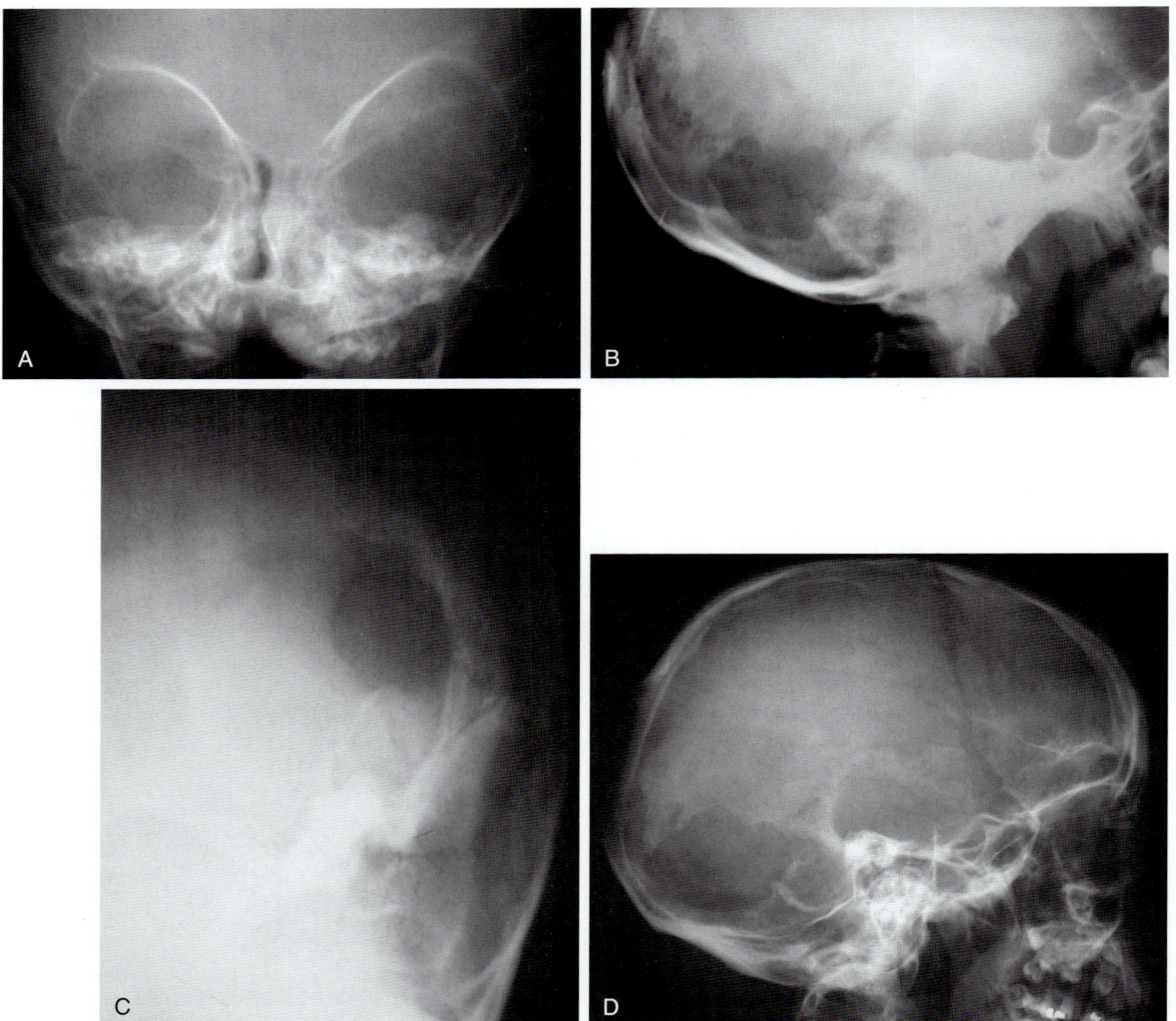

Figure 21-3 Skull changes of neurofibromatosis (NF) type 1. **A,** A frontal view of the orbits reveals an elevated sphenoid wing (bilateral) and hypoplasia of the left sphenoid bone. **B** and **C,** A 5-year-old boy with NF has a defect in the left lambdoid suture seen on lateral (**B**) and oblique (**C**) views. **D,** A lateral view of another child with NF who has a large skull defect seen in the left lambdoid suture. (Courtesy Peter Strouse, MD, Ann Arbor, MI.)

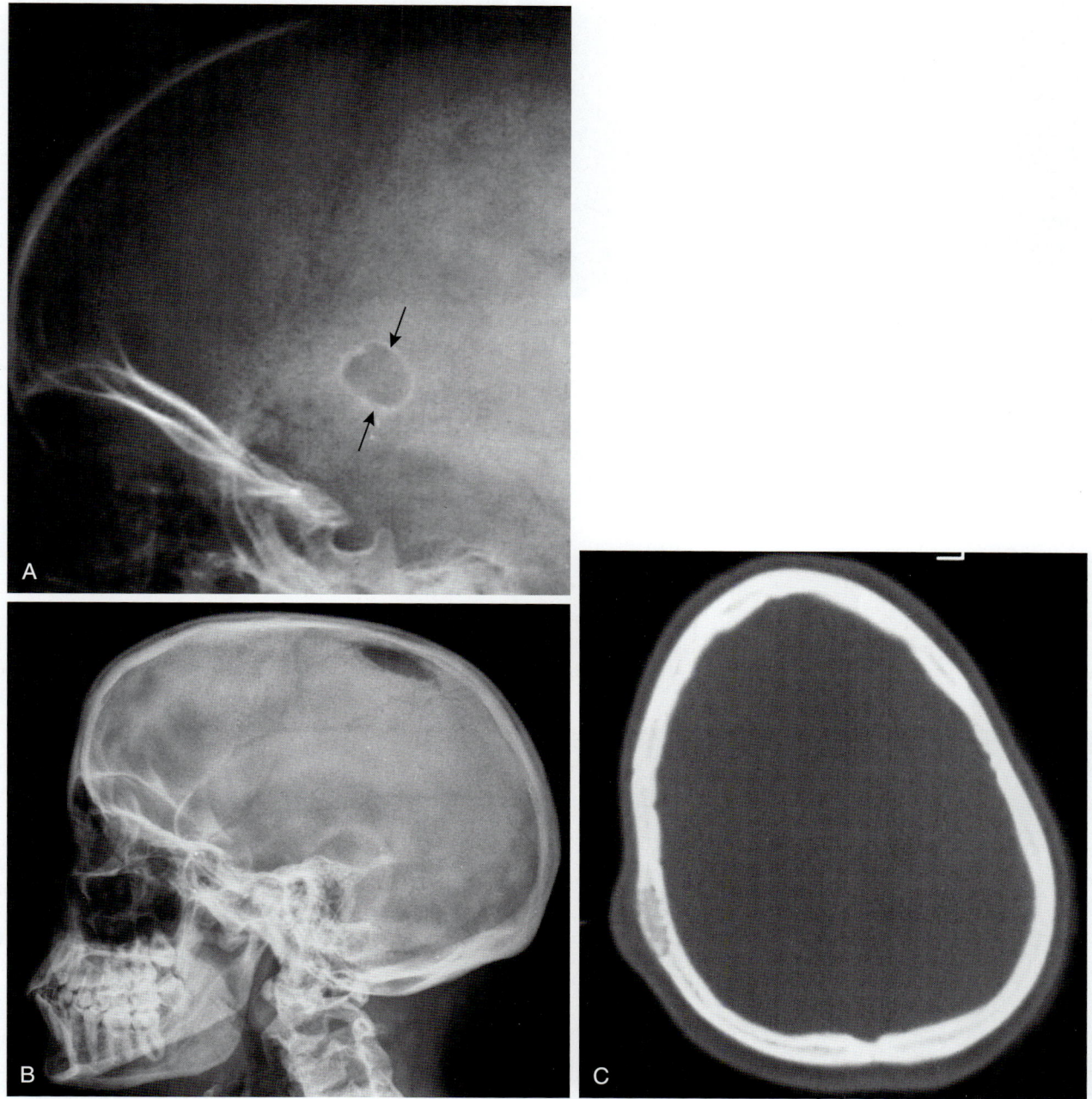

Figure 21-5   An epidermoid in a 1-year-old infant. **A,** Arrows point to a small oval defect in the parietal bone with a sharply defined sclerotic border. **B** and **C,** An epidermoid in another child shows that these lesions may not be as well demarcated by sclerotic edges (**B**). A computed tomography scan reveals the lesion and soft tissue swelling (**C**).

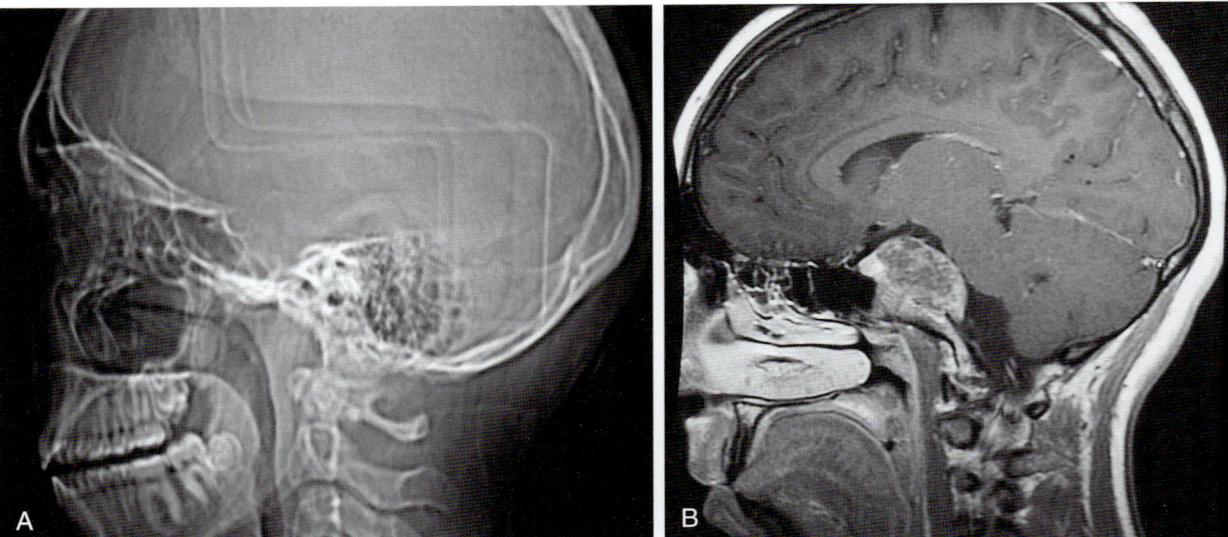

Figure 21-7   **A chordoma. A,** A computed tomography scout image reveals the absence of the clivus. **B,** A contrast-enhanced magnetic resonance image shows the huge enhancing chordoma, which is involving the clivus and sphenoid, pushing on the brainstem.

cell anemia. A malignant calvarial doughnut lesion caused by a metastatic carcinoma has been reported with features of a button sequestrum.[18]

Secondary Neoplasms

Secondary tumors of the calvarium are more common than primary tumors and include leukemia, neuroblastoma, small round cell tumors, and histiocytosis (Figs. 21-10 through

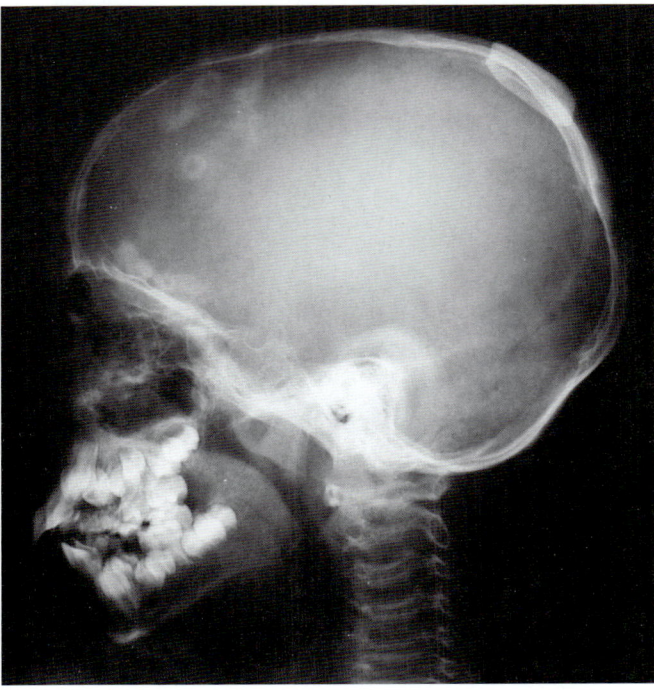

Figure 21-9   A calvarial doughnut lesion in a well child.

21-12 and e-Fig. 21-13). The differential diagnosis of a permeative pattern includes osteomyelitis.

Neoplasm-like Lesions

LANGERHANS CELL HISTIOCYTOSIS

LCH manifestations are addressed in more detail in Chapter 139; only their calvarial manifestations are presented here. Lesions in the skull are common, with a reported incidence of 28% in one large series.[19] The calvarium is affected more frequently than the skull base. Multiple lesions occur more frequently in children younger than 5 years. A solitary calvarial lesion in a child older than 5 years is likely to be associated with LCH of bone (Figs. 21-14 and 21-15). Lesions also occur in the mastoid portion of the temporal bone and adjacent petrous pyramids, in the sphenoid bone, and in the bones of the orbit.[20] Sphenoid bone involvement may be associated with diabetes insipidus. Exophthalmos may occur when the bones of the orbit are affected.[21]

Mandibular involvement with LCH is more common than maxillary involvement and begins characteristically in the molar areas of the alveolar processes, where focal destruction of bone results in a characteristic finding of "floating teeth." The teeth are frequently loose, and spontaneous shedding of teeth is common.

The radiographic hallmark of the disease is a "punched out" radiolucent defect with little or no adjacent reaction. Involvement of the external table to a greater degree than the internal table may produce a beveled edge. Lesions may extend intracranially and across sutures. LCH is the most common cause of a button sequestrum (which also may be seen in cases of infection, neoplastic disease, radiation necrosis, and a variety of other conditions). In the course of healing, the margins of the lesions lose their sharpness, and the disparity in opacity between the lesion and the adjacent bone diminishes to the point of disappearance.

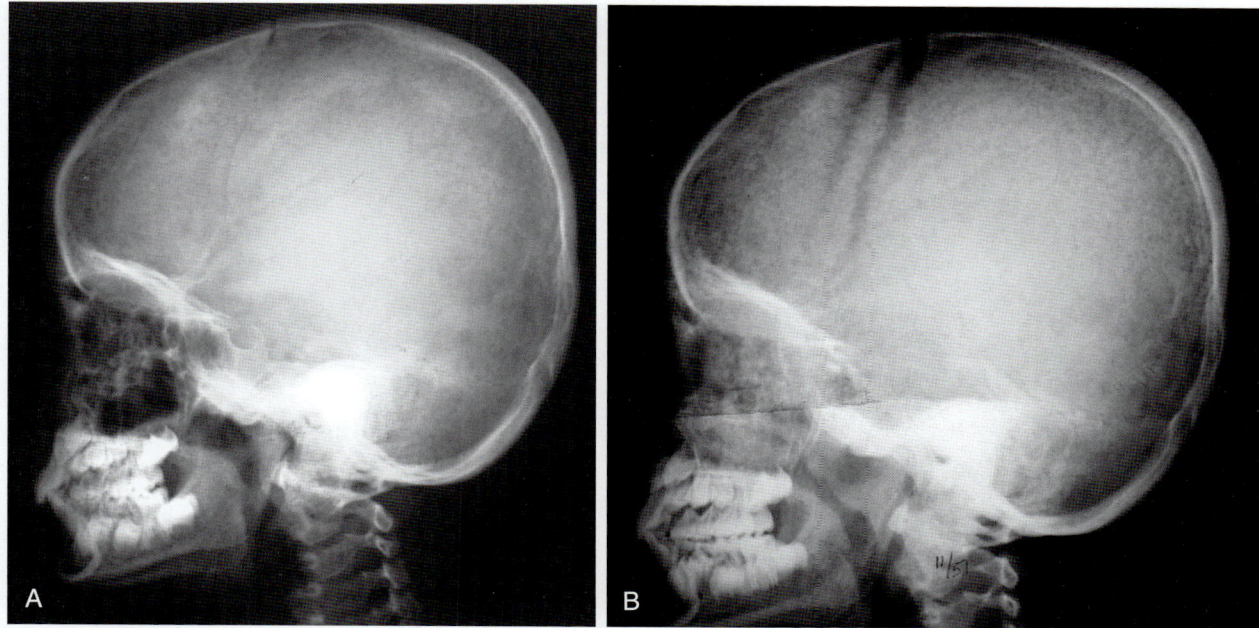

Figure 21-10 Leukemia. **A,** An initial radiograph shows a mottled "salt and pepper" appearance to the frontal region of the calvaria and some spiculation of bone over the parietal region. **B,** Radiographic evaluation in another child with leukemia shows much more florid inhomogeneity of the skull density and widened coronal sutures indicating increased intracranial pressure.

FIBROUS DYSPLASIA

Fibrous dysplasia of the calvarium in children usually involves the frontal, sphenoid, and ethmoid bones (Fig. 21-16)[22] and may manifest as painless progressive bony bulges or masses. Children rarely present with a change in vision or blindness as a result of compression of the orbital apex and ischemia of the optic nerve.[23]

CT findings of fibrous dysplasia consist of three types: the ground-glass pattern (56%), the homogeneously dense pattern (23%), and the cystic variety (21%).[24] The MR signal intensity of fibrous dysplasia is usually low on T1-weighted images and intermediate on T2-weighted images.[25,26] Fibrous tissue may demonstrate marked enhancement on MRI, simulating a tumor.

Infections of the Calvaria

OSTEOMYELITIS

Osteomyelitis of the skull is rare in children and is a complex disease with many different etiologies.[27] Infection at the pin site in children with halo insertion may occur when pins become loose.[28] Trauma is a common precursor.[29] Systemic diseases can alter the body's defense and predispose to infections. Bones adjacent to the paranasal sinuses may become infected from direct extension of sinusitis.

Hematogenous osteomyelitic foci may develop in the course of bacteremia, or the underlying bone may be infected by direct extension from cellulitis of the scalp or from compound fractures or bone flaps. Infection in the bone can spread inwardly to form epidural or subdural abscess, meningitis, or intracerebral inflammatory disease, or it can spread outwardly to form subgaleal or subcutaneous abscesses. Use of CT and MRI must be considered for identification of intracranial penetration.

During the early stages of osteomyelitis, the radiographic findings are negative. When areas of inflammatory necrosis of sufficient size develop, they can be identified as areas of diminished density involving the inner and outer tables and diploic spaces. These lesions may be single or multiple and are more common in the frontal and parietal bones than elsewhere. Localized osteomyelitis may spread by contiguity or through the diploic veins. Remote lesions first appear as fine lytic foci or rarefactions that enlarge and coalesce, sometimes giving rise to a moth-eaten rarefaction that involves the entire bone or even the entire calvarium. In infants, the avascular sutures act as barriers to spreading. The differential diagnosis of this permeative destructive pattern includes osteomyelitis, leukemia, metastatic neuroblastoma, and metastatic small round cell tumors (Ewing sarcoma, medulloblastoma, and retinoblastoma).[30] Clival osteomyelitis resulting from the spread of infection through the fossa navicularis magna has been reported after retropharyngeal abscess.[31] In chronic osteomyelitis, sclerotic changes usually are present; in disease resulting from paranasal sinusitis, the bony walls of the affected sinus often are sclerotic.

Infection of a cephalhematoma, usually after bacteremia or attempted needle aspiration, is not rare and may be associated with severe complications, such as osteomyelitis, septicemia, meningitis, and transverse venous sinus thrombosis.

The accuracy of diagnosing an infected cephalhematoma is poor because cephalhematomas without infection may demonstrate radiolucencies as they heal. CT is the best modality for showing bony erosion and destruction. MRI is superior for detecting the intracranial complications of venous sinus thrombosis and cerebellar hematoma or abscess.

Pott puffy tumor, described in 1760 by Sir Percival Pott, consists of a subperiosteal abscess and osteomyelitis of the frontal bone.[32,33] It may result from acute frontal sinusitis and trauma. The valveless diploic veins drain the sinuses, and

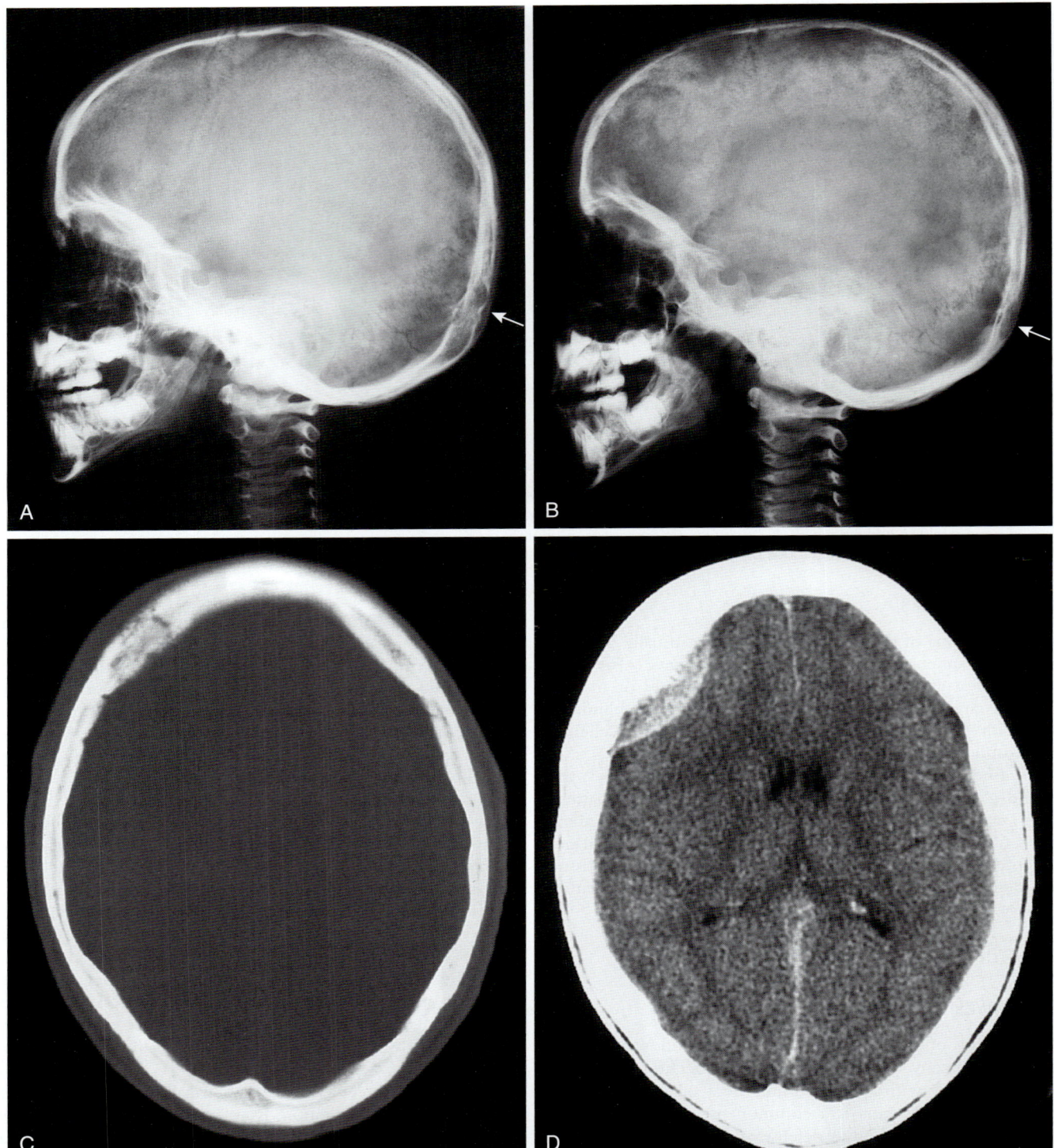

Figure 21-11 A metastatic neuroblastoma. **A** and **B,** Plain films in a child who presented with scalp pain and a destructive lesion in the occipital lobe. A mild "salt and pepper" change of the calvaria is present in (**A**), seen best in the frontal and occipital regions (*arrow*). This change is much more pronounced in **B**. **C** and **D,** A computed tomography scan in another patient. A permeative right frontal lesion is present, and brain imaging shows the enhancing epidural mass.

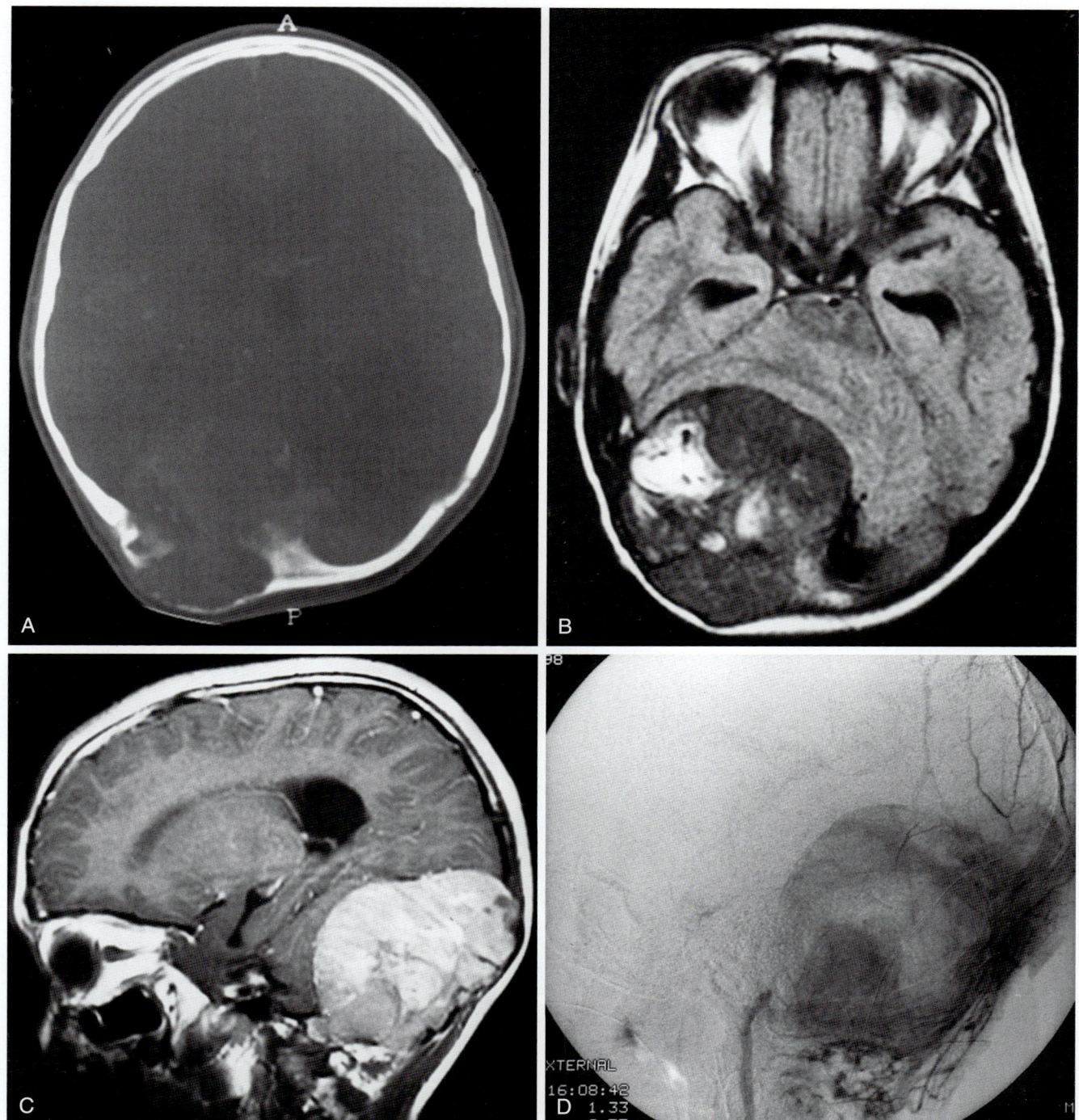

Figure 21-12 A metastatic neuroblastoma. **A,** An axial computed tomography scan shows a mass in the occipital region with bone destruction. Axial nonenhanced (**B**) and sagittal enhanced (**C**) magnetic resonance imaging scans show the extradural mass. **D,** Angiography shows that the mass is vascular.

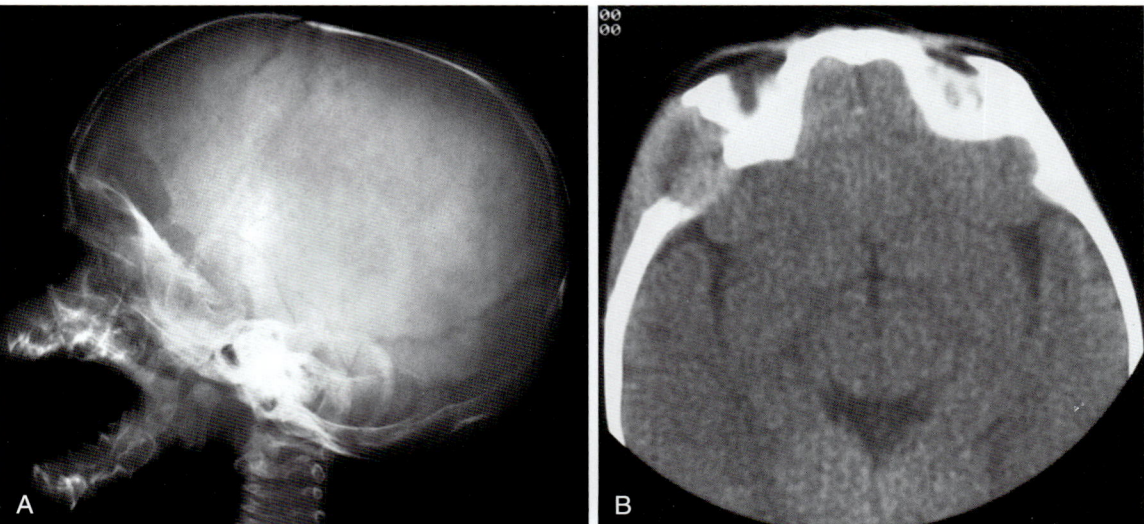

Figure 21-14   Langerhans cell histiocytosis. **A,** A lateral skull film shows a lytic, well-defined lesion in the frontal region just above the orbit. **B,** A computed tomography scan shows the bony destruction and soft tissue mass in this region. Note the beveled appearance with the greater destruction of the outer table.

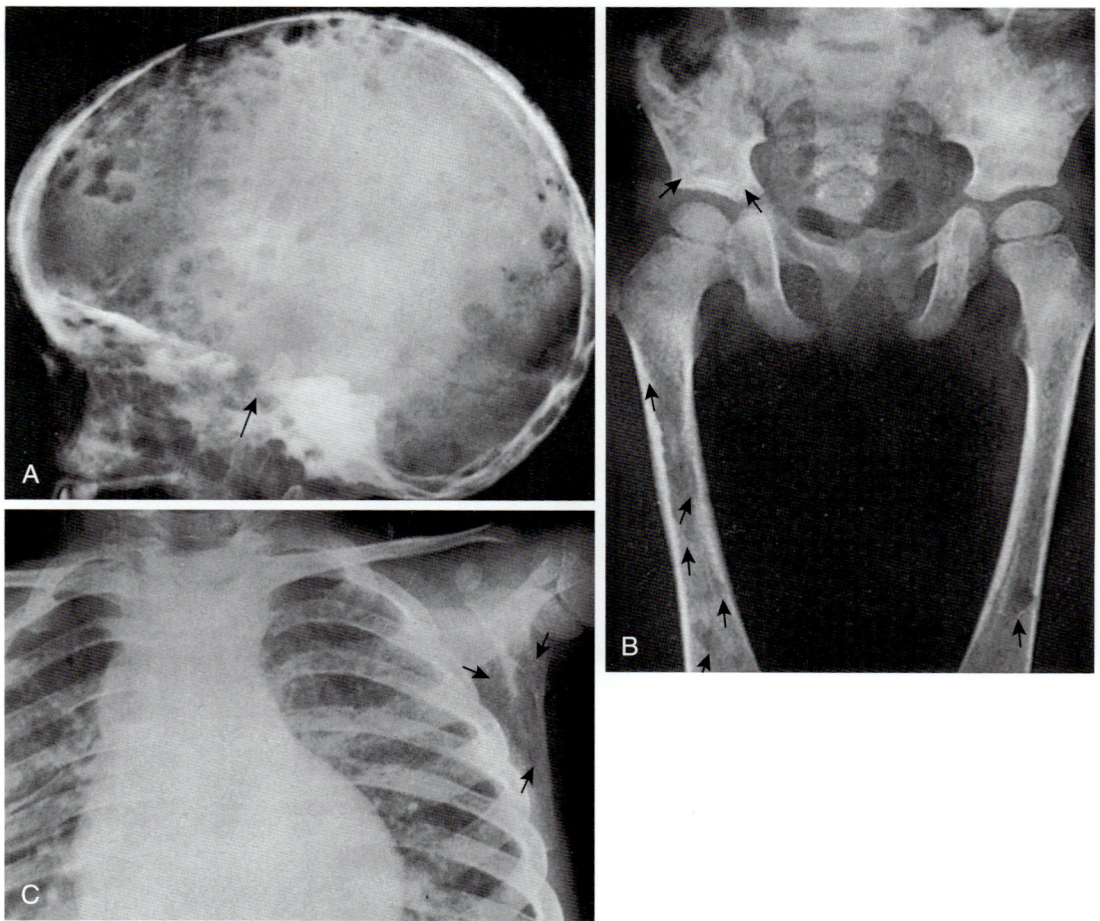

Figure 21-15   Langerhans cell histiocytosis in a 3½-year-old boy. **A,** A lateral skull radiograph shows numerous small and large rounded defects in the calvaria and base (*arrow*). An autopsy disclosed replacement of a large part of the body of the sphenoid. **B,** Large and small defects (*arrows*) in the ilia and femora; the latter show erosions of the cortex, which indicates their origin in the medullary cavity and not under the periosteum. **C,** Defects (*arrows*) in the scapula and infiltration of the lungs and pleura.

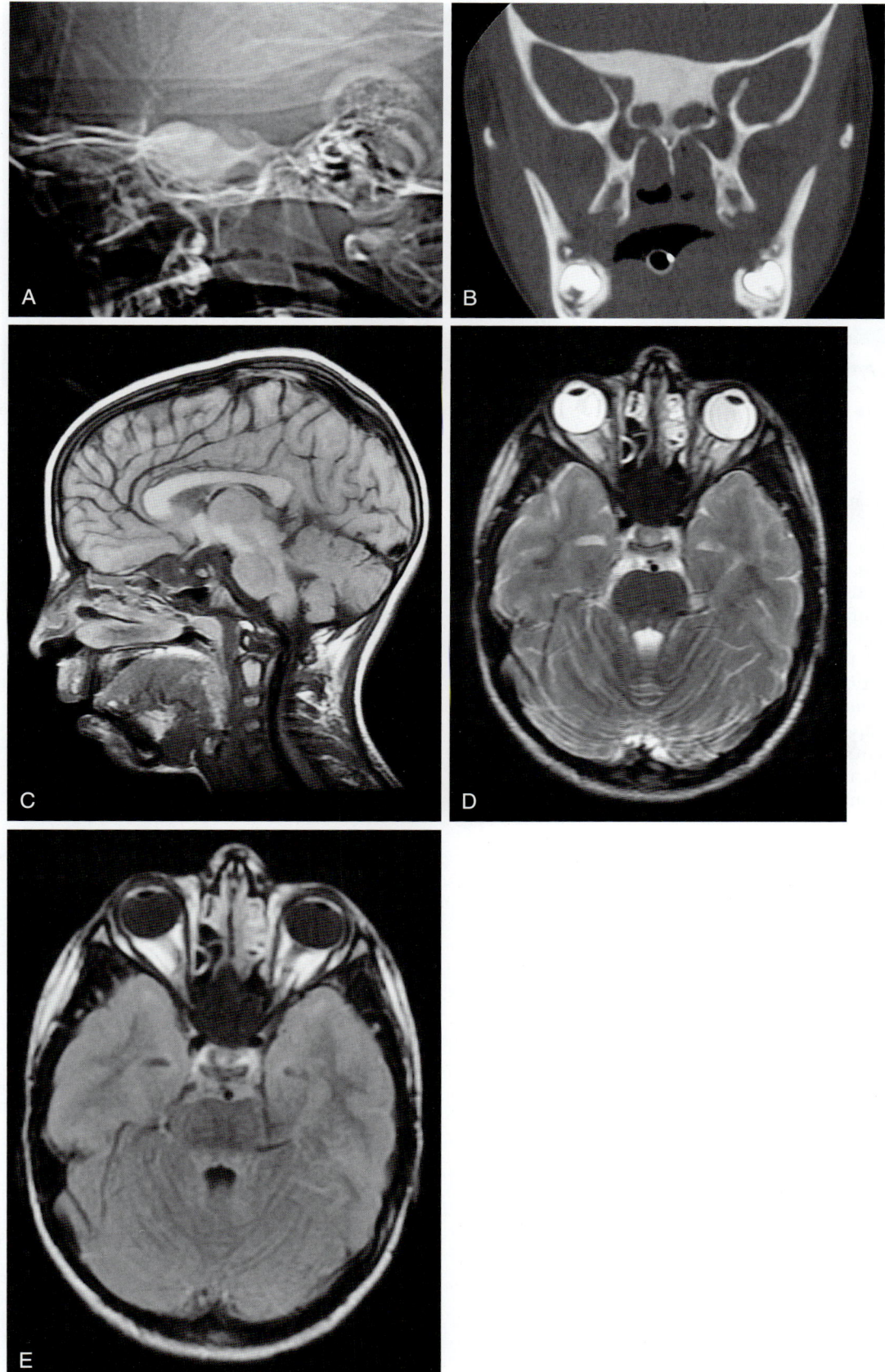

Figure 21-16 Fibrous dysplasia of the skull. **A**, A scout computed tomography (CT) film shows dense sphenoid bone. **B**, A coronal CT scan shows the extent of the lesion. **C, D,** and **E**, Magnetic resonance imaging shows the lesion to be hypointense on T1-weighted (**C**), T2-weighted (**D**), and fluid attenuated inversion recovery (**E**) sequences.

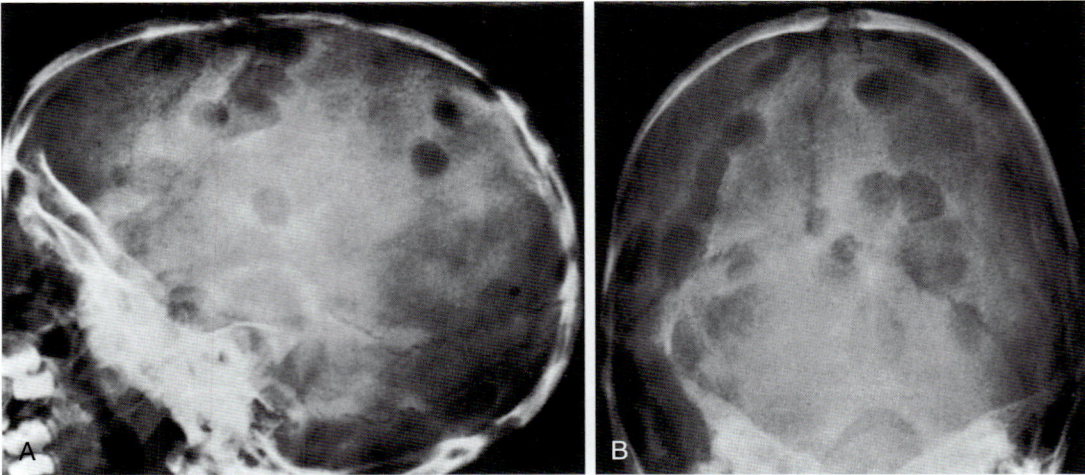

Figure 21-18 Multiple destructive tuberculosis foci in the calvaria of a 3-year-old girl. Lateral (**A**) and frontal (**B**) projections are shown.

septic emboli can lead to abscess formation (e-Fig. 21-17). Sonography may demonstrate a subgaleal abscess. CT and MRI may show frontal sinusitis, frontal osteomyelitis, and a subgaleal abscess.

Petrous apicitis (Gradenigo syndrome) must be considered in the setting of middle ear disease with headache, cranial neuropathy, and an elevated erythrocyte sedimentation rate. Characteristic CT and MRI findings include petrosal marrow T1 hypointensity, soft tissue abnormalities, and bone destruction. Cochlear implants are an increasing cause of mastoid inflammatory disease and osteomyelitis. Lytic lesions of the skull have been seen with cat scratch fever, and the frontal and sphenoid bones have been involved in chronic recurrent multifocal osteomyelitis.[34]

TUBERCULOSIS

Tuberculosis of the calvaria usually manifests as a painless subgaleal scalp swelling with a discharging sinus. The lesions are usually either small, circumscribed, punched-out lytic areas (Fig. 21-18); or spreading, circumscribed sclerotic areas; or a combination of the two.[35]

SARCOIDOSIS

Sarcoidosis of the diploic space is associated with large radiolucent patches in the frontal, parietal, and occipital bones (e-Fig. 21-19).[36]

SYPHILIS

The cranium can be involved in cases of infantile syphilis in association with severe syphilitic osteitis of the long bones. Destructive and productive changes may be present, usually in the parietal and frontal bones.

MYCOTIC OSTEOMYELITIS

The cranium sometimes is involved in chronic fungal infections, including actinomycosis, blastomycosis, coccidiomycosis, cryptococcosis, and candidiasis.[37] The radiographic appearance of the lesions is similar to that of tuberculous, syphilitic, and chronic purulent osteomyelitis, and diagnosis requires identification of the responsible organism. Underlying immunodeficiency often is present.[38]

Key Points

Primary neoplasms are rare in children. Most primary neoplasms are benign.

Secondary neoplasms are more common than primary neoplasms.

LCH can have many appearances.

Trauma and sinusitis are common precursors to osteomyelitis.

Pott puffy tumor consists of a subperiosteal abscess and osteomyelitis of the frontal bone.

Suggested Readings

Arico M, Egeler PM. Clinical aspects of Langerhans cell histiocytosis. *Hematol Oncol Clin North Am.* 1998;12:247-258.

Atkinson GO, Davis PC, Patrick LE, et al. Melanotic neuroectodermal tumour of infancy: MR findings and a review of the literature. *Pediatr Radiol.* 1989;20:20-22.

Calliauw L, Roels H, Caemaert J. Aneurysmal bone cysts in the cranial vault and base of the skull. *Surg Neurol.* 1985;23:93-98.

Koch BL. Imaging extracranial masses of the pediatric head and neck. *Neuroimaging Clin N Am.* 2000;10:193-214.

Lui YW, Dasari SB, Young RJ. Sphenoid masses in children: radiologic differential diagnosis with pathologic correlation. *AJNR Am J Neuroradiol.* 2011;32:617-626.

Miyazaki S, Tsubokawa T, Katayama Y, et al. Benign osteoblastoma of the temporal bone in an infant. *Surg Neurol.* 1987;27:277-285.

Posnick JC, Wells MD, Drake JM, et al. Childhood fibrous dysplasia presenting as blindness: a skull base approach for resection and immediate reconstruction. *Pediatr Neurosurg.* 1993;19:260-266.

References

Full references for this chapter can be found on www.expertconsult.com.

Chapter 22

The Mandible

THOMAS L. SLOVIS

Embryology

At birth, the mandible consists of two lateral halves united in the midline at the symphysis by a bar of cartilage (Fig. 22-1, e-Fig. 22-2, and Figs. 22-3 and 22-4). Bony fusion of the symphysis usually occurs before the second year, but segments of the fissures may persist beyond puberty. The body of the mandible is large at birth compared with the relatively short rami and poorly differentiated coronoid and condylar processes. The rami form an angle of about 160 degrees with the body at birth.

Formation of the dental buds is visible by 20 weeks' gestation. Beginning mineralization in the first molar tooth occurs between gestational weeks 33 and 34, and in the second molar tooth, it occurs between gestational weeks 36 and 37. In contrast to bone age, dental age is little affected by endocrine aberrations.

All or some of the teeth may be missing developmentally, as in persons with anhidrotic ectodermal dysplasia (Fig. 22-4).[1] Because infants and children with normal dentition seem to have a plethora of teeth in radiographs (deciduous and permanent dentitions), the condition may be recognized in a newborn by the lack of dental buds. Many diseases cause loss of dentition, and recognition of premature loss of teeth can lead to important diagnoses (Box 22-1).[2]

The opposite condition—too many teeth with little alveolar bone—can be seen in persons with cleidocranial dysplasia, who have marked delay in shedding of the deciduous teeth. Early tooth extraction has no effect on the subsequent eruption of the permanent dentition and may result in a lengthy edentulous period for the child.[3]

Anatomy

The mandible is the only freely movable bone of the face; it articulates with the temporal bone in the temporomandibular fossa anterior to the external auditory canal (see Fig. 22-3). The range of motion is free in all directions, and the condyle moves downward and forward in the articular fossa upon opening of the jaw.

The temporomandibular joint (see Fig. 22-3) is a complex joint in which a biconcave fibrous disk divides the articular space into upper and lower compartments.[4-6] Gliding movements occur in the upper compartment, whereas the lower compartment functions as a true hinge joint. The articulating bony surfaces are not covered by hyaline cartilage as in other joints, but by an avascular, fibrous tissue that is separated from the underlying bone of the condyle by growth cartilage.[7]

Diseases of the Mandible

Significant congenital malformations of the mandible are rare, with the most important being hypoplasia (micrognathia), which may be a cause of congenital stridor. The short, small mandible apparently causes a retrodisplacement of the tongue and obstruction to airflow (Fig. 22-5).

Micrognathia occurs in a variety of dysmorphic syndromes. The combination of cleft palate and hypoplasia of the mandible defines the Pierre Robin sequence radiographically. The Pierre Robin association is nonspecific and occurs with several genetic and drug-induced syndromes and some loosely associated anomalies, as well as an isolated symptom complex.[8] In the cerebrocostomandibular syndrome, it is associated with posterior rib defects, cleft palate, and, occasionally, mental retardation.[9]

Elongation of the body of the mandible and widening of its arc occur in conditions associated with an enlarged tongue, including lymphatic malformations and Beckwith-Wiedemann syndrome. Relative enlargement of the mandible is observed in several craniofacial syndromes. The angle of the mandible is markedly increased in persons with pyknodysostosis. Rare cases of hyperplasia of the coronoid process are observed; the enlargement impinges on the zygomatic arch and interferes with normal opening of the jaw. The temporomandibular joints frequently are involved in persons with juvenile rheumatoid arthritis. Rarely, the mandible may be partially duplicated.

Temporomandibular Joint Disorders

Disorders of the temporomandibular joint are infrequent but not rare.[10,11] Adventitious sounds on mandibular movement, muscle tenderness or pain, and deviation of the mandible during movement are the most common signs and symptoms. Magnetic resonance imaging (MRI) is the most precise imaging modality.[12,13]

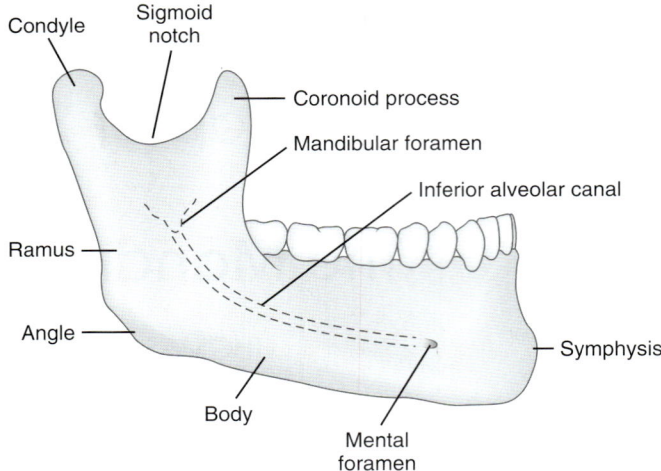

Figure 22-1 Important anatomic features of the normal mandible.

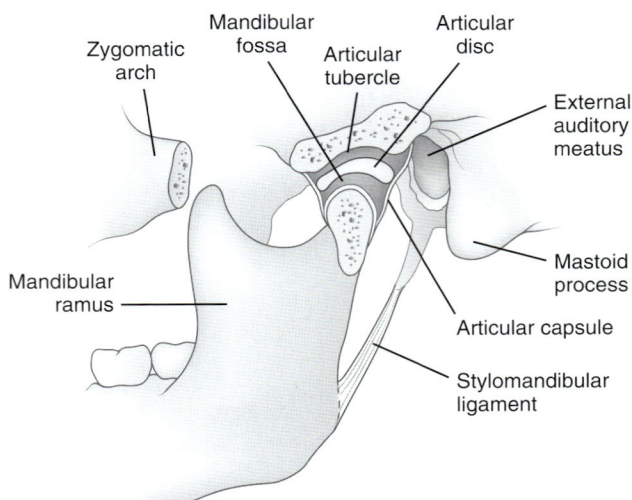

Figure 22-3 Anatomy of a normal temporomandibular joint. The zygomatic arch and a portion of the ramus of the mandible are cut away to expose the articular disk.

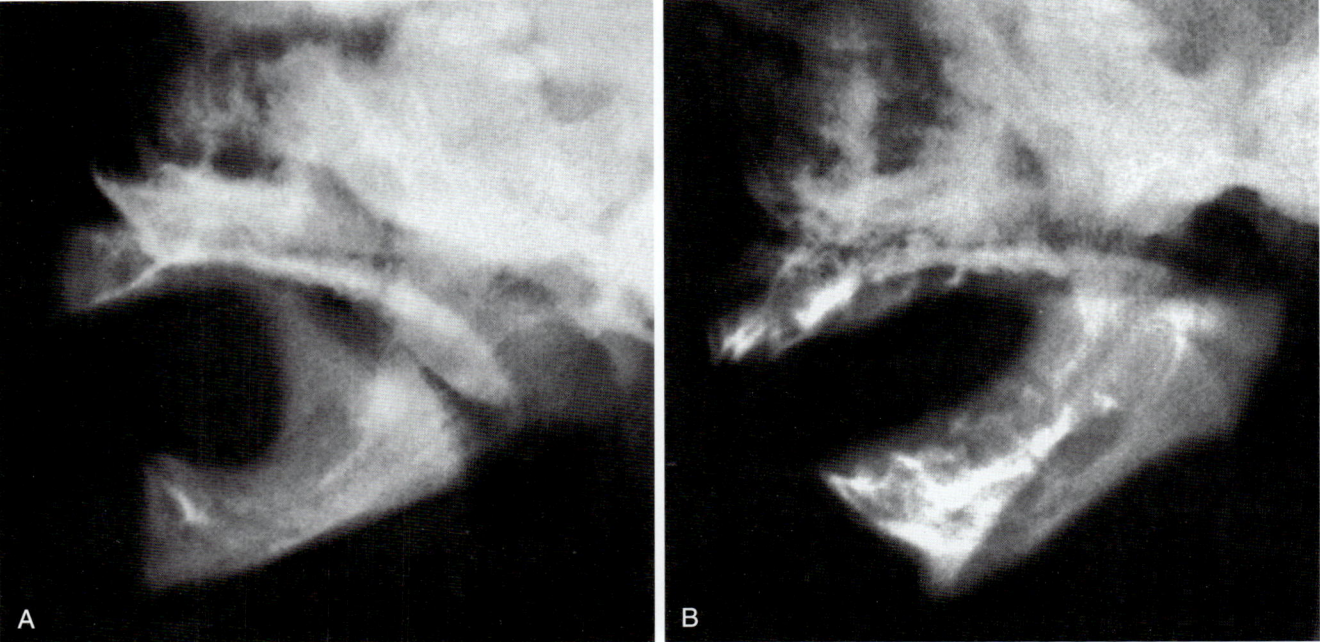

Figure 22-4 **A,** A mandible in an 8-week-old infant with hereditary ectodermal dysplasia shows failure of calcification of dental crowns and defective dental sacs. **B,** A radiograph of a normal 8-day-old newborn shows normal dental development in the neonatal period.

Box 22-1 Premature Loss of Primary or Permanent Teeth

Most Common

Hypophosphatasia
  Early-onset periodontitis
  • Secondary to any condition with impaired polymorphonuclear leukocyte function
  • Diabetes mellitus (usually poorly controlled)

Medications

Membrane ion chamber blockers
  Antiepileptic drugs
  Antihypertensive calcium antagonist
  Cyclosporine (alone or in combination with nifedipine)
  Steroids

Other Systemic Diseases

Human immunodeficiency virus
  Histiocytosis syndromes
  Acrodynia

Genetic Disorders

Down syndrome
  Chronic granulomatous disease
  Papillon-Lefèvre syndrome
  Chédiak-Higashi syndrome
  Ehlers-Danlos syndrome
  Wiskott-Aldrich syndrome

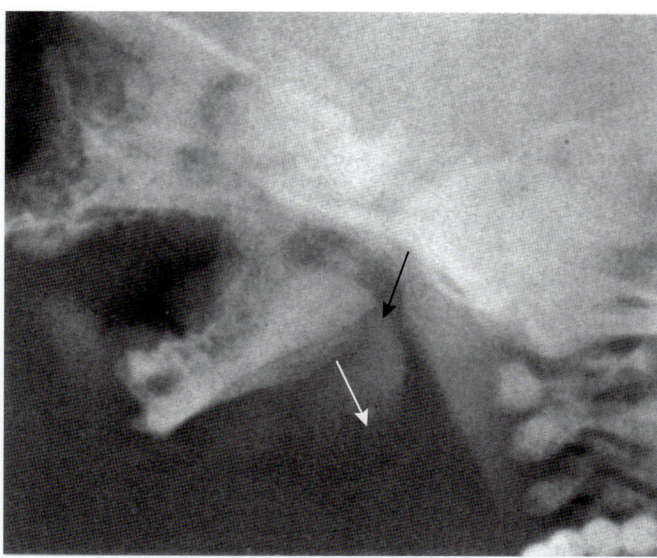

Figure 22-5 Hypoplasia of the mandible in a 1-day-old newborn—lateral projection. The short dorsoventral diameter of the mandible is evident; the tongue is displaced posteriorly and fills the greater part of the pharynx (*black arrow*). The displaced tongue impinged on the epiglottis and interfered with the flow of air to and from the larynx (*white arrow*).

Fractures

Direct trauma is the usual cause of fractures, although pathologic fractures occur in association with cysts, destructive inflammations, and neoplasms. More than half of traumatic fractures are found in the body of the mandible near the canine fossa. Fractures high in the ramus frequently are overlooked on standard radiographs but are clearly defined by computed tomography (CT) (Fig. 22-6) and panographic tomography (e–Fig. 22-7). Direct trauma is the usual cause, although pathologic fractures occur in association with cysts, destructive inflammations, and neoplasms. More than half of traumatic fractures are found in the body of the mandible near the canine fossa.

Vehicular trauma is responsible for 35% of mandibular fractures in children, and falls cause 28%. More condylar fractures are found in younger children (<9 years). During childhood, the mandible contains teeth in different stages of eruption, and the pattern of the alveolar bone predisposes it to fractures along the lines of the developing dental crypts. The lack of cortical bone and the relative excess of cancellous bone are responsible for the frequency of incomplete, greenstick fractures with minimal destruction of the bone or cartilage. The condylar neck usually breaks before the condyle itself because of the vascularity and thickness of the latter. During childhood, rapid union of mandibular fractures should be expected because of the rich blood supply, the high osteogenic potential of the periosteum, and the high local metabolic rate.[14] The radiographic criteria for healing of fractures in other bones are not applicable to mandibular fractures because strips of rarefaction may persist at the margins of the fracture long after satisfactory union has occurred.

Osteomyelitis

Osteomyelitis rarely occurs in the mandible because it has no metaphyseal–epiphyseal junction structures. Osteomyelitis generally occurs as a result of dental infection or local trauma (e–Fig. 22-8). The immature mandibular structure allows inflammation to extend easily and rapidly. Bone necrosis and sequestra formation are common; destructive changes may not be visible by conventional radiography until weeks after the onset of infection.[15] Hyperplastic changes usually predominate and have been confused with the manifestations of infantile cortical hyperostoses (Caffey disease).

Cysts, Neoplasms, and Neoplasm-like Disorders

Most primary mandibular cysts and neoplasms are of dental origin (Figs. 22-9 through 22-11, e–Fig. 22-12, and Box 22-2).[16] Cystic changes of the jaw may be a manifestation of the basal cell nevus syndrome, in which basal cell carcinomas, skeletal anomalies, ovarian and falx calcification, ovarian fibromas, and pits in the palms and soles also are present (see Fig. 22-9). The jaw cysts may manifest in

---

Box 22-2 Categorization of Jaw Lesions by Radiographic Appearance on Panoramic Radiographs

Well-circumscribed Lesions

Odontogenic origin
- Periapical granulosa
- Odontoma
- Dentigerous cyst
- Radicular cyst

Nonodontogenic origin
- Simple bone cyst
- Aneurysmal bone cyst
- Central giant cell granulosa
- Giant cell tumor

Poorly Circumscribed Radiolucent Lesions

Central hemangioma
Infection

Lesions of Mixed or Variable Appearance

Cemento-ossifying fibroma
Cementoma
Cemento-osseous dysplasia
Osteosarcoma
Non-Hodgkin lymphoma
Ewing sarcoma
Osteoma

Radiopaque Lesions

Chondrosarcoma
Fibrous dysplasia
Fibromatosis

From Gupta M, Kaste SC, Hopkins KP. Radiologic appearance of primary jaw lesions in children. *Pediatr Radiol.* 2002;32:153-168.

Text continued on page 231.

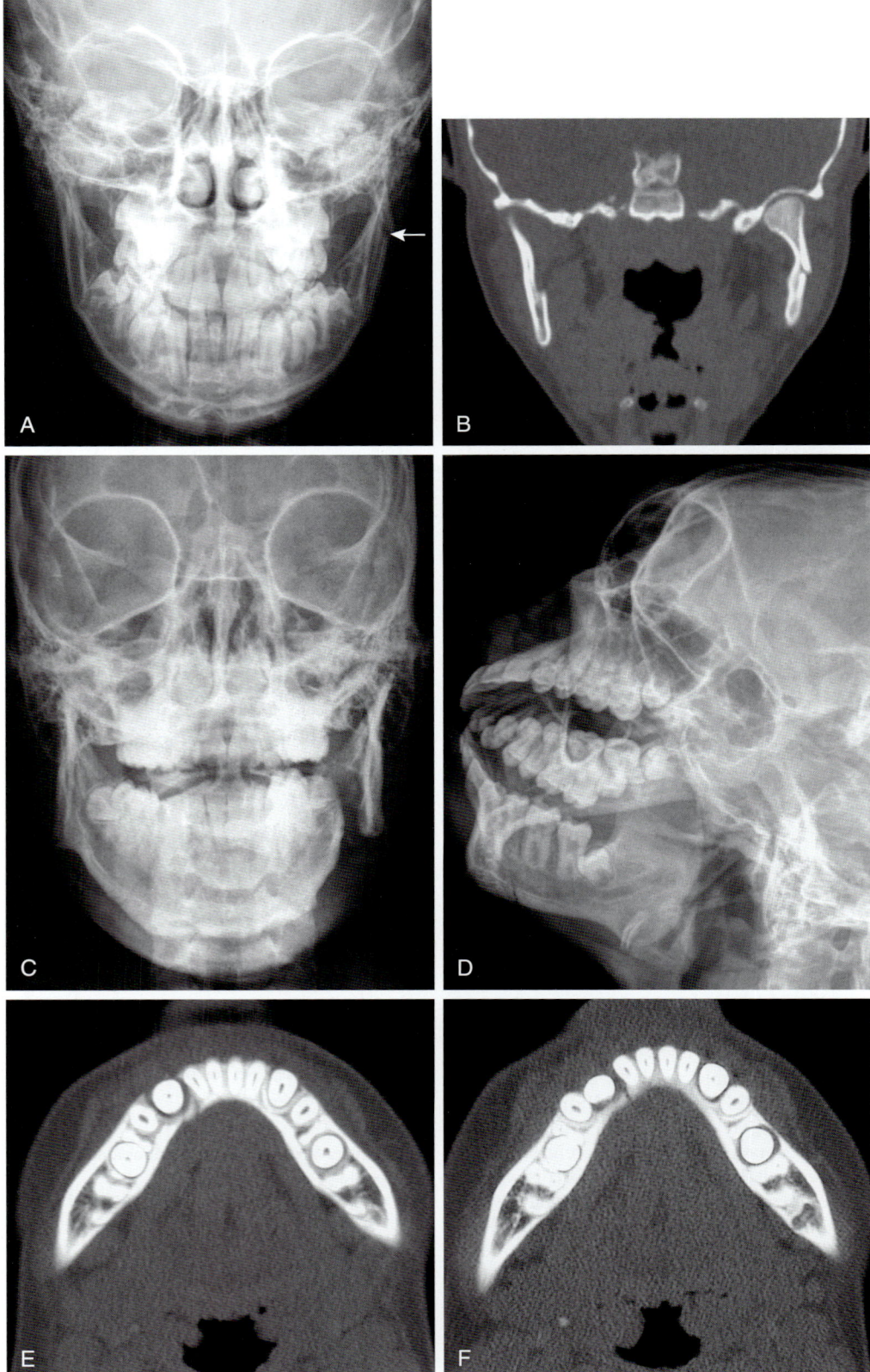

Figure 22-6   A fractured mandible. **A,** A 14-year-old patient with a subtle fracture of the left mandibular vertical ramus (*arrow*). **B,** Coronal computed tomography reconstruction shows the fracture. **C, D, E,** and **F,** A 14-year-old patient with an overt left mandibular fracture of the body and ramus junction and a subtle fracture through the right dentition.

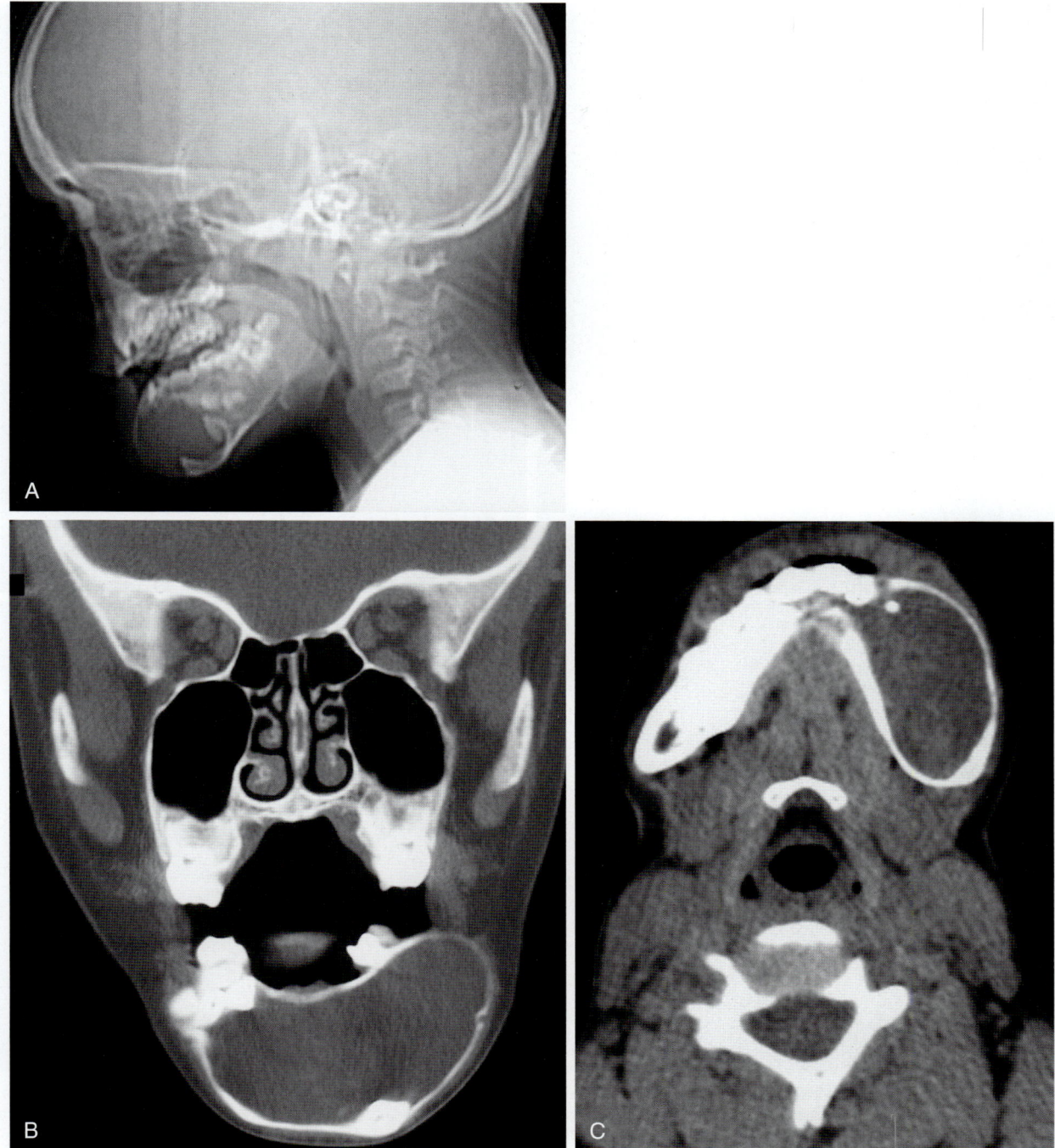

Figure 22-9 An 11-year-old patient with basal cell nevi syndrome. **A,** A skull radiograph from the computed tomography (CT) scout image reveals the large round lesion in the central portion (mentum) of the mandible deviating the dentition. **B,** A coronal nonenhanced CT scan shows that the lesion is homogeneous. **C,** An axial CT scan with soft tissue windows shows a deviation of dentition and the well-circumscribed lesion.

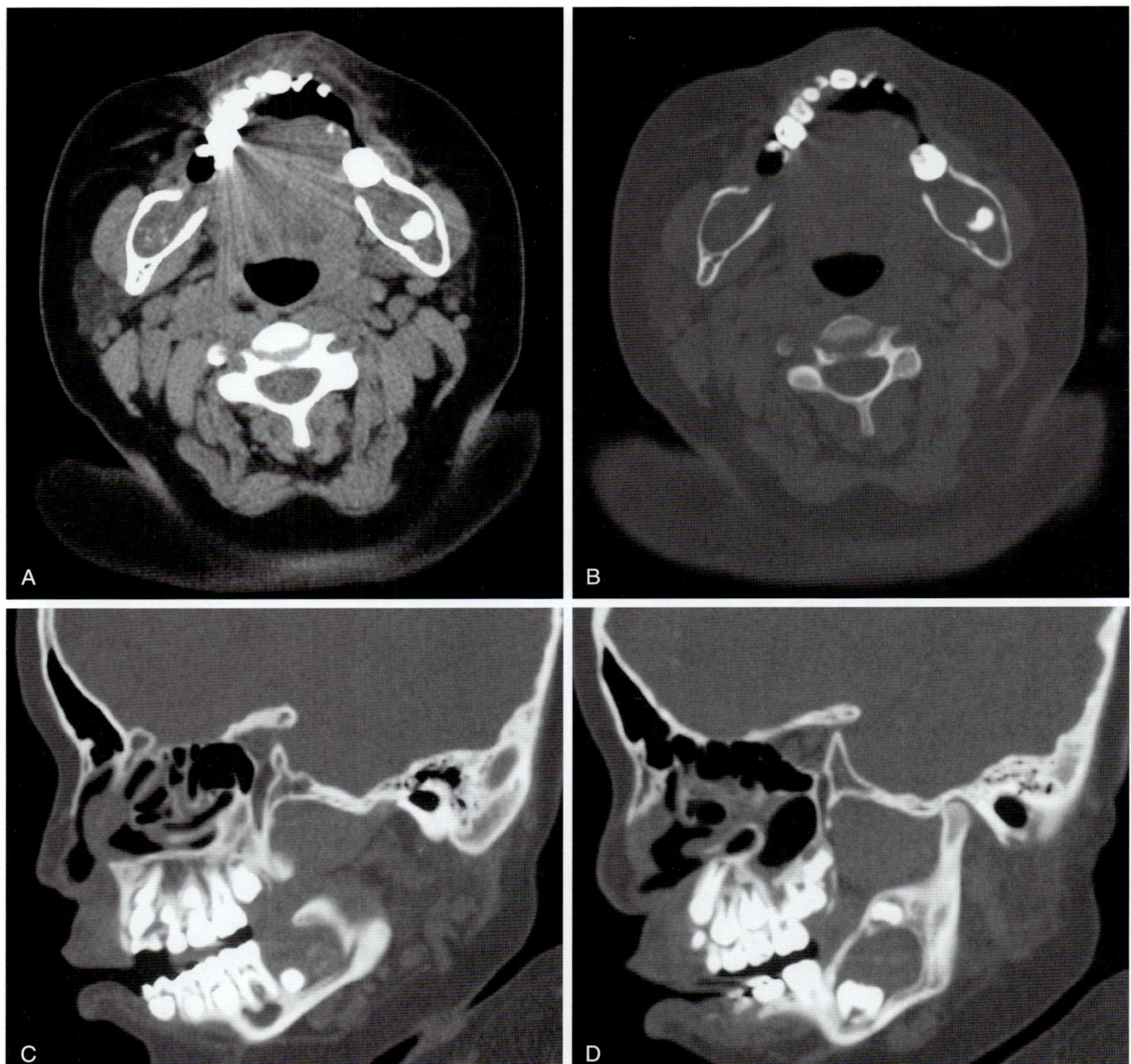

Figure 22-10 A 2-year-old patient with multiple odontogenic keratocysts. **A,** An axial scan shows bilateral lesions in the posterior aspect of the body of the mandible that are deviating the dentition. **B,** Bone windows show further the extent of remodeling on the mandible. **C** and **D,** Sagittal reconstruction reveals the isointense lesion and its effect on the teeth and the mandible.

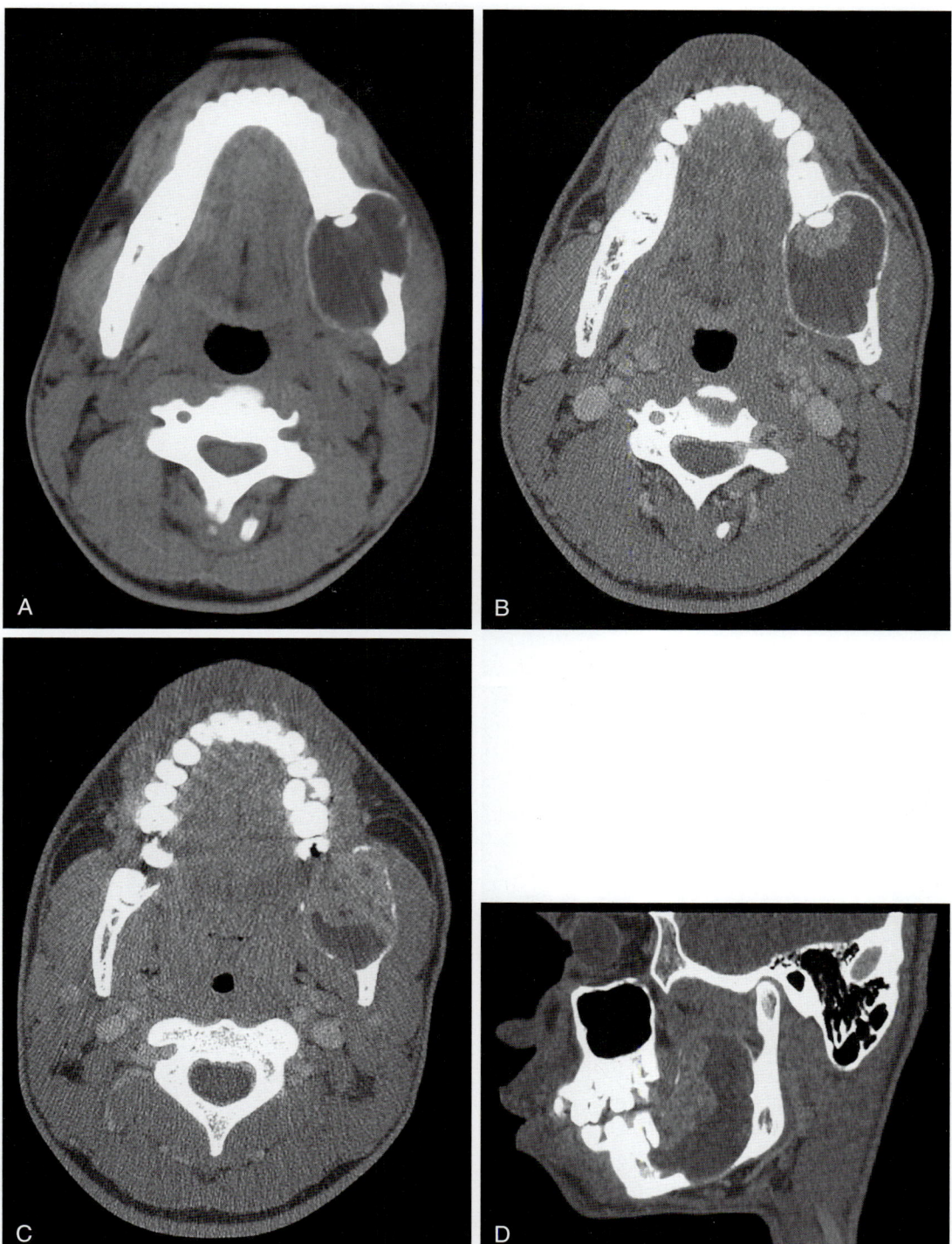

Figure 22-11 A 4-year-old patient with ameloblastoma of the left mandible. **A,** An axial computed tomography (CT) scan shows the large destructive lesion of the left mandible. **B,** Contrast-enhanced axial CT. With further windowing, the two components of the lesion are demonstrated: a more solid component anteriorly and a more cystic component posteriorly. **C,** A cut slightly inferior to that shown in **B** reveals the solid component. **D,** The sagittal reconstruction shows the effect on the mandible; solid and cystic components of the lesion are seen.

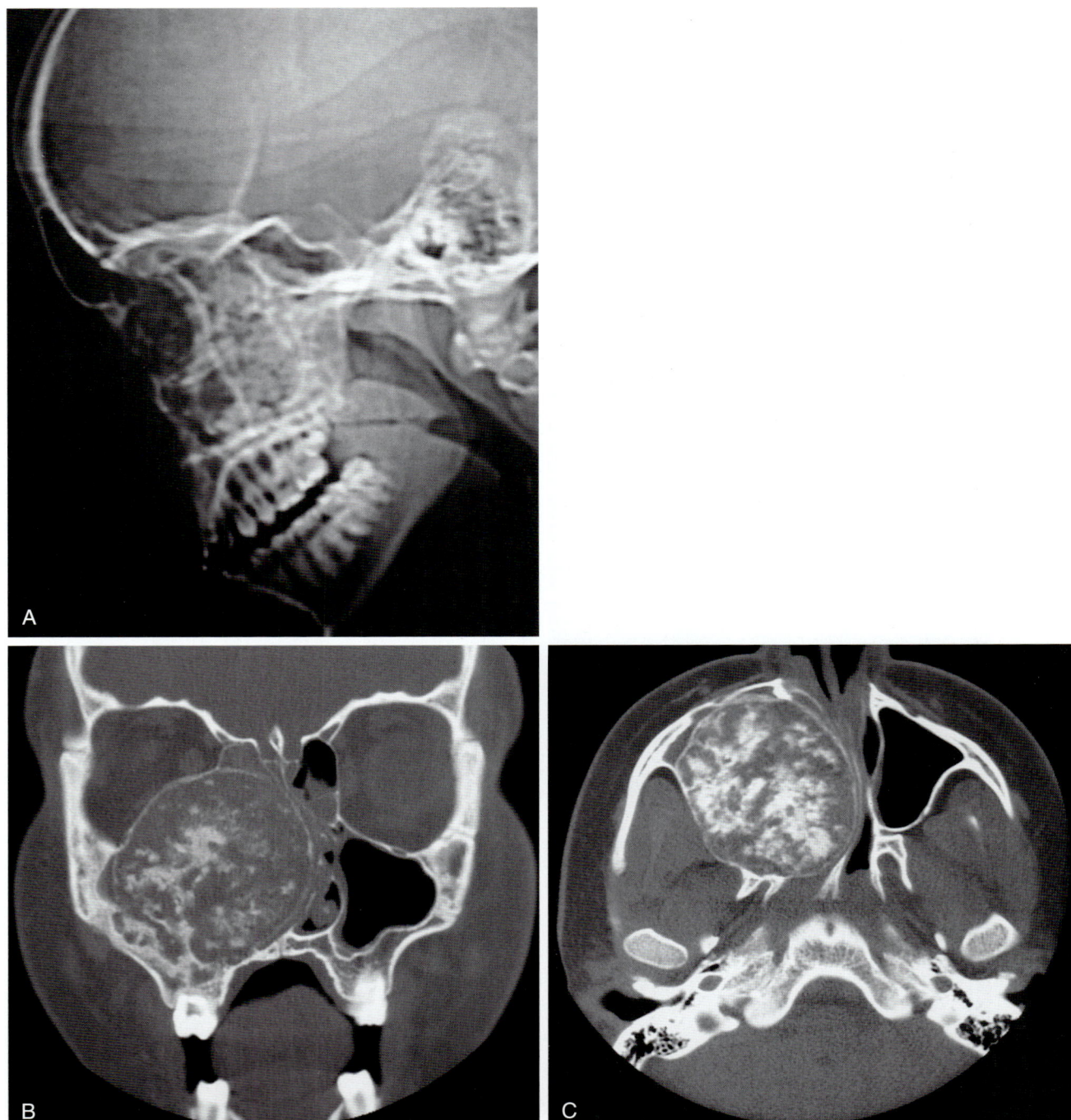

Figure 22-14 **Chondrosarcoma of the maxilla. A,** The lateral view of a computed tomography (CT) scout image reveals increased calcification of the midface. **B** and **C,** Coronal (**B**) and axial (**C**) CT scans show the cartilaginous matrix. This large lesion is destroying the right maxilla, invading the right maxillary sinus, and obstructing the right nasal passage.

childhood; the basal cell carcinomas develop only later. Dental root cysts result from proliferation of paradental epithelial cells in the periapical granulation tissue of local infection. Dentigerous cysts are formed by the excessive accumulation of fluid between the enamel and the dental capsule and show a well-formed dental crown without roots with its base adjacent to a large cystic structure that surrounds its upper portion (see Fig. 22-10).

Cystic adamantinomas or ameloblastomas result from the proliferation of ectopic ameloblasts derived from the enamel organ (see Fig. 22-11).[17] Composite odontomas have increased radiodensity (see e-Fig. 22-12). Osteomas and giant cell tumors resemble similar lesions elsewhere, but tissue diagnosis is necessary in all cases. Osteomas of the mandible and other cranial bones may be a manifestation of Gardner syndrome, which is associated with other connective tissue tumors and particularly polyposis of the large bowel. Benign osteoblastoma has been reported in the mandible. Giant cells, usually osteoclasts, are found in a variety of bone lesions in the jaws.[18] Radiographic findings alone do not provide adequate differential characteristics because radiographic, CT, and MRI patterns may be found in association with several different microscopic patterns (e-Fig. 22-13, Fig. 22-14, and e-Fig. 22-15).

The radiographic "floating teeth" of Langerhans cell histiocytosis (Fig. 22-16) are not pathognomonic, having been observed in metastatic neuroblastoma, lymphosarcoma, reticulum cell sarcoma, and Ewing sarcoma. Neuroblastoma is the most common metastatic disease to the mandible.[19] The common pathologic factor is a destructive process that affects the supporting alveolar structures of the teeth. Melanotic neuroectodermal tumor of infancy occurs most frequently in

the maxilla; however, occasionally it may arise in the mandible. In native children of equatorial Africa, Burkitt lymphoma of the jaw accounts for 30% to 50% of all lymphomas, but this frequency is rare in the non-African form of the disease.

Desmoblastic fibroma, chondrosarcoma, pseudotumors, and chondroid tumors also may occur in the mandible (see Fig. 22-14 and e-Fig. 22-15).

Familial Fibrosis of Jaws (Cherubism)

Cherubism is an autosomal-dominant condition characterized by asymptomatic facial swelling beginning about the third year of life. The mandible and maxilla are generally involved with multilocular cystic changes, but other facial bones are spared. Rarely, cystic lesions in the anterior ends of the ribs have been reported. Stretching of the skin as a result of maxillary involvement tends to pull the lower eyelids down, revealing a band of white sclerae between the eyelid and the iris (Fig. 22-17). This cherubic "eyes raised to heaven" expression has led to the term "cherubism." Dentition is seriously disturbed; deciduous and permanent teeth are shed prematurely and irregularly, and some of the molar and premolar teeth are congenitally absent.

During the first 2 to 3 years after onset, the swellings increase rapidly in size, then remain stationary until puberty, when spontaneous regression begins and continues through the second and third decades. Not all patients have the typical features and course; massive jaw swelling and similar dental abnormalities usually seem to be variants of the condition, because no other satisfactory diagnosis can be made.

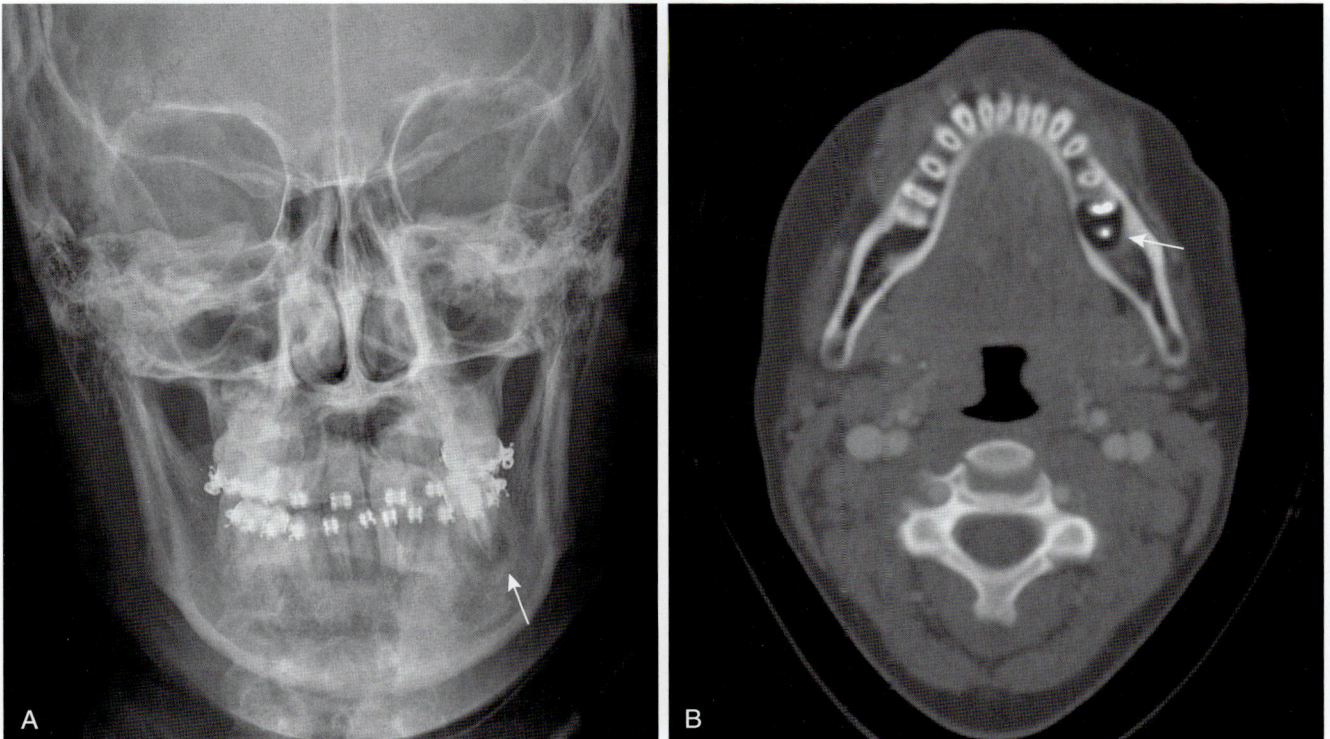

Figure 22-16 Langerhans cell histiocytosis. **A,** A radiograph of the skull reveals a lucent area (*arrow*) around a left molar. This area can represent an abscess, but in this case it is a floating tooth. **B,** An axial computed tomography scan shows the destructive lesion surrounding the tooth (*arrow*).

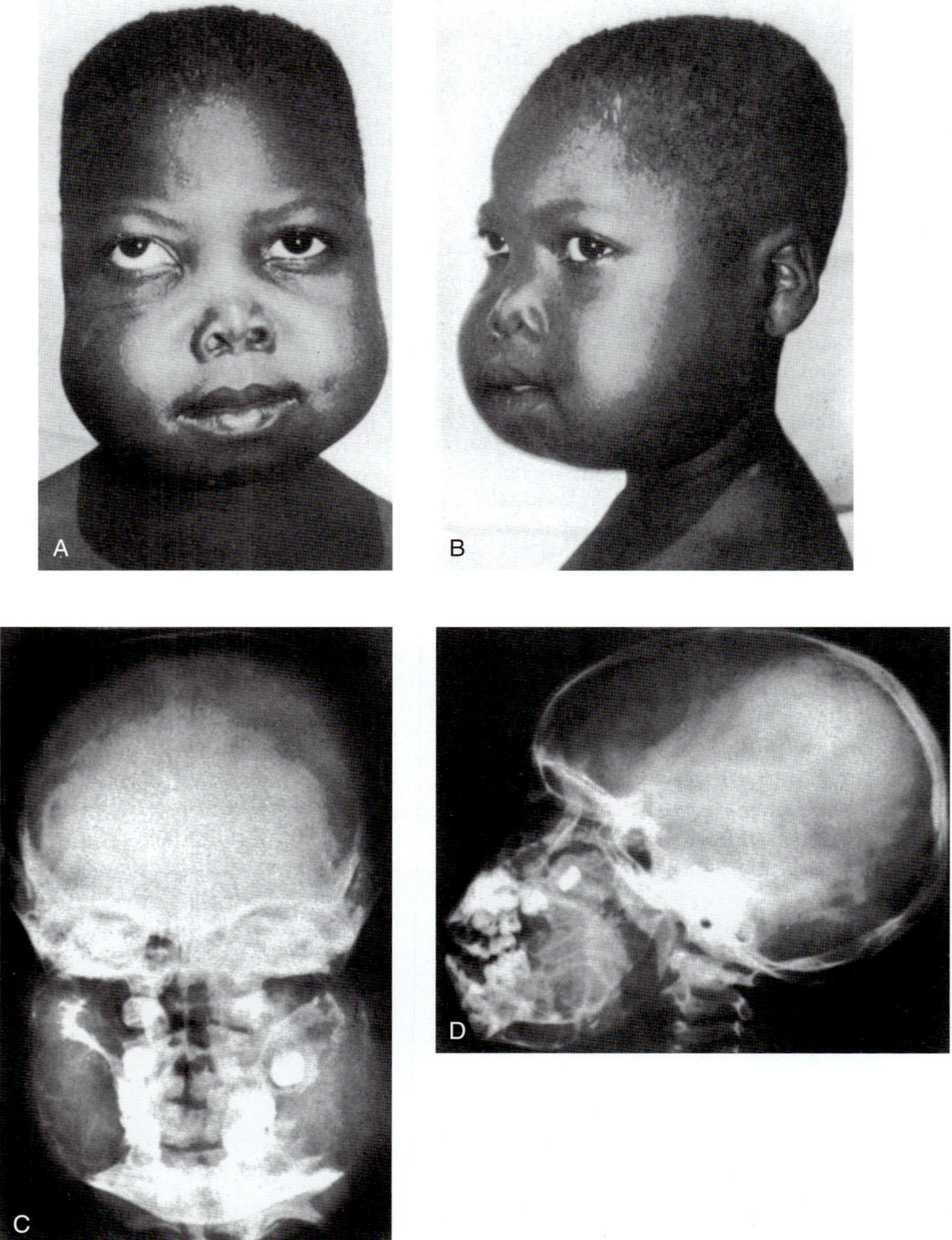

Figure 22-17   Familial fibrosis of the jaws (cherubism) in a 6-year-old boy whose two siblings and father were affected. **A** and **B,** Clinical photographs. Massive painless swelling extends to the preauricular level and obscures the normal external ears in the frontal view. The downward displacement of the lower lids explains the term cherubism ("eyes raised to heaven"). **C** and **D,** Frontal (**C**) and lateral (**D**) skull projections show cystic swelling of the mandible and, to a lesser degree, the maxilla. The teeth are displaced medially except for the unerupted left maxillary molar. The unerupted right molar and the swollen maxilla impinge on the right maxillary sinus, partially obliterating its cavity. The clouding of the left maxillary sinus extends to the left ethmoid, indicating bony involvement or ostial occlusion. (From Shuler RK, Silverman FN. Familial fibrous dysplasia of the jaws of "cherubism" in a Haitian family. *Ann Radiol.* 1965;8:45-52.)

Radiographs show diffuse swelling and multiloculated rarefaction of the mandible (see Fig. 22-17 and e-Fig. 22-18). The maxilla is also enlarged, with at least partial obliteration of the sinuses. CT can detect lesions of the upper jaws not observable in conventional radiographs, including involvement of the head of the condyle (e-Fig. 22-18).[20,21] Mandibular enlargement and some sclerosis may persist in later life.

Microscopic examination shows diffuse fibrosis of the affected bones, with replacement of bone by fibrous tissue that contains varying numbers of giant cells and blood vessels. Submandibular lymph nodes are usually enlarged, showing nonspecific hyperplasia on biopsy. No definite relationship with polyostotic fibrous dysplasia has been shown.

Mandibular Involvement in Generalized Diseases of the Skeleton

Rheumatoid arthritis affects the mandible in about 15% of cases because of the retardation of growth ventrally and caudally after temporomandibular arthritis. Deformity of the condyles and a prominent antegonial notch may be present. Because of the small size of the mandible, these patients have birdlike facies, and movements of the mandible are limited.

In persons with thalassemia, the changes in the mandible are similar to those in the calvarium and long bones and include expanded external contours, dilation of the medullary spaces, cortical atrophy, and generalized osteoporosis.

Fibrocystic changes in the mandible may be a feature of polyostotic fibrous dysplasia.

The disappearance of the lamina dura in persons with hyperparathyroidism was considered a pathognomonic radiographic sign of the disease. More experience has shown that the lamina dura also may be resorbed (in part or in toto) in persons with many other disorders, including rickets, leukemia, Cushing disease, Paget disease, idiopathic osteomalacia, idiopathic chronic familial hyperphosphatemia, and primary and metastatic malignancies, as well as after dental extractions. The bone of the alveolar processes is always affected when the lamina dura has disappeared; the lamina dura does not disappear in the presence of normal alveolar bone.[22] Mandibular involvement in infantile cortical hyperostosis is an important diagnostic feature of this condition.

Key Points

Formation of the dental buds is visible by 20 weeks' gestation.

In contrast to bone age, dental age is little affected by endocrine aberrations.

The temporomandibular joint allows gliding and hinge movements.

Vehicular trauma and falls account for most mandibular fractures.

Floating teeth are not specific for Langerhans cell histiocytosis.

No imaging modality has a high sensitivity for differentiating among the many unusual neoplasms of the mandible.

Suggested Readings

Bodner L, Woldenberg V, Bar-Ziv J. Radiographic features of large cystic lesions of the jaws in children. *Pediatr Radiol*. 2003;33:3-6.

Dunfee BL, Sakai O, Pistey R, et al. Radiologic and pathologic characteristics of benign and malignant lesions of the mandible. *Radiographics*. 2006;26:1751-1768.

Leuno AK. Natal teeth. *Am J Dis Child*. 1986;140:249-251.

References

Full references for this chapter can be found on www.expertconsult.com.

Chapter 23

Traumatic Lesions of the Skull and Face*

THOMAS L. SLOVIS

Congenital Depressions

Congenital depressions of the calvaria occur as a result of mechanical factors that occur before or during birth.[1] These depressions usually are visible by direct inspection, but radiographs often are obtained to search for associated fractures. During labor, depressions of the calvaria are caused by excessive localized pressure on the head by the bony prominences in the maternal pelvis, including the sacral promontory, pubic symphysis, and sciatic spines (e-Fig. 23-1). Application of forceps to the fetal head and traction with excessive force is another less common cause of congenital depressions that occurs during labor.

Severe cranial deformities also may develop during fetal life from sustained abnormal fetal positions (e-Fig. 23-2). Grooves in the calvarium and face may be caused by excessive pressure of an ectopic shoulder or limb. Lower and upper limb positions may be responsible and represent restrictions of the usual active movements of the fetus. Deformities also may arise as a result of pressure from amniotic bands.

Cranial depressions that are present at birth and are not associated with edema or hemorrhage of the underlying soft tissues usually are due to long-standing faulty fetal position rather than to a recent birth injury. Spontaneous elevation of prenatal depressions during the first year after birth without adverse residual effects have been reported.[1] Acute depressions as a result of the application of forceps, often called "ping-pong ball depressions," have been elevated by simple tangential digital pressure on opposite sides of the depression and by suction with a hand-operated breast pump.[2]

Caput Succedaneum

Caput succedaneum is a local swelling of the scalp that contains edema fluid and blood and usually is a result of pressure on the presenting head. The condition is recognized at birth and disappears after a few days. Local swelling of the scalp casts a shadow of water density on skull radiographs that

disappears without residual bone production or destruction. In rare cases, the hemorrhage can be so massive that associated shock occurs; in such cases, intracranial hemorrhage often is present.

Hemorrhage

Hemorrhage in the neonatal scalp may occur at three different levels: subcutaneous (as in caput succedaneum), subaponeurotic (subgaleal), and subperiosteal. More superficial bleeds cross suture lines and may extend widely into the face ventrally, onto the neck dorsally, and onto the zygomatic arches and mastoid processes laterally. Subgaleal hemorrhages also are known as cephalohematoceles and may contribute to the swelling and clinical findings in massive caput succedaneum. Subperiosteal hemorrhages are known as cephalhematomas. In contrast to the previous two conditions, cephalhematomas are confined sharply by the edges of the bones they overlie, and shells of bone form over them during resolution, arising from the elevated periosteum that covers them externally (Fig. 23-3). The usual cause of cephalhematomas is trauma to the fetal head during labor. Cephalhematomas also may develop after cephalic injuries during infancy and childhood. Fine linear fractures of the underlying bone may be found in the sites of cephalhematomas and are thought by some investigators to be the principal cause of bleeding of the pericranium. The incidence of cephalhematomas in two very large series of neonates was found to be 1.5% to 2.5%.[3,4] Associated fractures were found in 25% of the cephalhematomas studied radiographically.[3] The incidence of forceps delivery in the two studies was 75% and 33%, a probable explanation for the difference in the incidence of fracture-associated lesions.

Clinically, subperiosteal cephalhematomas appear as localized swellings, usually over the parietal and occipital bone (Fig. 23-4). The fresh lesions characteristically extend over the entire surface of the affected bone and are sharply limited at the edges of the bone where the periosteum is bound tightly to the membranous tissue of the sutures. The parietal bones are most often affected, but occipital lesions are common and may be confused with occipital meningoceles during the first days of life. Frontal cephalhematomas are very rare.

The radiographic findings vary with the age of the cephalhematomas. During the first 2 weeks, the lesion is

---

*This chapter originally was written by Dr. John Caffey and revised by Dr. Frederic Silverman. Although some of the images in this chapter appeared in the first edition in 1945, they are still the best available examples of clinical and radiographic imaging.

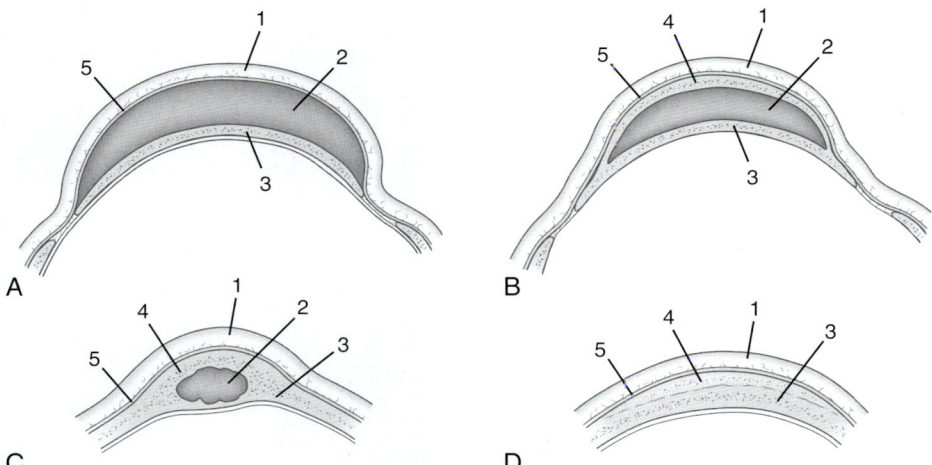

Figure 23-3 Diagrammatic sketches of anatomic changes that occur in a person with a cephalhematoma. **A,** A fresh subperiosteal hematoma. **B,** The healing phase, which shows a new shell of subperiosteal bone over the hematoma. **C,** Persistence of an organized hematoma in the diploic space. **D,** Persistent residual external thickening of the outer table after complete resorption of subperiosteal blood. **C** and **D** represent late residuals that may persist into adult life. *1,* Scalp; *2,* hematoma; *3,* normal calvaria; *4,* new subperiosteal bone; *5,* periosteum.

composed of fluid blood and casts a shadow of water density (Fig. 23-5). Near the end of the second week, bone begins to form under the elevated periosteum. It appears first at the margins, but soon the entire cephalohematoma is overlaid with a complete shell of bone (e-Fig. 23-6; see Fig. 23-5). Depending on their size, cephalhematomas clinically are gradually absorbed over 2 weeks to 3 months. The radiographic findings, in contrast, persist long after the clinical signs have disappeared (e-Fig. 23-7). The outer table usually remains thickened as a flat, irregular hyperostosis for several months and is gradually resorbed. Fresh cephalhematomas may become infected during bacteremia or needle aspiration.[5] Ultrasonography may be used for early diagnosis, thus

avoiding the use of radiation (Fig. 23-8). Associated fractures generally are of no clinical significance.

In some cases, the space between a new shell of bone and the inner table remains widened for many years, and the space originally occupied by the hematoma becomes filled with normal diploic bone (Fig. 23-9). In other cases, large and small cystlike defects persist in the sites of cephalhematomas (e-Fig. 23-10).[6] Infantile cephalhematoma occasionally persists into adult life, when symptomless large segments of bone production and destruction still may be visible in the calvarium (cephalhematoma deformans) (e-Fig. 23-11).[7] The possibility of a prior neonatal cephalhematoma should be considered in practically all lesions of parietal and occipital

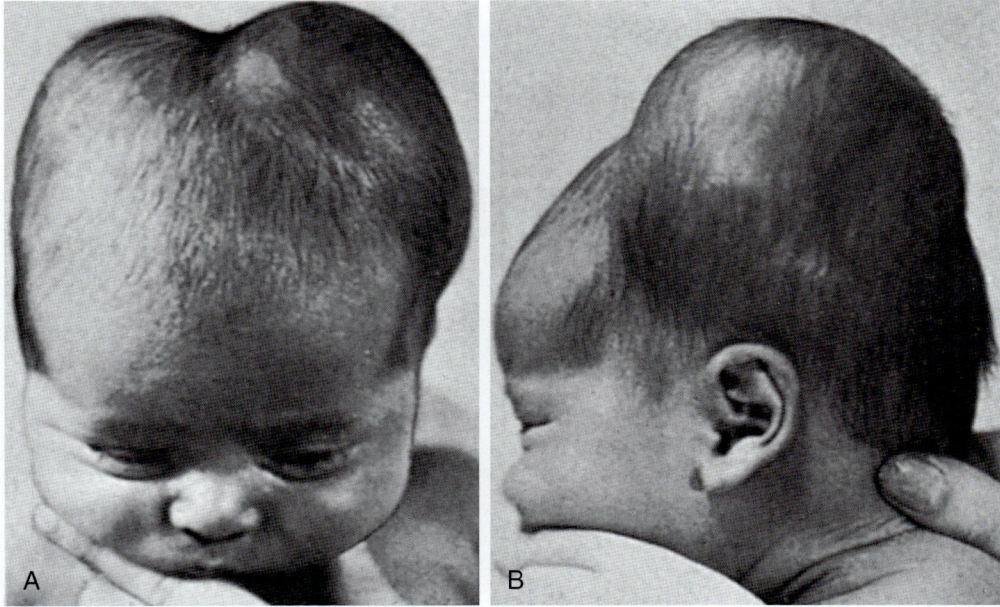

Figure 23-4 Bilateral parietal cephalhematomas in a 13-day-old neonate. Limitation of the edges of the tumors to the sutures is shown clearly at the sagittal, coronal, and lambdoid sutures. The deep furrow between the two parietal cephalhematomas is due to fixation of the periosteum at the sagittal suture. Frontal (**A**) and lateral (**B**) views are provided.

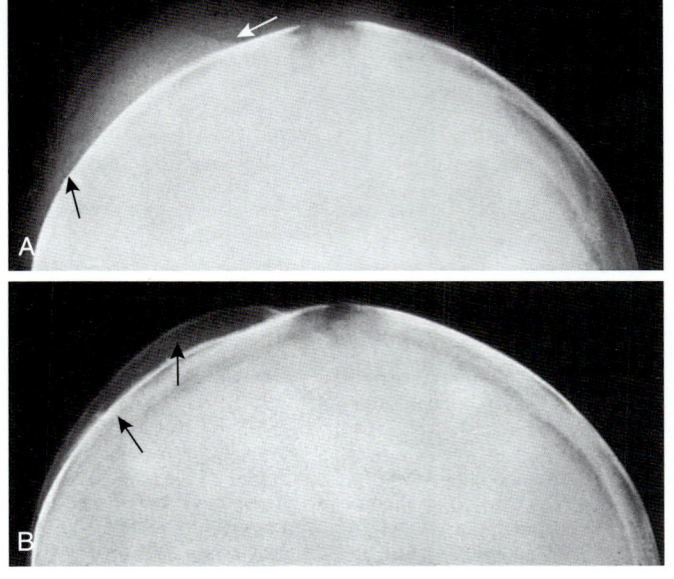

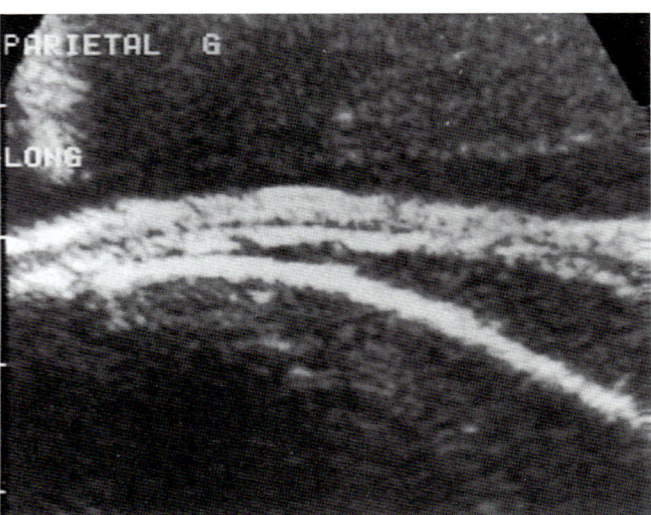

Figure 23-8   An ultrasound scan of the edge of a parietal cephalhematoma (compare with Fig. 23-3, *B*). The periosteum is raised by the sonolucent blood; its width and echogenicity result from subperiosteal bone formation that is too minimal to show on radiographs. (Courtesy Dr. Daniel Nussle, Geneva, Switzerland.)

Figure 23-5   A cephalhematoma. **A,** Rounded soft tissue swelling (*arrows*) of water density over the left parotid bone at age 7 days. **B,** The same skull at age 32 days shows a thin shell of newly formed subperiosteal bone (*upper arrow*) overlying the margin of the partially resorbed hematoma (*lower arrow*).

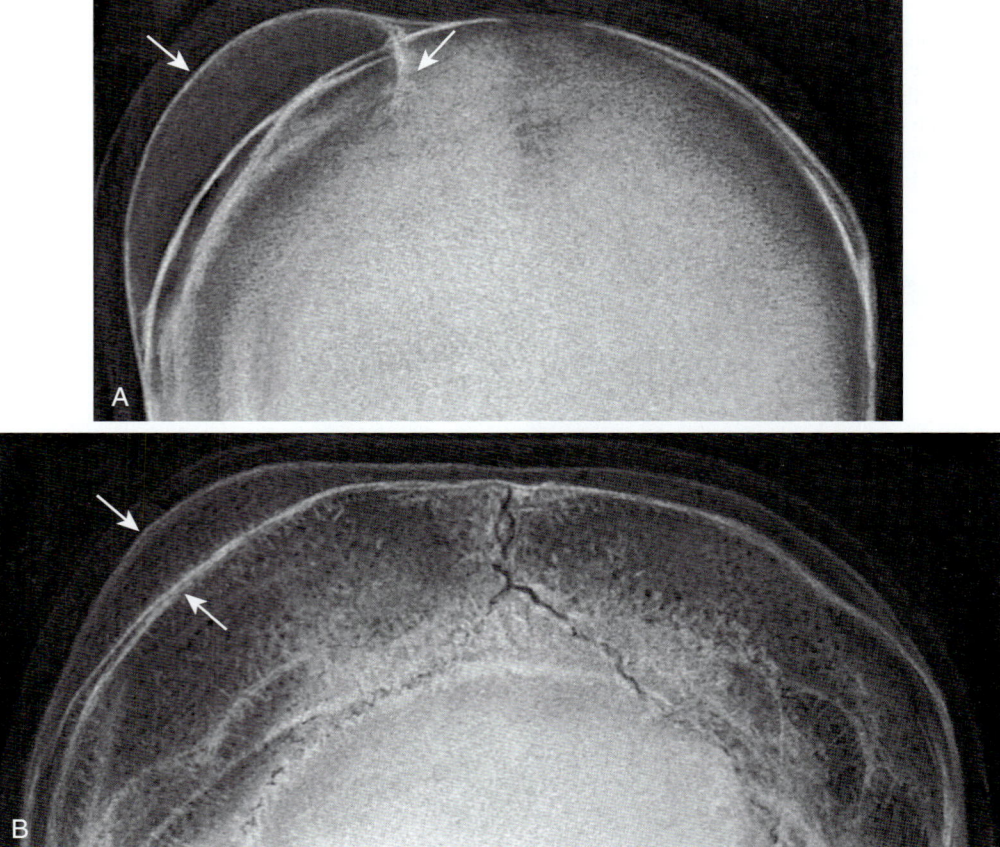

Figure 23-9   Radiographs show late residual thickening of the calvaria resulting from neonatal cephalhematoma. **A,** At 7 weeks of age, a large hematoma (*arrows*) is covered by a thin osseous shell on the right parietal bone. **B,** At 3 years and 11 months of age, a widening of the diploic space (*arrows*) occurs in the right parietal bone, where the neonatal hematoma was located.

bones in older infants, children, and adults. An adequate history of the state of the neonatal head should be taken before the final radiographic evaluation of lesions of the calvarium is made.

Subgaleal Hygroma

A subgaleal hygroma clinically may simulate a cephalhematoma or a caput succedaneum. Radiographically, the swellings in the parietal regions usually are associated with underlying fractures (Fig. 23-12). Trauma from use of obstetric forceps is a common cause of subgaleal hygromas. In older children, a subgaleal hygroma may result from hair-pulling in cases of child abuse or accidental entrapment of long hair in mechanical equipment. A subgaleal hematoma may occur without antecedent trauma in patients with coagulation abnormalities. The scalp swells because of the accumulation of cerebrospinal fluid (CSF), and usually some blood, beneath the epicranial aponeurosis. The abnormal fluid extends across the sutures, contrary to the pattern seen with cephalhematomas.

Cranial Fractures

NEONATES

Occasionally the skull vault is fractured during delivery. Fractures of the base are rare. Simple linear or fissure fractures are the rule, which appear as lines of diminished density on skull radiographs.

A 12% incidence of skull fractures, all depressed, was reported in a large series of head injuries sustained at birth.[8] Forceps were used in most of these deliveries. The fractures were almost all in the parietal and occipital bones. When clinical signs warrant intracranial evaluation, CT may be used in emergent situations, but MRI will provide more detailed brain evaluation.

INFANTS AND CHILDREN

Plain radiographic examination of the skull has little to offer in the management of nonabusive head trauma in infants and

---

Box 23-1 Criteria for Head Computed Tomography in Children with a Glasgow Coma Scale Score of 14

A. <2 Years Old
1. Altered mental status
2. Palpable skull fracture
3. Occipital, parietal, or temporal scalp hematoma
4. Loss of consciousness >5 seconds
5. Severe mechanism of injury
6. Not acting normally, per parent

B. >2 Years Old
1. Altered mental status
2. Signs of basilar skull fracture
3. Loss of consciousness
4. Vomiting
5. Severe mechanism of injury
6. Severe headache

Modified from Kuppermann N, Holmes JF, Dayan PS, et al. Identification of children at very low risk of clinically important brain injuries after head trauma: a prospective cohort study. *Lancet.* 2009;374: 1160-1170.

---

children. The presence or absence of a fracture neither correlates with the clinical situation nor affects management.[9-14] In a series of 256 children younger than 5 years who fell out of bed at home or in the hospital, only three skull fractures were found, and clinically these fractures were insignificant.[14] Serious injuries attributed to falls from a bed must be evaluated very carefully for possible child abuse factors (see Chapters 47 and 144).

The major indication for skull radiographs is suspected child abuse. Prospective study of a series of more than 7000 patients suggests that if certain clinical criteria are present singly or in combination, CT or MRI examination is warranted to evaluate for intracranial injury.[15-21] The selection criteria are (1) unconsciousness or a documented decreasing level of consciousness; (2) a history of a craniotomy with a shunt in place; (3) the probability of a skull depression or identification of a skull depression by probing through a laceration or a puncture wound; (4) blood in the ear or fluid

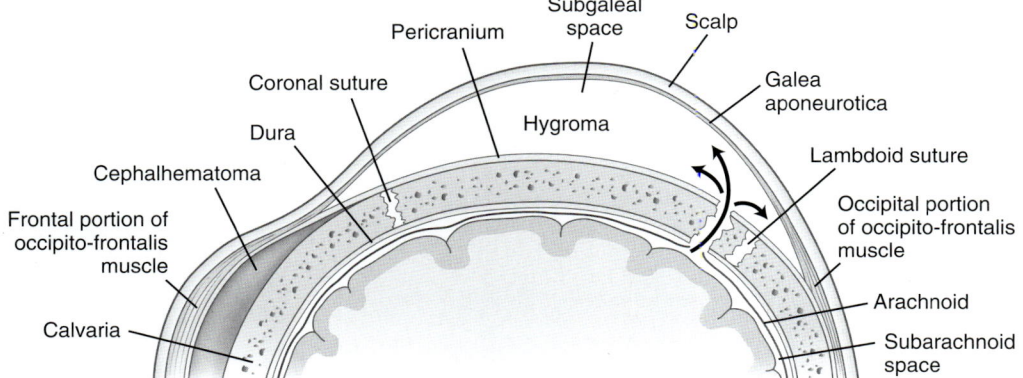

Figure 23-12 Course of flow of the cerebrospinal fluid after fracture of the calvaria. Tears of the arachnoid and dura internally and of the periosteum externally into the subgaleal (epicranial) space form a large subgaleal hygroma under the galea aponeurotica. (Modified from Epstein JA, Epstein BS, Small M. Subepicranial hygromas: a complication of head injuries in infants and children. *J Pediatr.* 1961;59:562-566.)

discharge from the ear; (5) CSF discharge from the nose; (6) ecchymosis behind the ear (Battle sign); (7) bilateral orbital ecchymoses; and (8) unexplained focal neurologic signs. If cephalhematoma, drowsiness, and age younger than 1 year were added as criteria, no fractures would have been missed in these series.

In a multi-institutional study in which more than 42,000 children with head trauma and a Glasgow Coma Scale score of 14 or 15 were evaluated, a negative predictive value of almost 100% and a sensitivity of greater than 96.8% were found when the criteria in Box 23-1 were absent. In the absence of these findings, no risk is posed to the patient when a CT scan is not obtained.

Depressed fractures of the skull occur most frequently when large vectors of force are involved, as in vehicular accidents or direct local trauma or after forceps deliveries in the neonate. Many fractures are compounded by associated lacerations or communication with the nasal or aural cavities, and the fractures often are comminuted. Dural tears are relatively common with depressed fractures, whereas extradural and subdural hematomas are far less common.[8]

When performing an examination for fractures in young patients in whom the cranial sutures are conspicuously visible, it is necessary to keep in mind the great normal variability of these structures (see Chapter 18). Sutures may widen radiographically as a possible disturbance of desmogenous ossification as a result of the long-term administration of prostaglandin E_1.[22] The observation of sutural widening during recovery from nutritional deprivation may involve similar mechanisms.[23] The linear shadows of diminished density arising from fractures must be differentiated from linear vascular markings, particularly those of the grooves for the middle meningeal artery and its branches. Whether or not the fractures are depressed, they may result in tears of dural sinuses, especially when located in areas through which they course. The position of the bone edges at the time of post-trauma examination may give no indication of how much displacement took place at the moment the fracture occurred. Oblique single-bevel fractures that interrupt the continuity of the inner and outer tables in different planes may be invisible or simulate two fractures in certain projections. In some cases, especially with depressed fractures, the edges of the fragments may overlap and cast linear shadows of increased density. CT is the optimal modality for evaluating the depressed fragments and their relation to the underlying brain (Fig. 23-13). Some of the radiographic characteristics of cranial fractures are shown in e-Figure 23-14, Figures 23-15 through 23-17, and e-Figure 23-18.

Linear fractures in infants and children generally heal with few or no sequelae. The relatively sharp margins become hazy, and obliteration of the fracture line itself may occur 3 to 6 months after the original injury. In some instances in which considerable comminution has occurred, bone may be resorbed locally, leaving a defect. If the dura has been disrupted at the time of the fracture, the bony edges of the fracture have a tendency to separate. Leakage of CSF from damaged underlying pia-arachnoid into the area of fracture can result in the development of a leptomeningeal cyst (a growing fracture of childhood).[24,25] The leptomeninges disappear from the inner surface of the torn dura and over the underlying brain. Cysts are thought to be most common in fractures that involve the sutures because the dura is tightly bound there and more likely to rupture when the bone edges separate. Cysts have been reported after vacuum extraction when too anterior a placement of the cup was followed by widening of one coronal suture.[26]

By transmitting the pulsations of the brain, the cyst causes pressure atrophy of bone that is unprotected by dura, and a large defect may develop after many months or years (Fig. 23-19). The progressive changes are shown schematically in Figure 23-20. Before the development of a cyst, it is probably the pulsating CSF that begins the erosion of the internal table. Progressive enlargement of the calvarial defect has given rise to the term "growing fracture." If the brain has been damaged by the trauma, a porencephalic cavity may underlie the calvarial defect. The scalloped margin of the defect results from differential erosion of inner and outer tables. Occasionally, an intradiploic cyst is present. These lesions generally occur after fractures in infancy and seldom are observed in fractures that occur after the fifth year.

Gas may accumulate in the soft tissues of the skull contiguous to fractures, usually through breaks in paranasal airspaces or pneumatic cells of the temporal bone. If air escapes from the sinuses externally into the subaponeurotic space of the scalp, the result is called "extracranial traumatic pneumocephalus." Air also may leak into the cranial cavity, causing internal pneumocephalus. Intranasal manipulations, a craniotomy, and erosions caused by inflammatory destruction and by pressure atrophy arising from expanding neoplasms may result in pneumocephalus. Intraventricular pneumocephalus has been observed as a result of a congenital defect in the roof of the nasal cavity. Cephalhematomas are limited by periosteum.

Text continued on page 243.

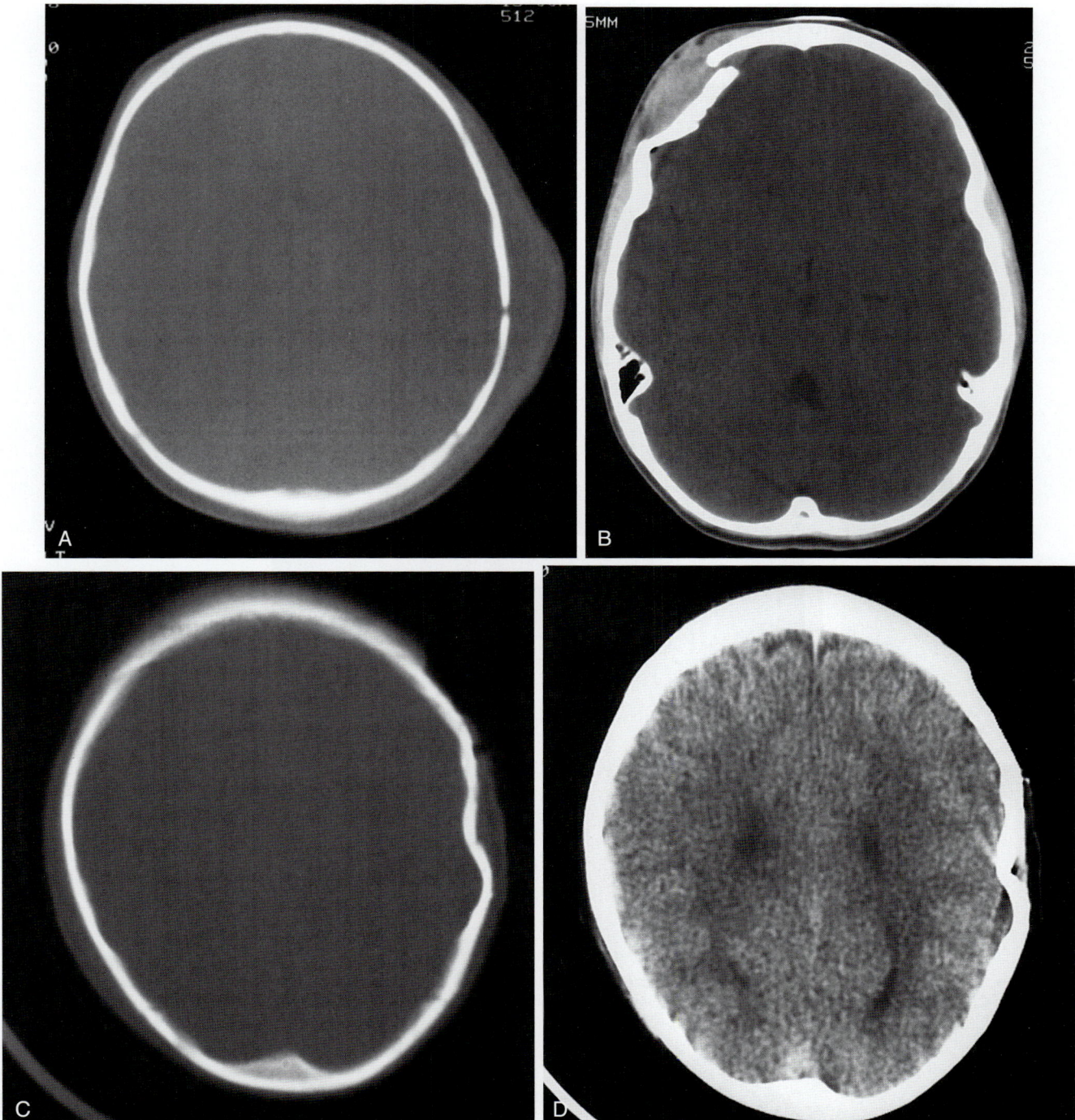

Figure 23-13 Computed tomography (CT) in evaluating calvaria and intracranial trauma. **A,** A CT scan with bone windows shows a large soft tissue hematoma and linear fracture in the left parietal region. **B,** A CT scan in another child shows a depressed right frontal fracture with a large external hematoma and a small epidural lesion anteriorly. Bone (**C**) and brain (**D**) windows reveal lack of any intracranial involvement, but the child has sustained a left parietal fracture and lacerations of the soft tissues of the left scalp.

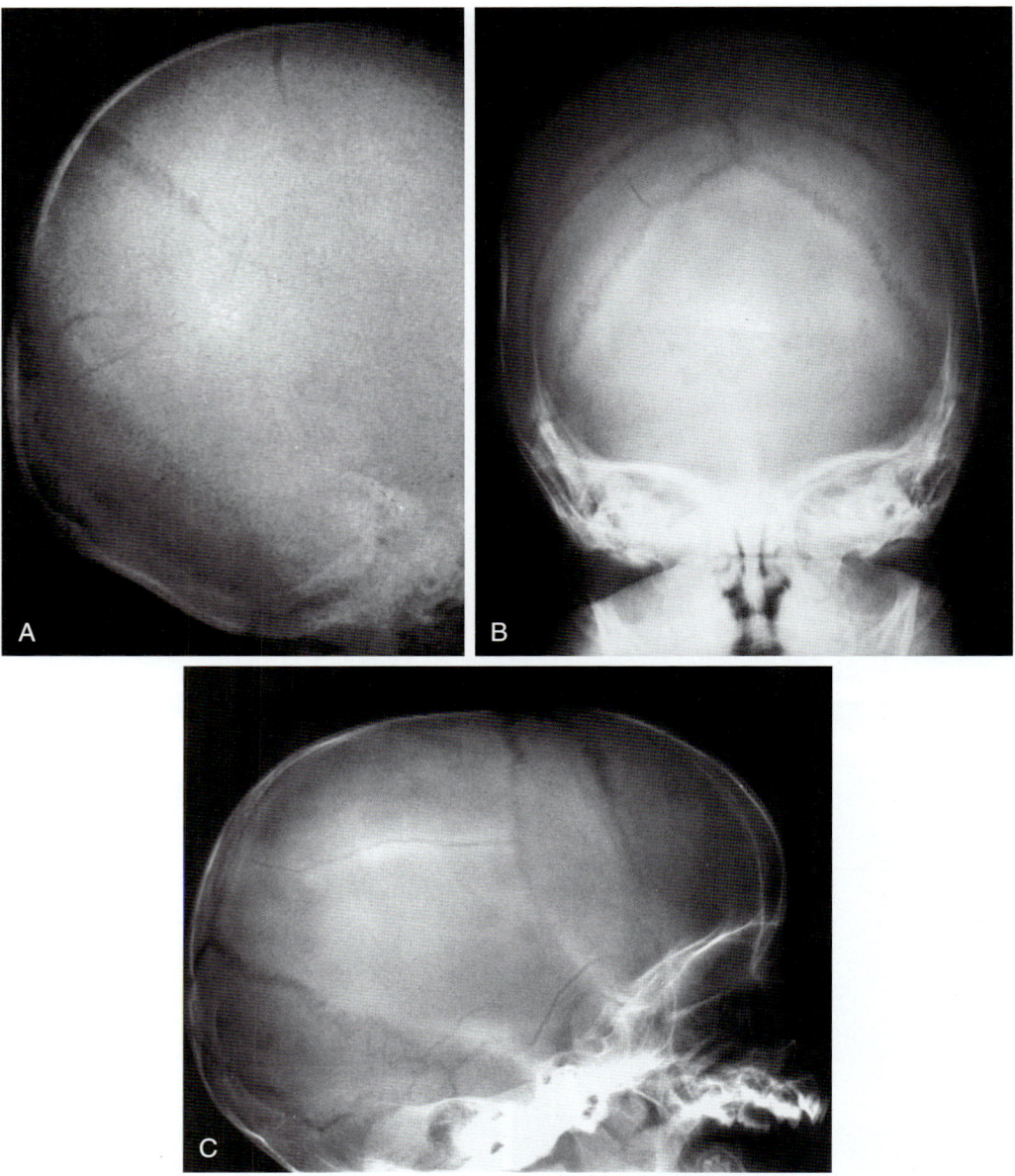

Figure 23-15 Linear fractures alone and with signs of increased intracranial pressure. **A,** Multiple fractures of the right parietal bone in a 9-month-old infant. **B** and **C,** A linear parietal fracture in another child, who also has diastatic sutures denoting increased intracranial pressure.

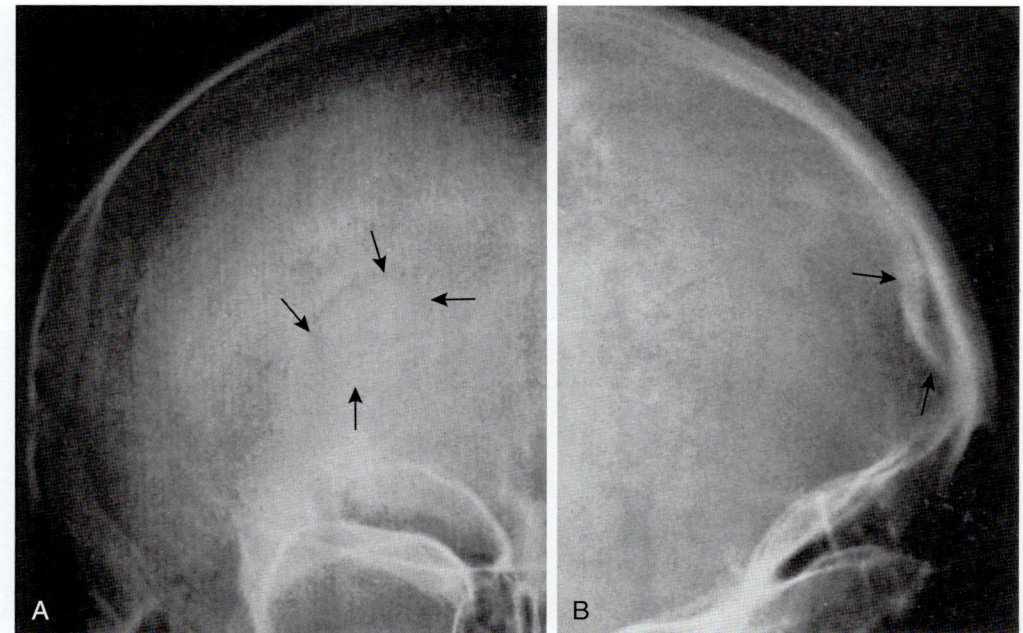

Figure 23-16 Depressed fracture of the frontal bone in a 9-year-old child. **A,** A posteroanterior projection with the fracture indicated by arrows. In the medial inferior segment, the arcuate shadow of diminished density is replaced by a curved linear shadow of increased density that is caused by overlapping of the fragments in this segment. **B,** A lateral projection clearly demonstrating the depression of the tables (*arrows*).

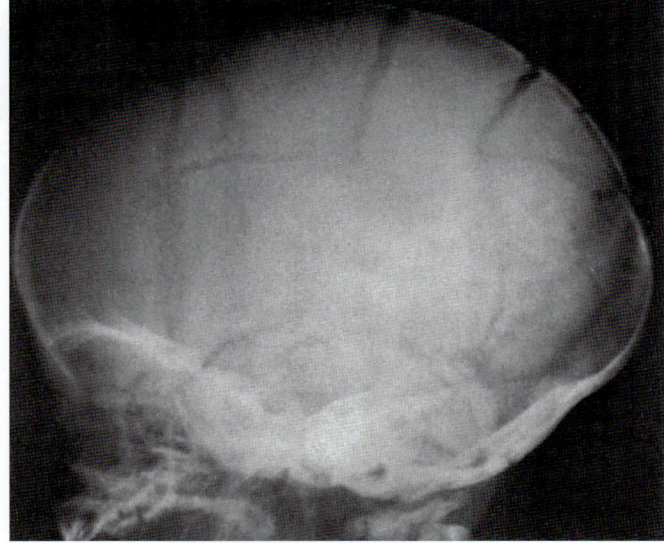

Figure 23-17 A case of nonaccidental trauma. Comminuted diastatic fractures of both parietal bones in a 2-month-old infant are shown. Both ocular fundi contained retinal hemorrhages, and bilateral subdural hematomas were present. The child had been severely beaten by the mother.

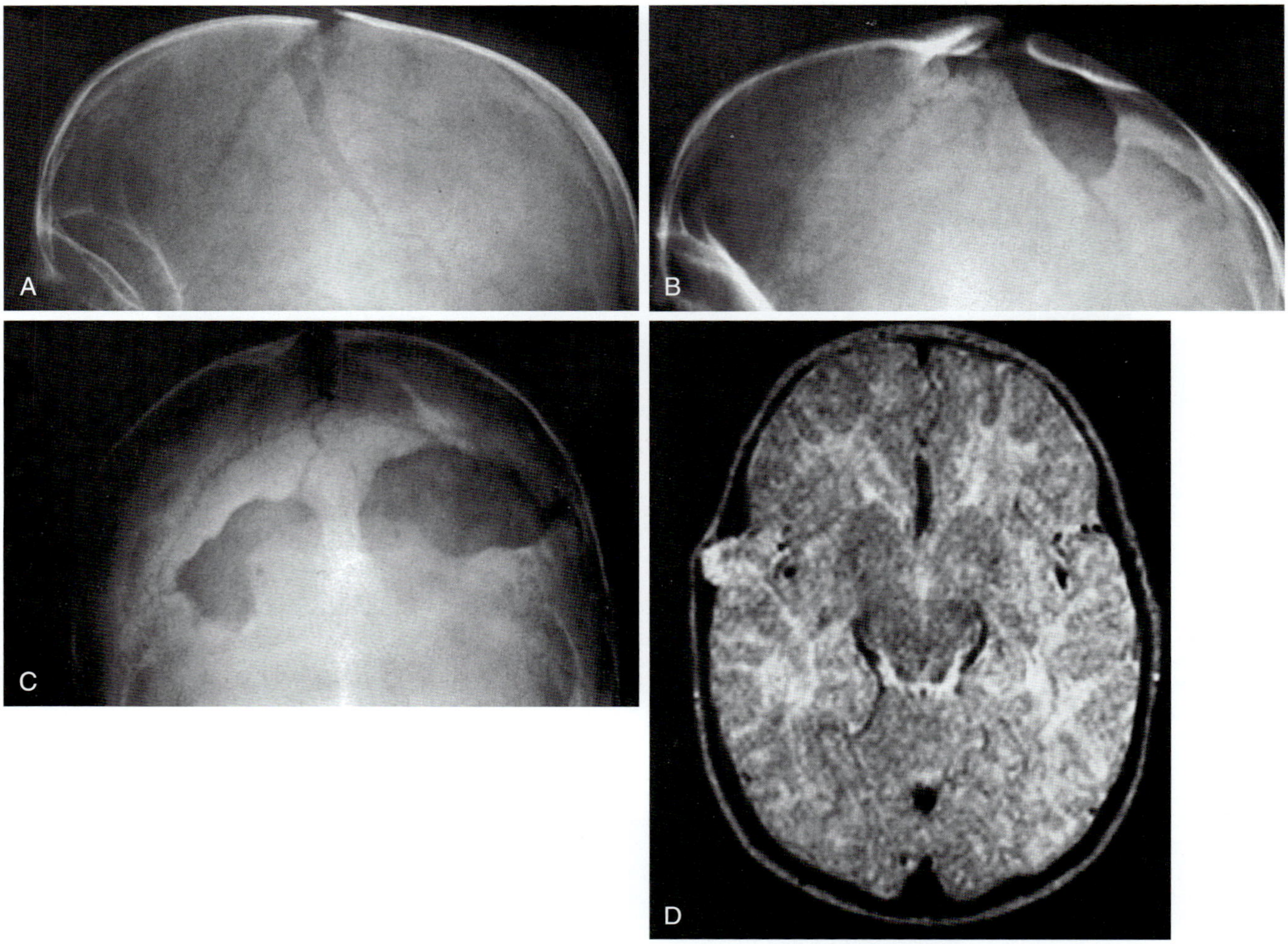

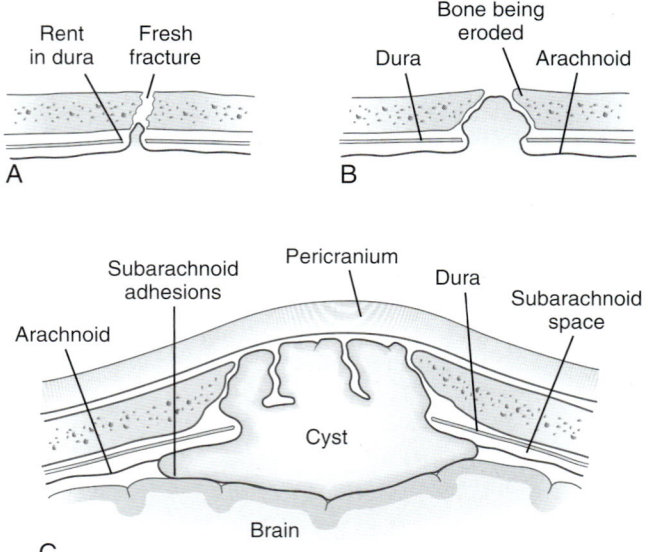

Figure 23-19 A pulsating leptomeningeal cyst with residual bilateral large defects in the calvaria. **A,** Diastatic bilateral comminuted parietal fractures after a head injury during infancy. Lateral (**B**) and frontal (**C**) projections 5 years later show large bilateral defects in the sites of the earlier parietal fractures. At surgery, the dura beneath the fractures was found to be torn. The bone on the margins of the defect is sclerotic and thickened. **D,** Magnetic resonance imaging in another child with a leptomeningeal cyst reveals herniation of the brain outward in the right parietal region. (**A, B,** and **C** Courtesy Walter E. Berdon, MD.)

Figure 23-20 A schematic drawing of the mechanism and progressive changes in the formation of a leptomeningeal cyst. **A,** Immediately after an injury occurs, fresh fractures of the parietal bone, a fresh rent in the underlying dura, and early protrusion of the arachnoid membrane into and through the fracture are seen. **B,** Lateral marginal erosion of bone and widening of the dural defect. **C,** Later incomplete cyst formation in the arachnoid as a result of adhesions, depression, and pressure atrophy of the underlying brain and leptomeninges and increases in bony and dural defects. (Courtesy Juan M. Taveras, MD.)

Key Points

Cranial fractures seldom correlate with the clinical situation or management except in cases of child abuse.

Plain radiographic examination of the skull has little to offer in the management of nonabusive head trauma in infants and children.

A leptomeningeal cyst (i.e., a growing fracture of childhood) is uncommon after 5 years of age.

References

Full references for this chapter can be found on www.expertconsult.com

Chapter 24

Embryology and Brain Development

MARVIN D. NELSON JR and THOMAS L. SLOVIS

The human brain undergoes four phases of development: (1) dorsal induction (primary and secondary neurulation), (2) ventral induction (patterning of the forebrain), (3) neuronal proliferation and migration, and (4) myelination. During the third week of embryogenesis, initiation of the central nervous system evolves with the development of the notochordal process. This derivative of ectoderm grows rapidly in length so that by 20 days it is converted from a hollow tube to a solid rod—the notochord (Fig. 24-1; e-Table 24-1). The notochord works with the axial mesoderm to induce the neural plate. The neuroepithelium of the neural plate begins the formation of the brain and spinal cord. It appears initially at the cranial end of the embryo and differentiates craniocaudally. At the beginning of the fourth week, the neural plate is composed of a broad cranial portion and a narrow caudal portion—the fetal brain and spinal cord.

Dorsal Induction

The process of neurulation or formation of the neural tube occurs when the lateral edges of the neural plate elongate to become neural folds and join together to form the neural tube (Fig. 24-2).[1] The process starts at the craniocervical region and proceeds superiorly and inferiorly. The space within the neural tube, the neural canal, initially is open at the cranial (or rostral) and caudal ends (cranial and caudal neuropores) and communicates with the amniotic cavity. The neuropores gradually decrease in size and close between the twenty-fourth and twenty-sixth day, apparently at multiple sites and not necessarily in a craniocaudal fashion.[1] The lowest portion of the spinal cord, the inferior sacral and coccygeal levels, are formed by a different process called secondary neurulation (see Chapters 40 and 43). Pluripotent tissue within the caudal eminence forms a solid neural cord; this neural cord forms a lumen that fuses with the neural tube (e-Fig. 24-3). This secondary process is not completed until the eighth week after fertilization of the ovum.[1]

Some neural crest cells (the population of neural cells arising at the lateral edge of the neural plate during neural tube formation) detach during neurulation and form many different tissues (e.g., melanocytes and chromaffin cells of the adrenal medulla), including the major components of the peripheral and autonomic nervous system (e-Table 24-2).[1]

Ventral Induction

The prechordal plate cephalic to the neural tube and notochord induces this stage of development. The three major divisions of the brain—the prosencephalon or forebrain, mesencephalon or midbrain, and rhombencephalon or hind brain—are more clearly differentiated during the rostral expansion of the neural tube (the formation of the primary brain vesicles).[1,2] During the fourth and fifth weeks, a series of brain foldings occur (brain flexures—midbrain, cervical, and later pontine) so that by the end of the fifth week, five secondary brain vesicles are present (Table 24-3). With further development, the prosencephalon becomes subdivided into the telecephalon and the diencephalon. The rhombencephalon subdivides into the metencephalon and myelencephalon. The mesencephalon does not divide. Within each of these five vesicles, the neural canal expands into a primary ventricle. The central canal of the spinal cord is continuous with the brain ventricles. The fate of these structures is shown in Table 24-3. The cranial nerve nuclei appear in the brainstem during the fifth week (see the next section).[1,2]

Neuronal Proliferation and Migration

During the period of morphologic development of the brain, cytodifferentiation occurs. Formation of the cerebral neocortex is a complex process with proliferation, migration, and differentiation varying in time from one site to another. Several patterns of neuronal migration occur, including (1) radial migration along the path of radial glial cells from the ventricles toward the surface and (2) tangential migration along transverse surfaces (e-Fig. 24-4).[1-3]

Although details of the migration process vary for each region of the brain, general principles include the following: (1) the ultimate migration is from deep (ventricle) to superficial regardless of trajectory differences; (2) the migration establishes layers of the cortex (Figs. 24-5 and 24-6); and (3) neurons of each later wave of migration pass through the preceding layers to form a more superficial layer.[4]

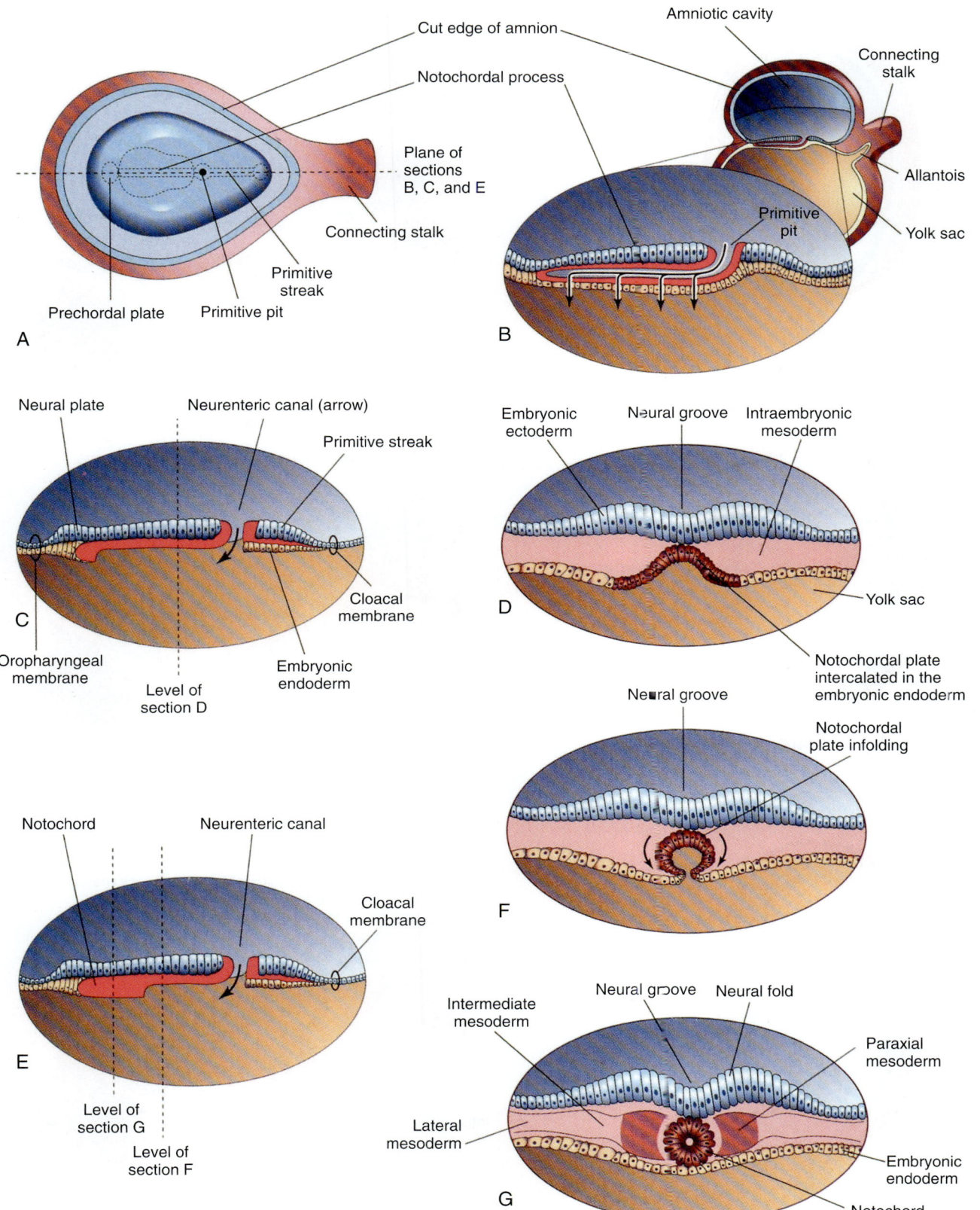

Figure 24-1 Further development of the notochord by transformation of the notochordal process. **A,** Dorsal view of the embryonic disc (about 18 days), exposed by removing the amnion. **B,** Three-dimensional median section of the embryo. **C** and **E,** Similar sections of slightly older embryos. **D, F,** and **G,** Transverse sections of the trilaminar embryonic disc shown in **C** and **E**. (From Moore KL, Persaud TVN. *Before we are born.* 5th ed. Philadelphia: WB Saunders; 1998.)

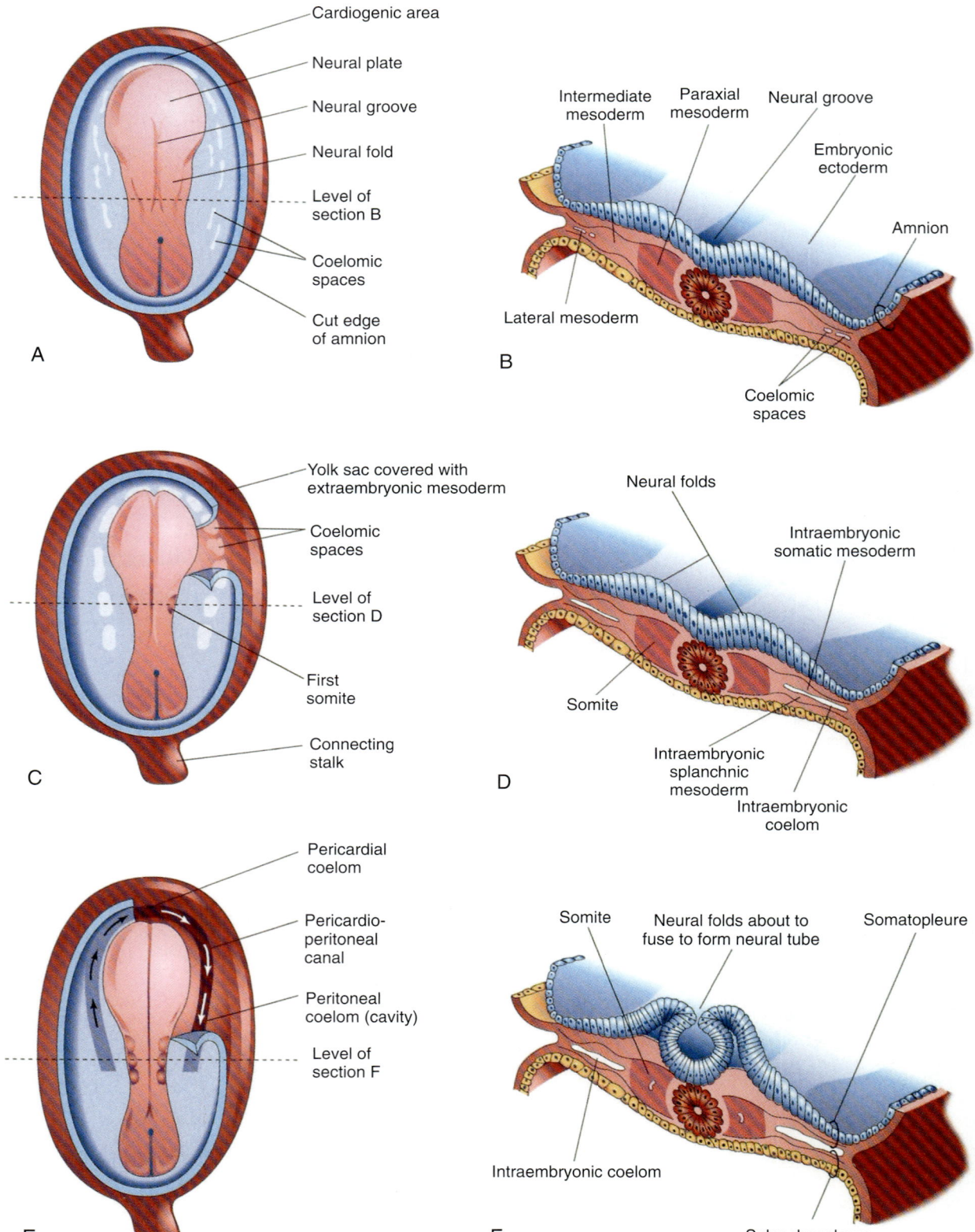

Cardiogenic area

Neural plate

Neural groove

Neural fold

Level of section B

Coelomic spaces

Cut edge of amnion

A

Intermediate mesoderm

Paraxial mesoderm

Neural groove

Embryonic ectoderm

Amnion

Lateral mesoderm

Coelomic spaces

B

Yolk sac covered with extraembryonic mesoderm

Coelomic spaces

Level of section D

First somite

Connecting stalk

C

Neural folds

Intraembryonic somatic mesoderm

Somite

Intraembryonic splanchnic mesoderm

Intraembryonic coelom

D

Pericardial coelom

Pericardio-peritoneal canal

Peritoneal coelom (cavity)

Level of section F

E

Somite

Neural folds about to fuse to form neural tube

Somatopleure

Intraembryonic coelom

Splanchnopleure

F

Figure 24-2 Drawings of embryos of 19 to 21 days, illustrating development of the somites and intraembryonic coetom. **A, C,** and **E,** Dorsal view of the embryo, exposed by removal of the amnion. **B, D,** and **F,** Transverse sections through the embryonic disc at the levels showing. **A,** Presomite embryo of about 18 days. **C,** An embryo of about 20 days, showing the first pair of somites. A portion of the somatopleure on the right has been removed to show the isolated coelomic spaces in the lateral mesoderm. **E,** A three-somite embryo (about 21 days) showing the horseshoe-shaped intraembryonic coelom, exposed on the right by removal of a portion of the somatopleure. (From Moore KL, Persaud TVN. *Before we are born.* 5th ed. Philadelphia: WB Saunders; 1998.)

Table 24-3

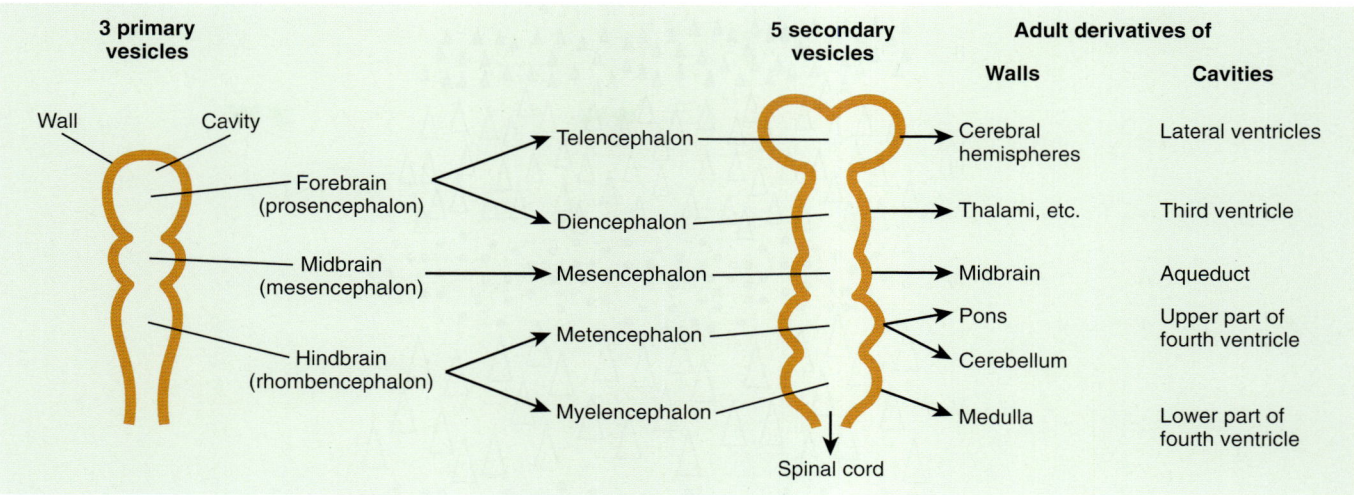

3 primary vesicles	5 secondary vesicles	Adult derivatives of Walls	Cavities
Forebrain (prosencephalon)	Telencephalon	Cerebral hemispheres	Lateral ventricles
	Diencephalon	Thalami, etc.	Third ventricle
Midbrain (mesencephalon)	Mesencephalon	Midbrain	Aqueduct
Hindbrain (rhombencephalon)	Metencephalon	Pons	Upper part of fourth ventricle
		Cerebellum	
	Myelencephalon	Medulla	Lower part of fourth ventricle

Spinal cord

From Moore KL, Persaud TVN. *Before we are born.* 5th ed. Philadelphia: WB Saunders; 1988.

During the tenth to twentieth weeks of gestation, neuronal genesis occurs. The proliferative cells of the ventricular level arising from the germinal matrix form waves of migrating neuroblasts and all precursor cells. After 20 weeks, only the glial cells are produced by this substance.[4] The germinal matrix eventually disappears by term but is significantly diminished by 32 weeks.[3] The subventricular zone produces neuroblasts after 20 weeks, and these neuroblasts migrate through the intermediate zone to form the cortical subplate.

Each new layer migrates through the preceding layer to become more superficial. The mature cortex has six layers, and neuronal migration concludes between 20 and 24 weeks' gestation. The subplate and cortical plate form the cortex, whereas the intermediate zone becomes the white matter (see Fig. 24-5). The germinal matrix also produces the glial cells, that is, astrocytes and oligodendrocytes.[4] The microglial cells are of mesodermal origin and are the resting tissue histiocytes of the brain. In contrast to cortical migration, glial cell migration and differentiation continues for more than 1 year after birth. Radial migration is the process whenever the radial glial cells provide a link between the ventricular zone of the neural tube and the pial surface, which provides a tract along which the neuroblasts migrate. Once the neuroblasts reach their destination, they detach from the radial glial tracts.[4]

Excessive cells of the fetal neurosystem ranging from 30% to 70% are produced when compared with the number of mature cells. These "surplus" cells undergo programmed death or apoptosis.

The steps of neurulation, cell proliferation, and migration are induced by multiple neurotransmitters, and genes

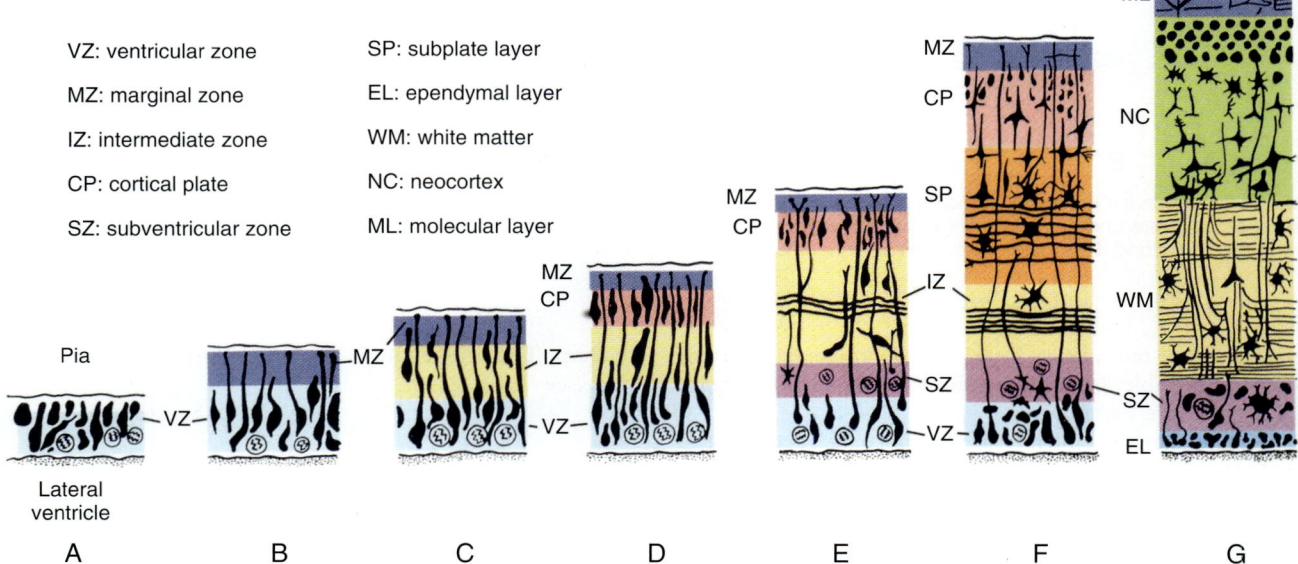

VZ: ventricular zone
MZ: marginal zone
IZ: intermediate zone
CP: cortical plate
SZ: subventricular zone
SP: subplate layer
EL: ependymal layer
WM: white matter
NC: neocortex
ML: molecular layer

Figure 24-5 Cytodifferentiation of the cerebral neocortex. Although the timing of neuroblast formation varies widely in different regions of the cerebral hemispheres, the general scheme illustrated here is typical for all regions. (From Larsen WJ. *Human embryology.* 2nd ed. New York: Churchill Livingstone; 1997.)

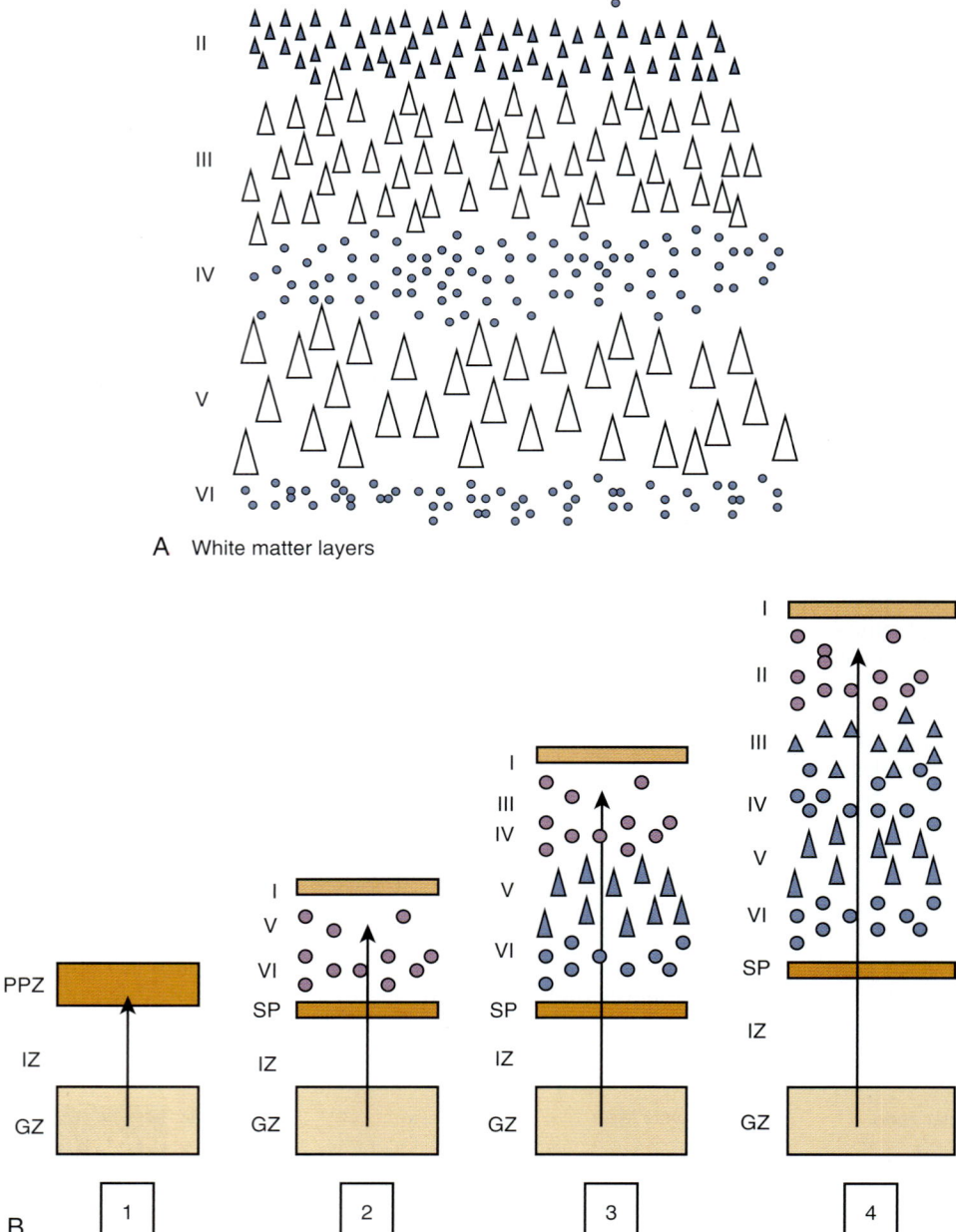

Figure 24-6 Schematic illustration of mammalian neocortical formation and neuronal migration. *Arrows* and *light gray circles* indicate migrating neurons; *black circles* and *triangles* represent postmigratory neurons. *GZ*, Germinative zone; *IZ*, intermediate zone (prospective white matter); *PPZ*, primitive plexiform zone; *SP*, subplate; *I*, cortical layer I or molecular layer; *II* or *VI*, cortical layers II to VI. (From Martin RJ, Fanaroff AA, Walsh MC, eds. *Fanaroff and Martin's neonatal perinatal medicine.* 8th ed. Philadelphia: Mosby Elsevier; 2006.)

controlling these transmitters have been identified. An example is found in e-Table 24-4, which shows the genetics of radial migrations in the cortex.[5]

The brainstem and spinal cord are similar in development. Two basal (ventral) columns and two alar (dorsal) columns are formed. These columns form a dorsal sensory and ventral motor configuration and are found in both the brainstem and spinal cord. The cranial nerves IX through XII come from the mesencephalon (medulla) and cranial nerves IV through VII form the metencephalon (pons) (see Table 24-3). The pons is largely composed of white matter tracts of the cere-

bellum. The cerebellum is also derived from the metencephalon (see Table 24-3).

Fetal Development in the Preterm Infant

The normal brain anatomy of the fetus is in many ways quite different from the normal anatomy of the term infant. The following differences are noted:

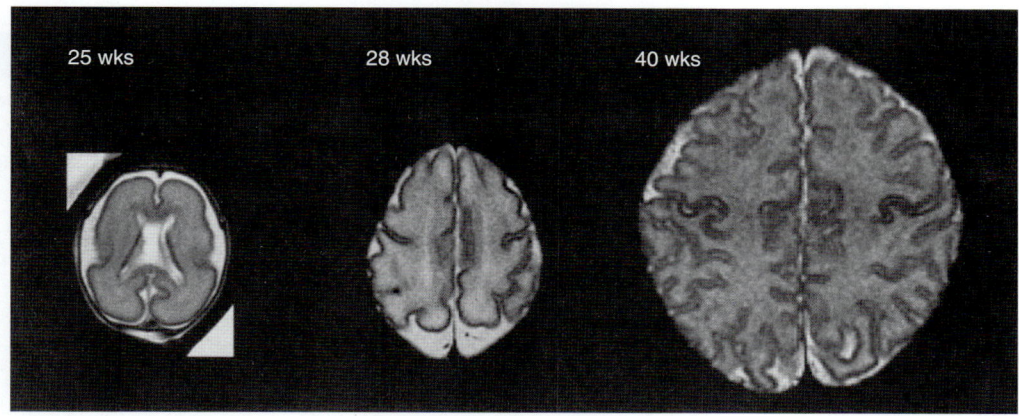

Figure 24-7   Cortical folding illustrated from 25 to 40 weeks' gestation by in vivo magnetic resonance imaging. T2-weighted images obtained at 25, 28, and 40 weeks' gestational age. (From Martin RJ, Fanaroff AA, Walsh MC, eds. *Fanaroff and Martin's neonatal perinatal medicine.* 8th ed. Philadelphia: Mosby Elsevier; 2006.)

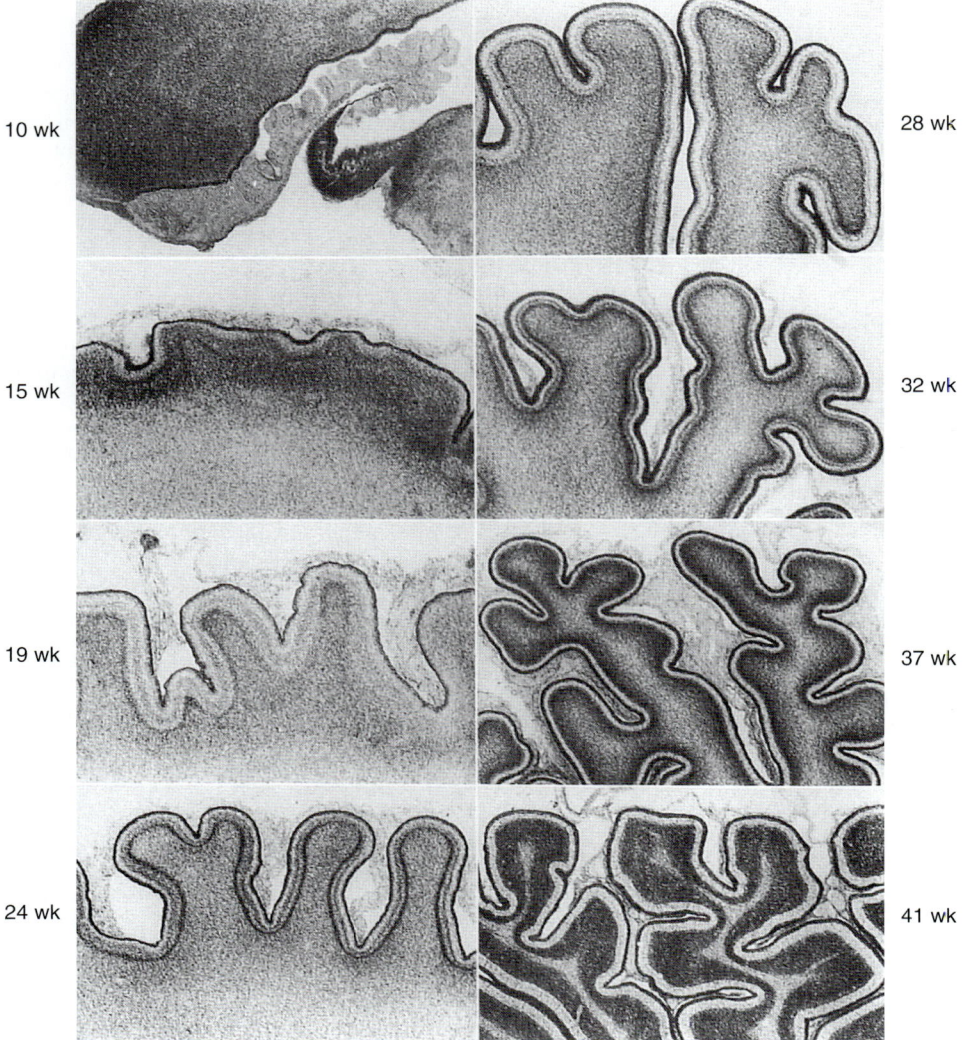

Figure 24-8   Morphologic appearance of the developing neocortex from 10 to 40 weeks. (From Gilbert-Barness, ed. *Potter's pathology of the fetus and infant.* Vol 2. St Louis: Mosby; 1997.)

Table 24-5

Sequence of Myelination Based on Histologic Analysis and Magnetic Resonance Imaging			
		Age for Detection of Myelin: Magnetic Resonance Imaging	
Anatomic Region	**Median Age for Detection of Myelin Histology**	**T1-Weighted Images**	**T2-Weighted Images**
Ventrolateral thalamus	28-30 wk	32 to 34 wk	
Posterior limb of internal capsule	38/44 wk*	38-40 wk	Posterior portion 40-48 wk Anterior portion 56-70 wk
Anterior limb of the internal capsule	50/87 wk	48-53 wk	70-90 wk
Central corona radiata	37/52 wk	28-56 wk	52-65 wk
Genu corpus callosum	50/53 wk	56-64 wk	64-72 wk
Splenium corpus callosum	54/65 wk	52-56 wk	56-64 wk
Occipital white matter			
Central	47/87 wk	52-60 wk	76-96 wk
Peripheral	56/122 wk	56-70 wk	90-102 wk
Frontal white matter			
Central	50/119 wk	52-64 wk	90-106 wk
Peripheral	72/119 wk	70-90 wk	96-114 wk

*The first number corresponds to earliest identification of some myelin tubules by microscopic examination of hematoxylin and eosin stained sections. The second number corresponds to mature myelin stained with blue dye by eye observation.
From Martin RJ, Fanaroff AA, Walsh MC, eds. *Fanaroff and Martin's neonatal perinatal medicine.* 8th ed. Philadelphia: Mosby Elsevier; 2006.

1. The fetal ventricles are large relative to the size of the brain and have a posterior (occipital) predominance that decreases after 25 weeks.
2. The fluid-filled spaces of the brain are large; subarachnoid spaces are increased in size relative to size of the brain, and the cisterna magna is larger than at term.
3. The germinal matrix, for aforementioned reasons, is quite large but decreases after 26 weeks.
4. Sulcation and gyration follow a predictable course (Figs. 24-7 and 24-8).[6]

The normal biochemical profile follows the type and amount of cells present in any given stage of development. This can be seen through the normal but different spectrographic patterns (e-Fig. 24-9).[3] Normal myelinization occurs via a defined order from the third trimester onward during the first year of life (Table 24-5).[7,8] Generally, myelination proceeds caudal to rostral and posterior to anterior.

Normal Anatomy

The result of these complex processes result in the mature brain and spinal cord. Neuroanatomic descriptions in detail are beyond the scope of this text, but many atlases of anatomy and imaging are available. Comparison of normal development with pathologic development will be discussed in Chapter 31.

Key Points

The neural tube differentiates into the brain and spinal cord. The neural crest gives rise to the peripheral and autonomic nervous system.

Neuronal migration proceeds from the periventricular to the superficial region of the brain along radial glial cells.

In general, myelination proceeds caudal to rostral and posterior to anterior.

References

Full references for this chapter can be found on www.expertconsult.com.

Chapter 25

Magnetic Resonance Spectroscopy and Positron Emission Tomography

ASHOK PANIGRAHY, SUNHEE KIM, and STEFAN BLUML

Most clinical magnetic resonance (MR) scanners now allow the addition of the magnetic resonance spectroscopy (MRS) modality, which can be used to assess cellular metabolism noninvasively and is the most accessible method for studying and monitoring neurometabolic disorders in patients (Table 25-1). The most important MRS method, proton or hydrogen (^{1}H) spectroscopy, is approved by the Food and Drug Administration (FDA) for general use in the United States and can be ordered by clinicians for their patients, if indicated. For the brain in particular, it has been proved that MRS provides additional clinically relevant information for several disease processes such as brain tumors, metabolic disorders, and systemic diseases.

Theoretical Background of Magnetic Resonance Spectroscopy

The signal used by magnetic resonance imaging (MRI) to create anatomic maps is generated primarily by the hydrogen nuclei, also known as protons (^{1}H), of water molecules (H_2O). In contrast, ^{1}H MRS analyzes the signal of protons attached to other molecules. Whereas for MRI only a single peak (water) is being mapped, the output of MRS is a collection of peaks at different radiofrequencies representing proton nuclei in different chemical environments, that is, the spectrum (Fig. 25-1 and Table 25-2). MRS can measure a variety of metabolites. Typical MR spectra of normal occipital gray matter is shown in Figure 25-1. The x axis, or chemical shift axis, is a measure of the frequency shift of a proton relative to a universally fixed reference substance (tetramethylsilane at 0 ppm). In spectra in vivo, the protons of water (usually not shown) resonate at 4.7 parts per million (ppm). The ppm scale has been selected instead of Hertz (Hz = sec^{-1}) because it is independent of the magnetic field strength. The y axis is a measure of the signal intensity, which is proportional to the concentration of a chemical.

Main Metabolites of the in Vivo Proton Spectrum

N-ACETYLASPARTATE

The most prominent peak of the ^{1}H spectrum is the resonance at 2.0 ppm from three equivalent protons of the acetyl group of the N-acetylaspartate (NAA) molecule (see Fig. 25-1). The role of NAA and its regulation in vivo are not well understood. In the normal brain, NAA is synthesized in neurons, diffuses along axons, and is broken down in oligodendrocytes. NAA is present in high concentrations only in normal neurons and axons,[1,2] and from an MRS perspective, it is a marker for adult type "healthy" neurons and axons. Proton spectra of any disease that is associated with neuronal or axonal loss will exhibit a reduction of NAA. Brain NAA increases rapidly as the brain matures, peaks at ≈10 to 15 years, and then decreases slightly over time as the number of neurons and axons declines even in the normal brain.[3]

TOTAL CHOLINE

The next prominent peak at 3.2 ppm is commonly referred to as choline or trimethylamines. Choline is a complex peak comprising several metabolites that contain choline, and therefore the term *total choline* (tCho) is used in this chapter. Compounds that contain choline are involved in the synthesis and breakdown of phosphatidylcholine (lecithin). Phosphatidylcholine is the major phospholipid component of eukaryotic cells, accounting for approximately 60% of total cellular phospholipids.

CREATINE

The second tallest peak in occipital gray matter spectra is *creatine* (Cr) at 3.0 ppm. For normal brain tissue, the Cr peak comprises contributions from free Cr and phosphocreatine in approximately equal proportions. Phosphocreatine is in rapid chemical exchange with free Cr and is used to replenish adenosine triphosphate (ATP) levels, if required. Like NAA, Cr levels also are low in the newborn.

MYO-INOSITOL

tCho, Cr, and NAA can be detected readily and quantified in long *echo time* (TE) MRS. Short TE acquisition methods are necessary for reliable quantitation of myo-inositol (mI), which is a little-known sugarlike molecule that resonates at 3.6 ppm in the proton spectrum. It has been identified as a marker for astrocytes and is an osmolyte.[4,5] mI also is involved in the metabolism of phosphatidyl inositol, a membrane phospholipid. Similar to choline, mI is altered in response to alteration of membrane metabolism or membrane damage.

Table 25-1

Common Indications for Pediatric Magnetic Resonance Spectroscopy	
Tumors	New tumor
	Evaluate progression
	Tumor vs. encephalitis/other lesions
Hypoxic ischemic injury	Patients at risk for cerebral malperfusion (congenital heart defects—status, postoperative)
	Status, postoperative cardiac arrest, apneic episodes
	Trauma, nonaccidental trauma
	Birth asphyxia
Other	New seizures, worsening seizures
	Unknown neurologic condition, altered mental state, developmental delay, global hypotonia
	Metabolic disorders, phenylketonuria
	Leukodystrophies—monitoring
	Liver problems/failure—preliver transplant

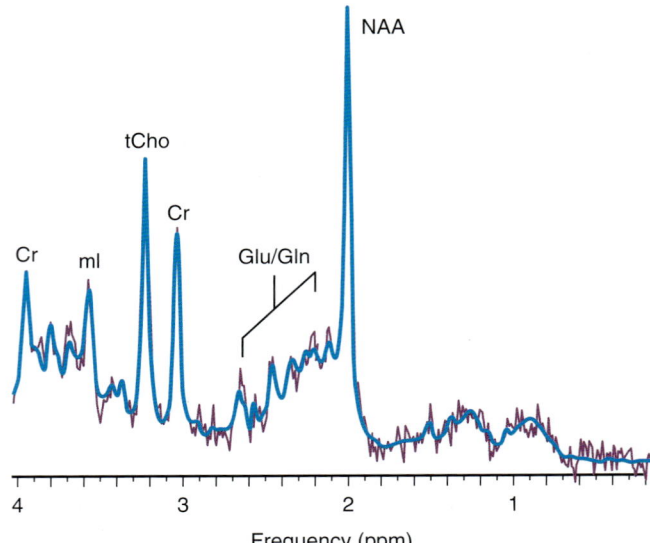

Figure 25-1 ¹H spectra of occipital gray matter acquired in a control subject. Magnetic resonance imaging uses the signal provided by the protons of the water to generate an anatomic map of the brain. In contrast, ¹H magnetic resonance spectroscopy uses the signal from the protons of chemicals to generate a biochemical fingerprint of a "region of interest." Spectra were acquired using a point resolved spectroscopy sequence with echo time of 35 ms. *NAA,* N-acetylaspartate; *Cr,* creatine; *tCho,* choline containing metabolites; *mI,* myo-inositol; *Glu,* glutamate; *Gln,* glutamine; *ppm,* parts per million.

Both tCho and mI are high in the newborn brain but decrease rapidly to normal levels within the first 12 to 24 months after birth.

LACTATE

Lactate is an important metabolite because it indicates anaerobic metabolism. Although lactate can be detected at pathologically elevated concentrations, in healthy tissue the lactate concentration is too low for routine detection with currently available methods. Lactate is the product of anaerobic glycolysis and increases when subsequent oxidation of lactate in the tricarboxylic acid cycle is impaired (for example, by lack of oxygen or mitochondrial disorders). Lactate also can increase in necrotic tissue and cysts. An elevation of lactate in "normal" appearing tissue would indicate global disruption or impairment of perfusion consistent with hypoxia and eventual poor outcome.[6-10]

Table 25-2

Summary of Chemicals Detectable with in Vivo Hydrogen Magnetic Resonance Spectroscopy			
	Long Name	**Role, Regulation, Location**	**Altered in Magnetic Resonance Spectrum When:**
NAA	N-acetylaspartate	Synthesized in neurons, diffuses along axons, broken down in oligodendrocytes, high in neurons and axons	Nonspecific but quantitative marker for neuronal/axonal damage
Cr	Creatine (creatine + phosphocreatine)	Synthesized in liver; functions as "battery" to replenish adenosine triphosphate levels	Abnormal in diseases of creatine synthesis, absent in cells that lack creatine kinase
tCho	Choline-containing metabolites	Involved in membrane synthesis and breakdown, osmolyte (GPC)	High in proliferative tumors, gliosis, leukodystrophies, low in hypoosmotic conditions, after radiation therapy
mI	Myo-inositol	High in astrocytes, osmolyte, sugarlike molecule, involved with phosphatidyl inositol (membrane lipid) metabolism	High in glial-based tumors (but low in glioblastoma multiforme), adrenoleukodystrophy, depleted in hepatic encephalopathy, low in other encephalitis (infections), liver disease
Glu	Glutamate	Excitatory neurotransmitter, high in neurons	High in seizures? Low in hepatic encephalopathy
Gln	Glutamine	Glutamate detoxification, osmolyte, high in glial cells, ammonia detoxification	High in hepatic encephalopathy, encephalitis (infections), ischemic-hypoxic injury
Lac	Lactate	End product of glycolysis, accumulates in cystic necrotic tissue, anaerobic metabolism indicator	Often high in tumors, (secondary) hypoxic-ischemic injury, mitochondrial disorders
Lip	Lipids	Membrane degeneration marker, necrosis marker	Aggressive tumors, infections, diseases associated with membrane breakdown
Glc	Glucose	Principle substrate for energy metabolism	Diabetes, disrupted energy metabolism
Tau	Taurine	Membrane stabilization?	Elevated in medulloblastoma and possibly other primitive tumors

LIPIDS AND MACROMOLECULES

The protons of the methyl groups ($-CH_3$) of lipid molecules resonate at 0.9 ppm, whereas protons of the methylene groups ($-CH_2-$) resonate at 1.3 ppm in the ^1H spectrum. Both resonances are broad and also may comprise contributions from other macromolecules. In normal tissue, the concentration of free lipids is small, and very little signal should be present in this part of the spectrum. Lipid signals increase upon breakdown of cell membranes and release of fatty acids. Lipids therefore are important markers for severe brain injury.

Magnetic Resonance Spectroscopy Methods

DATA ACQUISITION TECHNIQUES

Localized Single-Voxel Spectroscopy

Single-voxel MRS measures the MR signal of a single selected region of interest, whereas signal outside this area is suppressed. For single-voxel MRS, the magnetic field and other parameters are optimized to get the best possible spectrum from a relatively small region of the brain. Manufacturers generally provide point-resolved spectroscopy,[11,12]

stimulated echo acquisition mode,[13] and image-selected in vivo spectroscopy.[14] These sequences differ in how radiofrequency pulses and so-called gradient pulses are arranged to achieve localization. It is beyond the scope of this review to discuss details about localization methods; the interested reader is referred to the aforementioned publications.

2-Dimensional or 3-Dimensional Chemical Shift Imaging

With chemical shift imaging (CSI) approaches, multiple spatially arrayed spectra (typically more than 100 spectra per slice) from slices or volumes are acquired simultaneously. Slice selection can be achieved with a selective radiofrequency pulse, as for MRI (Fig. 25-2). When it is desired that the region of interest be limited to a smaller volume, for example, to avoid bone and fat from the skull, CSI is usually combined with point-resolved spectroscopy, stimulated echo acquisition mode, or image-selected in vivo spectroscopy, but with a significantly larger volume selected than for single-voxel MRS. CSI is a very efficient method for acquiring information from different parts of the brain. An important feature is that within the examined volume of interest, any region of interest can be selected *retrospectively* by a process termed *voxel shifting*.

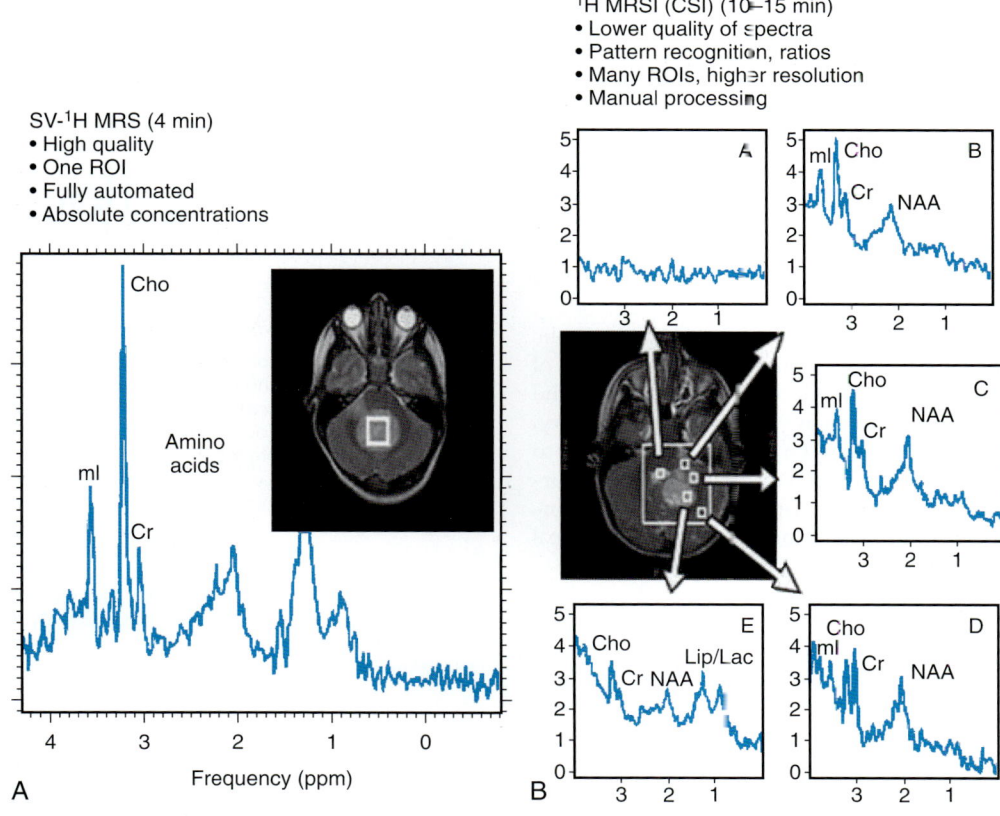

Figure 25-2 Differences between single-voxel (**A**) and multivoxel (**B**) acquisition. *Cho,* Choline; *Cr,* creatine; *CSI,* chemical shift imaging; *Lip/Lac,* lipid/lactate; *MRS,* magnetic resonance spectroscopy; *MRSI,* magnetic resonance spectroscopy imaging; *NAA,* N-acetylaspartate; *ppm,* parts per million; *ROI,* region of interest.

PARAMETERS

The most important parameter is the TE. Indeed, MRS can be separated into long TE and short TE methods. Long TE (typically >135 ms) has been easier to use in clinical practice because of a flat baseline and because three peaks (NAA, Cr, and tCho) can be unequivocally separated. Short TE MRS (≈30 ms) allows the detection of an increased number of metabolites and has a signal-to-noise advantage over long TE.

Clinical Applications

NEONATAL HYPOXIC-ISCHEMIC ENCEPHALOPATHY

In neonates with hypotensive injury, acute injury can be detected by MRS even when both diffusion imaging and conventional imaging are negative.[15-26] Within the first 24 hours of injury, MRS can detect elevated lactate levels in the cerebral cortex or basal ganglia, depending on the pattern of injury. Reduced NAA and elevated glutamate/glutamine levels usually are detected after 24 hours. NAA and lactate can be detected using either short echo (35 ms) or long echo (144 or 288 ms) time. MI, glutamate/glutamine, and lipids can be detected only during use of the short echo technique (Fig. 25-3). The lactate/NAA peak ratio, measured in deep gray matter, is an accurate prognosticator for neonatal hypoxic-ischemic encephalopathy,[27-36] whereas diffusion imaging can be limited by pseudonormalization of apparent diffusion coefficient in neonates.[37]

METABOLIC DISEASES AND WHITE MATTER DISORDERS

Readers are referred to an extensive review of the role of MRS in metabolic disease and white matter disease by Cecil and Kos.[38] Inborn errors of metabolism can present in the neonatal period. Leukoencephalopathies, which include a broad spectrum of inherited and acquired diseases that affect white matter, are associated with genetic enzyme defects that can lead to dysfunction and breakdown of myelin. These disease processes tend to present in infancy or childhood.

Metabolic disease may be classified as acquired metabolic disorders or inborn errors of metabolism. Some examples of acquired metabolic disorders include hyperbilirubinemia and hypoglycemia, both of which may result in brain injury. Inborn errors of metabolism can be classified broadly into organic acidemias, disorders of amino acid oxidation, disorders of fatty acid oxidation, primary lactic acidosis, mitochondria function, lysosomal storage disorders, and peroxisomal disorders.[39-42]

Some examples of organic acid disorders include methylmalonic acidemia and propionic aciduria. In these disorders, enzymatic defects occur in the conversion of valine, isoleucine, threonine, and methionine to propionic acid, succinic acid, and methylmalonic acid. Conventional MR findings include abnormal signal change corresponding to edema in both myelinated and unmyelinated structures. The edema in the myelinated structures is characterized by a vacuolating (or spongiform) myelinopathy, which can be seen in both amino acid and organic acid disorders. In vacuolating myelinopathy, water is trapped within vacuoles that can be found within

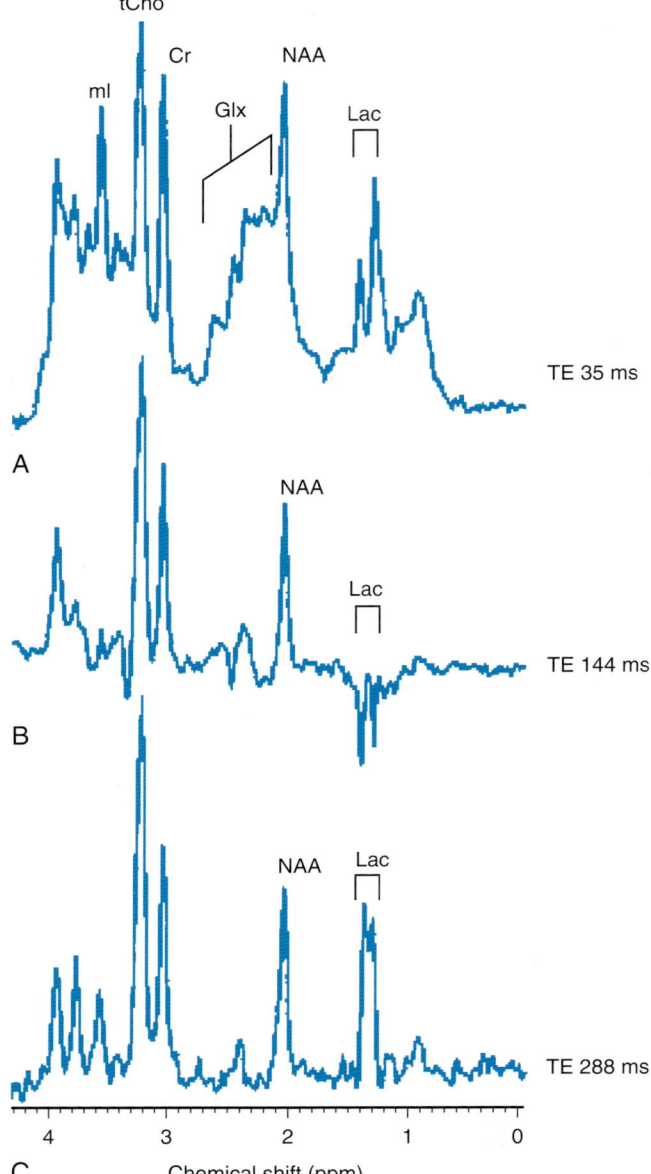

Figure 25-3 Comparison of magnetic resonance spectroscopy (MRS) of neonatal hypoxic-ischemic encephalopathy (acquired at multiple echo times (*TEs*)) with neonatal metabolic disease. **A-C** show single-voxel MRS at three different echo times in the basal ganglia of a hypoxic-ischemic term infant. Note the characteristic modulation of lactate (*Lac*). **A,** A spectrum acquired using short TE (35 ms), which shows a myo-inositol (*ml*) peak (left side of the spectrum), an elevated glutamine/glutamine (*Glx*) peak next to a reduced N-acetylaspartate (*NAA*) peak (middle spectrum), and an elevated lactate doublet next to a lipid peak (right side of the spectrum). **B,** A spectrum acquired using long TE (144 ms) that shows a lactate doublet peak inverted and reduced NAA, but nonvisualization of myo-inositol, glutamate, and lipids. **C,** A spectrum acquired using longer TE (244 ms) that is similar to 144 ms, except that the lactate doublet reverts to the other side of the spectrum.

the myelin sheath layers, resulting in restricted diffusion of water. MRS of these organic acid disorders detects reduction in mI and NAA levels and elevation of glutamine and lactate levels as a result of hyperammonia, ketoacidosis, and mitochondrial dysfunction.[39-43]

The classic phenotype of maple syrup urine disease is a disturbance in the metabolism of the essential amino acids leucine, isoleucine, and valine. Symptoms occur by the first week of life and include seizures, vomiting and dystonia, fluctuating ophthalmoplegia, and coma. Conventional MR findings include abnormal edema in the deep cerebellar white matter, brainstem tegmentum, posterior limb of the internal capsule, perirolandic white matter, and pre- and postcentral gyrus. The accumulation of abnormal branched-chain amino acids and branched-chain α-keto acids results in a peak at 0.9 ppm. Both the changes detected by diffusion imaging and MRS may normalize after treatment is started.[44,45]

Urea cycle defects are characterized by a total of five disorders that involve different defects in the biosynthesis of enzymes of the urea cycle, including ornithine carbamyl transferase deficiency, carbamyl phosphate synthetase deficiency, argininosuccinic aciduria, citrullinemia, and hyperargininemia.[46,47] In patients with these disorders, MRS can detect elevated glutamine levels resulting from hyperammonemia, which can be reversed with treatment.

Mitochondrial disorders are caused by defects of intracellular energy metabolism and result in decreased ATP production.[48-50] Leigh disease is a multisystem disorder in which the defect may be at different enzymatic mitochondrial levels, including the pyruvate dehydrogenase complex, cytochrome c oxidase, or ATP synthase. Conventional and diffusion imaging show abnormalities in signal intensity and mean diffusivity in the brainstem (pons, periaqueductal gray, substantia nigra, and medulla), the subthalamic nucleus, and the globus pallidus. MRS is used to detect lactate in these disorders. It should be noted, however, that an elevated lactate level is not specific for a mitochondrial disorder. Similarly, failure to detect lactate does not exclude the possibility of a mitochondrial abnormality.

Leukoencephalopathies can be classified in multiple ways, including (1) involvement of the primary cellular organelle; (2) biochemistry; and (3) location of primary involvement (periventricular, subcortical, white matter only, and gray and white matter). The MRS correlate of these white-matter disorders have been reviewed extensively by Cecil and Kos.[38] One of the most exclusive pathognomonic MRS diagnoses is that of Canavan disease. Canavan disease is an autosomal-recessive disorder arising from a deficiency of the enzyme aspartoacyclase (a cytosolic enzyme found in oligodendrocytes[51]) that results in an accumulation of NAA in the brain. MRS shows marked elevation of the NAA peak (Fig. 25-4).

PEDIATRIC BRAIN TUMORS

Posterior Fossa Lesions

Approximately 60% of all pediatric tumors arise from the posterior fossa. In most cases these tumors are grade IV medulloblastoma, grade I pilocytic astrocytoma, or (less frequently) grade II or III ependymoma. Occasionally, a cystic/necrotic medulloblastoma may have imaging characteristics that overlap with posterior fossa pilocytic astrocytoma (Fig. 25-5). Proton spectroscopy and diffusion imaging appear to be particularly useful for diagnoses. Taurine (Tau) elevation has been observed consistently by several groups in persons with a medulloblastoma[52-55] and is an important differentiator of medulloblastoma from other tumors of the posterior fossa.

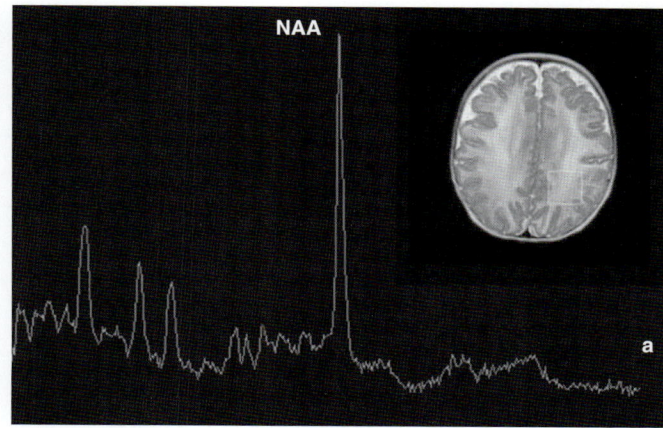

Figure 25-4 Elevated N-acetylaspartate (*NAA*) in a patient with Canavan disease.

A possible caveat is that in our institution we have observed that taurine levels are low in some desmoplastic nodular medulloblastoma variants. Medulloblastomas also have higher levels of choline than other posterior fossa tumors.[56,57] The hallmark of pilocytic astrocytomas is very low Cr concentrations, low mI, and low tCho concentrations, consistent with their low cellularity. Lipids also are low in pilocytic astrocytomas, but mean lactate levels are higher than in other tumors. Ependymomas have higher mI levels than do medulloblastomas or pilocytic astrocytomas; their choline levels are variable but generally fall between that of medulloblastomas and pilocytic astrocytomas.

Tumors Outside the Posterior Fossa

Approximately 40% of all pediatric brain tumors arise outside the posterior fossa. Medulloblastoma belongs to the group of *embryonal tumors*. Embryonal tumors outside the posterior fossa are central nervous system primitive neuroectodermal tumors or atypical teratoid/rhabdoid tumors. Preliminary data from our institution indicate that central nervous system primitive neuroectodermal tumors have metabolic profiles comparable with that observed in medulloblastomas, with prominent choline and taurine levels present. Atypical teratoid/rhabdoid tumors, on the other hand, appear to have a different metabolic pattern, with more moderate choline levels in some cases. Also, no evidence of taurine was seen in five cases studied at our institution. A pilocytic astrocytoma outside the posterior fossa may show a slightly more prominent mI signal, but the metabolic pattern otherwise is quite comparable with that of cerebellar pilocytic lesions.

Treatment Response

Conventional imaging does not reliably distinguish between recurrent/residual disease and postoperative changes or necrosis after radiation. Postradiation changes sometimes occur many months after therapy, and the correct diagnosis is a major challenge for the optimum management of pediatric patients. It is well known that spectroscopy is an important tool to assess response to therapy in pediatric and adult brain tumors.[58-64] Effective therapy causing cell death thus will result in generally reduced metabolite concentrations

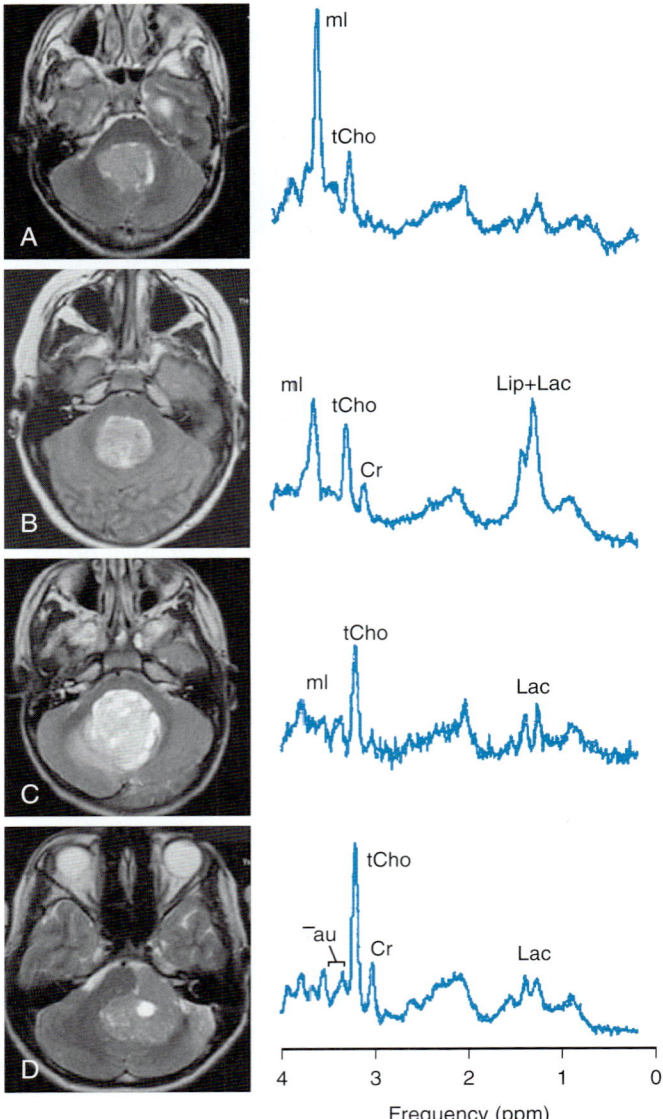

Figure 25-5 T2-weighted magnetic resonance (MR) images and MR spectra of posterior fossa tumors. **A,** Choroid plexus papilloma. **B,** Ependymoma (grade II). **C,** Pilocytic astrocytoma. **D,** Classic medulloblastoma. All spectra were acquired from lesions with no partial volume of surrounding tissue using a single-voxel point resolved spectroscopy sequence with a short echo time of 35 ms. Shown are the original unfiltered spectra (*thin line*) and the LCModel fits to the data (*thick line*) (Stephen Provencher Inc., version 6.1-G4). In all four cases presented, MR spectroscopy provided clues to the correct diagnosis, which was different from the impression of the routine anatomic MR image. *Cr,* Creatine; *Lac,* lactate; *Lip,* lipid; *ml,* myo-inositol; *tCho,* total choline; *Tau,* taurine.

(including tCho) and increased lipids because of the release of fatty acids from cell membranes. On the other hand, increasing levels of tCho (or tCho/NAA) are indicators for failed therapy and high risk for progressing disease.

NEOPLASIA VERSUS ENCEPHALITIS

Accurate initial diagnoses are needed not only to distinguish different types of tumors, but also to separate neoplastic from nonneoplastic disease. Multiple other focal lesions in the brain

may mimic brain tumors on conventional anatomic MRI. Some of these lesions include infectious or inflammatory lesions, infarcts, and demyelinating lesions (tumefactive demyelinating lesions). Because of a disrupted blood-brain barrier, these lesions can demonstrate avid contrast enhancement that can mimic conventional MRI characteristics of a malignant brain tumor. In a recent study,[65] it was shown that brain lesions resulting from *acute* encephalitis have a metabolic fingerprint that is significantly different from that of astrocytoma. We have found that mI levels are reduced in *acute* encephalitis cases (mostly viral) compared with neoplastic processes. Accurate noninvasive diagnosis of encephalitis is important because biopsies with the possibility of complications can be avoided.

HEPATIC ENCEPHALOPATHY

Hepatic encephalopathy refers to a broad spectrum of neurologic derangements associated with liver disease. MRS of hepatic encephalopathy typically demonstrates decreased levels of mI and choline and increased concentration of glutamate/glutamine (Glx) (Fig. 25-6). More recently, it has been demonstrated that MRS metabolites are correlated with plasma ammonia levels and the ratio of branched-chain to aromatic amino acids and can be useful to help establish a diagnosis of minimal hepatic encephalopathy in pediatric patients.[66]

Quantification in Positron Emission Tomography Imaging

Positron emission tomography (PET) is able to quantify radioactivity concentration within a given region of interest. Analysis of tracer activity and its distribution can provide meaningful information on available receptor binding sites or biochemical processes. Three categories of methods in analyzing data are available: (1) qualitative analysis (visual assessment), (2) semiquantitative assessment such as standardized uptake value (SUV) and lesion-to-background ratio, and (3) absolute quantitative analysis using nonlinear regression, Patlak graphical analysis, and simplified quantitative methods.[67] Qualitative analysis requires minimal effort but has the least accuracy, whereas an absolute quantification method requires more complex procedures such as compartmental kinetic modeling to measure the individual rate constant based on data from dynamic image acquisition and serial blood sampling. Because of its complexity and time-consuming nature, this method is impractical in most clinical settings.

In clinical fluorodeoxyglucose (FDG)-PET studies, SUV is the most commonly used semiquantitative parameter. SUV is defined by lesion concentration of tracer per injected dose of normalized patient body weight multiplied by a decay factor:

$$SUV = \text{Tissue activity concentration (MBq/mL)} \\ \text{(Injected dose (MBq/mL)/Body weight (g)} \\ \times \text{Decay factor of 18 F)}$$

Compared with kinetic modeling, the SUV calculation is simple (without any need for arterial blood sampling) and faster (without dynamic image acquisition). Tissue SUV is

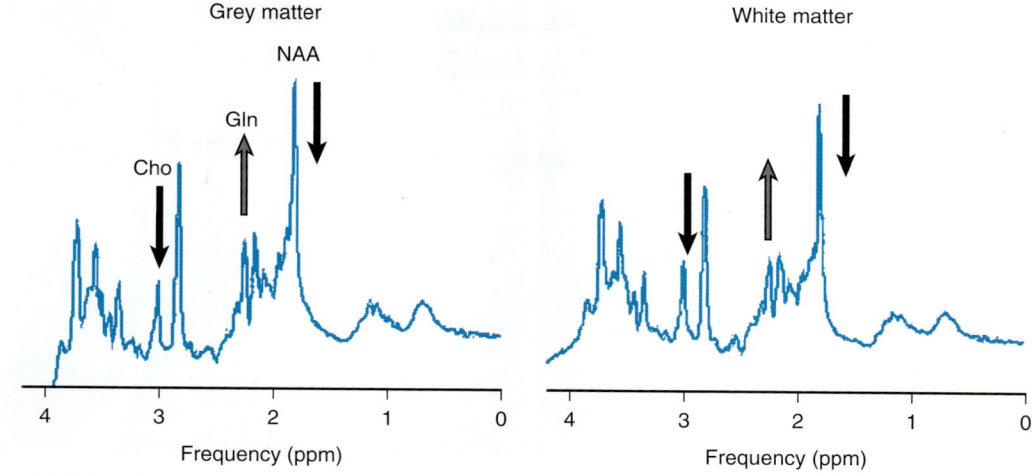

Figure 25-6 Hepatic encephalopathy in a pediatric patient with iron intoxication and acute liver failure. Magnetic resonance spectroscopy performed at 3T with point resolved spectroscopy and a time echo of 35 ms. Three voxel locations show an elevated glutamine (*Gln*) level, a reduced choline level, and a reduced myo-inositol level, indicating poor liver function. N-acetylaspartate (*NAA*) also is reduced, which may indicate neuronal/axonal loss/damage. Conventional magnetic resonance imaging was within normal limits. *ppm*, Parts per million.

known to have a linear relationship with the rate of glucose metabolism measured by kinetic modeling, with high correlation coefficients of up to 0.91.[68,69]

Positron Emission Tomography and Brain Development

Chugani et al[70] evaluated the functional development of the pediatric brain using FDG-PET. They reported that the metabolic pattern of a developing brain follows the order of anatomic, evolutional, and behavioral development. Increased glucose metabolism demonstrated in the visual cortex, sensorimotor cortex, and cerebellum is correlated with early visuospatial and sensorimotor function and primitive reflexes. It also is known that hypermetabolism in the basal ganglia is associated with developing movement and sensorimotor function.

The degree of glucose metabolism of infants is known to be significantly lower than that of adults based on the quantitative analysis of brain FDG-PET. The current hypothesis is that increased metabolism is associated with increased metabolic demands from neuronal plasticity development.[71] The metabolic level of the neonatal brains is about 30% that of adults, and it continues to increase with age. By the age of 3 years, the degree of metabolic activity exceeds that of adults, reaching its plateau between ages 4 and 9 years, with a value 1.3 times higher than that of healthy adults.[72] After this period, the metabolic activity continues to decrease to adult levels by the end of the second decade.[70] The overall degree of cortical metabolism significantly decreases with age, a consistent finding related to normal aging according to a study of 120 healthy volunteers between the ages of 17 and 79 years.[73]

The distribution of glucose metabolism of a pediatric brain becomes similar to that of young adults by the age of 1 year. The frontal lobe demonstrates more significant age-related metabolic changes compared with other parts of the brain. For the first 4 months of life, the frontal lobe has relatively low glucose levels, and the metabolic levels in this area gradually increase as frontal lobe–mediated cognitive function and complicated social interaction develops. A 38% decrease in whole-brain metabolism and a 42% decline in frontal lobe metabolism with aging based on linear regression analysis was demonstrated by Chawluk et al.[74] No significant differences in regional glucose metabolism were found between men and women.[73,75]

The remaining cortical areas such as the parietal, occipital, and temporal lobes have significant variations within and across age groups. The metabolic activity in the basal ganglia, thalami, hippocampi, cerebellum, visual cortices, and posterior cingulate gyrus is shown to remain stable at different ages,[73] whereas the metabolic activity in the brainstem increases with age.[73] Further studies are required to explain whether brain atrophy contributes to hypometabolism with aging.

Positron Emission Tomography in Pediatric Epilepsy

The PET tracer most widely used in clinical practice for evaluation of brain glucose metabolism to localize epileptogenic focus is fluorine-18-deoxyglucose (^{18}F-FDG). FDG-PET is better suited for capturing the interictal state of epilepsy rather than the ictal state because of its long uptake period (40 to 60 minutes). The typical pattern of PET glucose metabolism of an epileptic focus is hypometabolism of the ipsilateral temporal lobe with or without less severe hypometabolism in the extratemporal structures such as the frontal lobe, parietal lobe, and contralateral temporal lobe. When anatomic lesions are associated with epilepsy, the extent of hypometabolism is known to be greater than the size of the structural lesion.[76]

The pathophysiology of regional hypometabolism in interictal FDG-PET is not clearly known, although several hypotheses have been proposed, including neuronal cell loss, neuronal inhibition, and diaschisis associated with

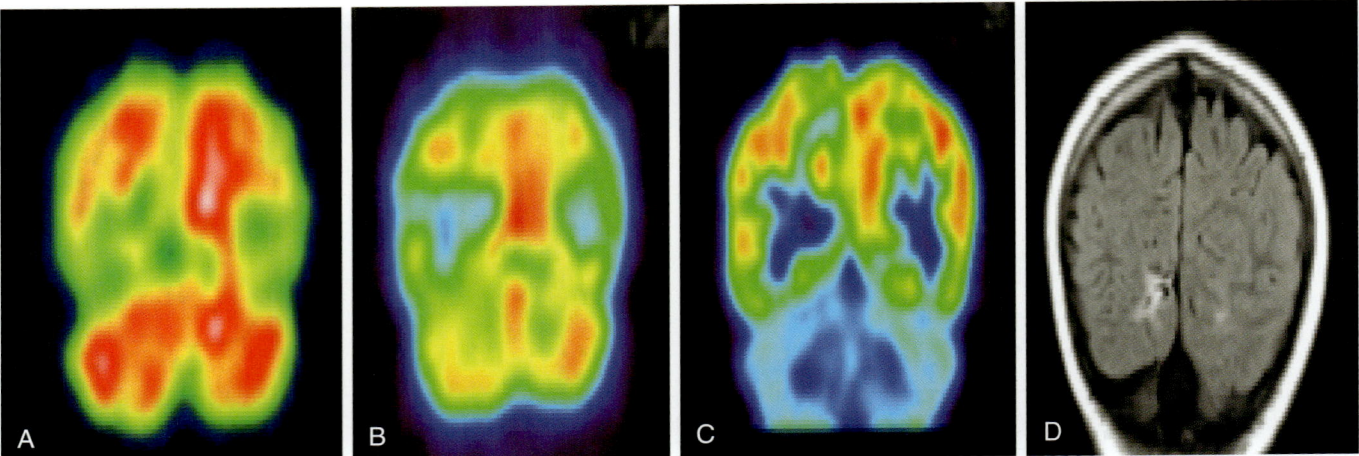

Figure 25-7 A 13-year-old girl with extratemporal lobe (right occipital) epilepsy with localizing epileptogenic focus shown in interictal single photon emission computed tomography (SPECT), positron emission tomography (PET), magnetic resonance imaging (MRI), and nonlocalizing ictal SPECT. **A,** An ictal SPECT scan demonstrates an asymmetric perfusion pattern with relative hypoperfusion in the right occipital lobe. No focal hyperperfusion is noted. **B,** An interictal SPECT scan demonstrates hypoperfusion in the right occipital lobe with an epileptogenic focus. **C,** A fluorodeoxyglucose-PET scan demonstrates hypometabolism in the right occipital lobe with an epileptogenic focus. **D,** An MRI fluid attenuated inversion recovery scan demonstrates hyperintensity in the right occipital lobe, suggesting an epileptogenic focus.

hippocampal neuronal loss[77] (Fig. 25-7). However, conflicting evidence also exists, such as temporal hypometabolism without neuronal loss or gliosis[78] and a poor correlation between metabolic change in the temporal lobe and hippocampal cell count.[79]

Additional proposed hypotheses to explain interictal hypometabolism include an inhibitory process and reduction in synaptic density. Findings of several studies suggested that this secondary inhibition or neuronal loss in the area surrounding the epileptic zone can cause larger and more extensive hypometabolism in FDG-PET[77,80,81] and hypoperfusion in single photon emission computed tomography (SPECT)[82] than the area of involvement seen on electroencephalography or a pathologic correlate. Further work needs to be performed to validate this mechanism. Interictal FDG-PET is known to be more sensitive than MRI in localizing epileptogenic foci in cases of both temporal and extratemporal epilepsy.[83]

About 29% of patients with partial or focal epilepsy have normal MRI findings.[84] Intracranial electroencephalography has limitations in this situation because of a lack of electrode targeting precision to the areas of suspected seizure origin. Lee et al.[85] have described the potential diagnostic role of FDG-PET and SPECT in the absence of anatomic findings, and they showed that the positive predictive value of FDG-PET and ictal SPECT in MRI-negative cryptogenic epilepsy was greater than 70%. The localization rates by FDG-PET in patients with normal MRI findings were 57% and 32%, as reported by Chugani et al.[86] and Swartz et al.,[87] respectively.

PET/CT Imaging of Pediatric Brain Tumors

Recently, the use of PET and radiopharmaceutical agents for PET for brain tumor imaging has increased. Currently the only radiotracer approved by the FDA is ^{18}F-FDG. In clinical practice, FDG-PET is being used as an adjunct tool in cases in which CT and MRI are unable to address a specific clinical question. The most common clinical indications of PET imaging include: (1) confirmation of the presence or absence of tumor; (2) help in establishing the grade of malignancy; (3) determination of the degree of treatment of the tumor or tumor response; and (4) distinguishing tumor recurrence from radiation necrosis[88] (Figs. 25-8 and 25-9). FDG-PET is known to be very sensitive in detecting high-grade gliomas. The high background uptake of FDG normally seen in the cortex results in less accurate detection of low-grade gliomas.[89] More recently, PET imaging has been integrated into pediatric multiinstitutional protocols of the Pediatric Brain Tumor Consortium, which will yield useful pediatric data.[90]

PET/MRI

Combined PET/MRI is a promising newer technology offering the potential application for novel molecular imaging with excellent soft-tissue differentiation, lack of ionizing radiation from the MRI component, and simultaneous anatomic and functional data acquisition.

Several approaches for conducting PET/MRI studies have been proposed, with the two machines currently approved by the FDA employing different strategies. The Philips Ingenuity TF (Philips Healthcare, Andover, MA) is designed as two separate scanners that share a rotating bed to keep mutual interference to a minimum, although it is not truly simultaneous acquisition. The Siemens Biograph mMR (Siemens Medical Solutions USA, Inc., Malvern, PA) uses PET detectors integrated between the MR body coil and the gradient coils, providing simultaneous acquisition.

The first PET/MRI studies in humans demonstrated an excellent simultaneous performance of both PET and MRI imaging without degrading image quality.[91,92] The diagnostic advantages of fused PET and MR images over PET/CT were shown by a 2006 study.[93] Moreover, PET/MRI is more

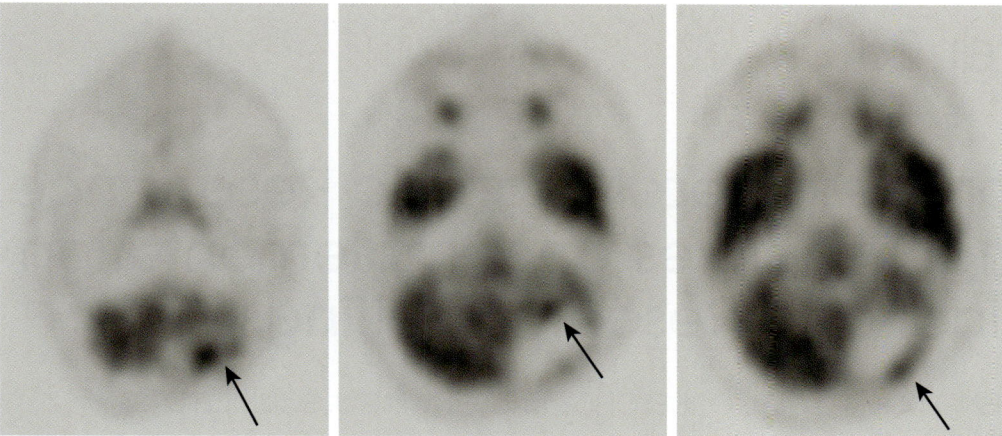

Figure 25-8   An 18-year-old male patient with a history of anaplastic ependymoma in the left cerebellum, after having multiple surgeries. A brain fluorodeoxyglucose–positron emission tomography scan demonstrates multiple areas of increased activity in the anterior and posterior resection margin consistent with malignant disease (*arrows*).

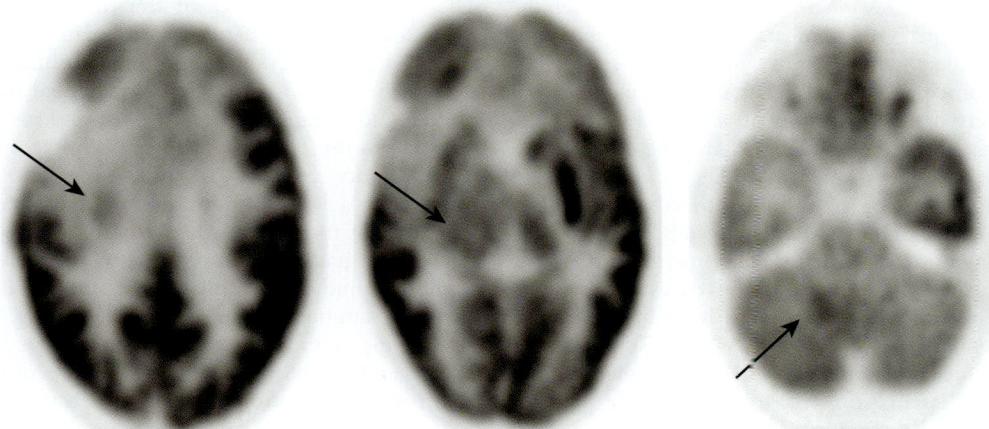

Figure 25-9   A 9-year-old boy with an anaplastic astrocytoma after undergoing resection in the right frontal lobe. Multiple areas of increased metabolic activity (*arrows*) are noted involving the right posterior medial frontal lobe, right basal ganglia, right thalamus, and the right cerebellum corresponding to areas of tumor infiltration seen with magnetic resonance imaging.

beneficial to pediatric patients because it entails much less radiation exposure compared with PET/CT.

Suggested Readings

Cecil KM, Kos RS. Magnetic resonance spectroscopy and metabolic imaging in white matter diseases and pediatric disorders. *Top Magn Reson Imaging.* 2006;17:275-293.

Panigrahy A, Nelson Jr MD, Bluml S. Magnetic resonance spectroscopy in pediatric neuroradiology: clinical and research applications. *Pediatr Radiol.* 2010;40(1):3-30.

References

Full references for this chapter can be found on www.expertconsult.com.

Chapter 26

Diffusion-Weighted Magnetic Resonance Imaging: Principles and Implementation in Clinical and Research Settings

JESSICA L. WISNOWSKI, RAFAEL C. CESCHIN, and VINCENT J. SCHMITHORST

Of the advanced magnetic resonance imaging (MRI) modalities, diffusion-weighted (DW) MRI has probably garnered the most excitement in both clinical and research settings during the past decade. Standard now in nearly every neuroimaging MR protocol, DW-MRI has demonstrated substantial clinical utility in the detection of acute ischemia, the differential diagnosis of intracranial lesions, and the evaluation of white matter. More recently, DW-MRI, or more specifically, diffusion tensor imaging (DTI) and other high-angular resolution diffusion imaging (HARDI) models, have been applied to the evaluation of normal developmental processes and pathology, particularly that which involves the white matter. Numerous postprocessing methods have been developed that not only allow for group level comparisons of the underlying "tissue microstructure" but also allow for estimation (and visual representation) of the underlying white matter "tracts." In this chapter, we will (1) review the underlying principles of DW-MRI acquisitions; (2) review basic diffusion-weighted imaging (DWI) acquisitions (DWI and its application in clinical settings); (3) review DTI models and postprocessing methods, with emphasis on the strengths and potential pitfalls in both clinical and research settings; and (4) review advanced diffusion imaging models (e.g., diffusion kurtosis imaging [DKI], HARDI, Q-ball, and diffusion spectrum imaging [DSI]). Further examples of the application of DW-MRI will be evident in numerous other chapters in this volume.

Underlying Principles of DW-MRI Acquisition

At its core, DW-MRI involves the application of two additional pulses of magnetic field gradient (called "diffusion-encoding" or "diffusion-sensitizing" gradients) to a T2-weighted sequence after the excitation pulse but before the readout. During the first gradient pulse, spin precession is accelerated in accordance with the spatial position of the individual water molecules; spins associated with water molecules with a high Z coordinate, for example, will precess more quickly after administration of a gradient pulse along the Z direction, whereas spins associated with water

molecules with a low Z coordinate will precess more slowly. Therefore the net effect of the first gradient pulse on the ensemble of spins is that the spins begin precessing at different rates and consequently "dephase," resulting in signal attenuation. The second gradient pulse is equal in direction, magnitude, and duration (δ) to the first and is either of opposite polarity (in the case of a gradient echo acquisition) or of the same polarity (in the case of a spin echo acquisition) but placed after a 180-degree refocusing pulse. Assuming that the spins do not move from their original locations, the effect of the second gradient pulse will be to precisely undo the effect of the first and thus "rephase" the spins so there is no longer any signal attenuation due to spin dephasing. However, under physiologic conditions, water molecules possess thermal energy and therefore will move a finite distance away from their original locations during the time between gradient pulses (Δ). Thus the rephasing is incomplete and the signal will be attenuated compared with the signal with no diffusion-sensitizing gradients.

Assuming that the movement of water molecules is not hindered by any form of barrier (so-called "free diffusion"), the mean squared distance that the spins will move over a given period is described by the Einstein-Smoluchowsky equation and is linearly proportional to the time (Δ) and to the self-diffusion coefficient D. The amount of attenuation is a function of the gradient strength G, gradient duration δ, time between gradient pulses Δ, and diffusion coefficient D. Typically G, δ, and Δ are combined to derive the "b-value"; the higher the b-value, the greater the signal attenuation in the resultant DW images (Fig. 26-1). In fact, signal attenuation is exponential, where S is the measured signal and S_0 is the signal in the absence of diffusion weighting. As a result, D (measured in mm²/s) can be estimated by obtaining DW images at different b-values or by obtaining images with and without diffusion weighting.

However, the diffusion of water molecules in the brain differs in two important respects from free diffusion. First, the diffusion of water is hindered by a variety of barriers, including axon sheaths and glial cell and astrocyte membranes. Hence the measured diffusion coefficient is not a self-diffusion coefficient and therefore is referred to as an *apparent* diffusion coefficient (ADC). Furthermore, the diffusion of water in the brain is not isotropic (i.e., independent

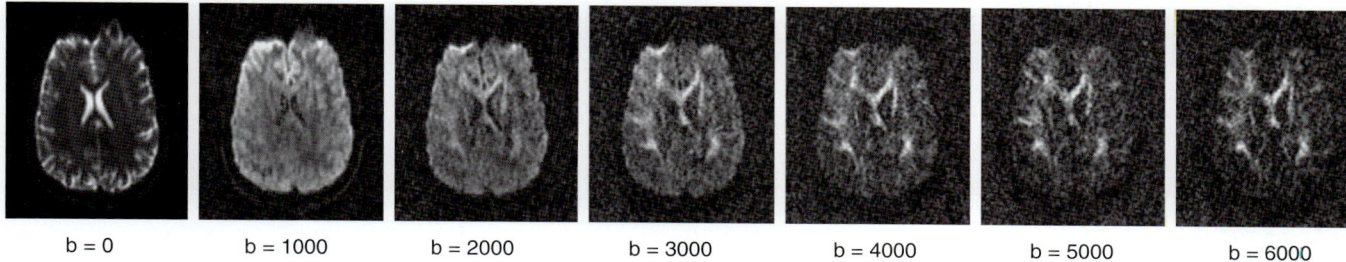

| b = 0 | b = 1000 | b = 2000 | b = 3000 | b = 4000 | b = 5000 | b = 6000 |

Figure 26-1   Changing b-value. Displayed are corresponding slices from a single subject imaged at multiple b-values. Notice how contrast between gray and white matter increases with the increasing b-value, whereas overall signal/noise ratio decreases. (Data courtesy Justin Haldar, University of Southern California, Department of Electrical Engineering.)

of direction). For instance, diffusivity along an axon direction will be larger than diffusivity perpendicular to the axon direction. Hence DW images often are obtained using a variety of gradient directions to infer information about the diffusivity of water molecules in different directions; the amount of attenuation in the DW images is dependent on the diffusion of water molecules only in the direction of the applied diffusion-encoding gradients.

It also is important to note that because DW measurements reflect an *attenuation* of signal at a given spatial location, maintenance of sufficient signal to noise in the resultant data is an inherent challenge in DWI. Moreover, the time needed to acquire data sufficient for some of the most advanced postprocessing techniques, which require acquisitions at many different gradient direction and b-values, is often well outside of what is typically feasible in clinical settings and in many pediatric populations. Thus in practice, most pediatric DW-MRI studies generally are limited to the more basic DW-MRI models (i.e., DTI, described in a later section of this chapter), although recent developments provide hope that other DW-MRI techniques soon will be clinically feasible.

Diffusion Weighting, Apparent Diffusivity, and Their Application in Clinical Settings

Clinically relevant information is available even from a single DWI acquisition. For instance, diffusion is restricted in regions of cytotoxic edema after a stroke, and these regions therefore will be hyperintense on DW images. However, typical DWI acquisitions are strongly T2-weighted, because a long echo time is necessary as a result of the time needed to apply the diffusion-sensitizing gradients. Therefore it is important to distinguish hyperintensity on DWI that represents true diffusion restriction from hyperintensity that reflects tissue T2 prolongation (often termed "T2 shine-through"). This differentiation usually is performed by the additional acquisition of an image without diffusion weighting (e.g., b = 0) and quantifying ADC on a pixel-by-pixel basis, which subsequently can be represented in gray scale as an ADC map. Additionally, instead of a single DW acquisition, three DW images typically are acquired using three orthogonal gradient directions, and the results are averaged to obtain *directionally averaged* DW images and ADC maps to minimize the effects of anisotropy. The directionally averaged ADC

map is proportional to the trace of the diffusion tensor (described later), and thus the DWI images and ADC maps often are referred to as "trace-weighted DWI" and "trace diffusion tensor maps," respectively (Fig. 26-2).

As previously noted, in the past two decades, trace DW images with corresponding ADC values have demonstrated remarkable clinical utility in the detection of acute cerebral ischemia, often before such injuries otherwise become apparent. In persons with ischemia, a critical drop in cerebral blood perfusion leads to energy failure, and more specifically, a failure of the Na+/K+−adenosine triphosphatase pumps in the cell membrane. This phenomenon, in turn, leads to an influx of sodium (and other ions) and water into the cell, causing the cell to swell (i.e., cytotoxic edema). Although other events also might contribute to the change in ADC, it has been suggested that ADC is most sensitive to a small change in the distribution of water between extracellular and intracellular environments, and thus ADC can be viewed as a marker of fluid-electrolyte homeostasis.

In addition to fluid homeostasis and intracellular water, DWI and ADC also are sensitive to the relative properties of water in the extracellular space. Thus DWI also is useful in the differential diagnosis of intracranial lesions. In lesions with high cellularity (e.g., high-grade tumors), the increased cellularity restricts water motion in the extracellular space, resulting in decreased ADC in the lesion (or in areas of the lesion with relatively higher cellularity). Accordingly, DWI often can distinguish high-grade tumors such as primitive neuroectodermal tumors from other lower grade pediatric brain tumors such as ependymomas or astrocytomas (Fig. 26-3).

Diffusion Tensor Imaging

Although three diffusion-sensitizing gradients are sufficient for calculating a directionally averaged ADC image, a minimum of six directions is needed to characterize diffusion anisotropy. Anisotropic diffusion is directionally dependent, as within white matter fiber bundles, and is distinguishable from isotropic diffusion, which is observed in free fluids (e.g., the lateral ventricles) (Fig. 26-4).

To calculate anisotropy, DTI models diffusion as a tensor quantity (a 3×3 matrix) on a voxel-by-voxel basis. Typically, the matrix is rotated such that anisotropy may be described in terms of three coordinate axes ("eigenvectors"), with the principal axis (the one corresponding to the largest "eigenvalue" λ_1, also known as $\lambda_{||}$, or axial diffusivity) being along

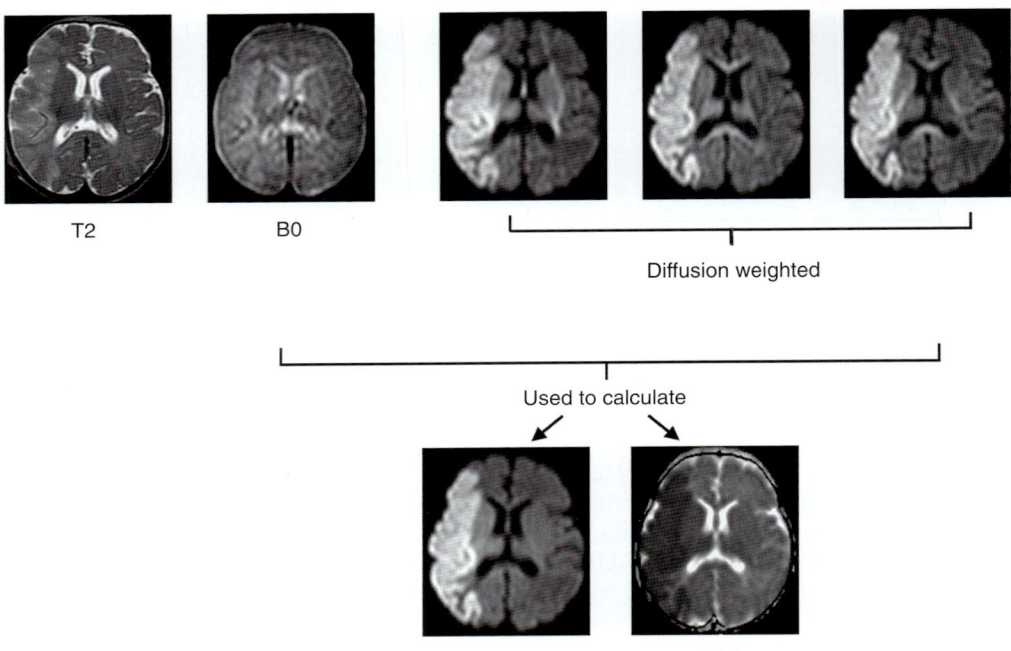

T2   B0

Diffusion weighted

Used to calculate

Trace DWI   ADC

Figure 26-2 Diffusion-weighted (DW) imaging demonstrated in a 3-week-old neonate with an acute stroke. **Top row,** Corresponding slices from an axial T2-weighted and DW-magnetic resonance imaging scan. In most protocols, three diffusion-encoding directions (rather than one) are acquired, averaged, and compared with the image without diffusion encoding (B0) to generate (*bottom row*) trace-weighted and apparent diffusivity maps that demonstrate areas of restricted diffusion as areas of high and low signal, respectively. Note that areas of directional anisotropy are visualized in each of the diffusion-encoding directions, but as a result of averaging, these areas are not apparent in the trace-weighted and apparent diffusion coefficient (*ADC*) maps.

the axis of preferred diffusion and the remaining two eigenvalues (λ_2 and λ_3) corresponding to vectors perpendicular to the principal axis. Eigenvalues λ_2 and λ_3 often are combined (averaged) to generate another metric referred to as radial diffusivity ($\lambda_\perp$). Importantly, although the 3×3 *diffusion tensor* may be ideal for estimating diffusion in a three-dimensional (3D) structure characterized by fiber bundles aligned in a single orientation, this model falls short if the underlying structure includes fiber bundles of different orientations (e.g., "crossing fibers"). Accordingly, potential pitfalls associated with DTI will be discussed in further detail later.

The most common anisotropy metric derived from DTI data is fractional anisotropy (FA). FA is a scalar metric (rather than a vector) and represents the degree of anisotropy at a

given voxel. It is calculated by comparing the estimated diffusion along each of the three eigenvalues in accordance with the following equation:

$$FA = \frac{\sqrt{(\lambda_1 - \lambda_2)^2 + (\lambda_2 - \lambda_3)^2 + (\lambda_3 - \lambda_1)^2}}{\sqrt{2(\lambda_1^2 + \lambda_2^2 + \lambda_3^2)}}$$

As can be determined from this equation, FA can range from 0 (when $\lambda_1 = \lambda_2 = \lambda_3$, i.e., isotropic diffusion) to 1 (when $\lambda_2 = \lambda_3 = 0$, i.e., fully anisotropic). In adults, typical white-matter values range between 0.9 and 0.4 depending on whether the measurement is obtained in a region where fiber bundles are heavily myelinated, tightly packed, and uniformly oriented (e.g., in the corpus callosum) or in a region where the organization deviates from that (such as in the vicinity of crossing fibers), respectively. FA values are much lower in neonates (ranging between 0.45 and 0.1) but rapidly increase toward the adult range in the first 2 years of life and then continue to increase at a much lower rate through adolescence into adulthood.[1-3]

Because of the higher water content in the neonatal brain and the fact that this increase in extracellular water is associated with increased diffusivity and increased signal attenuation in the setting of diffusion encoding gradients, neonates often undergo imaging at a lower b-value (e.g., b = 700 s/mm^2).

To further enhance the clinical utility of FA, FA often is combined with information regarding the direction of the principal eigenvector, yielding a color FA map (Fig. 26-5). The typical convention is to color pixels red when the principal eigenvector is in the left-right direction relative to the 3D coordinate space, green when the principal eigenvector

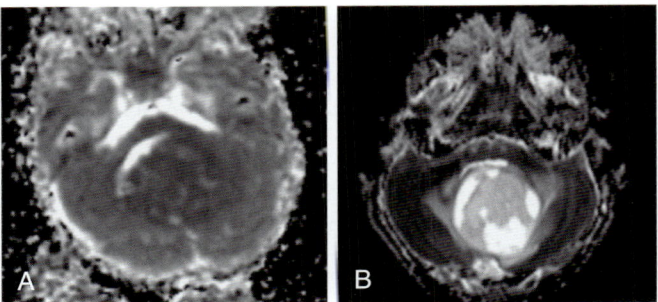

Figure 26-3 Apparent diffusion coefficient (ADC) and intracranial lesions. **A,** The ADC map demonstrates restricted diffusion in a tumor with high cellularity (a medulloblastoma). **B,** The ADC map demonstrates increased diffusion in a tumor with low cellularity (a pilocytic astrocytoma).

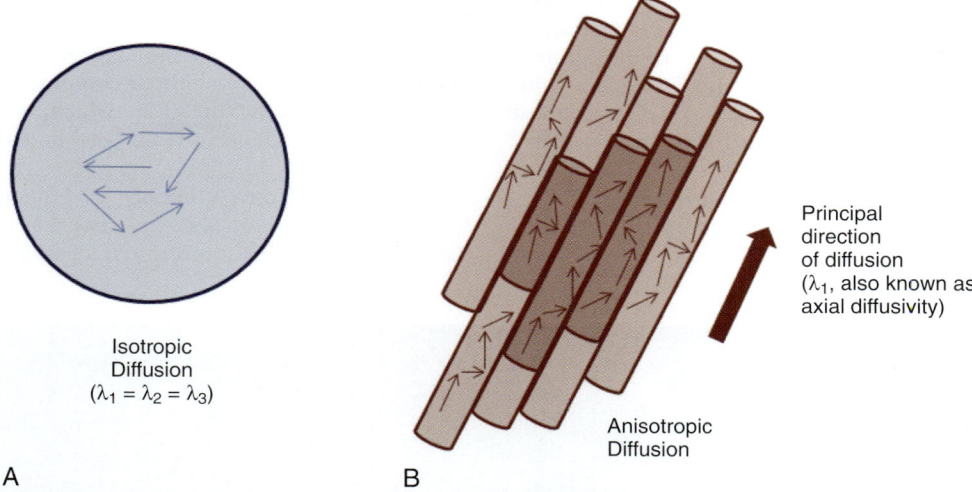

Figure 26-4 Isotropic and anisotropic diffusion. **A,** Isotropic diffusion is exemplified by free diffusion such as in a large glass of water. **B,** Anisotropic diffusion occurs when diffusion is greater in one direction compared with the others, such as in axons. By convention, the principal eigenvalue (λ_1) represents diffusion along the preferred axis.

is anterior-posterior, and blue when the principal eigenvector is inferior-superior.

MICROSTRUCTURAL INTEGRITY

The sensitivity of DTI to local ("microstructural") tissue properties has rendered the technique a popular instrument for investigating the neuroanatomic underpinnings of various conditions (e.g., traumatic brain injury, multiple sclerosis, white matter injury of prematurity, autism, and dyslexia, but also such areas as normal development, learning, and musical training) at the level of gray and white matter tissue micro-structure. Moreover, DTI sequences are readily available in most commercial MRI scanners, with the acquisition time necessary for a typical 30 to 60 direction DTI sequence being between 5 minutes to less than 15 minutes. Accordingly, DTI is not only feasible in most pediatric patients but also is a

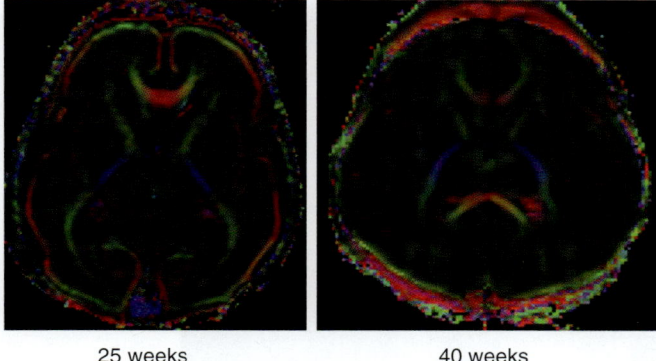

25 weeks   40 weeks

Figure 26-5 Color fractional anisotropy maps reconstructed from diffusion tensor imaging data acquired from a preterm neonate at 25 weeks and a term neonate at 40 weeks. By convention, voxels in which the principal eigenvector (λ_1) is in a left-right orientation (relative to the slice) are colored in red, voxels in which λ_1 is in an anterior-posterior orientation are colored green, and voxels in which λ_1 is in a superior-inferior orientation are colored blue. Note the presence of high anisotropy in the cortex of the neonate at 25 weeks and that, by term, the cortex has lower anisotropy than the adjacent white matter.

potential key to understanding the neuroanatomic basis for a wide range of conditions, many of which are not associated with visible changes on conventional T1- and T2-weighted imaging.

However, the precise interpretation for many of the differences in DTI measures of microstructure remains to be determined. Pioneering laboratory work by Sheng-Kwei Song and colleagues in mouse models demonstrated that myelin loss alone (without loss or degeneration of axons) results in an increase in radial diffusivity (RD), leaving axial diffusivity (AD) unchanged.[4] In contrast, direct axonal damage results in a decrease in AD.[5] Based on these findings, many researchers have drawn inverse conclusions on their own data—namely, that an increase in RD in a given white matter region reflects primarily damage to myelin, whereas a decrease in AD reflects primarily damage to axons. Unfortunately, the inverse conclusion is not necessarily valid. First, most of the laboratory work supporting the interpretation of AD and RD in relation to axonal pathology versus myelin has been carried out in the optic nerve, spinal cord, or corpus callosum.[4-6] These structures are unique in the central nervous system in that they contain fiber bundles essentially aligned along a single axis. In contrast, the cerebrum and even the brainstem have far fewer regions where the fiber bundles are organized along a single axis (it has been estimated that as many as 90% of white matter voxels in the cerebrum contain crossing fibers).[7] It is not known how altering myelination or axonal integrity along a single fiber bundle, in the setting of multiple crossing fibers, would alter AD or RD. Accordingly, in the cerebrum, given available knowledge at this point, a more appropriate interpretation may be "altered microstructure," with more specific conclusions being drawn from collateral information. However, this technique continues to show great promise.

TRACTOGRAPHY

Some of the increasingly common—and most important—questions that researchers and neuroradiologists have aimed to address with use of DTI concerns anatomic connectivity (e.g., "Which cortical and subcortical regions are connected, and by which fiber pathways?" "How strong are the connections between X and Y? ... in this population compared with that one?"). To address these types of questions, most researchers and clinicians begin by constructing a visual representation of the white matter fibers (or *tracts*). This task is carried out with use of computer algorithms that regard fiber tracts as a continuous trajectory derived from local (voxel or pixel) estimates of fiber orientation (e.g., eigenvectors;

Fig. 26-6). This technique is commonly known as *tractography*. It should be emphasized that no tractography method is capable of reconstructing axonal fibers or even fiber bundles. Rather, these methods compute trajectories or pathways represented by the data, which, it is hoped, parallel the predominant trajectories of the underlying axonal fiber bundles.

One of the most commonly used algorithms for tractography is known as *fiber assignment by continuous tracking* (also known as deterministic tractography).[8] This algorithm

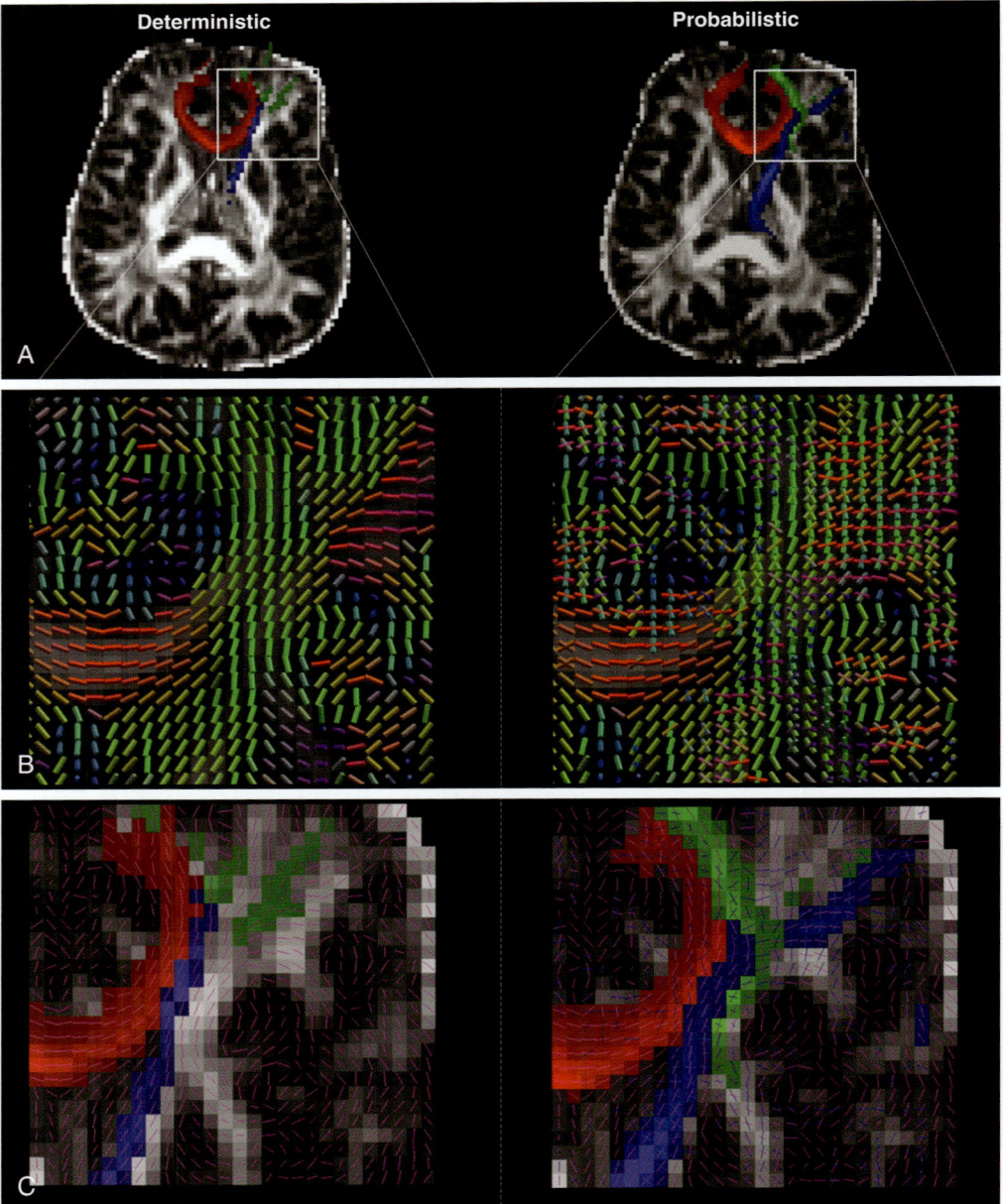

Figure 26-6 Deterministic and probabilistic tractography. **A,** The same seed and waypoints were used to track anterior thalamic radiation (blue), genu of corpus callosum (red), and inferior frontooccipital fasciculus using deterministic (left) and probabilistic (right) algorithms on the same dataset acquired on a single subject. **B,** In deterministic tractography, the direction of anisotropy is considered to be along the axis of a single, principal eigenvector, which is represented voxelwise in the image on the left. (Color convention is as described in Fig. 26-5.) In contrast, probabilistic tractography models anisotropy as a probability distribution and allows for a two-fiber solution, which is represented on the right, with the major axis being larger in scale compared with the minor axis. **C,** The difference in output is clearly visualized in the region of the crossing fibers where, on the left, deterministic tractography (principal eigenvector overlaid as pink lines) fails to yield as many tracks as the output from the probabilistic algorithm on the right (again, principal and secondary eigenvectors are overlaid in pink and blue, respectively).

proceeds from an initially determined point (seed region) and propagates pixel by pixel in the direction of the principal eigenvector until a predetermined lower FA threshold or maximal turning angle is reached, at which point the fiber path is terminated (see Fig. 26-6). The result is a *streamline*, a visual representation of anisotropic diffusion, and importantly, not an actual visual representation of axons or fiber bundles. Moreover, the number of streamlines originating from a particular seed region is directly proportional to the number of seed points within a given voxel, and accordingly, not directly related to the underlying anatomic connectivity. However, assuming the same number of seed points per given voxel are used across populations of interest (which, in most software packages, is not a number that can be manipulated by the operator), the number of streamlines can be considered a proxy for the underlying tissue microstructure, and accordingly, may be used as a metric in group-level comparisons.

One of the key limitations in tractography is that the mathematical model used to reconstruct DTI data assumes that a single fiber population exists in each voxel. However, at the resolution of a typical DTI acquisition (≥2 mm in each dimension), many voxels contain populations of fibers that are oriented in some manner other than parallel (from one third to 90%),[7,8] including fibers that are crossing, fanning, branching, or bottlenecking. This crossing fiber problem is a significant concern if one is trying to carry out tractography on DTI data. First, the main effect of crossing or other nonparallel fiber orientations on the principal eigenvectors is to decrease the principal eigenvalue. This effect, in turn, results in a decrease in FA, which can cause tractography algorithms to prematurely stop if the FA value has fallen below the predetermined threshold. Second, because the algorithm follows only the principal eigenvector, it may generate spurious streamlines (e.g., a streamline that propagates into a crossing region perpendicular to the principal eigenvector could be made to bend and then continue in the new direction).

One method to address limitations associated with using deterministic tractography and DTI parameters is to use the information derived from the diffusion tensor fit to generate a 3D probability distribution regarding the diffusion of water molecules instead of constraining the molecules to only move along the direction of the principal eigenvector. In this way, probabilistic tractography algorithms allow water molecules to follow more than one orientation when passing through a voxel in a crossing region. Current probabilistic algorithms allow for the modeling of uncertainty of two (or more) fiber directions at each voxel. Tracking is done by launching a high number of streamlines from a seed region, and at each voxel—instead of deterministically following the principal eigenvector—drawing from the previously determined 3D probability distribution to propagate the tracts. Coherent fiber orientation is preserved by following the sampled direction that is most closely parallel to the previous location's direction, as opposed to only following an arbitrary angle threshold. After a sufficient number of samples, the output is a probabilistic mapping of the uncertainty of fiber tracts at each voxel, with the dominant streamline surfacing as most probable (see Fig. 26-6). Notably, this method does not resolve the crossing-fiber problem with 100% certainty, but the resulting probabilistic map yields a much more robust estimate of the dominant fiber path when compared with

deterministic approaches.[9] Moreover, it also shows improvements in the rendering of the lateral corticospinal and corticobulbar tracts and the medial portion of the superior longitudinal fasciculus, which typically are not visualized by deterministic tractography. Figure 26-6 shows the comparison between deterministic and probabilistic algorithms in modeling fibers passing through a densely packed, high-fiber–crossing region of the brain. The probabilistic output shows significant improvement in delineating crossing fiber tracts, such as the inferior frontooccipital fasciculus and anterior thalamic radiation. Similar performance is noted in a single direction tract, as in the genu of the corpus callosum. Despite improved performance in modeling regions with crossing fiber tracts, probabilistic tractography still cannot completely overcome the limitation that the diffusion tensor model is not an adequate model for the underlying physiology in crossing fiber regions. This limitation requires more advanced approaches, as described in the next section.

ADVANCED DIFFUSION IMAGING TECHNIQUES

Advanced diffusion imaging techniques have been proposed to address the two major limitations of the DTI model: multiple/crossing fiber bundles and signal attenuation that deviates from an exponential decay with increasing b-value. Currently these approaches have found limited clinical use because of their greater acquisition time and the greater computational resources needed for data analysis. However, as technology continues to improve, such techniques likely will become available for clinicians on clinical MRI scanners.

To address the problem of crossing fibers, HARDI methods (sometimes called "Q-ball")[10,11] sample a much larger number of diffusion directions (e.g., 64 to 256) and then typical DTI acquisitions (e.g., ~30, although DTI analysis is possible with as few as 6). Thus more complicated models than a simple tensor may be used to model the physiology (for further detail, the interested reader is referred to references 11 to 14 for an introduction).[12-15] It is possible, with these techniques, to model two, three, or even more crossing fiber bundles. In conjunction with probabilistic tractography, this provides a very powerful technique to model brain structural connectivity, and success has been seen even in regions with a very high number of crossing fibers. Typically, higher b-values are used in HARDI acquisitions (~3000 s/mm^2) as opposed to those used in DTI (~1000 s/mm^2). The reason is that diffusion is more restricted in directions perpendicular to the axon for intraaxonal water molecules, as opposed to interstitial water molecules, because the distance to the axonal membrane is smaller. Therefore the use of a higher b-value will suppress the signal from interstitial water, leading to a "cleaner" profile of fiber directionality.

Because most voxels consist of a mix of interstitial and intraaxonal water, the signal attenuation will deviate from an exponential decay with respect to b-value at higher b-values as the relative contribution from each type of water molecule changes. One approach to quantifying this deviation is DKI, which involves acquisition of data at several b-values; the "kurtosis" quantities describe deviations from exponential decay. (For details about DKI acquisition and analysis, see reference 16.) Compared with DTI, DKI has been shown to be more sensitive to subtle tissue microstructural changes[17] and also has been found to yield additional information regarding pathologic changes in neural tissue, such as glioma grade discrimination.[18] In typical DKI acquisitions, however, the angular resolution is not as great as HARDI because acquiring data at additional b-values is performed in lieu of additional diffusion gradient directions.

Finally, the "ultimate" in DWI acquisition is when acquisitions are obtained both at multiple gradient directions and multiple b-values,[19] which will make possible a completely accurate specification of the water diffusion profiles, enabling the simultaneous modeling of crossing fiber bundles as well as nonexponential decay. This technique is called DSI or Q-space imaging. The acquisition demands are intense; a typical DSI protocol involves 512 separate DWI acquisitions, making the total acquisition time longer than 1 hour for typical DWI acquisition protocols.

Key Points

The diffusion of water is hindered by a variety of barriers, including axon sheaths and glial cell and astrocyte membranes.

The amount of attenuation in the DW images is dependent on the diffusion of water molecules only in the direction of the applied diffusion-encoding gradients.

In addition to fluid homeostasis and intracellular water, DWI and ADC also are sensitive to the relative properties of water in the extracellular space.

Because of the higher water content in the neonatal brain and because of the fact that this increase in extracellular water is associated with increased diffusivity and increased signal attenuation in the setting of diffusion encoding gradients, neonates often undergo imaging at a lower b-value (e.g., b = 700 s/mm²).

Tractography methods compute trajectories or pathways represented by the data, which, it is hoped, parallel the predominant trajectories of the underlying axonal fiber bundles.

Advanced diffusion imaging techniques address the two major limitations of conventional tractography: (1) multiple/crossing fiber bundles and signal attenuation that deviates from an exponential decay with increasing b-value.

Suggested Readings

Jones DK, Knösche TR, Turner R. White matter integrity, fiber count and other fallacies: the do's and don'ts of diffusion MRI. *Neuroimage.* 2012;pii:S1053-S8119 (12)01025-7, doi: 10.1016/j.neuroimage.2012.06.081 [E-pub ahead of print].

Roberts TPL, Schwartz ES. Principles and implementation of diffusion-weighted and diffusion tensor imaging. *Pediatr Radiol.* 2007;37:739-748.

References

Full references for this chapter can be found on www.expertconsult.com.

Chapter 27

Functional Magnetic Resonance Imaging

JAMES LEACH

Physiologic Basis of Functional Magnetic Resonance Imaging

Functional magnetic resonance imaging (fMRI) is based on the blood oxygen level–dependent (BOLD) contrast effect and neuronal activity–cerebrovascular flow coupling. Underlying the BOLD effect is the ability of MRI to differentiate magnetic properties of hemoglobin oxygenation states. Oxygenated blood (oxyhemoglobin) is diamagnetic, producing little susceptibility-related dephasing on MR signal. Deoxyhemoglobin is paramagnetic and elicits a more prominent effect on local field homogeneity and phase coherence, resulting in signal loss. Changes in the relative concentrations of oxyhemoglobin and deoxyhemoglobin in the vascular bed therefore result in changes in regional MR signal. The increase in cerebral blood flow that accompanies neuronal activity results in a relative increase in oxyhemoglobin concentration and a resultant localized increase in MR signal.[1] Although seemingly straightforward, the actual physiology underlying the BOLD response is complex and is the subject of ongoing research.[2] Many anatomic and physiologic changes occur during brain development that have the potential to alter the BOLD response in children compared with adults.[3,4-6] Despite these physiologic differences, the basic BOLD response in children is generally similar to that in adults,[3,7] albeit with some task-related differences.[8] Neonates and infants may exhibit significantly different BOLD responses than do older children and adults, complicating interpretation in this age group.[9-11]

Technical Considerations for fMRI Performance in Children

The requirements for fMRI performance include an MRI scanner with gradient hardware capable of performing fMRI useable sequences, stimulation/presentation hardware and software linked to the scanner to allow for synchronization of stimuli and MR imaging, hardware and software for documenting patient responses, and postprocessing software for producing activation maps. The small BOLD effect changes in MR signal typically are detected by echo planar imaging (EPI) T2*-sensitive gradient recalled echo techniques.

Because of increased signal to noise and sensitivity for BOLD contrast effects, 3T scanners are preferred for fMRI studies.[12,13]

Performance of useful clinical fMRI examinations in children requires specialized preparation and resources. Before the scheduled examination, the patient is assessed for underlying neurologic deficits, developmental level, and ability to complete the fMRI paradigms. Explanation of the MR procedure and fMRI paradigms to the patient and parents in a calm, child-centered environment is critical. Practicing the fMRI paradigms is important to maximize performance and to adapt the tasks for the patient's clinical and developmental level. Video presentations and mock scanners are highly useful in preparing children for the fMRI environment.[14,15] Patient comfort should be maximized.

Patient motion can influence fMRI performance in children.[14,16] Despite some ability to retrospectively correct for head motion, gross head movement typically results in unusable fMRI data. Head coil bite bars, inflatable head cushions, and forehead and chin straps may be used but can be difficult to implement. Head motion is more pronounced in younger children and in boys.[16] Older children and girls have a higher rate of successfully completed examinations.[14] With care and adequate preparation, most children presenting for clinical fMRI studies can complete fMRI examinations with multiple administered paradigms. The routine application of real-time fMRI processing can reduce the number of inadequate studies.[17]

Repeated samplings of the brain (one brain volume scan during each repetition time period) while the subject alternates between active cognitive and control tasks typically is performed (the fMRI "paradigm"). Typical fMRI paradigms require 3 to 7 minutes of imaging time for acquisition of 100 or more image volumes during three to five cycles of alternating behavior. Although many approaches are possible, clinical fMRI is most commonly performed in a "blocked-periodic" design in which blocks of task and control (baseline) conditions are administered sequentially.[18] The fMRI paradigm that is used ideally will result in activation of brain regions involved with the sensory, motor, or cognitive task presented, without activation in other regions. The proper choice of control and task conditions is important to allow this distinction and must be carefully matched to elicit detectable BOLD signal and isolate the function of interest.[19,20] For successful performance of fMRI examinations in children, utilization of age and developmentally appropriate paradigms is mandatory.[14,21]

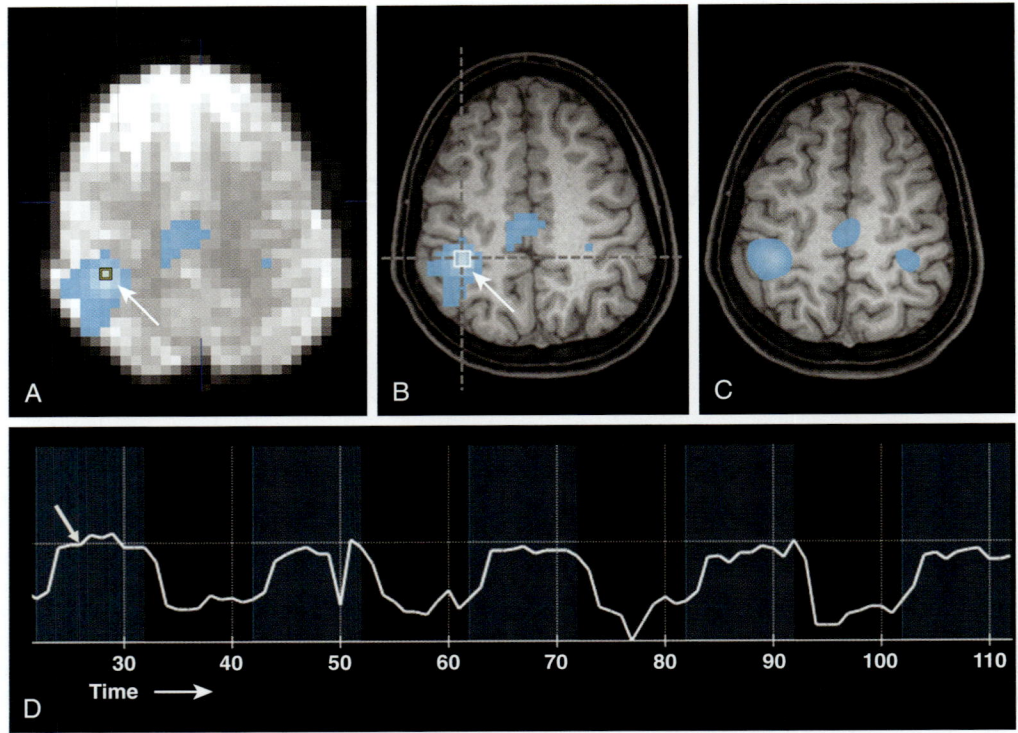

Figure 27-1 Example of bilateral finger tapping functional magnetic resonance imaging (fMRI) and the effect of smoothing on the appearance of fMRI statistical maps. **A,** A source echo planar image with an overlayed nonsmoothed statistical activation map. A single voxel region of interest (*arrow*) is located in the region of maximal statistical significance. **B,** A nonsmoothed fMRI statistical activation map overlayed onto a 1 mm isotropic T1-weighted image shows activation overlying the right central sulcus in the hand motor region (*arrow*). Overlay onto anatomic MRI images allows the spatial relationships of the fMRI activation areas to be appreciated and related to anatomy and pathology. **C,** An fMRI statistical activation map overlayed on a 1 mm isotropic T1-weighted image with smoothing applied to fMRI data. **D,** Actual signal intensity within a voxel of interest (*arrow* in **A**) during the fMRI paradigm. Blue time periods are during finger tapping. Black periods are times of rest. Note the delay in the signal increase (hemodynamic response, *arrow*) after task initiation.

Imaging processing is required for fMRI and should involve the interpreting radiologist. After acquisition of images during the fMRI paradigm, the images typically are processed to diminish EPI artifacts, correct for susceptibility-related distortions, limit effects from patient movement during the paradigm, align and transform the T2★ EPI images to a higher resolution anatomic dataset, and statistically analyze the images for BOLD signal changes between the task conditions on a voxel by voxel basis (the statistical map) (Fig. 27-1).[22] Increasingly, streamlined, clinically oriented options are being offered on most clinical MR systems or by a growing number of third-party vendors. The most common statistical tests used for clinical fMRI are the general linear model[21] and the cross-correlation method.[18] Determination of the optimum statistical threshold for use in individual clinical patients is a complex issue.[22,23] Evaluating fMRI studies at multiple different thresholds is important to maximize clinical effectiveness.

Clinical Applications of fMRI in Children

Although many indications for pediatric fMRI are undergoing active research evaluation, the most common clinical use of fMRI in children is for presurgical assessment of language and memory function for patients with intractable epilepsy and evaluation of potentially eloquent cortex in patients with brain lesions (e.g., tumors and cavernous malformations).

LIMITATIONS

Some fundamental concepts must be kept in mind when performing and interpreting fMRI studies in clinical patients.[24] For example, fMRI activation regions are not functionally specific, and lack of activation in a brain region does not indicate lack of critical brain function. The fMRI procedure is an indirect evaluation of neuronal function and relies on statistical mapping techniques that are not clinically standardized. The BOLD effect can be directly altered by pathologic states with changes in cerebrovascular autoregulation and neurovascular coupling,[25] including vascular steno-occlusion, tumors with high vascularity, and arteriovenous malformations.[25-27] Artifacts from regions of susceptibility effect (e.g., skull base, sinuses, hemorrhage, and prior surgery) may limit fMRI sensitivity. Sedation also can alter the BOLD response significantly.[28]

SENSORIMOTOR SYSTEM EVALUATION

The most common and reproducible application of fMRI in clinical patients is assessment of the sensorimotor system (Fig.

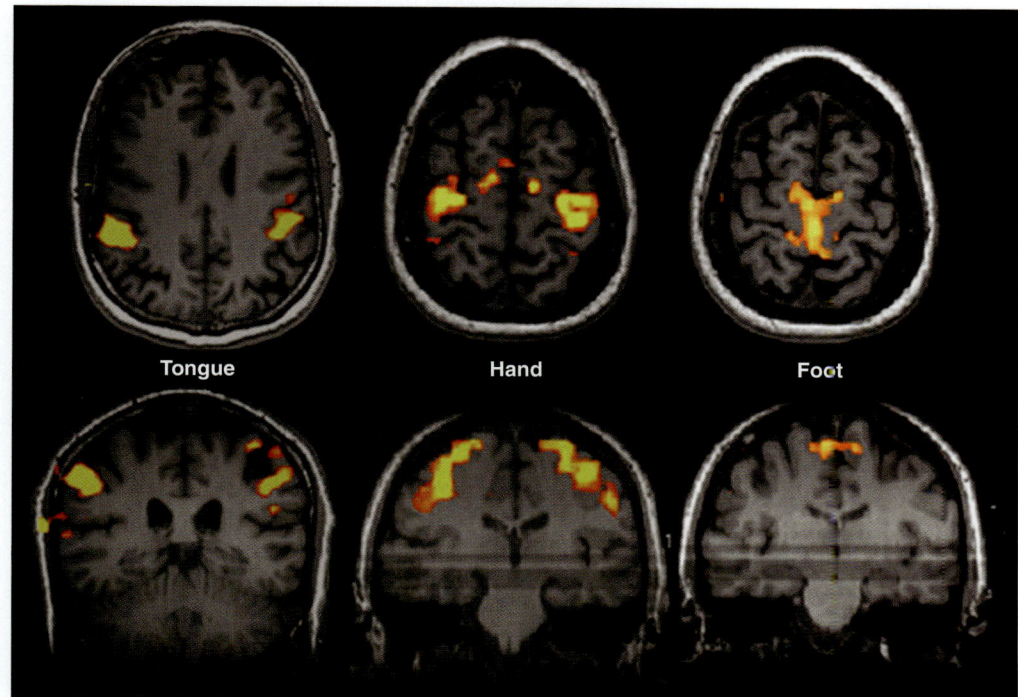

Figure 27-2   Examples of different motor paradigms useful for clinical functional magnetic resonance imaging. Tongue: Sequential tongue movement while the mouth is closed. Hand: Sequential bilateral finger tapping. Foot: Sequential bilateral foot flexion and extension. Typically performed clinical paradigms include sequential finger thumb opposition, hand grasping, wrist flexion and extension, foot flexion and extension, lip puckering, and tongue movement for motor strip assessment and tactile stimulation with brushes or air puffs for sensory component evaluation.

27-2).[24,29] The fMRI activation areas are somatotopically arranged along the central sulcus. Secondary regions including the supplementary motor area and premotor cortex often commonly are identified. Validation with direct electrocortical simulation (ECoS), the surgical gold standard, generally has been excellent,[30-33] with recent studies demonstrating nearly 100% concordance.[29] Sensorimotor fMRI evaluation is most useful when the normal anatomic relationships relating to the central sulcus are distorted by adjacent mass lesions;

fMRI can help guide operative approaches in these cases (Fig. 27-3). High success rates of motor fMRI (93%) in children undergoing surgery for epilepsy have been documented.[34]

LANGUAGE EVALUATION

Multiple clinical and fMRI studies have established that a left hemispheric dominance exists for semantic and phonological language functions in most persons. Most fMRI studies of

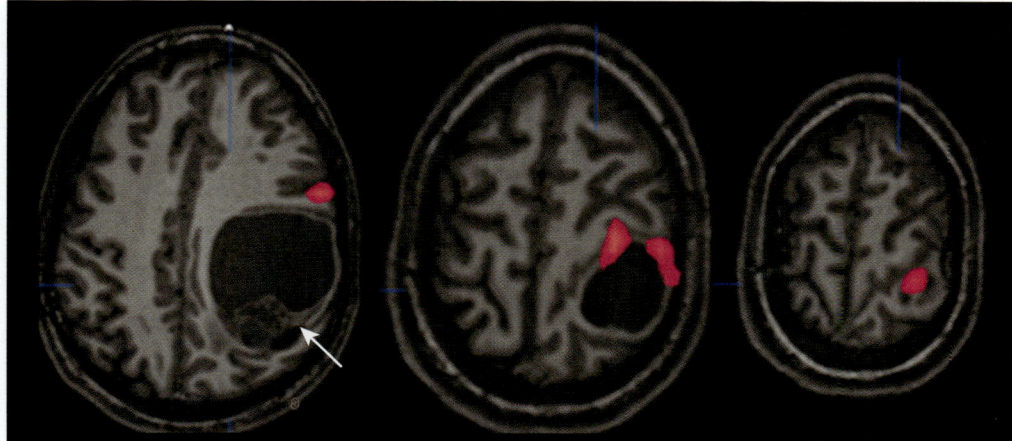

Figure 27-3   A 15-year-old boy with progressive right-sided motor weakness. Anatomic magnetic resonance imaging revealed a large cystic and solid mass within the left parietal lobe (*arrow*) that was markedly distorting normal anatomy; functional magnetic resonance imaging (fMRI) was requested to outline the location of the motor strip more definitively. An fMRI image obtained during right-sided sequential finger tapping demonstrates activation along the superior and anterior aspects of the mass. A posterior surgical approach was performed with gross total resection and no new deficit. Pathology revealed that the mass was an anaplastic ependymoma.

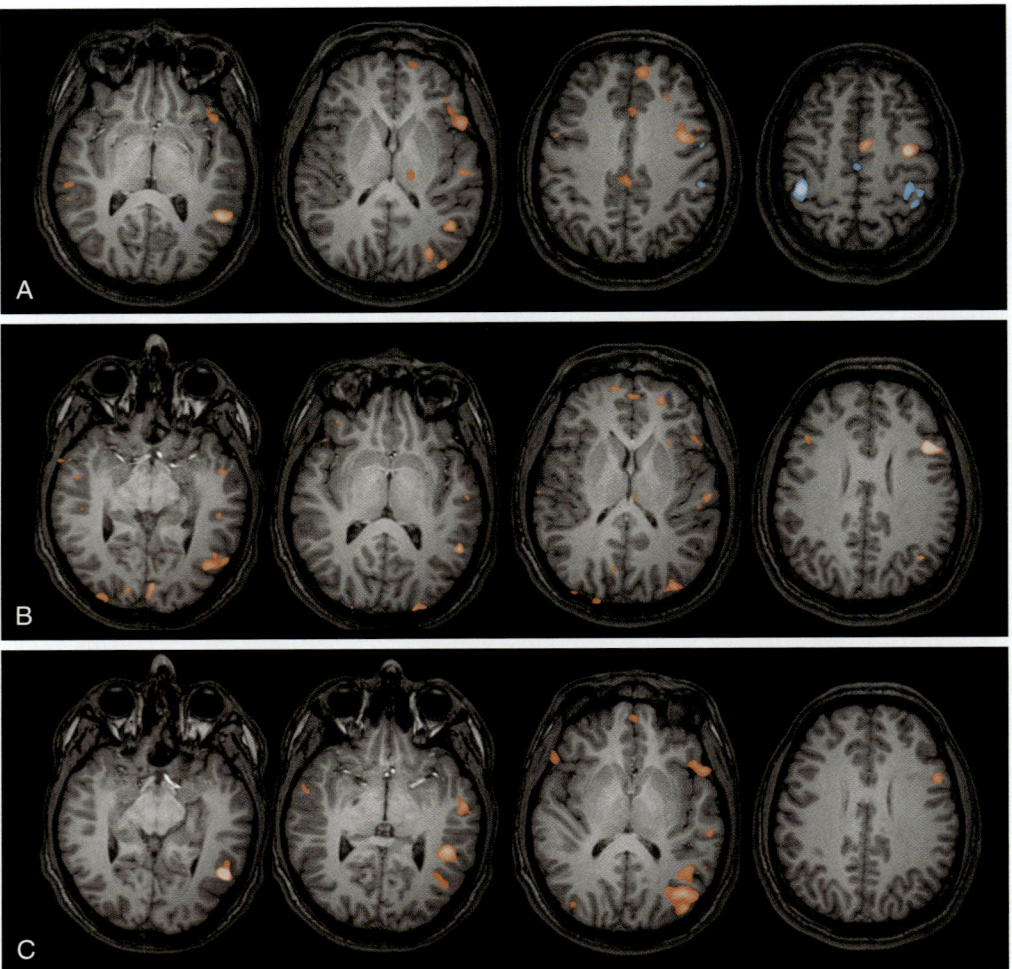

Figure 27-4 Examples of language functional magnetic resonance imaging (fMRI) paradigms in a 12-year-old right-handed girl with intractable epilepsy. **A,** Verb generation (control task: finger tapping). A statistical map of fMRI activation during verb generation (*orange areas*) demonstrates left lateralization, particularly in the left inferior frontal lobe and left temporal lobe, which is typical for this paradigm. Activation during finger tapping is noted along both central sulci in the hand motor regions, as well as the putative supplementary motor area in the midline. **B,** Semantic decision (control task: tone discrimination). A similar left lateralizing pattern is noted with robust inferior frontal and temporal parietal activation, which is typical for this paradigm. The semantic decision task provides an additional assessment of frontal and temporal language areas and has the added capability of allowing direct assessment of patient performance. **C,** Story processing (control task: backwards speech). Clear left lateralizing activation is noted in the temporal lobe. Left lateralizing inferior frontal activation also is noted. These paradigms together indicate typical left lateralization of language in this patient.

language lateralization in children have shown similar patterns of activation compared with adults, supporting the theory that language networks are established by early childhood. However, multiple cross-sectional and longitudinal fMRI studies have demonstrated changes in BOLD localization[20,35-39] with multiple language paradigms during development. In general, greater and more widespread activation is present in children compared with adults, which likely is related to differential brain maturation. Hemispheric language dominance is related to handedness, with approximately 95% of right-handed subjects being left hemispheric dominant for language, whereas approximately 20% of non–right-handed subjects (those who are ambidextrous or left handed) exhibit atypical (nonlateralizing or right-sided) hemispheric language dominance.[40] These findings should be kept in mind when interpreting language fMRI examinations in children.

Paradigms for Language Assessment

Multiple fMRI paradigms have been created to assess different aspects of language function (Fig. 27-4 and e-Fig. 27-5). It is important to utilize multiple language tasks in clinical patients to more fully define language processing.[20,41-43] The use of multiple tasks reduces the likelihood of nondiagnostic findings, improves inter-rater reliability, and helps in the confirmation of language laterality.[43] Three of the most studied paradigms in children are verb generation, semantic decision, and story processing (Fig. 27-2).

The verb generation task[35] (Fig. 27-4, *A*) involves the auditory presentation of a series of concrete nouns. The patient covertly (silently) generates as many verbs associated with the noun as possible. Control tasks include rest or bilateral sequential finger tapping.[35,36,44] The semantic decision task has been modified for children and involves the auditory presentation of single words (animal names)[41,45] (Fig. 27-4, B). The child makes a button press if the animal fits a target semantic property (e.g., "Does the animal walk on four legs?"). In the control condition, the patient listens to a series of tones for a specific tonal sequence. The story processing task[41,46,47] typically involves the auditory presentation of simple stories, each composed of sentences with specifically formulated complex syntactic constructions (Fig. 27-4, C). The control tasks are listening to various tonal sequences[20] or to identical periods of temporally reversed speech.[47] Other tasks such as linguistic prosody, read response naming, and auditory and reading sentence comprehension also have been used successfully with children.[41,48,49]

CLINICAL EXAMINATION INTERPRETATION

Interpretation of language fMRI in children can be difficult. Descriptions of language laterality and hemispheric dominance in clinical and research contexts typically have been described on the basis of a region of interest (ROI) "laterality" or "asymmetry" index (LI).[20,24] LI calculations are dependent on the statistical technique and threshold used for calculating activated voxels, ROI, and fMRI task.[50,51] They are more robust when ROIs targeted to typical language areas are used.[52,53] Use of multiple thresholds and fMRI tasks in individual patients to more completely assess language laterality is recommended.[50] Interestingly, visual assessment of lateralization in individual patients actually may be as good as ROI-based LI calculations.[49,54] Typically, fMRI examinations are interpreted in clinical patients as left hemispheric dominant (typical activation pattern), right hemispheric dominant, and bilateral or nonlateralizing language representation. Bilateral activation patterns can be problematic in evaluation of individual clinical patients because this fMRI pattern often cannot be conclusively interpreted.[50] Epilepsy,[55] perinatal stroke,[56] and a prenatally or perinatally acquired lesion[57] can effect language development and lead to altered lateralization of language function (e-Fig. 27-6).

VALIDATION OF LANGUAGE fMRI

The traditional method for determining language dominance before surgery has been the Wada or intracarotid amobarbital procedure (IAP). Another method of language mapping is direct ECoS either during surgery with the patient awake or with use of subdural grid electrodes.[58] The IAP is expensive, invasive, and more difficult to perform in children.[58,59] It carries with it a small but definite risk of complications,[59-61] and its invasive nature limits repeated assessments.[62] Although it provides lateralization information, the IAP cannot spatially localize language functions in the brain, which is an advantage for fMRI.

Correlation studies between fMRI and IAP for language lateralization consistently have shown an 85% to 90% concordance rate,[19,60,61,63,64] with the use of multiple tasks increasing the degree of concordance.[52,53] Discrepancies are most common in patients who exhibit atypical language lateralization, particularly patients with bilateral, nonlateralized representation.[62,63,65] Discordance between fMRI and the IAP also is more common in patients with neocortical epilepsy (a more common scenario in pediatric patients than in the adult

epilepsy population) and left temporal lobe seizure origin.[54] The few studies that have specifically compared language-based fMRI with the IAP in children have demonstrated concordance in 80% to 100% of patients.[62,66] Although fMRI may not be able to replace the IAP in all circumstances, routine fMRI can diminish IAP utilization significantly.

The fMRI procedure also has been used in an attempt to guide resections near eloquent language regions. Because fMRI will demonstrate areas of the brain that are associated with, but not necessarily essential to, a particular task, fMRI will always exhibit a lack of specificity for language mapping in this scenario. Few direct comparisons between language fMRI and ECoS for regional language mapping have been performed, and the results have been variable. The sensitivity of fMRI in identifying critical language areas as established by ECoS varies between 22% to 100%, with specificities of between 61% and 100%.[67] A recent detailed study in adult patients with a brain tumor found an overall fMRI sensitivity of 80% and a specificity of 78% for critical language areas compared with the results of ECoS.[68] Despite the variable reported correlations, fMRI may be very useful to guide intraoperative ECoS procedures and for counseling parents and children regarding surgery in eloquent areas.[17,69]

OTHER INDICATIONS

The fMRI procedure has been used to investigate a wide variety of clinical conditions in children, including the evaluation of reading and dyslexia, attention deficit–hyperactivity disorder, autism, and hearing loss,[70-72] to name a few. Clinical applications in these conditions are evolving, and at present, should be regarded as research tools. Assessment of memory by fMRI is possible and has begun to be assessed in clinical patients. Clinical research studies have been performed that correlate fMRI activation patterns with the IAP[73,74] and postoperative memory after temporal lobe resection in adults,[74] with encouraging results; however, evaluation of the application in pediatric patients is incomplete. The fMRI procedure, often in combination with other functional modalities (e.g., diffusion tensor imaging and magnetoencephalography), may allow for guidance during surgical access and resection using modern neuronavigation systems (functional neuronavigation).[75] Use of fMRI in conjunction with ECoS and frameless stereotaxy has been found to help facilitate tumor resection in children with a wide variety of lesions near eloquent cortical regions (e-Figs. 27-7 and 27-8).[76]

Future Techniques

Newer techniques of fMRI acquisition and processing hold promise to expand the utility of fMRI in children. These techniques include advanced connectivity analyses of fMRI data and fMRI performed in the so-called *resting state*.[77] Resting state fMRI analyses have begun to be used in evaluating the functional networks in the developing brain[78] and may have particular clinical use in identifying functionally important cortex and networks in patients in which task-based fMRI examinations are not feasible (e.g., in neonates, infants, and sedated patients). Although currently it is a research tool, initial clinical applications have been described in adults and children.[79,80]

Key Points

Clinical fMRI use in children primarily is used to assess eloquent brain regions before surgery relating to lesions or epilepsy.

Clinical fMRI in children requires special preparation and resources, as well as developmentally appropriate fMRI paradigms.

Somatosensory and language assessments are the most commonly performed fMRI examinations in clinical patients.

Standardization of fMRI paradigms and interpretation, as well as better validation and outcome studies, are needed in pediatric patients.

Newer techniques such as resting state fMRI hold promise to expand clinical fMRI applications to children who currently are unable to perform task-directed fMRI examinations.

Full references for this chapter can be found on www.expertconsult.com.

Suggested Readings

Holland SK, Vannest J, Mecoli M, et al. Functional MRI of language lateralization during development in children. *Int J Audiol.* 2007;46: 533-551.

Kotsoni E, Byrd D, Casey BJ. Special considerations for functional magnetic resonance imaging of pediatric populations. *J Magn Reson Imaging.* 2006; 23:877-886.

Leach JL, Holland SK. Functional MRI in children: clinical and research applications. *Pediatr Radiol.* 2010;40:31-49.

O'Shaughnessy E, Berl M, Moore E, et al. Pediatric functional MRI: issues and applications. *J Child Neurol.* 2008;23(7):791-801.

Wilke M, Holland SK, Myseros JS, et al. Functional magnetic resonance imaging in pediatrics. *Neuropediatrics.* 2005;34(5):225-233.

Chapter 28

Perfusion Imaging and Magnetoencephalography

ARASTOO VOSSOUGH

Perfusion Imaging

In the cerebrovascular literature, perfusion imaging refers to an all-encompassing term of various methods to measure hemodynamically derived functional parameters in the brain.[1,2] In radiology, the three most common parameters that are assessed and utilized clinically are cerebral blood volume (CBV), cerebral blood flow (CBF), and mean transit time (MTT). CBV refers to the amount (volume) of blood within a given mass of brain tissue at a given time and is measured in mL/100 g. CBF refers to the flow of blood through an area of the brain and is usually measured in mL/100 g of brain tissue per minute. MTT refers to the time it takes for blood to flow between the arterial inflow and venous outflow in the brain, that is, the time that blood spends in the cerebral capillary circulation, and is often measured in seconds. The general relationship between these three parameters is depicted by the central volume theorem:

$$CBV = CBF \times MTT$$

Evaluation of these various perfusion parameters can give us an understanding of the physiological state of the brain and cerebral vasculature in various disorders and help in patient management. Cerebral perfusion can be measured by a variety of methods including magnetic resonance imaging (MRI), computed tomography (CT), and nuclear medicine techniques. These techniques differ in terms of image acquisition duration, spatial resolution, the types of endogenous or exogenous tracers used, and their ability or accuracy in measuring different perfusion parameters.[1] The clinical applications of perfusion imaging include investigation of cerebrovascular disease, brain tumors, and the effect of other diseases on cerebral perfusion.

PERFUSION MRI

Perfusion MRI can be performed via the injection of dynamic gadolinium-based contrast material or without contrast material injection by tagging intravascular protons using MR labeling schemes (i.e., arterial spin labeling [ASL]).

Dynamic Susceptibility Contrast Perfusion MRI

Dynamic susceptibility contrast (DSC) perfusion MRI is based on susceptibility effects using T2-weighted or, more commonly, T2*-weighted images and is the most commonly studied and clinically used perfusion technique in assessment of brain masses and stroke. This method is based on the principle that the signal change that occurs during passage of a high-concentration bolus of gadolinium contrast material in the vessels causes a difference in susceptibility between the vessels that contain contrast material and brain tissue and that this signal change can be converted to a relaxation rate change proportional to the fraction of blood volume within each voxel.[3,4] Data generally are acquired during first-pass perfusion over approximately 1 minute, during which time a high-concentration bolus of gadolinium chelate is rapidly injected intravenously. Time-signal intensity curves drawn during this acquisition will show a rapid decline in signal as the contrast enters the brain, with return of the signal to near baseline after the first pass (Fig. 28–1). These measurements are used to construct a relative CBV map, and the time signal intensity curve can be used to derive other perfusion parameters by various mathematical methods.[1,5,6]

To provide adequate temporal resolution during dynamic contrast administration, most centers currently use gradient echo planar imaging sequences to perform clinical DSC perfusion MRI.[7-9] This technique is very sensitive to structures that cause magnetic field inhomogeneity such as blood, calcium, bone, metals, or air interfaces such as the skull base. The use of DSC imaging entails multiple technical considerations.[10,11] Accuracy of CBV maps can vary substantially depending on the acquisition and postprocessing methods used.[6] It is important to take into consideration the type of acquisition used in applying research results for characterization of lesions, because the results and thresholds may vary.[12] Derivation of the perfusion parameters also depends on the mathematical models used by the various processing software, and caution must be exercised in comparing results from different calculation methods.[13,14] Sometimes a small prebolus dose of contrast material is given before the actual DSC acquisition to correct for leakage and more accurate calculation of the perfusion parameters.[6,10]

DSC perfusion applications are used predominantly to assess cerebrovascular disease and in brain tumor management (e-Fig. 28–2). DSC perfusion can assess the ischemic penumbra in persons who have had an acute stroke and aid in the imaging triage and management of these patients.[15,16] DSC perfusion has been used in differentiation of brain tumors from other masslike lesions in the brain, preoperative grading of brain tumors, differentiation of primary from metastatic tumors, assessment of treatment response, and differentiation of radiation necrosis from a recurrent tumor.[1,17-23]

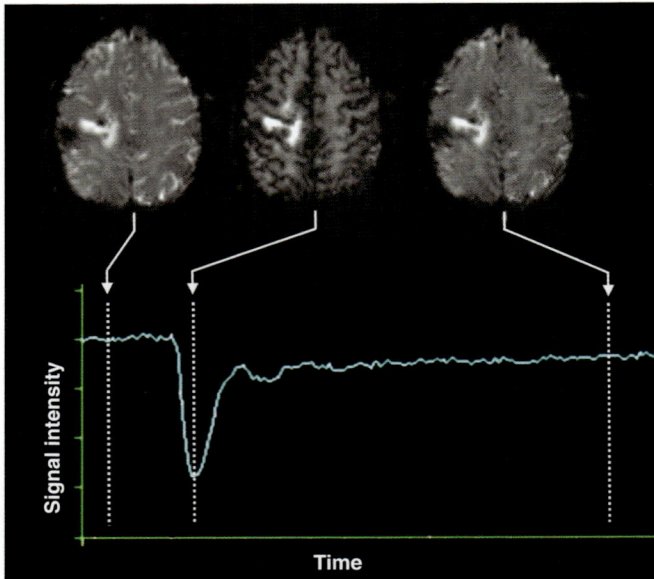

Figure 28-1 Acquisition of dynamic susceptibility contrast perfusion magnetic resonance imaging. Typically, a rapid echo planar acquisition is obtained through the head continuously over the course of approximately 1 or 1.5 minutes. A rapid injection of gadolinium-based contrast material is injected, which results in a transient dip in the signal intensity during the course of the first pass of contrast through the brain. After this first pass, the signal returns toward normal, although often not completely. A time-signal intensity curve is plotted before, during, and after the first pass bolus for each voxel, including brain tissue and vascular structures, which in turn is used to derive various perfusion parameters.

Arterial Spin Labeling Perfusion MRI

ASL perfusion imaging does not require exogenous contrast injection. It uses magnetically labeled arterial blood water as an endogenous flow tracer.[24] A general scheme of the ASL technique is illustrated in Figure 28-3. Two sets of images

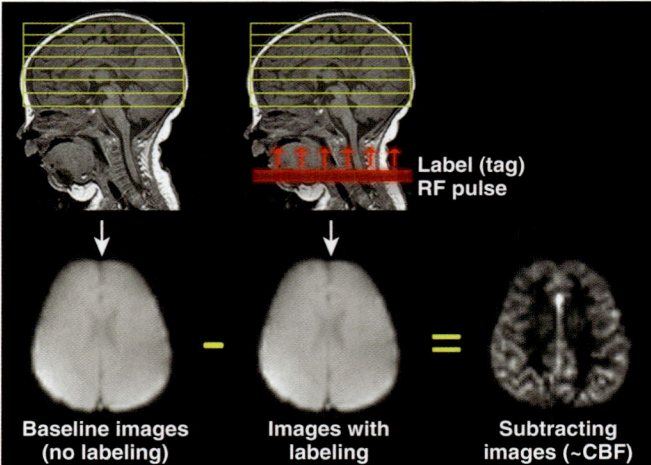

Figure 28-3 A schematic demonstration of the general principle of arterial spin labeling perfusion magnetic resonance imaging. Images of the head are obtained once without and once with labeling of blood water protons using a radiofrequency (RF) pulse. The labeled (or tagged) blood flows into the brain, and if the images without and with label are subtracted from each other, the difference image results from these labeled blood protons and is proportional to cerebral blood flow (CBF).

are obtained, one as a baseline image of the brain and the other after labeling (or tagging) blood arterial water protons in the neck using an inversion or saturation radiofrequency pulse. This second set is obtained after a short delay time that allows the labeled blood to flow into the imaging slices. If the baseline and postlabel images are subtracted from each other, the resulting subtracted image is proportional to blood flow that has entered the brain. Quantitative measures of CBF can then be derived from the subtracted images. Numerous schemes exist for ASL tagging and imaging; however, the details are beyond the scope of this chapter.[25] Typically, echoplanar or spiral nonechoplanar techniques are used for image acquisition. ASL imaging takes significantly longer than DSC perfusion MRI because the signal change resulting from the arterial spin label is very small (in the order of 0.5% to 3%), and therefore numerous signal averages need to be acquired to gain acceptable signal to noise. Imaging at 3 Tesla significantly increases the signal and quality of ASL images. Given the requirement for image subtraction and longer acquisition times, ASL perfusion is very sensitive to motion artifacts.

ASL has a number of potential advantages compared with exogenous contrast–based perfusion methods. ASL does not require rapid injection of a large bolus of contrast, which sometimes can be a problem in young children because of a lack of intravenous access and poor renal function. ASL has the potential to provide quantitative perfusion data and also can be repeated in the same imaging session if the child moves. The disadvantages of ASL perfusion include longer imaging times, sensitivity to patient motion, lack of an easy way to derive CBV and MTT parameters, and specific artifacts as a result of arterial transit delays between the labeling and imaging planes, for example, when blood passes through collateral circulation channels.

Applications of ASL perfusion include cerebrovascular disease, detection of changes during complicated migraine (Fig. 28-4), hypoxic-ischemic injury, depiction of hypoperfusion in mesial temporal sclerosis, and emerging applications in brain tumors.[26-32] Further work is needed to establish the role of ASL imaging in pediatrics.

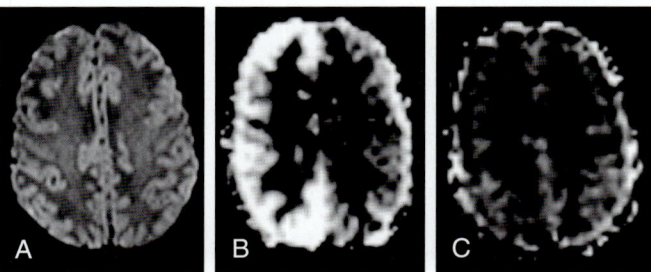

Figure 28-4 Arterial spin labeling (ASL) in a child with hemiplegic migraine. The patient presented with acute onset left-sided weakness in the face and both the upper and lower extremities, along with headache. Magnetic resonance imaging (MRI) was emergently performed to exclude an arterial ischemic stroke. No abnormality was found on diffusion-weighted imaging (**A**), but ASL perfusion MRI demonstrated increased cerebral blood flow in the right cerebral hemisphere (**B**). Two days later, the patient's symptoms have completely resolved and a repeat MRI demonstrated normal appearance of the brain on ASL perfusion imaging (**C**).

COMPUTED TOMOGRAPHIC PERFUSION IMAGING

Dynamic CT perfusion imaging bears some similarity to DSC perfusion MRI in that perfusion parameters are derived from a time–concentration curve obtained during continuous scanning of the first pass of a rapid injection of iodinated contrast material through the brain.[1,33,34] Quantitative maps of CBV, CBF, and MTT can be obtained. Dynamic CT perfusion imaging has the advantage of widespread availability and speed, which can be important in the setting of acute stroke or in patients with contraindications to MRI. CT perfusion imaging often is performed in conjunction with CT angiography in the evaluation of cerebrovascular disease. Although continuous scanning of the head for CT perfusion can lead to exposure to a high radiation dose, CT perfusion can be performed satisfactorily with 80 kVp and a low mA technique, which considerably decreases the radiation dose.[1,35] CT perfusion imaging has been studied extensively in the evaluation of patients with cerebrovascular disease, especially in the setting of acute ischemic stroke.[33,36] It can demonstrate the ischemic penumbra and tissues at risk and can be helpful in patient management (Fig. 28-5).[1,33]

OTHER PERFUSION IMAGING METHODS

Xenon CT perfusion uses stable nonradioactive Xenon gas inhaled over the course of a few minutes to act as a contrast agent for perfusion after crossing the blood-brain barrier. Xenon CT perfusion can produce accurate quantitative CBF measurements and even can be used to assess cerebrovascular reserve after a vasodilatory challenge in patients with occlusive or stenotic cerebrovascular disease.[1,37,38] Various nuclear medicine techniques also have been used to quantitatively assess cerebral perfusion. These techniques include positron emission tomography using $H_2^{15}O$, $^{15}O_2$, and $C^{15}O_2$ and single photon emission CT using ^{99m}Tc-HMPAO and ^{133}Xe. Xenon CT and nuclear medicine perfusion methods are not often performed in pediatric patients because of a lack of widespread availability and clinical expertise with these techniques and potential concerns about the radiation dose.

Magnetoencephalography

Magnetoencephalography (MEG) is a noninvasive technique that records magnetic fields produced by the electrical currents of neural activity in the brain. MEG signals arise from intracellular currents that flow from dendrites to the cell body.[39] These magnetic signals are extremely weak, on the order of 10 to 1000 femtoTesla,[40] requiring special sensors for detection. These magnetic fields induce electrical current in an array of special coils coupled to a superconducting

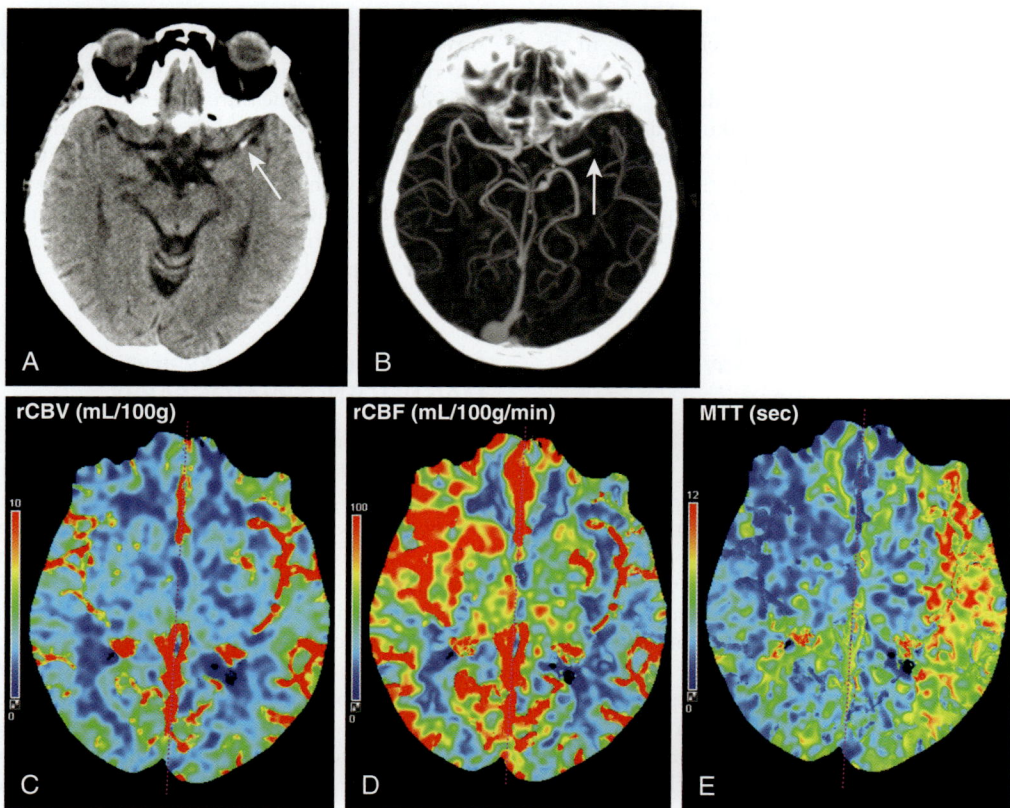

Figure 28-5 Computed tomography (CT) perfusion imaging in a patient with acute right-sided weakness and aphasia. Noncontrast CT examination (**A**) demonstrated a focus of high density (*arrow*) in the M1 segment of the left middle cerebral artery. No loss of gray white differentiation or edema was seen on CT at this time. CT angiography (**B**) showed an abrupt cutoff in the left middle cerebral artery (*arrow*). CT perfusion imaging done immediately after CT angiography showed no large change in relative cerebral blood volume (**C**), but the relative cerebral blood flow (**D**) was decreased and mean transit time (**E**) was elevated in the distribution of the left middle cerebral artery compared with the contralateral side.

quantum interference device.[40] Modern-day MEG machines typically have a few hundred sensor channels that surround the head (e-Fig. 28-6). Given the very weak magnetic fields generated by brain activity and the very high sensitivity of the superconducting quantum interference device sensors, MEG is very prone to interference from external magnetic sources, and thus siting in a highly shielded room is required to prevent electromagnetic contamination. MEG provides excellent temporal resolution (less than 1 ms), and compared with standard electroencephalography, it provides very good spatial resolution (down to 5 to 15 mm) in the detection of normal and abnormal brain waveforms. The most important clinical applications of MEG relate to evaluating epilepsy and presurgical functional mapping.

In a typical MEG examination, multiple sequential recordings are made via the various channels. The MEG waveform analysis results often are coregistered to a volumetric MRI of the head for source spatial localization of the abnormal waveforms or functional mappings. This combination of MEG with MRI is known as magnetic source imaging. For clinical purposes, when one uses the term MEG, it usually refers to magnetic source imaging with MRI coregistration. The registration of MEG and MRI typically is performed by using fiducial markers in predetermined regions, such as over the nasion and the right and left preauricular positions.[41] The same fiducial markers can be used for determining patient motion and motion correction, which is important for clinical interpretation. After acquisition of the MEG waveform data, various complex mathematical models and algorithms are used for source localization, along with the ability to provide information from a "virtual depth electrode" in the brain.[40,41]

Various artifacts almost always occur during an MEG examination. Muscle twitching, eye blinking, and cardiac electrical activity can cause changes in MEG waveforms. The presence of dental and orthodontic hardware, vagal nerve stimulators (even when turned off), and metallic piercings will cause artifacts on MEG as well.

MAGNETOENCEPHALOGRAPHY IN THE EVALUATION OF PATIENTS WITH EPILEPSY

The major goal in the presurgical evaluation of patients with epilepsy is identification of the epileptogenic or ictal onset zones.[42,43] It is hoped that surgical removal of this epileptogenic region will result in a seizure-free state (or at least a significant decrease in seizure frequency) with minimal postsurgical neurologic deficits. The excellent temporal and very good spatial resolution of MEG makes it a very useful tool in the evaluation of patients with epilepsy, especially those who are medically refractory. MEG evaluation typically is performed by passive interictal recording of spontaneous electromagnetic activity and discharges. Patients often are instructed to be sleep deprived overnight to increase interictal activity. In young children, typically 5 years or younger, or in patients with developmental delay or psychiatric issues, general anesthesia may be required to perform the MEG examination. The choice of anesthetic medication is important so as to avoid interference with the detection of epileptiform changes on MEG.[41]

MEG has the potential to be used in the following clinical scenarios in the evaluation of patients with epilepsy:

1. When no structural lesion is found on MRI in a patient with epilepsy, MEG results occasionally may be used to guide a targeted "second look" at the MRI for possible detection of subtle abnormalities that initially may have been difficult to identify
2. Confirmation of localization based on other methods, allowing surgery to proceed without long-duration invasive intracranial electroencephalographic (EEG) monitoring
3. More accurate spatial localization of the epileptogenic zone to decrease the extent of craniotomy and grid placement for invasive EEG monitoring
4. In patients with multiple structural lesions on MRI, determination of whether one of the lesions is primarily responsible for the patient's refractory seizures, indicating surgical feasibility
5. Determination of multiple epileptogenic zones, suggesting an unfavorable outcome or contraindication for surgery
6. Recurrence of epilepsy after surgery (Fig. 28-7)
7. Investigation of discrepancy between EEG and neuroimaging findings
8. Investigation of inconclusive EEG results
9. Delineation of eloquent cortex to aid presurgical decision making

Careful visual scrutiny of the source MEG waves is necessary to help determine the presence or absence of significant epileptiform activity or artifacts. Various automated software waveform analyses and statistical tests can be performed to determine the significance of the waveforms detected on MEG. One such measure is determining kurtosis, or "spikiness" of the waves, which can help in identifying areas of significant activity. The addition of MEG to the evaluation of patients with epilepsy has been shown to improve the quality of medical care and surgical outcomes after epilepsy and provides important nonredundant information in a significant proportion of patients.[42-45]

BRAIN FUNCTIONAL MAPPING USING MAGNETOENCEPHALOGRAPHY

The gold standard for functional mapping of eloquent cortex is intraoperative direct cortical stimulation and mapping. Noninvasive examinations such as functional MRI (fMRI) often are used for preoperative localization and mapping before resection of tumors, vascular malformations, and epileptogenic foci. The blood oxygenation level dependent response used in fMRI localization is a measurement of the hemodynamic response to neuronal activity rather than direct measurement of the neuronal activity (see Chapter 27). Many pathophysiologic processes are known to adversely affect and/or blunt the hemodynamic response measured with fMRI, such as arteriovenous malformations or some tumors. MEG can be used as another noninvasive method for functional identification of eloquent cortical regions.[46-48] Motor, somatosensory, and language areas typically are examined by MEG in the clinical setting. Auditory and visual centers also occasionally are investigated. Similar to fMRI, MEG recordings

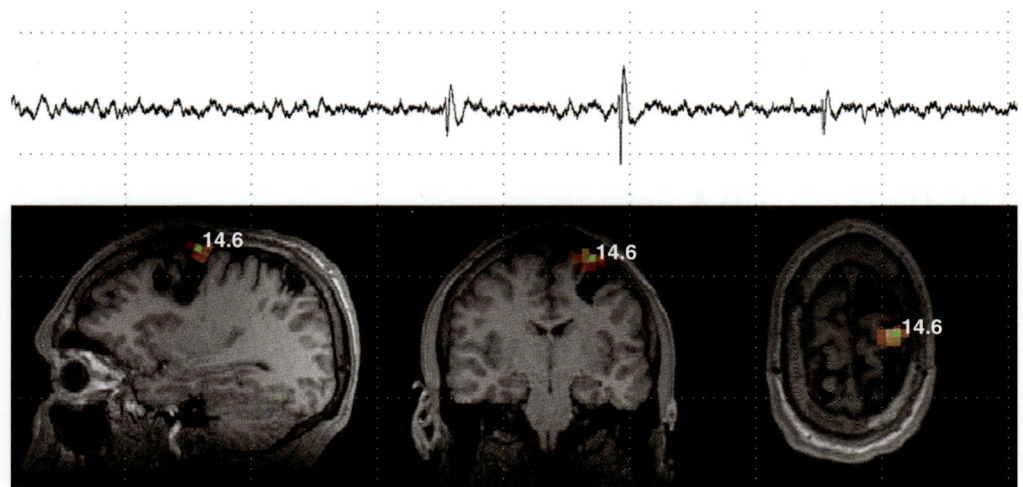

Figure 28-7 Magnetoencephalography (MEG) and magnetic source imaging in a patient with continued seizures even after epilepsy surgery. The patient had undergone multiple cortical resections after an extensive epilepsy workup and invasive cortical mapping a few years earlier. However, although some improvement in the frequency of seizures occurred, the patient continued to have medically refractory epilepsy. An interictal MEG shows multiple isolated spike and slow wave abnormalities during multiple recordings localized to a focus along the superomedial aspect of the site of surgical resection.

are used to evaluate responses to task performance and/or evoked stimulation.

Motor mapping can be performed with self-paced button pressing using left and right index fingers and recording the MEG response. Typically these motor actions result in event-related desynchronization (ERD) in the beta wave band, approximately 200 to 300 ms after the button press. Depending on the area of interest for motor mapping, occasionally other areas such as the great toes and elbows also could be used. Somatosensory testing can be performed with use of various stimuli while recording the MEG response as well. Alternatively, especially in patients who are sedated or anesthetized, somatosensory testing can be performed via painless electric stimulation of the median or tibial nerves. Typically, MEG activity at 20 ms after stimulus is used to map somatosensory function.

Language mapping is another area in which MEG can be useful, either in evaluation of language lateralization or localization. The language tasks used are similar to those used with fMRI; common language tasks in children may include picture naming, word recall, stem completion, and verb generation, among others. The tasks typically are displayed via a screen in front of the patient, with the operator giving audio instructions when they are needed. Similar to motor mapping, ERD associated with neuronal activity can be exploited for assessing language-related centers in the brain, approximately 400 to 500 ms before the patient's response.

After the functional mapping tasks and stimulations are performed, areas of target activity or statistically significant ERD are overlaid on volumetric MRI to visualize the functional areas mapped by MEG (e-Fig. 28-8). In small children and in patients who are anesthetized, it generally is not feasible to perform motor and language mapping. Somatosensory mapping only via median or tibial nerve stimulation may be a viable choice. The functional mappings performed by means of MEG are used in determining the feasibility and risks of surgery and occasionally in planning the surgical approach to lesions.

Key Points

Perfusion imaging includes a number of imaging techniques used to measure hemodynamically derived functional parameters in the brain.

DSC perfusion MRI provides measures of CBV, CBF, and MTT, which are useful in the imaging evaluation of cerebrovascular diseases and brain neoplasms.

ASL perfusion MRI is a noninvasive method that uses magnetically labeled arterial blood water as an endogenous tracer to measure CBF.

MEG is a robust and sensitive tool in the depiction of abnormal epileptiform activity in the brain and can be coregistered with MRI to localize these abnormal discharges in children with epilepsy.

MEG also can be used for presurgical functional mapping of motor, somatosensory, and language areas in the brain.

Suggested Readings

Chuang NA, Otsubo H, Pang EW, et al. Pediatric magnetoencephalography and magnetic source imaging. *Neuroimaging Clin N Am.* 2006;16: 193-210.

Schwartz ES, Dlugos DJ, Storm PB, et al. Magnetoencephalography for pediatric epilepsy: how we do it. *AJNR Am J Neuroradiol.* 2008;29: 832-837.

Wintermark M, Sesay M, Barbier E, et al. Comparative overview of brain perfusion imaging techniques. *Stroke.* 2005;36:e83-e99.

Wolf RL, Detre JA. Clinical neuroimaging using arterial spin-labeled perfusion magnetic resonance imaging. *Neurotherapeutics.* 2007;4:346-359.

Zaharchuk G. Theoretical basis of hemodynamic MR imaging techniques to measure cerebral blood volume, cerebral blood flow, and permeability. *AJNR Am J Neuroradiol.* 2007;28:1850-1858.

References

Full references for this chapter can be found on www.expertconsult.com.

Chapter 29

Prenatal Imaging

DOROTHY BULAS

Central nervous system (CNS) anomalies occur in 1.4 to 1.6 per 1000 live births and 3% to 6% of still births.[1] Whereas some anomalies can be detected as early as the first trimester (such as anencephaly), others may not develop until—or only become apparent—later in gestation.[2]

Ultrasound is the initial imaging modality used for the assessment of fetal CNS anomalies. When ultrasound is carefully performed using established guidelines, it can be very sensitive in evaluating the fetal brain.[3] Axial images are important for the assessment of biparietal diameter and head circumference measurements, ventricular size, and cerebellar configuration. Coronal and sagittal images can confirm the presence of the cavum septum pellucidum and corpus callosum. However, because of limitations from skull shadowing, fetal lie, maternal obesity, and oligohydramnios, evaluation of the fetal brain by ultrasound may be incomplete. When a fetal CNS anomaly is being considered, magnetic resonance imaging (MRI) is an adjunct that provides additional information.[4-7]

The multiplanar capability of MRI allows for the evaluation of the brain in any plane regardless of fetal lie, oligohydramnios, and overlying bone and gas. Single shot rapid acquisition with relaxation enhancement sequences decrease movement artifact. Slices as thin as 2 to 3 mm can be obtained and provide excellent anatomic detail. T1 sequences take longer to obtain and may require thicker slices for sufficient signal, but they are useful for detecting hemorrhage, calcification, and gliosis.

Advanced techniques include diffusion-weighted imaging, diffusion tensor imaging, and magnetic resonance (MR) spectroscopy.[8] The apparent diffusion coefficient normally decreases after 30 weeks' gestation,[9] but higher apparent diffusion coefficient values have been reported in high-risk fetuses.[10] Diffusion-weighted imaging can help detect hemorrhage and acute ischemia (Fig. 29-1). Diffusion tensor imaging measures the magnitude and direction of diffusion (fractional anisotropy). Although intrinsic anisotropy is low in the fetal brain, imaging improvements will help understand the onset and timing of delayed white matter connectivity.[11,12] Proton MR spectroscopy has advanced the investigation of fetal brain metabolism. Creatine and N-acetylaspartate peaks appear to have a progressive increase, whereas choline decreases in the third trimester.[13] Alterations in these peaks may help identify conditions associated with fetal compromise.

Ongoing enhancement of ultrafast MR sequences and postprocessing methodology has resulted in imaging techniques that can evaluate growth, organization, and remodeling processes that occur during fetal brain development.[14,15] Three-dimensional volumetric studies have demonstrated the value of quantitative assessment of brain growth in healthy versus high-risk fetuses. Fetuses with congenital heart disease have been shown to have impaired third-trimester brain growth compared with control subjects, offering a method to evaluate timing and progression of abnormal fetal brain growth.[16] Three-dimensional reconstruction of the fetal brain can provide cortical measures such as surface area and gyrification indices.

Although fetal MRI currently is performed with 1.5-Tesla (T) units, advanced imaging may turn to 3-T units to improve on these innovative techniques. Issues regarding increased specific absorption rate heating and movement artifacts currently limit the use of 3-T units. It is hoped that use of these advanced neuroimaging techniques will improve our ability to assess anomalies and provide methods for monitoring high-risk pregnancies, leading to improved counseling, planning of fetal intervention, and perinatal management.

Normal Development of the Fetal Brain

Knowledge of normal fetal morphology and development is important when evaluating anomalies. From 18 to 24 weeks' gestation, the brain is smooth, with minimal sulcation. The ventricles and extraaxial subarachnoid space, including the cisterna magna, are prominent until the third trimester[17] (Fig. 29-2).

Neuronal migration patterns can be documented by MRI.[18] Three layers are visualized, including the germinal matrix, cell sparse zone, and cortex. The germinal matrix has a low signal on T2-weighted images along the lateral ventricular walls and involutes from posterior to anterior after 28 weeks' gestation. The cell sparse zone represents migrating

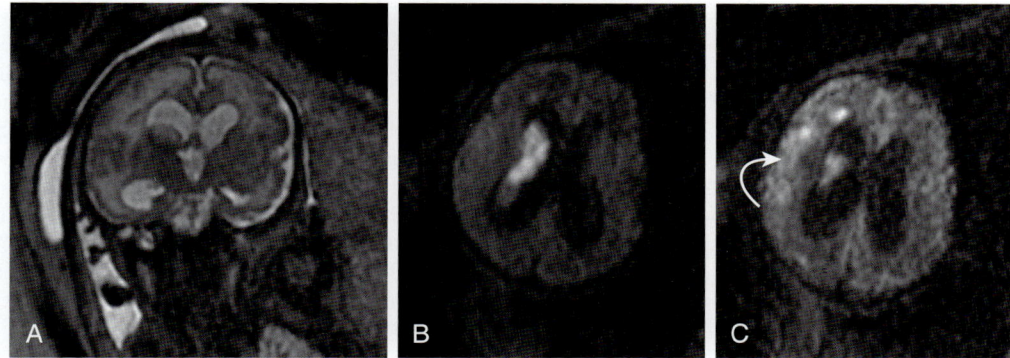

Figure 29-1   A fetus at 32 weeks' gestation with periventricular hemorrhagic infarction. **A,** A coronal single shot fast spin-echo T2-weighted magnetic resonance image shows moderate ventriculomegaly, intraventricular material, and an abnormal high signal in the right periventricular white matter. An axial diffusion-weighted sequence demonstrates increased diffusion signal within the lateral ventricle (**B**) and deep frontal white matter (**C,** *arrow*) consistent with intraventricular hemorrhage and a periventricular hemorrhagic infarct.

glial cells and eventually becomes the white matter. In the second trimester, the cortical ribbon is intermediate in signal.

The fetal cortical mantle follows a predictable course in maturation. Gyration progresses throughout the second and third gestation and can be used to assess gestational age (Box 29-1). By 32 weeks' gestation, extensive gyration and sulcation is present (Fig. 29-3).[17-19]

Fetal Ventriculomegaly

The fetal ventricles are prominent in relation to the brain parenchyma until the third trimester. After 25 weeks' gestation, the ventricles lose their colpocephalic configuration. Fetal ventriculomegaly is defined as an atrial measurement greater than 10 mm with separation of choroid from the medial wall (i.e., floating choroid). Ventriculomegaly can be due to obstruction, atrophy, maldevelopment, or, rarely, overproduction of cerebrospinal fluid. Ultrasound and MRI should be used to carefully assess for findings that suggest chromosomal anomalies (e.g., trisomy 13, 18, or 21), malformations (e.g., Chiari 2, Dandy-Walker, agenesis of the corpus

callosum [ACC], or holoprosencephaly), or destructive lesions (e.g., infarction or infection).[19-21]

The degree of ventriculomegaly has been shown to be associated with the incidence of live birth and survival beyond the neonatal period. With mild to moderate ventriculomegaly (10 to 15 mm), a close search for other anomalies and chromosome evaluation is important for further assessment. When ventriculomegaly is isolated, abnormal outcome can range from 10% to 25%. If other anomalies are present, outcome is worse, with only 50% to 80% of fetuses having a normal neurodevelopmental outcome.[22-24] In a large series evaluating fetal ventriculomegaly, motor outcomes were more severely affected than cognitive or adaptive outcomes, although prenatal atrial diameter was not consistently associated with postnatal developmental outcome.[25]

Agenesis of the Corpus Callosum

The corpus callosum forms between the eighth and twentieth week from genu to splenium. The rostrum forms last, between 18 to 20 weeks' gestation. Anomalies can be complete (ACC) or partial (hypogenesis). The corpus callosum may be difficult to visualize sonographically, particularly in

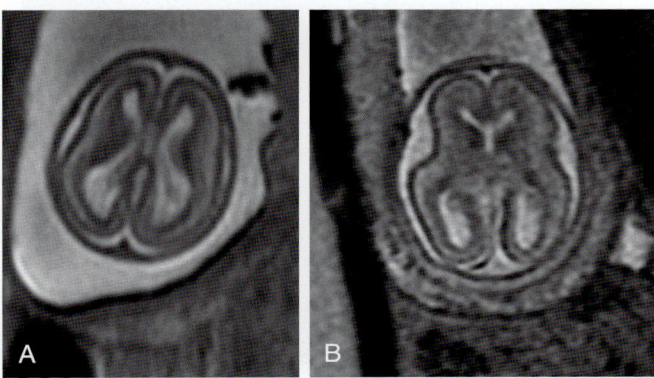

Figure 29-2   Normal development. An axial single shot fast spin-echo T2-weighted magnetic resonance image at 19 weeks' gestation (**A**) shows a smooth cortex, prominent ventricles, and subarachnoid space. Low-signal germinal matrix is present along the lateral ventricular walls. **B,** At 22 weeks' gestation, mild infolding of the sylvian fissure has occurred.

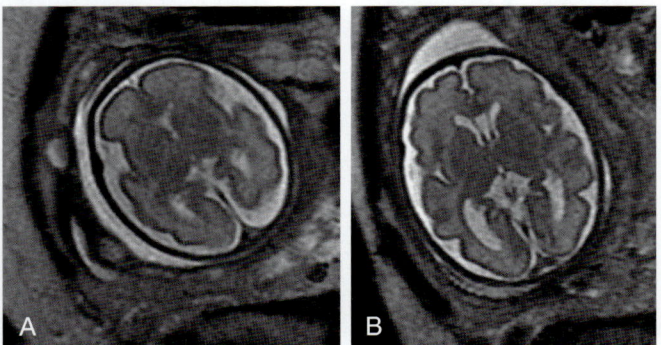

Figure 29-3   Progression of sulcation. **A,** An axial single shot fast spin-echo T2-weighted image at 28 weeks' gestation shows progression of the sulcation with involution of the germinal matrix. **B,** By 32 weeks' gestation, all primary sulcation is present.

the early weeks of gestation and/or with hypogenesis.[26] Sonographic and MR findings include colpocephaly of the occipital horns with parallel orientation of the lateral ventricles, an absent septum pellucidum, and a high-riding third ventricle (Fig. 29-4). Coronal images are particularly helpful in demonstrating the presence or absence of the cavum septum pellucidum and corpus callosum. With ACC, the frontal horns tend to be narrow with straight medial borders secondary to the bundles of Probst, which represent the callosal fibers that have not crossed the midline. The third ventricle may extend superiorly into an interhemispheric cyst. The cerebral convolutions have a radial arrangement on sagittal imaging. An associated lipoma may be present, which will be echogenic on ultrasound and isointense to gray matter on T2-weighted MRI (e-Fig. 29-5). If ACC is isolated, there is a 15% to 25% risk of a handicap and a 10% risk of aneuploidy. If associated anomalies are detected, such as Dandy-Walker malformation, cortical dysplasia, or encephalocele, the outcome is poorer.[27-29]

Neural Tube Defects

Cranial neural tube defects can be assessed by ultrasound and include anencephaly, iniencephaly (cervical dysraphism and fixed fetal head extension), Chiari 3 malformation (low occipital/high cervical encephalocele), and cranial encephaloceles (Fig. 29-6). MRI is particularly useful to further

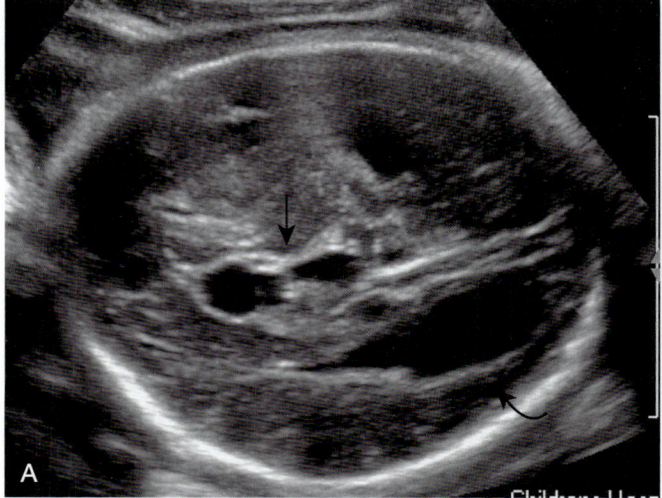

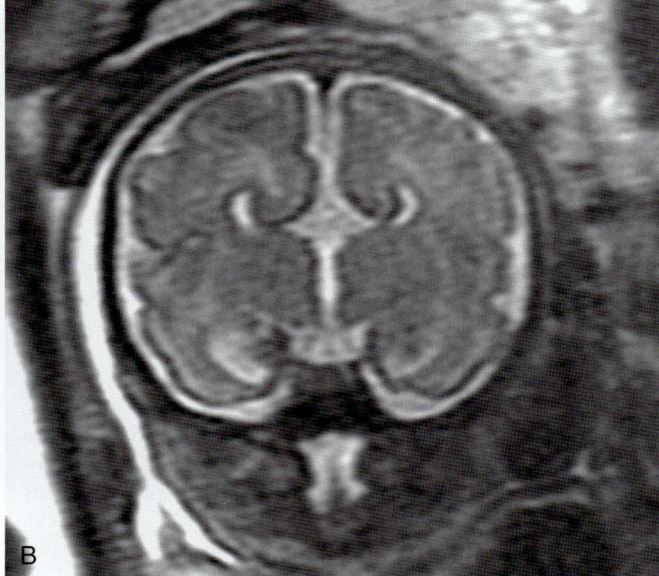

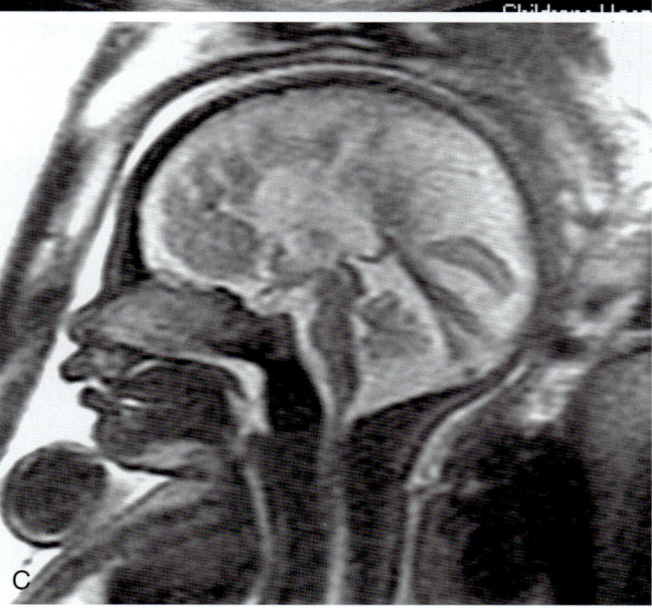

Figure 29-4 Agenesis of the corpus callosum. **A,** A transverse sonogram of the fetal brain shows dilatation of the occipital horns (*curved arrow*) and a high-riding third ventricle (*arrow*). **B,** A coronal T2-weighted image shows that the cavum septum pellucidum is absent, along with a high-riding third ventricle. The medial walls of the anterior horns are indented by the bundles of Probst. **C,** A sagittal T2-weighted image shows medial sulci radiating perpendicular to the expected course of the corpus callosum. The pericallosal sulcus is absent.

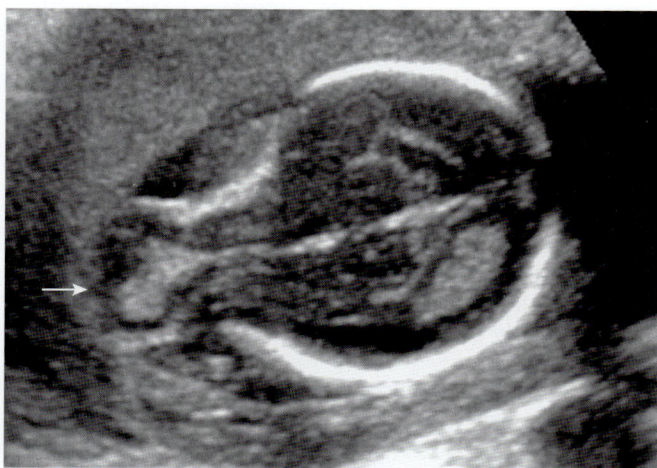

Figure 29-6 Encephalocele. An axial sonogram of the fetal brain at 16 weeks' gestation shows a frontal skull defect with brain contents herniated anteriorly (*arrow*).

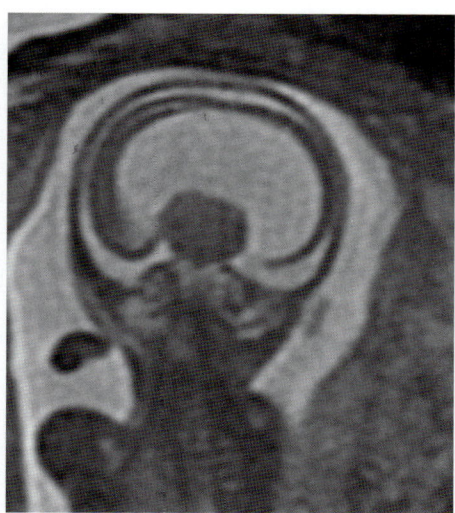

Figure 29-8 An example of 17-week gestation alobar holoprosencephaly. A coronal single shot fast spin echo T2-weighted magnetic resonance image of the fetal brain shows a single mantle of neural tissue with a monoventricle and fused thalami.

evaluate the amount of herniated brain and associated cranial anomalies.

Meningomyeloceles associated with Chiari 2 malformation are the most common neural tube defect. The cranial findings in fetuses with Chiari 2 malformation that are identified sonographically include a small or absent cisterna magna, cerebellar herniation (banana sign), frontal concavity (lemon sign), and ventriculomegaly.[30,31] MRI can further delineate the amount of brainstem and cerebellar herniation, beaking of the tectum, heterotopias, small subarachnoid space, and callosal dysgenesis. After fetal surgery, hindbrain herniation may reverse, decreasing the need for shunting postnatally.[32,33]

Holoprosencephaly

Failure of prosencephalic cleavage results in holoprosencephaly; septo-optic dysplasia is the mildest form, and alobar holoprosencephaly is the most severe form.[34] These anomalies are associated with several genetic syndromes such as Meckel-Gruber, Smith-Lemli-Opitz, trisomy 13 and 18, and teratogen exposure. Midline structures often are abnormal as well and can include proboscis, trigonocephaly, cyclopia, hypotelorism, and facial clefts (e-Fig. 29-7). Ultrasound can identify the most severe alobar form, but subtle cases of lobar holoprosencephaly may be difficult to diagnose, even with MRI.

Alobar holoprosencephaly is complete failure of division of the promesencephalic vesicle. A monoventricle is identified with "kissing choroid" by ultrasound. The thalami and basal ganglia are fused. The falx, corpus callosum, and interhemispheric fissure are absent (Fig. 29–8). With semilobar and lobar forms, a posterior interhemispheric fissure is present, with absence of the genu of the corpus callosum. Lobar holoprosencephaly may have a normally formed thalamus and callosal splenium. The anterior frontal lobes are fused and the frontal lobes typically are hypoplastic. The septum pellucidum and anterior falx are absent. Syntelencephaly is a variant in which the anterior parietal lobe or posterior frontal lobes are contiguous across the midline.[35,36]

Septo-optic dysplasia may be identified by the presence of ventricular dilation, an absent septum pellucidum, and flat roof of the frontal horns. Schizencephaly, heterotopias, and callosal dysgenesis often are associated with this sporadic anomaly and are better seen by MRI.[20]

Posterior Fossa Malformations

Malformations of the cerebellum and brainstem can be categorized by posterior fossa size: small, normal, or large. The cisterna magna is measured from the midline posterior aspect of the vermis to the inner occiput and normally measures between 3 to 10 mm. Although ultrasound can identify many posterior fossa anomalies, MRI is particularly useful in evaluating the vermis, brainstem, and location of the tentorium.[37-39]

When a small posterior fossa is noted, a Chiari malformation should be considered, with a close search for an associated meningomyelocele. The tentorium is low and the cisterna magna is small. The differential diagnosis includes cerebellar hypoplasia.

When the posterior fossa is normal in size, abnormalities include cerebellar/pontocerebellar hypoplasia and vermian dysgenesis (partial or total absence of the vermis) (e-Fig. 29-9). Rarely, rhombencephalosynapsis (agenesis of the vermis with fusion of cerebellum) can be identified prenatally. The fetal vermis is not completely developed until 18 weeks' gestation, and the fetal cerebellum continues to form in the third trimester, with cellular migration occurring through the first year of life, and thus mild cerebellar hypoplasia may be difficult to diagnose prenatally.[40-43] Volume measurements are available to aid in the diagnosis. Although pontocerebellar hypoplasia has a poor prognosis, the outcome for vermian dysgenesis is not as clear. In these cases, counseling must proceed cautiously and be correlated with associated anomalies and aneuploidy.

When the posterior fossa is enlarged, the differential diagnosis includes mega cisterna magna, Blake's pouch cyst,

Dandy-Walker malformation, or arachnoid cyst. Mega cisterna magna is a wide cistern (anteroposterior greater than 10 mm) with a normal vermis and cerebellum (e-Fig. 29-10). The tentorium is located in a normal position. Mega cisterna magna can be a normal finding, although it has been associated with aneuploidy. If no additional anomalies are found and chromosomes are normal, the outcome should be good.[44]

Blake's pouch cyst is a posterior protuberance of the inferior medullary velum into the cistern. This fluid collection is posterior inferior to the vermis and communicates with the fourth ventricle. The vermis typically is intact, with mass effect and elevation of the tentorium. The cyst does not communicate with the subarachnoid space.[45]

Dandy-Walker malformation is a retrocerebellar cyst that communicates with the fourth ventricle. The posterior fossa is enlarged, with an elevated tentorium. The vermis is incomplete, elevated, and rotated (Fig. 29-11). Hydrocephalus usually is present. Prognosis depends on the degree of vermian hypoplasia, brainstem hypoplasia, and associated anomalies such as ACC, heterotopias, and encephaloceles.

Arachnoid cysts can develop in the posterior fossa, causing an effect of the mass on the vermis, which otherwise is normally formed (e-Fig. 29-12). These cysts do not communicate with the fourth ventricle. The tentorium may be elevated. Symptoms can occur if hydrocephalus develops or the brainstem is compressed.

Cortical Development

Disorders of neuronal cell migration can be difficult to recognize in the fetal brain both by ultrasound and by MRI.[46,47] The cortex is poorly visualized by ultrasound, and whereas MRI demonstrates the cortical mantle relatively well, the cortex is not well developed in the second trimester. Thus a relatively smooth brain at 20 weeks that is normal can be indistinguishable from smooth pachygyria.

Abnormalities of cellular differentiation include unilateral megalencephaly and tuberous sclerosis (TS).[48] Subependymal hamartomas are present in up to 80% of patients with TS. Subependymal and subcortical tubers may be noted as intermediate-signal lesions on T2-weighted images and high-signal lesions on T1-weighted images in the third trimester (e-Fig. 29-13).

Neuronal heterotopias result when neurons fail to reach their destination at the cortical plate. Clusters can remain in the subependymal region or subcortical layer or form bands in the subcortical white matter. Subependymal heterotopias may be unilateral or bilateral, projecting as small lumps into the ventricles. The differential diagnosis includes hamartomas of TS and subependymal hemorrhage. Subcortical heterotopias are clumps of neurons and glial cells in the white matter that often are associated with ACC or neuroepithelial cysts. Associated microcephaly may not develop until the late third trimester or postnatally.

Agyria/pachygyria results from arrest of migration of neuroblasts with abnormal cortical lamination and failure of sulcation. Classic lissencephaly has few sulci, whereas pachygyria is less severe. In fetuses with cobblestone lissencephaly, cellular overmigration is present with hydrocephalus. Prenatally, ventricles typically are enlarged. Fetal MRI may show abnormal cortical sulcation in the third trimester (Fig. 29-14).[49]

Polymicrogyria is excessive folding of cerebral cortical cell layers with fusion of the gyral surface. It is common after cytomegalovirus infection in the second trimester and is

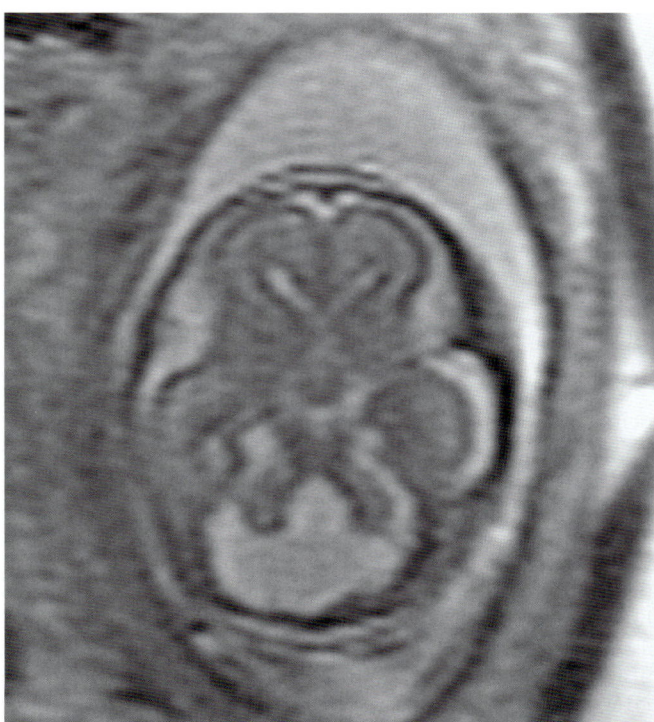

Figure 29-11 Dandy-Walker malformation. A saggital single shot fast spin-echo T2-weighted magnetic resonance image demonstrates an enlarged posterior fossa, hypoplastic elevated vermis, and retrocerebellar fluid collection connected to the fourth ventricle with elevated torcula.

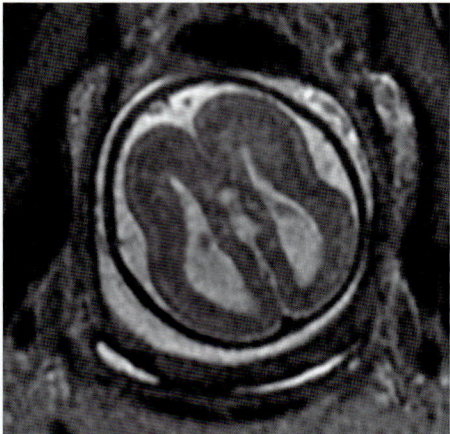

Figure 29-14 Lissencephaly. A single shot fast spin-echo T2-weighted image of a 36-week gestation fetus demonstrates an abnormal smooth surface with lack of gyri and sulci. The cortical and subcortical layers are disorganized. Colpocephaly is present with dilated atria. The infant was diagnosed with Miller-Dieker syndrome after delivery.

difficult to diagnose before the third trimester. Multiple small, irregular sulci may be noted with mild ventriculomegaly.

Interpreting fetal MR images can be challenging because structures are small and change with fetal maturation. Great care must be taken when performing and interpreting these studies. Prognosis of abnormalities can be varied, making counseling difficult, even when anomalies are well delineated. Long-term follow-up studies are necessary to provide accurate data. Ultrasound remains the screening modality of choice in the assessment of the fetal brain. However, when an anomaly is identified, MRI has become an important adjunct in the assessment of complex fetal CNS anomalies.

Key Points

Neuronal migration and gyration follows a predictable course throughout the second and third trimester.

Fetal ventriculomegaly outcome is variable. Associated anomalies and aneuploidy bode for a worse prognosis.

Because fetal vermis does not develop until 18 weeks' gestation and the cerebellum continues to form in the third trimester, vermian and cerebellar hypoplasia may be difficult to diagnosis accurately in the second trimester.

Cortical dysplasias may not be visualized in the second trimester.

Suggested Readings

Garel C. Fetal MRI: what is the future? *Ultrasound Obstet Gynecol.* 2008;31:123-128.

Garel C. *MRI of the fetal brain: normal development and cerebral pathologies.* Berlin: Springer-Verlag; 2005.

Limperopoulos C, Clouchoux C. Advancing fetal brain MRI. Targets for the future. *Semin Perinatol.* 2009;33:289-298.

Twickler DM, Reichel T, McIntire DD, et al. Fetal central nervous system ventricle and cisterna magna measurements by MRI. *Am J Obstet Gynecol.* 2002;187:927-931.

Vezina G. Congenital malformation of the brain: prenatal and postnatal imaging. *Semin Roentgenol.* 2004;39:165-181.

References

Full references for this chapter can be found on www.expertconsult.com.

Chapter 30

Neonatal Brain Injury

ANDRE D. FURTADO, JESSICA L. WISNOWSKI, MICHAEL J. PAINTER,
ASHOK PANIGRAHY, and P. ELLEN GRANT

Adverse events during the neonatal period (the first month of life) account for a large proportion of child deaths and permanent neurologic disability. Preterm neonates are particularly vulnerable to brain injury during the first weeks of life. Imaging has been used widely not only to diagnose and understand brain injury in neonates, but also to predict the neurodevelopmental outcome.[1] Because of its portability, cranial ultrasound is usually the first imaging modality to be performed and can be used serially to monitor the evolution of certain injuries. Ultrasound is usually sufficient for evaluation of germinal matrix hemorrhage (GMH) and intraventricular hemorrhage (IVH), hydrocephalus and serial assessment of ventricular size, cystic white matter injury of prematurity, and severe brain malformations. Ultrasound is less sensitive than computed tomography (CT) or magnetic resonance imaging (MRI) in the detection of small calcifications and is less sensitive than MRI in the detection of hypoxic-ischemic injury and subtle brain malformations. MRI also is excellent for the evaluation of punctate white matter lesions, which are seen in the setting of premature white matter. Because of the associated ionizing radiation, the use of CT is mainly restricted to instances in which there is a suspicion of skull fracture or to confirm the presence of intracranial calcifications, lesions that contain fat, and acute intracranial hemorrhage. MRI is the most sophisticated modality to evaluate the neonatal brain, and with advanced imaging techniques such as diffusion-weighted imaging (DWI), functional magnetic resonance imaging (fMRI), and magnetic resonance spectroscopy (MRS), it has the advantage of providing information regarding physiology, function, and metabolism. With the development of arterial spin labeling techniques, it is now possible to assess brain perfusion in the neonate without the use of intravenous contrast material.

Imaging Techniques

High-resolution images with good tissue contrast are essential for an adequate evaluation of the neonatal brain. Ultrasound provides high-resolution images of the neonatal brain, but it has limitations regarding visualization of deeper structures and the cerebellum. Because increased tissue contrast in CT usually is achieved at the expense of increased radiation dose, CT usually is performed with use of low radiation dose protocols and is reserved for a limited number of situations.

MRI is the imaging modality with the highest sensitivity for differentiating abnormalities from normal brain. Conventional MRI, including T1-weighted, T2-weighted, DWI, and gradient-echo sequences or susceptibility-weighted images provide the most useful diagnostic information. Sequences should be modified to optimize signal to noise for the neonatal brain. Structurally, the brains of preterm infants and neonates have much higher water content and much lower lipid content compared with brains of older children. This makeup of the brain stems from both the composition of the extracellular matrix and the extent of myelination, which begins along specific tracts in the third trimester of fetal gestation and continues well into the postnatal years. Importantly, these differences cause a lengthening of the T2-relaxation time with decreasing age, necessitating longer echo times for younger patients. Similarly, the T1 relaxation is longer for infants and young children and varies with the magnetic field strength. In general, this scenario results in the need for longer inversion times of T1-weighted scans in infants. Finally, the higher water content and lower anisotropy in infants necessitate a lower b-value to obtain sufficient signal to noise in DWI.

Dedicated neonatal MR head coils improve image contrast and resolution at the smaller field of view optimal for neonatal imaging.[2,3] These dedicated coils improve gray-white matter differentiation and provide better visualization of the brainstem and posterior fossa.

Patient Preparation, Safety, and Hazards

Ultrasound can be performed at the bedside and does not use contrast material or ionizing radiation. The only precaution with ultrasound is prevention of infection, which can be achieved with use of sterile gel and a probe cover. CT examination requires transportation of the neonate to the scanner; however, the scanning time is short. Contrast material is rarely needed and should be avoided in neonates because of their physiologic renal immaturity, which is present in the first few days to weeks after birth.

Because of the MR environment and length of most MRI examinations, MR safety is a particular concern for neonates. Before the MR examination, any patient, including neonates, should be screened for possible cardiac devices, implants, non–MR-compatible leads, or surgically implanted wires. The compatibility of any device must always be verified with the manufacturer. Additionally, Shellock and Kanal[3a] provide useful information about the attraction/deflection forces of many items exposed to static magnetic fields. Continuous monitoring and support for respiratory and cardiovascular functions can be achieved with MR-compatible equipment. Thermoregulation, which can be a particular concern for preterm neonates, can be supported through use of MR-compatible incubators and monitored through use of an MR-compatible temperature probe.

Increasingly, neonates undergoing MRI are scanned during natural sleep (i.e., "feed and bundle" procedures). Although acoustic noise and table vibration from the MR scanner may awaken an older infant (i.e., >3 months of age, a developmental stage at which infants normally begin to awaken to startling noises), young infants (<3 months) often tolerate even long MR protocols when imaging is performed during natural sleep. When imaging during natural sleep is not possible, neonates and older infants are scanned while sedated. Sedation should be performed only by properly trained and credentialed clinicians.

Germinal Matrix and Intraventricular Hemorrhage

The germinal matrix (GM) is a transient area of proliferation and migration of the neuronal and glial precursor cells located within the walls of the ventricles (ventricular/subventricular zones). The GM is highly vascular; it has thin-walled vessels with limited capability to compensate for hemodynamic and oxygen tension changes, which makes it susceptible to hemorrhage after hypoperfusion followed by reperfusion. GMH may extend into the lateral ventricles (IVH), and in severe instances, it may result in hydrocephalus. The choroid plexus also may hemorrhage, usually in association with GMH. During the end of the second trimester, the GM starts to involute. One of the last areas to involute is the ganglionic eminence located deep to the ependyma in the caudothalamic notch, a groove between the head of the caudate nucleus and the thalamus. After 34 weeks of gestational age, the GM matures, and hemorrhage becomes very unlikely to occur. Most infants with a small area of GMH are asymptomatic or demonstrate subtle signs that are easily overlooked. An unexplained drop in the hematocrit may occur with larger areas of bleeding.

Hemorrhagic brain injury of prematurity has been classified into four groups. Grade I is hemorrhage confined to the GM; grade II is GMH extending into the ventricles without evidence of ventricular dilatation; grade III is IVH with evidence of ventriculomegaly; and grade IV is IVH with an associated parenchymal infarction, as a result of congestion of the venous outflow (Table 30-1). Grades I and II of IVH have a low morbidity and mortality, whereas grades III and IV have higher mortality rates and a substantial risk of poor neurodevelopmental outcome among survivors (Fig. 30-1). Posthemorrhagic ventricular dilation can be managed with a temporizing neurosurgical procedure, including a ventricular reservoir, a subgaleal shunt, or a ventriculoperitoneal shunt.

Table 30-1

Classification of Germinal Matrix Hemorrhage/ Intraventricular Hemorrhage	
Grade	**Definition**
1	Hemorrhage confined to germinal matrix
2	Intraventricular without ventriculomegaly
3	Intraventricular with ventriculomegaly
4	Parenchymal hemorrhage related to venous infarction (not directly related to grades 1-3)

The cerebellum also has a GM, located in the granular layer. Hemorrhage into the immature cerebellum is an under-recognized complication of premature birth. Cerebellar hemorrhage often occurs concomitantly with supratentorial hemorrhage and is associated with high mortality and cerebral palsy. Cerebellar hemorrhage involving the medial part of the cerebellum (vermis) is particularly associated with cerebral palsy. Multiple periventricular and cerebellar hemorrhages may be a manifestation of an underlying clotting disorder.

Premature White Matter Injury

For more than a century, it has been recognized that the developing white matter is exceptionally vulnerable to injury during the second half of fetal gestation (i.e., the period during which preterm infants are born, and in most cases, survive beyond infancy). However, more recently it increasingly has been recognized that injury to the preterm neonate can involve many regions in the central nervous system (CNS), from gray matter (thalamus, cortex, and basal ganglia) to white matter to the brainstem and cerebellum. As a result, it has been argued that more comprehensive terms such as "encephalopathy of prematurity" should be used when referring to injury in the preterm neonate (see Suggested Readings). At the same time, the pattern of injury in preterm neonates has changed during the past several decades in parallel with advances in neonatal intensive care. Historically, cystic periventricular leukomalacia, characterized by multiple areas of cavitary necroses in the periventricular and deep white matter with surrounding astrogliosis, was a frequent observation, particularly among neonates who underwent autopsy. In the modern era, subtle changes in the white matter are more often observed on neuroimaging (e.g., "diffuse excessive high signal intensity") and at autopsy (e.g., gliosis) with or without accompanying microscopic (1 to 2 mm or less) necroses (visualized on MRI as punctate lesions with high T1-signal intensity in the periventricular and deep white matter).[4,5] A low concentration of lactate may be detected in preterm neonates and neonates who are small for gestational age using MRS and is often considered a "normal" finding unless it persists beyond term–equivalency or is associated with other findings (Fig. 30-2).

Several other pathologic and nonpathologic processes may be confused with brain injury of prematurity. Viral encephalitis may present with periventricular and/or subcortical lesions, which also may demonstrate reduced diffusivity. Metabolic disorders such as organic acidemia and neuromuscular disorders such as Fukuyama muscular dystrophy are other

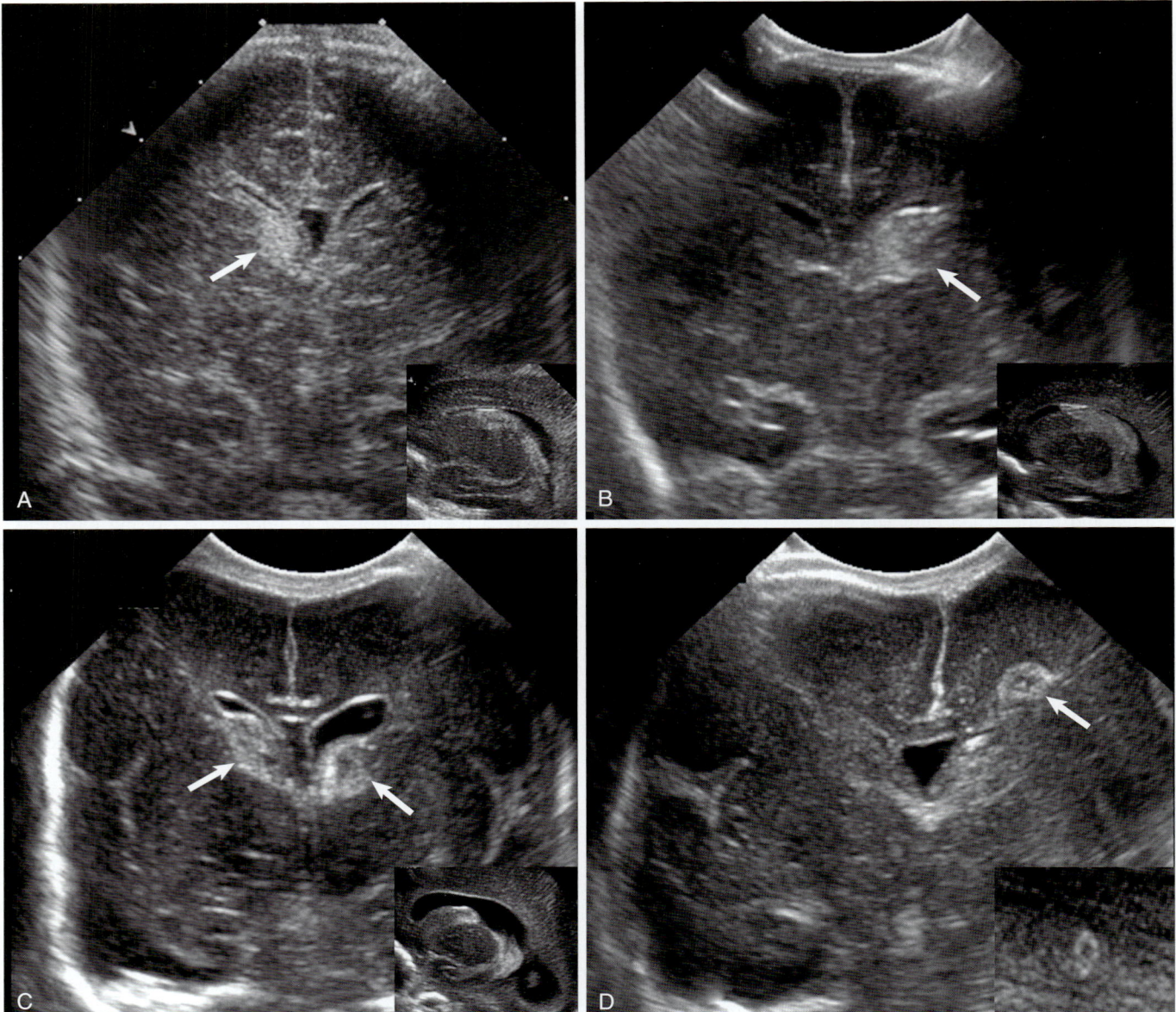

Figure 30-1   Ultrasound of germinal matrix hemorrhage. **A,** Grade 1, hemorrhage confined to the germinal matrix (*arrow*). **B,** Grade 2, germinal matrix hemorrhage extending into the ventricles (*arrow*). **C,** Grade 3, germinal matrix and intraventricular hemorrhage with ventriculomegaly (*arrows*). **D,** Intraparenchymal hemorrhage (*arrow*).

causes of increased T2 signal in the white matter. Signal abnormality involving the gray matter may be seen in organic acidemias, particularly propionic acidemia, and cortical dysplasia typically is present in persons with Fukuyama muscular dystrophy. Congenital periventricular cysts and coarctation of the frontal horns may be misdiagnosed as cystic white matter changes. The location of these anatomic variants is very characteristic and therefore is useful in distinguishing the variants from injury. Congenital periventricular cysts usually are located below the level of the ventricular angles, and the coarctation of the fontal horns is lateral to the ventricles and follows the normal contour of the ventricular wall.

As previously noted, ultrasound is most often the first neuroimaging modality used in the evaluation of a preterm neonate. Normal periventricular white matter is relatively

echogenic in preterm neonates. To be considered "normal" in a diagnostic setting, the echogenicity in the white matter must be bilaterally homogenous and symmetric. Asymmetry, heterogeneity, and focal areas of increased echogenicity relative to the choroid plexus are all considered to be a concern for abnormality. However, it also should be noted that transient hyperechogenicity in the periventricular white matter (i.e., less than 7 days) has been described in normal infants; accordingly, serial ultrasound often is performed before white matter injury is more definitively diagnosed. Abnormally increased periventricular echogenicity representing edema or hemorrhage most commonly occurs in the first week of life, and when present, the cystic changes develop at approximately 3 to 4 weeks of age. Ultrasound shows unilateral or bilateral linear hyperechoic hemorrhagic material in the

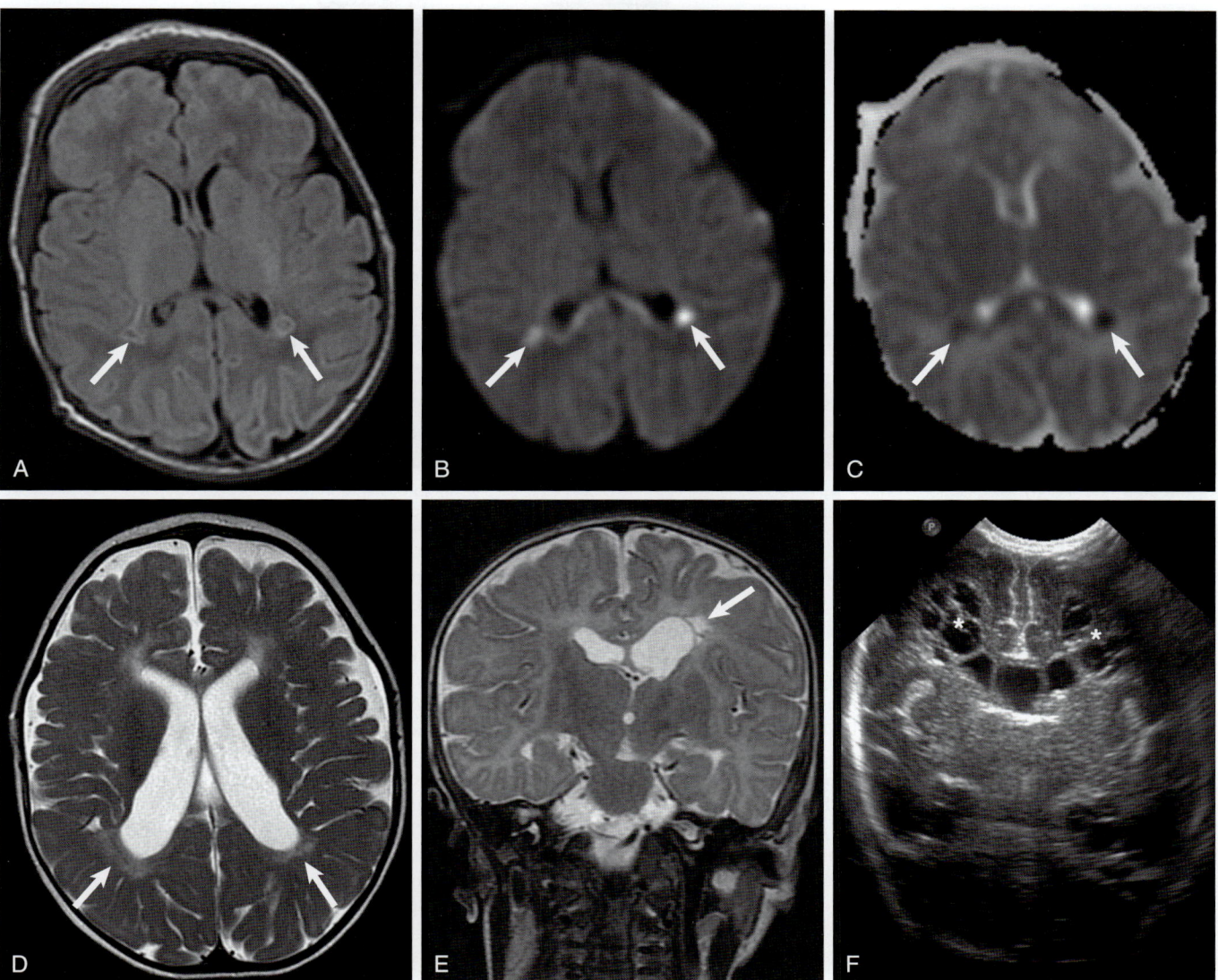

Figure 30-2 **White matter injury of prematurity.** Acutely, focal areas of necrosis with increased signal are seen on T1-weighted images (**A**), with restricted diffusion (**B**) and low apparent diffusion coefficient (*arrows*) (**C**). **D,** A different patient at 2 years of age has increased T2 signal and volume loss involving the periventricular white matter bilaterally (*arrows*). **E,** A unilateral white matter injury with small cysts (*arrow*) seen on T2-weighted imaging. **F,** A bilateral cystic white matter injury (*asterisks*) on cranial ultrasound.

region of the caudothalamic notch, choroid plexus, ventricles, and periventricular white matter. Ultrasound findings of extensive periventricular cystic lesions and white matter damage portends a poor prognosis, but normal ultrasound findings do not necessarily imply a normal neurodevelopmental outcome.

Hypoxic-Ischemic Encephalopathy

Brain damage in the term neonate is highly variable and depends on the severity and duration of insult. Moreover, the imaging findings vary dramatically in relation to the timing of imaging studies. Imaging before 72 hours may underestimate the severity because delayed cell death, such as apoptosis, peaks around 72 hours after the insult occurs. Therapeutic hypothermia, which typically is applied for 72

hours beginning within 6 hours of life, may further delay this process.

CENTRAL PATTERN OF HYPOXIC-ISCHEMIC ENCEPHALOPATHY

The central pattern of hypoxic-ischemic encephalopathy (HIE) usually occurs with profound asphyxia, when there is an abrupt interruption of the blood supply, depriving the neonatal brain of oxygen and glucose. Highly metabolic structures such as the thalami, basal ganglia, and brainstem are more vulnerable to hypoxia and ischemia, more specifically the ventral lateral thalami, posterolateral lentiform nuclei, posterior midbrain, hippocampi, lateral geniculate nuclei, and perirolandic cerebral cortex (Fig. 30-3).[5] Quadriparesis, choreoathetosis, seizures, mental retardation, and cerebral palsy have been associated with profound asphyxia.[6]

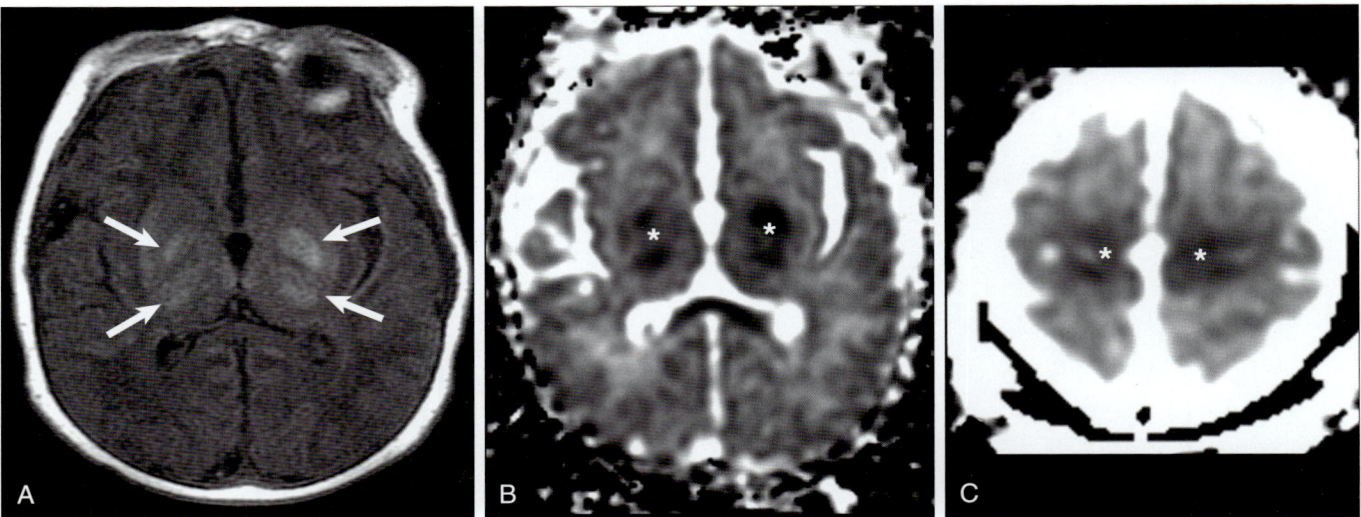

Figure 30-3 Central hypoxic-ischemic injury. **A,** Increased T1 signal in the globi pallidi and ventrolateral thalami bilaterally (*arrows*). **B** and **C,** Reduced apparent diffusion coefficient in the globi pallidi and thalami and in the regions of the perirolandic cortex bilaterally (*).

Ultrasound and CT have low sensitivity to detect early ischemic changes in the deep structures of the brain. The most common pattern on ultrasound is transient or persistent hyperechogenicity, which may progress to cavitation in the basal ganglia and thalami, particularly in the globus pallidus and ventral lateral nuclei of the thalamus. With more severe insults involving the cortex and subcortical white matter, ultrasound and CT may depict indirect evidence of edema, such as effacement of the sulci, loss of gray-white matter differentiation, and compressed lateral ventricles.

MRI is the imaging modality of choice for neonatal encephalopathy. MRS performed 24 hours after the insult is considered sensitive for hypoxic-ischemic brain injury. Elevated lactate and diminished N-acetyl-aspartate (NAA) are the most common MRS findings in neonates with neurologic and developmental abnormalities (e-Fig. 30-4). Lactate rises after the hypoxic-ischemic event, peaking at 3 to 5 days, whereas NAA starts to decline around the third day. Although a minimally elevated lactate level (lactate/choline ratio <0.15) may be detected in the normal neonatal brain at term, an increased lactate level relative to the total creatine peak in the basal ganglia provides an early indication of brain injury before changes may be apparent on conventional T1- and T2-weighted imaging. It has been suggested that resuscitation may rapidly clear lactate and that a secondary increase in lactate may occur after 12 to 24 hours. The metabolites tend to normalize after about day 5, although in some cases abnormal metabolite ratios persist. Persistently elevated lactate levels in the basal ganglia provide prognostic information about the severity of the brain injury and the subsequent neurodevelopmental outcome. False-negative MRS findings also may occur, with normal spectral findings but abnormal outcomes.

DWI is a sensitive technique for assessment of acute brain injury. DWI also shows deep gray matter and perirolandic gray matter lesions before they are seen with conventional MRI. If DWI is performed in the first few hours after the injury, it may underestimate the extent of the injury or even show normal results. Paralleling the clinical presentation of HIE, in which neonates may actually transiently improve before demonstrating a more permanent decline in neurologic functioning because of delayed cell death via apoptotic mechanisms, some patients demonstrate mild brain damage for the first few days and then proceed to demonstrate extensive brain involvement around 5 days after the injury. Apparent diffusion coefficient (ADC) values always evolve over time; they decrease initially after the injury, with the nadir around 3 to 5 days, and increase (via facilitated diffusion) later in the chronic phase. As ADC values increase, a point of transient "pseudonormalization" exists in which injured tissue can be misdiagnosed as "normal." Conventional MRI findings are usually unremarkable during the first few days but then begin to demonstrate first an increased T1-weighted signal and a decreased T2-weighted signal in the subacute period followed by an increased T2-weighted signal in the more chronic period. Evidence suggests that hypothermia therapy delays the onset of MR changes (in metabolic, diffusion, and conventional imaging) associated with injury and, in particular, delays the onset of pseudonormalization in the ADC signal.[7]

PERIPHERAL PATTERN OF HYPOXIC-ISCHEMIC ENCEPHALOPATHY

The peripheral pattern of HIE usually results from a period of decreased blood supply to the brain (rather than a near total and abrupt interruption) and is thought to develop as a result of a compensatory shunting of blood to vital brain structures, such as the brainstem, thalami, basal ganglia, hippocampi, and cerebellum, at the expense of less metabolically active structures, namely the cerebral cortex and white matter (Fig. 30-5). Therefore the brainstem, cerebellum, and deep gray matter structures generally are spared from injury in mild to moderate hypoxic-ischemic insults. More prolonged insults result in injury to the intervascular border (watershed) zones, which are relatively hypoperfused as a result of this shunting. Neurologic examination varies depending on the severity of the insult, from asymptomatic in mild cases to proximal extremity weakness or spasticity and cerebral palsy in persons who sustain severe insults.[6] Increasing severity of watershed-distribution injury is associated with impaired neurocognitive

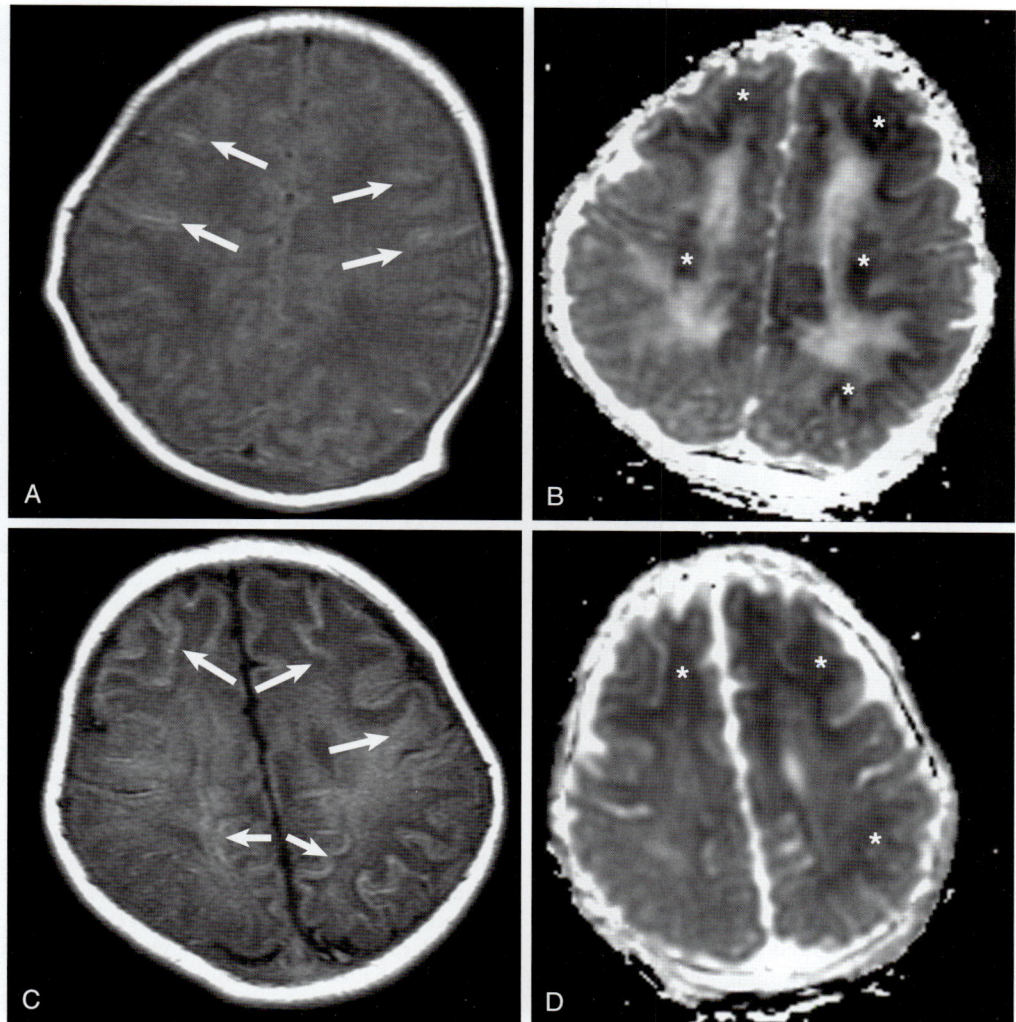

Figure 30-5 Peripheral pattern of hypoxic-ischemic injury. **A,** At day 2 after the ischemic event, subtle findings are seen on T1-weighted imaging (*arrows*), but reduced apparent diffusion coefficient (ADC), mainly involving the subcortical white matter, is marked (*) (**B**). **C,** At 7 days after the insult, T1-weighted images demonstrate progression on the areas of increased T1 signal, mainly involving the subcortical white matter (*arrows*), and less conspicuously reduced ADC (*) (**D**).

functioning, including language, visuoperceptual, and executive functioning impairments.

Ultrasound lacks sensitivity in assessing partial prolonged hypoxia-ischemia because it provides poor visualization of the triple watershed zone. CT also is not sensitive to the early changes but may show effacement of the gray-white junction, hypoattenuation with mass effect from acute edema, or hypoattenuation with volume loss in the watershed zone. Similar to central HIE, in the acute phase, MRI can detect lactate and restricted diffusion with corresponding low ADC values in the affected brain regions, which predominantly involve the cortex and underlying white matter along the parasagittal frontal-parietal cortex. With time, increased T2/fluid attenuated inversion recovery signal and mass effect related to edema may develop. Chronically, gliosis and volume loss mainly involving the deep portion of the gyri result in mushroom-shaped gyri, known as ulegyria, which sometimes is associated with an epileptogenic focus. Atrophic changes and gliosis predominately involve the subcortical white matter in the border zone between the

anterior and the middle cerebral arteries, in the parasagittal watershed zone, and in the parietal lobes at the border zone of the three major cerebral arteries, that is, the triple watershed zone.

Neonatal Arterial Infarction

Infarctions involving the vascular territory of a major artery, most commonly the middle cerebral artery (L>R), are more common in term than in preterm neonates. Symptoms are subtle and nonspecific, and many neonatal arterial infarcts may be unrecognized until motor or cognitive symptoms develop later in infancy or childhood. In the neonatal period, the most common presenting symptom is a focal motor seizure involving the contralateral limbs, which may secondarily generalize. Infarcts of the anterior and posterior cerebral arteries are underdetected because they may be asymptomatic and difficult to visualize on ultrasound. Several causes have been described, including sepsis, bacterial meningitis,

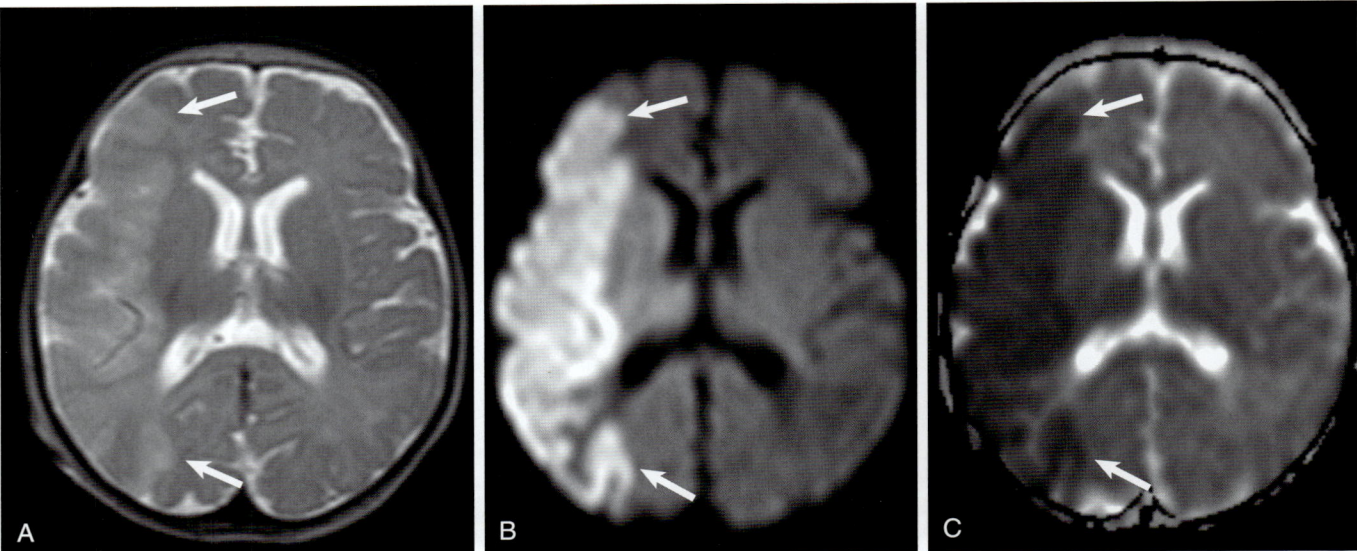

Figure 30-6   Ischemic infarct. **A,** A T2-weighted image shows a large ischemic infarct (*arrows*) involving the territory of the right middle cerebral artery, with corresponding restricted diffusion on diffusion-weighted imaging (*arrows*) (**B**) and low apparent diffusion coefficient values (*arrows*) (**C**).

inherited or acquired coagulopathies (heterozygosity for factor V Leiden and disseminated intravascular coagulation), and cardiac abnormalities, but often no specific cause is identified. Initial imaging shows a loss of gray-white matter differentiation, which in severe instances may be detected on ultrasound but is most readily visualized on MRI as increased signal on DWI with low ADC values (Fig. 30-6). Later (after 24 to 48 hours) the edema becomes apparent as increased echogenicity on ultrasound, hypoattenuation on CT, increased signal on T2-weighted MRI, and decreased signal on T1-weighted MRI. Although the high water content of the unmyelinated neonatal brain poses significant challenges for the detection of edema on CT or conventional MRI sequences, loss of gray-white matter differentiation frequently is present. This lack of contrast between the normal brain and the infarction is particularly relevant at 5 to 10 days after infarction when the ADC may be pseudonormalized. With time, ADC values increase (via facilitated diffusion); after a few weeks, volume loss and encephalomalacia become apparent. Hemorrhagic transformation of an ischemic stroke is rare in neonates, but increased signal on T1-weighted imaging along the cortex related to laminar necrosis is not uncommon. Interestingly, acutely after a perinatal ischemic infarct, hyperperfusion as demonstrated on arterial spin label sequences frequently is observed in the regions corresponding to areas of low ADC on diffusion-weighted MRI. Occasionally, focal areas of hyperperfusion also can be seen after seizures (epileptiform activity) in the neonate.

Neonatal Intraventricular and Parenchymal Hemorrhage

Term neonates may have IVH, parenchymal hemorrhage, and rarely GMH. In a large proportion of these cases, the source is not identified. The most common documented cause is cerebrovenous sinus thrombosis, followed by

coagulopathy, infection, hypoglycemia, vascular malformation, a tumor, and genetic disorders. A hemorrhagic and thrombotic screening is the first step in any neonate with intracranial hemorrhage. Additionally, confirmation of vitamin K administration and examination of alloimmune antibodies in the mother's blood should be obtained. Although hemorrhage may occur anywhere in the term neonatal brain, the thalamus and the choroid plexus are the most common locations. Rarely, hemorrhages occur in areas of residual GM. Blood degradation products without surrounding edema or hydrocephalus with chronic blood products in the first days of life are suggestive of intrauterine hemorrhage, which are most commonly caused by maternal factors such as anticoagulants, vasogenic agents (including illicit drugs), diabetes, and trauma. Less commonly, fetal conditions such as arteriovenous malformation (AVM) (vein of Galen malformation), congenital brain tumor, and genetic disorders may lead to prenatal hemorrhage.

Neonatal Cerebrovenous Sinus Thrombosis

Neonatal cerebrovenous sinus thrombosis (CVST) is a rare but devastating condition. It may be a result of trauma, increased hematocrit, sepsis, dehydration, cardiac failure, and thrombotic disorders such as factor V Leiden. The impaired venous drainage commonly results in cytotoxic edema, vasogenic edema, and parenchymal hemorrhage, and in more severe cases acute or chronic hydrocephalus. Although venous infarction can occur anywhere in the brain, the most characteristic locations are the thalami, resulting from thrombosis of the straight sinus and vein of Galen, and the bilateral parasagittal cortex and subcortical white matter, resulting from thrombosis of the superior sagittal sinus. Diffuse cerebral swelling with slitlike ventricles may be a result of extensive CVST.

The diagnosis of CVST may be achieved by demonstrating the thrombus or the lack of normal venous flow in the venous sinuses. Doppler ultrasound may detect superior sagittal sinus thrombosis in neonates, but it has limited sensitivity in evaluating the remainder of the venous system. Serial Doppler ultrasound is an easily performed and inexpensive alternative for monitoring sinovenous thrombosis. CT without contrast may demonstrate a hyperattenuating sinus in a large thrombus but has limited value for small thrombi. False-positive results can occur with unenhanced CT because of relative hyperattenuation of the normal blood of a neonate due to the high hematocrit and the adjacent hypoattenuating nonmyelinated brain tissue. Moreover, hyperattenuating subdural hematomas that are present in up to a third of the neonates can be misinterpreted as a thrombus. The demonstration of filling defects using CT venography is confirmatory of CVST. Beam hardening artifact from dense bone adjacent to the dural sinus and normal arachnoid granulations may mimic a filling defect. The normal dural sinus and veins have flow voids on unenhanced MRI. Phase-contrast MR venography and two-dimensional time-of-flight MR venography are specific for flow and are valuable in demonstrating obstruction. High signal on unenhanced MRI or lack of flow-related signal on two-dimensional time-of-flight MR venography can be related to thrombus or slow flow. Thin-slice images oriented perpendicular to the flow in the sinus with an abnormal signal is usually sufficient to correct for this "artifact." MR venography and contrast-enhanced MRI are complementary to unenhanced MRI to show the filling defect and to differentiate venous thrombosis from adjacent subdural hematoma. The best unenhanced conventional MR sequences for detection of sinus venous thrombosis are spin echo T1 and proton density images. Although full anticoagulation is controversial in the neonatal period, CVST is a medical emergency, and a definite diagnosis should be confirmed as soon as possible. When the aforementioned diagnostic modalities are inconclusive, digital subtraction angiography is the gold standard.

Vascular Malformations

Most vascular malformations are silent during the neonatal period but may be diagnosed prenatally or incidentally. A full description of all the major vascular malformations is beyond the scope of this chapter. Instead, we will focus on those that more commonly manifest in the neonatal period: cerebral (pial) vascular malformations, aneurismal malformation of the vein of Galen, and malformation of the dural sinuses.

ARTERIOVENOUS MALFORMATIONS

AVMs are abnormal thin-walled vessels that connect arteries to veins without intervening capillaries. Most cases of AVM manifest later in childhood or in early adulthood. Neonates with an AVM tend to present with systemic cardiac manifestations or seizures related to the parenchymal hypoperfusion. Macrocephaly and hydrocephalus related to abnormally increased venous pressure and spontaneous hemorrhage are less common in the neonatal period.

In symptomatic patients, early diagnosis and emergency endovascular embolization is important because progression to atrophy and leukomalacia may occur rapidly. Unenhanced CT is useful to detect acute hemorrhaging, but it lacks the sensitivity necessary to detect the underlying vascular malformation. CT angiography (CTA) involves significant radiation exposure but provides exquisite anatomic detail of a nidus (if present), feeding arteries, draining veins, and the presence of possible aneurysms. MR angiography (MRA) is excellent for the detection of hemorrhage and to delineate the AVM, although smaller vascular malformations may go undetected. The flow void seen in the tangled vessel of the nidus has been described as a "bag of black worms." High-resolution T1-weighted sequences are important to define the location of the nidus. Three-dimensional (3D) time-of-flight MRA has slightly less special resolution than does CTA, but it does not expose the neonate to radiation. Time-resolved MRA has less special resolution than 3D Time-of-flight (TOF) MRA and CTA, but it may provide sufficient information to differentiate feeding arteries and draining veins.

VEIN OF GALEN MALFORMATION

Malformations involving the vein of Galen are true congenital arteriovenous connections between thalamic perforating, choroidal, and anterior cerebral arteries with the embryonic median prosencephalic vein. Associated cardiovascular anomalies may be present, such as aortic coarctation and secundum atrial septal defect.[8] The most common clinical presentation is high-output cardiac failure. The prognosis is mainly related to the number of abnormal arteriovenous connections and the amount of associated parenchymal injury from arterial steal and hypoperfusion. The most common is the choroidal type with innumerous connections, which usually is fatal. The mural type with one to four connections has a better prognosis and is less likely to present in the neonatal period. This type usually presents during infancy as developmental delay, hydrocephalus, and seizures, or in older children as hemorrhage. Endovascular therapy is the treatment of choice. Prenatal and postnatal spontaneous thrombosis has been reported.

MALFORMATION OF THE DURAL SINUSES

Saccular malformations of the dural sinus are rare; when they occur, they are associated with thrombosis, likely related to slow flow. The neonatal venous system has poor capacity to establish collateral circulation, and the drainage to the cavernous sinus is not yet developed. The propagation of the venous thrombosis within a dural sinus malformation may cause venous infarcts. The treatment of choice is preventive anticoagulation.

Birth Trauma

Birth trauma is more common in vaginal delivery, particularly if forceps or vacuum extraction is used. The most common traumatic birth lesions are extracranial hematomas, skull fractures, osteodiastasis, and extraaxial hematomas. Parenchymal contusions or lacerations are very rare; however, infarcts, particularly in the setting of large extraaxial hematomas, may be observed.

EXTRACRANIAL HEMATOMAS

The major types of extracranial hematomas are subgaleal hematoma, caput succedaneum, and cephalohematoma (also see Chapter 23). Subgaleal hematomas may enlarge rapidly and lead to potentially life-threatening hypovolemia. Anemia, coagulopathy, metabolic acidosis, renal impairment, and skull fracture have been reported as predictors of poor outcome. Early recognition and management are essential. An extracranial hematoma is caused by rupture of the emissary veins between the dural sinuses and the scalp veins; the hemorrhage accumulates between the epicranial aponeurosis of the scalp and the periosteum. Upon imaging, extracranial hematomas appear as a hemorrhagic collection overlying the calvarium and crossing the sutures. They may extend underneath the attachments of the occipitofrontalis muscle to the orbital margins anteriorly, the temporal fascia laterally, and the nuchal ridge posteriorly.

Caput succedaneum and cephalohematomas are rarely associated with complications. Cephalohematomas are subperiosteal hemorrhages confined by cranial sutures. Cephalohematomas are not of clinical significance but may be associated with skull fracture and epidural hematomas. Blood degradation within a hematoma may cause mild jaundice. Typically, hematomas increase in size after birth, and a small proportion of them calcify. Caput succedaneum represents edema, which may be accompanied by hemorrhage, within the subcutaneous tissues. Caput succedaneum is common after vaginal delivery, particularly when vacuum extraction is used. Typically, resolution occurs within a few days without complications.

SUBDURAL HEMATOMAS

Small subdural hematomas, particularly in the posterior fossa or caudal to the occipital lobes, are not uncommon after vaginal births and have been described in up to 30% of neonates. Subdural hematomas are usually asymptomatic and occur as a result of a dural tear during vaginal delivery, characteristically involving the tentorium. Although most subdural hematomas are venous in origin, large subdural hematomas may be caused by arterial bleeding. Most lethal cases are related to large infratentorial hemorrhages with compression of the brainstem. Interhemispheric subdural hematomas related to tearing of the inferior sagittal sinus and subdural hematomas along the convexity related to tearing of cortical veins are less frequent than those involving the tentorium. Associated subarachnoid hemorrhage related to tearing of cortical veins is not infrequent. Large subdural hematomas may cause parenchymal infarction as a result of either impaired arterial supply or, more likely, obstruction of the venous drainage, leading to hemorrhagic venous infarction. Large subdural hematomas may interfere with cerebrospinal fluid (CSF) reabsorption and cause hydrocephalus. Subdural hematomas that are not evacuated undergo absorption or evolve into subdural hygromas, which can persist for several months.

Finally, subdural hematoma is the most common presentation of nonaccidental trauma, which should be considered in addition to late hemorrhagic disease of the newborn.

Congenital and Neonatal Infection

Neonatal brain infections are an important cause of severe long-term neurologic morbidity. Viral, bacterial, and parasitic infections may be transmitted to the fetus or newborn in utero (congenital), intrapartum, or postnatally. As a general rule, bacterial and fungal infections are most commonly transmitted intrapartum or postnatally, whereas toxoplasmosis, syphilis, rubella, and cytomegalovirus (CMV) are most commonly transmitted in utero. The transmission of herpes simplex virus infection and human immunodeficiency virus (HIV) may occur in utero, intrapartum, or postnatally.

BACTERIAL INFECTIONS

The most common bacterial neonatal brain infections are caused by group B streptococcus, *Escherichia coli*, *Streptococcus pneumoniae*, *Haemophilus influenzae* type B, and *Listeria monocytogenes*. Imaging should be performed in neonates with bacterial meningitis if a rapid response to treatment does not occur or if a focal neurologic deficit develops. Complications of meningitis include empyema, ventriculitis, hydrocephalus, infarction, venosinus thrombosis, cerebritis, or abscess. In uncomplicated meningitis, imaging is usually normal. Leptomeningeal enhancement may be seen as a result of vascular engorgement.

Ventricular enlargement resulting from impaired CSF absorption by fibrinous inflammatory exudate is the most common imaging finding in persons with meningitis and does not necessarily indicate ventriculitis. Ventriculitis usually presents with ependymal enhancement and sometimes with a pus-fluid level. Ventriculitis often is associated with hydrocephalus and sometimes with intraventricular abscess. Sterile subdural effusions are not uncommon in neonates with meningitis; however, in a very small percentage of cases (approximately 2%), empyemas develop. Subdural collection with a signal intensity different from that of CSF, peripheral enhancement sometimes with septa, and signal abnormality involving the brain parenchyma are suggestive of empyema. Cerebritis is not uncommon in autopsies of neonates with meningitis despite normal findings of in vivo imaging. When imaging findings are present, cerebritis appears as an area of vasogenic edema with or without patchy areas of enhancement and/or cortical enhancement that may resolve with treatment. If the infection progresses, the enhancing areas become more confluent, and later an abscess forms with restricted water diffusivity and an enhancing capsule. Neonatal *Citrobacter koseri* (diversus) meningitis is rare but often is complicated by formation of abscesses, with a predilection for the frontal lobes. Neonatal pneumocephalus also has been reported as a complication of *C. koseri* meningitis. *Citrobacter* meningitis usually has a poor neurologic outcome (e-Fig. 30-7).

FUNGAL INFECTION (CANDIDA)

Candida is a neonatal commensal fungus. Infection is caused by organisms that are already present in the intestine and other locations. The key risk factors are catheters and use of wide-spectrum antibiotics; premature infants are particularly susceptible. At first the inflammation consists of neutrophils, and later it consists of epithelioid cells and giant cells. It causes meningitis, multiple enhancing hemorrhagic microabscesses, macroabscesses, and extensive brain necrosis. Multiple macroabscesses within the subcortical and periventricular regions and basal ganglia are the most common imaging findings in the neonate; however, imaging findings may be normal.

HERPES SIMPLEX VIRUS TYPE 2 INFECTIONS

Women who have their first outbreak of herpes simplex virus type 2 genital herpes during pregnancy are at high risk of miscarriage or delivering a baby with a low birth weight. The infection can be passed to the neonate in utero or, most commonly, during birth. The most serious risk to the infant is herpes simplex virus type 2 encephalitis. Signs and symptoms in the newborn are nonspecific, with irritability, a high-pitched cry, fever, and poor feeding. Diagnosis is made via a viral culture or polymerase chain reaction (PCR) of the CSF. If the infection occurs early in pregnancy, it may cause hydranencephaly, basal ganglia calcifications, and microphthalmia (the classic TORCH pattern). Late pregnancy or intrapartum transmission involves the bilateral gray and white matter diffusely, which rapidly develops into whole brain necrosis. Multiple cortical hemorrhagic foci and sometimes leptomeningeal enhancement often are present. With time, cystic white matter changes develop (Fig. 30-8).[9]

ENTEROVIRUS AND PARECHOVIRUS INFECTION

Enterovirus and parechovirus belong to the family *Picornaviridae*. Enteroviruses are well known for causing neonatal hepatitis, myocarditis, and meningoencephalitis, which can lead to death or severe long-term morbidity. Parechoviruses recently have been reported as causing severe neonatal infection, including involvement of the CNS. The diagnosis is made by PCR; however, PCR for enterovirus does not detect parechovirus. Meningoencephalitis in the neonatal period causes extensive white matter abnormalities, which appear as hyperechogenicity on ultrasound, hypoattenuation on CT, increased signal on T2-weighted MRI images, and decreased signal on T1-weighted MRI images, with or

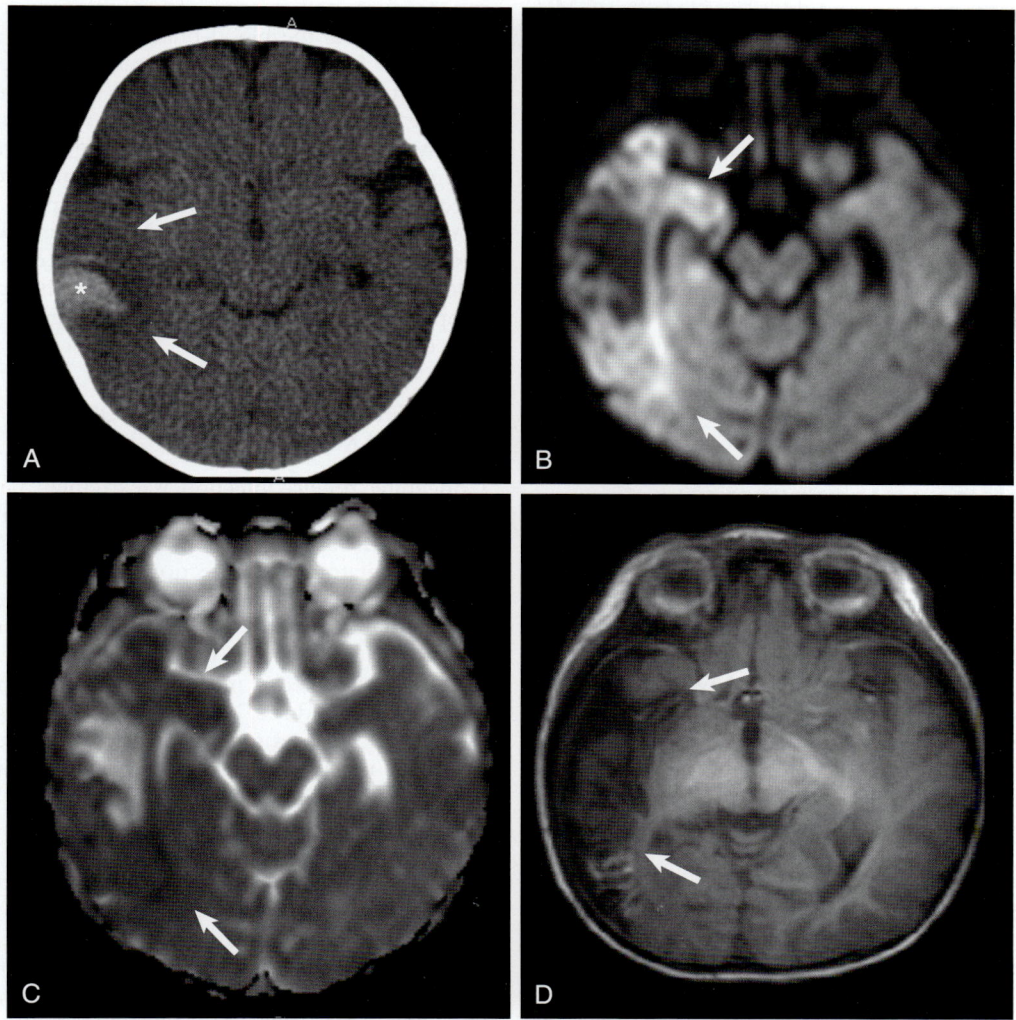

Figure 30-8 Herpes encephalitis. **A,** A noncontrast computed tomography (CT) image showing a large area of parenchymal edema in the right temporal lobe (*arrows*). A peripheral area of increased attenuation (*) represents confluent petechial hemorrhages. A subsequent magnetic resonance image demonstrates restricted diffusion on diffusion-weighted imaging (**B**) and low apparent diffusion coefficient values (*arrows*) (**C**). Of note, the medial temporal lobe, mainly the hippocampus, is usually spared in middle cerebral artery infarcts but is commonly involved in persons with herpes encephalitis. **D,** Thirty days after the first CT scan, encephalomalacia of the involved area is seen (*arrows*).

without restricted water diffusivity (e-Fig. 30-9). This pattern of injury easily may be misinterpreted as white matter injury of prematurity or as being caused by hypoxic–ischemic injury, particularly the partial prolonged type.[10]

CONGENITAL CYTOMEGALOVIRUS INFECTION

CMV is the most common congenital viral infection in the United States. Between 30% and 50% of women of child-bearing age in the United States have never been infected with CMV, and about 1% to 4% have a primary CMV infection during a pregnancy. The transmission rate to the fetus is about 33%. More than 5000 children each year experience permanent problems caused by CMV infection in the United States. Maternal antibodies, which protect the fetus from rubella and toxoplasmosis, do not prevent fetal transmission of CMV, but they do lessen the severity of the disease. Chorioretinitis occurs in 15% to 20% of cases. Diagnosis of CMV infection in the newborn is usually made via a urine culture. No cure exists for CMV infection. Treatment is primarily supportive.

The brain is the most commonly affected organ. CMV interferes with normal fetal brain development and is associated long-term with mental retardation, blindness, deafness, or epilepsy. Depending on the timing of infection during fetal development, neonates with congenital CMV may have microcephaly, predominately periventricular calcifications, ventriculomegaly, lissencephaly, polymicrogyria, cerebellar hypoplasia, dysplastic white matter, and porencephaly.[11] Other findings include intrauterine growth restriction, hepatosplenomegaly, cardiomyopathy, echogenic bowel, and hydrops. CT can detect and characterize diminutive periventricular and subependymal calcifications. CMV is also the leading infectious cause of sensorineural hearing loss; CT may demonstrate a Mondini malformation with an absent interscalar septum, a large vestibule, and an enlarged vestibular aqueduct.

CONGENITAL TOXOPLASMOSIS INFECTION

It is estimated that 400 to 4000 cases of congenital toxoplasmosis occur each year in the United States. In the first trimester, maternal infection is less likely to result in congenital infection (2% to 10%), but when it occurs, it is more likely to be severe or to result in abortion. Severe congenital toxoplasmosis meningoencephalitis is associated with intrauterine growth restriction, hydrocephalus, microcephaly, calcifications, porencephaly, or hydranencephaly. Maternal infection after 20 weeks of gestation has a much higher rate of transmission to the fetus (20% to 30%). The sequelae are generally less severe but still include blindness, epilepsy, and mental retardation.

Although the neurologic outcome is good in the absence of brain abnormalities, congenital toxoplasmosis may be unrecognized until late in infancy when infants present with seizures or other neurologic symptoms. Nonshadowing cerebral and hepatic calcifications are the most typical ultrasound findings. Intracranial calcifications may be periventricular or random in distribution. Other less specific imaging findings are subependymal cysts, echogenic lenticulostriate and thalamostriate arteries (candlestick sign), and cystic white matter changes. CT is sensitive for the detection and characterization

of cerebral calcifications and may demonstrate hydrocephalus and microcephaly. The ocular calcifications seen on CT may mimic retinoblastoma. Because of its high sensitivity and absence of ionizing radiation, MRI may be used serially throughout pregnancy to evaluate for the development of brain abnormalities. Acutely, the fetal brain abnormality consists of white matter signal abnormality such as loss of the intermediate zone layer in young fetuses. In fetuses with advanced gestational age, cystic lesions with a mural nodule are characteristic; however, MRI is not sensitive for small calcifications. After birth, calcifications, variable degrees of white matter dysplasia and gliosis, and cortical malformations all may be detected on MRI.

CONGENITAL HIV INFECTION

HIV transmission to the fetus or neonate occurs in utero, intrapartum, or postpartum via breast milk. Without treatment, about 30% of pregnant women with HIV pass the infection to their fetus. Intrapartum treatment with protease inhibitors, elective caesarean section, and avoiding breastfeeding decreases the transmission to the fetus to less than 2%. HIV penetrates the blood-brain barrier via macrophages (the so-called "Trojan horse") very early in the course of disease and incites a subacute encephalitis with perivascular mononuclear inflammatory cell infiltration. Neuroimaging findings usually are normal in neonates with HIV. The onset of neurologic decline generally occurs between 2 months to 5 years. Atrophy, delayed myelination, corticospinal tract degeneration, cervical lymphadenopathy, benign lymphoepithelial cysts in the parotid glands, aneurysms, opportunistic infections, progressive multifocal leukoencephalopathy, and CNS lymphoma are all associated late findings of congenital HIV infection.

CONGENITAL RUBELLA INFECTION (GERMAN MEASLES)

Congenital rubella infection is extremely rare as a result of vaccination and screening of pregnant women. The most common manifestation is rash, fever, and symptoms of an upper respiratory tract infection. Most people are exposed to rubella during childhood and develop antibodies to the virus and thus are immune. Rubella infection during early pregnancy can pass through the placenta to the fetus and cause serious birth defects, including heart abnormalities, mental retardation, blindness, and deafness. Imaging usually shows nonspecific findings such as microcephaly, ventriculomegaly, abnormal myelination, and calcifications, particularly of the basal ganglia.

CONGENITAL SYPHILIS INFECTION

Syphilis is a sexually transmitted bacterial infection that can be transferred from mother to fetus through the placenta. It is estimated that in up to 50% of cases of congenital syphilis, the neonate is born prematurely, is stillborn, or dies shortly after birth. Nevertheless, congenital syphilis rarely manifests with neurologic symptoms in the neonatal period. Only a few patients present with meningitis, choroiditis, hydrocephalus, or seizures. Severe ischemic-hemorrhagic lesions involving predominantly unilateral periventricular white matter, which are thought to be a result of endarteritis, have been reported in neonates. Other findings of congenital syphilis are generalized lymphadenopathy, hepatosplenomegaly, jaundice, and rash. The findings of CNS syphilis, such as leptomeningeal enhancement (particularly involving the basal meninges) and intraparenchymal mass (gumma), as well as frontal bossing, saddle nose deformity, mulberry molars, peglike upper frontal incisor, and saber shin, typically are observed later in infancy or childhood.

CONGENITAL VARICELLA INFECTION

The incidence of congenital varicella syndrome after maternal varicella infection during the first two trimesters is <1%. As with CMV and toxoplasmosis, intrahepatic and intracranial calcifications are very common. Intrauterine encephalitis, cortical atrophy, and porencephaly have been reported in cases of congenital varicella infection before 20 weeks of gestational age. Other possible fetal abnormalities are polyhydramnios, limb hypoplasia, and contractures, as well as paradoxical diaphragmatic motion as a result of unilateral paralysis. Neonates may demonstrate dysfunction of the autonomic nervous system (neurogenic bladder), hydroureter, esophageal dilation, aspiration pneumonia, and cutaneous lesions in a dermatomal distribution.[12]

CONGENITAL LYMPHOCYTIC CHORIOMENINGITIS VIRUS

Lymphocytic choriomeningitis virus (LCMV) primarily infects rodents, but it also can infect humans through inhalation of aerosolized particles of rodent urine, feces, or saliva; through ingestion of contaminated food; or through direct contact of open wounds to virus-infected blood. Human-to-human transmission may occur via the placenta or through solid-organ transplantation. The disease is usually mild in healthy individuals, but it may cause serious consequences to immunosuppressed persons and pregnant women. Miscarriage, birth defects, and long-term neurologic problems may result from congenital LCMV. LCMV causes chorioretinitis, ependymitis with ependymal calcifications, polymicrogyria, and microcephaly or hydrocephalus. These findings are similar to those of congenital toxoplasmosis and CMV; however, hepatosplenomegaly usually is not present in persons with LCMV.

Acquired Metabolic Disorders

KERNICTERUS (BILIRUBIN ENCEPHALOPATHY)

Kernicterus is caused by markedly elevated or sustained unconjugated hyperbilirubinemia. Kernicterus usually develops in the first week of life; however, it may occur as late as the third week. Severe hemolytic conditions, especially Rh hemolytic disease with hydrops fetalis, are the most common causes. Other risk factors include prematurity, polycythemia, resolving hematomas, sulphonamide (co-trimoxazole) administration, G6PD deficiency, and Crigler-Najjar and Gilbert syndromes. Although risk factors are usually present, kernicterus has been reported in otherwise healthy babies. Acutely, kernicterus manifests as lethargy, decreased feeding, hypotonia or hypertonia, a high-pitched cry, spasmodic torticollis, opisthotonus, the setting sun sign, fever, seizures, and even death. In severe cases, kernicterus results in a tetrad of movement disorder, auditory dysfunction, oculomotor impairments, and dental enamel hypoplasia of the deciduous teeth. Persons with mild cases are still at risk for isolated hearing loss or some degree of neurologic, cognitive, learning, and movement disorders.

Pathologically, kernicterus causes damage to the globi pallidi, subthalamic nuclei, and hippocampi (CA2 and CA3 regions). Ultrasound and CT are not sensitive in detecting early abnormalities in persons with kernicterus. On MRI, an increased signal initially is seen on T1-weighted images; this signal is inconsistent. Increased signal on T2-weighted images of affected areas develops later (Fig. 30-10), when hyperechogenicity may appear on ultrasound and hypoattenuation may appear on CT.[13] Restricted diffusion usually is not seen in persons with kernicterus unless it is associated with other conditions, such as hypoxia-ischemia. Conventional T1 spin echo images appear to be more reliable than 3D T1 spoiled gradient echo images, because the latter are associated with a high signal in normal subthalamic nuclei, which may cause false-positive results. A metabolite signature of acute

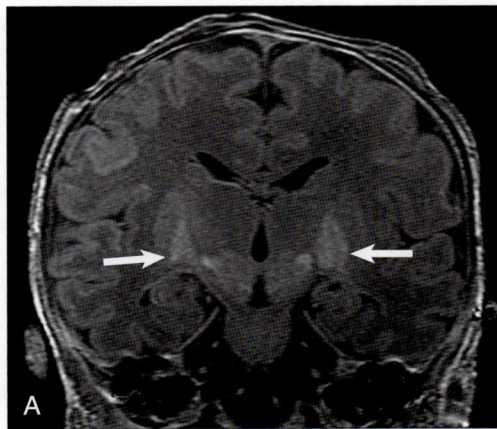
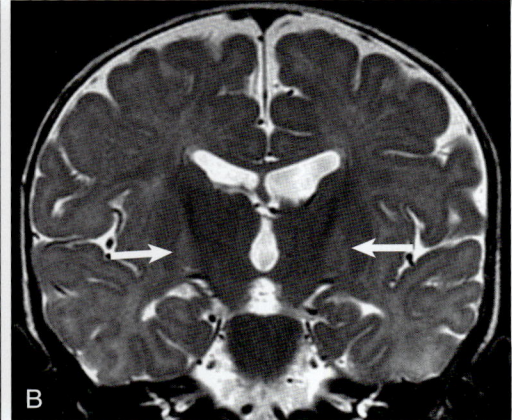

Figure 30-10 Kernicterus. **A,** An increased T1 signal is seen in the globi pallidi (*arrows*) at 1 week of age. **B,** An increased T2 signal (*arrows*) is seen 1 month later.

kernicterus has been proposed on MRS using an echo time of 35 ms with elevated ratios of taurine, glutamate, glutamine, and myo-inositol and a decreased ratio of choline relative to creatine with no significant elevation of lactate.

HYPOGLYCEMIA

Neonatal encephalopathy resulting from hypoglycemia typically occurs when glucose concentrations are less than 30 mg/dL in the term infant and less than 20 mg/dL in the preterm infant. The clinical presentation of neonatal hypoglycemia may be subtle, including stupor, jitteriness, seizures, respiratory abnormalities, and hypotonia. MRI is the imaging modality of choice, showing abnormalities in the posterior parietal and occipital cortex and adjacent white matter. Acutely, there is restricted diffusion on DWI as well as edema on T1- and T2-weighted imaging. MRS with an echo time of 30 ms exhibits an increased lactate-lipid peak and a decreased NAA peak in the involved areas. In the chronic phase, the involved areas evolve into encephalomalacia and atrophy. If the hypoglycemia is severe and prolonged, progression to diffuse brain damage occurs with involvement of the hippocampus, corpus striatum, and cerebellum.[14]

Inborn Errors of Metabolism

Inborn errors of metabolism present with signs and symptoms related to the involvement of one or more of the organ systems, including the CNS. Inborn errors of metabolism are classified into organic acidemia, disorders of amino acid oxidation, disorders of fatty acid oxidation, primary lactic acidosis, mitochondria function, lysosomal storage disorders, and peroxisome disorders (also see Chapter 33). Whereas some inborn errors of metabolism manifest immediately at birth (e.g., primary lactic acidosis, type 2 glutaric aciduria, long-chain acyl coenzyme A dehydrogenase, hydroxymethylglutaryl-CoA lyase, ornithine transcarbamylase, and carbamyl phosphatase synthetase deficiencies), in others, it takes a few days for signs and symptoms to develop (e.g., isovaleric acidemia, methylmalonic acidemia, propionic acidemia, nonketotic hyperglycinemia, citrullinemia, argininosuccinic aciduria, and maple syrup urine disease).

The inborn errors of metabolism that affect the nervous system exclusively (namely l-2-hydroxyglutaric aciduria, glutaric aciduria type 1, 4-hydroxybutyric aciduria, alphaketoglutaric aciduria, mevalonic aciduria, and N-acetylaspartic aciduria [Canavan disease]) present later in life and are not encountered in neonates. MRS can provide valuable information regarding specific metabolites in certain neonatal metabolic disorders: increased branched-chain amino acids (e.g., l-leucine, l-isoleucine, and valine) in persons with maple syrup urine disease, increased glycine in persons with nonketotic hyperglycinemia, and absence of creatine in persons with guanidinoacetate methyltransferase deficiency (also see Chapter 25).

ORGANIC ACID DISORDERS

Methylmalonic acidemia and proprionic aciduria are examples of organic acid disorders. These disorders cause ketoacidosis, often leading to severe acidosis, vomiting, tachycardia,

lethargy, seizures, coma, and death. In these disorders, edema is present in both myelinated and unmyelinated structures. The edema involving the myelinated white matter is related to vacuolating or spongiform myelinopathy, which acutely demonstrates restricted water diffusivity because the water is trapped within vacuoles. Findings on conventional imaging include edema with increased T2 signal and decreased T1 signal involving the white matter. In more severe cases, the deep gray structures may be involved, with a predilection for the globi pallidi in persons with methylmalonic acidemia and for the putamina and caudate nuclei in persons with proprionic aciduria. MRS detects a reduction in myo-inositol and NAA and an elevation of glutamine. Elevation of lactate as a result of hyperammonia, ketoacidosis, and/or mitochondrial dysfunction also may be present during an acute metabolic crisis.

AMINO ACID DISORDERS

Maple syrup urine disease results from an interruption of the metabolism of the essential amino acids leucine, isoleucine, and/or valine. The most severe form manifests in the first week of life with seizures, vomiting, dystonia, fluctuating ophthalmoplegia, and coma. The imaging findings are almost pathognomonic. Conventional MR shows edema in the deep cerebellar white matter, brainstem tegmentum, posterior limb of the internal capsule, perirolandic white matter, and precentral and postcentral gyrus. Restricted water diffusivity is seen acutely in the areas of vacuolating edema in the myelinated white matter. MRS shows a peak at 0.9 parts per million (ppm) related to the accumulation of abnormal branched-chain amino acids and branched-chain apha-ketoacids. The imaging findings by diffusion imaging and MRS may resolve with treatment.[15]

UREA CYCLE DISORDERS

Urea cycle enzyme defects include ornithine carbamyl transferase deficiency, carbamyl phosphate synthetase deficiency, argininosuccinic aciduria, citrullinemia, and hyperargininemia, resulting in hyperammonemia and elevation of glutamate. Cases with severe impairment of elimination of nitrogen waste products manifest as irritability, lethargy, poor feeding, hypothermia, and seizures during the neonatal period.

Imaging in the acute phase shows markedly diffuse vasogenic edema, predominantly in the unmyelinated white matter, with early involvement of the subcortical U fibers and relative preservation of the myelinated white matter. The underlying pathophysiology of the urea cycle defects is related to vasogenic edema, in contrast to vacuolating myelinopathy in persons with maple syrup urine disease. As a result, the mean diffusivity maps in the urea cycle defect will show increased signal intensity in the unmyelinated white matter. In some cases, the lentiform nuclei (particularly the globi pallidi), the posterior insular cortex, and the perirolandic cortex also may be involved with increased T1 signal. This presentation causes some overlap between the conventional imaging findings of urea cycle disorders and hypoxic-ischemic injury. However, involvement of the globi pallidi and putamina in urea cycle disorders is predominant as opposed to thalami in cases of hypoxia-ischemia. MRS in patients with urea cycle defects typically demonstrates increased levels of glutamate and glutamine and decreased levels of myo-inositol, NAA, choline, and creatine.

NONKETOTIC HYPERGLYCINEMIA

Nonketotic hyperglycinemia is caused by a defect of the glycine cleavage system, which is present in the liver, kidney, and brain, leading to the accumulation of glycine in blood, urine, and CSF. The diagnosis is established by calculating the CSF/plasma glycine concentration ratio. A value of greater than 0.08 is diagnostic. Confirmation of the diagnosis requires measurement of the activity of the glycine cleavage system in liver tissue. The neonatal (classic) form of nonketotic hyperglycinemia is far more common than the infantile, late-onset, or transient phenotypes. The neonatal form presents in the first days of life with encephalopathy, hypotonia, lethargy, seizures, and characteristic hiccups, which can progress rapidly to intractable seizures, coma, and respiratory failure. The outcome is invariably poor.

On MRI, abnormal myelination and a hypoplastic or dysgenic corpus callosum are seen, which progresses to diffuse cerebral atrophy. Increased T2 signal and restricted water diffusivity involving the myelinated portion of the posterior limb of the internal capsules, pyramidal tracts, middle cerebellar pedicles, and dentate nuclei have been reported. The underdevelopment of the corpus callosum is difficult to assess in the neonate because of its small size and lack of myelin, but it becomes evident later. Atrophy and delayed myelination also are common findings in other metabolic disorders, particularly in organic acidurias. MRS exhibits a large glycine peak at 3.55 ppm.

PEROXISOMAL DISORDERS

Peroxisomal disorders that manifest in the neonate are primarily a result of the failure to form viable peroxisomes (peroxisomal biogenesis disorders), resulting in multiple metabolic abnormalities. Zellweger syndrome and neonatal adrenoleukodystrophy are the most common peroxisomal disorders in the neonate, and both have pathognomonic findings on conventional MRI. Zellweger syndrome is characterized by delayed myelination, temporal and parietal polymicrogyria, and subependymal germolytic cysts adjacent to the frontal horns of the lateral ventricles. In contrast to Zellweger syndrome, neonatal adrenoleukodystrophy causes dysmyelination, mainly involving the occipital lobes, the splenium of the corpus callosum, and/or the cerebellum. Often these lesions demonstrate restricted water diffusion and peripheral enhancement. MRS in persons with Zellweger syndrome is not specific, showing a marked decrease in NAA levels in the gray and white matter, thalamus, and/or cerebellum, a decreased myo-inositol level in the gray matter if concomitant hepatic dysfunction is present, and in some cases, elevated glutamine levels.

MOLYBDENUM COFACTOR DEFICIENCY

Molybdenum cofactor deficiency is a rare, usually underrecognized, autosomal-recessive disorder caused by genetic mutation of the genes that produce enzymes essential for the formation of molybdenum cofactor. The absence of molybdenum cofactor leads to toxic levels of sulphite, which may be detected by hypouricemia, elevated urine sulfate, and elevated S-sulfocysteine. Clinically, molybdenum cofactor deficiency manifests in the first few days of life with seizures and encephalopathy and usually leads to death within months. Imaging shows edema and cystic changes involving predominantly the basal ganglia and severe volume loss of the gray and white matter. Reduced water diffusivity may be present in the affected areas.

MITOCHONDRIAL DISORDERS

Mitochondrial disorders are a group of diseases caused by enzymatic defects leading to primary lactic acidosis and decreased ATP production. Pyruvate transcarboxylase, pyruvate dehydrogenase, and cytochrome c oxidase deficiencies are the most common enzymatic defects leading to primary lactic acidosis in the neonatal period. MRI is the imaging modality of choice for its capability to detect areas of reduced water diffusivity and the presence of lactate typically associated with these disorders. Characteristically, areas of increased T2 signal and reduced water diffusivity are found in the brainstem, the subthalamic nucleus, and the globus pallidum. MRS detects elevated lactate levels in the areas with abnormal signal, as well as in the normal-appearing brain. It should be noted, however, that elevated lactate is not always indicative of a mitochondrial disorder, and nondetectable lactate levels do not preclude the possibility of a mitochondrial disorder. Sometimes specific peaks can be detected—for example, elevated succinate peak at 2.4 ppm in persons with succinate dehydrogenase deficiency and an elevated pyruvate peak at 2.36 ppm in persons with pyruvate dehydrogenase complex deficiency.

Key Points

MRI is the imaging modality with the highest sensitivity for differentiating abnormalities from normal brain.

The central pattern of HIE usually occurs with profound asphyxia, when an abrupt interruption of the blood supply occurs, depriving the neonatal brain of oxygen and glucose. The peripheral pattern of HIE usually results from a period of decreased blood supply to the brain.

Arterial infarctions are more common in term than in preterm neonates, and most frequently involve the middle cerebral artery and its branches.

Birth trauma is more common in vaginal delivery, particularly if forceps or vacuum extraction is used.

Small subdural hematomas are seen in up to 30% of vaginal births.

The most common bacterial neonatal brain infections are caused by group B streptococcus, *Escherichia coli*, *Streptococcus pneumoniae*, *Haemophilus influenzae* type B, and *Listeria monocytogenes*.

Continued

Kernicterus is caused by markedly elevated or sustained unconjugated hyperbilirubinemia.

Neonatal encephalopathy resulting from hypoglycemia typically occurs when glucose concentrations are less than 30 mg/dL in the term infant and less than 20 mg/dL in the preterm infant.

Inborn errors of metabolism are classified into organic acidemia, disorders of amino acid oxidation, disorders of fatty acid oxidation, primary lactic acidosis, mitochondria function, lysosomal storage disorders, and peroxisomal disorders.

Suggested Readings

Barkovich AJ. MR imaging of the neonatal brain. *Neuroimaging Clin N Am.* 2006;16(1):117-135, viii-ix.

Barkovich AJ. *Pediatric neuroradiology.* 5th ed. Philadelphia: Lippincott Williams & Wilkins; 2012.

Huang BY, Castillo M. Hypoxic-ischemic brain injury: imaging findings from birth to adulthood. *Radiographics.* 2008;28(2):417-439, quiz 617.

Rutherford MA. MRI of the neonatal brain (website): www.mrineonatalbrain.com. Accessed October 19, 2012.

Volpe JJ. The encephalopathy of prematurity—brain injury and impaired brain development inextricably intertwined. *Semin Pediatr Neurol.* 2009;16(4):167-178.

References

Full references for this chapter can be found on www.expertconsult.com.

Chapter 31

Congenital Brain Malformations

NANCY ROLLINS

With advances in magnetic resonance imaging (MRI) and molecular biology and the availability of mutant mouse models of human cortical malformations, many malformations of brain development have been reclassified.[1-3] Given the large number of congenital human brain malformations, the complexity of the molecular genetics, and the degree of anatomic variability, an in-depth discussion of some malformations is beyond the scope of this chapter. This chapter addresses malformations seen most often in clinical practice and those malformations that are less common but are distinctive and have a profound impact of early childhood development. The malformations presented here are grouped according to presumed dominant defect in embryologic or fetal development. Diffusion tensor imaging (DTI) is included in the diagnosis of malformations in which aberrant white matter tracts are a dominant feature.

A rudimentary description of relevant embryology is needed. Around 26 to 28 days after conception, the process of neurulation, in which the lateral edges of the neural plate elevate into neural folds, takes place.[1] The folds then fuse medially to form the neural tube. At the cranial end of the neural tube, the primitive brain vesicles form and include the prosencephalon, mesencephalon, and rhombencephalon.[1,2,4] The prosencephalon divides into the *telencephalon*, which gives rise to the cerebral hemispheres and the corpus striatum, and the *diencephalon*, which gives rise to the thalami and the hypothalamus. The cerebral peduncles and midbrain arise from the mesenchephalon. The rhombencephalon gives rise to the *metencephalon*, which forms the pons and cerebellum, and the *myelencephalon*, from which the medulla arises. Malformations of brain development may result from chromosomal aberrations, single gene mutations, teratogenic infections and agents, or ischemia.[1,3] However, in 70% of malformations, the etiology is identifiable.

Defects of Neurulation

CEPHALOCELES

Complete failure of closure of the cranial end of the neuropore results in *anencephaly*, in which the forebrain, skull, and scalp are absent. Affected patients die soon after birth and postnatal imaging is not usually indicated. Less severe disorders of neural tube closure result in meningoceles and encephaloceles, which are protrusions of the meninges or brain, respectively, through a congenital defect of the skull and dura; the latter occurs in about 1 per 5000 live births.[4] Encephaloceles tend to be midline. In the countries of the Western hemisphere, a predominance of posterior cephaloceles is seen, whereas in Asian children, encephaloceles tend to be anterior.[1] Frontal encephaloceles include interorbital frontal, nasofrontal, nasoethmoidal, and naso-orbital lesions. Interorbital frontal encephaloceles protrude through a defect in frontal bone (Fig. 31-1). Nasofrontal encephaloceles involve the region of nasal bridge, the floor of the anterior cranial fossa, or both (Fig. 31-2). Nasofrontal encephaloceles are also referred to as *nasal gliomas*, although they are not neoplastic. These masses of neuroglial tissue are categorized as *extranasal* (60%), *intranasal* (30%), or *mixed* (10%).[1,2,4] When telangiectasias occur on the skin overlaying an external nasal glioma, the lesion may be mistaken for a hemangioma. Often, hypertelorism is present with a broad nasal bridge. Intranasal glioma presents as an intranasal mass; biopsy should be avoided prior to imaging because of the risk of meningitis. With nasoethmoidal encephaloceles, frontal bone is intact. Neural tissue bulges into the ethmoid sinus through a defect in the floor of the anterior cranial fossa, and the nasal septum defines the posterior margin. A defect in the medial orbital wall results in a naso-orbital encephalocele, which protrudes into the orbit and produces unilateral exophthalmos. Other facial anomalies seen with anterior encephaloceles include a bifid nasal tip or complete midline splitting of the nose in an uncommon malformation known as *frontonasal dysplasia* (e-Fig. 31-3). Morning Glory syndrome includes midline facial defects, callosal agenesis, frontal encephaloceles, and characteristic eye anomalies.

Basal encephaloceles result from defects in the sphenoid bone (Fig. 31-4); the encephalocele herniates into the posterior nasopharynx anterior to the dorsum sella and may contain pituitary tissue, optic nerves, branches of the circle of Willis, or all (Fig. 31-5). Encephaloceles in the parietal bone range from large deforming "towering" lesions to small meningoceles (Fig. 31-6). Atretic encephaloceles or meningoceles present as small subcutaneous fibrofatty masses, which are often painful to palpation (Fig. 31-7). Occipital encephaloceles usually contain dysplastic cerebellar tissue alone or with the cerebral cortex (Fig. 31-8). Rarely, the brainstem may be within the encephalocele; this malformation is lethal.

Conditions and syndromes associated with encephaloceles include trisomy 13 and 18, amniotic band syndrome, Meckel-Gruber syndrome, dyssegmental dwarfism, Knobloch syndrome, Walker-Warburg (type II lissencephaly) syndrome, cryptophthalmos, and Voss syndrome. The prognosis depends

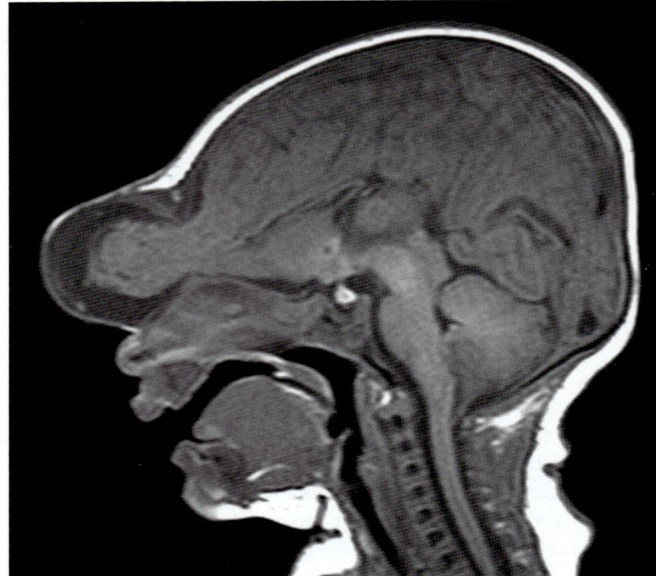

Figure 31-1   Frontal encephalocele. A sagittal T1 image shows agenesis of the corpus callosum associated with encephalocele at the glabella.

on the severity of associated brain anomalies and the amount of dysplastic brain contained within the encephalocele.[1,2,4]

Imaging   High-resolution MRI is performed soon after birth to define contents of the encephalocele, the severity of the malformation, and the frequent associated anomalies. These include callosal agenesis, anomalies of cortical formation, and variable anomalies of the cerebellum, diencephalon, and brainstem. Although dysplastic nonfunctional neural tissue is usually resected during closure of the encephalocele, major dural venous sinuses are preserved. Therefore, magnetic resonance venography is essential for diagnosing large occipital and midline parietal encephaloceles that may contain dural venous sinuses. Basal encephaloceles containing optic chiasm or nerves or pituitary tissue cannot be closed without

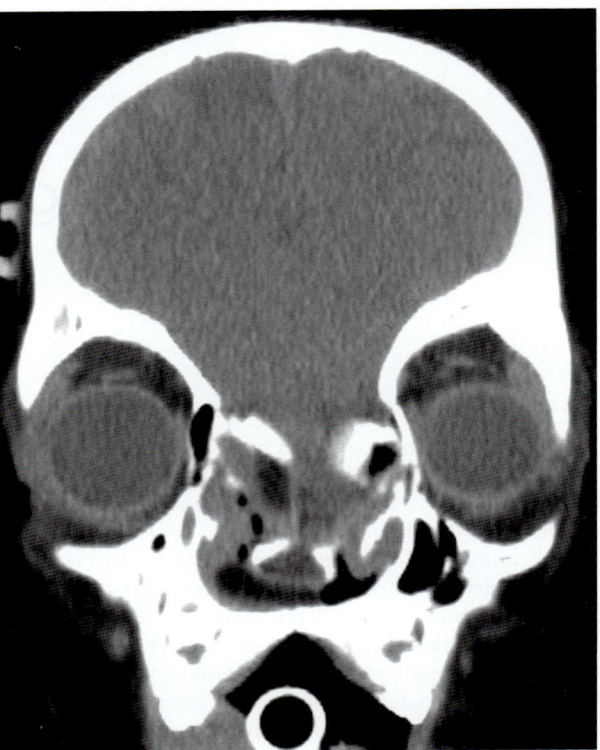

Figure 31-4   Basal encephalocele. A coronal reformatted computed tomography image shows the floor of the anterior cranial fossa is deficient, the nasal turbinates are disorganized, and marked hypertelorism exists.

sacrificing these structures. Affected patients are at risk for meningitis and cerebrospinal fluid (CSF) leakage into the nasophayrnx. The typical intracranial manifestations of atretic parietal encephaloceles include posterior tenting of the tectal plate, a persistent falcine sinus with or without atresia of the straight sinus, and expansion of posterior interhemispheric CSF. Hydrocephalus is common after closure of large parietal and occipital encephaloceles.

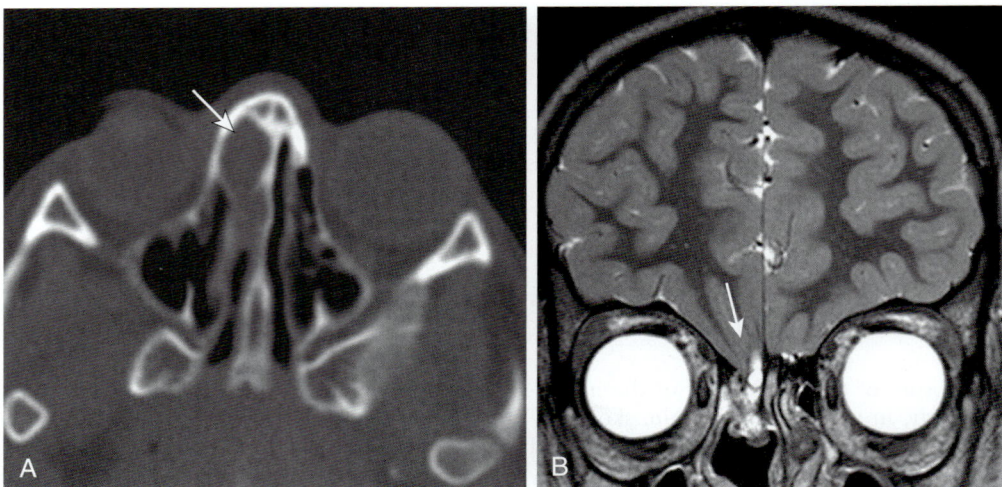

Figure 31-2   Incidental nasofrontal encephalocele found on head computed tomography done for trauma. **A,** Axial computed tomography shows a focally expansile lesion within the right ethmoid sinus (*arrow*). **B,** A high-resolution coronal T2 image shows the clinically occult defect in the right cribriform plate through which has herniated the frontal cortex (*arrow*).

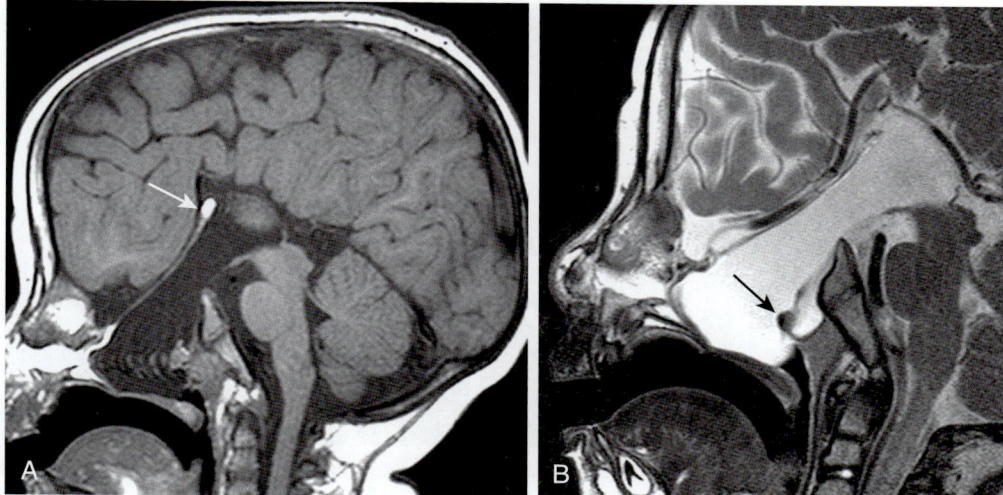

Figure 31-5 Basal encephalocele. **A,** A sagittal T1-weighted image shows callosal agenesis with a tiny lipoma (*arrow*). A large defect in the basisphenoid is seen. Note the apparent absence of the pituitary, floor of the third ventricle, and optic pathways. **B,** A high-resolution sagittal T2-weighted image shows the pituitary-hypothalamic structures (*arrow*) and optic pathways are contained within the encephalocele.

CHIARI II MALFORMATIONS

Clinical Presentation Chiari II malformations are the intracranial manifestations of posterior dysraphic defects such as myelomeningoceles. Neural tube defects have been reported with multiple chromosomal abnormalities, including trisomies 18, 13, and 9; triploidy; unbalanced translocations and deletions; and in Turner, DiGeorge, and velocardiofacial syndromes. The genes in the region of 22q11 have been implicated in the development of neural tube defects, although neural tube defects and the associated Chiari II malformation are probably caused by a combination of genetic polymorphisms and environmental factors, including dietary folate intake and maternal folate metabolism.[5]

The most commonly accepted unifying theory for the Chiari II malformation suggests that the failure of neural tube closure prevents the transient closure of the central canal, which is essential for the distension of the primitive ventricular system;[6] this results in the premature fusion of the mesenchymal components that form the calvarium, whereas the hindbrain manifestations result from leakage of CSF through the neural tube defect. The Chiari II malformation is associated with a wide range of brain malformations;[1,2,7,8] DTI shows disordered axonal migration, suggesting that the malformation is not explained by mechanical alterations caused by faulty CSF dynamics alone.[8] The Chiari II malformation is characterized by mesodermal dysplasia, small and dysplastic lower cranial nerve ganglia, deficient tentorium cerebelli,

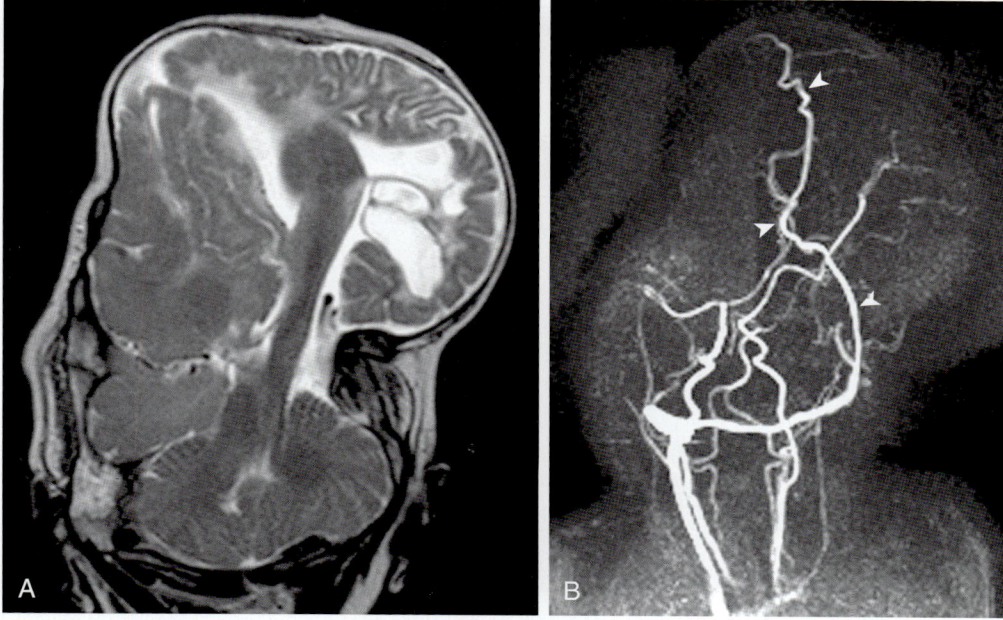

Figure 31-6 Parietal encephalocele. **A,** A coronal T2-weighted image shows extremely dysmorphic hemisphere and diencephalic structures contained within the massive parietal encephalocele. **B,** Coronal maximum-intensity projection from two-dimensional magnetic resonance venogram shows dysplastic dural sinuses (*arrowheads*) contained within the encephalocele.

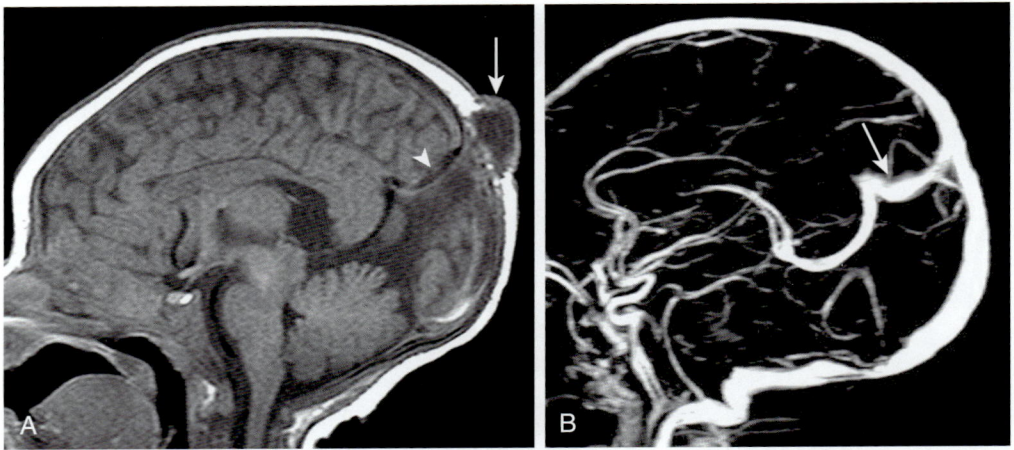

Figure 31-7 Atretic parietal meningocele. **A,** A sagittal T1-weighted image shows the small meningocele (*arrow*) over the parietal vertex. Focal expansion of the posterior interhemispheric subarachnoid space is shown (*arrowhead*). **B,** A sagittal image from a gadolinium-enhanced magnetic resonance venogram shows a persistent falcine sinus (*arrow*) draining the deep medullary venous system; no straight sinus is present.

hypoplastic and dysmorphic cerebellum, and thickened basal meninges.[6] As in holoprosencephaly (HPE), these anomalies are attributable to a defective or deficient mesenchyme, which presumably deprives the skull base, hindbrain, and rhombencephalon of normal inductive effects.[7] Clinical problems related specifically to the malformed hindbrain include apnea, aspiration, feeding difficulties, and recurrent respiratory infections.

Imaging The calvarial manifestations of the Chiari II malformation include a bifid frontal bone and luckenschadel, or lacunar, skull. The latter is a manifestation of the mesodermal dysplasia of the membranous skull and is caused by nonossified fibrous bone in the inner and outer tables of the skull, resulting in the apparent cranial scalloping (Fig. 31-9); the affected cranium ossifies and appears normal by 6 months of age. Luckenschadel is not the result of increased intracranial pressure and is not synonymous with "the beaten copper skull."

The intracranial stigmata of the Chiari II malformation are complex and variable; the hallmarks of the malformation are infratentorial. In the most severe forms, the foramen magnum is enlarged and the posterior cranial fossa is constricted, with effacement of CSF spaces; the cerebellum wraps around the ventral aspect of the brainstem (see Fig. 31-9), and the clivus and petrous ridges are concave. MRI shows caudal displacement of a dysplastic brainstem and a hypoplastic cerebellum into the upper cervical canal with "kinking" of the cervicomedullary brainstem (Fig. 31-10). The fourth ventricle is effaced and caudally displaced. The torcula and transverse sinuses are low lying, which presents a potential surgical hazard during decompressive suboccipital craniectomy, which may be performed for relief of symptomatic hindbrain compression. A "beaked" tectal plate is present, and a variably thickened massa intermedia may be so thick that the thalami appear virtually fused with partial atresia of the third ventricle.[1,7] Common supratentorial abnormalities include callosal dysgenesis, neuronal migration anomalies, and hydrocephalus.

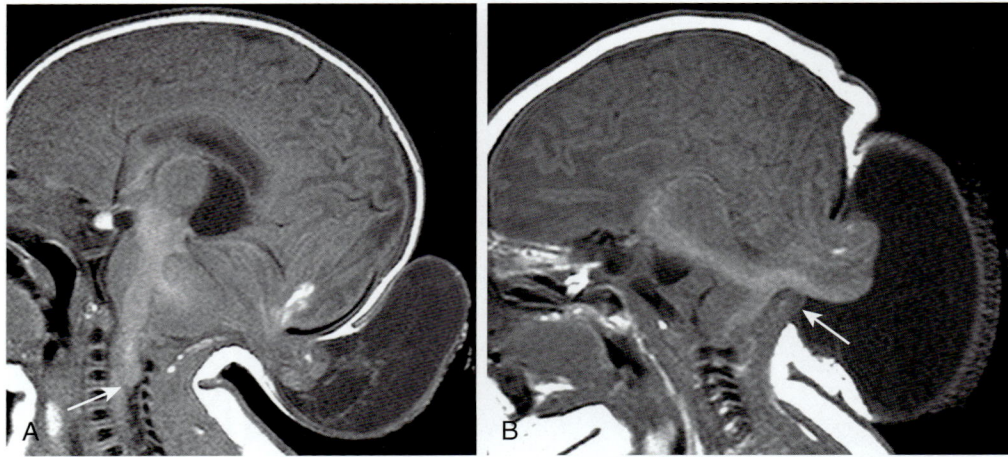

Figure 31-8 Occipital encephalocele. **A,** A sagittal T1-weighted image shows an occipital encephalocele containing cerebrospinal fluid and dysplastic cerebellum. A beaked tectal plate and kinking of the cervicomedullary brainstem (*arrow*), similar to that seen in the Chiari II malformation, are present. **B,** A sagittal T1-weighted image in a different patient shows a large cephalocele containing both cerebellar tissue and brainstem (*arrow*); the patient died after closure of the defect.

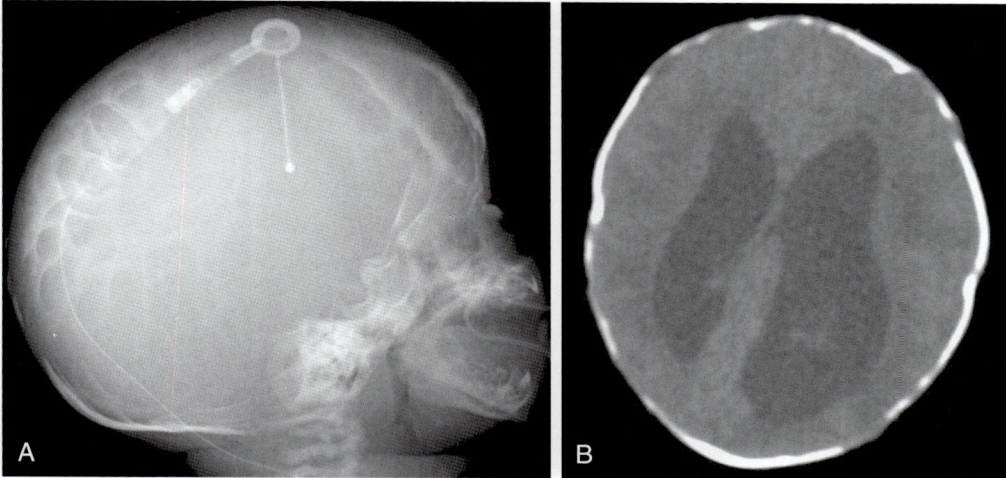

Figure 31-9 Luchenschadel. **A,** A skull radiograph shows a lacelike appearance to the cranium. **B,** Axial computed tomography shows scalloping of the inner and outer tables of the calvarium.

After ventricular shunt placement, the cerebral hemispheres drop away from the inner table of the skull, allowing interdigitations of the cortex across the midline under the hypoplastic falx and projection of the superior cerebellar vermis superiorly across a widened tentorial incisura. These findings are nonspecific manifestations seen after CSF diversion of severe congenital obstructive hydrocephalus. DTI of Chiari II malformations associated with more severe degrees of cerebellar hypoplasia shows absence of the dorsal transverse fibers at the level of the pons with preservation of the corticospinal tracts and mediolateral lemniscus fibers (Fig. 31-11). The cingulum may be anomalous, crossing the midline above the corpus callosum (Fig. 31-12). These alterations in axonal migration evident by DTI are difficult to appreciate with conventional MRI.

Chari III malformations are high cervical or low occipital encephaloceles.[9] The term *Chiari IV malformation* describes severe cerebellar hypoplasia in association with a neural tube defect. A better description of affected patients would be Chiari II malformation with cerebellar hypoplasia or aplasia (e-Fig. 31-13). Defects of neurulation have also been reported to coexist in patients with HPE; the latter malformation is considered a disorder of differentiation of the dorsal neural plate.[10,11] The coexistence of these malformations, traditionally considered disparate in embryologic timing and insult, may be explained, in part, by mutations in genes implicated in both developmental pathways.[12,13]

Disorders of Differentiation of Dorsal Neural Plate

HOLOPROSENCEPHALY

Clinical Presentation HPE is the most common anomaly affecting the ventral forebrain, resulting from a primary defect

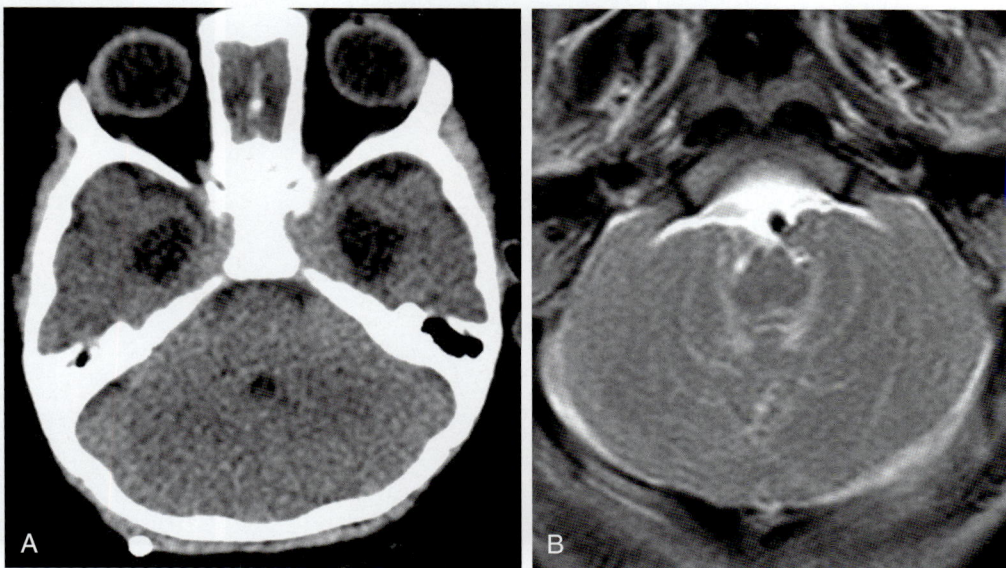

Figure 31-10 Chiari II malformation. **A,** Axial computed tomography showing a constricted posterior fossa, the fourth ventricle is small and low lying, and a paucity of cerebrospinal fluid exists. **B,** An axial T2-weighted image through the posterior fossa shows cerebellar tissue wrapping around the brainstem.

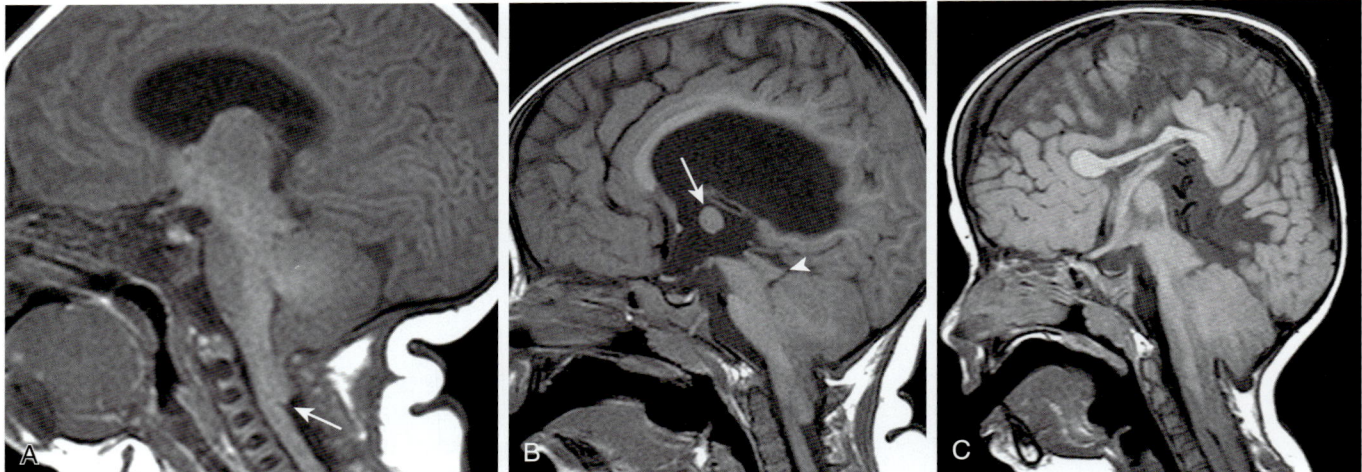

Figure 31-11 Chiari II malformation. **A,** A sagittal T1-weighted image shows a small cerebellum, the fourth ventricle caudally displaced, and a kink at the cervicomedullary junction (*arrow*). The brainstem is well-formed. **B,** A sagittal T1-weighted image in another patient shows that the cerebellum and brainstem are more hypoplastic and the tectal plate is distorted (*arrowhead*). Note the large massa intermedia (*arrow*) and hydrocephalus. **C,** Sagittal T1-weighted image in another patient shows the brainstem is hypoplastic with a beaked tectal plate. The cerebellum is dysplastic and caudally herniated. The fourth ventricle is inapparent.

in patterning and induction of the basal forebrain expressed around the fifth to sixth week of gestation, and occurs in 1 in 250 embryos and 1 in 8300 to 16,000 live births.[1,13,14] HPE is thought to be caused by a deficient or defective prechordal mesoderm, with failure of induction or abnormal fusion of normally paired and separate neo–cortex, caudates, and claustrum. The consequences of the inductive failure of the median and paramedian structures are most pronounced in the ventral forebrain and decline in severity from rostral to caudal and from medial to lateral. HPE is caused by a combination of genetic polymorphisms and environmental factors; the incidence of HPE is increased 200-fold in maternal diabetes mellitus. HPE is notable for its genetic heterogeneity. Mutations in single genes result in syndromic forms of HPE, triploidies of entire chromosomes (e.g., 13 and 18), deletions or duplications of regions of a chromosome, and copy number variants. At least 12 HPE loci that play some role in the midline of the developing nervous system have been

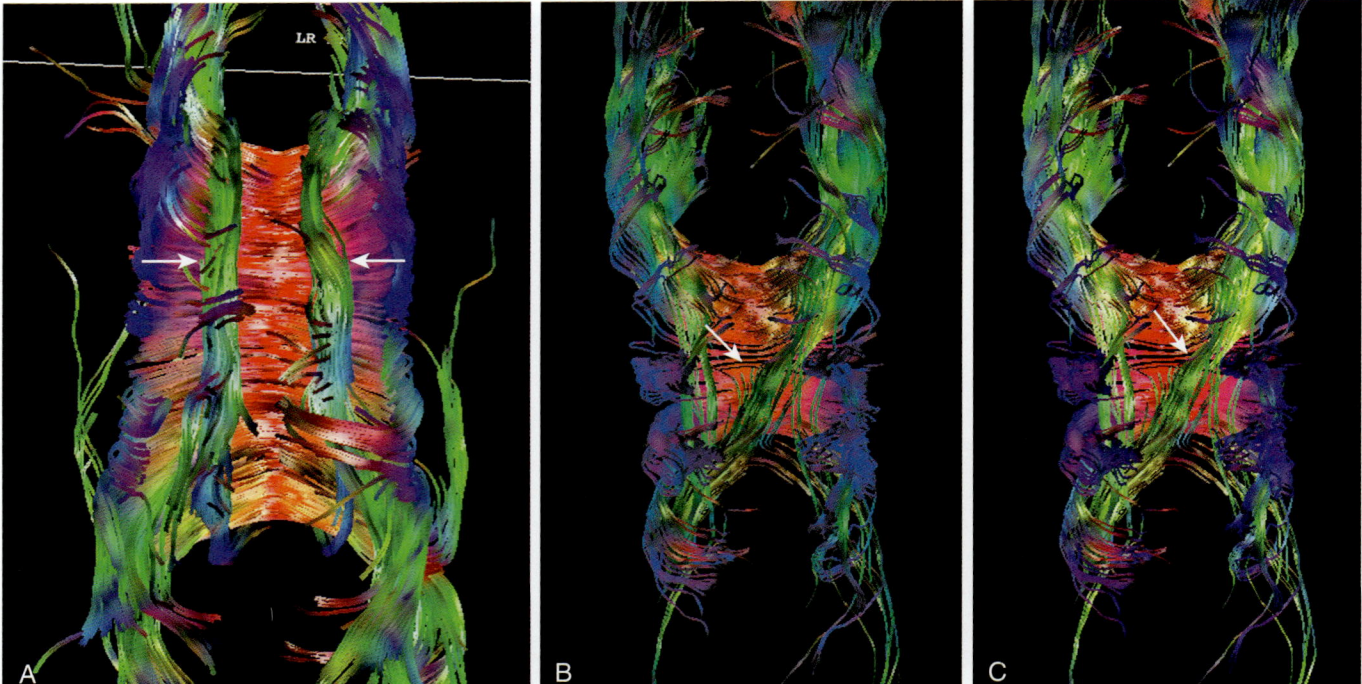

Figure 31-12 Diffusion tensor imaging in Chiari II malformation. **A,** Diffusion tractography from a normal patient shows paired cingula (*arrows*), which are association fibers of the outer limbic system, above the corpus callosum. The green orientation indicates the fibers are oriented back-to-front. By definition, association fibers do not cross the midline. **B,** In a patient with Chiari II malformation, diffusion tractography shows the left cingulum (*arrow*) is medially displaced. **C,** In another patient with Chiari II malformation, the right cingulum is absent, and the left cingulum (*arrow*) crosses the midline.

identified, including *Shh*, *Otx2*, *Emx*, *Pax*, *Nkx-2.2*, and some POU domain genes.[13] Although 24% to 45% of affected live-born individuals have chromosomal abnormalities, no known correlation exists between the type or severity of the holoprosencephalic defect and the specific mutation. In addition to controlling prosencephalic separation and differentiation, the inductive effects of the prechordal mesoderm also influence the corpus striatum, thalami, eyes, face, and cerebral vasculature.[13] The spectrum of associated facial anomalies range from flattening of the nasal bridge, hypotelorism without metopic synostosis, a single central maxillary incisor, cleft lip or palate to facial clefting, and cyclopia with a central proboscis.[15] More severe facial anomalies are seen with more severe variants of HPE, but mild facial anomalies may occur in the absence of brain anomalies. Clinical problems associated with HPE include developmental delay, seizures, hypothalamic and brainstem dysfunction with swallowing and respiratory problems, thermal instability, pituitary dysfunction, and erratic sleeping patterns.[13,15]

Imaging The hallmark of HPE is incomplete separation of the forebrain, absence of the anterior interhemispheric falx, and fusion of central gray nuclei. The septum pellucidum is absent. Considerable topographic variation exists in HPE, which is most often characterized as alobar, semilobar, or lobar.[13-19] The malformation represents a continuum, ranging from *overt hypotelorism*, with severe facial anomalies, to *mild hypotelorism*, with subtle fusion of basal forebrain and central gray nuclei. Hydrocephalus may be present.

ALOBAR HOLOPROSENCEPHALY

In this most severe form of HPE, separation between the cerebral hemispheres is completely lacking, with absence of the falx. The corpus callosum and septum pellucidum are absent, the central gray nuclei are fused, and the rudimentary single ventricle has a "U" configuration, which may communicate with a dorsal cyst (Fig. 31-14).[1,14,17]

SEMILOBAR HOLOPROSENCEPHALY

Relative preservation of the lateral and posterior cerebrum and the splenium exists in semilobar HPE. The posterior interhemispheric fissure and falx are present, whereas the hypoplastic frontal lobe is undivided. (Fig. 31-15).[1,13,16] Lack of formation of the frontal lobes results in an anterior position of the Sylvian fissures, termed a "wide Sylvian angle" by Barkovich et al.[17] The globus pallidi are absent or hypoplastic, and the caudate nuclei are fused, resulting in obliteration of or lack of formation of the septal region. The posterior limbs of the internal capsules are ventral to partially or totally fused thalami. The hippocampus is virtually always present, although usually incompletely or abnormally developed. A dorsal cyst may be present (e-Fig. 31-16).

LOBAR HOLOPROSENCEPHALY

In this mildest form of HPE, hypoplasia of the frontal poles is present, along with agenesis of the septal pellucidum and incomplete separation of the basal forebrain, which is best depicted with high-resolution coronal images. The posterior frontal, parietal, and occipital lobes are more normally

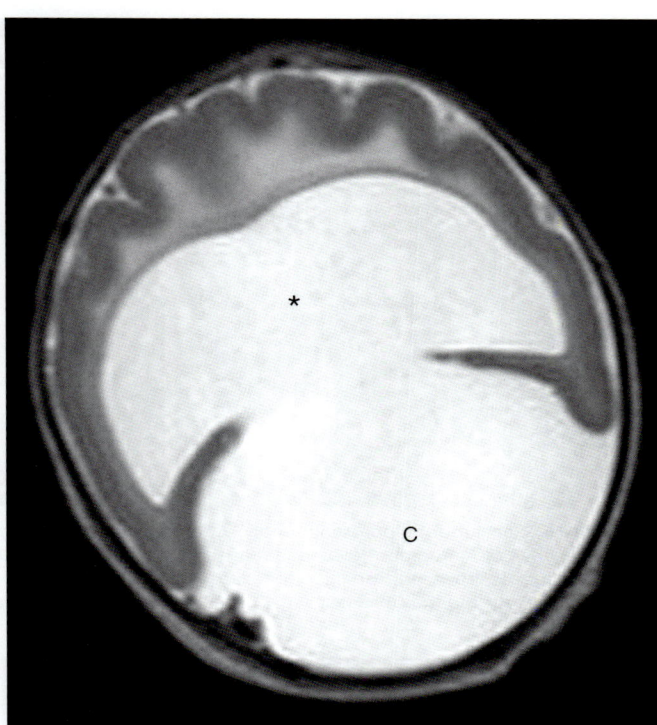

Figure 31-14 Alobar holoprosencephaly. An axial T2-weighted image shows a mantle of parenchyma anteriorly without any midline separation with an associated monoventricle (*asterisk*) and a large dorsal cyst (*C*).

formed.[1,14,17] The callosal body and splenium are preserved (Fig. 31-17).

Syntelencephaly (Middle Frontal Variant)

The middle frontal variant is an unusual variant of lobar HPE characterized by separation of the frontal and occipital poles, fusion of the middle portions of the cerebral hemispheres (Fig. 31-18), preservation of portions of the commissural fibers of the corpus callosum, and neuronal migration anomalies; thalamic fusion is variable.[18,19]

SEPTO-OPTIC DYSPLASIA

Clinical Presentation Septo-optic dysplasia (SOD) is considered along the continuum of disorders of ventral forebrain differentiation.[20] Patients typically present in early childhood with nystagmus, optic nerve atrophy, short stature because of growth hormone deficiency, or panhypopituitarism without diabetes insipidus. Affected patients are at risk for Addisonion crisis from subclinical adrenal insufficiency, which may become clinically apparent only during illness or severe stress. Most cases of isolated SOD are sporadic.

Imaging SOD is characterized by absence of the septum pellucidum and variable optic nerve hypoplasia (e-Fig. 31-19). The neurohypophysis is often ectopic or may be absent, in which case the pituitary stalk may be interrupted. However, agenesis of the septum pellucidum may be isolated with

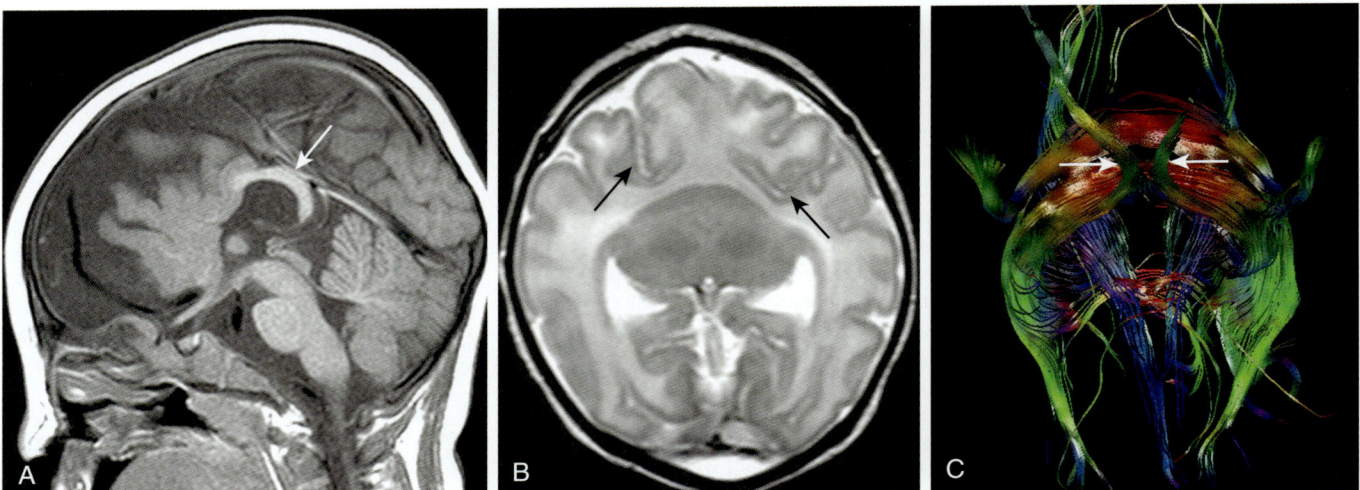

Figure 31-15 Semilobar holoprosencephaly. **A,** A sagittal T1-weighted image shows underdeveloped frontal lobes with midface hypoplasia. The splenium (*arrow*) of the corpus callosum is formed. **B,** An axial T2-weighted image shows failure of separation of the frontal lobes; the caudate and thalami are fused. Arrows indicate the anomalous anterior position of the Sylvian fissures. **C,** Diffusion tractography. The brain is viewed from the inferior aspect; arrows indicate the optic pathways. The red fibers are midline extensions of anomalous association fibers.

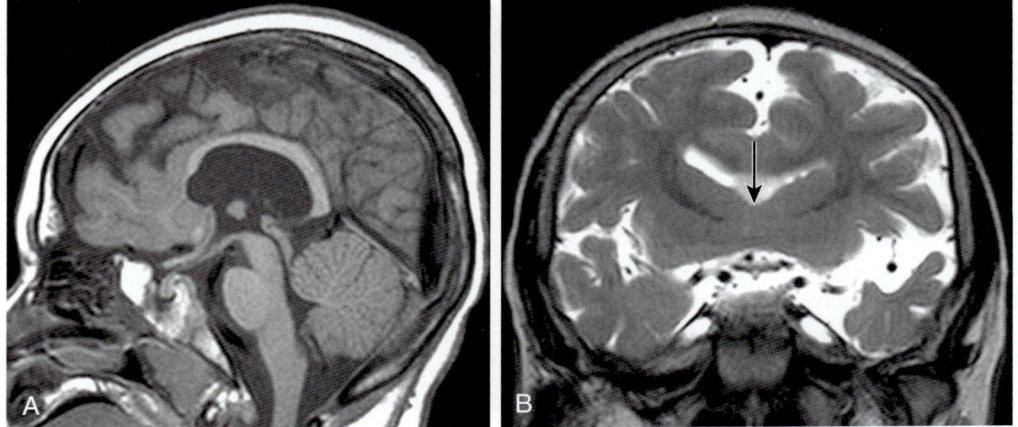

Figure 31-17 Lobar holoprosencephaly. **A,** A sagittal T1-weighted image shows that the rostrum and genu of the corpus callosum are deficient; the body and splenium are formed, but thin. **B,** On the coronal T2-weighted image, the subfrontal region is unseparated (*arrow*).

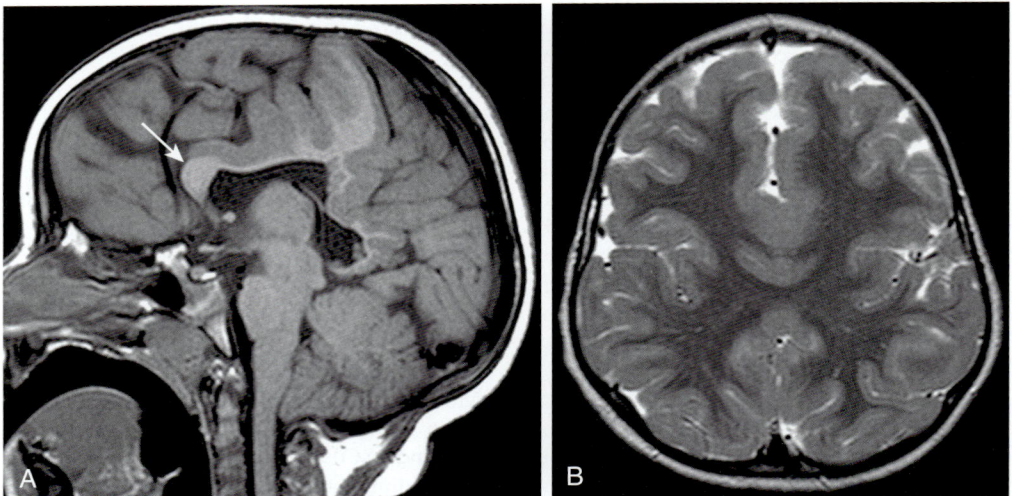

Figure 31-18 Middle frontal variant of holoprosencephaly. **A,** A sagittal T1-weighted image shows that the callosal genu (*arrow*) is formed; the callosal body appears formed but is hypoplastic. Partial fusion of the frontal lobes is seen. **B,** An axial T2-weighted image shows fusion of cortex and white matter across the midline in the middle frontal region.

normal optic pathways and intact neuroendocrine function. Absence of the septal leaves results in downward displacement of the fornices into the third ventricle. SOD is associated with multiple malformations, such as schizencephaly, neuronal migration anomalies, and neural tube defects.

CALLOSAL AGENESIS OR DYSGENESIS

Complete or partial malformation of the corpus callosum has an incidence of 1 in 4000.[21] Normal corpus callosal development requires a precise sequence of cellular proliferation and migration, axonal growth and guidance, and midline glial development and patterning. Disruptions in this sequence may result from gene mutations, genetic polymorphisms, intrauterine infections, ischemia, and toxins.[21]

The telencephalic commissures normally develop in a predictable sequence.[1,21] The anterior commissure (AC) forms around 55 days after conception, arising from the primitive hippocampal formations and ultimately connecting the anterior temporal lobes. Approximately 3 weeks later, the initial interhemispheric migration of pioneering callosal axons occurs, aided by the "glial sling," which consists of primitive subependymal glial cells. The "glial wedge" is composed of radial glial cells that guide callosal axons across the midline and then repel the axons away from the midline into the contralateral hemisphere.[1,21] After crossing the midline, callosal axons grow into the contralateral hemisphere; their ultimate destination mirror-images their region of origin and is within the same cortical layer from which the axon arose.[21,22] The crossing axons follow a rostrocaudal gradient with the callosal rostrum forming before the splenium; formation of the splenium is complete by around 85 days after conception. Many of the crossing axons undergo programmed cell death after reaching their final destination; this apoptosis commences during the second trimester, with pruning of axonal axons continuing after birth.[1,22]

Imaging   The corpus callosum is the largest of the three telencephalic commissures, which include the anterior and hippocampal commissures. The AC is a variably-sized tract embedded in the cranial aspect of the lamina terminalis, which demarcates the anterior wall of the third ventricle and connects the anterior temporal lobes. The hippocampal commissure is a thin sheet of white matter connecting the two crura of the fornices and is not routinely visualized on MRI of the normal brain. Absence of the corpus callosum, AC, and hippocampal commissure is described as "complete commissural agenesis," although some portion of the corpus callosum may be preserved (Fig. 31-20).[1,2,22,23] Preservation of the AC in the absence of the corpus callosum and hippocampal commissure is "callosohippocampal agenesis" (e-Fig. 31-21), whereas the anterior and hippocampal commissures may be preserved, which results in "isolated callosal agenesis" (e-Fig. 31-22). Callosohippocampal agenesis is the most common malformation, although it might be argued these classifications are somewhat academic. The AC may be enlarged. On MRI, the sulci over the mesial surface of the frontal lobes have a radial configuration, and the lateral ventricles have a characteristic parallel orientation. Absence of the temporal segments of the cingulum results in dilatation of the temporal horns. Hypoplasia of association fibers connecting the occipital and temporal lobe allows

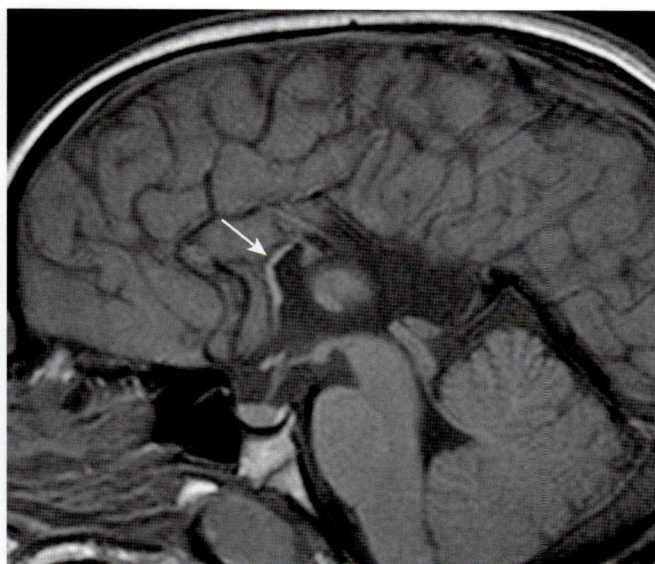

Figure 31-20   **Near total callosal agenesis.** The callosal remnant contiguous with the superior aspect of the lamina terminalis (*arrow*), which demarcates the anterior wall of the third ventricle, may represent the ventral hippocampal commissure, which normally involutes.

dilatation of trigones of the lateral ventricles referred to as *colpocephaly*. When the axons fail to cross the midline and remain in their hemisphere of origin, they course along the medial aspect of the lateral ventricle, forming the longitudinal callosal bundles of Probst, which are thought to function as association fibers connecting regions of cortex within the same hemisphere (e-Fig. 31-23). Callosal agenesis may be associated with an interhemispheric diencephalic pseudocyst (e.g., high-riding third ventricle), or interhemispheric cysts that do not communicate with the ventricles (see e-Fig. 31-23). By DTI, the rudimentary cingulum and fornices are fused to the bundles of Probst (Fig. 31-24). In patients with preservation of a portion of the corpus callosum, diffusion tractography suggests the existence of aberrant connections between regions of cortex and subcortical structures in some patients, and heterotopic hemispheric connections that exist in such a manner that a frontal lobe may be connected with the contralateral parietal or occipital lobe (e-Fig. 31-25). These aberrant callosal fibers have been termed "asymmetric sigmoid bundles" and have also been reported in patients with a fully formed but abnormally shaped corpus callosum (e-Fig. 31-26).[24,25]

Callosal agenesis may be an isolated anomaly or associated with a myriad of other malformations, including aqueductal stenosis, Chiari II malformations, and malformations of cortical, brainstem, and cerebellar development.[21-25] Numerous syndromes are associated with complete or partial agenesis of the corpus callosum. Aicardi syndrome is a rare sporadic X-linked dominant malformation seen in females, with an incidence of less than 1 in 200,000 births. Affected males have Klinefelter syndrome (XXY). Clinical findings include profound developmental delay, infantile spasms, microophthalmia, coloboma, short philtrum, flat nose, and large ears. Imaging shows callosohippocampal agenesis, interhemispheric cysts, gray matter heterotopias, polymicrogyria (PMG), and cerebellar malformation. Ocular abnormalities include

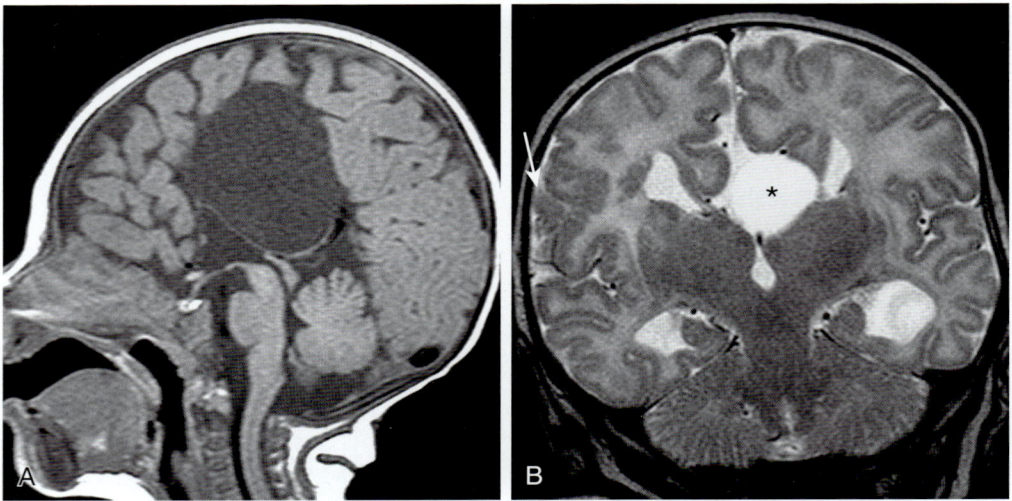

Figure 31-24 Corpus callosal agenesis with interhemispheric cyst. **A,** A sagittal T1-weighted image shows a large interhemispheric cyst, which does not communicate with the ventricular system. **B,** A coronal T2-weighted image in another patient, the interhemispheric cyst (*asterisk*) represents a "high-riding" third ventricle. Note the cortical dysplasia (*arrow*) in the right cerebrum.

chorioretinic lacunae and coloboma. CRASH syndrome (*c*orpus callosum agenesis, *r*etardation, *a*dducted thumbs, *s*pastic paraplegia, and *h*ydrocephalus) is caused by mutations in the L1 cell adhesion molecule gene that codes for a transmembrane cell adhesion protein involved in axonal migration.

CALLOSAL HYPOPLASIA

The corpus callosum may be incompletely formed, diffusely hypoplastic, or segmentally deficient (e-Fig. 31-27).[23] Partial callosal agenesis is usually characterized by absence of the splenium and dorsal body, with relative preservation of the genu and the rostral body. Diffuse callosal hypoplasia is characterized by diffuse thinning, whereas segmental callosal hypoplasia involves an intermediate portion of the corpus callosum. The segmental defects may result from a secondary callosal destruction or injury to regional white matter.

Callosal lipomas are rare and are thought to result from abnormal differentiation of pluripotential mesenchymal tissue. Most cases are associated with agenesis or incomplete formation of the corpus callosum. Anterior lipomas are more common than posterior. The lipoma itself may be an incidental finding and may be seen with a fully formed corpus callosum (Fig. 31-28).

MICROCEPHALY VERA

Microcephaly is a nonspecific diagnosis defined by head circumference greater than 3 standard deviations below normal for age and gender and, as such, is a descriptor rather than a specific entity. Microcephaly may be caused by prenatal infections or intrauterine or perinatal insult or may be part of a syndrome. Microcephaly vera ("true" microcephaly) is an autosomal-recessive trait typically not associated with seizures.[26] About 15% of patients with microcephaly vera have normal neurodevelopmental outcomes. MRI shows diffuse undersulcation of the brain, which may be subtle; brain structures are otherwise normal.

ENCEPHALOCLASTIC OR DESTRUCTIVE LESIONS

The term *hydrancephaly* describes near-complete to total absence of the cerebral hemispheres, with preservation of the brainstem, central gray nuclei, and the cerebellum and is thought to be caused by an intrauterine ischemic insult.[1] Remnants of the inferior frontal, anterior temporal, or occipital lobes may exist (Fig. 31-29). Affected patients appear neurologically normal at birth because of the intact brainstem. The hydrocephalus in hydrancephaly results from aqueductal stenosis.

The differential diagnosis of hydrancephaly is aqueductal stenosis with severe hydrocephalus. In the latter conditions,

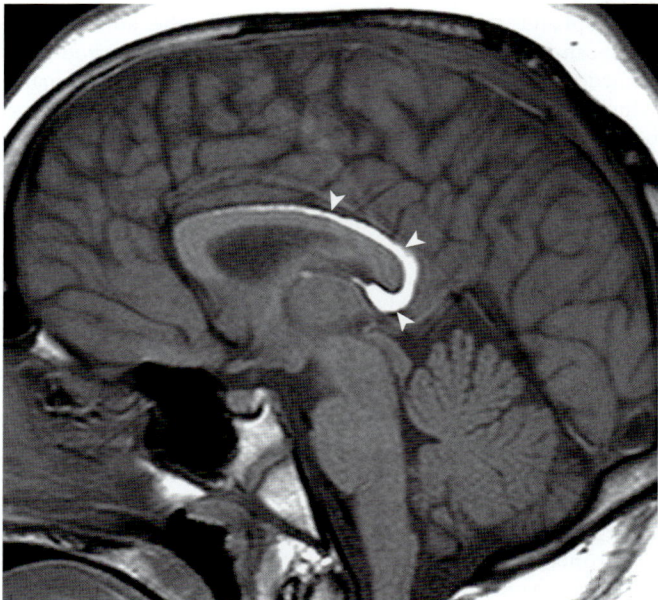

Figure 31-28 Callosal lipoma. A sagittal T1-weighted image shows a hyperintense lipoma (*arrowheads*) with a normally formed corpus callosum.

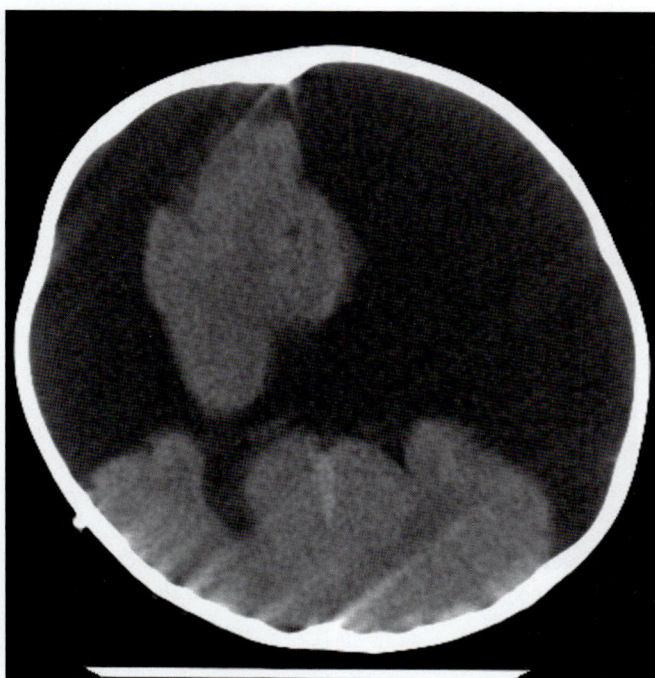

Figure 31-29 Hydrancephaly with preservation of portions of cerebral cortex.

CSF diversion results in variable reexpansion of the cerebral cortex, whereas shunt placement in patients with hydrancephaly serves to limit the ultimate size of the cranium but does not affect the appearance of the rudimentary cerebral cortex. CSF diversion is done in patients with hydrancephaly and hydrocephalus to prevent massive enlargement of the head resulting from production of CSF by preserved choroid plexus with aqueductal stenosis.

Other encephaloclastic lesions include porencephaly, which are CSF-containing spaces that usually communicate with the ventricular system. Porencephaly may occur from intrauterine vascular insult, trauma, infection, and nontraumatic hemorrhage. Unlike schizencephalic defects, porencephalic defects are not lined with dysplastic grey matter.

Neuronal Migration Anomalies or Anomalies of Cortical Development

These malformations include a wide spectrum of developmental malformations of the cortex caused by disruption of neuronal cell proliferation, migration, and organization.[3,26,27] Neuronal proliferation occurs in the germinal matrix along the subependymal layer of the walls of the lateral ventricles during week 7 of gestation. Around week 8, the neurons begin to migrate from the germinal zone to the surface of the brain along bipolar radial glial fibers, which provide scaffolding for neuronal migration. A smaller population of neurons also migrates orthogonal to the radial glial cells. Neurons in cortical layer 1 are the first to reach the cortex, followed by those destined for layers 5, 4, 3, and 2 in an "inside out" sequence. At the completion of migration, the cortex becomes organized with synaptic contacts, which develop between neurons throughout the six-layered cortex. Disruptions of neuronal proliferation, migration, and organization may result from infections such as cytomegalovirus (CMV), toxoplasmosis, intrauterine ischemic insults, toxins, radiation exposure, or genetic anomalies, or from no known cause. Affected patients have seizures, developmental delay, and variable focal neurologic deficits. The resulting malformation depends on which process is disrupted:

- Disorders of proliferation include *microlissencephaly*, in which neuronal proliferation is diffusely decreased; *hemimegancephaly*, in which proliferation is increased; and *focal cortical dysplasia* (FCD), in which proliferation is abnormal.
- Disorders of migration include *type I* or *classic lissencephaly* (LIS1), in which neuronal migration is diffusely decreased; *type II cobblestone lissencephaly*, in which diffuse overmigration of neurons occurs; and *gray matter heterotopias*, in which migration is focally ectopic.
- Disorders of organization include *PMG* and *schizencephaly*.

MICROLISSENCEPHALY

Clinical Presentation Patients with microlissencephaly have severe microcephaly at birth, with dysmorphic craniofacial features, abnormal genitalia, and arthrogryposis.[26] These patients suffer from seizures and have developmental delay that is pervasive and profound. The mode of inheritance is thought to be autosomal recessive, related in some patients to mutations of the *RELN* gene. Congenital infections are known to cause microlissencephaly, especially CMV.

Imaging The diagnosis of is made on the basis of a diffusely thinned cerebral mantle, with abnormal sulcation consisting of agyria-pachygyria (Fig. 31-30), variable callosal agenesis, and variable hypoplasia of the brainstem and cerebellum. Type A (Norman-Roberts syndrome) is microlissencephaly without infratentorial anomalies, and type B (Barth syndrome) is microlissencephaly with severe cerebellar and brainstem hypoplasia. Milder forms of microlissencephaly are referred to as *microcephaly with a simplified gyral pattern*; the cortex is usually of normal thickness.

HEMIMEGALENCEPHALY

Clinical Presentation Hemimegalencephaly is hamartomatous overgrowth of a cerebral hemisphere or lobe of the brain.[1,2,28] It occurs as an isolated anomaly or with neurocutaneous syndromes such as epidermal nevus syndrome, Proteus syndrome, unilateral hypomelanosis of Ito, neurofibromatosis type I, Klippel-Trenaunay syndrome, and tuberous sclerosis. The malformation is thought to arise from faulty neuronal proliferation prior to radial neuroblast migration. Hemispherectomy is required for relief of the severe intractable epilepsy.

Imaging MRI shows diffusely enlarged hemisphere or lobe (Fig. 31-31), with abnormal sulcation pattern that may include PMG, lissencephaly, and gray matter heterotopias. The regional white matter is thickened and gliotic. A hallmark is enlargement of the ipsilateral ventricle that becomes

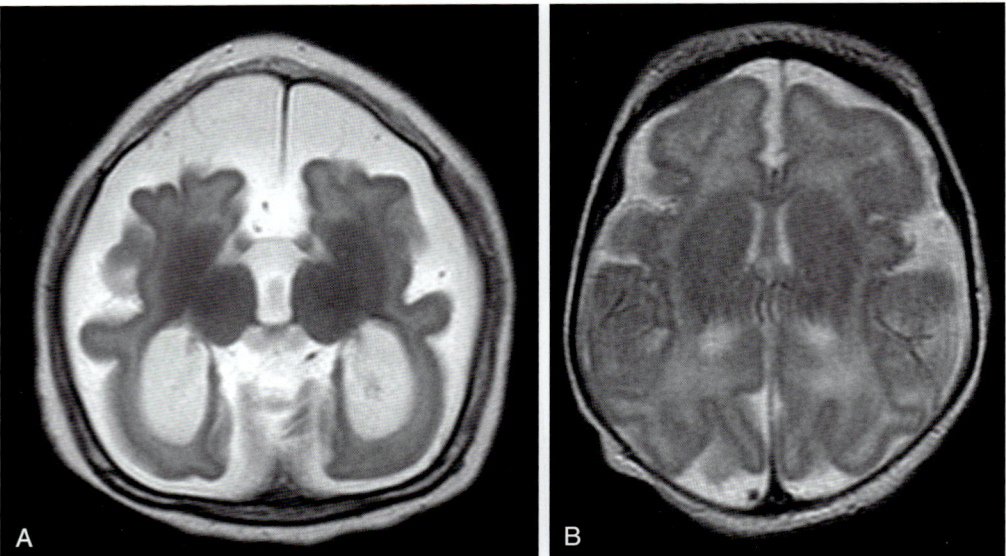

Figure 31-30 Microlissencephaly. **A,** The brain is diffusely undersulcated with callosal agenesis and dilated ventricles. **B,** Marked microcephaly is associated with severe cerebellar and brainstem hypoplasia.

more pronounced with age with expansion of the overlaying hemicranium.

FOCAL CORTICAL DYSPLASIA

The most common clinical presentation of FCD is medication-resistant focal epilepsy.[29,30] FCD is probably caused by mutations in multiple genes, but unlike lissencephaly and periventricular nodular heterotopias, FCD is not associated with a known single genetic mutation.[29,30] The histologic hallmark of FCD is lack of normal cortical lamination. FCD is classified into types I, II, and, more recently, type III, based on cortical laminar structure, cytoarchitectural disruption, cell composition, and the presence of associated destructive brain lesions.[30] Type I FCD has alterations in cortical layering, with distortion of the normal radial cortical lamination and lack of the normal six-layered neocortex; by definition, type I FCD has no balloon cells. Type II FCD is characterized by cortical dyslamination and dysmorphic neurons with or without balloon cells. FCD Type III is found in association with encephaloclastic lesions such as traumatic brain injury, perinatal ischemia, Rasmussen encephalitis, or low-grade tumors.[30]

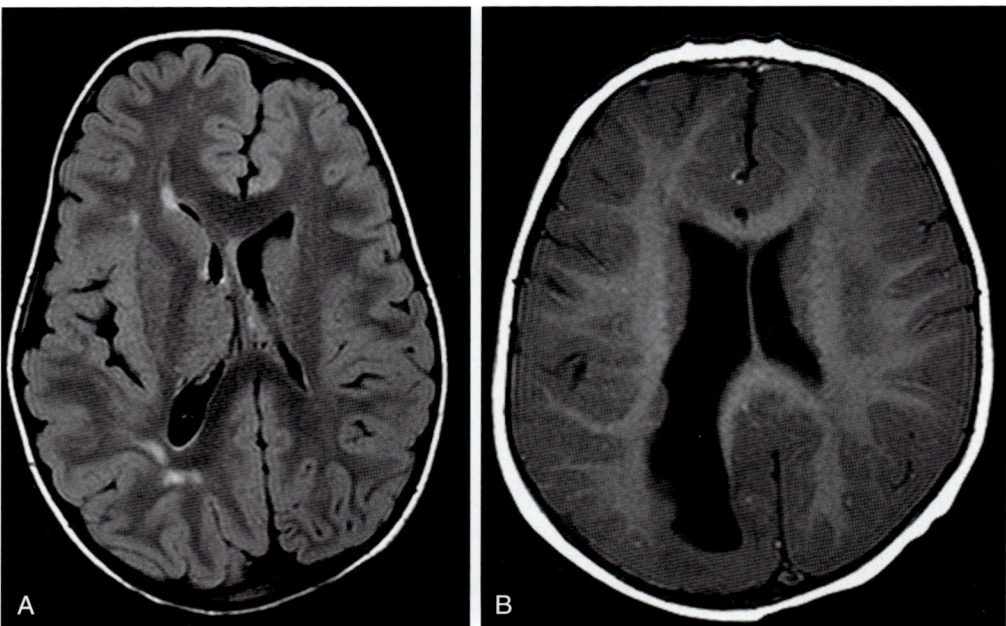

Figure 31-31 Hemimegancephaly. **A,** The hemimegancephaly is lobar, with sparing of the right frontal lobe. The right occipital horn is dilated, and expansion of the right hemicranium and pachygyria, as well as periventricular grey matter heterotopias, are seen. **B,** In this patient, the entire right cerebrum is affected. The white matter is thickened and focally gliotic.

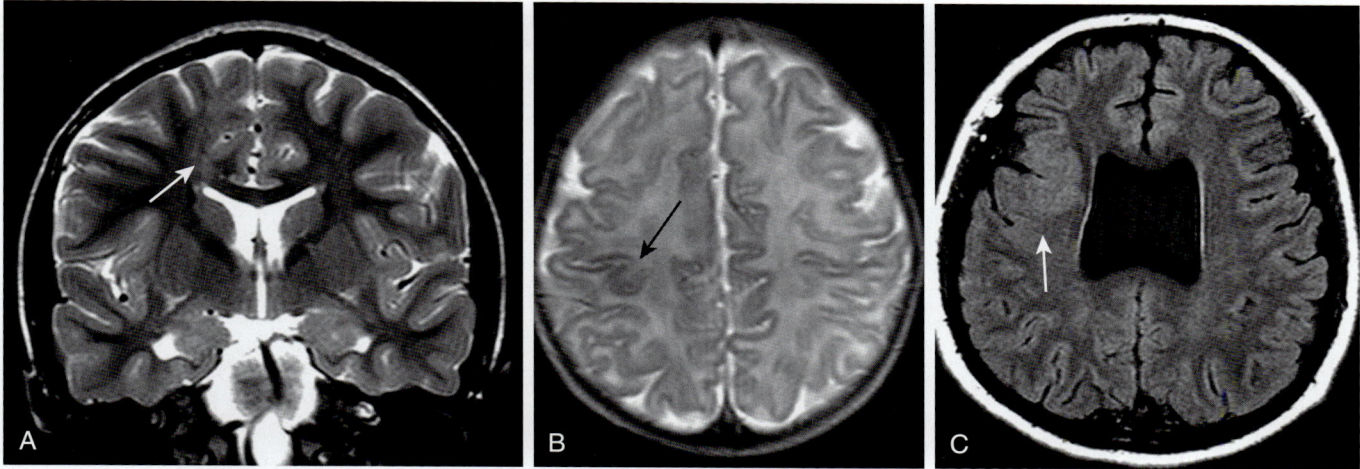

Figure 31-32   The variable appearance of focal cortical dysplasia. **A,** On the coronal T2-weighted image and axial fluid-attenuated inversion recovery images, focal thickening of left parasagittal cortex (arrow) is seen. **B,** The small area of dysplastic cortex (arrow) was seen only on the T2 image in this neonate with seizures. **C,** Right frontal cortical dysplasia (arrow) with absence of the septum pellucidum. Focal expansion of the overlying subarachnoid space has occurred, and anomalous superficial cortical veins may simulate a vascular malformation.

Imaging Identification of FCD requires high-resolution MRI, using T1-weighted, T2-weighted, and FLAIR (fluid-attenuated inversion recovery) sequences (Fig. 31-32); the diagnostic accuracy of MRI is increased with scrutiny of thin sections of the region of brain suspected of harboring the epileptogenic focus. Findings of type I FCD include focal cortical thickening, often within the depth of a sulcus, and blurring of the gray–white junction. FCD may be clinically occult and found on MRI performed for reasons other than seizures or may be associated with seizures and variable cognitive impairment. The most common histopathologic finding in surgical specimens removed from patients with cryptogenic epilepsy (e.g., epilepsy in which no lesion is identifiable by imaging) is type I FCD.[29,30]

Type II FCD is more readily apparent with MRI, especially in the presence of balloon cells. MRI shows increased T2 signal within the subcortical white matter underlying abnormal gyri and is often best seen on T2-weighted and FLAIR images. The radial extension of balloon cells and ectopic neurons into the deep white matter constitutes the "transmantle sign" of FCD and may be the sole visible evidence of FCD.[29] The differential diagnosis of type II FCD is low-grade tumor. Although type II FCD may be suggested on the basis of MRI findings, overlap exists in imaging findings between type I and II, and the ultimate diagnosis is based on histopathology.[30]

GRAY MATTER HETEROTOPIAS

Gray matter heterotopias are ectopic neurons resulting from mutations in the genes that code for proteins involved in neuronal migration (Fig. 31-33). Periventricular nodular heterotopias are gray matter heteropias along the walls of the lateral ventricles. These are nodular masses of normal neurons and glial cells devoid of laminar organization and are intrinsically epileptogenic. The seizures result from hyperexcitable circuitries between the ectopic neurons and the overlaying cortex.[31,32] The clinical impact depends on the amount and location of the heterotopias and on the degree of extension to the overlying cortex. Bilateral heterotopias are associated with more severe and generalized seizure activity and cognitive delay compared with unilateral heterotopias.[33]

Imaging MRI shows variable-sized nonenhancing nodules along the ependymal surface of the lateral ventricles (see Fig. 31-33) that have the same signal intensity as the cortex on all sequences.[33] The nodules may be single, multiple, isolated, or associated with other malformations.

Disorders of Neuronal Migration

TYPE I (CLASSIC) LISSENCEPHALY

LIS1 is caused by disruption of the migration of neuroblasts from the ventricular surface to the pial surface, which normally occurs between 10 and 14 weeks' gestational age.[34-38] LIS1 includes lissencephalies with defined genetic abnormalities, isolated lissencephalies without any identifiable genetic defect, and lissencephalies associated with syndromes of multiple malformations.[33-37] Mutations resulting in isolated LIS and Miller-Dieker syndrome (MDS) map to chromosome 17p13.3, which, along with mutations in the double cortin (*DCX*) gene, accounts for about 70% of LIS1. The *DCX* and Aristaless-related homeobox (*ARX*) genes are X-linked. The less common Reelin (*RELN*) gene maps to chromosome 7 and the α-tubulin 1a (*TUBA1A*) gene to chromosome 12. LIS1 occurs in 1 in 500,000 live births, with gender predominance only in the less common X-linked forms. Histopathology of LIS1 shows inversion of cortical laminar architecture; the normal six-layered cortex is replaced with a thick four-layered cortex. In the lissencephalic brain, layer I is a superficial molecular layer. Deep under layer I is layer II, which is a layer of pyramidal cells resembling the fifth and sixth layers of the normal neocortex, followed by a sparse cellular layer (layer III) and a thick band of disorganized

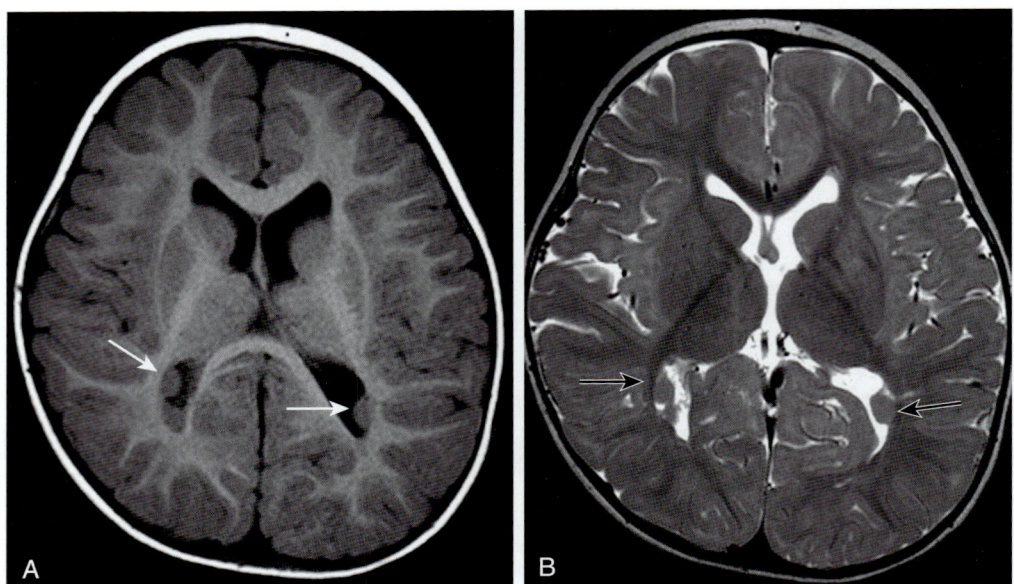

Figure 31-33 Periventricular gray matter. **A** and **B,** The periventricular gray matter heterotopias (*arrows*) have the same signal intensity as the cortex.

neurons of variable size (layer IV), which extends into the regional white matter.

Clinical Presentation The hallmarks of LIS1 are profound mental retardation, with a normal–small head size, intractable seizures, hypertonia, and hyperreflexia. Patients with isolated lissencephaly have normal facial structures, whereas patients with MDS have LIS1 with abnormal facies: wrinkled skin over the glabella and frontal suture, prominent occiput, narrow forehead, downward slanting palpebral fissures, and small nose and chin. Males with *DCX* mutation have classic LIS1 as seen on MRI, whereas females with *DCX* mutation have variable cognitive delay without seizures and subcortical band heterotopias (SBH) as delineated by MRI. The presence of an unexplained seizure disorder or cognitive problems in the mother of a male child with lissencephaly should trigger a screening MRI of the mother for possible SBH. Females with *ARX* mutation have ambiguous genitalia without lissencephaly; males have lissencephaly with ambiguous genitalia (*XLAG*) syndrome. Lissencephaly caused by *RELN* mutation is associated with congenital lymphedema.[33-37]

Imaging The phenotypic expression of lissencephaly caused by LIS1 is similar in males and females and consists of a markedly thickened cerebral cortex, which may be diffuse (Fig. 31-34) or most pronounced posteriorly (Fig. 31-35); and Sylvian fissures fail to occur.[1,2,36-38] The thickened cortex shows a highly organized pattern, as shown by DTI, because of the persistence of the radial pattern of the neurons in arrested migration.[39] The lissencephalic pattern in males with *DCX* mutation is similar to L1S1 and more severe anteriorly. Females with *DCX* mutation have SBH or "double cortex."[37,38] MRI shows bands of heterotopic neurons within the cerebral white matter between a normal-appearing cortex and the ventricles (Fig. 31-36).[40] *MDS* and the *ARX* mutation are associated with more severe lissencephaly posteriorly. With LIS1 mutations of *MDS* and *DCX*, the pons may be normal or mildly hypoplastic; severe cerebellar and pontine

hypoplasia suggest a *RELN* mutation. MRI abnormalities described in the rare mutations of the *TUBA1A* gene include classic lissencephaly, with brainstem dysplasia and cerebellar hypoplasia.

TYPE II COBBLESTONE LISSENCEPHALY (CONGENITAL MUSCULAR DYSTROPHY)

The cobblestone type II lissencephalies (dystroglycanopathies) result from excessive neuronal migration, in contrast to LIS1, in which neuronal migration is deficient.[41] Dystroglycan is a glycoprotein in the extracellular matrix receptor of muscle and the central nervous system (CNS), which mechanically stabilizes the muscle sarcolemma against contraction-stretch stress and which also plays a role in signal transduction during cell migration. Dystroglycan requires the addition of glycosol groups to function; the CNS manifestations of the defective glycosylation are overmigration of neurons through the defective glial–pial limiting membrane into the subarachnoid space, resulting in a cobblestone appearance to the surface of the brain. The malformation includes variable pachygyria and PMG, with a thickened cortex that lacks the normal six-layered architecture, fibroglial proliferation of the leptomeninges, and focal interhemispheric fusion.

Clinical Presentation The clinical presentation of the cobblestone lissencephalies is congenital muscular dystrophy (CMD), which comprises a heterogeneous group of inherited disorders presenting with diffuse symmetric hypotonia at birth or in infancy.[1,41] CMD is categorized as (1) CMD without CNS abnormalities, and (2) CMD with CNS abnormalities; the latter includes Fukuyama (FCMD), muscle-eye-brain disease (MEBD), and Walker–Warburg syndrome (WWS).[41] Depending on the specific syndrome, affected patients also have psychomotor retardation, seizures, micro-ophthalmia, optic nerve hypoplasia, and colobomas. Scoliosis and contractures develop during early childhood. Death often results from

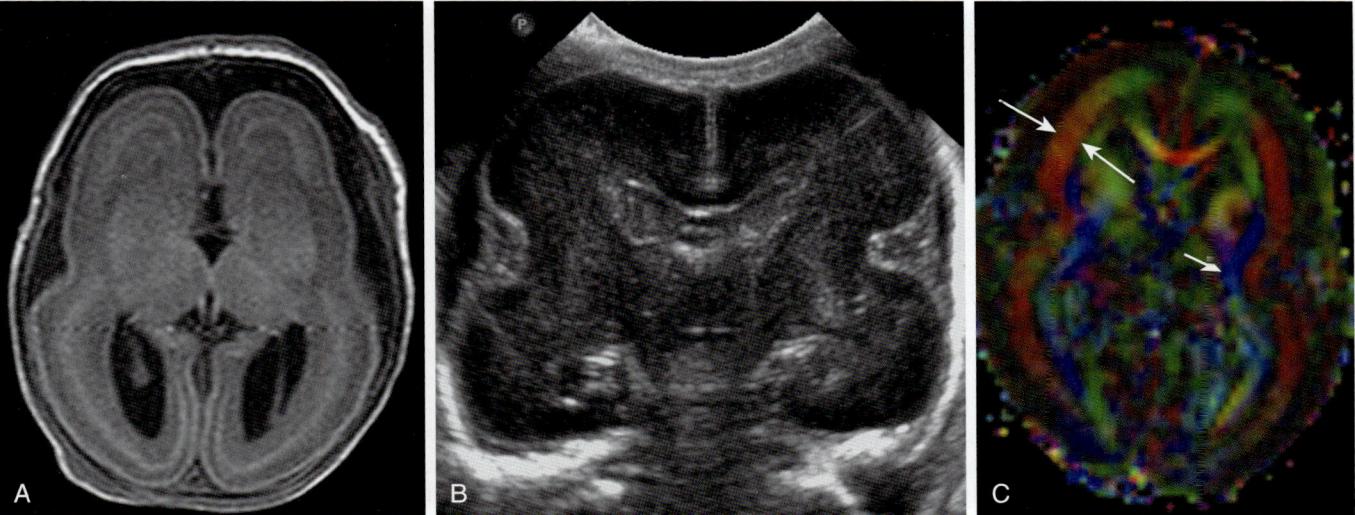

Figure 31-34 Classic lissencephaly caused by undermigration of neurons. **A,** A T2-weighted fluid-attenuated inversion recovery image from a term neonate shows abnormally thickened laminated cerebrum with no sulcation. **B,** A cranial sonogram shows that the Sylvian fissures are unapposed, which is abnormal for a term infant. The undersulcated appearance suggests the brain of an extremely preterm infant. **C,** An axial color map from diffusion tensor imaging shows thick bands of brushlike fibers (*long arrows*) caused by the neurons arrested during radial migration. The blue fibers (*short arrow*) are projection fibers that are vertically oriented.

respiratory failure, caused by chest wall rigidity and weakness of the diaphragm or aspiration, or from cardiomyopathy. The specific diagnosis is made on the basis of clinical findings, serum creatine kinase, neuroimaging, muscle and skin biopsy, and molecular genetic testing.[41]

FCMD is an autosomal-recessive disorder most common in Japan, where the incidence approaches 3 in 100,000 individuals.[41] The syndrome results from mutations in the *FKTN* gene on chromosome 9, which codes for the protein fukutin, which interacts with α-dystroglycan in the extracellular

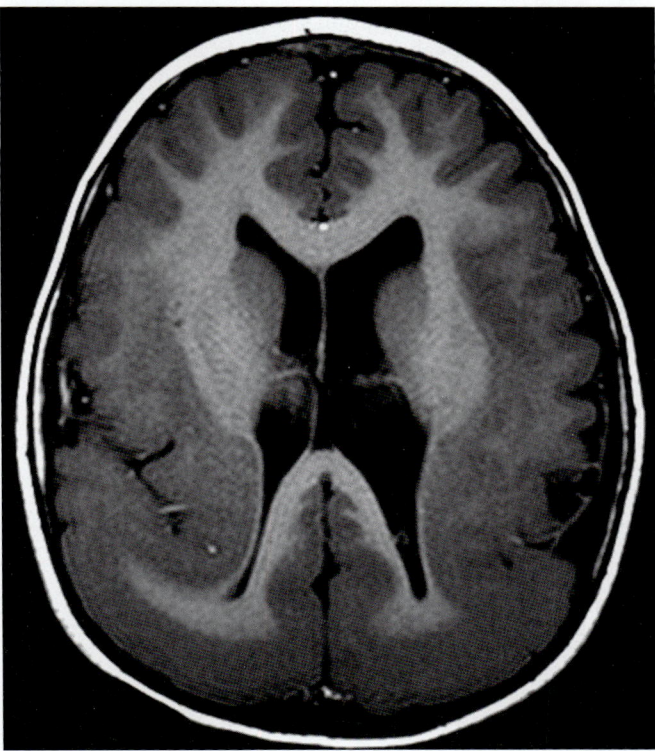

Figure 31-35 Incomplete lissencephaly. More severe involvement is seen posteriorly, which is typical of the Miller-Dieker syndrome and the rare *ARX* gene mutation.

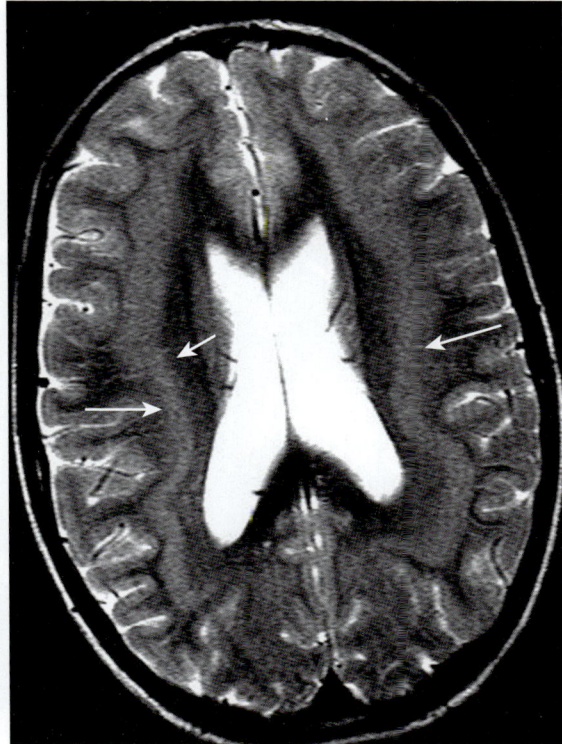

Figure 31-36 Subcortical band heteropia in a female with the double-cortin (*DCX*) gene mutation. Arrows indicate the symmetric bands of gray matter interposed between the superficial cortex and the deep white matter.

matrix. MEB disease is an autosomal-recessive disorder, which is rare outside of Finland and is caused by mutations in the *POMT1*, *POMT2*, *POMGnT1*, *fukutin*, and *FKRP* genes; phenotypes may overlap with FCMD. WWS is the most severe form of CMD with CNS manifestations and is also associated with mutations in the *POMT1*, *POMT2*, *fukutin*, and *fukutin-related protein* genes.[41]

Imaging MRI abnormalities are less severe in FCMD than in WWS and MEBD.[41] In mild cases of FCMD, the cerebrum may be relatively normal or have a simplified gryal pattern. More severe malformations have variable pachygyria and PMG; the white matter is gliotic with cysts. Neurons may be seen lining the ependymal surface of the ventricle, contrasted on T2-weighted images by hyperintense signal of the CSF and the abnormal white matter (e-Fig. 31-37). The lateral ventricles are enlarged. The cerebellum consistently shows small cysts with variable PMG. The most severe cerebellar hypoplasia is seen with WWS, which is also associated with occipital encephalocele (Fig. 31-38). The brainstem is usually normal in FCMD, hypoplastic in MEBD, and small and kinked posteriorly in WWS. Hydrocephalus is rare in FCMD, common in MEBD, and almost invariable in WWS; the hydrocephalus may mask the malformation.[41]

DERANGED NEURONAL ORGANIZATION (POLYMICROGYRIA, SCHIZENCEPHALY)

Clinical Presentation PMG results from disruption of normal terminal neuronal migration and organization and is defined by excessive convolutions of the cerebral cortex.[42-45] PMG may be unilateral and focal or bilateral and diffuse; bilateral patterns are most often frontoparietal and peri-Sylvian. The severity of seizures and developmental impairment correlates with the location and severity of the malformation. Focal PMG may be clinically occult or associated with seizures that are often medically uncontrollable. Bilateral peri-Sylvian PMG is associated with epilepsy, delayed development, strabismus, dysphagia and speech problems, and paresis. PMG may be isolated or associated with known disorders, including callosal agenesis, Aicardi syndrome, Joubert syndrome, FCMD, and Zellweger spectrum. Bilateral peri-Sylvian PMG is X-linked, whereas frontoparietal PMG maps to chromosome 16. At least 11 mutations in the G protein–coupled receptor 56 (*GPR56*) gene have been identified in bilateral PMG. PMG may also occur from CMV infection and intrauterine ischemic injury.[42,43]

Imaging MRI shows increased cortical thickness and irregularity at the cortex–white matter junction (Fig. 31-39). The pattern of the PMG appears to differ with location.[44] The appearance of the PMG may change with brain maturation, and microgyri obvious in unmyelinated brain may be less conspicuous as myelination progresses.

Schizencephaly results from congenital clefts in the cerebral hemisphere, which extend from the pial surface to the ventricles.[46] Affected patients may present with seizures, motor deficits, or both or may be asymptomatic. Larger or bilateral defects are associated with poorer neurodevelopmental outcome.[1,2]

Imaging The lips of the defects may be in apposition (closed lip) or separated (open lip). The clefts are lined with dysplastic gray matter, which extends the full length of the cleft (Fig. 31-40). Discontinuity of the ventricular ependyma and the subpial membrane in open-lip schizencephaly results in communication between the lateral ventricles and the subarachnoid space. The pulsations of the CSF may cause remodeling and outward expansion of the calvarium overlaying the open cleft. The septum pellucidum is absent in most cases of schizencephaly involving the frontoparietal regions. Unilateral schizencephaly is often associated with contralateral peri-Sylvian cortical dysplasia.[46]

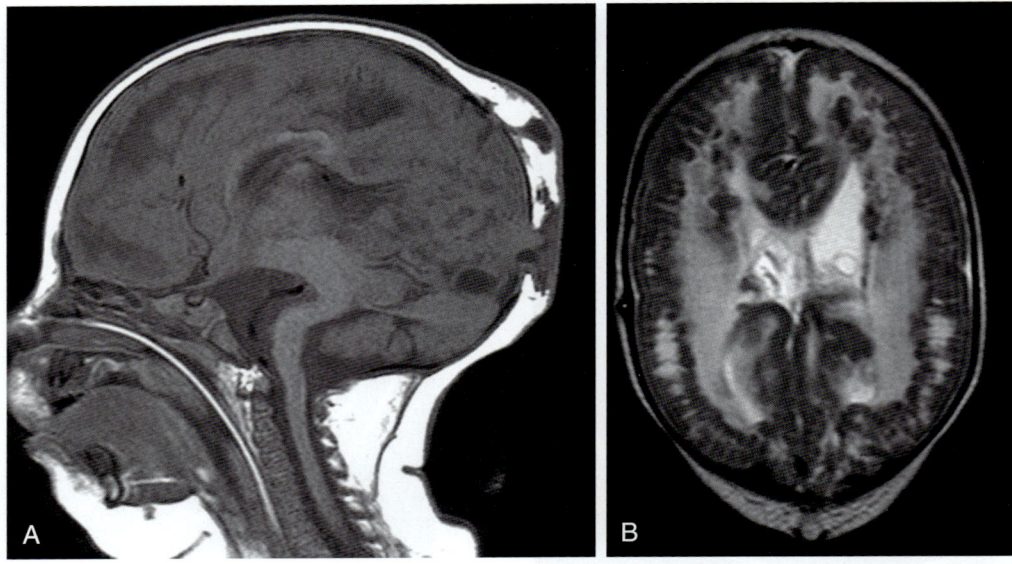

Figure 31-38 Walker-Warburg lissencephaly is the most severe form of congenital muscular dystrophy with central nervous system involvement. **A,** A sagittal image shows the typical cerebellar hypoplasia and dorsal beaking of the brainstem. Small parieto-occipital meningoceles are present. **B,** An axial T2-weighted image showing the cobblestone appearance at the grey-white junction. The patient required shunt placement at birth for associated hydrocephalus.

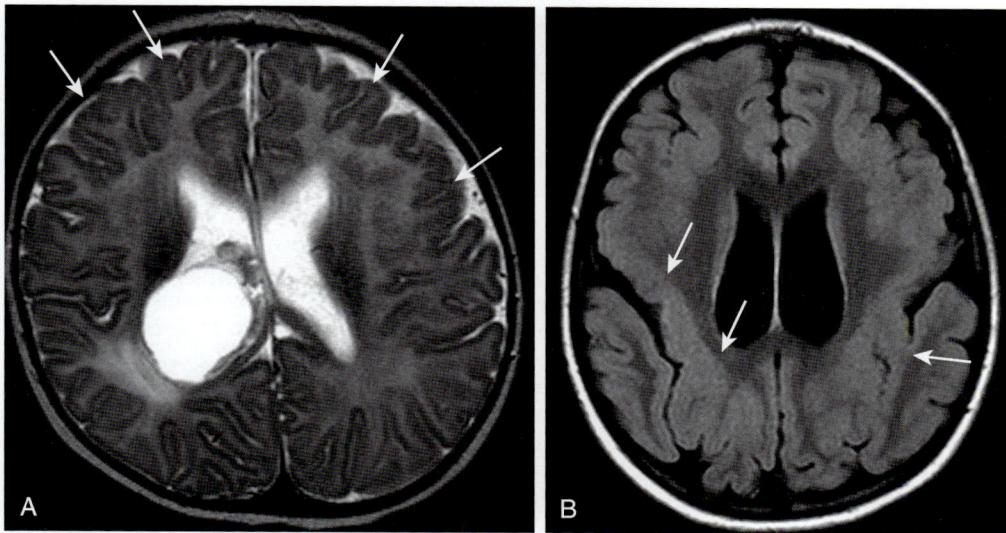

Figure 31-39   Variants of polymicrogyria. **A,** Bifrontal polymicrogyria (*arrows*) with a choroid plexus cyst in the right lateral ventricle. **B,** Peri-Sylvian polymicrogyria (*arrows*) on T2-weighted fluid-attenuated inversion recovery image.

Hindbrain and Cerebellar Malformations

BRAINSTEM MALFORMATIONS

Brainstem malformations may be classified into four groups based on embryology and genetics.[47]

1. Group I comprises malformations resulting from defects in early differentiation of the neural tube (e.g., Chiari II).
2. Group II comprises generalized malformations affecting the brainstem, the cerebellum, the cerebrum, or all. These include type I lissencephalies with cerebellar hypoplasia, CMDs with CNS involvement (cobblestone lissencephaly), CMV, and so on
3. Group III includes localized malformations affecting the brainstem and the cerebellum. The hallmark of these disorders is deficient or defective formation of cranial nerve nuclei, resulting in problems with ocular movement and lid control, facial palsy, neurosensory hearing loss, or all.
4. Group IV includes combined brainstem hypoplasia and atrophy in degenerative disorders of prenatal onset.

Malformations in which the brainstem is the predominant or only structure affected (group III) are uncommon. Conventional MRI is useful in the diagnosis of brainstem

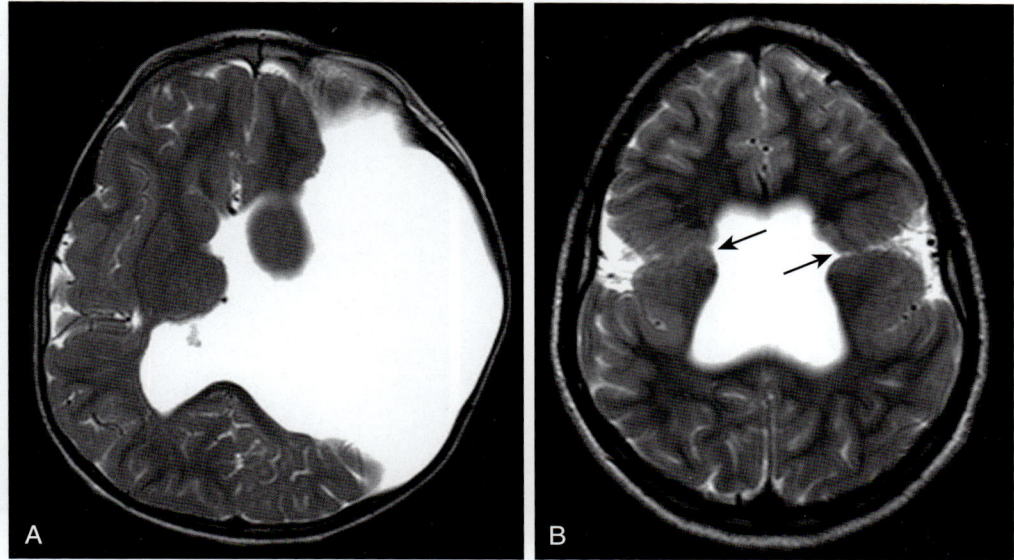

Figure 31-40   Schizencephaly. **A,** Bilateral closed lip schizencephalic defects (*arrows*) are associated with agenesis of the septum pellucidum. **B,** Large open lip defect is also associated with septal agenesis; the expansion of the left hemicranium is caused by the pulsations of the underlying cerebrospinal fluid.

malformations in which brainstem surface morphology and size are affected, although DTI provides more information about the internal derangement of white matter tracts from defective or deficient axonal guidance and neuronal migration. The Chiari I malformation is included here for convenience, although it is not considered a true brainstem malformation.

JOUBERT SYNDROME AND RELATED DISORDERS

Clinical Presentation   Joubert syndrome is a rare malformation that is usually autosomal recessive; it involves one of multiple genes involved in ciliary function integral to chemical signaling during neuronal and axonal migration. The clinical syndrome is characterized by hypotonia, episodic hypoventilation, and hyperventilation, which tend to improve with age; truncal ataxia, which develops during early childhood; and oculomotor apraxia, nystagmus, pigmentary retinopathy, endocrinopathies, and abnormal facial features, including ptosis, hypertelorism, and low-set ears. Joubert syndrome and related disorders (JSRD) describes the constellation of clinical problems associated with Joubert syndrome, which are diverse. The marked clinical variability probably results in underdiagnosis.

Imaging   The diagnosis of Joubert syndrome is made on the basis of characteristic MRI findings, which include hypoplasia of the superior vermis, with enlargement of the superior aspect of the fourth ventricle and the superior cerebellar peduncles.[48-50] The molar tooth sign (Fig. 31-41), seen on an axial image through the pontomesencephalic junction, is also seen in a number of cerebello-oculo-renal disorders. DTI of Joubert syndrome shows variable absence of transverse pontine fibers; the decussating fibers of the superior cerebellar peduncles are absent.[50] In addition to the clinical variability of JSRD, considerable variability also exists in the appearance of the brainstem.

HORIZONTAL GAZE PALSY WITH PROGRESSIVE SCOLIOSIS

Clinical Presentation   Horizontal gaze palsy with progressive scoliosis (HGPPS) is the expression of mutation of the *ROBO3* gene that codes for proteins involved in axonal guidance and neuronal migration.[51,52] Expression of the defective gene appears to be limited to decussating fibers in the brainstem. Patients with HGPPS tend to be cognitively normal but have congenital nystagmus and are unable to perform lateral eye movements because of lack of decussating fibers in the brainstem. Progressive scoliosis develops during early childhood.

Imaging   MRI shows hypoplasia of the pons, which is partially divided by a midsagittal cleft (e-Fig. 31-42). Facial colliculi are absent, the inferior olivary nuclei are prominent, and the medulla lacks the normal dorsal convexities. DTI of HGPPS shows hypoplasia of the ventral transverse pontine fibers and absence of the dorsal transverse pontine fibers, small middle and superior cerebellar peduncles, and decussating fibers of the superior cerebellar peduncle within the midbrain.[51] The appearance of the brainstem by diffusion imaging in HGPPS is similar to that of other less well-characterized brainstem malformations.

PONTINE TEGMENTAL CAP DYSPLASIA

Pontine tegmental cap dysplasia is a rare brainstem malformation associated with variable developmental delay, ataxia, restricted horizontal gaze, failure initiating fast eye movements, facial weakness, deafness, and swallowing problems, which reflect deficient lower cranial nerves.[53]

Imaging   MRI shows pontine hypoplasia; the ventral surface is flattened, and ectopic tissue protrudes dorsally into the fourth ventricle, which is referred to as the tegmental "cap."

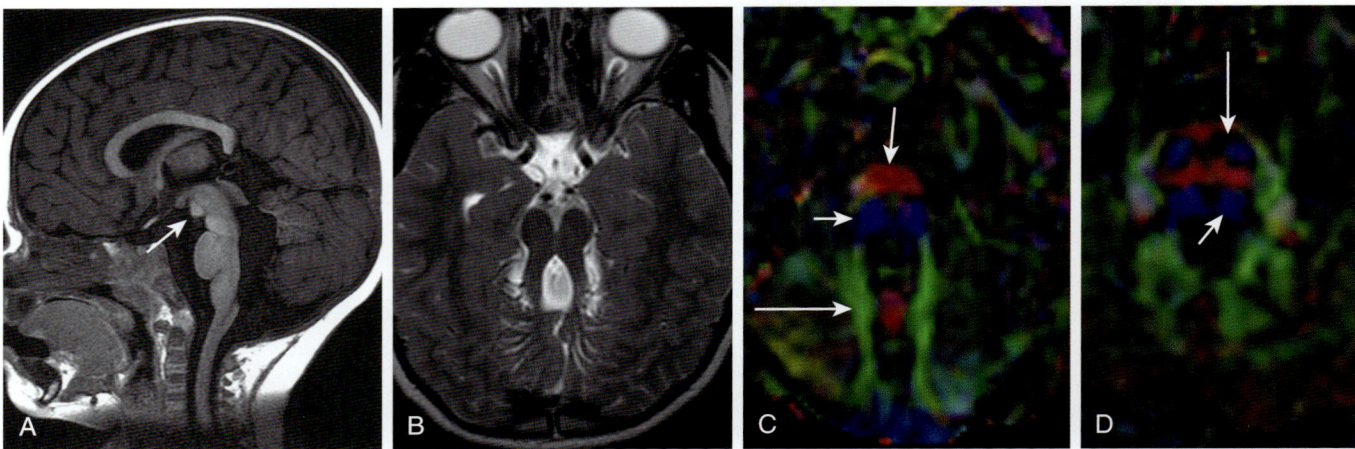

Figure 31-41   Joubert syndrome. **A,** A sagittal image shows an elongated mesencephalon with a ventral bulge (*arrow*). The roof of the fourth ventricle is dilated, and the superior cerebellar vermis is underdeveloped and dysplastic. **B,** An axial T2-weighted image shows the classic "molar tooth deformity." **C** and **D,** An axial color map from diffusion tensor imaging shows a single ventrally positioned transverse fiber bundle. The vertically oriented (*blue*) tracts consist of the corticospinal tracts (*long arrows*) and mediolateral lemniscus bundles (*short arrows*), which in a normal brainstem (*D*) are separated by a second transverse pontine fiber bundle.

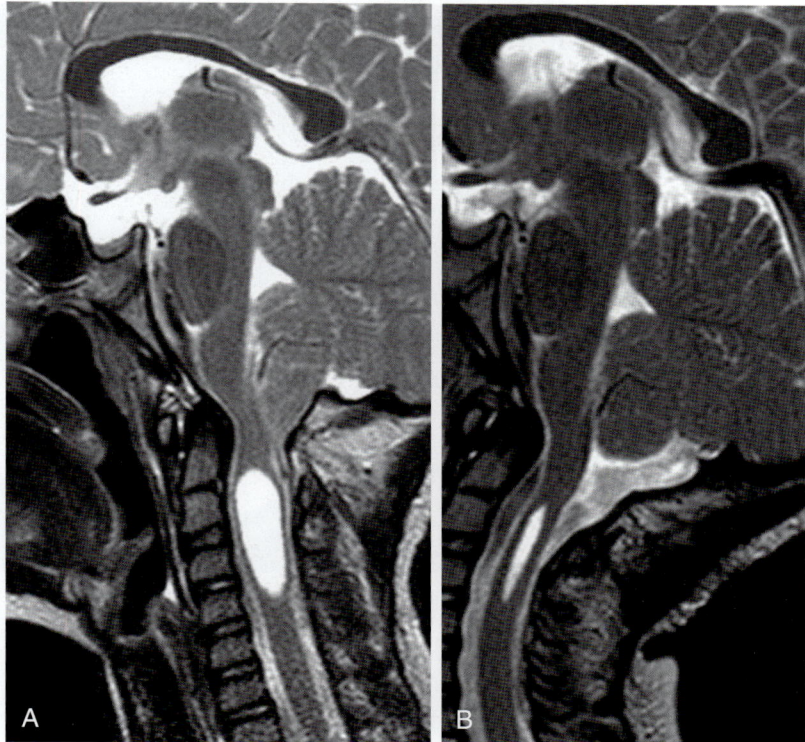

Figure 31-43 Chiari I malformation. **A,** A focally expansile cervical cord syrinx is present. **B,** The syrinx is collapsed after a decompressive suboccipital craniectomy was done.

The superior cerebellar vermis is hypoplastic, which, along with the elongated and laterally misplaced superior cerebellar peduncle, results in a molar tooth–like deformity. As shown by DTI, the tegemental cap is composed of transversely oriented ectopic pontine fibers. DTI also shows the absence of the normal decussations of the superior and middle cerebellar peduncles.[54] The pattern of white matter tract abnormalities, as shown by DTI, is similar to those reported in some cases of JSRD.

CHIARI I

The Chiari I malformation is not associated with defective neural tube closure, and Chari I "malformations" may be acquired or spontaneously resolve. Chiari I malformation is defined as downward displacement of cerebellar tonsils below the foramen magnum.[55-57] Although many patients with Chiari I malformations are asymptomatic, some patients experience suboccipital headaches, neck pain, ataxia, dysmetria, nystagmus, and dysequilibrium because of brainstem or cerebellar compression, upper extremity weakness and pain caused by cervical cord myelopathy, or both. Treatment of a symptomatic Chiari I malformation with or without syrinx is a suboccipital decompressive craniectomy, with or without duraplasty. In many centers, cerebellar tonsils are also resected.

Imaging The Chiari I malformation is defined by cerebellar tonsils greater than 6 mm below the posterior lip of the foramen magnum. In symptomatic patients, the low-lying tonsils disrupt CSF flow across the foramen magnum, which predisposes to syringomyelia in the thoracic or cervical spinal cord (Fig. 31-43). Flow of CSF across the foramen magnum

is further impaired when the odontoid is elongated and dorsally angulated or with any significant basilar invagination. The dynamic significance of the low-lying tonsils is best depicted using single-slice, multiple-phase, peripheral, or cardiac-gated two-dimensional phase contrast in the sagittal and axial planes with a velocity encoding of 5 centimeters per second (cm/s). Obstruction of CSF flow results in abnormal bidirectional movement of the hindbrain across the foramen magnum, which is seen as changes in signal intensity on the phase contrast sequence. In patients with Chari I malformations, increased intracranial pressure, caused by a tumor or hydrocephalus resulting in secondary tonsillar herniation, should be excluded with screening images through the brain (Table 31-1).

Table 31-1

Comparison of Chiari I and II Malformations

Chiari I	Chiari II
Headache and neck pain increased by cough or Valsalva maneuver; dysarthria, dysphagia, downbeat nystagmus, upper extremity weakness or numbness	Brainstem dysfunction; swallowing or feeding difficulties, stridor, apnea, weak cry, nystagmus
Downward herniation of cerebellar tonsils resulting in compression of cervicomedullary brainstem; impeded cerebrospinal fluid flow	Downward herniation of dysplastic lower brainstem and cerebellar vermis
Brain usually normal	Callosal dysgenesis, neuronal migration anomalies, hydrocephalus
Syringomyelia in 30%-70%	

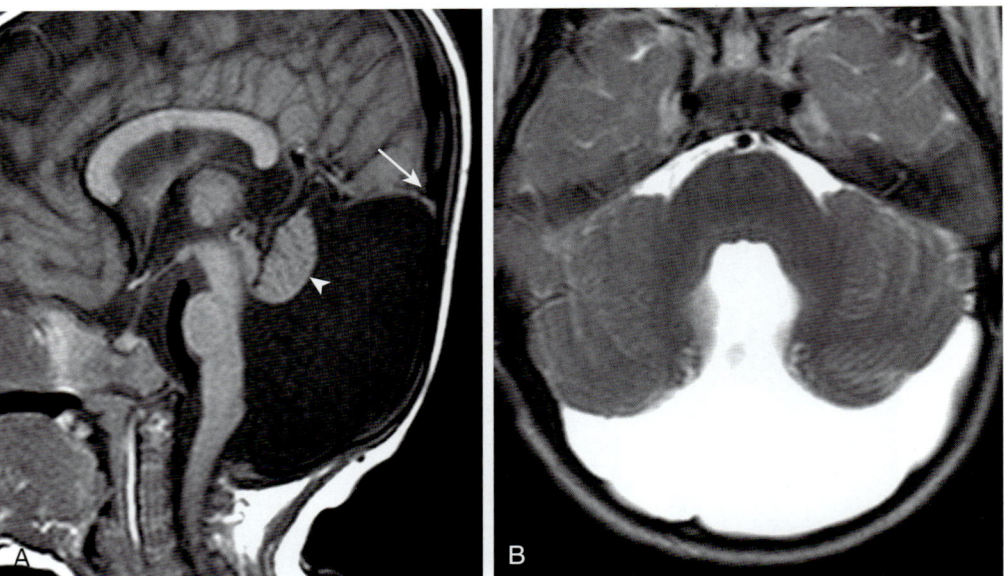

Figure 31-44   Dandy-Walker malformation. **A,** A sagittal T1-weighted image shows that the cerebellum (*arrowhead*) is hypoplastic and the torcula (*arrow*) is elevated. Note the hypoplastic pons. **B,** An axial T2-weighted image shows absence of the inferior vermis; the large retrocerebellar fluid collection communicates with the dilated fourth ventricle.

CEREBELLAR MALFORMATIONS

This section addresses malformations of the cerebellum in which the cerebellum is hypoplastic or dysplastic but will not address cerebellar atrophy, a classification proposed by Patel and Barkovich.[58] Cerebellar hypoplasia is defined by a small cerebellum with fissures of normal size compared with the folia. Cerebellar dysplasia describes disorganized development and includes an abnormal folial pattern, cerebellar gray matter heterotopias, which may be generalized involving cerebellar hemispheres and vermis, or focal and limited to a hemisphere or vermis. The latter would include the isolated inferior vermian hypoplasia often suggested by fetal MRI. Cerebellar hypoplasia includes the Dandy–Walker continuum and isolated focal cerebellar hypoplasia.

DANDY-WALKER CONTINUUM

The Dandy-Walker continuum includes the Dandy-Walker malformation and the Dandy-Walker variant.[59] The Dandy-Walker malformation is defined by complete or partial agenesis of the vermis, cystic dilatation of the fourth ventricle, and an enlarged posterior fossa with cranial displacement of the torcula (Fig. 31-44) and is often associated with supratentorial hydrocephalus. Associated anomalies occurring in 70% of patients include an abnormal or absent corpus callosum, callosal lipoma, and neuronal migration anomalies. The Dandy-Walker variant is defined as inferior vermian hypoplasia with nonobstructive cystic dilatation of the fourth ventricle; the posterior fossa is normal or somewhat enlarged (Fig. 31-45). In contrast to the Dandy-Walker continuum, the posterior fossa arachnoid cyst (Fig. 31-46) and mega cisterna magna (Fig. 31-47) are associated with a fully formed cerebellum. Retrocerebellar arachnoid cysts cause anterior displacement of the fourth ventricle and the cerebellum. The mega cisterna magna consists of enlarged retrocerebellar CSF spaces with no mass effect.

CEREBELLAR DYSPLASIA

Cerebellar dysplasia may be isolated or associated with other anomalies. The affected cerebellar tissue may be hypoplastic (Fig. 31-48) or hyperplastic (Fig. 31-49).

RHOMBENCEPHALOSYNAPSIS

This is a relatively rare major malformation in which the cerebellum is incompletely divided into two hemispheres. Clinical problems vary, depending on the severity of associated malformations. Isolated rhomboencephalosynapsis may

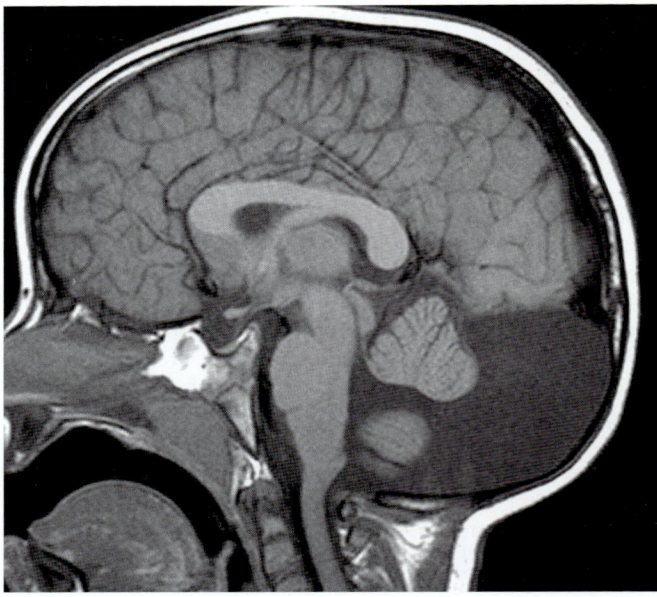

Figure 31-45   Dandy-Walker variant; a continuum in the spectrum.

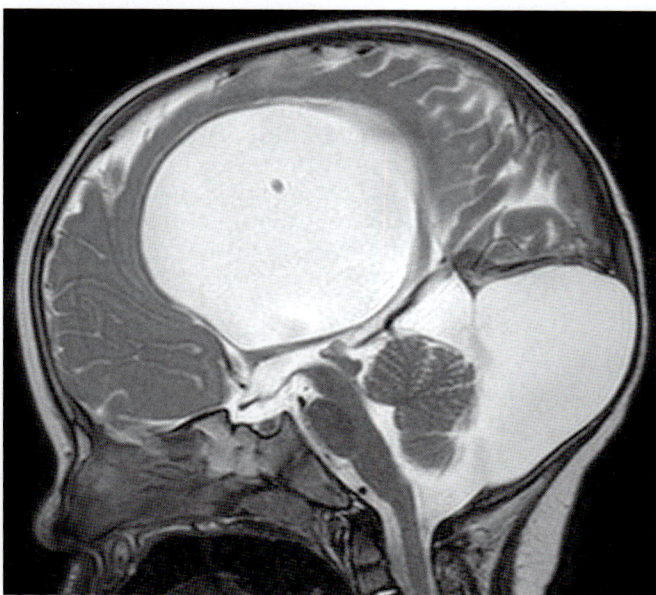

Figure 31-46 Retrocerebellar arachnoid cyst. A sagittal T2-weighted magnetic resonance imaging scan shows that the cerebellum is fully formed. Associated agenesis of the septum pellucidum and hydrocephalus are seen.

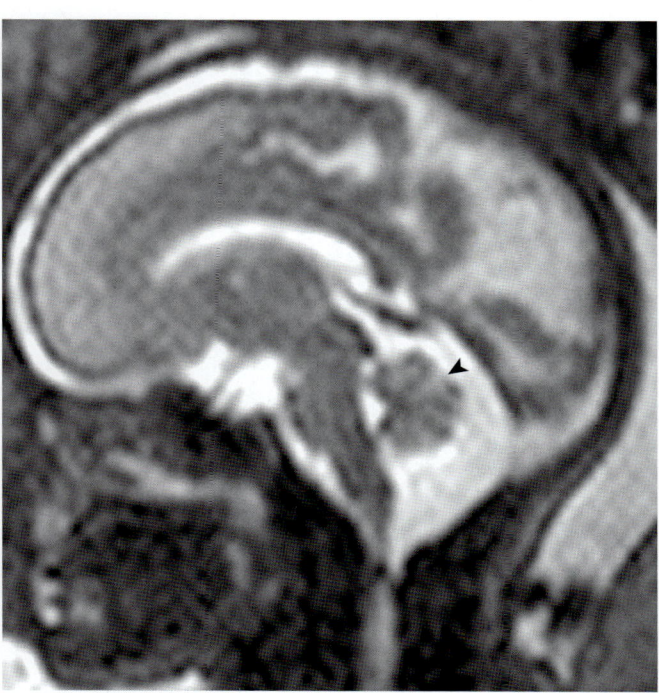

Figure 31-47 Mega cistern magna. A sagittal T2-weighted prenatal magnetic resonance imaging scan shows prominent posterior fossa cerebrospinal fluid space with a normal inferior cerebellar vermis (*arrowhead*).

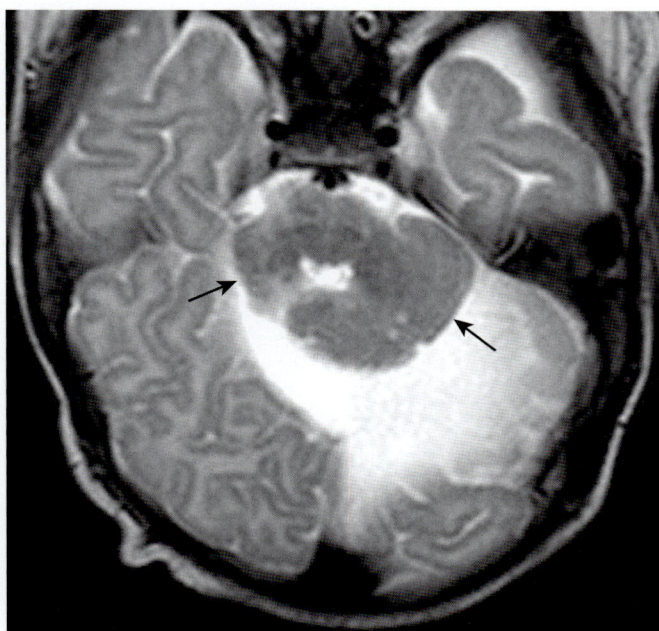

Figure 31-48 Cerebellar dysplasia. An axial T2-weighted image shows hypoplastic and malformed cerebellar hemispheres (*arrows*).

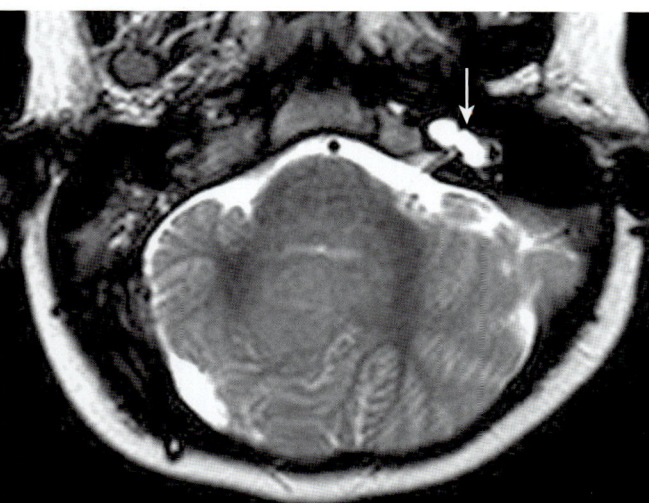

Figure 31-49 Cerebellar dysplasia. An axial T2-weighted image shows right cerebellar hyperplasia with dysplastic folia and malformed membranous labyrinth on the left inner ear (*arrow*).

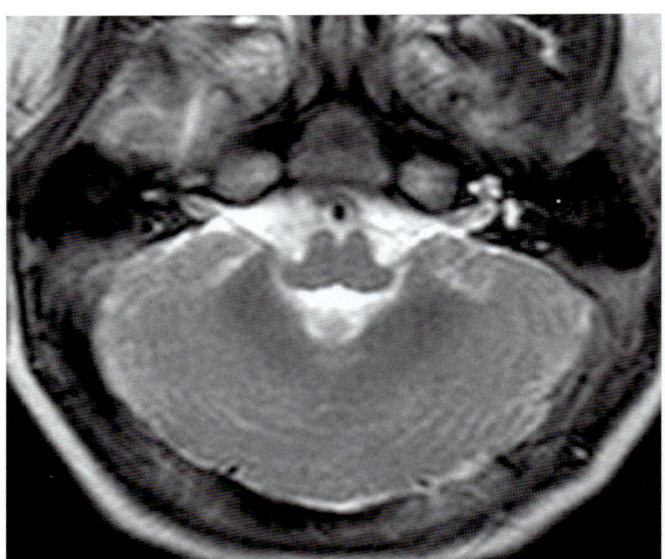

Figure 31-50 Rhomboencephalosynapsis. An axial T2-weighted image shows fusion of the cerebellar hemispheres.

be associated with normal cognition or behavioral disorders, hypotonia, and ataxia.

Imaging The cerebellar hemispheres are fused (Fig. 31-50). Associated brainstem abnormalities include fusion of the colliculi, atresia or dilatation of the fourth ventricle, and abnormalities of lower cranial nerves and the medulla. The corpus callosum may be hypoplastic or absent, and failure of formation of diencephalic structures with thalamic fusion, hydrocephalus, and malformations of cortical development may exist.

References

Full references for this chapter can be found on www.expertconsult.com.

Chapter 32

Hydrocephalus

GIULIO ZUCCOLI and GAYATHRI SREEDHER

Hydrocephalus means "water in the brain." It is the end result of many different processes that lead to enlarging ventricles with compression of brain parenchyma and subarachnoid spaces, which in turn leads to raised intracranial pressure (ICP). The active enlargement of cerebrospinal fluid (CSF) space in the ventricles eventually leads to loss of brain tissue if the fluid is not diverted. By convention, ventriculomegaly associated with increased ICP is termed "hydrocephalus." It is crucial to differentiate it from ex vacuo enlargement of the ventricles as a result of volume loss or from congenital anomalies with associated ventriculomegaly.

Hydrocephalus is one of the most common sequelae of any insult to a child's central nervous system (CNS). Hydrocephalus occurs in 1 in 2000 live births and is associated with one third of all CNS malformations. Since the 1970s, the incidence of spinal dysraphism related to hydrocephalus has declined.[1] Reasons include maternal folate therapy, which has resulted in fewer patients with spinal dysraphism, and vaccinations, which have diminished the number of patients with meningitis and its complications.

Physiology of Cerebrospinal Fluid

CSF appears in response to degeneration of the primitive mesenchyma that surrounds the brain. Although the precise timing of CSF formation is not clear, CSF circulation from the ventricles to the subarachnoid space does not occur until after formation of the fourth ventricle outlet foramina at the ninth to tenth week of gestation.

Approximately 60% of CSF is produced by the choroid plexus, and the remainder is produced extrachoroidally, possibly across parenchymal capillaries or by the ependyma itself. The rate of CSF production in adults by the choroid plexus is approximately 500 mL per 24 hours. Normal CSF volume in an adult is estimated to be approximately 150 mL. The CSF volume in a neonate is approximately 50 mL. However, using volumetric magnetic resonance imaging (MRI), a CSF volume of 150 mL has been found within the neonatal subarachnoid space, with an additional 100 to 120 mL within the spinal subarachnoid space.

The sites of CSF absorption remain controversial. It is widely accepted that arachnoid villi are one of the major sites in adults and older children.[2] The arachnoid villi (pacchionian granulations) are not developed in children until the closure of the fontanels. Various studies also have suggested that a portion of CSF drains through the perivascular and perineural spaces into the lymphatic system.[3] In neonates, most CSF absorption may occur through the lymphatic and venous system.[4]

Mechanisms of Hydrocephalus

Several theories have been used to explain the pathophysiology of hydrocephalus. Two widely accepted theories include the bulk flow theory and the Greitz model (hydrodynamic theory).

CLASSIC BULK FLOW THEORY

According to the classic bulk flow theory, hydrocephalus occurs as a result of imbalance between the production and the absorption of CSF. An obstruction inside the ventricular system proximal to fourth ventricle foramina of Luschka and Magendie causes obstructive hydrocephalus, whereas an obstruction outside the ventricular system causes communicating hydrocephalus.

Increased CSF production is rare and may occur with choroid plexus papilloma. Decreased CSF uptake occurs as a result of obstruction to the bulk flow anywhere along the CSF pathway. The common sites of obstruction along the CSF pathway are the foramen of Monro, the aqueduct of Sylvius, the fourth ventricle outlet foramina, the basal cisterns, and the arachnoid villi.

HYDRODYNAMIC MODEL FOR CSF CIRCULATION

The hydrodynamic model is based on the concept that the absorption of CSF occurs through the capillaries in the CNS rather than through the arachnoid granulations and villi.[3] The skull is a nonelastic housing for brain tissue; blood, CSF, and brain tissue are almost incompressible. As stated by the Monro-Kelly doctrine, the total volume of arteries, veins, CSF, and brain confined within the skull cavity and dura mater is constant, and any increase in volume in one or more compartments causes a decrease in volume in the others. Skull and dura mater are more elastic. The elasticity of these structures plays a pivotal role in the hydrodynamic theory of hydrocephalus. During cardiac systole, the expansion of the intracranial arteries increases the ICP, causing CSF displacement into the spinal canal and an increase in the venous outflow. During cardiac diastole, inflow of CSF from the spinal canal occurs, which causes elevation of pressure in the subarachnoid space. Thus increased pressure is present in the CSF spaces during the entire cardiac cycle, which in turn compresses the venous outlets, causing an increase in outlet resistance and venous "counter" pressure. This pressure is necessary to keep the intracerebral veins sufficiently distended to accommodate the normal cerebral flow.

Imaging

COMPUTED TOMOGRAPHY AND MAGNETIC RESONANCE IMAGING

Computed tomography (CT) and MRI are used as primary modalities to assess ventricular size. Ultrasound of the head is used as the initial study in infants with macrocephaly. Several parameters can help differentiate between hydrocephalus and ex vacuo dilatation of ventricles from cerebral atrophy in infants (Box 32-1).

The most reliable sign of hydrocephalus is enlargement of the anterior and posterior recesses of the third ventricle (Fig. 32-1); this phenomenon does not occur in ex vacuo ventricular enlargement. The disproportionate enlargement of the recesses occurs because the thin hypothalamus and cisterns surrounding these recesses provide relatively little resistance to expansion. In contrast, the body of the third ventricle is restricted by the rigid thalami, which provide more resistance to expansion. The anterior recesses (i.e., the chiasmal and infundibular recesses) expand earlier than the posterior recesses (i.e., the pineal and suprapineal recesses), which is best appreciated on midsagittal MRI.[5] On axial CT, dilation of the anterior recesses of the third ventricle is detected when the third ventricle is larger at the level of the optic chiasm than at the middle of the ventricle.

The enlargement and inferior displacement of the anterior recesses may cause flattening of the pituitary gland with erosion of the dorsum sella, giving the classic plain film appearance of increased ICP in older children and adults. The recesses may compress the infundibulum, resulting in hypothalamic-pituitary dysfunction. Enlargement of the suprapineal and pineal recesses may displace the pineal gland inferiorly and occasionally elevates the vein of Galen. A large diverticulum of this recess may compress the tectum inferiorly and shorten it in the rostrocaudal direction, mimicking a neoplasm.

Commensurate dilation of the temporal horns with the lateral ventricles also is a strong indicator of hydrocephalus.

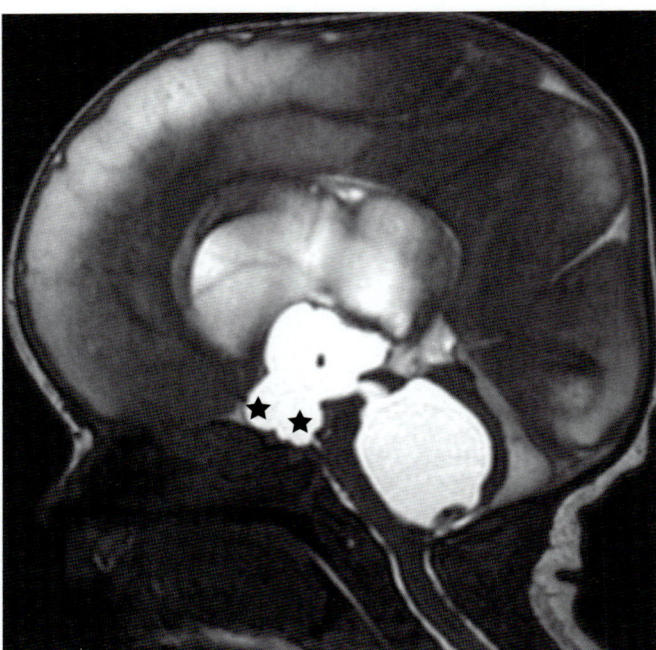

Figure 32-1 Obstructive hydrocephalus. A midline sagittal balanced steady-state free precession image demonstrates the dilatation of the chiasmatic and infundibular recess of the third ventricle (*stars*). A dilated fourth ventricle also is noted in this patient with fourth ventricular outflow obstruction (an entrapped fourth ventricle) from neonatal hemorrhage.

The dilation of the temporal horns is best viewed on coronal T2-weighted images. The choroidal fissure is enlarged, and the hippocampus is compressed and displaced inferomedially (Fig. 32-2). Studies have suggested that temporal horns dilate less than the bodies of the lateral ventricles in generalized atrophy.[6] This finding may be related to the small size of the temporal lobes and to their relatively small volume of white matter.

In ex vacuo dilatation of ventricles associated with cerebral atrophy, the superior and inferior walls of temporal horns remain parallel and are smaller than the lateral ventricle body. The hippocampus is normally placed, and the choroidal fissures are not enlarged. The sylvian fissure is enlarged in patients with temporal lobe atrophy, and in these patients, temporal horn enlargement cannot be used to distinguish hydrocephalus from ex vacuo ventriculomegaly.

The mamillopontine distance is measured on MRI from the anterior root of the mamillary body to the top of the pons parallel to the anterior mesencephalon. The normal average distance is 3.8 mm.[5] The floor of the third ventricle as seen on sagittal MRI is usually concave downward. With enlargement of the third ventricle, it becomes straightened or convex downward, resulting in reduction of the mamillopontine distance (e-Fig. 32-3).

The ventricular angle (e-Fig. 32-4) measures the divergence of the frontal horns.[6] Concentric enlargement of the frontal horns in a patient with hydrocephalus causes diminution of this angle, as seen on axial or coronal images. This concentric dilation produces an enlargement of the frontal horn radius with a rounded configuration of the frontal horns, or a "Mickey Mouse ears" appearance.

Box 32-1 Imaging Characteristics of Hydrocephalus*

Enlargement of the third ventricle, particularly the anterior and posterior recesses

Commensurate dilation of the temporal horn with the lateral ventricles

Narrowing of the mamillopontine distance

Narrowing of the ventricular angle

Widening of the frontal horn radius

Periventricular interstitial edema

Effacement of cortical sulci

*Listed in order of diagnostic value.
From Barkovich AJ. Hydrocephalus. In: Barkovich AJ, ed. *Pediatric neuroimaging*. 4th ed. Philadelphia: Lippincott Williams & Wilkins; 2005:663.

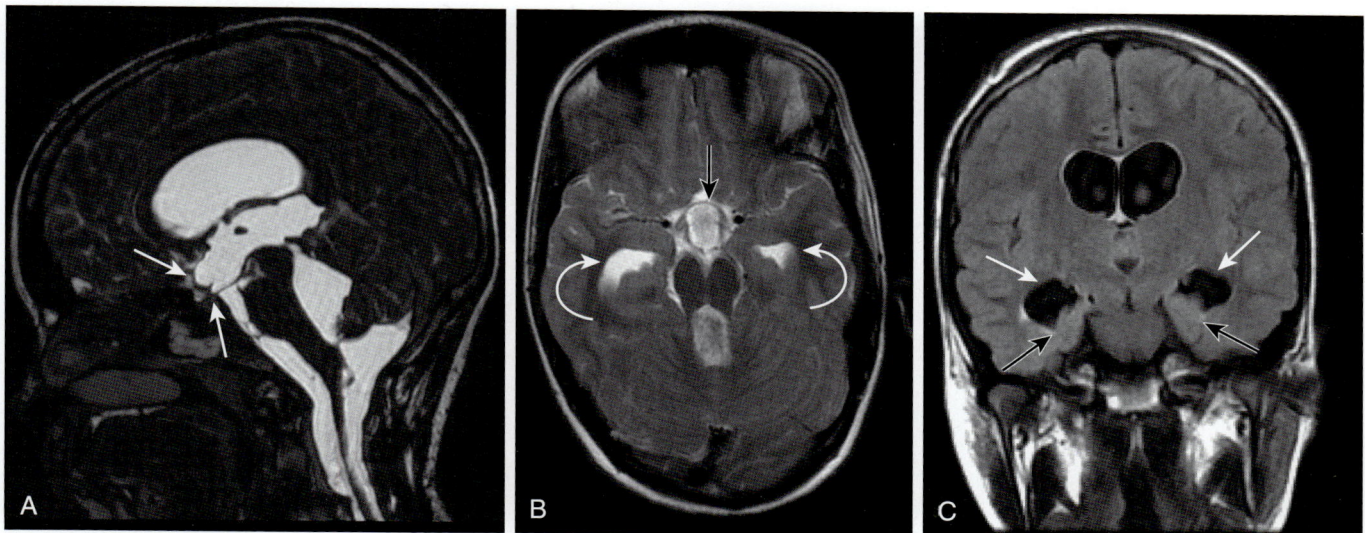

Figure 32-2 Magnetic resonance imaging findings in a patient with hydrocephalus. **A,** A midsagittal T1-weighted image in a 10-year-old girl with obstructive hydrocephalus demonstrates dilation of the chiasmatic and infundibular recesses (*arrows*). **B,** An axial fluid-attenuated inversion recovery image shows dilated anterior recess of the third ventricle (*straight arrow*). The temporal horns also are dilated (*curved arrows*), with a surrounding increase in signal suggestive of increased transependymal cerebrospinal fluid resorption. **C,** A coronal T2-weighted image shows the characteristic dilation of the temporal horns (*white arrows*) with enlargement of the choroidal fissure and inferomedial displacement of the hippocampus (*black arrows*).

Enlargement of the ventricles disproportionate to enlargement of the cortical sulci favors a diagnosis of hydrocephalus. However, this parameter is not reliable in children, especially in the first years of life, because patients with communicating hydrocephalus and atrophy have enlargement of both of the fluid spaces. In addition, the sizes of the ventricles and the subarachnoid spaces may vary tremendously, as seen in infants with benign macrocephaly. Therefore it is important to evaluate ventricular size in conjunction with the patient's neurologic evaluation and serial head circumference measurements. A large or rapidly enlarging head would favor a diagnosis of hydrocephalus, whereas a small or diminishing head circumference would suggest atrophy.

The presence of periventricular interstitial edema is indicative of hydrocephalus (Fig. 32-5). With elevation of pressure within the ventricles, the normal centripetal flow toward the ventricles is reversed. The CSF is forced out through the ependyma into the surrounding extracellular spaces to be absorbed by alternative routes. This increase in periventricular fluid constitutes interstitial edema. It is best recognized on MRI with fluid-attenuated inversion recovery and proton density sequences. It is more difficult to appreciate on T2-weighted images because of the bright signal from the ventricles. Periventricular interstitial edema is difficult to appreciate in neonates and young infants because it is masked by a bright signal from immature myelin, with its high water content. On CT, periventricular interstitial edema is seen as hypoattenuation in the periventricular region, with indistinct ventricular margins.

A CSF "flow void" in the third ventricle, aqueduct of Sylvius, and fourth ventricle may be accentuated in persons with hydrocephalus as a result of hyperdynamic flow, although the specificity of this finding is unclear (e-Fig. 32-6).

Hydrocephalus causes mass effect and distortion of adjacent brain structures. Stretching, upward displacement, and smooth, uniform thinning of the corpus callosum occurs as a result of lateral ventricular enlargement. Corpus callosum thinning also occurs with atrophy, but typically it is not elevated superiorly and may not be uniformly thin, as seen with hydrocephalus.

Marked hydrocephalus may lead to the formation of atrial diverticula, which is herniation of the ventricular wall through the choroidal fissure of the ventricular trigone into the supracerebellar and quadrigeminal cisterns. Diverticula may cause compression and distortion of the tectum and may mimic arachnoid cysts in the region of the quadrigeminal cistern.[7]

MRI in persons with hydrocephalus frequently involves utilization of three-dimensional balanced steady-state free precession (SSFP). This sequence is particularly useful in demonstrating arachnoid membranes, intraventricular cysts, and aqueductal stenosis.

Qualitative and quantitative CSF analysis can be performed using phase-contrast cine MRI. The technique is useful in demonstrating pulsatile flow at the craniocervical junction (Fig. 32-7), aqueduct of Sylvius, and across a surgically created third ventriculostomy.[18]

ULTRASOUND

Ultrasound of the head is a useful initial examination for evaluation of macrocephaly in infants if the anterior fontanelle is open. Transcranial Doppler techniques may be helpful in identifying infants with raised ICP and may help determine the need for shunt placement. With elevated ICP, arterial flow tends to be reduced during diastole, resulting in elevated pulsatility of arterial flow. Many researchers have demonstrated elevated resistive indices in infants with raised ICP and a subsequent decrease on ventricular tapping. These results, however, have not been uniformly reproducible.[8-10]

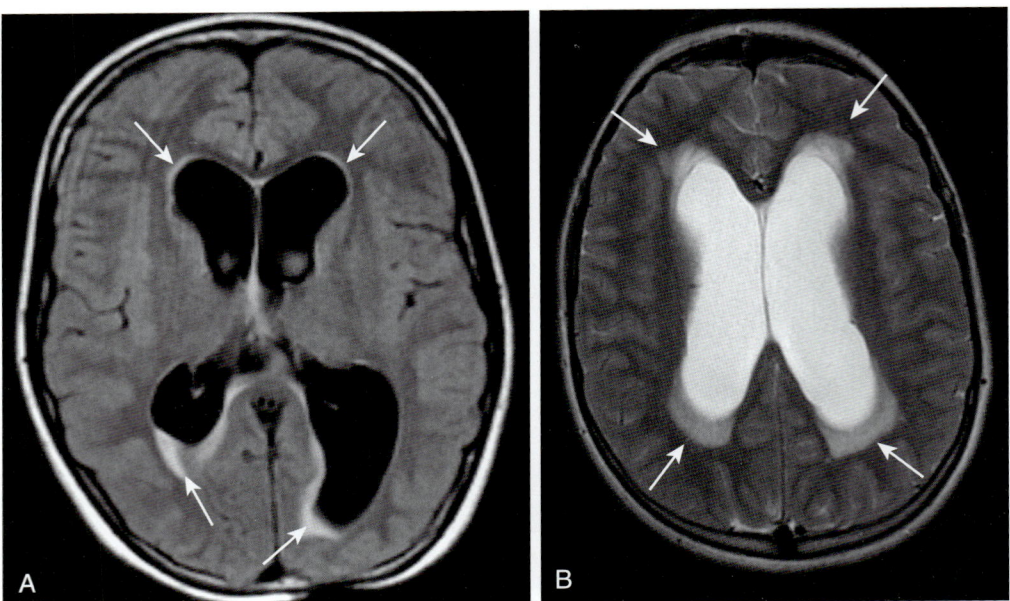

Figure 32-5   Hydrocephalus. **A,** An axial fluid-attenuated inversion recovery sequence at the level of the lateral ventricles demonstrates characteristic transependymal flow of cerebrospinal fluid (CSF) and periventricular hyperintensities. **B,** An axial T2-weighted image in a different patient demonstrates increased transependymal flow of CSF characteristic of hydrocephalus.

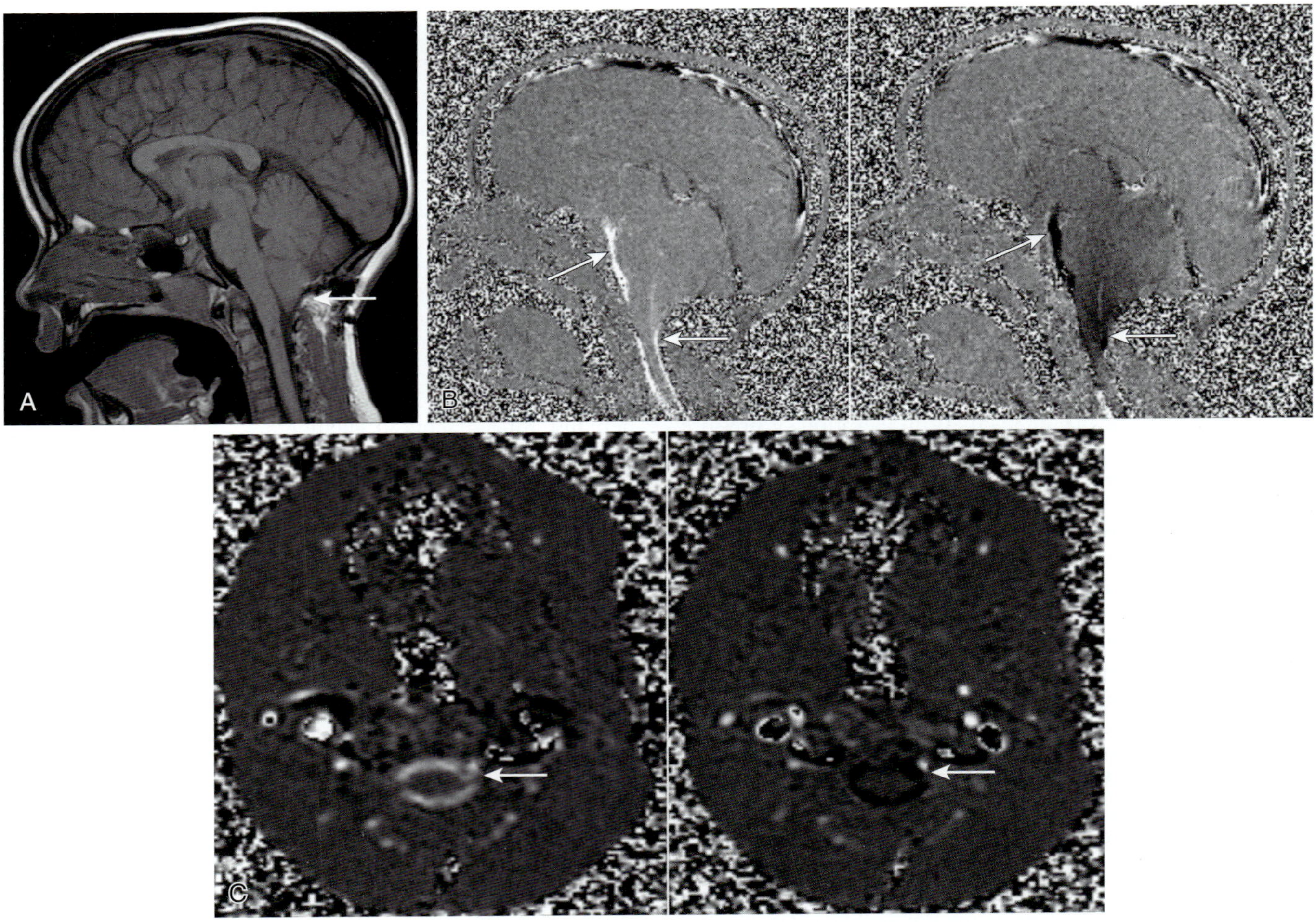

Figure 32-7   Phase-contrast cine magnetic resonance (MR) imaging. Images are acquired throughout the cardiac cycle and demonstrate pulsatile cerebrospinal fluid (CSF) motion. **A,** A midsagittal T1-weighted image shows the presence of a Chiari 1 malformation (*arrow*). **B,** A sagittal cine phase-contrast MR image demonstrates pulsatile CSF flow in the prepontine cistern and craniocervical junction (*arrows*). **C,** An axial phase-contrast MR image demonstrates pulsatile CSF flow at the foramen magnum (*arrows*). CSF flow velocity can be measured using dedicated software.

PLAIN RADIOGRAPHS

The changes related to elevated ICP on a plain radiograph of the skull depend on the age of the child. In children up to 8 or 10 years of age, sutural diastasis may occur within a few days of elevated pressures (e-Fig. 32-8). After 12 to 13 years of age, sutural diastasis is uncommon early, and the first sign of long-standing hydrocephalus may be erosion of the sellar cortex caused by enlargement of the third ventricular anterior recesses. The anterior part of the base of the dorsum is the earliest to be eroded, but the erosion may spread to involve the sella floor.

NUCLEAR MEDICINE CISTERNOGRAM

Occasionally, radionuclide cisternography is helpful in diagnosing communicating hydrocephalus if other imaging studies and a neurologic examination are equivocal. Indium–111–labeled diethylenetriaminepentaacetic acid is injected intrathecally via a lumbar puncture. The opening CSF pressure is determined at the time of injection. Planar and single-photon emission CT imaging is performed at 4 and 24 hours, and if needed, at 48 hours. The protocol involves collection of urine for 4 hours after injection of the isotope to calculate the percentage of isotope excreted in the urine. The interpretation of the cisternogram is based on three pieces of information—the CSF opening pressure, the percentage of isotope excreted in the urine, and the images obtained:

1. The normal opening CSF pressure should be in the range appropriate for the age of the child (infants, 0 to 5 mm Hg; children, 5 to 10 mm Hg; and older children and adults, 10 to 15 mm Hg). Elevated pressures suggest hydrocephalus.
2. The percentage of isotope excretion is normally in the range of 40% to 50%. If the excretion measures below this level, the study result is abnormal.
3. In a normal cisternogram, the tracer enters the basal cisterns, and by 24 hours it is seen over the cerebral convexities, where it is absorbed by the arachnoid granulations. If the tracer enters the ventricular system and persists for more than 24 hours, it is indicative of communicating hydrocephalus.

The first two pieces of information are most useful. The results from imaging should be interpreted cautiously.

Etiologies of Hydrocephalus

NEWBORNS AND INFANTS

The common etiologies for ventriculomegaly are listed in Box 32-2.

Infants with ventriculomegaly typically present with macrocephaly. It is critical and often difficult to differentiate between ventriculomegaly caused by communicating hydrocephalus, which requires shunting, and ventriculomegaly related to benign extraaxial fluid of infancy, which does not require intervention. These infants therefore should be assessed clinically for other signs of elevated ICP, such as dilated scalp veins, bulging fontanelles, and sutural diastasis. They may have ocular signs and spasticity in the lower extremities as a result of disproportionate stretching of the corticospinal tracts arising from the motor cortex leg area by

---

Box 32-2 Causes of Ventriculomegaly in the Newborn and Infant

Ventriculomegaly without Elevated Intracranial Pressure

Mild ventriculomegaly associated with benign extraaxial fluid of infancy

Ex vacuo dilation of ventricles as a result of atrophy

Congenital anomalies: corpus callosal anomalies, lissencephalies, holoprosencephaly

Ventriculomegaly with Elevated Intracranial Pressure

Intraventricular hemorrhage

Infection

Congenital anomalies: myelomeningocele, Dandy-Walker malformation, aqueductal stenosis, X-linked hydrocephalus, vein of Galen malformation

Thrombosis of dural venous sinuses or other causes of obstruction to venous drainage

Tumor

---

the enlarged ventricles. Infants with macrocephaly should be evaluated with imaging to assess for ventricular dilation. Ultrasound is the most common initial modality used to obtain images of infants with macrocrania.

In persons with communicating hydrocephalus, the ventricles typically are disproportionately larger than the subarachnoid spaces. At times, the two conditions cannot be differentiated on imaging. The imaging findings should always be interpreted in the context of the clinical history and serial head circumference measurements. Infants with communicating hydrocephalus usually have other signs of raised ICP and an abnormal neurologic examination. When the imaging findings and clinical examination are equivocal, a CSF cisternogram may help to differentiate between the two conditions. Rarely, the issue needs to be resolved by the gold standard of invasive ICP monitoring.

Benign Extraaxial Collections of Infancy

The most common cause of macrocephaly in infants is benign extraaxial collections of infancy. This condition has been called benign enlargement of subarachnoid spaces in infancy, benign external hydrocephalus, benign macrocrania, and benign subdural effusion of infancy. These infants typically present between 2 and 6 months of age with increased head circumference; they have normal neurologic development with no clinical signs of raised ICP. The head circumference is above the 95th percentile and stabilizes along a curve parallel to the 95th percentile by 18 months of age. The subarachnoid spaces are mildly enlarged and return to normal size by 18 to 24 months of age. The CSF spaces are disproportionately larger, with the ventricles only mildly prominent. This condition likely represents a transient communicating hydrocephalus from a delay in maturation of the arachnoid villi.

Imaging demonstrates mild prominence of the subarachnoid spaces along the frontoparietal convexities, the cortical sulci, the sylvian fissures, and the anterior interhemispheric fissures (Fig. 32-9). The ventricles typically are normal or mildly enlarged. The extraaxial fluid is most frequently symmetric (but may also be asymmetric), have the same signal intensity as CSF, and have no mass effect. If the fluid

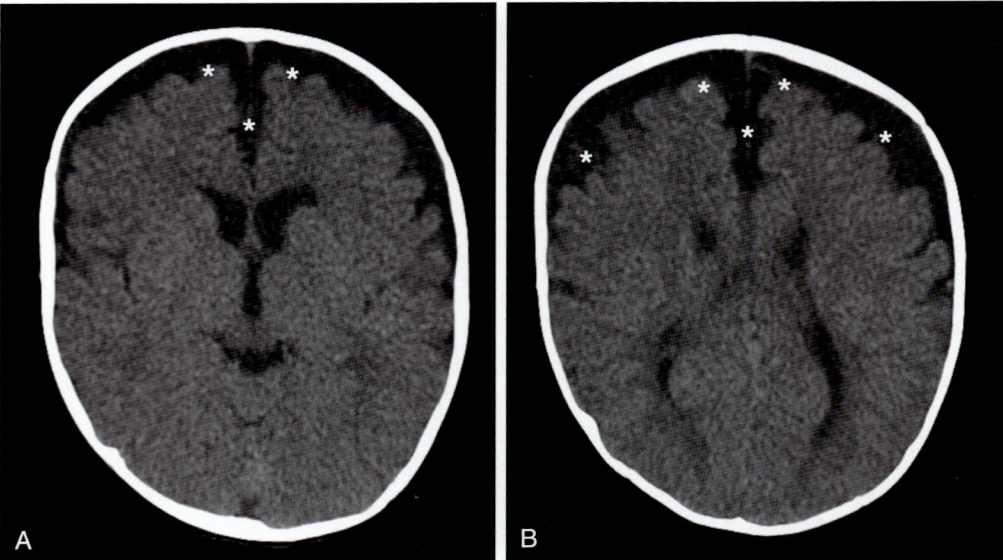

Figure 32-9 Benign extraaxial collections of infancy. **A** and **B,** Axial computed tomography shows prominent extraaxial fluid spaces and an interhemispheric fissure (*asterisks*). The ventricles are also mildly prominent.

collection is of higher attenuation than CSF, is asymmetric, or exerts mass effect on adjacent structures, MRI should be performed to evaluate for blood products from a subdural hematoma. At our institution, we use proton density MRI to distinguish benign extraaxial collections and extraaxial hematomas. Extraaxial hematomas are brighter than CSF on proton density sequences. Both MRI and ultrasound can help differentiate between subarachnoid fluid and a subdural hematoma. With enlarged subarachnoid spaces, the cortical veins course through the fluid and lie adjacent to the inner table of the calvarium. If the subdural space is enlarged, the cortical veins should be displaced away from the inner table toward the cerebral cortex. The signal intensity of chronic subdural hematoma also differs from that of CSF on MRI.[11] It has been questioned whether enlarged CSF spaces may make these patients more susceptible to subdural hemorrhage from minor trauma, which occurs in children with arachnoid cysts.

The diagnosis of benign extraaxial collection of infancy is a diagnosis of exclusion. Other causes of prominent CSF subarachnoid spaces include congenital anomalies, communicating hydrocephalus, infection, hypercortisolism, dehydration, cerebral atrophy, and drugs (parenteral nutrition and chemotherapy).

OLDER CHILDREN

Common causes of ventriculomegaly in older children are listed in Box 32-3. Because of the inability of their cranium to expand as quickly as in infants and young children, older children with hydrocephalus have a more acute presentation. They may have the classic triad of headache, vomiting, and lethargy. Children who have chronic hydrocephalus as a result of slowly expanding lesions typically present with persistent morning headaches and intermittent vomiting. Papilledema often is encountered. Focal neurologic deficits from the primary lesion and pyramidal tract signs, which are more marked in the lower extremities, may be present.

Hypothalamic-pituitary dysfunction also may develop as a result of compression of these structures by enlarging anterior recesses of the third ventricle.

Normal Pressure Hydrocephalus

Intermittent high CSF pressures with consequent reduced cerebral blood flow may lead to brain damage and can lead to hydrocephalus if concomitant reduction in the compliance in the cranial cavity occurs (Greitz model), which is the postulated pathogenesis for normal pressure hydrocephalus. The loss of compliance is believed to be due to damage to arachnoid membranes or loss of dural elasticity. Normal pressure hydrocephalus is mainly a disease of adults, with pediatric cases seen in association with a history of meningitis or intraventricular bleeding. CSF volume is displaced at the craniovertebral junction during systole, and the venous stroke volume is decreased. Intracranial CSF pulse pressure is increased (although mean CSF pressure is normal), commensurate with reduced compliance in the meninges.

The CSF pressure assessed at lumbar puncture is normal. Upon imaging, fast flow at the aqueduct is seen on phase-contrast cine MRI.

Box 32-3 Causes of Ventriculomegaly in Older Children

Ventriculomegaly without Elevated Intracranial Pressure
Ex vacuo dilation as a result of atrophy
Congenital anomalies

Ventriculomegaly with Elevated Intracranial Pressure
Infection
Trauma
Tumors: direct pressure or leptomeningeal metastases
Delayed identification of congenital abnormality

Assessment of Children with Ventricular Shunts

METHODS OF SHUNTING

Different methods have been used for CSF shunting, with the goal to decrease ICP by providing an alternative pathway for CSF absorption. The shunt catheters have a proximal intracranial segment connected in series to a valve and distal tubing. The proximal catheter may be inserted through the occipital, frontal, or posterior temporal approach. The placement of the ventriculostomy catheter is optimal if the tip and the side holes of the catheter are not in direct contact with the choroid plexus. This technique minimizes the chances of tissue ingrowth and occlusion of the proximal catheter. The distal catheter may be placed in various locations, including the peritoneal cavity, pleural cavity, central veins or right atrium, and gallbladder. The peritoneal cavity is the overwhelmingly favored location. The only relative contraindications to its use are active intraperitoneal infection, significant risk of future peritoneal infections, severe adhesions, and previous failure of peritoneal shunts.

SHUNT MALFUNCTION

Hemorrhage from insertion of the proximal catheter occurs in approximately 1% of patients (Box 32-4). It is even more common when an old catheter is removed. Neuronal injury may result in focal deficits if the catheter traverses the internal capsule. Seizures can occur and are more common with catheters placed through a frontal approach. With lumbar catheters, there is a 5% reported risk of radiculopathy and a 1% risk of myelopathy.

It is an axiom in pediatric medicine that when a child with a ventricular shunt has a medical problem, the shunt is the cause of the problem until proven otherwise. The causes of shunt malfunction can be divided broadly into two categories: (1) mechanical shunt failure involving the shunt apparatus and (2) shunt infection. The most common time for the shunt to fail is in the first 6 months after insertion. Multiple studies indicate that patients younger than 6 months are at a higher risk of shunt malfunction. The overall 1-year failure rate is 40% for patients with a corrected median age of 55 days and 30% in older age groups.

Mechanical Shunt Failure

The leading cause of shunt malfunction is mechanical failure. Obstruction is most common at the proximal end and can

---

Box 32-4 Complications of Catheter Insertion

Intracranial hemorrhage

Damage to neuronal tissue

Pneumocephalus: air lock in the shunt

Altered cerebrospinal fluid flow dynamics: loculated fourth ventricle

Slit ventricles

Subdural hematoma

Meningeal fibrosis

Craniosynostosis

Box 32-5 Abdominal Complications of a Distal Shunt Catheter

Acute abdomen

Ascites

Cerebrospinal fluid: enteric fistula

Inflammatory pseudotumor of the mesentery

Inguinal hernia

Intrahepatic abscess

Omental cyst

Perforation of the bowel

Perforation of the gallbladder

Pseudocyst

Small bowel obstruction

Umbilical fistula

Ureter obstruction

Volvulus

From Martin AE, Gaskill SJ. Cerebrospinal fluid shunts: complication and results. In: McLone DG, ed. *Pediatric neurosurgery: surgery of the developing nervous system*. 4th ed. Philadelphia: WB Saunders; 2001.

---

result from occlusion by brain parenchyma, choroid plexus, a protein plug, or tumor cells.[12] Disconnection may occur at any point in the shunt apparatus, but it is most frequent at the site of connection between the valve and the peritoneal catheter and at sites of increased mobility (i.e., the lateral neck) (e-Fig. 32-10). The shunt tubing may migrate to a variety of sites.

The distal catheter has its own unique set of complications (Box 32-5), which are best evaluated with abdominal imaging. Pseudocysts may occur at the distal end, with or without infection, causing impairment of CSF absorption.

Chronic shunt placement may alter CSF flow dynamics, resulting in isolated ventricles. An isolated fourth ventricle may occur with shunting of a noncommunicating hydrocephalus. Upon shunting, enlarged lateral ventricles collapse, resulting in obstruction of the aqueduct of Sylvius that becomes irreversible over time. The CSF being produced in the fourth ventricle cannot be drained from above (because of obstruction at the aqueduct) or below (because of the original outlet obstruction), causing progressive dilation of the fourth ventricle (e-Figs. 32-11 and 32-12).

Other chronic complications include subdural hematomas, which occur because of rapid decompression of the ventricular system before the brain parenchyma can expand to fill the cranial vault. Meningeal fibrosis, although rare, may occur, possibly as a reaction to a chronic subdural hematoma. The meninges show profuse enhancement on postcontrast images. Craniosynostosis is a rare complication occurring only in patients who undergo placement of a shunt before 6 months of age.

Shunt Infections

Shunt infections remain an important and distressing cause of shunt failure, with an overall infection rate of 5% to 10%. The rate of infection in infants is much higher (10% to 20%). Most infections present within 2 months of surgery, indicating that they occur during surgery. Shunt infection also can occur from other abdominal surgical procedures, such as bladder augmentation and gastrostomy tube placement.

EVALUATION OF SHUNT MALFUNCTION

The diagnosis of shunt malfunction is based primarily on the presenting clinical signs and symptoms. Plain radiographs of the shunt and CT of the head are the primary radiologic investigations for evaluating shunt malfunction.

Plain radiographs of the entire shunt are obtained with frontal and lateral views of the skull and with frontal views of the chest and abdomen. These radiographs help assess shunt discontinuity or migration. Calcification along the tubing is common in old shunts, which are prone to fracture (see e-Fig. 32-10). Abdominal complications such as mass effect from pseudocyst formation, bowel perforation, and adhesions resulting in bowel obstruction also are evaluated on plain radiographs. If preperitoneal placement of distal tubing is suspected, a lateral radiograph should be obtained.[13]

Imaging of the head, typically with CT, is performed to assess changes in the shape and size of the ventricles, as well as any other collections or loculated compartments. One problem is that CT usually is obtained only when the patient is sick, and thus there is no valid baseline comparison when the patient is well. The position and course of the catheter can be assessed on CT. Dilation of ventricles compared with previous images is the clearest sign of shunt malfunction. However, some patients with shunt malfunction may demonstrate little if any enlargement, and some patients may have small ventricles. Therefore the ventricular size alone, especially in the absence of previous studies, may be misleading. Enlarged ventricles are seen in approximately 70% of patients with mechanical obstruction and in 30% of those with a shunt infection.

The advantages of CT are that it is widely available and relatively inexpensive, and it allows quick examination and a reproducible assessment of ventricular size and catheter position. However, even a single CT study exposes children to potentially harmful levels of radiation, and children with

hydrocephalus are usually exposed to multiple CT procedures, further increasing their cancer risk.

MRI is an alternative to CT for shunt evaluation with limited steady-state gradient-recalled sequence and balanced SSFP sequences (Fig. 32-13). Fast MRI sequences such as single-shot or half-Fourier T2-weighted sequences and T1-weighted spoiled gradient sequences reduce the scan time dramatically, decreasing or eliminating the need for sedation. These sequences provide reliable visualization of the catheter and superior anatomic detail.[14]

The subset of symptomatic patients with little or no change in ventricular size, or with small ventricles, may benefit from shunt tapping and, rarely, from a shuntogram. Tapping of the shunt is also helpful for CSF sampling if a shunt infection is suspected. Free flow of CSF may indicate adequate patency of the proximal catheter. Manometric measurements also can be performed. A shuntogram can be performed by injecting contrast material into the valve chamber at the time of shunt tapping and taking radiographs at 1 and 15 minutes. Peritoneal spilling of contrast material proves patency of the distal tubing. The results of the shuntogram may be inconclusive in patients with partially obstructed shunts. Shunt injection studies are more helpful in diagnosing distal malfunction. A 25% to 40% rate of false-positive results is found in patients with proximal malfunction (i.e., failure of proximal CSF to pass through the distal tubing despite patent tubing). Similarly, radioisotope studies occasionally are used to assess shunt patency and obtain physiologic information about CSF flow through the shunt.

In general, small ventricles in a child with a shunt are good, and large ventricles are bad. Approximately 1% to 5% of patients with very small, or slit, ventricles become symptomatic with acute or chronic headaches, nausea, vomiting, and lethargy. These patients have been lumped together under the term "slit ventricle syndrome" (e-Fig. 32-14). This terminology is confusing because it has been used for multiple clinical entities.[15] At one end of the spectrum is a child with small ventricles who is very sick as a result of intracranial hypertension. At the other end of the spectrum is an

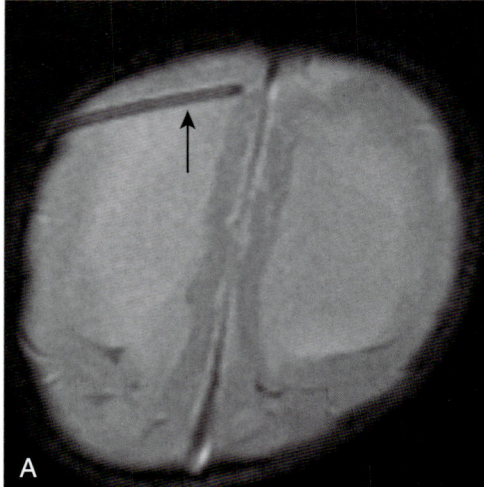
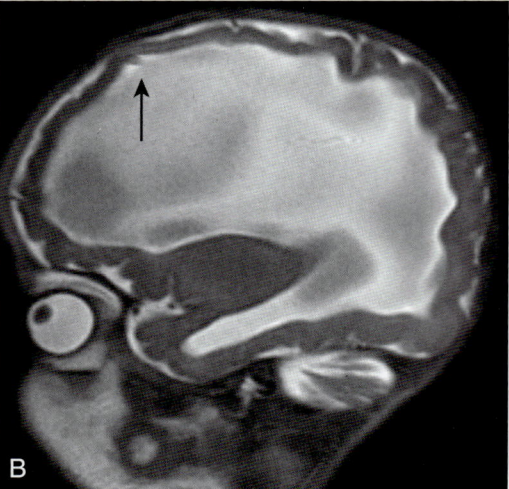

Figure 32-13   **A,** An axial steady-state gradient sequence demonstrates the course of the catheter in the right lateral ventricle. **B,** A sagittal balanced steady-state free precession sequence demonstrates the tip of the catheter within an enlarged lateral ventricle (*arrow*).

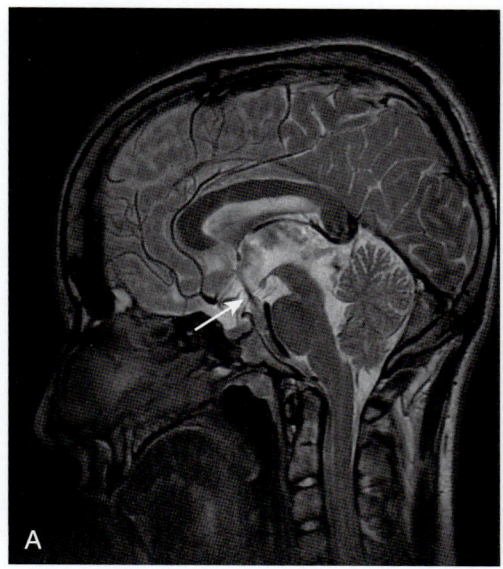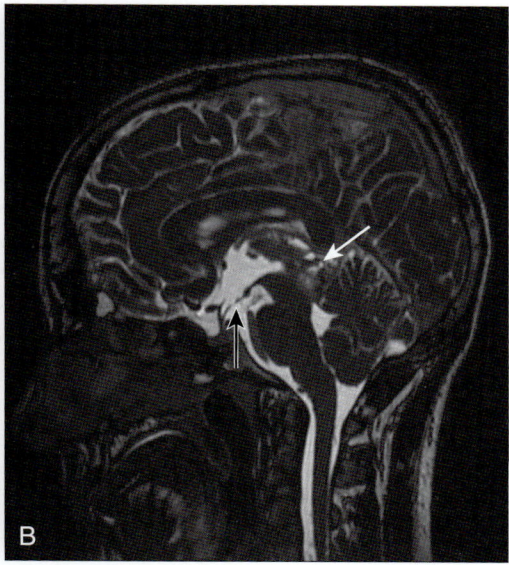

Figure 32-15   Third ventriculostomy. **A,** A midsagittal T2-weighted image through the third ventricle at 2-mm section thickness and 512 × 512 matrix demonstrates the flow void through the ventriculostomy in a patient affected by a tectal tumor. **B,** A midsagittal balanced steady-state free precession image shows the ventriculostomy defect (*dark arrow*) and the tectal tumor (*white arrow*).

asymptomatic child with a harmless and inconsequential CT finding.

Endoscopic Third Ventriculostomy

During the past decade, the treatment of hydrocephalus with endoscopic procedures has received renewed enthusiasm. The major attraction is to give children with hydrocephalus freedom from lifelong dependency on external shunts and their numerous inherent complications. Endoscopic third ventriculostomy is most often used for obstructive hydrocephalus, with a success rate of 60% to 70%. The technique involves use of an endoscope to perforate the floor of the third ventricle just anterior to the mammillary bodies, thereby establishing communication between the ventricles and cisterns. Endoscopic fourth ventricular aqueductoplasty, with or without stent placement, has been described as an alternative method when ETV is not feasible.[16] This approach is especially useful in patients with a trapped fourth ventricle.

On postoperative imaging (Fig. 32-15), a gradual decrease is seen in the size of the ventricles over months to years. This finding is contrary to imaging with external shunts, when a rapid reduction in the size of the ventricles is seen. The third ventricle responds early and decreases in size over 3 months, whereas the lateral ventricles decrease over 2 years. Thus it is difficult to assess for third ventriculostomy patency on the basis of ventricular size.[17]

Fast spin echo T2-weighted sequences are sensitive in assessing patency of the third ventriculostomy. Midline sagittal images show hypointensity in the region of the ventriculostomy as a result of CSF-related flow-void if the ventriculostomy is patent. Balanced SSFP images also can demonstrate closure of the ventriculostomy by the absence of a defect but may not detect CSF flow voids.

Phase contrast cine MRI is helpful to assess the patency of the ventriculostomy.[18] With use of cardiac gating, phase contrast images can demonstrate the pulsatile flow of CSF through the ventriculostomy and determine flow velocity. A caveat of phase contrast cine MRI is the presence of turbulent or pulsatile flow as a result of third ventricular floor motion (e-Fig. 32-16).

> ### Key Points
>
> Hydrocephalus is one of the most common sequelae of any insult to a child's CNS.
>
> The most common cause of macrocephaly in infants is benign extraaxial collections of infancy.
>
> Ultrasound of the head is a useful initial examination if the anterior fontanelle is open. After fontanelle closure, CT or MRI is required for evaluation of the ventricular system and shunts.
>
> The most reliable sign of hydrocephalus is enlargement of the anterior and posterior recesses of the third ventricle.

Suggested Readings

Barkovich AJ, Raybaud C, eds. *Pediatric neuroimaging.* 5th ed. Philadelphia: Lippincott Williams & Wilkins; 2012.

Blount JP, Campbell JA, Haines SJ. Complications in ventricular cerebrospinal fluid shunting. *Neurosurg Clin N Am.* 1993;4:633-656.

Li V. Methods and complications in surgical cerebrospinal fluid shunting. *Neurosurg Clin N Am.* 2001;12:685-693.

Martin AE, Gaskill SJ. Cerebrospinal fluid shunts: complications and results. In: Cheek WR, ed. *Pediatric neurosurgery: surgery of the developing nervous system.* 3rd ed. Philadelphia: WB Saunders; 1994.

Maytal J, Alvarez LA, Elkin CM, et al. External hydrocephalus: radiologic spectrum and differentiation from cerebral atrophy. *AJR Am J Roentgenol.* 1987;148:1223-1230.

Schmidek HH, ed. *Schmidek & Sweet operative neurosurgical techniques: indications, methods and results.* 4th ed. Philadelphia: WB Saunders; 2000.

References

Full references for this chapter can be found on www.expertconsult.com.

Chapter 33

Inherited Metabolic and Neurodegenerative Disorders

GIULIO ZUCCOLI, HANNAH CROWLEY, and KIM M. CECIL

Inherited Metabolic Brain Disorders

Inherited metabolic brain disorders produce changes in brain metabolism and structure as a result of genetic mutations affecting enzyme function, protein, and mitochondrial expression. Clinically, children with metabolic brain disorders often present with nonspecific symptoms, such as hypotonia, seizures, and developmental delay, which often makes diagnosis difficult. A combination of neurologic symptoms with and without visceral manifestation and age at onset of symptoms often are important factors indicating an underlying inherited metabolic brain disorder. The diagnosis traditionally has been accomplished by laboratory analyses of biologic specimens (i.e., urine or blood) and tissue (muscle or fibroblast) biopsy. However, the increased availability of imaging studies incorporating advanced techniques, specifically magnetic resonance imaging (MRI) with diffusion-weighted imaging (DWI) and MR spectroscopy (MRS), offers more diagnostic features, thereby improving the ability to recognize disease patterns and classify patients for metabolic and genetic investigations with candidate diseases prioritized from imaging and clinical features. Although the number of metabolic brain disorders is significant, neuroradiologists should be able to recognize the features of the key disorders outlined in this chapter.

Because these disorders generally are progressive, the classification of neurodegenerative features also is used appropriately as imaging findings worsen—for example, cortical volume loss, gliosis, and hypomyelination. The generic term "hypomyelination" is used to describe abnormal myelination, whether it is improperly formed or altered after formation, because distinguishing demyelination from dysmyelination is a pathologic analysis, not one that can be distinguished objectively by imaging alone. Because these diseases frequently or primarily involve the white matter, they often are put into a general category of leukodystrophy. The known leukodystrophies are genetic diseases involving defects in oligodendroglia function and myelinogenesis. The term "leukodystrophy" describes a chronic, progressive, destructive process of the white matter within the central nervous system (CNS) characterized by a metabolic disorder of myelin sheath formation and maintenance. It belongs to a larger group of so-called degenerative processes of the nervous system. These disorders often are characterized by a slow but progressive loss of nervous system structures. The clinical course is progressive and typically includes mental retardation with signs of long tract dysfunction, such as pyramidal and cerebellar disturbances with abnormal conduction of visual auditory and somatic sensory input as measured by evoked potentials.

In young children, more heavily T2-weighted sequences with a repetition time of 2500 to 3000 msec and time to echo (TE) of 100 to 200 msec should be obtained, especially in children younger than 5 years. It is difficult to evaluate the degree of myelination in children younger than 2 years because the normal myelination process does not begin until the fifth month of fetal gestation and proceeds rapidly during the first 2 years of life. Fluid-attenuated inversion recovery (FLAIR) imaging may be misleading before 18 months of age because it sharpens the difference between myelinated and even physiologically unmyelinated white matter. By 2 years of age, 90% of all the white matter fiber tracts have become myelinated, but myelination is incomplete, and some variability exists in the meeting of various milestones. In children younger than 2 years, the destructive process may not be adequately demonstrated on T2-weighted images. However, by 2 years of age and older, a destructive process in which there is hyperintensity of the white matter fibers on long T2-weighted images is demonstrated in the leukodystrophies instead of the normal hypointensity. In recent reports, contrast enhancement has been helpful because many of the newly recognized leukodystrophies have disruption of the blood-brain barrier. The end-stage appearance of all the leukodystrophies on computed tomography (CT) or MRI is marked generalized volume loss. Most leukodystrophies involve the central white matter in a symmetric fashion; Canavan disease is the exception. Patients with delayed myelination or symmetrically abnormal myelination from an earlier insult may have an imaging appearance similar to an early leukodystrophy, making radiologic diagnosis less accurate. Symptoms in these children may be similar to those in children with a leukodystrophy.

DWI provides information about the gross mobility of water. Cytotoxic and myelinic edema can produce a hyperintense signal of diffusion-weighted images. To distinguish this signal from a hyperintense signal arising from T2 weighting, an apparent diffusion coefficient (ADC) map can be generated easily. On an ADC map, cytotoxic and myelinic edema generates a hypointense signal, indicating a restriction of water diffusion. Diffusion tensor imaging holds the promise of providing microstructural details about the white matter by revealing the magnitude and direction of water movement along the axons. As myelination is detected, water molecules demonstrate reduced diffusivity and increased diffusion anisotropy. Abnormal myelin can be quantitated from changes in these properties using measures such as mean diffusivity and fractional anisotropy.

MRS is useful in the evaluation of metabolic diseases in children because many laboratory studies that test for systemic metabolic diseases often do not reveal abnormalities, especially when the metabolic derangements are within localized regions of the brain. When CNS involvement is demonstrated on anatomic MR images, the MRS spectrum is usually abnormal. In some metabolic disorders, abnormalities are observed in the MRS spectrum in the absence of anatomic MR abnormalities, that is, creatine deficiency syndromes.

In the evaluation of a possible metabolic disorder, acquiring both short- and long-echo spectra offers the most diagnostic utility. The use of a short echo time allows for the detection of metabolites with faster T2 decay, especially glutamine/glutamate and myo-inositol (mI). The long-echo spectra have a flatter baseline, which is important for the detection of lactate, a double resonance at 1.3 ppm. Identification of lactate within cerebral tissue typically reflects mitochondrial impairment and should raise suspicion of mitochondrial disease, with confirmation by a muscle biopsy and possibly laboratory analyses of serum or cerebrospinal fluid (CSF). Mitochondrial enzyme systems are involved in many key cell metabolic pathways—oxidative phosphorylation, oxidation of fatty acids and amino acids, and processes involved in the Krebs cycle and part of the urea cycle. Abnormal lactate accumulation detected in patients with mitochondrial disorders can reflect the following mechanisms: (1) a high degree of nonoxidative glycolysis resulting from impaired oxidative energy metabolism, (2) the use of anaerobic metabolism by infiltrating macrophages, and (3) damage to or loss of viable neuroaxonal tissue.

This chapter includes as a reference a large listing of metabolic brain diseases encountered in the imaging setting (see Tables 33-1 to 33-10). For convenience, the recognized metabolic or genetic defect and the patterns of inheritance are summarized. However, because of space limitations, the following discussion will address only the most commonly encountered of these rare disorders.

Lysosomal Storage Diseases

Many neurodegenerative diseases are characterized by the accumulation of nondegradable molecules in cells or at extracellular sites in the brain. One such family of diseases is lysosomal storage disorders, which result from defects in various aspects of lysosomal function. The lysosomes are intracellular organelles responsible for degrading lipids, proteins, and complex carbohydrates. In most lysosomal disorders, the genetic mutation resulting in the absence or partial deficiency of an enzyme or protein is known and functionally understood. For most of the lysosomal diseases, the substrate for the defective enzyme builds up, leading to intralysosomal storage. Although the diseases are complex, mechanical disruption of the cell as a result of the storage of nondegradable material leads to cellular dysfunction. In general, the pathology primarily involves neuronal dysfunction rather than loss, with the exception of differential loss of Purkinje cells that characterize several storage diseases, including Niemann-Pick disease type C and the massive cell loss that occurs in the neuronal ceroid lipofuscinoses (NCLs). It is not known whether the storage material affects cellular function only when it begins to accumulate in extralysosomal sites or if problems in cell homeostasis are triggered while the material is still confined to the lysosome.

Text continued on page 336.

Table 33-1

Summary of Metabolic Disorders Encountered in the Pediatric Neuroimaging Setting: Adrenoleukodystrophy—Argininosuccinate Lyase Deficiency					
Disorder	**Gene Name; Abbreviation (Locus)**	**OMIM**	**Mode of Inheritance**	**Primary Classification**	**Primary Defect**
Neonatal adrenoleukodystrophy	*PTS1* and Peroxin genes	202370	Autosomal recessive	Peroxisomal	Deficiency in oxidizing VLCFA
X-linked adrenoleukodystrophy	Adrenoleukodystrophy; *ALD/ABCD1* (Xq28)	300100	X-linked	Peroxisomal	Inability to oxidize VLCFA into shorter chain fatty acids
Alexander disease	Glial fibrillary acidic protein; *GFAP* (17q21.31)	203450	Autosomal dominant	Leukodystrophy	Presence of Rosenthal fibers, glial fibrillary acid proteins in astrocytes
Alpers disease	Nuclear encoded mitochondrial DNA polymerase-gamma; *POLG* (15q26.1)	203700	Autosomal recessive	Mitochondrial	Respiratory chain abnormalities
Argininemia (arginase deficiency)	Arginase; *ARG1* (6q23.2)	207800	Autosomal recessive	Urea cycle	Defect encoding enzyme *ARG1*
Argininosuccinate lyase deficiency	Argininosuccinate lyase; *ASL* (7q11.21)	207900	Autosomal recessive	Urea cycle	Defect encoding enzyme *ASL*

OMIM, Online Mendelian Inheritance in Man Database; *VLCFA,* very-long-chain fatty acid.
Adapted From Cecil KM. MR spectroscopy of metabolic disorders. *Neuroimaging Clin North Am* 2006;16:87-116; used with permission. Data from The Johns Hopkins University, Online Mendelian Inheritance in Man (OMIM), McKusick-Nathans Institute for Genetic Medicine, Johns Hopkins University (Baltimore, MD) and the National Center for Biotechnology Information, National Library of Medicine (Bethesda, MD), 2000. Available at http://www.ncbi.nlm.nih.gov/omim/. Accessed October 2012.

Table 33-2

Summary of Metabolic Disorders Encountered in the Pediatric Neuroimaging Setting: Biotinidase Deficiency—Citrullinemia

Disorder	Gene Name; Abbreviation (Locus)	OMIM	Mode of Inheritance	Primary Classification	Primary Defect
Biotinidase deficiency	Biotinidase gene; BTD (3p25.1)	253260	Autosomal recessive	Organic or amino acid	Biotinidase deficiency with elevated lactate, b-hydroxyisovalerate
Canavan disease	Aspartoacylase; ASPA (17p13.2)	271900	Autosomal recessive	Leukodystrophy	Enzyme deficiency; aspartoacylase deficiency; inability to metabolize NAA into aspartate and acetate
Carbamoyl phosphate synthetase I deficiency	Carbamoyl phosphate synthetase I; CPS1 (2q34)	237300	Autosomal recessive	Urea cycle	Defect encoding enzyme; CPS1 enzyme deficiency; catalyzes first committed step in the urea cycle
Cerebrotendinous xanthomatosis	27-sterol hydroxylase: CYP27 (2q35)	213700	Autosomal recessive	Lysosomal	Enzyme deficiency—sterol 27-hydroxylase
Childhood ataxia with diffuse CNS hypomyelination (vanishing white matter)	EIF2B1-5 (12q24.31, 14q24.3, 1p34.1, 2p23.3, 3q27)	603896	Autosomal recessive	Leukodystrophy	Gene defect in eukaryotic translation initiation factor (mRNA translated into proteins)
Citrullinemia, classic (argininosuccinate synthetase deficiency)	Argininosuccinate synthetase; ASS (9q34.11)	215700	Autosomal recessive	Urea cycle	Gene defect encoding enzyme argininosuccinate synthetase

CNS, central nervous system; mRNA, messenger ribonucleic acid; NAA, N-acetylaspartate; OMIM, online Mendelian Inheritance in Man Database.
Adapted From Cecil KM. MR spectroscopy of metabolic disorders. Neuroimaging Clin N Am 2006;16:87-116; used with permission. Data from The Johns Hopkins University, Online Mendelian Inheritance in Man (OMIM), McKusick-Nathans Institute for Genetic Medicine, Johns Hopkins University (Baltimore, MD) and the National Center for Biotechnology Information, National Library of Medicine (Bethesda, MD), 2000. Available at http://www.ncbi.nlm.nih.gov/omim/. Accessed October 2012.

Table 33-3

Summary of Metabolic Disorders Encountered in the Pediatric Neuroimaging Setting: Cockayne Disease—Creatine Deficiency

Disorder	Gene Name; Abbreviation (Locus)	OMIM	Mode of Inheritance	Primary Classification	Primary Defect
Cockayne disease	Excision-repair cross-complementing group 8 gene; ERCC8 (5q12.1)	216400	Autosomal recessive	Miscellaneous	Defective DNA repair
Congenital muscular dystrophies	Fukuyama: fukutin; FCMD (9q31.2)	253800	Autosomal recessive	Congenital muscular dystrophy	Defect in dystrophin-associated proteins
	Merosin-deficient: laminin alpha-2-gene; LAMA2 (6q22.33)	607855	Autosomal recessive	Congenital muscular dystrophy	Absence of merosin in muscle
	Duchenne: dystrophin DMD (Xp21.2-p21.1)	310200	X-linked recessive	Congenital muscular dystrophy	Absence of dystrophin in muscle
Creatine deficiency—creatine transporter defect	SLC6A8 (Xq28)	300036	X-linked	Miscellaneous	Creatine transport impaired to the brain
Creatine deficiency—arginine:glycine amidinotransferase deficiency	AGAT (15q21.1)	602360	Autosomal recessive	Miscellaneous	Creatine synthesis impaired
Creatine deficiency—guanidinoacetate methyltransferase deficiency	GAMT (19p13.3)	601240	Autosomal recessive	Miscellaneous	Creatine synthesis impaired

DNA, Deoxyribonucleic acid; OMIM, online Mendelian Inheritance in Man Database.
Adapted From Cecil KM. MR spectroscopy of metabolic disorders. Neuroimaging Clin N Am 2006;16:87-116; used with permission. Data from The Johns Hopkins University, Online Mendelian Inheritance in Man (OMIM), McKusick-Nathans Institute for Genetic Medicine, Johns Hopkins University (Baltimore, MD) and the National Center for Biotechnology Information, National Library of Medicine (Bethesda, MD), 2000. Available at http://www.ncbi.nlm.nih.gov/omim/. Accessed October 2012.

Table 33-4

Summary of Metabolic Disorders Encountered in the Pediatric Neuroimaging Setting: Ethylmalonic Aciduria—Hydroxyglutaric Aciduria

Disorder	Gene Name; Abbreviation (Locus)	OMIM	Mode of Inheritance	Primary Classification	Primary Defect
Ethylmalonic aciduria	ETHE1 (19q13.31)	602473	Autosomal recessive	Organic or amino acid	Ethylmalonic aciduria with cytochrome c oxidase deficiency in skeletal muscle; lactic acidemia
Galactosemia	GALT (9p13.3)	230400	Autosomal recessive	Miscellaneous	Defect encoding galactose-1-phosphate uridyltransferase
Globoid cell leukodystrophy (Krabbe disease)	Galactocerebrosidase; GALC (14q31.3)	245200	Autosomal recessive	Lysosomal	Enzyme deficiency—galactocerebroside beta-galactosidase deficiency
Glutaric aciduria	Type I glutaryl-CoA-dehydrogenase; GCDH (19p13.2)	231670	Autosomal recessive	Organic or amino acid	Enzyme deficiency altering metabolism of lysine, hydroxylysine, tryptophan
Glutaric aciduria	Type II multiple acyl CoA-dehydrogenase genes (19q13.41, 15q24.2-q24.3, 4q32.1)	231680	Autosomal recessive	Organic or amino acid	Disorder of fatty acid, amino acid, and choline metabolism
Homocystinuria	Cystathionine b-synthase; CBS (21q22.3)	236200	Autosomal recessive	Organic or amino acid	Increased urinary homocystine and methionine
L-Hydroxyglutaric aciduria	L2HGDH 14q21.3	236792	Autosomal recessive	Organic or amino acid	Uncertain

OMIM, Online Mendelian Inheritance in Man Database.
Adapted From Cecil KM. MR spectroscopy of metabolic disorders. *Neuroimaging Clin N Am* 2006;16:87-116; used with permission. Data from The Johns Hopkins University, Online Mendelian Inheritance in Man (OMIM), McKusick-Nathans Institute for Genetic Medicine, Johns Hopkins University (Baltimore, MD) and the National Center for Biotechnology Information, National Library of Medicine (Bethesda, MD), 2000. Available at http://www.ncbi.nlm.nih.gov/omim/. Accessed October 2012.

Table 33-5

Summary of Metabolic Disorders Encountered in the Pediatric Neuroimaging Setting: Isovaleric Acidemia—Ketothiolase Deficiency

Disorder	Gene Name; Abbreviation (Locus)	OMIM	Mode of Inheritance	Primary Classification	Primary Defect
Isovaleric acidemia	Isovaleryl CoA dehydrogenase; IVD (15q15.1)	243500	Autosomal recessive	Organic or amino acid	Accumulation of isovaleric acid
Juvenile Huntington disease	Huntington; HTT (4p16.3)	143100	Autosomal dominant	Miscellaneous	Neural cell death from production of quinolinic acid
Kearns-Sayre syndrome	Various mitochondrial deletions	530000	Mitochondrial	Mitochondrial	Lactic acidosis, decreased Co-Q
Kernicterus	Uridine diphosphate-glucuronosyltransferase; UGT1A1 (2q37.1)	237900	Autosomal recessive	Miscellaneous	Hyperbilirubinemia
b-Ketothiolase deficiency	Acetyl-Co-A-acetyltransferase 1; ACAT1 (11q22.3)	203750	Autosomal recessive	Organic or amino acid	Increased urinary 2-methyl-3-hydroxybutyric acid
Leigh syndrome	Nuclear and mitochondrial-encoded genes involved in energy metabolism	256000	Autosomal recessive, mitochondrial	Mitochondrial	Lactic acidosis
Leukoencephalopathy with brainstem and spinal cord involvement with elevated lactate	DARS2 (1q25.1)	611105	Autosomal recessive	Leukodystrophy	
Lowe disease	Phosphatidylinositol polyphosphate 5-phosphatase; OCRL (Xq25-q26)	309000	X-linked recessive	Organic or amino acid	

OMIM, Online Mendelian Inheritance in Man Database.
Adapted From Cecil KM. MR spectroscopy of metabolic disorders. *Neuroimaging Clin N Am* 2006;16:87-116; used with permission. Data from The Johns Hopkins University, Online Mendelian Inheritance in Man (OMIM), McKusick-Nathans Institute for Genetic Medicine, Johns Hopkins University (Baltimore, MD) and the National Center for Biotechnology Information, National Library of Medicine (Bethesda, MD), 2000. Available at http://www.ncbi.nlm.nih.gov/omim/. Accessed October 2012.

Table 33-6

Summary of Metabolic Disorders Encountered in the Pediatric Neuroimaging Setting: Maple Syrup Urine Disease—Molybdenum Cofactor Deficiency

Disorder	Gene Name; Abbreviation (Locus)	OMIM	Mode of Inheritance	Primary Classification	Primary Defect
Maple syrup urine disease	Mutations in the catalytic subunit genes of the branched chain alpha ketoacid dehydrogenase complex; BCKD, DBT, DLD (19q13.2, 7q31.1, 6q14.1, 1p21.2)	248600	Autosomal recessive	Organic or amino acid	Defect in the genes of the branched chain alpha ketoacid dehydrogenase blocking oxidative decarboxylation
MELAS	Multiple mitochondrial genes	540000	Mitochondrial	Mitochondrial	Lactic acidosis
Menkes disease	Cu(2+) transporting ATPase, alpha polypeptide; ATP7A (Xq21.1)	309400	X-linked recessive	Mitochondrial	Low copper
Metachromatic leukodystrophy	Arylsufatase A; ASA/ARSA (22q13.33)	250100	Autosomal recessive	Lysosomal	Decreased arylsulfatase A, ARSA activity
Methylmalonic aciduria	Methylmalonyl-CoA mutase; MUT (6p12.3)	251000	Autosomal recessive	Organic or amino acid	Defect in methylmalonyl-CoA mutase; disorder of methylmalonate and cobalamin metabolism
Molybdenum cofactor deficiency	Molybdenum cofactors; MOCS1 (6p21.3); MOCS2 (5q11.2); gephyrin GPHN (14q23.3)	252150	Autosomal recessive	Miscellaneous	Increased urinary sulfite, taurine, and xanthine

ATPase, Adenosine triphosphatase; *MELAS*, mitochondrial encephalomyopathy, lactic acidosis, and strokelike symptoms; *OMIM*, online Mendelian Inheritance in Man Database.
Adapted From Cecil KM. MR spectroscopy of metabolic disorders. *Neuroimaging Clin N Am* 2006;16:87-116; used with permission. Data from The Johns Hopkins University, Online Mendelian Inheritance in Man (OMIM), McKusick-Nathans Institute for Genetic Medicine, Johns Hopkins University (Baltimore, MD) and the National Center for Biotechnology Information, National Library of Medicine (Bethesda, MD), 2000. Available at http://www.ncbi.nlm.nih.gov/omim/. Accessed October 2012.

Table 33-7

Summary of Metabolic Disorders Encountered in the Pediatric Neuroimaging Setting: Mucopolysaccharidoses (MPS)

Disorder	Gene Name; Abbreviation (Locus)	OMIM	Mode of Inheritance	Primary Classification	Primary Defect
MPS IH—Hurler	MPS1 (4p16.3)	607014	Autosomal recessive	Lysosomal	a-L-Iduronidase deficiency
MPS II—Hunter	MPS2 (Xq28)	309900	X-linked recessive	Lysosomal	Iduronate sulfatase deficiency
MPS III—San Fillipo	MPS3A (17q25.3)	252900	Autosomal recessive	Lysosomal	Heparan sulfate deficiency
	MPS3B (17q21.2)	252920	Autosomal recessive	Lysosomal	N-Acetyl-a-D-glucosaminidase, a-Glucosamine-N-acetyltransferase, N-acetylglucosamine-6-sulfate sulfatase
MPS IV—Morquio	MPS4A (16q24.3)	253000	Autosomal recessive	Lysosomal	N-Acetylgalactosamine-6-sulfate sulfatase, B galactosidase
MPS IS—Scheie	IDUA 4p16.3	607016	Autosomal recessive	Lysosomal	a-L-Iduronidase
MPS VI—Maroteaux-Lamy	MPS6 5q14.1	253200	Autosomal recessive	Lysosomal	Arylsulfatase B
MPS VII—Sly	MPSVII 7q11.21	253220	Autosomal recessive	Lysosomal	b-Glucuronidase

OMIM, Online Mendelian Inheritance in Man Database.
Adapted From Cecil KM. MR spectroscopy of metabolic disorders. *Neuroimaging Clin N Am* 2006;16:87-116; used with permission. Data from The Johns Hopkins University, Online Mendelian Inheritance in Man (OMIM), McKusick-Nathans Institute for Genetic Medicine, Johns Hopkins University (Baltimore, MD) and the National Center for Biotechnology Information, National Library of Medicine (Bethesda, MD), 2000. Available at http://www.ncbi.nlm.nih.gov/omim/. Accessed October 2012.

Table 33-8

Summary of Metabolic Disorders Encountered in the Pediatric Neuroimaging Setting: Neuronal Ceroid Lipofuscinosis—Phenylketonuria

Disorder	Gene Name; Abbreviation (Locus)	OMIM	Mode of Inheritance	Primary Classification	Primary Defect
Neuronal ceroid lipofuscinosis	CLN3 (16p11.2)	204200	Autosomal recessive	Lysosomal	Defects involve lysosomal function
Niemann-Pick type C	NPC1 (18q11.2)	257220	Autosomal recessive	Lysosomal	Defective cholesterol esterification due to a deficiency of sphingomyelinase
Nonketotic hyperglycinemia	Multiple genes (GLDC (9p24.1), GCSH (16q23.2), AMT (3p21.31))	605899	Autosomal recessive	Amino aciduria	Defective mitochondrial enzyme involved in glycine cleavage
Ornithine transcarbamylase deficiency	Ornithine carbamoyltransferase; OTC (Xp11.4)	311250	X-linked recessive	Urea cycle	Gene defect encoding enzyme ornithine carbamoyltransferase
Pantothenate kinase (Hallervorden-Spatz)	Pantothenate kinase; PANK (20p13)	234200	Autosomal recessive	Mitochondrial	Iron deposition in globus pallidus, caudate, and substantia nigra
Pelizaeus-Merzbacher	Proteolipid protein; PLP (Xq22.2)	312080	X-linked	Leukodystrophy	Duplication or deficiency of PLP gene results in altered myelin
Phenylketonuria	Phenylalanine hydroxylase (12q23.2)	261600	Autosomal recessive	Amino aciduria	Phenylalanine hydroxylase deficiency

OMIM, Online Mendelian Inheritance in Man Database.
Adapted From Cecil KM. MR spectroscopy of metabolic disorders. *Neuroimaging Clin N Am* 2006;16:87-116; used with permission. Data from The Johns Hopkins University, Online Mendelian Inheritance in Man (OMIM), McKusick-Nathans Institute for Genetic Medicine, Johns Hopkins University (Baltimore, MD) and the National Center for Biotechnology Information, National Library of Medicine (Bethesda, MD), 2000. Available at http://www.ncbi.nlm.nih.gov/omim/. Accessed October 2012.

Table 33-9

Summary of Metabolic Disorders Encountered in the Pediatric Neuroimaging Setting: Propionic Aciduria—Sandhoff Disease

Disorder	Gene Name; Abbreviation (Locus)	OMIM	Mode of Inheritance	Primary Classification	Primary Defect
Propionic aciduria	Propionic-CoA carboxylase; PCC (3q22.3)	232050	Autosomal recessive	Organic or amino acid	Defect in propionic-CoA carboxylase
Pyruvate decarboxylase deficiency	E1-alpha polypeptide of pyruvate dehydrogenase; PDHA1 (Xp22.12)	312170	X-linked	Mitochondrial	Defect in first of 3 enzymes in PDH-glycolysis and TCA cycle
Pyruvate dehydrogenase deficiency	Multiple genes of the pyruvate dehydrogenase complex	Multiple	Multiple	Mitochondrial	Defect in enzymes coupling glycolysis and TCA cycle for conversion of pyruvate to acetyl-CoA
Refsum disease	Infant: PEX1 7q21.2, PXMP3 8q21.11, PEX26 22q11.21 Adult: PHYH 10p13, PEX7 6q23	266510, 266500	Autosomal recessive	Peroxisomal	Phytanic acid oxidase deficiency
Ribose 5-phosphate isomerase deficiency	Ribose 5-phosphate isomerase deficiency; RPIA 2p11.2	608611	Autosomal recessive	Leukodystrophy	Deficiency in ribose 5-phosphate isomerase
Salla disease	SLC17A5 (6q13)	604369	Autosomal recessive	Lysosomal	Defect in sialic acid transport at the lysosomal membrane
Sandhoff disease	Hexosaminidase; HEXB 5q13.3	268800	Autosomal recessive	Lysosomal	Defect in beta subunit of hexosaminidase A and B isoenzymes

OMIM, Online Mendelian Inheritance in Man Database; CoA, coenzyme A; PDH, pyruvate dehydrogenase; TCA, tricarboxylic acid.
Adapted From Cecil KM. MR spectroscopy of metabolic disorders. *Neuroimaging Clin N Am* 2006;16:87-116; used with permission. Data from The Johns Hopkins University, Online Mendelian Inheritance in Man (OMIM), McKusick-Nathans Institute for Genetic Medicine, Johns Hopkins University (Baltimore, MD) and the National Center for Biotechnology Information, National Library of Medicine (Bethesda, MD), 2000. Available at http://www.ncbi.nlm.nih.gov/omim/. Accessed October 2012.

Table 33-10

Summary of Metabolic Disorders Encountered in the Pediatric Neuroimaging Setting: Sjögren-Larsson Syndrome—Zellweger Syndrome

Disorder	Gene Name; Abbreviation (Locus)	OMIM	Mode of Inheritance	Primary Classification	Primary Defect
Sjögren-Larsson syndrome	Fatty aldehyde dehydrogenase (17p11.2)	270200	Autosomal recessive	Lysosomal	Fatty alcohol oxidation failure
Succinate semialdehyde dehydrogenase deficiency	Succinic semialdehyde dehydrogenase; SSADH (6p22.3)	271980	Autosomal recessive	Organic or amino acid	Succinic semialdehyde dehydrogenase deficiency with 4-hydroxybutyricaciduria
Tay-Sach disease	Hexosaminidase A; HEXA 15q23	272800	Autosomal recessive	Lysosomal	Defect in alpha subunit of hexosaminidase A
Vacuolating megaencephalic leukoencephalopathy (with subcortical cysts, MLC)	MLC1 (22q13.33)	604004	Autosomal recessive	Leukodystrophy	Uncertain
Walker-Warburg syndrome	POMT1 9q24.13,	236670	Autosomal recessive	Congenital muscular dystrophy	Elevated creatine kinase; defective glycosylation of alpha-dystroglycan
Wilson disease	ATP7B (13q14.3)	277900	Autosomal recessive	Miscellaneous	Defect in copper transport
Zellweger syndrome	several genes involved in peroxisome biogenesis	214100	Autosomal-recessive	Peroxisomal	Decreased dihydroxyacetone phosphate acyltransferase (DHAP-AT) activity

OMIM, Online Mendelian Inheritance in Man Database.
Adapted From Cecil KM. MR spectroscopy of metabolic disorders. *Neuroimaging Clin N Am* 2006;16:87-116; used with permission. Data from The Johns Hopkins University, Online Mendelian Inheritance in Man (OMIM), McKusick-Nathans Institute for Genetic Medicine, Johns Hopkins University (Baltimore, MD) and the National Center for Biotechnology Information, National Library of Medicine (Bethesda, MD), 2000. Available at http://www.ncbi.nlm.nih.gov/omim/. Accessed October 2012.

Lysosomal disorders typically are inherited as autosomal-recessive traits; they usually afflict infants and young children, involve brain pathology, and are untreatable. However, adult-onset forms exist. The collective frequency of lysosomal storage diseases is estimated to be approximately 1 in 8000 live births, with some occurring at high frequency in select populations. The common biochemical hallmark of these diseases is the storage of macromolecules in the lysosome.

Lysosomal disorders primarily affecting gray matter include the gangliosidoses, mucopolysaccharidoses, and NCLs. Two of the more common lysosomal disorders, metachromatic leukodystrophy (MLD) and Krabbe disease, demonstrate abnormalities in white matter. However, broader involvement of gray and white matter often occurs in later stages of lysosomal disease progression.

GANGLIOSIDOSES

The gangliosidoses are divided into two groups, referred to as GM1 and GM2. In the GM1 group, the primary enzyme deficiency is that of β-galactosidase. For the GM2 group, an abnormal accumulation of gangliosides is the result of a hexosaminidase deficiency.

GM1 Gangliosidosis

Three types of GM1 gangliosidosis exist: type I (infantile), type II (late infantile/juvenile), and type III (adult). An intermediate form between infantile and juvenile has been reported.[1] The clinical presentation of GM1 gangliosidosis typically occurs in infancy; its features include seizures, decerebrate posturing, pitting edema of the face, hypotonia, developmental delay, hepatosplenomegaly, macrocephaly, and cherry red spots involving the macula of the retina. Additional features include broad digits, kyphoscoliosis, skeletal dysplasia with widening of the metabphyses, and dermal pigmentary lesions.[2] The course is progressive, with death common within 2 years of life. A juvenile form presents during the second year of life with progressive ataxia but without many features of the infantile variety.

The underlying deficiency of β-galactosidase results in accumulation of GM1 ganglioside in both gray and white matter of the cerebrum, brainstem, cerebellum, and spinal cord. Results of cerebral MRI initially are normal, with subsequent loss of cortical gray matter. Secondary changes to the white matter manifest later and typically exhibit an abnormal, nonspecific, patchy, hyperintense T2 signal within the centrum semiovale. Hypointensity of the thalami on T2-weighted images also has been reported.[3]

GM2 Gangliosidosis

The most common forms of GM2 gangliosidoses include Tay-Sachs disease and Sandhoff disease. Tay-Sachs disease arises with β-N-acetylhexosaminidase-A isoenzyme deficiency in Jewish children of eastern European descent. Onset is usually before the age of 1 year with irritability, hypotonia, seizures, blindness, and cherry-red spots on the macula in 90% of patients. Death usually results by 2 to 3 years of age. Sandhoff disease is attributed to a deficiency of A and B isoenzymes of hexosaminidase. The clinical course is similar to that of Tay-Sachs disease. There is visceral involvement, including hepatomegaly and cardiac and renal tubular abnormalities. Brain MRI in the early stages demonstrates increased T2 signal in the basal ganglia, particularly with the enlarged caudate nuclei. Later, cortical and deep gray matter volume loss occurs with patchy increases in T2 signal in the white matter. Thalamic involvement is more reflective of Sandhoff disease. In adult-onset Sandhoff disease, lower motor neuron involvement has been reported. Whereas cerebellar atrophy may vary, it does not appear to be correlated with clinical severity.[4] In persons with Tay-Sachs disease, the thalami may be hypointense on T2-weighted images and hyperintense on T1-weighted images because of calcium deposition. It has been reported that T2-weighted hyperintensity in cerebral matter is indicative of abnormal myelin production and active demyelination.[5] Asymmetrical swelling and high T2 intensity in the white matter and basal nuclei of the right hemisphere has been reported. Elevated levels of cytokines have been reported, possibly indicating inflammation as a contributing factor to the progression of gangliosidosis.[6] In the B1 variant of GM2 gangliosidosis, the bilateral thalami may appear hyperdense/hyperintense on CT/T1-weighted MRI and show a T2-hypointense signal in the ventral thalami and a hyperintense signal in the posteromedial thalami. Other findings in this variant include involvement of the medullary lamellae, bilateral T2 hyperintense/swollen basal ganglia, diffuse white matter hyperintensity on T2-weighted images, and brain atrophy in later stages.[7]

MUCOPOLYSACCHARIDOSES

The mucopolysaccharidoses are the best known of the lysosomal abnormalities affecting predominately gray matter. The primary metabolic defect in this group of disorders is a failure to break down sulfates (dermatan, heparan, and keratan); thus mucopolysaccharides fill up and overburden the lysosomes within histiocytes of the brain, bone, skin, and other organs. Glycosaminoglycans accumulate with target organs such as the bone, liver, and brain. Eight subtypes have been defined; however, six distinct forms are now recognized within this classification scheme, based on which metabolite is involved. The six are referred to as Hurler (IH), Hunter (II), Sanfilippo (III), Morquio (IV), Maroteaux-Lamy (VI), and Sly (VII), with the classic prototypical disease being that of Hurler. Coarse facial and bony features, as well as complex skeletal manifestations, are well-known clinical characteristics for all of these disorders. Without treatment, death usually comes within the first decade of life.

All of these diseases are autosomal recessive except type II, Hunter, which is an X-linked recessive condition. Hydrocephalus is common, probably as a result of plugging of the pacchionian granulation.

Cerebral MRI demonstrates two major abnormalities:
1. Diffuse patches of hyperintensity on T2-weighted images resulting from accumulation of mucopolysaccharide in neurons and astrocytes and degenerative effects on myelin
2. Prominent cystic or perivascular spaces resulting from metabolic accumulation within histiocytes located in perivascular areas, which is the most characteristic imaging feature; reversal of these changes after bone marrow transplantation has been reported

Spinal stenosis is especially common in Morquio and Maroteaux-Lamy variants but may be demonstrated in other variants. Typical bullet-shaped vertebral bodies are characteristic (Fig. 33-1).

For the mucopolysaccharidoses, proton MRS reveals a broad resonance at 3.7 ppm, which is attributed to a composite of mucopolysaccharide molecules. After bone marrow transplantation, the resonance at 3.7 ppm decreases in the brain of some patients, which may aid in determining the efficacy of the therapy. N-acetylaspartate (NAA) levels may improve in response to treatment.

NEURONAL CEROID LIPOFUSCINOSES

NCL is a disorder or group of disorders characterized by striking volume loss of brain parenchyma. NCL, which can be divided into six subtypes based on age at onset, is one of the most common neurodegenerative syndromes, with an incidence of 1 per 25,000 live births. The various subtypes are associated with different mutations in the CLN genes and have similar clinical manifestations occurring at different ages. These manifestations include seizures and abnormal eye movements, with subsequent vision loss, dementia, hypotonia, and speech and motor deficits. CSF neurotransmitter abnormalities also have been reported in patients with NCL.[8] At pathology, these disorders are characterized by distinctive granular inclusions in neuronal lysosomes, called granular osmiophilic deposits. Imaging findings follow behind the clinical presentation in all but the infantile form of NCL and are dominated by progressive cerebral and cerebellar volume loss. Later stages of disease are characterized by development of a band of hyperintense signal in the periventricular white matter on T2-weighted images. In palmitoyl protein thioesterase-1 related NCL, isolated, symmetric dentate nucleus hyperintensities have been reported in early stages on T2-weighted images.[9] Proton MRS has shown progressive decreases in NAA and relative increases in mI in persons with NCL.

METACHROMATIC LEUKODYSTROPHY

In persons with MLD, the primary metabolic defect is a deficiency in the enzyme arylsulfatase A, resulting in the accumulation of cerebroside sulfate within the lysosome. MLD has four subtypes: congenital, late infantile, juvenile, and adult. The late infantile subtype is the most common and presents from around 14 months to 4 years of age. The early presentations are an unsteady gait that progresses to severe ataxia and flaccid paralysis, dysarthria, mental retardation, and decerebrate posturing. Gallbladder involvement has been reported, possibly appearing before the onset of neurologic symptoms. Intestinal involvement also has been reported, specifically polypoid masses in one patient.[10]

Histologic analysis of the abnormal nervous tissue demonstrates a complete loss of myelin (demyelination) followed by axonal degeneration. Metachromatic granules are reported within engorged lysosomes in white matter and neurons and on peripheral nerve biopsies. Oligodendrocytes are reduced in number, and areas of demyelination predominate throughout the deep white matter region. Early sparing of the subcortical arcuate white matter fibers ("U" fibers) occurs until late in the disease process. An inflammatory response typically is absent, which accounts for a lack of enhancement in this

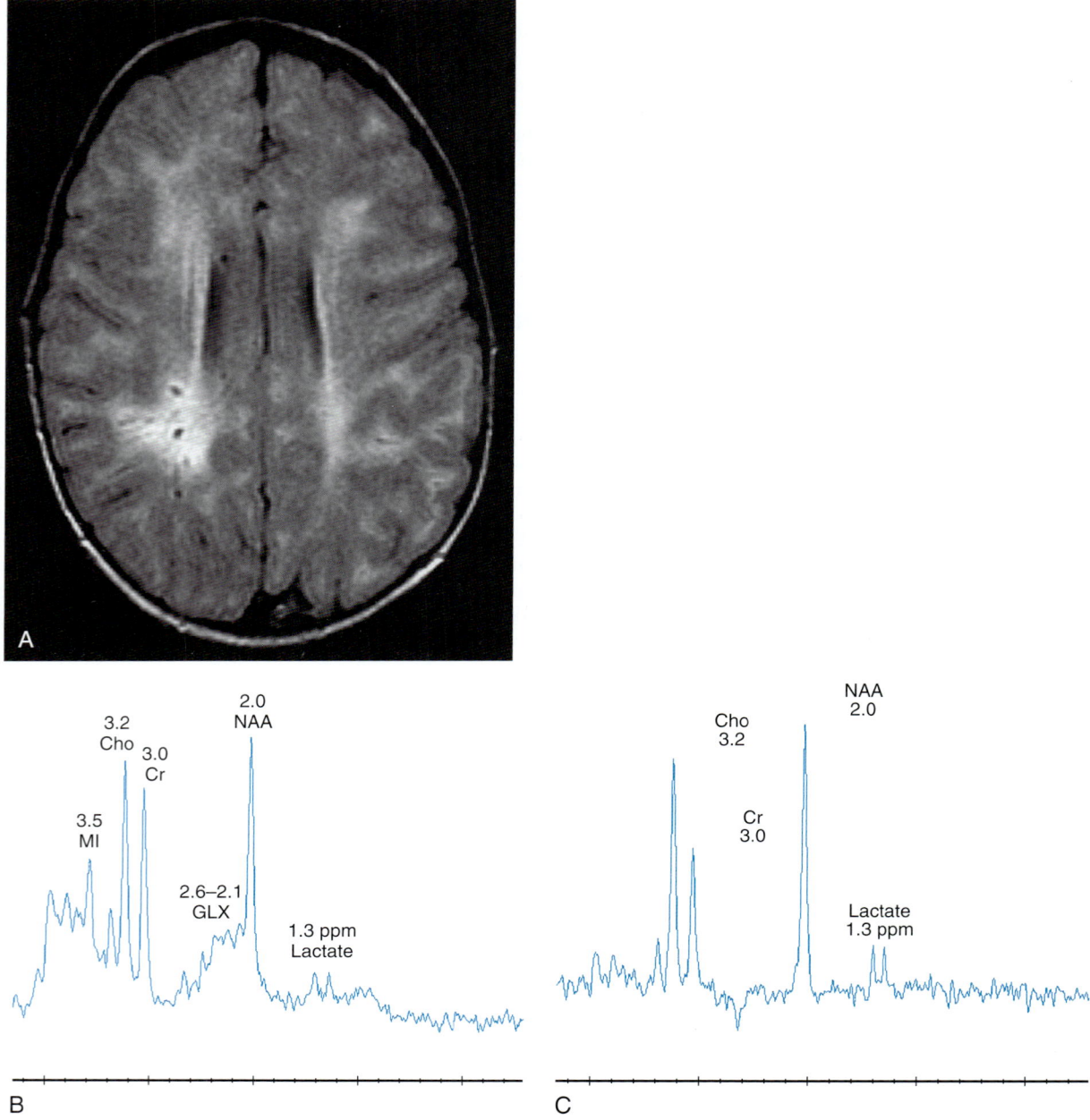

Figure 33-1   A 2-year-old boy with Hunter syndrome, mucopolysaccharidoses, type II. Select axial fluid-attenuated inversion recovery (**A**), short echo (time to echo (TE) 35 msec) magnetic resonance spectroscopy (MRS) (**B**), and long echo (TE 288 msec) MRS (**C**) images are shown. The patient underwent scanning within months of a stem cell transplant. Prominent perivascular spaces are demonstrated with a diffuse, abnormal, hyperintense signal throughout the periventricular and subcortical white matter. The spectra demonstrate diminished N-acetylaspartate levels with elevated lactate, which may reflect histiocytic cell infiltration of the perivascular spaces and brain parenchyma. (From Cecil KM. MR spectroscopy of metabolic disorders. *Neuroimaging Clin N Am*. 2006;16:87-116; used with permission.)

disorder, but eventually, even myelinated white matter is replaced by astrogliosis and scarring. The corpus callosum is involved before significant progression, whereas subcortical white matter remains unaffected until the disease has progressed; atrophy is a late sign. Demyelination also can be seen in the posterior limbs of the internal capsule, descending pyramidal tracts, and the cerebellar white matter.[11] Thalamic changes may be common in primary MLD, and isolated cerebellar atrophy may be seen in some atypical later-onset variants. On T2-weighted images, there is marked hyperintensity of the white matter fiber tracts involving the cerebral hemispheres that may extend to the cerebellum, brainstem, and spinal cord. The findings further demonstrate diffuse deep white matter involvement with relative sparing of subcortical white matter. The findings initially are focal and patchy, but later, a diffuse, hyperintense T2 signal of the centrum semiovale develops. Two distinct white matter appearances have been noted that mimic what was previously considered to be pathognomonic of Pelizaeus-Merzbacher disease (PMD). Punctate areas of hypointensity ("leopard skin" appearance) and radiating patterns of linear tubular structures of T2 hypointensity ("tigroid" appearance) are seen, with areas of relatively normal–appearing white matter within the areas of demyelination. On T1-weighted images, the white matter fibers may be isointense with, or hypotense to, gray matter (Fig. 33-2).

Proton MRS studies have demonstrated reduced NAA, which is expected with neuroaxonal loss, but they also have revealed disturbances in glial cell metabolism associated with elevated mI and choline. The levels of NAA in white matter have been found to correlate with motor function in children with MLD.[12]

GLOBOID CELL LEUKODYSTROPHY (KRABBE DISEASE)

Globoid cell leukodystrophy (Krabbe disease) arises from a deficiency in the enzyme β-galactocerebrosidase, leading to the accumulation of cerebroside and galactosylsphingosine, which induces apoptosis in the oligodendrocyte cell lines. Globoid cell leukodystrophy, an autosomal–recessive disorder, has a frequency of 2 in 100,000 in a series reported from Sweden. It is seen predominantly in young children; however, the infantile form is the most common. Onset of symptoms usually begins between 3 and 5 months after birth with

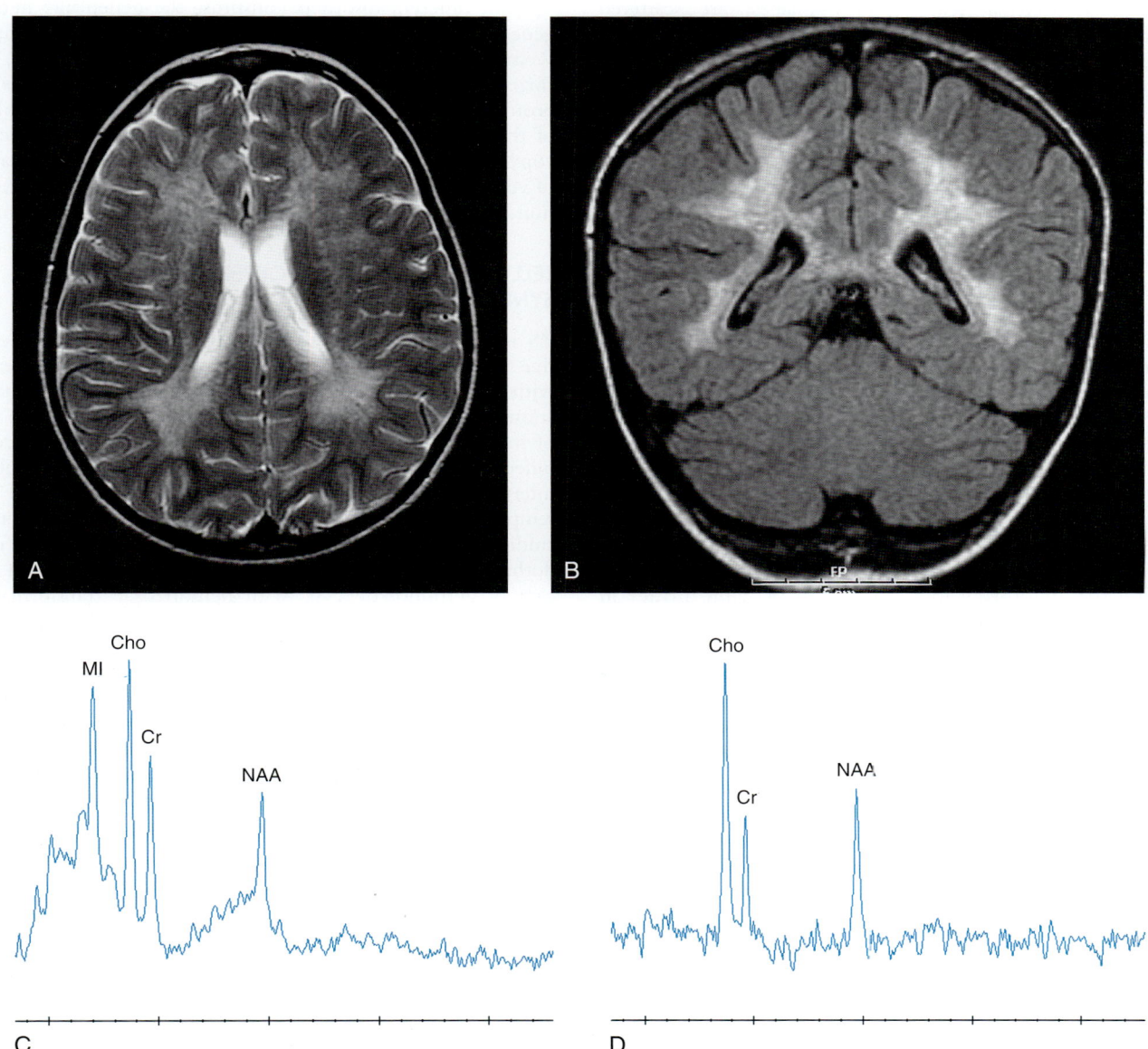

Figure 33-2 A 7-year-old boy with metachromatic leukodystrophy. Select axial T2-weighted (**A**), coronal fluid-attenuated inversion recovery (**B**) with left parietal white matter short echo magnetic resonance spectroscopy (MRS) (**C**) and long echo MRS (**D**) images reveal an abnormal hyperintense signal in the periventricular white matter throughout the cerebrum, sparing the subcortical U fibers. The signal has a "tigroid" appearance on T2-weighted images. The spectra demonstrate significant elevations of choline and myo-inositol with diminished N-acetylaspartate reflecting neuroaxonal loss, demyelination, and glial activation. (From Cecil KM. MR spectroscopy of metabolic disorders. *Neuroimaging Clin N Am.* 2006;16:87-116; used with permission.)

irritability. The disease continues to progress, with development of symptoms mimicking encephalitis with motor deterioration and atypical seizures. At the end stage of the disease, the child is in a vegetative state with decerebrate posturing. Elevated CSF protein has been reported, to a larger extent in adult phenotypes than in phenotypes affecting younger people.[13] Positional ocular flutter has been reported in one patient with infantile Krabbe disease.[14] In nerve conduction studies, the severity of abnormalities appears to correlate with the severity of clinical symptoms.[15]

The disease involves predominantly the white matter of the cerebral hemispheres, cerebellum, and spinal cord. Pathologic changes include a marked toxic reduction in the number of oligodendrocytes. Multinucleated cells that appear to be globoid, as well as reactive macrophages, are scattered throughout the white matter region. Hypomyelination may be extensive and eventually leads to gliosis and scarring in the white matter region. Gray matter involvement in the basal ganglia region also can be found with punctate calcification.

Delayed myelination may be the first finding noted on MRI in infants with this disorder. In infantile Krabbe disease, MRI findings may be normal, but as the disease progresses, classic Krabbe features emerge; this phenomenon is probably related to the immature myelination.[16] The appearance of Krabbe disease on MRI is featured as one of either two patterns. A patchy hyperintense periventricular signal on T2-weighted images, consistent with hypomyelination, eventually may evolve into a more diffuse pattern in the white matter. In this form, involvement of the thalami with a hyperintense T2 signal often is present as well. A second pattern is a patchy low signal on T2-weighted images in a similar distribution to the hyperdense regions seen on CT, which is suspected to represent a paramagnetic effect from calcium deposition in the region. Additional early changes include increased density in the distribution of the thalami, cerebellum, caudate heads, and brainstem that may precede the abnormally low attenuation of white matter in the centrum semiovale. Symmetric enlargement of the optic nerves also has been described in persons with Krabbe disease, which is presumed to reflect accumulation of proteolipid in globoid cells. The distal optic nerves are primarily involved; however, a case has been described with proximal prechiasmatic enlargement of the nerves.[17] At times, changes within the cerebellar white matter also have been reported, with hyperintensity on T2-weighted images. The findings within the spinal cord are visualized as atrophic changes. Diffuse volume loss and periventricular white matter abnormalities predominate in the latter stages of this disease (Fig. 33-3).

Proton MRS demonstrates the reduced NAA expected with neuroaxonal loss but also has revealed disturbances in glial cell metabolism associated with hypomyelination. In addition to a reduced NAA level, elevated levels of choline and mI also have been reported in this condition, which is consistent with the general neurodegenerative pattern as seen on proton spectroscopy.

DWI also has been applied in a limited number of patients with Krabbe disease. Loss of diffusion relative anisotropy was noted in the hyperintense areas as seen on T2-weighted images, which preceded those signal changes.

Peroxisomal Disorders

Peroxisomes are organelles within a cell that contain enzymes responsible for critical cellular processes, including biosynthesis of membrane phospholipids (plasmalogens), cholesterol, and bile acids; conversion of amino acids into glucose; oxidation of fatty acids; reduction of hydrogen peroxide by catalases; and prevention of excess oxalate synthesis. Peroxisomal disorders are subdivided into two major categories: (1) peroxisomal biogenesis disorders (PBDs) that arise from a failure to form viable peroxisomes, resulting in multiple metabolic abnormalities, and (2) disorders resulting from the deficiency of a single peroxisomal enzyme.

Four different disorders constitute the genetically heterogeneous PBD group: Zellweger syndrome (ZS), infantile Refsum disease, neonatal adrenoleukodystrophy (ALD), and rhizomelic chondrodysplasia punctata. X-linked ALD is the prototypical peroxisomal disorder in which the morphology of the organelle is found to be normal on electron microscopy, but a single enzyme defect leads to the accumulation of very-long-chain fatty acids and progressive CNS deterioration in the form of a chronic progressive encephalopathy.

ZELLWEGER SYNDROME (CEREBROHEPATORENAL SYNDROME)

ZS is an autosomal-recessive disease characterized by defective peroxisomal functions. Infants are symptomatic early, with hypotonia, seizures, large liver size, and limb and facial anomalies that are easily recognizable at birth. A diffuse lack of myelination throughout the white matter is noted, combined with cortical dysplasia. The gyri are broad, with shallow intervening sulci found mainly in the anterior frontal and temporal lobes but also over the convexities in the periolandic area. The presence of a germinolytic cyst in the caudothalamic groove is common in persons with ZS, and one case of germinolytic cysts with hemorrhagic transformation has been reported.[18] In one case, signal abnormality suggestive of demyelination was identified almost solely in the bilateral corticospinal tracts, in particular in the brainstem with concomitant motor losses.[19] Variants of ZS also have been described that do not follow the typical prototype but demonstrate many common features to ZS. Clinical overlap may occur with other conditions, including neonatal ALD, infantile Refsum disease, and hyperpipecolic acidemia. Death usually comes with many of these conditions within the first two years of life (e-Fig. 33-4).

MRS performed in older patients with ZS and Refsum disease reveals similar features, with dramatic lipid and choline elevations, minor mI elevations, and reduced NAA levels for sampled white matter. For rhizomelic chondrodysplasia punctata, two studies report elevations of mobile lipids, mI–glycine, and acetate and reduced choline levels as consistent with a deficiency in plasmalogen biosynthesis. In contrast to ZS, infantile Refsum disease, and neonatal ALD, rhizomelic chondrodysplasia punctata does not feature liver disease, which is significant to account for the mI differences. To detect mI levels, a short echo technique (i.e., TE ≤35 msec) must be used to recognize a resonance appearing at 3.5 ppm. For MRS performed at 1.5 T, the mI resonance normally is

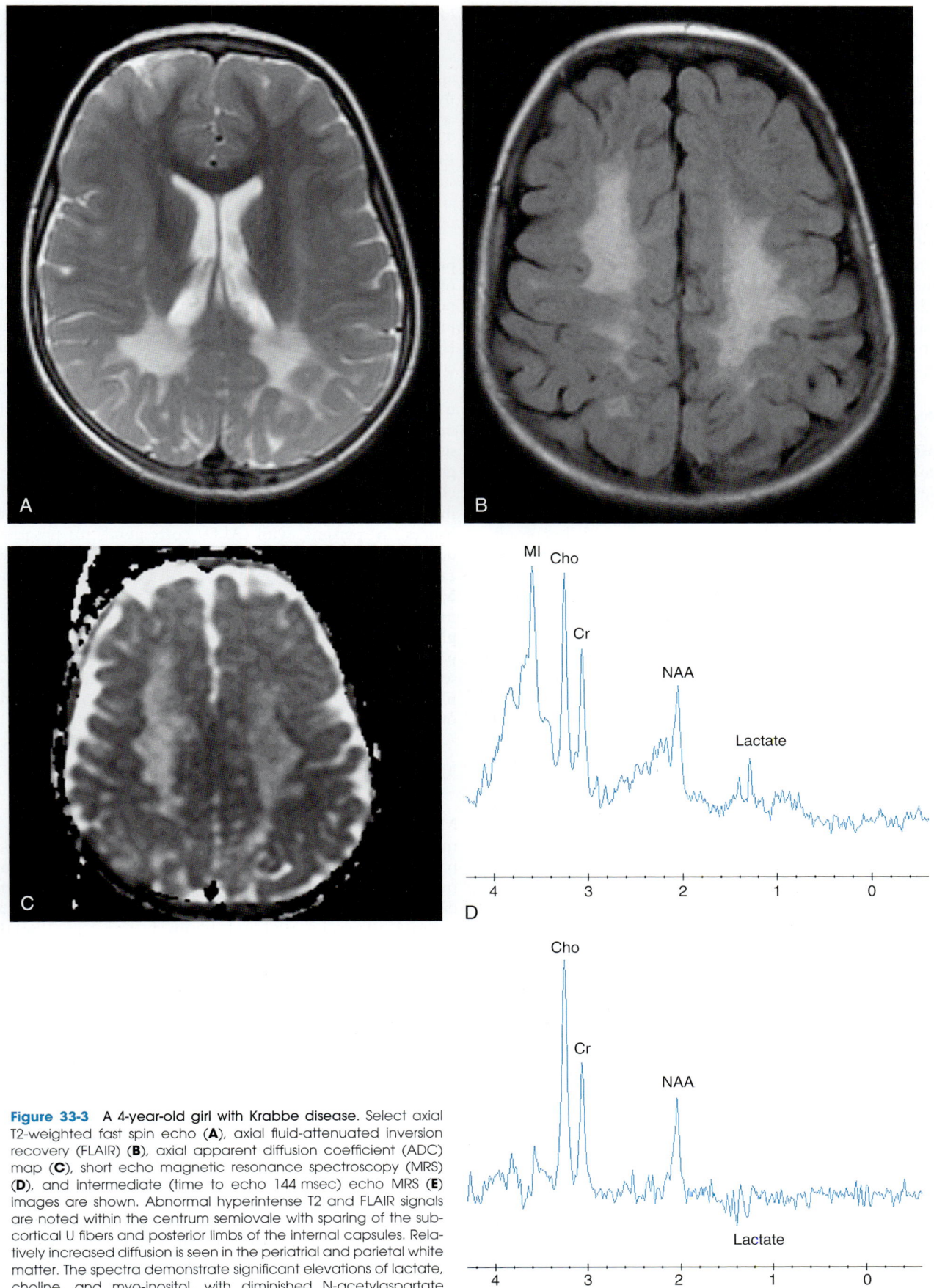

Figure 33-3 A 4-year-old girl with Krabbe disease. Select axial T2-weighted fast spin echo (**A**), axial fluid-attenuated inversion recovery (FLAIR) (**B**), axial apparent diffusion coefficient (ADC) map (**C**), short echo magnetic resonance spectroscopy (MRS) (**D**), and intermediate (time to echo 144 msec) echo MRS (**E**) images are shown. Abnormal hyperintense T2 and FLAIR signals are noted within the centrum semiovale with sparing of the subcortical U fibers and posterior limbs of the internal capsules. Relatively increased diffusion is seen in the periatrial and parietal white matter. The spectra demonstrate significant elevations of lactate, choline, and myo-inositol, with diminished N-acetylaspartate reflecting neuroaxonal loss, demyelination, and glial activation.

distinct, with four of the molecule's six methine protons magnetically indistinguishable, thereby coresonating at the same location (3.5 ppm). However, increased spectral dispersion inherent at higher field strengths (3 T) now produces two distinct resonances (3.5 and 3.6 ppm) for the four protons, effectively reducing the signal by half. Normal mI levels visually appear lower at higher field strengths in contrast to 1.5 T. Although some reports have found improved detection of mI at high field strength arising from increased signal/noise ratio, it may be problematic depending on the acquisition conditions. The usage of phased array coils with parallel imaging offers tremendous advantages for imaging. Unfortunately, in the clinical setting, inadequate methods currently exist for optimally combining the elements of the phased array coil for single voxel spectroscopy applications. A single coil element with inadequate signal averaging can provide a low signal-to-noise ratio, thereby limiting the ability to detect mI.

NEONATAL ADRENOLEUKODYSTROPHY

Neonatal ALD is characterized by the presence of multiple recognizable enzyme deficiencies with grossly normal but deficient numbers of peroxisomes. Specific conditions include pipecolic and phytanic acidemia and a deficiency of plasmalogen synthetase. This condition also presents with hypotonia in the first months of life but without many of the facial features of ZS. Cortical abnormalities in the form of a dysplasia can be found in this condition, as well as hypomyelination in cerebral white matter (Fig. 33-5).

ADRENOLEUKODYSTROPHY

X-linked ALD is the prototypical peroxisomal disorder in which the morphology of the organelle is found to be normal on electron microscopy but a single enzyme defect, acyl-CoA synthetase, along with a failure of incorporation into cholesterol esters for myelin synthesis, leads to the accumulation of very-long-chain fatty acids and progressive CNS deterioration in the form of a chronic progressive encephalopathy. This "classic" form of ALD is an X-linked disorder with a clinical onset between the ages of 5 to 7 years that includes behavioral problems, followed by a rapidly progressive decline in neurologic function and death within the ensuing 5- to 8-year period. The first indication of this condition may include mental status changes or a decline in school performance, progressing to subtle alterations in neurocognitive function, and ultimately resulting in severe spasticity and visual deficits, leading finally to a vegetative state and death. Childhood cerebral ALD, although rare, can present with raised intracranial pressure (ICP) and an elevated level of CSF protein.[20]

X-linked ALD has been described with a typical appearance on CT and MRI with predominately posterior involvement that, over time, progresses from posterior to anterior into the frontal lobes and from the deep white matter to the peripheral subcortical white matter. On CT, the involvement appears as symmetrical low attenuation in a butterfly distribution across the splenium of the corpus callosum, surrounded on its periphery by an enhancing zone (inflammatory intermediate zone). Three zones are readily distinguished on MR: an inner zone of astrogliosis and scarring corresponds to the low density zone seen on CT that appears hypointense on T1-weighted images and hyperintense on T2-weighted sequences; an intermediate zone of active inflammation that appears isointense on T1-weighted images and isointense or hypointense on T2-weighted images; and an outer zone of active demyelination that appears minimally hypointense on T1-weighted images and hyperintense on T2-weighted scans. Enhancement after administration of gadolinium is demonstrated within the intermediate zone of active inflammation and may disappear as the first change after bone marrow transplantation (Fig. 33-6).

Patients with X-linked ALD who are evaluated with proton MRS demonstrate abnormal spectra within regions of abnormal signal, as well as white matter that appears normal. The spectral profile for normal-appearing white matter of neurologically asymptomatic patients is characterized by slightly elevated concentrations of composite choline compounds, with an increase of both choline and mI reflecting the onset of demyelination. Markedly elevated concentrations of choline, mI, and glutamine in affected white matter suggest active demyelination and glial proliferation. A simultaneous reduction of the concentrations of NAA and glutamate is consistent with neuronal loss and injury. An elevated lactate level is consistent with inflammation and/or macrophage infiltration. The more severe metabolic disturbances in persons with ALD correspond to progressive demyelination, neuroaxonal loss, and gliosis leading to clinical deterioration and, eventually, death. The detection of MRS abnormalities before the onset of neurologic symptoms may help in the selection of patients for bone marrow transplantation and stem cell transplantation. Stabilization and partial reversal of metabolic abnormalities is demonstrated in some patients after they undergo therapies. The spectral profiles can be used to monitor disease evolution and the effects of therapies.

Mitochondrial Diseases

Mitochondrial diseases generally refer to disorders of the mitochondrial respiratory chain, the only cellular metabolic pathway under control by both the mitochondrial genome (mtDNA) and the nuclear genome (nDNA). Mitochondrial diseases demonstrate impaired respiratory chain function and reduced adenosine triphosphate production. The mtDNA mutations can be divided into two categories: those that impair mitochondrial protein synthesis *in toto* and those that affect respiratory chain subunits. Disorders attributed to mtDNA mutations follow lax rules of mitochondrial genetics. However, disorders arising from nDNA mutations are governed by Mendelian genetics. The disorders attributed to mutations in nDNA are more abundant because most respiratory chain subunits are nucleus-encoded and the correct assembly and functioning of the entire respiratory chain require numerous steps. The clinical phenotypes of nDNA-related mitochondrial disorders tend to be uniform, whereas both the spectrum and severity of clinical manifestations associated with mtDNA-related disorders are extremely variable. Marked genotype-phenotype variability is characteristic of mtDNA-related disorders. The clinical diversity observed in patients with mtDNA-related disorders can be partially explained by heteroplasmy, the coexistence of mutant and

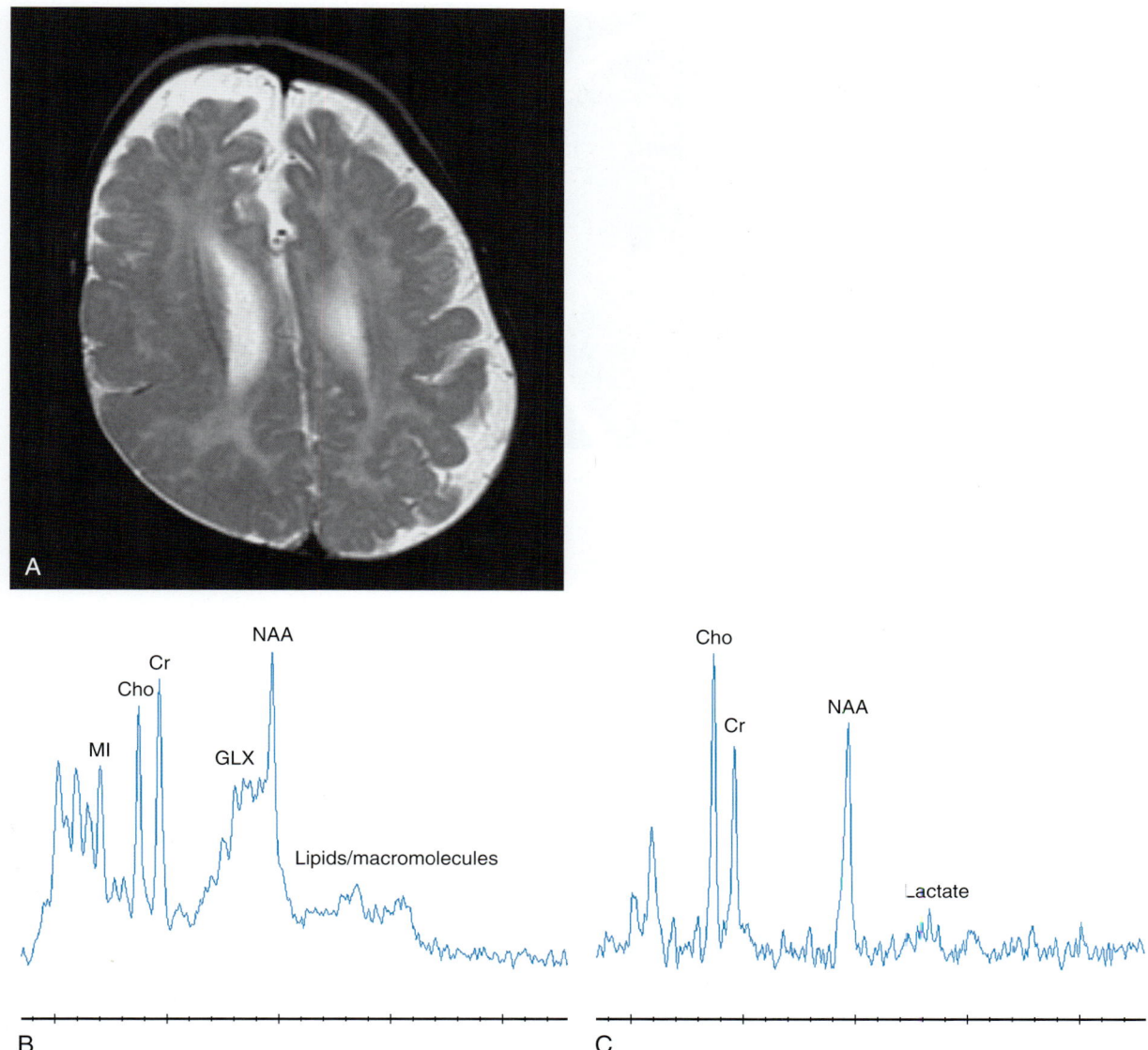

Figure 33-5 **A 12-month-old boy with neonatal adrenoleukodystrophy.** Axial T2-weighted (**A**), short echo magnetic resonance spectroscopy (MRS) (**B**), and long echo MRS (**C**) images are shown. The imaging reveals an abnormal hyperintense signal within the central white matter and an abnormal cerebral gyral pattern consistent with polymicrogyria. The lateral ventricles and extraaxial spaces are prominent in size with a thin corpus callosum. The spectroscopy performed in the left parietal cortex and white matter reveals elevated glutamate and glutamine with a slightly elevated lactate signal and reduced N-acetylaspartate levels. (From Cecil KM. MR spectroscopy of metabolic disorders. *Neuroimaging Clin N Am.* 2006;16:87-116; used with permission.)

wild-type mtDNA within a cell. Only when the proportion of mutant genomes exceeds a particular level is the disease expressed (threshold effect).

KEARNS-SAYRE SYNDROME

A group of clinical syndromes arising from mtDNA rearrangements, either deletions or duplications, includes Kearns-Sayre syndrome, Pearson syndrome, and progressive external ophthalmoplegia. A brief discussion about Kearns-Sayre syndrome is presented.

Kearns-Sayre syndrome is a mitochondrial cytopathy characterized by external ophthalmoplegia, retinal pigmentary

degeneration, and conductive hearing block. Ragged red fibers indicative of a defect in the respiratory chain of mitochondria are demonstrated on muscle biopsy, in common with mitochondrial encephalomyopathy, lactic acidosis, and strokelike symptoms (MELAS) and myoclonic epilepsy with ragged red fibers (MERRF) syndromes. The heart is often affected, causing conduction defects, which progress to heart block, manifesting as heart failure.[21] Choroid plexus failure also has been reported.[22] Cerebral MRI demonstrates diffuse, patchy areas of hyperintensity on T2-weighted images. In the presence of calcification, both the basal ganglia and dentate regions also may show hyperintense T1-weighted signal. On T2/FLAIR images, bilateral involvement of the thalamus,

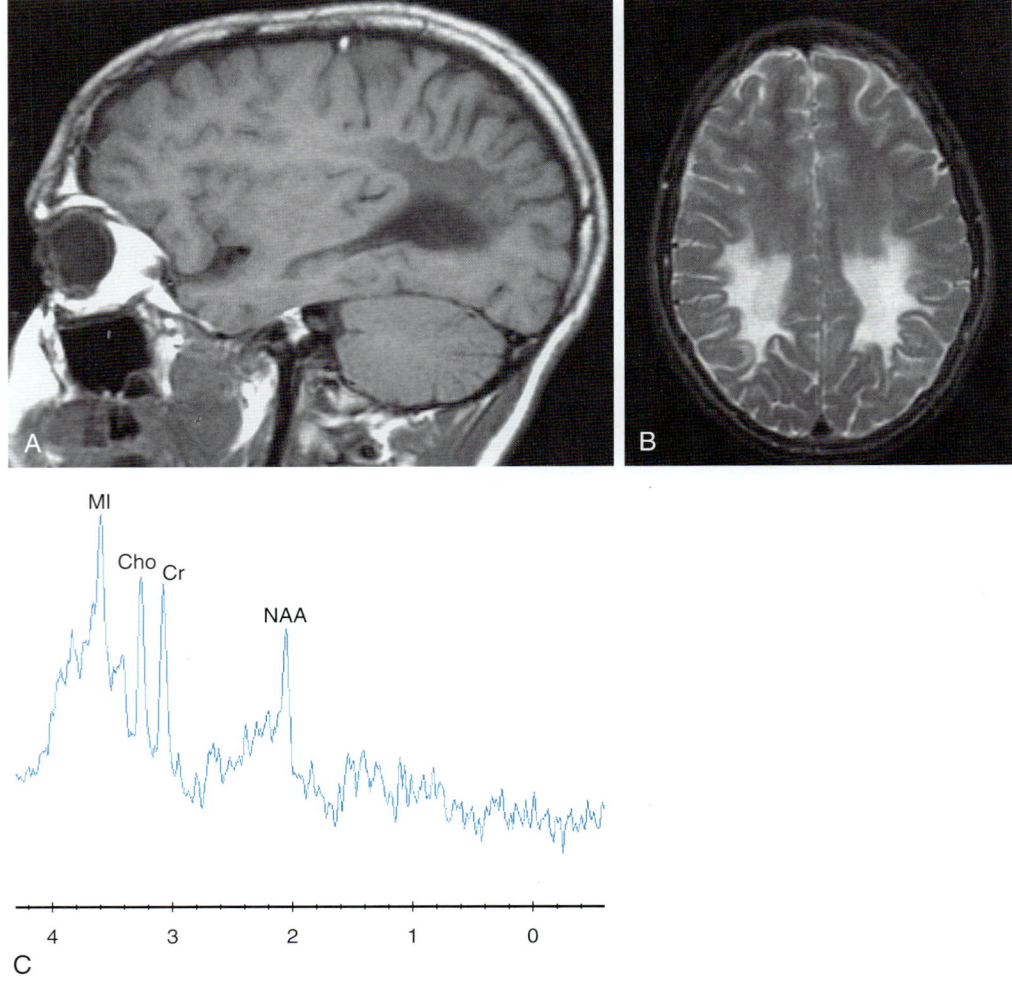

Figure 33-6 A 16-year-old boy with X-linked adrenoleukodystrophy, 8 months after a bone marrow transplant. Sagittal T1-weighted (**A**), axial T2-weighted (**B**), and short echo magnetic resonance spectroscopy (**C**) images are shown. The imaging demonstrates an abnormal signal in the posterior portion of the cerebrum. The spectra sampled in the right posterior parietal white matter reveals a diminished N-acetylaspartate level with an elevated myo-inositol level. Imaging and spectroscopy reflected disease stability for this patient.

basal ganglia, and brainstem are observed. Cerebral and, more frequently, cerebellar atrophy often are observed.[23] Ocular myopathy characterizes some patients affected by Kearns-Sayre syndrome (e-Fig. 33-7).

MELAS SYNDROME

Several clinical syndromes arising from point mutations in mtDNA are encountered. The most noticeable are MELAS syndrome, MERRF syndrome, neurogenic weakness and ataxia with retinitis pigmentosa syndrome, and Leber hereditary optic neuropathy. MELAS syndrome often is caused by an A3243G point mutation in tRNA-leu[UUR] or the *MTTL1* gene (80% of cases). Other phenotypes can result in the A3243G point mutation (e.g., maternally inherited deafness and diabetes). The clinical presentation of MELAS syndrome resembles that of cerebral infarction; however, the "infarcts" are affected without the usual arterial stroke patterns. Age of onset is usually between 2 and 11 years. The basal ganglia and parietal and occipital lobes are most commonly involved. Cerebral

MRI demonstrates areas of hyperintensity on T2-weighted images with volume loss presenting as a late development.

Proton MRS has been used to aid diagnosis of mitochondrial disorders, with the assumption that elevation of lactic acid is a primary feature. However, positive lactate at spectroscopy does not necessarily equal the presence of a mitochondrial disorder, and the absence of lactate on MRS does not rule out a defect in mitochondrial function. Proton MRS in patients with MELAS syndrome can demonstrate variable results as strokelike lesions emerge and evolve. Proton MRS details energy failure with increased lactate and decreased creatine. Elevation of lactate in the acute and subacute stages typically is observed, with subsequent declines in NAA and creatine, consistent with neuroaxonal injury that may or may not be reversible. It has been reported that both increase of lactate peaks in MRS and state of hyperperfusion in continuous arterial spin labeling images are both indicative of active lesions.[24] Reports have shown that MELAS syndrome is differentiated from ischemic stroke because of its longer ADC decline. Another distinctive characteristic of MELAS

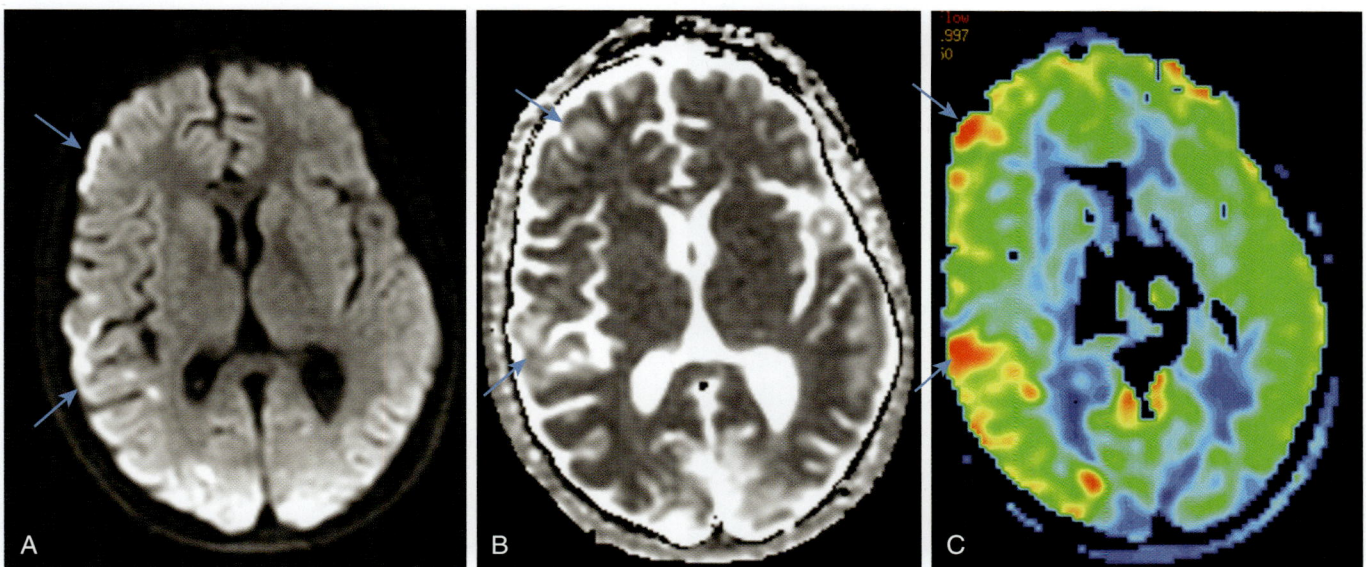

Figure 33-8 A 13-year-old boy affected by mitochondrial encephalomyopathy, lactic acidosis, and strokelike symptoms. Select axial diffusion-weighted imaging (**A**), an axial apparent diffusion coefficient map (**B**), and an axial arterial spin labeling color map (**C**) are shown. Scattered foci of vasogenic edema corresponding to increased perfusion are identified in the acute phase of the disease in the right cerebral hemisphere.

syndrome is the gradual spread of the core of the edematous lesion, a contributing factor to the prolonged ADC decline[25] (Fig. 33-8).

LEIGH SYNDROME (SUBACUTE NECROTIZING ENCEPHALOMYELOPATHY)

Disorders arising from defects in nDNA are numerous; however, the most commonly encountered syndrome is Leigh syndrome. The genetic defect of Leigh syndrome can arise from several sources, including pyruvate dehydrogenase complex deficiency, complex I deficiency, complex V deficiency with adenosine triphosphatase 6 mutation, and cytochrome oxidase deficiency with *SURF1* mutation. This group of disorders characteristically presents at 3 months to 2 years of age but may begin with symptoms of hypotonia in the newborn period or even in adulthood. Clinical signs include ophthalmoplegia, cerebellar signs, and spasticity, which are slowly progressive. Other features include psychomotor regression, extrapyramidal signs, blindness, nystagmus, respiratory compromise, or cranial nerve palsies. Onset of symptoms within the first years of life typically portends a rapid downhill course. A later onset of symptoms is generally associated with slower progression (Fig. 33-9 and e-Fig. 33-10).

Pathologically, this syndrome involves both gray and white matter of the brain and spinal cord. Common sites of anatomic involvement include the basal ganglia, specifically the globus pallidus and putamina, and the thalami, midbrain, pons, cerebellum, and medulla. Pathologic changes include spongiform degeneration, demyelination, and vascular compromise/proliferation.

An abnormal low signal on T1-weighted images or a high signal on T2-weighted images in the basal ganglia, periaqueductal gray matter, and brainstem/cerebellum are characteristic of this group of disorders. Bilateral symmetric lesions in the basal ganglia (globus pallidus and putamen) characterized by a hypointense signal on T1-weighted images and a hyperintense signal on T2-weighted images is highly suggestive of this condition and should prompt further clinical investigation for signs of lactic acid in the serum or CSF. Late involvement may manifest as regions of an abnormal hyperintense signal on T2-weighted images in the centrum semiovale.

Proton MRS images obtained from the basal ganglia, occipital cortex, and brainstem show elevations in lactate, which are most pronounced in regions where abnormalities are seen with routine T2-weighted MRI. Proton MRS images in regions of abnormal MRI signal also reveal a decrease in the NAA/creatine ratio and an increase in the choline/creatine ratio, representing neuronal loss and breakdown of membrane phospholipids. Some evidence indicates that a reduction of lactate levels may correlate with response to therapy, such as dichloroacetate and coenzyme Q10.

PANTOTHENATE KINASE-ASSOCIATED NEURODEGENERATION

Pantothenate kinase-associated neurodegeneration, also called neurodegeneration with brain iron accumulation (NBIA), is caused by mutations in the gene that encodes pantothenate kinase 2 (*PANK2*). *PANK2* is necessary for the production of coenzyme A in mitochondria. Other similar mutations result in atypical presentations of the same syndrome. "Classic" NBIA has an early onset of disease in infancy, with rapid progression of gait impairment, development of choreoathetoid movements, rigidity, dysarthria, and cognitive decline. Dystonia is a prominent feature of this disorder. All of these clinical manifestations reflect the impact of the disease upon the basal ganglia and striatum. Atypical NBIA has a later presentation with slower progression (Fig. 33-11).

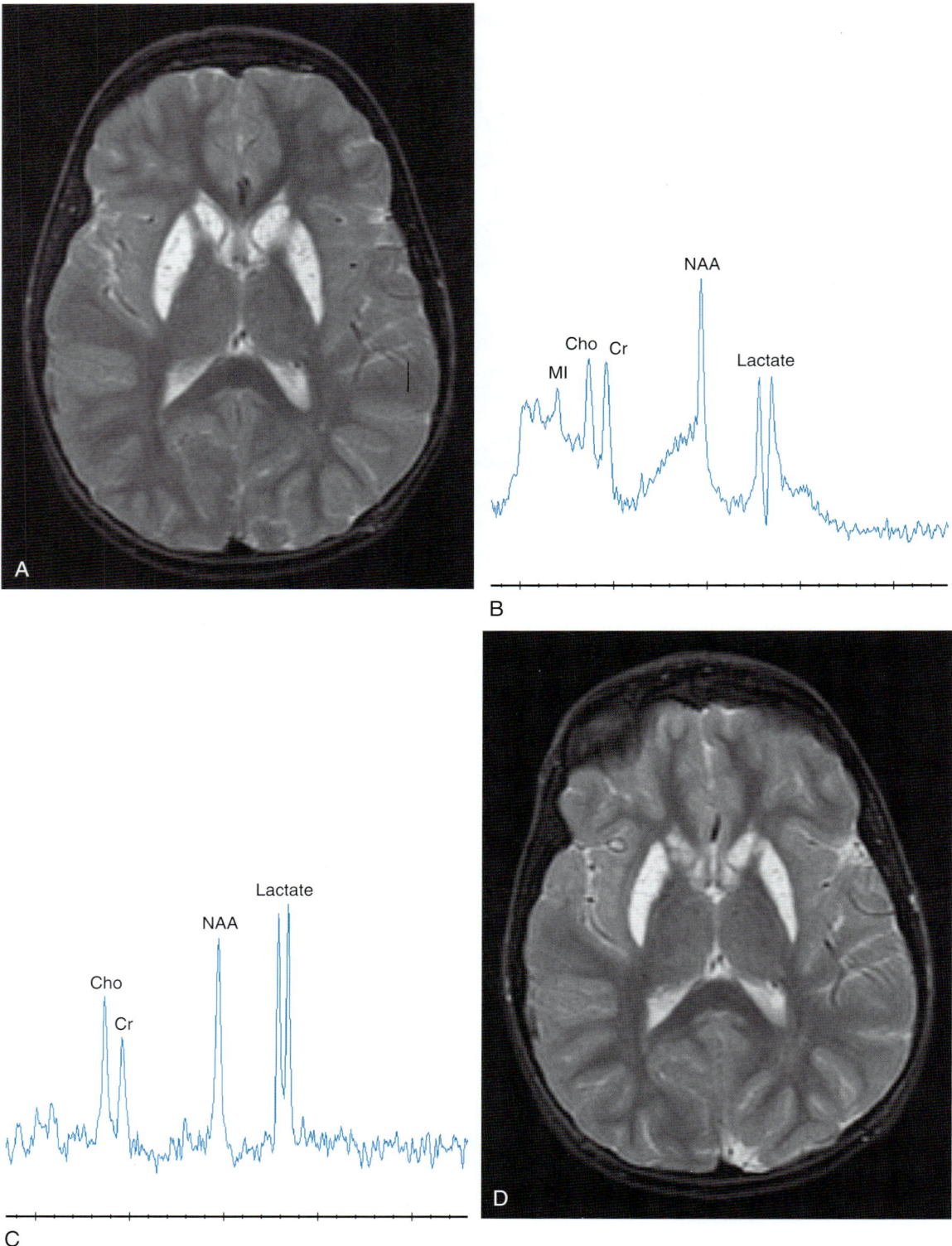

Figure 33-9 A complex I deficiency with magnetic resonance examinations in an 8-year-old girl acquired approximately 3 months apart. Axial T2-weighted (**A**), short echo magnetic resonance spectroscopy (MRS) (**B**), and long echo MRS (**C**) images were obtained. The imaging reveals a pattern characteristic of "Leigh syndrome" with an abnormal hyperintense signal bilaterally within the caudate and globus pallidus. The MRS image acquired in the left basal ganglia at a period of clinical exacerbation caused by febrile illness demonstrates a dramatic elevation of lactate compared with her routinely observed levels as shown in axial T2-weighted (**D**), short echo MRS (**E**), and long echo MRS (**F**) images. The spectra acquired 3 months later demonstrates a significant reduction in lactate. A comparison of the imaging data is unremarkable between the examinations. The dramatic elevation of lactate revealed on MRS in **B** and **C** corresponds to worsening clinical symptoms (seizures and leg stiffening). The lactate levels observed in **E** and **F** are typical and consistent with this mitochondrial defect. (From Cecil KM. MR spectroscopy of metabolic disorders. *Neuroimaging Clin N Am.* 2006;16:87-116; used with permission.)

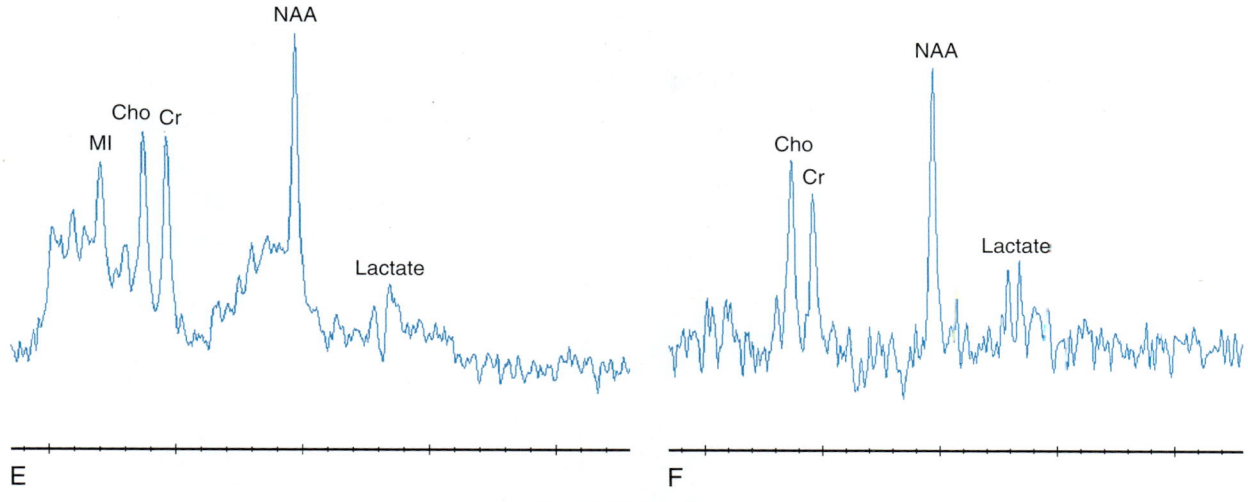

Figure 33-9, cont'd.

MENKES DISEASE

Menkes disease (also known as trichopoliodystrophy or kinky-hair syndrome) is an X-linked recessive mitochondrial cytopathy. The disease may commence in utero and has been recognized at birth. It appears in males with the clinical features of hypotonia, seizures, spastic quadriplegia, and profound retardation with sparse, fragile hair that is easily broken. Growth failure and microcephaly are common. Absorption of copper from the gastrointestinal tract is decreased. The defective intracellular binding and membrane transport of copper are related to an abnormal metallothionein, a copper-binding protein. Decreased activity of copper-dependent enzymes is found in the liver, brain, and white cells.

Plain radiographs may demonstrate wormian bones in the skull, rib fractures, and metaphyseal infarctions in long bones. Neuroimaging findings include cerebral volume loss and subdural collections, and cerebral angiography shows dilated and tortuous vessels within the circle of Willis. Basal ganglia lesions have been reported in advanced stages; however, a

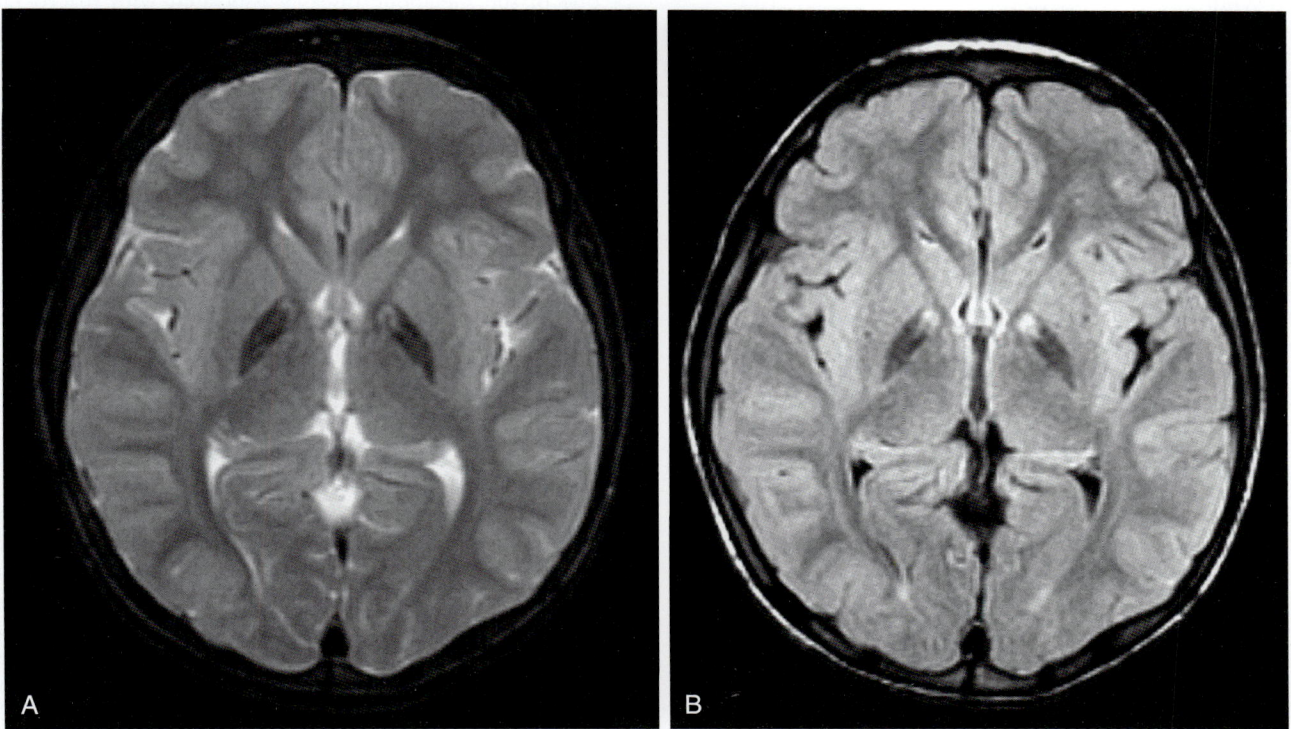

Figure 33-11 A 6-year-old girl with pantothenate kinase-associated neurodegeneration or neurodegeneration with brain iron accumulation, traditionally referred to as Hallervorden-Spatz syndrome. Axial T2-weighted (**A**) and axial fluid-attenuated inversion recovery (**B**) images are shown. An abnormal hypointense signal is demonstrated bilaterally in the globus pallidus.

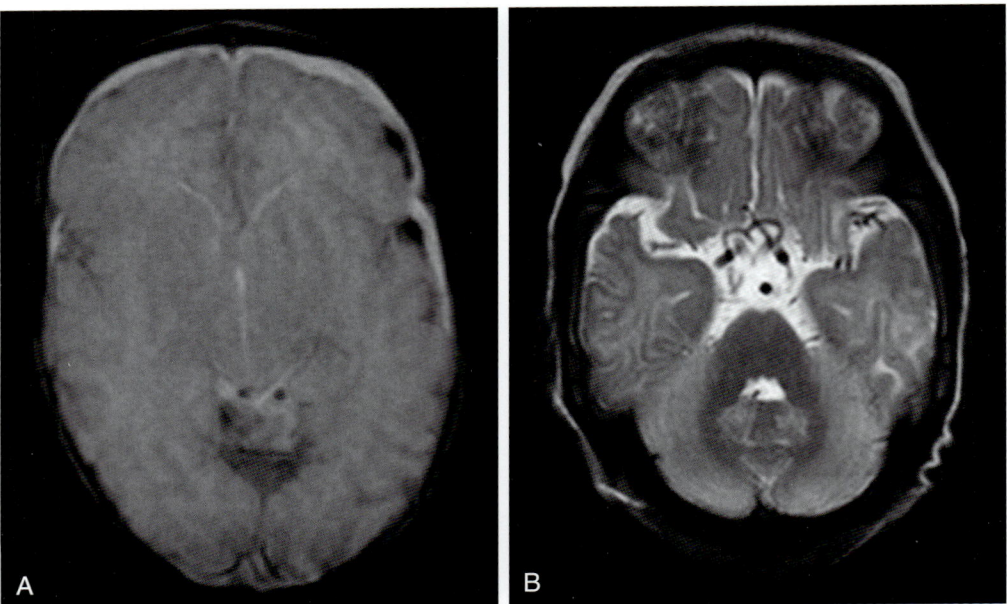

Figure 33-12 Menkes disease in a male patient. **A,** Axial multiple planar gradient recalled images reveal bilateral subdural collections with evidence of hemorrhage at 6 weeks. **B,** An axial T2-weighted image at the cerebellum at 4 months.

case documented basal ganglia involvement in a patient in the early stages of Menkes disease.[26] A hyperintense signal within white matter on T2-weighted images indicates a lack of myelination with this disorder, but this finding may be related to a relative lack of blood flow as a result of the vascular involvement. The combination of extracerebral collections and metaphyseal infarctions may simulate battered child syndrome (Fig. 33-12).

Organic and Amino Acid Disorders

Many disorders of organic acid metabolism affect mitochondrial function, and as such, they demonstrate imaging features similar to those of mitochondrial disorders. Two key disorders are glutaric aciduria and methylmalonic acidemia. Myelin formation is dependent on amino acids. Defects in amino acid metabolism lead to failure of formation and maintenance of normal myelin. Disorders primarily of amino acid metabolism include phenylketonuria, maple syrup urine disease (MSUD), homocystinuria/hyperhomocysteinemia, and non-ketotic hyperglycinemia.

GLUTARIC ACIDURIA

Glutaric aciduria type I is an organic aciduria resulting from deficiency of the enzyme glutaryl-CoA dehydrogenase, which is involved in the metabolism of hydroxylysine, lysine, and tryptophan. It is autosomal recessive in origin. Presentation may be acute with encephalopathy or chronic with multiple neurologic abnormalities, including hypotonia, ataxia, dysmetria, and delayed achievement of milestones.

Brain MRI demonstrates hyperintensity on T2-weighted images in the basal ganglia, especially the putamen, but also in the caudate nucleus and globus pallidus. Myelination is delayed. Bilateral temporal arachnoid cysts and enlarged

frontotemporal spaces with subdural hematomas may be found. As a consequence, this rare disorder is sometimes considered as a differential diagnosis in children with nonaccidental trauma. The development of T2 prolongation in the basal ganglia and periventricular white matter would support the diagnosis of glutaric aciduria type I in such cases. The enlargement of extraaxial spaces makes glutaric aciduria type I one of the metabolic diseases associated with macrocrania. Unlike in Alexander disease and Canavan disease, the macrocrania does not reflect megalencephaly. Enlargement of the sylvian fissure has been correlated with severity of the enzyme deficiency. Acute striatal necrosis is the main cause of death during infancy; it can be visualized as usually symmetric, strokelike signal hyperintensity on T2-weighted and diffusion-weighted MRI, bilateral striatal lucency on CT, or a sharp decline of fluorodeoxyglucose uptake on positron emission tomography.[27] Prenatal MRI has been shown to be useful in identifying GA1, revealing focal reduction of the anterior pole of both temporal lobes with widening of the liquoral space[28] (Fig. 33-13).

METHYLMALONIC AND PROPRIONIC ACIDEMIAS

Methylmalonic acidemia results from a deficiency in methylmalonyl CoA mutase, an enzyme required for the conversion of methylmalonic CoA to succinyl CoA, which is necessary for the proper metabolism of the amino acids methionine, threonine, isoleucine, and valine. The high levels of methylmalonic acid resulting from the enzyme deficiency inhibit succinate dehydrogenase, which disrupts aerobic metabolism in the mitochondria. A relatively milder form of the disease is caused by deficiency of the cobalamin coenzyme. Propionic aciduria is a result of a deficiency in propionyl-CoA carboxylase and presents in a similar fashion (e-Fig. 33-14).

Epilepsy is common in patients with methylmalonic acidemia, and cardiac involvement, including cardiomyopathy,

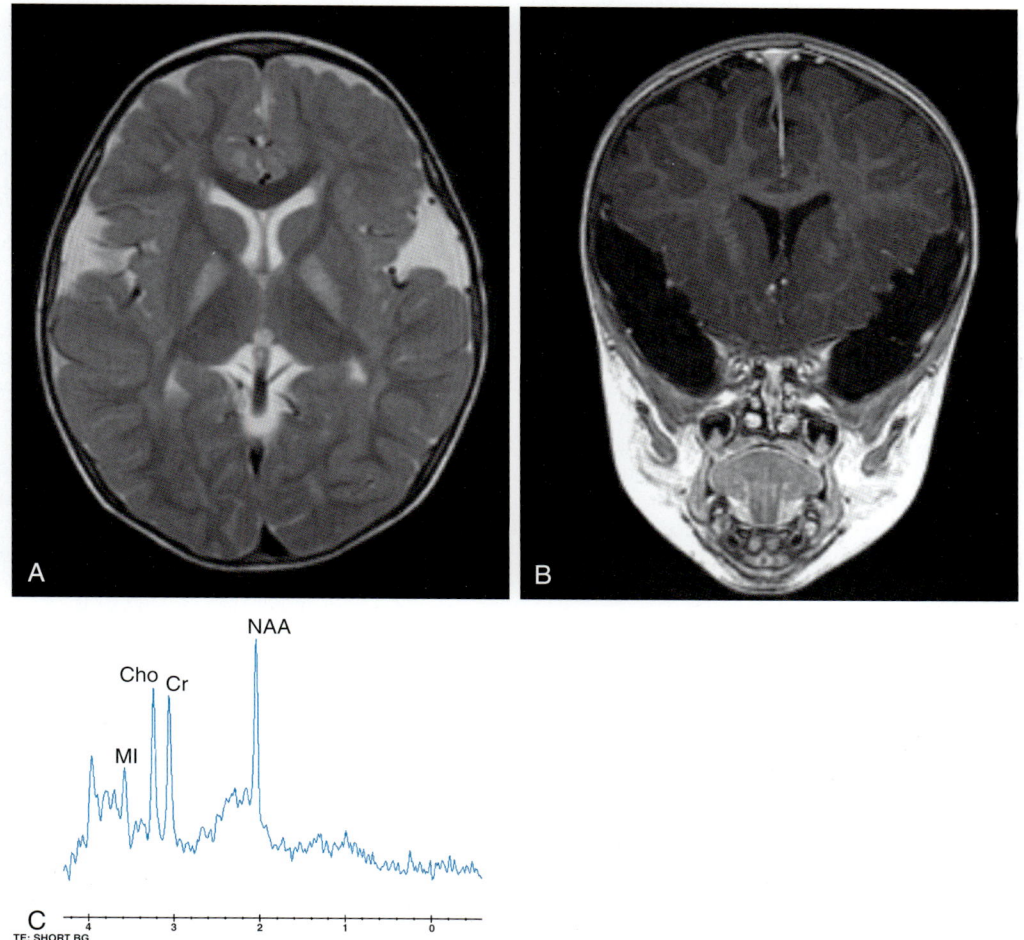

Figure 33-13   Glutaric aciduria I in a 22-month-old boy. **A,** An axial fast spin echo T2-weighted image demonstrates a hyperintense signal bilaterally within the globus pallidus. **B,** A coronal spoiled gradient echo image features the prominent symmetric, bilateral widening of the sylvian fissures with frontotemporal hypoplasia. **C,** A short echo (time to echo 35 msec) magnetic resonance spectroscopy image acquired within the basal ganglia demonstrates an elevation of choline.

arrhythmias, carnitine deficiency, and structural heart disease, have been reported.[29,30] Hyperglycemia also has been reported.[31] On imaging, parenchymal volume often is decreased, with delays in myelination. Optic neuropathy also has been reported.[32] Like other mitochondrial-based syndromes, the organic acidemias have a strong tendency to cause lesions in the basal ganglia, most particularly the globus pallidus. Lesions in the globus pallidus are striking in their stereotypical appearance from patient to patient. Affected areas will appear low in attenuation on CT and hyperintense on T2-weighted MRI. Strokelike episodes similar to MELAS occasionally may be encountered. DWI will show restricted diffusion in affected regions. Proton MRS has shown decreases in NAA and elevation of lactate levels. Lactate elevation also can be found in the CSF, which is important for narrowing the differential diagnosis.

PHENYLKETONURIA

Phenylketonuria is an autosomal-recessive disorder resulting from enzyme deficiencies (phenylalanine hydroxylase, dihydrobiopterin reductase, and dihydrobiopterin biosynthesis) that impair the ability to convert phenylalanine to tyrosine, thereby producing the accumulation of neurotoxic acids. Its frequency is on the order of 1:14,000 live births.

Brain MRI appearances initially demonstrate symmetric hyperintense areas on T2-weighted images in the periatrial white matter. Extension occurs into the optic radiations and periventricular frontal white matter with more severe involvement and contrast enhancement. In untreated patients, it has been reported that diffuse white matter pathology is evidence of hypomyelination; however, white matter abnormalities in patients who are treated early are indicative of intramyelinic edema.[33] Hyperintensity in multiple areas on T1-weighted images has been reported, corresponding to subcortical parenchymal calcification.

White matter alterations revealed on MRI studies in patients with phenylketonuria correlated to blood phenylalanine concentrations and to brain phenylalanine concentrations measured by proton MRS. MRS may demonstrate an abnormal peak at 7.30 ppm resulting from elevated phenylalanine. Interindividual variations of blood-brain barrier phenylalanine transport constants and variations of the individual brain phenylalanine consumption rate are responsible for the patient differences.

MAPLE SYRUP URINE DISEASE

MSUD is a rare autosomal-recessive disorder caused by defective oxidative decarboxylation of three branched-chain amino acids: valine, isoleucine, and leucine. The accumulation of metabolites in the urine leads to the characteristic odor, which resembles that of maple syrup. Although cerebral imaging findings initially may be unremarkable, diffuse cerebral edema develops with subsequent residual areas of hyperintensity in the dorsal brainstem and pons. Proton MRS of the brain appears to be useful for examining patients who have MSUD in different metabolic states. The accumulation of abnormal branched-chain amino acids and branched-chain alpha-ketoacids appear as a broad peak at 0.9 ppm accompanied by an elevated lactate level. The presence of cytotoxic or intramyelinic edema as evidenced by restricted water diffusion on DWI, with the presence of lactate on spectroscopy, could imply cell death. However, in the context of metabolic decompensation in MSUD, it appears that changes in cell osmolarity and metabolism can reverse completely after metabolic correction. Classification of MSUD includes a form that is responsive to thiamine (Fig. 33-15).

NONKETOTIC HYPERGLYCINEMIA

Nonketotic hyperglycinemia occurs when a metabolic defect impairs the conversion of glycine to serine, resulting in an accumulation of glycine within the CNS. The toxic effects of an elevated glycine level present in the neonatal period as lethargy, hypotonia, myoclonus, and seizures that may lead to an unresponsive state with apnea. Prognosis is poor, with few patients surviving beyond the neonatal period.

Pathology in nonketotic hyperglycinemia is characterized by vacuolation, astrocytosis, and demyelination, also called vacuolating myelinopathy. Because these changes only occur in myelinated white matter, in the neonate they are restricted to the dorsal limbs of the internal capsule, dorsal brainstem, pyramidal tracts in the coronal radiata, and lateral thalamus. A long tractlike lesion involving the spinal cord has been reported in persons with late-onset disease.[34] On MR, these areas will show a hyperintense signal on T2-weighted images and restricted diffusion on DWI. Volume loss ensues and may be present at birth as a result of the toxic effects of glycine in utero. Proton MRS can detect the accumulated glycine itself, as a distinct resonance at 3.55 ppm. In patients with nonketotic hyperglycinemia, elevated cerebral glycine can be measured with proton MRS. Using long echo times, such as 288 ms, MRS reveals glycine at 3.5 ppm. With use of short echo times, the resonance at 3.5 is a composite of mI and glycine. Select metabolite ratios (NAA, mI, and glycine) appear to correlate with the patient's course (Fig. 33-16).

Primary Disorders of White Matter (Leukodystrophies)

The term "leukodystrophy" generally is reserved for conditions that are both progressive and genetically determined. Although these conditions eventually may involve and alter gray matter, the primary features affect the white matter.

CANAVAN DISEASE

Canavan disease is an autosomal-recessive disorder arising from a deficiency of the enzyme aspartoacylase, which results in the accumulation of NAA acid in the brain. Three clinical subtypes—infantile, juvenile, and adult—are recognized. The most common is the infantile type, which usually presents within the first 6 months of life with hypotonia, irritability, and enlarging head size, leading to spasticity, blindness, choreoathetoid movement, and myoclonic seizures.

The diagnosis is made by demonstrating increased amounts of NAA in the urine and plasma. On histologic examination, the disease is seen to begin in a peripheral location, involving the U fibers of the subcortical white matter of the cerebral hemispheres. Later, the abnormality involves the deep white matter structures of both cerebral hemispheres, and eventually it extends to the cerebellum and spinal cord. The involvement of the U fibers of the white matter is diffuse, with evidence of vacuoles within the subcortical white matter and extending into the adjacent cortex.

The MRI findings are related to the myelin degeneration of the white matter tracts. The first change detected is hyperintensity on T2-weighted images of the subcortical U fibers. Eventually there is diffuse involvement of all the white matter fiber tracts in both cerebral hemispheres. In the later stages of the disease, volume loss of the cerebral hemispheres occurs. Enlarged perivascular spaces, likely reflecting spongiform degeneration of the white matter, has been described in one patient.[35] MRS demonstrates marked elevation of the NAA peak, which is diagnostic for Canavan disease (Fig. 33-17).

ALEXANDER DISEASE

Missense mutations in the gene encoding for glial fibrillary acidic protein (GFAP) are found in all three clinical variants (infantile, juvenile, and adult) of Alexander disease. In brain biopsy specimens, Rosenthal fibers label extensively for GFAP upon immunocytochemistry. The mutations in Alexander disease are heterozygous and dominant, and accordingly most cases are sporadic. The most commonly encountered variant of Alexander disease is the infantile form, which presents in the first 2 years of life with megalencephaly and developmental delay and frequently with seizures. Children with the infantile form of the disease rarely survive to the second decade. The juvenile form presents after 4 years of age with speech and swallowing difficulties, ataxia, and spasticity. Progression is slower, with a more prolonged survival. Adult-onset disease has a more variable clinical presentation and occasionally is diagnosed incidentally at autopsy.

The diagnosis traditionally has been performed via a brain biopsy. The predominant histologic feature is a considerable amount of Rosenthal fibers within the white matter. Most commonly, the disease begins in the periventricular white matter, usually involving the frontal lobes and then extending into the parietotemporal and then the occipital regions. Eventually, involvement of the cerebellar white matter and spinal cord occurs. CSF oligoclonal bands have been reported in the adult-onset variant.[36]

The MRI findings demonstrate macrocephaly with hyperintensity on T2-weighted images involving the white matter areas, which commonly is seen in the frontal areas with

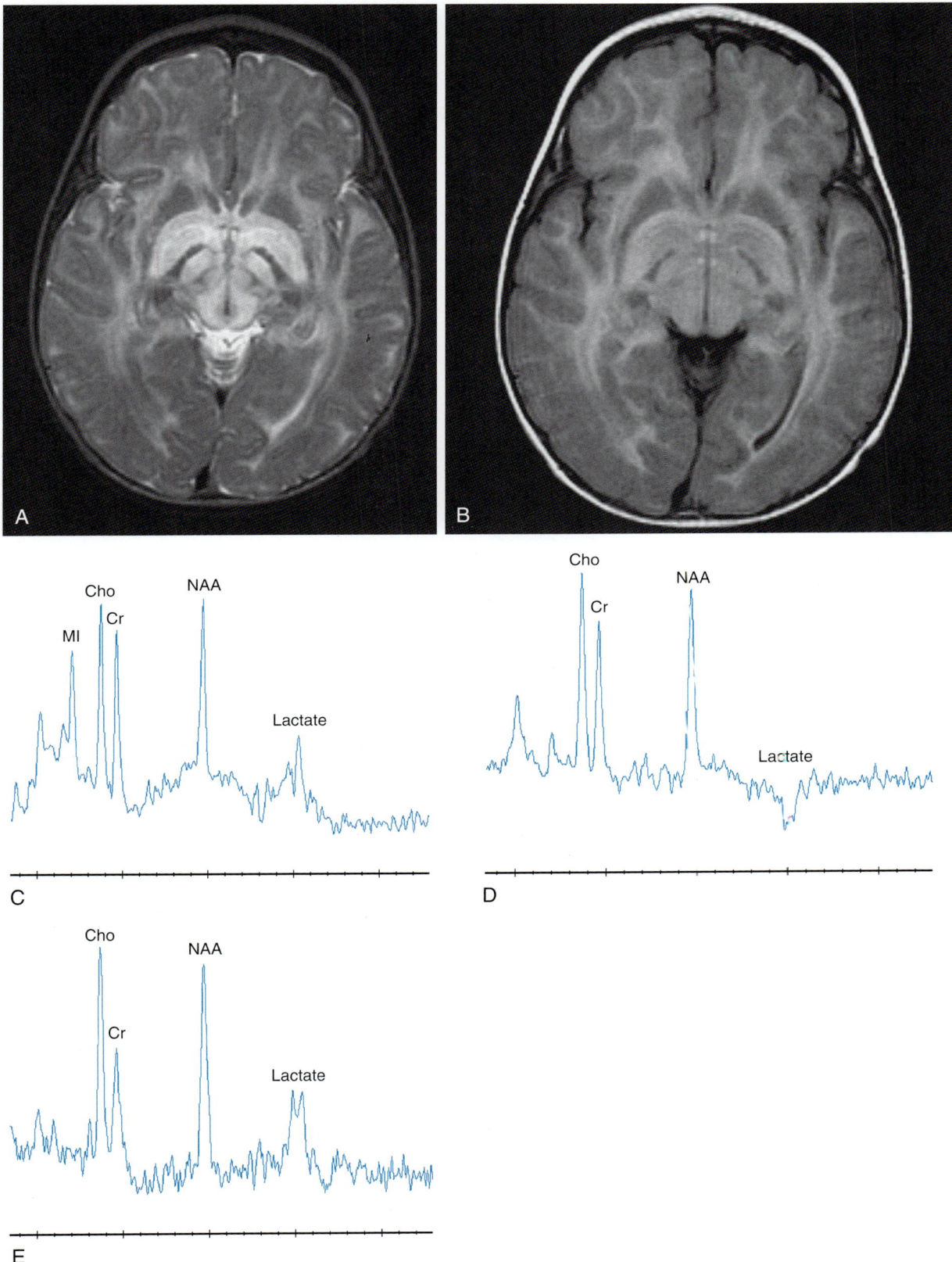

Figure 33-15 An infant with maple syrup urine disease. Axial T2-weighted (**A**), axial fluid-attenuated inversion recovery (**B**), short echo magnetic reso-nance spectroscopy (MRS) (**C**), intermediate echo MRS (**D**), and long echo MRS (**E**) images reveal an abnormal signal within the brainstem, internal capsule, and globus pallidus. On short echo MRS, a composite of branched chain amino acids (0.9 ppm) with lactate (1.35 ppm) is inverted on inter-mediate echo and upright on long echo MRS. Notice the reduced signal intensity associated with the inversion at time to echo (TE) 144 with partial restoration of the signal intensity at TE 288. (From Cecil KM. MR spectroscopy of metabolic disorders. *Neuroimaging Clin N Am.* 2006;16:87-116; used with permission.)

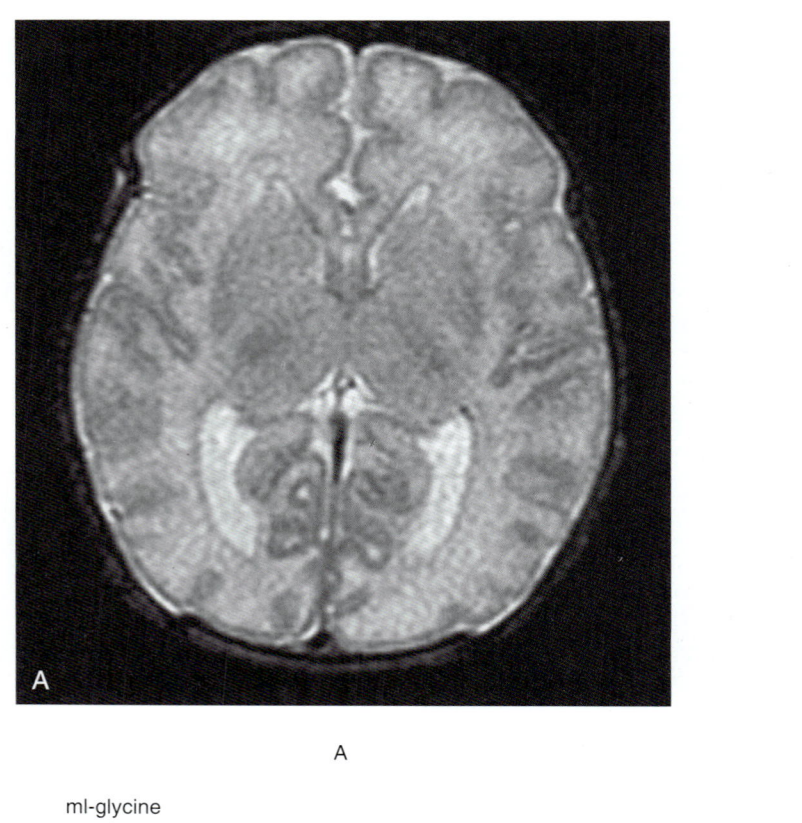

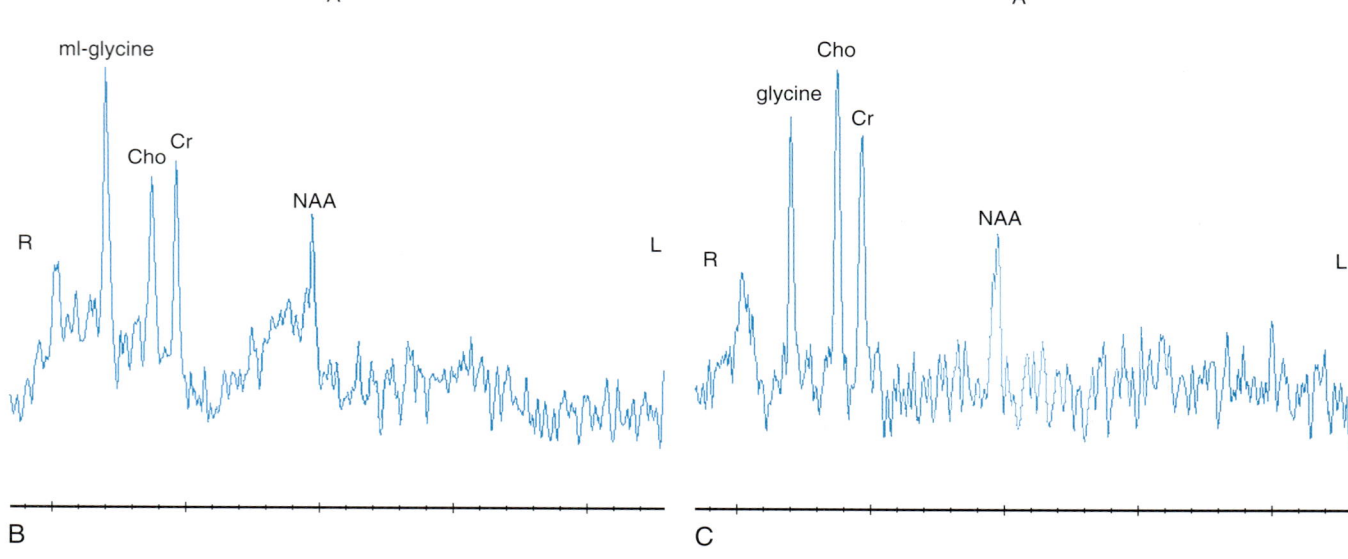

Figure 33-16 A neonate with nonketotic hyperglycinemia. Axial T2-weighted (**A**), short echo magnetic resonance spectroscopy (MRS) (**B**), and intermediate (144 msec) MRS (**C**) images are shown. The short echo spectrum demonstrates a composite myo-inositol and glycine resonance at 3.5 ppm. The intermediate echo demonstrates glycine. (From Cecil KM. MR spectroscopy of metabolic disorders. *Neuroimaging Clin N Am.* 2006;16:87-116; used with permission.)

progression posteriorly to involve other parts of the cerebral hemispheres. According to van der Knapp et al.,[37] the findings of frontal predominance, a periventricular rim of high-T2/low-T1 signal, involved central gray matter and brainstem, plus enhancement of portions of the involved areas are very characteristic of this disease (Fig. 33-18).

van der Knapp et al[38] identified five characteristics of Alexander disease on MRI that can be applied to suspected cases to make a presumptive diagnosis. These characteristics are (1) extensive cerebral white matter changes with frontal predominance, (2) a periventricular rim with a high signal on T1-weighted images and a low signal on T2-weighted images, (3) signal abnormalities with swelling or volume loss in the basal ganglia and thalami, (4) brainstem signal abnormalities, and (5) contrast enhancement of one or more of the following structures: ventricular lining, periventricular rim of tissue, white matter of the frontal lobes, optic chiasm, fornix, basal ganglia, thalamus, dentate nucleus, or brainstem structures. Although many of these abnormalities may be seen in other leukodystrophies, the association of four or more appears to be relatively specific for Alexander disease. The extent and pattern of contrast enhancement and the

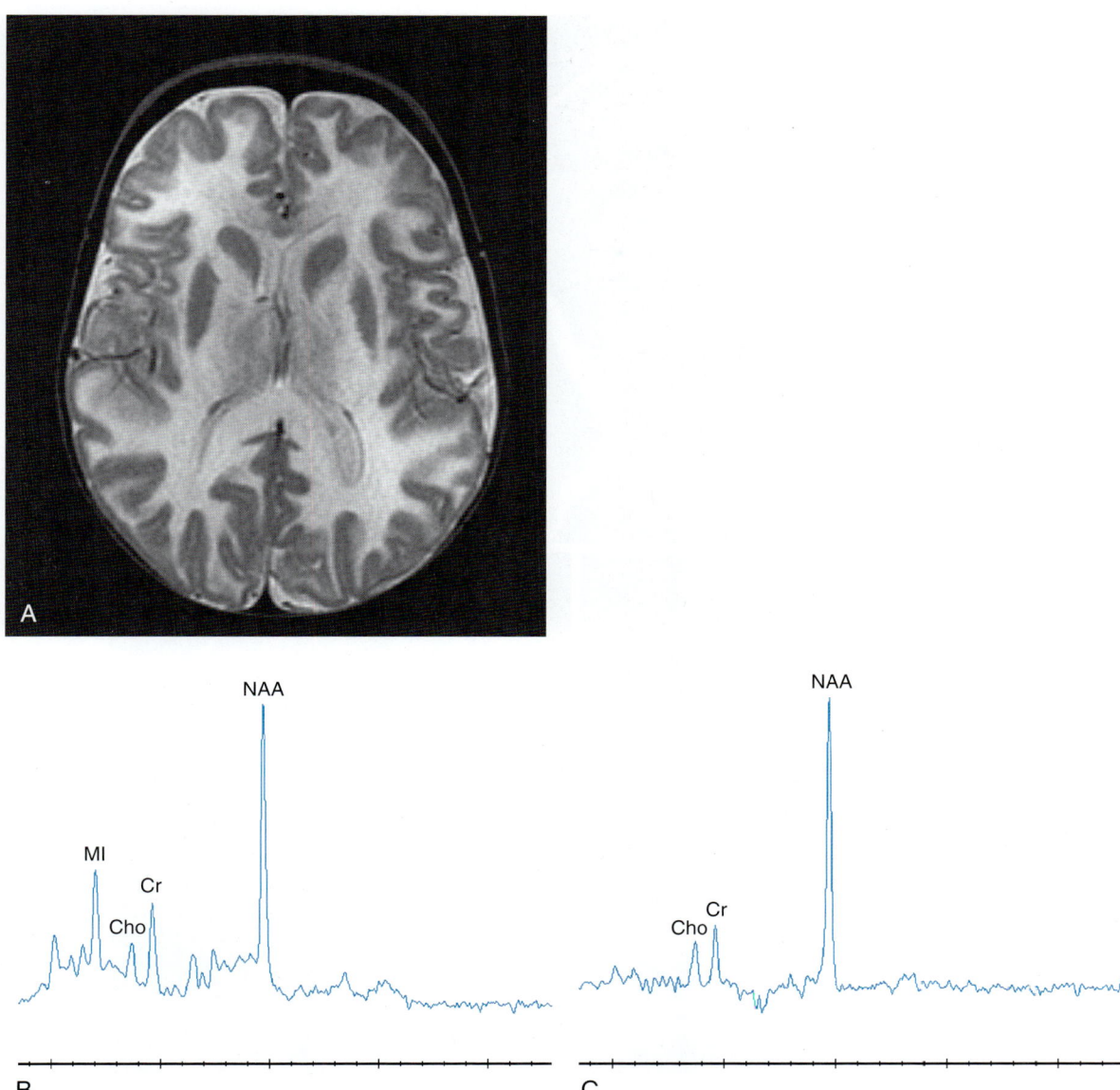

Figure 33-17 A 12-month-old girl with Canavan disease. Select axial T2-weighted (**A**), short echo magnetic resonance spectroscopy (MRS) (**B**), and long echo MRS (**C**) images are shown. Diffuse hypomyelination is revealed on the T2-weighted image. Elevated N-acetylaspartate (NAA) is the key feature with secondary myo-inositol elevation representing gliosis. Because of the deficiency in aspartoacylase, NAA accumulates in the mitochondria, impairing myelin synthesis. (From Cecil KM. MR spectroscopy of metabolic disorders. *Neuroimaging Clin N Am.* 2006;16:87-116; with permission.)

distinctive periventricular rim of abnormal signal are not encountered in many other processes. This leukodystrophy is one of the few in which the administration of contrast material provides specific additional information that can lead to the correct diagnosis by imaging.

Brockmann et al.[39] used localized proton MRS to assess metabolic abnormalities in gray and white matter, basal ganglia, and cerebellum of four patients with infantile Alexander disease identified with heterozygous de novo mutations in the gene-encoding GFAP. Elevated concentrations of mI in conjunction with normal or increased choline compounds in gray and white matter, basal ganglia, and cerebellum point to astrocytosis and demyelination. Neuroaxonal degeneration, as reflected by a reduction of NAA, was most pronounced in cerebral and cerebellar white matter.

MEGALENCEPHALIC LEUKOENCEPHALOPATHY WITH SUBCORTICAL CYSTS

Megaloencephalic leukoencephalopathy with subcortical cysts typically presents in infancy or childhood with macrocrania, developmental delay, seizures, and motor disability. MRI demonstrates widespread signal abnormalities throughout the white matter, with sparing of deep structures. Cysts typically are identified in the subcortical temporal lobes and less frequently in the frontal, parietal, or occipital lobes. Despite the extensive abnormalities on imaging, many affected patients achieve a high level of normal function. The genetic source of the condition has been traced to a gene on the long arm of chromosome 22 (22q13.33), the *MLC1* gene. The disease is inherited in an autosomal-recessive pattern, and

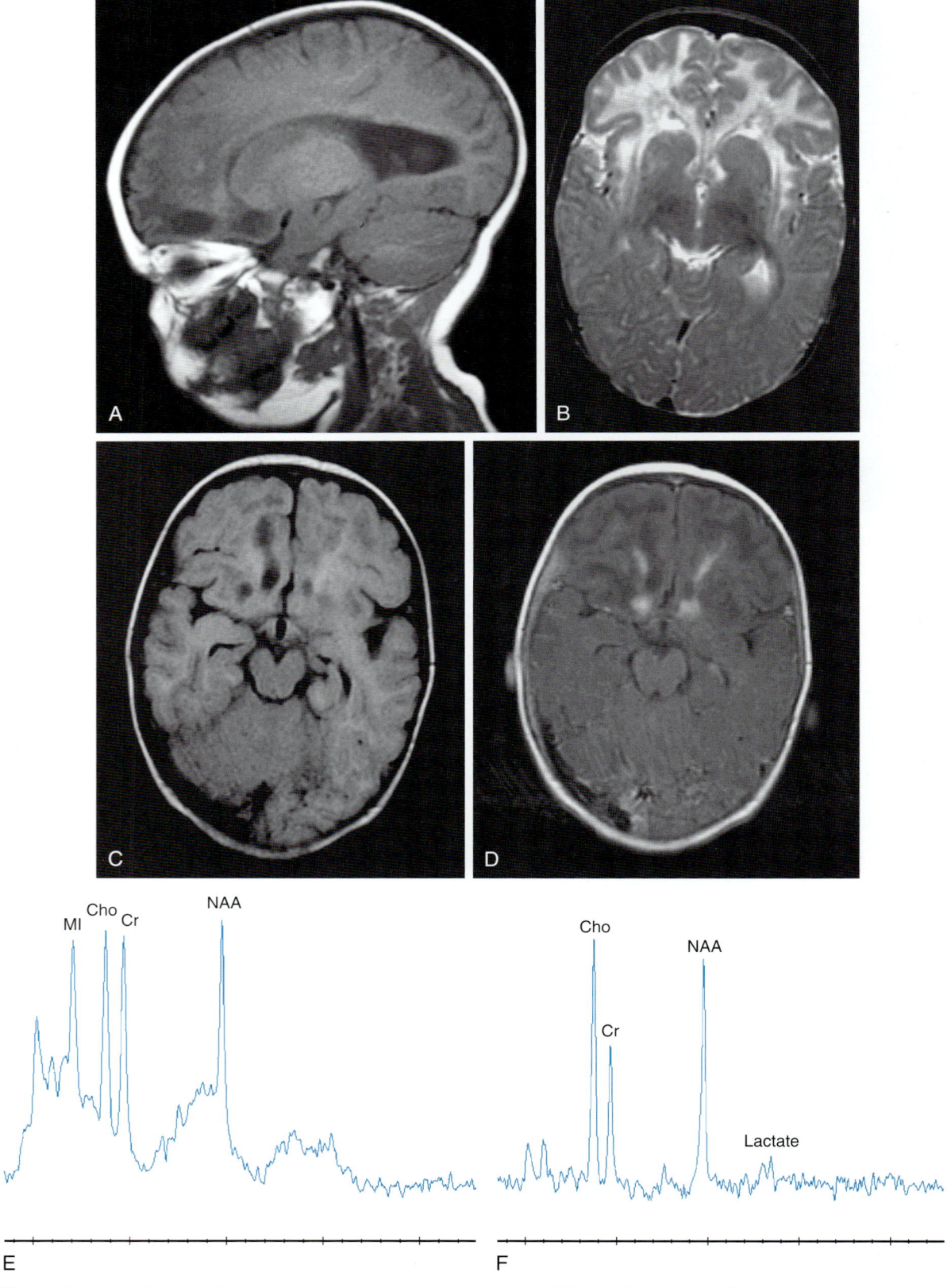

Figure 33-18 An 8-month-old girl with Alexander disease. Select sagittal T1-weighted (**A**), axial T2-weighted (**B**), axial fluid-attenuated inversion recovery (FLAIR) (**C**), axial T1-weighted postcontrast (**D**), short echo magnetic resonance spectroscopy (MRS) (**E**), and long echo MRS (**F**) images were acquired in the frontal white matter. The deep frontal and periventricular white matter demonstrate a hypointense T1-weighted and hyperintense T2-weighted signal. The frontal lobe cavitations are revealed on the FLAIR image with hypointense signal and demonstrate enhancement at the borders. Volume enlargement of the caudate heads is seen. Decreased N-acetylaspartate with lactate, choline, and myo-inositol elevations representing macrophage infiltration, demyelination, and astrocytosis are indicated from the MRS image.

because of the variable phenotype, identification of a single case should prompt further investigation and genetic counseling (e–Fig. 33–19).

LEUKOENCEPHALOPATHY WITH BRAINSTEM AND SPINAL CORD INVOLVEMENT AND ELEVATED WHITE MATTER LACTATE

Leukoencephalopathy with brainstem and spinal cord involvement and elevated white matter lactate recently has been described based on the MRI characteristics. Initial childhood development is generally unremarkable; the onset of presentation for leukoencephalopathy with brainstem and spinal cord involvement and elevated white matter lactate occurs in childhood with motor deterioration. The MRI pattern is quite distinct. The progressive white matter abnormalities spread from the periventricular region outward with sparing of the subcortical U fibers. The corpus callosum is affected with posterior preference. The pyramidal tracts are affected over their entire length from the posterior limb of the internal capsule and brainstem into the lateral corticospinal tracts of the spinal cord. The sensory tracts are involved from the dorsal columns in the spinal cord, the medial lemniscus through the brainstem up to the level of the thalamus, and the corona radiata above the level of the thalamus. The cerebellar involvement progresses over time to the point of significant volume loss. Clinical severity and the extent of neurologic abnormalities on MRI do not appear to correlate[40] (e–Fig. 33–20).

GALACTOSEMIA

Galactosemia is the result of a deficiency in galactose-1-phosphate uridyl transferase, which is an enzyme essential for the metabolism of galactose. It presents in infants soon after the introduction of cow's milk into the diet. Clinical features include failure to thrive, hepatomegaly with jaundice, vomiting and diarrhea, cataracts, increased ICP, and mental deterioration. It can be identified by the presence of increased reducing substances in the stool. Neurologic dysfunction is the result of hypoglycemia and the accumulation of galactose, galactose-1-phosphate, and galactitol in the brain and eye. In adult forms, low bone density often is observed.[41]

On CT, diffuse low attenuation of white matter mimicking diffuse edema often is present. The most consistent early finding on MRI is a delay in myelination, which may appear as persistence of a hyperintense signal in the peripheral white matter on T2-weighted images. These signal abnormalities may be more widespread in older children as a result of demyelination. Patchy areas of focal increased signal on T2-weighted images also have been reported and are thought to represent damaged areas of white matter. Eventually a pattern of mild cerebral or cerebellar volume loss is found.

Brain edema may occur in infants with galactosemia and has been associated with accumulation of galactitol.

CREATINE DEFICIENCY

Inborn errors of creatine metabolism, specifically defects in creatine synthesis and transport, recently have been reported. In many brain structures, including the cortex and basal ganglia, arginine glycine amidinotransferase (AGAT) and guanidinoacetate methyltransferase (GAMT) are expressed in a disassociated way rather than being coexpressed, leading to the thought that guanidinoacetate must be transported from AGAT to GAMT.[42] Proton MRS clinical studies have led to the discovery of three creatine deficiency syndromes: creatine transporter deficiency syndrome, AGAT deficiency, and (3) GAMT deficiency. Several patients have been found to have a markedly diminished or absent creatine signal with proton MRS. If proton MRS reveals the absence of creatine in the brain, serum and urine creatine assessments may give a preliminary indication of whether there is a synthesis defect (diminished creatine) or a transport defect (elevated creatine). In cases of synthesis defects, proton MRS can monitor increasing brain creatine concentration with oral supplementation, which offers improvement of some symptoms but not recovery of normal function (Fig. 33–21).

Miscellaneous White Matter Disorders

PELIZAEUS-MERZBACHER DISEASE AND DISORDERS OF MYELIN PROTEOLIPID PROTEIN

PMD is condition that manifests as a primary defect in myelin formation. It is the prototypical hypomyelination syndrome, in that the imaging appearance is of an otherwise normal brain that is severely delayed in its formation of myelin.

Mutations or duplications of the gene-encoding myelin proteolipid protein (PLP; Xq22.2) produce variable clinical manifestations resulting from alterations in this gene. Spastic paraplegia type 2 is characterized by lower limb spasticity alone. Persons with "complicated" spastic paraplegia type 2 exhibit cerebellar ataxia, nystagmus, and a pyramidal syndrome. The more severe phenotypic manifestations traditionally have been categorized as PMD and result in alterations of multiple functional systems, with symptoms including nystagmus and compromises in respiratory function, with associated severe disability and morbidity.

The classic descriptions of PMD divide it into several different subtypes. The most common presentation is that of the slowly progressive "classic" form that presents in infancy with early nystagmus ("dancing eyes"), poor head control, spasticity, ataxia or extrapyramidal movement disorders, and severe developmental delay. These findings slowly progress, usually leading to death in late adolescence or young adulthood. A second pattern (connatal, or the Seitelberger type) begins in the neonatal period and is more rapidly progressive, with death typically occurring in the first decade.

Imaging demonstrates a marked delay in myelination from the onset. Whereas many metabolic or neurodegenerative processes are associated with delayed myelination, the absence of other imaging findings is characteristic of the early stages of the PLP gene disorders. On CT, hypomyelination can be appreciated as diffuse low attenuation of white matter. The characteristic normal progression of myelination as detected by MRI in the first 2 years of life is well documented in multiple texts. T1-weighted images show a steady development of shortening (bright signal) in white matter tracts as they acquire myelin during the first 10 to 12 postnatal months. A similar advance of T2 shortening (dark signal) can be seen during the 6- to 24-month time frame. This steady progression is entirely

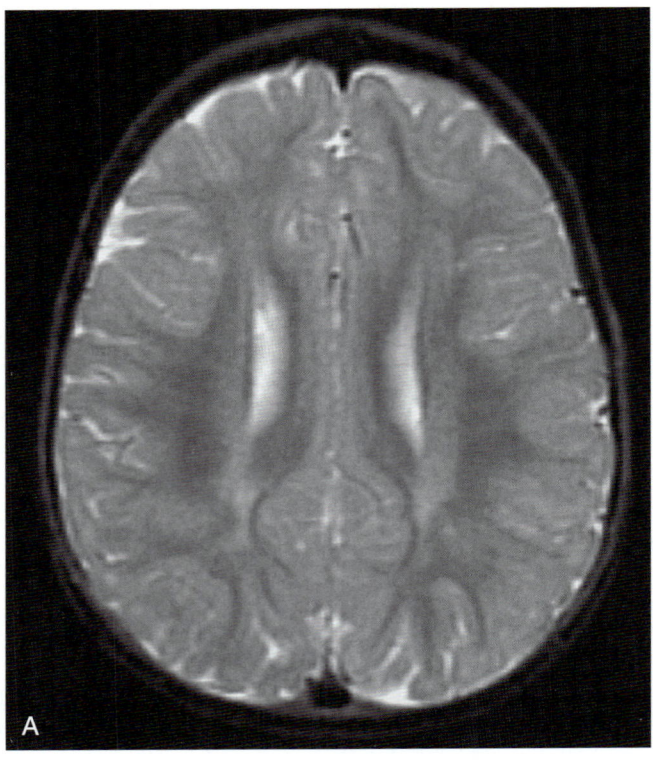

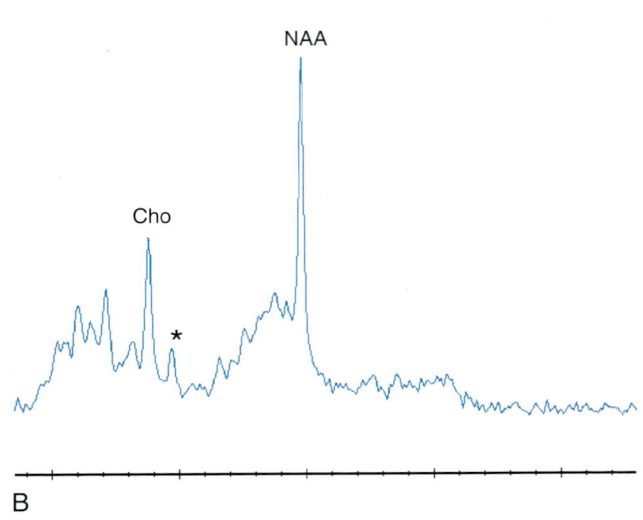

Figure 33-21   A 2-year-old boy with a known mutation of the creatine transporter. Axial T2-weighted (**A**) and short echo magnetic resonance spectroscopy (**B**) images reveal an abnormal signal within the periventricular white matter, representing hypomyelination. Short echo spectroscopy reveals a marked reduction of creatine signal (*asterisk*).

absent or severely slowed in persons with the *PLP* gene disorders. Myelination that does occur tends to be patchy, without the characteristic predictable distribution within the white matter tracts. In the later stages of disease, white matter volume may decrease, with thinning of the corpus callosum and excess mineralization in the basal ganglia.

Diffusion tensor imaging has been reported to be effective for detecting subtle changes in the microstructure of the white matter, such as abnormal myelination, even when findings of MRI and MRS are normal.[43]

Diminished values of NAA and mild elevations of choline have been reported when MRS is performed in patients with PMD, indicating axonal injury and secondary gliosis. Plecko et al.[44] found heterogeneous cerebral metabolite patterns in patients with PMD and Pelizaeus-Merzbacher–like disease, indicating a mixture of unspecific changes as a result of primary hypomyelination and secondary gliosis and demyelination. However, neither MRI nor MRS provided unique patterns to allow differentiation between patients with PMD and Pelizaeus-Merzbacher–like disease.

Other Disorders Affecting the Basal Ganglia

HUNTINGTON DISEASE

Huntington disease (HD) is an autosomal-recessive degenerative disorder that is uncommon in children, with most cases presenting after the fourth decade. HD is characterized by a movement disorder. Cerebellar symptoms, seizures, rigidity,

and mental retardation are common. Caudate volume loss is demonstrated on MRI, although cortical changes also may be detected.[45] Bilateral areas of hyperintensity may be seen in the basal ganglion on T2-weighted images. Global atrophy in persons with HD shows a disproportionate relationship to caudate involvement.[46] In pre-HD, gray matter change has been reported to be specific to regions consistent with basal ganglia-thalamocortical pathways, whereas white matter changes were much more generalized.[47] White matter diffusivity abnormalities also have been reported in the corpus callosum and external/extreme capsules.[48] In premanifest gene carriers, the white matter pathway of the sensorimotor cortex is impaired.[49] Changes in the hypothalamic region have been reported in prodromal HD and appear to be one of the earliest evident features of this disease.[50]

FAHR DISEASE

Fahr disease comprises a group of disorders that have basal ganglia calcification. Mental deterioration and growth retardation have been described. Cerebral MRI demonstrates areas of signal void within the basal nuclei and dentate nuclei on T1- and T2-weighted images. The appearances correlate with the areas of calcification on CT. Transcranial sonography also has been reported to be useful for visualizing calcifications of the basal ganglia.[51]

WILSON DISEASE

Hepatolenticular degeneration, or Wilson disease, is inherited in an autosomal-recessive fashion and is a result of an inborn error in copper metabolism. Ceruloplasmin, the serum transport protein for copper, is deficient, with resultant copper deposition in various sites. This disease typically presents in young adults with chronic hepatic insufficiency and neurologic deterioration. Copper fails to be excreted in the bile and thus accumulates in the body, especially in liver, brain, kidney, and red blood cells. The clinical presentation is primarily that of extrapyramidal signs, hepatic insufficiency, and the presence of Kayser-Fleischer corneal rings. Either the hepatic toxicity or the neurologic findings may predominate. Neurologic dysfunction begins with changes in mentation, abnormalities in speech or language, and difficulty swallowing, all of which may progress with time.

On CT, the basal ganglia are typically low in attenuation, especially the globus pallidus and putamen arising from copper accumulation. Volume loss of these structures eventually follows. The white matter also may appear low in attenuation, with volume loss eventually leading to compensatory dilatation of the lateral ventricles. On MRI, the basal ganglia are hyperintense on T1-weighted images and the first echo of the T2-weighted sequence, as seen with other causes of hepatic dysfunction. These same regions typically are hyperintense on T2-weighted images early in the course of the disease, but the hyperintense signal may decrease late in the disease associated with an increase in signal on the T1-weighted images. The white matter demonstrates progressive increase in T2-signal as a result of demyelination and gliosis. Corpus callosum abnormalities also have been reported.[52] The presence of signal changes involving the basal ganglia, thalami, and brainstem; the "face of giant panda" sign; midbrain tectal plate signal changes; or central pontine myelinolysis-like changes all can be considered to be diagnostic of Wilson disease.[53]

Key Points

Clinical Features Suggestive of a Metabolic or Neurodegenerative Disorder

Loss of developmental milestones or unexplained developmental delay

Predisposing conditions are absent

Basal ganglia symptoms such as hypotonia and hypertonia

Progressive features of encephalopathy

An unexplained clinical course inconsistent with imaging findings

General Imaging Features of a Metabolic or Neurodegenerative Disorder

Progressive changes with time coupled with clinical progression

Progressive hypomyelination

Symmetric involvement of white matter tracts

Pervasive and symmetric involvement of white and gray matter

Contrast enhancement appears in later stages of the disease course

---

Clinical Indications for Incorporating MRS into the Imaging Evaluation

Developmental regression or a condition that is progressive (as opposed to static)

Feeding difficulties

Parental consanguinity

Previously affected siblings

Family history of mental retardation

Multiple organ involvement

Delayed myelination on conventional anatomic images

Genetic Origins of Select Mitochondrial Disorders

Deletions in mtDNA
    Kearns-Sayre syndrome

Mitochondrial DNA point mutations
    Adenosine triphosphate 6 mutation
    Maternally inherited myopathy/cardiomyopathy
    MELAS
    MERRF
    Multiple inherited subcutaneous lipomatosis
    Leber hereditary optic neuropathy

Nuclear DNA abnormalities
    Infantile cytochrome oxidase deficiency

Leigh syndrome

Mitochondrial myopathy, peripheral neuropathy, gastrointestinal encephalopathy

---

Suggested Readings

Dali C, Hanson LG, Barton NW, et al. Brain N-acetylaspartate levels correlate with motor function in metachromatic leukodystrophy. *Neurology.* 2010;75(21):1896-1903.

Ergül Y, Nişli K, Sagygili A, et al. Kearns-Sayre syndrome presenting as somatomedin C deficiency and complete heart block. *Turk Kardiyol Dern Ars.* 2010;38(8):568-571.

Kamate M, Hattiholi V. Normal neuroimaging in early-onset Krabbe disease. *Pediatr Neurol.* 2011;44(5):374-376.

Miller E, Widjaja E, Nilsson D, et al. Magnetic resonance imaging of a unique mutation in a family with Pelizaeus–Merzbacher disease. *Am J Med Genet A.* 2010;152A:748-752.

Toscano M, Canevelli M, Giacomelli E, et al. Transcranial sonography of basal ganglia in calcifications in Fahr disease. *J Ultrasound Med.* 2011; 30(7):1032-1033.

References

Full references for this chapter can be found on www.expertconsult.com.

Chapter 34

Infection and Inflammation

AVRUM N. POLLOCK, STEPHEN M. HENESCH, and LUCY B. RORKE-ADAMS

Bacterial, viral, fungal, and parasitic organisms are all causative factors in neurologic infection. Brain infection manifests as encephalitis, cerebritis, and meningitis. *Encephalitis* refers to diffuse infection of the brain parenchyma, whereas *cerebritis* is a more focal parenchymal infection. *Meningitis* refers to infection of the pia, arachnoid, and dural membranes, as well as the cerebrospinal fluid (CSF). Ventriculitis is often present in cases of meningitis. Infectious complications most often include abscess, empyema, or both. Infection in the setting of tumor often presents a diagnostic conundrum.

Imaging of central nervous system (CNS) infection is most often initially performed by means of computed tomography (CT) to assess for the possibility of hydrocephalus or increased intracranial pressure prior to the preparation of a lumbar puncture. Nonspecific parenchymal hypoattenuation indicative of edema on CT is sometimes appreciated in cases of more focal infection. CT is superior in the evaluation of bone erosion and destruction. Magnetic resonance imaging (MRI) is warranted in the assessment of infectious complications such as abscess, empyema, vasculitis, and ischemia in the setting of a worsening clinical condition or lack of clinical improvement despite appropriate therapy. Infection is most often manifested on MRI by abnormal hyperintense signal on T2-weighted (T2W), proton density, and fluid-attenuated inversion–recovery (FLAIR) sequences, with corresponding hypointense signal on T1-weighted (T1W) sequences. Post-contrast T1W images are essential in the evaluation for infectious collections and meningeal enhancement. Magnetic resonance venography (MRV) sequences may detect associated venous sinus thromboses. Diffusion-weighted imaging (DWI) may assist in localizing abscess collections, infection associated with ischemia, or both and may at times help distinguish lymphoma from abscess, especially in immunocompromised patients. DWI may also demonstrate lesions earlier than conventional sequences in viral infections such as herpes and West Nile virus (e-Fig. 34-1). Magnetic resonance spectroscopy has shown promise in distinguishing pyogenic abscesses from those caused by atypical organisms, with the former often demonstrating the presence of amino acids and lack of choline.

Bacterial Infections

Nearly two thirds of cases of bacterial meningitis in the United States occur in children. Routes of transmission include hematogenous, direct traumatic, congenital routes, as well as direct extension from adjacent sinus or mastoid disease (Figs. 34-2 through 34-4 and e-Fig. 34-5). Imaging plays a key role in determining the course of treatment for bacterial infection. It is essential to distinguish between focal cerebritis (Fig. 34-6), which tends to respond to antibiotics, and abscess, which often requires surgical intervention. Hypoattenuation on CT, indicative of edema, and corresponding hyperintense T2W and hypointense T1W signal on MRI, with patchy nonspecific postcontrast enhancement, are typical imaging characteristics of cerebritis. Mild to moderate mass effect is often present. Sequential imaging is essential in the assessment of the response to antibiotics as well as for progression to an abscess. Progression from cerebritis to abscess generally takes 1 to 2 weeks but may progress more quickly in neonates. *Citrobacter, Serratia*, and *Proteus* are the most common causes of neonatal brain abscess. *Citrobacter* and *Serratia* infection may cause medullary vein thrombosis and associated hemorrhage (Fig. 34-7). In general, abscesses tend to be situated at gray-white matter junctions, where the diameter of the end arterioles decreases (Fig. 34-8). Opportunistic organisms are common in immunocompromised neonates.

Differential diagnostic considerations of a peripherally contrast-enhancing fluid-filled structure in the brain includes infectious abscess and tumor. On DWI, abscesses will appear hyperintense (and dark on apparent diffusion coefficient, indicating restricting material within the capsule. On both MRI and CT, abscesses tend to have smooth regular inner margins and are often thinner walled along their medial edge than along their lateral margins. Intraventricular rupture of an abscess portends a poor outcome. Spectroscopy of abscesses is notable for the presence of amino acids and lactate (Fig. 34-9) and the absence of normal metabolite peaks. In neonates, ultrasonography may depict a hypoechoic abscess with peripheral hyperechogenicity, which may contain dependent echogenic debris.

Bacterial meningitis is the most common form of pediatric CNS infection. Although not diagnosed by imaging, imaging is warranted if a diagnosis is unclear, persisting seizures are present, and symptoms persist despite treatment. It is more common in preterm infants and full-term infants within the first month of life. The subarachnoid space tends to resist infection in older children, making meningitis in this age group a rarity. Most cases of neonatal meningitis in the United States are caused by group B *Streptococcus* (Fig. 34-10) and *Escherichia coli*. Other less common organisms (e.g., *Serratia*, enterococci, and *Listeria*) tend to inflict more extensive

Text continued on page 366.

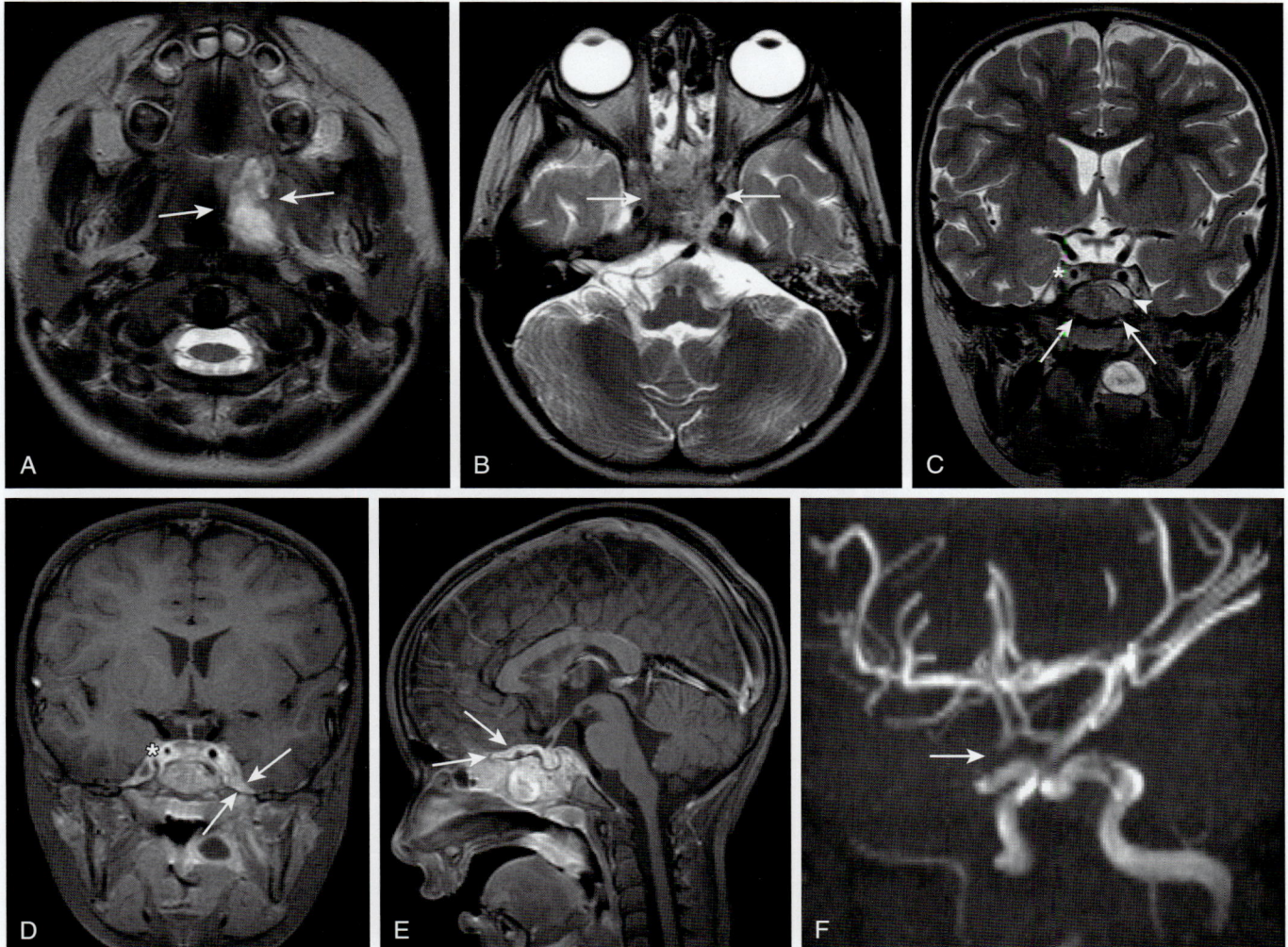

Figure 34-2 **Parameningeal spread of retropharyngeal infectious process or abscess.** A 3-year-old female child with retropharyngeal abscess, now with fever, headache, emesis, and left sixth nerve palsy. Axial T2-weighted images at the level of the adenoids (**A**) and sphenoid bone (**B**) and coronal T2 (**C**) images, coronal (**D**) and sagittal (**E**) postcontrast T1, as well as three-dimensional time-of-flight magnetic resonance angiography (MRA) in the left anterior oblique projection (**F**) were obtained. Note the inflammatory process within the left retropharyngea region (*arrows in* **A**). Note the abnormal marrow signal within the sphenoid bone (*arrows in* **B** *and* **C**). In addition, note the abnormal soft tissue seen extending superior to the sphenoid bone on the coronal T2 sequence (arrowhead in **C**). Corresponding abnormal contrast enhancement is seen along the region of the skull base and planum sphenoidale seen on the postcontrast images (*arrows in* **D** *and* **E**). Note the diminution in size of the right internal carotid artery (*asterisks in* **C** *and* **D**) with corresponding narrowing of the right supraclinoid carotid artery on the right on the MRA (*arrows in* **F**). (Ccse courtesy of Kim M. Cecil, Ph.D. Department of Radiology, Cincinnati Children's Hospital.)

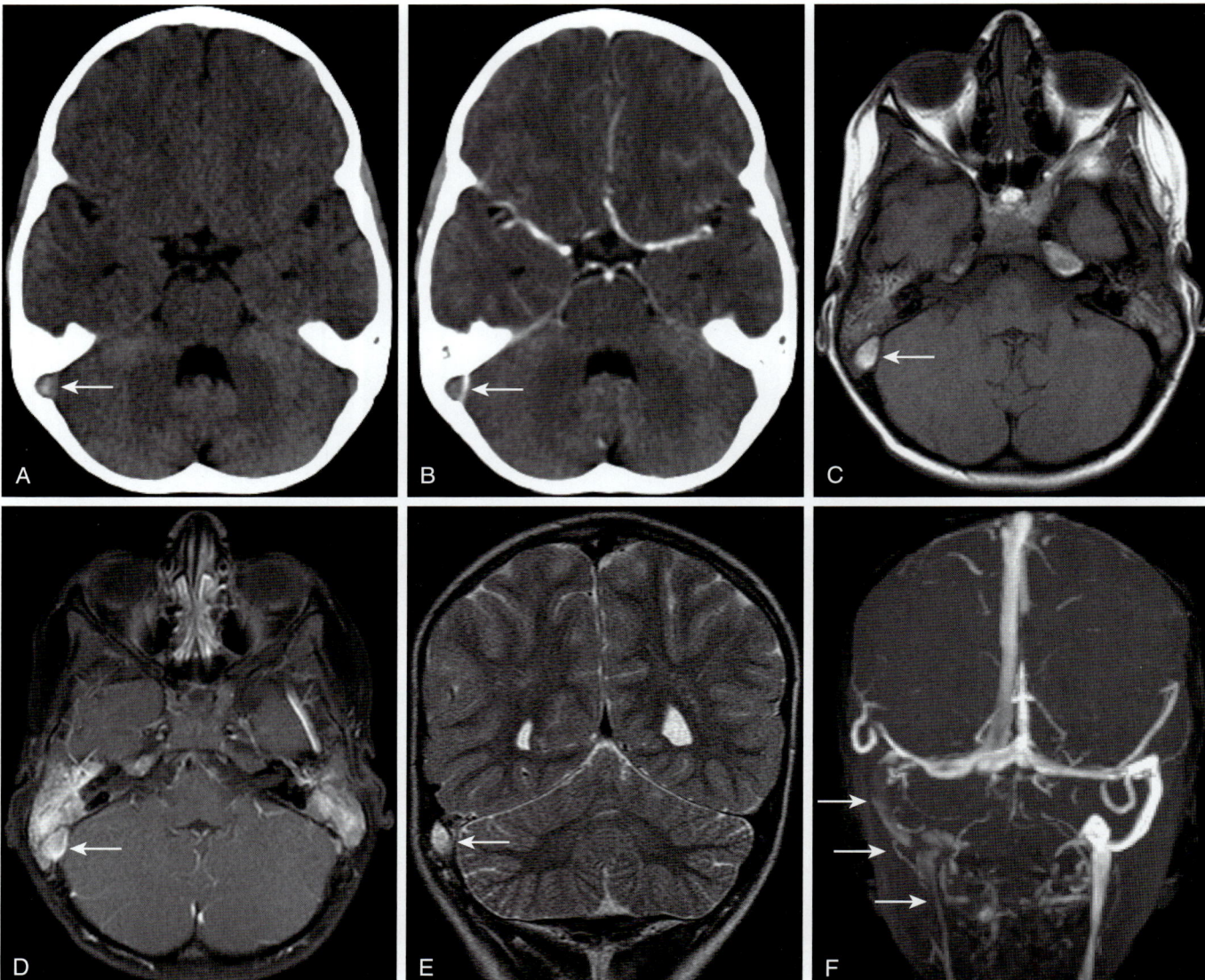

Figure 34-3 **Transverse sinus thrombosis associated with otomastoiditis or middle ear disease.** A patient with otitis media, headache, and papilledema. Axial noncontrast (**A**) and contrast-enhanced (**B**) computed tomography (CT) of the head through the level of the posterior fossa, axial magnetization transfer T1 precontrast (**C**) and postcontrast (**D**) magnetic resonance imaging scans, coronal T2 (**E**) and coronal multiple intensity projection image from a three-dimensional time-of-flight magnetic resonance venogram (MRV) (**F**) were obtained. Note the dense appearance within the right transverse sinus on the noncontrast CT study (*arrow in* **A**), with corresponding lack of contrast filling on the postcontrast CT study (*arrow in* **B**). Corresponding T1 shortening is seen on the precontrast magnetic resonance image (*arrow in* **C**), with corresponding abnormal signal on the postcontrast images in keeping with clot or slow flow within the region of the right transverse sinus or sigmoid sinus (*arrow in* **D**). Corresponding T2 prolongation is seen on the coronal T2 image (*arrow in* **E**). Note the striking asymmetry of flow within the right posterior fossa dural venous system or internal jugular vein on the right on the three-dimensional time-of-flight MRV (*arrows* **F**).

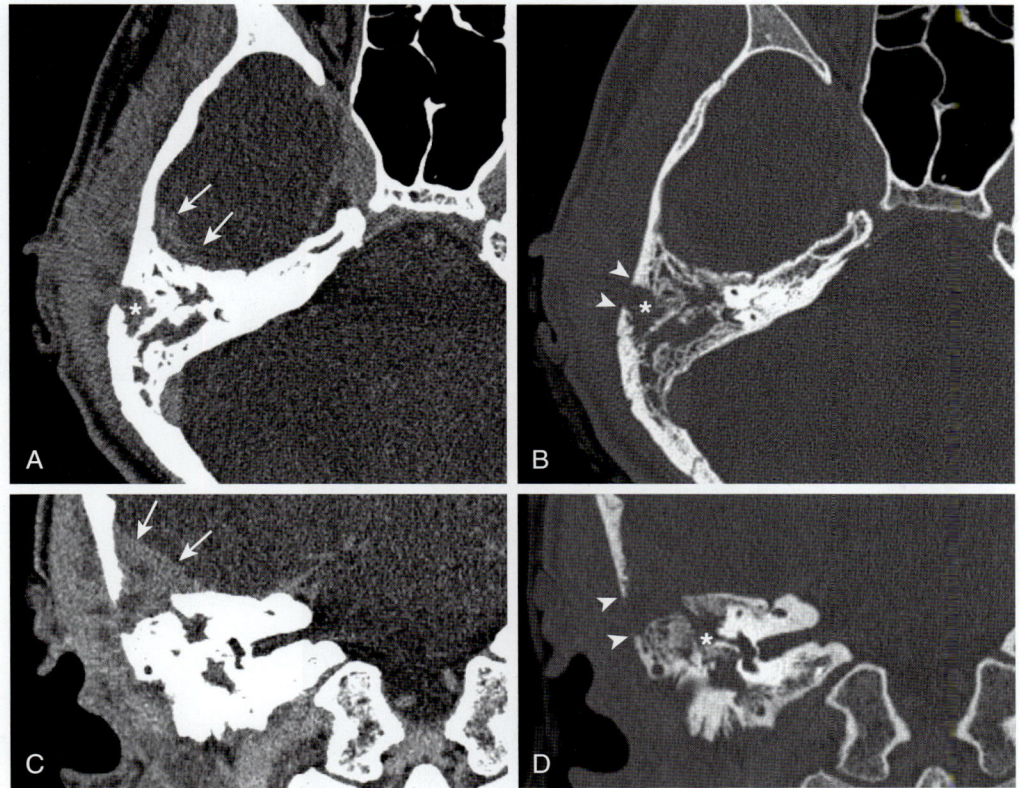

Figure 34-4 **Mastoiditis with associated epidural abscess.** A 17-year-old male with 5-month history of otitis media, now with severe right-sided mastoid pain. Axial postcontrast computed tomography images through the right mastoid region, including soft tissue (**A**) and bone windows (**B**), and direct coronal images from the same study obtained on soft tissue (**C**) and bone windows (**D**) were obtained. Note the abnormal soft tissue opacification within the right mastoid region (*asterisks in* **A** *and* **B**). Associated abnormal soft tissue swelling is seen along the external surface of the skull or scalp, with an abnormal soft tissue component seen extending intracranially (*arrows*), corresponding to epidural abscess formation. Bony resorption or breakdown is seen within the mastoid cortex laterally (*arrowheads*). In addition, note the erosion of the lateral semicircular canal (*asterisk in* **D**).

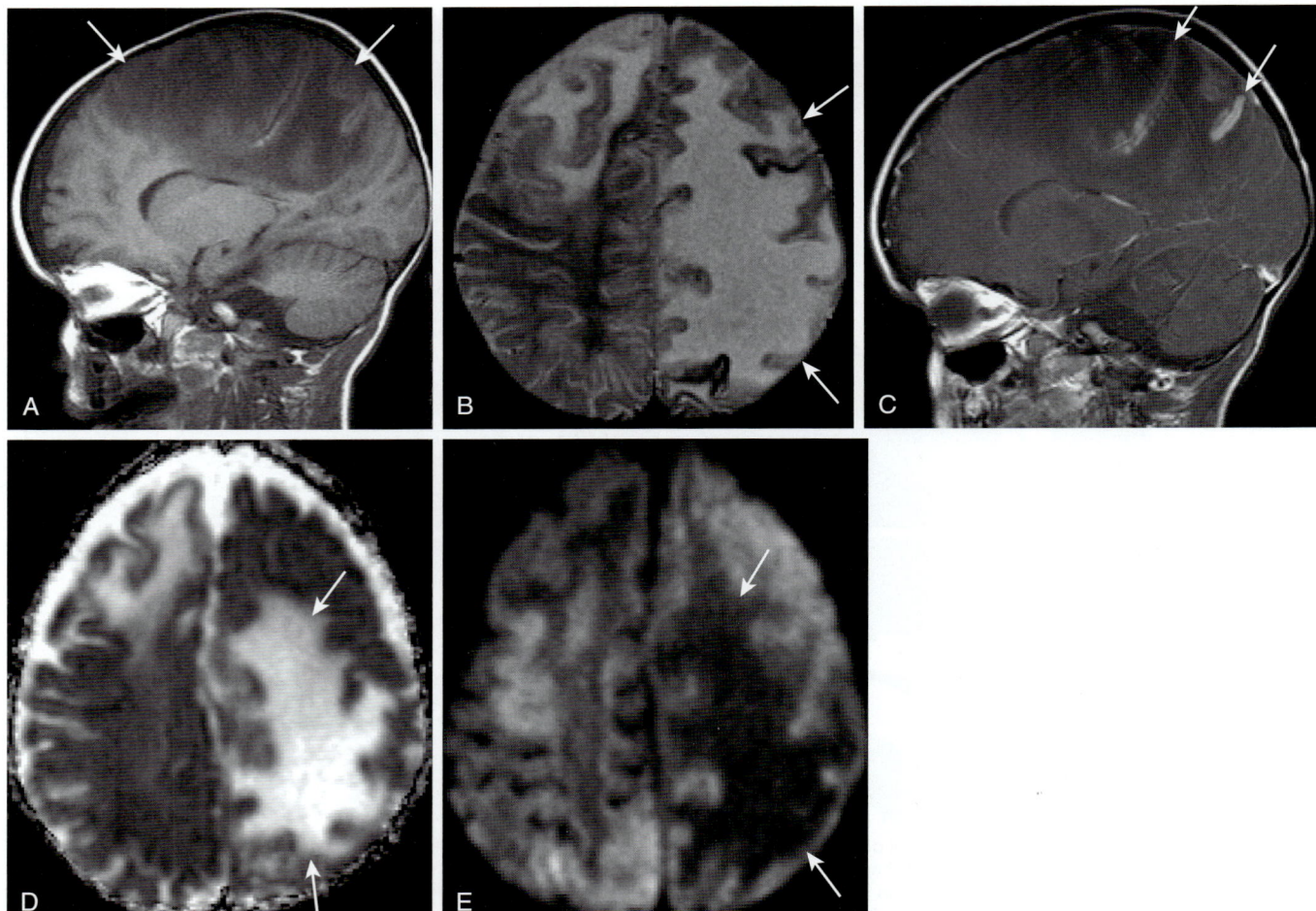

Figure 34-6 Cerebritis. A 2-year-old male with *Staphylococcus aureus* bacteremia, persistent fevers, and new-onset of hypertension. **A** and **B,** Sagittal T1-weighted and axial T2-weighted images demonstrate T1 and T2 prolongation (*arrows*). **C,** Sagittal postcontrast spin echo images show mild cortical enhancement (*arrows*) **D,** An axial diffusion-weighted imaging shows increased signal (*arrows*). **E,** The corresponding decreased signal indicates restricted diffusion on apparent diffusion coefficient image.

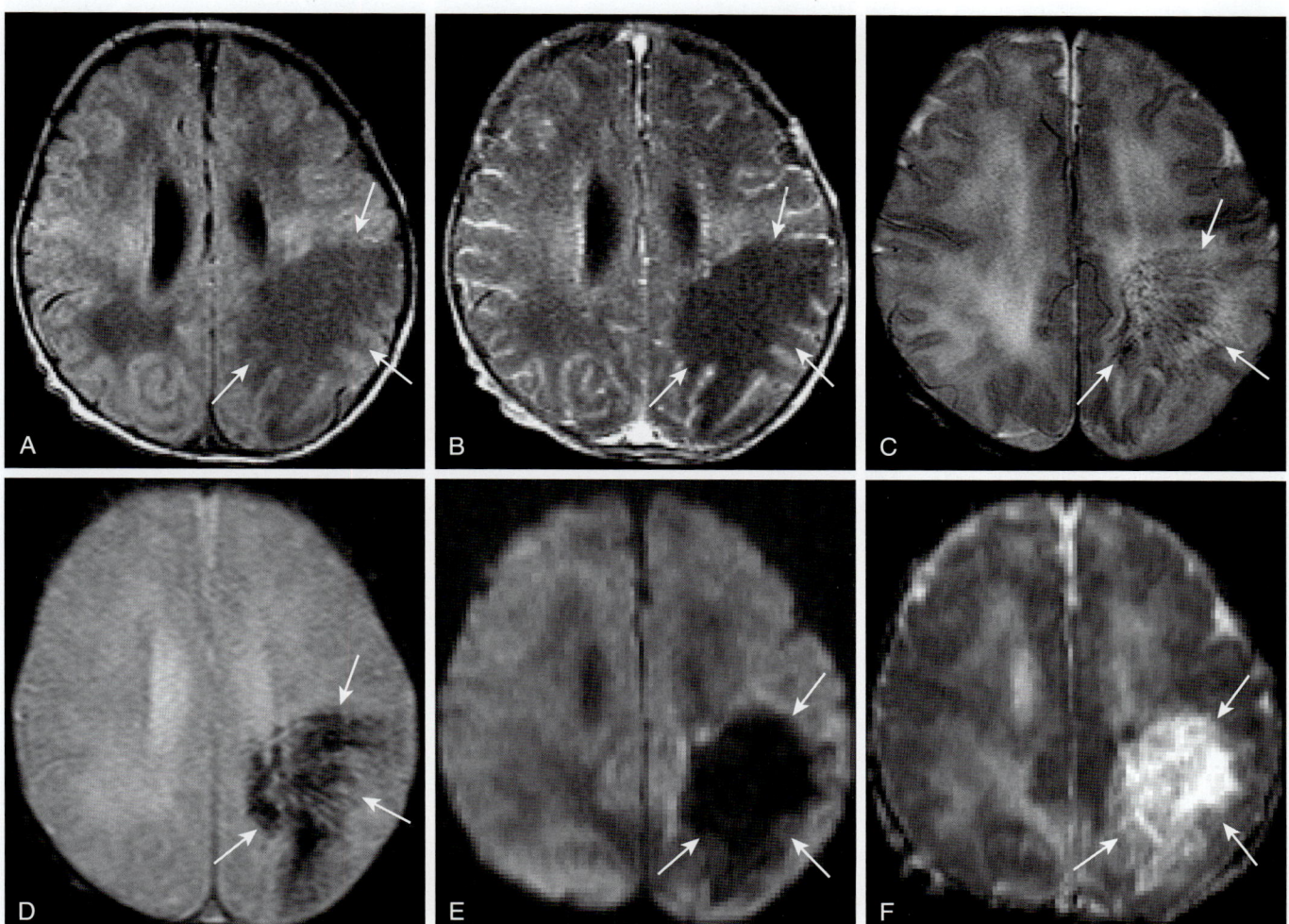

Figure 34-7   Citrobacter infection with secondary venous thrombosis. A 7-day-old full-term female neonate with seizures, and gram-negative sepsis, as well as increased white blood cell count on lumbar puncture. Axial precontrast and postcontrast T1, (**A** and **B**, respectively), axial T2 (**C**), axial gradient echo (**D**), as well as axial diffusion-weighted imaging and apparent diffusion coefficient maps (**E** and **F**, respectively) were obtained. Note the area of T1 prolongation within the left posterior frontal parietal region (*arrows* **A** *and* **B**), corresponding to areas with linear signal voids on both T2 and gradient echo sequences (*arrows in* **C** *and* **D**), corresponding to distended medullary veins. Note the absence of diffusion restriction and the presence of increased diffusion in the corresponding area on the diffusion-weighted sequences (*arrows in* **E** *and* **F**).

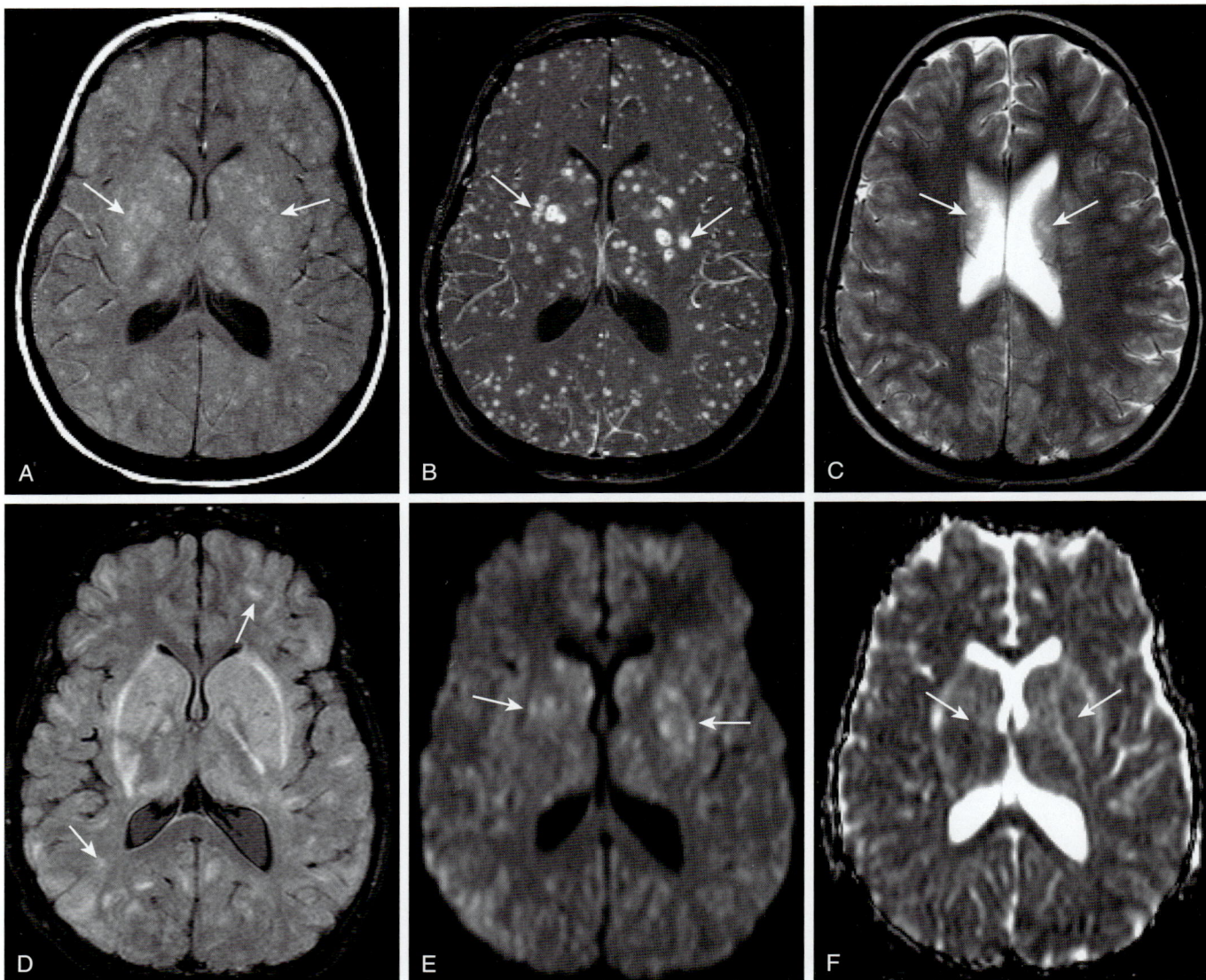

Figure 34-8 *Streptococcus viridans* **abscesses.** A 12-year-old female child with acute myelogenous leukemia and mental status changes. Axial T1 magnetization transfer (MT) images, precontrast and post contrast (**A** and **B**), axial T2 and fluid-attenuated inversion recovery (FLAIR) (**C** and **D**), and axial diffusion-weighted imaging with apparent diffusion coefficient maps (**E** and **F**) were obtained. Note the areas of T1 shortening on the precontrast MT image (*arrows in* **A**), and the corresponding marked gadolinium enhancement within multiple bilateral intraparenchymal nodules of differing size (*arrows in* **B**). T2 prolongation is noted on the axial T2 and FLAIR sequences in some corresponding areas (*arrows in* **C** *and* **D**), but this is markedly less conspicuous than on the postcontrast images. Subtle restricted diffusion is noted in some of the nodular areas, specifically within the region of the basal ganglia bilaterally corresponding to the largest lesions seen on postcontrast images (*arrows in* **E** *and* **F**).

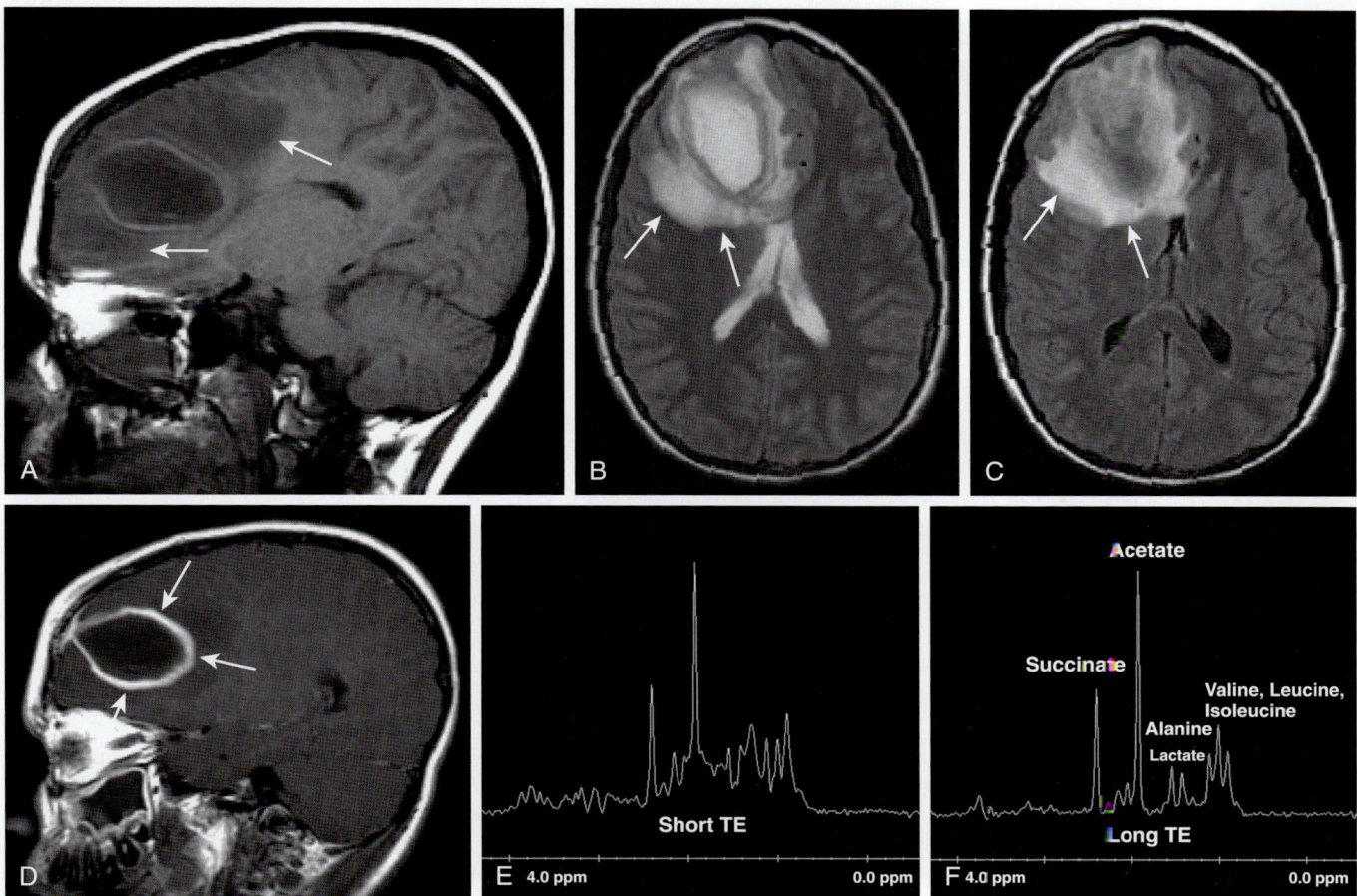

Figure 34-9 **Cerebral abscess.** Patient with seizures and fever. Sagittal T1 (**A**), axial T2 (**B**), axial fluid-attenuated inversion-recovery (**C**), postcontrast sagittal spin echo images (**D**), as well as short TE and long TE spectroscopic images (**E** and **F**, respectively) were obtained. Note the areas of T2 prolongation (**B** and **C**), with some central low signal intensity (**C**) in the region of abscess with surrounding vasogenic edema. Thick, rindlike enhancement of the periphery of the right frontal abscess is seen (*arrows in* **D**). Spectroscopic images demonstrate abnormal amino acid peaks at around 1 part per million (ppm), and a doublet lactate peak deflected upward at 1.33 ppm.

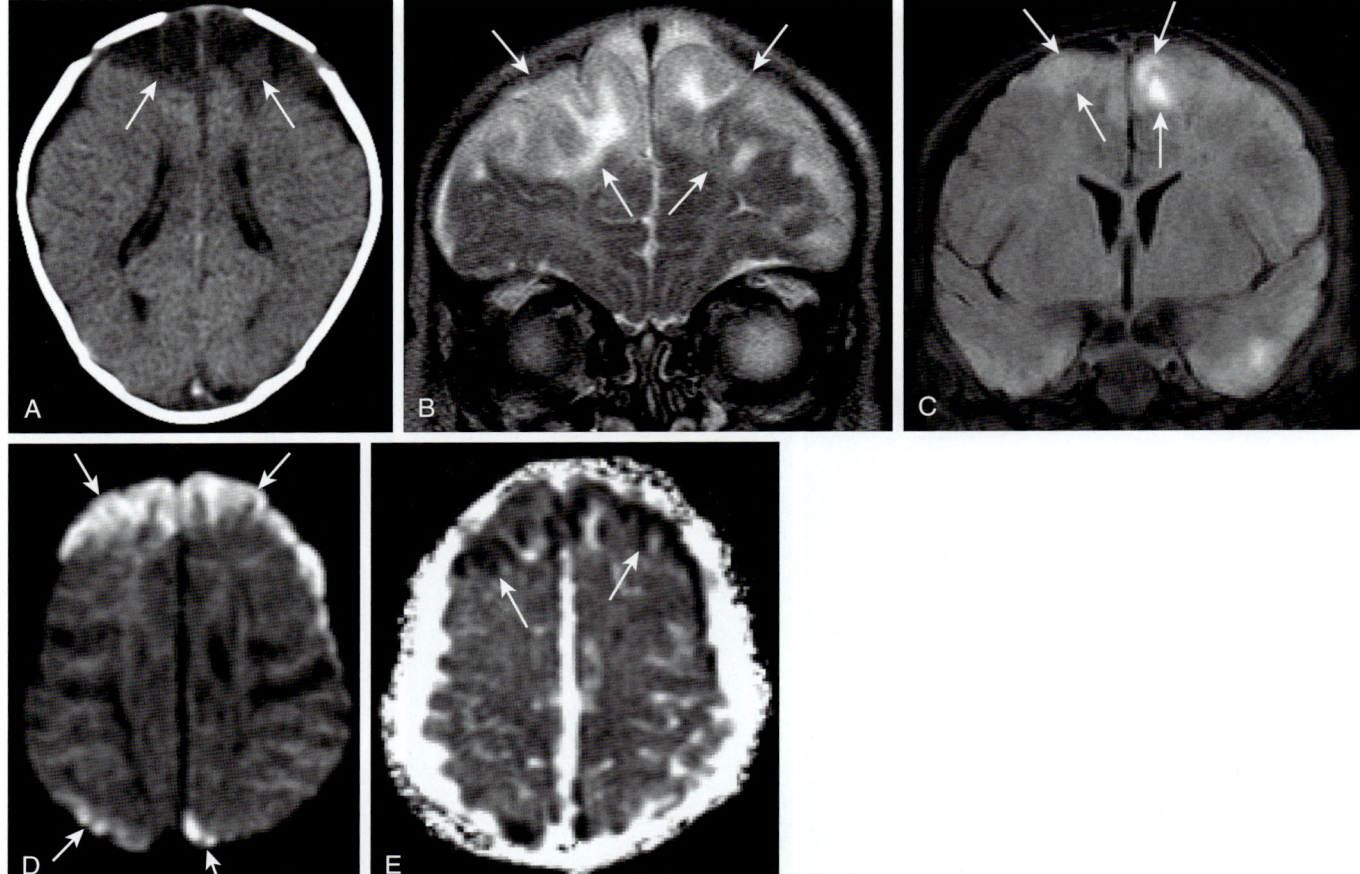

Figure 34-10 Group B *Streptococcus* **meningitis.** A 10-week-old female baby with group B *Streptococcus* sepsis and meningitis. Axial noncontrast computed tomography of the head (**A**), coronal T2 (**B**) and fluid-attenuated inversion recovery (FLAIR) (**C**) magnetic resonance imaging scans, diffusion-weighted imaging, and apparent diffusion coefficient map (**D** and **E**, respectively) were obtained. Note the low attenuation within the frontal lobes bilaterally (**A**). Corresponding T2 prolongation and abnormal increased FLAIR signal (*arrows*) are seen (**B** and **C**, respectively). In addition, restricted diffusion is evident within the frontal and parietal regions bilaterally (*arrows in* **D** *and* **E**), indicating ischemic changes secondary to meningitis.

destruction. In infants older than 1 month, the most common causative organisms are *Haemophilus influenza* type B, *Streptococcus pneumonia* (Fig. 34-11), *Neisseria meningitides*, and *Escherichia coli*. Complications of meningitis include cerebritis, abscess, empyema, hydrocephalus, venous thrombosis, infarction (venous and arterial), ventriculitis (e-Fig. 34-12), mycotic aneurysms (Fig. 34-13), and sensorineural hearing loss (Fig. 34-14).

TUBERCULOSIS INFECTION

CNS infection with *Mycobacterium tuberculosis* (tuberculosis [TB]) differs clinically and radiographically from pyogenic infection. Other granulomatous and fungal organisms are rare in the pediatric age group and often present with similar imaging characteristics as those in TB. The pathogenesis of tuberculous meningitis is different from that of other bacterial meningitides. Hematogenous dissemination of tuberculous bacilli is believed to occur about 1 week following the infected inhalation. Hematogenous spread to the CNS may produce miliary TB (rare in children), but more typically produce tuberculomas in the meninges, the brain

(at the gray-white junction), spinal cord, or, rarely, the choroid plexus. After a variable period, organisms from one or more of these foci are discharged into the CSF or subarachnoid space causing meningitis. Isolated meningeal tuberculomas tend to localize in the region of the Sylvian fissures, but meningitis is typically most severe in the basal cisterns. This leads to secondary complications, including cranial nerve palsies, secondary infarction consequent to vasculitis, and hydrocephalus secondary to blockage of fourth ventricular outlet foramina. Clinical presentation ranges from personality change and anorexia to coma and death, with nuchal rigidity being the most common presenting clinical sign. Pathologically, tuberculous exudate fills the subarachnoid spaces. Most of the affected patients demonstrate hydrocephalus.

On CT, exudate within the cisterns is manifested by its greater than CSF attenuation. On contrast-enhanced MRI, marked subarachnoid and cisternal enhancement is seen on T1W sequences (e-Fig. 34-15), with T2W images demonstrating obscuration of the cisterns caused by the hyperintense signal within these affected regions. Microinfarctions are not uncommon. Tuberculomas often occur at gray-white junctions

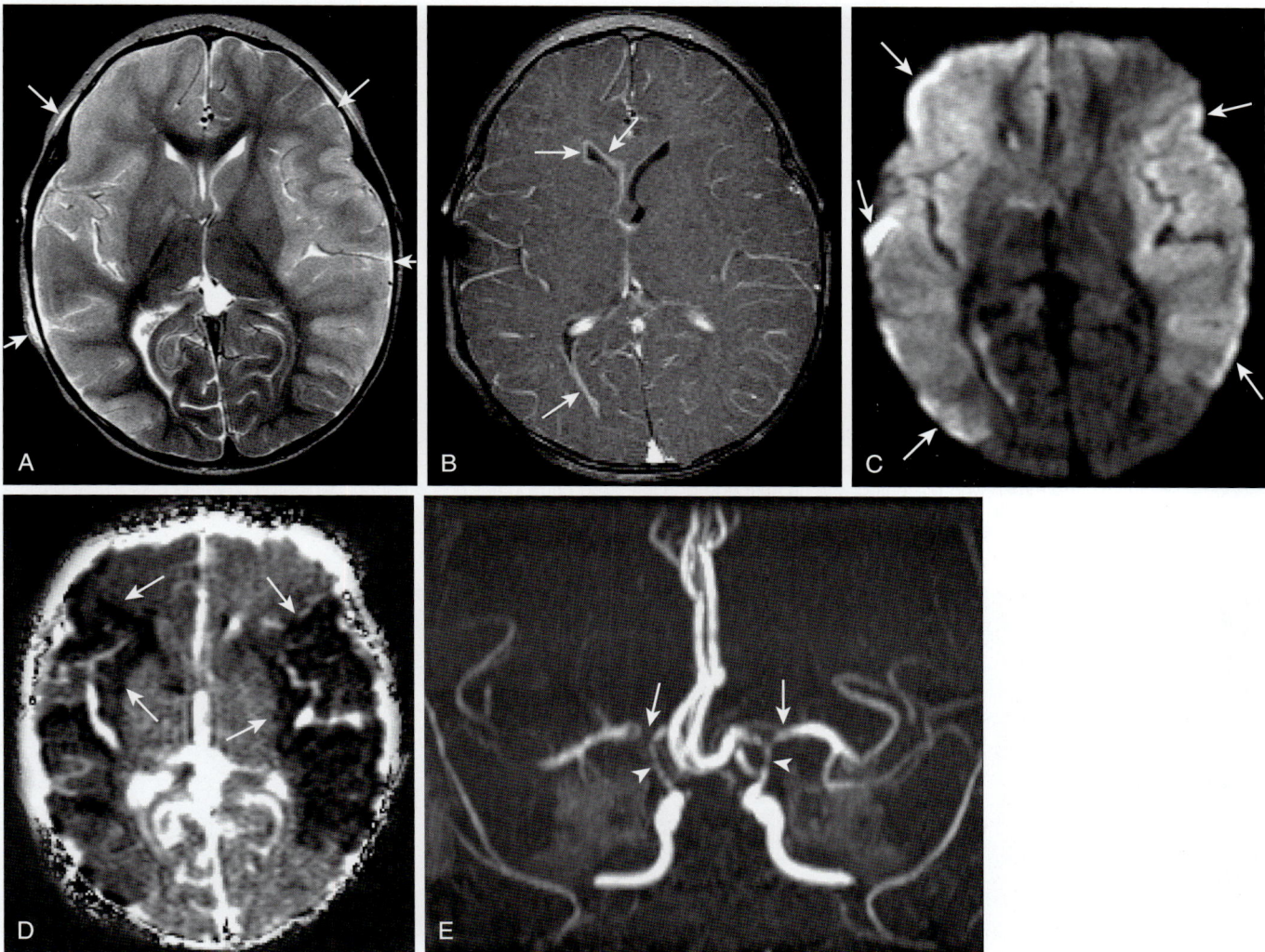

Figure 34-11 **Pneumococcal meningitis with infarctions.** An 11-month-old female with ventriculostomy and mental status changes, with suspected meningitis. Axial T2 (**A**), axial postcontrast T1 (**B**), axial diffusion-weighted imaging, apparent diffusion coefficient maps (**D** and **E**, respectively), and three-dimensional time of flight (TOF) magnetic resonance angiogram (**E**) were obtained. Diffuse T2 prolongation is seen within the cerebral cortex bilaterally (*arrows in* **A**), with associated abnormal enhancement along the ventricular lining (*arrows in* **B**) in keeping with ventriculitis. Note the marked restricted diffusion within both hemispheres (*arrows in* **C** *and* **D**), indicating cytotoxic edema secondary to infection. Bilateral middle cerebral artery narrowing, right greater than left (*arrows in* **E**), and narrowing of the supraclinoid carotid arteries bilaterally (*arrowheads in* **E**) are seen.

and are more common above the tentorium cerebelli. On CT, they demonstrate high attenuation and ring enhancement (Fig. 34-16), whereas on MRI, they demonstrate hyperintense T1W and hypointense T2W signals and enhance uniformly or peripherally when less than and greater than approximately 2 cm, respectively. The rare tuberculous abscess may be differentiated from a tuberculoma by its central hyperintense T2W signal and more pronounced associated vasogenic edema. Although DWI is not particularly helpful in making a diagnosis, lipid detection on spectroscopy has been reported in some cases.

LYME DISEASE

Lyme disease is the most common tickborne disease in the United States and Europe. More than 1 in 5 cases has been reported in children or adolescents. This multisystemic disorder involves the neurologic system in approximately one fifth of affected children, manifesting as lymphocytic meningitis, meningoencephalitis, pseudotumor cerebri-like syndrome, or cranial neuropathy. It is unclear whether the mechanism of CNS involvement is a result of direct invasion by the *Borrelia burgdorferi* organism or an autoimmune phenomenon.

CT scans are usually normal in Lyme disease, although focal areas of hypoattenuation have been reported. Focal T2W hyperintense white matter lesions are seen in about 1 in 4 neurologically affected patients. Contrast-enhanced MRI may show leptomeningeal enhancement, with or without enhancement of the affected nerves, in children with cranial neuropathy (Fig. 34-17).

CYSTICERCOSIS

Although cysticercosis is not very common in the United States, it often presents in immigrants from endemic regions. Presenting symptoms of neurocysticercosis include seizures,

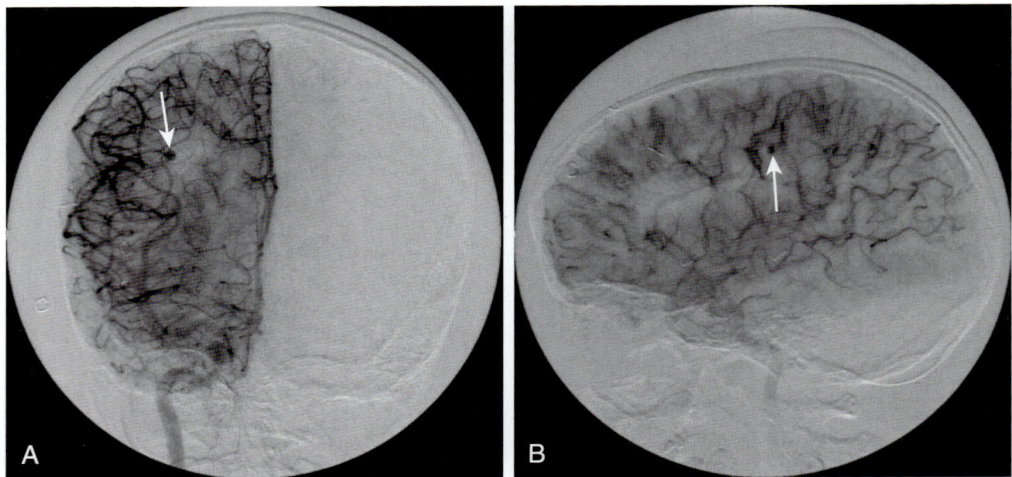

Figure 34-13   Mycotic aneurysm of right middle cerebral artery distribution. A 9-year-old male child with complex congenital heart disease and subacute bacterial endocarditis who presented with hemorrhage and left-sided hemiparesis and a normal angiogram 2 weeks prior to the present study. Frontal (**A**) and lateral (**B**) views from digital subtraction angiography demonstrate a small outpouching from a right middle cerebral artery branch on the right (*arrows*), indicating a mycotic aneurysm.

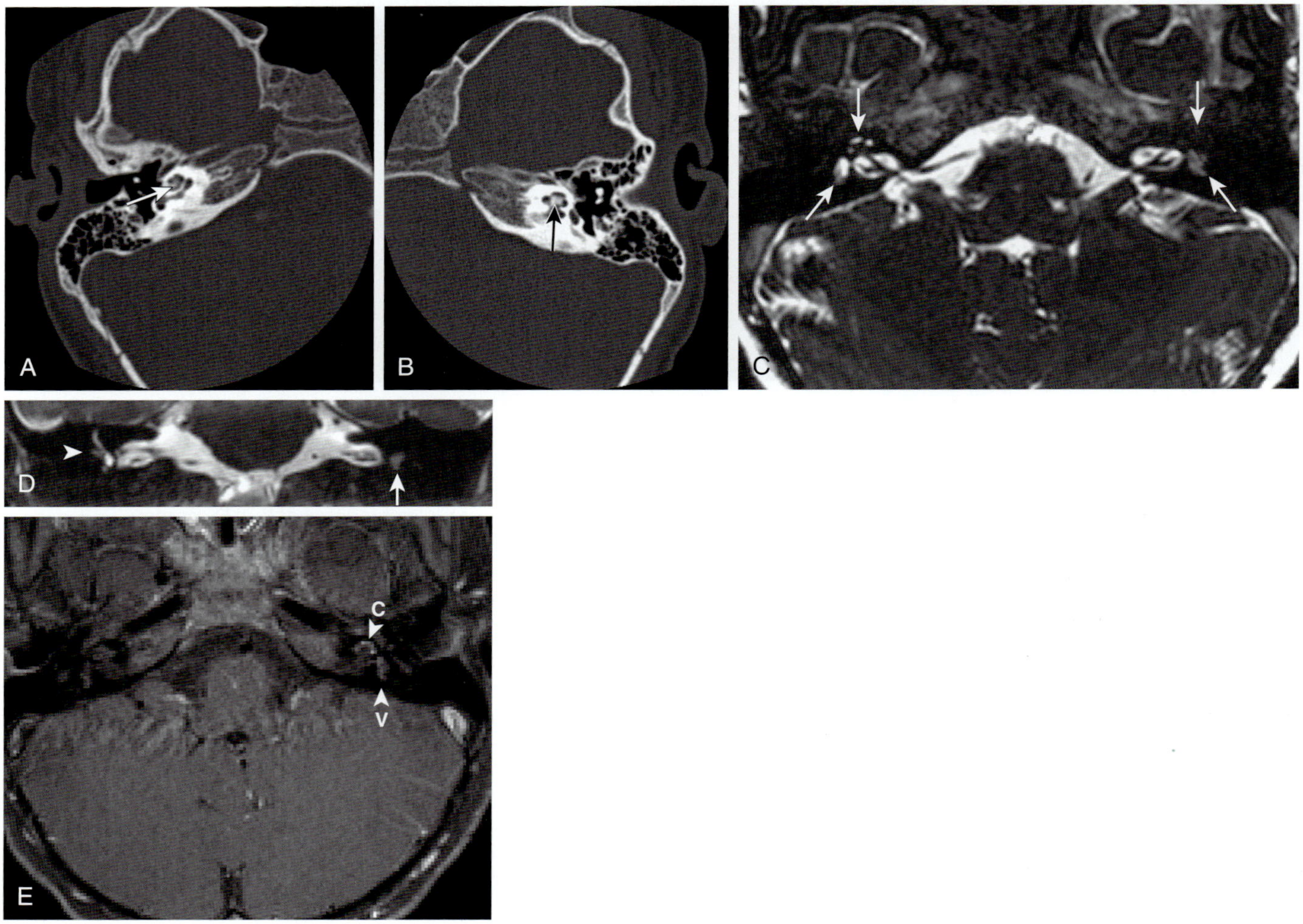

Figure 34-14   Labyrinthitis ossificans. A patient with bilateral sensorineural hearing loss following bacterial meningitis. Axial high-resolution computed tomography images through the right (**A**) and left (**B**) temporal bones were obtained. In addition, high-resolution magnetic resonance imaging constructive interference in steady-state images were obtained through the region of the internal auditory canals bilaterally (**C**) and were reconstructed in the coronal plane (**D**). In addition, high-resolution fat-suppression T1-weighted postcontrast images were obtained through the region of the internal auditory canals (**E**). Note the ossification of the membranous labyrinth bilaterally, left greater than right (*arrows in* **A** *and* **B**). Corresponding T2 signal dropoff is most marked on the left side (*arrows in* **C** *and* **D**). Note the blunting of the right lateral semicircular canal (*arrowhead in* **D**). In addition, fairly avid contrast enhancement is seen within the membranous labyrinth of the cochlea and vestibule, left greater than right (*arrowheads in* **E**) (*c, cochlea; v, vestibule*).

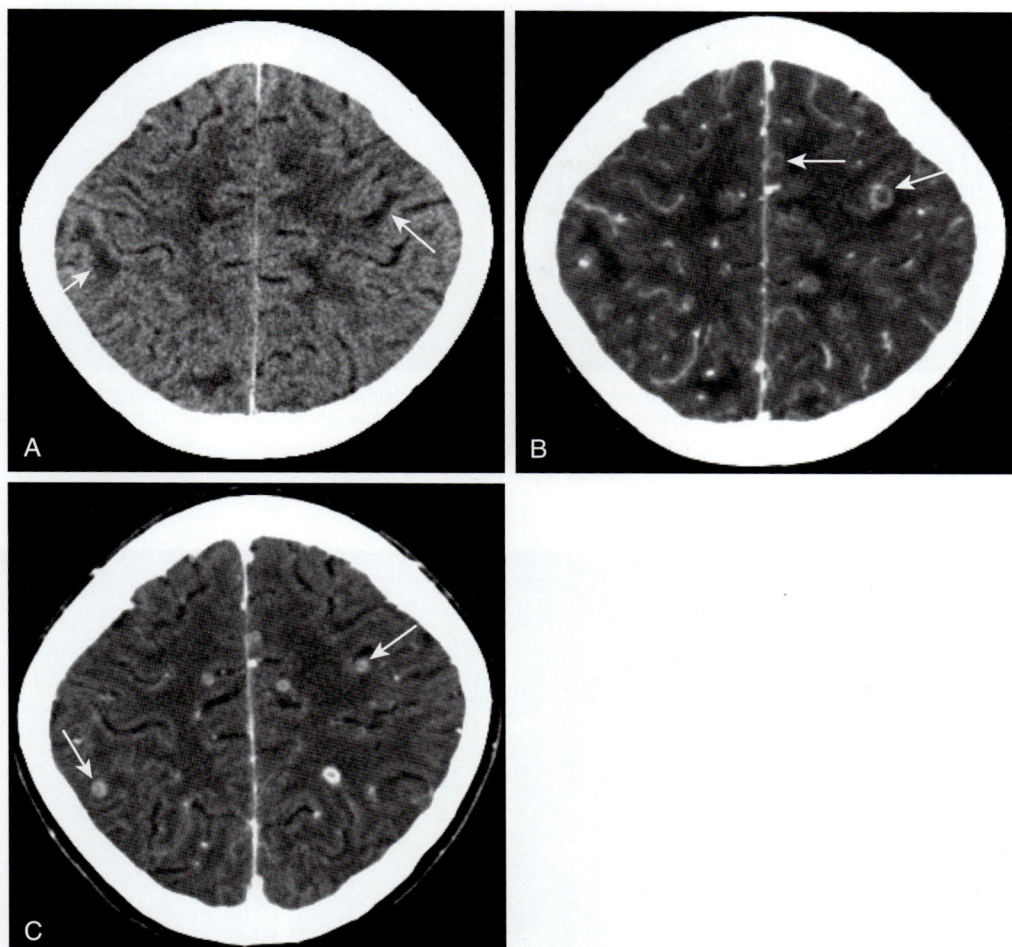

Figure 34-16 Tuberculosis microabscesses. A 13-year-old female child with headaches, vomiting, and vertigo. The purified protein derivative test was positive, and chest radiography was abnormal. Axial noncontrast computed tomography (CT) of the head (**A**) and corresponding contrast-enhanced CT from the same date (**B**), as well as postcontrast image from 1 month follow-up (**C**) were obtained. Note the areas of low attenuation at the gray-white matter junction (*arrows in* **A**). Multiple ring enhancing lesions are noted at the gray-white matter junction (*arrows in* **B** *and* **C**), corresponding to multiple tuberculosis microabscesses.

developmental delay, and hydrocephalus. The most common form, parenchymal cysticercosis, is caused by an inflammatory reaction secondary to the death of the parasite. Focal lesions are cystic and solid, and demonstrate peripheral enhancement and calcification, respectively. They are most often situated in the cortex, the gray-white matter junction, or both areas (Fig. 34-18). Parenchymal lesions follow CSF signal intensity on DWI, which helps differentiate them from pyogenic abscesses. The typical calcification seen in adults is not always seen in children. Surrounding inflammatory reaction demonstrates hyperintense signal abnormality on T2W imaging. Intraventricular cysterci often cause obstructive hydrocephalus, and thin-slice T1W imaging best depicts the causative intraventricular scolex (Fig. 34-19). The leptomeningeal form of cysticercosis mimics the radiographic appearance of TB, with marked subarachnoid postcontrast enhancement. Subarachnoid granulomata mimic their parenchymal counterparts. Hydrocephalus and vasculitis are common associated findings. Large racemose cysts are most often found in the cerebellopontine angle, Sylvian fissures, and in the basilar and suprasellar cisterns. Multiple coexisting forms of cysticercoids are a clue to the diagnosis. On MRI, clusters of cysts are most commonly depicted.

Viral Infections

All viral CNS infections produce inflammation and neuronal necrosis to a greater or lesser extent. Some viruses such as herpes simplex and Coxsackie may also produce white matter necrosis, whereas the primary inflammatory process involves the parenchyma. Usually, a meningeal inflammatory reaction or even ventriculitis occurs. In general, acute viral infection typically causes marked edema, causing hyperechogenicity on ultrasonography, hypoattenuation on CT, and hyperintense signal on T2W and FLAIR sequences. Restricted diffusion is the earliest imaging sign of viral encephalitis, and DWI should be performed when viral infection is suspected. Fortunately, differences in presentation and location help suggest one viral etiology over another. Viral-like syndromes with autoimmune associations such as acute disseminated encephalomyelitis (ADEM) and posttransplantation lymphoproliferative disorders

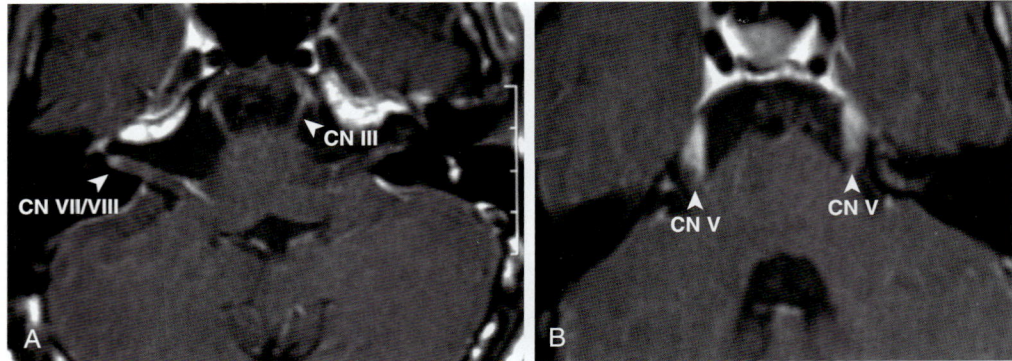

Figure 34-17 **Lyme disease.** A 15-year-old male child with multiple cranial nerve neuropathies and suspected tuberculosis exposure. Axial postcontrast T1 images were obtained through the posterior fossa. Note the symmetric abnormal contrast enhancement along the cranial nerves (CN).

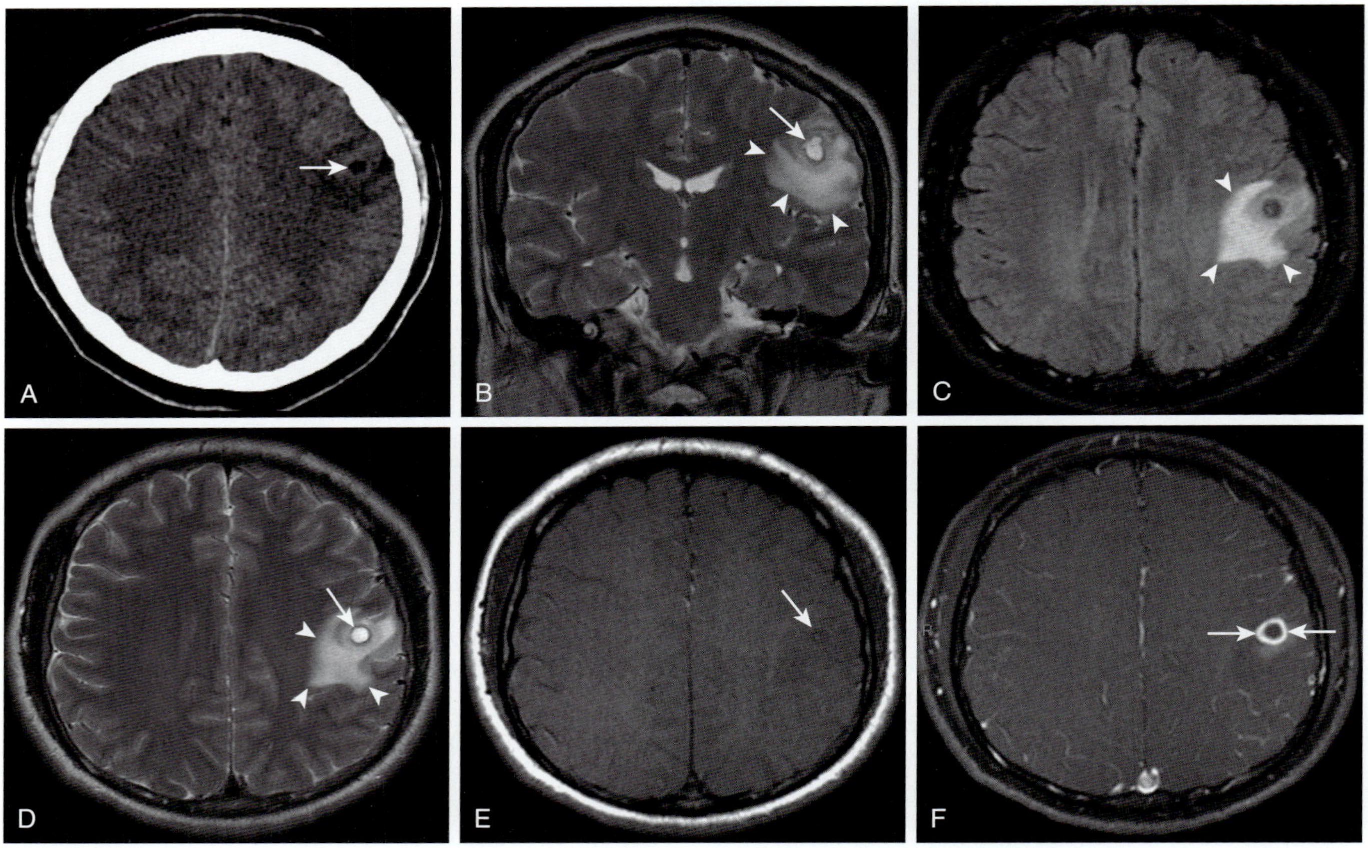

Figure 34-18 **Cysticercosis.** History of ingestion of uncooked pork. Axial noncontrast computed tomography (**A**) shows an area of decreased attenuation (*arrows*). Coronal T2 (**B**), axial fluid-attenuated inversion recovery and T2 sequences (**C** and **D**, respectively), and axial precontrast and postcontrast magnetization transfer T1-weighted magnetic resonance images (**E** and **F**) were obtained. Corresponding cystlike T2 prolongation is seen within the center of this region identified on coronal and axial T2 images (*arrows in* **B** *and* **D**), with surrounding vasogenic edema (*arrowheads in* **B**, **C** *and* **D**). In addition, a subtle area of T1 shortening is seen within the center of the lesion (*arrow in* **E**) corresponding to the scolex. Note the thick reactive rim enhancement around the area of the parasite (*arrows in* **F**).

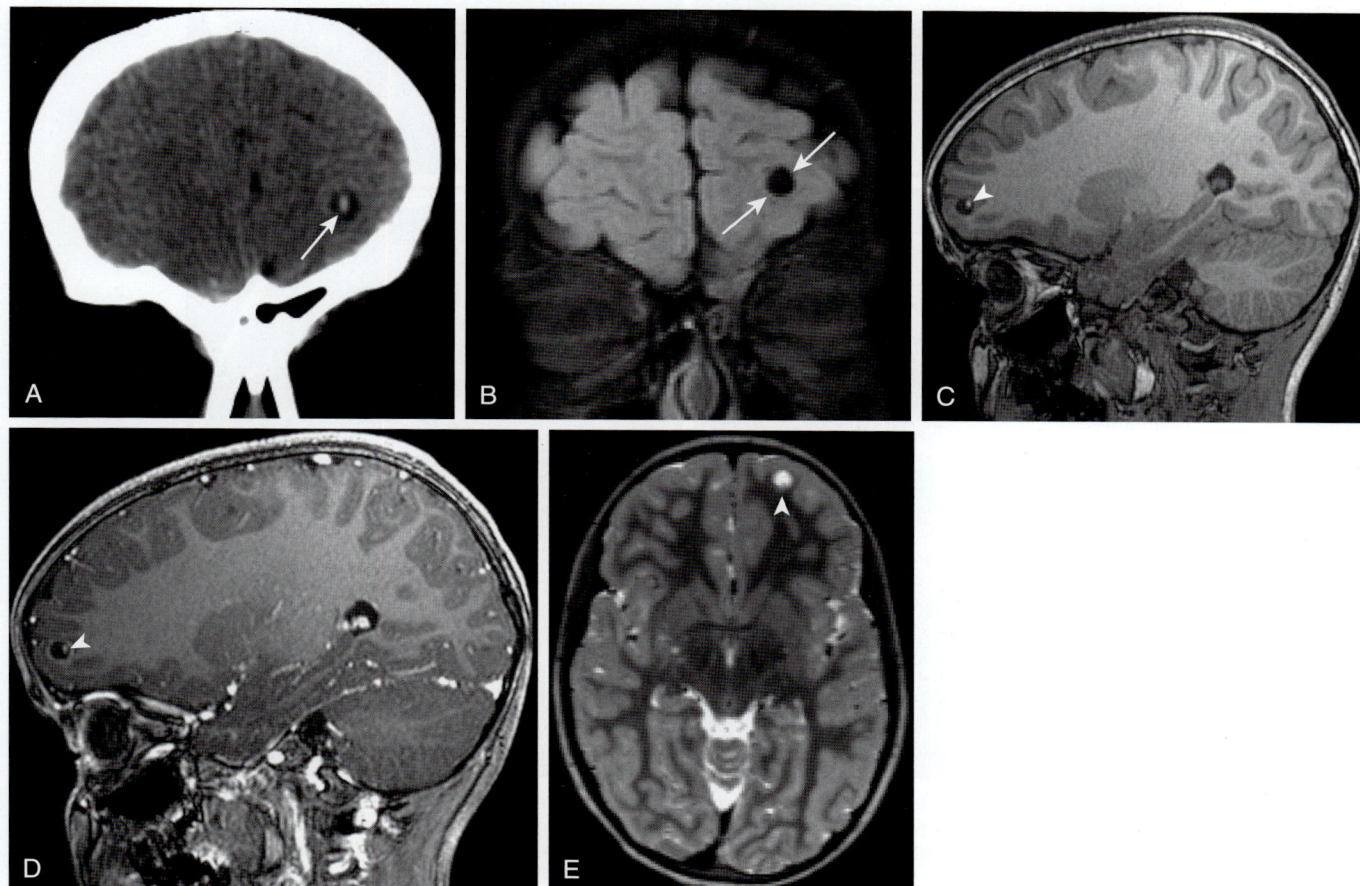

Figure 34-19   Cysticercosis. A 7-year-old female child with left frontal cystic lesion. Coronal non-contrast computed tomography of the head (**A**), coronal fluid-attenuated inversion–recovery (**B**), sagittal precontrast and postcontrast three-dimensional (3D) spoiled gradient images through the level of the left frontal lobe (**C** and **D**), and reconstructed axial 3D T2 weighted magnetic resonance images through the same area (**E**) were obtained. Note the area of high attenuation within the center of the lesion (*arrows in* **A**), corresponding to the scolex. This is seen to be within a cystic rim (*arrows in* **B**). Note the bright appearance of the scolex (*arrowheads in* **C** *and* **D**) and the subtle area of T2 shortening at the base of the cyst within the frontal lobe (*arrowheads in* **E**).

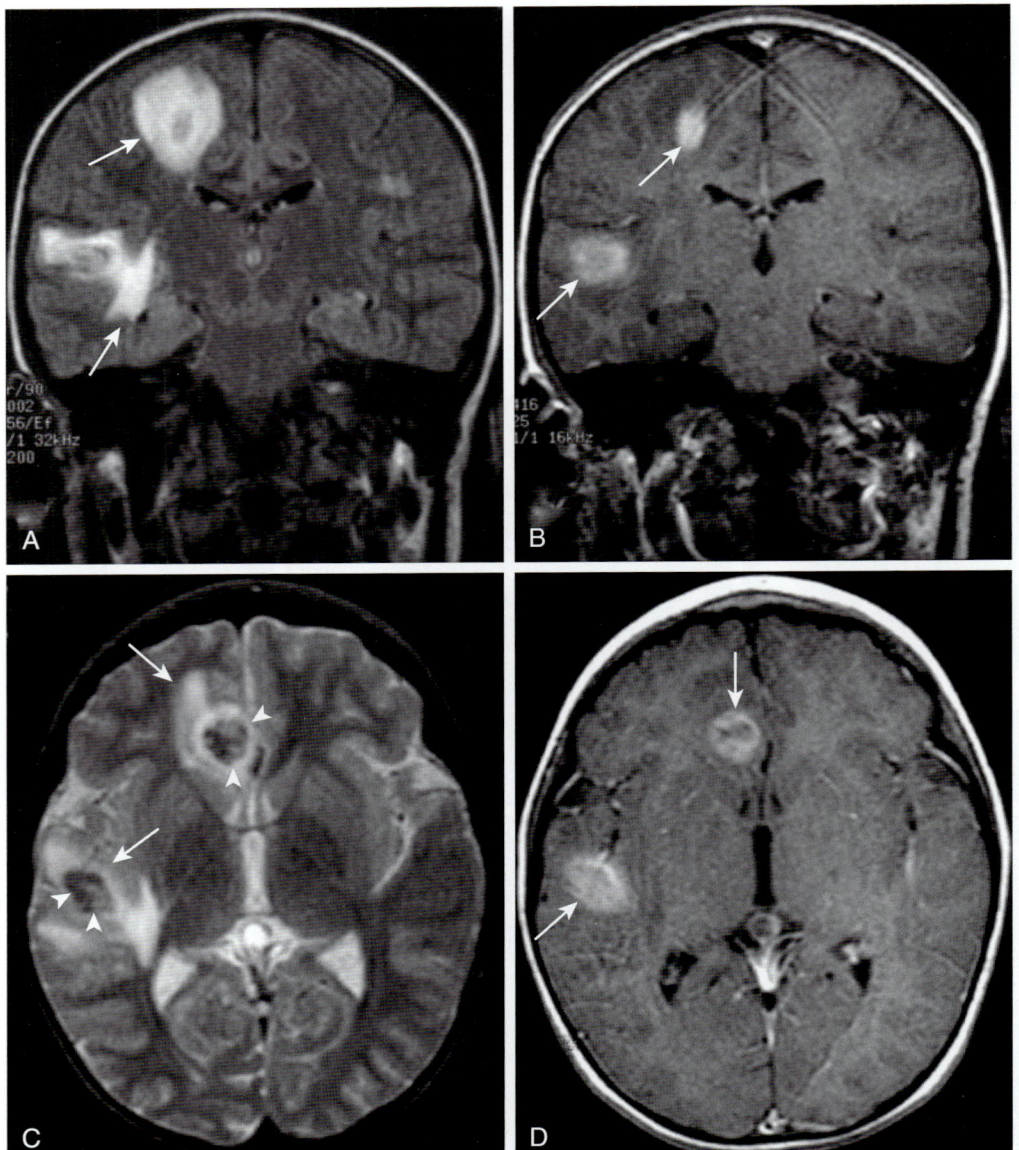

Figure 34-20 Posttransplantation lymphoproliferative disease. A 7-year-old male child, following heart transplantation, now with headache and visual changes. Coronal fluid-attenuated inversion recovery (**A**), coronal postcontrast T1 (**B**), axial T2 (**C**), and axial postcontrast T1 images (**D**) were obtained. Note the multiple areas of T2 prolongation within the right cerebral hemisphere (*arrows in* **A** *and* **C**). Central T2 shortening suggests an element of hemorrhage (*arrowheads in* **C**). In addition, avid contrast enhancement is evidenced on the postcontrast images (*arrows in* **B** *and* **D**).

(Fig. 34-20) often demonstrate imaging characteristics similar to those of viral infections.

HERPES SIMPLEX VIRUS TYPE I

Herpes simplex virus type 1 (HSV-1), as opposed to the prenatally or perinatally acquired HSV type 2 (HSV-2), is a spontaneous infection most often caused by reactivation of an orofacial herpes infection. HSV-1 CNS infection occurs in all ages but has a pediatric predominance. Early symptoms of fever and malaise may progress to seizures and hemiparesis. Restricted diffusion on MRI is the earliest radiologic manifestation, with unilateral or bilateral medial temporal lobe hyperintense signal on T2W and FLAIR sequences and more

heterogeneous restricted diffusion appearing several days later (Fig. 34-21). CT findings of low attenuation within the temporal lobe and insular cortex do not manifest until several days following the onset of symptoms. Leptomeningeal and cortical contrast enhancement, as well as foci of calcification hemorrhage, or both, may also be present.

HUMAN IMMUNODEFICIENCY SYNDROME

In the United States, greater than 90% of children with human immunodeficiency virus (HIV) are infected as a result of maternal transmission to the fetus. CNS imaging manifestations of congenital HIV include atrophy as well as basal ganglia and subcortical calcifications (Fig. 34-22). Superinfection and

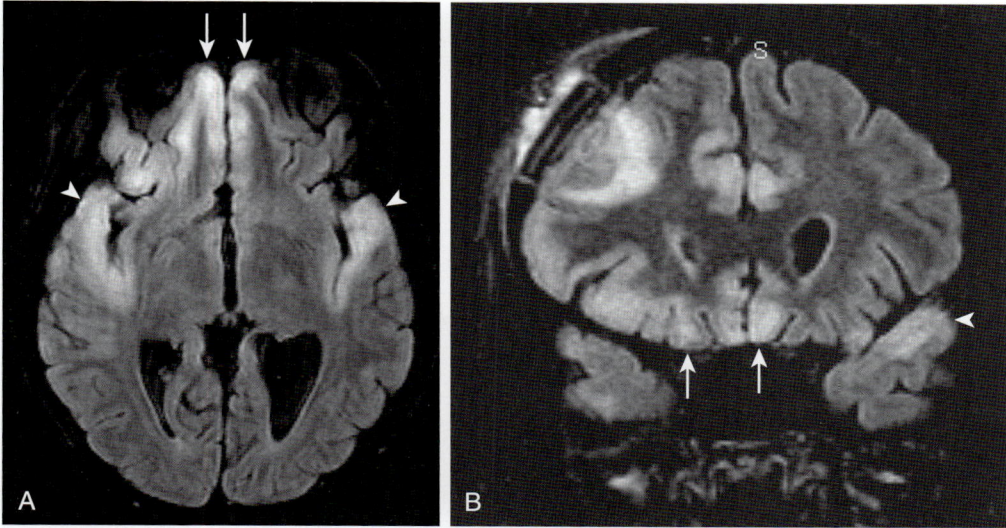

Figure 34-21 Herpes simplex virus (HSV). A patient with seizures and decreased level of consciousness. Axial (**A**) and coronal fluid-attenuated inversion recovery (**B**) images show abnormal signal intensity within both frontal lobes (*arrows*) and temporal lobes (*arrowheads*) indicative of HSV encephalitis. The bilateral temporal lobe involvement is a clue to the underlying causative agent.

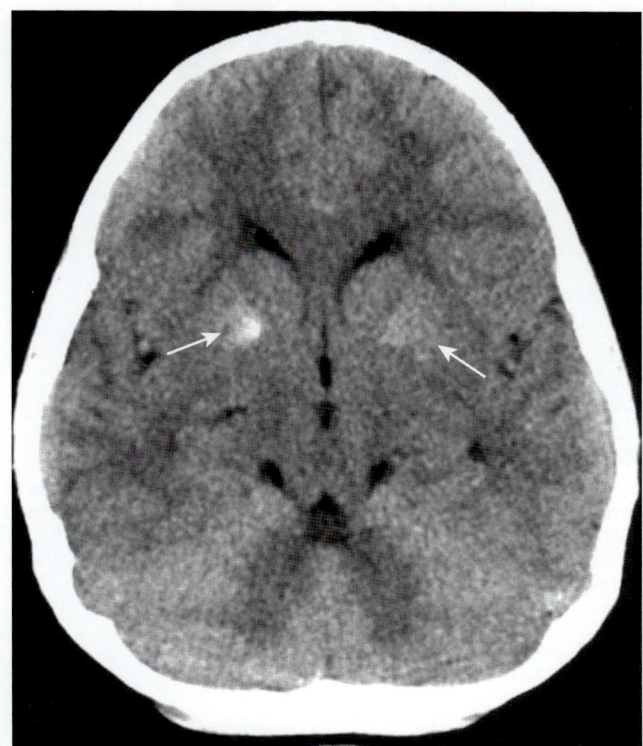

Figure 34-22 Human immunodeficiency virus (HIV) calcifications on computed tomography. A 9-year-old male child with known HIV infection. Noncontrast computed tomography of the head was obtained to the level of the basal ganglia. Note the calcific areas within the basal ganglia bilaterally (*arrows*), right greater than left, not uncommonly seen in patients with HIV.

neoplasm, not uncommon in adults with HIV, are seldom seen in children. Progressive multifocal leukoencephalitis (PML) caused by the John Cunningham polyomavirus, is radiologically identical to its presentation in adults. PML demonstrates white matter hypoattenuation on CT, as well as hyperintense signal on T2W and FLAIR sequences. These lesions characteristically lack mass effect and do not enhance following contrast administration. HIV infection may also lead to vasculitis (Fig. 34-23).

ACUTE DISSEMINATED ENCEPHALOMYELITIS

ADEM is a monophasic perivascular inflammatory and demyelinating disorder that often affects both the brain and the spinal cord, following a vaccination or viral infection. Lesions are generally hyperintense on T2W sequences and have corresponding hypointensity or isointensity on T1W sequences. MRI characteristics of ADEM (Fig. 34-24) are variable, with enhancement patterns, ranging from solid or ringlike enhancement to no enhancement at all, in lesions that range from small to large and which affect gray matter, white matter, or both. A clinical history of a recent viral illness, vaccination, or both is the key to properly diagnosing these lesions.

SUBACUTE SCLEROSING PANENCEPHALITIS

Subacute sclerosing panencephalitis is believed to represent a response to reactivation of the measles virus years after an infection. MRI reveals cortical and basal ganglia predominant hyperintense signal on T2W and FLAIR sequences.

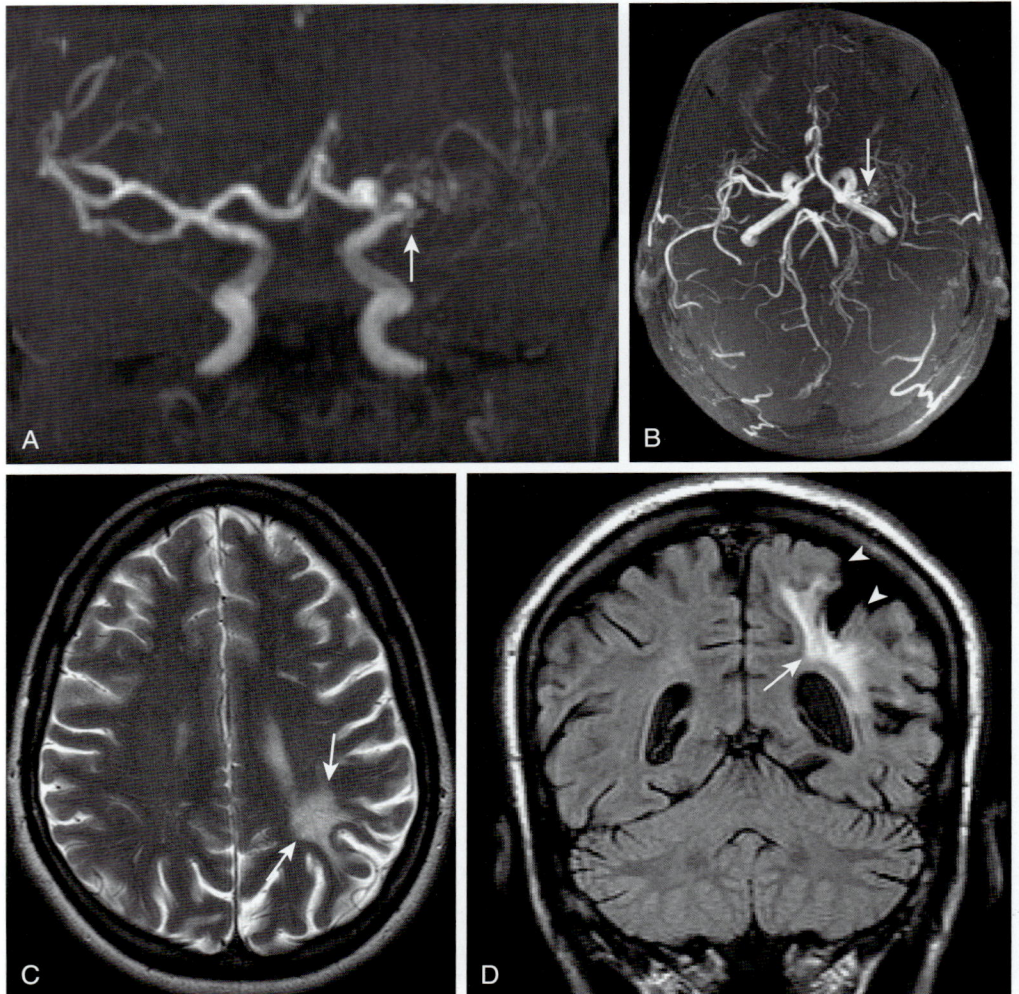

Figure 34-23   Human immunodeficiency virus (HIV) vasculitis. An 18-year-old female with HIV and right hemiplegia. Coronal and collapsed cranio-caudad view of the intracranial circulation from a three-dimensional time-of-flight magnetic resonance angiogram (MRA) (**A** and **B**, respectively), axial T2 (**C**), and coronal fluid-attenuated inversion recovery (**D**) magnetic resonance imaging scans were obtained. Note the marked narrowing of the left middle cerebral artery on the time-of-flight MRA (*arrows in **A** and **B***). Corresponding T2 prolongation is seen within the left parietal subcortical white matter (*arrows in **C** and **D***), corresponding to gliosis. Associated overlying cortical volume loss is also seen (*arrowheads in **D***).

RASMUSSEN ENCEPHALITIS

Rasmussen encephalitis is one of the leading causes of intractable epilepsy in children, which presents between 1 and 15 years of age and is characterized by seizures, progressive hemiplegia, and progressive psychomotor deterioration. It is characteristically localized to one hemisphere. Initial imaging studies are normal, but MRI later demonstrates hemispheric atrophy and hyperintense signal on T2W and FLAIR sequences in the frontal and temporal lobes, predominantly within the white matter and basal ganglia.

CONGENITAL INFECTIONS

Transplacental and less often transvaginal transfer of infection to the fetus is often the result of TORCH (**t**oxoplasmosis, **o**ther, **r**ubella, **c**ytomegalovirus, **h**erpes) infection (Fig. 34-25). Insults occurring during the first two trimesters most often

manifest as severe congenital malformations. Those occurring during the third trimester often result in destructive lesions.

CYTOMEGALOVIRUS

Cytomegalovirus (CMV) is the most common serious viral infection to affect newborns in the United States, occurring in nearly 1% of all live births. Up to 25% of infected infants develop neurologic or developmental abnormalities, including microcephaly, hearing impairment, chorioretinitis, and seizures, in the first year of life. Neonatal ultrasonography in affected patients often demonstrates nonspecific mineralizing vasculopathy of the basal ganglia (e-Fig. 34-26). MRI and CT demonstrate the sequelae of infection in the third trimester as periventricular calcification, hemorrhage, or both; ventricular and sulcal prominence; and periventricular and subcortical white matter changes (Figs. 34-27 and 34-28). Intrauterine infection with this virus is associated with

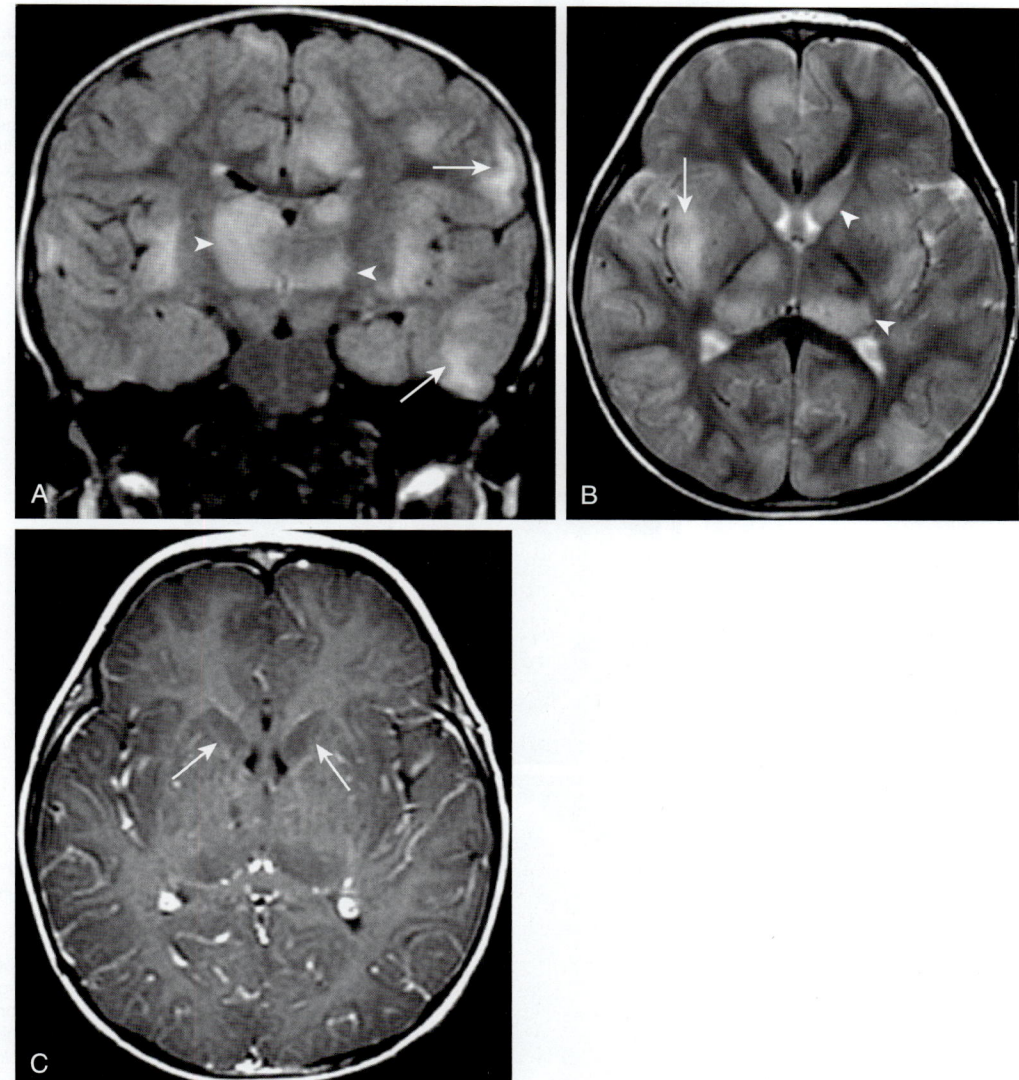

Figure 34-24 **Acute disseminated encephalomyelopathy.** A 22-month old male child with lethargy, hypotonia, ataxia, and decreased righting reflexes preceded by an antecedent upper respiratory illness. Coronal fluid-attenuated inversion recovery (**A**), axial T2 (**B**), and axial postcontrast T1 (**C**) magnetic resonance images were obtained. Note the patchy bilateral subcortical white matter T2 prolongation (*arrows in* **A** *and* **B**), as well as abnormal T2 prolongation within the central gray structures (*arrowheads in* **B**). No significant contrast enhancement, however, is seen, and the central gray structures appear to standout in relief on the postcontrast images (*arrows in* **C**) likely secondary to abnormal T1 prolongation.

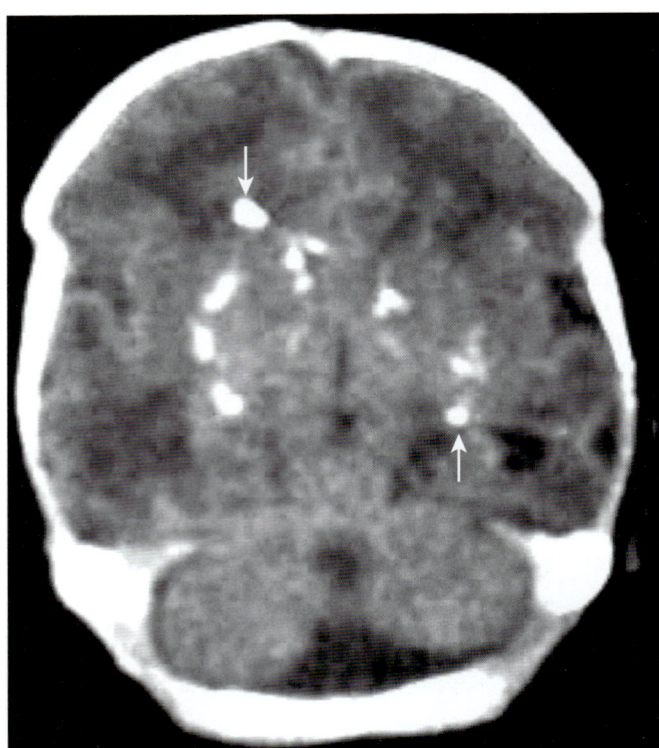

Figure 34-25 TORCH (toxoplasmosis, other, rubella, cytomegalovirus, herpes) infection on computed tomography. A female neonate with seizures and questionable intracranial hemorrhage. Noncontrast computed tomography of the head demonstrates multiple scattered punctate calcifications (*arrows*) seen bilaterally, slightly greater on the right than on the left, in a more random fashion than is expected with cytomegalovirus infection. This likely represents calcification from another TORCH type infection, such as toxoplasmosis.

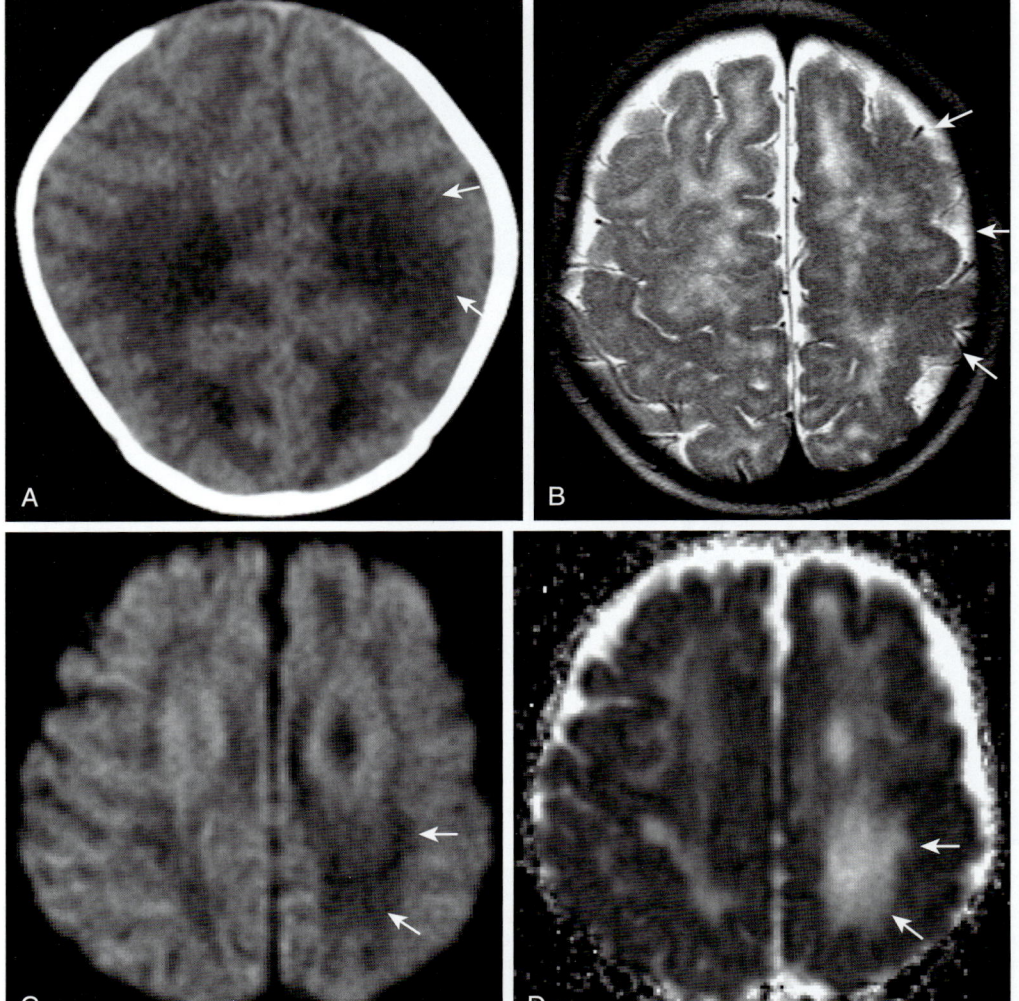

Figure 34-27 Cytomegalovirus (CMV). Child with congenital CMV, pale left optic nerve, and failed hearing test. Axial noncontrast computed tomography of the head (**A**), axial T2 magnetic resonance imaging (**B**), and axial diffusion-weighted imaging and apparent diffusion coefficient map (**C** and **D**, respectively) were obtained. Note the abnormal low attenuation within the white matter (*arrows in* **A**). Abnormal sulcation of the left hemisphere indicates associated polymicrogyria (*arrows in* **B**). Note the increased diffusion within the corresponding white matter, left greater than right (*arrows in* **C** *and* **D**).

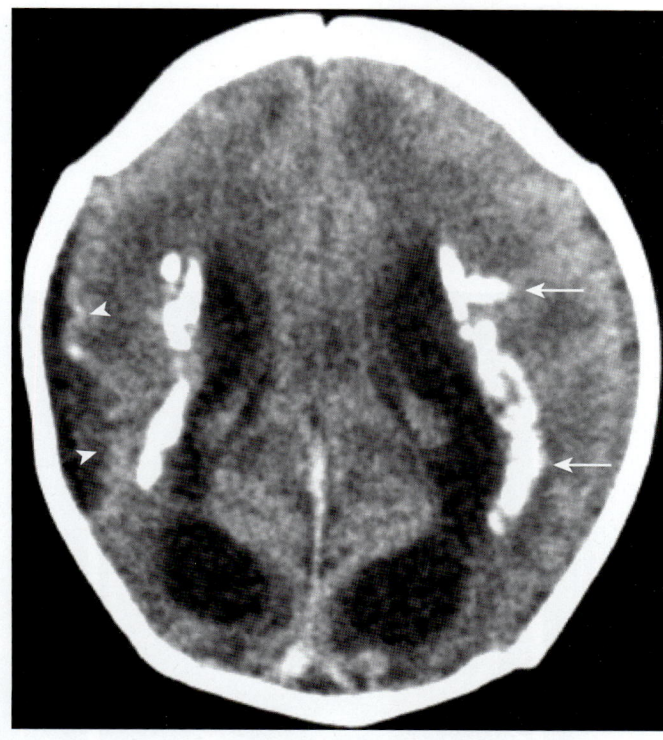

Figure 34-28 Cytomegalovirus. A 1-day-old infant with congenital with cytomegalovirus infection. Noncontrast computed tomography of the head demonstrates bilateral areas of periventricular confluent calcifications (*arrows*). Note the abnormal sulcal pattern of the right hemisphere indicating associated polymicrogyria (*arrowheads*).

polymicrogyria, especially in the region of the Sylvian fissures.

TOXOPLASMOSIS

Symptomatic congenital infection with *Toxoplasma gondii* is far less common compared with CMV. Principle clinical findings include hydrocephalus, abnormal CSF, bilateral chorioretinitis, and intracranial calcifications. Fetal infection before 20 weeks leads to severe neurologic signs; infection between 20 and 30 weeks leads to a more variable outcome. Beyond 30 weeks, CT manifestations often include intracerebral and periventricular calcifications, which are nearly identical to the distribution in children affected by CMV, and is rarely accompanied by ventricular dilatation. Cortical abnormalities typical with CMV are most often absent in cases of toxoplasmosis.

HERPES SIMPLEX VIRUS TYPE 2

Most cases of neonatal HSV-2 are contracted transvaginally as the baby passes through the birth canal. Neonatal CNS herpetic infection is believed to occur in approximately 1 in 10,000 births. CNS manifestations generally present between 2 to 4 weeks of life and include meningoencephalitis with seizures, lethargy, and fever. Sequelae include mental retardation, severe neurologic deficits, or even death, secondary to virulent destruction of the brain. The disease may

produce ischemic infarction of parts or all of the brain, necrosis, atrophy, encephalomalacia, demyelination, and gliosis (Fig. 34-29). Watershed distribution ischemia is also fairly common in areas remote from the primary herpetic lesions. MRI-restricted diffusion, which may be multifocal or limited to the temporal lobes, brainstem, or cerebellum, is the first radiologic sign of herpetic brain destruction. CT in early disease is either normal or demonstrates subtle areas of low attenuation. Later, patchy white matter low attenuation on CT and corresponding hyperintense signal on T2W imaging with rapid progression is demonstrated. Meningeal enhancement reflects the extent of the disease. Also of note is classic persisting hyperattenuation of cortical gray matter on CT, and corresponding T1 and T2 shortening on MRI. Eventually, diffuse cerebral and cerebellar (in about 50% of cases) atrophy and encephalomalacia ensue (Fig. 34-30). It should be noted that HSV-1 encephalitis, which affects older children and adults, is different from neonatal herpes infection.

CONGENITAL RUBELLA, VARICELLA, AND SYPHILIS

Congenital rubella is rare in Western countries and now has an incidence in the United States of about 1 in 1,000,000 births. Congenital varicella is also rare; even when the pregnant mother contracts varicella zoster virus, the fetus is most often not affected. Congenital syphilis is unlikely to cause neurologic symptoms in the neonatal period.

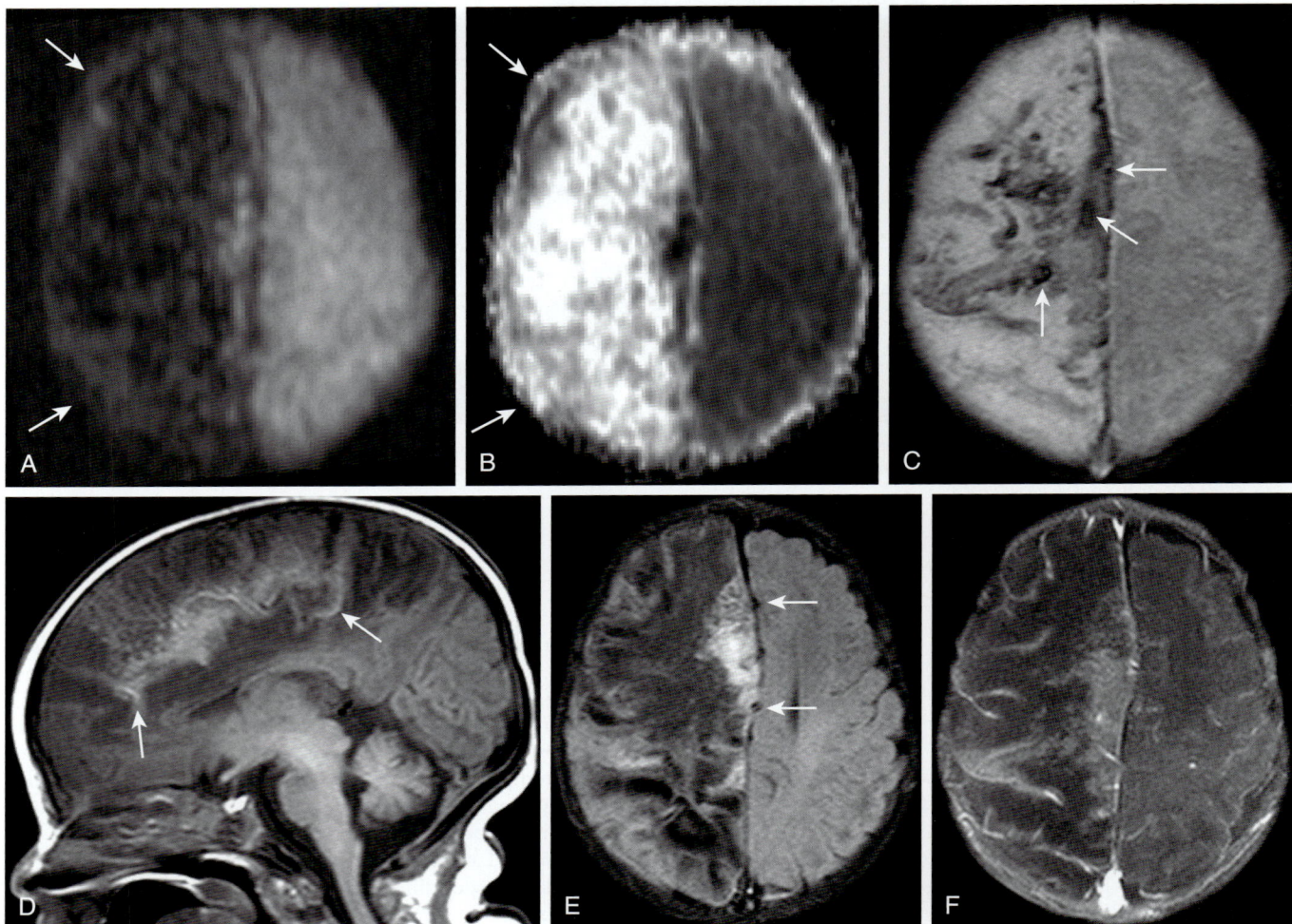

Figure 34-29 Herpes simplex virus (HSV) cerebritis or encephalitis (hemorrhagic type). A 1-month-old female infant with several days' history of seizures and positive HSV culture from recent cerebrospinal fluid sample. Diffusion-weighted imaging and apparent diffusion coefficient map (**A** and **B**, respectively), axial gadolinium-enhanced (**C**), sagittal T1 (**D**), axial fluid-attenuated inversion recovery (**E**), and axial postcontrast fat-suppression T1-weighted (**F**) images were obtained. Note the increased diffusion throughout the right cerebral hemisphere (*arrows in* **A** *and* **B**). Corresponding T2* effect is seen within the superior right cerebral hemisphere corresponding to hemorrhage (*arrows in* **C**). Corresponding T1 shortening is seen near midline sagittal T1-weighted image (*arrows in* **D**) corresponding to mineralization. Note the mass effect caused by edema of the right cerebral hemisphere (*arrows in* **E**), and the paucity of contrast enhancement (**F**).

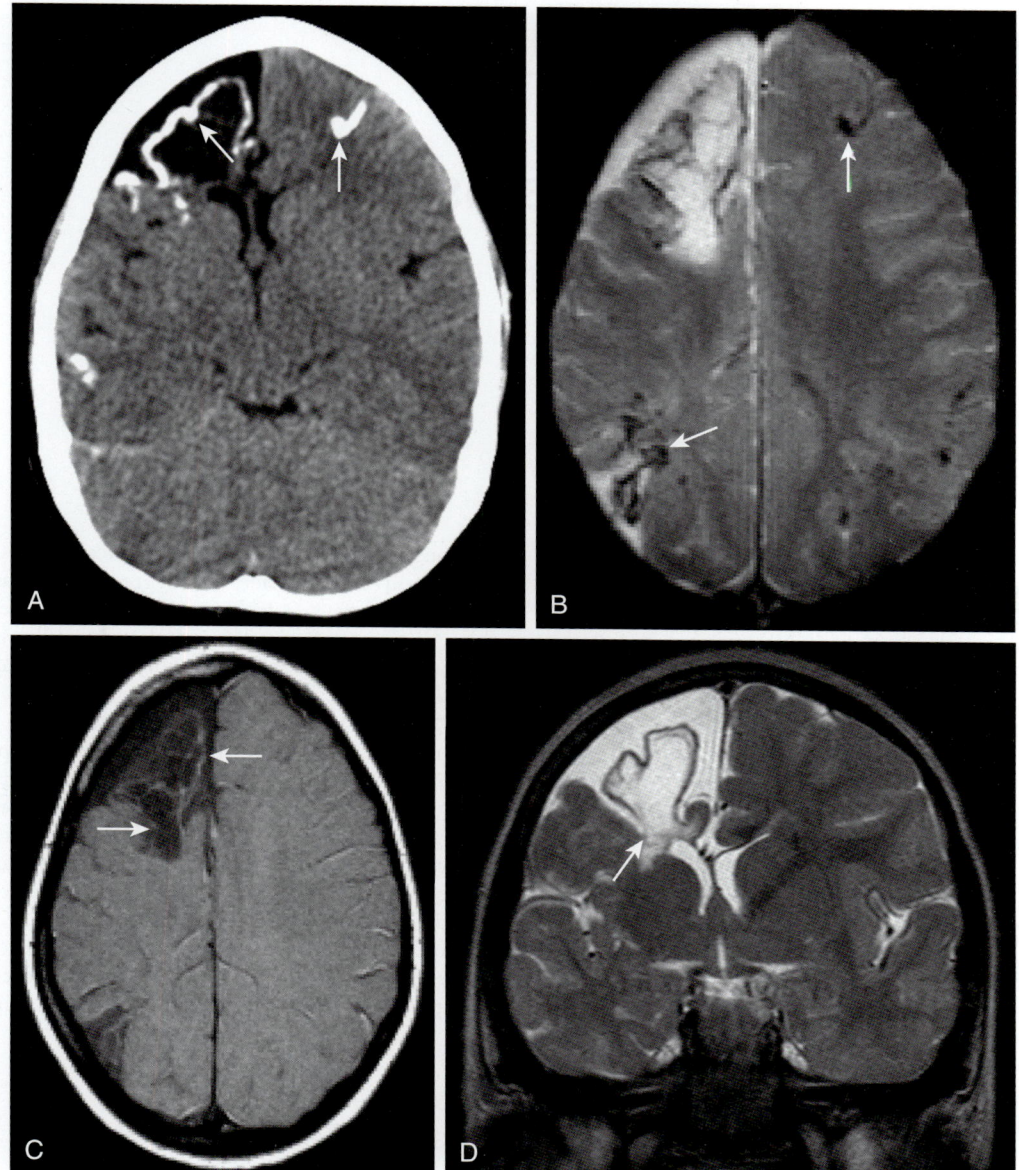

Figure 34-30 Herpes simplex virus (HSV) (chronic changes). A 5-year-old female child with fulminant hepatic failure, renal failure, and lethargy with a prior history of HSV encephalitis. Axial noncontrast computed tomography of the head (**A**), axial gadolinium-enhanced sequence from magnetic resonance imaging (**B**), axial magnetization transfer (MT) T1-weighted (**C**) and coronal T2 magnetic resonance image (**D**) were obtained. Note the bilateral calcification seen within both hemispheres (*arrows in* **A**), with corresponding areas of T2* effect within both cerebral hemispheres (*arrows in* **B**) indicating mineralization. Note the slight T1 shortening effect on the MT T1 sequence (*arrows in* **C**), corresponding to mineralization. Volume loss is seen within the frontal lobe and associated T2 prolongation on the coronal T2 sequence (*arrows in* **D**).

Suggested Readings

Barkovich AJ, Raybaud C. *Pediatric neuroimaging.* 5th ed. Philadelphia, PA: Lippincott Williams and Wilkins; 2011.

Gasparetto EL, Cabral RF, da Cruz LC, Jr., et al. Diffusion imaging in brain infections. *Neuroimaging Clin North Am.* 2011;21(1):89-113.

Hedlund GL, Boyer RS. Neuroimaging of postnatal pediatric central nervous system infections. *Semin Pediatr Neurol.* 1999;6:299-317.

Murthy SN, Faden HS, Cohen ME, et al. Acute disseminated encephalomyelitis in children. *Pediatrics.* 2002;110:E21.

Nickerson JP, Richner B, Santy K, et al. Neuroimaging of pediatric intracranial infection—part 2: TORCH, viral, fungal, and parasitic infections. *J Neuroimag.* 2012;22(2):e52-e63.

Chapter 35

Pediatric Brain Neoplasms

SANJAY P. PRABHU and TINA YOUNG POUSSAINT

Brain tumors are the most common solid pediatric tumors and are the leading cause of death in children from solid tumors.[1] The estimated incidence of all childhood primary brain and central nervous system (CNS) tumors is 4.8 cases per 100,000 person-years.[2] Approximately 4150 new cases of childhood primary nonmalignant and malignant brain and CNS tumors were diagnosed in the United States in 2011.[3] Nearly 50% of brain tumors in children older than 1 year arise in an infratentorial location. However, in neonates, infants, and children up to the age of 3 years, supratentorial tumors are more common.[3]

Etiology

The etiology of pediatric brain tumors, an area of research beyond the scope of this chapter, requires an understanding of genetic alterations, signaling systems, and molecular genetics and pathways. Although no one risk factor explains more than a small percentage of childhood brain tumors, therapeutic doses of ionizing radiation to the head for brain tumors and radiation for leukemia,[4,5] as well as certain genetic syndromes, are known risk factors in the pediatric population. Among the congenital syndromes associated with brain tumors are neurofibromatosis types 1 and 2, Gorlin syndrome (basal cell nevus syndrome), tuberous sclerosis, Turcot syndrome, von Hippel-Lindau syndrome, and Li-Fraumeni syndrome.[6]

Imaging

The wide availability of computed tomography (CT) for diagnosing patients who present acutely, particularly in the emergency department setting, has produced several advantages, including its ability to detect a sizable mass lesion, identify the effect of a mass, and check for ventricular enlargement, lesional hemorrhage, calcification, and osseous involvement.

Because of its superior soft tissue resolution, multiplanar capability, and lack of ionizing radiation, magnetic resonance imaging (MRI) with contrast is the modality of choice in determining lesion size, location, and characterization. And although contrast enhancement typically reflects disruption of the blood-brain barrier, the degree of contrast enhancement does not always correlate with tumor grade. For example, benign tumors (e.g., choroid plexus papillomas and pilocytic astrocytomas) can enhance avidly, whereas anaplastic astrocytomas may not enhance at all.[7]

MRI also is used to assess tumor response and progression and monitor treatment effects. Essential to optimal treatment planning is accurate staging of the tumor that confirms whether the tumor has spread through the neural axis. Intraoperative MRI is being used in some centers to guide both conventional and minimally invasive tumor resection. As these systems are refined, they are expected to form the standard of care at many medical centers.[8]

After surgical resection, imaging is used to determine the presence of residual tumor and to evaluate postoperative complications such as hemorrhage or ischemia.

Role of Advanced Imaging Techniques

Advanced imaging techniques such as magnetic resonance (MR) diffusion, MR spectroscopy, MR perfusion, and positron emission tomography (PET) are used to complement structural imaging, providing insight into tumor physiology.

Diffusion-Weighted Imaging

Contrast on diffusion-weighted images (DWI) reflects the mean distance traveled by free water protons in tissue as a result of Brownian motion.[9,10] Diffusion occurs freely in the direction of white matter tract orientation and is restricted in orthogonal planes. DWI can assess the properties of diffusion occurring within a particular voxel, which is expressed as the apparent diffusion coefficient (ADC). A markedly decreased ADC usually correlates well with increased tumor cellularity in brain neoplasms. Vasogenic edema and necrosis show an increased ADC.[7,11,12] ADC values are interpreted in conjunction with structural MRI sequences. Diffusion tensor imaging (DTI), an adaptation of DWI, acquires diffusion data in six or more directions to establish the direction and magnitude of water diffusion.

DWI also can be extremely useful in the postoperative period, when low ADC values at the surgical margins or within the resection cavity may be indicative of ischemia or abscess. This technique typically is used in conjunction with conventional MRI, which helps exclude artifact from hematoma.[13] Further, DTI aids in identifying patterns of tumor interaction with white matter fiber tracts (i.e., the extent of deviation, edema, infiltration, and destruction),[14] and when used in conjunction with volumetric data, it effectively guides surgical resection and predicts possible postoperative deficits resulting from white matter tract damage (e-Fig. 35-1). Reduced fractional anisotropy (FA), which is a measure of the directional diffusivity of water made using DTI, has been found in the white matter of patients with a medulloblastoma, even in the absence of abnormalities on structural sequences.[15] Decreased FA values have been shown to correlate with the age at which radiation was administered and with poor academic performance among school-age patients.[16] FA thus may be considered a noninvasive biomarker to monitor effects of radiotherapy.[16]

Magnetic Resonance Spectroscopy

Magnetic resonance spectroscopy (MRS) is a noninvasive in vivo technique that provides metabolic information beyond structural imaging sequences. It enables detection and quantification of abnormal metabolites in the brain and can help identify tumor tissue, differentiate tumor types, and separate active tumor from radiation necrosis or scar formation. MRS can be performed with most standard MRI scanners, typically by incorporating either the point resolved spin echo or stimulated echo acquisition mode techniques. Simultaneous acquisition of MRS from multiple voxels increases spatial resolution; this procedure is known as "chemical shift imaging" or MR spectroscopic imaging.[17]

Normal metabolites detected in the brain include N-acetylaspartate (NAA), a neuronal marker; choline, a cell membrane marker; and creatine, a marker of energy metabolism. Myoinositol, a glial marker, can be optimally assessed with short echo time MRS techniques.

Most brain tumors are characterized by the presence of increased choline/creatine and decreased NAA/creatine ratios, indicating loss of neuroaxonal integrity and increased cell membrane turnover. The presence of lactate in the tumor suggests an anaerobic process with impaired energy metabolism.[18] In general, high-grade tumors have higher choline/creatine and lower NAA/creatine ratios than do low-grade lesions. In rapidly growing malignant tumors, necrotic areas may contain lipid resonances.[19] However, in pediatric patients, we frequently (and paradoxically) see elevated levels of choline and lactate in pilocytic astrocytomas, a low-grade tumor.[20]

The presence of specific metabolites such as alanine (an inverted doublet at 1.44 ppm) in meningiomas (e-Fig. 35-2) and taurine (peak at 3.3 to 3.4 ppm) in primitive neuroectodermal tumors (PNETs) may help narrow the differential diagnosis.[21,22] Citrate is a tricarboxylic acid cycle intermediate metabolite that has been described in pediatric brain tumors and is found at particularly high levels in pontine gliomas.[23]

In one study of grade 2 astrocytomas, citrate was significantly more prominent in tumors that progressed.[24]

Perfusion-Weighted imaging

Perfusion-weighted imaging measures cerebral hemodynamics at the microcirculation level. Parameters measured by perfusion-weighted imaging include cerebral blood volume (CBV), cerebral blood flow, and mean transit time. Of these, the CBV, defined as the volume of blood in an area of brain tissue expressed in mL/100 g, is the most commonly used parameter in evaluation of brain tumors.[25] Lower grade astrocytomas have relatively lower regional CBV than do higher-grade tumors such as anaplastic astrocytomas and glioblastomas[26] (e-Fig. 35-3). However, low-grade pediatric pilocytic astrocytomas can have a high relative cerebral blood volume.[27]

Three main techniques are available to measure perfusion within the brain: T2$\star$ dynamic susceptibility contrast imaging, T1-weighted dynamic contrast-enhanced MR perfusion, and arterial spin labeling (ASL).

The most widely available technique is T2$\star$-weighted dynamic susceptibility contrast imaging, which consists of a rapid bolus of intravenous (IV) paramagnetic contrast agent followed by a rapid acquisition of echo-planar images during the first pass of contrast material through the capillary bed. As the contrast medium is delivered, it goes through the tissues and results in a signal drop proportional to the blood volume during the first pass. Routine use of this technique in children requires the use of rapid contrast medium injection and power injectors, as well as strategies to overcome problems associated with large-bore IV catheter placement, especially in infants.[28]

ASL uses endogenous blood as a tracer. The two major types of ASL, pulsed and continuous, are now widely available on clinical scanners. A third type, pseudocontinuous ASL, has just recently been introduced for clinical use. ASL has shown promise for hemodynamic evaluation of brain tumors,[29,30] but data in children are limited at this time.

Functional MRI

Functional MRI (fMRI) is a technique that essentially relies on two physical principles, namely, that oxyhemoglobin is diamagnetic and deoxyhemoglobin is paramagnetic in nature. Because of the relative increased blood flow and consequent increased utilization of oxygen within the activated portions of the brain, the MR signal, in this case known as the "blood oxygen level dependent signal," or BOLD, is measurably different compared with other parts of the brain. The primary value of fMRI is in localizing the eloquent areas in the brain controlling language, motor skills, and memory. This information helps provide surgical guidance.[31] More detailed information can be found in Chapter 27.

Single PET and PET

The assessment of regional cerebral blood flow by single PET has been largely replaced by MR perfusion and fMRI techniques in recent years.

The role of PET in the evaluation of pediatric brain tumors is to determine metabolic activity at diagnosis, assess response to therapy, and distinguish treatment effect versus tumor recurrence. Fluorine-18-deoxyglucose (^{18}F-FDG) is the most commonly used isotope for PET studies in children. PET scanning using other labeled agents such as the amino acid analogues [^{11}C] methionine and [^{11}C] tyrosine have shown promise in detecting low-grade tumors in adults, although their diagnostic value in children has not yet been established.[32] These amino acid analogues are incorporated via amino acid transport pathways into tumor proteins, and therefore uptake reflects tumor protein synthesis.[33,34]

Other isotopes still at the investigational stage include cell proliferation agents (e.g., ^{18}F-fluorothymidine) and cell hypoxia imaging agents (e.g., ^{18}F-fluoromisonidazole and ^{62}Cu-labeled diacetyl-bis [N4-methylthiosemicarbazone]).

Specific Tumors

CLASSIFICATION OF PEDIATRIC BRAIN TUMORS

The differential diagnosis is effectively limited by classifying tumors by location, describing the appearance of the lesion on conventional MRI, and applying advanced imaging techniques (Box 35-1).

TUMORS OF THE CEREBRAL HEMISPHERES

Astrocytomas

The modified World Health Organization (WHO) classification of CNS tumors divides astrocytomas into low grade (grades I and II) and high grade (grades III and IV).[35] Grading of astrocytomas by the WHO criteria is predictive of patient survival.[35]

Pilocytic astrocytomas are grade I WHO tumors; they account for 20% to 30% of all childhood brain tumors.[36] Pilocytic astrocytomas typically arise in the first two decades of life. The most common locations of these tumors are in the optic pathways, hypothalamus, thalamus, basal ganglia, cerebral hemispheres, cerebellum (Fig. 35-4), and brainstem. Patients with neurofibromatosis type 1 (NF1) have an increased risk of the development of pilocytic astrocytomas, including optic pathway tumors. Patients with NF1 who have optic pathway tumors tend to have a better long-term prognosis than do patients without NF1 who have optic pathway tumors.[37]

On CT and MRI, a grade I astrocytoma usually is a well-defined lesion that demonstrates contrast enhancement of its solid component. Cystic components may be present. The presence of increased ADC values within these lesions helps to distinguish them from higher grade astrocytomas.

Rarely, pilocytic astrocytomas can present with diffuse leptomeningeal spread, which most often is seen in association with the diencephalic syndrome (discussed later in this chapter) or with the pilomyxoid variant of astrocytomas. Pilomyxoid astrocytomas have an indolent course, but their propensity for slow-growing, persistent recurrences makes them difficult to treat.[38]

Gross total resection of pilocytic astrocytomas is often curative, but micrometastases and recurrences may occur.

Box 35-1 Classification of Pediatric Brain Tumors Based on the Location of the Tumors

Tumors of the Cerebral Hemispheres
- Astrocytoma (World Health Organization grade I-IV)
- Supratentorial primitive neuroectodermal tumor
- Atypical teratoid/rhabdoid tumor
- Supratentorial ependymoma
- Thalamic astrocytoma
- Dysembryoplastic neuroepithelial tumor
- Meningioangiomatosis
- Germinoma
- Choroid plexus tumors—papilloma and carcinoma
- Neuronal and mixed neuronal-glial tumors (including desmoplastic infantile ganglioglioma)

Sellar and Suprasellar Tumors
- Craniopharyngioma
- Chiasmatic/hypothalamic glioma
- Hypothalamic hamartoma
- Pituitary adenoma
- Germ cell tumors
- Langerhans cell histiocytosis
- Rathke cleft cyst
- Arachnoid cyst
- Dermoid/epidermoid cyst

Posterior Fossa Tumors

Intraaxial
- Medulloblastoma
- Cerebellar astrocytoma
- Brainstem neoplasm
- Atypical teratoid rhabdoid tumor
- Ependymoma
- Teratoma
- Hemangioblastoma

Extraaxial
- Dermoid
- Epidermoid
- Teratoma
- Schwannoma
- Meningioma
- Skull base neoplasms

Parameningeal Tumors
- Osseous, chondroid, or myeloid origin
- Other mesenchymal origin tumors
- Tumors from notochordal elements
- Metastatic disease, including leptomeningeal disease from dissemination of primary brain tumors

Pineal Region Tumors
- Germ cell tumors
- Pineal parenchymal tumors
- Tumors of supporting tissues of the pineal gland or adjacent structures

---

Supratentorial High-Grade Gliomas

High-grade gliomas in children are significantly less common than are low-grade lesions, which account for up to 20% of all hemispheric gliomas.[39,40]

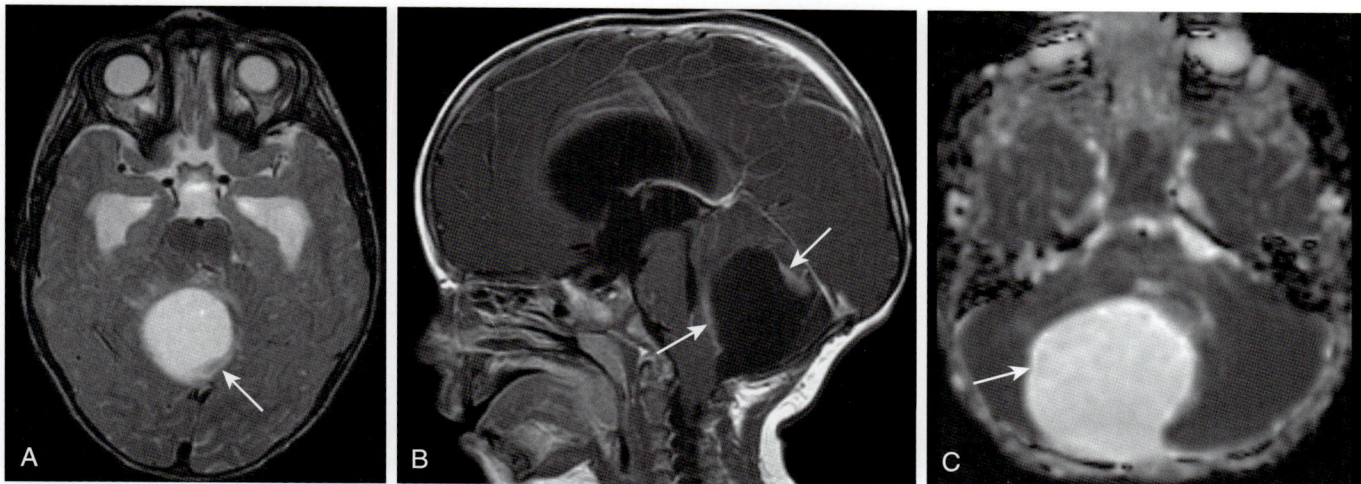

Figure 35-4 A cerebellar astrocytoma. **A,** An axial T2-weighted image shows a large cystic mass centered in the right cerebellar hemisphere with small solid components along the posterior and anterior aspects (*arrow*). **B,** A postcontrast sagittal T1-weighted image shows the solid components (*arrows*) along the anterior and posterior margins that enhance after paramagnetic contrast administration. **C,** An apparent diffusion coefficient map shows increased diffusion within the lesion (*arrow*) consistent with the relatively low cellularity within the lesion.

On CT, these lesions demonstrate heterogeneous enhancement and density with edema, occasional hemorrhage, mass effect, and ill-defined margins. On MRI, these lesions have heterogeneous signal intensity (Fig. 35-5). They typically are hypointense on T1-weighted images and hyperintense on T2-weighted images with surrounding white matter edema. They show effect of the mass on surrounding structures and demonstrate irregular enhancement with necrosis and hemorrhage similar to that seen on CT.

Aggressive surgical resection with preservation of neurological function, followed by radiotherapy directed at the tumor bed, remains the cornerstone of treatment of pediatric malignant gliomas.[41] The addition of chemotherapy has been shown to improve survival compared with surgery and radiotherapy alone.[40] The overall prognosis for children with supratentorial malignant gliomas remains poor, however, with 5-year progression-free survival rates of around 30%.[40]

Supratentorial PNETs

Although supratentorial PNETs are relatively rare, these tumors are more common in the first decade of life, with peak incidence from birth to 5 years of age.[42] They account for 5% of all supratentorial tumors in childhood. At

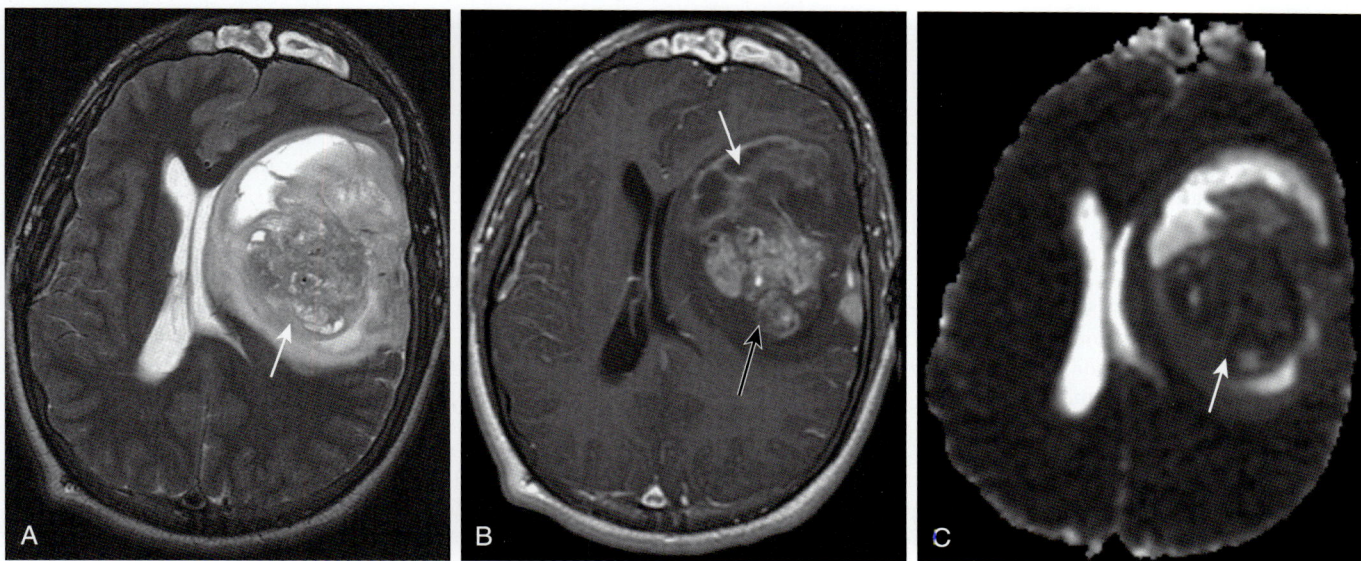

Figure 35-5 A supratentorial high-grade glioma. **A,** An axial T2-weighted image shows a large heterogeneous mass (*arrow*) in the left frontal, temporal, and parietal lobes with marked mass effect, subfalcine herniation, surrounding edema, and rightward midline shift. **B,** A postcontrast T1-weighted image shows heterogeneous enhancement of the solid components of the tumor (*black arrow*) and nonenhancing components anteriorly (*white arrow*), suggestive of necrosis. **C,** An apparent diffusion coefficient map reveals decreased diffusion within the solid component (*arrow*), indicating high cellularity.

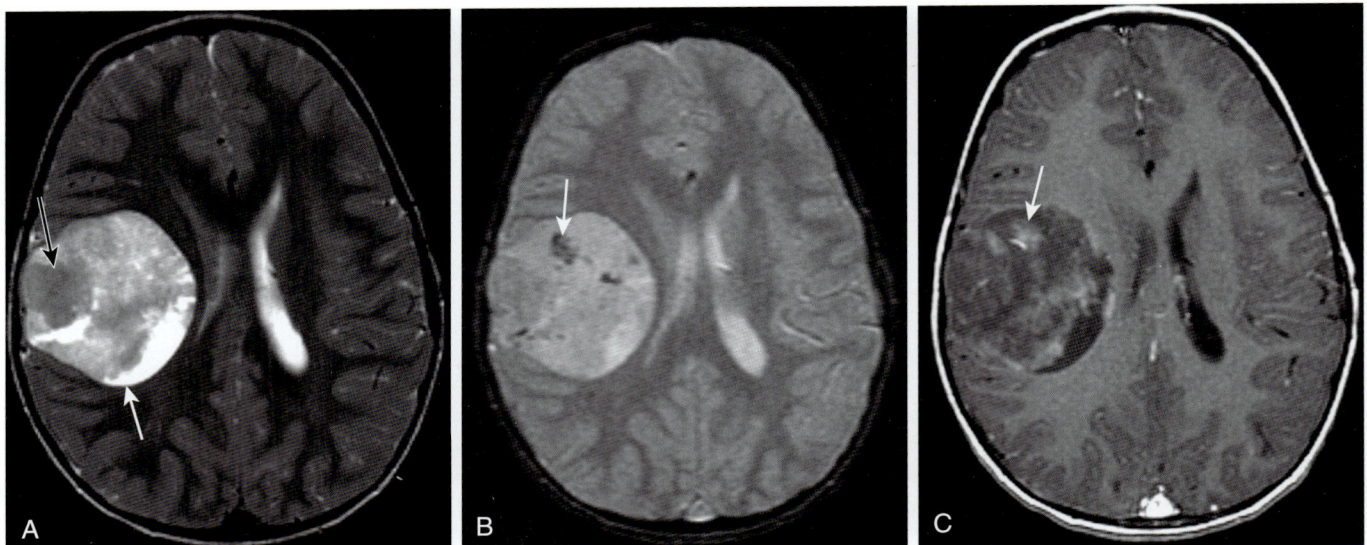

Figure 35-6 A supratentorial primitive neuroectodermal tumor. **A,** An axial T2-weighted image shows a well-defined, large, heterogeneous mass lesion in the right cerebral hemisphere with a predominant solid T2-hypointense component (*black arrow*) and smaller areas of T2 prolongation (*white arrow*). **B,** An axial gradient-recall echo image shows scattered foci of susceptibility (*arrow*) suggestive of calcification or blood products within the lesion. **C,** An axial postcontrast T1-weighted image shows patchy heterogeneous enhancement within the lesion (*arrow*).

presentation they often are large and fairly well defined, occurring either in the cerebral hemispheres or in the lateral ventricles. They may be solid and homogenous or heterogeneous with cyst formation.[43] Calcification often is seen on CT. Heterogeneous contrast enhancement is seen along with regions of necrosis.

On MRI, solid areas have restricted diffusion and T2-hypointense areas (Fig. 35-6), reflecting high nuclear-to-cytoplasm ratio, increased cellularity, and increased CBV values. Necrosis and hemorrhage also can occur in these lesions.

Supratentorial Ependymoma

Ependymomas constitute approximately 10% of all intracranial tumors in children.[44] Of these, supratentorial ependymomas typically occur in children younger than 6 years and account for up to 40% of all ependymomas.[45] These tumors are thought to arise from embryonic rests of ependymal tissue trapped in the developing cerebral hemispheres.[46] Ependymomas are heterogeneous and often contain calcification and cystic areas. They are hypointense on T1-weighted images and isointense to hyperintense to gray matter on T2-weighted images. Moderate to avid enhancement of the soft tissue components of the tumor is seen, intermixed with poorly enhancing or nonenhancing areas.[47]

CHOROID PLEXUS TUMORS

Choroid plexus tumors account for approximately 3% of pediatric brain tumors.[48] Of these, 10% to 20% arise in the first decade of life and 80% occur in the first 2 years of life, including a considerable number of tumors diagnosed in utero.[49] Choroid plexus papillomas account for the vast majority of choroid plexus tumors (up to 85%), with the remainder being choroid plexus carcinomas.

These tumors typically occur in the trigone of the lateral ventricles in children, as opposed to adults, in whom they occur in the fourth ventricle. On CT, choroid plexus papillomas are lobulated masses that typically are isodense to hyperdense, may have punctate calcifications, and enhance avidly and homogenously. On MRI, they are homogeneous, enhancing intraventricular masses that are hypointense on T1-weighted images and predominantly hyperintense on T2-weighted images (Fig. 35-7).

Choroid plexus carcinomas may be hyperdense on CT, reflecting increased cellularity. These tumors almost always invade the adjacent brain through the ventricular wall and cause vasogenic edema.[50] They are characterized by areas of heterogeneous signal intensity on both T1- and T2-weighted images because of hemorrhage and necrosis. MRS may help distinguish between papillomas and carcinomas. The myoinositol level is significantly lower and the choline level is significantly higher in choroid plexus carcinomas than in choroid plexus papillomas.[51]

Spinal drop metastases can occur in both choroid plexus papillomas and carcinomas, although they are seen more frequently in carcinomas.

SELLAR AND PARASELLAR TUMORS

Craniopharyngiomas

Craniopharyngiomas are slow-growing, benign, nonglial tumors arising in the sellar and parasellar regions. They constitute between 3% and 10% of all pediatric brain tumors.[44] Craniopharyngiomas are classified as WHO grade I tumors and arise from ectodermal remnants of the Rathke pouch with a bimodal incidence in the first and fifth decades of life. The adamantinous type is more common in children, whereas the squamous-papillary variant tends to occur in adults.[44] Although histologically craniopharyngiomas are benign, they

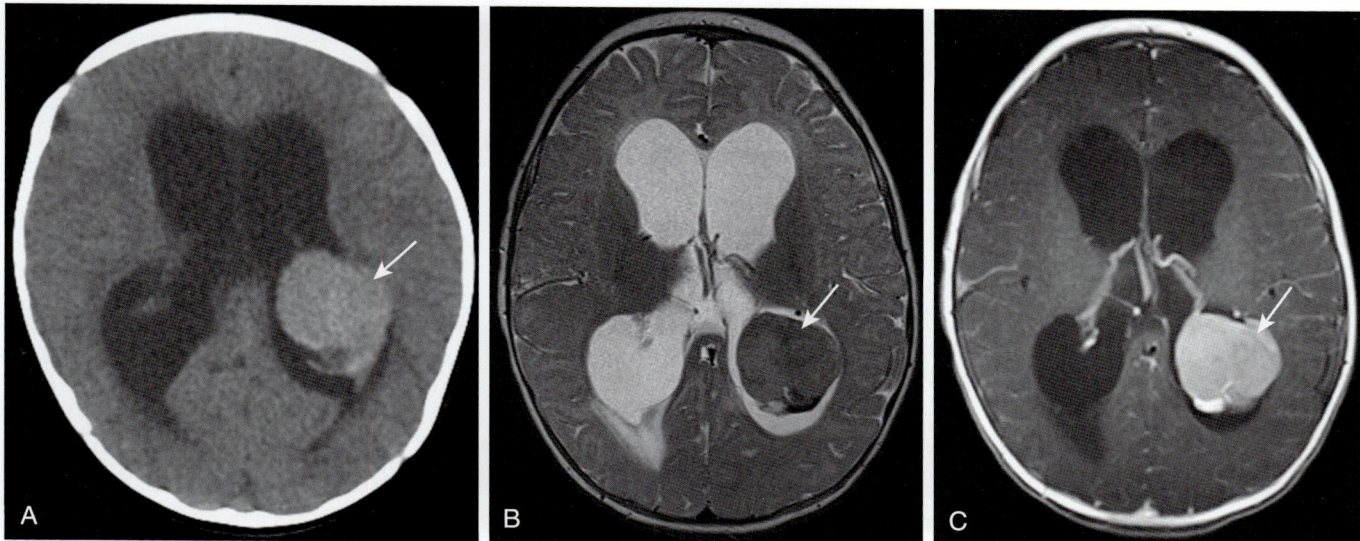

Figure 35-7 A choroid plexus papilloma. **A,** Axial noncontrast computed tomography shows a lobulated hyperdense mass in the left lateral ventricle (*arrow*). **B,** An axial T2-weighted image shows that the mass in the left lateral ventricle is hypointense compared with the brain parenchyma (*arrow*). **C,** An axial postcontrast T1-weighted image shows homogenous enhancement of the lesion (*arrow*) after administration of contrast material.

can invade surrounding structures, eliciting a gliotic response that makes resection challenging.

The imaging appearance of craniopharyngiomas reflects their mixed cystic and solid nature, with 90% having calcification and 90% having a cyst formation. On MRI, high signal intensity on both T1- and T2-weighted images is seen in areas with high protein content (Fig. 35-8) or in lesions that show evidence of subacute hemorrhage. Hypointensity on T1-weighted images can be seen reflecting the presence of keratin in some of the cysts. CT often is used to demonstrate calcification, which is important for diagnosis and surgical planning. Surgical treatment remains the mainstay, with radiotherapy having a role in cases that are not amenable to gross total resection. Recurrence-free, 5-year survival is close to 87% but falls to less than 50% with subtotal resection.[52]

Follow-up imaging is directed toward identifying recurrence, second tumors, and associations with moyamoya syndrome.

Chiasmatic/Optic Pathway/ Hypothalamic Gliomas

Optic pathway gliomas are low-grade pilocytic astrocytomas (WHO grade I) that represent 15% of supratentorial tumors.[53] Although sporadic lesions are not uncommon, a strong association of optic nerve gliomas with NF1 exists; bilateral optic nerve tumors are virtually pathognomonic of NF1.[54] Twenty percent to 50% of optic gliomas occur in patients with NF1, whereas the prevalence of optic pathway gliomas in the NF1 population is between 1.5% and 19%.[54] The tumors may involve the optic nerves, optic chiasm, optic tracts, lateral

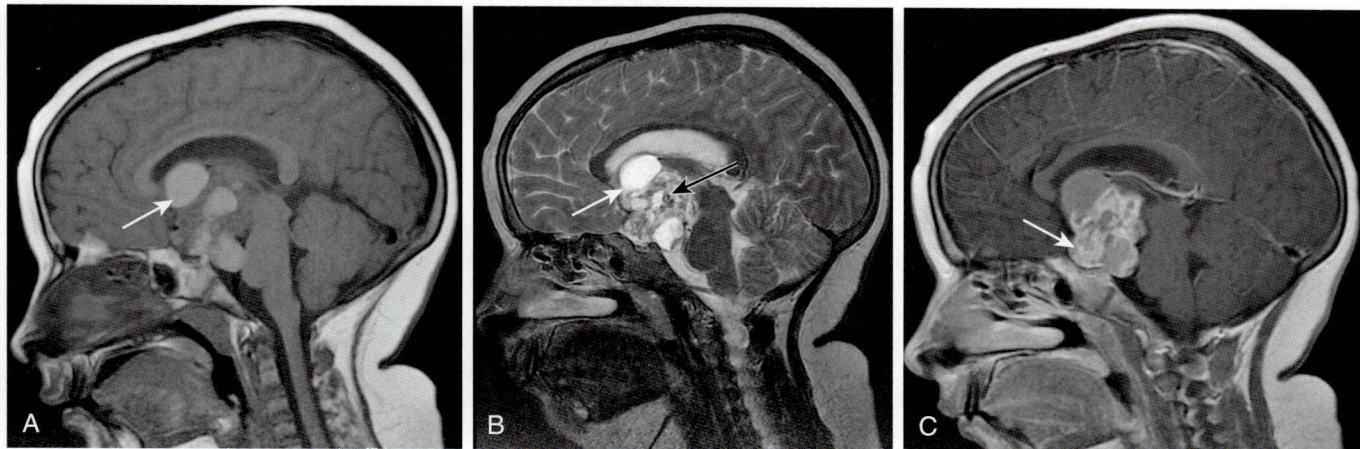

Figure 35-8 A craniopharyngioma. **A,** A sagittal T1-weighted image shows a large suprasellar lesion containing solid and cystic components with T1 shortening within the cystic components (*arrow*) consistent with proteinaceous content. **B,** A sagittal T2-weighted image shows T2 hyperintensity within the cystic components (*white arrow*) and scattered hypointensity consistent with foci of calcification (*black arrow*). **C,** A sagittal postcontrast T1-weighted image shows avid enhancement of the solid component (*arrow*).

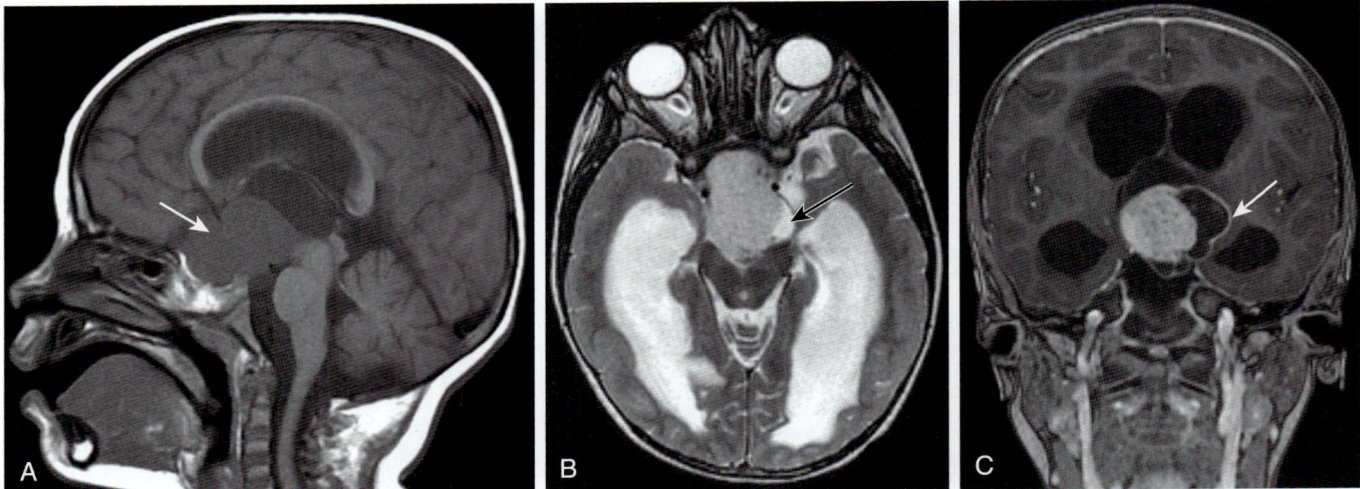

Figure 35-9 A chiasmatic/hypothalamic glioma. **A,** A sagittal T1-weighted image shows a large lobulated suprasellar mass (*arrow*) in the region of the optic chiasm with superior extension into the third ventricle and pontine cistern. **B,** An axial T2-weighted image shows that the lesion is hyperintense compared with brain parenchyma and that a more hyperintense cystic component is present along its superior and right aspects (*black arrow*). **C,** A coronal T1 postcontrast image shows marked enhancement of the central solid component and peripheral enhancement of the cystic components (*arrow*).

geniculate bodies, and/or optic radiations. Tumors in children with NF1 reportedly are less aggressive than those in children without NF1.[55]

Optic pathway gliomas are usually isointense to hypointense on T1-weighted images (Fig. 35-9). On T2-weighted images, the lesions demonstrate mixed signal intensity; intense enhancement also is common. Use of coronal and axial fat-suppressed thin-section postcontrast T1-weighted images and inversion recovery or T2 images with fat saturation enables optimal visualization of the optic pathways.[56]

Diencephalic syndrome may be seen in a small percentage of patients with hypothalamic/chiasmatic astrocytomas who present with failure to thrive. These tumors often are larger, occur at a younger age, are more aggressive than others at presentation, and they may seed throughout the cerebrospinal fluid (CSF) pathways.[57]

POSTERIOR FOSSA TUMORS

Medulloblastoma

Medulloblastomas are the most common posterior fossa tumors of childhood, accounting for nearly 38% of all posterior fossa tumors and approximately 15% to 20% of all pediatric brain tumors. Medulloblastoma is a heterogeneous disease, with histopathologic and molecular variants that have distinct biological behaviors.[58] Medulloblastomas can be separated on the basis of their histopathologic features into the classic type and four variants, including desmoplastic/nodular; medulloblastoma with extensive nodularity; anaplastic medulloblastoma; and large cell medulloblastoma.[35] Children who have medulloblastomas with extensive nodularity and desmoplastic/nodular medulloblastomas generally have a better outcome than do children with classic tumors. Patients with large cell and anaplastic medulloblastomas do not fare as well because these tumors behave aggressively and typically are resistant to most therapies.[58] Medulloblastomas are characterized by major molecular subgroups that are based on various signaling pathways, including the Shh (sonic

hedgehog pathway) variant; Wnt (Wingless); ERBB2 (receptor kinase family); and non-Shh/Wnt subtypes.[58,59]

Medulloblastomas usually arise in the midline within the vermis and grow into the fourth ventricle, resulting in obstructive hydrocephalus. In older patients and in those with the desmoplastic subtype, they are localized to the cerebellar hemispheres.[60] Medulloblastomas usually are hyperdense masses on CT (Fig. 35-10, *A*); on MRI, they characteristically are T1 and T2 hypointense relative to gray matter with homogeneous enhancement (Fig 35-10, *B* and *C*). Elevated taurine content on MRS has been reported in persons with a medulloblastoma.[20] The incidence of CSF dissemination at diagnosis is between 20% and 30%.[61]

Treatment of medulloblastomas consists of surgery, radiation therapy, and chemotherapy. Conventional risk stratification is based on the age of the patient, the extent of the tumor at the time of diagnosis, and completeness of surgical resection.[62] High-risk features include younger age at diagnosis, incomplete resection or postoperative tumor residuum greater than 1.5 cm^2, and metastatic disease.[63] More recently, the presence of anaplasia on histopathology, ERBB2 positivity, and classification into the c-Myc and non–Wnt/Shh molecular subgroups have emerged as potential biomarkers of a poor prognosis.[59,64]

Tectal Gliomas

Patients with tectal gliomas present with symptoms of obstructive hydrocephalus caused by the growth of these lesions adjacent to the aqueduct of Sylvius. Tectal gliomas can be diagnosed on the basis of imaging findings alone. Although imaging appearance is similar to that of pilocytic astrocytomas that appear elsewhere in the cerebral hemispheres, tectal gliomas usually do not enhance after contrast enhancement (Fig. 35-11). They may require CSF diversion procedures to relieve hydrocephalus but usually do not require biopsy or resection. Careful observation suffices for slowly progressing asymptomatic tumors. Rarely, tumors larger than 10 cm may require surgical debulking and/or chemotherapy.[65,66]

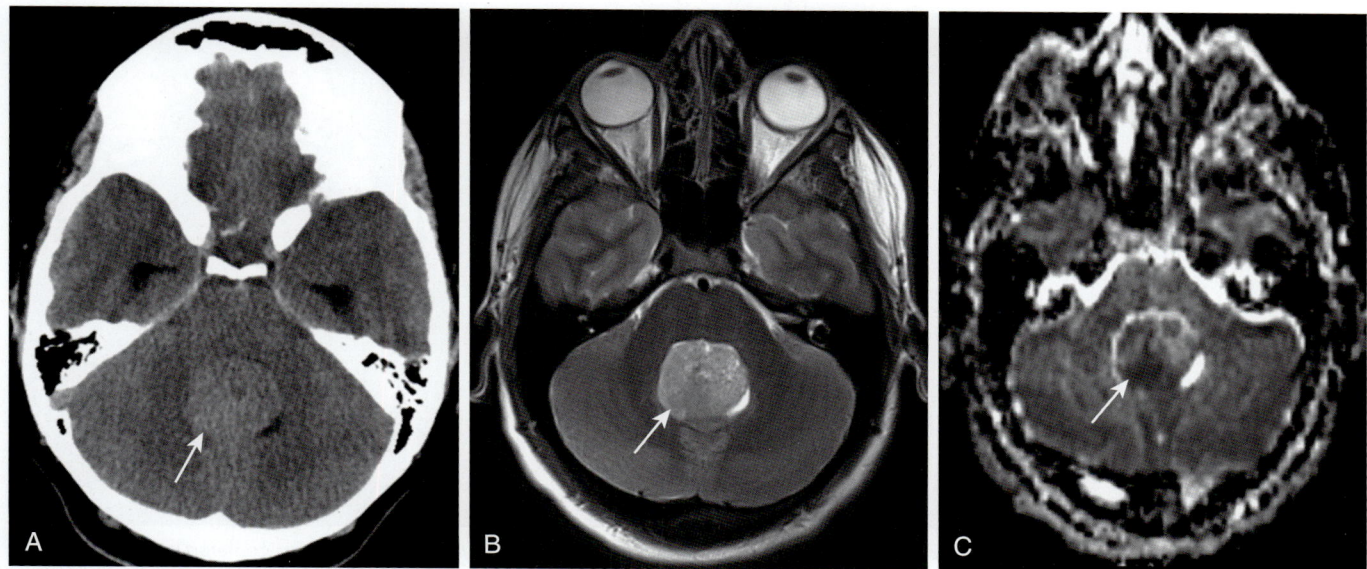

Figure 35-10   A medulloblastoma. **A,** Axial noncontrast computed tomography shows a rounded mass (*arrow*) hyperdense to cerebellar white matter in the fourth ventricle. **B,** An axial T2-weighted image shows a solid mass centered in the cerebellum close to the midline (*arrow*). The mass is hypointense on the T2-weighted images. **C,** An apparent diffusion coefficient map shows restricted diffusion in parts of the mass (*arrow*), indicating high cellularity.

Brainstem Gliomas

Brainstem tumors account for up to 12% of all brain tumors in children.[3] Four types are described on MRI: focal, dorsal exophytic, cervicomedullary, and diffuse intrinsic brainstem glioma.

Diffuse Intrinsic Brain Stem Gliomas (Diffuse Pontine Gliomas)

Diffuse intrinsic brainstem gliomas account for up to 85% of all brainstem gliomas. They typically are centered in the pons and hence also are called diffuse pontine gliomas. Because persons with these tumors have a poor long-term survival, they are the focus of numerous clinical trials.[67]

Because of their location in the brainstem, these lesions previously were considered inoperable. However, with advances in neurosurgical techniques and new molecular analyses using very small amounts of tissue, biopsy of some of these lesions is now being reconsidered.[68]

On CT, pontine gliomas are hypodense or isodense. On MRI, these tumors are isointense to hypointense on

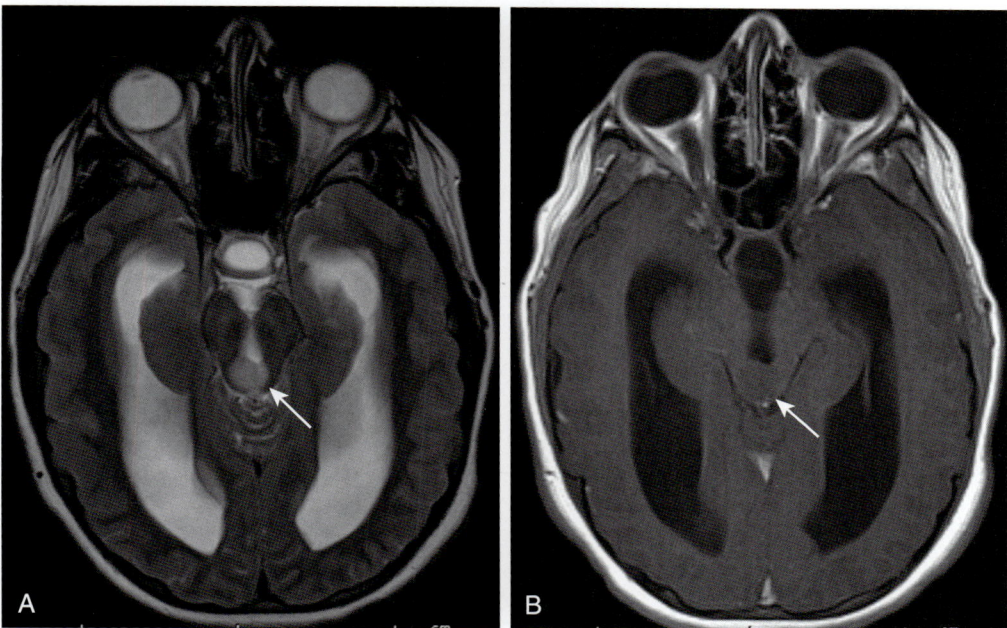

Figure 35-11   A tectal plate glioma. **A,** An axial T2-weighted image shows a hyperintense lesion (*arrow*) involving the tectum that is causing obstruction of the aqueduct. **B,** An axial postcontrast T1-weighted image shows the mass is T1-isointense to brain parenchyma (*arrow*) and does not enhance after administration of contrast material.

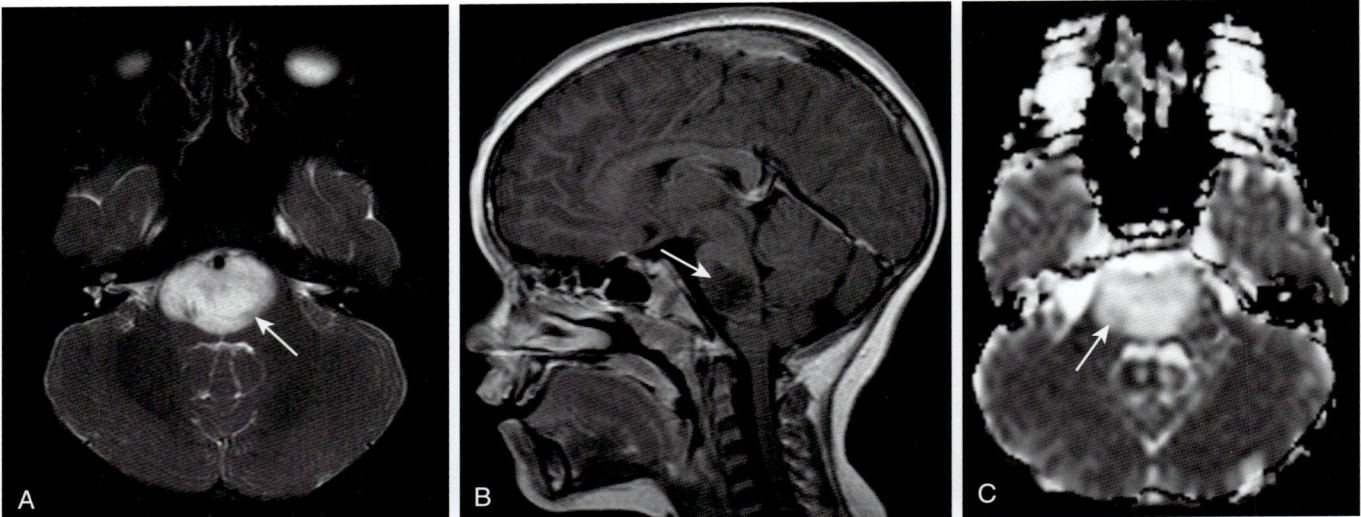

Figure 35-12. A diffuse intrinsic brainstem glioma. **A,** An axial T2-weighted image shows a rounded, hyperintense mass centered in the pons (*arrow*) surrounding the basilar artery and narrowing the pontine cistern. **B,** A postcontrast sagittal T1 image shows that the lesion does not enhance (*arrow*) after administration of contrast material. **C,** An apparent diffusion coefficient map shows increased diffusion within the lesion (*arrow*), a typical finding at initial presentation.

T1-weighted images and hyperintense on T2-weighted images (Fig. 35-12, *A*). Enhancement is minimal or absent at presentation in most patients (Fig. 35-12, *B*), but in the later stages of tumor progression, diffuse enhancement and necrosis may be present. Calcification or hemorrhage is rare.

MR spectroscopy has a potential value in determining tumor treatment response or failure. Decreases in choline : creatine and choline : NAA values are seen within responding tumors after initiating radiotherapy.[69] A recent MRS study has shown that increased choline : NAA on single voxel spectroscopy and increased maximum choline : NAA on chemical shift imaging are predictive of a shorter period of survival over time.[70]

On diffusion images, these tumors have increased ADC values (Fig. 35-12, *C*) and reduced FA at presentation, with reduced ADC after initiation of radiotherapy.[67,71,72] Increased ADC values are thought to be a result of a larger extracellular volume, possibly arising from a combination of vasogenic edema and a lower number of tumor cells.[73] Tumor enhancement generally is associated with a shorter survival time, lower tumor diffusion values (and thus increased cellularity), and a smaller drop in diffusion values after radiotherapy.[67] Diffusion tensor imaging depicts tracts that initially are infiltrated,[74] although not fully disrupted. Improved visualization of white matter tracts is apparent after radiation. As the tumor progresses, complete loss of anisotropy results; this effect may be due to tract infiltration or to possible tract disruption.[71] Survival in pediatric patients whose pontine glioma shows ^{18}F-FDG uptake of 50% or more on PET imaging is poorer than in children whose tumor demonstrates less than 50% of ^{18}F-FDG uptake.[75] Intense tracer uptake in the tumors, compared with gray matter, also suggests a decreased rate of survival.[75] Higher ^{18}F-FDG uptake within the tumor is associated with enhancement on MR images. Increased tumor cellularity, as reflected by restricted MRI diffusion, may be correlated with increased ^{18}F-FDG uniformity throughout the tumor.[75]

These tumors usually respond initially to radiation therapy, which has improved the median overall survival rate from weeks to months.[76] Unfortunately, adjuvant therapies (e.g., radiation sensitizers, differentiation agents, cytotoxic drugs, and molecularly targeted drugs) have not resulted in significantly improved patient outcomes.[76,77]

Atypical Teratoid Rhabdoid Tumor

Atypical teratoid/rhabdoid tumors (ATRTs) are highly malignant tumors with a peak incidence between birth and 3 years.[78] These tumors account for almost 10% of CNS tumors in children and approximately 1% to 2% of all pediatric brain tumors.[79] Nearly 60% of these tumors are seen in the posterior fossa at the cerebellopontine angle. However, supratentorial ATRTs also are seen frequently at additional sites in the CNS such as the spine, pineal, and suprasellar regions.[80]

ATRTs have been identified as being pathologically distinct entities from medulloblastomas and PNETs. This finding is supported by evidence of deletions or loss of material at chromosome 22q11.2, identification of the tumor suppressor gene *hSNF5/INI-1*, and germline and somatic mutations of *INI-1* in approximately 75% of cases of CNS ATRTs.[79]

Imaging appearances of ATRTs are similar to those of medulloblastomas; namely, they are isointense on T1-weighted images and have hypointense signal intensity on T2-weighted images (e-Fig. 35–13). Cystic areas are common. Because of their high cellularity, T2 hypointensity often is seen in the solid areas and is associated with restricted diffusion. Hemorrhage and calcification are not uncommon (e-Fig. 35–13, *A*).[81] Imaging of the entire neuroaxis is important, because subarachnoid spread throughout the CNS with spinal drop metastases is common, with frequency ranging between 25% and 46%.[82,83] ATRT survival rates historically have ranged from 0.5 to 11 months.[84] In recent years, the prognosis for these patients has improved with the availability of

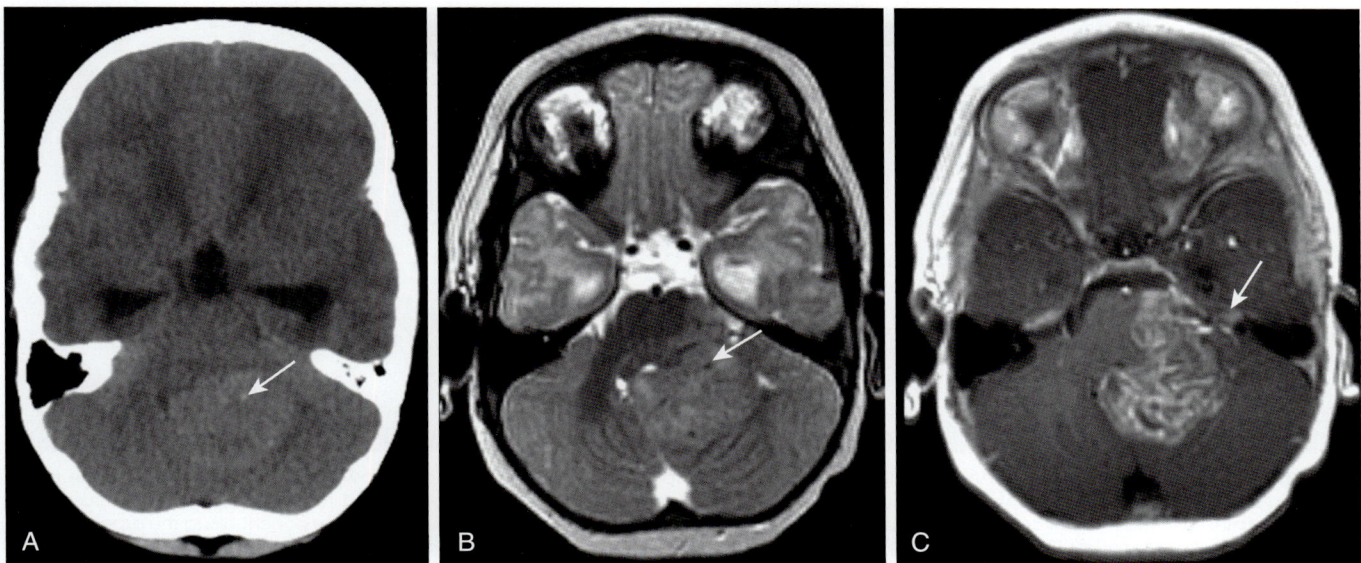

Figure 35-14 **An ependymoma. A,** An axial noncontrast computed tomography image shows a hyperdense mass lesion occupying the fourth ventricle and extending through the left foramen of Luschka. Note several tiny punctate areas of calcification (*arrow*). **B,** An axial T2-weighted image shows that the lesion (*arrow*) is isointense compared with gray matter. **C,** An axial postcontrast T1-weighted image shows heterogeneous enhancement of the lesion and its extension toward the left foramen of Luschka (*arrow*).

multimodality treatments. A small number of survivors of relapsed disease have been reported.[83,85]

Infratentorial Ependymomas

Infratentorial ependymomas constitute 8% to 15% of posterior fossa tumors in children. They arise from the ventricular ependymal lining and grow out of the fourth ventricle via the foramina of Luschka and Magendie into the cerebellopontine angles and cisternal spaces around the brainstem and cervicomedullary junction. These tumors are hypointense on T1-weighted images and isointense to gray matter on T2-weighted images. Up to 50% contain foci of calcification (Fig. 35-14, *A*). These lesions demonstrate heterogeneous enhancement on MRI (Fig. 35-14, *B* and *C*). Disseminated disease is present in 7% to 15% of patients with ependymomas at diagnosis.[86] In the posterior fossa, ependymomas demonstrate significantly higher ADC values than do medulloblastomas and lower ADC values than in astrocytomas.[87] These variations in ADC values may help differentiate tumors preoperatively and enable more effective treatment planning.

Among all prognostic factors, the extent of surgical resection is the most important. Complete surgical resection followed by other treatments has shown >80% disease-free survival after 3 years of follow-up.[88,89] Older age at presentation, along with favorable histologic grading, also may contribute to a better prognosis.[90]

PINEAL REGION TUMORS

Pineal tumors constitute between 3% and 8% of all pediatric brain tumors.[91] Pineal region tumors are divided into four categories: germ cell tumors, pineal cysts, pineal parenchymal tumors, and tumors of tissues supporting the pineal gland or adjacent structures (such as pineal gliomas, dermoids, and epidermoids).

Germ Cell Tumors

The most common tumors of the pineal region are germ cell tumors, of which 65% are pure germinomas.[92] Other variants such as nongerminomatous germ cell tumors, mixed germ cell tumors, teratomas and embryonal cell carcinomas, yolk sac tumors, and choriocarcinomas constitute the remainder.

Germinomas are hyperdense on CT and enhance homogenously. On MRI, these lesions have homogenous signal intensity that is isointense to gray matter on all sequences, with intense enhancement (Fig. 35-15). These tumors grow anteriorly into the floor of the third ventricle and may infiltrate the thalami and midbrain. Spinal dissemination is common (in up to 36% of cases).[93]

Imaging appearances of nongerminomatous germ cell tumors are nonspecific, with intratumoral cysts and calcifications being a relatively common finding. Teratomas are heterogeneous and contain fat, cysts, and calcification; they also demonstrate variable enhancement. The presence of hemorrhage is more suggestive of a choriocarcinoma.

Pineal Parenchymal Tumors

Pineocytomas are well-differentiated tumors that retain morphologic features of the pineal parenchymal cells. They are slow-growing tumors that are circumscribed but nonencapsulated. Pineocytomas are more commonly solid tumors, although cystic variants also have been described. Solid tumors are either T1 hypointense or isointense to gray matter and T2 hyperintense. Enhancement is homogeneous, and calcification is common. Cystic variants often are indistinguishable from pineal cysts.[94]

Pineoblastomas are malignant tumors that resemble PNETs, but they are distinct from PNETs in other locations because of their photosensory differentiation.[95] On MRI, these lesions are hypointense to isointense on T1-weighted

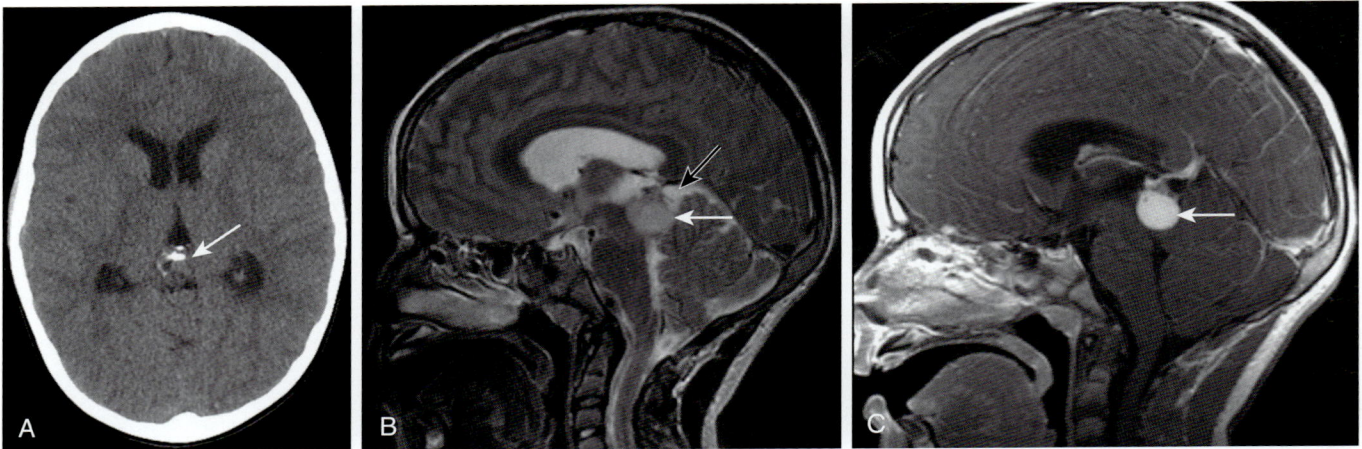

Figure 35-15 A pineal germinoma. **A,** An axial unenhanced computed tomography image shows a partially calcified lesion (*arrow*) in the pineal region. Note the presence of hydrocephalus resulting from third ventricular obstruction. **B,** A sagittal T2-weighted image shows a rounded mass (*white arrow*) hyperintense to gray matter centered in the pineal region. Note the presence of a cystic T2-hyperintense component along the superior aspect (*black arrow*). **C,** A postcontrast T1-weighted image shows homogeneous enhancement of the solid component (*arrow*) of the lesion.

images and demonstrate variable low, high, or mixed signal on T2-weighted images (e-Fig. 35-16). Pineoblastomas have lobulated contours, enhance homogenously, and calcify less often than pineocytomas. The "exploded pineal pattern" of calcification (characterized by peripheral displacement of pineal gland calcification) is more typical of pineal parenchymal tumors, effectively differentiating them from germ cell tumors.[96] Pineoblastomas are resected surgically with adjuvant craniospinal radiation and multiagent chemotherapy. The prognosis is relatively poor.[97]

Conclusion

Advances in neuroimaging coupled with the advances in molecular biology and neurosurgery during the past decade have improved our ability to detect, diagnose, characterize, and treat pediatric CNS tumors. It is important to recognize the typical features of each of these tumors on imaging studies, because recognition of the typical features forms the basis for further management. Accurate characterization of a tumor at presentation and its relation to eloquent areas of the brain can help plan immediate and, in some cases, long-term management. Our ability to make rapid and more accurate diagnoses of CNS tumors of childhood, design treatment regimens tailored to the individual patient, and enable improved assessment of treatment response and early detection of recurrence hinges, to a great extent, on continued technological improvements in imaging.

References

Full references for this chapter can be found on www.expertconsult.com.

Chapter 36

Cerebrovascular Disorders

RICHARD L. ROBERTSON and AMY R. DANEHY

Stroke is defined as a neurologic deficit persisting for more than 24 hours. Stroke may be caused by either cerebral ischemia or intracranial hemorrhage. The estimated annual incidence of stroke in children ranges from 2 to 13 per 100,000 person years and is among the top 10 causes of death in childhood.[1]

The presentation of stroke in children is sometimes heralded by the abrupt onset of a focal neurologic deficit, but often, especially in infants and young children, the symptoms are nonspecific and the diagnosis of stroke is frequently delayed. Although many children who have had a stroke recover completely, more than 75% will have a perceptible persistent neurologic deficit, and more than 40% will have major neurologic sequelae.[2]

Unlike adults, in whom hypertension, diabetes, smoking, and hypercholesterolemia are frequently identified as risk factors for the development of stroke, cerebrovascular arteriopathy, vascular anomalies, aneurysms, congenital heart disease, sickle cell disease, and hematologic abnormalities are among the most common predisposing conditions in children.[1] More than half of all strokes in children are ischemic, caused either by an intrinsic vasculopathy or emboli from a remote source.[2] Vascular malformations, aneurysms, and venous sinus thrombosis are the most common causes of hemorrhagic stroke. This chapter focuses on intrinsic vascular abnormalities as causes of ischemic and hemorrhagic pediatric stroke.

Arteriopathy

Ischemic stroke in children has an annual incidence of between 2 and 3 per 100,000 children in the United States.[3] The causes of ischemic stroke in children are diverse and include a variety of cerebrovascular entities in approximately 70% of children, such as arterial dissection, moyamoya disease or syndrome, sickle cell disease, isolated angiitis of the central nervous system or vasculitis, coagulopathy, or other known source; the remainder of cases are idiopathic in origin. More than one risk factor may be present. Twenty-five percent of children with ischemic stroke have coexistent cardiac disease.[2] Metabolic disorders, such as mitochondrial diseases and hyperhomocysteinemia, should be considered in the differential diagnosis of ischemic stroke in children, especially if the distribution of the infarction does not conform to an arterial territory.

The most common symptoms of ischemic stroke in children are hemiplegia, seizures, fever, dysphagia, headache, and altered level of consciousness. Headache and seizures are especially common in chronic ischemic conditions such as moyamoya disease.[4]

Imaging The imaging features of ischemic stroke in children are variable and depend on the underlying cause. In acute arterial dissection, an end arterial distribution infarction is often present on computed tomography (CT) or magnetic resonance imaging (MRI). By contrast, in proximal, chronic steno-occlusive disease such as moyamoya disease (Fig. 36-1), infarctions may be absent, conform to an arterial territory, or lie within the border zones between the major vascular territories. In chronic multivessel steno-occlusive disease, there may be a shift in the location of the vascular border zones because of differential involvement of the various branches of the circle of Willis.

Noninvasive vascular imaging such as computed tomographic angiography (CTA) or magnetic resonance angiography (MRA) typically shows an abrupt vascular cutoff with dissection and thromboembolic stroke. In moyamoya disease, stenosis or occlusion of the supraclinoid segment of the internal carotid and proximal middle or anterior cerebral artery is usually present, with numerous collateral vessels in the basal ganglia at certain stages of the disorder.[5] Vasculitis causes irregular narrowing of medium or small vessels and is inconsistently demonstrated on CTA or MRA.[6] Catheter angiography remains the gold standard for the imaging diagnosis of cerebrovascular disease in children and should be considered whenever a small vessel vasculitis is suspected or when surgical treatment is contemplated.

Vascular Anomalies

Vascular anomalies are disorders of vascular development. Although congenital, they may only become symptomatic many months or years after birth. Intracranial vascular malformations are classified according to the vascular channels

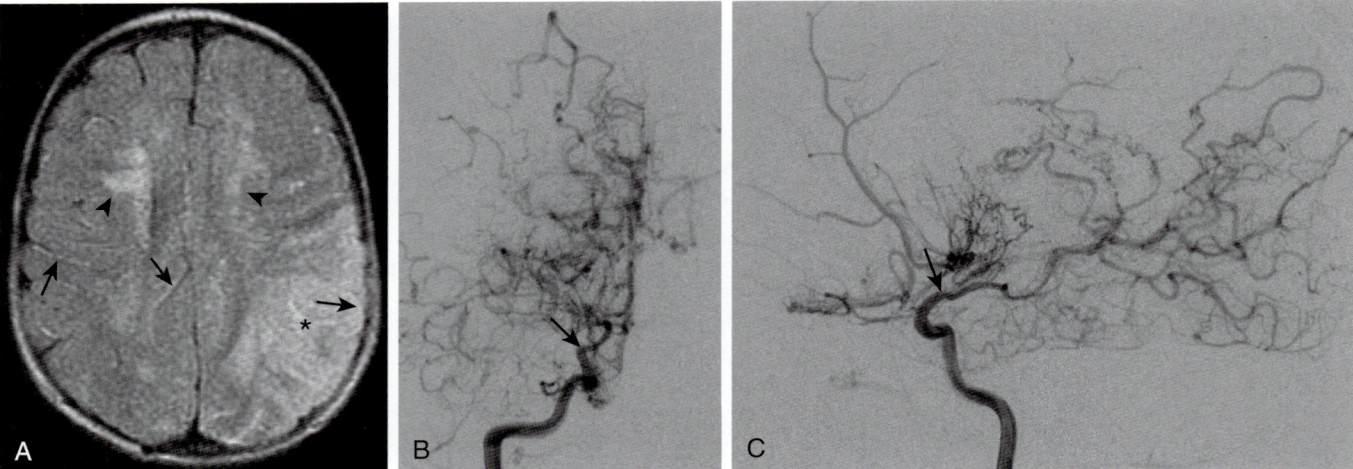

Figure 36-1 A 2½-year-old child presenting with new-onset right-sided hemiplegia and imaging findings of moyamoya disease. **A,** Axial fluid-attenuated inversion recovery magnetic resonance imaging scan shows a subacute infarct involving the left middle cerebral artery–posterior cerebral artery watershed territory (*asterisk*). There is periventricular white matter T2 prolongation due to chronic ischemic change (*arrowheads*). Linear sulcal signal abnormality is demonstrated bilaterally, consistent with slow flow (*arrows*) in leptomeningeal vessels. **B,** Frontal projection from digital subtraction angiogram shows severe steno-occlusive changes involving the distal right internal carotid artery (*arrow*), with occlusion of the middle and anterior cerebral arteries and multiple basal collaterals. **C,** Lateral projection again shows the distal tapering and occlusion of the supraclinoid internal carotid artery (*arrow*), multiple basal collaterals, and anterior shift of the posterior cerebral territory through pial collaterals to supply the posterior portions of the middle and anterior cerebral territories.

involved and the hemodynamics of the lesion (high-flow vs. low-flow).[7]

HIGH-FLOW VASCULAR ANOMALIES

High-flow vascular anomalies occur when there is an abnormal connection between an artery and a vein that bypasses the normal arteriolar–capillary network. In arteriovenous fistula (AVF), the supplying artery communicates directly with the draining vein through a macroscopic fistula. In arteriovenous malformation (AVM), the supplying artery

connects with the draining vein through a plexiform network of abnormal vessels, termed the *nidus*. Both AVF and AVM are further subdivided, on the basis of anatomic location, into dural, subarachnoid (vein of Galen malformation), pial, or parenchymal (Figs. 36-2, 36-3, and 36-5; e-Fig. 36-4).[7,8]

High-flow vascular malformations may produce symptoms and signs in several ways.[7,9,10] The presence of an abnormal connection between a supplying artery and a draining vein allows for potentially rapid blood flow through the anomaly. In the absence of venous outflow obstruction, the malformation may cause high-output cardiac failure due to the lack of

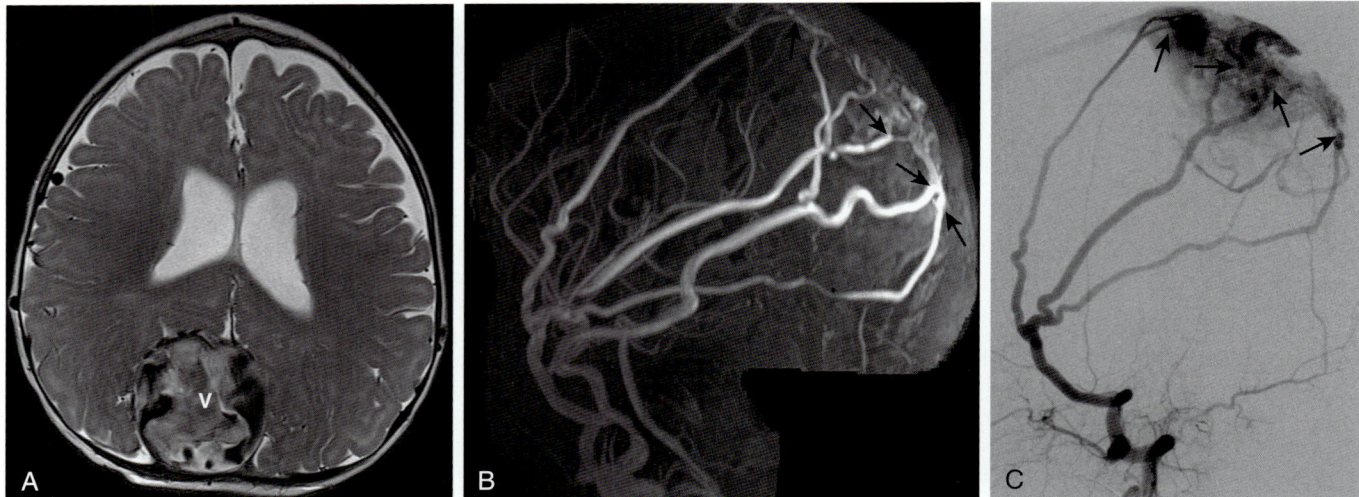

Figure 36-2 Five-month-old girl presenting with vomiting, lethargy, macrocephaly, and scalp vein distension with pulsating veins from dural arteriovenous fistula. **A,** Axial T2-weighted image shows an enlarged, partially thrombosed superior sagittal sinus (*V*). Also noted are prominent middle meningeal arterial branches along the dural surface bilaterally. **B,** Maximum intensity projection reconstruction of the two-dimensional coronal magnetic resonance imaging venogram shows bilaterally enlarged middle meningeal arteries with fistulae (*arrows*) to the dilated, partially thrombosed superior sagittal sinus. **C,** Digital subtraction angiogram—lateral projection demonstrates the dural arteriovenous fistulae with the markedly enlarged middle meningeal artery branches directly communicating through several fistulae (*arrows*) with the superior sagittal sinus near the torcular herophili.

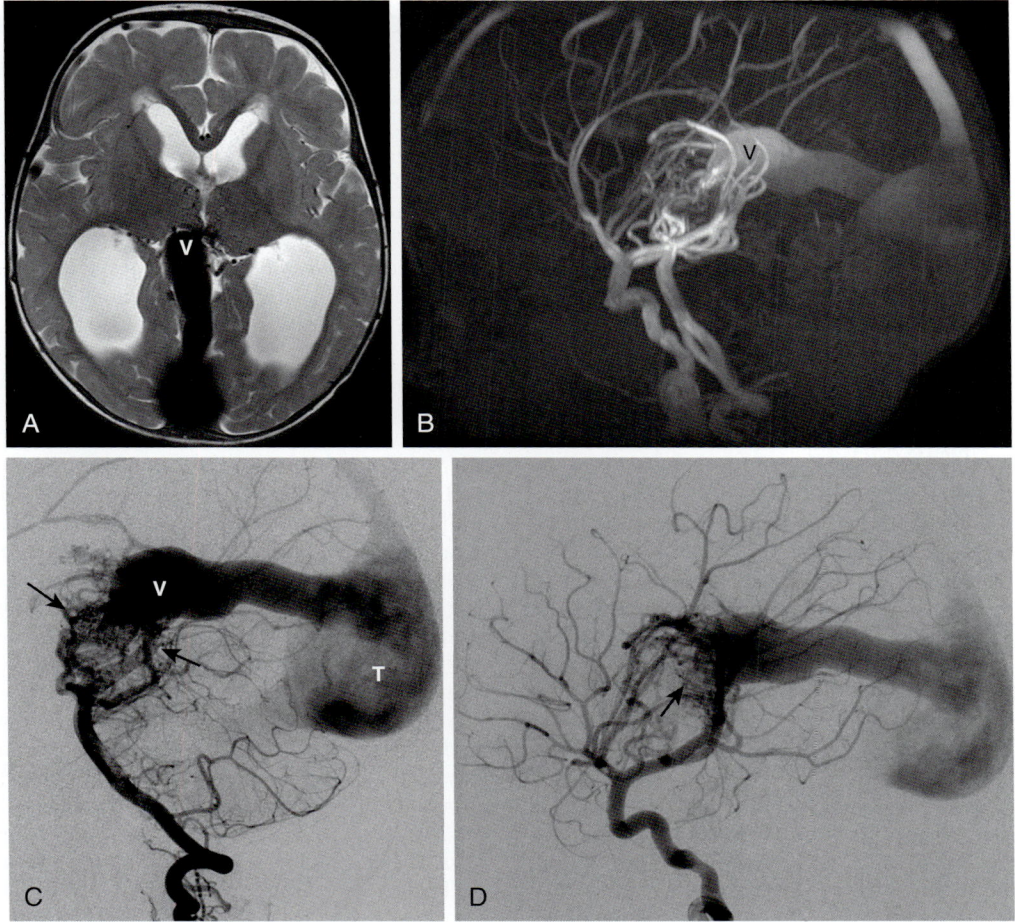

Figure 36-3 A 12-month-old child presenting with macrocephaly and developmental delay. Magnetic resonance imaging (MRI) revealed a vein of Galen malformation. **A,** Axial T2-weighted image shows a dilated median vein of the prosencephalon (*V*). The straight sinus and torcular herophili are enlarged. Multiple small serpinginous signal voids are present medially between the thalami from enlarged branches from a primitive arterial arcade. Hydrocephalus is present from venous hypertension. **B,** Sagittal maximum intensity projection from an MRI angiogram confirms a high-flow arteriovenous connection with marked flow related enhancement in the varix and draining sinuses. **C,** Digital subtraction angiogram—lateral view of the left vertebral artery injection shows enlarged left vertebral, basilar, and posterior cerebral arteries supplying a primitive arterial arcade with a vascular nidus of abnormal vessels draining into the enlarged prosencephalic vein. **D,** Lateral view of the right internal carotid artery injection demonstrates additional anterior circulation supply to the malformation (*arrow*).

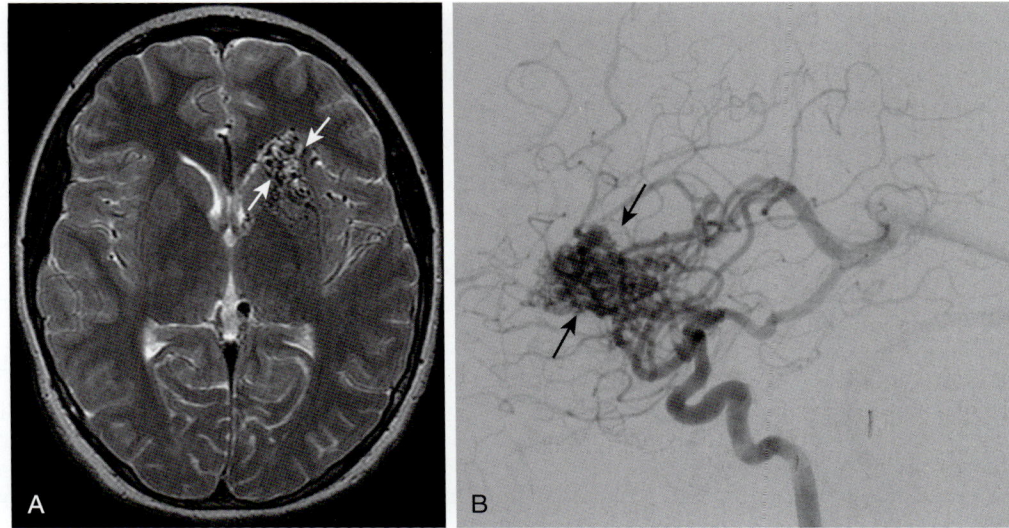

Figure 36-5 An 11-year-old girl presenting with severe headache, vomiting, and left leg weakness is found to have intraventricular hemorrhage and left frontal arteriovenous malformation. **A,** Axial T2-weighted image shows multiple signal voids in the left inferior frontal lobe involving the caudate head and basal ganglia. **B,** Lateral projection of a cerebral angiogram demonstrates the large vascular nidus (*arrows*) with early opacification of the internal cerebral veins and straight sinus.

regulation of blood flow through the normal arteriolar and capillary network. The lower resistance through the malformation may result in diversion of blood away from the normal brain parenchyma ("steal" phenomenon), producing cerebral ischemia. High-flow malformations also expose the draining veins to arterial pressure, which may cause progressive stenosis of the vein, termed *high-flow venopathy*. High-flow venopathy may be a cause of seizures or cerebral atrophy due to impaired tissue perfusion from a diminished arterial-venous pressure gradient. Hydrocephalus can develop from increased venous pressures, that result in impaired resorption of cerebrospinal fluid (CSF) (see Fig. 36-3, *A*). Elevated venous pressure can also result in the development of a varix that predisposes to hemorrhage.

DURAL HIGH-FLOW ANOMALIES

Dural AVF or AVM comprise a meningeal arterial supply with dural venous sinus drainage and often present in the prenatal or immediate postnatal period as a cause of fetal or neonatal heart failure (see Fig. 36-2).[7,10,11] The anomalies may include a single or multihole fistula or complex malformation. The abnormal connections are frequently located either in the vicinity or in the torcular herophili or involve dural venous sinuses that drain into the torcular herophili.

VEIN OF GALEN MALFORMATIONS

Vein of Galen malformations (VOGMs) consist of AVF or AVM deriving arterial supply from a primitive choroidal arcade and venous drainage through an aneurysmally dilated median vein of the prosencephalon, the embryologic precursor to the vein of Galen (see Fig. 36-3).[7,11,12] The symptoms, signs, and age at presentation associated with VOGMs depend on the angioarchitecture of the anomaly and the degree of venous outflow obstruction. VOGMs with numerous connections between the supplying arteries and the draining vein and without venous outflow obstruction typically produce congestive heart failure in the fetus or neonate due to the shunting of blood through the malformation. Chronic ischemic brain injury occurs from poor brain perfusion caused by arterial steal. Intracranial hemorrhage can occur from rupture of the varix. VOGMs with fewer arteriovenous connections often present later in infancy or childhood with hydrocephalus or brain atrophy caused by progressive stenosis of venous outflow and impaired parenchymal perfusion caused by a decreased arteriovenous pressure gradient (see Fig. 36-3).

PIAL HIGH-FLOW ANOMALIES

Pial AVF and AVM comprise a pial arterial supply with cortical venous drainage (see e-Fig. 36-4).[7] Pial AVFs or AVMs are rarely detected in the neonate and usually come to medical attention in late infancy or early childhood. The fistulous connections occur along the surface of the brain, resulting in marked dilation of the unsupported superficial cortical draining veins. The anomalies may consist of only a single-hole fistula or may be mixed AVF and AVM. Pial AVF or AVM may be asymptomatic for long periods, being discovered only incidentally on imaging performed for other reasons, or the high-flow anomaly may be a cause of catastrophic intracranial hemorrhage.

PARENCHYMAL HIGH-FLOW ANOMALIES

Intraparenchymal AVMs, like pial anomalies, derive their arterial supply from either the anterior or posterior cerebral circulation (see Fig. 36-5). Parenchymal AVMs usually present after infancy, most often as a cause of intracranial hemorrhage.[7,9,10] The angioarchitecture of these anomalies is often less complex than that of similar malformations in adults, although extensive lobar malformations are occasionally encountered. Intranidal aneurysms and varices occur commonly; however, aneurysmal dilation of the supplying arteries is much less frequent than in adults.

Imaging   Imaging in high-flow vascular malformations is directed toward delineation of the vascular anomaly and demonstration of complications. Dural and VOGM AVFs or AVMs may be diagnosed in utero on either obstetrical sonography or fetal MRI.[7,8,11] Fetal ultrasound or MRI of dural AVF or AVM shows an off-midline vascular mass with enlarged meningeal arteries. Fetal ultrasound or MRI of VOGM demonstrates a midline vascular mass, with obvious increased flow in the supplying arteries and draining veins on color Doppler examination. In dural AVF or AVM as well as VOGM, fetal cardiomegaly and congestive heart failure with hydrops may be present. In addition to showing the vascular mass, fetal and postnatal MRI scans may show T1 shortening in the white matter, indicating chronic ischemic brain injury. Postnatal CT is now used less frequently to evaluate high-flow anomalies in the neonate but may show chronic ischemic brain injury with loss of gray/white matter contrast and parenchymal calcification, in addition to the vascular anomaly.

Treatment of dural malformations and VOGMs is typically performed via an endovascular approach.[9,10,13] Successful treatment of the anomaly requires occlusion of the arteriovenous connection. AVFs may be treated by placement of coils across the lesion, whereas closure of AVMs requires obliteration of the nidus and is best accomplished by using a liquid embolic agent.[10,13] Pial and parenchymal malformations are often treated with endovascular embolization, surgical resection, or combined preoperative embolization, followed by surgical resection.[9,10,13] Malformations that are not surgically accessible may be treated by using endovascular techniques or focused radiation therapy, including proton beam treatment.[14,15]

LOW-FLOW VASCULAR ANOMALIES

Low-flow vascular anomalies include capillary telangiectasias, cavernomas, and developmental venous anomalies (DVAs).[16-21] Each of these entities consists of a malformed, endothelial-lined, blood-filled vascular structure.

Capillary Telangiectasia

Capillary telangiectasias are composed of dilated capillaries and are found most frequently within the pontine tegmentum (e-Fig. 36-6).[16-18] Capillary telangiectasias are usually clinically silent and are noted incidentally on imaging performed for other reasons. Rare cases of pontine hemorrhage in which no cause is determined may be caused by capillary telangiectasia.

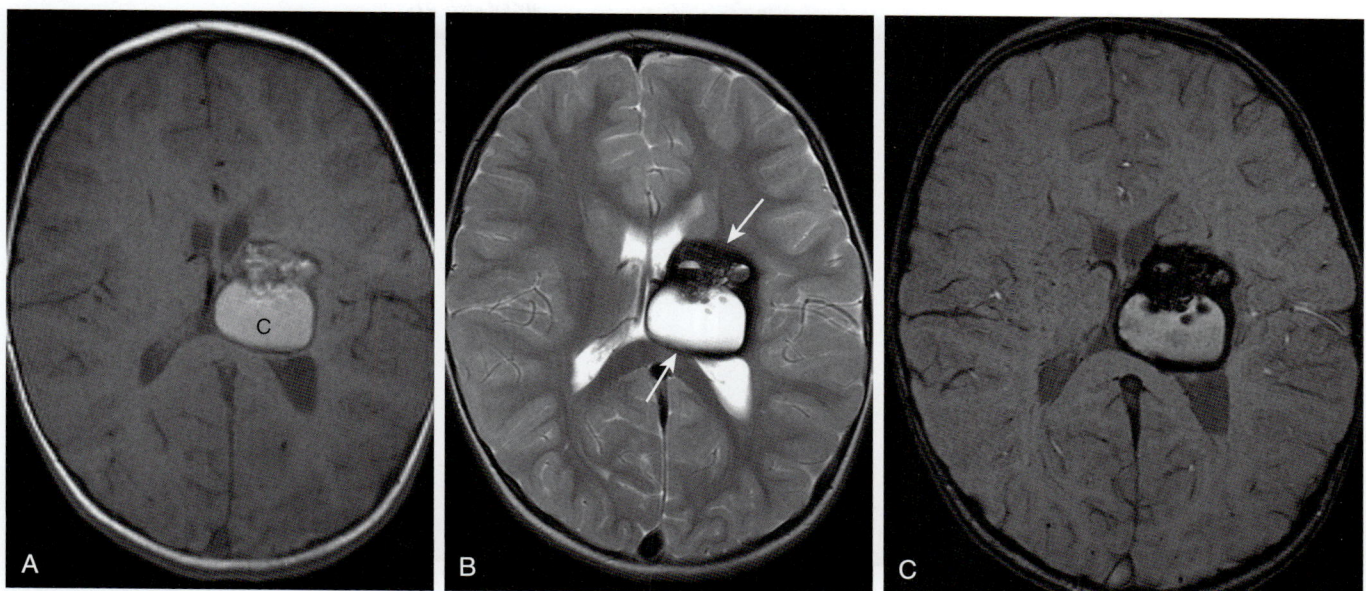

Figure 36-7 A 3-year-old presenting with early left hand preference and speech delay. Magnetic resonance imaging revealed a large cavernoma involving the left basal ganglia and the thalamus. **A,** Axial T1-weighted image reveals a large heterogeneous lesion with areas of T1 shortening suggestive of blood products. **B,** Axial T2-weighted image demonstrates a low signal intensity rim of hemosiderin (*arrows*) surrounding the lesion. **C,** Susceptibility-weighted sequence demonstrates "blooming" of the susceptibility artifact from hemosiderin.

Imaging On imaging, capillary telangiectasia is typically not apparent on noncontrast imaging or appears as a faint focus of T2 prolongation without an associated mass effect. Following the administration of contrast, subtle enhancement is seen.

Cavernoma

Cavernomas are localized collections of venous blood.[18-21] Cavernomas can occur in isolation (Fig. 36-7) but may also occur very close to DVAs, which suggests a venous origin. Cavernomas may be single or multiple; when multiple, they may be familial, or they may develop in response to radiation therapy for treatment of neuro-oncologic disease.[8,21] Cavernomas may be discovered incidentally on imaging or may produce symptomatic intracranial hemorrhage or symptoms due to the mass effect. Pediatric cavernomas behave more aggressively compared with their adult counterparts and are two to three times more likely to hemorrhage.[21]

Imaging On imaging, small cavernomas are typically occult or very subtle on spin-echo imaging but appear as foci of signal voids on long echo, gradient echo, or susceptibility-weighted imaging because of the presence of the magnetic susceptibility effects from associated blood products (see Fig. 36-7).[8] Larger lesions are centrally hyperintense on T1-weighed and T2-weighted imaging, with a hypointense rim from the deposition of hemosiderin around the margin of the lesion. Cavernomas are usually found within the brain parenchyma but are occasionally superficial and exophytic, simulating an extra-axial mass.

Developmental Venous Anomaly

DVAs are abnormal veins typically draining normal brain parenchyma. The usual appearance of a DVA is of a cluster of medullary veins radially arranged around the end of an abnormally dilated collecting vein (Fig. 36-8).[19,22] DVAs may be small or provide the entire venous drainage for a cerebral lobe or hemisphere. DVAs are usually asymptomatic and discovered incidentally but are occasionally associated with intracranial hemorrhage, especially when associated with a cavernoma. Intracranial DVAs may be seen in association with venous malformation or other vascular anomalies of the scalp and face.[22] DVAs are occasionally identified in association with cortical malformations in the evaluation of seizures.[23]

Imaging On contrast-enhanced CT or MRI, DVAs are seen as multiple enhancing medullary veins draining into a single collecting vein; an appearance often referred to as the *caput medusa* (see Fig. 36-8). DVAs are also visible on catheter angiography and should opacify with contrast at the same time as normal intracerebral veins.[19,22]

Aneurysms

Intracranial aneurysms in children are a heterogeneous group of diseases and differ in many respects from aneurysms in adults.[24-26] Aneurysms are much less common in children than in adults. Pediatric aneurysms account for less than 5% of all aneurysms and are rare in the first year of life.[25,27,28] Intracranial aneurysms in children are more likely to be fusiform, involve the posterior circulation, and be larger at the time of presentation than in adults.[25] Symptoms of mass effect are at

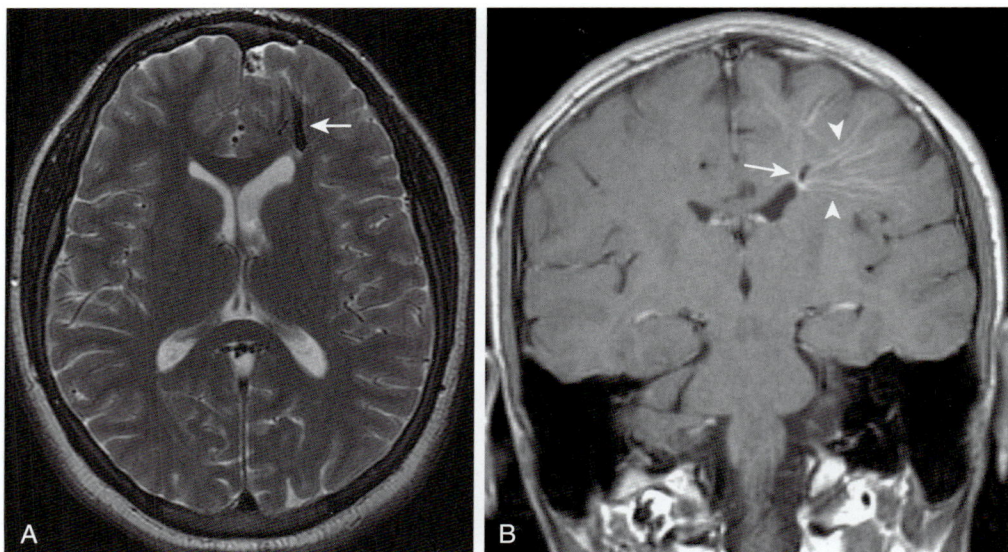

Figure 36-8 A 15-year-old with remote history of trauma presenting with increasing headaches. **A,** Axial T2-weighted magnetic resonance imaging scan shows a prominent intraparenchymal dilated vein in the anterior left frontal lobe (*arrow*). **B,** Postcontrast coronal T1-weighted images shows the cluster of radially arranged medullary veins (*arrowheads*), the "caput medusa," associated with the abnormally dilated collecting vein (*arrow*) of a developmental venous anomaly.

least as common as those from subarachnoid hemorrhage. Aneurysms in children, especially those that are giant or fusiform, may also be discovered incidentally on neuroimaging performed for unrelated reasons. Unlike in adults, in whom aneurysms show a female predominance, in children, boys are more likely to be affected than girls.[25] Comorbidities such as collagen vascular disease, polycystic kidney disease, dwarfism, moyamoya disease, and infections are present with roughly 25% of intracranial aneurysms in children.[25,29]

Saccular aneurysms, the most common form in adults, tend to occur at vessel bifurcations and are believed to be caused by chronic hemodynamic stress on the vessel wall (Fig. 36-9).[25] However, because of the time required for vascular stresses to have an effect, saccular aneurysms are much less common in children. Saccular aneurysms tend to occur most frequently at the origin of the posterior communicating artery but are also found at the origin of the anterior communicating artery and basilar artery bifurcation in children. Saccular aneurysms can cause subarachnoid hemorrhage but can also present with symptoms of local mass effect.

Fusiform aneurysms can be congenital or caused by vessel dissection.[25,30] Common sites of involvement in children include the supraclinoid internal carotid artery, the proximal

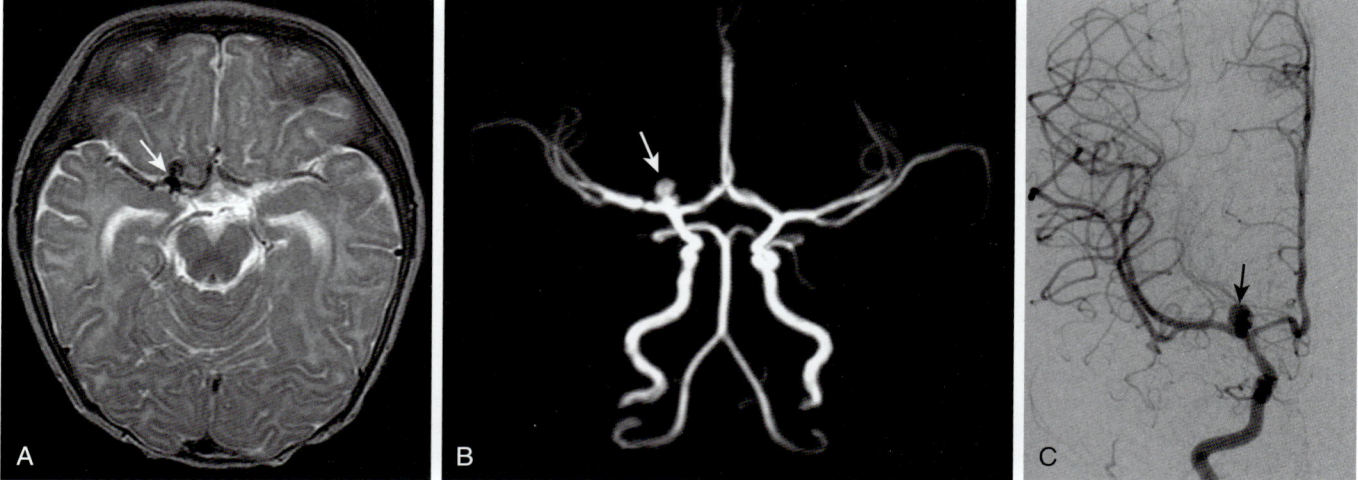

Figure 36-9 A 5-month-old girl who presented with new-onset seizure is found to have aneurysmal subarachnoid hemorrhage on computed tomography. **A,** Axial T2-weighted magnetic resonance imaging demonstrates a region of signal void (*arrow*) near the right internal carotid artery–middle cerebral artery bifurcation. **B,** Time-of-flight magnetic resonance angiography demonstrates flow-related enhancement in a lobulated saccular aneurysm (*arrow*) involving the proximal M1 segment of the right middle cerebral artery. **C,** The saccular aneurysm (*arrow*) is confirmed on the frontal view from a right internal carotid artery injection on catheter angiography.

middle cerebral artery, and the basilar artery. Fusiform aneurysms are more likely to result in symptoms due to mass effect (e-Fig. 36-10) but can also result in subarachnoid hemorrhage, particularly when vessel dissection is the underlying cause.

Mycotic aneurysms tend to occur along distal vascular segments.[24,25] Aneurysms caused by infections are likely to lead to subarachnoid hemorrhage and may increase in size or number rapidly in children. Posttraumatic aneurysms may also occur in distal vascular segments.

Imaging   CT is often the first neuroimaging study performed when an intracranial aneurysm is suspected. Subarachnoid, intraventricular, or parenchymal hemorrhage may be seen on non–contrast-enhanced CT. In giant aneurysms, a hyperdense mass in proximity to the parent artery is typically evident.[8] CTA with dynamic imaging during the intravenous administration of contrast with multidimensional reformatting may be used to delineate the relationship of the aneurysm to the parent vessel, the size of the neck of the aneurysm, intra-aneurysmal thrombus, and potential collateral vessels, all factors important in treatment planning.

MRI and MRA are also frequently used in the evaluation of intracranial aneurysms.[8] On MRI, the aneurysm may appear as a localized signal void, adjacent to an intracranial vessel or as a fusiform expansion of the vascular signal void. Giant aneurysms may have a lamellated appearance, with alternating areas of T1 shortening and signal void because of the presence of both thrombus and intra-aneurysmal flow. Artifacts from vascular pulsation may be present adjacent to the aneurysm in the phase encode direction of the images (e-Fig. 36-10, *A*). MRA can be used, in a similar fashion to CTA, to visualize the features of the aneurysm relevant to endovascular or surgical treatment planning. Unlike CTA, MRA does not use ionizing radiation and can therefore be performed without the administration of intravenous contrast; however, it is often limited by flow artifacts in high-flow lesions.

Catheter angiography remains the gold standard for the evaluation of intracranial aneurysms and is often performed with the intent of endovascular treatment during the procedure.[22,26] Catheter angiography, especially when combined with rotational imaging, generally shows the anatomic features of the aneurysm as clearly as, or better than, CTA and has the advantage of providing information on the hemodynamics of the aneurysm.

Key Points

Pediatric stroke can be caused by either cerebral ischemia or intracranial hemorrhage.

The presenting symptoms of stroke in children are frequently nonspecific, which often results in delay in diagnosis and initiation of therapy.

The majority of children with stroke will have a persistent neurologic deficit on follow-up.

Ischemic infarctions may be in an arterial territory or in a vascular border zone distribution, depending on the nature of the underlying vasculopathy.

Vascular anomalies are classified on the basis of hemodynamics, angioarchitecture, and anatomic location.

Aneurysms are less common in children than in adults and may come to clinical attention because of either subarachnoid hemorrhage or symptoms of local mass effect.

Suggested Readings

Amlie-Lefond C, Bernard TJ, Buillaume S, et al. Predictors of cerebral arteriopathy in children with arterial ischemic stroke: Results of the International Pediatric Stroke Study. *Circulation.* 2009;119:1417-1423.

Carvalho KS, Garg BP. Arterial strokes in children. *Neurol Clin.* 2002;20:1079-1100.

Jordan LC, Hillis AE. Hemorrhagic stroke in children. *Pediatr Neurol.* 2007;36:73-80.

Niazi TN, Klimo P, Anderson RC, et al. Diagnosis and management of arteriovenous malformations in children. *Neurosurg Clin North Am.* 2010;21:443-456.

References

Full references for this chapter can be found on www.expertconsult.com.

Chapter 37

Stroke

P. ELLEN GRANT and KATYUCIA DE MACEDO RODRIGUES

Stroke is an important cause of mortality and long-term neurologic morbidity in children. In the pediatric age group, it is defined as a cerebrovascular event occurring between 14 weeks of gestation and 18 years of life. It ranks among the top 10 causes of death in children,[1] with the highest incidence observed in the perinatal period. It occurs in approximately 25 per 100,000 live births in the neonatal population and in 2 to 3 per 100,000 in children between 30 days and 18 years. Recurrence is estimated to be around 3% to 5% in neonates and ranges from 20% to 40% in older children. Among those who survive, more than 50% progress to the development of permanent neurologic or cognitive sequelae.[2] The required treatment and rehabilitation programs usually result in a large economic burden to the family and society (Box 37-1).

The reported incidence of pediatric stroke has been on the rise, perhaps because of increased awareness among medical professionals, but also because of improved diagnostic imaging techniques. In the past, infectious processes such as meningitis often were found, but today congenital heart disease, sickle cell anemia, extracranial carotid dissection, and thrombophilia constitute most cases. Even though it often is possible to identify more than one risk factor, in approximately 50% of cases, a definite cause remains undetermined. Clinical management of children who have had a stroke remains controversial, despite the fact that treatment algorithms have been established for adults.

Fetal Stroke

Fetal stroke occurs between 14 weeks of gestation until the onset of labor. Because of the lack of maternal or otherwise detectable fetal symptoms, the true incidence of fetal stroke is unknown; usually it is only diagnosed incidentally by antenatal ultrasound performed late in the second trimester or in the third trimester. Sometimes a fetal stroke is detected only during the neonatal period or later in life when developmental delays become perceptible.

Maternal, placental, and fetal risk factors have been reported, but in more than 50% of cases, no obvious cause is found. The common maternal conditions associated with fetal stroke are alloimmune thrombocytopenia, diabetes, anticoagulant or antiepileptic therapy, and trauma. Placental factors include placental hemorrhage, abruption, and thromboemboli.[3] It is unclear whether coagulopathy is a risk factor, but a case of fetal protein C deficiency has been reported.

Intraparenchymal hemorrhage, cerebral cavitary lesions, and ventriculomegaly are common findings on antenatal ultrasound. These findings are not specific for the type of stroke; however, the location of the injury and the distribution (arterial or venous) may suggest an underlying mechanism. Acute injury and small ischemic lesions can be difficult to detect with ultrasound.

Once an abnormality is found on a prenatal ultrasound examination, fetal magnetic resonance imaging (MRI) usually is performed; it is the imaging modality of choice for assessing fetal brain injury (Fig. 37-1). Hemorrhagic lesions have been reported in more than 90% of cases, compared with porencephalic cysts, which are reported in 10% of cases. Arterial ischemic stroke (AIS) typically involves the major arterial territories, most commonly the middle cerebral artery (MCA). Arterial ischemic insults occurring in the second trimester can cause cortical disorganization, resulting in polymicrogyria. If fetal hemorrhagic strokes are similar in origin to the vast majority of preterm and term hemorrhages, it is likely that many fetal hemorrhagic strokes are venous strokes. When tissue destruction occurs as a result of a fetal stroke, the type of tissue response identified on postnatal imaging can help determine the time of the intrapartum event. Porencephalic cysts lack a surrounding astroglial response and develop with injuries between 22 and 27 weeks of gestation. Thereafter, cystic encephalomalacia with gliosis is seen on pathology and MRI. Unlike in neonates and adults, diffusion-weighted imaging (DWI) may not be reliable in predicting the approximate date of an event.[4]

Finally, although a fetal stroke is often subclinical, strokes identified by prenatal screening are typically large and result in death or an adverse neurodevelopmental outcome in more than three quarters of cases.

Perinatal or Neonatal Stroke

Perinatal or neonatal stroke is an event that occurs between the late third trimester and the first month of life. The pathophysiology is complex and typically multifactorial. Recently, prothrombotic abnormalities of the coagulation pathway have been of particular interest because of the evolving role and potential use of antithrombotic agents for both treatment and prevention.[5]

It is important to differentiate ischemic stroke from hypoxic-ischemic injury, even though both can coexist, because management and prognosis can be different.

Box 37-1 Causes of Pediatric Stroke

Arterial Ischemic Stroke
Cardiac
- Congenital heart disease
- Valvular heart disease
- Neoplasm, myxomas
- Cardiac surgery
- Myocarditis, cardiomyopathy

Cerebral Vasculopathy
- Infection (e.g., meningitis)
- Collagen vascular disease (e.g., systemic lupus erythematosus, giant cell arteritis, Takayasu arteritis, Kawasaki arteritis)
- Primary angitis of the central nervous system
- Viral infection (e.g., varicella)
- Trauma, dissection

Disorders of Coagulation
- Protein C or S deficiency
- Antithrombin III deficiency
- Anticardiolipin antibodies
- Lupus anticoagulant
- Dysfibrinogenemia
- Polycythemia and hyperviscosity

Moyamoya Disease
- Idiopathic/familial (Japanese)
- Secondary (e.g., sickle cell disease)
- Neurofibromatosis type 1
- Radiation vasculopathy

Inborn Errors of Metabolism
- Fabry disease
- Hyperhomocysteinemia
- Ehlers-Danlos syndrome (type IV)

Sinovenous Thrombosis
- Infection of the head and neck
- Dehydration
- Hypercoagulable states
- Chemotherapeutic agents
- Iatrogenic

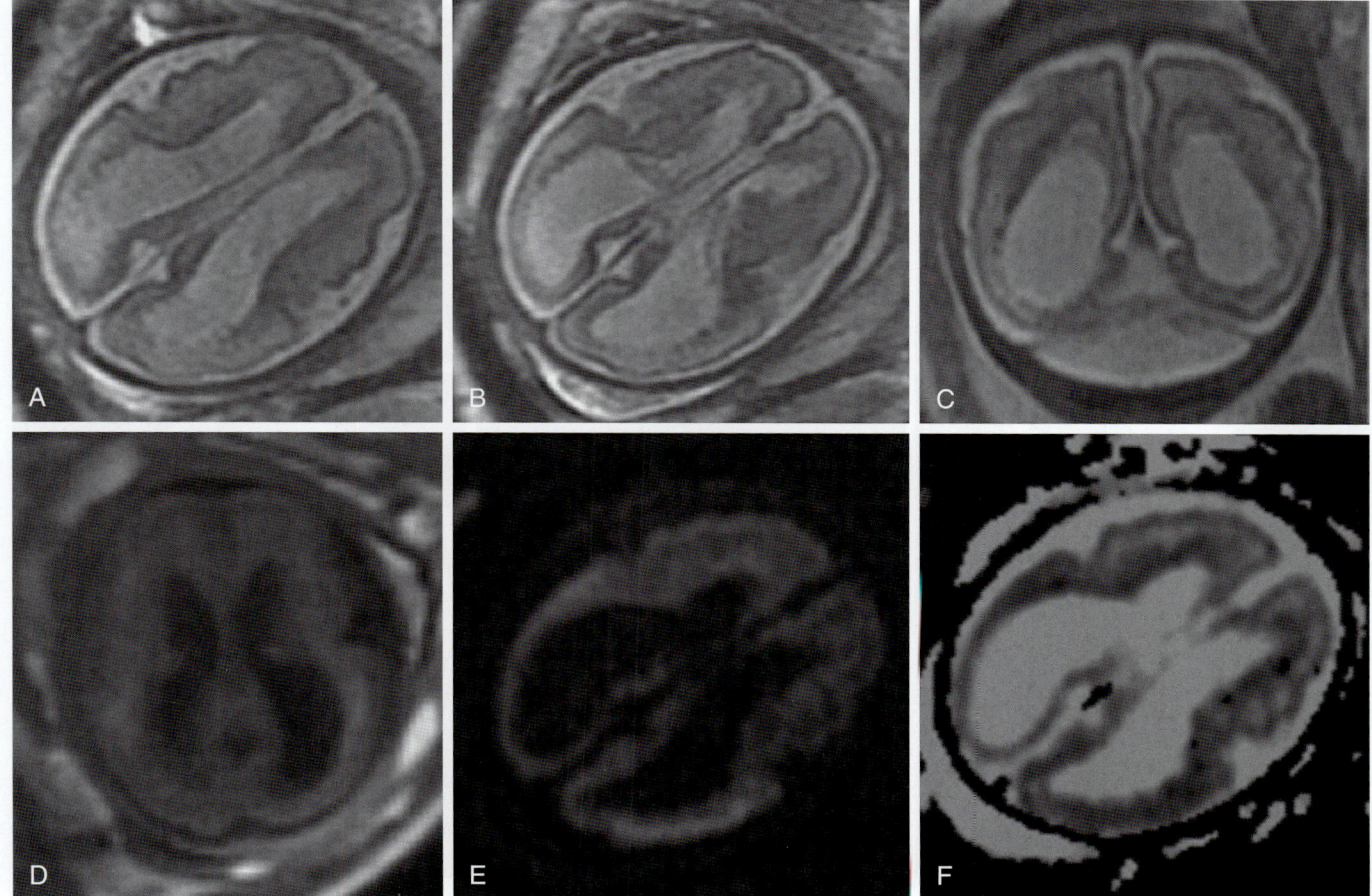

Figure 37-1 Fetal stroke. A 30-year-old woman underwent a magnetic resonance imaging scan after fetal ventriculomegaly was found on a routine prenatal ultrasound at 29 weeks' gestational age. **A, B,** and **C,** T2-weighted images show dilatation of the lateral ventricles associated with T2 prolongation, thinning, and irregularity of the periatrial white matter. **D,** T1-weighted image. **E,** Diffusion-weighted image. **F,** Apparent diffusion coefficient map. Reduced diffusion also is observed within the periventricular white matter, suggesting evolving ischemic necrosis.

ARTERIAL ISCHEMIC STROKE

Perinatal AIS leads to focal ischemic necrosis in an arterial distribution, most commonly in the MCA territory. The cause is undetermined in more than half of all cases. In the remainder of cases, the source of the thromboemboli may be an intracranial or extracranial vessel, the heart, or the placenta. An increased incidence of dehydration and sepsis also is found, along with cardiac and coagulation disorders.[2] AIS may be clinically subtle, and newborns often present with seizures without encephalopathy 2 to 3 days after birth. At the time of clinical presentation, ultrasound of the head can be have false-negative results. Computed tomography (CT) can detect hemorrhage and areas of advanced infarction but also may have false-negative results. Furthermore, ionizing radiation exposure is discouraged in neonates. Acute AIS is easily identified on MRI as regions of bright signal on DWI and decreased signal on apparent diffusion coefficient (ADC) maps within a vascular territory. The reduction in ADC values results from the presence of acute ischemic necrosis and the associated physiologic changes, such as cellular swelling, increased tortuosity of the extracellular space, decreased intracellular cytosolic streaming, and increased intracellular viscosity. The reduction in ADC can persist for up to 2 weeks, being more conspicuous during the first 4 days.[6]

On T2-weighted images, subtle loss of gray-white matter differentiation often is identified, although it may be negative within the first hours after clinical presentation. MR angiography (MRA) may be helpful in excluding complete occlusion of a major intracranial artery, but turbulent or fast flow often can result in signal dropout, which generates a concern for partially occlusive thrombus in this clinical context. Cerebral perfusion can be obtained using arterial spin labeling. This technique uses arterial blood water magnetically labeled by a radiofrequency pulse to obtain cerebral blood flow measurements; it does not require intravenous injection of contrast media (see Chapter 28). This technique can be particularly useful in determining the presence of reperfusion in areas of abnormal ADC (Fig. 37-2).[7]

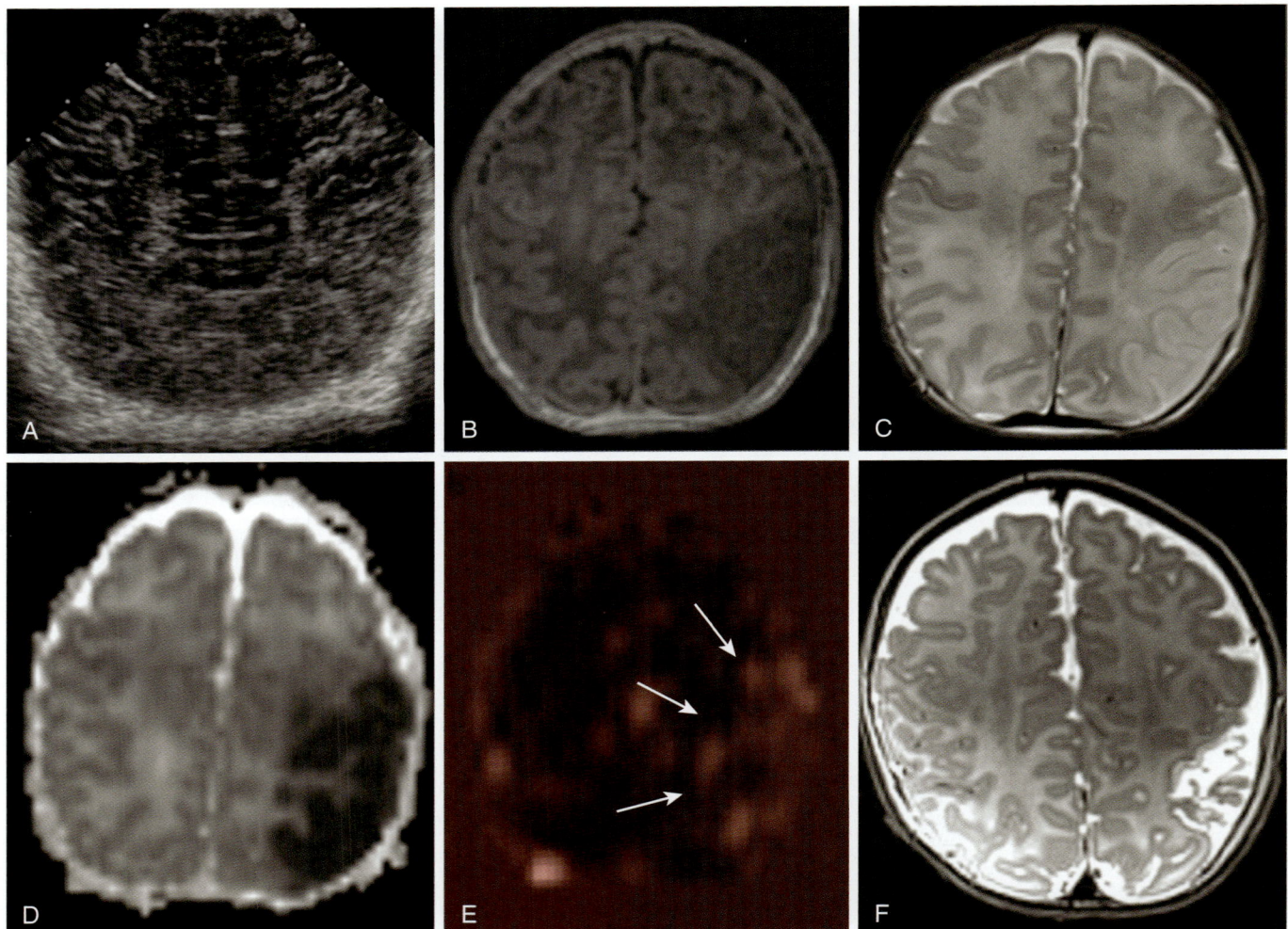

Figure 37-2 **Neonatal stroke.** A 1-day-old full-term infant with seizures. **A,** Ultrasound of the head shows normal cerebral architecture. A magnetic resonance imaging scan performed 10 hours later shows edema (**B,** T1-weighted image; **C,** T2-weighted image) and decreased diffusion (**D,** apparent diffusion coefficient map) involving gray and white matter in the left middle cerebral artery (MCA) territory. Perfusion-weighted images demonstrate relative increased blood flow in the same region (*arrows* in **E,** arterial spin labeling). A follow-up T2-weighted image at 3 months (**F**) shows encephalomalacic changes and volume loss within the area of the prior MCA territory infarct.

Ultrasound of the head combined with color and pulsed Doppler imaging remains a useful technique to evaluate the circle of Willis, in particular the regions of signal loss on MRA. If an intraluminal clot is identified or confirmed, bedside Doppler imaging can be used to monitor for recanalization and decreases in resistive indices that may occur as a result of secondary hyperperfusion.

In two thirds of patients, neurologic deficits with hemiplegia develop if the posterior limb of the internal capsule, motor strip, or basal ganglia is involved on the initial studies.

On long-term follow-up, regions of AIS can evolve into regions of volume loss, glial scarring, or cystic encephalomalacia, depending on the severity of the injury.

AIS also can develop as a result of bacterial meningitis as inflammatory cells infiltrate the vessel wall, leading to foci of necrosis that incite thrombosis of the arteries or veins coursing through the infected space (Fig. 37-3).

VENOUS STROKE

Venous strokes are associated with vasogenic edema, hemorrhage, and ischemic necrosis in a venous distribution. A venous stroke can occur as a result of transient mechanical or thrombotic occlusion of a vein or venous sinus. Newborns present with nonspecific symptoms related to increased intracranial pressure, lethargy, or seizures. A significant proportion of neonatal sinovenous thrombosis (SVT) is classified as idiopathic, but risk factors include dehydration, sepsis, asphyxia, maternal diabetes, and thrombophilia.[8] Isolated SVT has a good prognosis, except in rare cases when the deep venous system becomes involved.

CT may show a hyperdense clot in the involved vein or venous sinus and can identify intraventricular hemorrhage seen with involvement of the deep venous system. MRI is the preferred modality for confirming the diagnosis and

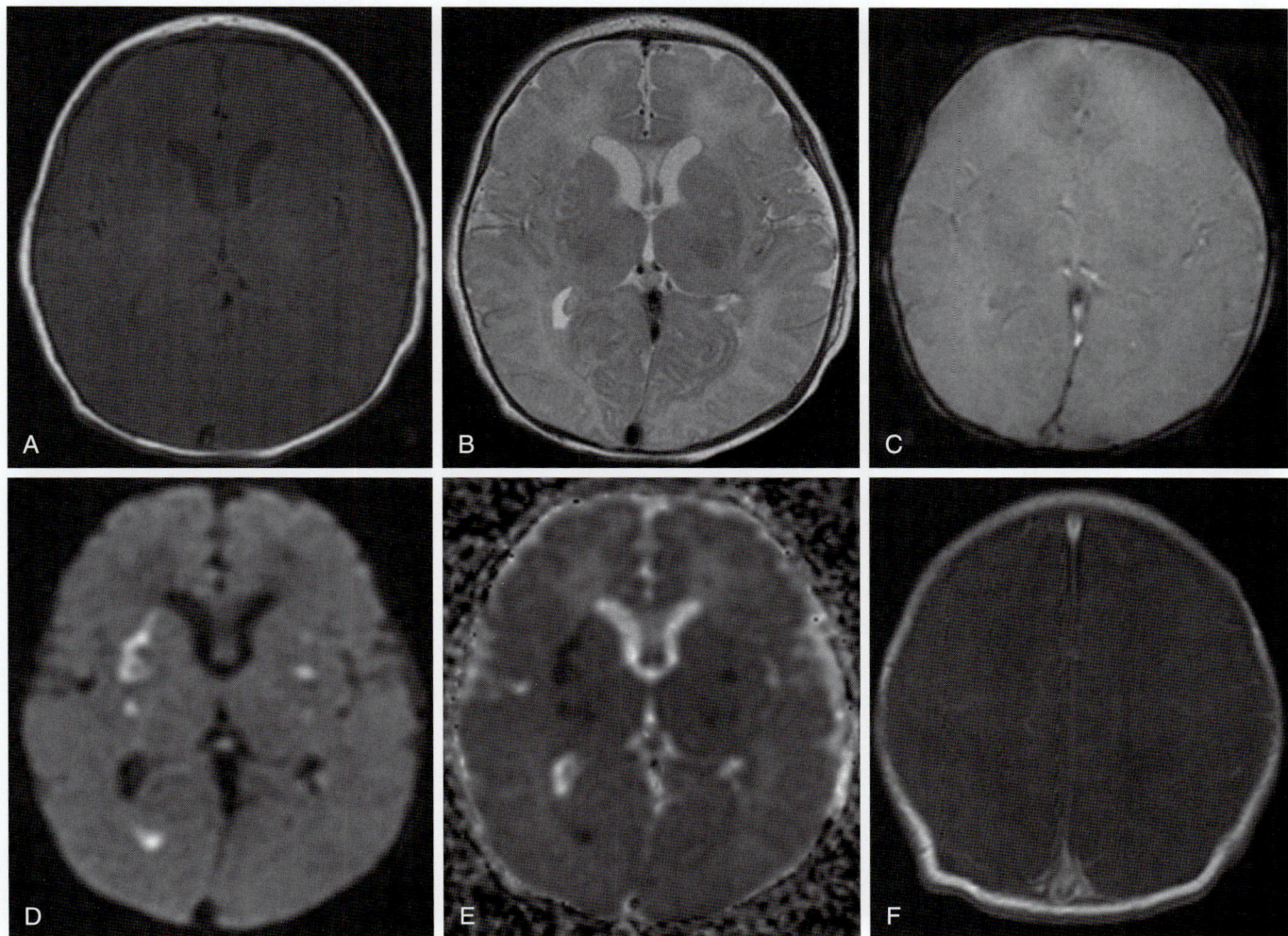

Figure 37-3 Postinfectious arteritis. A 5-day-old girl with group B streptococcus meningitis (**A,** T1-weighted image; **B,** T2- weighted image; **C,** T2 planar gradient recalled; **D,** diffusion-weighted image; **E,** apparent diffusion coefficient map; **F,** postcontrast T1-weighted image). Small regions of T2 signal abnormality and bilateral foci of decreased diffusion are seen within the basal ganglia and thalami, consistent with ischemic necrosis. In addition, material isointense to gray matter is layered dependently within the atria of the right lateral ventricle, which demonstrates decreased diffusion, but no evidence is seen of a susceptibility artifact on multiple planar gradient recalled images, suggesting pyogenic material. Subtle, scattered prominence of leptomeningeal enhancement also is seen along the cortical surfaces.

determining the presence and extent of the associated brain injury. T2* gradient-echo or susceptibility-weighted images are particularly useful in demonstrating the thrombus as a region of "blooming" in the venous system and detecting intraparenchymal hemorrhage (Fig. 37-4 and Boxes 37-2 and 37-3). On follow-up examinations, brain parenchyma affected by a venous stroke can show atrophy or can almost completely resolve, depending on the severity and duration of the injury.

Ultrasound can be used to visualize the echogenic clot at the bedside and to monitor its evolution. It also can be used to screen for additional complications, such as hydrocephalus as a result of intraventricular hemorrhage.

Childhood Stroke

The incidence of childhood stroke based on imaging findings is estimated to be 2.4 cases per 100,000 patient population.[9] Cerebrovascular insults in children can be categorized as AIS or SVT.

ARTERIAL ISCHEMIC STROKE

In more than half of childhood cases of AIS, the precise etiology is never determined. In the remaining cases, a variety of pathologies are found, including thromboembolism (from

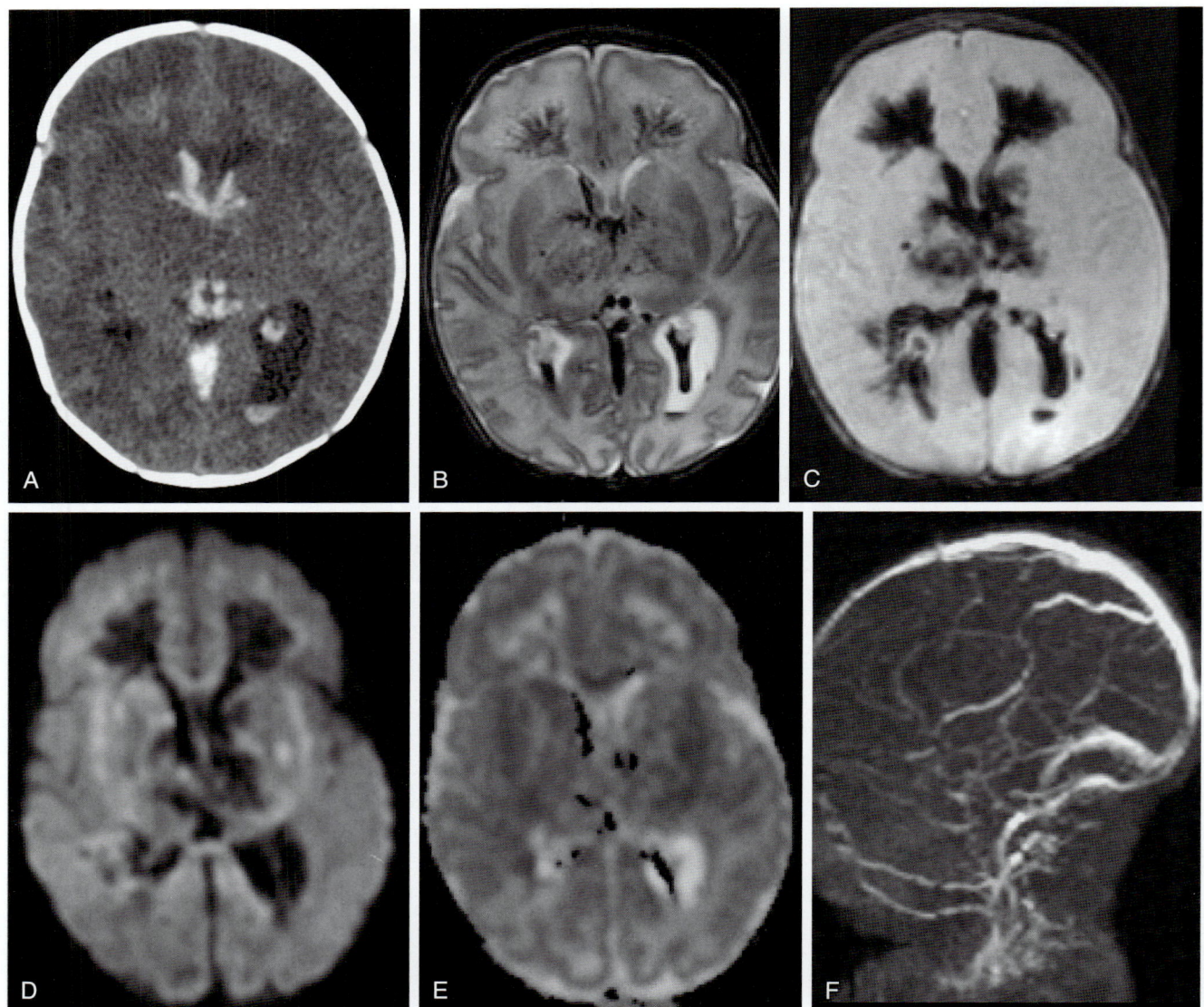

Figure 37-4 **An 11-day-old newborn with seizures for 24 hours.** An axial computed tomography (CT) scan (**A**), T2-weighted magnetic resonance (MR) image (**B**), susceptibility sequence (**C**), diffusion-weighted image (DWI) (**D**) with apparent diffusion coefficient (**E**), and two-dimensional time-of-flight MR venography (MRV) (**F**) from CT shows hyperdense clots involving the deep venous system with extensive cerebral edema. MR imaging with MRV confirms lack of enhancement of the entire deep venous system, consistent with thrombosis with extension into the perimedullary veins. Extensive edema is present involving the deep gray nuclei and white matter with associated bithalamic and intraventricular hemorrhage. On DWI, the cerebral edema shows both decreased and increased diffusion, consistent with a combination of cytotoxic and vasogenic edema. Factor V Leiden mutation was the cause of the hypercoagulable state.

Box 37-2 Cerebral Infarction: Computed Tomographic Findings

Hyperacute Infarct (<12 hours)

Normal (50%-60%)

Hyperdense artery (25%-50%)

Acute (12-24 hours)

Low-density basal ganglia

Loss of gray–white interfaces (insular ribbon sign, obstruction of cortex–medullary white matter border)

Sulcal effacement

1-3 Days

Increasing mass effect

Wedge-shaped low-density area that involves both gray and white matter

Hemorrhagic transformation may occur (basal ganglia and cortex are common sites)

4-7 Days

Gyral enhancement

Mass effect and edema persist

1-8 Weeks

Contrast enhancement persists

Mass effect resolves

Transient calcification can occur (pediatric strokes)

Months to Years

Encephalomalacic change, volume loss

Calcification is rare

Data from Osborn AG. *Diagnostic neuroradiology: a text atlas.* St Louis: Mosby-Year Book; 1994.

stenotic arteries necessitates blood transfusion to prevent stroke.[12] Brain MRI is usually performed to evaluate children with sickle cell anemia presenting with seizures or motor or sensory deficit.

Moyamoya disease accounts for approximately 6% of AIS incidence in Western countries. Moyamoya disease is a progressive vasculopathy causing stenosis of intracranial arteries with a predilection for terminal portions of the internal carotid arteries (Fig. 37-5). It can be associated with neurofibromatosis type 1, radiation vasculitis, Down syndrome, and SCD; if the cause remains undetermined, it is referred to as moyamoya disease. Collateral formation from the lenticulostriate vessels and thalamoperforators lead to a classic "puff-of-smoke" appearance on angiography. MRI can demonstrate loss of the normal flow void in the distal carotid branches on T2-weighted images, as well as development of abnormally

Box 37-3 Cerebral Infarction: Magnetic Resonance Imaging Findings

Immediate

Absence of normal flow void

Intravascular contrast enhancement

Low apparent diffusion coefficient

Perfusion alterations

<12 Hours

Anatomic alterations on T1-weighted image

Sulcal effacement

Gyral edema

Loss of gray-white interface

12-24 Hours

Hyperintensity develops on T2-weighted image

Meningeal enhancement adjacent to infarct

Mass effect

1-3 Days

Intravascular and meningeal enhancement begins decreasing

Early parenchymal contrast enhancement

Signal abnormalities striking on T1- and T2-weighted images

Hemorrhagic transformation may become evident

4-7 Days

Striking parenchymal contrast enhancement

Hemorrhage apparent in 25%

Mass effect and edema begin to diminish

Intravascular and meningeal enhancement disappear

1-8 Weeks

Contrast enhancement often persists

Mass effect resolves

Decrease in abnormal signal on T2-weighted image sometimes noted (fogging effect)

Hemorrhagic changes evolve, become chronic

Months to Years

Encephalomalacic changes, volume loss in affected vascular distribution

Hemorrhagic residua (hemosiderin/ferritin)

Data from Osborn AG. *Diagnostic neuroradiology: a text atlas.* St Louis: Mosby-Year Book; 1994.

intracranial or extracranial vessels, cardiac disorders such as congenital or acquired heart disease, intracardiac shunts, and procedures), arteriopathy (arterial dissection, moyamoya disease, vasculitis, sickle cell disease [SCD] arteriopathy, post-varicella angiopathy, and idiopathic focal cerebral arteriopathy), and hypercoagulable states (protein C or S deficiency, antithrombin III, and factor V Leiden mutation).[10,11]

SCD, a common risk factor for stroke in children, increases the risk of having a stroke approximately 200 to 400 times. The rigid, sickle-shaped red blood cells lead to vascular occlusion. Additionally, adherence to the vessel wall damages the intima and media, resulting in fibrosed and stenotic vessels. Proximal MCA or distal internal carotid artery branches are the most commonly involved vessels. In approximately 5% to 8% of patients with SCD, symptomatic cerebrovascular disease develops, and in about 20% of cases, a clinically silent stroke also may develop.

On imaging, acute infarction is usually superimposed on a diseased brain with atrophy and chronic changes. MRA commonly shows irregular stenotic arteries involving the anterior circulation with leptomeningeal collaterals, often longstanding. CT angiography (CTA) use is limited because iodinated contrast predisposes to sickling crises. Low osmolar agents should be used when iodinated contrast is deemed necessary, along with transfusion and hydration to reduce the risk of complications. Biannual screening with transcranial Doppler imaging is routinely performed, and abnormally elevated time-averaged mean velocities (>200 cm/sec) from

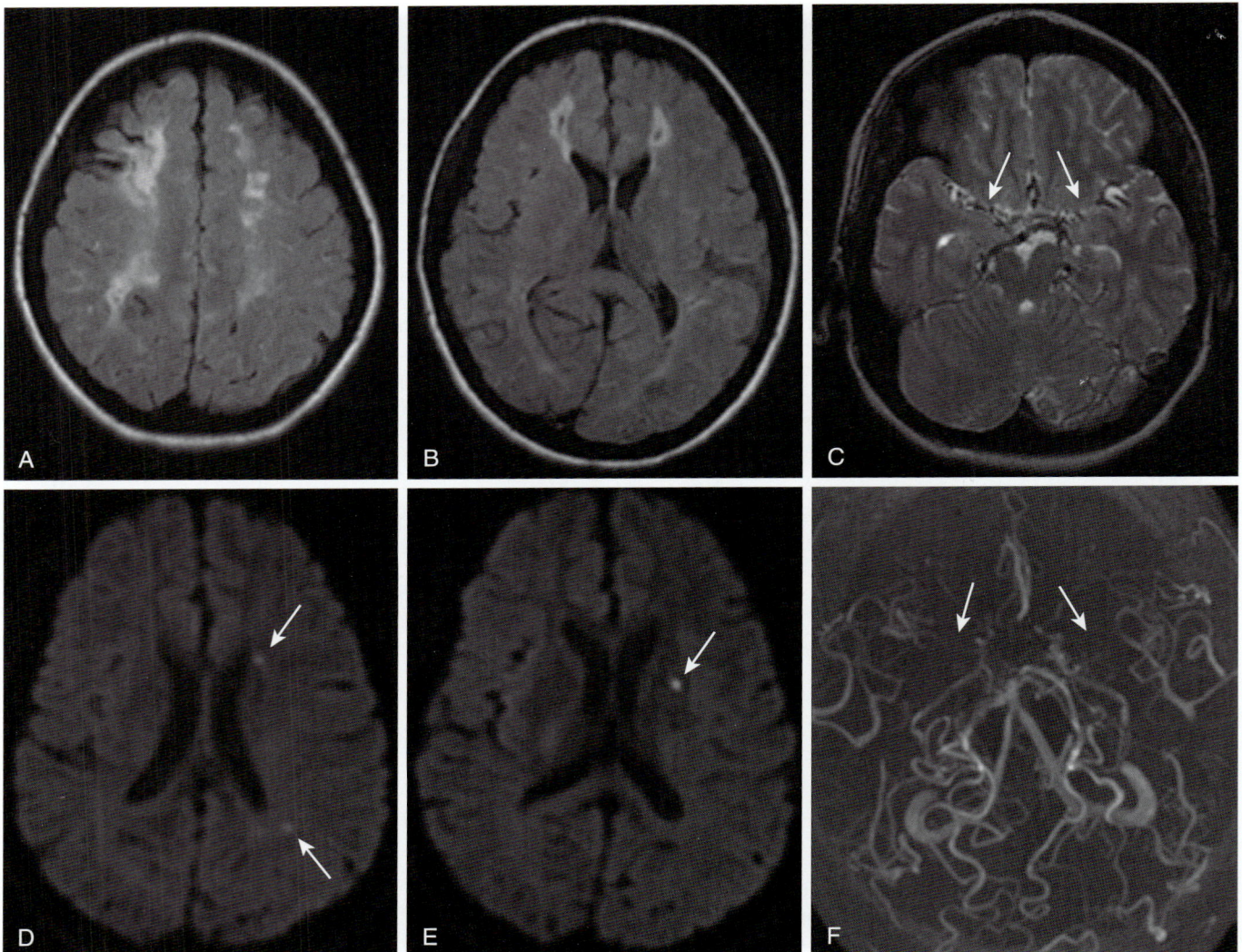

Figure 37-5 **Moyamoya disease.** A 16-year-old girl with a history of sickle cell disease and multiple cerebrovascular accidents has new onset right-sided numbness. Axial fluid attenuated inversion recovery images (**A** and **B**) demonstrate multiple small areas of old infarcts surrounded by gliosis in a watershed distribution. A T2-weighted image (**C**) shows prominence of extraaxial vessels (*arrows*), suggesting collateral circulation. Diffusion-weighted images (**D** and **E**) show tiny foci of decreased diffusion (*arrows*), compatible with small acute ischemic strokes. Magnetic resonance angiography (**F**) shows lack of flow related enhancement of the supraclinoid internal carotid arteries and middle cerebral arteries (*arrows*).

large and irregular collateral vessels. Fluid attenuated inversion recovery images often show increased signal in distal vessels with decreased flow. Carotid stenosis also can be observed on MRA, but its severity can be overestimated because of slow and turbulent flow.[13] Postcontrast MRA and, in particular, CTA can improve accuracy. DWI demonstrates acute areas of ischemic necrosis, whereas perfusion imaging and arterial spin labeling can demonstrate peripheral areas of delayed cerebral flow.

Arterial dissection may occur spontaneously or after trauma. Arterial dissection leads to formation of an intramural thrombus, which can propagate and embolize distally, or it can lead to vascular occlusion. The common locations are at the junction between relatively fixed and mobile segments of arteries and among the intracranial arteries; the supraclinoid internal carotid artery often is affected. T1-weighted fat-saturated sequences performed from the aortic arch to the cavernous sinus can demonstrate concentric hyperintense

signal because of methemoglobin in the vessel wall in the subacute phase. If the dissection is recent, close inspection of the images is necessary to rule out isointense concentric wall thickening. If MRA is degraded by flow artifacts, CTA can be performed (Fig. 37-6). The angiographic findings are abrupt segmental narrowing with an intimal flap, a beaded appearance, or pseudoaneurysm formation.[14]

Mitochondrial disorders usually involve multiple systems, but the strokelike events that appear as focal neurologic deficits of abrupt onset can mimic and be clinically indistinguishable from AIS. Mitochondrial injuries do not follow the vascular boundaries, and on MRI, the ADC values are typically normal to elevated, as opposed to the classically low values seen with AIS[6] (see Chapter 33).

The presence of transient neurologic symptoms in patients with migraine also can simulate stroke. Migraine with aura has been associated with increased risk for stroke in the adult population, and the literature includes some case reports of

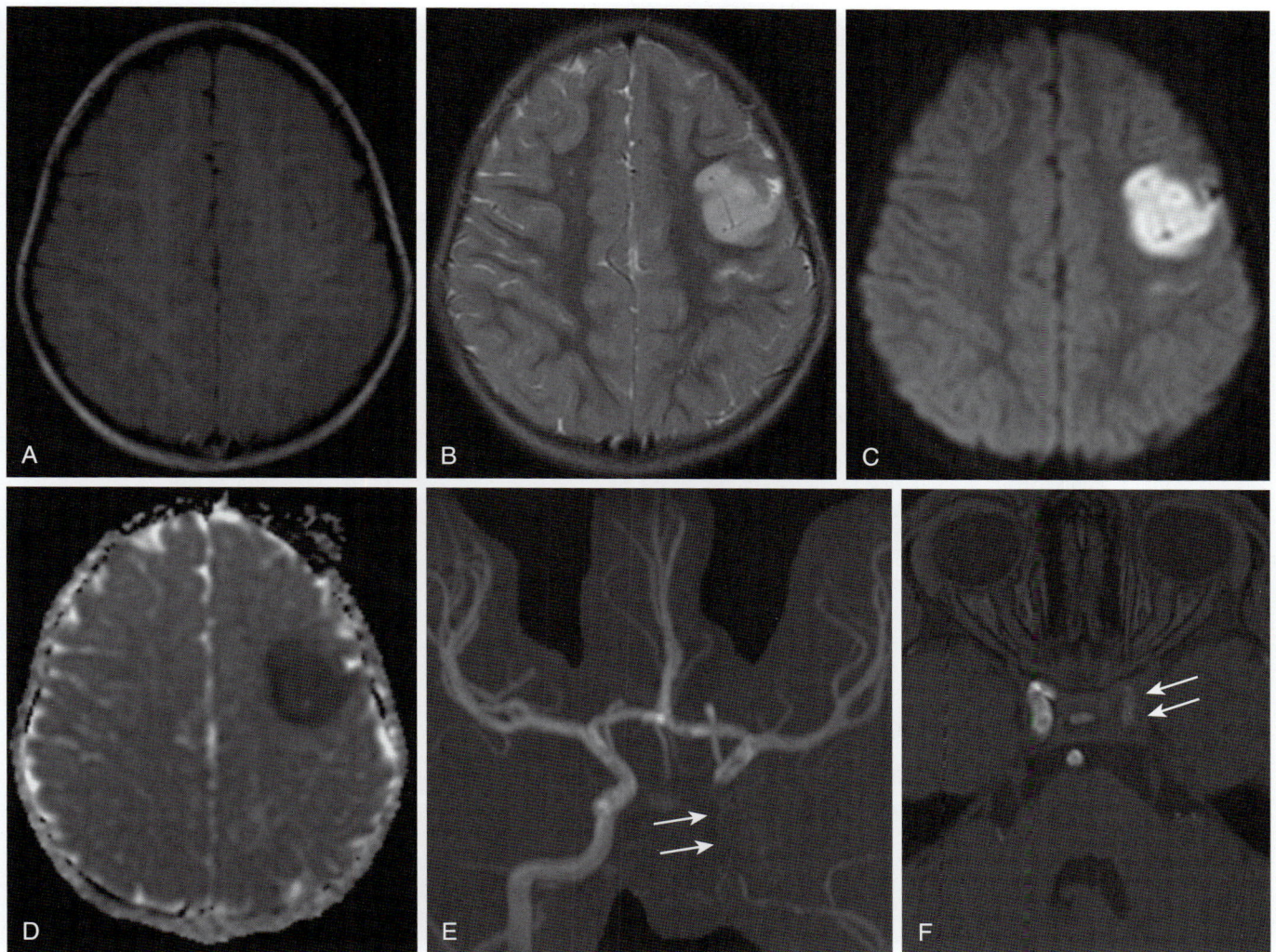

Figure 37-6 Carotid dissection. A 3-year-old girl with right facial drop and right upper extremity weakness after blunt trauma to the neck. A magnetic resonance imaging scan shows evidence of cortical and subcortical edema within the left frontal lobe (**A**, T1-weighted image; **B**, T2-weighted image) with reduced diffusion associated (**C**, diffusion-weighted image; **D**, apparent diffusion coefficient map) compatible with ischemic infarction. Maximum intensity projection magnetic resonance angiography (MRA) shows absence of flow within the left internal carotid artery (*arrows* in **E**). An MRA source image (**F**) shows irregular and diminutive flow signal within the cavernous segment of the left carotid artery (*arrows*).

migrainous infarct in adolescents. The association between these two entities is thought to be related to a dysfunction of cerebral arteries during migraine bouts (Fig. 37-7).[15]

VENOUS STROKE

In children, SVT is the primary cause of venous stroke. Dehydration, complicated otitis media, and sinusitis are the major risk factors in older children. Less commonly, a pro-thrombotic disorder, trauma, or medication is the identified cause. If the superficial cortical veins are involved, SVT leads to regional cerebral edema, which has a good prognosis. SVT is demonstrated as hyperdensity on CT and variable signal intensity on conventional MRI sequences. MRI with susceptibility-weighted images, DWI, MR venography, and postcontrast volumetric T1 imaging are the sequences of choice. DWI is helpful for determining whether vasogenic edema or ischemic necrosis is present. Postcontrast volumetric T1 images provide direct visualization of filling defects in the venous system and allow secondary evaluation of regions of signal dropout on MR venography.[16] Identification of the clot on susceptibility sequences is the best confirmation of SVT. If MRI is equivocal, CT venography can give a better delineation of the venous system, at the expense of radiation exposure (Fig. 37-8).

Summary

Stroke is a well-established entity in infants and children, where it is an important cause of morbidity and mortality. It can be a challenging diagnosis, despite imaging advances, because the diagnosis often is unsuspected and imaging is typically is ordered only in the subacute to chronic phase. In addition, the common presence of complex etiologies in children who have had a stroke is in marked contrast to the

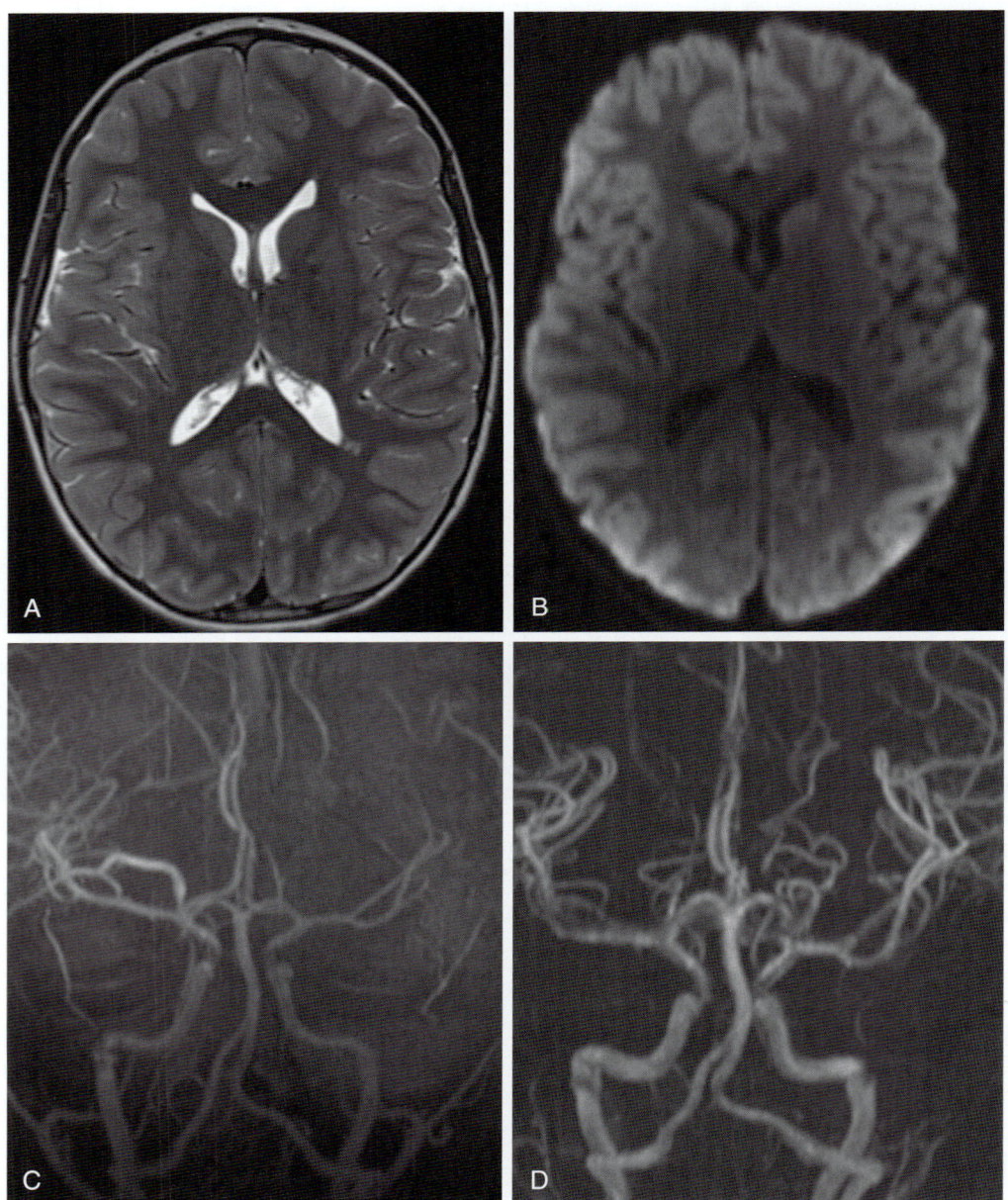

Figure 37-7 Vasospasm. A 7-year-old boy has headache, ataxia, and confusion. A T2-weighted image (**A**) and diffusion-weighted image (**B**) are unremarkable. Magnetic resonance angiography (MRA) (**C**) demonstrates asymmetry of the intracranial vascularity with left middle cerebral artery branches less prominent than the contralateral side. Follow-up MRA (**D**) 21 hours later shows significantly improved visualization of the distal M3 and M4 segments of the left middle cerebral artery.

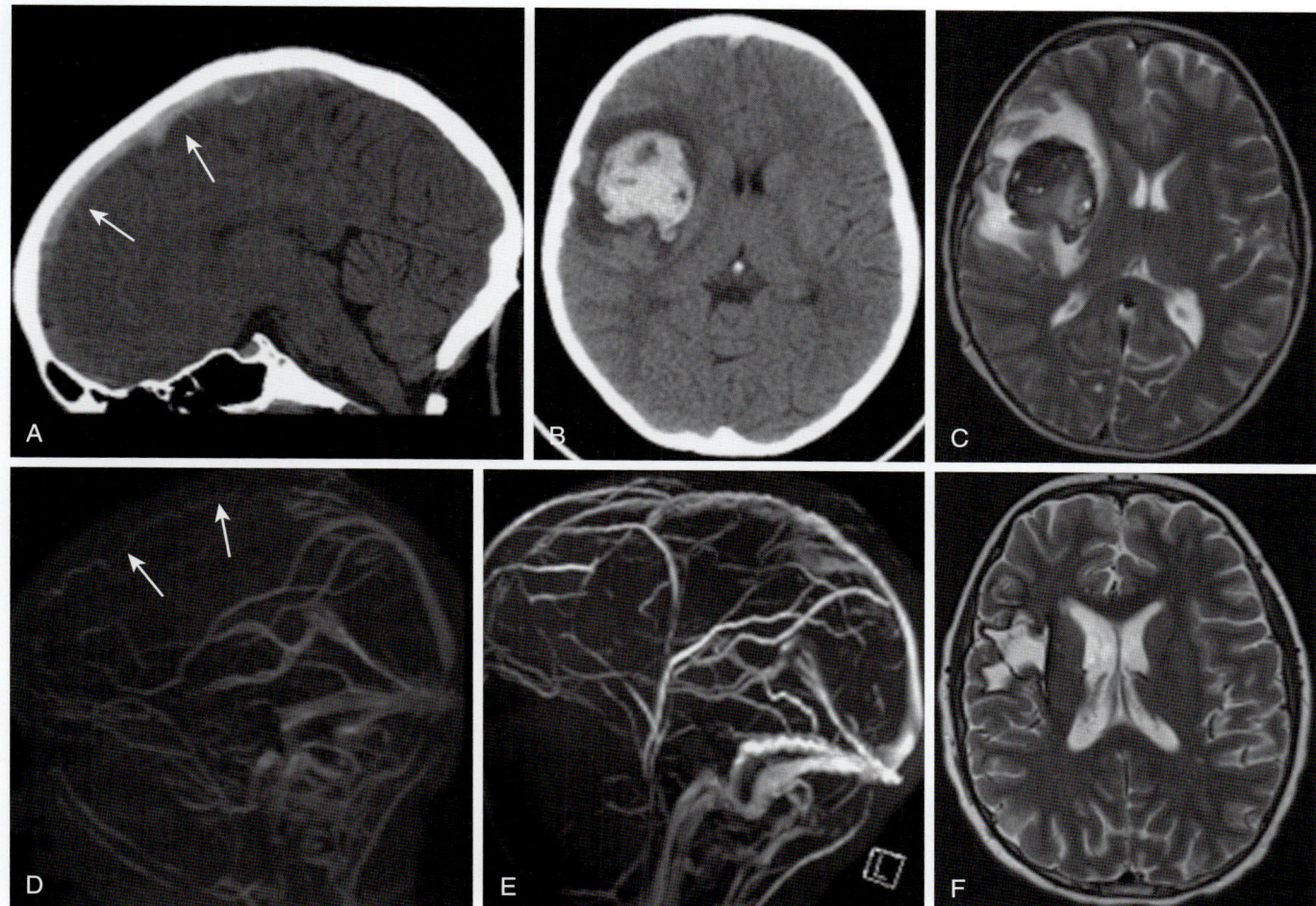

Figure 37-8 **Hemorrhagic venous infarct.** An 11-year-old boy with acute lymphocytic leukemia, status postinduction, presented with nausea, vomiting, left upper limb weakness, and left facial weakness. A computed tomography (CT) scan in the sagittal view (**A**) shows hyperdense material compatible with a clot within the superior sagittal sinus (*arrows*). An axial view CT image (**B**) and T2-weighted magnetic resonance (MR) image (**C**) demonstrate a large intraparenchymal hemorrhage in the right frontoparietal region consistent with hemorrhagic venous infarct, associated with effect of a mass causing effacement of the right lateral ventricle and mild leftward midline. Surrounding edema also is noticed. MR venography (MRV) (**D**) shows lack of flow-related enhancement of the superior sagittal sinus (*arrows*). A follow-up scan 1 year later (**E**) shows a patent superior sagittal sinus on MRV (**E**), as well as encephalomalacic changes on a T2-weighted image in the area of the previous hemorrhagic venous infarct (**F**).

situation in adults, in whom stroke is almost always a result of atherosclerotic vascular disease. Management remains controversial in many situations because of the lack of understanding of etiology and the future risk of recurrent stroke. Increased awareness of the different types and causes of pediatric stroke is necessary to facilitate early diagnosis, intervention, and prevention in high-risk children. Pediatric stroke also is an area in need of extensive clinical research to help understand the many complex pathophysiologies and outcomes and to determine the optimal treatment strategy for each type of stroke.

Suggested Readings

Jackson BF, Porcher FK, Zapton DT, et al. Cerebral sinovenous thrombosis in children: diagnosis and treatment. *Pediatr Emerg Care.* 2011;27(9): 874–880.

Mackay MT, Wiznitzer M, Benedict SL, et al. Arterial ischemic stroke risk factors: the International Pediatric Stroke Study, International Pediatric Stroke Study Group. *Ann Neurol.* 2011;69(1):130–140.

Rodrigues K, Grant PE. Diffusion-weighted imaging in neonates. *Neuroimaging Clin N Am.* 2011;21(1):127–151.

References

Full references for this chapter can be found on www.expertconsult.com.

Chapter 38

Neuroimaging in Pediatric Epilepsy

ELKA MILLER and ELYSA WIDJAJA

Epilepsy is a common pediatric neurological disorder. In North America, the overall annual incidence of epilepsy is approximately 50 per 100,000 persons. The incidence is highest for children younger than 5 years and for elderly persons.[1,2] Children are at higher risk for the development of epilepsy than are adults. Atypical, idiopathic, and focal epilepsy, as well as epileptic syndromes, require evaluation with magnetic resonance imaging (MRI). In approximately 30% of children with epilepsy, the disease becomes refractory to medical therapy.[3] In children with refractory epilepsy, neuroimaging is critical for identification of an epileptogenic substrate that is responsible for the epilepsy, particularly in children undergoing surgery. Patients without a lesion (that is, patients who have normal MRI findings) have been reported to have poorer outcomes of epilepsy surgery compared with patients who have a lesion identified upon neuroimaging.[4] Epileptogenic substrates include malformations of cortical development (MCDs), developmental tumors, anoxic-ischemic injuries, prior cerebrovascular disease, neurocutaneous syndromes, and Rasmussen encephalitis. Concurrent lesions such as MCD, hippocampal sclerosis, and developmental tumors can occur in approximately 13% to 20% of cases.[5,6] Another important role of imaging in children with intractable epilepsy is to identify the location of eloquent cortex and white matter tracts as part of the presurgical evaluation (see Chapter 27).

The MRI epilepsy protocol should include volumetric T1-weighted imaging, T2-weighted imaging, fluid attenuated inversion recovery (FLAIR), proton density, and inversion recovery sequences in at least two orthogonal planes, covering the entire brain. Volumetric gradient echo T1-weighted acquisitions with 1- to 1.5-mm section thickness provide excellent gray/white matter contrast and are useful for better anatomic delineation. This sequence can be reformatted into any orthogonal or nonorthogonal plane without the penalty of increased scan time and can be used for anatomic integration of functional data, stereotactic electrode placement, and neuronavigation.[7-9] In persons with temporal lobe epilepsy, the coronal plane should be acquired perpendicular to the long axis of the hippocampus. Injection of contrast material does not improve the detection of a lesion but may help characterize a lesion once it is found. In cases in which an epileptogenic focus is not identified, further evaluation with dedicated higher resolution MRI, image postprocessing, or additional imaging techniques including diffusion tensor imaging, magnetic resonance spectroscopy, and functional imaging with interictal positron emission tomography (PET) or ictal/interictal single photon emission computed tomography (SPECT), along with magnetoencephalography, may help in identifying a lesion or the epileptogenic zone.[10,11]

Malformations of Cortical Development

MCDs are a major cause of drug-resistant epilepsy,[12] in particular focal cortical dysplasia (FCD), hemimegalencephaly, and tuberous sclerosis. Other MCDs such as lissencephaly, gray matter heterotopia, polymicrogyria, and schizencephaly also are associated with epilepsy.[13-16]

FOCAL CORTICAL DYSPLASIA

Overview FCD is an MCD that is intrinsically epileptogenic. It is one of the most common causes of intractable epilepsy in children and accounts for up to 39% of surgical cases.[17,18] The mechanism of epilepsy is still unclear. Possibilities include abnormal firing from the dysplastic neurons rather than from balloon cells,[19] dysfunction of synaptic circuits with abnormal synchronization of the neuronal population, and abnormal organization of the inhibitory interneurons.[20] Numerous classifications of FCD have been proposed.[13,21-23] Recently, a consensus classification has been proposed by the International League Against Epilepsy (Table 38-1).[24]

Imaging FCD can be located in any cortex of the cerebral hemisphere and can have variable size, from one gyrus to more than one lobe. The MRI features of FCD are increased cortical thickness, blurring of the cortical–white matter junction, increased T2 or FLAIR signal in the cortex and subcortical white matter, high T1 signal in the cortex, and an abnormal sulcation and gyration pattern. Taylor FCD or FCD type IIB more commonly involves the extratemporal cortex and is more likely to demonstrate a high T2 and FLAIR signal that tapers toward the ventricle.[21,25,26] Non-Taylor FCD (type I FCD and mild MCDs) is more likely to be located in the temporal lobe and to demonstrate hypoplasia or atrophy of the white matter and mild increased signal. FCD, in particular non-Taylor FCD, is associated with hippocampal sclerosis.[27] The MRI appearance of FCD may change with brain maturation. Longitudinal MRI studies in infants with FCD have shown that findings of the early study

Table 38-1

Histopathologic Classification of Focal Cortical Dysplasia	
Type	**Description**
FCD type I (isolated)	Type Ia: FCD with abnormal radial cortical lamination Type Ib: FCD with abnormal tangential cortical lamination Type Ic: FCD with abnormal radial and tangential lamination
FCD type II (isolated)	Type IIa: Cortical dyslamination and dysmorphic neurons without balloon cells Type IIb: Cortical dyslamination and dysmorphic neurons with balloon cells
FCD type III (associated with principal lesion)	With associated lesion Type IIIa: Hippocampal sclerosis Type IIIb: Epilepsy-associated tumors Type IIIc: Vascular malformation Type IIId: Other lesion

FCD, Focal cortical dysplasia.
From Blumcke I, Thom M, Aronica E, et al. The clinicopathologic spectrum of focal cortical dysplasias: a consensus classification proposed by an ad hoc Task Force of the ILAE Diagnostic Methods Commission. *Epilepsia.* 2011;52(1):158-174.

may be normal but later imaging may demonstrate a high T2 signal in the white matter, a high T1 signal in the cortex, and blurring of the cortical/subcortical white matter junction.[28] The high signal in the white matter may be a result of abnormal myelination, either because of the underlying disease or as a result of seizures. Thus even when the MRI findings appear normal in a neonate or an infant with refractory partial seizures or infantile spasm, a repeat study is recommended (Fig. 38-1).[28] In contrast to the high T2/FLAIR signal in the white matter of FCD in children, the white matter adjacent to the dysplastic cortex may demonstrate a low T2 and high T1 signal in neonates and infants, which is thought to be secondary to early white matter myelination as a result of repeated seizures.[29]

Treatment Good seizure control or a seizure-free outcome is achieved in up to 50% to 70% of patients with FCD after surgical resection of the FCD.[30-32] This outcome compares favorably with the outcome of patients who have hippocampal sclerosis[33] and a low-grade neoplasm.[34] The reported surgical outcomes of persons with subtypes of FCD are variable. Authors of some studies reported a better surgical outcome in persons with Taylor FCD,[21,35,36] whereas other authors reported better surgical outcomes in persons with other subtypes of FCD, including type I FCD and mild MCD.[37,38] Differences in outcomes of persons with subtypes of FCD may in part be related to the preponderance of type I FCD and mild MCD in the temporal lobe.[37]

HEMIMEGALENCEPHALY

Overview Hemimegalencephaly is an MCD that is characterized by one hemisphere being larger than the contralateral side. It may be sporadic or it may be associated with a variety of syndromes, including proteus syndrome, epidermal nevus

syndrome, hypomelanosis of Ito, linear nevus sebaceous syndrome, neurofibromatosis type I, and tuberous sclerosis. The sporadic form is considered a hemispheric variant of FCD.[39] On histology, the appearance is similar to FCD with abnormal gyration of the cortex, dyslamination, blurring of the gray/white matter junction, giant neurons in both gray and white matter, and balloon cells in 50% of cases. The most common clinical presentation is early intractable epilepsy; other clinical presentations include hemiparesis, hemianopia, and mental retardation.

Imaging The affected hemisphere is larger than the contralateral side. The cortex is dysplastic and thick, with broad gyri and shallow sulci (e-Fig. 38-2). The ipsilateral lateral ventricle may be enlarged. The ipsilateral white matter demonstrates variable signal changes, depending on the age of the patient. Neonates and infants usually demonstrate a high T1 and low T2 signal in the white matter suggestive of early myelination, whereas in older children the white matter shows a low T1 signal and a high T2 signal with associated cystic changes and calcification.[40-42] With recurrent seizures or status epilepticus, the enlarged hemisphere later may become atrophic.[43]

Treatment and Follow-up An early functional hemispherectomy or hemispherotomy may be required as a result of severe intractable epilepsy that is refractory to medications.

TUBEROUS SCLEROSIS COMPLEX

Overview and Imaging Tuberous sclerosis complex is an autosomal-dominant neurocutaneous syndrome characterized by multisystem involvement including the brain, eyes, heart, kidney, skin, and lung. Seizures occur in 80% to 90% of patients, and seizures are intractable in 25% to 30% of patients.[44] Children with medically refractory epilepsy usually have multiple cortical/subcortical tubers that exhibit broad gyri, a thick cortex, and an abnormal signal in the cortex and subcortical white matter. The cortical/subcortical tubers occasionally may demonstrate calcification and cystic degeneration. A combination of structural and functional imaging such as fluorodeoxyglucose (FDG)-PET, ictal/interictal SPECT, and magnetoencephalography can be used to identify the epileptogenic tubers[45-48] (Fig. 38-3). Cerebellar tubers also occur and more commonly are seen in patients with a high cerebral tuber burden. The subependymal nodules often calcify. Another manifestation of tuberous sclerosis complex is subependymal giant cell astrocytomas, which commonly occur near the foramen of Monro.

Sturge-Weber Syndrome

Overview and Imaging Sturge-Weber syndrome, or encephalotrigeminal angiomatosis, is a phakomatosis characterized by a facial capillary vascular malformation or "port wine stain" in the territory of the trigeminal nerve, ipsilateral leptomeningeal angiomatosis, and angiomatosis of the choroid of the ipsilateral eye. Seizures usually are the initial neurological manifestation in the first year of life. Children with early onset of epilepsy are more likely to have hemiparesis, status epilepticus, and developmental delay compared with persons

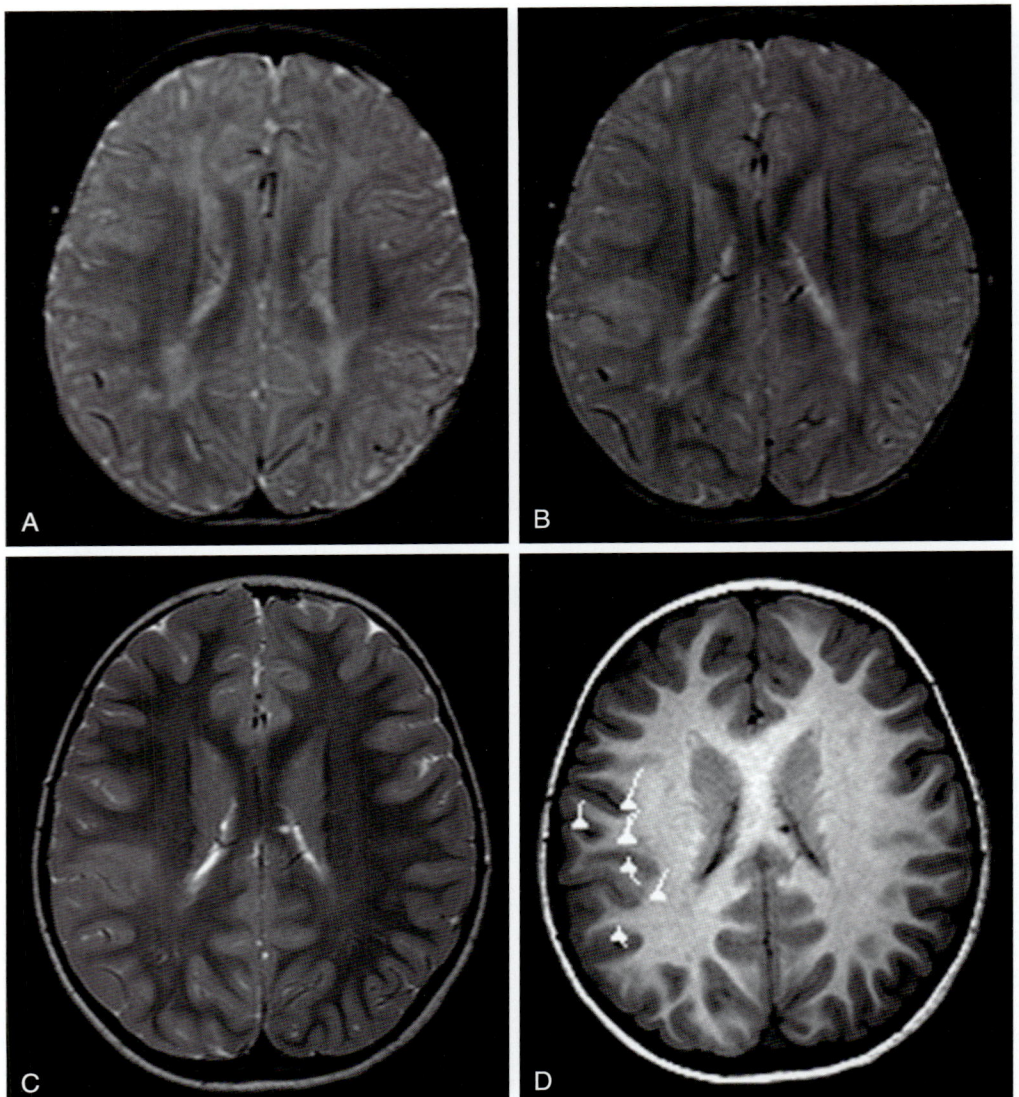

Figure 38-1 A 5-year-old girl with focal cortical dysplasia. An axial T2-weighted image at 12 months (**A**) does not show a lesion. However, at 19 months (**B**) and 5 years of age (**C**), axial T2-weighted images demonstrate an abnormal signal in the cortex and subcortical white matter that is associated with blurring of the gray/white matter junction. **D,** Magnetoencephalography projected onto an axial T1-weighted image demonstrates that the dipoles, indicative of the epileptogenic zone, are located in and around the lesion. Surgical resection of the lesion and epileptogenic zone confirms the presence of focal cortical dysplasia type IIB.

whose seizures start later in life.[49] Imaging findings include leptomeningeal angiomatosis, enlargement of the choroid plexus, parenchymal atrophy, calvarial changes, and calcification (Fig. 38-4). Leptomeningeal angiomatosis and choroid plexus hyperplasia appear earlier in the course of the disease, whereas atrophy and calcification usually are evident later. Contrast-enhanced MRI is considered the most sensitive sequence for depicting leptomeningeal enhancement and revealing subtle bilateral hemispheric involvement, compensatory venous drainage, enlarged choroid plexus in the atria, and cerebellar and eye involvement.[50-52]

Treatment Medical therapy is the first line of treatment for controlling seizures. Surgical lobectomy or hemispherotomy also may be indicated in cases in which seizures are refractory to medical therapy.

Mesial Temporal Sclerosis

Overview and Imaging Mesial temporal sclerosis is encountered less frequently in children than in adults.[53-56] The etiology of hippocampal sclerosis is unknown, but a link with febrile seizures has been suggested.[57,58] Hippocampal sclerosis is characterized by neuronal loss and gliosis in the hippocampus.[59] MRI features include atrophy and increased T2 and FLAIR signal in the hippocampus (Fig. 38-5).[59-62] Other findings include loss of interdigitations of the hippocampal head,[63] atrophy of the ipsilateral mamillary body and fornix,[64] dilatation of the ipsilateral temporal horn, volume loss of the temporal lobe, and atrophy of the collateral white matter between the hippocampus and collateral sulcus.[62] Functional imaging with FDG-PET usually reveals hypometabolic

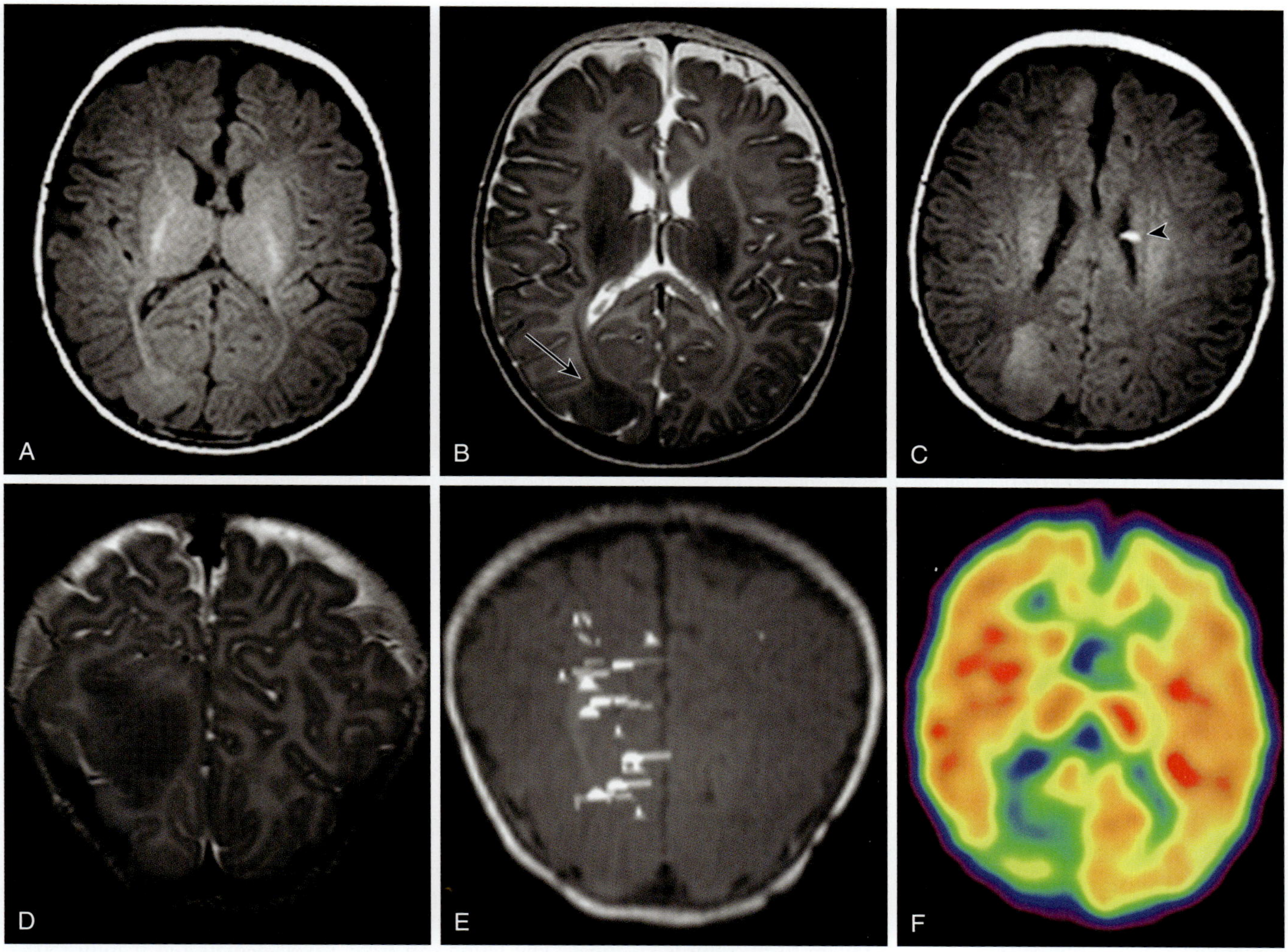

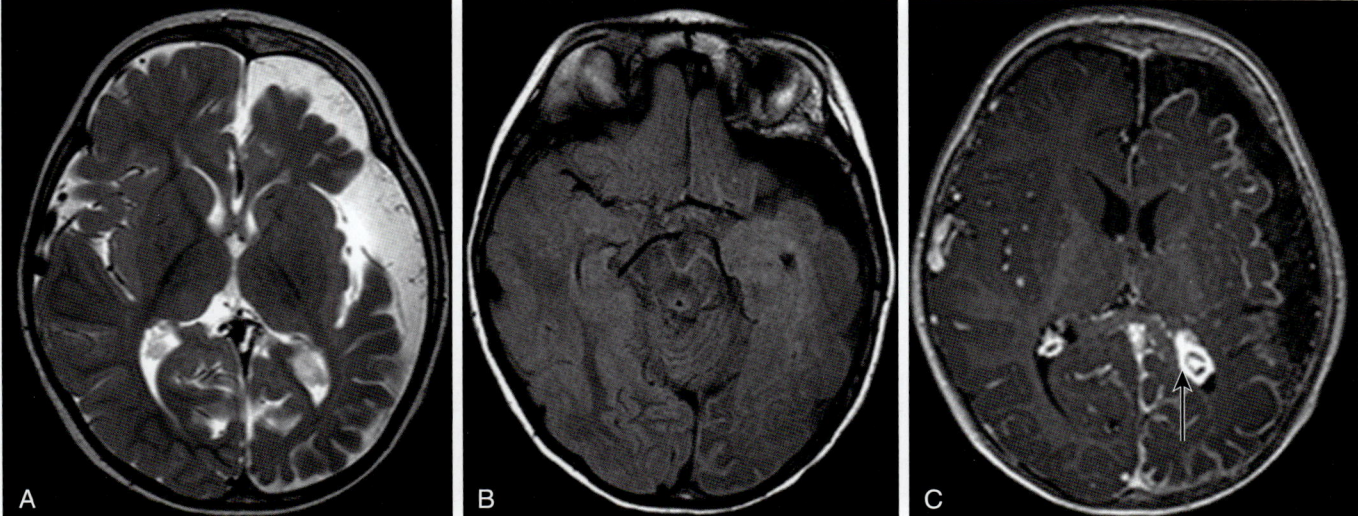

Figure 38-3 A 3-month-old with tuberous sclerosis complex and right occipital lobe intractable epilepsy. Axial T1-weighted images (**A** and **C**), an axial T2-weighted image (**B**), and a coronal T2-weighted image (**D**) indicate several cortical/subcortical tubers in the right frontal and occipital lobes (*arrow*) that demonstrate a high T1 and lower T2 signal. Several subependymal nodules also are present (*arrowhead*). **E,** Magnetoencephalography dipoles projected onto a coronal T1 image demonstrate a dipole cluster in the right occipital lobe. **F,** A fluorodeoxyglucose positron emission tomography study shows hypometabolism (*blue* and *green*) that is more extensive than the right occipital tuber.

Figure 38-4 A 15-month-old boy with Sturge-Weber syndrome. An axial T2-weighted image (**A**) and an axial fluid attenuated inversion recovery (FLAIR) image (**B**) show volume loss in the left cerebral hemisphere with enlargement of subarachnoid spaces and a high FLAIR signal in the left cerebral sulci. **C,** An axial T1-weighted postcontrast image shows pial enhancement over the left cerebral hemisphere, as well as an enlarged choroid plexus in the left trigone (*arrow*).

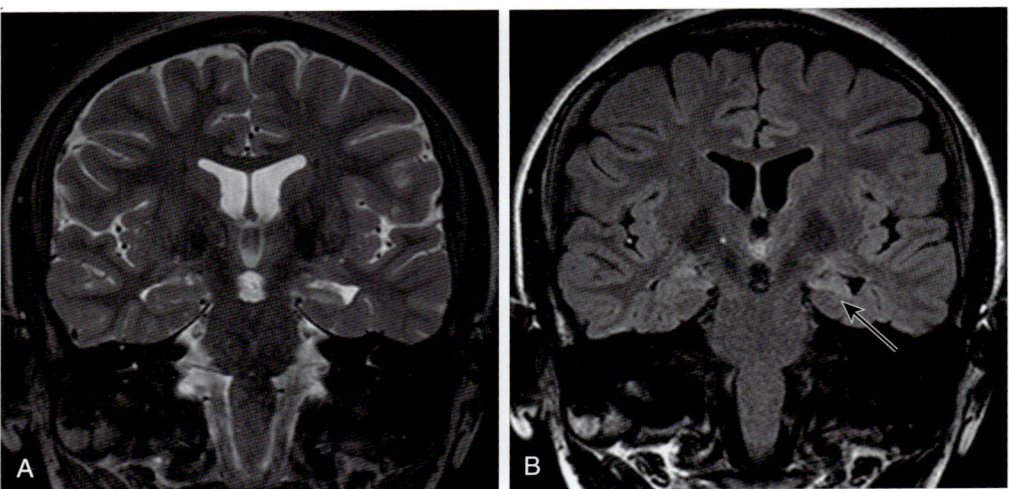

Figure 38-5   An 11-year-old girl with left mesial temporal sclerosis. A coronal T2-weighted image (**A**) and a coronal fluid attenuated inversion recovery (FLAIR) image (**B**) demonstrate a high T2 and FLAIR signal that is associated with volume loss in the left hippocampus (*arrow*).

activity that is larger than the hippocampus abnormality[65,66] and can identify mesial temporal metabolic abnormalities in patients with normal MRI.[67]

Treatment and Follow-up   In patients who have medically refractory epilepsy, surgery offers good seizure control in 70% to 90% of cases.[68-71]

Epilepsy-Associated Developmental Tumors

Epilepsy-associated tumors may account for up to two thirds of the surgical pathologic substrate[72-75] in epilepsy surgery. These tumors originate in and develop from the cortex and present clinically with seizures. Tumors associated with epilepsy usually are associated with benign biological behavior and a low proliferation index. Only a small percentage of these tumors may undergo malignant transformation.[76] The tumors include gangliogliomas, gangliocytomas, desmoplastic infantile gangliogliomas, dysembryoplastic neuroepithelial tumors (DNETs), pleomorphic xanthoastrocytomas (PXAs), and low-grade astrocytomas.[77] FCD may be present concurrently.

GANGLIOGLIOMA

The most common clinical presentation of gangliogliomas is seizures, which often are complex, partial, and medically intractable.[78] Tumors are larger in children than in adults,[79] and they are located mostly in the temporomesial (50%) or temporolateral (29%) location.[80] Gangliogliomas are composed of glia and neurons and may present as a solid mass in 43% of cases, a cyst in 5% of cases, and a mixed lesion in 52% of cases.[76,81] Because they are cortical, they may cause remodeling of the adjacent bone. Most gangliogliomas (38%) are hypodense on computed tomography (CT), but isodense (15%), hyperdense (15%), or mixed density masses (32%) can be found,[82] and calcification is seen in 30% to 50% of cases.

On MRI, the solid part of the tumor may appear hypointense or isointense to gray matter on T1-weighted images and hyperintense on T2-weighted images (Fig. 38-6). Enhancement is present in up to 60% of cases; it can be nodular, ringlike, or solid. Gangliocytomas, a variant of gangliogliomas without any glial component, affect older children and young adults. On MRI, a gangliocytoma may demonstrate a low T1 and a high T2 signal and show enhancement.[83,84]

DYSEMBRYOPLASTIC NEUROEPITHELIAL TUMOR

A DNET is a pathologically benign supratentorial cortical tumor that shows predilection for the temporal lobes (in 62% to 86% of cases).[85] DNETs also frequently affect the frontal lobes. The lesion can have a well-demarcated margin (50%), or the margins may be slightly blurred. The tumor may be associated with broadening of the gyri, effacement of the sulci, distortion of the ventricles, and remodeling of the overlying skull.[85,86] On CT, a DNET tends to be hypodense with a cystic appearance.[87] Calcification has been reported in 20% to 36% of cases.[86] On MRI, a DNET demonstrates a low T1 and a high T2 signal, often with a multicystic and "bubbly" appearance,[85] and it may have a thin rim of high signal on a FLAIR sequence (Fig. 38-7).[88,89] Approximately one third of cases shows nodular, patchy, or ring enhancement. The tumor may extend to the ventricle in 30% of cases. Hemorrhagic changes are rare but have been described.[88,90]

PLEOMORPHIC XANTHOASTROCYTOMA

PXA is a rare localized glioma of astrocytic origin affecting children and young adults.[91] It is mostly temporal (49%) and less commonly parietal, frontal, and occipital in location.[92,93] Upon imaging, a PXA appears as a large hemispheric cystic and solid mass close to the cortex. CT shows that the tumor is predominantly hypodense with a mixed-density enhancing nodule. Upon MRI, the cystic portion of the tumor is isointense to CSF, and the solid tumor is hypointense to isointense to gray matter on T1-weighted images and hyperintense to isointense on T2-weighted images. Enhancement of the

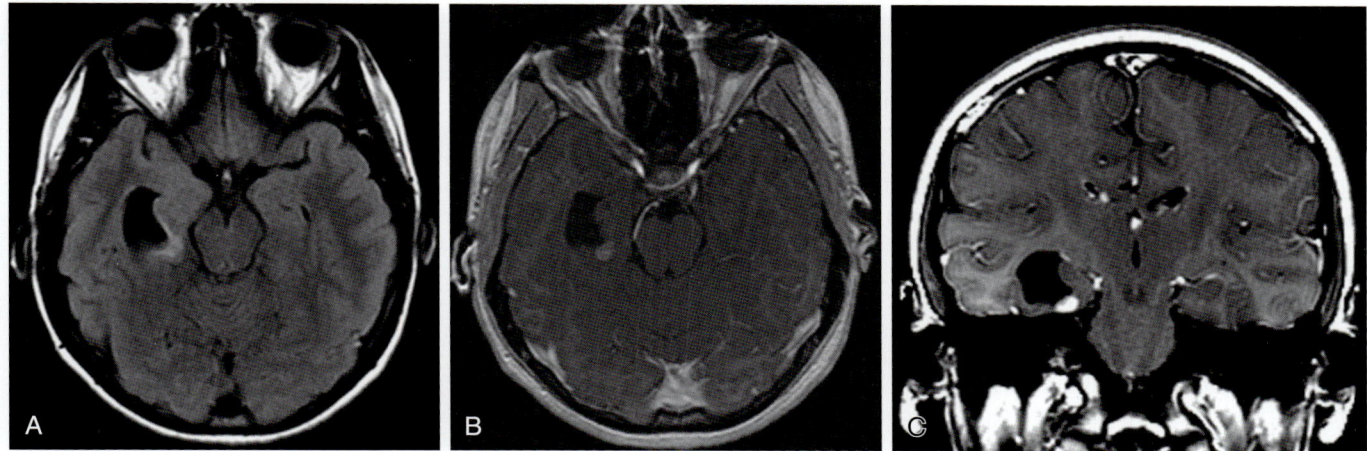

Figure 38-6 A 16-year-old girl with a ganglioglioma. An axial fluid attenuated inversion recovery image (**A**), an axial image (**B**), and a coronal T1-weighted postcontrast image (**C**) show a cystic tumor with a mural enhancing nodule in the right mesial temporal lobe.

nodular solid component and the adjacent meninges is seen ("dural tail") (e-Fig. 38-8).[94] PXA may be associated with FCD.[95,96]

Treatment and Follow-up Patients with a ganglioglioma have the best surgical outcome with respect to epilepsy control compared with other types of epilepsy-associated tumors.[74,80,97] DNETs have a less favorable seizure outcome compared with gangliogliomas, which could be related to longer duration of epilepsy, incomplete resection of the tumor, or the presence of FCD beyond the margins of the resected DNET.[97-99] The prognosis of patients with PXA is generally good, but the tumor may recur, and malignant degeneration occurs in 20% of cases.[100]

HYPOTHALAMIC HAMARTOMA

Overview and Imaging Hypothalamic hamartoma, also known as hamartoma of the tuber cinereum, is a congenital malformation of the hypothalamus that may be asymptomatic or may manifest with precocious puberty or gelastic seizures.[101] Intrahypothalamic hamartomas that invade the third ventricle are associated with early occurrence of epilepsy, whereas the parahypothalamic hamartomas that do not involve the third ventricle more commonly present with central precocious puberty.[102,103] MRI demonstrates a mass at the tuber cinereum that is T1 hypointense relative to the gray matter, T2 isointense or hyperintense relative to gray matter, and hyperintense on FLAIR. No enhancement occurs, and no calcification is seen (e-Fig. 38-9). Careful examination of the hypothalamic region on MRI is needed because hamartomas can be small and nonpedunculated.

Treatment and Follow-up The first-line treatment is medical therapy with hormonal therapy and antiepileptic medications. However, if the hamartoma becomes refractory to medical treatment, surgical resection or radiosurgery are considered.[104]

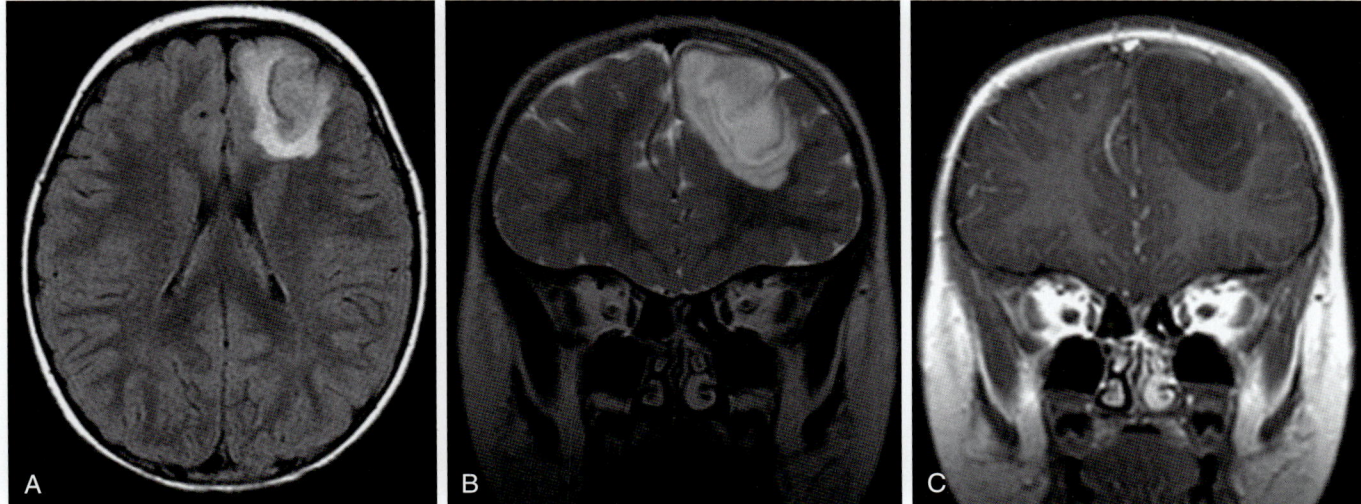

Figure 38-7 A 4-year-old boy with a dysembryoplastic neuroepithelial tumor. An axial fluid attenuated inversion recovery (FLAIR) image (**A**), a coronal T2-weighted image (**B**), and a gadolinium-enhanced coronal T1-weighted image (**C**) demonstrate a well-defined tumor in the right frontal lobe involving the cortex and white matter. The tumor extends to the margin of the frontal horn of the left lateral ventricle. The tumor has a rim of high FLAIR signal and does not show enhancement.

Rasmussen Encephalitis

Overview and Imaging Rasmussen encephalitis is a rare, chronic, progressive encephalitis characterized by severe refractory epilepsy and unilateral brain atrophy.[105] Clinically, seizures begin abruptly in previously healthy children and include partial seizures and epilepsia partialis continua. With disease progression, hemiparesis or hemiplegia and cognitive decline develop. The disease might have an autoimmune basis.[106-108] The histological findings include chronic encephalitis with lymphocytic infiltrations and perivascular cuffing; in the later stage of the disease, nonspecific findings such as atrophy and gliosis with minimal inflammatory cellular infiltrate are found.[109] In the acute stages, findings of MRI can be entirely normal[110,111] or demonstrate cortical swelling with a low T1 and hyperintense T2 and FLAIR signal, with no enhancement. With disease progression, MRI shows progressive volume loss and a progressive abnormal signal in the white matter and cortex (Fig. 38-10).[112] Rasmussen encephalitis is predominantly a unilateral disease, and the frontal and temporal lobes more commonly are involved.

Treatment and Follow-up Treatment options include medical treatment such as intravenous immunoglobulin, plasmapheresis, or immunosuppressive medications. However, functional hemispherectomy or hemispherotomy is frequently necessary for seizure control and to prevent progression of cognitive impairment and spread of seizures to the contralateral hemisphere.

Cavernomas

Overview and Imaging In children, seizures are the most common symptom of cavernomas at presentation.[113-115] Cavernomas are more commonly supratentorial (80%) and can have variable size. On MRI, cavernomas have a combination

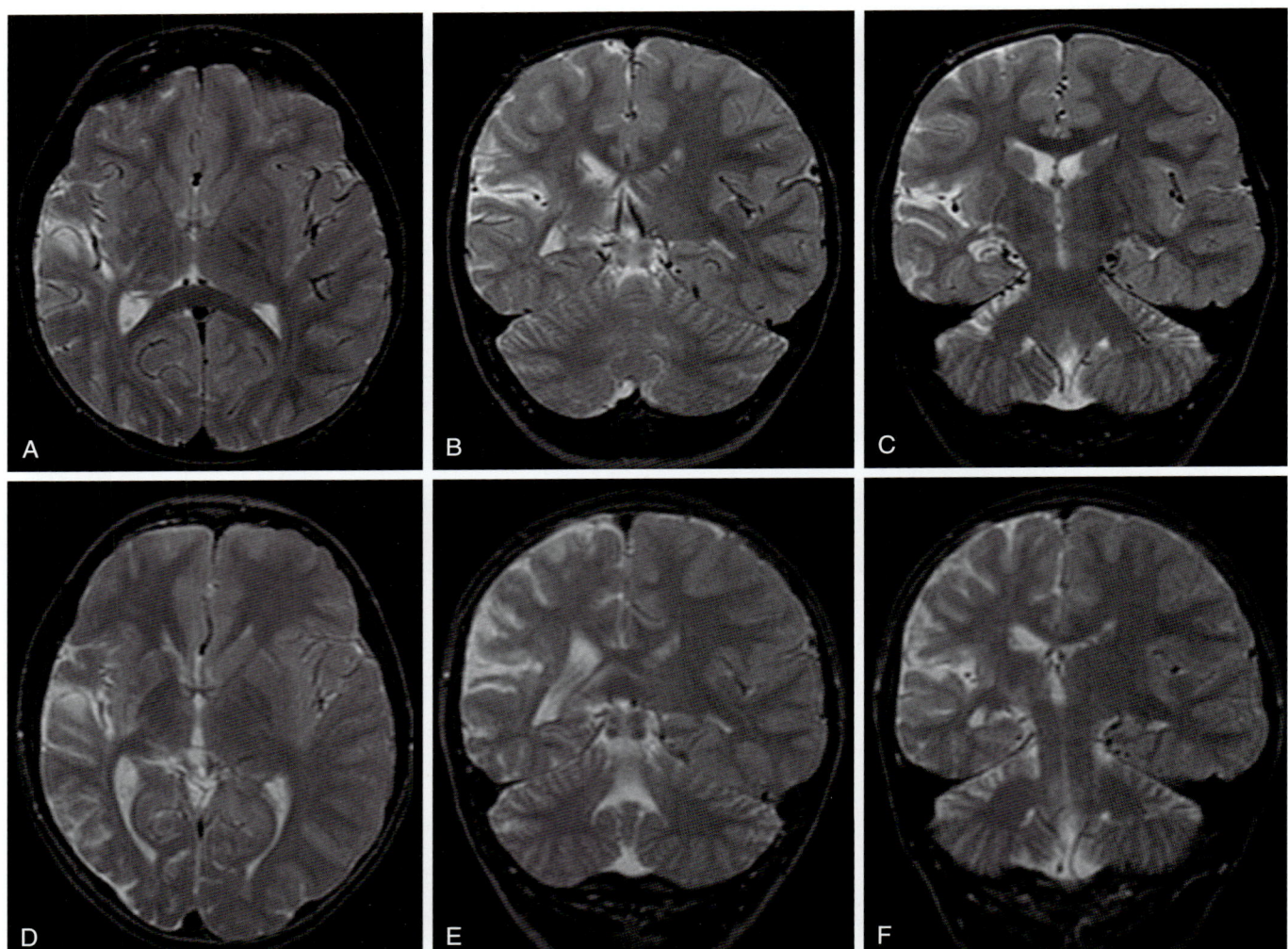

Figure 38-10 A 5-year-old boy with Rasmussen encephalitis presenting with epilepsia partialis continua. At presentation (**A**, **B**, and **C**), axial and coronal T2-weighted images demonstrate mild volume loss in the right Sylvian and temporal lobe. Three years later (**D**, **E**, and **F**), axial and coronal T2-weighted images demonstrate progressive volume loss in the right Sylvian, temporal, and parietal lobes with ex vacuo dilation of the right lateral ventricle.

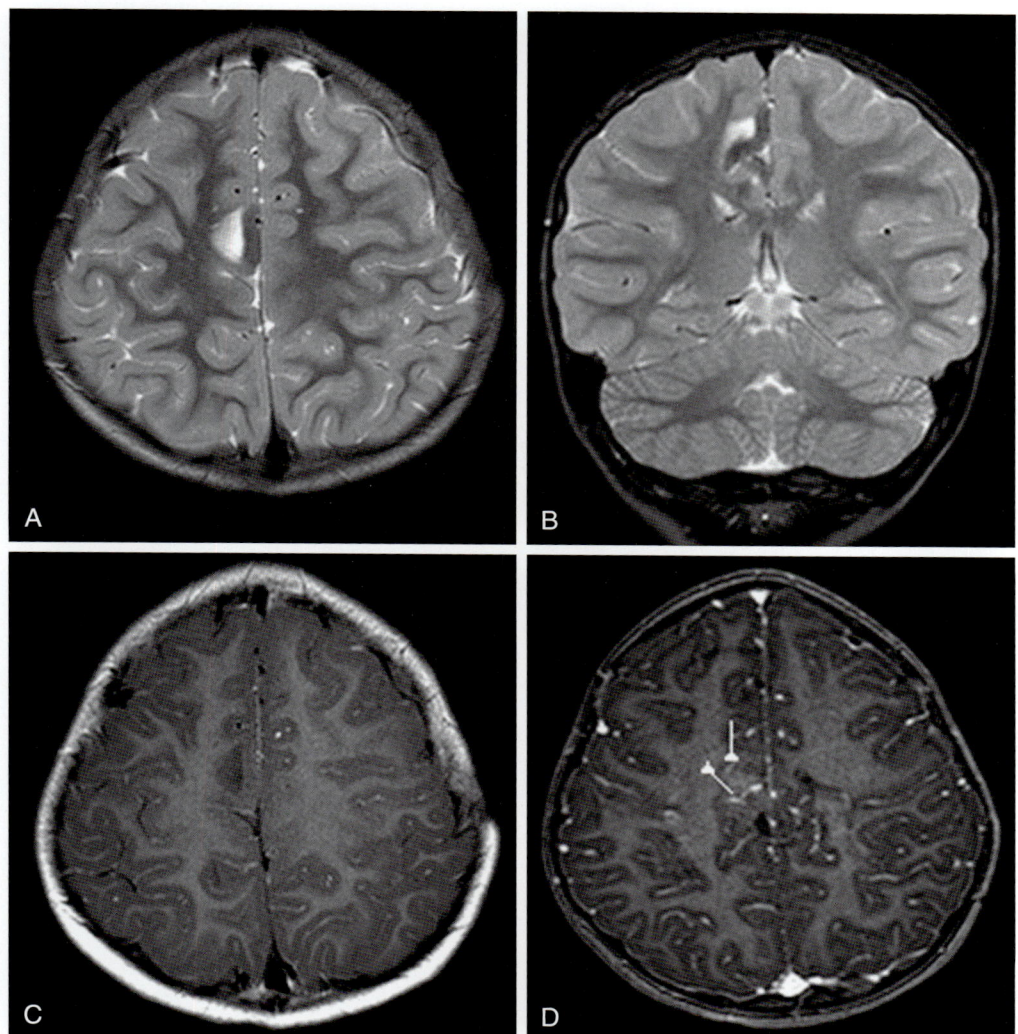

Figure 38-11 A 5-year-old boy with meningioangiomatosis and right frontal lobe epilepsy. An axial image (**A**) and a coronal T2-weighted image (**B**) show a low T2 signal in the cortex and a high T2 signal in the subcortical white matter of the lesion in the right mesial frontal lobe. **C,** An axial T1-weighted postcontrast image shows no enhancement of the lesion. **D,** Magnetoencephalography dipoles projected onto an axial T1-weighted postcontrast image show dipoles around the lesion.

of mixed high and low T1 and T2 signals surrounding the hemosiderin rim,[116] and they are best depicted on T2★ gradient echo imaging. Calcification may be seen on CT.

Treatment Cavernomas that present with refractory epilepsy should be treated surgically. The longer the duration of preoperative seizures, the greater the likelihood of continued seizures postoperatively.[117,118]

Meningioangiomatosis

Overview and Imaging Meningioangiomatosis is a rare lesion characterized by vascular proliferation involving the cortex and leptomeninges. The lesion can be sporadic or can occur in association with neurofibromatosis type 2. Sporadic lesions are solitary and typically present with refractory epilepsy. Lesions associated with neurofibromatosis type 2 often are multiple.[119] On CT, the lesion is hypodense and may contain calcification. On MRI, the cortex may have a hypointense

T1 and T2 signal as a result of calcification, and the subcortical white matter may have a hyperintense T2 signal. Enhancement may be seen after the administration of contrast material (Fig. 38-11). Meningioangiomatosis may mimic other disorders such as tumors, FCD, and arteriovenous malformation.[120] Treatment is surgical resection. However, patients with meningioangiomatosis tend to have poorer outcome with respect to seizure control compared with patients who have tumors or hippocampal sclerosis.[121]

Conclusion

Neuroimaging plays a crucial role in identifying anatomic lesions responsible for epilepsy and can assist in localizing the eloquent cortex and white matter tracts for presurgical planning. In persons with MRI-negative epilepsy, functional imaging with PET, SPECT, and magnetoencephalography may help localize the epileptogenic zone and also can assist in detecting subtle lesions.

WHAT THE CLINICIAN NEEDS TO KNOW

- If a lesion is present, what is the lesion?
- What is the extent of the lesion? For example, is it focal or diffuse, or does it involve a unilateral hemisphere or bilateral hemispheres?
- Where is the lesion located? Is the lesion close to eloquent brain areas?
- Determine if dual pathology is present. For example, in cases of low-grade tumors or FCD in the temporal lobe, does hippocampal sclerosis coexist?

Key Points

In approximately 30% of patients with epilepsy, the disease becomes refractory to medical therapy, and surgery may be necessary to control seizures in some of these patients. It is essential to identify a lesion on neuroimaging, because identification of a lesion has an impact on the surgical outcome.

A wide range of brain abnormalities can cause epilepsy. In children, the two most common causes of intractable focal epilepsy are MCDs and developmental tumors. Hippocampal sclerosis is less common in children compared with the adult population with intractable focal epilepsy.

Dual lesions can occur in approximately 15% of patients.

Meticulous review of MRI is necessary to identify subtle lesions such as FCD. MRI should be reviewed with knowledge of the clinical information, including seizure semiology and electroencephalographic findings.

In patients with MRI-negative epilepsy, functional imaging with ictal PET, ictal/interictal SPECT, and magnetoencephalography may help localize the epileptogenic zone.

Suggested Readings

Colombo N, Salamon N, Raybaud C, et al. Imaging of malformations of cortical development. *Epileptic Disord*. 2009;11(3):194-205.

Duncan JS. Epilepsy and imaging. *Brain*. 1997;120:339-377.

Rastogi S, Lee C, Salamon N. Neuroimaging in pediatric epilepsy: a multimodality approach. *Radiographics*. 2008;28(4):1079-1095.

Knowlton RC. Multimodality imaging in partial epilepsies. *Curr Opin Neurol*. 2004;17:165-172.

Widjaja E, Raybaud C. Advances in neuroimaging in patients with epilepsy. *Neurosurg Focus*. 2008;25(3):E3.

Reference

Full references for this chapter can be found on www.expertconsult.com.

Chapter 39

Trauma

ANDRE D. FURTADO, AJAYA R. PANDE, and VERA R. SPERLING

Incidence and Etiology

Head trauma and resulting traumatic brain injury (TBI) are the most common causes of morbidity and mortality in children. Head trauma alone, or in combination with injuries to other organs, is responsible for 50% of deaths in children from the ages of 1 to 14 years. Approximately 475,000 cases of TBI occur each year among infants, children, and adolescents younger than 14 years in the United States. Half of the cases occur in children younger than 5 years. Infants and children younger than 4 years and adolescents between 15 and 19 years of age are the two pediatric age groups at highest risk for TBI. Across the age groups, boys are more frequently injured than are girls (2:1). Motor vehicle accidents, especially car-versus-pedestrian accidents, are the most common causative events; they are responsible for approximately 30% of TBI cases.

In infants younger than 2 years, the most common causes of head trauma are falls, collision of the head with an object, the infant being dropped, and nonaccidental trauma (NAT). NAT accounts for more than 80% of deaths from head trauma in this group. Skull fractures, subdural hematomas, cerebral edema, and parenchymal contusions are common injuries before the age of 2 years. In children between 3 and 14 years of age, falls, sporting activities, all-terrain vehicle and motor vehicle accidents (when the child is a passenger, pedestrian, or cyclist), and assaults are the most common causes of head trauma. Fractures and parenchymal contusions are the most common injuries in this group. In older adolescents (>14 years), diffuse axonal injury (DAI) related to motor vehicle accidents predominates.

Birth trauma related to cephalopelvic disproportion, large gestational weight, atypical presentation, and the use of forceps or vacuum extraction is discussed in Chapter 23.

Imaging in Pediatric Head Trauma

COMPUTED TOMOGRAPHY

In general, computed tomography (CT) is the initial imaging modality used to evaluate patients with known or suspected head trauma to detect potentially life-threatening conditions that may require immediate surgical intervention. CT is widely available, easy to obtain, and can be performed quickly. It can be used with all manner of life-support and monitoring equipment. The advantages of multidetector CT scanners are a shorter scanning time and the ability to rapidly provide multiplanar and three-dimensional (3D) images. These advances have increased the sensitivity of CT in detecting the sequelae of head trauma, particularly skull base and temporal bone fractures. CT angiography (CTA) is useful in the evaluation of traumatic vascular injury and has the relative advantage of speed and fewer flow-related artifacts compared with magnetic resonance angiography (MRA).

Limitations of CT include low contrast in the immature brain, which decreases its sensitivity in detecting edema in infants, and beam hardening artifact, which may partially obscure small extraaxial collection or subtle cortical contusions adjacent to bone, particularly in the posterior fossa and skull base. Although advances in CT scanners have improved their sensitivity in detecting TBI, CT is known to underestimate the degree and extent of traumatic parenchymal injuries when compared with MR imaging (MRI). Nonetheless, acute imaging findings on CT have been proposed as criteria for grading and predicting outcome in persons with TBI (the Marshall Classification and subsequent modifications by Maas et al.).[1]

CT has been used liberally in children with scalp contusions. Recently, the exposure of children's brains to excessive radiation has become a concern after Pearce et al.[2] demonstrated that children exposed to radiation to the head from CT scans have an increased risk of the development of brain tumors many years later. For patients with a minor head injury (Glasgow Coma Scale [GCS] score of 13 to 15), clinical guidelines are available regarding indications for obtaining a CT scan of the head, such as the New Orleans Criteria, the Canadian CT Head Rule, and guidelines from the Pediatric Emergency Care Applied Research Network, with high sensitivity for detecting injuries that require neurosurgical intervention.[3] The American College of Radiology also publishes Appropriateness Criteria for imaging in the setting of head trauma, including a special section for children younger than 2 years in whom clinical assessment and criteria are less reliable than for older children.[4]

Adaptive statistical iterative reconstruction is a reconstruction technique that reduces image noise and improves low-contrast detectability and image quality. It provides higher diagnostic performance at a lower dose with no loss of image sharpness, noise, and artifacts.[5]

MAGNETIC RESONANCE IMAGING

Because of its more limited availability and longer scanning times, MRI generally is a secondary modality in the evaluation of acute head trauma. MRI usually is performed in the subacute and chronic phases when the findings on CT do not correlate with the patient's clinical condition, or when patients have unexpected neurologic deterioration or are not responding as expected. MRI offers the advantages of direct multiplanar imaging and greater overall sensitivity and specificity for the detection of TBI. It is particularly useful in the detection of small extraaxial hematomas, nonhemorrhagic intraaxial contusions, edema, brainstem injury, posterior fossa abnormalities, and DAI.[6] Contraindications to MRI include incompatible vascular clips, metallic implants, ocular foreign bodies, and most pacemakers.

Specific MRI sequences are invaluable in the evaluation of TBI. Fluid attenuation inversion recovery sequence (FLAIR) uses an inversion recovery pulse with a long inversion time that nulls signal from cerebrospinal fluid (CSF). FLAIR is sensitive for delineation of foci of signal abnormality adjacent to the ventricles and subarachnoid space.

T2* gradient-echo sequence (GRE) uses a pair of bipolar gradient pulses instead of a refocusing 180-degree pulse to enhance magnetic susceptibility caused by magnetic field distortion. Susceptibility-weighted imaging (SWI) is a technique that uses the signal loss from out-of-phase protons with different magnetic susceptibilities. SWI is more sensitive than GRE for detection of blood products such as deoxyhemoglobin, methemoglobin, and hemosiderin.[7]

Diffusion-weighted imaging (DWI) assesses the diffusion of water protons with use of a bipolar gradient pulse. The normal diffusion of water protons along the gradient reduces the MR signal. Areas of restricted diffusion will retain the MR signal and represent acute cerebral injury in persons with ischemia/hypoxia, trauma, metabolic disorders, and infection. Reduced diffusion is present in lesions with a low nucleus-cytoplasm ratio. DWI is susceptible to the intrinsic T2* signal of the tissue because it is a gradient sequence, known as the T2 shine-through effect. To separate the DWI signal from T2 shine through, the apparent water diffusion coefficient (ADC) is calculated by acquiring images with different gradient duration and amplitude (b-values), thus eliminating the T1 and T2* values.[8] Diffusion tensor imaging (DTI) assesses the anisotropy of the brain tissue by evaluating differences in the direction of diffusion of water molecules in normal and abnormal tissues and provides information about the orientation and integrity of the white matter tracts.

MRA and MR venography, which usually are performed without intravenous contrast material using the time-of-flight technique, are useful if a vascular injury is suspected.

MR spectroscopy (MRS) assesses the distribution and quantification of naturally occurring molecules within the central nervous system (see Chapter 25). Various techniques are available. The most commonly used technique is the point-resolved spectroscopy sequence. Both short time to echo (TE) and long TE acquisitions can be obtained. All acquisitions provide sensitive, noninvasive analysis of brain metabolites and cellular biochemical changes. Decreased N-acetyl aspartate (NAA) has been reported to correlate with abnormal neuropsychological function tests in persons with TBI.[9]

Perfusion MRI of the brain can be assessed either through a dynamic T2/T2* acquisition during a bolus injection of intravenous contrast material or with unenhanced techniques such as arterial spin labeling and blood–oxygen level dependent sequences (see Chapters 27 and 28). Perfusion MRI provides the cerebral blood volume, cerebral blood flow, and mean transit time in targeted areas of the brain.

Magnetization transfer imaging (MTI) relies on the principle that protons bound in macromolecules of tissues exhibit T1 relaxation coupling with protons in the aqueous phase or water. When an off-resonance saturation pulse is applied, it selectively saturates the protons that are bound in macromolecules. These protons subsequently exchange longitudinal magnetization with free water protons, leading to a reduction in the detected signal intensity. The magnetization transfer ratio (MTR) may provide a quantitative index of the structural integrity of tissue. Animal models of rotational acceleration suggest that quantitative MTI offers increased sensitivity to detection of histopathologically proven damage, such as axonal swelling, compared with conventional MRI. Although the precise mechanism for MTR reduction is incompletely understood for mild head trauma, the extent of the abnormality usually increases as the MTR value decreases. Abnormal MTR also has been found in normal-appearing white matter on MRI and is an apparent predictor of poor outcome.[10] Functional MRI has shown changes in regional brain activation in patients with TBI and has been used for assessment of clinical outcome of these patients.

OTHER IMAGING MODALITIES

Magnetoencephalography (MEG) detects the magnetic waves that are created by the electric current along the axons. The advantage of MEG over electroencephalography is that the magnetic waves are less susceptible to distortion caused by the skull than the electric currents (see Chapter 28). This method of imaging has found that brain dysfunction is present in a significantly greater number of patients with minor head trauma and postconcussive syndrome than is shown by MRI or electroencephalography. This method shows excessive abnormal low-frequency magnetic activity, which provides objective evidence of brain injury in these patients that correlates with the degree of symptomatic recovery.

Single-photon emission CT can detect abnormalities in cerebral blood flow; however, alterations in cerebral blood flow are not always associated with traumatic lesions on imaging. A negative initial single-photon emission CT scan after trauma seems to be a strong predictor of a favorable clinical outcome. A worse prognosis is associated with large lesions, multiple lesions, and lesions in the brainstem, temporal lobes, parietal lobes, or basal ganglia.

Positron emission tomography (PET) measures the cerebral metabolism of various substrates (see Chapter 25). Fluorodeoxyglucose is the primary substrate used in the measurement of glucose metabolism, which should correspond to neuronal viability. PET can be used in patients with DAI to determine the extent of damage and prognosis. PET also has been helpful in delineating the extent of reversibility of lesions. The major limitation of PET is the inability to distinguish functional abnormalities from structural damage.

Classification and Mechanisms of Head Injury

Based on different mechanisms of trauma and the associated injuries, the sequelae of head trauma can be classified into direct injury related to impact loading forces and indirect injury related to acceleration/deceleration and rotational forces. Direct injury may be subclassified into penetrating and nonpenetrating closed head injury (CHI). Moreover, brain injury in persons with a CHI may result directly from the impact (coup), or it may happen indirectly (contrecoup). The most common sequelae of direct head injury are scalp hematoma, skull fracture, direct brain contusion caused by a fracture and inward deformation of the skull, brain contusion caused by movement against the rough surface of the skull base, indirect (contrecoup) brain contusion diagonal to the site of impact, stretching and laceration of the brain parenchyma, subarachnoid hemorrhage (SAH) as a result of parenchymal injury, and epidural and subdural hematomas caused by direct vascular injury beneath the site of impact. Nonimpact, acceleration/deceleration injuries are the result of forces of translation (linear), acceleration/deceleration, and rotational and angular acceleration causing shear-strain forces on axons, neurons, and blood vessels. These injuries include contusions, DAI, deep gray matter injury, brainstem injuries, intraparenchymal hematomas as a result of vascular injury, and extraaxial hematomas. The axons are most vulnerable, and the blood vessels are the most resistant to injury from acceleration/deceleration forces (Fig. 39-1).[11]

Based on the GCS, head injuries are classified as mild (GCS score 13 to 15), moderate (GCS score 9 to 12), and severe (GCS score 3 to 8). Most head trauma results in mild injury; the risk of death from minor head injury in childhood approaches 0%. Moderate head injury in children has a similar rate of occurrence as in adults but a lower mortality rate. Severe head injury occurs less frequently in children compared with adults and has a significantly lower mortality rate. The exception is in infants younger than 2 years, who have a higher mortality rate from severe head injuries. This higher mortality rate is partially attributed to the occurrence of NAT in this age group.[12]

SCALP HEMATOMA

A scalp contusion often results in subcutaneous edema. If the contusion is of sufficient severity to cause a hemorrhage, a hematoma is formed under the skin. Scalp hematomas usually resolve without complication, with the exception of subgaleal hematomas in infants, which pose the risk of life-threatening hypovolemia. The size and location of the contusion and the patient's age are important factors when evaluating a patient with a scalp contusion, because large scalp hematomas (particularly involving the parietal or temporal regions in infants younger than 12 months) are associated with an increased risk of skull fracture and intracranial injury.

SKULL FRACTURES

The likelihood of intracranial injury increases significantly when a skull fracture is present in a child. However, the absence of a skull fracture does not preclude intracranial injury and has little prognostic significance in pediatric head trauma. The skull of a younger child is thinner and more pliable than the adult skull. Therefore children have a higher incidence of both skull fractures and traumatic intracranial injury without the presence of a fracture, particularly between the ages of 6 months to 2 years. The parietal and occipital

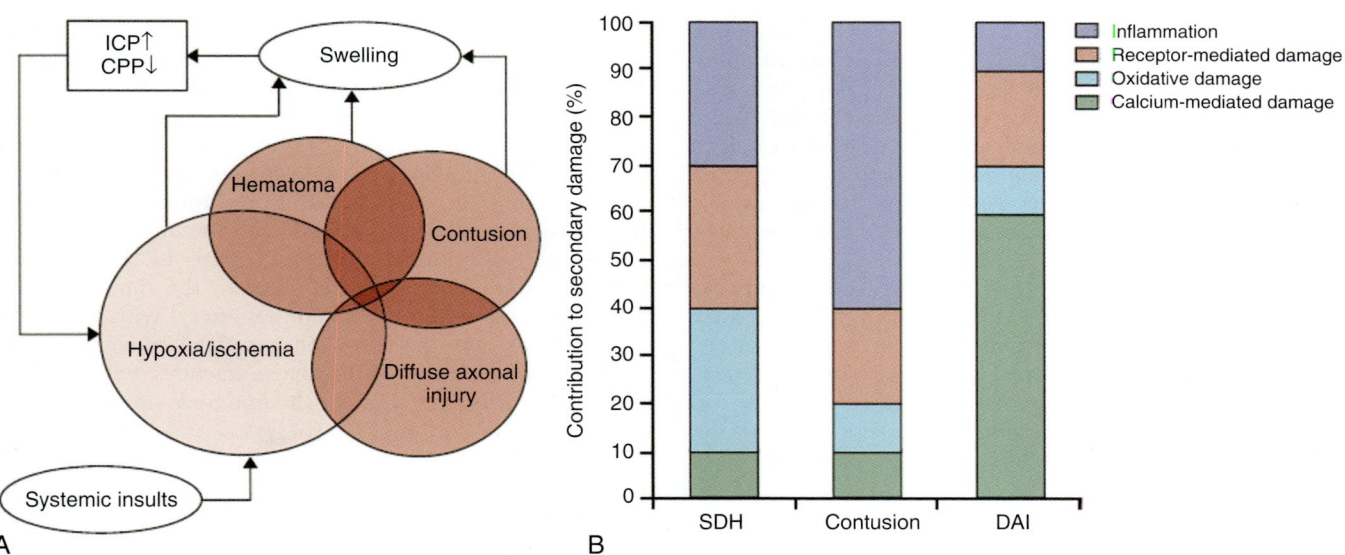

A   B

Figure 39-1 Components of traumatic brain injury and the importance of different pathophysiological mechanisms. *CPP,* Cerebral perfusion pressure; *DAI,* diffuse axonal injury; *ICP,* intracranial pressure; *SDH,* subdural hematoma. (From Maas AIR, Stocchetti N, Bullock R. Moderate and severe traumatic brain injury in adults. *Lancet Neurol* 2008;7:728-741.)

bones are most commonly involved, followed by the frontal and temporal bones. Falls and motor vehicle accidents account for most skull fractures in children.

Fractures in infants may be linear, depressed, diastatic, compound (stellate or "egg shell"), "ping pong" (buckled), or penetrating. In this age group, fractures are usually the result of a fall from the arms of a caregiver, or they result from an object striking the head. Fractures tend to pass through points of weakness and course toward a suture, synchondrosis, foramen, or canal. As the calvarium becomes more mature, comminuted fractures may occur.

Linear calvarial fractures are more frequent in all age groups, followed by depressed or comminuted calvarial fractures and basilar fractures. Linear fractures usually heal without complication. Complex fractures in which the dura mater is torn may be complicated by herniation of the pia and arachnoid layers, creating a leptomeningeal cyst. The CSF pulsations lead to progressive erosion of skull around the fracture, known as a "growing fracture," which appears as an angular or linear lytic lesion in the skull with scalloped margins (see Chapter 23). Underlying brain contusion is not uncommon.

Depressed fractures are comminuted skull fractures in which broken bones are displaced inward by at least the thickness of the skull. Depressed skull fractures usually result from blunt force trauma to the head and may result in increased intracranial pressure (ICP), epidural hematoma, and parenchymal contusion or laceration. Depressed fractures usually are treated surgically to prevent complications and also for cosmetic reasons. Fractures displacing the dural sinuses often are treated conservatively because of the potential risk of fatal hemorrhage with intervention (e-Fig. 39-2). Depressed fractures are categorized as compound fractures when a laceration of the overlying scalp is present and as penetrating fractures when an underlying dural tear is present, allowing potential communication between the external environment and the brain. Fractures that communicate with the paranasal sinuses, middle ear, or the mastoid air cells within the intracranial compartment are considered compound fractures. Pneumocephalus indicates the presence of a compound fracture (e-Fig. 39-3). The most serious complications of compound skull fractures are CSF leak and infection. Increased risk factors for infection include visible contamination (hair, skin, fat, or bone), a meningeal tear, and delayed treatment for more than 8 hours after the initial injury. A rare type of compound skull fracture is the elevated skull fracture, which occurs when the fracture is elevated outward above the outer table of the skull.

Diastatic skull fractures involve the cranial sutures. Although diastatic fractures usually involve the lambdoid suture in newborns and infants, they may involve any suture in any age group. The normal suture becomes widened, measuring more than 2 mm. Asymmetric sutures, even if they are less than 2 mm in width, should raise suspicion for a diastatic fracture. An overriding suture is indicative of a diastatic fracture.

Fractures involving the skull base are associated with increased risk of vascular or cranial nerve injury. Basilar fractures most commonly involve the temporal bone, causing bleeding into the middle ear and mastoid air cells. Temporal bone fractures are classified according to their orientation to the long axis of the temporal bone as longitudinal, transverse,

or complex. This classification is helpful in determining the risk of complications. Longitudinal fractures represent the majority (70% to 90%) and may be associated with facial nerve injury, incudostapedial dissociation, and pneumocephalus. Transverse temporal bone fractures are less common but have a higher risk of permanent injury to the facial nerve and vestibulocochlear nerve, as well as cochlear disruption, causing facial paralysis, sensorineural hearing loss, and perilymph fistula, respectively. Temporal bone fractures involving the petrous apex or the carotid canal are associated with increased risk of carotid dissection, occlusion, pseudoaneurysm, and/or jugular vein injury.

Studies report a sensitivity of 94% to 99% for the detection of linear or depressed skull fractures with routine radiographis of the calvarium. These radiographs usually are obtained in suspected cases NAT as part of a skeletal survey to document additional areas of injury. Standard CT has a lower overall sensitivity for the detection of linear fractures parallel to the plane of imaging. Images and 3D CT reconstructions often are diagnostic in difficult cases. CT has a relatively high degree of sensitivity for the detection of depressed and basilar skull fractures and fractures of the facial bones, sinuses, and orbits. In children, skull fractures typically heal in 6 to 8 weeks but may remain radiographically apparent for 1 year.

EXTRAAXIAL AND INTRAVENTRICULAR HEMORRHAGE

Epidural Hematoma

Epidural hematoma is uncommon in infants and slowly increases in incidence with age, reaching a peak in adulthood. The etiology of epidural hematomas in children is different from that in adults. In younger children, venous epidural hematomas are more common than the arterial epidural hematomas. Tearing of a dural venous sinus, typically the transverse or sigmoid sinus, or an emissary or diploic vein are common causes of venous epidural hematomas. The typical locations of venous epidural hematomas are in the posterior fossa and occipital region from laceration of the transverse or sigmoid sinus, in the middle cranial fossa from injury of the sphenoparietal sinus or middle meningeal veins, and in the parasagittal area from a tear of the superior sagittal sinus. In older children and adolescents, arterial hematomas are more common. The vascular groove for the middle meningeal artery is relatively shallow, with the dura more adherent to the calvarium in children. Trauma to the calvarium causing inward deformity can separate the dura from the inner table and injure the meningeal artery, with hematoma accumulating over the temporal or parietal convexities (Fig. 39-4). The incidence of associated fractures with epidural hematomas is slightly less in children than in adults (83% vs. 93%).

The clinical presentation of epidural hematomas in children typically includes an absence of loss of consciousness at the time of injury, with a lucid interval within the first 24 hours. Several factors are associated with a poor outcome in children with epidural hematomas, including absence of an immediate lucid period, the presence of additional intracranial injuries, and delayed diagnosis and surgical intervention, if indicated.

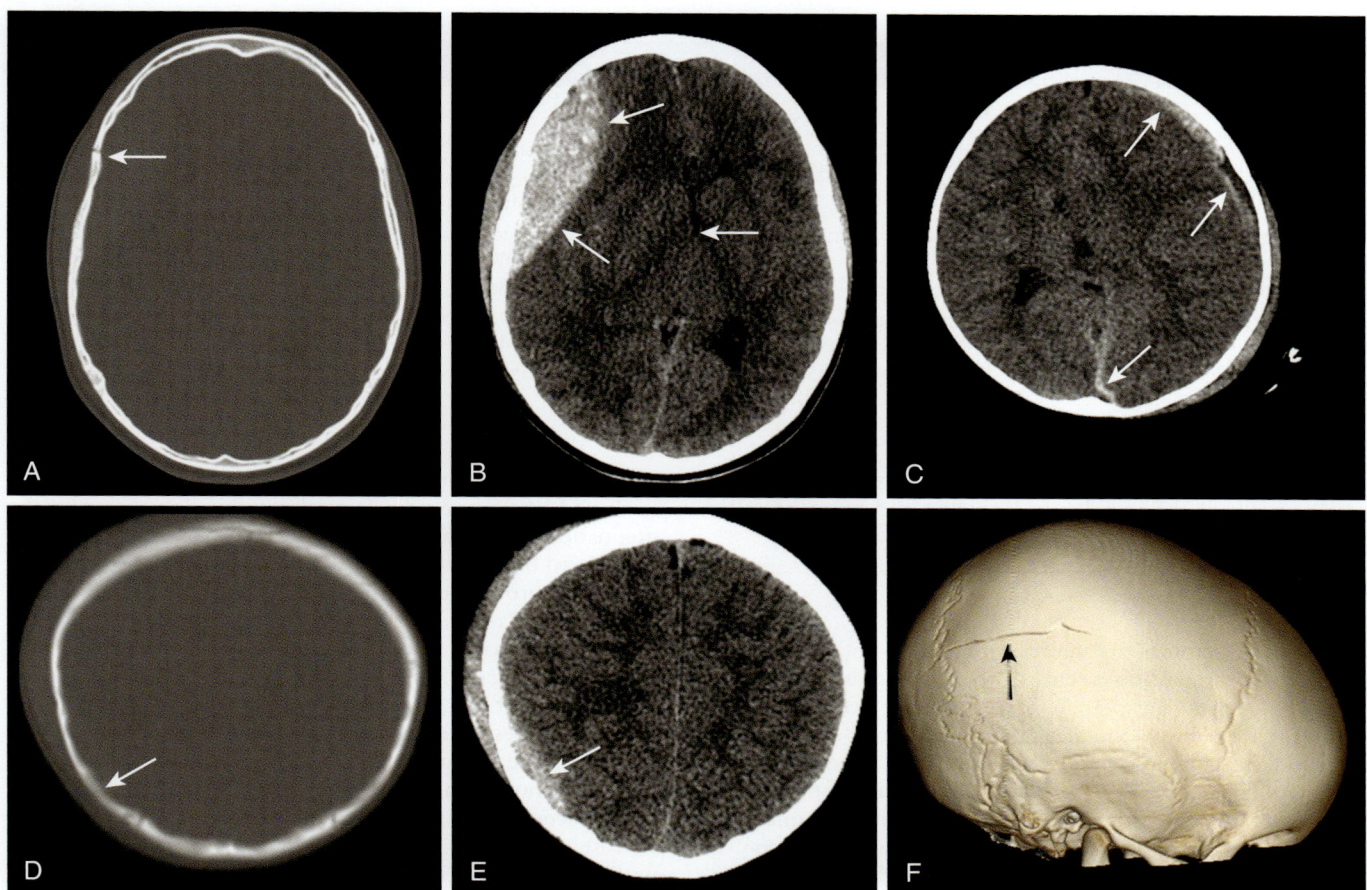

Figure 39-4 Skull fractures and extraaxial hematomas. Unenhanced computed tomography images showing a pterional fracture (*arrow*) (**A**) and a large acute epidural hematoma with a contralateral midline shift (**B**). **C,** In contrast to the acute epidural hematoma, a hyperacute mixed attenuation left frontal subdural hematoma extending to the left occipital lobe is shown (*arrows*). **D,** A skull fracture parallel to the image plane appears as focal hypoattenuation (*arrow*). **E,** An acute epidural hematoma adjacent to the fracture (*arrow*) in the same patient as in part **D. F,** The fracture that is poorly visualized on axial images is well demonstrated on three-dimensional volume rendering (*arrow*).

Epidural collections do not cross suture lines because of periosteal attachments, but they do cross over the falx and tentorium. Posterior fossa epidural hematomas may extend into the supratentorial compartment, whereas subdural hematomas are confined to one compartment. Moreover, epidural collections adjacent to the frontal bones may cross the midline over the superior sagittal sinus, whereas subdural hematomas extend along the falx. These features are much more reliable in differentiating epidural hematomas from subdural hematomas than is a biconvex or lentiform shape, which may not always be present. Venous epidural hematomas frequently are concave, particularly in the posterior fossa. Venous epidural hematomas are usually larger and carry an overall worse prognosis compared with arterial epidural hematomas because of their delayed presentation.

On CT, acute epidural hematomas have increased attenuation with progression to intermediate attenuation in the subacute phase and decreased attenuation, possibly with enhancing membranes, in the chronic phase. Mixed attenuation may represent active bleeding, hypercoagulable states, a dural tear with mixed CSF and blood in the epidural space, or layering serum as a result of clot retraction. Active bleeding may produce a "swirl" effect within the collection. If the mass effect of an epidural hematoma appears disproportionate to the size of the collection, underlying edema related to parenchymal contusion should be suspected.

On MRI, the signal characteristics of extraaxial collections are more variable than on CT and depend on several factors such as the patient's hematocrit, local partial pressure of oxygen, pH level, protein concentration, and the strength of the magnetic field. The signal changes over time of intracranial hematomas have been mainly studied for parenchymal hemorrhages and subdural hematomas in adults.

The aging of extraaxial hematomas based on signal characteristics in children has not been validated. The evolution of epidural and subdural hematomas follows a similar pattern (Table 39-1). In contrast to parenchymal hematomas, the hypointense rim on T1- and T2-weighted images representing hemosiderin is rarely seen in extraaxial hematomas because of the absence of a blood-brain barrier.

MRI is useful in distinguishing small epidural from subdural hematomas, in which the displaced dura is visualized as a thin, uniform line of hypointense signal on intermediate and T2-weighted sequences. The inner membrane of a

Table 39-1

Magnetic Resonance Imaging Appearance of Blood at Different Stages at 1.5 Tesla			
	T1	**T2**	**Gradient Echo**
Hyperacute (4-6 hours)	Isointense	Hyperintense	Hypointense
Acute (7-72 hours)	Isointense	Central hypointensity and peripheral hyperintensity	Hypointense
Early subacute (4-7 days)	Peripheral hyperintensity and central isointensity	Hypointense with some central hyperintensity	Hypointense
Late subacute (1-4 weeks)	Hyperintense	Hyperintense	Hypointense
Early chronic (months)	Peripheral iso intensity to hypointensity and central hyperintensity	Peripheral hypointensity and central hyperintensity	Hypointense
Late chronic (months to years)	Hypointense	Hypointense	Hypointense

subacute or chronic subdural hematoma may have a similar appearance, but the membrane is thicker and more irregular in contour.

Subdural Hematoma

Subdural hematomas are more common in infants than in older children and adolescents. Typically, subdural hematomas result from shear-strain forces causing stretching and tearing of bridging veins that traverse the inner layer of the dura and the arachnoid membrane. In infants, subdural hematomas are bilateral in 80% to 85% of cases. The most common causes of subdural hematomas are accidental trauma and NAT, shunt placement or overshunting with intracranial hypotension, and blood dyscrasias. Most subdural hematomas in infants younger than 2 years are caused by child abuse. Other findings suggestive of NAT include additional signs of unreported physical trauma, a history of trauma inconsistent with the severity or type of injury, interhemispheric subdural hematomas, subdural hematomas at different stages of blood degradation, and the presence of retinal hemorrhages.

Clinically, infants with subdural hematomas are asymptomatic or may present with vomiting, poor feeding, irritability, a bulging fontanelle, and increasing head circumference. Older children more commonly present with the classic signs of raised ICP, headache, altered level of consciousness, increased systemic blood pressure with decreased heart rate, irregular respiration, asymmetric pupils (anisocoria), and hemiparesis. Large subdural hematomas may manifest with anemia as a result of blood loss.

Subdural hematomas are most commonly located over the frontal, parietal, and temporal lobes. Posterior fossa subdural hematomas, which account for approximately 10% of cases, usually are a result of tearing of the dural sinuses or tentorium. In contrast to epidural hematomas, subdural collections cross sutures but do not cross the falx or tentorium. The normal falx is hyperdense on CT, but it is very thin with a smooth contour. Irregularity or thickening is suggestive of a subdural hematoma.

The CT imaging characteristics of subdural hematomas depend on the age of the hematoma. Hyperacute hematomas representing unclotted blood show attenuation similar to flowing blood in the dural sinuses. After a few hours, an acute subdural hematoma demonstrates increased attenuation related to clotted blood. The hyperattenuating acute blood clot may be mixed with blood from active bleeding, serum

from clot retraction, or CSF resulting from a tear in the arachnoid (see Fig. 39-4). Typically within 1 to 3 weeks, the attenuation of a subacute hematoma decreases and becomes isodense to brain parenchyma. After 2 to 3 weeks, the attenuation of a chronic hematoma becomes similar to that of CSF. The hematoma may be difficult to see during the subacute and chronic phases, and associated signs of mass effect will indicate its presence, such as effacement of the adjacent sulci, displacement of the gray-white matter junction, compression of the ventricles, or herniation. If the presence of a hematoma is questionable, intravenous contrast material can be administered to show enhancing inner and outer membranes that are not seen in the acute phase. If the size of the collection increases or if the attenuation values appear greater than expected or are heterogeneous, rebleeding should be suspected. The development of a fluid-fluid level in the chronic phase also is suggestive of rebleeding. The membranes calcify in up to 3% of cases.

MRI is more sensitive than other modalities for the detection of subdural hematomas, particularly when their attenuation is similar to that of the brain parenchyma or of CSF on routine T1 and T2 sequences. Proton-density and FLAIR sequences are the most sensitive for detection of subdural hematomas that are isointense to CSF on T1- and T2-weighted images. The appearance of subdural hematomas on MRI also varies, depending on the phase and organization of the blood products. The evolution of the signal characteristics of subdural hematomas are the same as those previously described for epidural hematomas.

Subdural hygromas are caused by laceration of the arachnoid with accumulation of CSF in the subdural space. Subdural hygromas may occur either alone or in combination with acute hemorrhage after trauma. Subdural hygromas generally manifest 3 to 5 days after injury and are often bilateral (~50% of cases). Hygromas differ from chronic subdural hematomas that are isointense to CSF on T1- and T2-weighted images because they follow the CSF signal in all sequences, including FLAIR and proton-density sequences.

SUBARACHNOID AND INTRAVENTRICULAR HEMORRHAGE

Traumatic intraventricular hemorrhage is related either to shearing of subependymal veins or decompression of a parenchymal or subarachnoid hematoma into the ventricles. The most common location of injury to the subependymal veins is along the anterior corpus callosum, posterior fornix, or septum pellucidum. Traumatic SAH is usually a result of damage of pia-arachnoid vessels and associated parenchymal injury. It is seen in approximately 18% to 25% of pediatric CHI cases. The amount of blood in the subarachnoid space is typically small and rarely persists for more than 1 week. If a patient has a large SAH without parenchymal damage or extraaxial hematomas, the possibility of an underlying aneurysm or arteriovenous malformation that bled prior to the trauma may be considered. SAH may obstruct the normal CSF resorption at the level of the pacchionian granulations and result in communicating hydrocephalus.

CT is the imaging modality of choice for acute SAH and intraventricular hemorrhage, showing increased attenuation blood within the sulci (Fig. 39-5), layering along the interhemispheric fissure and the tentorium, and in the ventricles. The most common location of traumatic SAH is in the posterior interhemispheric fissure and along the tentorium. Although the normal falx is relatively hyperdense on CT, hyperdense material insinuating into the cerebral sulci is indicative of SAH. Initially, SAH is detected adjacent to the source of bleeding. With time, SAH accumulates in the basal cisterns (particularly the interpeduncular cistern) and Sylvian fissures, over the convexities, and in the occipital horns of the lateral ventricles.

MRI is more sensitive than CT in detecting small amounts of SAH, showing increased signal on FLAIR sequences. GRE and SWI sequences are less sensitive than FLAIR, but the

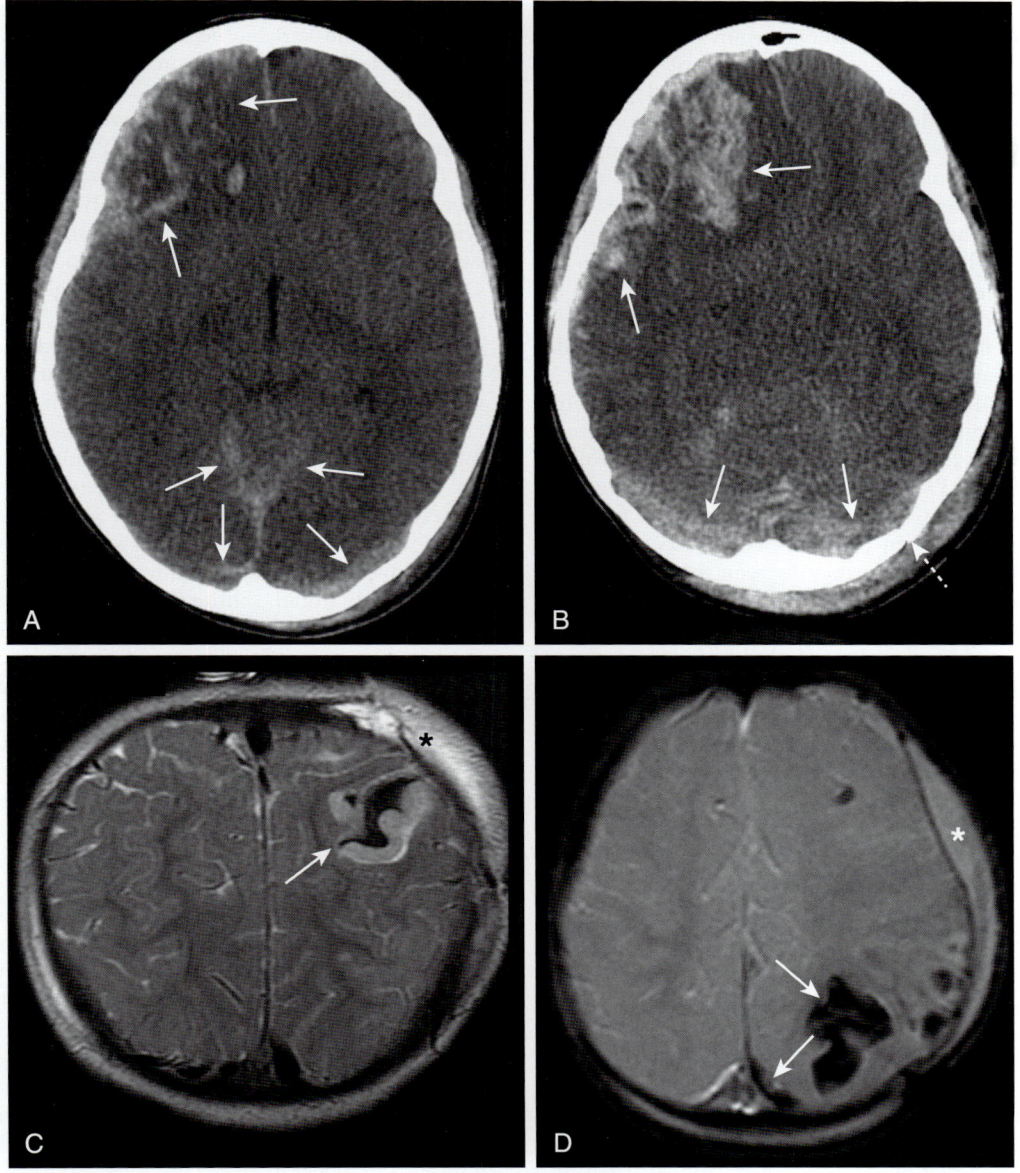

Figure 39-5 Parenchymal contusion, subarachnoid hemorrhage, and laceration. Unenhanced computed tomography images (**A** and **B**) showing a contrecoup right frontal and temporal contusion with associated subarachnoid hemorrhage. In the occipital region, acute bilateral subdural hematomas are present, along with a left occipital fracture and a large scalp hematoma from the primary impact (*broken arrow*). A magnetic resonance imaging T2-weighted image (**C**) and susceptibility-weighted image (**D**) show a typical perenchymal laceration with a hematoma (*arrows*). Also note postcraniectomy findings (*asterisks*).

demonstration of hypointensity on these sequences confirms the presence of blood. Although extensive or recurrent SAH is rare in children, it may lead to superficial siderosis as a result of the presence of hemosiderin in macrophages along the leptomeninges. Vasospasm resulting from traumatic SAH is very rare in children.

TRAUMATIC PARENCHYMAL INJURY

Contusion and Laceration

A brain contusion is a bruise of the parenchyma. The cortex is invariably involved, with variable involvement of the underlying white matter. Brain contusions are twice as common in children as in adults. Brain contusion may occur at the site of impact (coup), diagonally opposite the site of the impact (contrecoup), along the rough calvarial surfaces in the anterior temporal and orbitofrontal regions (acceleration/deceleration), and against the free margins of falx cerebri, tentorium, and foramen magnum (in cases of herniation). Brain edema develops over the first 1 to 2 days and is maximal 3 to 5 days after the initial injury. Approximately 50% of brain contusions are hemorrhagic. Hemorrhage occurs in the Virchow-Robin spaces, perpendicular to the pial surface, and may extend into the subarachnoid space. With increasing severity, the microhemorrhages coalesce into more focal hematomas, which usually develop 2 to 4 days after the injury. The presence of focal parenchymal hematomas has been associated with an adverse outcome. After approximately 1 month, the contused areas evolve into encephalomalacia and associated volume loss.

CT shows hypoattenuation with loss of the gray-white matter differentiation and effacement of the sulci. Hemorrhagic foci appear as areas of increased attenuation involving the cortex (see Fig. 39-5). The attenuation of acute focal parenchymal hematomas increases during the first few days as the clot retracts and then decreases with subsequent proteolysis. Cortical enhancement may be seen for 1 to 2 weeks as a result of proliferation of immature capillaries that lack a blood-brain barrier.

MRI is the imaging modality of choice for parenchymal contusion. In the first hours after the injury when overt edema is not apparent, DWI is the most sensitive sequence for detecting parenchymal contusion, as well as shear injury. After 1 to 2 days, the contused areas appear hyperintense on FLAIR and T2-weighted images related to edema, and the microhemorrhages or focal confluent hemorrhages appear hypointense on T2 GRE or SWI images (e-Fig. 39-6). High signal intensity on T1-weighted images may be seen in the subacute phase, related to the presence of methemoglobin. FLAIR is insensitive to parenchymal contusion in neonates and infants because of the low contrast with the unmyelinated white matter. T2-weighted images are particularly useful in these cases showing loss of gray-matter differentiation and hyperintensity relative to the normal brain.

Lacerations of brain parenchyma are the result of a greater mechanical force that causes tearing of tissue, extending from the cortex into the white matter. Although lacerations are characteristic of penetrating or perforating injury, they also occur in CHI or near a fracture. They are associated with a variable degree of hemorrhage (see Fig. 39-5). The hematoma may rapidly increase in size after the injury, and follow-up imaging in the first 24 to 48 hours is recommended. The most typical locations for parenchymal laceration are the inferior frontal and anterior temporal lobes. Lacerations also may occur in the corpus callosum and brainstem in association with DAI. Lacerations in the pontomedullary junction and cerebral peduncles presumably are related to hyperextension injury. Cerebellar contusions usually are associated with occipital fractures and most frequently involve the inferior cerebellar hemispheres and cerebellar tonsils.

Diffuse Axonal Injury

DAI is one of the most devastating types of TBI and the most common cause of posttraumatic neurologic and cognitive disability and a vegetative state. DAI is more common in children than previously recognized, with infants being particularly susceptible. Different parts of the brain have different consistencies depending on cell morphology, cell concentration, and variable degrees of fixation. DAI results from rapid acceleration/deceleration, resulting in angular and rotational forces that stretch the axons, causing damage to the axonal cytoskeleton, resulting in swelling. Subsequent calcium influx into injured axons is thought to cause further damage.

The degree of impairment of consciousness is usually more severe than with other primary injuries. Patients may present with immediate loss of consciousness and coma. Clinical symptoms often are disproportionate to imaging findings, and CT findings may be normal. Although high-speed motor vehicle accidents are the most common cause of DAI, it also may be caused by any head trauma, including relatively minor trauma. The mechanism of shear-strain injury in infants younger than 12 months is different from the pattern in older children and adults; the incidence of hemorrhagic lesions in infants seems to be lower. The dominant histologic abnormality in infants predominantly is related to hypoxia, which acutely leads to brain swelling and sometimes death. In later stages, extensive encephalomacia and volume loss occur.

All imaging modalities underestimate the extent of DAI. As previously noted, diffuse brain damage may not be evident on CT. Reports have found that CT of acute CHI reveals abnormalities in only 20% to 50% of patients with axonal shear injuries, primarily because of their small size and frequent initial nonhemorrhagic nature. The typical CT findings of DAI include discrete foci of increased or decreased attenuation, which are usually bilateral, less than 1 cm in size, and are oriented in an axis that parallels the tracts. DAI is most commonly located in the subcortical white matter, near the gray-white matter junction of the frontal and temporal lobes, posterior corpus callosum (most commonly the posterior body and splenium), and brainstem (dorsolateral midbrain and upper pons). An important indirect sign of axonal injury involving the corpus callosum is the presence of intraventricular hemorrhage from shearing of the adjacent subependymal veins (Fig. 39-7). With increasing severity, involvement of the internal and external capsules, basal ganglia, thalami, cerebellum, and parietal and occipital lobes occurs. CT also demonstrates diffuse brain edema in infants with severe shear-strain injury. Within 2 to 3 weeks, encephalomalacia and volume loss develop.

MRI is more sensitive than other modalities in detecting shear injuries. In patients in whom DAI is suspected, imaging should be performed at least 3 to 7 days after injury because cellular necrosis and edema are maximal at this time. Fast spin

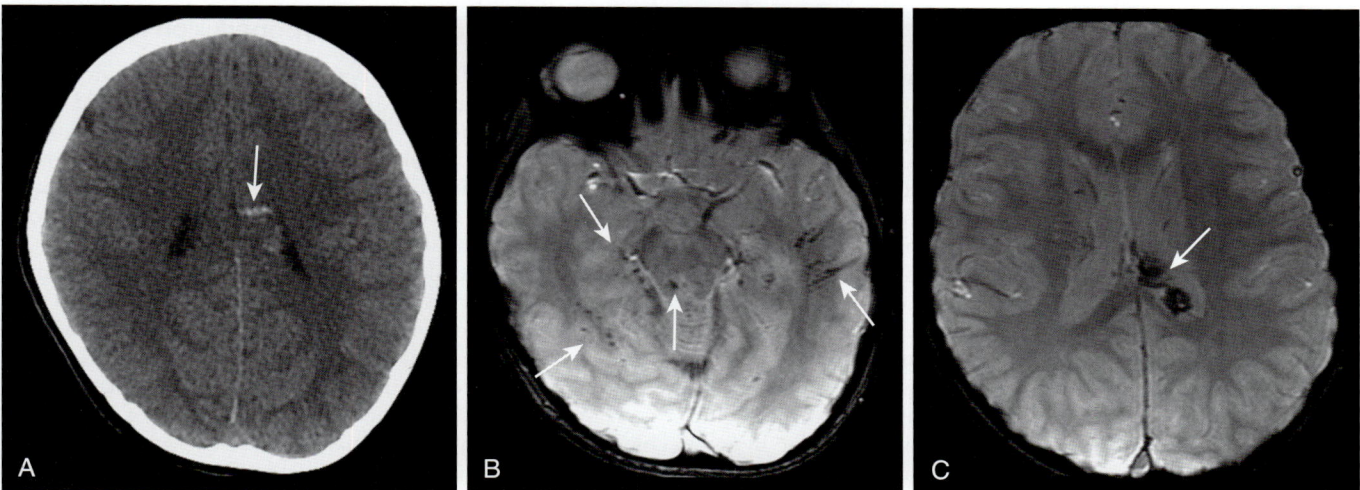

Figure 39-7 Diffuse axonal injury. **A,** An unenhanced computed tomography image with hyperdense foci in the region of the corpus callosum compatible with a shear injury (*arrow*). **B** and **C,** A magnetic resonance susceptibility-weighted imaging sequence shows multiple susceptibility foci of hypointensity/blooming (*arrows*) consistent with parenchymal (**B**) and intraventricular (**C**) hemorrhage.

echo imaging is less sensitive to DAI than is conventional spin echo imaging.

MRI using SWI and T2★ sequences detects DAI in approximately 30% of patients with mild head injury and an initially normal CT scan. DAI is visualized as multiple small, round, ovoid, or elliptical areas of decreased T1 signal, increased T2 and FLAIR signal, and abnormal DWI signal. Hemorrhagic lesions cause susceptibility effect, with hypointensity on T2★ and SWI (see Fig. 39-7). Initial nonhemorrhagic lesions may convert to hemorrhagic foci with time, showing typical evolution of signal characteristics of blood, with increasing size as a result of hemorrhage and edema. DWI depicts additional lesions that exhibit facilitated or, most commonly, restricted diffusion. ADC values decrease over a longer period, ~18 days, after injury, which is beyond the usual time frame for cytotoxic edema related to ischemia.[13]

A reduction in fractional anisotropy has been shown with DTI in early imaging in patients with TBI; this reduction is not apparent with other imaging, including DWI. DTI with 3D fiber tracking has been shown to visualize acute axonal shearing injuries and may have prognostic value for cognitive and neurologic sequelae after TBI.

MTI can show the extent of these lesions to a greater degree. The MTR provides a quantitative index of the magnetization transfer effect and may be viewed as a measure of the structural integrity of tissues. The detection of abnormal MTR in normal-appearing white matter may predict a poor patient outcome. With MTI, the MTR can be derived and can quantitatively measure the structural integrity of tissues. It is more sensitive than T2-weighted images in detecting histologic axonal damage in animal models. Associations have been found between MTI abnormalities and neurologic and cognitive deficits. MRS also can quantify the damage after DAI with decreased NAA, increased choline, and increased glutamate and glutamine levels.

A grading scheme for DAI based on the severity of head trauma and the location of the lesions has been proposed, with mild trauma resulting in more superficial lesions and increasingly severe trauma resulting in involvement of deeper

structures. Although DAI is rarely fatal, a greater number of lesions correlates with poorer outcomes. Patients with widespread MRI findings or brainstem injuries usually show no significant neurologic recovery.

Deep Gray Matter Injury

Deep gray matter injury, which usually occurs in severely or fatally injured patients, constitutes less than 5% of all primary intraaxial injuries. This type of injury is found in the thalami, basal ganglia, upper brainstem, and regions around the third ventricle from shear-strain forces disrupting small perforating vessels. The vascular injury can lead to ischemic injury and infarctions with hemorrhagic or nonhemorrhagic lesions. Patients who survive have profound neurologic deficits. CT is usually normal but can show small foci of petechial hemorrhage. FLAIR is the most sensitive MRI sequence for nonhemorrhagic deep gray matter injury, showing foci of hyperintense signal. Other sequences give the expected signal changes of blood products if the lesions are hemorrhagic.

Brainstem Injury

Although primary and secondary brainstem injury is uncommon in the pediatric population, it likely underestimated because CT remains the initial imaging modality of choice in children with head trauma. Clinically, patients with a brainstem injury do not follow the expected course of recovery, warranting further evaluation with MRI.

Primary injuries include brainstem contusion, brainstem shear injury, and the rare pontomedullary separation. Secondary lesions include hypoxic-ischemic injury and Duret hemorrhages. Secondary brainstem injuries cause death in almost 50% of cases of head injury caused by blunt trauma.

Primary brainstem injury can occur from direct forces or, more commonly, indirect forces. This type of injury characteristically involves the dorsal lateral midbrain and superior pons. Less frequent involvement is seen in the lateral midbrain or cerebral peduncle, and infrequent involvement is seen in the periaqueductal region of the midbrain. The lesions involving the periaqueductal region may show hemorrhage and ischemia on MRI related to secondary shear-strain forces on perforating vessels of the brainstem. Indirect forces resulting in brainstem injury can have associated DAI in the corpus callosum and deep white matter of the cerebrum. Although rare, direct forces have been found to result in injury to the upper midbrain from impaction against the free edge of the tentorium. The association of this type of injury with DAI is variable. Pontomedullary separation is a tear of the brainstem at the ventral pontomedullary sulcus as a result of hyperextension forces. This injury is often associated with craniocervical dislocation and is usually fatal.

Secondary brainstem injury can be caused by mechanical forces on the upper midbrain resulting in transtentorial herniation, global injury related to hypoxia-ischemia, or hypoperfusion injury related to hypotension. Transtentorial herniation may be a result of many etiologies, including generalized edema, increased ICP, and intraaxial and extraaxial hematomas. If the cause of transtentorial herniation can be treated, its sequelae have the potential to be reversed. Prolonged compression of the brainstem often results in irreversible injury, typically involving the central brainstem. Brainstem injury related to hypoxia is usually a terminal event.

The tegmentum of the midbrain and the anterior pons are most commonly involved in secondary brainstem injury and can show areas of hemorrhage, infarction, and necrosis. Duret hemorrhages typically are seen in the central pons. They are always seen in association with downward herniation and usually are caused by damage to the medial pontine perforating branches of the basilar artery. The basilar artery is relatively tethered by the circle of Willis, and caudal displacement of the brainstem results in stretching and ultimately laceration of the perforating arteries. The hemorrhage also can result either from vessel wall rupture caused by hypoxic injury or from venous infarction.

Diffuse Brain Swelling and Hypoperfusion Injury

Diffuse brain swelling has been reported to occur in 21% of cases of head trauma in the pediatric age group and is 3.5 times more common in this group, particularly in infants and young children, compared with adults. In head trauma in children, two conditions produce similar but distinguishable imaging patterns of diffuse brain swelling: increased blood volume and axonal shear injury.

After a young child sustains a traumatic injury, the immature vasoregulatory system responds with vasodilation and increased blood flow, resulting in a hyperemic state and subsequent diffuse cerebral swelling or edema. In addition, the release of excitatory amines also causes vasodilation and increased blood volume, and the redistribution of intracranial blood from pial to intraparenchymal vessels seems to contribute further to the hyperemic state. On CT, axonal shear injury in the early stage can have an imaging appearance similar to that of cerebral edema.

The imaging findings in both conditions primarily affect the cerebrum with loss of the gray-white interface, diffuse homogeneously decreased attenuation, and effacement of the basal cisterns and ventricles on CT. The decreased attenuation can cause the circulating blood to appear hyperdense on CT and give a "pseudo-SAH" appearance, and the cerebellum may appear relatively hyperdense in contrast to the edematous cerebral hemispheres ("white cerebellar sign," Fig. 39-8).

DWI, MRS, and SWI are helpful in differentiating the two conditions. Increased blood flow and interstitial fluid (vasogenic) edema have increased diffusion on DWI (a hypointense DWI signal and a hyperintense ADC signal), whereas acute axonal shear injury with cytotoxic edema shows restricted diffusion (a hyperintense DWI signal and a hypointense ADC signal). DTI also has been found to show decreased anisotropy, providing detection of neuronal injury

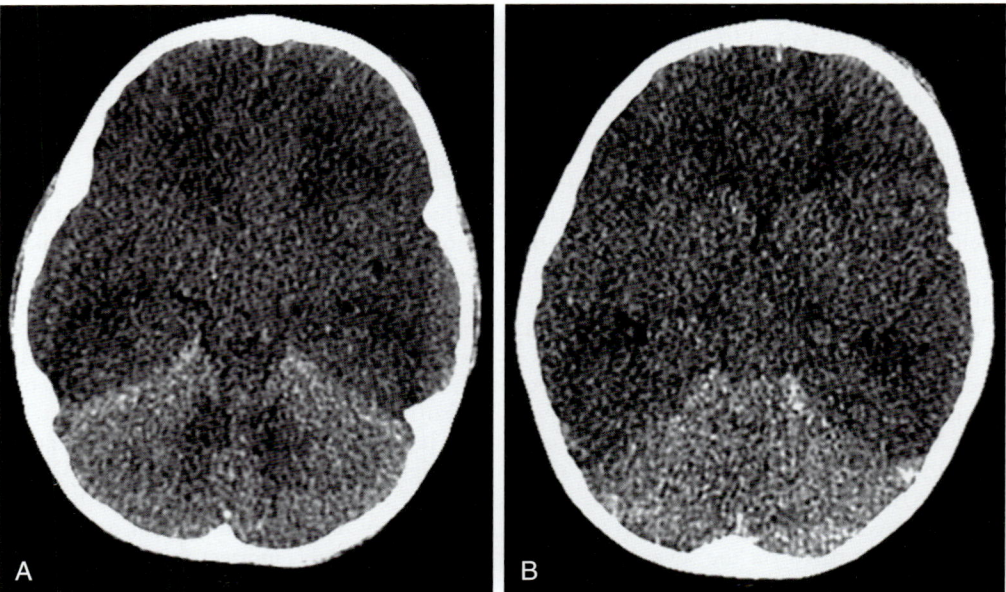

Figure 39-8 White cerebellum sign. **A** and **B,** A noncontrast computed tomography image showing a diffuse decrease in attenuation of cerebral parenchyma, with a relatively increased attenuation of the cerebellum.

earlier than conventional DWI. MRS shows decreased NAA levels and increased lactate, choline, and neurotransmitter levels as a result of neuronal (axonal) injury in persons with acute DAI, with metabolites near normal early in the course of cerebral edema. This spectral pattern with axonal injury predicts a poor prognosis. SWI has a high sensitivity for the detection of hemorrhagic lesions and is useful in the evaluation of DAI. Additionally, significant axonal injury leads to evidence of volume loss on follow-up studies, whereas the brain returns to a normal appearance with cerebral edema if significant neuronal damage is not present.

Progressive edema and increased ICP can result in transtentorial, subfalcine, and tonsillar herniation, with subsequent vascular complications, which leads to death in 7% of pediatric cases. Overall, these complications occur less frequently in children than in adults.

Hypoperfusion injury in persons who have sustained a trauma may be due to many etiologies, including severe cerebral edema, hypotension, and shock. This pattern also shows a diffuse loss of gray-white interface; however, relative preservation of the extraaxial spaces and basal cisterns occurs, and ventricles appear relatively normal. Restricted diffusion is present in persons who have a hypoperfusion injury, in contrast to the presence of increased diffusion in persons with vasogenic edema. Distinguishing the three described patterns of injury by imaging has significant clinical implications because the therapy is vastly different for each of the conditions.

The "reversal sign" is a striking CT pattern in children who have had significant anoxic-ischemic injury in which there is decreased attenuation of the cortex diffusely with relative preservation of the attenuation of the thalami, brainstem, and cerebellum. Although children with a diffuse edema pattern have an overall higher mortality rate than do children with the reversal sign, its presence also portends a poor prognosis.

Sequelae of Trauma

Sequelae of trauma may manifest early or as long-term complications. Posttraumatic edema, vascular injuries, and infarction typically manifest acutely. Encephalomalacia and neurologic and cognitive disability occur as the long-term sequelae of trauma. Seizures and hydrocephalus may manifest early or have a delayed onset.

Pediatric traumatic vascular injury is less common in children than in adults. Traumatic arterial dissection may result in infarction (Fig. 39-9). Vasospasm, vascular thrombosis, compression of a vessel from a hematoma, and hypoperfusion also can cause infarction. Intracranial carotid dissection, pseudoaneurysms after skull base fractures, and carotid cavernous fistula are less common sequelae following trauma. Intraoral trauma as a result of a fall with an object in the mouth is the most common cause of extracranial carotid artery injury in children.

Dissection of the vertebral arteries is unusual in children. Dissection occurring at C1-C2 level may be predisposed by the presence a bony bridge over the vessel on the atlas known as the arcuate first neural foramen, which is an anatomic variant.

Venous injury involving the dural venous sinuses is more common as a result of birth trauma and often is accompanied by fractures, subdural hematomas, or epidural hematomas. Thrombosis of the venous sinuses can be related to injury to the epithelial lining, compression as a result of intracranial bleeding or an adjacent fracture, or increased ICP.

CTA can be used for the diagnosis of possible vascular injury in skull base fractures and the diagnosis of possible vascular injury such as laceration, occlusion, dissection, pseudoaneurysm, or arteriovenous fistula.

Pneumocephalus following trauma can be located within any of the extraaxial spaces or within the ventricles and is generally self-limiting, although tension pneumocephalus with mass effect may necessitate urgent surgical evacuation.

CSF leaks can be evaluated with use of CT or radionuclide cisternography or with high-resolution CT alone. High-resolution long T2-weighted MRI also can demonstrate sites of CSF leak.

Infection is an uncommon sequela of trauma and may be seen in penetrating injuries. It can present as meningitis, empyema within the epidural or subdural spaces, cerebritis, or intracranial abscess.

Nonaccidental Trauma

More than five children die each day in the United States as a result of abuse and neglect, with many cases likely unreported. Head injury after NAT is one of the leading causes of mortality and morbidity in infants and children. Radiologic findings are an integral part of the workup and diagnosis of NAT (see Chapter 144). Head injuries in these infants and children include skull fractures, intracranial and retinal hemorrhages, and parenchymal brain injury such as contusions, edema, ischemia, and infarction.

Clinical presentation and findings often may be nonspecific, and children may present with irritability, lethargy, or seizures without external manifestations of injury. Imaging findings therefore may provide the first clue to the diagnosis of NAT. As in other cases of trauma or in the acute clinical presentation of altered mental status, CT is often the initial imaging modality, with MRI used to further define the extent of injury and to look for potential craniocervical injury.

Subdural hematomas are common in NAT because of the most common mechanism of injury. Rotational forces on the head tear the bridging veins in the extraaxial space. Bleeding into the subarachnoid space may coexist and is seen in the sulci and basal cisterns. The epidural hemorrhages seen in infants and young children who have sustained accidental trauma are uncommon in those who have sustained NAT.

Most acute subdural hematomas have high density on CT, but this finding is variable, especially when dilution is present as a result of mixing with CSF from a dural tear. A hematocrit layering effect may be seen. As hematomas age, they gradually become lower in attenuation. Isodense subdural hematomas can be differentiated from prominent subarachnoid spaces by the peripheral location of the veins in the extraaxial space and a more medial location noted when a subdural hematoma is present.

On MRI, the signal intensity of parenchymal injuries varies with time, and when correlated with other clinical findings, it can be helpful to clinicians and child advocacy services. However, the precise aging of parenchymal lesions and extraaxial hematomas should be undertaken with caution.

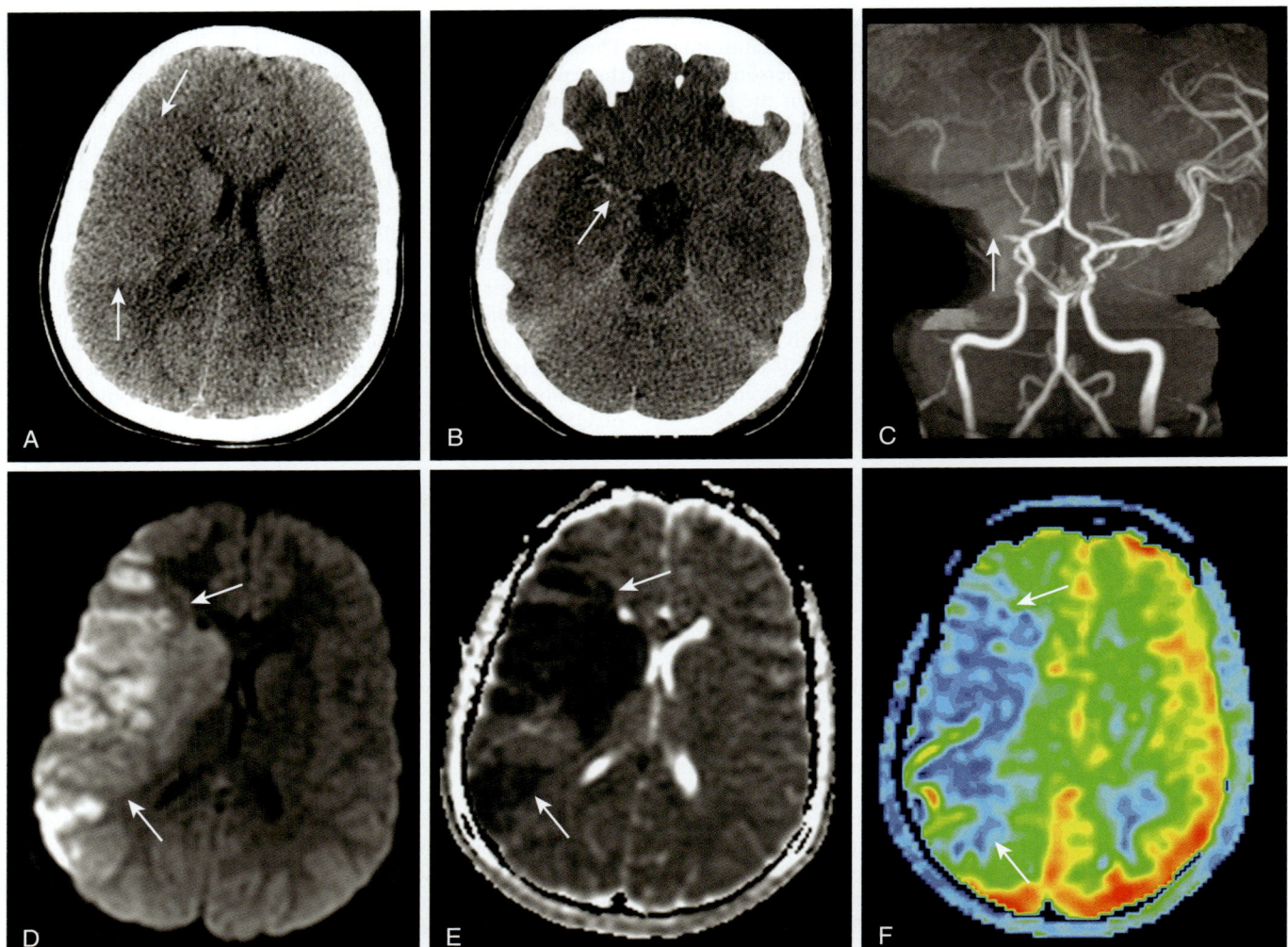

Figure 39-9 Traumatic dissection of the right middle cerebral artery (MCA). **A,** An unenhanced computed tomography (CT) image of the brain at the level of the lateral ventricles demonstrates poor gray-white matter differentiation in the right frontal lobe (*arrows*). **B,** An unenhanced CT image at the level of the circle of Willis and midbrain demonstrates the "hyperdense MCA sign" (*arrow*). **C,** Occlusion of the right MCA (*arrow*) on three-dimensional time-of-flight magnetic resonance angiography. **D** and **E,** Restricted diffusion and low apparent diffusion coefficient values (*arrows*). **F,** An arterial spin label perfusion image showing decreased cerebral blood flow in the right MCA territory (*arrows*).

CT hyperdensity is the only reliable indicator of age (Fig. 39-10). Subdural hematomas in infants younger than 2 years and subdural hematomas of different ages are highly suspicious for NAT. Retinal hemorrhages are a cardinal manifestation of NAT (Fig. 39-11). The severity of retinal hemorrhages and their extension to the periphery of the retina correlates with the likelihood of NAT and the severity of associated brain injury.

Mortality and morbidity in children with NAT often are due to parenchymal injury. Hypoxic ischemic injury and brain edema as a result of the trauma are more common than are primary parenchymal contusions and DAI. Hypoxic ischemic injury is more often diffuse, and although the exact mechanism is unclear, it is most likely related to hypoperfusion.

Imaging findings show a diffuse loss of gray-white matter differentiation with sparing of the basal ganglia. Severe insults show more extensive brain edema, and the basal ganglia and the posterior fossa structures may be involved. Hypoxia resulting from strangulation involves the territory of the anterior circulation as a result of compression of the carotid vessels with relative sparing of the vertebral circulation. MRI and DWI are useful to delineate the full extent of ischemic injury, and MRS may demonstrate neuronal loss by demonstrating a decrease in the neuronal marker NAA and an increase in lactate, indicating anaerobic metabolism in the affected areas of the brain (see Fig. 39-11).

A multidisciplinary approach should be used in the diagnosis of NAT when radiologic findings are suspicious or inconsistent with the provided clinical history. Certain metabolic disorders such as glutaric aciduria type 1, an inherited autosomal-recessive metabolic disorder that can present with subdural hematomas, should be considered in the differential diagnoses. Congenital or acquired coagulopathies can give rise to intracranial hemorrhage or vascular thrombosis. Birth injury can be associated with intracranial hemorrhage in

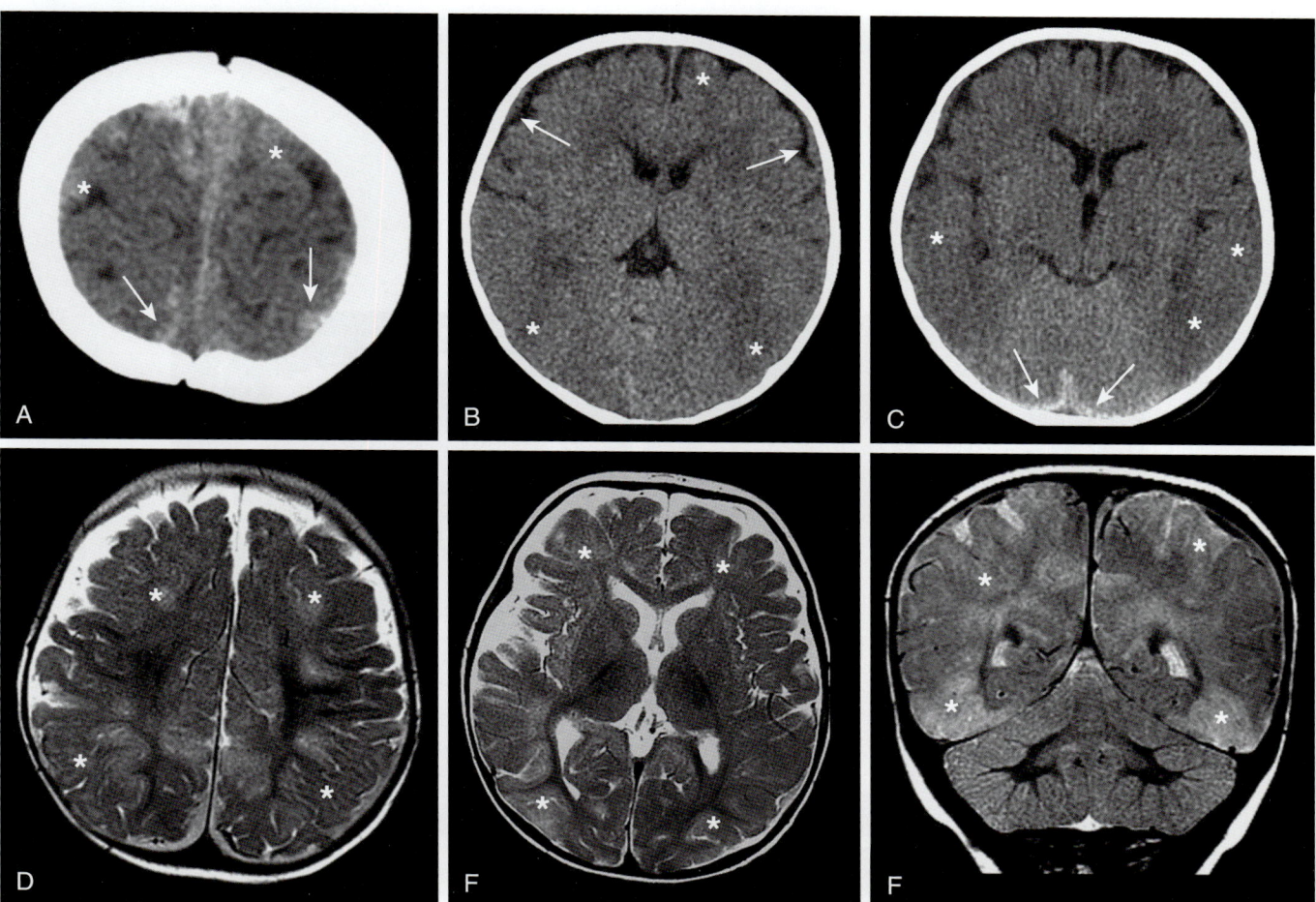

Figure 39-10 Nonaccidental trauma. **A, B,** and **C,** An unenhanced computed tomography image demonstrates multiple areas of loss of gray-white matter differentiation (*) and bilateral acute and subacute subdural hematomas. **D, E,** and **F,** Magnetic resonance imaging T2-weighted images show the extent of the parenchymal injury with multifocal areas of cortical and subcortical injury (*asterisks*).

infants, which generally resolves within a month. Severe forms of meningoencephalitis can present with extraaxial collections and parenchymal hemorrhage.

Vigilance, familiarity with the radiologic findings, communication with the referring physician, relevant clinical history, and recommendation for further imaging, if needed, all aid in the diagnosis of NAT.

Prognosis

Children are more likely than adults to recover from focal brain injury and have a higher likelihood of survival after severe injury. However, children seem to be more vulnerable to long-term cognitive and behavioral dysfunction after diffuse brain injury. Some degree of learning disability is found in 50% of survivors of head trauma, with severe motor, sensory, cognitive, and behavioral deficits present in many patients. Overall, children younger than 6 years have the worst prognosis, likely because of the increased risk and prevalence of shear injury in the relatively immature brain. Ultimately, functional outcome depends on how many neurons are preserved after injury. The location and extent of injury and the ability of existing neurons to reorganize their connections to recover function are critical.

Summary

Head trauma is a frequent cause of morbidity and mortality in the pediatric population. A wide spectrum of traumatic head injuries occurs in children, many of which are unique to the pediatric population. The type of injury primarily depends on the mechanism of injury, the force sustained, and the age of the patient. Newer imaging modalities are useful in the evaluation of these patients and have the potential to predict recovery and outcome.

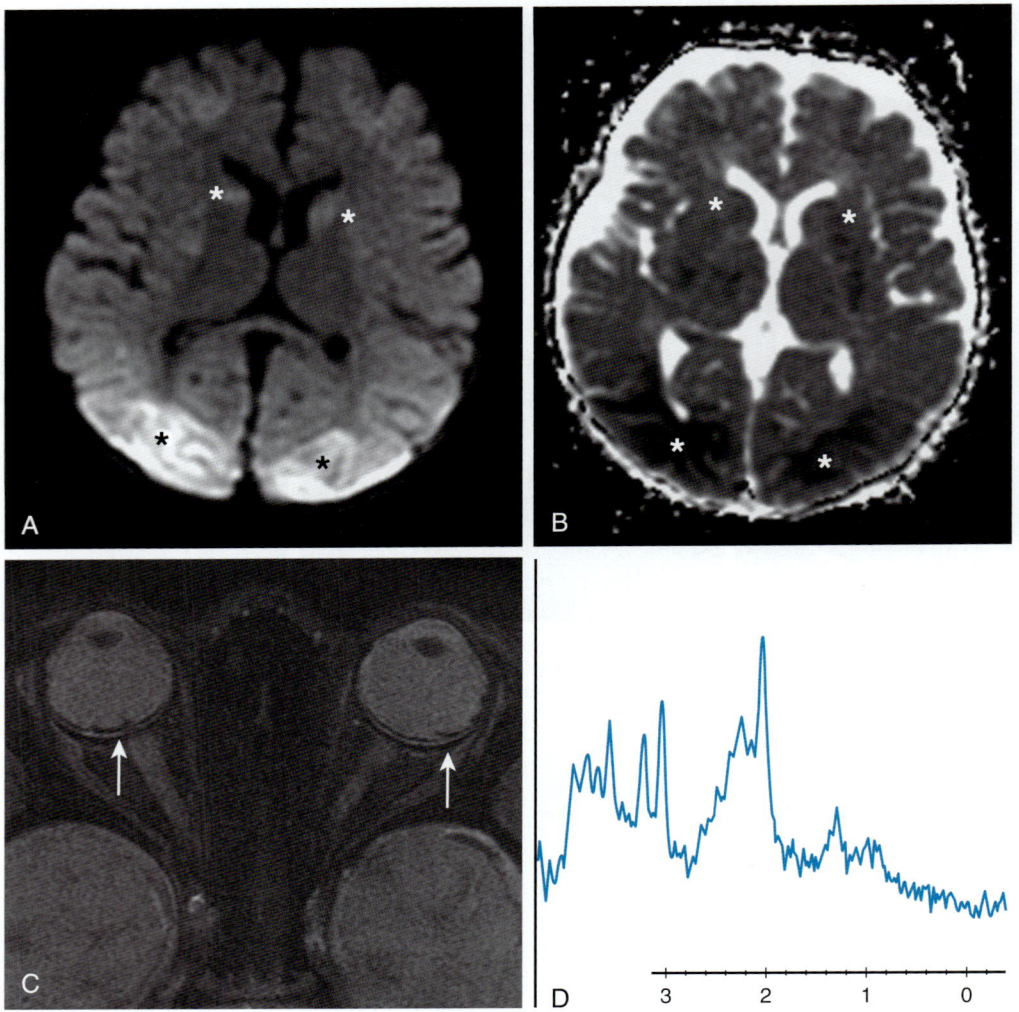

Figure 39-11   Nonaccidental trauma. **A** and **B,** Magnetic resonance imaging (MRI) diffusion-weighted imaging (DWI) sequences show multiple areas of restricted diffusion that are more pronounced in the bilateral occipital lobes and the head of the caudate nuclei seen (*asterisks*) on DWI (**A**) and apparent diffusion coefficient (**B**). **C,** A high-resolution MRI susceptibility-weighted imaging sequence shows susceptibility related to retinal hemorrhages bilaterally (*arrows*). **D,** MR spectroscopy at level occipital lobes demonstrates a decreased N-acetylaspartate level (2.0 ppm) and elevated lactate and lipid (0.8 to 1.2 ppm) and glutamate/glutamine (2.2-2.4 ppm) levels.

Key Points

Head trauma and resulting TBI are the most common causes of morbidity and mortality in children.

In general, CT is the initial imaging modality used to evaluate patients with known or suspected head trauma.

The risk of death from minor head injury in childhood approaches 0%.

The likelihood of intracranial injury significantly increases when a skull fracture is present in a child. The absence of a skull fracture, however, does not preclude intracranial injury and has little prognostic significance in pediatric head trauma.

In younger children, venous epidural hematomas are more common than arterial epidural hematomas.

A brain contusion is a bruise of the parenchyma. The cortex is invariably involved, with variable involvement of the underlying white matter.

DAI is one of the most devastating types of TBI and is the most common cause of posttraumatic neurologic and cognitive disability.

Diffuse brain swelling and hypoperfusion injury is more common in children and can be differentiated using DWI, MRS, and SWI techniques.

Children are more likely than adults to recover from focal brain injury and have a higher likelihood of survival after severe injury. However, children seem to be more vulnerable to long-term cognitive and behavioral dysfunction after sustaining a diffuse brain injury.

Suggested Readings

Barkovich AJ. *Pediatric neuroradiology*. 5th ed. Philadelphia: Lippincott Williams & Wilkins; 2012.

Provenzale JM. Imaging of traumatic brain injury: a review of the recent medical literature. *AJR Am J Roentgenol*. 2010;194(1):16-19.

Tortori-Donati P, Rossi A. *Pediatric neuroradiology: brain, head, neck and spine*. New York: Springer; 2005.

References

Full references for this chapter can be found on www.expertconsult.com.

Chapter 40

Embryology, Anatomy, and Normal Findings

LISA H. LOWE, PETER WINNINGHAM, and SAMI ABEDIN

Embryology

The spinal cord forms in three stages beginning in the third gestational week when the notochord induces surrounding ectoderm to differentiate into neuroectoderm.[1] The first stage, neurulation, involves progression from neural plate to neural groove to neural tube.[1] The notochord transforms into the nucleus pulposus of the intervertebral disks.[2] The second stage, canalization, involves formation of cysts within the caudal cell mass that gradually coalesce and fuse to the distal neural tube to form the primitive spinal cord. The third stage, retrogressive differentiation, involves programmed cell death leading to regression of the primitive distal spinal cord to form the fetal conus, filum terminale, and ventriculus terminalis[1,2] (Fig. 40-1).

The vertebral bodies develop from somites that have been converted through signaling molecules to form sclerotomes.[3] The caudal and cranial portions of adjacent sclerotomes fuse to become single vertebral bodies. Failure of this process leads to congenital vertebral segmentation anomalies such as block or hemivertebrae (Fig. 40-2).[4,5]

Anatomy and Physiology

The spinal cord is larger in the cervical and lumbar regions than in the thoracic region. Paired dorsal and ventral nerve roots arise from each level, and the spinal cord itself is held in place by the lateral dentate ligaments. The distal end of the spinal cord and the thecal sac typically extend to the L2-L3 disc space and the S2 level, respectively.

Although 5% of humans have differing numbers of vertebrae, most often people have 7 cervical, 12 thoracic, and 5 lumbar vertebral bodies, as well as 5 sacral and 4 coccygeal segments.[6] Running craniocaudal are the anterior and posterior longitudinal ligaments, supraspinous and interspinous ligaments, and ligamentum flavum.

Vascular supply to the spine is largely via paired segmental arteries. These arteries arise directly from the aorta in the thoracic and lumbar regions, from the vertebral arteries in the cervical region, and from the lateral sacral arteries in the sacrum. The segmental and radicular arteries supply the bony vertebrae and the spinal nerves.

The arterial supply to the spinal cord is via the single, midline anterior spinal artery and the paired posterior spinal arteries. The anterior spinal artery originates from bilateral branches of the intradural segments of the vertebral arteries and courses along the ventral surface of the spinal cord. Similarly, the posterior spinal arteries arise from the intradural vertebral arteries, but course along the dorsal surface of the spinal cord.[7] Radicular artery branches contribute to the cord arterial supply at multiple points. One particularly large branch, the artery of Adamkiewicz, typically enters the spinal canal between the T9 and T12 levels and can be recognized by its characteristic proximal hairpin turn.[8]

NORMAL FINDINGS

The pediatric spine is imaged with plain radiographs, ultrasonography, computed tomography (CT), and magnetic resonance imaging (MRI), depending on the age of the child and indication for the examination. Radiographs and CT are used to screen for osseous anomalies and acute conditions such as trauma. In neonates, spine sonography and MRI are the most frequently used modalities. Spine ultrasonography is the ideal screening study for infants younger than 6 months because it provides excellent resolution and does not expose patients to radiation. It is able to provide sufficient characterization of spinal anomalies to determine if intervention is required, if MRI is needed acutely, or if further imaging can be delayed. In older infants and children, MRI is the study of choice for evaluation of the spine.

The indications for spine ultrasonography include screening neonates with multiple congenital anomalies, screening complicated dimples with skin stigmata, and evaluating soft tissue masses that suggest possible underlying closed (occult) spinal dysraphism, as well as determining the cause of failed lumbar puncture and localizing fluid for possible additional attempts at lumbar puncture.[9,10] High-risk skin stigmata include atypical dimples (>5 mm) located above the gluteal crease (>2.5 mm from the anus), dimples in which the bottom cannot be visualized, and those with skin stigmata such as a hairy patch, hemangioma, a mound of soft tissue, skin tag, or tail.[11] In anomalies requiring surgery and dimples draining cerebrospinal fluid, urgent MRI is the initial study of choice.[12,13] Additionally, MRI is helpful to further

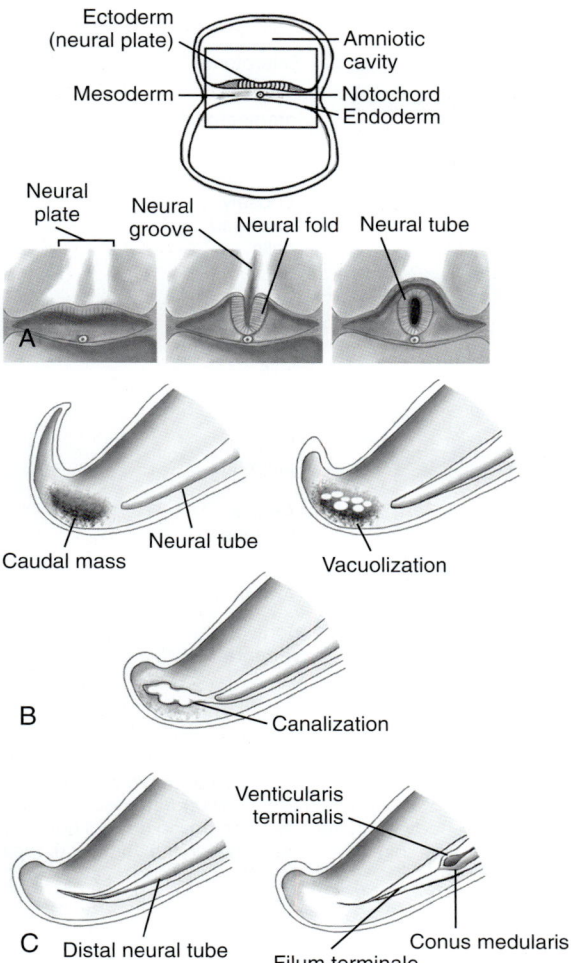

Ectoderm (neural plate)
Amniotic cavity
Mesoderm
Notochord
Endoderm

Neural plate   Neural groove   Neural fold   Neural tube

A

Caudal mass   Neural tube

Vacuolization

B

Canalization

Venticularis terminalis

C   Distal neural tube   Filum terminale   Conus medullaris

Figure 40-1 Embryological development of the spinal cord. **A,** Neurulation schematic illustrates progression from neural plate to groove to neural tube. **B,** Canalization schematic depicts coalescence of cysts within the caudal cell mass that fuse to the distal neural tube. **C,** A retrogressive differentiation schematic reveals the process of programmed cell death forming the conus medullaris and filum terminale.

characterize anomalies found on ultrasound and is best performed immediately prior to therapeutic intervention.[9]

The location of the conus medullaris is usually determined by counting down from the twelfth rib, as well as up from the lumbosacral junction.[11,12,14] In some cases, one may need to count down from the cervical level as well.[13] If the conus level is still uncertain, follow-up ultrasound may be considered. Rarely, an immediate determination is important in patient management, in which case a BB can be placed at the level of the tip of the conus (as determined by ultrasound) and a radiograph of the entire spine obtained for further clarification.[15]

Spine sonography requires knowledge of normal anatomy and variants that may simulate pathology to prevent unnecessary referral for MRI. The tapering spinal cord forming the conus medullaris, and the layering cauda equina nerve roots are easily seen within the hypoechoic cerebrospinal fluid (Fig. 40-3). The spinal cord and nerve roots often are observed pulsating (oscillating) with the cardiac cycle, which can be documented with cine or on M mode ultrasound. However,

this motion is "variably present" in the newborn.[15] The normal filum terminale, an echogenic linear structure that extends from the conus medullaris to the distal thecal sac, should be homogeneous in echogenicity and thickness throughout its length, measuring less than 1 to 1.5 mm. The conus medullaris is normally located at or above the superior end plate of L3.[16] Recent reports indicate that infants with isolated borderline low conus position extending to the midbody of L3 on spine ultrasound are normal and will meet normal developmental milestones.[17] A conus tip below the midbody of L3 is abnormal.[16] Occasionally, determination of conus level on ultrasound and marked radiographs are not clear and MRI is needed to clarify.

Normal variants to be aware of include the ventriculus terminalis, filar cysts, a prominent filum terminale, a pseudosinus tract, a cauda equina pseudomass, and a dysmorphic coccyx. The ventriculus terminalis, which is seen mostly in children younger than 5 years, and occasionally in adults, involves persistence of the normal fetal terminal ventricle. It is characterized by contiguity with the central spinal canal, which expands within the conus medullaris to form a small space containing fluid (Fig. 40-4). It must be distinguished from a syrinx, which is typically larger and may grow over time.

Filar cysts are midline, fusiform, well defined hypoechoic fluid spaces located in the cauda equina immediately below the conus medullaris, and are of uncertain origin (Fig. 40-5). They are seen on ultrasound in 11.8% of infants, typically are not seen on MRI, and lack pathologic description, indicating that they may be structural pseudocysts.[18] When seen on ultrasound in isolation, they are of no clinical significance.[18]

The normal filum terminale may cause confusion because it is often more prominent than the rest of the cauda equina. It is distinguished by its normal thickness (<1 to 1.5 mm) and midline anatomic location (e-Fig. 40-6). A prominent filum must be distinguished from a fibrofatty filum and a filar lipoma, which are suspected when focal hyperechogenicity and thickening (>2 mm) of the filum terminale are seen (Fig. 40-7).[19] A fibrofatty filum may be incidental but has also been described as part of the "tight filum terminale syndrome," the symptoms of which may develop at any age and include lower extremity weakness, spasticity, foot deformities, bladder dysfunction, scoliosis, and back pain.[20]

A pseudomass due to nerve root clumping may be seen when infants undergo sonography are in the decubitus position. This finding is easily evaluated by showing resolution of the "mass" when the infant undergoes repeat scanning in the prone position. Pseudosinus tracts, or fibrous cords of echogenicity extending from the base of dimples to the coccyx, are a frequent normal variant seen on modern high-quality spinal ultrasound (Fig. 40-8). These tracts do not drain or contain fluid, do not have an associated mass, and must be distinguished from true dermal sinus tracts. True sinus tracts, which often drain cerebrospinal fluid and are associated with an increased risk of meningitis, are attributed to incomplete disjunction of the cutaneous ectoderm from the neuroectoderm.[21] A final normal variant, the misshapen or dysmorphic coccyx, is a common ultrasound finding that may be discovered on physical examination when a "mass" is palpated.[22] Although the variety and degree of dysmorphic coccygeal shapes may be impressive, the finding is of no clinical significance (e-Fig. 40-9).

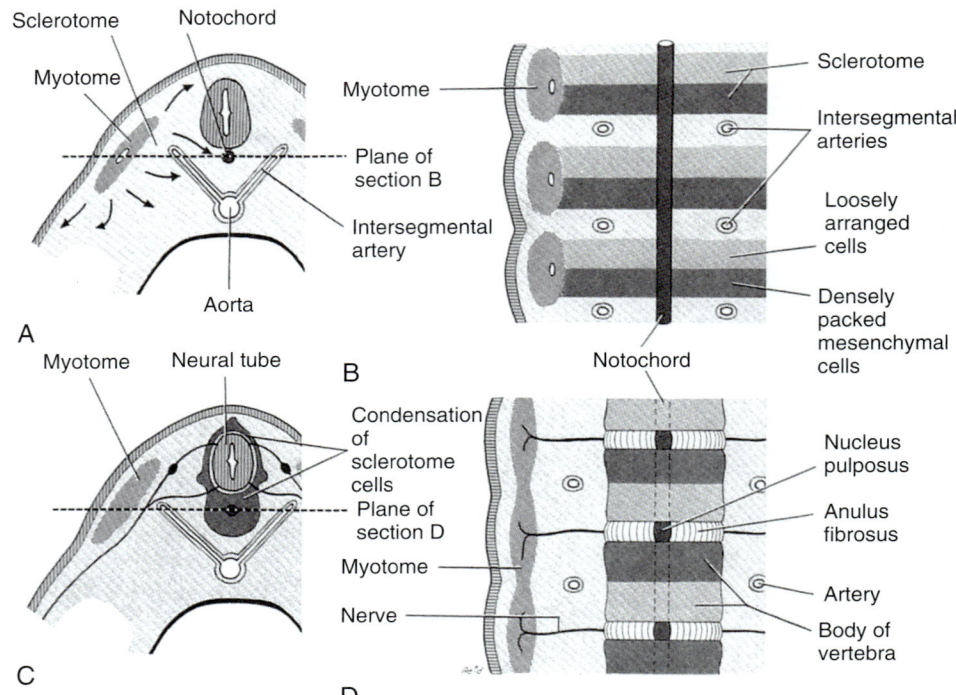

Figure 40-2 **Embryological development of the vertebra. A,** A partial transverse section through a 4-week embryo shows arrows indicating the spread of mesenchymal cells from the sclerotome region of the somite on the right. **B,** A diagrammatic frontal section of this embryo showing that the condensation of sclerotome cells around the notochord consists of a cranial area of loosely packed cells and a caudal area of densely packed cells. **C,** A partial transverse section through a 5-week embryo shows the condensation of sclerotome cells around the notochord and the neural tube, which forms a mesenchymal vertebra. **D,** A diagrammatic frontal section illustrates that the vertebral body forms from the cranial and caudal halves of two successive sclerotomes. The intersegmental arteries now cross the bodies of the vertebrae, and the spinal nerves lie between the vertebrae. The notochord is degenerating except in the intervertebral disk, where it persists as the nucleus pulposus. (From Moore KL. *The developing human: clinically oriented embryology.* 4th ed. Philadelphia: Saunders; 1988:338.)

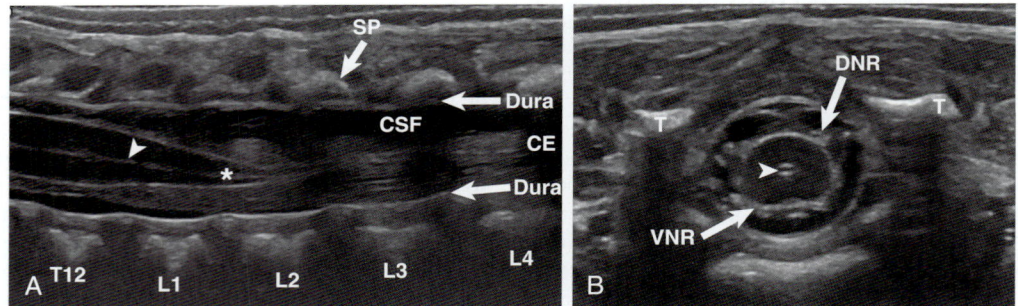

Figure 40-3 **A normal spine sonogram in a 1-day-old male with multiple congenital anomalies.** Longitudinal (**A**) and transverse (**B**) images demonstrate the normal anatomy. Note the dura, central echo complex (*arrowheads*) and conus medullaris (*asterisk*). Other labeled structures include the vertebra (T12-L4); SP, spinous processes; CE, cauda equina; CSF, cerebrospinal fluid; T, transverse processes; VNR, ventral nerve roots; and DNR, dorsal nerve roots.

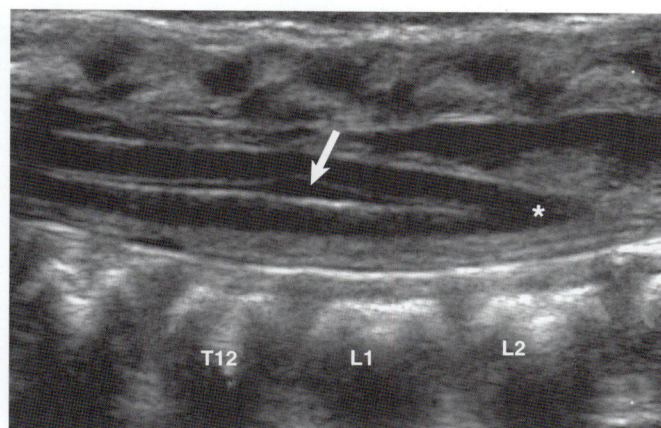

Figure 40-4 Ventriculus terminalis in a 3-month-old girl with a deep dimple. Longitudinal sonography demonstrates focal distension of the distal central spinal canal (*arrow*) in the lumbar cord just above the conus medullaris (*asterisk*).

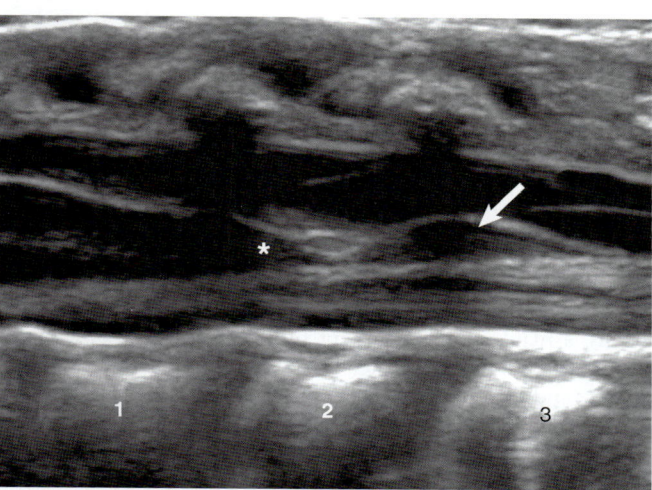

Figure 40-5 A filar cyst in a 6-week-old male with an asymmetric gluteal crease. A longitudinal sonogram shows a fusiform, midline hypoechoic "cyst" (*arrow*) just below the conus medullaris (*asterisk*).

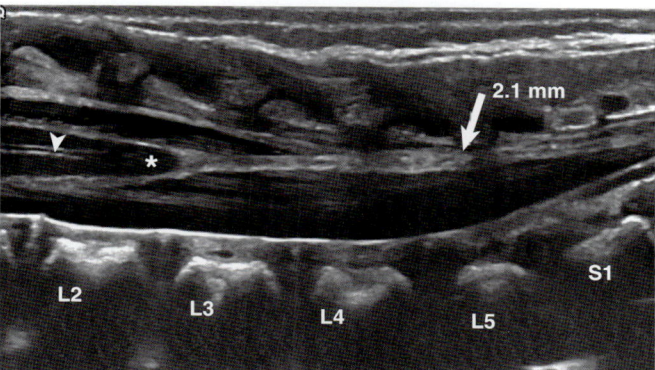

Figure 40-7 Fatty filum in a 2-day-old male with VATER syndrome. A longitudinal sonogram shows a subtle focus of increased echogenicity and thickening of the filum (*arrow*) as it extends from the conus medullaris to the distal thecal sac. The filum measures 2.1 mm. Also note the normal central echo complex (*arrowhead*).

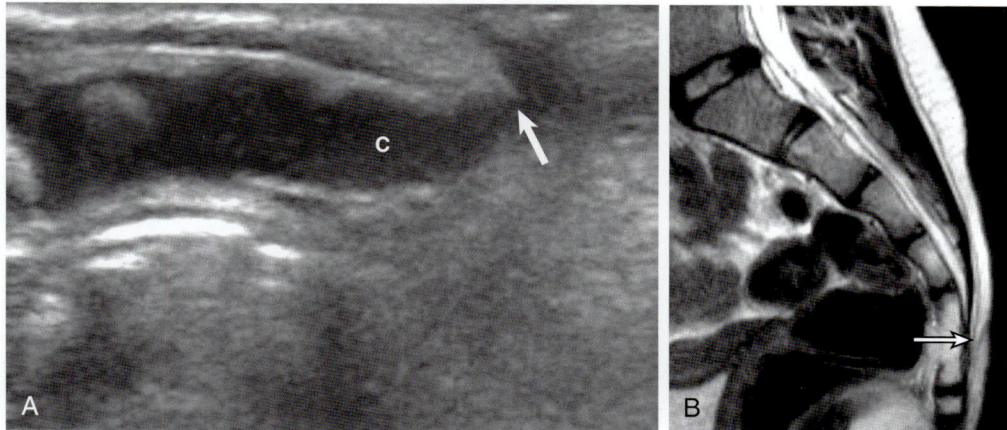

Figure 40-8 A pseudosinus tract in a 3-month-old girl with a deep dimple in the gluteal crease. **A,** A longitudinal sonogram identifies the normal hypoechoic coccyx (*C*) with a cordlike hypoechoic pseudotract (*arrow*) extending to the skin dimple. **B,** Follow-up magnetic resonance imaging at age 6 months confirms the uncomplicated pseudosinus tract (*arrow*).

Key Points

Spine ultrasonography and MRI are the imaging modalities of choice for the pediatric spine.

Imaging requires knowledge of normal anatomy and normal variants, especially those seen on ultrasound, to prevent improper referral for unnecessary imaging and workup.

Normal variants to remember include ventriculus terminalis, a filar cyst, a prominent filum terminale, a "pseudomass" due to positional nerve root clumping, a pseudosinus tract, and a dysmorphic coccyx.

Suggested Readings

Bulas D. Fetal evaluation of spine dysraphism. *Pediatric Radiology.* 2010;40(6):1029-1037.

Johanek AJ, Lowe LH, Moore AW. Sonography of the neonatal spine: Part 1, normal anatomy, imaging pitfalls and variations that may simulate disorders. *Am J Roentgenol.* 2007;188:733-738.

Johanek AJ, Lowe LH, Moore AW. Sonography of the neonatal spine: part 2, Spinal disorders. *Am J Roentgenol.* 2007;188:739-744.

References

Full references for this chapter can be found on www.expertconsult.com.

Chapter 41

Spinal Cord Imaging Techniques

PAUL THACKER and LISA H. LOWE

Pediatric spinal cord imaging is a complex and interesting area that relies heavily on ultrasound in infants younger than 6 months of age and magnetic resonance imaging (MRI) thereafter.[1,2] Other imaging modalities such as plain radiography, myelography, computed tomography (CT), and nuclear scintigraphy serve a limited role but can provide useful adjunctive information in cases with a specific question.

Plain Radiography

Radiographic spine series typically include frontal and lateral radiographs of the cervical, thoracic, or lumbar region. Additional oblique radiographs may be added depending on the clinical indication. Plain radiographs have limited utility as a primary imaging tool in the evaluation of spinal cord but may demonstrate indirect evidence of underlying cord abnormalities and prompt performance of additional cross-sectional imaging. Nowhere else is this more true than in the setting of acute trauma.[3] Although some studies have concluded that CT should be the initial study in acute trauma screening, radiography continues to be the mainstay for screening patients with trauma. Radiography also may be performed to screen older children with various spine-related complaints such as chronic back pain and torticollis. Subtle findings such as posterior vertebral body scalloping, widening of the neural foramina, or widening of the central canal may suggest underlying pathology (Fig. 41-1).[4]

Contrast Radiography

Contrast radiography is a term that includes angiography with biplane and triplane fluoroscopy and conventional myelography. As with plain radiography, contrast radiography has a limited role in the evaluation of spinal cord pathology. Largely, conventional myelography has been supplanted by MRI. CT myelography is useful in rare, specific clinical circumstances such as when patients cannot undergo MRI because of an implanted prosthesis, for example, cochlear implants or pacemakers.[5] In such patients, myelography with or without CT can provide useful information about the spinal cord and thecal sac.

The role of conventional angiography in pediatric spinal imaging is as a secondary or tertiary modality to define vascular anatomy in preparation for treatment of dural fistulas and arteriovenous malformations, both of which are extremely rare in children.[2]

Computed Tomography

Like plain and contrast radiology, CT plays a limited role in direct spinal cord imaging. However, CT has the advantages of speed, availability, improved contrast resolution compared with radiography, limited operator independence, and the capability for multiplanar and three-dimensional reformations. It provides superior sensitivity and specificity in delineating osseous anomalies compared with other modalities and can indicate the need for additional spinal cord imaging (Fig. 41-2).[3] Finally, as previously stated, CT and CT myelography can be performed in children who are unable to undergo MRI, thus allowing identification and characterization of mass lesions, calcifications, and areas of hemorrhage.[5]

Spinal CT technique typically includes a high-resolution, 3-mm, bone and/or soft tissue algorithm obtained axially. The 3-mm slice images are reformatted to submillimeter axial images and then reformatted in the sagittal and coronal planes if desired. An intravenous and, rarely, intrathecal contrast agent may be added for specific clinical indications.

Ultrasound

Ultrasonography is a well-established method for evaluation of the neonatal spinal canal and its contents.[1,6] The predominately cartilaginous and incompletely ossified spinal arches in infants serve as a superb acoustic window for transmission of the ultrasound beam. However, with progressive ossification, the acoustic window diminishes, allowing limited visualization of the spinal cord between the spinous processes.[6] Although this limited acoustic window persists into adulthood, the spinal cord becomes difficult to adequately visualize on a routine basis in infants older than 6 months of age.[1]

Spinal ultrasound is performed with a high-frequency 7- to 12-MHz linear-array transducer or 8- to 10-MHz

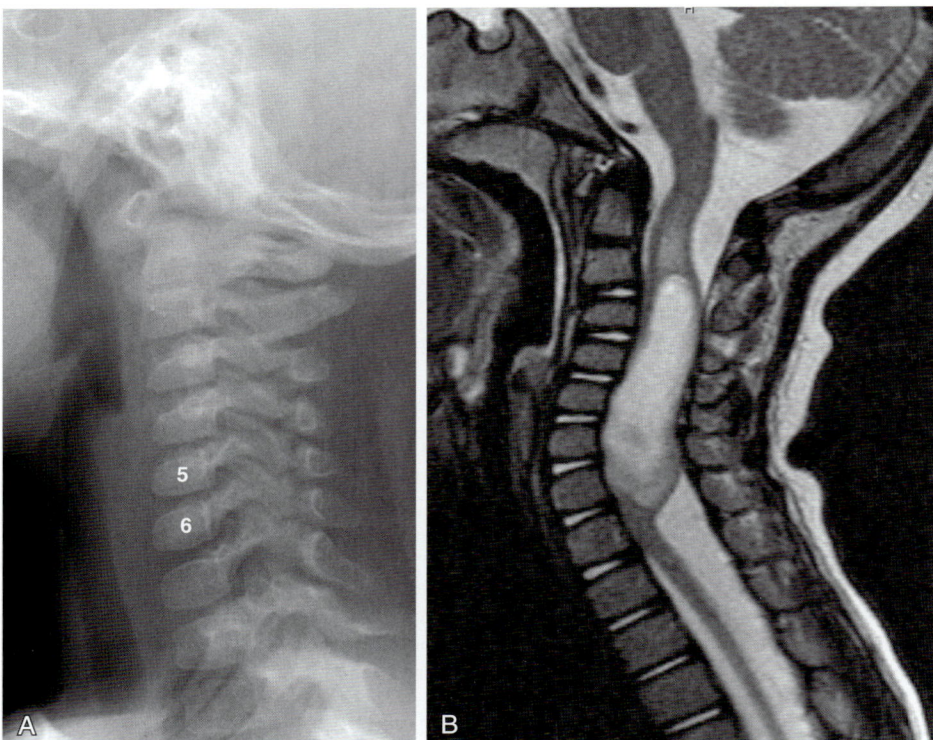

Figure 41-1   A cervical cord astrocytoma on a plain radiograph and magnetic resonance imaging in a 1-year-old girl with persistent torticollis. **A,** A lateral cervical spine radiograph shows subtle posterior vertebral body scalloping causing C5 and C6 to take on an abnormal square shape compared with the normal adjacent rectangular vertebral bodies. **B,** A sagittal T2-weighted magnetic resonance image confirms expansion of the cervical spinal canal because of a T2-hyperintense mass within the cervical cord. Note T2 bright cord edema above and below the mass.

curved-array transducer.[1] Newborns undergo imaging while prone in the longitudinal (sagittal) and transverse (axial) planes from the craniocervical junction through the conus medullaris and cauda equina (Fig. 41-3). Paramedian scanning may be useful in some patients with partially ossified vertebra.[1] The vertebral bodies are carefully numbered by counting down from either the lowest rib and/or the craniocervical junction, and numbering is confirmed by counting up from the lumbosacral junction.[1,7] This dual technique of numbering allows one to avoid misdiagnosing a low-lying, possibly tethered spinal cord. Real-time cine loops are obtained routinely as part of the examination in order to demonstrate the normal rhythmic movement of the cauda equina nerve roots during the cardiac cycle.[1]

Indications for spine ultrasound include screening for dysraphism and low conus position (possible tethered cord) in newborns with multiple congenital anomalies, as well as evaluation of midline dimples located above the gluteal crease more than 2.5 cm from the anus; dimples with associated skin stigmata (e.g., a hairy patch, hemangioma, pigmented area, skin tag, or tail); and deep dimples in which the bottom cannot be visualized on physical examination.[7]

Magnetic Resonance Imaging

OVERVIEW

Overall, MRI is the primary modality for imaging the pediatric spinal cord because of its superior tissue contrast characteristics.[2] MRI not only affords detailed evaluation of the

spinal cord but also provides assessment of the surrounding soft tissues and osseous structures. Additional evaluation of cerebrospinal fluid flow characteristics are possible with phase contrast cerebrospinal fluid cine imaging, which most often is used to assess obstruction by Chiari 1 malformations at the craniocervical junction[8] (Fig. 41-4). Bone marrow changes in a variety of disorders also may be assessed with conventional T1- and T2-weighted sequences.[4,9] Lastly, MRI can be used as a secondary or tertiary modality for defining abnormalities identified on prenatal or antenatal ultrasonography, conventional radiography, and CT.[2,4]

INDICATIONS

The indications for spinal MRI in the pediatric population are numerous. Some of the more common indications include evaluation of known or suspected masses, inflammatory processes, posttraumatic spinal injuries, metastatic spread of an intracranial primary neoplasm, characterization of spinal dysraphisms, and dimples draining fluid.[2,4,10]

PEDIATRIC IMAGING CHALLENGES

MRI is technically the most complicated of all modalities used in pediatric spine assessment. It is particularly challenging when performed in infants, neonates, and younger children who often are unwilling or unable to cooperate for the entire examination. In these patients, it is crucial to properly use methods to control patient motion, such as swaddling, sleep deprivation, and sedation, to avoid diminished image

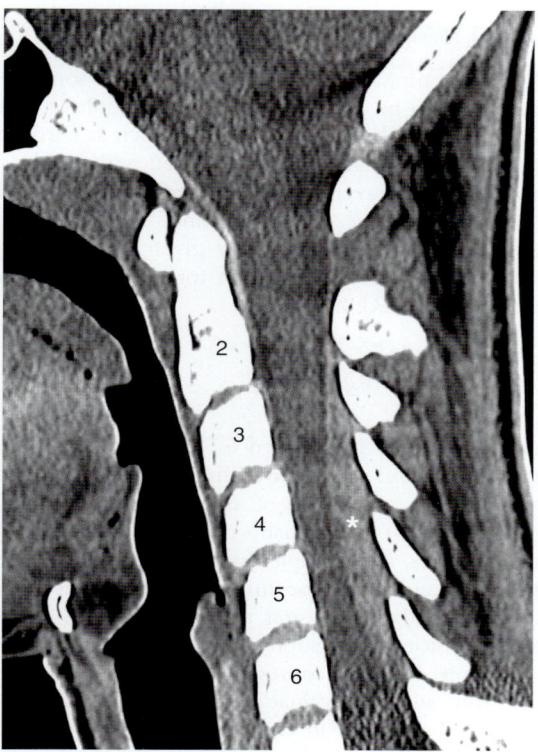

Figure 41-2 An epidural hematoma on computed tomography (CT) in a 15-year-old athlete with sudden arm pain and weakness. A sagittal cervical spine CT image demonstrates a posterior hyperattenuated fluid collection (*asterisk*) compressing the spinal cord from C3 to C6. Magnetic resonance imaging (not shown) was obtained for further evaluation and followed by surgical drainage.

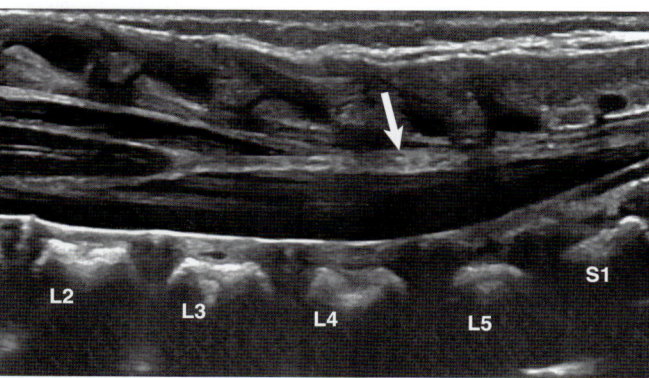

Figure 41-3 Fatty filum on ultrasound in a neonate with VATER syndrome. A longitudinal sonogram reveals a normally positioned conus medullaris at L2-L3. Focal hyperechoic fat within the filum terminale (*arrow*) is noted. The child had normal development at 2 years of age.

quality.[2] Various sedation techniques have been used over the years, ranging from oral and intravenous drugs administered by the attending radiologist to general anesthesia performed by the anesthesiologist. No single recipe works for all patients and in all circumstances. Thus the sedation approach that is used will depend on the resources available at the institution performing the examination.

To produce high-quality magnetic resonance (MR) spinal examinations in children, various technical challenges must be overcome. Because of the small spinal cord volume, a smaller field of view and higher imaging matrix with thin sections and decreased or no interslice gap must be used.[11,12]

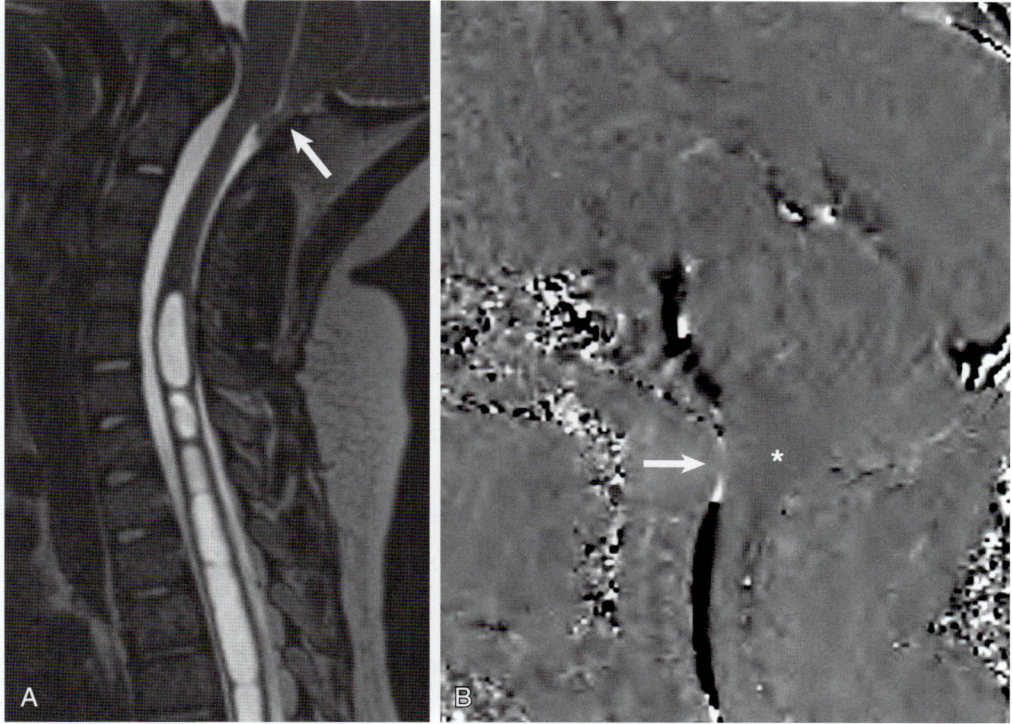

Figure 41-4 A Chiari 1 malformation on magnetic resonance imaging with cerebrospinal fluid (CSF) cine in a 6-year-old boy with levothoracic scoliosis. **A,** A sagittal isometric heavily T2-weighted image reconstructed along the scoliotic curve shows the cerebellar tonsils extending into the posterior aspect of the upper cervical spinal canal (*arrow*) and a large multiseptated cervicothoracic syrinx **B,** A phase-contrast CSF cine (velocity encoded to 5 cm/s) image reveals decreased flow across the foramen magnum (*arrow*) and slight cerebellar tonsil motion (*asterisk*).

Because adjusting these technical parameters will result in a reduction of the signal-to-noise ratio (SNR), an increased number of excitations and thus longer imaging time is mandated. With longer imaging times, patient and physiologic motion become more of an issue, even with proper sedation. Technical advances useful in overcoming this issue include application of flow-compensation (gradient moment nulling), respiratory gating, and saturation bands.[11,13]

HIGH FIELD STRENGTH MRI

With the increased utilization of 3-Tesla (T) MRI scanners, the inherent signal-to-noise issues encountered at 1.5 T may be overcome by using a higher field strength. When using the same scanning parameters, 3 T provides superior image quality and detail compared with 1.5 T.[14] The improved image detail possible at 3 T is a direct result of the higher SNR compared with the lower field strength. The surplus of SNR can also be used in children to decrease imaging times without changing image quality, thus reducing sedation times and increasing MRI throughput.[13,14]

Although it is useful in the spine, high field strength MRI is not without its own limitations, including increased magnetic susceptibility artifact, increased chemical shift artifact, and increased specific absorption rate.[13,14] Higher field strengths markedly increase magnetic susceptibility artifact from metallic objects, as well as from tissue-bone and tissue-air interfaces. This effect can be compensated for, to some degree, by increasing the band width. Chemical shift artifacts also increase with increasing field strength, degrading standard spin echo images. This effect too can be compensated for by increasing the bandwidth, but at a cost of decreasing SNR. Finally, the increased specific absorption rate at higher field strength is a potential limiting factor at 3 T, although standard specific absorption rate values are rarely exceeded with routine imaging.[14]

COIL SELECTION

Surface coils are the standard practice, and higher channel numbers will provide increasing image quality. Only coils directly aligned with the region of interest should be turned on during scanning.[15]

MRI PARAMETERS

Standard pediatric spinal MR sequences include, at a minimum, axial and sagittal T1 imaging and axial and sagittal T2 imaging with or without fat saturation.[2,10] Coronal T2 sequences often are routinely performed, as they are particularly helpful in patients with scoliosis or paraspinal lesions. Isometric sequences allow volumetric imaging with curved reformations in the evaluation of severely scoliotic patients.[16,17] Recently, diffusion weighted imaging (e-Fig. 41-5) has been used in the spine to differentiate dermoids and epidermoids from arachnoid cysts.[5,11] Although use of diffusion tensor imaging has been popular in the pediatric brain, thus far it has not been used routinely in the pediatric spine.

CONTRAST MATERIAL

Gadolinium contrast enhancement occurs in some lesions, allowing them to be better visualized as a result of increased tissue contrast.[18] Although many lesions, such as cord transection and infarction, can be fully evaluated without the use of a contrast agent, intravenous gadolinium is administered routinely when assessing neoplastic and inflammatory processes.[2,10] In addition, it is variably given on a case by case basis, depending on the indication for the examination and the unenhanced MRI findings.

Nuclear Scintigraphy

Nuclear scintigraphy has limited use in the evaluation of the pediatric spinal cord and surrounding structures. Other than very rare use in assessment of shunt patency and cerebral spinal fluid leaks, it occasionally is used to evaluate adjacent osseous structures, for example, gallium scanning for vertebral osteomyelitis and bone scanning for metastatic disease. However, with the increasing utilization of high-resolution positron emission tomography with ^{18}F-2-fluorodeoxyglucose, positron emission tomography imaging may develop a larger role in the evaluation of spinal cord disorders, particularly in tumors in which treatment response can be assessed.[19]

Key Points

Ultrasound is able to provide detailed evaluation of the pediatric spinal cord up to approximately 6 months of age, after which time vertebral ossification obscures visualization of anatomic detail.

MRI is the primary imaging modality for pediatric spinal cord evaluation because of its superior soft tissue contrast resolution.

Recent advances in MRI techniques allow for the use of higher field strength and modern imaging sequences to fully evaluate pediatric spinal pathology.

Suggested Readings

Lowe LH, Johanek AJ, Moore CW. Sonography of the neonatal spine: part 1, normal anatomy, imaging pitfalls, and variations that may simulate disease. *AJR Am J Roentgenol.* 2007;188(3):733-738.
Lowe LH, Johanek AJ, Moore CW. Sonography of the neonatal spine: part 2. Spinal disorders. *AJR Am J Roentgenol.* 2007;188(3):739-744.
Vertinsky AT, Krasnokutsky MV, Augustin M, et al. Cutting-edge imaging of the spine. *Neuroimaging Clin N Am.* 2007;17(1):117-136.

References

Full references for this chapter can be found on www.expertconsult.com.

Chapter 42

Prenatal Imaging

ERIN SIMON SCHWARTZ and DAVID M. MIRSKY

Vast improvements have been made in the diagnosis and therapy of fetal anomalies as a result of advances in imaging and surgical technology. Nowhere is this more applicable than in the fetal spine. Ultrasonography is the primary imaging modality for fetal evaluation and helps distinguish normal spine development from abnormal spine development while providing valuable information about spinal anomalies. Magnetic resonance imaging (MRI) is complementary to ultrasonography for assessment of spinal malformations, as it has the advantage of better detection and depiction of associated central nervous system (CNS) and non-CNS anomalies that may have a significant impact on postnatal neurologic function and quality of life.

The major lesion of the CNS currently amenable to fetal diagnosis and intervention is open spinal dysraphism, commonly referred to as *myelomeningocele* (MMC); this lesion is a significant driving force behind the use of highly detailed prenatal imaging. The osseous detail and real-time evaluation of lower extremity configuration, position, and motion detectable with ultrasonography, combined with soft tissue and parenchymal assessments with the use of MRI, provide the maternal-fetal medicine specialist and pediatric neurosurgeon with highly detailed anatomic information. Because the surgery is not without risk to the mother and the fetus, obtaining extremely accurate information is essential for determining surgical appropriateness and presurgical planning. When significant congenital anomalies are present outside of the CNS, information about associated spinal abnormalities is valuable for counseling and parental decision making regarding the management of the pregnancy, labor, and delivery or interruption of the pregnancy.

Imaging Techniques

The accuracy of identifying spinal anomalies during nontargeted screening ultrasonography varies, depending on the skill and experience of the operator. The accuracy of a referral center performing detailed targeting studies for a suspected neural tube defect (elevated maternal serum α-fetoprotein) is close to 100%. A detailed protocol should be performed. Because fetuses with open neural tube defects typically have Chiari II malformations, the fetal brain should be scanned initially. A small cisterna magna with rounded small cerebellum is termed the "banana sign" and is 99% sensitive in the diagnosis of a Chiari II malformation (Fig. 42-1). The frontal bones may be concave, and this is termed the "lemon sign." This sign is less specific and may be present in 1% to 2% of normal fetuses and may resolve by the third trimester. Ventriculomegaly may be present. Axial and longitudinal views of the spine should be obtained. Spine ossification progresses from 10 to 22 weeks' gestation. By 16 weeks' gestation, neural arch ossification is complete to L5. By 19 weeks, S1 is completely ossified, and by 22 weeks, S2 is ossified. Splayed pedicles are best visualized in the transverse plane. An overlying sac may be imaged in transverse and longitudinal planes, with higher-frequency transducers showing cord tethering and placode contents (Fig. 42-2).

Fetal MRI is typically performed on 1.5 Tesla (T) magnets, although some centers are now performing fetal MRI at 3.0 T. A surface coil (torso, cardiac, or body phased-array) is used to maximize image quality. A standard localizer sequence generally facilitates quick identification of fetal position. This is used to guide the initial imaging plane, which should be appropriately aligned with the fetal anatomy in question. Subsequent imaging sequences are prescribed in orthogonal planes with respect to the fetal spine, each adjusted from the preceding image set, to account for changes in fetal position.

Ultrafast sequences are used to minimize image degradation by maternal and fetal movements. T2-weighted images provide most of the diagnostic information for the examination: single-shot fast spin echo (SSFSE) or half-Fourier acquisition single-shot turbo spin echo (HASTE) sequences at minimal slice thickness (2 to 4 mm). Fast T1-weighted gradient echo imaging is frequently attempted but seems to show satisfactory contrast resolution and signal-to-noise ratio only after approximately 26 weeks' gestation. Extremely rapid gradient echo, echo planar imaging, with its high sensitivity to paramagnetic susceptibility may be used to identify osseous and vascular structures and hemorrhage. Diffusion-weighted imaging is increasingly being used to assess for acute ischemia.

Open Spinal Dysraphism

ETIOLOGY

Abnormalities in neurulation may result from defects in disjunction, the process by which the neural tube separates from the overlying ectoderm. A large site of complete failure of disjunction may result in MMC. Prenatally, the findings of

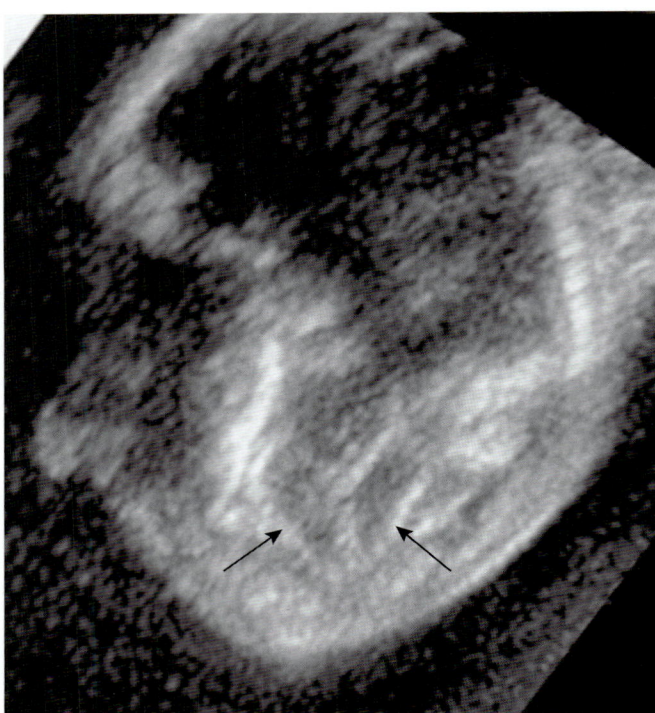

Figure 42-1 **Banana sign.** An axial ultrasonographic image through the posterior fossa in a 21-week fetus with a Chiari II malformation shows the crowding of the cerebellum around the brainstem that has been termed the "banana sign" (demarcated by arrows).

MMC are clearly detectable with ultrasonography and MRI. In the presence of elevation of the neural placode, secondary to expansion of the subarachnoid space, the lesion is referred to as MMC (Fig. 42-3). This is distinguished from myeloschisis, also known as *myelocele*, where an open neural tube defect exists, but the subarachnoid space is not expanded, and the neural placode remains within the confines of the dysraphic spinal canal (Fig. 42-4). MMC occurs during the formation of the primitive neural tube (neurulation) in the third week of gestation, when a localized failure of neural tube closure occurs. This failure may occur anywhere along the length of the spinal cord, but it is most common in the lumbar region. The resulting lesion is an open spinal canal with a flat neural placode instead of a cylindrical spinal cord. Imaging reveals the failure of neurulation in the MMC as a posterior osseocutaneous defect. When present, the expansion of the subarachnoid space is readily apparent (see Fig. 42-3). The neurologic deficits sustained by the fetus are postulated to occur in stages—a "two-hit" hypothesis. The first "hit" is the original defect in neurulation that creates the dysraphism and any associated myelodysplasia. The second "hit" is the secondary chemical or physical trauma (or both) to the neural tissue as a result of its exposure to the intrauterine environment.

A unified theory regarding the pathogenesis of the associated Chiari II malformation was postulated by McLone and Knepper, who suggested that the open spinal canal and associated free drainage of cerebrospinal fluid (CSF) promote collapse of the primitive ventricular system and cause lack of expansion of the rhombencephalic vesicle, from which the posterior fossa develops. This lack of distention leads to an abnormally small posterior fossa and subsequent herniation and other associated malformations in the brain. The Chiari II malformation is a pancerebral anomaly, affecting broad areas of the brain. Abnormalities include herniation of the medulla, cerebellar tonsils, and vermis through the foramen magnum; a small posterior fossa; "beaking" of the tectum of the midbrain; an enlarged massa intermedia of the thalami; partial or complete callosal dysgenesis; and structural changes in the skull (Fig. 42-5). Migrational abnormalities, particularly subependymal gray matter heterotopia, also are commonly seen. The cause of hydrocephalus in patients with MMC is frequently debated. Current theories include mechanical obstruction secondary to anatomic changes associated with the Chiari II malformation and dysfunctional CSF absorption. Clinically, hydrocephalus may not be present at birth but may become apparent after early postnatal closure of the defect.

TREATMENT

Prenatal repair of MMC has been performed in the United States for over 10 years. The initial intent was to preserve distal neurologic function by covering the exposed spinal cord. Although early results may have suggested some improvement in distal sensorimotor function, prenatal repair serendipitously led to a reduction in hindbrain herniation and a possible decreased need for ventricular shunting.

Ultrasound examination of fetuses with MMC at 18 weeks' gestational age frequently shows lower limb movements that correlate with the movements of unaffected fetuses, suggesting that loss of motor function in these patients

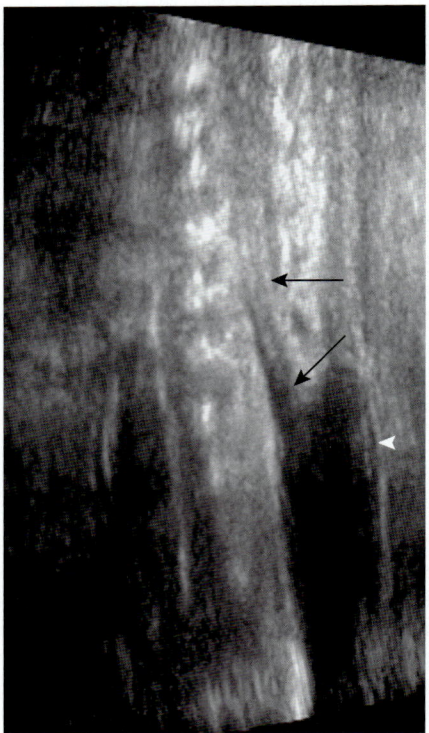

Figure 42-2 **Myelomeningocele.** Longitudinal ultrasonography through the lumbosacral spine in a 20-week fetus shows the defect in the posterior elements, with the abnormally low spinal cord extending to the level of the defect (*arrows*).

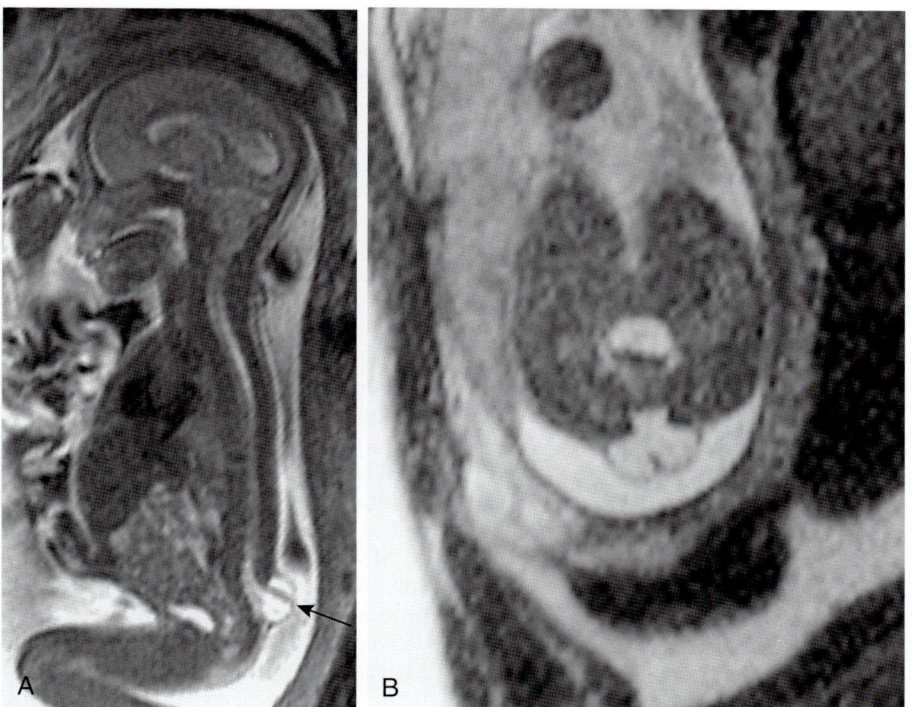

Figure 42-3 Myelomeningocele. **A,** A sagittal half-Fourier acquisition single-shot turbo spin echo (HASTE) magnetic resonance image in a 21-week fetus with a small myelomeningocele sac protruding at the lumbosacral junction level. The neural tissue can be readily identified traversing the sac (*arrow*). Note the Chiari II malformation findings. **B,** An axial HASTE image at the lumbosacral level shows the expanded subarachnoid space protruding through the wide posterior element deficiency. Note the neural placode outside the confines of the canal, traversing the sac.

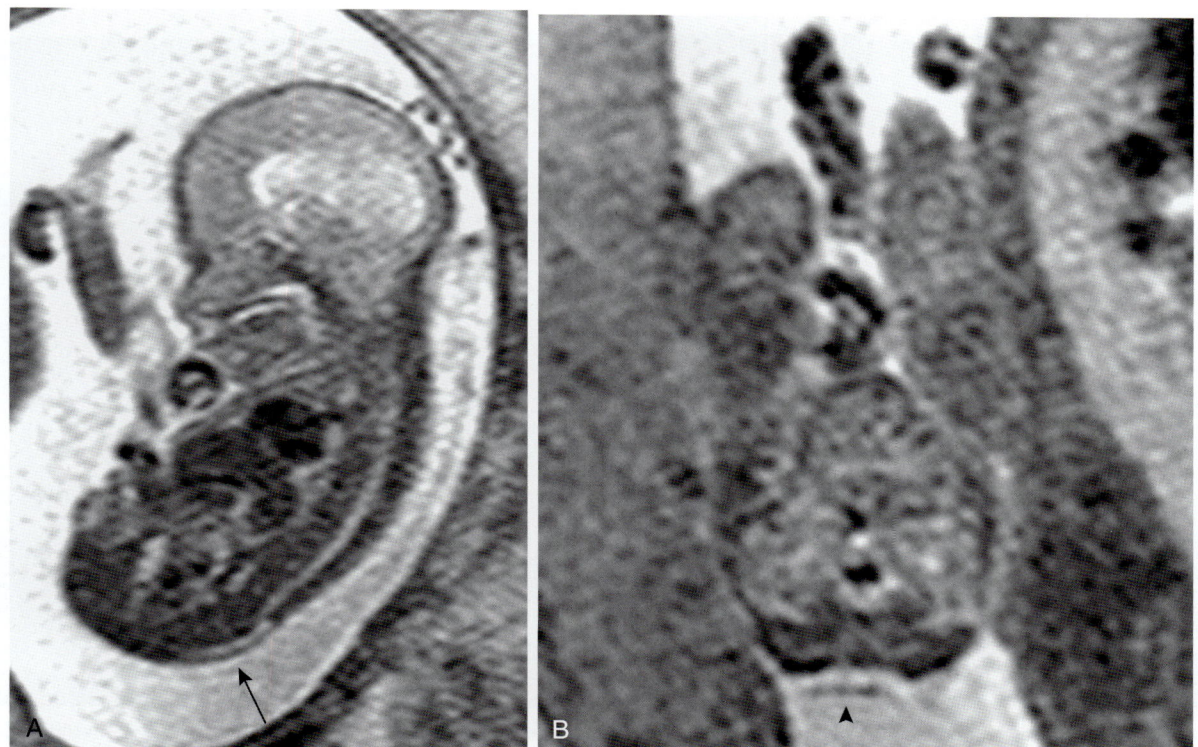

Figure 42-4 Myeloschisis. **A,** A sagittal half-Fourier acquisition single-shot turbo spin echo (HASTE) image of the spine in a 19-week fetus with a posterior spinal defect. The placode remains within the spinal canal (*arrow*). **B,** An axial HASTE image at the lumbosacral level shows the wide posterior element deficiency and neural placode within the confines of the broad canal (*arrowhead*).

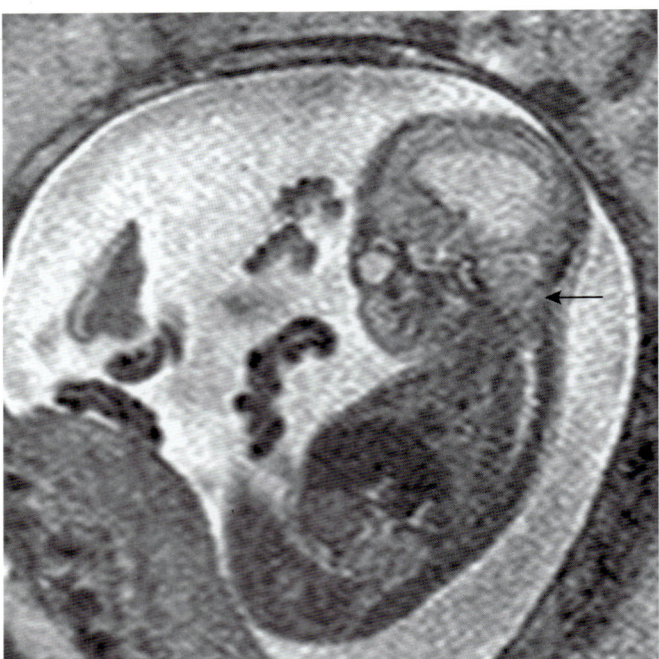

Figure 42-5 Chiari II malformation. A sagittal half-Fourier acquisition single-shot turbo spin echo image at the craniocervical junction in a 19-week fetus shows the hindbrain herniation and funneling of the posterior fossa of the Chiari II malformation (*arrow*). Note the ventriculomegaly and loss of the supratentorial subarachnoid spaces.

may occur later in gestation. Perhaps the most compelling argument for in utero repair of MMC comes from the lesser degrees of neurologic deficits in many of the forms of closed spinal dysraphism in which the neural elements remain covered by skin (e.g., lipomyelomeningocele). The first report on fetal surgery in humans, by Adzick and colleagues, suggested that intrauterine repair of MMC results in improvements in neurologic function and hindbrain herniation. These findings recapitulated experiment results and prompted the first large multicenter trial to determine the role of fetal surgery in fetuses with MMC.

The Management of Myelomeningocele Study trial found that fetuses who underwent in utero repair of MMC demonstrated superior standardized test scores for motor skills and that twice as many children were walking independently at 30 months of age compared with those randomized to postnatal surgery. Additionally, prenatal repair led to a reduction in hindbrain herniation (Fig. 42-6), and these children were half as likely to require ventricular shunting.

MMC is generally not a fatal disease in utero or postnatally, and most prenatally diagnosed infants survive to lead productive lives. Fetal surgery is associated with premature delivery and its attendant complications, including fetal loss. Maternal complications may range from uterine rupture and hemorrhage to deep venous thrombosis. Despite this, hundreds of mothers and fetuses have undergone prenatal repair of MMC and, as a result of the multicenter study, prenatal repair is now considered the standard of care in the United States.

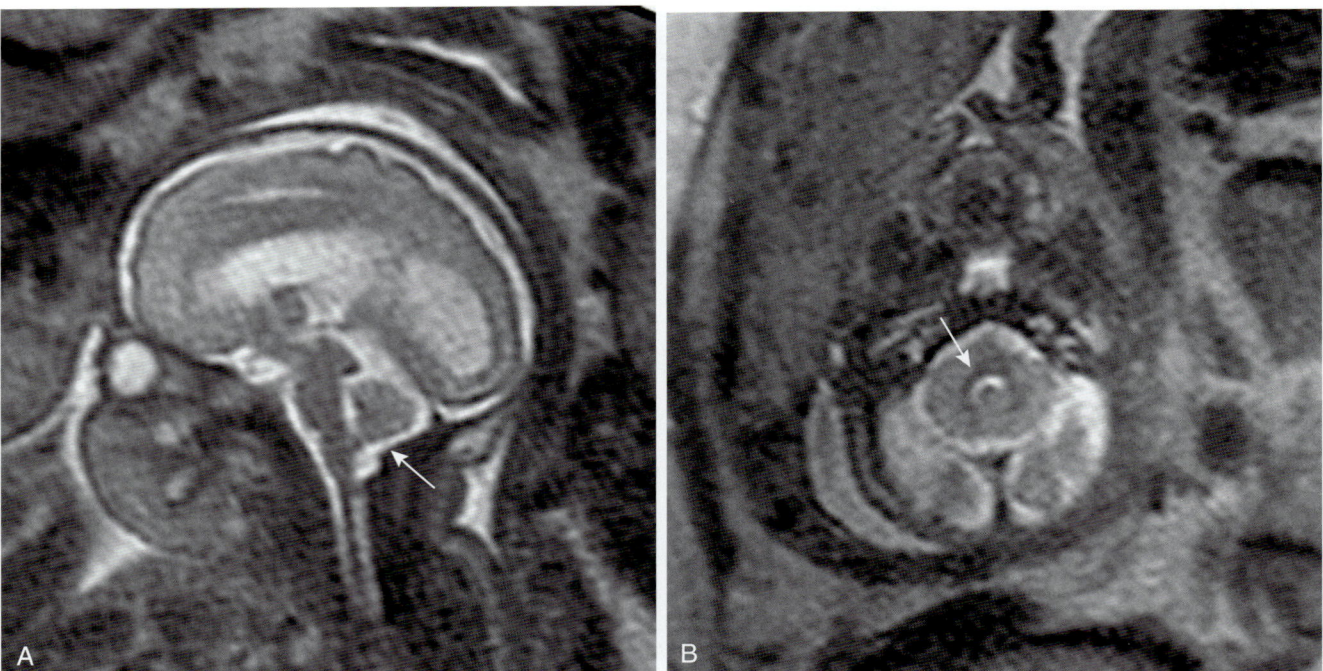

Figure 42-6 Reversal of hindbrain herniation after fetal myelomeningocele repair. **A,** A sagittal half-Fourier acquisition single-shot turbo spin echo (HASTE) magnetic resonance image of the same fetus as in Figure 42-5 reveals the dramatic improvement in the appearance of the brain 6 weeks after surgery. The hindbrain herniation has resolved, with return of the posterior fossa subarachnoid spaces (*arrow*). The supratentorial subarachnoid spaces are now normal, but the ventricles remain enlarged. **B,** An axial HASTE image through the posterior fossa shows the now normal appearance of the fourth ventricle (*arrow*).

Closed Spinal Dysraphism

Many other spinal anomalies may be recognized in utero. Although none are candidates for prenatal surgery at this time, it is important to recognize these anomalies and distinguish them from MMC to allow for proper patient counseling.

Spinal dysraphism, particularly the terminal myelocystocele, is frequently seen in association with systemic anomalies, most commonly anomalies of the genitourinary and lower gastrointestinal systems (cloacal anomalies). This is likely caused by the relative proximity of the caudal cell mass to the cloaca. The caudal cell mass is the origin of the conus medullaris, filum terminale, and lower lumbar and sacral nerve roots. A high index of suspicion should be maintained for lower spinal anomalies when cloacal anomalies are present. The reverse also is true. Constellations of anomalies that commonly have associated congenital spinal malformations include the OEIS (omphalocele, exstrophy, imperforate anus, spinal anomalies), VACTERL (vertebral, anal atresia, cardiac, tracheal, esophageal, renal, limb), and Currarino triad (sacral hypogenesis, anorectal malformations, presacral teratoma or meningocele). The vertebral anomalies seen with OEIS and VACTERL are most commonly hemivertebrae or butterfly vertebrae, which may be detected prenatally if they distort the spinal alignment; however, they are generally difficult to diagnose in utero. More severe anomalies have been reported as well. The association of the notochord with the induction of visceral organ formation is a likely explanation of the associations between congenital vertebral and spinal cord anomalies and thoracic or abdominal anomalies, including the VACTERL association and congenital diaphragmatic hernia.

LIPOMYELOMENINGOCELE

Premature disjunction of the cutaneous ectoderm from the neuroectoderm allows mesenchyme to contact the inner portion of the developing neural tube. As the tube begins to close, the mesenchyme is induced to become fat, the presence of which may interfere with neurulation. This may result in lipomyelomeningocele–lipomyeloschisis. These lesions are skin covered and consequently not associated with the Chiari II malformation or abnormal elevation of maternal serum or amniotic fluid α-fetoprotein and acetylcholinesterase (markers of an open neural tube). A small lipomyelomeningocele may be harder to detect with screening ultrasonography but should be apparent with MRI, particularly later in the second trimester and in the third trimester (Fig. 42-7). As in the case of MMC, the distinction between lipomyelomeningocele and lipomyeloschisis lies in the location of the placode–lipoma interface with respect to the plane of the back. The expansion of the subarachnoid space characterizes the lipomyelomeningocele, but in contrast to MMC, it is much less common than its flat counterpart. The placode in the lipomyelomeningocele is much more likely to be deformed, being rotated toward the lipoma and away from the protrusion of the meninges. This poses an additional problem for the pediatric neurosurgeon performing postnatal repair because the spinal nerve roots are similarly deformed, with shortened roots on the side of the lipoma, which tether the cord. The elongated roots on the side of the meninges

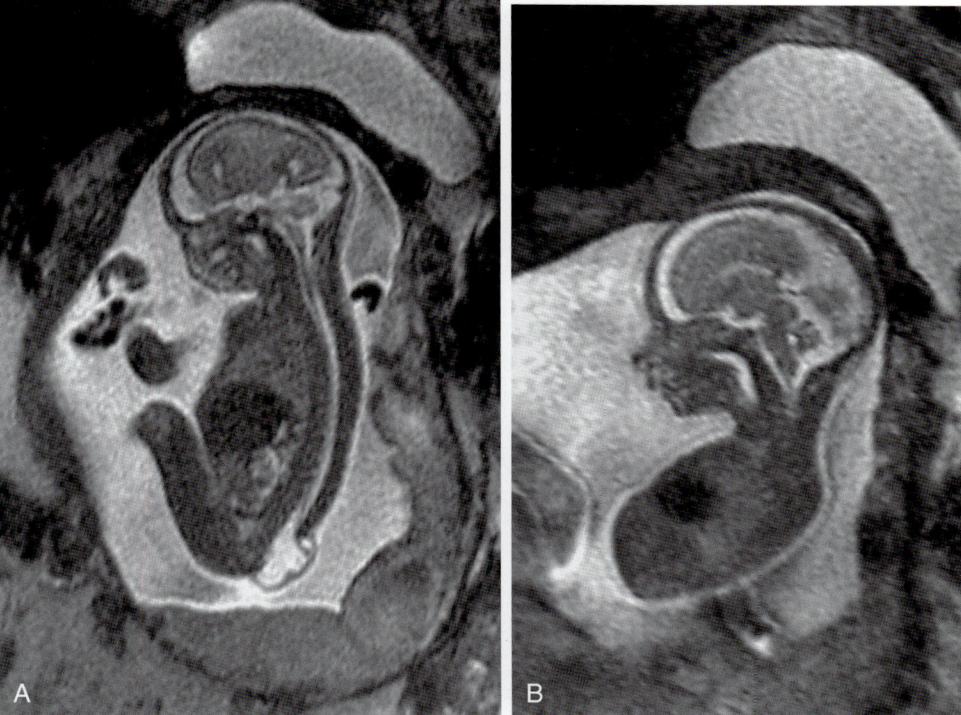

Figure 42-7 Lipomyelomeningocele. **A,** A sagittal half-Fourier acquisition single-shot turbo spin echo (HASTE) magnetic resonance image of a 21-week fetus shows a large lumbosacral defect with neural tissue traversing the sac. The sac appears slightly thicker walled than that of a myelomeningocele, although correlation with open neural tube defect markers is required. **B,** An axial HASTE image through the midline of the brain shows normal morphology, including a normal corpus callosum. No Chiari II malformation is present.

must be carefully negotiated as the surgeon attempts to access the placode–lipoma interface.

SPLIT CORD MALFORMATION

Split cord malformation (SCM) is a developmental abnormality of the notochord. It is not always possible on imaging to distinguish between diastematomyelia (spinal cord and canal splitting) and diplomyelia (spinal cord and canal duplication). As such, SCM is the preferred terminology.

The spinal cord is focally split into two hemicords, often asymmetrically (Fig. 42-8). This may involve the entire anteroposterior aspect of the cord or a portion of the spinal cord, the latter being quite rare. Each hemicord contains a central canal, and at least one dorsal horn and one ventral horn, from which nerve roots arise. An osseous septum between dual dural tubes (type I) or fibrous septum within a single dural tube (type II) separates the hemicords. Occasionally, no intervening septum exists in the type II lesion. SCM most commonly occurs in the lumbar region, and the type I is frequently associated with vertebral body anomalies. Cervicothoracic junction lesions may be more common than is currently reported because they are often asymptomatic owing to the absence of spinal cord tethering.

Type I SCM is readily recognized with fetal imaging (see Fig. 42-8). An often subtle alteration in spinal alignment from the associated anomalous vertebral bodies should be a clue that a spinal anomaly is present. When present, the osseous septum may appear on ultrasonography as an echogenic structure traversing the spinal canal. Echo planar MRI techniques may be valuable in assessing for the osseous septum, which commonly tethers the spinal cord, and is significant in determining the extent of postnatal surgical intervention. The simple fibrous septum or cord duplication without intervening septum (type II) may be difficult to visualize prenatally, particularly when imaging is performed in the second trimester. SCM is present in 40% of MMC, although this most commonly involves only duplication or splitting of the

placode, which may be impossible to detect prenatally. It is imperative to search for SCM when MMC is encountered because the spinal cord may remain tethered by the septum after MMC repair.

TERMINAL MYELOCYSTOCELE

This rare malformation may represent a severe manifestation of the persistent terminal ventricle, resulting from an inability of CSF to escape from the neural tube during its formation. The marked dilation of the distal central canal is also referred to as the *terminal ventricle of the spinal cord*, which herniates through a posterior lumbosacral spinal defect. The leptomeninges herniate around the bulbous distal spinal cord (Fig. 42-9). With prenatal imaging, terminal myelocystocele may sometimes be distinguished from the MMC with close attention to the morphology and wall thickness of the protruding sac, the absence of Chiari II malformation, and the lack of elevation of maternal serum and amniotic fluid markers of an open neural tube defect. A degree of downward displacement of the cerebellar tonsils through the foramen magnum and reduction of the infratentorial and supratentorial subarachnoid spaces may develop late in gestation with a large terminal myelocystocele, but this should not be mistaken for the Chiari II malformation.

MENINGOCELE

The simple posterior meningocele is characterized by a meningeal-lined CSF sac, which protrudes through a posterior osseous spinal defect (Fig. 42-10). The spinal cord does not enter the sac, although it may be associated with hypertrophy of the filum terminale or spinal cord tethering. Its etiology is not well understood, but some postulate that CSF pulsations cause the meninges to herniate through a focal posterior osseous defect. Most commonly encountered in the thoracic spine, these anomalies rarely may be present in utero and must be differentiated from thoracic MMC. Similar to

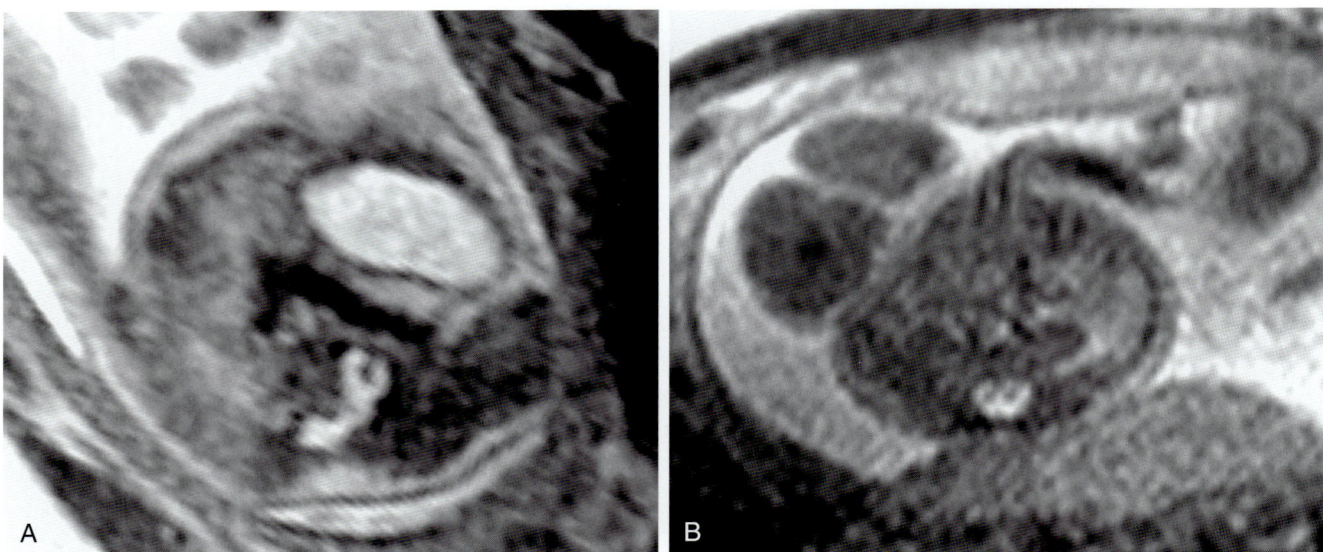

A   B

Figure 42-8 Split cord malformation. **A,** An axial half-Fourier acquisition single-shot turbo spin echo (HASTE) image through a type I split cord malformation. The osseous septum traversing the two canals is visible. **B,** An axial HASTE image through a type II split cord malformation. No septum is visible between the two hemicords.

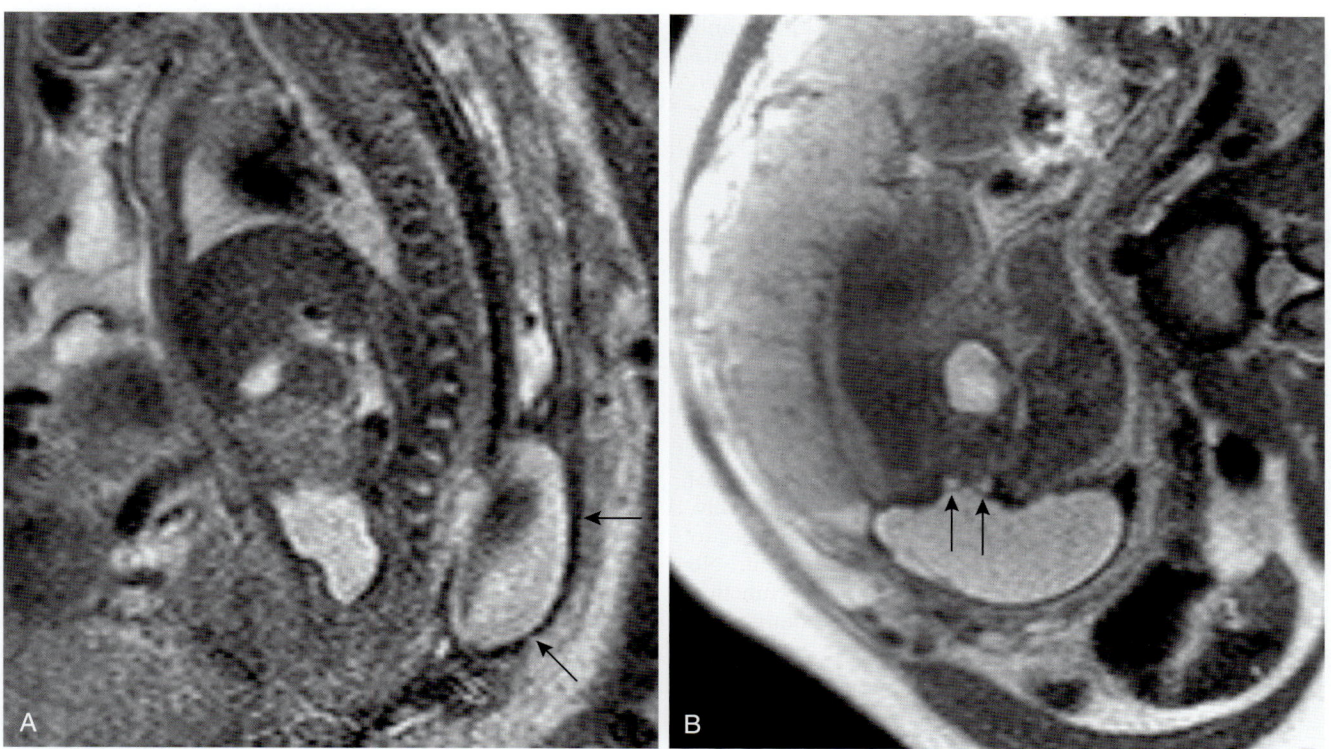

Figure 42-9   **Terminal myelocystocele. A,** A sagittal half-Fourier acquisition single-shot turbo spin echo (HASTE) magnetic resonance image in a 32-week fetus shows the thick-walled posterior sac (*arrows*) protruding through a focal lower lumbar osseous defect. **B,** An axial HASTE image through the osseous defect and large sac shows the distal spinal cord (*arrows*) splitting around the dilated central canal.

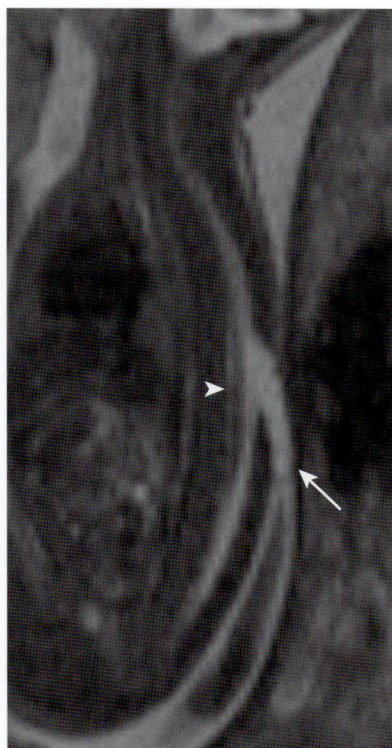

Figure 42-10   Dorsal meningocele. A sagittal half-Fourier acquisition single-shot turbo spin echo magnetic resonance image in a 22-week fetus shows the sac protruding through the posterior osseous defect (*arrow*). Note the spinal cord traversing, and not entering, the sac (*arrowhead*).

the terminal myelocystocele and lipomyelomeningocele, these skin–covered (closed) lesions do not have an associated Chiari II malformation, and the maternal serum or amniotic fluid does not contain markers of an open neural tube defect.

CAUDAL REGRESSION SYNDROME

Caudal regression syndrome represents a wide spectrum of anomalies, ranging from coccygeal or lumbosacral hypogenesis to frank sirenomelia. Infants of mothers with diabetes are the most susceptible, and the incidence is 1 : 7500 live births. This entity may be diagnosed prenatally, by a single lower extremity in the most extreme form to an absence or reduction in number of lower vertebral segments in lesser degrees of involvement. The less severe forms may not be detectable prenatally.

The lower extent of the spine determines the type of caudal regression and the severity of the clinical and imaging findings. The more severe form is diagnosed (type I) when the spine ends at or above the S1 level. The lowest formed level may even be in the midthoracic region. The spinal cord terminates abnormally high, with an abrupt, blunted tip, rather than the smooth taper that should be seen with a normal conus medullaris. Associated deformation of the cauda equina is common, with anterior and posterior separation of nerve roots. A spine terminating at or below the S2 level (type II) contains many fewer malformations, although the distal–most portion of the conus medullaris would not be present, resulting in a blunted appearance. Typically, the spinal cord is tethered by a tight filum terminale or filum lipoma.

In unusual cases of mild caudal regression syndrome, only the tip of the conus medullaris may be absent, and the spinal cord may not be tethered. It is not expected that these findings would be detectable prenatally. This complex continuum is also associated with syndromes, including OEIS, VACTERL, and the Currarino triad.

SEGMENTAL SPINAL DYSGENESIS

Segmental spinal dysgenesis is a rare entity in which a focal segment of the lumbar or thoracic spine is agenetic or markedly hypogenetic. The spinal cord at this level is segmentally disrupted, the distal spinal cord is often abnormally large (but may be more normal), and a sharply angled focal kyphosis develops after birth. Some authors believe that segmental spinal dysgenesis falls within the caudal regression spectrum and that the morphology depends on the level of notochordal disruption. If the notochordal development is affected distally, caudal regression syndrome ensues, but if the lesion occurs more proximally, segmental spinal dysgenesis is seen. No known treatment is currently available to improve function in this condition, although postnatal surgical decompression has been reported to prevent worsening neurologic function.

Key Points

Careful attention to morphology in the prenatal evaluation of spinal dysraphism may aid in distinguishing between entities with similar features (i.e. MMC, lipomyelomeningocele, and meningocele).

Prenatal surgical repair has become an accepted standard of care for the treatment of MMC in the United States.

Suggested Readings

Adzick NS, Thom EA, Spong CY, et al. A randomized trial of prenatal versus postnatal repair of myelomeningocele. *N Engl J Med.* 2011; 364(11):993-1004.

Glenn OA, Barkovich AJ. Magnetic resonance imaging of the fetal brain and spine: an increasingly important tool in prenatal diagnosis, part 1. *AJNR Am J Neuroradiol.* 2006;27(8):1604-1611.

Glenn OA, Barkovich AJ. Magnetic resonance imaging of the fetal brain and spine: an increasingly important tool in prenatal diagnosis: part 2. *AJNR Am J Neuroradiol.* 2006;27(9):1807-1814.

Griffiths PD, Paley MN, Widjaja E, et al. In utero magnetic resonance imaging for brain and spinal abnormalities in fetuses. *BMJ.* 2005; 331(7516):562-565.

Rossi A, Gandolfo C, Morana G, et al. Current classification and imaging of congenital spinal abnormalities. *Semin Roentgenol.* 2006;41(4):250-273.

Bibliography

Adzick NS, Sutton LN, Crombleholme TM, et al. Successful fetal surgery for spina bifida [letter]. *Lancet.* 1998;352:1666-1675.

Bruner JP, Tulipan N, Paschall RL, et al. Fetal surgery for myelomeningocele and the incidence of shunt-dependent hydrocephalus. *JAMA.* 1999;282:1819-1825.

Dias MS, McLone DG. Hydrocephalus in the child with dysraphism. *Neurosurg Clin North Am.* 1993;4:715-726.

Hasan SJ, Keirstead HS, Muir GD, et al. Axonal regeneration contributes to repair of injured brainstem-spinal neurons in embryonic chick. *J Neurosci.* 1993;13:492-507.

Heffez DS, Aryanpur J, Rotellini NA, et al. Intrauterine repair of experimental surgically created dysraphism. *Neurosurgery.* 1993;32: 1005-1010.

Inagaki T, Schoenwoif GC, Walker ML. Experimental model: change in the posterior fossa with surgically induced spina bifida aperta in mouse. *Pediatr Neurosurg.* 1997;26:185-189.

Johnson MP, Sutton LN, Rintoul N, et al. Fetal myelomeningocele repair: short-term clinical outcomes. *Am J Obstet Gynecol.* 2003;189:482-487.

Korenromp MJ, van Gool JD, Bruinese HW, et al. Early fetal leg movements in myelomeningocele [letter]. *Lancet.* 1986;1:917-918.

Larsen WJ. *Human embryology.* 2nd ed. New York: Churchill Livingstone; 1997.

Levine D, Barnes PD, Madsen JR, et al. Central nervous system abnormalities assessed with prenatal magnetic resonance imaging. *Obstet Gynecol.* 1999;94:1011-1019.

McLone DG, Knepper PA. The cause of Chiari II malformation: a unified theory. *Pediatr Neurosci.* 1989;15:1-12.

Meuli M, Meuli-Simmen C, Hutchins GM, et al. The spinal cord lesion in human fetuses with myelomeningocele: implications for fetal surgery. *J Pediatr Surg.* 1997;32:448-452.

Paek BW, Farmer DL, Wilkinson CC, et al. Hindbrain herniation develops in surgically created myelomeningocele but is absent after repair in fetal lambs. *Am J Obstet Gynecol.* 2000;183:1119-1123.

Pilu G, Falco P, Perolo A, et al. Ultrasound evaluation of the fetal neural axis. In: Callen P, ed. *Ultrasonography in obstetrics and gynecology.* 4th ed. Philadelphia, PA: Saunders; 2000:277-306.

Sutton LN, Adzick NS, Bilaniuk LT, et al. Improvement in hindbrain herniation demonstrated by serial fetal magnetic resonance imaging following fetal surgery for myelomeningocele. *JAMA.* 1999;282: 1826-1831.

Tulipan N, Bruner JP, Hernanz-Schulman M, et al. Effect of intrauterine myelomeningocele repair on central nervous system structure and function. *Pediatr Neurosurg.* 1999;31:183-188.

Tulipan N, Hernanz-Schulman M, Lowe LH, et al. Intrauterine myelomeningocele repair reverses preexisting hindbrain herniation. *Pediatr Neurosurg.* 1999;31:137-142.

Walsh DS, Adzick NS, Sutton LN, et al. The rationale for in utero repair of myelomeningocele. *Fetal Diagn Ther.* 2001;16:312-322.

Chapter 43

Congenital Abnormalities of the Spine

KEVIN R. MOORE

Embryology and Developmental Anatomy

Formation of the spine begins early in gestation, commencing at the end of the second gestational week with formation of the Hensen node and continuing into the beginning of the third week with the appearance of the neural plate during gastrulation. The notochordal process forms at day 16 or 17, with transient communication of the amnion through the notochordal canal to the yolk sac and through the neurenteric canal of Kovalevsky. The spine develops in a mostly orderly progression, and the vertebral axis and spinal cord develop synchronously. The rostral spinal cord (to about the level of S2) forms by the process of primary neurulation, whereas the caudal spinal cord (below the S2 level) forms by secondary neurulation, also referred to as *canalization and retrogressive differentiation*. Most congenital spinal anomalies can be explained by one or more events going awry during these processes.

The neural tube folds and closes at the end of the third gestational week, during primary neurulation; this leaves temporary cranial and caudal openings called *neuropores*. Normal neural tube closure by day 25 to 27 signals the end of primary neurulation. Meanwhile, the neural tube separates from the overlying ectoderm during the related process of dysjunction. If dysjunction occurs prematurely, perineural mesenchyme is permitted access to the neural groove and ependymal lining. This mesenchyme may differentiate into fat and prevent complete neural tube closure, which leads to the lipomatous malformation spectrum. If dysjunction fails to occur (nondysjunction), an ectodermal–neuroectodermal tract forms that prevents mesenchymal migration. Nondysjunction results in posterior dysraphism, producing the open neural tube defect spectrum of myelomeningocele (MMC), dorsal dermal sinus, and myelocystocele.

The neuroepithelial cells (neuroblasts) around the inner neural tube form the mantle layer, which produces the spinal cord gray matter. The outermost layer forms the marginal layer, which subsequently myelinates to produce the spinal cord white matter. The central neuroepithelial cells differentiate into ependymal cells along the central canal. Neural crest cells along each side of the neural tube form the dorsal root ganglia (DRG), autonomic ganglia, Schwann cells, leptomeninges, and adrenal medulla.

Concurrent with the neural tube folding during primary neurulation, spinal cord development below the caudal neuropore commences within the pluripotent tissue at the caudal eminence in the process of secondary neurulation. The initially solid cell mass canalizes and becomes contiguous with the rostral neural tube that was formed by primary neurulation. By day 48, a transient ventriculus terminalis appears in the future conus. If this persists after birth, it is noted incidentally as a normal variant ventriculus terminalis ("fifth ventricle"), usually of no clinical significance (see Chapter 40). Failure of proper secondary neurulation leads to caudal spine anomalies in the caudal regression, tethered cord, or sacrococcygeal teratoma (SCT) spectra in addition to terminal myelocystocele and anterior sacral meningocele (ASM).

By the third gestational month, the spinal cord extends the entire length of the developing spinal column. In fact, the more rapid elongation of the vertebral column and dura relative to the cord produces the apparent ascent of the cord during the remainder of gestation. Most importantly, the conus should be at adult level soon after birth, and persistent cord termination below L2–L3 after the first month of life in a full-gestation infant is probably abnormally low-lying.

Occurring simultaneously with spinal cord development is vertebral formation. During neurulation, the notochord induces the surrounding paraxial mesoderm derived from the primitive streak to form paired somite blocks (myotomes, sclerotomes). The myotomes form the paraspinal muscles and skin cover, and the sclerotomes divide into medial and lateral formations to produce the vertebral bodies, intervertebral disks, meninges, spinal ligaments (medial), and posterior spinal elements (lateral). Failure of correct notochordal induction leads to incomplete splitting of the neural plate from the notochord, producing the split notochord syndromes (neurenteric cyst and diastematomyelia [DSM]).

From day 24 until the fifth week, sclerotomal resegmentation commences, during which a horizontal sclerotomal cleft appears in the vertebra, and the caudal half of one vertebra combines with the rostral half of the vertebra below to form a "new" vertebral body. The notochord within the vertebral body degenerates, and the intervertebral notochord remnant becomes the intervertebral disk nucleus pulposus. Between days 40 and 60, the vertebrae undergo chondrification followed by subsequent ossification at distinct centers within the vertebral body and arches. This process continues past birth and into young adulthood. Ossification begins in the lower thoracic and upper lumbar regions and diverges cranially and caudally. In the cervical region, the vertebral primary ossification centers appear after the neural arch centers, beginning in the lower cervical spine (C6, C7) and proceeding rostrally. Aberrances occurring during the chondrification and ossification process produce myriad segmentation and fusion anomalies (SFAs; hemivertebrae, butterfly vertebrae, block vertebrae).

Spinal Dysraphism

Congenital spinal anomalies are classified both by clinical appearance (presence or absence of back mass) and by embryologic origin. Because the embryologic approach is easier to conceptualize, it will be emphasized here.

Spinal dysraphism is a broad term that encompasses a variety of disorders that have as a common feature abnormal dorsal spine formation; it is defined as incomplete or absent fusion of midline mesenchymal, bony, and neural structures. This term refers to large spinal defects, and not to the common spina bifida occulta, in which there is only a small cleft within a spinous process or a minor incomplete fusion of laminae at L5 or S1. Use of the term *spina bifida occulta* is strongly discouraged in favor of the preferred term *incomplete posterior element fusion,* because this finding is generally incidental and without clinical significance.

The osseous abnormalities associated with true spinal dysraphism may involve multiple vertebrae. *Spina bifida* (Latin, "cleft into two parts") is characterized by incomplete neural arch fusion with absence of all or parts of the affected posterior elements (laminae and spinous processes). Associated segmentation anomalies of the vertebral bodies—such as hemivertebrae, butterfly vertebrae, and block vertebrae—may be present.

Children with spinal dysraphism may come to medical attention with a back mass, abnormal cutaneous manifestations, gait disturbance, and bowel and bladder incontinence. Classically, spinal dysraphism is classified into two categories, based on the clinical presence or absence of a back mass. The first category is spinal dysraphism with back mass that is *not covered by skin* (e.g., spina bifida aperta or cystica, MMC,

myelocele); the second is spinal dysraphism with *skin-covered* back mass (e.g., lipomyelomeningocele [LMMC], myelocystocele, dorsal meningocele).

Abnormalities of Primary Neurulation

Primary neurulation abnormalities result from premature dysjunction, nondysjunction, or a combination of both.

PREMATURE DYSJUNCTION

Premature dysjunction of the neural tube from overlying ectoderm permits perineural mesenchyme to access the neural groove and ependymal lining. This mesenchyme differentiates into fat and prevents complete neural tube closure, resulting in skin-covered lipomatous malformations with or without posterior spinal dysraphism. The most commonly observed anomalies are lipomyelocele (LMC), LMMC (Fig. 43-1), and intradural spinal lipomas (Fig. 43-2).

An LMC is a skin-covered, closed dysraphism anomaly in which the neural placode is complexed with a lipoma that is contiguous with the subcutaneous fat through a dysraphic defect, attaching to and tethering the cord. An LMMC is an LMC with enlargement of the subarachnoid space that displaces the neural placode outside of the spinal canal. In both cases, syringomyelia is a common associated finding. LMC and LMMC account for 20% to 56% of occult spinal dysraphism and 20% of skin-covered lumbosacral masses. LMMC is not affected by maternal folate metabolism, unlike the less common MMC.

One important imaging point is that the neural placode is frequently rotated; this foreshortens the roots on one side, predisposing them to stretch injury, and it lengthens the roots on the other side, rotating them into the surgeon's field of view and making them more prone to injury. Magnetic

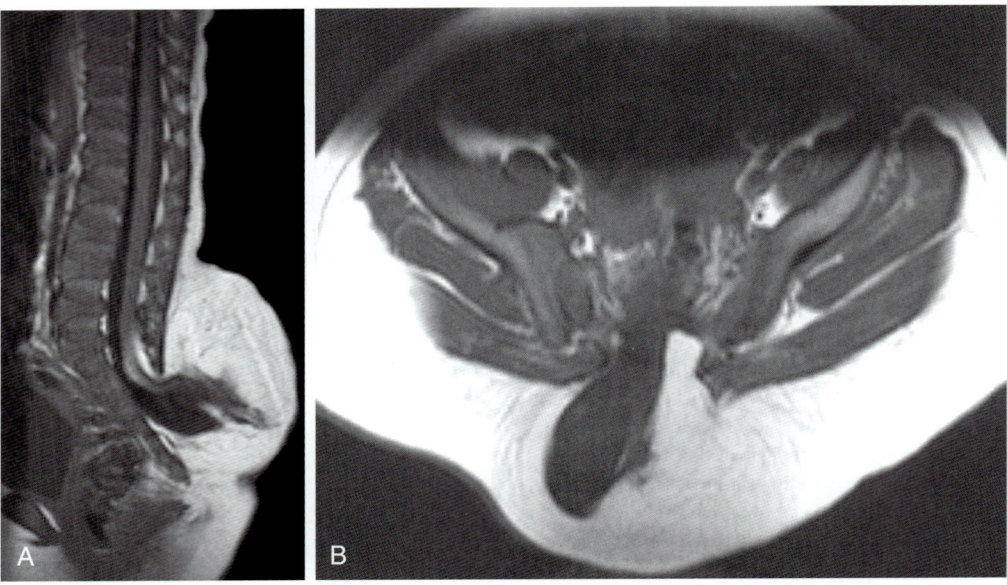

Figure 43-1   Lipomyelomeningocele. Sagittal (**A**) and axial (**B**) T1-weighted magnetic resonance (MR) images demonstrate a typical lipomyelomeningocele, with a low-lying cord tethered into a large lipomatous malformation contiguous with the subcutaneous fat through a posterior dysraphic defect.

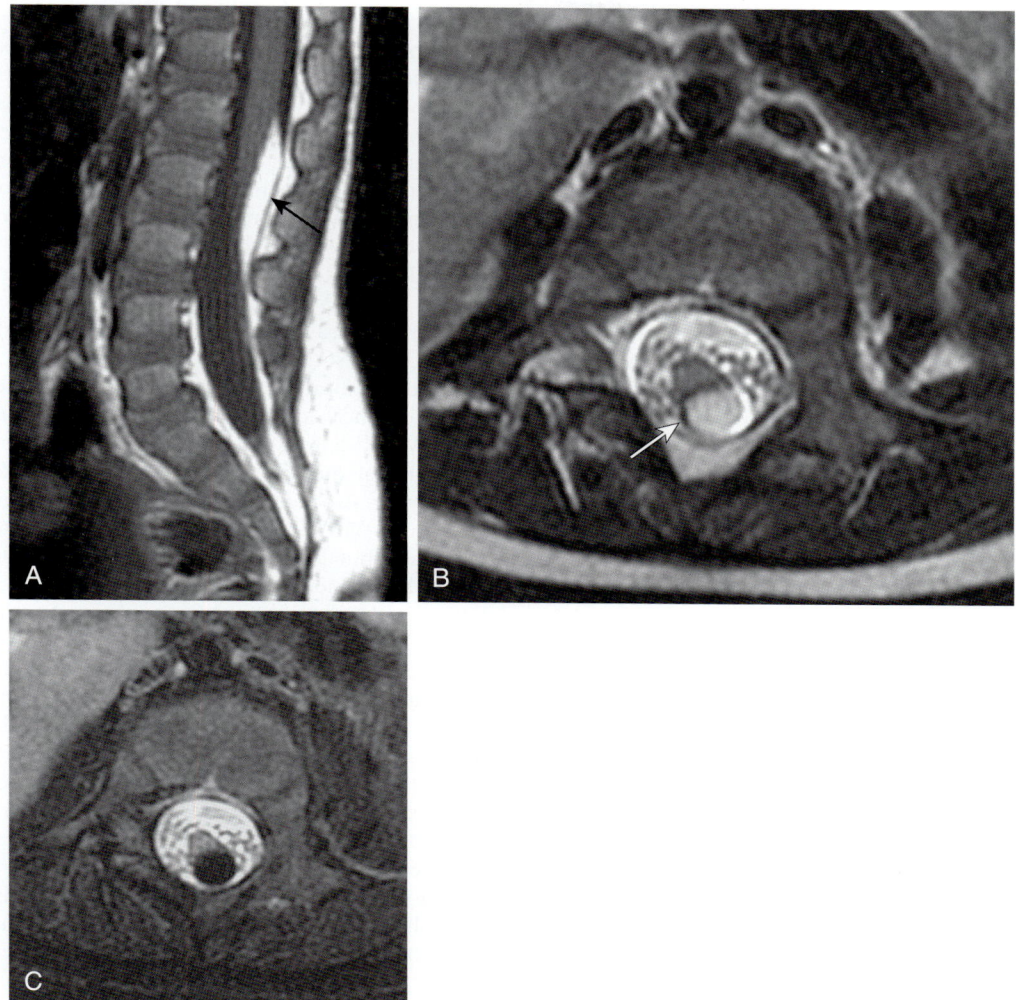

Figure 43-2 Juxtamedullary (subpial) spinal lipoma. **A,** Sagittal T1-weighted magnetic resonance (MR) image shows a small subpial intradural lipoma (*arrow*) adherent to the dorsal conus surface. **B,** Axial T2-weighted MR image confirms direct contiguity of the neural placode with the lipoma. Note chemical shift artifact (*arrow*) in the frequency encoding direction, indicating fat. **C,** Axial fat-saturated T2-weighted MR image confirms fat content by homogeneous signal loss within the lipoma.

resonance imaging (MRI) best delineates the critical anatomy and facilitates the search for the associated sacral dysgenesis, segmentation anomalies, or visceral organ anomalies. Early surgery can arrest or prevent neurologic deficits, and progressive deterioration after untethering prompts a search for retethering (mean time to retether, 52 months) or for other previously undiagnosed congenital spinal anomalies.

The spinal lipoma is subdivided into intradural (juxtamedullary, subpial) and terminal lipomas. *Intradural lipomas* are most common in the cervicothoracic or thoracic spine and most commonly occur near the conus. They are more often dorsal than ventral, are variable in size, and grow proportionally with the infant. Neurologic symptoms are representative of the lipoma level and usually progress slowly. More distal lipomas within the filum or at the filum insertion (terminal lipoma) may also occur with tethered cord symptoms. A focal sacral dysraphism is frequently seen in terminal lipoma.

MRI is the imaging modality of choice for lipoma diagnosis and treatment planning. A lipoma follows fat signal on all sequences, assisting differentiation from dermoid or proteinaceous cysts. Spinal lipoma and dermal sinus are

occasionally detected concurrently, so a dedicated search for multiple nondysjunction or premature dysjunction anomalies is always merited.

The fatty filum (filum fibrolipoma) is an exception to the previously described clinical presentations. It is common, occurs in up to 4% to 6% of people, and is seldom symptomatic. When it does produce symptoms, they are those of a tethered cord. It is always prudent to search for other occult anomalies before ascribing responsibility for neurologic symptoms to the fatty filum.

All lipomatous lesions may be asymptomatic, but frequently they produce the clinical symptoms of tethered spinal cord. For simplicity, some authorities lump all premature dysjunction disorders that feature abnormal fat together under the unifying term *lipomatous malformation*. Given the overlap of neurologic symptoms and imaging appearance between LMMC and lipoma, this simplified classification is plausible. In all cases, it is critical to assess how much fat is present and where it is located, the status and level of the spinal cord involved, the levels and extent of spinal dysraphism, and the presence or absence of other visceral or neuraxial anomalies for treatment planning because symptomatic patients usually require lipoma resection and cord untethering. Multiplanar MRI is the best modality for preoperative planning and for follow-up after symptom recurrence.

NONDYSJUNCTION

In contrast to lipomatous malformations, anomalies that result from nondysjunction occur when the neural tube fails to dissociate from adjacent cutaneous tissue. The simplest and least extensive variation is the dorsal dermal sinus, which occurs when a single connection persists and forms a fibrous cord from a skin dimple to the dural sac, conus, or central spinal cord canal. It is important to distinguish *dermal sinus* from its clinically asymptomatic mimic, *simple coccygeal dimple* (Fig. 43-3). In this mimic, the low sacral or coccygeal sinus originates from a low skin dimple and attaches to the coccyx via a short fibrous tract. These dimples are nearly always found within the intergluteal cleft, never communicate with the spinal canal, and require no treatment. Simple coccygeal dimples are the most common reason for newborn spinal ultrasound imaging.

Conversely, the true congenital dorsal dermal sinus tract (DST; Fig. 43-4) usually has an atypical dimple at the ostium that is larger (> 5 mm), often asymmetric, and remote (> 2.5 cm) from the anus. It may also be found in combination with other cutaneous anomalies, such as a hair patch or vascular lesion. The most common DST location is in the lumbosacral spine, followed by the occiput. In all dermal sinus cases, there is some degree of focal dysraphism, which may be as subtle as a bifid spinous process. The sinus tract cord is epithelial-cell lined and may or may not be canalized. When patent, it exposes the patient to an elevated risk of meningitis. It is critical to look for this anomaly in all patients

with atypical skin dimples, cutaneous back lesions, or lipomas. Additionally, 30% to 50% of DSTs may have an associated dermoid or epidermoid cyst. These patients should be imaged with MRI. The best MRI sequence is usually a sagittal T1-weighted MR image, windowed widely so that the hypointense tract is visualized as a gray cord immersed in bright fat that passes inferiorly and ventrally to the lumbodorsal fascia; it then turns upward to ascend within the spinal canal, often tenting the dorsal dura at the point of entry. Dermal sinuses are surgically excised to prevent meningitis and to untether the spinal cord.

More extensive nondysjunction produces the MMC lesion (Fig. 43-5) associated with maternal folate deficiency. Infants come to medical attention with an open, red, weeping skin defect on the back that features protruding neural elements. Most MMC lesions are either lumbosacral or thoracolumbar, but cervical and thoracic MMCs occur. Lesion level and severity of associated hydrocephalus determine the patient's prognosis. MMCs are linked to methylenetetrahydrofolate-reductase mutations with abnormal folate metabolism. *PAX3* paired box gene derangements and trisomy 13 or 18 (14% of fetuses with neural tube defect) are also described. These gene derangements and folate metabolism abnormalities are postulated to interfere with carbohydrate molecule expression on the neuroectodermal surface, which causes neural tube closure to fail. Prevalence in the United States is 2 in 10,000 live births, and it is more common in females by a ratio of 3:1. The prevalence of MMC decreased 23% between 1995 to 2004, which was attributed to more widespread folate fortification of food.

Associated orthopedic and neuraxial anomalies are common, and Chiari II malformation is universally present. Complications of the Chiari II malformation are the major cause of death in these patients. MMC patients should have

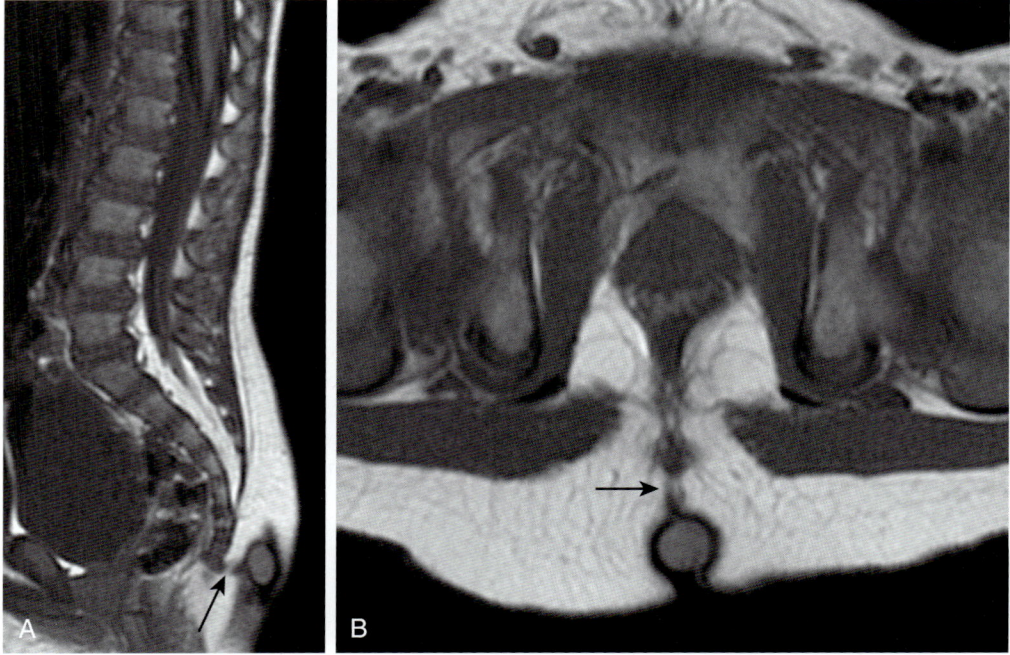

Figure 43-3 Simple sacrococcygeal dimple. Sagittal (**A**) and axial (**B**) T1-weighted magnetic resonance images demonstrate a low sacral dimple within the intergluteal cleft, marked by a hyperintense vitamin E capsule. The short fibrous tract (*arrow*) that extends from the dimple to the coccyx tip confirms the diagnosis.

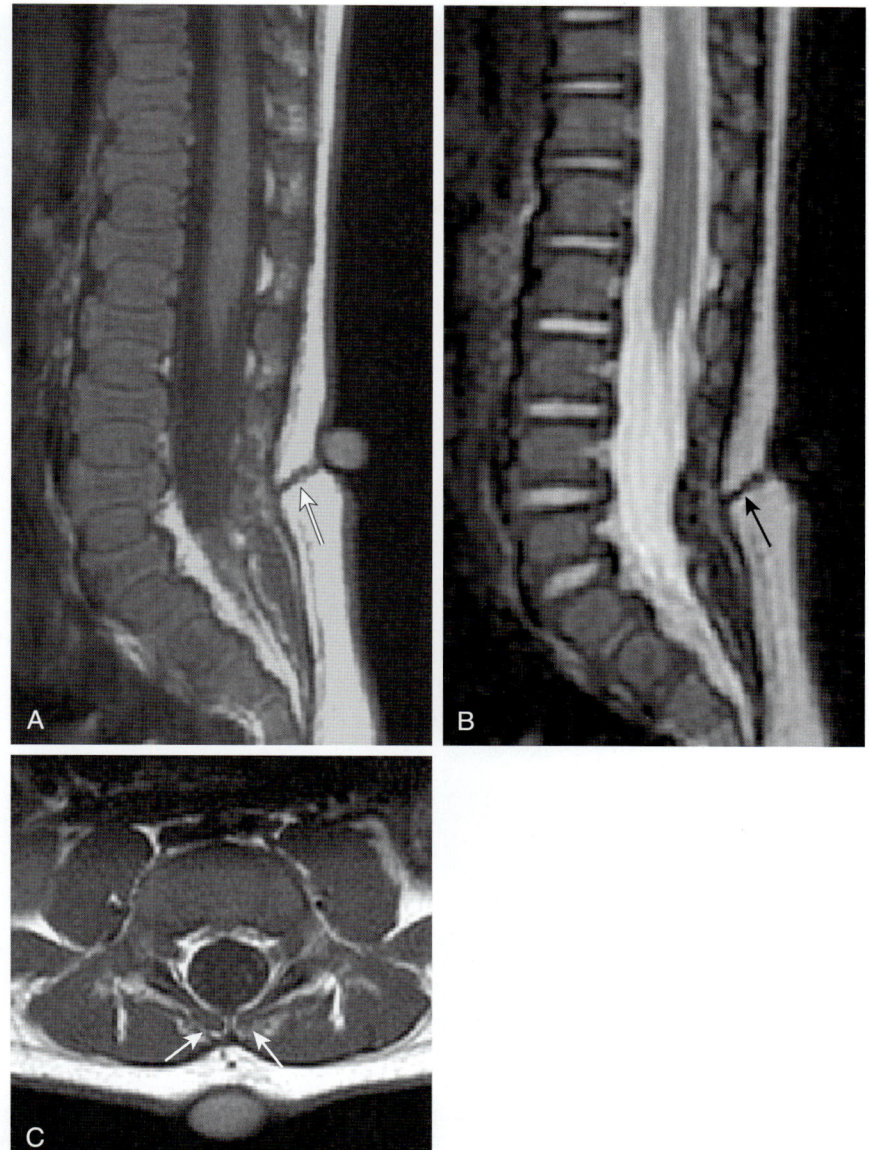

Figure 43-4 **Dorsal dermal sinus.** Sagittal T1- (**A**) and T2-weighted magnetic resonance (MR) images (**B**) demonstrate a low-lying spinal cord tethered by a dorsal dermal sinus tract (*arrows*). The skin opening is marked by a vitamin E capsule. Axial T1-weighted MR image (**C**) confirms the tract accessing the dural sac through a bifid spinous process (*arrows*).

a stable neurologic deficit following MMC closure, and a progressive or new neural deficit should prompt an imaging search for other occult spinal abnormalities, such as DSM, or complications of MMC repair, such as cord tethering, dural ring constriction, spinal cord ischemia, or syrinx. MRI is the best modality for postoperative imaging in the clinical context of progressive deficits. Rarely is imaging before MMC closure indicated.

Anomalies of the Caudal Cell Mass

Caudal cell mass anomalies are a diverse group of anomalies that result from aberrant secondary neurulation, postulated to be an insult to the caudal cell mass before the fourth gestational week. Most cases are sporadic, although a dominantly inherited defect in the *HLXB9* gene has been described. The mothers of 15% to 20% of these infants are diabetic, the offspring of 1% of diabetic mothers are afflicted, and an association has been found with VACTERL syndrome (*v*ertebral, *a*nal atresia, *c*ardiac, *t*racheal, *e*sophageal, *r*enal, *l*imb), omphalocele, bladder extrophy, imperforate anus, and the Currarino triad. The range of severity is substantial, from clinically unapparent mild dysgenesis to absence of the lower body.

Hypogenesis or agenesis of the caudal cell mass produces caudal regression syndrome (CRS; Fig. 43-6). Two types are described. The more severe CRS, type 1, features a foreshortened terminal vertebral column, high-lying wedge-shaped conus termination, and more severe associated visceral and orthopedic anomalies. The less severe CRS, type 2, has a low-lying tethered spinal cord with milder associated

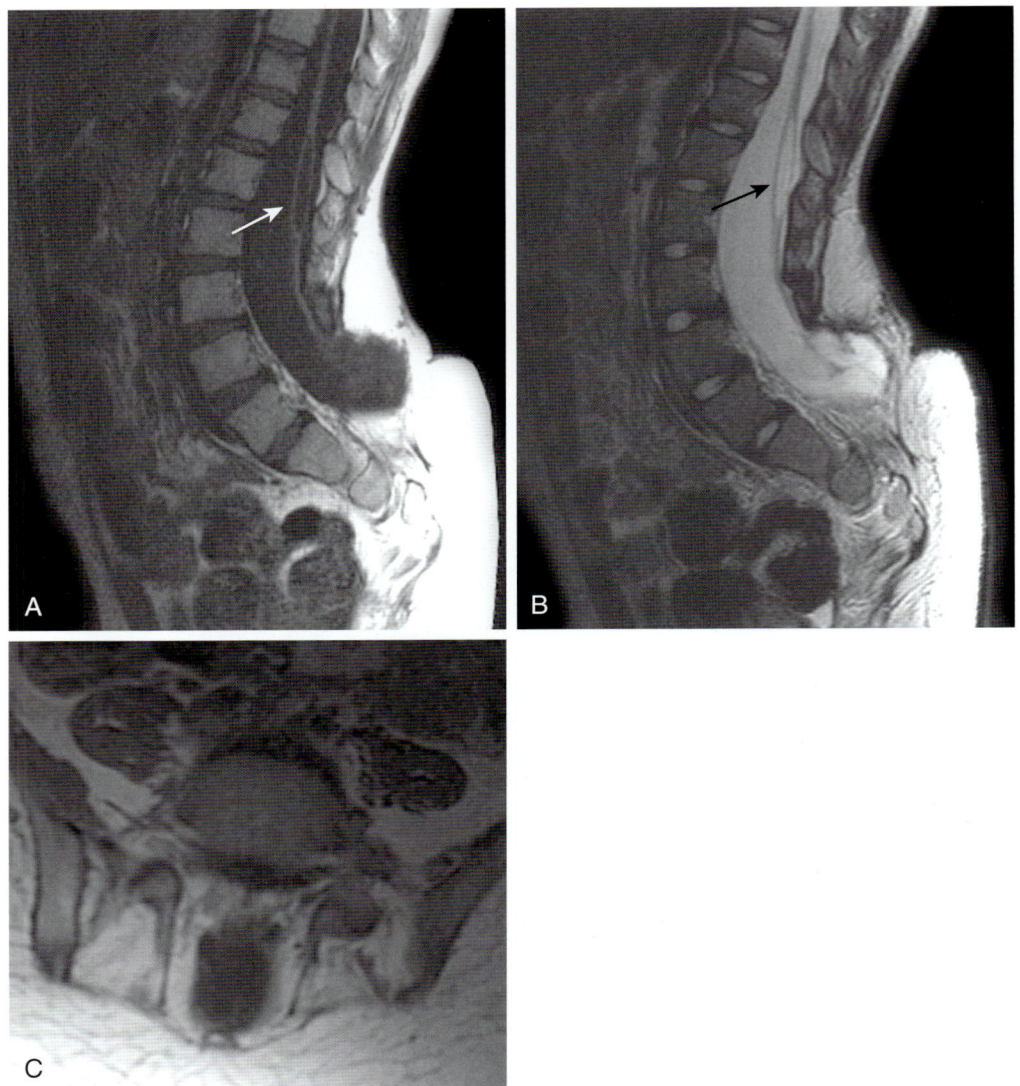

Figure 43-5 **Myelomeningocele.** Sagittal T1- (**A**) and T2-weighted (**B**) magnetic resonance (MR) images show the postoperative appearance of the spine after myelomeningocele closure. The large dysraphic defect is now covered with skin, and the attenuated distal spinal cord is scarred into the closure. A small syrinx is present (*arrow*). Axial T1-weighted MR image (**C**) reveals the protrusion of the distal sac through parallel dysraphic posterior elements.

malformations. In general, the higher the cord termination, the more severe the sacral anomalies. The most severe CRS presentations are lumbosacral agenesis, in which the spine terminates at the lower thoracic level, and severe sacral dysgenesis, with fused lower extremities in a "mermaid" configuration (sirenomyelia). In contrast, the mildest CRS cases may manifest merely as a missing terminal sacral segment identified on imaging that is clinically asymptomatic. CRS is associated with myriad other visceral abnormalities, including renal or pulmonary hypoplasia and anorectal malformations. Other commonly associated spinal malformations include open dysraphism, vertebral SFAs, and split-cord malformations.

Segmental spinal dysgenesis (SSD) is a very rare dysraphic anomaly characterized by segmental thoracolumbar or lumbar vertebral and spinal cord dysgenesis or agenesis. Congenital thoracic or lumbar kyphosis is characteristic, with a palpable dorsal bone spur located at the gibbous apex. The upper spinal cord is normal, but the cord segment below the dysgenetic segment is bulky, thickened, and low-lying. The spinal canal proximal and distal to the dysgenetic level is of normal caliber. Some authors believe that SSD and CRS represent different phenotypes along a single malformation spectrum, and that spinal morphology depends on the level of developmental disruption. If development is affected distally, CRS results, but if the lesion occurs more proximally, SSD is observed.

Perhaps the most common entity within the caudal cell mass dysplasia spectrum is tethered cord syndrome (TCS), which manifests clinically as gait spasticity, low back and leg pain that is worse in the morning, lower extremity sensory abnormalities, and/or bladder difficulties. TCS patients are most likely to come in during periods of rapid somatic growth. TCS refers strictly to patients with a low-lying cord and thickened filum, not those with other spine and cord abnormalities, although in fact those patients may be similar

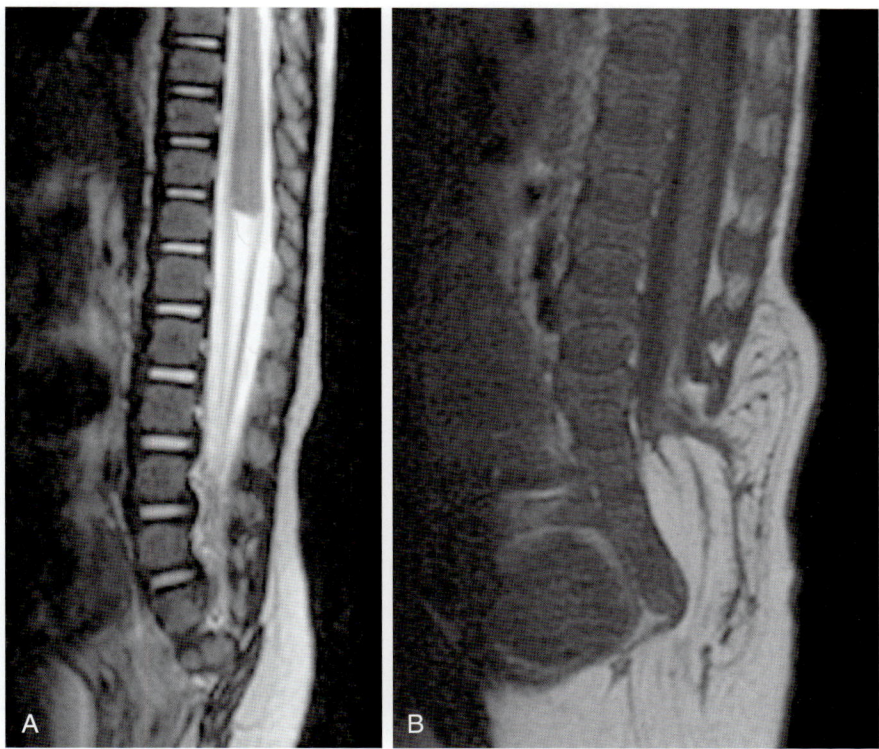

Figure 43-6 Caudal regression syndrome (CRS). Sagittal T2-weighted image (**A**) shows the typical appearance of type 1 CRS, with severe sacral dysplasia and the characteristic wedge-shaped high conus termination. Sagittal T1-weighted magnetic resonance image (**B**) contrasts the appearance of type 2 CRS (with a less severe sacral dysgenesis) with an elongated spinal cord that inserts distally into a terminal lipoma.

in clinical presentation and may be considered "tethered." It is important to consider TCS a distinct clinical diagnosis, with imaging relegated to the role of preoperative planning rather than establishing the primary diagnosis. On imaging, TCS manifests either as a taut spinal cord without definitive conus or a low-lying conus (Fig. 43-7). The filum is frequently thickened and shortened, and an associated terminal lipoma may be present. Symptomatic patients may benefit from surgery, but it is crucial to exclude other associated anomalies before surgery.

Two other important rare presentations of caudal cell mass dysplasia are the ASM and the terminal myelocystocele. ASM features a large anterior meningocele outpouching that traverses an enlarged sacral foramen and produces a presacral cystic mass. This may be clinically mistaken for a SCT and may prompt neuroimaging. Most ASMs are sporadic, but a minority show an inherited predisposition within the Currarino triad or in syndromes that feature dural dysplasia, such as neurofibromatosis type 1 (NF1) and Marfan syndrome. As with other caudal cell mass dysplasias, additional congenital abnormalities may be found, such as anorectal malformations, caudal dysgenesis, and dermoid or epidermoid cysts. Fortunately, imaging is highly characteristic in the more common simple form, with a presacral cystic mass that connects to the thecal sac through an enlarged sacral neural foramen (Fig. 43-8). Complex ASMs with fat or neural elements are also recognized by their extension through the neural foramen. Terminal myelocystocele is a very rare malformation that manifests as a hydromyelic spinal cord that traverses a meningocele to terminate in a skin-covered myelocystocele

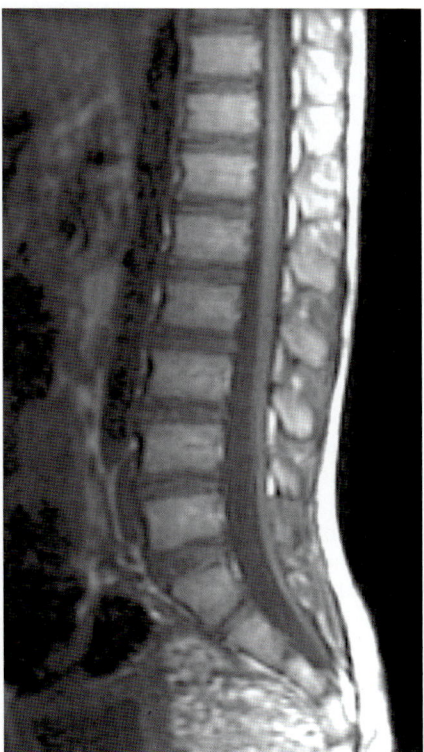

Figure 43-7 Tethered cord syndrome. Sagittal T1-weighted magnetic resonance image reveals an elongated spinal cord, indistinguishable from the filum, inserting into the terminal thecal sac.

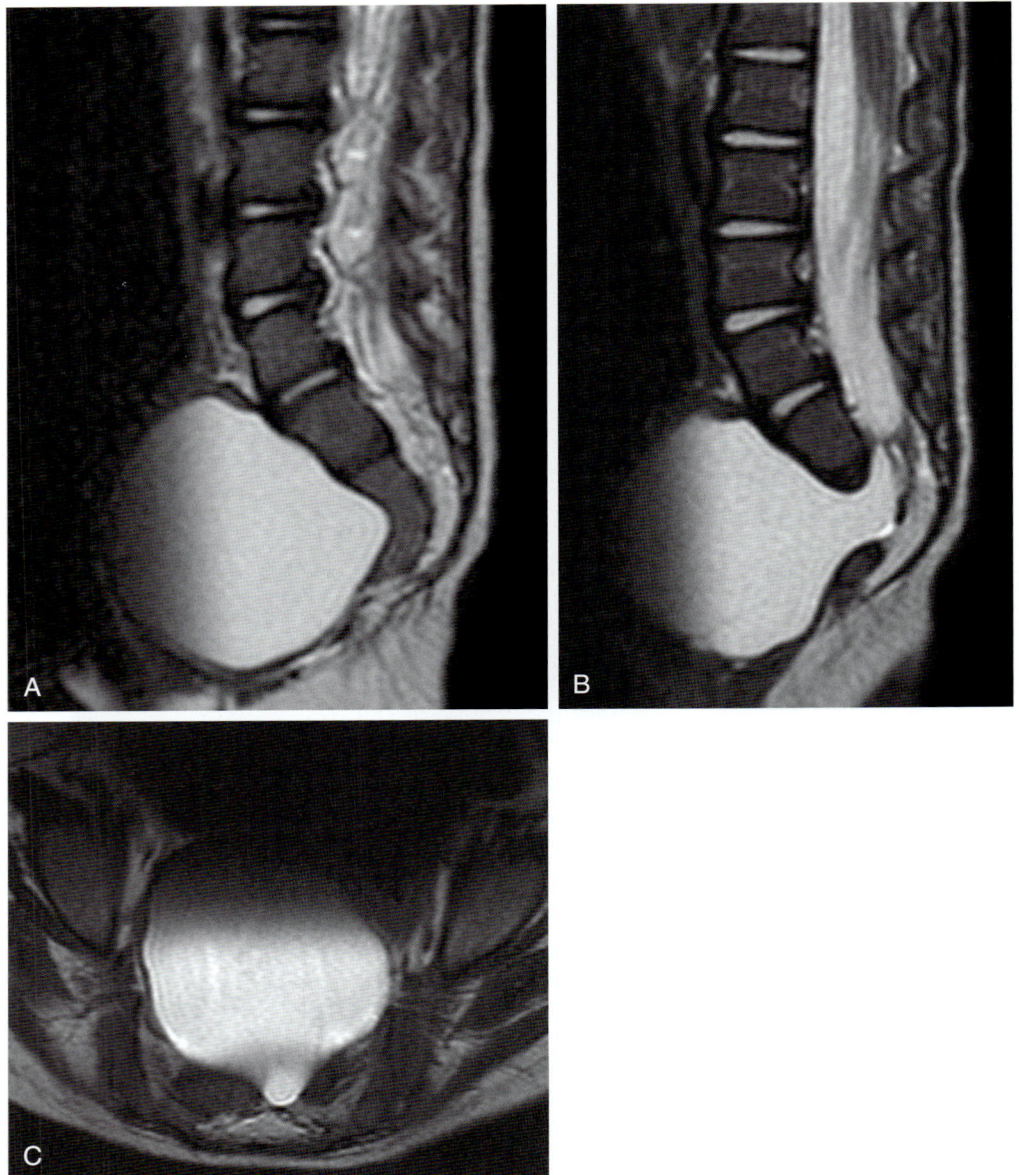

Figure 43-8 **Anterior sacral meningocele.** Sagittal T2-weighted magnetic resonance (MR) image (**A**) in the midline shows the characteristic scimitar shape of the sacrum. Parasagittal (**B**) and axial (**C**) T2-weighted MR images confirm a typical, simple, anterior sacral meningocele that appears as a presacral cyst contiguous with the thecal sac through an enlarged left sacral neural foramen.

(e-Fig. 43-9). These abnormalities are rarely imaged, until the infant survives the commonly associated anorectal and visceral anomalies that drive early management and produce most of the morbidity and mortality. Infants with terminal myelocystocele may be neurologically intact at birth but subsequently lose neurologic function.

Finally, if the primitive streak incompletely regresses and leaves a caudal totipotential cell rest remnant, an SCT (Fig. 43-10) may result. SCTs demonstrate tissue from all three cell layers and contain varying proportions of mature and immature elements. These are surgically graded, according to the American Academy of Pediatrics (AAP) classification, based on proportion of internal (pelvic) and external components; prognosis is determined by the AAP grade and by the presence or absence of mature or malignant components.

External tumors, mature elements, and younger patient age predict a better outcome. The surgeon must resect the coccyx to prevent recurrence. Fetal and early infancy morbidity and mortality are related mostly to cardiac failure from intratumoral shunting and associated visceral anomalies, whereas later mortality is related to lesion malignancy.

MRI is the best modality for preoperative planning and staging for all caudal cell mass anomalies. Computed tomography (CT) has a more limited role, such as in screening for visceral organ anomalies or evaluating bones. Ultrasonography may be helpful for initial newborn screening, because it can be performed portably in the newborn nursery or intensive care nursery, thereby eliminating transport issues in unstable infants, but it usually does not provide all the necessary information for surgical planning.

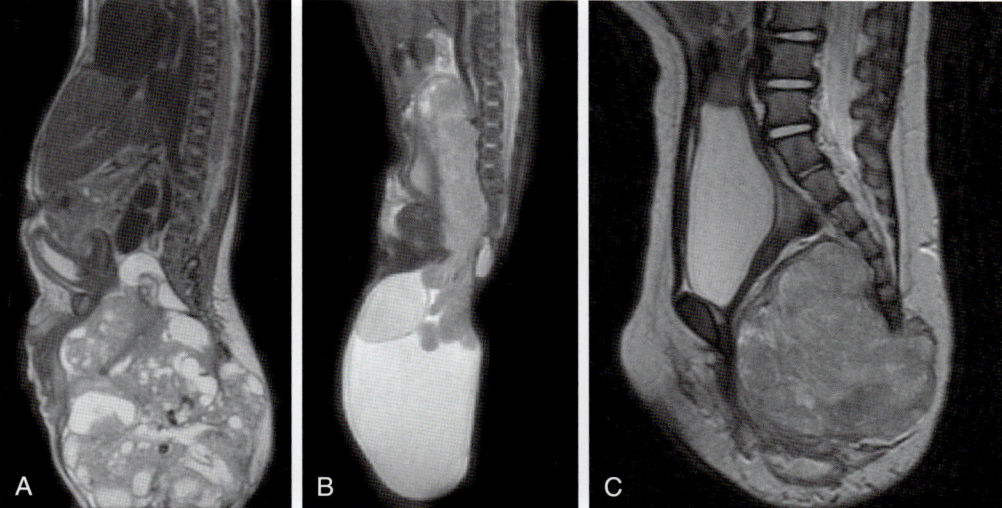

Figure 43-10 Sacrococcygeal teratoma. Sagittal T2-weighted magnetic resonance images in three different infants show large, mixed cystic and solid pelvic masses confirmed pathologically as sacrococcygeal teratomas. The proportions of internal and external tumor produce diagnoses of grade 1 (**A**), grade 2 (**B**), and grade 3 (**C**) using the American Academy of Pediatrics classification.

Anomalies of Notochord Development

Neurenteric cyst (e-Fig. 43-11) consists of an intraspinal cyst lined by enteric mucosa, and it is most common in the thoracic spine, followed by the cervical spine. Such cysts putatively arise from an abnormal connection between primitive endoderm and ectoderm that persists beyond the third embryonic week. Whereas normally the notochord separates ventral endoderm (foregut) and dorsal ectoderm (skin, spinal cord) during embryogenesis, in a neurenteric cyst, a separation failure "splits" the notochord and hinders the development of mesoderm, which traps a small piece of primitive gut within the developing spinal canal. This gut remnant may become isolated, forming a cyst, or it may maintain connections with gut or skin (or both); this produces the spectrum of fistulas and sinuses that constitute the spectrum of dorsal-enteric spinal anomalies. The most severe malformations remain in communication through the primitive vertebral osseous canal of Kovalevsky, but even mild cases usually show some vertebral segmentation anomalies on close inspection. Multiplanar MRI best demonstrates the cyst and its relationship to the spinal cord, as well as connections to the mediastinal or abdominal viscera. CT, particularly with multiplanar and three-dimensional reformats, optimally demonstrates osseous vertebral anomalies for preoperative planning.

DSM arises from an aberrant process similar to that of the neurenteric cyst and results in a splitting of the spinal cord into two hemicords, each with one ventral and one dorsal root. The hemicords may be symmetric, or they may be asymmetric, known as partial DSM; one or both may feature hydromyelia or be tethered. The much rarer (perhaps mythical) *diplomyelia,* or duplicated spinal cord, is the only other differential entity to consider; it occurs probably in the context of a duplicated spinal axis, and many authorities think it most likely represents a very severe DSM rather than true spinal cord duplication.

Because the notochord influences vertebral development, vertebral segmentation anomalies are very commonly associated with DSM. Therefore important factors for preoperative planning include the presence (type 1 DSM; Fig. 43-12) or absence (type 2 DSM; Fig 43-13) of an osseous or fibrous spur and whether the cords reside in separate or single dural tubes (see also Chapter 42). Occasionally in type 2 DSM, a nerve root or roots may become adherent to the dura and may tether the spinal cord, producing the meningocele manqué. DSM may be isolated or found in conjunction with other spinal anomalies, particularly MMC, thus it is critical to search for DSM before any spinal anomaly repair or scoliosis correction. A patient with MMC whose symptoms progress after surgical closure is a relatively common presentation of undiagnosed DSM. Cutaneous abnormalities such as skin dimples or discoloration, vascular lesions, or hair patches are sometimes present and can guide attention to the most likely level of DSM.

Other Congenital and Developmental Anomalies

Other uncommon but important congenital spinal anomalies whose etiology is not definitively known include the simple dorsal meningocele and the lateral meningocele.

Dorsal meningoceles (e-Fig. 43-14) by definition occur dorsally, most often over the lumbosacral spine, and feature a skin-covered meningocele devoid of neural elements that protrudes through a posterior dysraphic defect. In practice, however, it is not uncommon to find a dysplastic nerve root or other neural tissue within a meningocele.

Lateral meningoceles (e-Fig. 43-15) manifest as paraspinal masses filled with cerebrospinal fluid that are contiguous with the thecal sac and extend through the neural foramen, with adjacent pedicular and foraminal osseous remodeling. They are generally "simple," but some may contain fat or neural

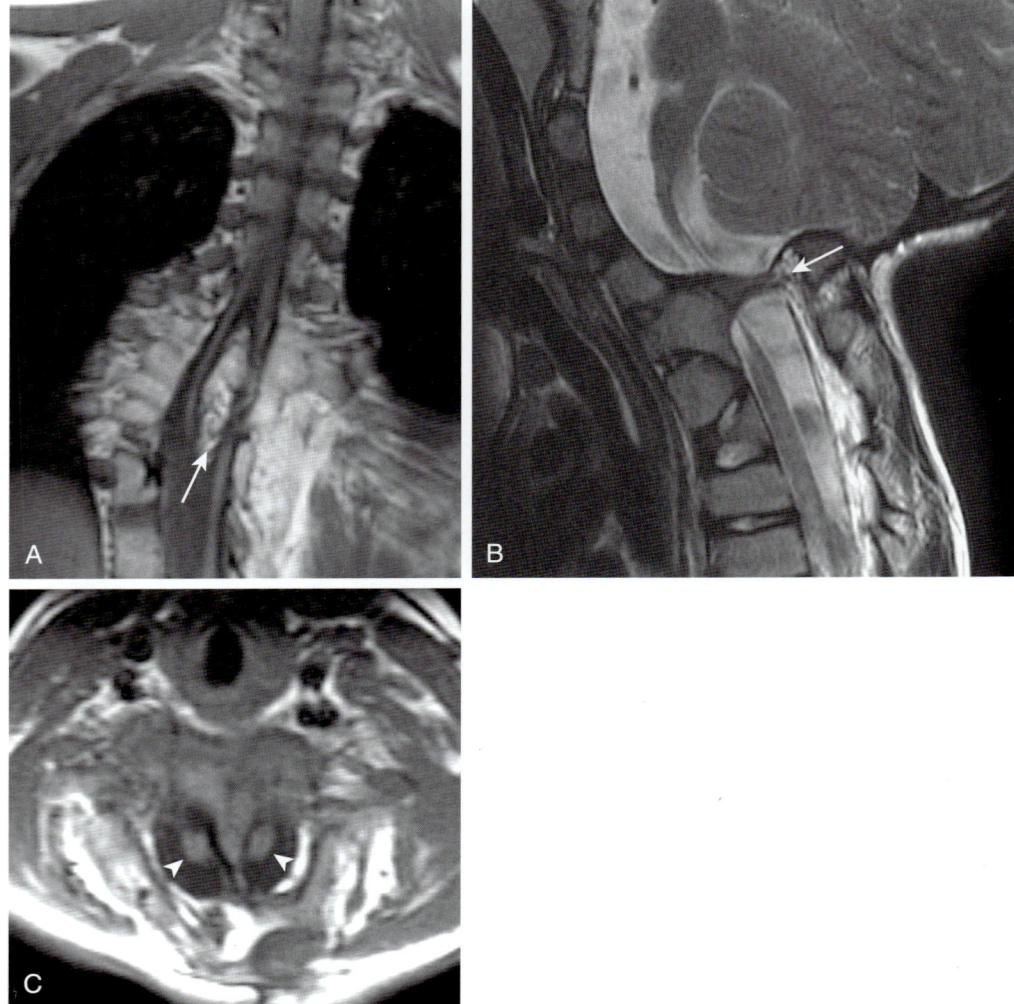

Figure 43-12 Diastematomyelia (DSM) type 1. Coronal (**A**) T1-weighted magnetic resonance (MR) images in a patient with type 1 DSM show a large ossified spur (*arrow*) that splits the thoracic spinal cord. Numerous vertebral segmentation anomalies with posterior rib fusions are present. Sagittal T2- (**B**) and axial T1-weighted (**C**) MR images of a different patient show a type 1 cervical DSM with ossified spur (*arrow* in *B*) and two hemicords (*arrowheads* in *C*).

tissue and are then better termed "complex." Important associations include Marfan syndrome and NF1.

In both anomalies, multiplanar MRI is the best modality to demonstrate the soft tissue components. CT is helpful for clarifying the osseous anatomy, and usually this is done before surgery. If MRI is contraindicated or inconclusive, CT myelography can demonstrate the meningocele and confirm its continuity with the dural sac.

Vertebral Formation and Segmentation Anomalies

Anomalies of vertebral formation and segmentation arise from aberrancies in vertebral column formation. These are generally divided into anomalies that result from either partial or total failure of vertebral formation (Fig. 43-16) and failure to correctly segment after vertebral formation (vertebral

segmentation failure; e-Fig. 43-17). The abnormal vertebra may be supernumerary, or it may replace a normal vertebral body. Abnormal *PAX1* expression is a postulated etiology in the development of segmentation anomalies, and other visceral and neuraxis anomalies are also commonly identified. More severe SFAs tend to have a higher incidence of concurrent visceral organ or other neuraxis anomalies. The degree and location of vertebral formation failure predicts morphology; unilateral chondral center deficiency and failure of ossification produces a hemivertebra, whereas central failure of ossification centers to unite produces a butterfly vertebra. Conversely, vertebral segmentation failure presents with composite or "block" vertebra and posterior element fusions (Fig. 43-18). Not surprisingly, block vertebrae frequently coexist with hemivertebrae and butterfly vertebrae (Fig. 43-19), leading many to lump these various vertebral anomalies together into the working term SFAs. Many clinical syndromes prominently feature SFAs, including Klippel-Feil and Jarcho-Levin (spondylothoracic dysplasia) syndromes.

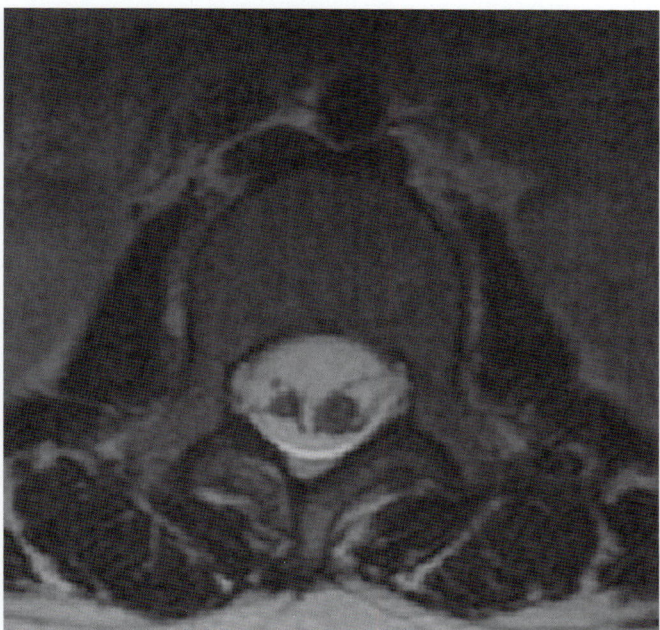

Figure 43-13 **Diastematomyelia type 2.** Axial T2-weighted magnetic resonance image in a patient with type 2 Diastematomyelia shows the spinal cord split into two hemicords within a single dural tube. No fibrous or osseous septum was identified.

Therefore SFAs are not findings that confirm a specific disorder, but rather they are imaging markers that prompt further consideration of a possible syndromic process.

Conclusions

Pediatric congenital spinal anomalies demonstrate myriad variations and are potentially confusing. However, with

understanding of simplified spinal embryology and anatomy, it is usually possible to identify a few characteristic features that permit a more specific diagnosis and alert for other possible associated anomalies.

Key Points

The conus is normally at adult level (L2 or above) soon after birth.
LMC and LMMC account for 20% to 56% of occult spinal dysraphism and 20% of skin-covered lumbosacral masses.
The simple coccygeal sinus that originates from a low sacral dimple found within the intergluteal cleft never communicates with the spinal canal.
The offspring of 1% of diabetic mothers have a caudal cell mass anomaly.
TCS is a specific clinical entity that usually presents during periods of rapid somatic growth.
MRI is the best modality for preoperative planning and staging of caudal cell anomalies.
Anomalies that reflect failure of vertebral formation and vertebral segmentation failure frequently coexist.

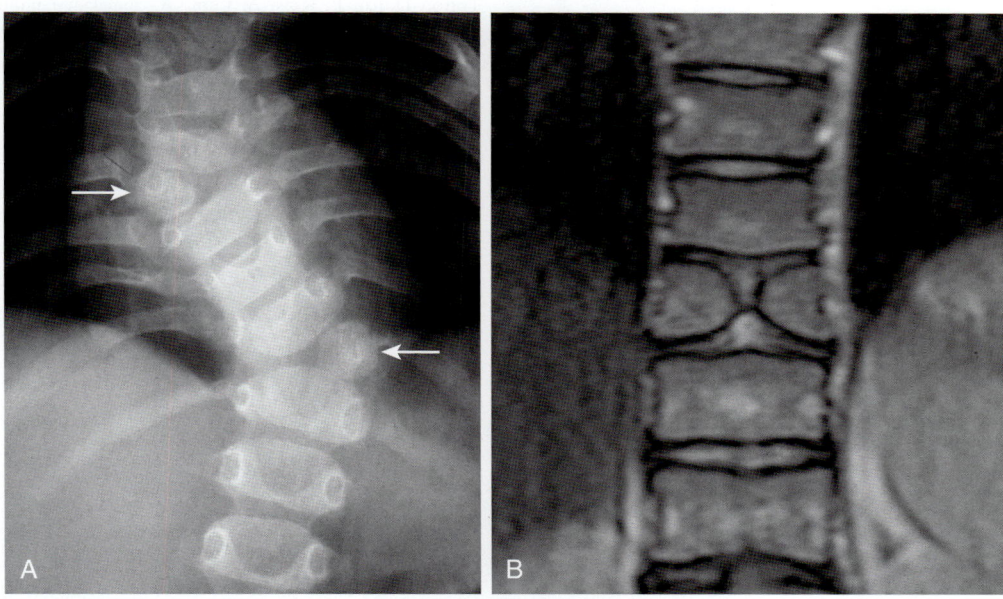

Figure 43-16 **Failure of vertebral formation. A,** Frontal radiography demonstrates balanced thoracic hemivertebrae (*arrows*) detected during evaluation of congenital scoliosis. **B,** Coronal T2-weighted magnetic resonance image shows a classic butterfly vertebra. Both of these may coexist with each other and with malformations of vertebral segmentation failure.

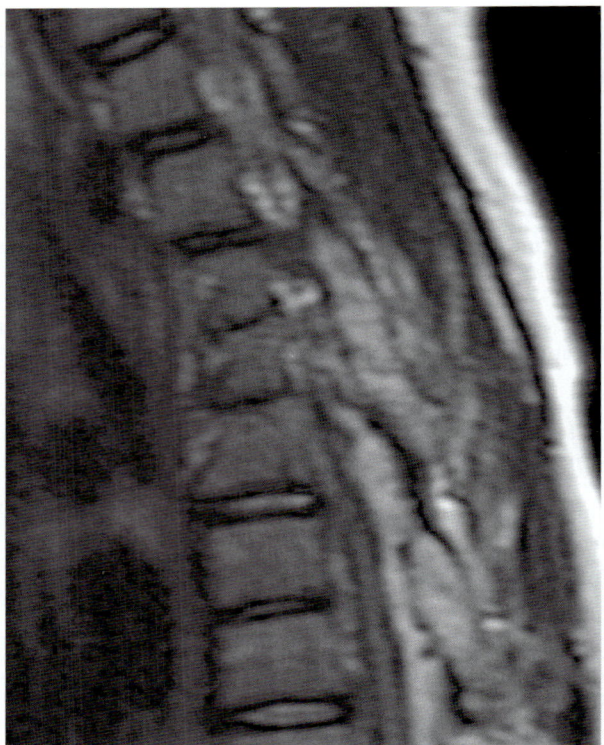

Figure 43-18 Posterior element segmentation failure with fusion. Sagittal T2-weighted image shows a multilevel pedicular and facet bar associated with vertebral segmentation failure at the same levels.

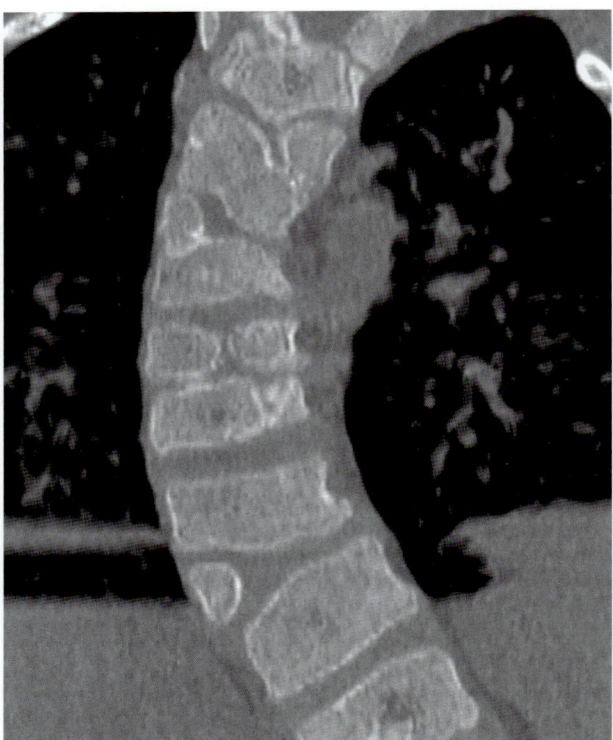

Figure 43-19 Coexistent vertebral segmentation and vertebral formation failure anomalies. Coronal computed tomography image in a patient with VACTERL syndrome (**v**ertebral, **a**nal atresia, **c**ardiac, **t**racheal, **e**sophageal, **r**enal, **l**imb), shows multiple combinations of both segmentation and formation failure with resultant congenital dextroscoliosis.

Suggested Readings

Giampietro PF, Dunwoodie SL, Kusumi K, et al. Progress in the understanding of the genetic etiology of vertebral segmentation disorders in humans. *Ann NY Acad Sci.* 2009;1151:38-67.

Pang D, Dias MS, Ahab-Barmada M. Split cord malformation: part I. A unified theory of embryogenesis for double spinal cord malformations. *Neurosurgery.* 1992;31:451-480.

Pang D. Sacral agenesis and caudal spinal cord malformations. *Neurosurgery.* 1993;32:755-778; discussion 778-779.

Rufener SL, Ibrahim M, Raybaud CA, et al. Congenital spine and spinal cord malformations—pictorial review. *AJR Am J Roentgenol.* 2010;194(suppl 3):S26-S37.

Tortori-Donati P, Rossi A, Biancheri R, et al. Magnetic resonance imaging of spinal dysraphism. *Top Magn Reson Imaging.* 2001;12:375-409.

Tortori-Donati P, Rossi A, Cama A. Spinal dysraphism: a review of neuroradiological features with embryological correlations and proposal for a new classification. *Neuroradiology.* 2000;42:471-491.

Chapter 44

Infections of the Spine and Spinal Cord

AVRUM N. POLLOCK and STEPHEN M. HENESCH

Spinal infections in children are uncommon. Etiologies include direct and indirect (hematogenous) inoculation by bacterial, viral, parasitic, and fungal agents. Direct bacterial infectious inoculation may occur as a result of trauma, instrumentation, or via a preexisting congenital sinus tract or area of spinal dysraphism (i.e., a meningocele). In recent years, Lyme disease (Fig. 44-1) caused by a *Borrelia burgdorferi* infected tick bite has emerged as a cause of spinal cord infection, especially in the Northeastern United States. Mosquito-borne West Nile virus (Fig. 44-2), with cases initially appearing along the east coast of the United States, has since been discovered nationwide and also has emerged as a more recent spinal cord infectious agent. Tuberculosis (TB) of the spinal cord usually occurs in the thoracic region in children (Fig. 44-3) and manifests as an intramedullary tuberculoma, most often seen in patients with acquired immunodeficiency syndrome or other types of immunocompromise. TB is most prevalent in India, but it is also widespread in Africa and in Southeast Asia. Cysticercosis (Fig. 44-4) is the most common parasitic infection encountered within the spinal cord. It occurs after ingestion of uncooked pork infected with *Taenia solium* and is most prevalent in South America and Southeast Asia. Gnathostomiasis (Fig. 44-5) is caused by the nematode *Gnathostoma spinigerum,* which is acquired by ingesting contaminated fish or meat and presents clinically with myeloradiculitis. It is endemic in Southeast Asia and virtually unknown in North America, other than in persons with infections that are acquired abroad.

Inflammation related to infection and resultant neurologic deficit are frequently how spinal cord infections manifest, prompting imaging for diagnostic answers. Magnetic resonance imaging (MRI) is the gold standard examination for the evaluation of spinal cord infection. In general, abnormalities present with hyperintensity on fluid-sensitive (T2-weighted) sequences and with variable enhancement on postgadolinium T1-weighted sequences. Like infections elsewhere, increase in cord caliber often occurs as a result of an increase in water content and edema. Rare related hemorrhages can at times be better elucidated with use of gradient echo sequences.

Discitis and Osteomyelitis

Disc space infection often coexists with vertebral osteomyelitis in children as a result of hematogenous spread through capillary tufts in vertebral body endplates and vascular channels of immature intervertebral disc spaces. Contrast-enhanced MRI is the study of choice and should be performed without delay in suspected cases (Fig. 44-6). Although infection can occur at any level, the midlumbar spine is most often affected. *Staphylococcus aureus* represents the most common etiologic organism. Worldwide, organisms such as TB are not uncommon etiologies. The first radiographic sign of infection is irregularity of the vertebral body endplates. The affected disc space is usually narrowed and demonstrates low signal intensity on T2-weighted MR sequences. Edema and postcontrast enhancement in adjacent vertebral body endplates indicate the presence of associated osteomyelitis and possible disc space abscess. Complicated cases demonstrate epidural and paravertebral abscess or phlegmon, which are well elucidated by MRI. Signs of late infection include vertebral body collapse and spinal deformity (Fig. 44-7). After treatment, vertebral body and disc space findings may persist for up to 24 and 34 months, respectively. Chronic recurrent multifocal osteomyelitis is the most severe form of chronic nonbacterial osteomyelitis and is of uncertain etiology. Although chronic recurrent multifocal osteomyelitis most commonly affects the metaphyses of long bones and the medial clavicles, vertebral column and pelvic involvement can occur.

Guillain-Barré Syndrome

Since the eradication of poliomyelitis, Guillain-Barré syndrome (GBS) (Fig. 44-8), or acute inflammatory demyelinating polyradiculoneuropathy, has become the most common cause of acute motor paralysis in children. It is believed to arise from an abnormal T-cell response precipitated by a preceding infection. Infectious etiologies include Epstein-Barr virus, cytomegalovirus, hepatitis, varicella, *Mycoplasma pneumonia*, and *Campylobacter jejuni.* MRI often shows thickening of the cauda equina and intrathecal nerve roots, as well as anterior predominant nerve root gadolinium enhancement, even beyond the period of the initial presentation. Imaging findings have been described to be 83% sensitive for acute GBS and are present in 95% of typical cases. Chronic inflammatory demyelinating polyneuropathy (Fig. 44-9) is thought to be a chronic form of GBS that shares in these imaging characteristics, but it often shows marked nerve root thickening.

Text continued on page 468.

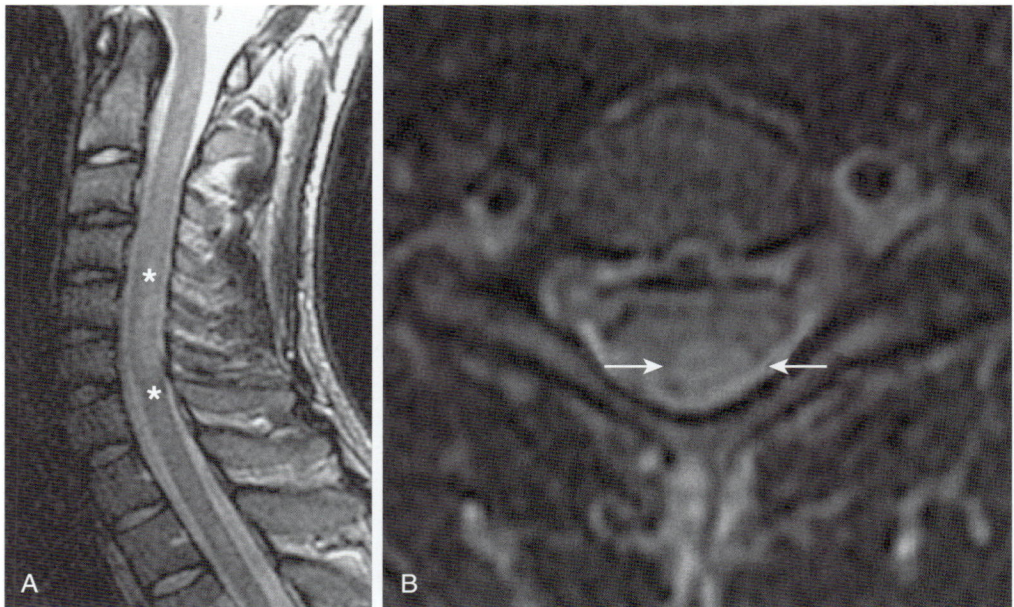

Figure 44-1 An adult who was bitten by a tick and infected with Lyme disease. Sagittal (**A**) and axial (**B**) T2-weighted images of the cervical spine demonstrate T2 prolongation (*asterisks* in **A** and *arrows* in **B**) within the dorsal spinal cord at the level of C5/C6 as a result of demyelination. (Case courtesy Gul Moonis, MD, Beth Israel Deaconess Medical Center, Division of Neuroradiology.)

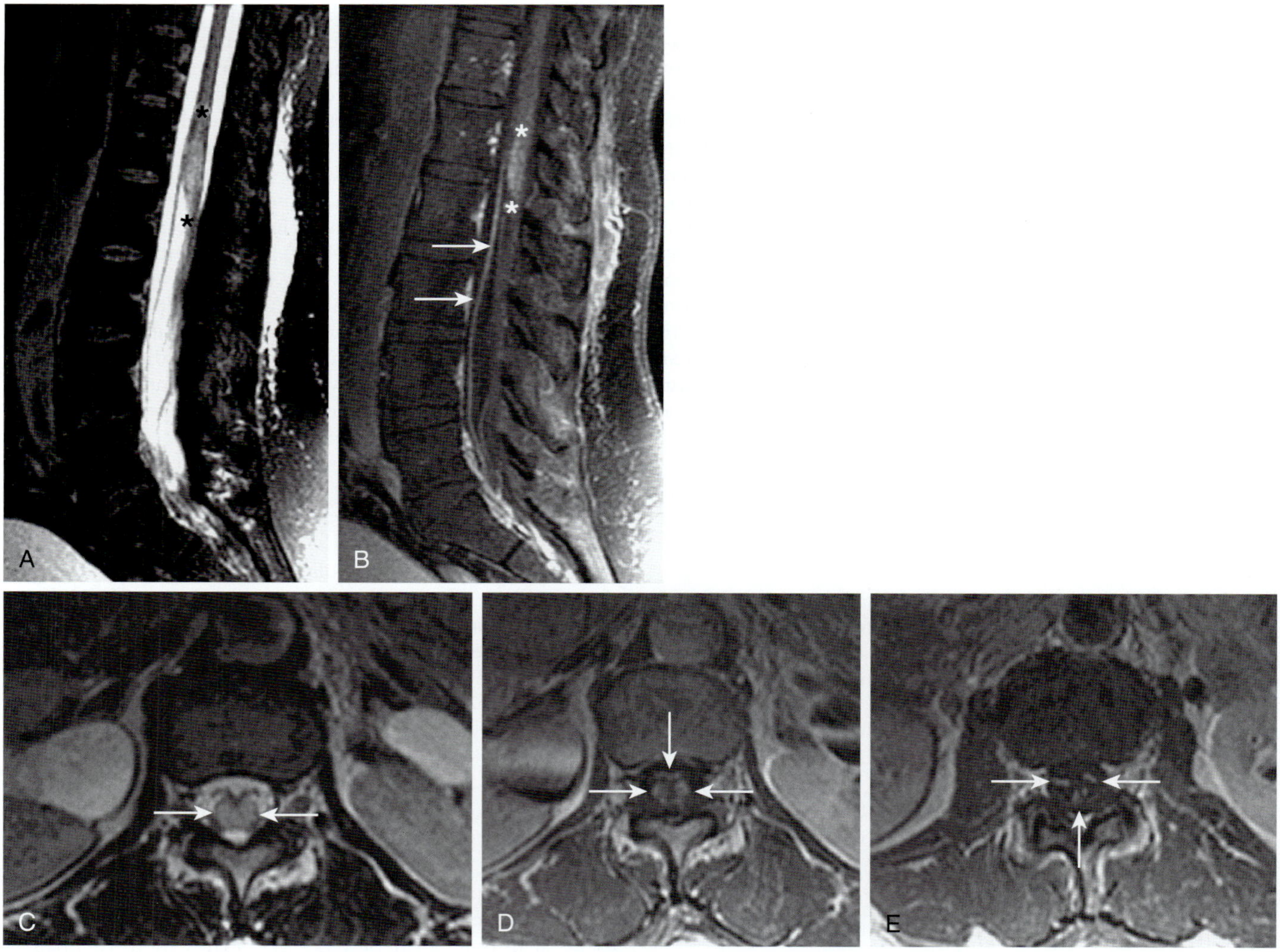

Figure 44-2 An adult patient who was bitten by a mosquito and infected with West Nile virus. Sagittal and axial T2-weighted images (**A** and **C**, respectively), and sagittal (**B**) and axial (**D** and **E**) postgadolinium T1-weighted images of the lumbar spine demonstrate T2 prolongation (**A**, *asterisks*, and **C**, *arrows*) within the distal spinal cord/conus medullaris, as well as contrast enhancement of the distal cord (**B**, *asterisks*)/conus medullaris (**D**, *arrows*) and within the cauda equina (**E**, *arrows*) as a result of viral myeloradiculitis. (Case courtesy Gul Moonis, MD, Beth Israel Deaconess Medical Center, Division of Neuroradiology.)

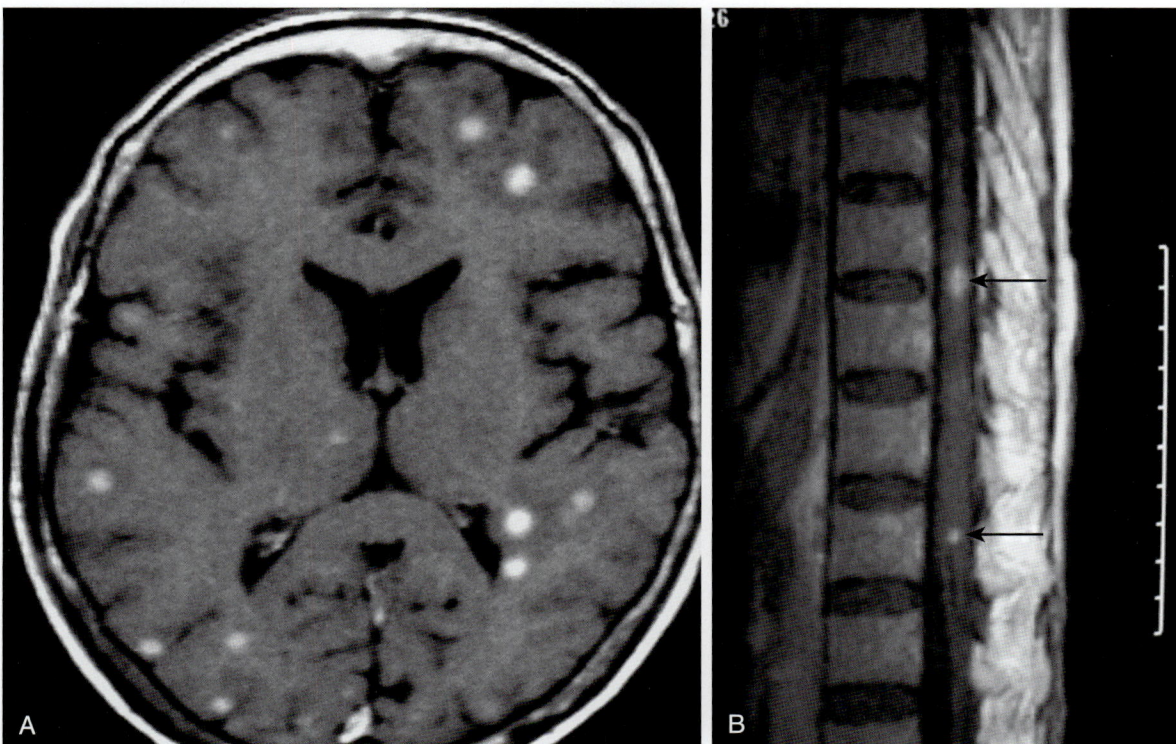

Figure 44-3 An adult patient with tuberculosis exposure. Axial postcontrast T1-weighted magnetic resonance imaging of the brain (**A**) and thoracic spine (**B**) demonstrate multiple enhancing intraaxial nodules corresponding to tuberculomas (*arrows* in **B**). (Case courtesy Drs. Pranjal Goswami, Nirod Medhi, and Pratul Kr. Sarma of Primus Institute in Guwahati, India.)

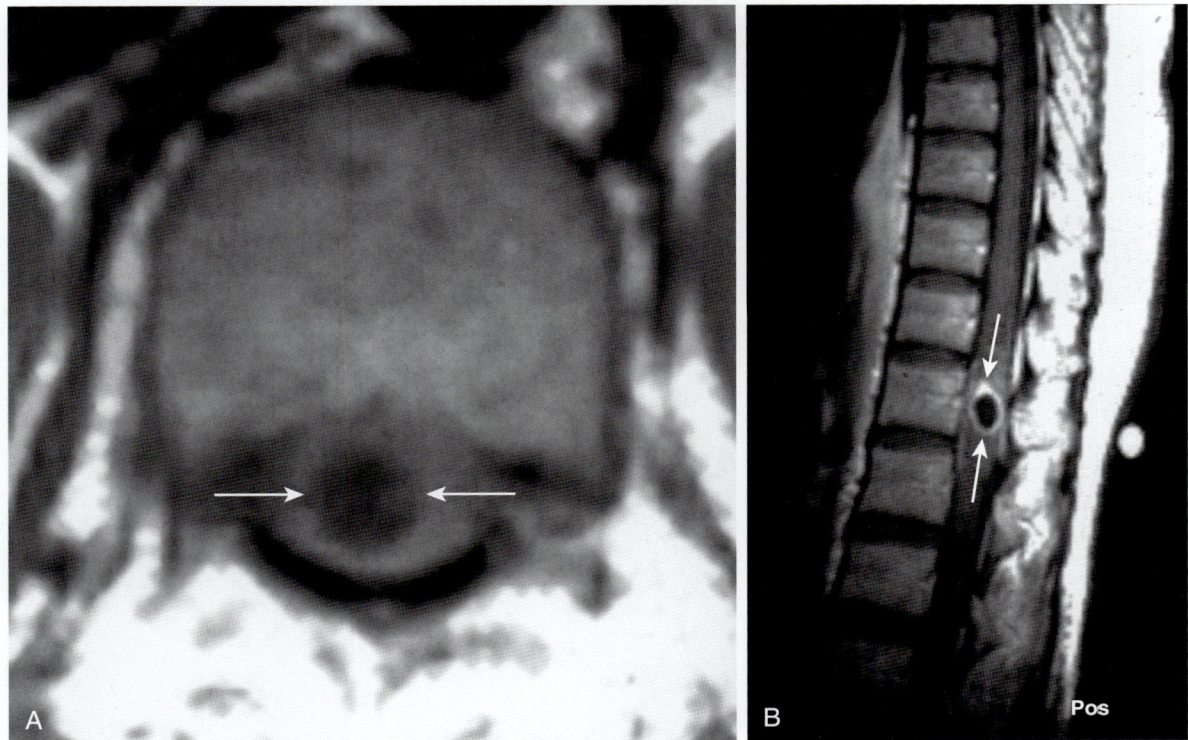

Figure 44-4 A 20-year-old man who presented with paraparesis that developed over a few weeks was found to have cysticercosis. An axial T1-weighted image (**A**) and a sagittal postcontrast T1-weighted image (**B**) of the thoracic spine demonstrate central T1 prolongation within the spinal cord proper (*arrows* in **A**), with corresponding rim enhancement on the postcontrast image (*arrows* in **B**). (Case courtesy Dr. Manu Shroff of the Hospital for Sick Children in Toronto, Canada.)

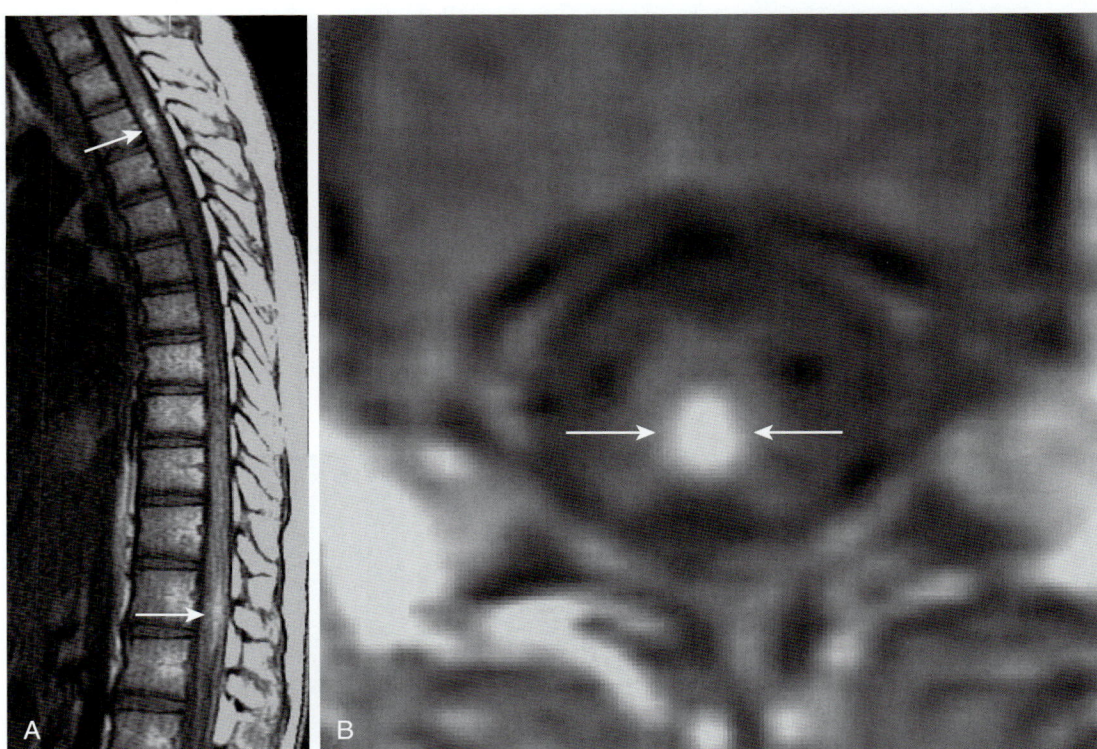

Figure 44-5 A 17-year-old boy from Thailand with gnathostomiasis. Sagittal (**A**) and axial (**B**) postcontrast T1-weighted images of the thoracic spine demonstrate enhancing nodules (*arrows* in **A** and **B**) within the spinal cord proper as a result of a parasitic infection. (Case courtesy Dr. Jiraporn Laothamatas of Mahidol University, Bangkok, Thailand.)

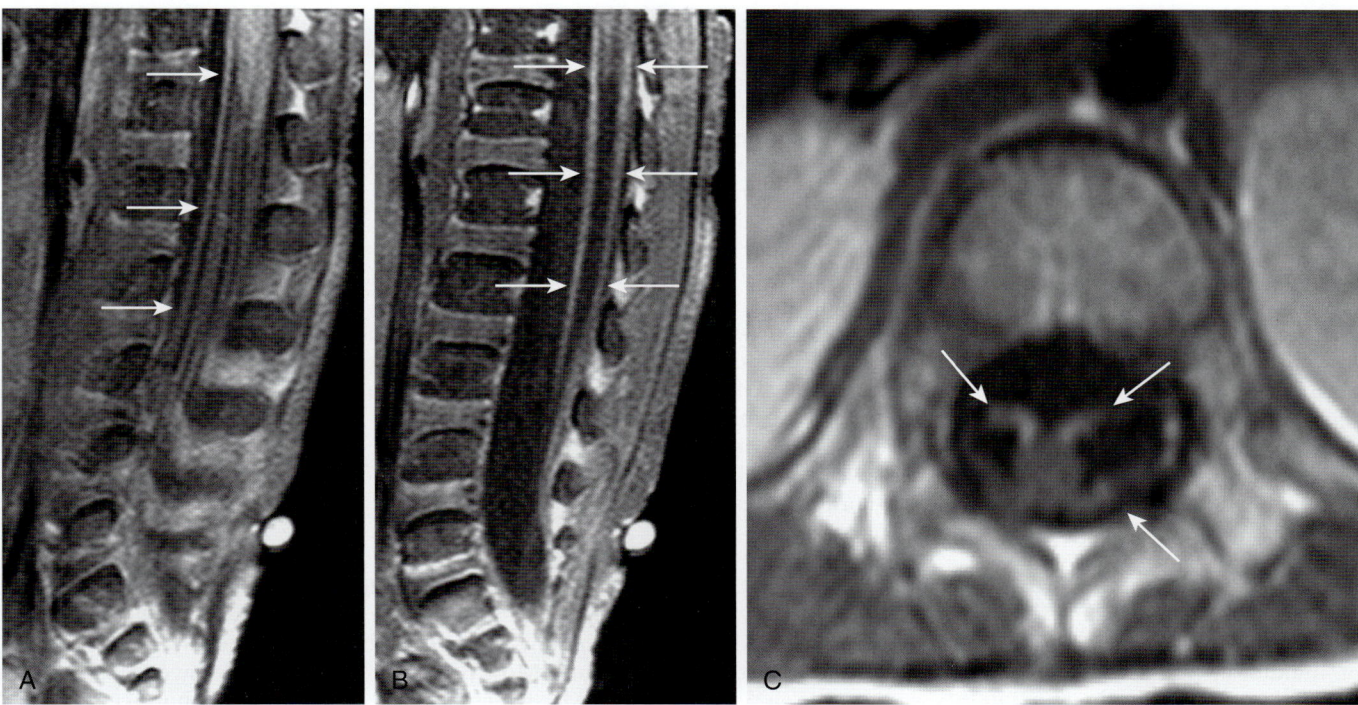

Figure 44-8 A patient who was unable to ambulate had Guillain-Barré syndrome. Sagittal off-midline and midline postgadolinium T1-weighted fat-saturated images through the lumbar spine (**A** and **B**), and axial postcontrast T1-weighted images through the conus medullaris and proximal lumbar nerve roots (**C** and **D**) demonstrate extensive contrast enhancement of nerve roots (*arrows*), particularly anteriorly, typical of Guillain-Barré syndrome.

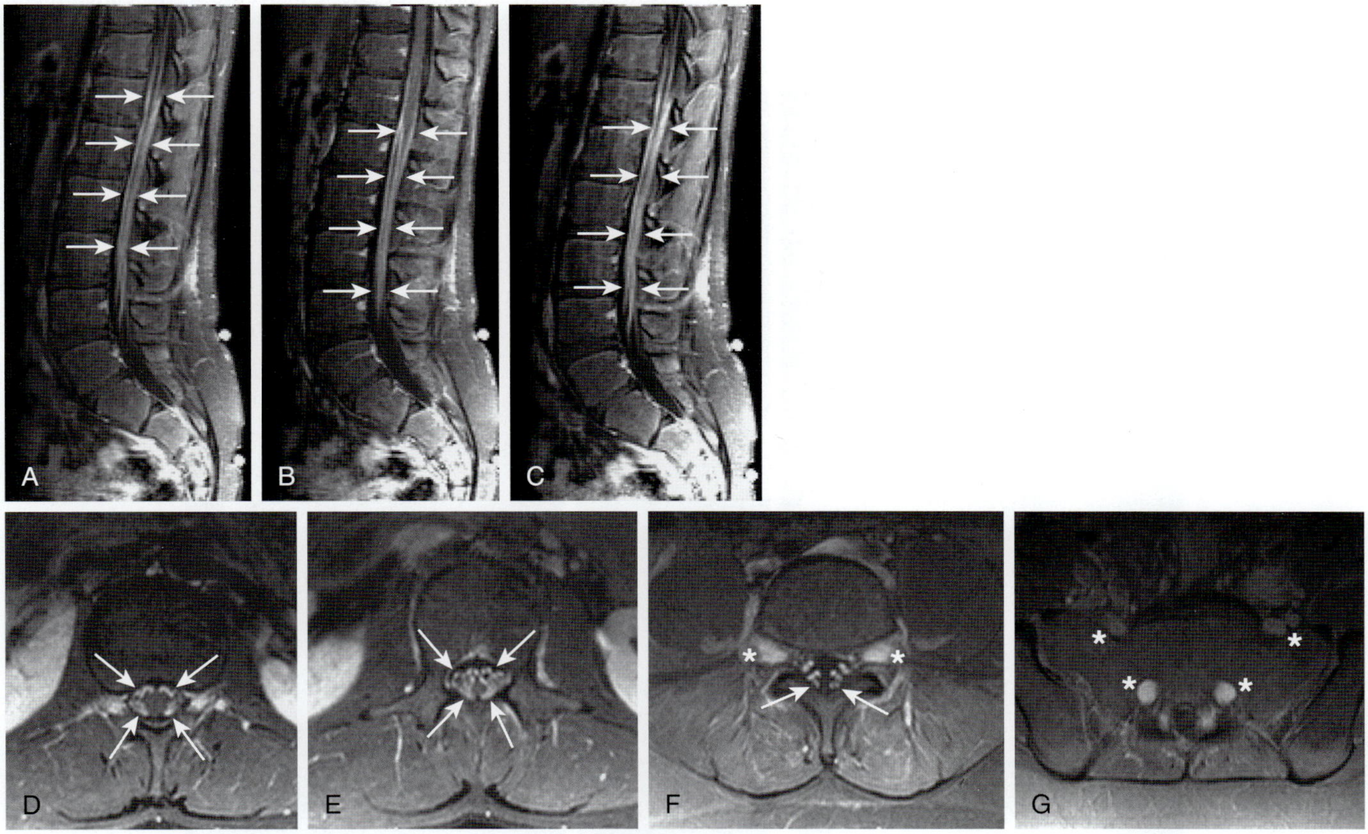

Figure 44-9 A 13-year-old boy with peripheral neuropathy and gait disturbances was found to have chronic inflammatory demyelinating polyneuropathy (CIDP). Sagittal fat-saturated T1-weighted images off-midline to the right, at midline, and off-midline to the left (**A, B,** and **C,** respectively) and axial postcontrast T1-weighted fat-saturated images through the lower thoraco-lumbar junction, conus medullaris, proximal nerve roots, and distal nerve roots (**D, E, F,** and **G,** respectively) demonstrate marked enhancement of the spinal nerve roots (*arrows*), with expansion of the nerve roots seen as they exit the neural foramina, best seen in **F** and **G** (*asterisks*). This enlargement and enhancement is typical of CIDP.

Transverse Myelitis

Transverse myelitis (TM) is an inflammatory condition that traverses a focal area of the spinal cord. In children, it most often occurs after the age of 10 years. The midthoracic spine is most often affected, and patients present with symmetrical bilateral sensory and motor deficits related to the affected regions. Although viral etiologies are believed to be the leading infectious cause of TM, as many as 60% of cases are thought to be idiopathic in nature. In most cases, a specific viral etiology is never determined. Vasculitides seen with autoimmune diseases such as lupus erythematosus also have been described as potential etiologies. TM manifests on MRI (Fig. 44-10) with increased T2 signal, encompassing more than two thirds of the spinal cord's diameter on fluid-sensitive (T2-weighted) sequences, extending along several vertebral segments, with variable enlargement of the cord as a result of edema and variable degrees of contrast enhancement.

ACUTE DISSEMINATED ENCEPHALOMYELITIS

Acute disseminated encephalomyelitis is a monophasic focal or multifocal, perivascular inflammatory, and demyelinating disorder, which often presents after a vaccination or viral infection. These lesions often present as a diagnostic dilemma in which the differential diagnosis also includes neoplasm of the spinal cord and can in isolation often be indistinguishable from the demyelinating lesions of multiple sclerosis (MS). Normal apparent diffusion coefficients within the corpus callosum (brain) may aid in diagnosing acute disseminated encephalomyelitis, as opposed to MS, which classically demonstrates abnormal callosal apparent diffusion coefficients. A clinical history of a recent viral illness and/or vaccination is the key to properly diagnosing these lesions. Lesions generally are hyperintense on T2-weighted sequences and have corresponding hypointensity or isointensity on T1-weighted sequences (Fig. 44-11). Contrast enhancement is variable, with enhancement patterns including solid or ringlike enhancement to no enhancement at all in lesions that range from small to large, and which affect gray matter, white matter, or both. These lesions often show dramatic response to plasmapheresis, corticosteroids, and immunoglobulin therapies, with consequent improvement or resolution of the imaging findings.

Multiple Sclerosis

Although it is much more prevalent in the adult population, MS also is seen in the pediatric age group. The presentation and diagnosis in children mimics that seen in adults. Viral and immune diseases are believed to be the most common etiologies. Most patients affected by MS have spinal lesions. Spinal MS, which has a cervical cord predominance, is associated with concomitant brain lesions in 80% of cases, making brain imaging essential when it is a differential consideration. MS can involve the white as well as gray matter, and it usually manifests as eccentrically situated lesions involving the dorsolateral aspect of the spinal cord. The concomitant

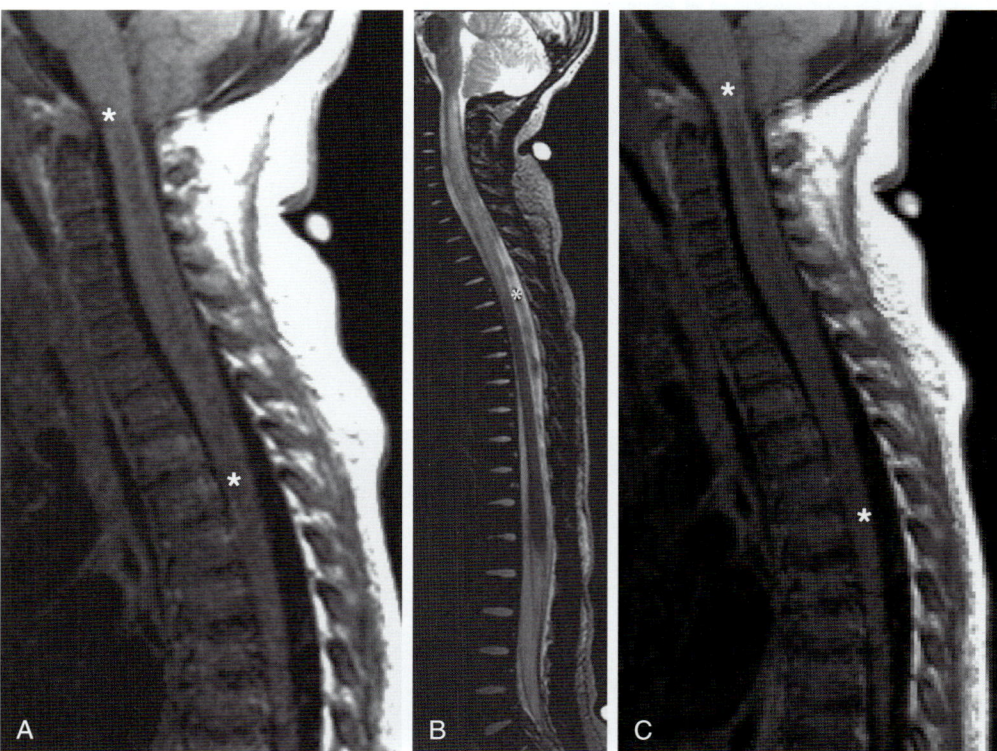

Figure 44-10 Fever and rapidly ascending paralysis in a 17-month-old boy with transverse myelitis. Sagittal T1-weighted (**A**), sagittal T2-weighted (**B**), and sagittal postgadolinium T1-weighted (**C**) images demonstrate the diffuse T1 (**A**) and T2 (**B**) prolongation (*asterisks*) of the entire cervical and upper thoracic spinal cord, with associated expansion of the cervical cord. No associated contrast enhancement is noted (**C**) (*asterisks*).

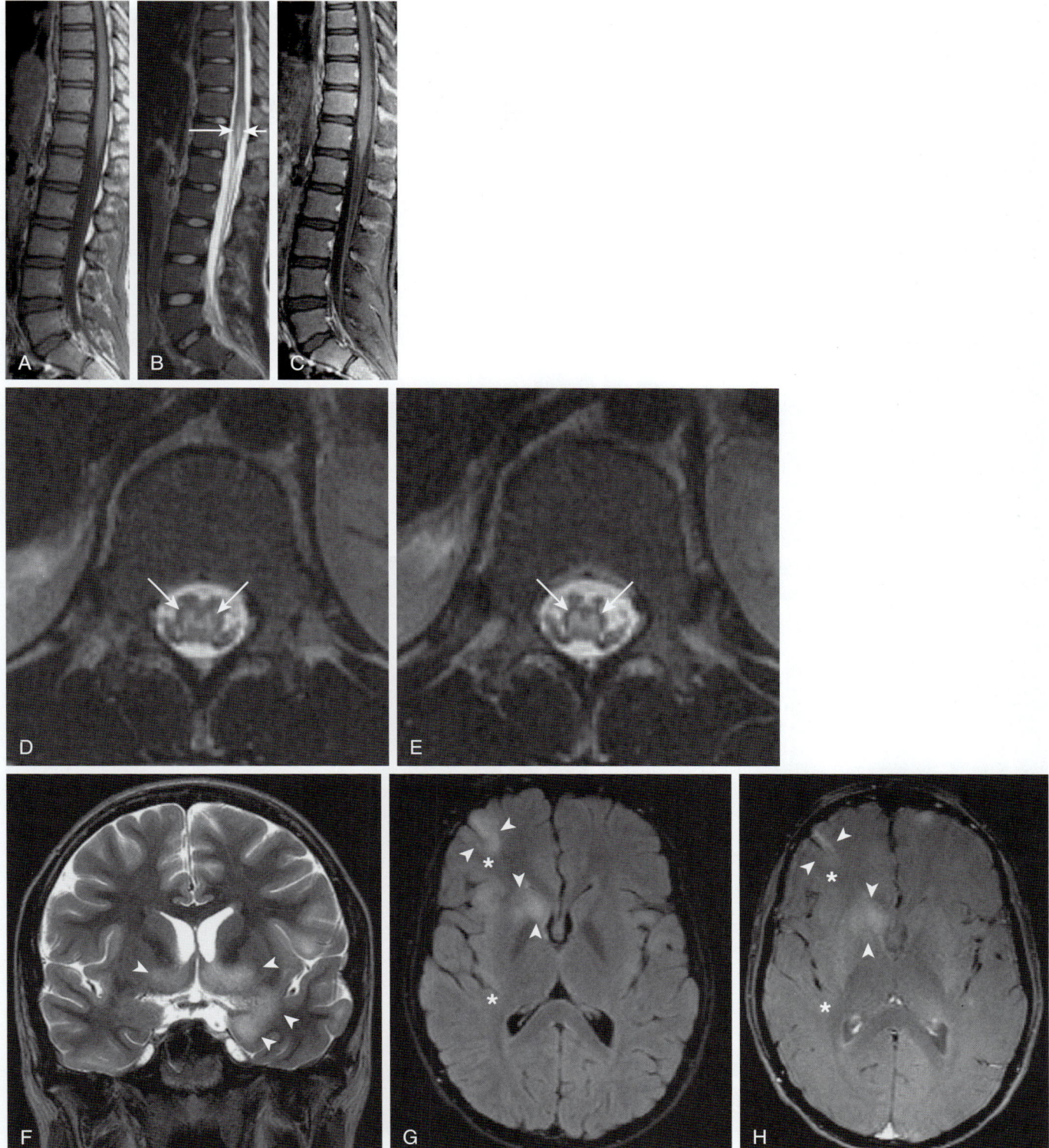

Figure 44-11   A 16-year-old boy with a history of constipation, urinary retention, and lower extremity weakness and numbness was found to have acute disseminated encephalomyelitis (ADEM). Sagittal T1-weighted, sagittal T2-weighted, and sagittal postgadolinium T1-weighted images (**A, B,** and **C,** respectively), axial T2-weighted images through the lower thoraco-lumbar region (**D** and **E**), a coronal T2-weighted image of the brain (**F**), an axial fluid attenuated inversion recovery image through the brain (**G**), and an axial postcontrast magnetization transfer T1-weighted image through the brain (**H**) were obtained. Note the nonexpansive T2 prolongation (*arrows*) of the central spinal cord (**D** and **E**). In addition, areas of T2 prolongation are seen within the brain (**F** and **G**), with involvement of both superficial gray and deep gray structures (*arrowheads*), including the right insula (*asterisks*), in keeping with changes of ADEM.

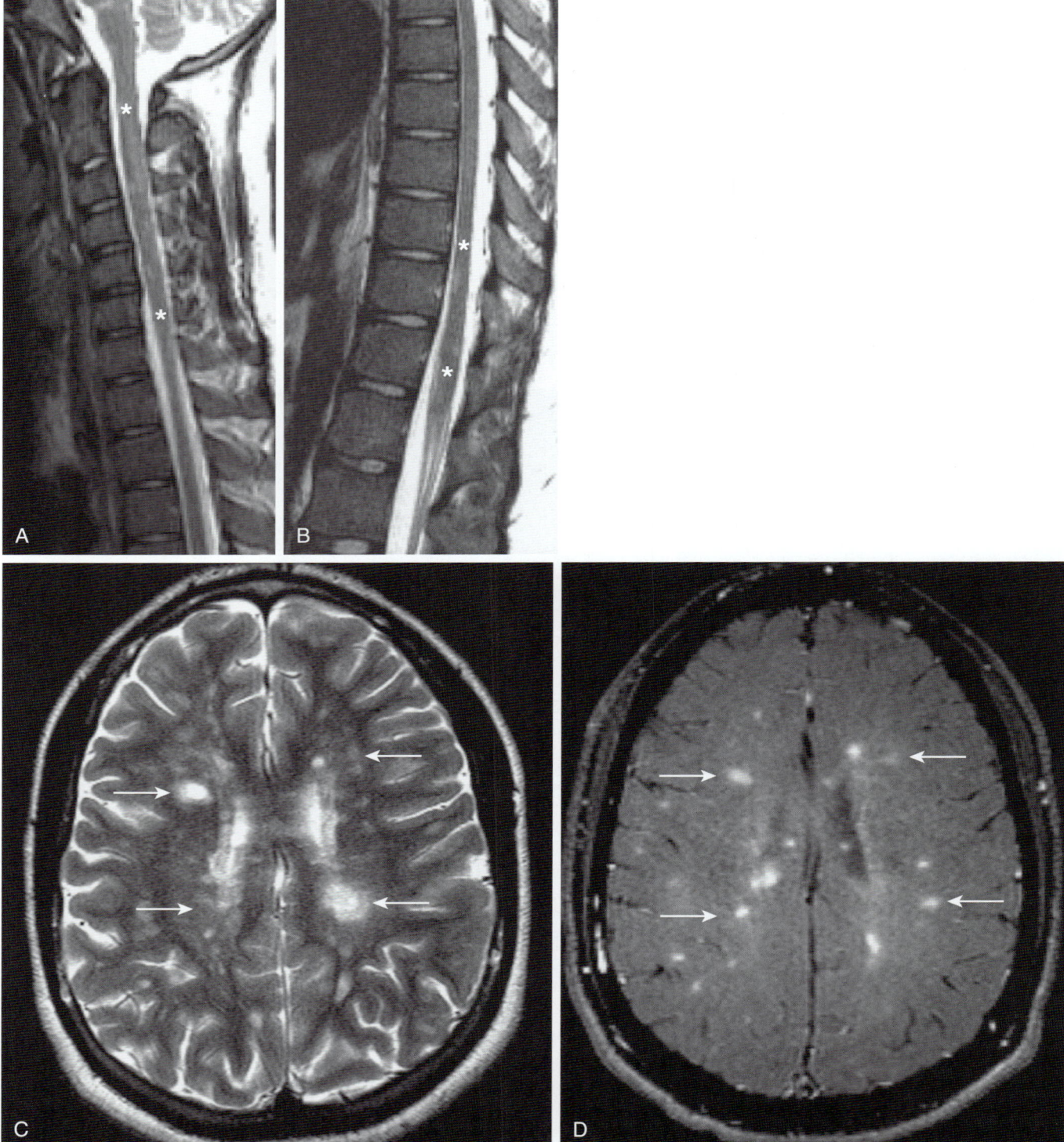

Figure 44-12 A child with sensory changes and decreased vision was found to have multiple sclerosis (MS). Multiplanar T1- and T2-weighted images of the cervical and thoracic spinal cord and the brain were obtained, including sagittal T2-weighted images through the cervical and thoracic regions (**A** and **B**), as well as an axial T2-weighted image of the brain (**C**) and an axial postcontrast T1-weighted MT image of the brain (**D**). Note the nonexpansive T2 prolongation (*asterisks*) of the spinal cord (**A** and **B**). This finding is associated with multiple areas of T2 prolongation (*arrows,* **C**) within the deep white matter of the cerebrum, running perpendicular to the lateral ventricles (the so-called Dawson fingers), associated with enhancement (*arrows,* **D**), suggesting acuity to the demyelinating plaques, which is typical of the findings seen with MS.

presence of optic neuritis, in addition to spinal cord involvement, constitutes what was previously known as Devic disease, now referred to as neuromyelitis optica. MRI, although nonspecific, is the gold standard in the diagnosis of MS and is seen to demonstrate disease in most patients presenting with clinical symptoms compatible with MS. MS lesions within the spinal cord usually span less than two vertebral bodies in length and demonstrate hypointense signal on T1-weighted images and a corresponding hyperintense signal on T2-weighted images (Fig. 44-12). Prompt contrast (gadolinium) enhancement occurs in active lesions. Fast short tau inversion imaging recovery sequences have greater sensitivity for lesion detection when compared with fast spin echo sequences.

Suggested Readings

Arabshahi B, Pollock AN, Sherry DD. Devic disease in a child with primary Sjögren syndrome. *J Child Neurol.* 2006;21(4):285-286.

Brown R, Hussain M, McHugh K, et al. Discitis in young children. *J Bone Joint Surg Br.* 2001;83:106-111.

Cameron ML, Durack DT. Helminthic infections. In: Scheld WM, Whitley RJ, Durack DT, eds. *Infections of the central nervous system.* Philadelphia: Lippincott Williams & Wilkins; 1997.

Choi KH, Lee KS, Chung SO, et al. Idiopathic tranverse myelitis: MR characteristics. *Am J Neuroradiol.* 1996;17(6):1151-1160.

Coskun A, Kumandas S, Pac A. Childhood Guillain-Barré syndrome. MR imaging in diagnosis and follow-up. *Acta Radiol.* 2003;44(2):230-235.

Dagirmanjian A, Schils J, McHenry MC. MR imaging of spinal infections. *Magn Reson Imag Clin North Am.* 1999;7:525-538.

Ferguson WR. Some observations on the circulation in fetal and infant spines. *J Bone Joint Surg Am.* 1950;32:640-648.

Fischer GW, Popich GA, Sullivan DE, et al. Discitis: a prospective diagnostic analysis. *Pediatrics.* 1978;62:543-544.

Fuchs PM, Meves R, Yamada HH. Spinal infections in children: a review. *Int Orthop.* 2012;36(2):387-395.

Goh C, Phal PM, Desmond PM. Neuroimaging in acute transverse myelitis. *Neuroimaging Clin N Am.* 2011;21(4):951-973.

Hughes RA, Rees JH. Clinical and epidemiological features of Guillain-Barré syndrome. *J Infect Dis.* 1997;176:S92-S98.

Iyer RS, Thapa MM, Chew FS. Chronic recurrent multifocal osteomyelitis: review. *AJR Integrative Imaging.* 2011;196(suppl 2):S87-S91.

Kesselring J, Miller DH, Robb SA. Acute disseminated encephalomyelitis. MRI findings and the distinction from multiple sclerosis. *Brain.* 1990;113(pt 2):291-302.

Khanna G, Sato TS, Ferguson P. Imaging of chronic recurrent multifocal osteomyelitis. *Radiographics.* 2009;29(4):1159-1177.

Kincaid O, Lipton HL. Viral myelitis: an update. *Curr Neurol Neurosci Rep.* 2006;6(6):469-474.

MacDonnell AH, Baird RW, Bronze MS. Intramedullary tuberculomas of the spinal cord: case report and review. *Rev Infect Dis.* 1990;12:432-439.

Mahboubi S, Morris MC. Imaging of spinal infection of children. *Radiol Clin North Am.* 2001;39:215-222.

Mendonca RA. Spinal infection and inflammatory disorders. In: Atlas SW, ed. *Magnetic resonance imaging of the brain.* 3th ed. Philadelphia: Lippincott Williams & Wilkins; 2002.

Noseworthy JH, Lucchinetti C, Rodriguez M, et al. Multiple sclerosis. *N Engl J Med.* 2000;343(13):938-952.

Rocca MA, Mastronardo G, Horsfield MA, et al. Comparison of three MR sequences for the detection of cervical cord lesions in patients with multiple sclerosis. *AJNR Am J Neuroradiol.* 1999;20(9):1710.

Ryan MM. Guillain-Barré syndrome in childhood. *J Paediatric Child Health.* 2005;41(5-6):237-241.

Shalmon B, Nass D, Ram Z, et al. Giant lesions in multiple sclerosis—a diagnostic challenge. *Harefuah.* 2000;138:936-939.

Singh S, Alexander M, Korah IP. Acute disseminated encephalomyelitis: MR imaging features. *AJR Am J Roentgenol.* 1999;173:1101-1107.

Sithinamsuwan P, Chairangsaris P. Images in clinical medicine. Gnathostomiasis—neuroimaging of larval migration. *N Engl J Med.* 2005;353(2):188.

Straus Farber R, Devilliers L, Miller A, et al. Differentiating multiple sclerosis from other causes of demyelination using diffusion weighted imaging of the corpus callosum. *J Magn Reson Imaging.* 2009;30(4):732-736.

Chapter 45

Spinal Tumor and Tumorlike Conditions

LISA H. LOWE and SETH GIBSON

Spinal Neoplasms

Overview Spinal tumors occur predominantly in young or middle-aged adults and tend to be less common in children. The most common presentation is 3 to 6 months of pain, gait disturbance, change in spinal curvature, motor weakness, and bowel and bladder dysfunction. In the setting of acute trauma, peritumoral edema may cause paresis or paralysis. In this chapter, general concepts regarding spinal neoplasms will be discussed, followed by specific anatomic categories of lesions. Categories will include neoplasms located in the intramedullary, intradural extramedullary, or extradural compartments.[1]

Imaging The imaging features of spinal neoplasms are often nonspecific, and findings overlap. Familiarity with age at diagnosis, key imaging findings, and associations can narrow the differential diagnosis, as summarized in Table 45-1.

Although osseous spinal erosion can occur as a late finding with pediatric spinal cord tumors, plain radiographs are of limited utility. Unenhanced computed tomography (CT) is helpful in imaging primary osseous lesions, but it is not useful in cord evaluation. Instead, magnetic resonance imaging (MRI) is the study of choice to characterize and define spinal cord lesions. Differentiating intramedullary (within the cord) versus extramedullary (outside of the cord) location is important and can be accomplished with multiplanar MRI. Intramedullary lesions show cord expansion, whereas extramedullary lesions will be separate from the cord in at least one plane.

Intraoperative ultrasound may be used to determine tumor location and borders during exposure and resection. Baseline postoperative MRI is deferred for at least 12 weeks because surgical changes make early postoperative scans difficult to interpret.[2]

Treatment The goal with benign, noninfiltrative spinal neoplasms is complete excision of both the solid tumor and associated syrinx cavities. If any portion of the neoplasm infiltrates the cord, surgical success decreases. Adjuvant radiation therapy and chemotherapy may be used, but the prognosis with an infiltrative, malignant lesion is dismal.[3]

Typically, a laminectomy is performed to gain access to the spinal cord lesion. Myelotomies are performed in the midline between the posterior columns or along the dorsal root entry zone. The tumor must be centrally debulked. Electrophysiologic monitoring techniques can be helpful as the periphery of the tumor is approached to prevent damage to the lateral columns of the spinal cord. The wound is closed when the tumor has been removed to its interface with normal-appearing spinal cord and the associated syrinx cavity has been carefully inspected for additional tumor deposits.[3]

Prognosis Preoperative neurologic deficits may persist postoperatively, but most tumors can be removed without new long-term disabilities. If complete tumor excision is not possible with histologically benign pediatric intramedullary gliomas, adjuvant radiation therapy is preferentially avoided because of adverse effects on the immature spinal cord and spinal column. Residual and recurrent tumor deposits often remain static for years or grow very slowly. Symptomatic recurrences can be managed by operating again.

Surgical management is considered with extradural tumors to establish a pathologic diagnosis with biopsy, to decompress the spinal cord in the setting of progressive myelopathy, for reconstruction in cases of spinal instability, and with an attempted radical resection for cure. Most childhood spinal epidural lesions are responsive to radiation or chemotherapy.[4]

Intramedullary Neoplasms

Overview Pediatric intramedullary tumors occur most commonly in the cervicothoracic cord.[5] Nonspecific symptoms often lead to a delay in diagnosis and vary with the age of the child. Younger children may present with spinal pain (dull and aching) or root pain, rigidity, persistent unexplained torticollis, and muscle spasm. Older children may present with gait disturbance and/or progressive scoliosis. Extremity weakness and paresthesias are common as well.[6] A subset of patients may present with symptoms of increased intracranial pressure (ICP) and hydrocephalus.

ASTROCYTOMA

Overview and Origin Up to 60% of intramedullary tumors in children are astrocytomas, and the cervical cord is most commonly involved.[3] Spinal astrocytomas usually occur in children around 10 years of age, with an equal sex predilection. Spinal astrocytomas are rarely seen in neonates and infants and may present with irritability, torticollis, and loss or absence of developmental milestones. Symptoms often are protracted.[6] Astrocytomas arise from astrocytes and range

Table 45-1

Pediatric Spinal Neoplasms: Location, Key Imaging Features, and Other Comments

Location	Neoplasm	Key Imaging Features	Other Comments
IM	Astrocytoma	Cervical most common Tend to be eccentric within cord ± syrinx Cystic with enhancing nodule	10 years of age Treatment: surgical debulking ± chemotherapy and radiation
	Ependymoma	Tend to be central within cord; cervical most common Hemosiderin cap on T2-weighted MRI Drop metastases	13-14 years of age If multiple lesions are present, consider NF2 Treatment: surgery ± radiation and chemotherapy
	Ganglioglioma	Similar appearance to ependymoma	7 years; associated with NF2 Treatment: surgical resection
	Hemangioblastoma	Cystic lesion with an enhancing mural nodule Flow voids	Associated with von Hippel–Lindau disease Treatment: surgery
EM	Leptomeningeal metastasis	Lumbosacral involvement Variable in size and number of lesions	Common with ependymomas, medulloblastomas, higher-grade astrocytomas Treatment depends on primary lesion
	Nerve sheath tumor (schwannoma, neurofibroma)	Expansion of intervertebral foramina Posterior vertebral body scalloping Target sign	Associated with NF1 and NF2 Treatment: typically conservative; rarely, debulking
	Meningioma	Isointense on noncontrast imaging Homogeneous, vigorous enhancement	Teenagers; multiple lesions in setting of NF2 Treatment: surgical resection
ED	Primary osseous lesion		
	Osteoblastoma	Posterior element, solid, expansile, enhancing mass	10-30 years; 40% occur in spine Treatment: surgical resection
	Aneurysmal bone cyst	Posterior element, expansile, multicystic, fluid-fluid levels	10-30 years; 20% occur in spine Treatment: embolization, surgical curettage, and packing
	Osteoid osteoma	Posterior element lucent nidus with marked surrounding enhancement, ± central calcification	90% <25 years of age; 10% occur in spine Treatment: radiofrequency ablation
	Lymphoma	Vertebral body lesion with little or no loss of height; single > multiple	Spinal involvement with systemic disease; rarely primary lesion Treatment: chemotherapy
	Leukemia	Vertebral body lesion with slight loss of height; multiple > single	Spinal involvement with systemic disease Treatment: chemotherapy
	Langerhans cell histiocytosis	Vertebral body lesion(s) with severe loss of height (vertebra plana) and soft tissue mass; single > multiple	Ranges from single osseous lesion (histiocytosis X) to systemic disease Treatment: usually chemotherapy
	Neuroblastoma		
	Sacrococcygeal teratoma	Paraspinous (adrenal is most common) mass encasing vessels with calcifications	1-5 years of age Treatment: chemotherapy and surgery

ED, Extradural (50%); *EM,* extramedullary (15%-20%); *IM,* intramedullary (30%-35%); *MRI,* magnetic resonance imaging; *NF1,* neurofibromatosis type 1; *NF2,* neurofibromatosis type 2.

from benign (grade I) to malignant (grade IV).[7] Spongioblastomas and pilocytic astrocytomas are at the benign end of the spectrum, and high-grade astrocytomas and glioblastoma multiforme tumors are at the malignant end of the spectrum.

Spinal astrocytomas may be cystic, mixed cystic and solid, solid, or contain necrotic components. Malignant astrocytomas can mimic spinal vascular malformations as a result of hypervascularity with possible intratumoral hemorrhage. Lesion size varies from focal to involvement of the entire spinal cord (a holocord tumor), which usually is seen during the first year of life.[8]

Imaging Contrast-enhanced spinal MRI is critical to the identification of small tumors with associated syringohydromyelia and to detect subarachnoid seeding. Key features of astrocytomas include cord expansion, eccentric location, hypointense to isointense appearance on T1-weighted imaging, heterogeneous hyperintensity on T2-weighted imaging, and variable enhancement, sometimes of a mural nodule, on postcontrast images (Figs. 45-1 and 45-2). T2 heterogeneity depends on the presence of solid, cystic, and necrotic components.[5]

EPENDYMOMA

Overview and Origin Up to 30% of intramedullary tumors in children are ependymomas. Ependymomas present in an older age group than do astrocytomas (at age 13 or 14 years), with a slight female predilection.[3] Ependymomas originate from ependymal cells within the central spinal cord or filum terminale, and they frequently span multiple segments. Holocord involvement, as with astrocytomas, is possible.[9] A variety of histologic subtypes of ependymomas exist, with cellular ependymoma the most common. Myxopapillary ependymoma occurs exclusively in the lower cord and filum terminale. Surgical management of the myxopapillary subtype is difficult because of varied physical consistency of the lesion and relationship to surrounding structures. When

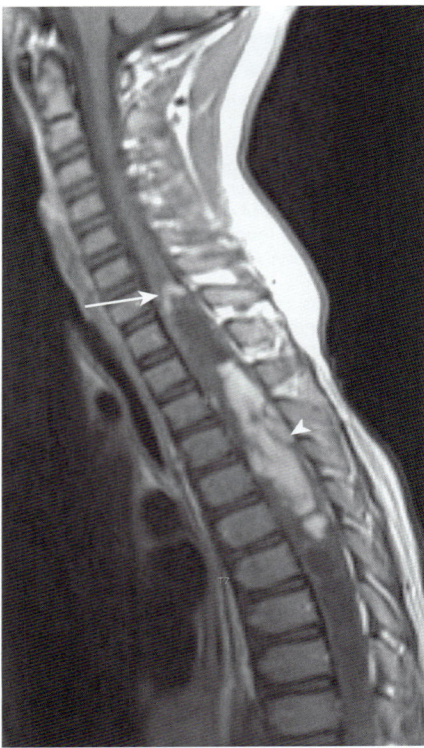

Figure 45-1   An astrocytoma in an 8-year-old boy with back pain. A sagittal T1-weighted contrast-enhanced image demonstrates an intramedullary cystic mass with dorsal nodular (*arrowhead*) and peripheral cranial (*arrow*) enhancement.

occurring in the cauda equina, this subtype may be associated with subarachnoid hemorrhage, back pain, lower extremity weakness, numbness, pain, and even bowel and bladder incontinence.[10]

Imaging   Ependymomas are distinguished by the findings of central cord location, cord expansion, heterogeneous signal intensity on all sequences, and a T2 hypointense hemosiderin cap along the cranial or caudal aspects of the tumor (Figs. 45-3 and 45-4). Contrast-enhanced spinal MRI is useful in the evaluation of small drop metastasis, a common feature of ependymomas.[11,12] The presence of metastatic spread to the brain with resultant hydrocephalus can be evaluated with cranial MRI. Multiple ependymomas should prompt consideration of neurofibromatosis type 2 (NF2).[13]

GANGLIOGLIOMA

Overview and Origin   Gangliogliomas contain both astrocytic and neuronal components. They present in the first three decades with an average presentation age of 12 years.[5,14]

Imaging   Gangliogliomas may be solid, cystic, calcified, or hemorrhagic. They demonstrate heterogeneous signal intensity on all sequences.[15] Notable imaging features include a lack of peritumoral edema, even when large in size, and associated adjacent osseous erosion (Fig. 45-5). Given this lesion's similar appearance to an ependymoma on MRI and its association with patients who have NF2, it should be included in the differential diagnosis when ependymoma is a diagnostic consideration.[14]

HEMANGIOBLASTOMA

Overview and Origin   Hemangioblastomas are most commonly intramedullary, but they can be pial, subpial, or combined intramedullary-extramedullary.[16] The presence of this lesion should prompt consideration of von Hippel–Lindau disease, and an appropriate workup should be initiated. Treatment includes chemotherapy and surgical resection.[17,18]

Imaging   Hemangioblastomas frequently are cystic masses with variable T1 signal intensity depending on the proteinaceous content of the cyst fluid, T2 hyperintensity, variable enhancement of mural nodules, and a syrinx in up to 50% of patients (Fig. 45-6). Flow voids are produced by the arterial supply and draining veins of the lesion. Associated hemorrhage and peritumoral edema are common.[19]

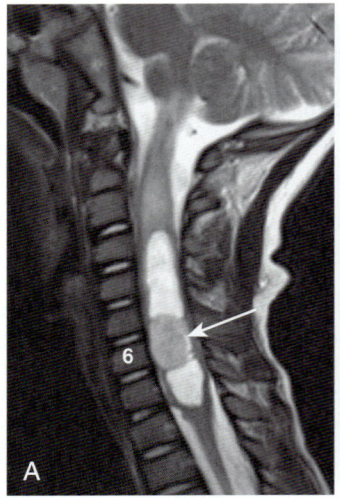
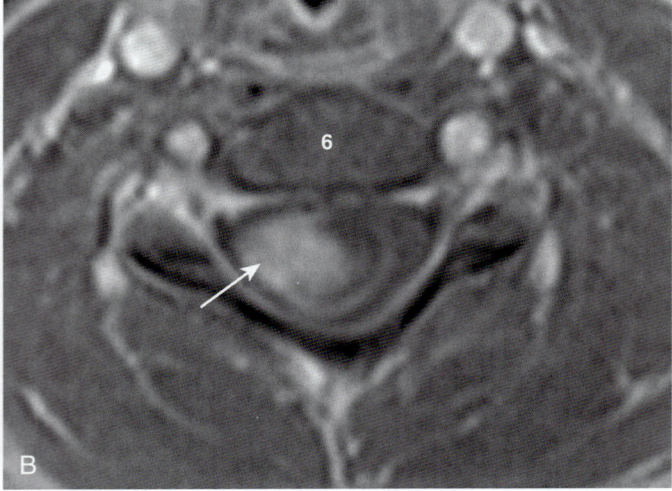

Figure 45-2   An astrocytoma in a 6-year-old boy with pain and decreased use of his right arm. **A,** A sagittal T2-weighted image shows an intramedullary cystic cervical cord mass with an enhancing mural nodule (*arrow*). Note T2 bright cord edema above the mass. **B,** An axial T1-weighted image with contrast through the enhancing nodule shows that the lesion is eccentric.

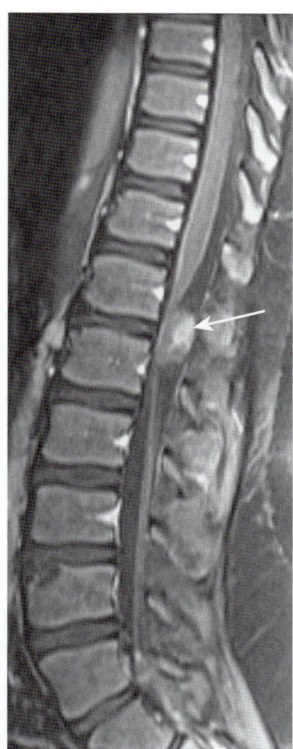

Figure 45-3 An ependymoma in an 11-year-old boy with unexplained altered mental status. A sagittal T1-weighted image with fat suppression demonstrates an extramedullary heterogeneously enhancing mass (*arrow*) at T12-L1 displacing the nerve roots ventrally.

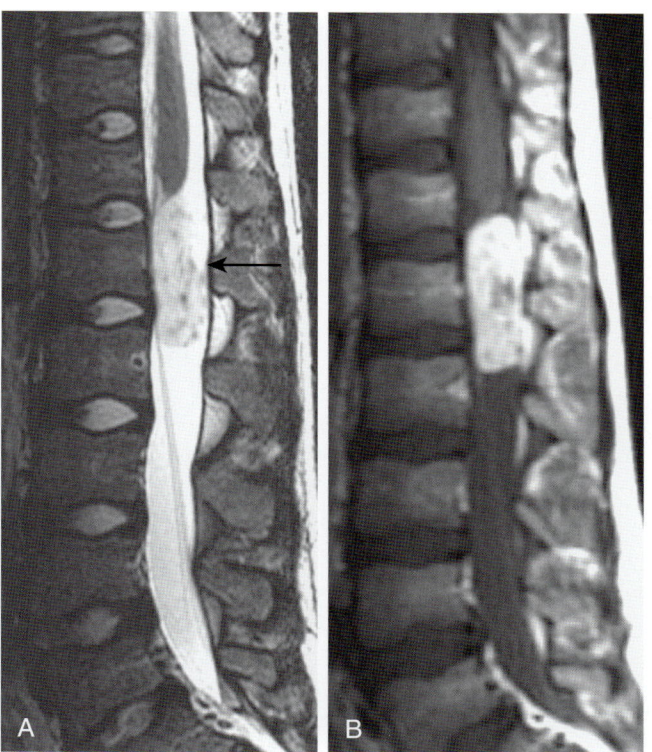

Figure 45-4 A myxopapillary ependymoma in an 11-year-old girl with back pain. **A,** Sagittal T2-weighted imaging demonstrates a hyperintense, well-defined mass with internal flow voids arising just below the conus medullaris (*arrow*). **B,** A sagittal contrast-enhanced T1-weighted image confirms a mass and shows avid enhancement.

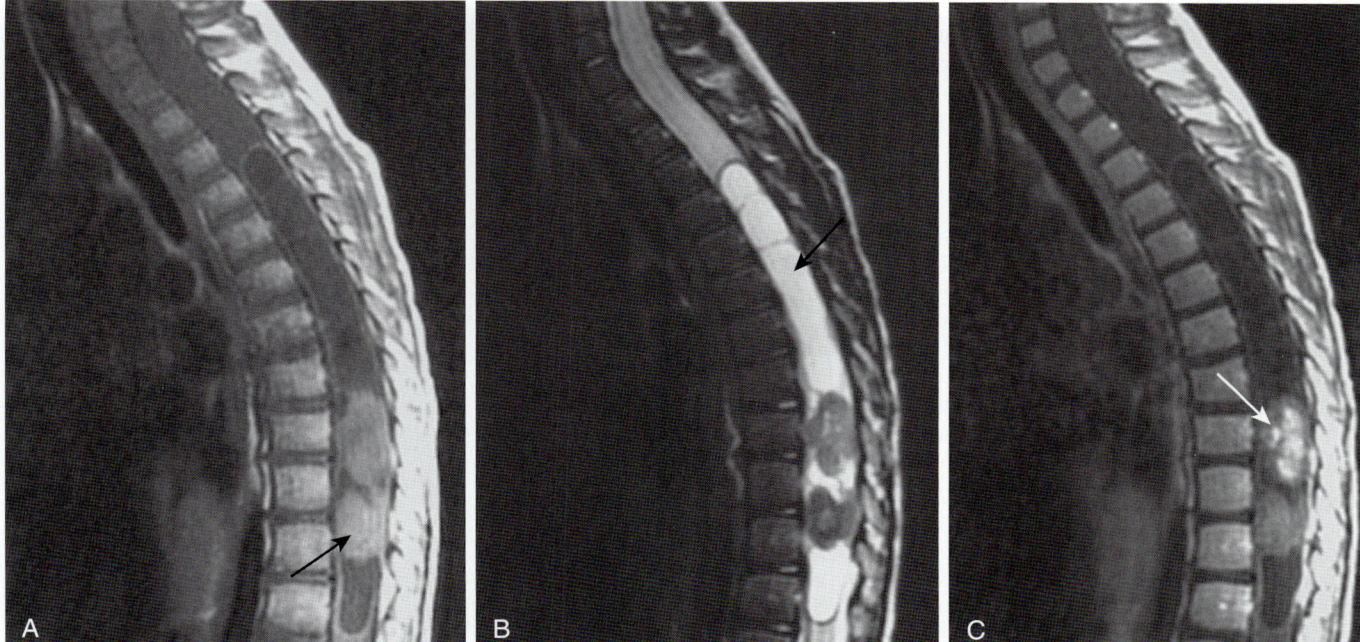

Figure 45-5 Ganglioglioma. **A,** A sagittal T1-weighted image shows a holocord tumor. Rounded hyperintense elements seen at the thoracolumbar junction were found at the time of surgery to represent hemorrhagic components of the tumor (*arrow*). **B,** A sagittal fat-suppressed T2-weighted magnetic resonance (MR) image shows the hemorrhagic components of the lesion as hypointense masses. Note the tumor cyst in the midthoracic cord (*arrow*). **C,** A sagittal postenhanced T1-weighted MR image shows enhancement of the caudal tumor (*arrow*).

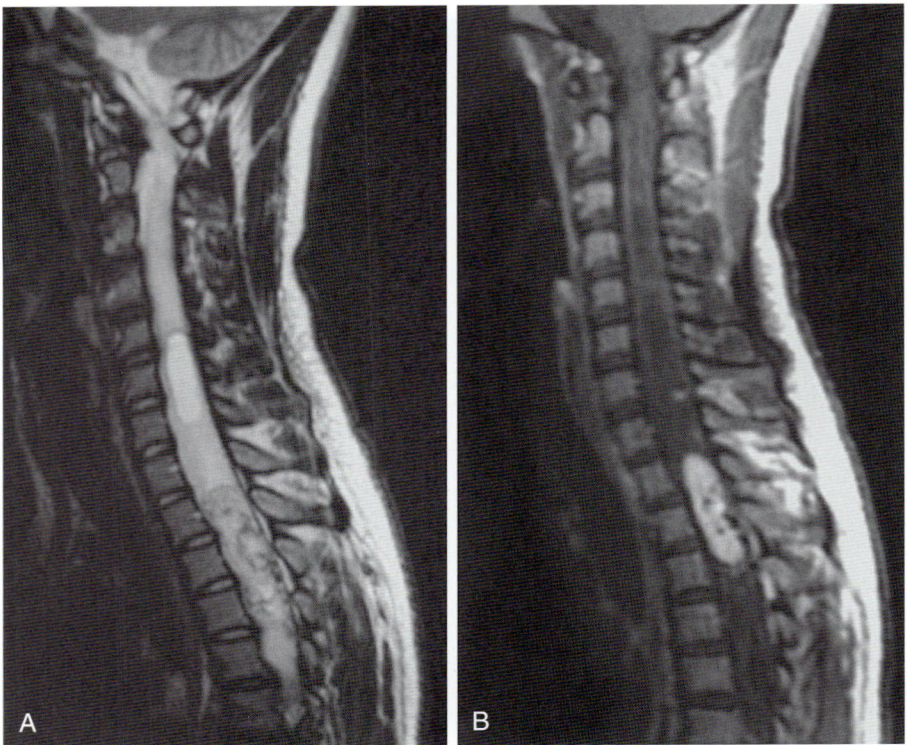

Figure 45-6   A hemangioblastoma in a 14-year-old child with von Hippel–Lindau disease. **A,** A sagittal T2-weighted image shows a cystic component superior to the heterogeneous lesion within the spinal cord. The heterogeneous lesion has flow voids. **B,** A sagittal contrast-enhanced T1 sequence shows marked enhancement of the tumor and multiple small, bright foci of other hemangioblastomas in the cystic portion of the cord mass. A cystic component with a low signal again is seen.

Intradural-Extramedullary Neoplasms

Overview   Intradural-extramedullary spinal neoplasms in children include a variety of lesions such as neurofibromas/schwannomas, meningiomas, and leptomeningeal metastases.

NERVE SHEATH TUMORS

Overview and Origin   The two main spinal nerve sheath tumors are neurofibromas and schwannomas, with the focus in this chapter on neurofibromas.[20] Neurofibromas may be derived from an intermediate cell or from a combination of Schwann cells and perineural fibroblasts. Most spinal neurofibromas are intradural-extramedullary lesions. The two morphologic types are fusiform (arising from a single nerve fascicle) and plexiform (involving multiple nerve branches). The lesions may be single, multiple, or diffuse. Neurofibromas usually are encountered in children with neurofibromatosis type 1 (NF1), but they may occur as an isolated lesion.[21]

Imaging   Neurofibromas have a variable T1 signal, are T2 hyperintense, and enhance after administration of contrast material. Diffuse neurofibromas may extend along the paraspinal region. Key imaging features of neurofibromas include remodeling and expansion of the intervertebral foramina, which is indicative of slow indolent growth, and a target appearance (central low signal with peripheral high signal) on T2-weighted images (Fig. 45-7). Rib erosion may be seen,

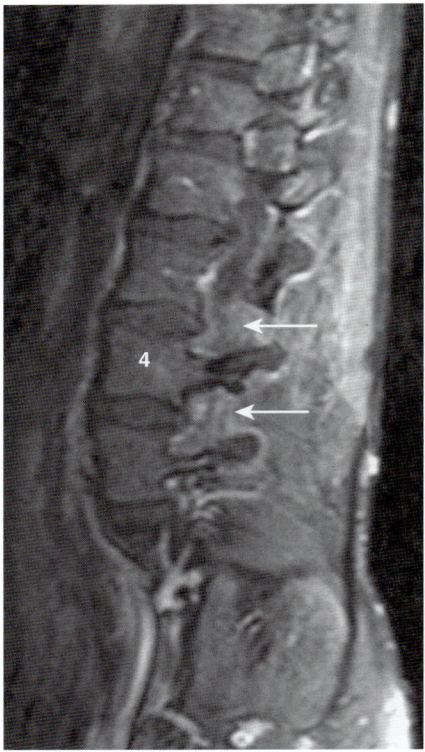

Figure 45-7   A plexiform neurofibroma in 13-year-old girl with neurofibromatosis type 1 and scoliosis. Sagittal T1-weighted, fat-suppressed imaging with contrast demonstrates expansion of the neural foramina at multiple contiguous levels in the lumbar spine (*arrows*).

and when it is severe over a long length of the rib, it may cause "ribbon ribs." Malignant degeneration into a neurofibrosarcoma is uncommon but should be considered in large lesions with bone destruction or necrosis.

MENINGIOMA

Overview and Imaging Meningiomas of the spinal cord are rare in childhood.[22] When they are seen in patients with NF2, they may occur intracranially and intraspinally. Meningiomas are T1 hypointense to isointense, T2 hyperintense, and uniformly enhance after administration of contrast material (Fig. 45-8). Areas of hypointensity may be due to calcification.[23]

LEPTOMENINGEAL METASTASES

Overview and Origin Metastatic spread to the spinal canal most commonly occurs via the cerebrospinal fluid (CSF) as a result of drop metastases from primary supratentorial and posterior fossa brain neoplasms, such as medulloblastoma, ependymoma, and atypical teratoid–rhabdoid tumors.[24]

Imaging CSF metastases may be solitary, multiple, or diffuse, coating the spinal cord and nerve roots. Metastatic nodules may range in size from 1 to 2 mm to 1 to 2 cm and may block CSF flow (Fig. 45-9). The most common site is the distal thecal sac in the lumbosacral area, followed by the thoracic, and finally the cervical spine.[22] To avoid false-positive MRI examinations, the spinal cord should be scanned

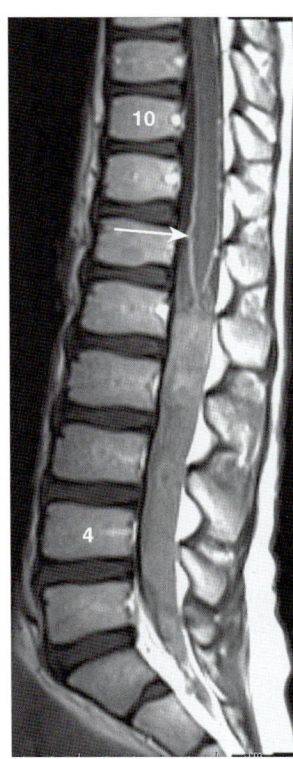

Figure 45-9 Leptomeningeal metastases in a 9-year-old girl with an atypical rhabdoid teratoid tumor who has undergone radiation. A sagittal contrast-enhanced T1-weighted image demonstrates leptomeningeal enhancement (*arrow*) of the spinal cord from the lower thoracic cord to the conus medullaris. Extensive solid tissue enhancement from L1-L5 fills the distal thecal sac.

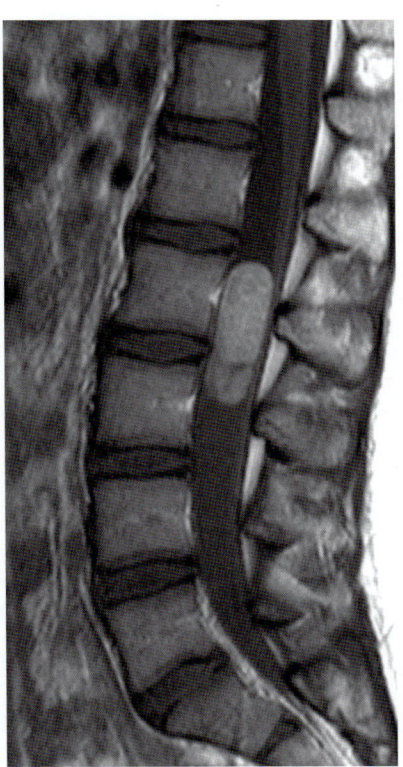

Figure 45-8 Meningioma in a 15-year-old girl with leg and back pain. Sagittal contrast-enhanced fat-suppressed T1-weighted image shows a well-defined enhancing mass in the lumbar spinal canal.

before surgery for newly diagnosed brain tumors with a propensity to spread via the CSF. If preoperative MRI is not feasible, MRI should be delayed for 4 to 6 weeks after surgery to avoid confusion and possible false positve results.[11]

Extradural Tumors

Overview Most childhood extradural neoplasms arise in the vertebral bodies or the paravertebral soft tissues and invade the spinal canal via the intervertebral foramina, such as neuroblastomas and sacrococcygeal teratomas. Primary osseous lesions, such as aneurysmal bone cysts, lymphoma, and Ewing sarcoma, as well as metastatic lesions, also may involve the vertebra and, secondarily, the spinal canal. Imaging is used to determine the extent of spinal involvement, the degree of neural element compression, and the degree of destabilization of the spinal column by destruction of osseous elements.[12,25]

NEUROBLASTOMA

Overview and Origin Tumors of neural crest cell origin include neuroblastomas, ganglioneuroblastomas, and ganglioneuromas. Neuroblastoma is by far the most common extracranial solid neoplasm, usually presenting between 1 and 5 years of age. Neuroblastomas are classified as primitive neuroectodermal tumors (PNETs) when they involve the central nervous system.

Neuroblastomas originate from neuroblasts along the sympathetic chain and arise most commonly from the adrenal gland. Metastatic involvement of the spine can be to bone or sympathetic chain ganglia, may be single or multilevel, or may extend into the epidural space with spinal cord compression. Larger lesions may have areas of hemorrhage and necrosis. Metastatic involvement of bone, bone marrow, liver, lymph nodes, and skin can be present. Ganglioneuroblastoma and ganglioneuroma are progressively less malignant forms of neuroblastoma that are composed of a mixture of mature ganglion cells and nerve fibers. They usually are well encapsulated and have a similar imaging appearance to neuroblastoma, although they are smaller and better defined.

Imaging Neuroblastomas are paraspinal soft tissue masses, often with intraspinal extension. The lesion is hypointense to isointense on T1-weighted imaging compared with the spinal cord, demonstrates subtle hyperintensity on T2-weighted imaging, and has variable enhancement after administration of contrast material (Fig. 45-10). Hypointense areas on T1- and T2-weighted imaging may indicate calcifications. Fat-suppressed T2-weighted imaging is important to determine the extent of disease. Imaging to evaluate for extension across the midline is important in staging.[1]

SACROCOCCYGEAL TERATOMAS

Overview and Origin Sacrococcygeal teratomas (SCTs) are neoplasms derived from all three germinal layers. These

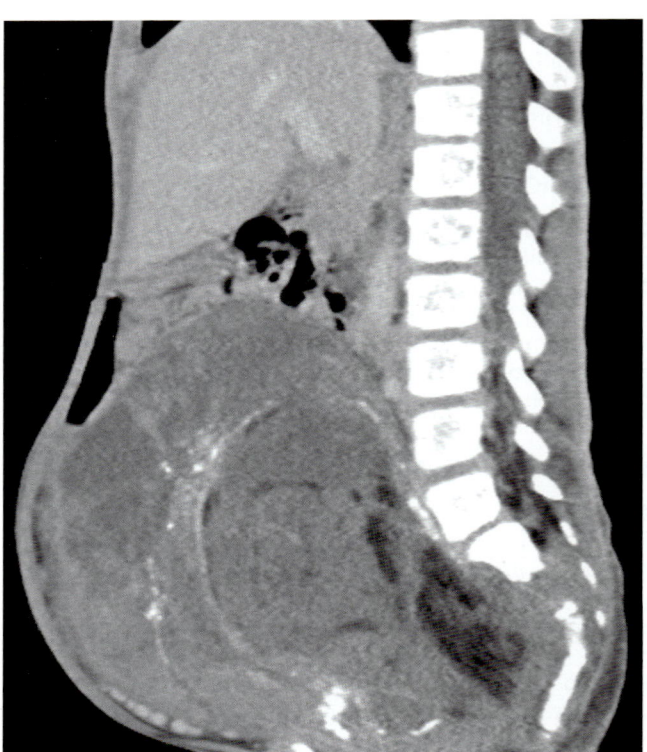

Figure 45-11 Sacrococcygeal teratoma, type 4, in a 6-day-old female with an abdominal mass. Sagittal reconstructed contrast-enhanced CT image shows a large mass anterior to and invading the sacrum. The heterogeneous mass contains low-attenuation fat mixed with soft tissue and scattered calcifications.

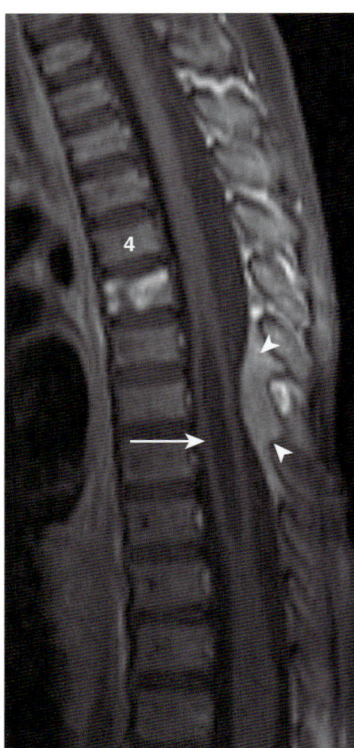

Figure 45-10 A metastatic neuroblastoma in a 2-year-old boy with leg weakness, vomiting, and diarrhea. A sagittal T1-weighted, fat-suppressed image demonstrates an enhancing metastatic lesion in the T5 vertebral body, a syrinx from T5-T11 (*arrow*), and a hyperintense, enhancing dorsal epidural lesion (*arrowheads*). A primary right adrenal mass was found but is not shown.

neoplasms may contain neural elements, squamous and intestinal epithelium, skin appendages, teeth, and calcium. Four types of SCTs are found; type 1 is external, type 2 is predominantly external with a small intrapelvic portion, type 3 is predominantly intrapelvic with a small external component, and type 4 is completely intrapelvic. All four types may present as an extradural mass and may be associated with sacrococcygeal bony erosions. SCTs can be cystic, mixed cystic-solid, or solid lesions. Lesions are more likely to have a favorable prognosis in younger patients, in female patients, when they are mostly cystic masses, when they are less heterogeneous masses, when more calcifications are present, and when they are type 1 (external). SCTs may be benign or malignant.

Imaging CT is used to demonstrate osseous destruction of the sacrum and coccyx, as well as calcification within the lesion. Cystic components of SCT are T1 hypointense and T2 hyperintense. The MR signal of hemorrhagic components will depend on the age of the hemorrhage. Solid components may enhance after administration of contrast material (Fig. 45-11).

The location of the SCT in relationship to the gluteal fold helps to differentiate this lesion from back masses associated with spinal dysraphic conditions. Specifically, SCTs typically extend below the gluteal fold, and masses associated with spinal dysraphism typically extend above the gluteal fold.[26]

Lymphoma and Leukemia

Overview and Origin Lymphoma involves the spine less commonly than it does other reticuloendothelial system structures, such as lymph nodes. Single or multiple vertebral bodies may be involved, especially with non–Hodgkin type lymphoma (Fig. 45-12). A diffuse dural infiltration, a localized dural-based mass, a primary osseous mass with spinal canal extension, or spinal cord masses may be present. Single or multiple vertebral levels may be involved. Epidural deposits from leukemia more commonly produce clinical symptoms in children than in adults, with myelogenous leukemia more likely presenting as a focal mass (Fig. 45-13).[27]

Imaging Epidural involvement in patients with lymphoma and leukemia is usually isointense on noncontrast T1-weighted imaging. Homogeneous enhancement is seen after administration of contrast material. A key imaging feature suggesting lymphoma or a myelogenous leukemic mass is slightly low signal on T2-weighted images, along with lack of vertebral compression or other osseous destruction.[28]

LEPTOMENINGEAL MELANOSIS

Overview Neurocutaneous melanosis is a rare, nonfamilial phakomatosis caused by melanocyte proliferation within the epidermis and leptomeninges. It is a nonfamilial disease characterized by large cutaneous pigmented nevi and melanosis of the leptomeninges. A forme fruste may occur in which

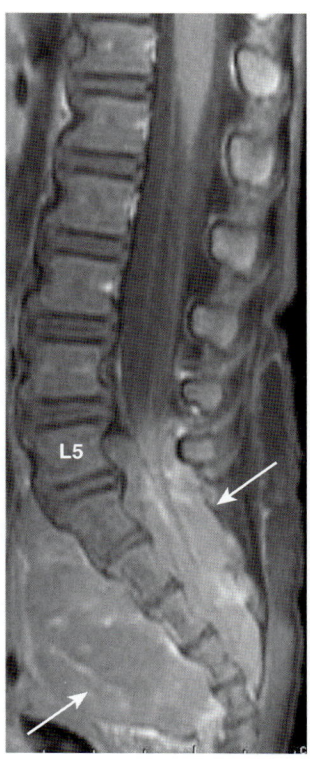

Figure 45-13 Megakaryocytic leukemia in a 1-year-old boy with thrombocytopenia. A sagittal T1-weighted, contrast-enhanced, fat-suppressed image identifies an enhancing mass arising from the sacrum with extensive lumbosacral epidural involvement (*arrows*).

only leptomeningeal involvement is present without cutaneous manifestations. In the pediatric population, leptomeningeal involvement may present with signs of raised ICP and hydrocephalus.

Imaging The most common appearance is diffuse leptomeningeal thickening and enhancement after administration of contrast material, as can be seen with leptomeningeal metastases. Although leptomeningeal metastatic disease is more common than leptomeningeal melanosis, the presence of melanin, which is seen as hyperintense signal on noncontrast T1-weighted images, should prompt consideration of this disease (Fig. 45-14). T1 hyperintense melanin deposits most commonly involve the hippocampus and brainstem.[29]

EXTRADURAL BONY LESIONS

Overview Numerous vertebral osseous abnormalities may extend outside of the spine and produce extradural mass effect. Lesions in the spine tend to arise either from the posterior elements or the vertebral body. Common posterior element lesions include osteoid osteomas, aneurysmal bone cysts, and osteoblastomas. Common primary pediatric vertebral masses include Ewing sarcoma, lymphoma, Langerhans cell histiocytosis, and metastatic disease such as neuroblastoma, leukemia, and PNET.

Imaging The imaging appearance of extradural bony masses varies depending on the specific type of lesion. Unlike with most spinal tumors, CT plays a greater role in the imaging

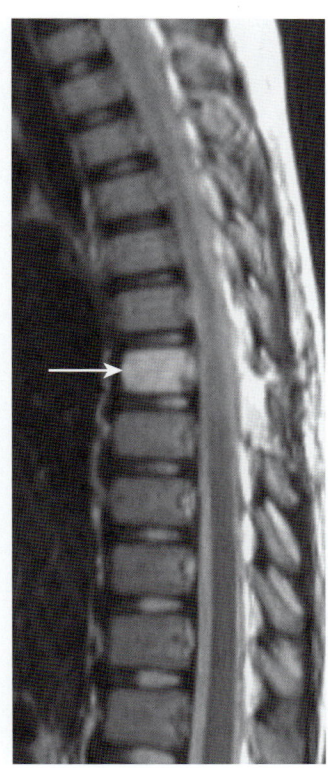

Figure 45-12 Burkitt lymphoma in a 5-year-old boy with back pain, paresthesias, and urinary retention. A sagittal T2-weighted image demonstrates a hyperintense T7 vertebral body lesion. Note postsurgical changes of the posterior elements.

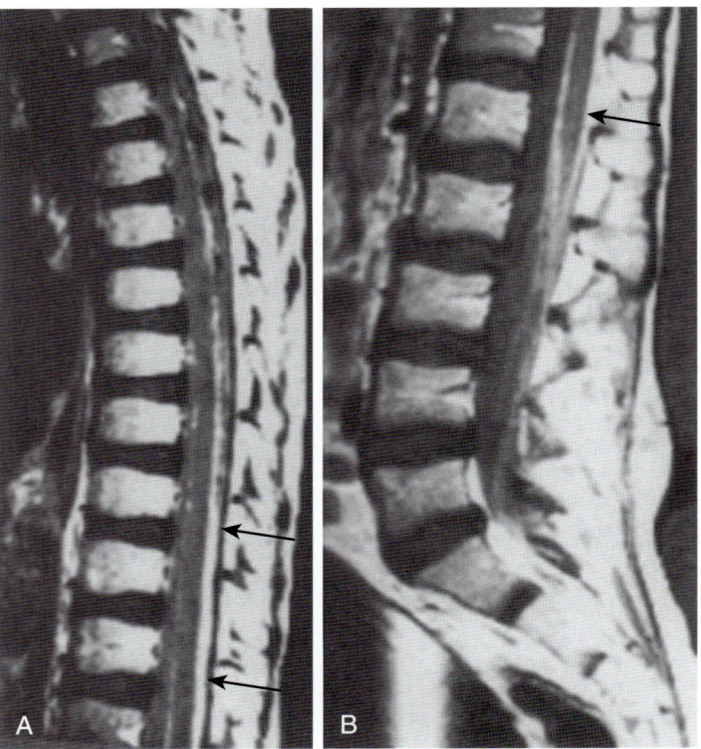

Figure 45-14   A postgadolinium sagittal T1-weighted magnetic resonance image of a patient with leptomeningeal melanosis showing diffuse enhancement (*arrows*) of the leptomeninges of the thoracic (**A**) and lumbosacral (**B**) spinal cord.

of osseous masses and neoplasms and is complimentary to MRI. Posterior element lesions, which include osteoid osteomas, have a focal sclerotic nidus surrounded by a lucent halo on CT and show a "double density sign" on nuclear bone scintigraphy. On MRI, these lesions show impressive surrounding edema. Aneurysmal bone cysts classically appear as an expansile, multilocular lesion with fluid-fluid levels due to internal hemorrhage and debris (Fig. 45-15). Osteoblastomas are expansile solid masses of the posterior elements and rarely have internal fluid levels (Fig. 45-16). Focal vertebral body lesions, as may be seen with Ewing sarcoma and lymphoma, tend to cause T1 hypointense, T2 hyperintense marrow signal with enhancement after administration of contrast material in a single vertebra with little loss of vertebral body height. Similar features are less often seen with multiple vertebral body involvement.[30]

Key Points

The differential diagnosis of spinal neoplasms in children can be limited by first determining the compartment of the lesion (intramedullary, intradural-extramedullary, or extradural).

The most common pediatric spinal cord mass is an astrocytoma, which is a long segment intramedullary, often eccentric, mass that may be partially cystic or have an enhancing nodule.

The second most common pediatric spinal cord neoplasm is an ependymoma, which is an intramedullary, often central, mass that may have a hemosiderin cap.

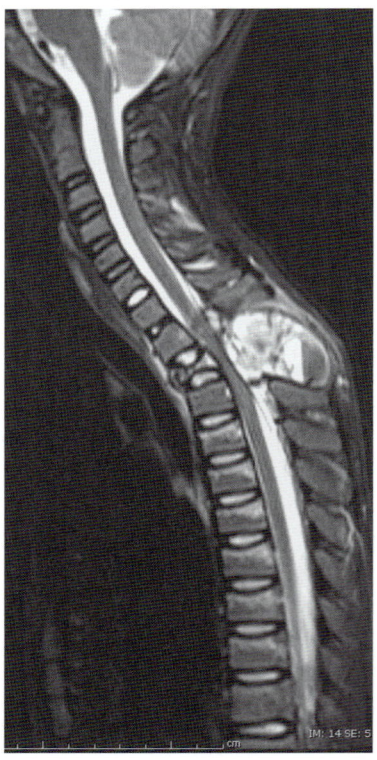

Figure 45-15   An aneurysmal bone cyst in a 10-year-old girl with back pain. A sagittal T2-weighted image demonstrates a multiloculated, expansile lesion with fluid levels in the T3 posterior elements. Compression of T3 causes effacement of the adjacent spinal canal.

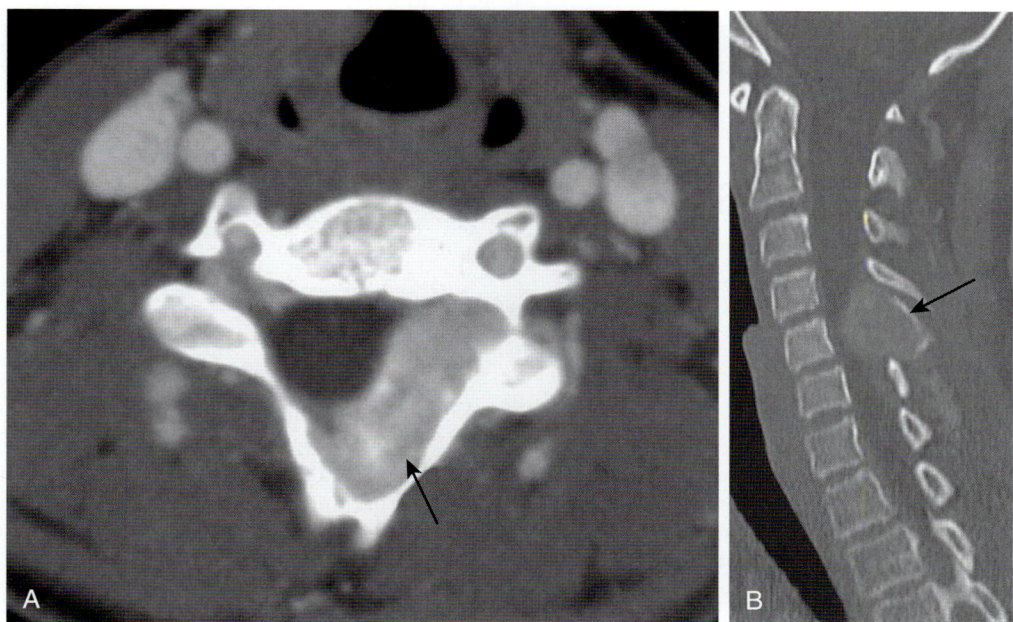

Figure 45-16   Osteoblastoma in 14-year-old boy with left neck pain and paresthesias. **A,** Axial contrast-enhanced computed tomography (CT) soft tissue windows demonstrate an enhancing epidural lesion (*arrow*) with rightward cord displacement. **B,** A sagittal cervical spine CT image demonstrates an expansile mass arising from the posterior element of C5 (*arrow*).

Suggested Readings

Crawford JR, Zaninovic A, Santi M, et al. Primary spinal cord tumors of childhood: effects of clinical presentation, radiographic features, and pathology on survival. *J Neurooncol.* 2009;95:259-269.

Jallo GI, Freed D, Epstein F. Intramedullary spinal cord tumors in children. *Childs Nerv Syst.* 2003;19:641-649.

Rossi A, Gandolfo C, Morana G, et al. Tumors of the spine in children. *Neuroimaging Clin N Am.* 2007;17(1):17-35.

References

Full references for this chapter can be found on www.expertconsult.com.

Chapter 46

Vascular Lesions

SARAH S. MILLA and LISA H. LOWE

Vascular lesions of the spine are uncommon in the pediatric population. The most common vascular lesions include fast-flow lesions such as arteriovenous malformations (AVMs) and arteriovenous fistulas (AVFs). Less common are venous (formerly "cavernous") malformations and spinal cord infarcts. Several syndromes are associated with spinal cord AVMs and AVFs, including hereditary hemorrhagic telangiectasia (Osler-Weber-Rendu), neurofibromatosis, and Parkes-Weber, Cobb, and CLOVES (congenital, lipomatous, overgrowth, vascular malformations, epidermal nevi, and spinal/skeletal anomalies or scoliosis) syndromes.[1,2] Pediatric spinal AVMs and AVFs presenting at less than 2 years of age are especially likely to occur in association with syndromes such as hereditary hemorrhagic telangiectasia.[1,3] However, recent reports have indicated that the association between Klippel-Trénaunay syndrome and AVMs may be erroneous. In a review of 208 patients with Klippel-Trénaunay syndrome, none was found to have spinal AVMs, as has been reported previously.[4] Further review revealed that many patients previously reported in the literature as having Klippel-Trénaunay syndrome and spinal AVMs likely had CLOVES syndrome.[5] This finding underscores the issues surrounding variable and inconsistent classification of pediatric vascular lesions.

Classification

Vascular lesions of the spine have undergone various classifications,[1,6-10] in part because of the complexity of their diagnosis and features. The term "spinal arteriovenous shunt" is used to encompass both types of high-flow lesions (AVMs and AVFs). Because AVMs and AVFs are found in various locations (i.e., intramedullary, intradural extramedullary, and extradural sites) with variable feeding vessels, structural features, drainage, and hemodynamic changes, additional subclassifications have been proposed.[6,8,9] On the basis of histopathologic discoveries, pediatric vascular anomalies increasingly have been classified using the International Society for the Study of Vascular Anomalies (ISSVA) system first published by Mulliken and Glowacki.[3,11,12] This system, which allows for correlation between lesion histology, clinical presentation, and treatment, is now used widely by pediatric subspecialists including dermatologists, interventional radiologists, plastic surgeons, and neurosurgeons.[10] The ISSVA classification system divides lesions into two broad categories neoplasms and vascular anomalies.[10-12] Vascular anomalies are further divided into slow/low (venous and/or lymphatic components) and fast/high (arterial components) flow lesions.[3] This chapter discusses pediatric vascular anomalies, including fast-flow vascular anomalies such as AVMs and AVFs, and slow-flow venous (formerly "cavernous") malformations. Spinal cord infarcts are also discussed in this chapter although as neither neoplasms nor vascular malformations, and they fall outside the ISSVA system.

Arteriovenous Malformations

Overview and Etiology AVMs are high-flow congenital communications between arteries and veins that result in arteriovenous shunting, causing the involved vessels to become enlarged and tortuous.[12] AVMs contain a nidus (a Latin word meaning "nest"), or vascular network, that communicates between the arteries and veins. The high-flow dynamics within the AVM predisposes the involved arteries to aneurysm and veins to variceal formation.[10] AVMs can be characterized further by the location of the nidus (within the spinal cord or on the cord surface), as well as by morphology of the nidus (the central, tightly formed "glomus" type or the diffuse, typically extensive, extramedullary "juvenile" or "metameric" type). In the pediatric population, the glomus spinal cord fast-flow AVM is the most common. In one large pediatric series, twice as many children had AVMs as had AVFs.[6] AVMs may occur anywhere along the spine in approximate proportion with each segment, including 30% to 40% cervical and 60% to 70% thoracolumbar.

Clinical Presentation The initial clinical presentation varies from acute paraparesis to slowly progressive myelopathy with weakness, sensory loss, and bowel and bladder dysfunction. Hemorrhage is more commonly seen in children (78%) compared with adults, especially in cervical cord AVMs. Children present acutely because of an arteriovenous malformation hemorrhage in 56% of cases.[6]

Imaging Magnetic resonance imaging (MRI) is the best noninvasive modality for initial diagnosis and follow-up of a spinal arteriovenous shunt.[6,13] Imaging findings of spinal cord AVMs include tortuous dilated vessels that can be within or on the surface of the cord. Hemorrhage has a variable appearance on T1-weighted and T2-weighted images depending on chronicity. T2-weighted images may demonstrate spinal cord edema and expansion.[3] MRI also documents the presence of cord cavitation, atrophy, and venous thrombosis. Images obtained after administration of gadolinium may reveal cord enhancement, which is attributed to venous stasis, ischemia, or spinal cord infarction[1] (Fig. 46-1). Distinguishing normal physiologic cerebrospinal fluid (CSF) pulsation and flow (particularly in the dorsal extramedullary midthoracic region) from vascular abnormalities requires optimization of spine imaging, which may include switching the phase and frequency encoding directions to decrease the effect of physiologic CSF pulsation. Computed tomography has a limited role in imaging AVMs but may document bony changes often seen in large, diffuse metameric-type lesions. Although MRI is excellent for the initial diagnosis, spinal angiography remains the gold standard for diagnosis and delineation of AVMs.

Treatment   Endovascular embolization is the primary line of treatment for fast-flow vascular anomalies, with the exception of lesions at the conus, which are managed surgically.[1,3,6] In cases in which complete embolization or resection are not possible because of an unacceptable risk of morbidity or mortality, the goal of treatment is to reach a hemodynamic equilibrium between the lesion and the spinal cord that will reduce the risk of ischemia and hemorrhage.[14,15]

Prognosis   A spectrum of outcomes may occur depending on the lesion location, presentation, and treatment.[15] The severity of symptoms at the time of diagnosis is directly related to patient outcome, with most symptoms persisting partially or completely after treatment.[14]

Arteriovenous Fistula

Overview and Etiology   The term AVF is used to describe a fast-flow lesion with a direct artery to vein fistula without a focal nidus, which is seen with AVMs. It is thought that AVFs likely are an acquired deformity resulting from microvascular injury and reparative healing, leading to an abnormal communication between an artery and vein.[8,16] In a large pediatric and adult series, a higher percentage of multiple spinal cord fistulas was present in pediatric patients (46%) compared with adults (27%).[6] AVFs are divided by location into two groups, spinal cord and spinal dural. Spinal cord AVFs are perimedullary in location and one third as common as AVMs in children. Spinal dural AVFs are extremely rare in the pediatric population.[6]

Clinical Presentation   The clinical presentation of AVFs is similar to AVMs, including slowly progressive weakness, sensory loss, and bowel and bladder dysfunction due to venous congestion, venous hypertension, and resultant myelopathy. However, AVFs hemorrhage less than AVMs, and acute presentations are uncommon.[6]

Imaging   Imaging findings of spinal cord AVFs are virtually identical to spinal cord AVMs in the pediatric population.[1] Dural AVFs, which are common in adults, are uncommon in children.[6]

Treatment   Because each spinal AVF is unique, treatment must be tailored to the specific lesion, taking into account location, size, number of fistula formation sites, and associated symptoms.[3] Therapies are the same as for other fast-flow anomalies, including endovascular embolization, microsurgical resection, radiation therapy (used rarely), or a combination of these therapies.[1,3,17] Endovascular embolization has the advantage of being less invasive than the other therapies, but the feeding arteries may not be accessible, and thus open surgery may be needed in some cases.[18]

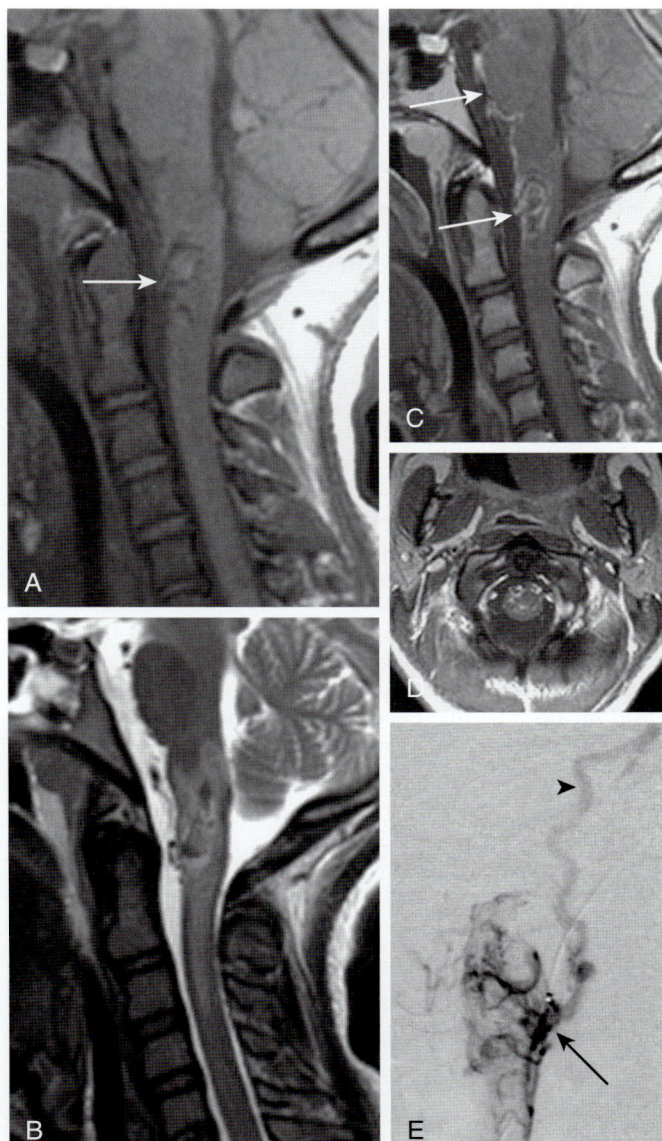

Figure 46-1   Arteriovenous malformation in a 14-year-old girl with sudden onset of severe headache, left-sided weakness, and loss of consciousness. Head computed tomography (not shown) revealed intraventricular hemorrhage. **A,** A sagittal T1-weighted image shows a hypointense lesion with subtle foci of high signal hemorrhage (*arrow*). **B,** A sagittal T2-weighted image confirms low-signal central hemorrhage with hyperintense surrounding edema. **C** and **D,** Postcontrast T1-weighted sagittal and axial images demonstrate enhancing superficial serpiginous vessels and peripheral intramedullary enhancement (*arrows*). **E,** A catheter angiogram injection of the vertebral artery reveals an intramedullary nidus (*arrow*) with arterial supply from anterior and lateral spinal artery contributors. Venous drainage is toward the jugular bulb via a recurrent perimedullary vein (*arrowhead*).

Prognosis Early diagnosis of AVFs is essential to preserve neurological function. Patient outcome is proportional to the severity of symptoms at the time of diagnosis. Patients who are nonambulatory and those with poor bladder or bowel function before treatment are unlikely to regain neurological functions after therapy.[17,18]

Venous (Cavernous) Malformations

Overview Slow-flow venous (cavernous) malformations (VMs), also previously termed cavernous angiomas and cavernomas, are congenital vascular malformations made up of dysmorphic venous vascular spaces lined by a single layer of endothelial cells with no intervening neural tissue.[19] According to the ISSVA classification system, VMs of the spinal cord have been reclassified as slow-flow vascular anomalies. Similarly, venous vertebral anomalies were previously misclassified as hemangiomas, although they are neoplastic. Pathologically, the cells of this lesion are anomalous vessels that do not divide and undergo mitosis because they are not neoplasms. Unfortunately, some classification systems still refer to this malformation as a neoplasm, which may lead to confusion.[8] The term venous (cavernous) VM, rather than the misnomer cavernoma, should be used to avoid confusion with a true neoplasm. Spinal cord VMs are less common than similar lesions found in the brain, with one study showing that 5% of pediatric VMs are located within the spine.[20]

Etiology The specific etiology of spinal VMs is unclear. However, the presence of multiple brain and/or spinal VMs in any pediatric patient at presentation should prompt a careful history and genetic analysis. Associated mutations predisposing patients to multiple VMs have been found on chromosomes 3 and 7, with an autosomal-dominant variable penetrance pattern of inheritance.[20] Deep venous anomalies are associated with sporadic VMs in up to 40% of cases.

Patients who previously have undergone radiation therapy, typically of the craniospinal axis, are predisposed to the development of a VM. Approximately 12% to 16% of pediatric patients have multiple lesions.[20,21]

Clinical Presentation The clinical presentation of VMs is a result of hemorrhage and ranges from nearly asymptomatic to severe neurologic symptoms. Pediatric patients are more likely to have a sudden clinical onset compared with adults, with up to 75% of children presenting acutely with hemorrhage.[20]

Imaging MRI findings of spinal cord VMs are similar to their intracranial counterparts, with T1-weighted signal heterogeneity within the lesion caused by blood products of varying age. On T2-weighted imaging, a hypointense rim representing hemosiderin is typical, with an internal heterogeneous T2 signal. Cord edema may be seen if recent hemorrhage has occurred (Fig. 46-2). On T2★ gradient recalled echo imaging and more recently reported susceptibility weighted imaging, a prominent blooming effect is noted because of the susceptibility effect of hemorrhage degradation products.[22] Susceptibility imaging has been shown to be significantly better than T2★ gradient imaging at detecting hemorrhage.[22] Distinguishing a spinal cord VM from other pathologies can be difficult in some cases but usually is based on identification of the classic rim of hemosiderin along the lesion margins and the absence of other morphologic features that would suggest a neoplasm, such as an enhancing mass.[19] Because VMs are very slow-flow lesions, they typically are not seen on catheter angiography.

Treatment Asymptomatic VMs and those located in delicate regions are treated conservatively in many cases rather than with endovascular techniques. Although symptomatic venous malformations located elsewhere in the body often are treated initially with sclerotherapy, this treatment is not an option

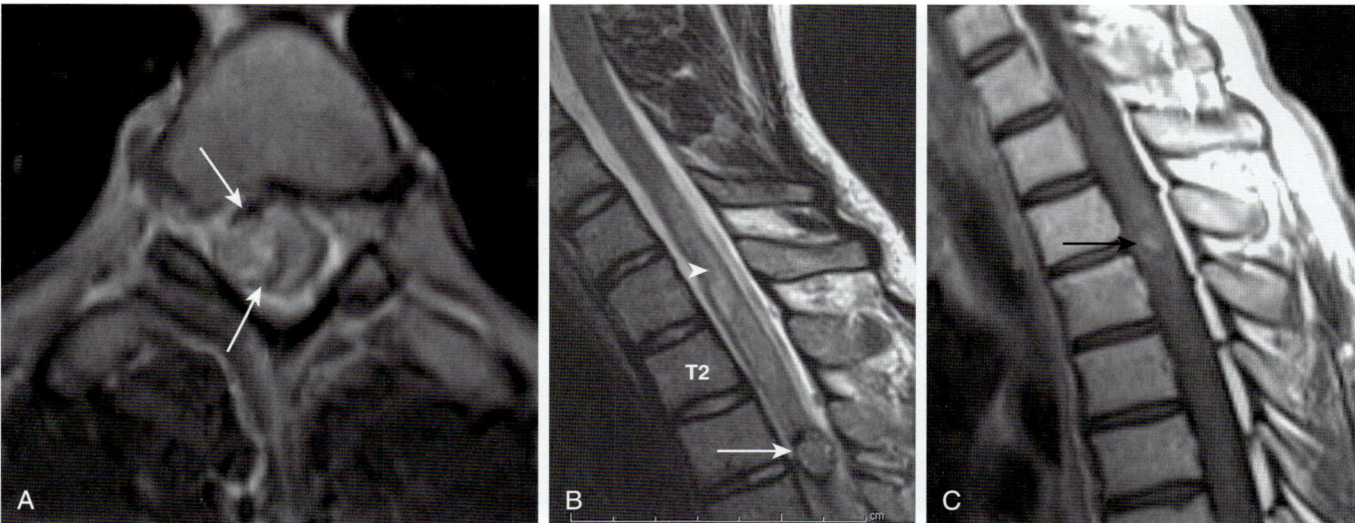

Figure 46-2 Venous (cavernous) malformation in a 16-year-old boy with arm weakness. **A** and **B,** Axial and sagittal T2-weighted images demonstrate a centrally hyperintense intramedullary lesion with a hypointense rim (*arrows*). Central bright signal cord edema is noted proximally as well (*arrowhead*). **C,** A postcontrast T1-weighted image shows no enhancement. Central hyperintense hemorrhage within the lesion (*arrow*) also was seen on precontrast T1-weighted images (not shown).

for intramedullary spinal cord lesions. Instead, patients with symptomatic spinal cord lesions may undergo surgical resection or, rarely, radiotherapy when the lesions are found in hard-to-reach locations.[19,21]

Prognosis The immediate postoperative outcome after VM resection in one study showed that 11% of patients had worse symptoms, 83% were the same, and 6% were improved. At 5-year follow-up, the percentages of patients who were the same and improved were 68% and 23%, respectively,[23] showing a moderate response to treatment.

Spinal Cord Infarction

Overview Infarction of the spinal cord is uncommon, particularly in children. The most vulnerable region of the spinal cord is the anterior half, which is supplied by the single anterior spinal artery. The posterior spinal cord is supplied by paired paramedian posterior spinal arteries, allowing more extensive collateral circulation.

Etiology Trauma and infection (e.g., meningitis) are the most common causes of cord infarction in children.[24] Other causes of spinal cord infarction include thrombotic and/or embolic phenomena from cardiac disease, hypercoagulable states, umbilical arterial lines, or fibrocartilaginous embolization, as well as hypoperfusion and cardiac arrest.[24,25] Fibrocartilaginous embolization is well described in dogs in the veterinary literature, and rarely occurs in humans. Fibrocartilaginous embolization is believed to result from vertical disc herniation and embolization of the nucleus pulposus. The mechanism by which disc fragments enter the spinal artery is unclear, and some authors do not subscribe to this causality.[25,26]

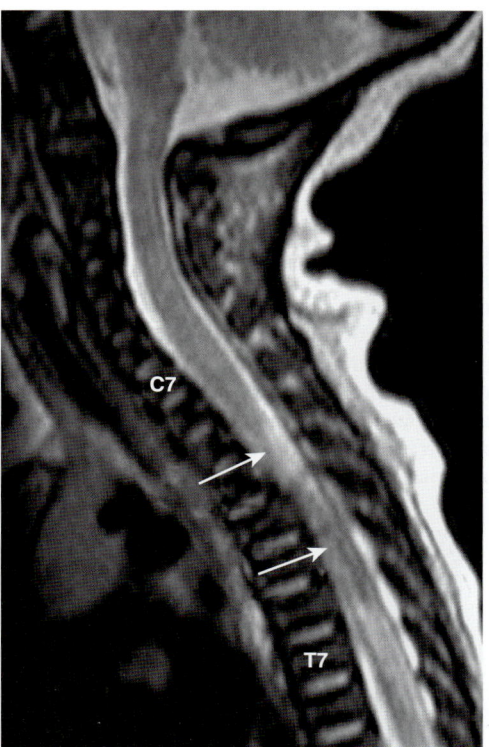

Figure 46-3 A thoracic spinal cord infarct in a newborn boy with paraplegia as a result of a traumatic delivery. Sagittal T2-weighted magnetic resonance image reveals a large region of heterogeneous signal intensity (*arrows*) due to cord transection. Proximal hyperintense edema also is seen. Labeled are the seventh cervical (C7) and thoracic (T7) vertebrae.

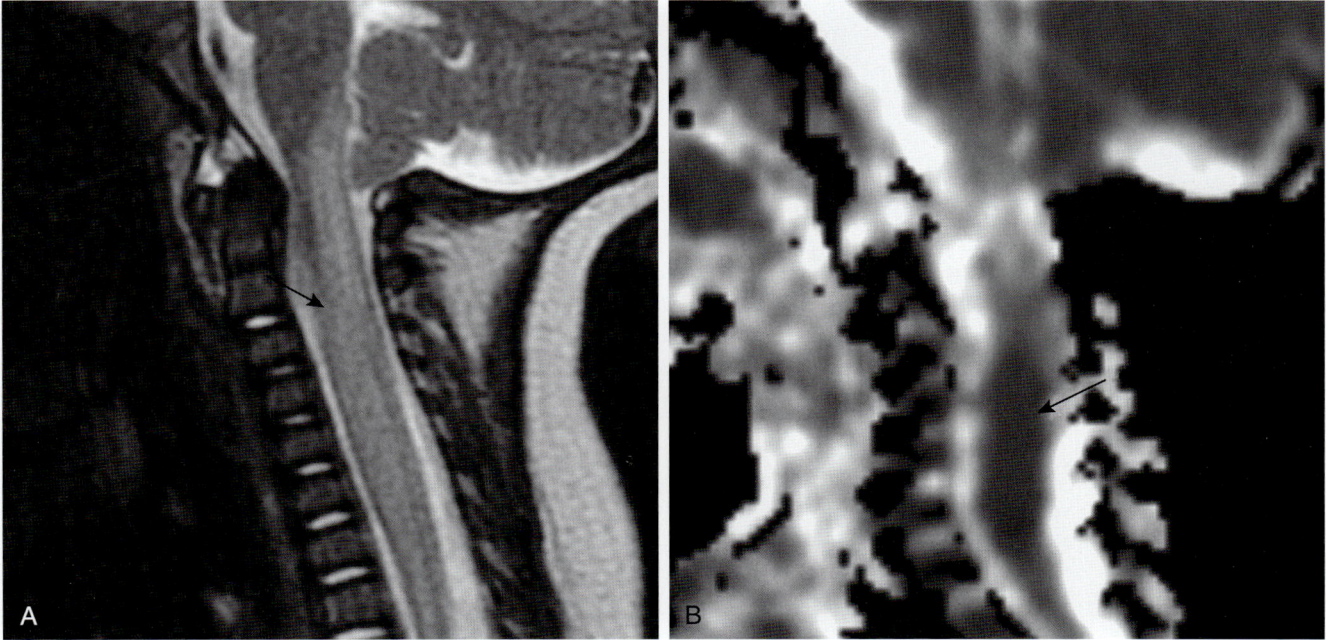

Figure 46-4 Cord ischemia as a result of infection from herpes simplex virus type 6. **A,** A sagittal fast spin echo T2-weighted magnetic resonance image shows T2 hyperintensity and cord swelling as a result of edema (*arrow*). **B,** An apparent diffusion coefficient map of a sagittal echo planar diffusion-weighted image shows hypointensity representing cytotoxic cord edema (*arrow*). The findings are consistent with necrotizing myelitis.

Clinical Presentation Spinal cord infarction most often presents with acute paraparesis or quadriparesis depending on the level of cord involvement.[26]

Imaging Because the single anterior artery supplies the anterior two thirds of the spinal cord, infarction often shows anterior cord involvement of both gray and white matter, seen as T1-weighted hypointensity and T2-weighted hyperintensity (Fig. 46-3). T2-weighted hyperintensity may not be seen initially if MRI is performed in a hyperacute setting. Cord edema and swelling can be seen acutely, and contrast enhancement can occur in the subacute (>5 days) phase.[27] Current MRI techniques allow diffusion imaging of the spinal cord as a supplement to standard sequences to confirm ischemia[27,28] (Fig. 46-4). In the differential diagnosis of cord infarction is transverse myelitis, which is more common than cord infarction in children (see Chapter 44).[29] Isolated involvement of the spinal cord gray matter suggests an infectious or postinfectious autoimmune process rather than infarction. Fibrocartilaginous embolization may be suspected when the infarct is located in the lumbar spine in association with adjacent disc disease (Fig. 46-5). Careful review of the patient's history, spinal fluid analysis, and the anatomic distribution of signal abnormality in spinal gray and/or white matter may be helpful to distinguish cord infarct from transverse myelitis.[24,29]

Treatment Supportive care is largely the only treatment for spinal cord infarct due to fibrocartilaginous embolization. Methylprednisone may be given in the acute setting to help limit cord edema, but its utility is questionable.[25,29]

Prognosis The outcome of cord infarction depends on the initial symptoms. Unfortunately, symptoms such as paraparesis and paraplegia seen at presentation often persist.[25,26]

Summary

Spinal vascular lesions in children are rare but have significant neurologic presentations and sequelae. Diagnosis of such a lesion should prompt evaluation for an underlying syndrome or genetic predisposition. Advances in histopathologic knowledge have allowed development of the ISSVA classification system, which improves correlation between the type of pediatric vascular anomaly, lesion treatment, and outcome. Newer imaging techniques can help characterize fast-flow spinal cord arteriovenous shunts, as well as slow-flow vascular lesions and spinal cord infarcts.

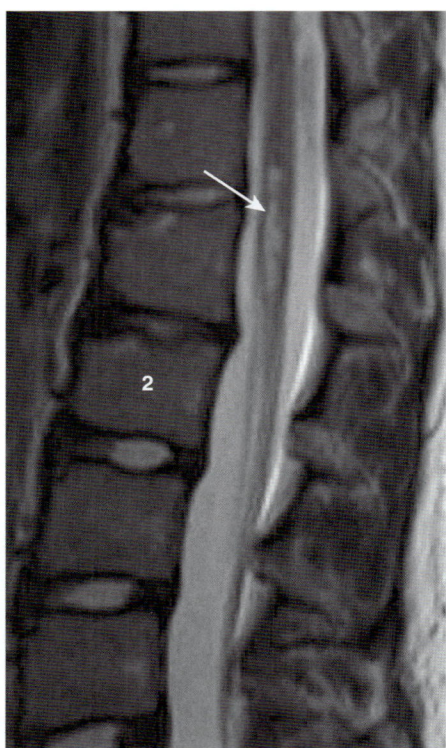

Figure 46-5 A lumbar spinal cord infarct in a 13-year-old girl with pain and leg weakness for 2 weeks, possibly fibrocartilaginous in etiology. Sagittal T2-weighted magnetic resonance image reveals a well-defined region of oblong hyperintensity (*arrow*). Irregularity at the anterior superior margin of L1 and L2 are consistent with Schmorl nodes.

Suggested Readings

Bemporad JA, Sze G. Magnetic resonance imaging of spinal cord vascular malformations with an emphasis on the cervical spine. *Neuroimaging Clin N Am.* 2001;11:111-129.

Boo S, Hartel J, Hogg JP. Vascular abnormalities of the spine: an imaging review. *Curr Probl Diagn Radiol.* 2010;39(3):110-117.

Mulliken JB, Glowacki J. Hemangiomas and vascular malformations in infants and children: a classification based on endothelial characteristics. *Plast reconstr Surg.* 1982;69:412-422.

Nagib MG, O'Fallon MT. Intramedullary cavernous angiomas of the spinal cord in the pediatric age group: a pediatric series. *Pediatr Neurosurg.* 2002;36:57-63.

Nozaki T, Nosaka S, Miyazaki O. Syndromes associated with vascular tumors and malformations: a pictorial review. *Radiographics.* 2013;33(1):175-195.

References

Full references for this chapter can be found on www.expertconsult.com.

Chapter 47

Trauma

LISA H. LOWE and PETER WINNINGHAM

Mortality of spine-related trauma in children is higher than in adults and is estimated at 25% to 32%.[1] Fortunately, children with incomplete neurologic lesions fare better compared with adults, with up to 90% having partial recovery and 60% having full recovery.[1,2]

Etiology

Motor vehicle accidents (MVAs), followed by falls and sports injuries, are the most common causes of pediatric spinal trauma. Young athletes are at higher risk for developing stress-related injuries than are adult athletes.[3] Gunshot injuries accounted for 22% of injuries in one study of 277 pediatric patients with spinal trauma.[4] Congenital spine anomalies such as os odontoideum, block vertebrae, Klippel-Feil syndrome, and Down syndrome increase the risk of cervical spinal injury. Nerve root avulsion with pseudomeningocele formation may result from birth trauma, MVAs, or less often, penetrating injury (Fig. 47-1).[5]

Younger children are more susceptible to upper cervical injuries compared with adults because of their relatively large-sized, heavy craniums and weaker neck muscles.[6] This anatomy causes a more cranial fulcrum of movement at C2-C3 in younger children versus C5-C6 in older children and adults.[1] Injuries in younger children, especially those under 8 years, differ from those in older children. Because of greater mobility and laxity of ligaments in the cervical spine of younger children, they tend to have higher cervical injuries (occiput to C3). These injuries are more likely associated with a neurologic deficit and to extend through synchondroses.[7]

SCIWORA

The unique biomechanical properties of young children, including their large-sized heads and higher fulcrum of motion, causes increased occurrence of spinal cord injury without radiographic abnormality (SCIWORA). The acronym SCIWORA was popularized in the early 1980s to describe children with clinical symptoms of cervical cord trauma and normal radiographs.[8] With the introduction of magnetic resonance imaging (MRI), injuries in children with SCIWORA could be visualized and the general prognosis predicted on the basis of the findings.[9,10] MRI allows for the diagnosis of SCIWORA by easily showing the findings of cord contusion, including hypointensity on T1-weighted imaging and hyperintensity on T2-weighted imaging, cord hemorrhage, or cord transaction (Fig. 47-2).[11] The presence of normal cord signal suggests the child will make a complete recovery, whereas intramedullary hemorrhage and transection portend a poor prognosis.[8]

Atlanto-Occipital Disassociation

Because of their relatively small occipital condyles and more horizontal atlanto-occipital joint orientation, young children are at increased risk for atlanto-occipital disassociation.[2,9,12] Devastating spinal cord injury often occurs, and many cases are fatal. A diagnosis is made by measuring a condylar gap greater than 5 mm (Kaufman condylar gap) or a basion to axis interval (BAI) of greater than 12 mm (Fig. 47-3).[2] One pitfall is that in children younger than 13 years, the BAI is less reliable.[12] Some helpful measurements to evaluate pediatric cervical spine trauma are listed in Table 47-1.[13] Atlanto-occipital dissassociation requires urgent stabilization.

Atlas or Jefferson Fracture

Compression loading forces on the cervical spine can result in a C1 burst fracture, or Jefferson fracture. This injury is most common in adolescents from MVAs and diving accidents. Jefferson fractures show between one and four defects in the C1 ring. The fracture may be stable or unstable, depending on whether or not the transverse ligament is intact or ruptured, respectively. A single defect in the ring is typically stable, whereas three or four defects are typically unstable.[9] A dens to C1 lateral mass distance of greater than 8 mm suggests instability. Forty percent of Jefferson fractures have an associated C2 fracture.[12] Lateral cervical spine radiographs are of little value, and the diagnosis is made on the open-mouth odontoid view by showing offset of the lateral masses of C1 on C2 (Fig. 47-4).[13] Pitfalls to avoid include rotation of the head on the open-mouth view that may cause the lateral mass to appear slightly laterally displaced, hypermobility in young children that may lead to minimal normal lateral displacement of C1 on C2 and finally, the normal developmental bilateral offset of the C1 lateral masses that may occur

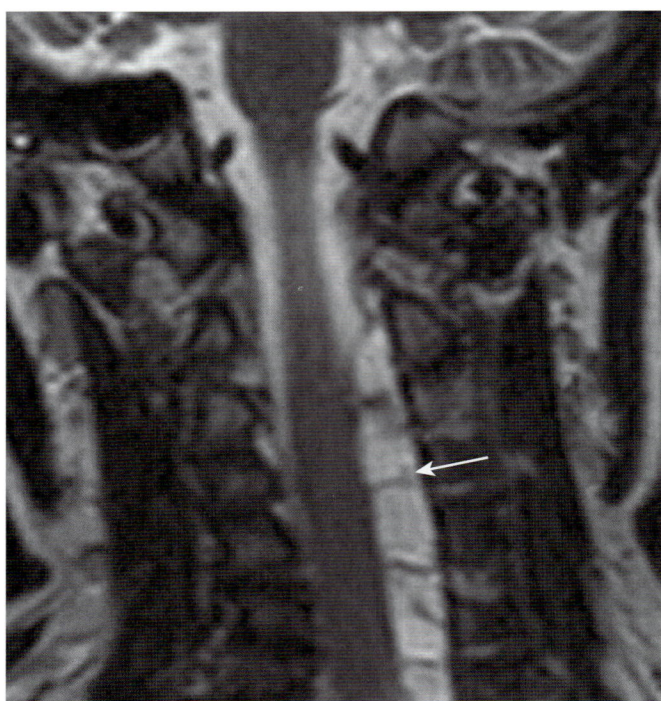

Figure 47-1   Avulsed nerve roots in a 13-year-old girl unable to use her left arm after an all-terrain vehicle accident. A coronal T2-weighted magnetic resonance image shows an extensive intradural cerebral spinal fluid collection (*arrow*) shifting the spinal cord (*C*) to the right due to C2 to T1 nerve root avulsions.

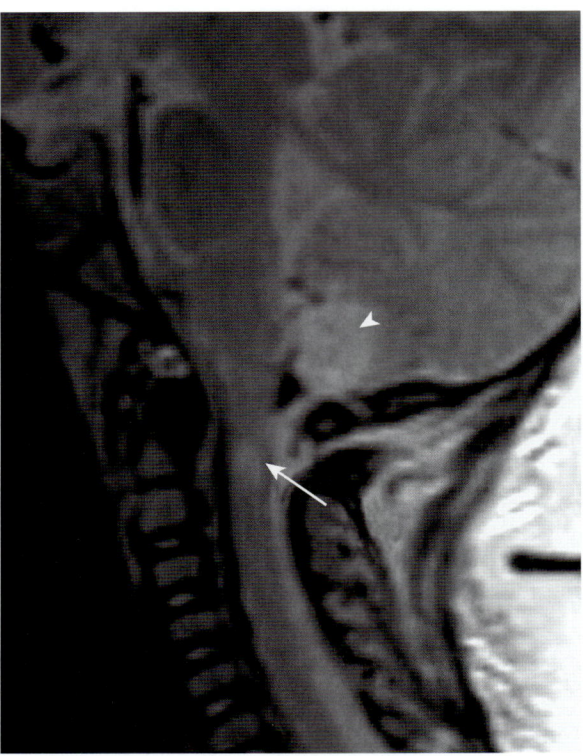

Figure 47-2   Spinal cord injury without radiographic abnormality (SCIWORA) in a 6-year-old boy with paraplegia after a fall from a horse and normal cervical spine radiographs. Sagittal magnetic resonance image of the craniocervical junction reveals hyperintense T2 contusions within the cervical spinal cord (*arrow*) and the inferior cervical vermis (*arrowhead*). Note T2 dark hemorrhage in the cerebral spinal fluid at the level of the foramen magnum just below the vermian contusion.

in children under 2 years of age because of the differential growth of C1 versus C2.[9]

Atlantoaxial Rotatory Force Injury

The atlantoaxial joint is responsible for 50% of normal range of motion of the neck. Temporary ligamentous laxity following infection or surgery in the head and neck because of hyperemic, inflamed synovial tissues with secondary contractures causes mild atlantoaxial rotatory subluxation (AARS), or Grisel syndrome. A similar situation, sometimes referred to as "wry neck," occurs in normal children who simply

awaken with a stiff neck and are unable to turn their head to one side.[9] Grisel syndrome and wry neck represent a mild form of C1 on C2 rotatory subluxation that is caused by muscle spasm and is self-limiting. With frank rotatory dislocation, children present with torticollis, holding their heads in a peculiar "cock robin" position, head rotated to one side and tilted to the other.[2] The duration of subluxation is proportional to the risk of recurrence. When rotatory injury is fixed, the term *atlantoaxial rotatory fixation (AARF)* may be

Table 47-1

Cervical Spine Measurements Useful in Evaluation of Pediatric Trauma			
Imaging Sign	**Definition**	**Normal**	**Injury**
Predental distance	Distance between posterior inferior C1 arch to anterior dens	Age 0-8years: <5 mm Age 8+ years: <3 mm Flexion/extension: <2 mm change	C1-C2 ligamentous injury
C1-C2 interspinous interval	Distance between C1-C2 spinous processes	<12 mm	C1-C2 ligamentous injury
Basion dens interval	Distance between basion to superior tip of dens	<12 mm	Atlanto-occipital distraction
Condylar gap	Distance between occipital and C1 condyles	<5 mm	Atlanto-occipital distraction
Dens to C1 lateral masses	Distance from dens to bilateral lateral C1 masses	Must be symmetric right to left >8 mm suggests instability	AARS,[1] AARF,[2] Jefferson fracture
Posterior cervical line	Line between C1 and C3 anterior spinous process cortex	Anterior spinous process cortex of C2 is missed by >1.5 mm	Hangman fracture

AARS, atlantoaxial rotatory subluxation; AARF, atlantoaxial rotatory fixation.

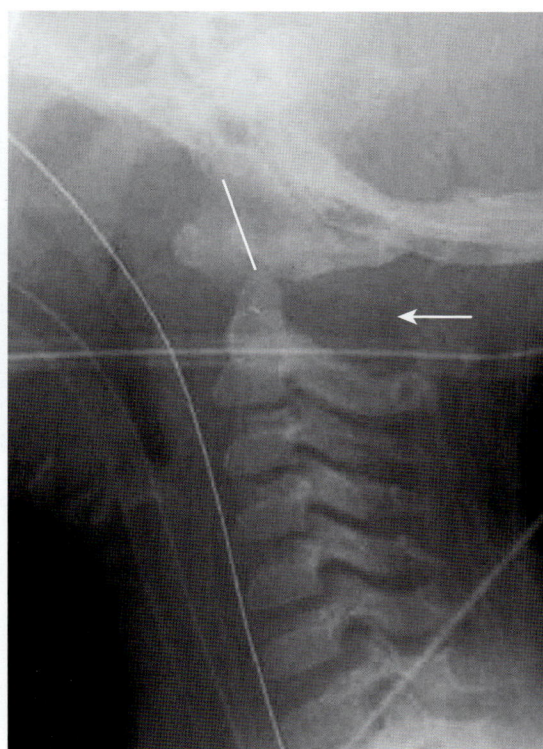

Figure 47-3 Atlantoaxial disassociation in a 5-year-old unrestrained girl after a motor vehicle accident. Lateral cervical spine radiograph demonstrates abnormally increased basion to dens distance of 15 mm (*white line*). The C1-C2 interspinous distance is also increased at greater than 12 mm (*arrow*).

Table 47-2

Fielding Classification of Atlantoaxial Rotatory Subluxation	
Type	**Description**
I	Rotatory displacement of C1 on dens without anterior displacement; most common type
II	3-5 mm of anterior C1 displacement with rotation centered on the lateral facets possibly disrupting the transverse ligaments
III	>5 mm anterior C1 displacement with rotation centered on lateral facets possibly disrupting the transverse ligament, alar ligament, and facet capsule
IV	Posterior C1 displacement on C2 of both lateral facets; rarely seen in adults with rheumatoid arthritis

applied. Atlantoaxial rotatory force injury is classified into four types, according to Fielding and Hawkins (Table 47-2).[14] Mild rotatory anomalies may be treated with muscle relaxers and physical therapy, but more aggressive management may include traction and, rarely, surgery, to prevent osseous fusion at C1-C2.[2] An imaging diagnosis of AARS is suggested by the presence of asymmetry in the dens to C1 lateral mass distance on open–mouth odontoid radiographs and computed tomography (CT) scans (Fig. 47-5). CT signs of rotatory disorders include loss of articulation of the occiput and C1 as well as sclerosis on both sides of the joint with impending fusion (Fig. 47-6).

Odontoid (Dens) Fractures

Dens fractures, or odontoid fractures, are common in all age groups. The rigid, upright nature of dens makes it susceptible to a variety of flexion, loading, and extension forces.[9] In young children, the odontoid is separated from the body of C2 by a cartilaginous synchondrosis, which fuses between the ages of 5 and 7 years.[9] The presence of the synchondrosis in infants and young children allows fractures to occur frequently through this growth plate, but fortunately, these fractures heal readily (Fig. 47-7). However, in adults, these fractures often interfere with blood supply to the odontoid, causing the fractures to be complicated by nonunion or pseudoarthroses.[1] Dens fractures are classified into three types, with only type 2 being unstable. Type 1 is through the tip of the dens, type 2 is through the base of the dens, and type 3 is through the body of C2.[2,9]

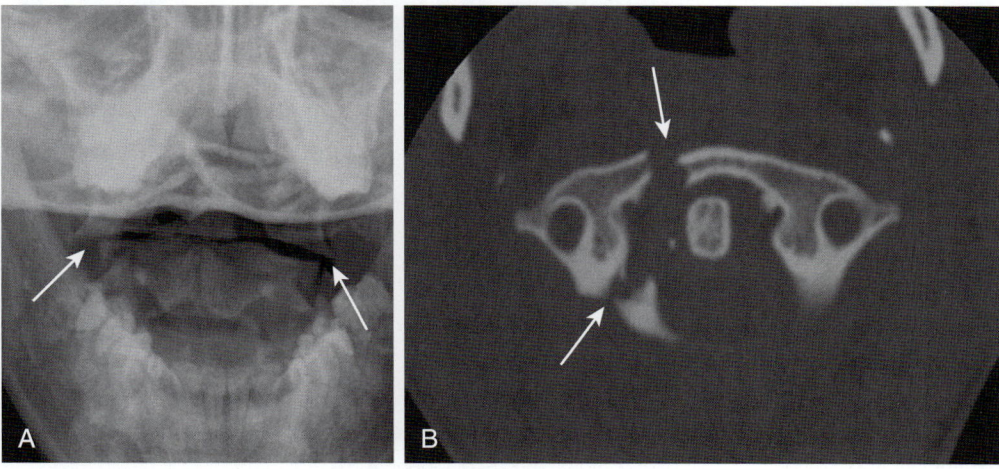

Figure 47-4 Jefferson fracture in an adolescent with unspecified trauma. **A,** Open-mouth odontoid view shows asymmetric bilateral offset of the lateral masses of C1 on C2 (*arrows*). **B,** An axial computed tomography image reveals fracture lucencies in the right anterior and posterior C1 arches (*arrows*).

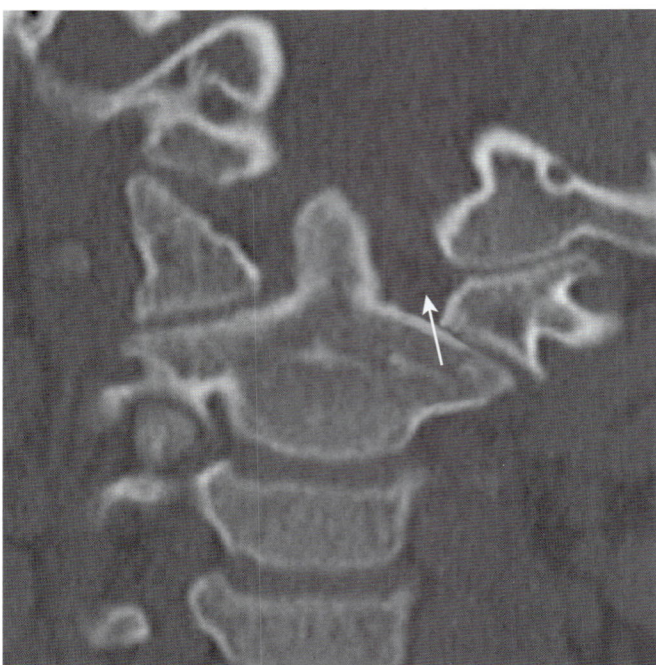

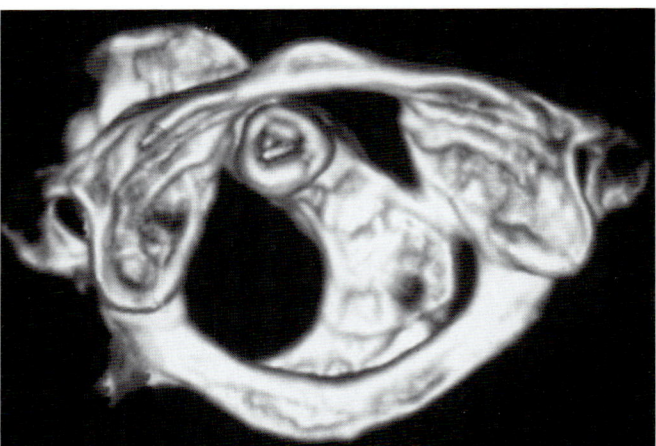

Figure 47-6 Atlantoaxial rotatory fixation (Fielding type 1) in a 15-year-old girl with rigid torticollis for 4 weeks following spinal manipulation. An axial three-dimensional cervical computed tomography image reveals rotation of C1 on C2 with loss of articulation of the condyles, but without anterior displacement of C1. Note normal distance between C1 and dens, which indicates a Fielding type 1 injury.

Figure 47-5 Atlantoaxial rotatory subluxation in a 13-year-old girl with torticollis for 2 weeks and no history of infection or trauma. A coronal reconstructed cervical spine computed tomography image shows widening of the atlantodental distance on the left (*arrow*) compared with the normal right side. This distance widened and narrowed when turning the head to the left and the right, respectively (*dynamic CT not shown*).

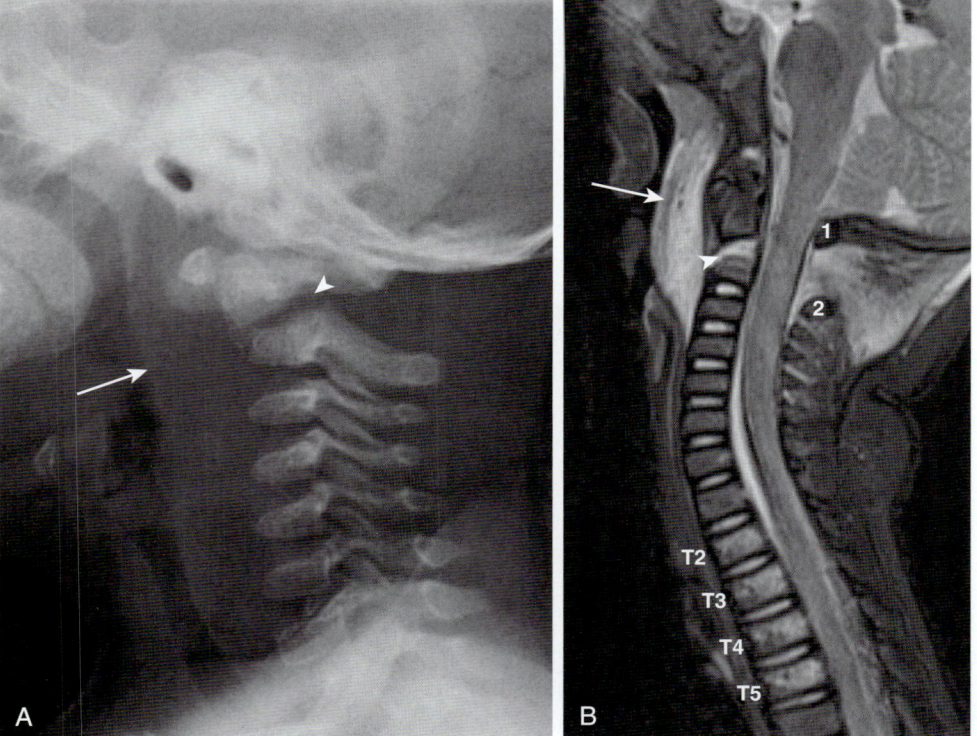

Figure 47-7 Odontoid fracture in a 12-month-old girl after a motor vehicle accident. **A,** Lateral cervical radiograph shows prevertebral soft tissue swelling (*arrow*), widening of the C2 synchondrosis (*arrowhead*), and anterior subluxation of the dens on the body of C2. **B,** Sagittal T2-weighted fat suppressed magnetic resonance image confirms the radiographic findings and also reveals additional vertebral contusions as hyperintense marrow signal of T2-T5. Ligamentous injury is seen as increase in the C1-C2 interspinous interval, which is filled with T2 bright soft tissue edema.

A pitfall to consider when searching for odontoid fractures is the presence of an os odontoideum, an oval or round ossicle of variable size with a smooth cortical border located in the expected position of the odontoid process. Small os odontoideums at the tip of the dens may be normal variants of no significance; however, when they are large enough to extend below the annular ligament, they could be unstable and susceptible to traumatic injury.[9] The etiology is controversial, but they are likely both posttraumatic and congenital in origin.[2,15]

Hangman Fracture

Hyperextension forces may cause fractures through the C2 pars intraarticularis, known as the *hangman fracture*. Often, these fractures are more complex in morphology being associated with combined flexion and extension forces in the same patient.[9] The C2 fracture lucency is diagnostic but may be difficult to visualize on neutral lateral radiographs (Fig. 47-8). It is more easily detected with flexion views. Application of the posterior cervical line (see Table 47-1) is helpful to diagnose the injury.[9] Hangman fractures may be unilateral or bilateral, in which case they are stable or unstable, respectively. In infants, one must be aware of the pitfall of congenital defects of C2 being confused with a hangman fracture. Congenital defects are distinguished by smooth, sclerotic, narrow margins. When hangman fractures are caused by airbag injuries, a high association with facial fractures exists.[9,16]

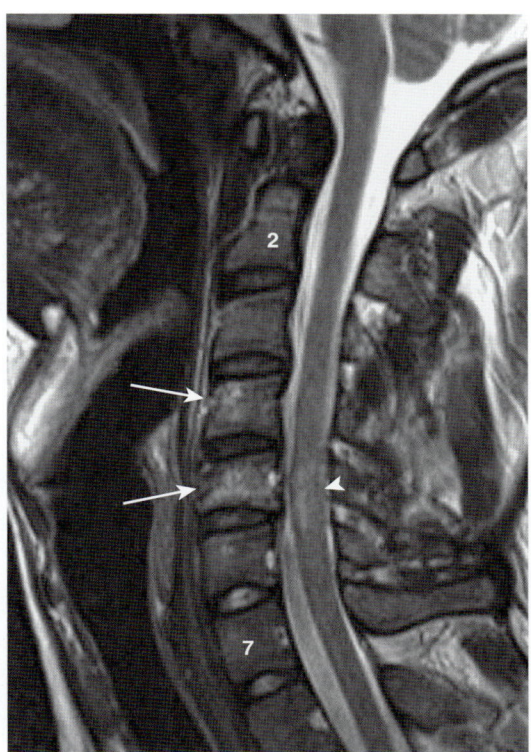

Figure 47-9 *Cervical spine compression fractures and cord contusion in a 17-year-old male after an all-terrain vehicle accident.* A sagittal T2-weighted magnetic resonance image shows hyperintense signal and decreased height of the anterior C4 and C5 vertebral bodies (*arrows*). T2 bright signal cord contusion is seen at the C5 level (*arrowhead*).

Thoracic and Lumbar Spine Fractures

Cervicothoracic junction injury is associated with breech deliveries, many of which present as SCIWORA or brachial plexus injuries, as previously discussed.[2] Associated findings also include T1 and T2 transverse process fractures.

Lower thoracic and upper lumbar spine injuries are most often caused by MVAs, with up to 50% having associated small bowel injury from seat-belt trauma.[2,17] Common lower thoracic and lumbar fractures include anterior column compressions, which are typically stable, and posterior column burst fractures, which are typically unstable (Fig. 47-9). Burst fractures occur with axial compression forces, causing endplate fracture extending into the anterior and posterior column (Fig. 47-10). Chance or seatbelt fractures are caused by flexion injury with horizontal extension through the posterior vertebral body, pedicles, and spinous processes (Fig. 47-11).[2]

Spondylolysis

Spondylolysis may be a congenital deformity or an acquired stress fracture extending through the pars interarticularis. It is thought to be most likely caused by repetitive flexion and extension in the adolescent spine and is often seen in

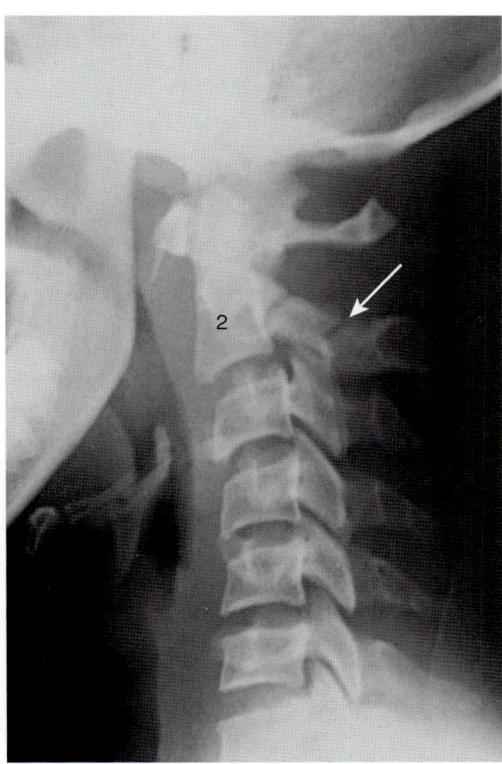

Figure 47-8 *Hangman fracture in a 15-year-old boy after an accidental fall.* A lateral cervical spine radiograph identifies lucency through the C2 posterior elements (*arrow*).

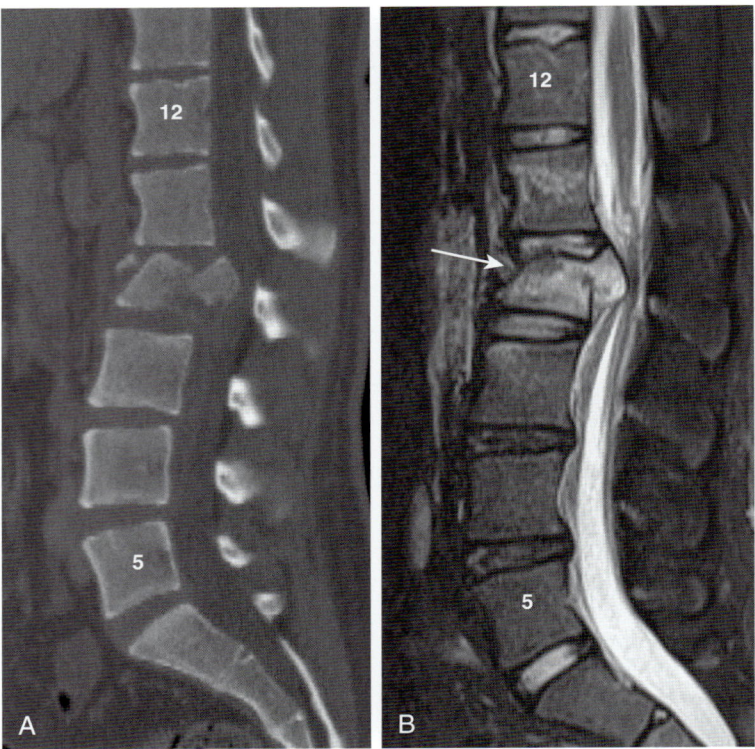

Figure 47-10 Burst fracture in a 16-year-old male with leg pain and weakness after a motor vehicle accident. **A,** A sagittal reformatted computed tomography image identifies a comminuted L2 fracture with a retropulsed fragment in the spinal canal. **B,** A sagittal FLAIR (fluid attenuated inversion recovery) magnetic resonance image confirms the fracture with retropulsed fragment compressing the cauda equina (*arrow*). In addition, T2 bright signal contusions in the adjacent L1 and L3 vertebral bodies are present.

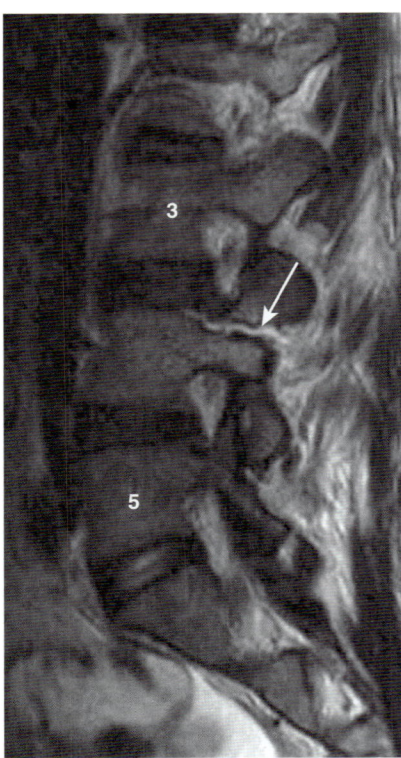

Figure 47-11 Chance fracture in a 5-year-old-boy unable to move his legs after a motor vehicle accident. A sagittal T2-weighted magnetic resonance image shows a horizontal fracture through the superior end-plate and pedicles of L4 (*arrow*). Associated surrounding T2 bright soft tissue edema is also seen.

athletes, having been reported in 11% of female gymnasts.[18] Lucency extends through the pars on radiography and CT, with MRI showing T2 bright signal in stress reactions and acute cases. Spondylolysis without spondylolisthesis is treated conservatively. Spondylolisthesis may require orthopedic stabilization depending on severity.

Spinal Cord Contusions and Transections

Spinal cord contusions and transections are a continuum of cord injuries that occur alongside fractures, ligamentous injuries, or both. Contusions are thought to occur secondary to shearing injuries, with rupture of the small intramedullary vessels resulting in focal petechia and edema, which, in some cases, progress to larger areas of hemorrhage in the cord and vascular compromise.[17] Complete cord transection, which has a very poor prognosis, typically results from extreme distraction or severe transverse shear injury (Fig. 47-12).[10]

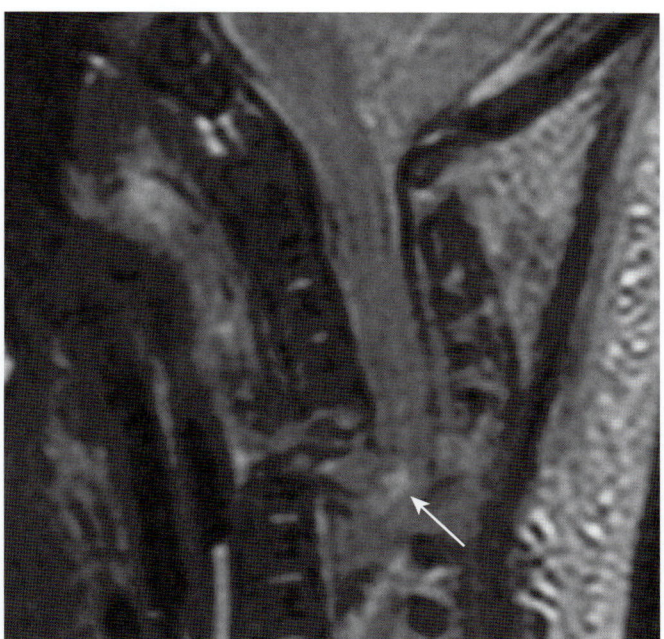

Figure 47-12   Cord transection in a newborn with distractive birth injury. A sagittal short tau inversion recovery magnetic resonance image shows disruption of the cervical vertebral column at C5-C6, transection of the spinal cord, and focal hyperintense signal within cord consistent with hyperacute edema and hemorrhage (*arrow*).

Key Points

The unique anatomy and physiology of infants and young children result in higher likelihood of upper cervical injury with greater risk of permanent morbidity.

MRI has become increasingly used to detect and characterize spinal cord and spinal ligament injuries such as SCIWORA.

In the evaluation of spinal cord injury, MRI is able to determine the extent of intramedullary hemorrhage, which correlates with patient outcome.

Suggested Readings

Egloff AM, Kadom N, Vezina G, et al. Pediatric cervical spine trauma imaging: a practical approach. *Pediatr Radiol.* 2009;39:447-456.

Gore PA, Chang S, Theodore N. Cervical spine injuries in children: attention to radiographic differences and stability compared to those in the adult patient. *Semin Pediatr Neurol.* 2009;16:42-58.

Lustrin ES, Karakas SP, et al. Pediatric cervical spine: normal anatomy, variants, and trauma. *Radiographics.* 2003;23:539-560.

References

Full references for this chapter can be found on www.expertconsult.com.

SECTION 4

Respiratory System

Embryology, Anatomy, and Normal Findings

MARY P. BEDARD, ERIC L. EFFMANN, and EDWARD Y. LEE

From a structural and functional perspective, the respiratory system is most logically considered as having conducting and gas exchange components, with the bifurcating airways and accompanying pulmonary arteries (PAs) conducting air and blood to peripheral capillary-lined airspaces for gas exchange. Clements and Warner[1] and more recently Bush[2] encourage consideration of the lung as a set of branching trees that include the airways, the pulmonary vasculature (arterial and venous), the systemic vasculature (arterial and venous), and the lymphatics. This approach assists the radiologist in understanding accurate descriptions of each of these components in congenital malformations and other pathologic processes. This chapter reviews the developmental biology and clinical anatomy of the respiratory system.

Developmental Biology

AIRWAYS

The neonatal airway is composed of the nose, pharynx, larynx, trachea, and bronchi. The nasal structures, which are derived from ectoderm, begin developing during the fourth week of gestation.[3,4] The olfactory placodes, which are evident as early as the third fetal week, eventually become the nasal pits, which separate into paired medial and lateral boundaries of the nasal walls. The medial portion of the nasal wall fuses during the formation of the nasal septum and central upper lip. The medial and lateral nasal processes fuse with the maxillary processes of the mandibular arch. The nasal cavity extends posteriorly, thinning the oronasal membrane, which eventually ruptures to form the choanae. Persistence of the oronasal membrane leads to choanal atresia.[3,5]

Incomplete closure of the foramen caecum during the third week of fetal development leads to the formation of gliomas or nasal encephaloceles. Neural tissue remains attached to epidermal elements, preventing normal migration of mesenchymal elements that will form the cartilaginous structures of the midface. This process leads to the presence of a bony defect through which brain tissue may herniate (e-Fig. 48-1). Gliomas have lost their central nervous system attachment, although 15% have a fibrous stalk connecting to the subarachnoid space. Encephaloceles maintain their central nervous system connection.[5]

Nasal dermoid cysts are benign masses with ectodermal and mesodermal elements. They present as masses on the dorsum of the nose and may have a fistulous opening on the skin or a sinus tract extending into the deep nasal elements. Nasal dermoid cysts are the result of faulty closure of the foramen caecum with invagination of dermal tissue between the developing nasal bones and cartilage.[5]

The larynx, trachea, and bronchi embryologically arise from a ventromedial diverticulum of the foregut that is known as the laryngotracheal groove. The proliferation of the laryngeal mesenchyme results in the arytenoid swellings that grow toward the tongue, converting the primordial glottis into a T-shaped laryngeal inlet. By 8 weeks, the larynx is usually sufficiently formed. In the infant, the larynx is high in location, with its inferior border located at the C4 level. During childhood, the lower border of the larynx descends and eventually reaches its adult location at the C6-C7 level by age 15 years. Functions of the larynx include breathing, phonation, and protection of the lower airway against aspiration.[4,6,7]

The laryngotracheal groove grows caudally, forming the trachea. It lies ventral and parallel to the dorsal foregut, which eventually becomes the esophagus. The separation of the trachea and esophagus progresses cranially and is complete by 6 weeks' gestation. The endodermal lining will produce the epithelium and glandular structures of the trachea, whereas the connective tissue, cartilage, and smooth muscle come from the surrounding splanchnic mesenchyme.[4,6,7] Faulty separation of the trachea and esophagus gives rise to esophageal atresia/tracheoesophageal fistula. Disproportionate growth of the esophagus at the expense of the trachea may give rise to tracheal stenosis or, in the most severe form, tracheal agenesis.

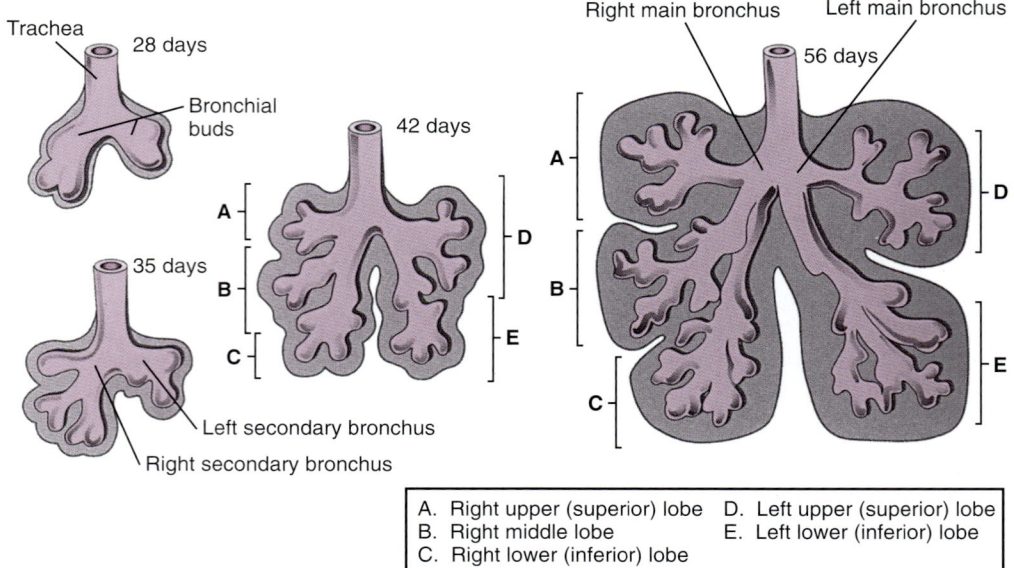

Trachea
28 days
Bronchial buds
42 days
35 days
A
B
C
D
E
Left secondary bronchus
Right secondary bronchus

Right main bronchus   Left main bronchus
56 days
A
B
C
D
E

A.	Right upper (superior) lobe	D.	Left upper (superior) lobe
B.	Right middle lobe	E.	Left lower (inferior) lobe
C.	Right lower (inferior) lobe		

Figure 48-2 Progressive stages in the development of the bronchi and lungs. (From The respiratory system. In: Moore KL, Persaud TVN, eds. *Before we are born: Essentials of embryology and birth defects.* 5th ed. Philadelphia: WB Saunders; 1998:247. Reprinted with permission.)

LUNGS

The lung bud arises from the caudal end of the laryngotracheal groove by the end of the fourth week and soon divides into two bronchial buds.[4,8,9] The bronchial buds grow laterally into the pericardioperitoneal canals. Early in the fifth week, the connection of the bronchial buds to the trachea enlarges to form the main stem bronchi. The right main stem bronchus bifurcates into a superior secondary bronchus, supplying the right upper lobe and an inferior secondary bronchus. The inferior bronchus subdivides into two bronchi, supplying the right middle and lower lobes. The left main stem bronchus divides into two secondary bronchi that supply the upper and lower lobes of the left lung. The bronchi continue to divide, and all airway divisions are complete by 16 weeks' gestation (Fig. 48-2). Cartilage appears at 10 weeks in the trachea and is found in the segmental bronchi by 16 weeks. Unequal growth of the lung buds can lead to the development of unilateral pulmonary agenesis or hypoplasia. Prolonged oligohydramnios or space-occupying thoracic lesions are associated with pulmonary hypoplasia.[4,8]

Lung development has been divided into five stages (Table 48-1). The embryonic (26 to 52 days) and pseudoglandular (52 days to 16 weeks) stages have been described previously. During the canalicular stage (17 to 28 weeks), the bronchi and terminal bronchioles become larger. The capillary bed begins to approximate the future air spaces, and gas exchange is possible. Type I and type II pneumocytes can be identified in the fetal lung by 20 to 22 weeks, but the capillary-alveolar interface is not adequate for extrauterine survival until 23 to 24 weeks of gestation.[4,8,9] The saccular stage (29 to 36 weeks) is characterized by the development of terminal air sacs with flattening of the epithelium in the distal air spaces. The type II pneumocytes produce surfactant, which is stored as lamellar bodies. During the alveolar stage (36 weeks to infancy), the size and number of alveoli increase. When birth occurs at full term, it is estimated that 50 million alveoli are present.

Alveolar development continues postnatally, and the mature human lung ultimately has 300 million alveoli (Table 48-2).

Surfactant

Surfactant is composed of phospholipids, protein, and neutral lipids (e-Fig. 48-3). Surfactant lines the alveoli and decreases surface tension, which leads to decreased work of breathing and stabilizes the terminal air spaces, especially at low lung volumes.[10] Surfactant can be detected as early as 24 to 26 weeks' gestation, although mature surfactant usually is not present until 34 to 36 weeks' gestation. Surfactant maturation can be affected by a variety of substances. Insulin delays surfactant maturation, whereas other substances, such as glucocorticoids and thyroid hormone, accelerate it.[11] Administration

Table 48-1

Classification of Phases of Human Intrauterine Lung Growth

Phase	Time of Occurrence	Significance
Embryonic	26-52 days	Development of trachea and major bronchi
Pseudoglandular	52 days to 16 wk	Development of remaining conducting airways
Canalicular	17-28 wk	Development of vascular bed, framework of acinus; flattening of epithelium
Saccular	29-36 wk	Increased complexity of saccules
Alveolar	36 wk to term	Presence and development of alveoli

From Thurlbeck WL. Lung growth and development. In Thurlbeck W, Churg AM, eds. *Pathology of the lung.* 2nd ed. New York: Thieme Medical Publishers; 1995;38.

Table 48-2

Changes in Lung Size With Growth				
	30 Weeks' Gestation	Full Term	Adult	Fold Increase After Birth
Lung volume	25 mL	150-200 mL	5 L	23
Lung weight	20-25 g	50 g	800 g	16
Alveolar number	—	50 m	300 m	6
Surface area	0.3 m²	3-4 m²	75-100 m²	23
Surface area/kg		0.4 m²	1 m²	2.5
Alveolar diameter	32 μm	150 μm	300 μm	22
No. of airways	24	23-24	22-24	22
Tracheal length		26 mm	184 mm	7
Main bronchi length		26 mm	254	10

From Hodson WA: Normal and abnormal structural development of the lung. In Polin RA, Fox WW, eds. *Fetal and neonatal physiology*, ed 2, Philadelphia, 1998, WB Saunders, p 1037.

of glucocorticoid to mothers 24 to 48 hours before preterm delivery accelerates surfactant maturation and results in a significant decrease in the incidence and severity of hyaline membrane disease (HMD). HMD is the result of surfactant deficiency and is characterized clinically by cyanosis, tachypnea, and retractions within a few hours of delivery. Tracheal instillation of exogenous surfactant can ameliorate the natural course of HMD significantly.[12]

Fetal Lung Liquid

The fetal lung is filled with fluid during gestation. This fluid is produced by pulmonary epithelial cells, and its composition is different from that of amniotic fluid.[13] As the fetus matures, surfactant can be found in this lung fluid. Fetal lung liquid is under higher pressure than amniotic fluid, and efflux of lung liquid into the amniotic fluid occurs, which is the basis of amniotic fluid analysis for surfactant to determine fetal pulmonary maturity.

Removal of liquid from the lung begins shortly before delivery and continues for several hours after delivery. The major routes for clearance of fetal lung fluid are pulmonary circulation and lymphatics. Delayed clearance of fetal lung fluid results in mild to moderate respiratory distress and is seen more commonly in infants delivered by cesarean section. This disorder is known as transient tachypnea of the newborn.

PULMONARY VASCULATURE/CIRCULATION

The fetal lung is the only organ that does not perform its postnatal function before birth. No reason exists for cardiac output to go to the fetal lungs because all gas exchange occurs via the placenta. Oxygenated blood returns to the fetus via the umbilical vein to the inferior vena cava (IVC) and right atrium (RA). Approximately two thirds of the IVC return entering the right atrium crosses the foramen ovale into the left atrium. The remaining one third of the IVC return and all of the superior vena cava (SVC) return enter the right ventricle. Most of the right ventricle output crosses the

ductus arteriosus (DA) into the aorta. These shunts at the foramen ovale and DA result in most of the fetal cardiac output bypassing the lungs (Fig. 48-4).[14]

At delivery, the pulmonary circulation undergoes dramatic changes. The lungs expand with air, the partial pressure of oxygen rises, and the umbilical cord is clamped. These changes result in a decrease in pulmonary vascular resistance, ductal constriction, and functional closure of the foramen ovale. The fetal shunts are functionally closed and all of the blood entering the RA passes through the lungs. In term and near-term infants, this process may go awry with the persistence of high pulmonary vascular resistance and continued shunting of blood away from the lungs via the foramen ovale and DA. This mechanism results in hypoxemia and is known as persistent pulmonary hypertension of the newborn. It usually is seen in infants with underlying respiratory disease or infection or in infants with perinatal stresses such as asphyxia or hypoglycemia. Management of persistent pulmonary hypertension of the newborn currently is aimed at treating the underlying disease and dilatation of the pulmonary vasculature. Inhalation of nitric oxide often results in relaxation of the pulmonary vasculature with improved oxygenation. Infants who do not respond to conventional treatment or administration of nitric oxide frequently require extracorporeal membrane oxygenation.

THE DIAPHRAGM

The diaphragm is derived from four embryonic components: the septum transversum, the pleuroperitoneal membranes, the

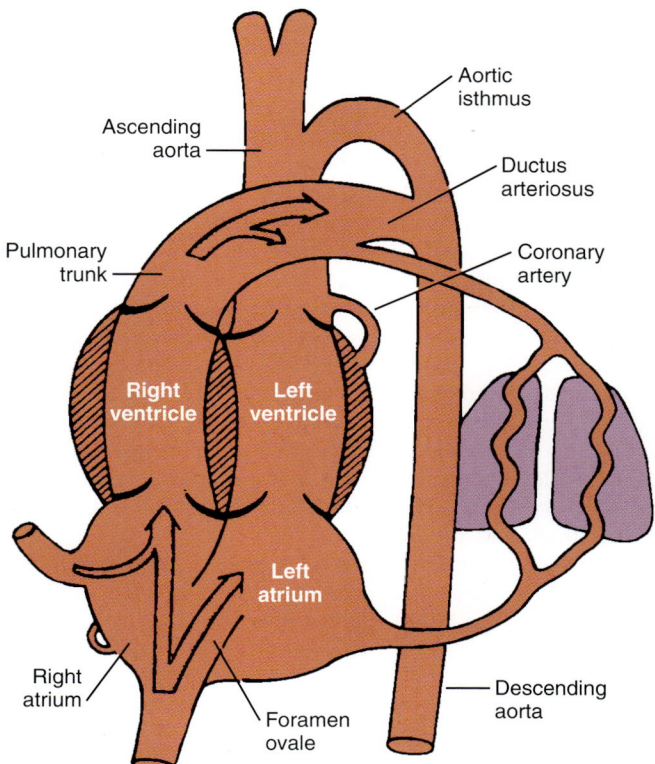

Figure 48-4 Diagrammatic representation of the fetal circulation. (From Teitel DF, Iwamoto HS, Rudolph AM. Effects of birth-related events on central blood flow patterns. *Pediatr Res.* 1987;22:558. Reprinted with permission.)

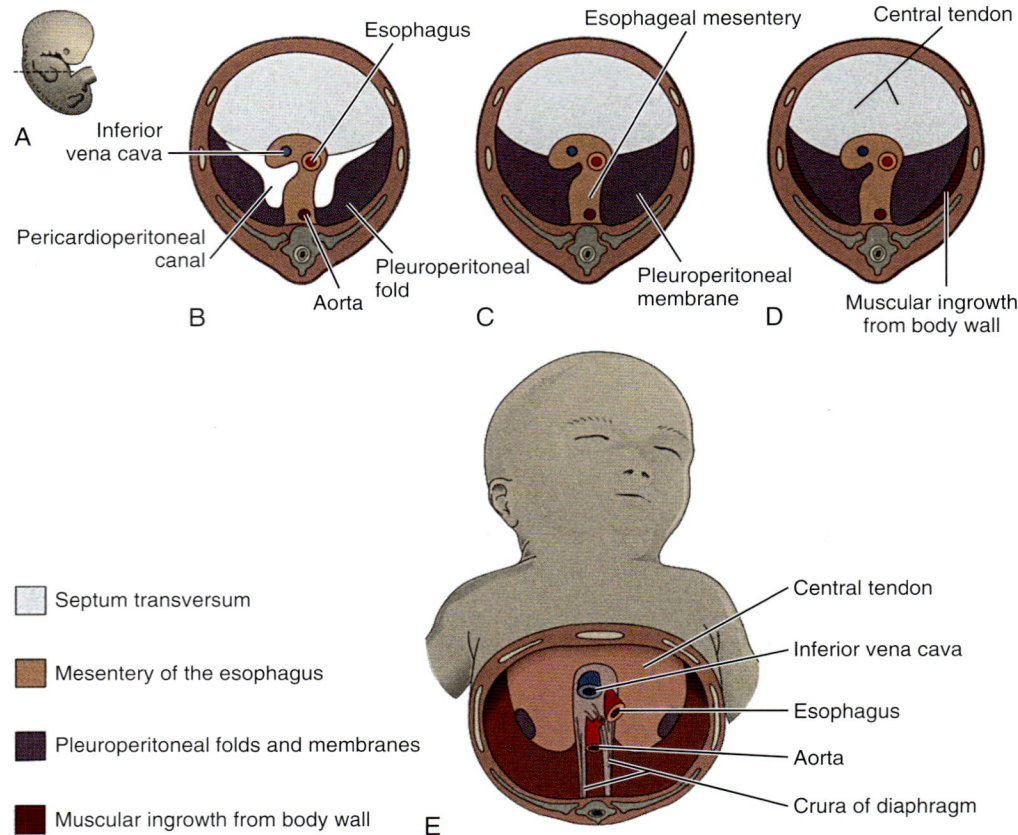

Figure 48-5 Development of the diaphragm. **A,** A sketch of the lateral view of an embryo at the end of the fifth week (actual size) indicating the levels of sections **B** to **E. B, C, D,** and **E,** The developing diaphragm as viewed inferiorly. (From Body cavities, mesenteries, and diaphragm. In: Moore KL, Persaud TVN, eds. *Before we are born: essentials of embryology and birth defects.* 5th ed. Philadelphia: WB Saunders; 1998:189. Reprinted with permission.)

dorsal mesenteric of the esophagus, and the lateral body walls (Fig. 48-5).[15,16] The septum transversum is the precursor of the central tendon of the diaphragm. The septum transversum grows from the ventrolateral body wall and forms a semicircular shelf that separates the heart from the liver and partially separates the pericardial cavity from the peritoneal cavity.

The pleuroperitoneal folds develop as the result of progressive narrowing of the opening between the pleural cavities and the pericardium. These pleuroperitoneal folds become pleuroperitoneal membranes. The pleuroperitoneal membranes extend ventromedially until they fuse with the septum transversum and the dorsal mesentery of the esophagus, separating the pleural and peritoneal cavities. This fusion obliterates the pleuroperitoneal canals that are present on each side of the esophagus. The right pleuroperitoneal canal closes earlier than does the left.

Between the ninth and twelfth weeks of gestation, the enlarging lungs and pleural cavities "burrow" into the body walls. This process forms the muscular and costal components of the diaphragm.

Clinical Anatomy

AIRWAYS

Basic airway anatomy to the level of the terminal bronchiole (the last purely conducting, i.e., nonalveolated, airway) is not

substantially different in children compared with adults except in size. The right lung has three lobes, and the left lung has two lobes (Fig. 48-6). The pleural fissures separating the lobes of the lungs often are anatomically incomplete. Portions of the fissures occasionally are radiographically visualized as fine lines in healthy infants. The lungs are subdivided further into 8 to 10 segments on the left and 10 on the right, each served by a segmental bronchus (Figs. 48-7 and 48-8).[17-19]

The trachea, which is the largest of the conducting airways, is a fibromuscular tube lined principally by ciliated columnar epithelium and mucous cells. The trachea is supported by 16 to 20 cartilaginous rings, which are incomplete posteriorly, where the tracheal wall is composed of fibrous, muscular, and elastic tissue. The trachea extends from the cricoid cartilage at the C4 level to the carina near the T4 level at birth and at a lower level with age. The right main bronchus originates from the trachea at an angle of 32 ± 5.5 degrees and the left at an angle of 51 ± 9.5 degrees from birth to 2 years of age. A tracheal cross-sectional area has been analyzed by computed tomography (CT) and grows predictably with age.[20,21] The cross-sectional shape may vary considerably in the normal population and depending on the phase of respiration.[22]

The bronchi are conducting airways that consist of the first 11 branching generations after the carina. The first four bronchial generations (through the segmental branches) are strongly supported by cartilaginous plates that aid in keeping

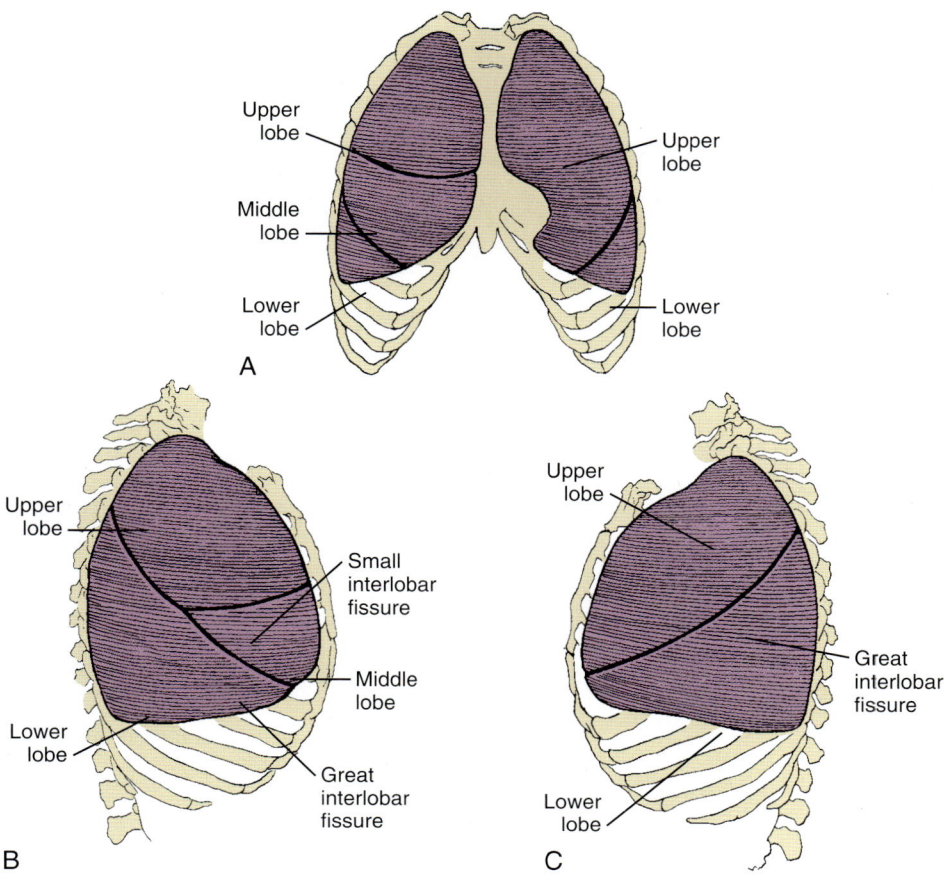

Figure 48-6 Lobes and fissures of normal lungs. **A,** Frontal aspect of both lungs. **B,** Lateral aspect of the right lung. **C,** Lateral aspect of the left lung.

the bronchi patent. The smaller cartilaginous bronchial branches, from the fifth to the eleventh generation, double in number with each branching generation and decrease in size down to approximately 1 mm in diameter (Fig. 48-9).[23] They are in a common fibrous sheath with an accompanying pulmonary arterial branch.

The bronchioles are the conducting airways that extend to the sixteenth generation and lack cartilage in their walls. They are dependent for their patency on the support of the surrounding lung parenchyma. As the lung expands, the bronchioles dilate. The last purely conducting branch of the airway is the terminal bronchiole, which gives rise to three generations of respiratory bronchioles, each giving rise to progressively greater numbers of alveoli. The alveoli and the alveolar ducts and sacs that give rise to them constitute the pure gas-exchange portion of the lung (see Fig. 48-9).

THE RESPIRATORY PORTION OF THE LUNGS

The number of alveoli rapidly increases after birth by a process of septation of the primary saccules distal to the terminal bronchioles. Most alveoli are formed in the first 2 years of life, and the process is complete by 8 years of age, after which the lungs continue to grow by enlarging the dimensions of all lung structures.

The two subunits of the peripheral airspaces that are most important to the radiologist are the acinus and the secondary lobule. The alveolus, which in an adult averages approximately 200 to 300 mm in diameter, is just below the limits of visibility. The acinus is the unit of lung peripheral to the terminal bronchiole and consists of a cluster of 50 to 400 alveoli. It occasionally is visible in the pediatric lung and typically ranges in diameter from 1 to 2 mm in infants younger than 1 year old to 7 to 9 mm in adolescents and adults (Fig. 48-10 and e-Fig. 48-11).[24]

The secondary pulmonary lobule is a cluster of about 3 to 24 acini that are separated from other lobules by interlobular septa composed of fibrous tissue. The secondary lobules and their septa are much better developed in the periphery of the lung than in the center. The mean diameter of the secondary lobule at birth is 3 mm, and by 12 years it measures 15 mm (see e-Fig. 48-11).[24] The pulmonary veins and lymphatics course through the interlobular septa, and the PAs and bronchioles are positioned centrally within the lobule (see Fig. 48-10). Thickened septa are visible in chest radiographs as Kerley B lines and on high-resolution CT (Fig. 48-12).

Multiple imaging modalities have been used to determine prenatal and postnatal lung volumes and growth. Accurate prenatal lung volumetry is currently possible using three-dimensional ultrasonography[25-27] and magnetic resonance imaging (MRI).[28,29] Total lung capacity and its subcomponents (i.e., tidal volume, vital capacity, functional residual capacity, and residual volume) increase with age. Linear or planometric measures from posteroanterior and lateral chest radiographs of children[30,31] obtained in inspiration may

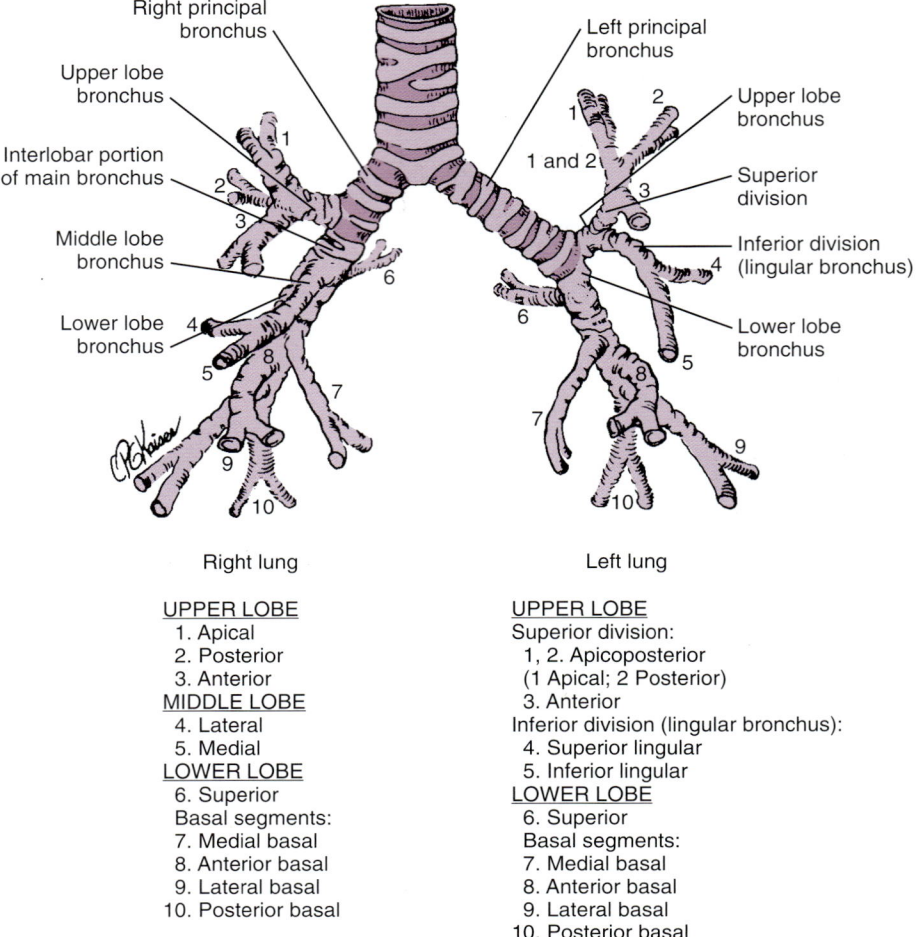

Right principal bronchus
Left principal bronchus
Upper lobe bronchus
Interlobar portion of main bronchus
Middle lobe bronchus
Lower lobe bronchus
Upper lobe bronchus
1 and 2
Superior division
Inferior division (lingular bronchus)
Lower lobe bronchus

Right lung

UPPER LOBE
1. Apical
2. Posterior
3. Anterior
MIDDLE LOBE
4. Lateral
5. Medial
LOWER LOBE
6. Superior
Basal segments:
7. Medial basal
8. Anterior basal
9. Lateral basal
10. Posterior basal

Left lung

UPPER LOBE
Superior division:
1, 2. Apicoposterior
(1 Apical; 2 Posterior)
3. Anterior
Inferior division (lingular bronchus):
4. Superior lingular
5. Inferior lingular
LOWER LOBE
6. Superior
Basal segments:
7. Medial basal
8. Anterior basal
9. Lateral basal
10. Posterior basal

Figure 48-7 The tracheobronchial tree with the segmental bronchi identified by name and number. (From Rosse C, Gaddum-Rosse P. *Hollingsched's textbook of anatomy.* 5th ed. Philadelphia: Lippincott-Raven; 1997:447.)

reliably estimate total lung capacity in children. In recent years, computerized automatic lung volume measurement tools available in most three-dimensional workstations can provide accurate volumetric measurement of lung volume from an axial CT dataset obtained with multidetector CT.[32-34]

A study of 50 subjects (birth to 17 years) undergoing CT with carefully controlled breath holding found substantial variability in lung expansion between subjects, but the size of the airway wall and lumen, as well as arterial areas, were exponentially related to the subject's height.[33] In a study of normal lung volume ranges as a function of age and sex in 1050 boys and girls with normal chest CT scans obtained during quiet breathing (e-Fig. 48-13), it was found that children younger than 8 years had a relatively narrow lung volume range.[32] The ranges broadened considerably in older children, likely reflecting a considerable variation in response to breath-holding instructions. Mean CT density decreases with age and increases in an anterior to posterior gradient in a quietly breathing supine child.[35] Patient age, anterior versus posterior location, and apical versus basal location are significant predictors of regional lung density at inspiratory and expiratory volumes.[36]

Collateral ventilation can occur across pulmonary segments because no pleurae separate them. It also may occur between lobes when fissures are incomplete. There are three routes of collateral ventilation: (1) alveolar pores of Kohn (2- to 10-mm circular apertures in the alveolar walls); (2) canals of Lambert (epithelial-lined tubular structures between preterminal, terminal, or respiratory bronchioles and the alveoli surrounding them); and (3) direct small airway anastomoses.[18] Collateral ventilatory pathways are less well developed in young infants than in older children and adults.

PULMONARY VASCULATURE/CIRCULATION

The lung has a dual blood supply consisting of a pulmonary arterial and a systemic arterial supply. The main PA arises from the right ventricle distal to the pulmonic valve and forms a segment of the left heart border before it bifurcates at the level of the carina. The left PA curves superiorly and posteriorly to the left hilum anterior to the left main bronchus, where it divides into two branches. The lower branch is directed posteriorly and crosses over the left upper lobe bronchus, descending parallel with but lateral to the left lower lobe bronchus. This vessel gives branches to the lingual

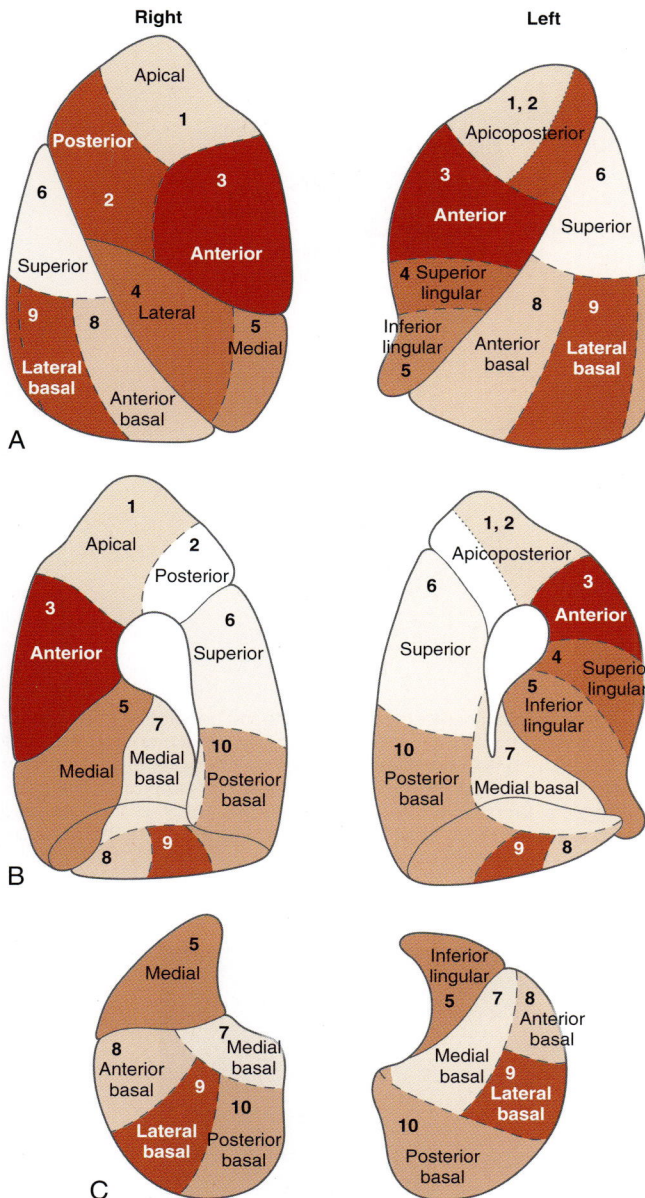

it, giving branches, in order, to the middle lobe, the superior segment of the lower lobe, and four branches to the basilar segments of the right lower lobe.

In the lung parenchyma, the pulmonary arterial branches travel and divide with the bronchial branches, although they also give off unaccompanied supernumerary branches. There are approximately 23 divisions of airway branching and approximately 28 divisions of pulmonary arterial branching. These vessels can be visualized on high-resolution CT to about the level of the sixteenth generation, which is a few millimeters from the pleural surface and corresponds to the level of the terminal bronchioles, allowing identification of the secondary pulmonary lobule (the parenchyma supplied by three to five or more terminal bronchioles). The arterioles continue to divide until they form a dense capillary network surrounding the alveolus. This network consists of 280 billion capillary segments with a total blood volume of 140 mL; pulmonary blood volume can nearly double during exercise.[37]

The primary role of the pulmonary circulation is to transport deoxygenated blood from the heart to the alveolar capillaries, where oxygenation occurs, and then transport oxygenated blood through the pulmonary veins back to the left atrium. The pressure in the pulmonary circuit is about one sixth that of the systemic circuit; total pulmonary blood flow is determined primarily by cardiac output, although the control of pulmonary blood flow is complex and also depends on the relative systemic and pulmonary pressures, gravity, and local pulmonary factors. Large numbers of lung capillaries normally are not perfused or are only minimally perfused, which allows for increased arterial flow without increased pulmonary arterial pressure. Gravity is an important determinant of regional pulmonary blood flow, with the more dependent regions receiving a greater volume of blood. The smaller, muscular, pulmonary arterial branches vasoconstrict under conditions of hypoxia in an attempt to maintain the ventilation-perfusion balance. When lung disease becomes severe enough, this protective mechanism is overwhelmed, and poorly ventilated alveoli are perfused, which results in right-to-left shunting and systemic desaturation. Hypoxemia and accompanying acidosis increase pulmonary vascular resistance, which leads to right ventricular hypertrophy and eventually to cor pulmonale.

The vast pulmonary capillary bed serves the function of gas exchange. Its endothelial cell lining has important metabolic functions and is quite sensitive to toxins, including high oxygen concentrations. When endothelial cells are damaged, increased permeability pulmonary edema often results.

The pulmonary venous radicles arise distal to the capillary meshwork and travel in the interlobular septa, which form the walls of the secondary pulmonary lobules; the veins do not accompany the PA and bronchial branches. They drain toward the hilum and gradually increase in size. Usually two large pulmonary veins are found on each side. The upper lobe veins are more vertical in orientation, and the lower ones are more horizontal before they enter the left atrium. The right superior vein is located posterior to the SVC and anterior to the right interlobar PA. The left superior pulmonary vein is located anterior to the left main PA and is just anterior to the left upper lobe bronchus. The right inferior branch enters the left atrium anterior to the right lower lobe bronchus, and the left inferior pulmonary vein enters the left

Figure 48-8 The bronchopulmonary segments as seen on the surface of the lungs. **A,** Lateral surface. **B,** Medial surface. **C,** Base or diaphragmatic surface. (Adapted from Boyden EA. *The segmental anatomy of the lungs.* New York: McGraw-Hill; 1955; and from Rosse C, Gaddum-Rosse P. *Hollingsched's textbook of anatomy.* 5th ed. Philadelphia: Lippincott-Raven; 1997:457.)

segment, to the superior segment of the lower lobe, and to the basilar segments. The smaller superior branch divides, and its branches parallel the bronchial divisions to the upper lobe. The right PA is almost horizontal and divides into its two major branches while still within the pericardium. It lies posterior to the ascending aorta and SVC and anterior to the right main bronchus. The main upper lobe branch, the truncus anterior, ascends anterior to the right upper lobe bronchus and subdivides into three branches that parallel the three segmental bronchi to the right upper lobe. The largest branch of the right PA is the interlobar artery, which passes anterior to the bronchus intermedius and descends lateral to

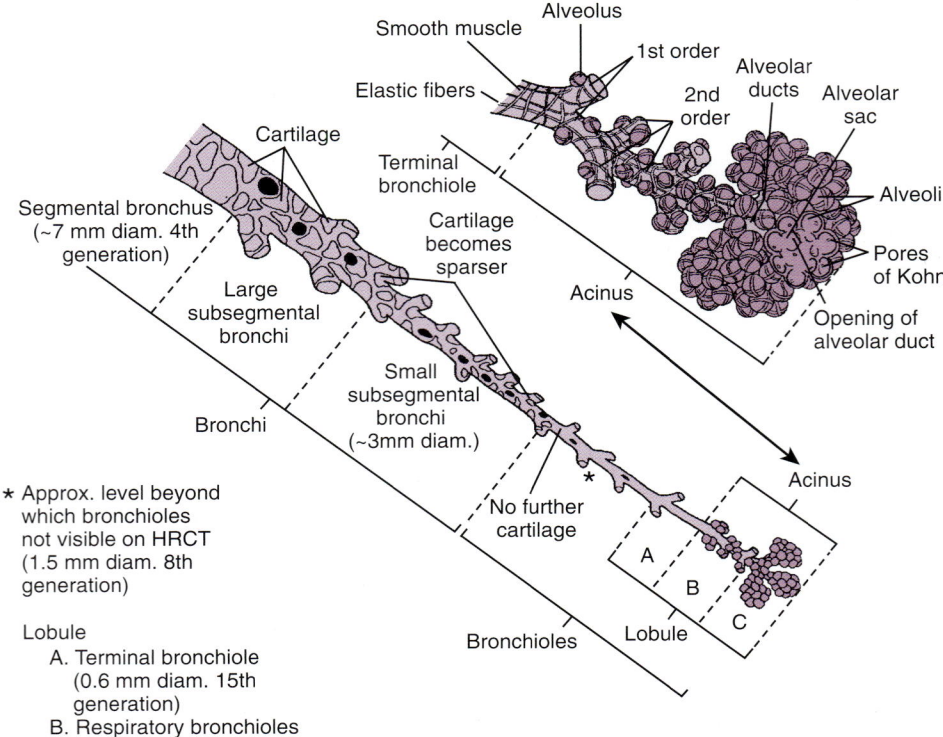

Figure 48-9 **Bronchial generations.** The bronchi and airways from the fourth generation (the segmental bronchus) to the last generation (the alveolar sacs and alveoli) are represented. Bronchi contain cartilage within their walls, to the level of small (3-mm diameter) subsegmental branches. They are readily visible on high-resolution computed tomography (HRCT). Bronchioles, which do not contain cartilage but rather an extensive network of fibers within their walls, are seen only to the eighth generation, which corresponds to a diameter of about 1.5 mm. Beyond the eighth generation, the bronchiolar walls are not visible by high-resolution CT unless they are abnormal. The terminal bronchioles are the sixteenth-generation bronchioles and conduct air into the lobules. Beyond the terminal bronchioles, four to eight respiratory bronchioles lead to distal acini. Respiratory bronchioles are characterized by the presence of outpouchings representing alveolar ducts and terminal groupings of alveolar sacs. (From Armstrong P. The normal chest. In: Armstrong P, Wilson AG, Dee P, et al, eds. *Imaging of diseases of the chest.* 3rd ed. London: Mosby; 2000:26.)

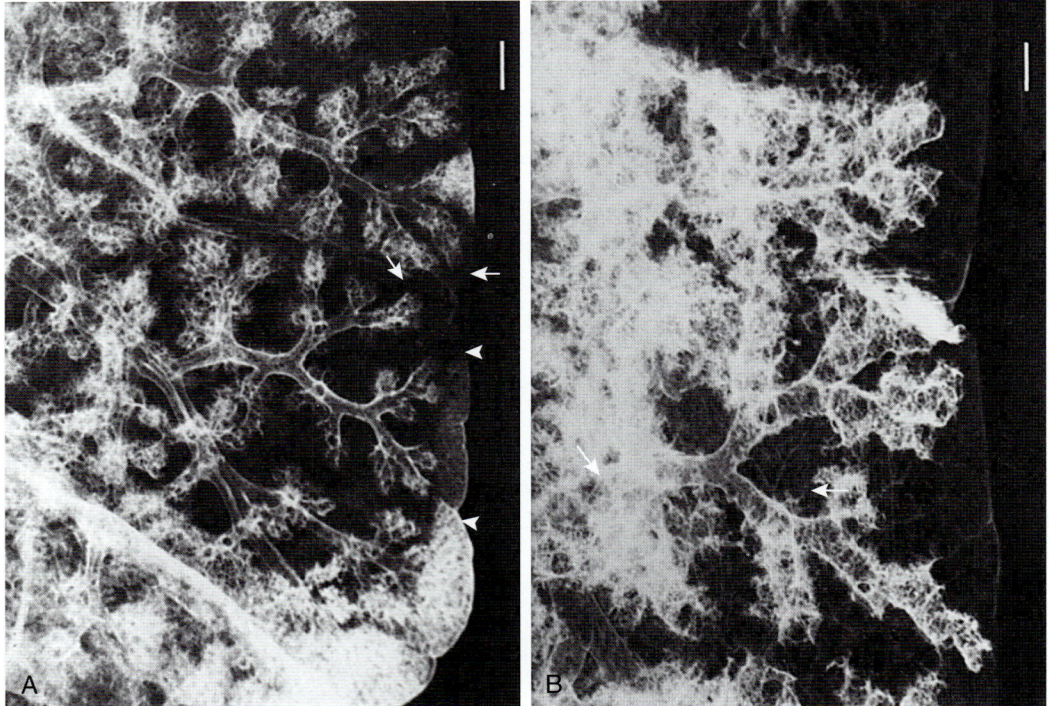

Figure 48-10 **Acinar and secondary lobular anatomy in children.** Radiographs of selected sections of human lung obtained from postmortem examination and prepared by silver nitrate bronchoacinography. **A,** The lung from a 2-month-old infant showing the diameter of one acinus extending between the terminal bronchial and acinar surface (*arrows*). A subjacent underfilled secondary lobule is delimited by interlobular septa (*arrowheads*). **B,** The lung from a 19-year-old adult showing a mean acinar diameter (*arrows*) that is considerably larger. Both images are at the same magnification, with the marker bar (*upper right*) equal to 1 mm (corrected for specimen shrinkage). (From Osborne DRS, Effmann EL, Hedlund LW. Postnatal growth and size of the pulmonary acinus and secondary lobule in man. *AJR Am J Roentgenol.* 1983;140:449).

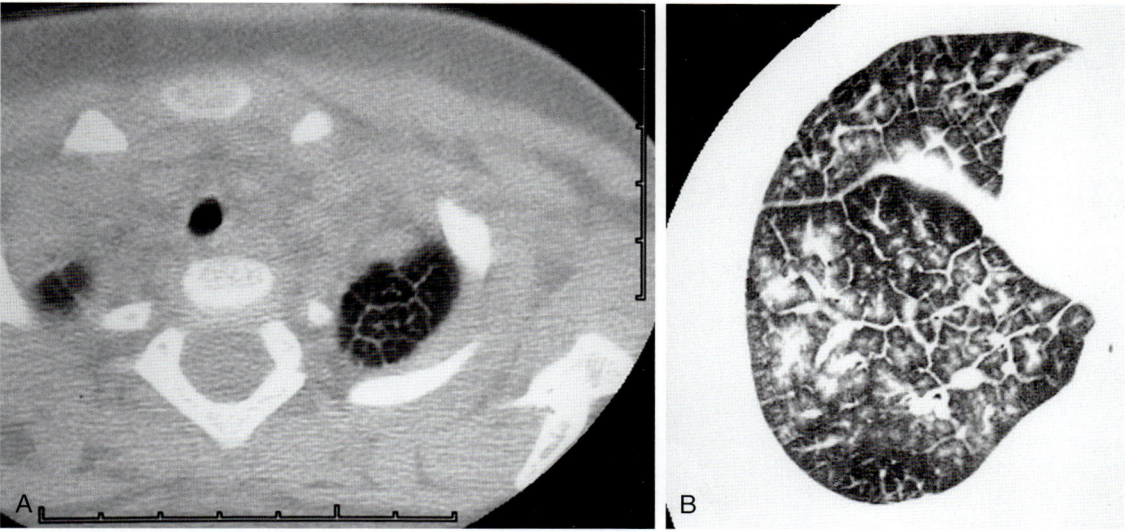

Figure 48-12 Secondary lobular septal thickening in two patients. **A,** A 1-year-old child with Noonan syncrome showing polygonal-shaped secondary lobules in the left lung apex. Respiratory motion degraded lower sections, which also showed patchy septal thickening. **B,** A 15-year-old girl with mixed connective tissue disease shows moderately severe septal thickening and patchy distribution of ground-glass opacities within some lobules.

atrium at a point just anterior to the descending aorta and posterior to the left lower lobe bronchus.

The systemic circulation to the lung is via two to four (most commonly one right and two left) bronchial arteries that are branches of the thoracic aorta. These vessels provide nourishment to the airways and central mediastinum. In the presence of PA obstruction, collateral circulation to the pulmonary capillaries can develop through precapillary anastomotic channels.

LYMPHATICS

Pulmonary lymphatics are essential to removal of initial fetal lung liquid and to the removal of protein and water outside the vascular space.[38,39] This fluid is returned to the circulation via the right lymphatic duct and the thoracic duct. Lymphatic vessels travel beside blood vessels in the bronchovascular spaces and in the connective tissues of the pleura. No lymphatics are present within the alveolar walls, but juxta-alveolar lymphatics represent the initial part of the lung lymphatic system. Enlargement of lymphatic channels in secondary lobular septa may be visualized on chest radiography and with CT (see Fig. 48-12).

Key Points

The number of alveoli increases sixfold from birth to adulthood.

Persistence of the pleuroperitoneal canal beyond 6 weeks of gestation leads to the development of a diaphragmatic hernia.

Two clinically useful subunits of airspace disease are the acinus and secondary lobule. The acinus is the unit of lung peripheral to the terminal bronchiole and consists of 50 to 400 alveoli, whereas the secondary lobule is a cluster of 3 to 24 acini separated by interlobular septa.

The peripheral pulmonary vasculature divides and accompanies bronchial branching. It may be visualized to at least the sixteenth generation of division within a few millimeters of the peripheral surface and corresponds to the level of the terminal bronchioles.

Suggested Readings

Bluestone CD, Stool SE, et al, eds. *Pediatric otolaryngology.* 4th ed. Philadelphia: Saunders; 2003.

Hansell DM, Armstrong P, Lynch DA, et al. The normal chest. In: Hansell DM, Armstrong P, Lynch DA, et al, eds. *Imaging of diseases of the chest.* 5th ed. Philadelphia: Mosby; 2010.

Polin RA, Fox WW, Abman SH, eds. *Fetal and neonatal physiology.* 3rd ed. Philadelphia: Saunders; 2004.

Webb WR, Müller N, Naidich DP. Normal lung anatomy. In: Webb WR, Müller N, Naidich DP, eds. *High resolution CT of the lung.* 4th ed. Philadelphia: Lippincott; 2009.

References

Full references for this chapter can be found on www.expertconsult.com.

Chapter 49

Imaging Techniques

HYUN WOO GOO, LAURA A. DRUBACH, and EDWARD Y. LEE

Overview

Various imaging modalities—conventional radiography, fluoroscopy, ultrasound, computed tomography (CT), magnetic resonance imaging (MRI), and nuclear medicine studies—currently are available and are used to assess the pediatric respiratory system in clinical practice. The presence of air in the airways and lungs can be beneficial and challenging with regard to imaging the respiratory system. Although having abundant air in the respiratory system is beneficial when performing conventional radiography, fluoroscopy, and CT, it complicates assessment of the respiratory system with ultrasound and MRI.

When answers to specific clinical questions are sought, radiologists and clinicians ideally should work together to select appropriate imaging modalities. Up-to-date knowledge about the advantages and disadvantages of each imaging modality should be carefully considered when making a selection because the imaging techniques for the pediatric respiratory system are continuously evolving. Furthermore, the imaging techniques should be tailored to the individual pediatric patient for optimal results. This chapter discusses indications, contraindications, benefits, risks, and other relevant issues pertaining to each imaging modality currently being used.

Conventional Radiography

Conventional radiography is the creation of a projection image with the use of x-rays to view parts of the human body. This primary, cost-effective imaging method currently is the modality used most frequently and widely in clinical practice for evaluation of the respiratory system in pediatric patients. Conventional radiography is associated with a very low level of ionizing radiation exposure (in the range of 0.01 to 0.02 mSv for chest posteroanterior [PA] radiography).[1,2] Soft tissue neck study and chest radiography, the two conventional radiographic imaging techniques used most frequently to assess the pediatric respiratory system, are discussed in the following sections.

SOFT TISSUE NECK STUDY

Inspiratory stridor resulting from an upper airway obstruction is the most frequent indication of a soft tissue neck study in pediatric patients.[3] The common causes of inspiratory stridor include croup, epiglottitis, a foreign body, and an upper airway mass in infants and children. To obtain optimal diagnostic quality, the neck of the patient should be extended and images should be obtained at full inspiration. The standard soft tissue neck radiographic views consist of both an anteroposterior (AP) view and a lateral view. An additional expiratory lateral view of the neck subsequently may be obtained for assessment of subglottic stenosis, which can be beneficial in differentiating a fixed large airway disorder (e.g., subglottic stenosis) from a dynamic large airway disorder (e.g., tracheomalacia).

Use of the high kilovoltage technique with added filtration and coned magnification may facilitate visualization of the upper airway and adjacent soft tissue. Immobilization may be necessary for infants and young children (<5 years) who may not be able to follow verbal instructions. However, pediatric patients with respiratory distress should not be immobilized, especially in a position that may further aggravate the airway obstruction. For instance, the upright position is preferred and the supine position is contraindicated in the setting of acute epiglottitis. When necessary, careful manual immobilization of the head and neck during the study by the child's parents or by an experienced technologist may be considered. A clinician should accompany the child with respiratory distress, and an emergency kit should be ready for immediate use in the examination room. In most conditions resulting in upper airway obstruction in pediatric patients, a soft tissue neck study usually is sufficient to make the diagnosis. However, when the underlying cause of upper airway obstruction is not evident, fluoroscopy, CT, or MRI may be necessary as a next step in the imaging evaluation.

CHEST RADIOGRAPHY

Chest radiography is the imaging study obtained most frequently to evaluate the respiratory system in pediatric patients. Immobilization is usually required in uncooperative infants and young children (<5 years) to achieve consistent image quality by decreasing motion artifacts and position deviations.[4] Chest radiography is obtained during quiet inspiration in uncooperative infants and young children and during full inspiration in cooperative older pediatric patients. The standard chest radiographic views consist of the AP view in infants and young children (<5 years) and both the AP and PA views in older children, in addition to a lateral view. AP, PA, and lateral views of the chest can be obtained with the patient in the supine or erect position. Exposure parameters of the chest radiography should be appropriately optimized. However, unnecessary radiation to nonthoracic structures such as the lower neck, proximal upper extremity, and upper abdomen should be avoided by using appropriate collimation and shielding.[5,6]

In contrast to a radiographic screen–film system, image acquisition and display are decoupled in digital radiography, which allows increased versatility of image manipulations.[7,8] One of the most commonly used image processing techniques in digital chest radiography is unsharp mask filtering or edge enhancement, which facilitates the detection of thoracic fine linear abnormalities or structures such as pneumothorax, vascular catheters, and the interlobar fissures, even in newborns.[9] Recently, optimization of digital radiographic techniques has been emphasized to reduce potentially unnecessary overexposure to pediatric patients.[6,10] The increased likelihood of overexposure in digital radiography, the so-called *dose creep,* is attributed not only to the lack of a standardized exposure index but also to the difficulty in recognizing overexposed radiographs by radiologic technologists and radiologists. Fortunately, a new standardized exposure index for digital radiography was proposed recently.[11]

Optimized techniques of digital chest radiography in children often are different from those in adults. For instance, automatic exposure control and grids are not particularly helpful in small pediatric patients. Additional views such as expiratory, decubitus, and oblique views sometimes are necessary to clarify abnormalities detected on standard AP or PA views or to solve unanswered clinical questions. Expiratory views may be used to confirm air trapping due to an underlying airway obstruction. The lateral decubitus view generally is used to detect freely shifting pleural effusion or air; it is used infrequently to demonstrate an air–fluid level in an intraparenchymal cavitary lesion. In addition, the lateral decubitus view may be used to demonstrate air trapping in the dependent lung or to clarify poorly defined lung opacities in the nondependent lung in uncooperative infants and young children.[12,13] Oblique views may be helpful for evaluating rib, soft tissue, hilar, carinal, and peripheral lung abnormalities.

Fluoroscopy

Fluoroscopy can be used to evaluate dynamic large airway and lung abnormalities, such as airway obstruction, air trapping, and diaphragmatic palsy/paralysis. Use of fluoroscopic techniques and equipment should be optimized to minimize exposure of both pediatric patients and operators to harmful ionizing radiation by following the "imaging gently" and "step lightly" principles.[14]

FLUOROSCOPY-GUIDED AIRWAY STUDY

A fluoroscopy-guided airway study may be helpful in demonstrating dynamic airway abnormalities, such as laryngomalacia, tracheomalacia, obstructive sleep apnea, and vocal cord dysfunction syndrome.[15-17] Additionally, a fixed airway disorder such as stenosis or stricture also can be identified and differentiated from a dynamic airway disorder. Compared with endoscopic procedures for evaluating large airways, a fluoroscopy-guided airway study generally is inexpensive and less invasive.[18] In recent years, the diagnostic role of the fluoroscopy-guided airway study has begun to be replaced by dynamic airway CT with a low radiation dose technique.[19] Dynamic airway CT is more accurate than a fluoroscopy-guided airway study for evaluation of the location, degree, and extent of both the dynamic and fixed airway abnormalities. Furthermore, dynamic airway CT can provide additional information about other intrathoracic structures, which is a valuable benefit.[19]

Ultrasound

Ultrasound is a valuable and widely used imaging modality for evaluating the lungs and pleura, particularly in pediatric patients, because it is widely available, relatively easy to perform, and does not expose patients to radiation.[20,21] Its real-time evaluation capability and portability are important additional benefits. Furthermore, crucial information regarding associated vascular structures or underlying blood flow also can be obtained with color Doppler ultrasound.[20,21] Although chest radiography or CT is the main imaging modality of choice for evaluating the lungs and pleura, the complementary use of ultrasound may provide clinically relevant information in patients with certain conditions.[20,21]

EVALUATION OF LUNGS

The main clinical indication for ultrasound of the lungs in pediatric patients is to characterize a peripheral lung opacity (i.e., parenchymal versus pleural disease) that has been detected with chest radiography.[20] Frequent underlying etiologies include atelectasis, consolidation, lung necrosis, a lung abscess, congenital lung lesions, and a primary or metastatic lung neoplasm (Fig. 49-1).[20,21] For evaluation of these abnormalities, conventional chest radiography should be carefully reviewed to localize the area of interest so the clinical question can be specifically answered with the ultrasound evaluation.[20,21] Ultrasound evaluation of the lungs typically is performed with the patient in the supine or upright position. However, to improve the visualization in some selected situations, the lateral decubitus view or the supraclavicular and/or suprasternal notch view may be beneficial. Optimal views can be achieved by placing a pillow or blanket on the dependent side or behind the shoulder to help extend the neck of the patient.[20]

The choice of ultrasound transducer depends primarily on three factors: the age of the patient, the size of the patient, and the location of the abnormality.[20,21] Although curved or linear array transducers typically are used to evaluate peripheral lung opacity, transducers that are smaller in size, such as sector or vector transducers, may be necessary for imaging in infants or young children who have a small available acoustic window (such as between the ribs). High-frequency transducers (e.g., 7.5 to 15.0 MHz) are helpful in evaluating the chest in infants and young children who do not have a substantial amount of subcutaneous fat because they provide higher resolution ultrasound images with a limited ability for soft-tissue penetration.[20] Conversely, use of low-frequency transducers (e.g., <5 MHz) may be necessary when evaluating older children who have a large amount of subcutaneous fat because these transducers provide better soft tissue penetration, although the ultrasound image resolution is decreased.[20] Color Doppler ultrasound is useful for evaluating lung lesions with underlying vascular structures in cases of pulmonary sequestration or blood flow in cases involving a neoplasm.

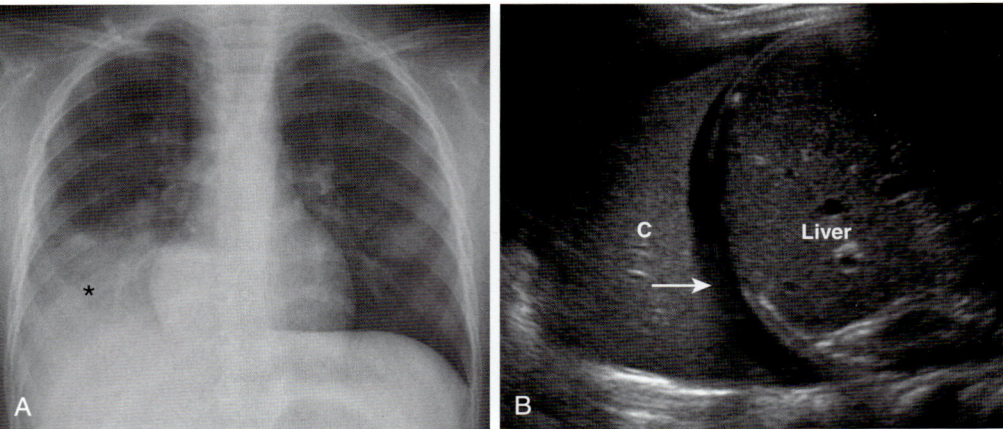

Figure 49-1 Plain radiography and ultrasound in a 3-year-old girl with fever, cough, and respiratory distress. **A,** Frontal chest radiograph shows an opacity (*asterisk*) projecting over the right lower lung zone. **B,** Longitudinal ultrasound view of the right hemithorax demonstrates a consolidated lung (*C*), small effusion (*arrow*), and liver.

EVALUATION OF PLEURA

Ultrasound can be useful in differentiating pleural fluid from atelectasis and/or consolidation when the diagnosis is equivocal on the basis of conventional radiography. Furthermore, ultrasound is more sensitive and accurate than conventional radiography or CT for characterizing pleural fluid, which may be simple or complex (Fig. 49-2).[20] Ultrasound evaluation of patients in both the erect and lateral decubitus positions can be useful for differentiating between freely flowing and loculated pleural fluid. In addition, ultrasound can visualize the internal debris, septations, and pleural thickening often associated with parapneumonic collections. Such complex pleural effusion often requires a drainage procedure that can be facilitated with the guidance of ultrasound.

Computed Tomography

CT is a valuable cross-sectional imaging study for evaluating pediatric airways and lungs, mainly because its images provide excellent air-tissue contrast. The development of multidetector CT (MDCT), which can provide a short scan time with a decreased rate of sedation, has increased the role of CT in the assessment of pediatric airways and lungs.[22] Respiratory motion artifacts often degrade CT image quality in infants and young children who breathe freely during the scan. These artifacts can be reduced with the use of general anesthesia, and controlled ventilation.[23,24] These techniques also can be used to control either the inspiratory or expiratory phases of respiration.[23-25] In addition, recently introduced high-pitch dual-source spiral CT scanning is very helpful in reducing motion artifacts on chest CT scans of children who breathe freely during the procedure.[26]

Reducing the CT radiation dose while maintaining diagnostic image quality is of critical importance in pediatric patients because of the greater radiosensitivity and longer life expectancy of children, coupled with increasing CT use. Low-dose, body size–adapted chest CT protocols using variable tube voltages and tube currents have been established, usually on the basis of body weight.[27,28] However, several recent studies have demonstrated that cross-sectional

dimensions provide better CT dose adaptation to body habitus.[29-31] A practical pediatric chest CT protocol based on a volume CT dose index individually determined by cross-sectional area and mean density of the body recently was developed for daily clinical use.[32] The tube current always should be modulated if applicable because this modulation allows the CT dose to be reduced substantially without degrading image quality.[33-35] Electrocardiogram-triggered sequential scanning may be used in CT of the chest in children to achieve fewer motion artifacts and a lower radiation dose.[24,36]

The image quality of CT of the chest in children may be further improved by adjusting kilovolt levels and reconstruction algorithms as follows: a low kilovolt level for enhanced CT and a high kilovolt level for unenhanced CT, a high-frequency reconstruction algorithm for lung evaluation, and

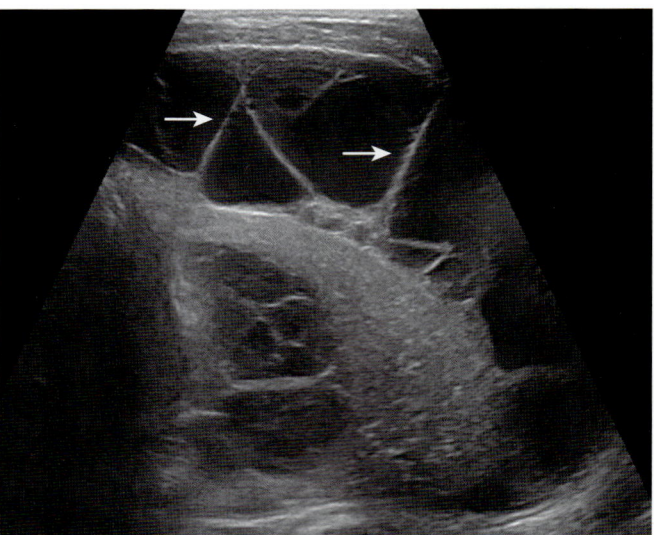

Figure 49-2 Ultrasound for pleural fluid in a 5-year-old boy with recurrent pneumonia in the right lung. A longitudinal ultrasound view of the right hemithorax shows a complex pleural effusion with thick septations (*arrows*).

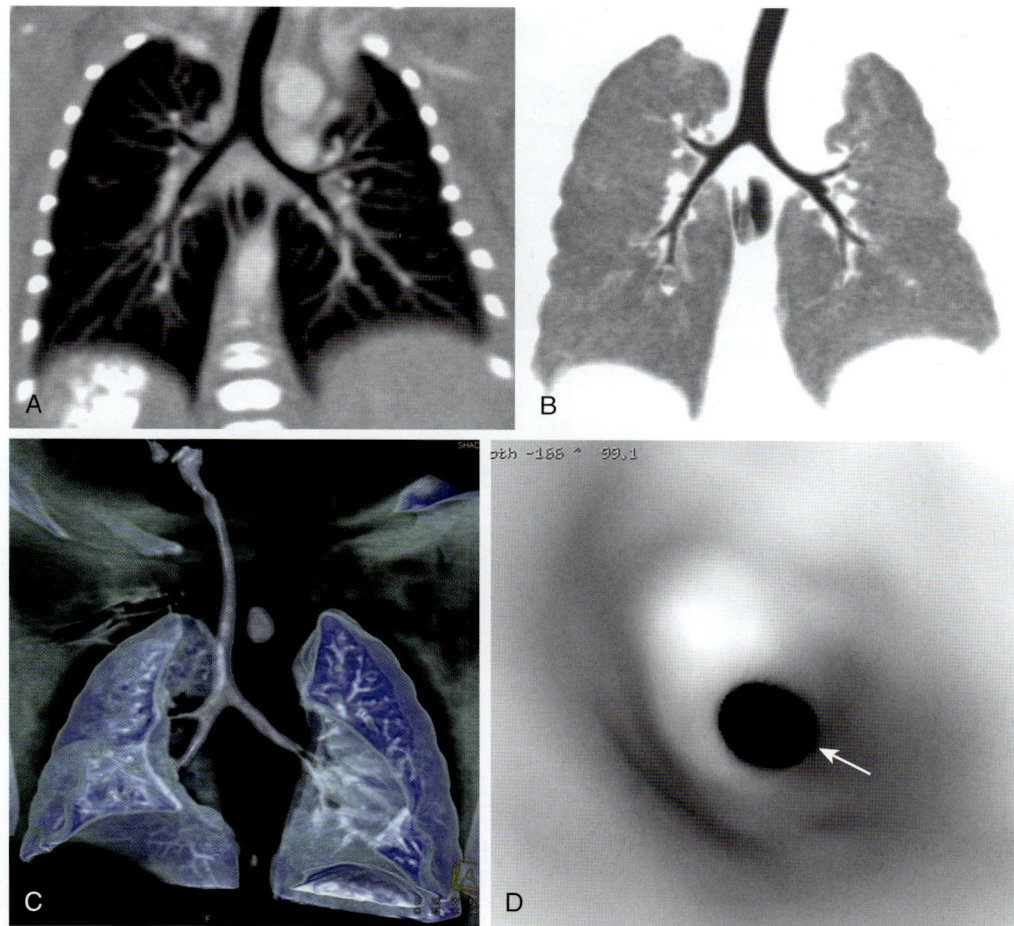

Figure 49-3   Multiplanar reformatted and three-dimensional (3D) computed tomography (CT) imaging. **A,** A coronal thin-slab CT image shows normal relationships between the airway and the pulmonary artery, indicating the thoracic situs solitus. **B,** A coronal minimum-intensity projection CT image shows anatomic details of the central airways. **C,** A volume-rendered CT image shows the 3D appearance of the lungs and airways. **D,** A virtual bronchoscopic image providing an endoscopic view of the trachea shows a concentric narrowing (*arrow*) from a tracheal web.

a standard reconstruction algorithm for mediastinal evaluation. In addition to axial CT images, postprocessed and reconstructed images such as multiplanar reformatted (MPR) and three-dimensional (3D) images considerably increase diagnostic accuracy of pediatric chest CT (Fig. 49-3).[37] CT scanning with thinner collimation (<1 mm) offers better quality MPR and 3D images. Various visualization techniques including maximum intensity projection, minimum intensity projection, volume rendering, and virtual bronchoscopy can help further visualize thoracic abnormalities (see Fig. 49-3).

EVALUATION OF AIRWAYS

Anatomic details of the pediatric airways can be imaged with CT.[38,39] However, small airways distal to the subsegmental level (i.e., airways <0.5 to 1.5 mm in diameter) often are invisible on CT because of their size. CT is less invasive than bronchoscopy in evaluating pediatric airways and provides cross-sectional imaging without superimposition. Various airway abnormalities, including fixed or dynamic obstruction, bronchiectasis, and wall thickening, can be diagnosed with CT. MRI may be used to evaluate large airways with comparable diagnostic accuracy, but MRI is clearly inferior to

CT in evaluating small airways because of lower spatial resolution and a lower signal/noise ratio.

Static Airway CT Study

A static airway CT study is performed mainly to assess a fixed airway narrowing or stenosis. Axial CT data are acquired in infants and young children while they breathe freely and in older children while they hold their breath at the end of an inspiration (Fig. 49-3, *C*). Anatomic details of the airway typically are well visualized, even in free-breathing studies, because of the fast scan speed of MDCT (>16 row MDCT). The extent and cause of airway abnormalities can be better evaluated with MPR and 3D CT images than with axial CT images alone.

Dynamic Airway Computed Tomographic Study

A paired inspiratory and expiratory CT study is performed primarily for the dynamic evaluation of a large airway disorder, most commonly tracheobronchomalacia.[19] Expiratory CT is performed with the low radiation dose technique to minimize the dose delivered during this dual-phase study

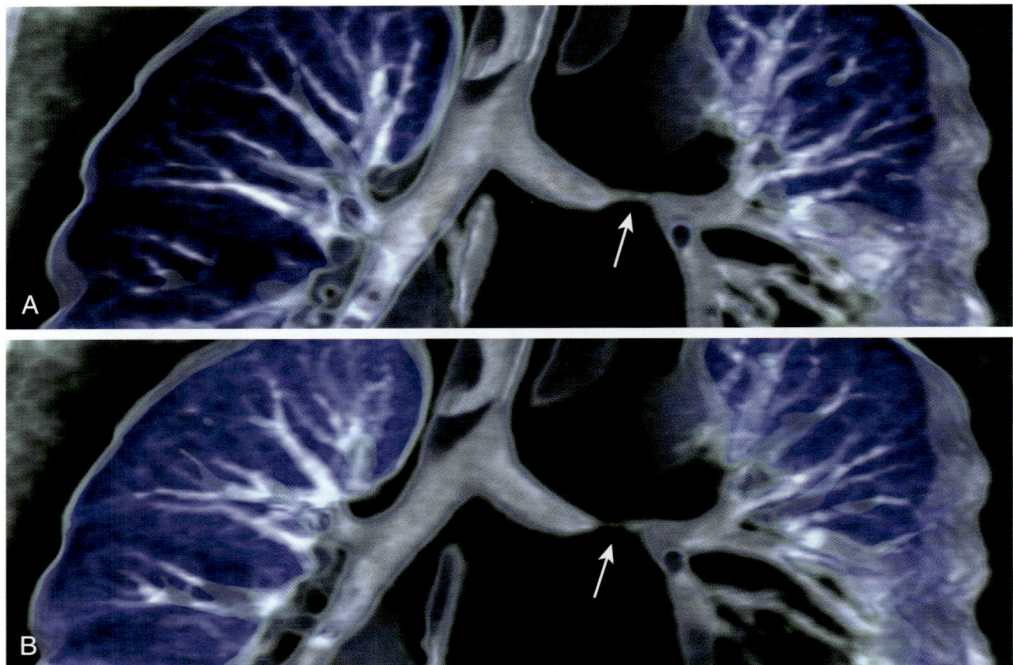

Figure 49-4 Four-dimensional airway computed tomography study. **A,** Peak inspiration **B,** Peak expiration. A fixed narrowing (*arrow*) is noted at the distal left main bronchus.

(Table 49-1). The resultant effective dose from this paired study typically is in the range of 3.5 to 7.5 mSv.[19] Expiratory CT can be obtained with two different respiratory maneuvers: (1) holding the breath at the end of an expiration during end-expiratory CT and (2) forced exhalation during dynamic expiratory CT. In uncooperative infants and young children, general anesthesia with intubation, controlled ventilation, or respiratory triggering can be used.[19,23,24,39]

Cine Airway Computed Tomographic Study

In cine airway CT, axial sequential scans are acquired continuously at predefined noncontiguous slices with high resolution and use of the low radiation dose technique throughout the respiratory cycle.[40] This technique allows changes in the cross-sectional area and shape of the airway to be demonstrated throughout the entire respiratory cycle, thus making the diagnosis of tracheobronchomalacia possible. To achieve the high temporal resolution required for cine airway CT, the fastest gantry rotation speed is used. The total scan time should be tailored to a range of one to two respiratory cycles to minimize the radiation dose. As a result, the radiation dose of cine airway CT is quite low—in the range of 0.2 mSv to 0.3 mSv.[24] Cine airway CT is performed in infants and young children as they breathe freely or with a coughing maneuver in cooperative older children.[19,41] Coughing exaggerates the expiratory collapse of the airway because it elicits a higher intrathoracic extra-airway pressure than does normal or forced exhalation, and thus it is the preferred technique for a cine airway CT study. In addition to dynamic airway evaluation, cine airway CT also can be used to detect trapping of air in the lung, which often is a secondary sign of underlying small airway disease.[40]

Four-Dimensional Airway Computed Tomographic Study

Increased longitudinal coverage (e.g., 4 cm for 64-section CT and 16 cm for 320-section CT) of modern MDCT makes a four-dimensional (4D) airway CT study feasible.[42] As in a cine airway CT study, an axial sequential CT scan is continuously acquired without table movement throughout the respiration cycle in 4D airway CT. The major difference from cine airway CT is the real–time volumetric coverage of almost the entire central airway in infants and young children (Fig. 49-4).

Table 49-1

Tube Current and Kilovoltage by Patient Weight for Central Airway Multidetector Computed Tomography		
Weight (kg)	**Tube Current (mAs) Inspiration/Expiration**	**Kilovoltage**
<10	40/20	80
10-14	50/25	80
15-24	60/30	80
25-34	70/35	80
35-44	80/40	80
45-54	90/40	90
55-70	100-120/40	100-120

From Lee EY, Boiselle PM. Tracheobronchomalacia in infants and children: multidetector CT evaluation, *Radiology.* 2009;252(1):7-22.

For tube current and kilovoltage by patient weight for end-expiratory multidetector computed tomography (MDCT) examination, mAs should be reduced by 50% to a maximum of 40 mAs while maintaining the same level of kilovoltage for end-inspiratory MDCT examination.

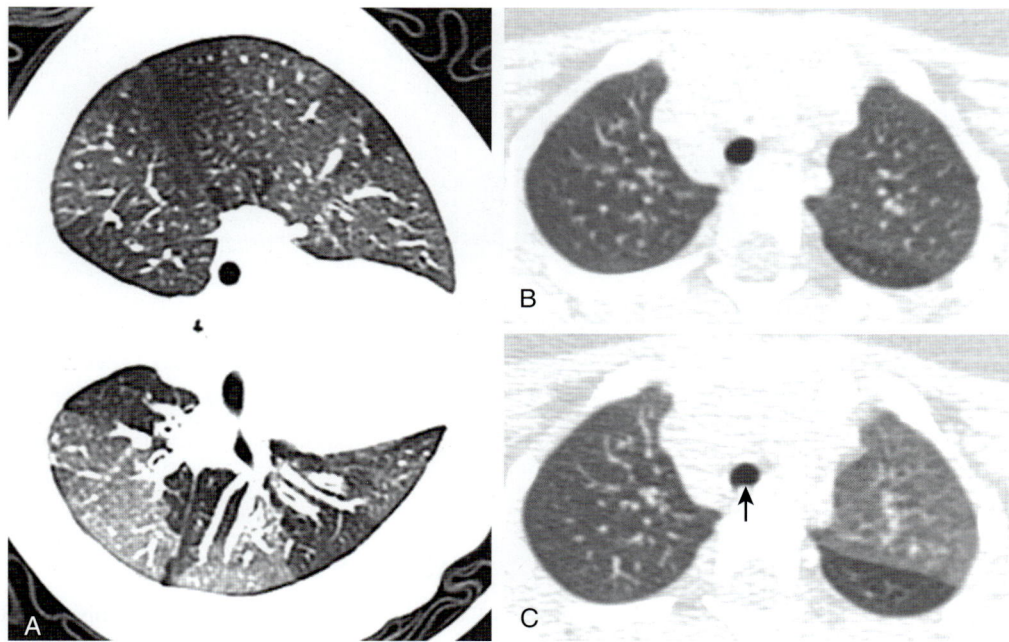

Figure 49-5 Expiratory computed tomography (CT) techniques in children breathing freely. **A,** A left side down lateral decubitus CT scan shows geographic hyperlucent areas due to trapping of air, the so-called mosaic lung attenuation, in the dependent left lung of a child with bronchiolitis obliterans. Inspiratory **(B)** and expiratory **(C)** cine CT images show the normal left upper lobe and the abnormal right upper and left lower lobes with trapping of air. The normal posterior indentation of the trachea (*arrow*) is noted at expiration **(C)**.

EVALUATION OF LUNGS

CT is valuable in evaluating not only the air spaces (which may be either opaque or hyperlucent) but also interstitial and vascular abnormalities and parenchymal nodules or masses in the lung. In addition, mediastinal, hilar, and chest wall abnormalities also can be assessed. However, soft tissue contrast resolution of CT is inferior to that of MRI. Furthermore, MRI is better than CT in evaluating intraspinal and paraspinal regions. However, expiratory CT is necessary to identify air trapping accurately.[40,43]

To obtain proper expiratory CT data, patient cooperation is required. In uncooperative infants and young children, lateral decubitus CT may be used as an alterative.[44] In this position, dependent and nondependent lungs show different lung volumes that mimic inspiration and expiration, respectively (Fig. 49-5, *A*). However, a potential drawback of the lateral decubitus CT technique is the need to change the position of the patient, which may awaken the patient, thus making interpretation difficult because of considerable respiratory misregistration between the dependent and nondependent lungs and exaggerated respiratory motion artifacts in the nondependent lung. Cine CT in the supine position can overcome some of the limitations of lateral decubitus CT (Fig. 49-5, *B* and *C*).[40] Recently, dual-energy chest CT has been used in pediatric patients to assess regional lung perfusion and ventilation.[45-51] By using 3D CT data, quantitative analysis to determine lung volume or density can be performed.

Routine Chest Computed Tomographic Study (Without or with Intravenous Contrast)

Routine chest CT is performed without or with intravenous administration of an iodinated contrast agent, depending on the clinical questions being addressed. As previously mentioned, tube voltage should be determined with the use of an iodinated contrast agent. High tube voltage should be used for an unenhanced chest CT scan, whereas low tube voltage should be selected for an enhanced chest CT scan. The use of precontrast and postcontrast (dual-phase) chest CT should be avoided in pediatric patients as much as possible to minimize exposure to radiation. Virtual unenhanced CT imaging using the dual-energy technique may substitute for real unenhanced CT imaging, thus reducing radiation dose.[51]

High-Resolution Computed Tomographic Study

High-resolution CT (HRCT) originally was developed in the 1980s as a special technique in which noncontiguous thin sections, approximately 1 mm in slice thickness, are acquired at 7- to 20-mm intervals depending on the size of the patient.[52] To illustrate fine details of the lung anatomy and pathology, a high spatial frequency reconstruction algorithm is used. This classic HRCT study has been used principally as a follow-up imaging study of diffuse lung abnormalities, such as interstitial lung disease or cystic fibrosis, while delivering a very low radiation dose. The recent development of MDCT allows contiguous thin sections of the entire lung to be viewed with a reasonably low radiation dose and MPR capabilities, which changes the technical concept of HRCT of the lung. MDCT with thin collimation (<1 mm), single spiral CT scanning can provide both thick sections (for a routine chest CT with standard reconstruction algorithm) and thin sections (for HRCT of the lung with high spatial frequency reconstruction algorithm) without additional scanning radiation exposure. It has been reported that reconstructed HRCT images from volumetric MDCT acquisition have significantly less motion artifact than images obtained with

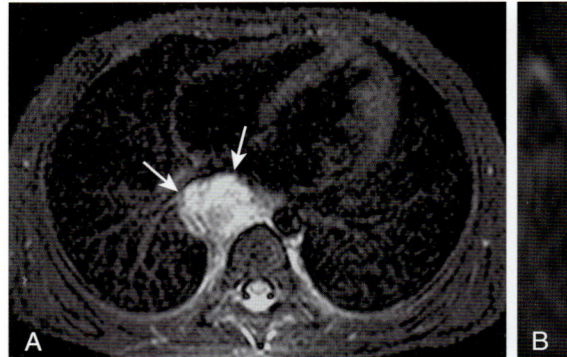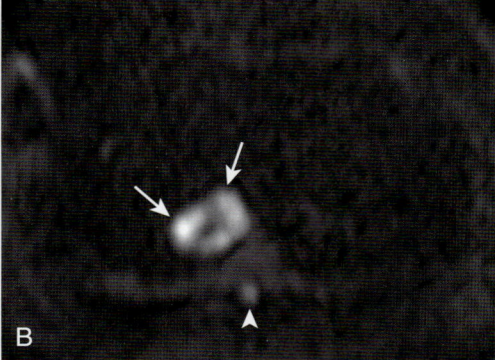

Figure 49-6 Diffusion-weighted magnetic resonance imaging (MRI). **A,** Axial T2-weighted chest MRI using a short tau inversion recovery sequence shows a metastatic neuroblastoma involving a paraesophageal lymph node (*arrows*). **B,** On axial diffusion-weighted MRI (b-value, 800 s/mm²), hyperintense areas are predominant in the lesion (*arrows*), indicating restricted water diffusion or hypercellularity. Of note, the normal spinal cord (*arrowhead*) appears modestly hyperintense.

traditional axial HRCT acquisition in pediatric patients.[52-55] Nonetheless, the classic HRCT technique still may be used in pediatric patients because of the overall decreased radiation with this CT technique compared with MDCT volumetric data acquisition.

Magnetic Resonance Imaging

Chest MRI has inherent limitations because of the low signal-to-noise ratio of the lung, cardiac and respiratory motion artifacts, and susceptibility artifacts that occur at air-tissue interfaces in the lung. A lengthy examination time is another important disadvantage of MRI, leading to a greater requirement for sedation in pediatric patients. However, recent technical advances in MRI, such as parallel imaging and multi-channel body-array coils, allow substantial reduction of examination time. In addition, vector electrocardiogram triggering, respiratory triggering, and navigator gating may be used separately or together to suppress motion artifacts.

Lack of ionizing radiation exposure and excellent soft tissue contrast are advantages of MRI. Different tissue characteristics can be evaluated with T1- and T2-weighted imaging and, more recently, balanced steady-state free precession imaging. Fat saturation may be added to the pulse sequence if necessary. The use of gadolinium contrast agents can further improve tissue characterization on T1-weighted imaging. In addition, a variety of functional thoracic assessments including perfusion, ventilation, and respiratory mechanics can be performed with MRI.[56,57] Water diffusivity or cellularity of thoracic masses may be evaluated with diffusion-weighted imaging (Fig. 49-6). Hyperpolarized gas MRI allows excellent static and dynamic visualization of the lung and airway and may overcome the limitations of proton MRI of the thorax. However, hyperpolarized gas MRI has markedly limited availability, which is the main obstacle to clinical use and the primary reason it remains in the research realm. It should be noted that chest MRI examination cannot be performed in some circumstances (e.g., when contraindications for MRI exist, such as the presence of a permanent cardiac pacemaker, the presence of a cardioverter defibrillator, or claustrophobia).

EVALUATION OF AIRWAYS

Central airways and their relationships to adjacent cardiovascular structures can be assessed with noncontrast black–blood MRI (Fig. 49-7).[58] Tracheobronchomalacia can be diagnosed with real-time dynamic airway MRI. However, it is preferable to perform airway evaluations with CT. The delineation of peripheral small airways on MRI is somewhat limited because of relatively low spatial resolution.

EVALUATION OF LUNGS

Despite the inherent limitations of lung MRI that were previously mentioned, a study showed that lung nodules of a diameter larger than 3 to 4 mm can be detected with MRI with use of 1.5T systems.[59] Contrast–enhanced time-resolved magnetic resonance angiography offers not only

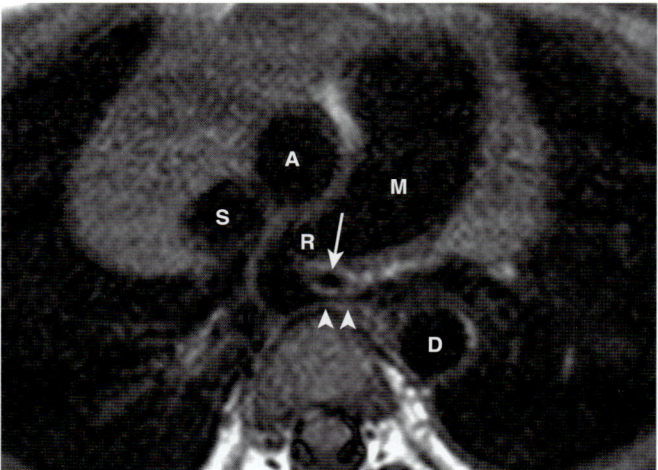

Figure 49-7 Black-blood magnetic resonance imaging (MRI). An axial T1-weighted, electrocardiogram-triggered chest MRI using spin-echo echo-planar imaging and the black-blood technique shows an intimate relationship between the left pulmonary artery sling and congenital tracheal stenosis (*arrow*), the so-called "sling-ring" complex. Note a severe focal stenosis (*arrowheads*) of the left pulmonary artery between the trachea and the spine. *M,* main pulmonary artery; *R,* right pulmonary artery; *A,* ascending aorta; *D,* descending aorta; *S,* superior vena cava.

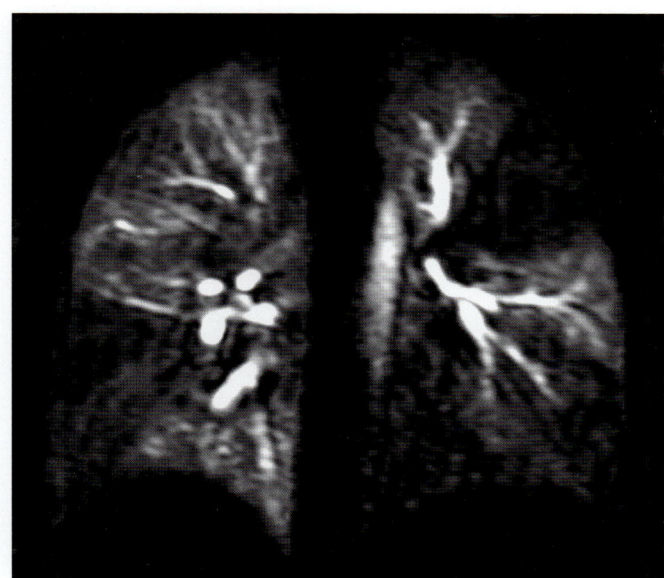

Figure 49-8 Contrast-enhanced lung perfusion magnetic resonance imaging. A coronal image obtained from time-resolved magnetic resonance angiography shows maximal contrast enhancement in the normal lung areas and multiple lung perfusion defects. The signal outside the lung is suppressed by means of subtraction.

anatomic details of pulmonary vessels but also hemodynamics of pulmonary circulation. Because contrast bolus timing is not needed and less motion artifact occurs because of high temporal resolution (e.g., <1 second for the entire lung), time-resolved MR angiography often replaces static high-resolution MR angiography in pediatric patients.[60] Lung perfusion MRI can be obtained with either the contrast-enhanced or non–contrast-enhanced technique (Fig. 49-8). Real-time dynamic chest MRI with the patient breathing freely may be used to demonstrate normal and abnormal respiratory dynamics.[61] Regional ventilation may be assessed with oxygen-enhanced MRI or hyperpolarized gas (^{3}helium or ^{129}xenon) MRI. Diffusion-weighted imaging using hyperpolarized gas enables calculation of the size of peripheral air spaces. Hyperpolarized xenon MRI has an additional capability of assessing diffusing capacity in the lung. A preliminary study recently reported a promising free-breathing proton MRI technique without any contrast agents that demonstrated both lung perfusion and lung tissue density in a single data acquisition by means of Fourier decomposition.[62] Although MRI may provide anatomic and functional information of the lung without radiation, CT generally is preferred in pediatric patients, mainly because of its high spatial resolution.

Nuclear Medicine Studies

Many nuclear medicine techniques have an important advantage over anatomic imaging methods in some clinical settings because they have the ability to evaluate physiologic processes. Several radionuclide techniques are commonly are used to evaluate pediatric diseases of the respiratory system or chest wall, as listed in Table 49-2. Most nuclear medicine studies are performed with an intravenous injection of a radiopharmaceutical agent. The biodistribution and subsequent route of clearance of the tracer determine the amount and organ distribution of radiation exposure to the patient. Many nuclear medicine procedures carry inherently higher radiation exposure to the patient than plain film radiographic procedures, but the radiation exposure is comparable to or less than that accompanying CT examinations. It is important to use the lowest possible injected tracer dosage that allows good-quality images to be recorded. Although accepted standard adult radiopharmaceutical dosages often are established, dosage determination in children is best calculated on the basis of weight, which in turn is derived from the adult reference administered activity.[63] In recent years, considerable efforts have been made to ensure that pediatric dosages are as low as possible while remaining practical. Current recommendations are presented in Table 49-2.

The acquisition time for nuclear medicine images often is quite long compared with radiographic techniques, and gentle immobilization and distraction is necessary in small children. Sedation during nuclear medicine imaging studies is seldom necessary, but occasionally is required during lengthy imaging sessions. Currently available nuclear medicine studies that are used to assess thoracic disorders in pediatric patients include the lung perfusion and ventilation study, salivagram, neuroendocrine imaging study, bone scan, and positron emission tomography, which are discussed in the following sections.

LUNG PERFUSION AND VENTILATION STUDY

Lung perfusion imaging, although largely supplanted by CT techniques for the diagnosis of pulmonary embolus, remains an important technique for the evaluation of lung physiology

Table 49-2

Recommended Administered Activities Based on the North American Consensus Guidelines for Administered Radiopharmaceutical Activities in Children and Adolescents			
Radiopharmaceutical Agent	**Recommended Administered Activity**	**Minimum Administered Activity**	**Maximum Administered Activity**
^{99m}Tc macroaggregated albumin	If ^{99m}Tc is used for ventilation, 2.59 MBq/kg (0.07 mCi/kg) If no ^{99m}Tc ventilation study is performed, 1.11 MBq/kg (0.03 mCi/kg)	14.8 MBq (0.4 mCi)	
^{99m}Tc methylene diphosphonate	9.3 MBq/kg (0.25 mCi/kg)	37 MBq (1.0 mCi)	
^{123}I metaiodobenzylguanidine	5.2 MBq/kg (0.14 mCi/kg)	37 MBq (1.0 mCi)	370 MBq (10.0 mCi)
Fluorine 18-labeled deoxyglucose	3.7-5.2 MBq/kg (0.10-0.14 mCi/kg)	37 MBq (1.0 mCi)	

Modified from Gelfand MJ, Parisi MT, Treves ST. Pediatric radiopharmaceutical administered doses: 2010 North American consensus guidelines, *J Nucl Med.* 2011;52:318-322.

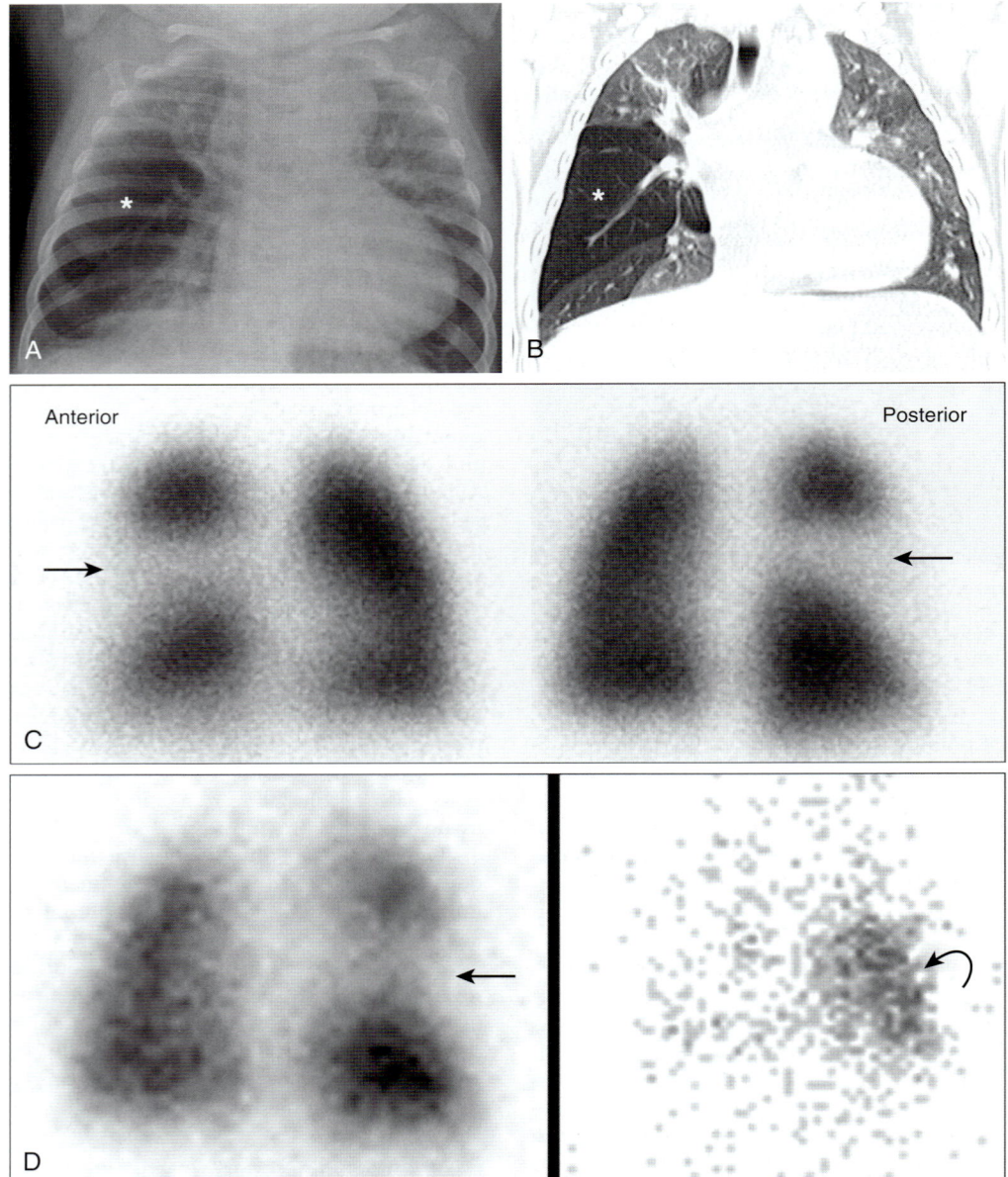

Figure 49-9 Multimodality imaging of a 7-month-old girl with congenital lobar emphysema. **A,** A frontal chest radiograph shows hyperlucency (*asterisk*) in the right mid to lower lung zone. **B,** A coronal lung window computed tomography image demonstrates hyperinflation and oligemia of the right middle lobe (*asterisk*), consistent with congenital lobar emphysema. **C,** A perfusion lung scan shows no perfusion to the right middle lobe (*arrow*) on the anterior view (*Anterior*) and posterior view (*Posterior*). **D,** A posterior image from a ventilation scan on the left showing initial decreased ventilation to the right middle lung (*straight arrow*) with air trapping in the same area of the later images on the right (*curved arrow*).

and pathology. The incidence of pulmonary embolism in the pediatric population is lower than in the adult population, but occasionally perfusion imaging is used with patients who have significant risk factors to evaluate for an embolus when a contraindication to the administration of radiographic contrast material exists. Nuclear ventilation and perfusion imaging is much more commonly used to evaluate relative function in diseases in which knowledge of physiology helps to guide clinical care. Both relative ventilation and perfusion can be quantitated, which permits treatment planning and follow-up evaluation in a variety of clinical entities such as lung malformations resulting from congenital lobar emphysema

and congenital pulmonary airway malformations (Fig. 49-9). The quantitative analysis of relative lung perfusion and ventilation also is useful in preoperative cases before pneumonectomy to evaluate for the estimated postsurgical lung capacity.[64]

Patients with congenital heart disease frequently undergo ventilation and perfusion imaging to quantitate relative perfusion between the right and left lung at baseline and after catheter intervention (Fig. 49-10).

The perfusion study is performed with technetium-99m (^{99m}Tc) macroaggregated albumin (MAA). The dosage in pediatrics is based on patient weight (Table 49-2). In cases

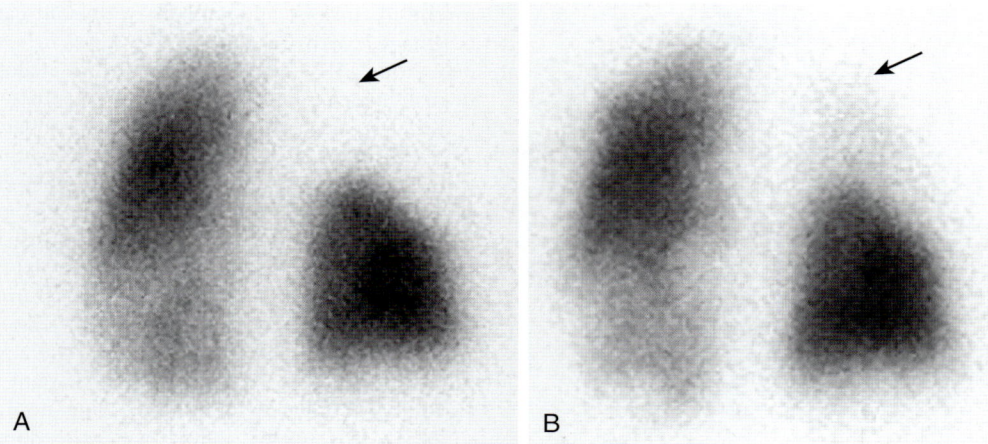

Figure 49-10   Nuclear medicine perfusion imaging in a 20-year-old man with tetralogy of Fallot. **A,** A posterior view of the lung scan shows decreased perfusion to the right upper lung (*arrow*). **B,** After placement of a right upper pulmonary artery stent, the perfusion study now shows some perfusion to the right upper lung (*arrow*).

of congenital heart disease when differential lung perfusion is evaluated, a specially prepared radiopharmaceutical agent with a low concentration of particles of MAA is recommended. The tracer is always injected with the patient supine so a hydrostatic gradient is not present from lung apex to base. Imaging can be performed with the patient either upright or supine, but supine imaging typically is performed in children. If imaging is being performed to evaluate pulmonary physiology, typically only anterior and posterior planar views are acquired. The differential lung perfusion is then calculated by drawing a region of interest around each lung and calculating the geometric mean (i.e., the square root of the product of anterior and posterior views) of counts in each lung. If the perfusion scan is being performed to evaluate for a pulmonary embolism, additional anatomic information is recorded, with a standard of eight planar images (i.e., anterior, posterior, left and right lateral, right anterior oblique, left anterior oblique, right posterior oblique, and left posterior oblique views). Alternatively, single photon emission computed tomography (SPECT) imaging of the lungs can be performed. When evaluating for a possible pulmonary embolus, a correlation should be made with a chest radiograph obtained within 24 hours of the study.

The ventilation study can be performed either with a radioactive gas (xenon-133) that demonstrates air flow or a radio aerosol (^{99m}Tc diethylenetriaminepentaacetic acid [DTPA]) that localizes in alveoli without significant large airway deposition. Xenon-133 gas has the principle photon energy of 81 keV, which is lower than ^{99m}Tc and thus the ventilation images must be acquired first. The DTPA aerosol study uses the same ^{99m}Tc label as MAA perfusion imaging, but much less aerosol tracer activity localizes in the lungs than is present with the intravenous MAA injection. Thus both xenon and aerosol ventilation imaging must be performed before the perfusion agent is administered.

Xenon-133 gas is administered by inhalation. The recommended dose is 10 to 20 mCi. The dynamic nature of the xenon study limits the projections that can be obtained, and thus imaging typically is acquired in the posterior view with a single-head camera. If a dual-head camera is used,

simultaneous anterior and posterior imaging can be acquired. The presence of the anterior detector over the child's face and thorax can cause the patient to become anxious, and thus in young children only the posterior image typically is acquired.

^{99m}Tc DTPA aerosol is administered via a shielded nebulizer; the child inhales long enough to accumulate sufficient aerosol in the lung for imaging. The aerosol remains in the lungs long enough for imaging to be performed in multiple projections, matching those acquired with perfusion imaging. When SPECT perfusion imaging is performed, SPECT aerosol images also can be acquired for meaningful comparison.

SALIVAGRAM

Radionuclide evaluation for salivary aspiration (i.e., a salivagram) offers a safe and easily performed test with minimal radiation exposure to the patient. The sensitivity of the salivagram has been reported to range between 26% and 73%.[65-67] The salivagram can be performed with the administration of a small drop (approximately 100 μL) of ^{99m}Tc sulfur colloid (300 μCi [11.1 MBq]) that is placed in the oral cavity while the patient is lying in a supine position in the imaging bed. After administration of the radiopharmaceutical agent, the patient is allowed to swallow normally and posterior planar imaging of the mouth, chest, and upper abdomen is obtained dynamically for 60 minutes. Imaging is acquired using a low-energy, high-resolution or ultra–high-resolution collimator, with consecutive dynamic images recorded every 30 seconds for a total of 120 frames. A positive salivagram for aspiration shows the radiopharmaceutical agent entering the bronchi (Fig. 49-11).

NEUROENDOCRINE IMAGING STUDY

Neuroendocrine tumors can be imaged very effectively with use of iodine-123–labeled metaiodobenzylguanidine (^{123}I MIBG). The two tumors most commonly evaluated with this tracer are pheochromocytomas and neuroblastomas (Fig. 49-12). Although other tumors such as ganglioneuromas,

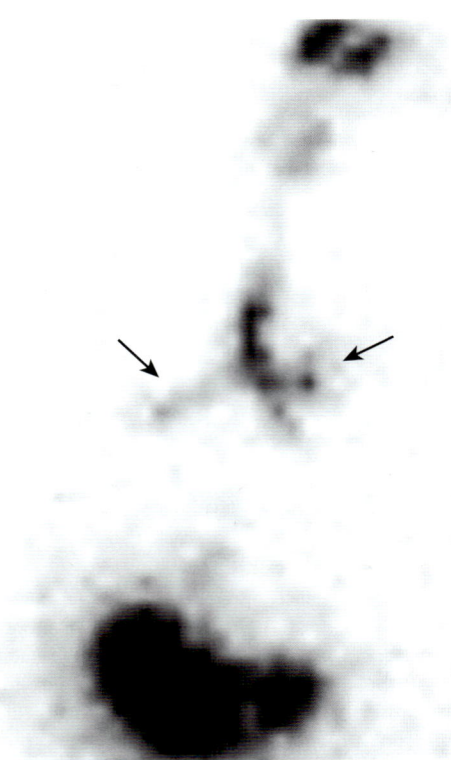

Figure 49-11 Salivagram. A posterior view of the neck, chest, and upper abdomen shows bilateral aspiration into the proximal bronchi (*arrows*).

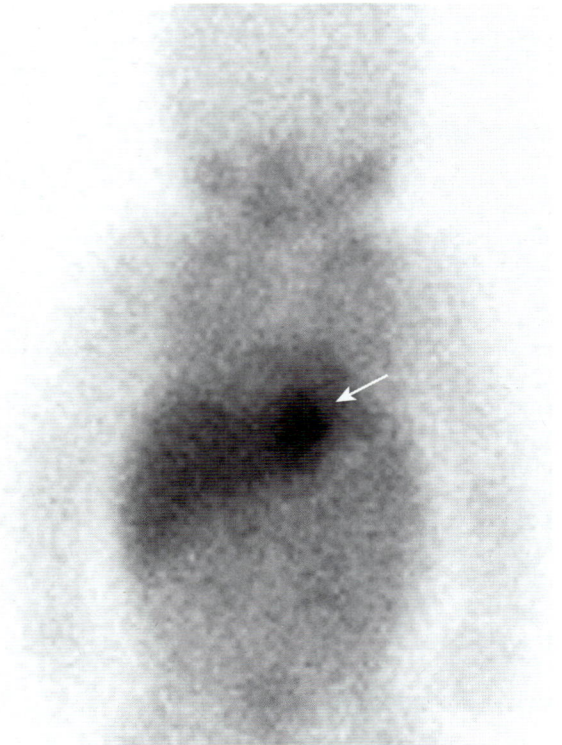

Figure 49-12 Neuroendocrine tumor imaging in a 4-week-old girl with a left-sided thoracic mass that was first detected on prenatal imaging. A ^{123}I metaiodobenzylguanidine study shows intense uptake by the mass (*arrow*). The patient underwent surgical resection of the mass. The histology result was consistent with neuroblastoma.

carcinoid tumors, and medullary thyroid carcinoma also can be imaged with this tracer, they show a lower sensitivity of detection. MIBG is a norepinephrine analog, and its uptake in malignancy can be used both to evaluate a primary tumor and metastasis at presentation and to evaluate tumor response after treatment. It is important to review the patient's medications before imaging because a number of pharmaceutical agents have the potential to block the tumor uptake of MIBG. These agents include preparations that contain ephedrine and its derivatives, along with neuroleptic drugs, tricyclic antidepressants, and central nervous system stimulants. The MIBG dose always contains a small amount of unlabeled radioiodine that will localize within the thyroid gland, thus increasing local radiation exposure. Patient radiation dosimetry can be reduced by administering nonradioactive iodine to block this uptake before the procedure. The increased circulating nonradioactive iodine reduces subsequent extraction of radioactive iodine and is easily achieved by administering a strong solution of potassium iodide (1 drop three times a day) beginning 1 day before the injection and continuing for 3 days after the tracer injection.

The recommended dosage of ^{123}I MIBG is 5.2 MBq/kg (0.14 mCi/kg). In cases of suspected pheochromocytoma, the tracer should be administered slowly, and the patient's blood pressure should be monitored during and after tracer administration, because rare hypertensive reactions have been reported.

The ^{123}I MIBG scan is performed the day after the intravenous administration of tracer. Whole-body planar imaging is performed, including lateral skull images, and SPECT of the neck, thorax, abdomen, and pelvis is obtained.

Another radiopharmaceutical agent used to image neuroendocrine tumors is indium-111–labeled pentetreotide (Octreoscan), a somatostatin receptor imaging agent. Pentetreotide is useful in imaging a wide variety of neuroendocrine tumors that express a high density of somatostatin receptors, such as carcinoid tumors. The dosage is 100 μCi/kg (3.7 MBq/kg), with a minimun of 1 mCi (37 MBq), and a maximum of 6 mCi (222 MBq). Imaging is performed 24 hours after administration with planar and SPECT images of the torso.

BONE SCAN

A bone scan is used frequently in the evaluation of the thoracic skeleton, such as in the evaluation of chest wall pain (Fig. 49-13). ^{99m}Tc-labeled methylenediphosphonate is the most common radiopharmaceutical agent used for bone scans. This tracer is administered intravenously, and imaging is performed from 2 to 4 hours after administration, using a whole body sweep (anterior and posterior) or individual images of the area of interest. SPECT imaging also can be performed. This technique is particularly useful in the evaluation of the ribs and spine. When evaluating a patient for suspected osteomyelitis, initial blood flow images are recorded immediately after the administration of tracer, in addition to the standard delayed imaging.

POSITRON EMISSION TOMOGRAPHY

Positron emission tomography (PET) is useful in evaluating many primary and metastatic intrathoracic tumors in pediatric patients (Fig. 49-14). Pediatric tumors commonly evaluated adequate accumulation of the tracer in the tumor. Images of the torso or of the entire body can be obtained according to the indication of the study. Several elements of patient preparation for the study are important. Because FDG is taken up competitively with glucose, the patient must fast (i.e., no solid food and nothing to drink except water) for at least 4 hours before the PET scan. The patient must not receive any form of glucose, including intravenous fluids containing glucose, for at least 4 hours before administration. The blood glucose level is measured routinely at the time of tracer administration and should be between 50 mg/dL and 200 mg/dL. Patients who are diabetic and/or dependent on insulin should take their diabetic medication and/or insulin 2 hours before the examination with a small amount of juice and dry toast or plain crackers. The patient should avoid any strenuous exercise 24 hours before the study because such exercise might lead to an increase in muscle uptake that hinders the interpretation of the study.

Another important aspect of pediatric PET studies is the high incidence of metabolically active brown fat activation compared with the adult population. The presence of brown fat increases the number of equivocal studies.[68] Warming patients at 24° C before and during the FDG uptake phase decreases the incidence of brown fat activation significantly.[69]

In the evaluation of tumors, PET provides an advantage over anatomic imaging because it detects viable tissue. Use of PET in the evaluation of Hodgkin lymphoma has been shown to increase the detection of metastases when compared with CT alone.[70]

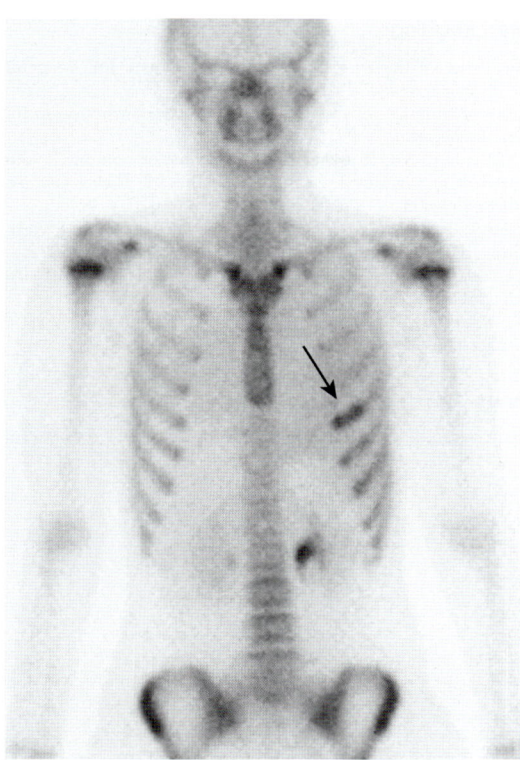

Figure 49-13 A bone scan of a 14-year-old with left-sided chest pain. The planar anterior view of the chest shows increased uptake in the left anterior fifth rib (*arrow*). A biopsy of this rib lesion was consistent with Ewing sarcoma.

with PET include Hodgkin lymphoma, non-Hodgkin lymphoma, rhabdomyosarcoma, osteosarcoma, Ewing sarcoma, neuroblastoma, and other less common malignancies.

The recommended dosage of fluorine 18-labeled deoxyglucose (FDG) is 150 µCi/kg (5.55 MBq) (minimum 500 µCi [18.5 MBq] and maximum 10 mCi [370 MBq]). Imaging is performed about 60 minutes after the injection to allow

WHAT THE CLINICIAN NEEDS TO KNOW

- Available imaging modalities for the pediatric respiratory system
- Advantages and disadvantages of each imaging modality
- Optimization of imaging techniques

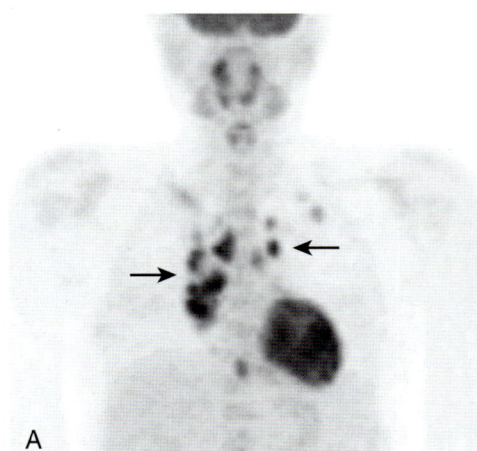
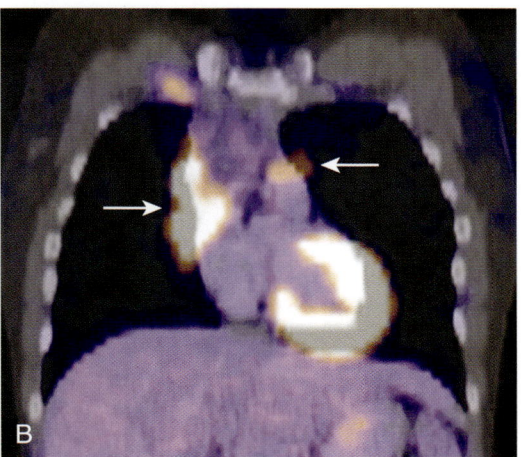

Figure 49-14 Positron emission tomography (PET) imaging in a 19-year-old with newly diagnosed Hodgkin disease. **A,** A coronal PET image shows multiple sites of abnormal uptake in the anterior mediastinum (*arrows*). **B,** Fusion of a PET and computed tomography (CT) image shows the abnormal area of uptake corresponding to the enlarged lymph nodes on CT (*arrows*).

Key Points

The presence of air in the airways and lungs is beneficial and sometimes challenging with regard to imaging of the respiratory system.

Up-to-date knowledge regarding imaging techniques is essential to achieve optimum diagnostic performance and to choose an appropriate imaging method for evaluation of the pediatric respiratory system.

Imaging parameters should be tailored to each individual pediatric patient for optimal results.

Risks related to diagnostic imaging, such as radiation exposure, the use of a contrast agent, and sedation, should be minimized.

Suggested Readings

Goo HW. State-of-the-art CT imaging techniques for congenital heart disease. *Korean J Radiol.* 2010;11:4-18.

John SD, Swischunk LE. Stridor and upper airway obstruction in infants and children. *Radiographics.* 1992;12:625-643.

Lee EY, Greenberg SB, Boiselle PM. Multidetector computed tomography of pediatric large airway diseases: state-of-the-art. *Radiol Clin North Am.* 2011;49(5):869-893.

Lee EY. Advancing CT and MR imaging of the lungs and airways in children: imaging into practice. *Pediatr Radiol.* 2008;38:S208-S212.

Treves ST, Baker A, Fahey FH, et al. Nuclear medicine in the first year of life. *J Nucl Med.* 2011;52(6):905-925.

Willis CE. Optimizing digital radiography of children. *Eur J Radiol.* 2009;72:266-273.

References

Full references for this chapter can be found on www.expertconsult.com.

Chapter 50

Prenatal Imaging and Intervention

DOROTHY BULAS and EDWARD Y. LEE

With the advances in high-resolution ultrasonography and magnetic resonance imaging (MRI), thoracic lesions are now commonly detected before birth. The most common congenital thoracic lesions include congenital diaphragmatic hernia (CDH); congenital bronchopulmonary malformations, which represent a group of lung anomalies, including congenital pulmonary airway malformation (CPAM), bronchopulmonary sequestration (BPS), and congenital lobar overinflation (CLO); and congenital hydrothorax. Additionally, congenital high airway obstruction (CHAOS), which is caused by obstruction or absence of the trachea, may also present in utero. Pulmonary hypoplasia, agenesis, and aplasia are less common and discussed in Chapter 53.[1-4]

In a fetus, the clinical importance of these lesions lies primarily in the mass effect on surrounding structures. This may result in compression of the airway, blood vessels, lymphatics, and lung with development of pleural effusions, polyhydramnios, hydrops, and pulmonary hypoplasia. The outcome depends on the timing of secondary effects and the severity of pulmonary hypoplasia. With improvements in fetal imaging, fetal intervention has also advanced. Masses that resulted in hydrops in the past were typically lethal. Now these masses may be amenable to fetal intervention including maternal steroids, intrauterine cyst aspiration, fetal thoracentesis, thoracoamniotic shunts, laser therapy, sclerotherapy, and in utero fetoscopic or open fetal surgery.[5-9]

In maternal-fetal surgery, the greatest responsibility is to the mother, who is an innocent bystander in the maldevelopment occurring in utero. She must be aware of the risks and benefits for herself and her infant and has the potential to undergo an operation that has no direct benefit to her. The limiting factor of invasive fetal therapy continues to be preterm labor despite advances in uterine relaxation. Almost all fetuses that undergo fetal therapy are still delivered prematurely. Women who have undergone open fetal surgery have been able to have normal children subsequently, although delivery of subsequent pregnancies requires cesarean section. Thus, invasive fetal therapy is limited to circumstances in which it may be predicted with reasonable certainty that the fetus or infant would not survive without fetal intervention.[7]

Common Congenital Thoracic Lesions in Fetus

CONGENITAL DIAPHRAGMATIC HERNIA

Etiology The diaphragm develops in the fourth week of gestation with fusion of four components. By 8 weeks, the pleural–peritoneal cavity separates. There is caudal migration with final diaphragmatic positioning by 12 weeks. The most common CDH occurs secondary to failure of fusion of the left pleuroperitoneal membrane to the remaining primitive diaphragm (Bochdalek hernia). The bowel returns to the abdomen by the 10th week of gestation and may begin to herniate into the chest if a diaphragmatic defect is present.

CDH occurs in 1:3000 to 1:4000 live births. They occur on the left in 88%, the right in 10%, and bilaterally in 2%. Herniation occurs by the second trimester and affects early lung development on the contralateral and ipsilateral sides. CDH is typically sporadic. However, a 15% to 45% incidence of associated anomalies is seen. Rare familial cases and syndromes have been described.[10] The presence of a major malformation significantly increases the mortality rate. Thus, close assessment of additional anomalies, fetal echocardiography, and karyotyping are important for appropriate counseling.

Imaging The diagnosis of CDH in fetuses may be missed ultrasonographically, particularly when the stomach is not herniated into the chest.[11,12] In these cases, mediastinal shift may be the first finding to suggest the diagnosis. Ultrasonographic evaluation should characterize the location of the diaphragmatic defect and the amount of herniated organs. Coronal and sagittal images help locate the defect, whereas axial images are important to assess the amount of mediastinal deviation. Contralateral lung volume should be measured. Ipsilateral lung tissue should be looked for but typically is too compressed to be visualized. The stomach and gallbladder are identified, and the location above or below the diaphragm is noted.

Herniation of the liver into the chest is associated with a poorer outcome and thus is important to determine. This may be difficult ultrasonographically because the liver and lung may have a similar echotexture. An abnormal course of the umbilical, hepatic, and portal veins may help confirm this finding.[13] With left CDH, the left lobe of the liver typically herniates into the anterior chest. If the stomach is adjacent to the anterior chest wall, liver herniation is unlikely. With right-sided hernias, the liver is more posterior in the chest. At times, small bowel loops may mimic lung cysts, making it difficult to differentiate it from CPAM. Color Doppler of the superior mesenteric artery may be helpful in confirming herniation of bowel loops by following the vessel into the chest. Associated anomalies, particularly cardiac, should be searched for.

Fetal MRI protocol should include T2-weighted images in all three planes and T1-weighted breath hold gradient recalled echo images in the coronal plane to assess for liver and meconium positions (Fig. 50-1). Meconium-filled bowel loops are low signal on T2-weighted images and high signal on T1-weighted images, making location of the bowel easy. The liver is high signal on T1-weighted images and intermediate signal on T2-weighted images, also making it easy to separate from bowel and adjacent lung (e-Fig. 50-2). MRI is most helpful in the evaluation of right and bilateral CDH.[14,15] In these cases, with the stomach often located below the diaphragm in the abdomen, it may be difficult to differentiate a CPAM from a CDH by ultrasound. MRI easily distinguishes abdominal contents within the chest from cystic lesions and provides specific information on hernia content, size of diaphragmatic defect, and amount of ipsilateral and contralateral lung.

One goal of fetal imaging is to predict outcome when counseling patients. Survival rates range from 40% to 90% with an overall mortality reported to be 70% to 80%.[16] Currently, no single finding or measurement has been shown to be an absolute indicator of postnatal outcome. Indications for poor prognosis include large mediastinal shift and liver herniation.[17] With liver herniation, the survival rate has been reported to be approximately 50%, whereas fetuses without herniation may have up to 90% survival.[14,18,19] Additional findings such as intrathoracic location of the stomach, asymmetric size of cardiac ventricles, and polyhydramnios also may indicate a worse prognosis. Syndromes associated with CDH, for example, Fryns syndrome, have a poorer prognosis (e-Fig. 50-3).[10] The presence of additional anomalies also affect outcome. Bilateral CDHs are typically fatal.

The degree of lung hypoplasia has prognostic value, but the best way to quantify this remains unclear. Measurement of the lung-to-head ratio adjusts for fetal size and gestational age and estimates the amount of residual contralateral lung.[19-22] The cross-sectional area of the lung at the level of the four-chamber view of the heart is measured ultrasonographically and expressed as a ratio of lung cross-sectional area over head circumference. With a low lung-to-head ratio, the outcome is poor; with a high ratio, the outcome is more favorable. At the extremes, if the ratio is less than 0.6, mortality is 100%, and if the ratio is greater than 1.4, the survival rate is 90%.

Multiple other methods have been attempted by MRI to quantify lung hypoplasia.[23-27] Total lung volumes may be compared with expected lung volumes for age. A lung volume of greater than 25 cm³ suggests a favorable prognosis, whereas less than 18 cm³ suggests a poor outcome. A ratio of observed to predicted lung volume less than 25% suggests a poor outcome.[26,27] Estimated expected lung volume is calculated by measuring fetal thoracic volume and then

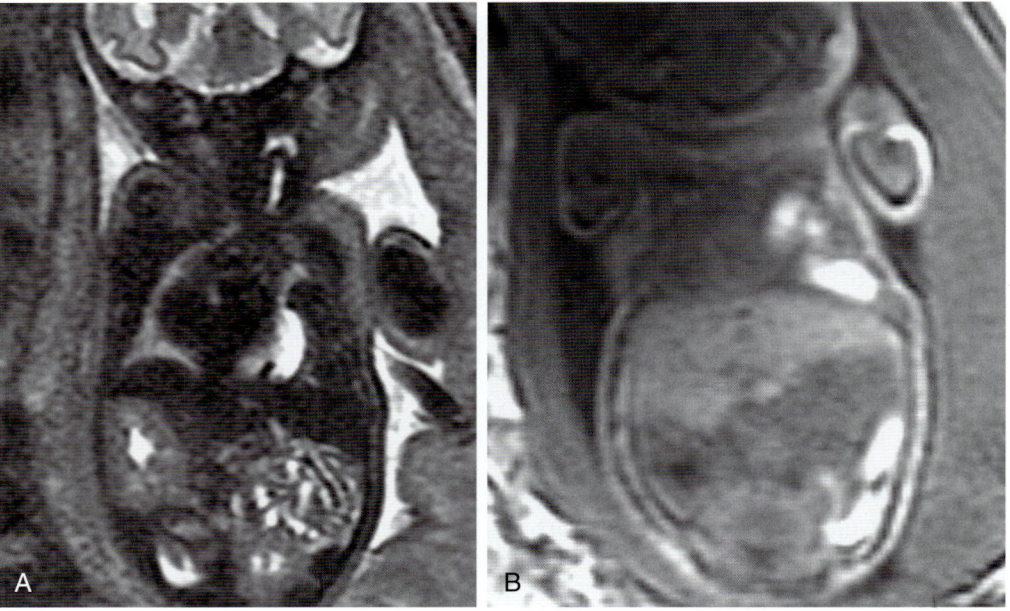

Figure 50-1   Left congenital diaphragmatic hernia. **A,** A coronal single-shot fast spin echo T2-weighted magnetic resonance image at 32 weeks' gestation demonstrates deviation of the heart to the right. High-signal fluid-filled stomach and low-signal meconium are herniated into the left chest. The liver appears infradiaphragmatic. **B,** A coronal gradient recalled echo T1-weighted image shows high signal meconium-filled colon herniated into the left hemithorax. The intermediate signal liver is infradiaphragmatic.

subtracting mediastinal volume. The lung volume of the fetus with a CDH is then measured and divided by this expected lung volume to give the percent predicted lung volume. Percent predicted lung volume of less than 15% has a 40% rate of survival compared to 100% if greater than 15%.[28] Other studies have suggested, however, that calculated lung volume is not predictive of outcome.[22,29,30]

Infants with CDH may develop pulmonary hypertension, and this may be predicted by the modified McGoon index. From ultrasonographic or MRI measurements, the right and left pulmonary artery diameters are added, which is then divided by the aortic diameter. If the value is less than 0.8, the risk of developing pulmonary hypertension is high; if the value is greater than 1.0, the risk is low.[31]

Treatment and Follow-up A wide spectrum of severity after birth exists in infants with the same anatomic defect, with some most likely to live and others most likely to die. The severity of pulmonary hypoplasia is determined by the timing of when the abdominal contents moved into the thorax and how much they compressed the developing lung. It is also known that esophageal obstruction from herniation and kinking of the gastroesophageal junction of the stomach produces polyhydramnios. To help these pregnancies, the fetal lung needs to be made to grow larger before birth, or a way has to be devised to support lung function after birth. Extracorporeal membrane oxygenation (ECMO) may support lung function for several weeks until the lungs grow and pulmonary hypertension resolves. To help lungs have more space to grow in utero, open fetal surgical diaphragmatic repair has been attempted. Most fetuses with CDH with their liver in the thorax are not amenable to traditional antenatal surgical repair because the umbilical vein kinks when the liver is returned to the abdomen. Open surgery worked fairly well for fetuses with livers "down" (below the diaphragm). For fetuses with livers "up" (above the diaphragm), however, this approach has failed. However, the National Institutes of Health (NIH) sponsored prospective fetal surgical trial showed no improvement in survival in fetuses with their livers "down."[32]

The history of fetal intervention for CDH has evolved from surgically invasive procedures to less invasive fetoscopic techniques.[29,33,34] It was noted that fetuses with laryngeal or tracheal atresia have larger than normal lungs. This led to animal experimentation that revealed that when the trachea was occluded and fetal lung fluid egress blocked, lung growth was stimulated. In utero tracheal occlusion, initially by application of an external tracheal clip and now by fetal bronchoscopic insertion of an occlusive balloon, has been performed to allow lungs to grow.[35] At delivery, the EXIT (ex-utero intrapartum treatment) procedure is performed to remove the tracheal clip or balloon prior to separation from the placenta. The efficacy of this endoscopic approach has had mixed results. An NIH-sponsored randomized trial in the United States failed to show a significant advantage. Temporary tracheal occlusion via fetoscopy is now being attempted in some centers, with a suggestion of early favorable results. Currently, the standard of care includes supportive care after term delivery with high-frequency ventilation and ECMO, if needed, with some centers advocating an EXIT-to-ECMO approach for high-risk fetuses.[36]

CONGENITAL PULMONARY AIRWAY MALFORMATION

Etiology CPAM, previously known as congenital cystic adenomatoid malformation, is the most common congenital lung abnormality, representing 30% to 47% of lung masses diagnosed in utero. CPAM is a hamartomatous lesion characterized by abnormal growth of terminal bronchioles containing cystic and solid tissue. It is currently thought that maldevelopment of the airways results in obstructive dysplastic changes.[37-39] Typically unilobular (85% to 95%), CPAMs may be multilobular and bilateral. They contain multiple microcysts or macrocysts lined by respiratory epithelium. Usually, a communication with the tracheobronchial tree exists, with blood supplied from pulmonary arteries.

Stocker's classification of CPAM includes five different types.[40] This is based on cyst size and underlying histologic resemblance to the bronchial tree and airspaces. Adzick described a classification based on fetal imaging appearance and gross anatomy: (1) macrocystic CPAM (multiple large cysts >5 mm with slow growth and favorable prognosis); and (2) microcystic CPAM (cysts <5 mm with solid appearance which have the highest risk for developing hydrops).[41]

Imaging Ultrasonographic appearance of CPAM depends on histology. With macrocystic CPAM, multiple nonconnecting cysts are seen. Often, a single lobe is affected, although multiple lobes and bilateral CPAM have been reported. Microcystic CPAMs are homogeneously echogenic and usually more echogenic than the adjacent lung.[42] Doppler shows flow from PAs in contradistinction to BPS, in which the vascular supply is from the aorta. Hybrid lesions with mixed features of CPAM (macrocysts) and BPS (aortic supply) are common. If the echogenicity of the CPAM is similar to adjacent lung, mass affect may be the only finding to suggest the diagnosis.[43]

MRI is useful in delineating the lung mass and amount of residual normal lung. The lung malformation is typically of high signal with macrocysts and intermediate signal with microcysts (Fig. 50-4).[44] The high signal masses sometimes are difficult to differentiate from the surrounding normal lung, particularly in the later weeks of gestation when normal lung signal increases. When bilateral, differentiation from CHAOS must be made. In these cases, MRI is useful in showing the fetal airway obstruction. In cases of congenital lobar emphysema, high signal lung that respects the anatomic boundaries of a normal lobe may be seen.

Prognosis of CPAM is typically favorable with spontaneous decrease in size in up to 90% of cases.[45-47] Although some masses may appear to resolve completely prenatally, computed tomography (CT) after delivery often identifies a residual mass. Theories as to the reason for the resolution include decompression into the bronchial tree, outgrowth of blood supply, or vascular pedicle torsion.

Treatment and Follow-up Rapidly growing CPAM, either solid or with a large dominant cyst, have a higher incidence of hydrops and are associated with a poorer outcome. Hydrops results from the severe mediastinal shift causing venous outflow obstruction and ultimately fetal cardiac failure. If no

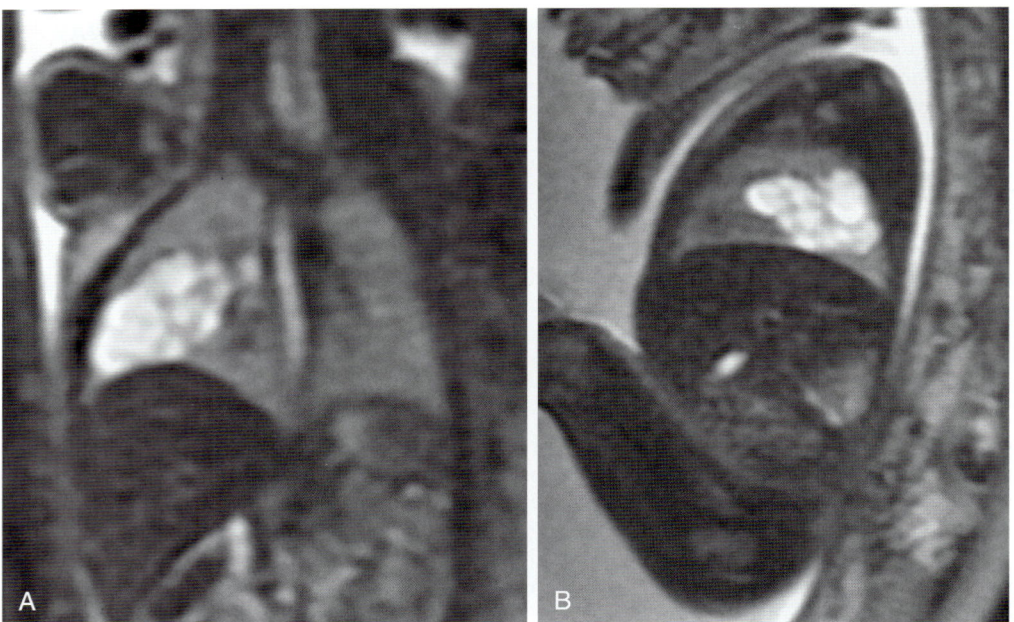

Figure 50-4   Macrocystic congenital pulmonary airway malformation. Coronal (*A*) and sagittal (*B*) single-shot fast spin echo T2-weighted magnetic resonance images demonstrate a multicystic high signal mass involving the posterior right lower lobe. No significant mass affect is seen.

hydrops exists, the outcome is excellent, with greater than 95% survival. If hydrops develops, the fetus will die without intervention.[5,48] The greatest period of growth of a CPAM is from 20 to 26 weeks' gestation.[48] Lesions that are largely solid in nature and rapidly increasing in size are at most risk for causing hydrops.

Crombleholme and colleagues developed a measure of mass volume divided by head circumference, termed *cystic adenomatoid malformation volume ratio* (CVR) in an attempt to predict which of the fetuses would progress to hydrops. The lung mass volume is determined using the ellipse formula (length × width × anteroposterior diameter ÷ 2), which is then divided by the head circumference. If the CVR is greater than 1.6, the risk is high for the development of hydrops. Fetuses with CVR less than 1.6 without a dominant cyst have less than a 3% risk of developing hydrops.[48]

If hydrops develops after 32 weeks' gestation, delivery is recommended. In fetuses that develop hydrops in the second trimester, fetal therapy has been beneficial. In fetuses with solid lesions, in utero resection of the lung mass has been lifesaving.[49,50] If the lesion has macrocysts, aspiration, thoracoamniotic shunting, and laser therapy have been attempted. In some centers, steroids have been used in an attempt to decrease the risk of hydrops.[5]

After delivery, if the infant is symptomatic, immediate resection is required. The need for resection if the infant is asymptomatic has been debated. Even if the chest radiograph appears normal, CT scans typically show a residual CPAM. (Fig. 50-5).[51,52] Residual cysts may develop air trapping or pneumothorax. Recurrent infections may occur. Rhabdomyosarcoma and bronchioalveolar carcinoma developing from CPAM has been reported.[53-57] Surgical resection is still advocated in asymptomatic patients despite no long-term outcome studies.

BRONCHOPULMONARY SEQUESTRATION

Etiology   BPS is abnormal pulmonary tissue with no connection with the normal tracheobronchial tree and systemic arterial blood supply from the aorta.[58] Typically located in the left posteroinferior thorax, BPS have been found infradiaphragmatically and within the diaphragm and may mimic a suprarenal neuroblastoma (Fig. 50-6).[59]

The two types of BPS are extralobar and intralobar BPS. Extralobar sequestration has a separate pleural covering and has systemic venous drainage via the azygous system or inferior vena cava. Intralobar sequestration has no separate pleura with venous drainage via the pulmonary veins. Both types receive arterial blood supply from the systemic circulation, usually the aorta.

Extralobar sequestration has a higher association with anomalies, including CDH, eventration, and foregut anomalies. Hybrid lesions are relatively common with CPAM masses associated with system arterial supply (see Fig. 50-5).[60] These may regress size. Rarely, these masses can present with effusions or hydrops.

Imaging   On ultrasonography, prenatal appearance is typically a solid triangular echoic mass in the lower hemithorax adjacent to the diaphragm.[61] Hybrid lesions may have a cystic component.[62] Systemic vascular supply should be searched for, typically branching from the aorta below the diaphragm. Color and power Doppler are helpful in identifying the vessel but may be difficult to demonstrate.

On MRI, BPS is homogeneous intermediate high signal on T2-weighted images. Vascular supply may be suggested by a low signal line coursing to the mass but also may be difficult to identify prenatally.

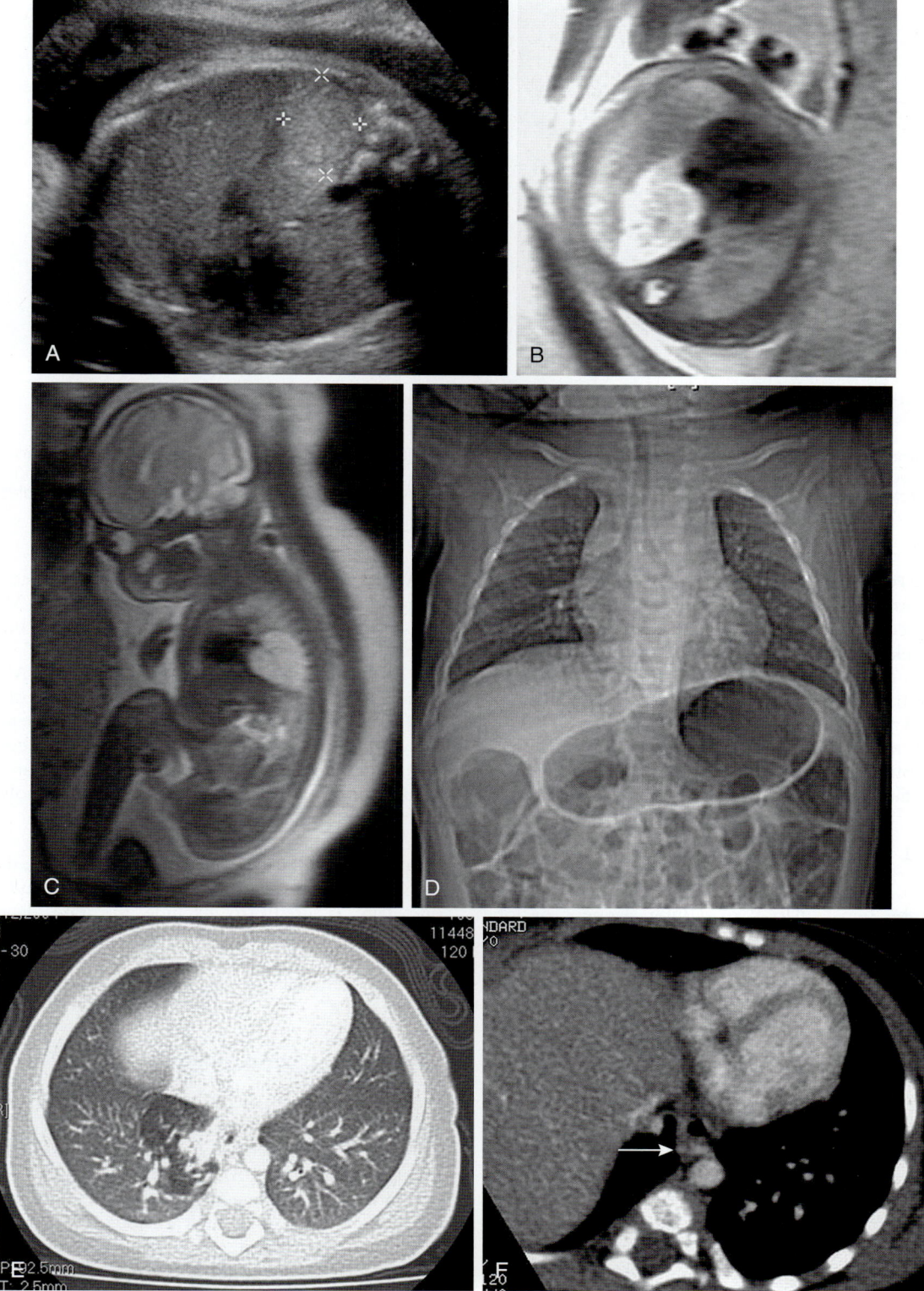

Figure 50-5 Hybrid congenital pulmonary airway malformation-sequestration. **A,** An axial sonogram shows an echogenic mass in the right lower hemithorax. **B** and **C,** Single-shot fast spin echo T2-weighted magnetic resonance images in the coronal (*B*) and sagittal (*C*) planes confirm the presence of a high signal mass in the right lower lobe. At delivery, the infant had no respiratory symptoms. **D,** A scout computed tomography (CT) scan of the chest at 3 weeks' gestational age shows no evidence of a residual lung mass. **E,** An axial CT scan demonstrates a hyperlucent lesion in the right lower lobe. **F,** A mediastinal reformatted image shows a feeding vessel (*arrow*) coursing from the aorta. At surgery, a congenital pulmonary airway malformation with a systemic feeding vessel was resected.

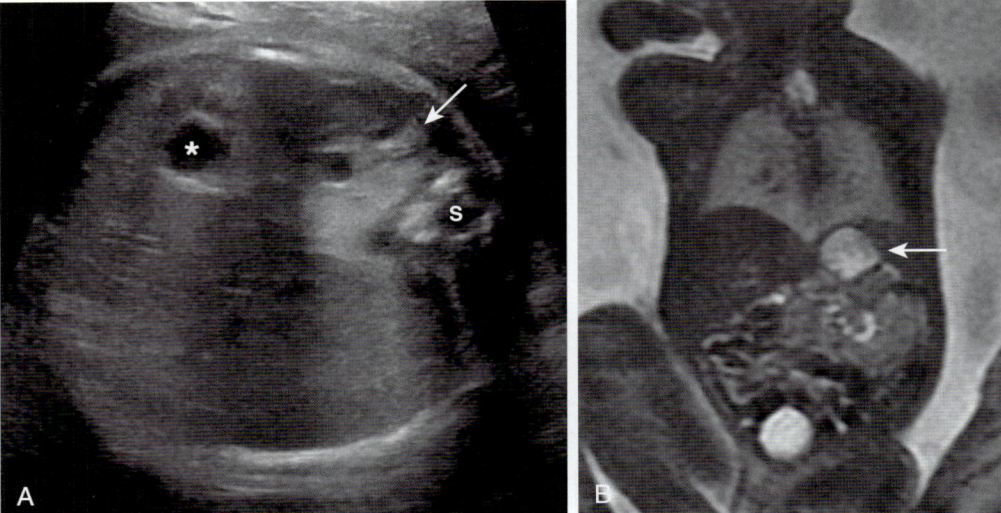

Figure 50-6 Infradiaphragmatic sequestration. **A,** An axial sonogram of a fetus of 26-week gestational age demonstrates a mixed cystic and solid mass (*arrow*) adjacent to the spine (*S*) and posterior to the stomach (*asterisk*). **B,** A coronal single-shot fast spin echo T2-weighted magnetic resonance image demonstrates a high signal mass below the diaphragm (*arrow*). The systemic feeding vessel was difficult to document prenatally.

Treatment and Follow-up Prognosis is typically favorable with only rare reports of associated hydrops.[63,64] If hydrops develops after 32 weeks' gestation, early delivery is recommended. Before 32 weeks, in utero surgical resection may be considered. Lesions may seem to resolve in utero but are typically present on postnatal CT. Postnatal CT with contrast enhancement or MRI is useful in identifying the feeding systemic vessel. Symptoms depend on the size of the mass. Because BPS may become infected, elective surgery is recommended even if the infant is asymptomatic.[65]

CONGENITAL LOBAR OVERINFLATION

Etiology CLO, also known as *congenital lobar emphysema*, is characterized by hyperinflation of a lung segment or lobe with normal pulmonary vascular supply. Microscopically, the alveoli are dilated but not maldeveloped.[2,3,37,39] The alveolar walls are intact, thus the preference of using the term *overinflation* rather than *emphysema*. Two subgroups of CLO seem to exist. The first group presents with respiratory distress postnatally with overinflation secondary to cartilage anomalies, absent bronchial cartilage, or extrinsic compression of the airway by bronchogenic cysts or pulmonary artery.[65] The obstructed airway results in air trapping. This group most commonly affects the left upper lobe, then right upper and middle lobes.[66] The second group of CLO is now recognized more frequently prenatally. These cases of segmental or lobar hyperinflation are often associated with bronchial atresia, often in the lower lobes.[67-69]

Imaging With the use of ultrasonography, CLO is often recognized in the second trimester as a homogeneously hyperechoic mass. No macrocysts are present. The hyperechogenicity is felt to be secondary to accumulation of fluid within the alveoli.[67] By the third trimester, the mass often becomes isoechoic and difficult to differentiate from adjacent normal lung. Mediastinal deviation may be the only clue that a CLO is present.

With MRI, the mass is of high signal compared with adjacent lung on T2-weighted MR images. Mass effect on the adjacent lower signal normal lung may be noted. The diaphragm often is flattened.

Differential of CLO from microcystic CPAM or sequestration may be difficult prenatally both by ultrasound and MRI. One useful differentiation is the assessment of vascularity with Doppler; normal pulmonary vessels course through CLO, with no systemic feeders (Fig. 50-7). Rarely, the mediastinal shift is severe enough to result in polyhydramnios, hydrops, and pulmonary hypoplasia.[70-72]

Treatment and Follow-up Prognosis is typically favorable. As with other fetal lung masses, follow-up ultrasonography prenatally is useful to exclude the rare development of ascites, skin thickening, and polyhydramnios. Diagnosis may be confirmed by following delivery with radiography and CT.[71,72] Postnatal surgery is performed if the child is symptomatic.

CONGENITAL HYDROTHORAX

Etiology Fetal pleural fluid may develop without an associated mass and is considered abnormal at any gestational age.[73,74] The fluid collection may be unilateral or bilateral. The incidence is 1:15,000 births. Chylothorax is the most common cause of congenital hydrothorax and may be caused by thoracic duct anomalies. Lesions associated with pleural effusions include masses (CDH, CPAM, BPS), lymphangiectasia, cardiac anomalies, Turner syndrome, trisomy 21, cystic hygroma, and TORCH (toxoplasmosis, other [congenital syphilis and viruses], rubella, cytomegalovirus, and herpes simplex virus) infection. Thorough evaluation is required to identify associated anomalies. Overall mortality is reported to be as high as 50%. Outcome is best if the effusion is unilateral. Primary chylothorax may resolve spontaneously (22%). If effusions progress to hydrops, mortality increases owing to the development of pulmonary hypoplasia.

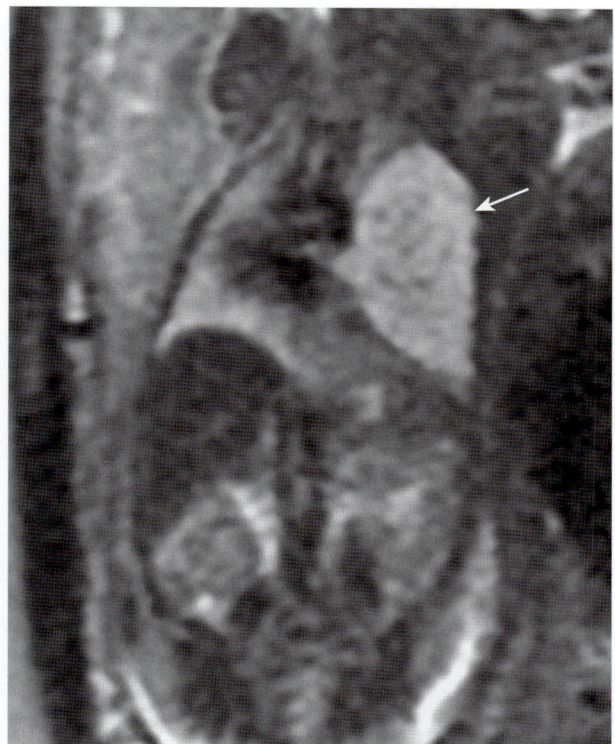

Figure 50-7   Congenital lobar overinflation. A coronal single-shot fast spin echo T2-weighted magnetic resonance image of a fetus of 25-week gestational age demonstrates a high signal homogeneous left upper lobe (*arrow*). Pulmonary vessels can be seen coursing through the parenchyma.

Imaging   Ultrasonography demonstrates anechoic fluid in the pleural space. MRI shows high signal fluid surrounding lung parenchyma. MRI may be useful in identifying a cause for the hydrothorax such as an underlying CPAM or BPS (Fig. 50-8).

Treatment and Follow-up   If the effusion is small, conservative observation is appropriate. If the effusion is large, and the infant is less than 32 weeks' gestational age, fetal thoracentesis and thoracoamniotic shunting are potential prenatal treatment options, although reaccumulation of fluid is frequent.

CONGENITAL HIGH AIRWAY OBSTRUCTION

Etiology   CHAOS is caused by obstruction or absence of the trachea. This rare entity may be the result of laryngotracheal atresia, tracheal stenosis, or a thick web. Aberrant pulmonary budding off the foregut is present. Most have a connection with the esophagus. An association with other anomalies, including Fraser syndrome and DiGeorge syndrome, exists.

Imaging   With ultrasonography, both lungs are seen to be symmetrically enlarged and echogenic as a result of fluid trapping. The heart is compressed, and the diaphragms are flattened. Hydrops may develop. Increase or decrease in amniotic fluid may occur.[75-77] MRI shows abnormally large high signal lungs on T2-weighted images. Diaphragmatic eversion is present (Fig. 50-9). Identification of a fluid-filled trachea and bronchi confirms the diagnosis. Differential diagnosis includes bilateral CPAM.

Treatment and Follow-up   EXIT delivery with airway control is the current management of choice in fetus with CHAOS. The prognosis is typically poor.[78,79]

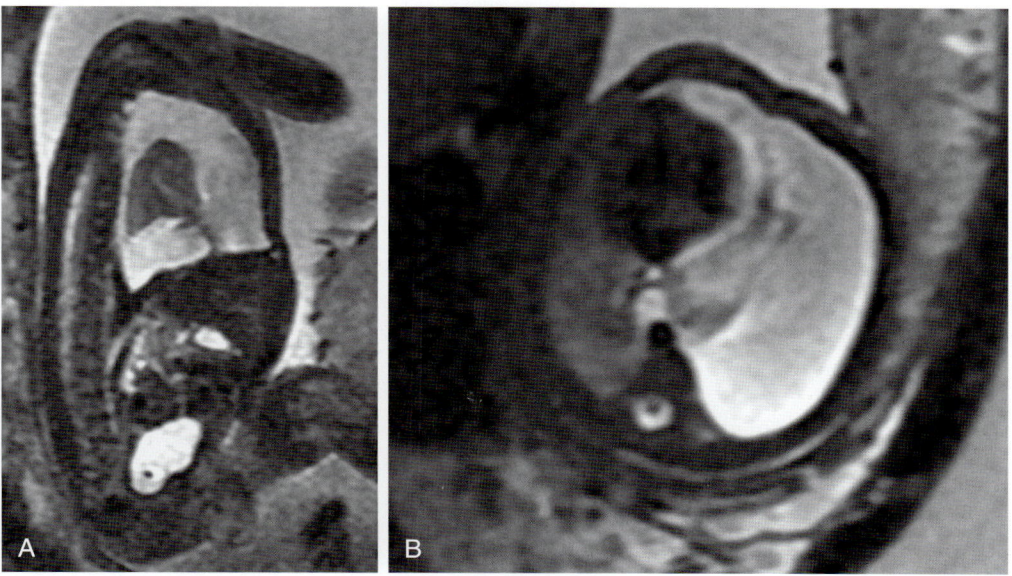

Figure 50-8   Pleural effusion. **A,** A sagittal single-shot fast spin echo T2-weighted magnetic resonance image shows a large pleural effusion with compression of the underlying lung parenchyma. **B,** An axial single-shot fast spin echo T2-weighted image of the chest demonstrates the severity of the mediastinal shift and compression of the contralateral lung.

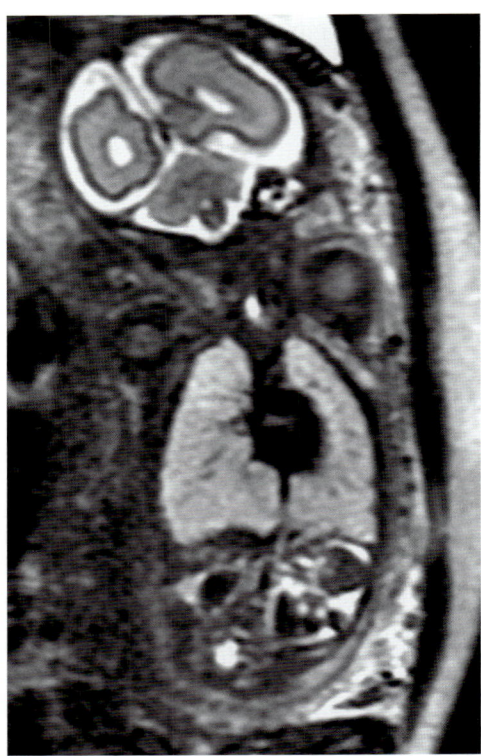

Figure 50-9 Congenital high airway obstruction secondary to tracheal stenosis. Coronal T2-weighted image of a 27-week-old fetus demonstrates abnormally enlarged high signal lungs. The diaphragms are flattened. Mild ascites is present.

WHAT THE CLINICIAN NEEDS TO KNOW

1. The most common fetal chest abnormalities include CDH, congenital bronchopulmonary malformations, and congenital hydrothorax.
2. Accurate prenatal diagnosis of fetal chest lesions aids in the planning of potential fetal intervention, mode of delivery, and postnatal care.
3. In a fetus with CDH, low lung-to-head circumference ratio and liver herniation into the chest suggest a worse outcome.
4. Prognosis of congenital bronchopulmonary malformations is typically excellent. However, if hydrops develops prenatally, the outcome is poor without intervention.
5. Chylothorax is the most common cause of congenital hydrothorax.

Suggested Readings

Adzick NS. Management of fetal lung lesions. *Clin Perinat.* 2009;36: 363-376.

Barth RA. Imaging of fetal chest masses. *Pediatr Radiol.* 2012;42(suppl 1):862-873.

Daltro P, Werner H, Gasparetto T, et al. Congenital chest malformations: a multimodality approach with emphasis on fetal MR imaging. *Radiographics.* 2010;30(2):385-395.

Deshmukh S, Rubesova E, Barth R. MR assessment of normal fetal lung volumes: a literature review. *AJR.* 2010;194:W212-W217.

Epelman M, Kreiger PA, Servas S, et al. Current imaging of prenatally diagnosed congenital lung lesions. *Semin Ultrasound CT MR.* 2010; 31:141-157.

Kline-Fath B. Current advances in prenatal imaging of congenital diaphragmatic hernia. *Pediatr Radiol.* 2012;42(suppl 1):S74-S90.

References

Full references for this chapter can be found on www.expertconsult.com.

Chapter 51

Upper Airway Disease

BERNARD F. LAYA and EDWARD Y. LEE

Upper airway disease is a common problem in the pediatric age group. Affected children usually present with acute respiratory distress associated with stridor, apnea, or even acute pulmonary edema. Some children may present with a more chronic course of clinical symptoms characterized by recurrent chest infections or obstructive sleep apnea, which can lead to growth retardation, chronic respiratory failure, cor pulmonale, and even death.[1]

Children with upper airway obstruction usually present with stridor, a harsh respiratory noise caused by turbulent air passing through a narrowed airway. Timing of stridor in relation to the respiratory cycle can indicate the location of the narrowing. Inspiratory stridor usually results from obstruction above the level of the glottis, whereas expiratory stridor is characteristic of intrathoracic obstructions. Biphasic stridor suggests obstruction in the area between the glottis and subglottis or fixed/critical obstruction at any level.[2]

Although a thorough history and physical examination may narrow differential diagnostic considerations of upper airway disease in the pediatric population, imaging evaluation plays an important role in establishing the diagnosis, localizing the anatomic area of abnormality, and defining the extent of disease. Frontal and lateral radiographs of the airway and fluoroscopy have been mainstays in upper airway evaluation. Advances in cross-sectional imaging techniques approaching near endoscopic detail have been developed to more accurately demonstrate airway anatomy.[3] For practical purposes, the discussion of pathology in this chapter is divided into the supraglottic, glottic, and subglottic regions.

Supraglottic Abnormalities

LARYNGOMALACIA

Etiology Laryngomalacia is abnormal laxity of the pharyngeal tissues that causes the epiglottis, arytenoids, and aryepiglottic folds to involute and partially obstruct breathing during inspiration. The underlying cause of laryngomalacia is attributed to the immaturity of the laryngeal cartilages and muscles, which allows the larynx and the supralaryngeal structures to collapse.[1-4] Laryngomalacia accounts for more than 75% of cases of congenital stridor and is the most common cause of symptomatic partial upper airway obstruction in infants.[5] The stridor typically improves when the infant is agitated or active and becomes worse when the infant is at rest.

Imaging The diagnosis of laryngomalacia can be established with use of airway fluoroscopy, although laryngoscopy is the diagnostic procedure of choice.[6] The characteristic imaging finding in patients with laryngomalacia consists of downward and posterior bending of the epiglottis and anterior buckling of the aryepiglottic folds, which narrow and eventually obliterate the upper airway (Fig. 51-1). Although airway fluoroscopy appears to be reliable because of its high specificity, it has low sensitivity, and thus negative findings of a fluoroscopic study require further diagnostic evaluation in the setting of a high clinical suspicion of laryngomalacia.[7]

Treatment and Follow-up In most infants with laryngomalacia, stridor resolves during the first year of life. However, potentially serious complications, including airway obstruction and sudden death, also may occur. In severe or life-threatening cases, the following surgical treatment options currently are available: supraglottoplasty, an incision in the aryepiglottic folds, epiglottopexy, and tracheostomy.[8]

EPIGLOTTITIS

Etiology Acute bacterial epiglottitis is a potentially serious cause of upper airway obstruction in children. It is characterized by inflammation and swelling of the epiglottis and the aryepiglottic folds but also can affect the false cords and the subglottic region.[9] Epiglottitis usually is attributed to *Haemophilus influenzae*, although other bacteria including *Streptococcus, Staphylococcus, Moraxella,* and *Pseudomonas* also have been implicated.[10] Because *Haemophilus influenzae* is now preventable by immunization, the incidence of epiglottitis has substantially diminished, although vaccine failures do occur.[11] Epiglottitis typically occurs in preschool children between 3 and 6 years of age, but it also can occur in adults.[12] Epiglottitis usually has a sudden onset with no history of a preceding upper respiratory tract infection. Affected children typically appear toxic with acute stridor, dysphagia, fever, restlessness, drooling, and increased respiratory distress in the recumbent position. Epiglottitis is a life-threatening disease that requires potential emergent intubation.

Imaging Epiglottitis usually is diagnosed with radiography, and endoscopy is obtained for confirmation. A lateral radiograph reveals swelling and marked enlargement of the epiglottis that resembles the shape of a thumb (Fig. 51-2).

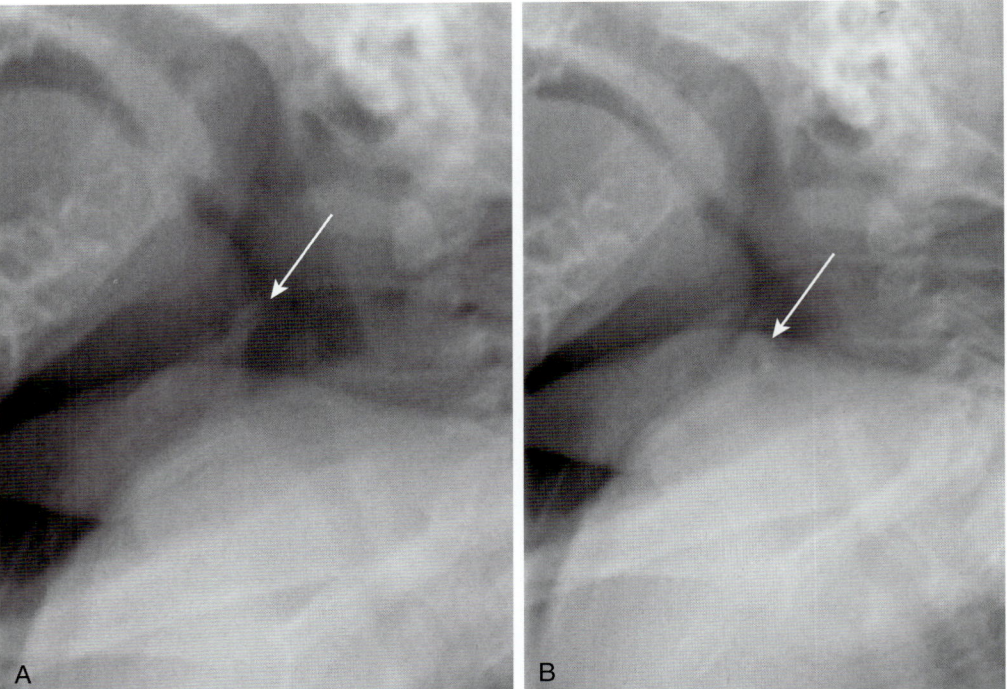

Figure 51-1   Laryngomalacia in a 3-month-old boy with stridor. **A,** Still image from an airway fluoroscopic study demonstrates the normal position of the epiglottis (*arrow*). **B,** Still image from an airway fluoroscopic study shows laxity of the epiglottis with posterior, downward movement obstructing the airway (*arrow*) consistent with laryngomalacia.

Associated thickening of the aryepiglottic folds also occurs. Inflammation extends into the glottis and subglottic regions, causing a steeple or funnel configuration of the airway on frontal views. Because of the potentially rapid progression of the condition, which can lead to sudden and complete obstruction of the upper airway, radiographs should be obtained expeditiously with minimal manipulation of the neck. When undergoing imaging, patients should remain upright in their position of maximal comfort. Conditions that mimic bacterial epiglottitis in children include caustic ingestion, angioneurotic edema, chemical or thermal injury, an abscess, and epithelial cyst, among others. The omega epiglottis with prominent lateral folds is a normal variant and should not be misinterpreted as epiglottitis. In such cases, the aryepiglottic folds remain thin.[13]

Treatment and Follow-up   Antibiotic therapy is a mainstay of treatment, and steroids are administered to some pediatric patients with epiglottitis. Direct laryngoscopy with intubation is performed to secure the airway in severely affected patients.[10]

Glottic Abnormalities

LARYNGEAL ATRESIA

Etiology   Laryngeal atresia, a rare congenital malformation, is usually fatal. The malformation is caused by nondevelopment of the sixth branchial arch during embryogenesis, resulting in failure of the larynx and the trachea to recanalize. Typical

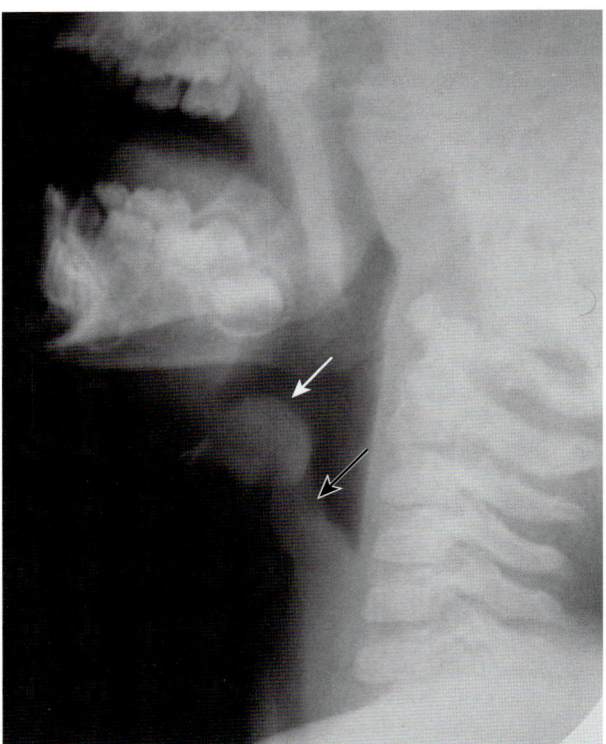

Figure 51-2   Epiglottitis in a 5-year-old boy with respiratory distress and drooling. A lateral soft tissue neck radiograph shows a markedly thickened epiglottis (*white arrow*), which is referred to as the "thumb" sign. The aryepiglottic folds (*black arrow*) also are thickened.

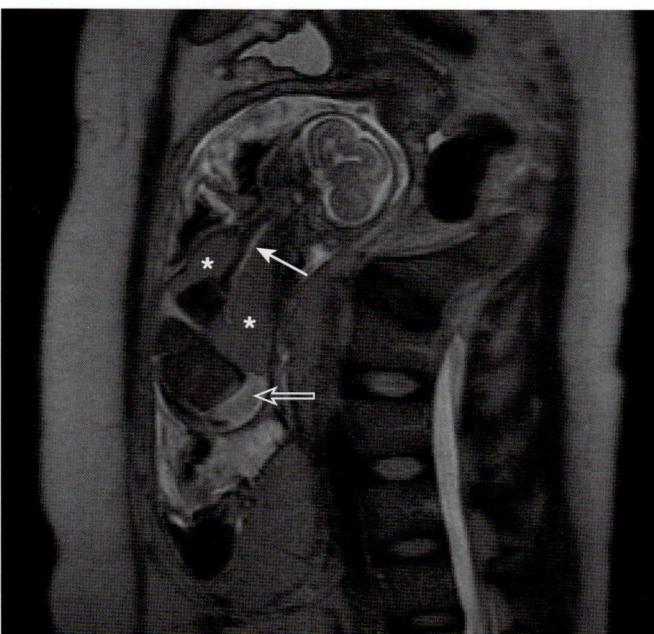

Figure 51-3 Congenital high airway obstruction syndrome in a 20-week-gestation fetus. A half Fourier acquisition single-shot turbo spin echo sequence of a fetal magnetic resonance imaging scan demonstrates a dilated, fluid-filled trachea up to the mid neck (*solid arrow*), enlarged hyperintense lungs (*asterisks*) with inversion of both hemidiaphragms, and ascites (*open arrow*). (Courtesy of Andrew Mong, MD, Philadelphia, PA.)

presentation of affected patients with laryngeal atresia at birth is severe respiratory distress despite strong respiratory effort. Associated anomalies include a tracheoesophageal fistula, esophageal atresia, urinary tract abnormalities, limb defects, and low-set ears.[14]

Imaging Laryngeal atresia can be diagnosed with use of prenatal ultrasound by identifying the signs of congenital high airway obstruction syndrome, such as hyperechogenic lungs, a flattened or inverted diaphragm, a dilated and fluid-filled trachea, fetal hydrops, and polyhydramnios.[15] Fetal magnetic resonance imaging (MRI), which correlates highly with prenatal ultrasound, can detect laryngeal atresia with the advantage of having a capability to identify the level of obstruction in most cases (Fig. 51-3).[16]

Treatment and Follow-up The treatment of laryngeal atresia focuses on prompt airway intervention at delivery after an accurate prenatal diagnosis, which may allow survival of infants with this otherwise fatal condition. An emergent tracheostomy is required immediately upon birth to secure an airway. Repair of laryngeal atresia requires laryngotracheal reconstruction.

LARYNGEAL WEB

Etiology A congenital laryngeal web is an uncommon condition caused by faulty embryogenesis of the laryngotracheal groove. This web is a band of varying thickness, usually located anteriorly at the level of the cords, which obliterates the anterior commissure. A congenital laryngeal web occasionally occurs just below the true cords. Affected infants

present with a weak or absent cry, varying degrees of stridor, and respiratory distress, and they often may have concomitant abnormalities such as subglottic stenosis.[1]

Imaging A definitive diagnosis of laryngeal web can be provided by direct laryngoscopy, but imaging evaluation plays a role in diagnosis. Plain radiography and fluoroscopy can demonstrate that the abnormality is in the glottis region, but no definitive radiographic findings exist.[5] Computed tomography (CT) with multiplanar imaging and three-dimensional reconstructions can provide precise information with respect to the exact location of the web, its thickness, and its extent (Fig. 51-4). Furthermore, CT is able to visualize the structures beyond the area of obstruction, which is a limitation of laryngoscopy.[17]

Treatment and Follow-up The primary goals of treatment for a congenital laryngeal web are to provide a patent airway and achieve a sufficient voice quality. Treatment depends on the thickness and extent of the abnormality. Surgical procedures include laryngotracheal reconstruction, laryngofissure and placement of a stent or keel, and endoscopic lysis with application of mitomycin C.[18,19]

LARYNGOCELE

Etiology A laryngocele is an abnormal dilatation of the laryngeal saccule, which is a narrow blind pouch arising from the anterior end of the laryngeal ventricle, extending superiorly into the paralaryngeal space, and bounded laterally by the thyroid cartilage.[20] A laryngocele may be congenital or acquired. Laryngoceles occur more often in males than in females. In neonates and young children, a laryngocele is likely congenital and is contingent upon the presence of a saccular dilatation of the ventricular appendage. Increased laryngeal pressure may cause the sac to distend, at times extending into the aryepiglottic fold.[21]

A laryngocele is classified as internal if it lies within the larynx and external if it protrudes through the thyrohyoid membrane. The most common type is mixed. As the laryngocele communicates with the larynx, it normally contains air but may be filled with mucus or fluid.[22] An acquired laryngocele may develop in older children or adults who experience increased intralaryngeal pressure, such as glass blowers, persons who play wind instruments, or persons with a chronic cough.

Imaging In the past, anteroposterior (AP) and lateral soft tissue neck radiographs, linear tomography, and contrast laryngoscopy were used to identify laryngoceles.[21] However, CT and/or MRI have replaced those older imaging techniques in recent years.[20] On CT or MRI, a laryngocele typically is a well-defined structure of air or near-water density value in a characteristic location, with a smooth surface and lack of mucosal abnormality (Fig. 51-5). The exact location and extent of upper airway narrowing due to a laryngocele also can be well evaluated with CT or MRI.

Treatment and Follow-up Endoscopic marsupialization is sufficient to treat most internal laryngoceles. When an external component exists, an open surgical approach may be necessary to remove the lesion completely.[9]

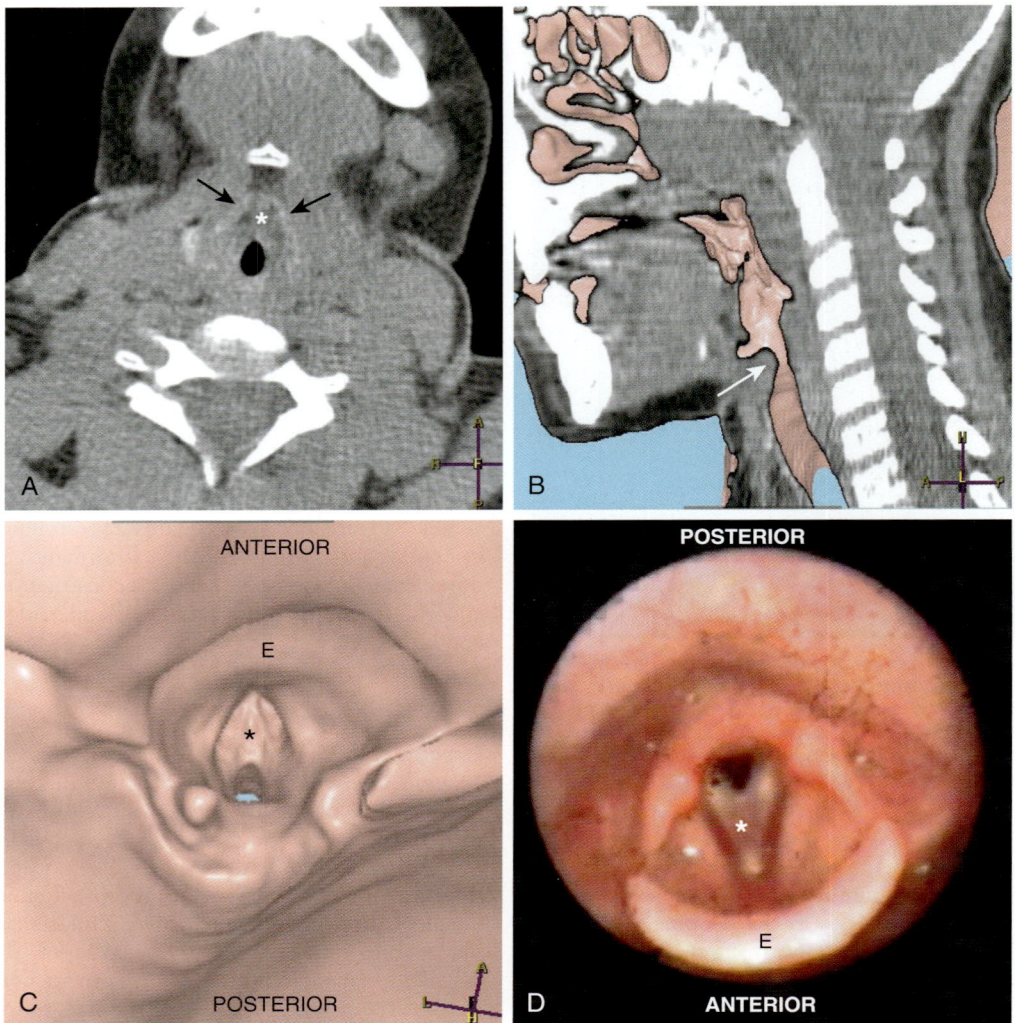

Figure 51-4 Laryngeal web. **A,** An axial computed tomography (CT) scan of the neck at the level of the larynx and the thyroid cartilage (*black arrows*) demonstrates the laryngeal web (*asterisk*). **B,** A sagittal virtual endoscopic view superimposed on a sagittal reformatted CT image shows the laryngeal web (*arrow*). A virtual endocsopic view (**C**) and corresponding larygoscopy (**D**) demonstrate the laryngeal web (*asterisk*). The epiglottis (*E*) is well demonstrated on these images. (Courtesy of Suleymen Men, MD, Izmir, Turkey.)

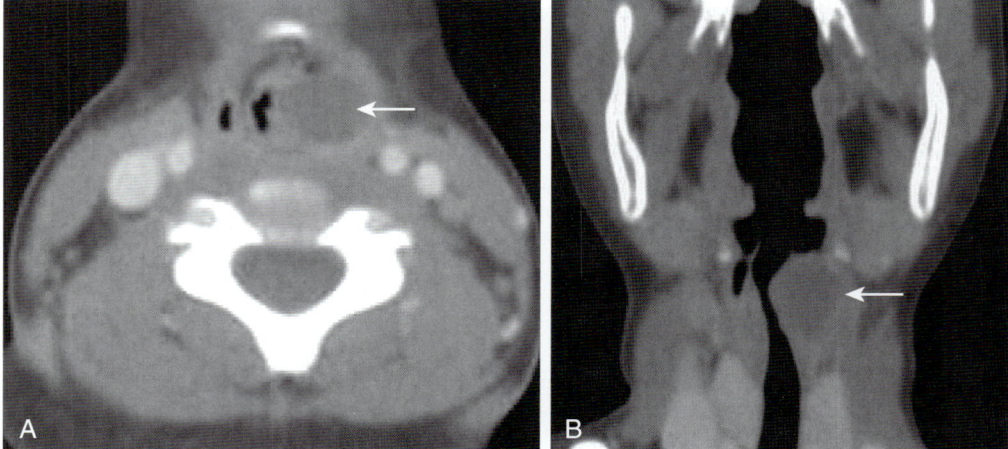

Figure 51-5 A laryngocele in a 5-year-old boy with chronic stridor. An axial computed tomography scan (**A**) with coronal reconstruction (**B**) of the upper airway reveals a well-demarcated fluid-filled rounded structure (*arrow*) adjacent to the left laryngeal ventricle compatible with a laryngocele. Also noted is a marked narrowing of the upper airway.

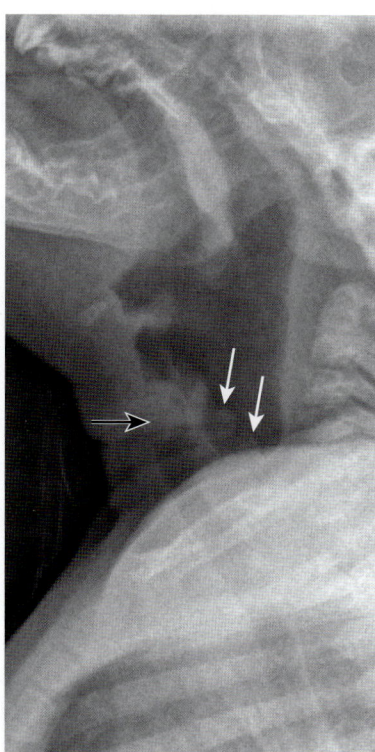

Figure 51-6 Recurrent respiratory papillomatosis in a 4-year-old boy. A lateral soft tissue radiograph demonstrates a rounded soft tissue mass in the laryngeal region (*black arrow*). Nodular soft tissue densities also are noted along the aryepiglottic folds (*white arrows*). (Courtesy Elizabeth H. Ey, MD, Dayton, OH.)

RECURRENT RESPIRATORY PAPILLOMATOSIS

Etiology Recurrent respiratory papillomatosis (RRP) is the most common benign neoplasm to affect the larynx in children.[23] It is the proliferation of benign squamous papillomas in the aerodigestive tract, usually involving the larynx. RRP tends to recur, spreads throughout the aerodigestive tract, and can even undergo malignant transformation. The etiology of RRP is infection of the upper airway with human papillomavirus types 6 and 11.[24] Vertical transmission occurring during delivery through an infected birth canal is presumed to be the major mode of transmission in children.[25]

Change in voice (e.g., hoarseness, weak cry, and aphonia) and stridor are the most common symptoms in patients with RRP. Less common presenting symptoms include chronic cough, recurrent pneumonia, failure to thrive, dyspnea, dysphagia, and acute respiratory distress, especially in infants with an upper respiratory tract infection.[26] The age of symptom onset typically ranges from neonates to 6 years. RRP can mimic other diseases including croup, tracheomalacia, or asthma. This diagnosis should be considered in children when other common pediatric airway diseases either do not follow the expected natural history or do not respond to treatment.[27]

Imaging On plain radiographs, RRP typically appears as an irregular filling defect in the glottis (Fig. 51-6). It also can extend into the subglottic region and seed peripherally in the

respiratory tract, resulting in pulmonary nodules or nonspecific lung parenchymal changes.[1] A confirmatory diagnosis of RRP is made by direct laryngoscopy and biopsy for tissue diagnosis.[27]

Treatment and Follow-up Carbon dioxide laser surgery, antiviral therapy, and other adjuvant regimens have been tried, but none of them have proved to be completely successful in treating RRP. Recurrences are very common.[26]

Subglottic Abnormalities

SUBGLOTTIC STENOSIS

Etiology Subglottic stenosis is a narrowing of the subglottic airway that can be either congenital or acquired. In pediatric patients, congenital subglottic stenosis is due to faulty recanalization of the fetal laryngeal lumen, whereas the acquired type usually is the result of prolonged endotracheal intubation.[1] Because of improved management of neonates who require ventilatory support, the incidence of neonatal subglottic stenosis has diminished substantially.[28] Stridor is the most common presentation. However, an infant or child with a mild degree of congenital or acquired subglottic stenosis may remain asymptomatic until an upper respiratory tract infection results in aggravation of the subglottic airway narrowing.[4]

Imaging Endoscopy is the reference standard for diagnosis, but imaging plays an important role in the evaluation of subglottic stenosis. Plain radiograph and fluoroscopy, which show fixed narrowing of the subglottic airway, usually enable diagnosis. However, CT with virtual bronchoscopy and MRI can be useful in assessing the exact site and length of stenosis and the airway distal to the area of narrowing (Fig. 51-7).[4,29]

Treatment and Follow-up The two major treatment options currently available for subglottic stenosis are endoscopic dilatation and surgical reconstruction.[30]

CROUP

Etiology Viral croup or laryngotracheobronchitis is the most common cause of upper airway obstruction in children from 6 months to 3 years of age. Parainfluenza and influenza virus are the two most common etiologic agents for viral croup. They induce a reactive inflammatory response, which results in subglottic edema and subsequent upper airway narrowing. Clinically, viral croup is characterized by a low-grade fever and varying degrees of inspiratory stridor, barking cough, and hoarseness.[4,31]

Imaging Although the diagnosis of viral croup is mainly clinical, airway studies often are obtained for diagnostic confirmation and exclusion of other causes of acute stridor, such as epiglottitis. On a frontal radiograph, the lateral walls of the subglottic larynx normally are convex or shouldered. Mucosal edema in viral croup narrows this space, which results in a loss of lateral convexity, creating a "steeple" shape below the vocal cords (Fig. 51-8). The narrowing can extend 5 to 10 mm below the vocal cords. The steeple sign is not specific for croup and may be seen in some children with epiglottitis.

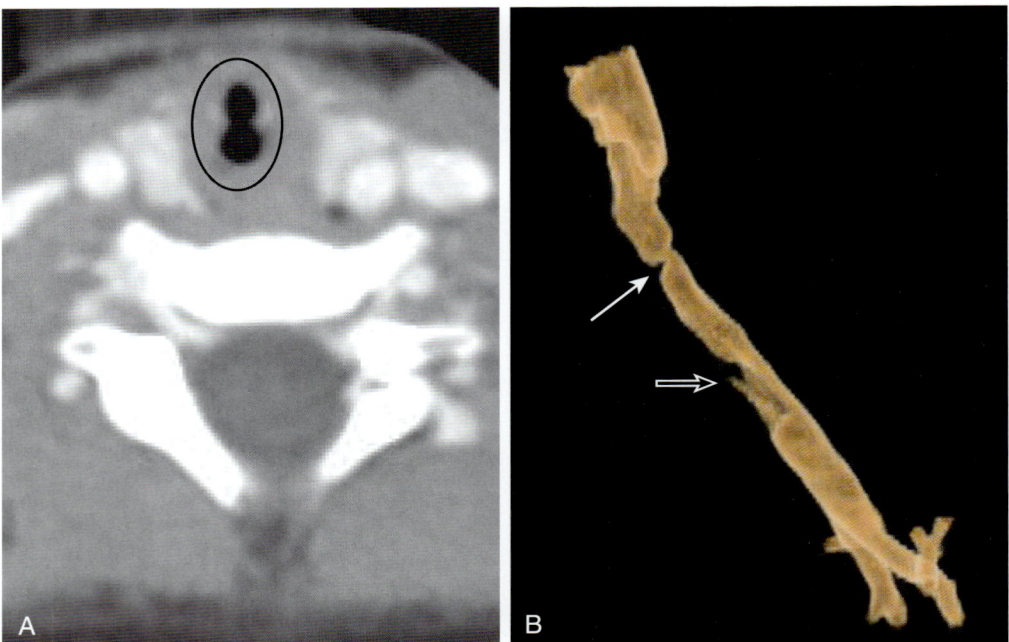

Figure 51-7 Subglottic stenosis in a 2-year-old girl, a former premature infant who had undergone chronic intubation. **A,** Axial neck computed tomography demonstrates severe transverse narrowing of the subglottic trachea (*circled*). **B,** An external surface volume-rendered reconstruction shows severe subglottic stenosis (*solid arrow*) and a defect from the tracheostomy tube (*open arrow*).

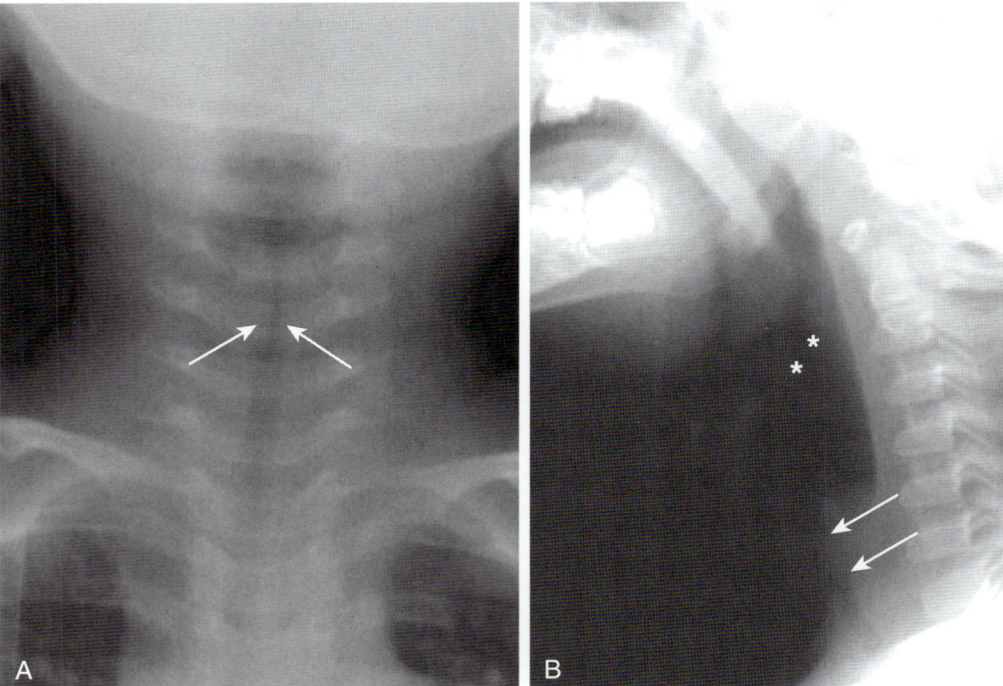

Figure 51-8 Croup in a 1-year-old girl with stridor. **A,** A frontal soft tissue neck radiograph demonstrates a "steeple" appearance of the subglotttic trachea (*arrows*). **B,** A lateral soft tissue neck radiograph shows a dilated hypopharyngeal region (*asterisks*), as well as haziness and narrowing of the subglottic region (*arrows*).

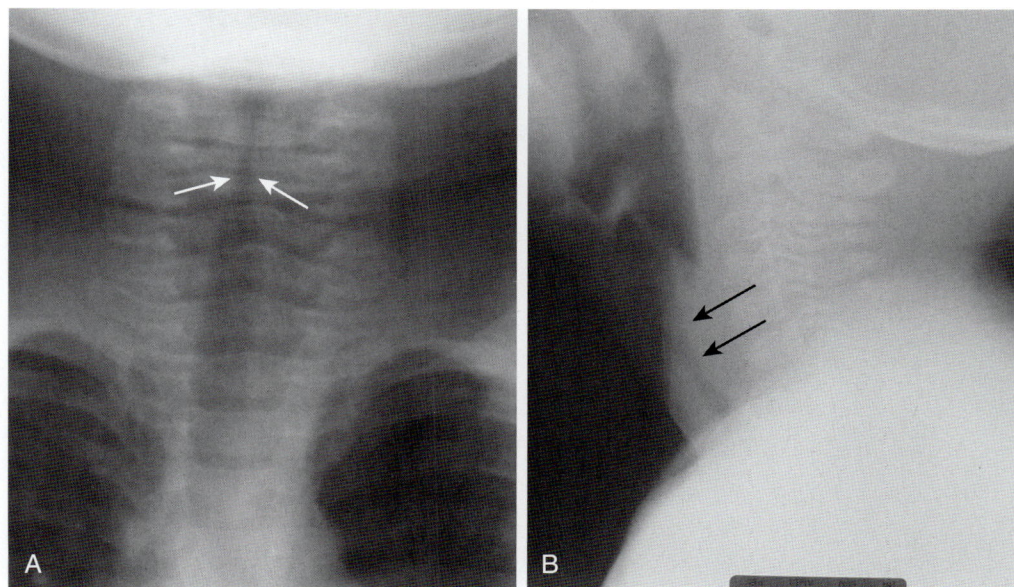

Figure 51-9 Bacterial tracheitis in a 7-year-old girl with a high fever, cough, and stridor. **A,** A frontal soft tissue neck radiograph shows subglottic tracheal narrowing (*arrows*). **B,** A lateral soft tissue neck radiograph shows haziness of the subglottic tracheal region with irregularity of the posterior tracheal wall (*arrows*).

Furthermore, it can be absent in children affected with viral croup. On lateral radiographs, the hypopharynx often is over-distended, and the subglottic region is hazy or indistinct as a result of narrowing of the airway by mucosal edema. The epiglottis, aryepiglottic folds, and prevertebral spaces are normal in persons with viral croup.[1-4]

Treatment and Follow-up   In most pediatric patients with viral croup, the disease is mild and self-limited. Depending on the severity of disease, steroids and nebulized epinephrine have been administered to treat patients.[31]

BACTERIAL TRACHEITIS

Etiology   Bacterial tracheitis is a potentially life-threatening cause of upper airway obstruction. Bacterial tracheitis also has been referred as membranous croup, pseudomembranous croup, bacterial croup, purulent tracheobronchitis, and membranous laryngotracheobronchitis. The common etiologic bacteria include *Staphylococcus, Moraxella, Streptococcus,* and *Haemophilus* species, although it is not unusual for a bacterial infection to coexist with viral disease.[32,33] The bacterial infection causes an inflammatory response that produces thick adherent mucopurulent exudates, ulceration, and sloughing of the laryngeal, tracheal, and bronchial mucosa. Such bacterial infection eventually results in various degrees of upper airway obstruction.[32,33] Affected children usually are pre-school- to school-aged children and are sicker than those affected with viral croup. Affected children usually present with a history of viral respiratory illness, rhinorrhea, cough, fever, and sore throat that may be present up to a week. These clinical symptoms in children with bacterial tracheitis often progress to high fever, a toxic appearance, and severe upper airway obstruction with hoarseness, cough, stridor, and tachypnea.[32-34] A definitive diagnosis of bacterial tracheitis is made on the basis of the history and physical examination,

combined with findings from laboratory and bronchoscopic evaluation.[34]

Imaging   Typical radiographic findings of bacterial tracheitis on the frontal radiograph of the cervical airway is narrowing of the subglottic airway. On lateral radiographs of the upper airway, diffuse haziness and marked irregularity of the anterior wall of the trachea may be seen, which is referred to as the "candle-dripping sign" (Fig. 51-9).[32,35] Opaque linear streaks or filling defects, membranes, or plaquelike irregularities can be seen within the airway. Chest radiograph abnormalities are common in children with bacterial tracheitis, with at least 50% showing concomitant findings of pneumonia.[35]

Treatment and Follow-up   When managing symptomatic children with bacterial tracheitis, a patent airway should be established to treat acute respiratory failure.[33] Antibiotic therapy usually is initiated, and laryngoscopy may be required for endoscopic removal of the obstructing purulent secretions and membranes.

RETROPHARYNGEAL CELLULITIS/ABSCESS

Etiology   Retropharyngeal cellulitis/abscess is a serious and occasionally life-threatening pyogenic infection with the potential to encroach on the upper airway. It occurs as a consequence of infections of the nasopharynx, paranasal sinuses, or middle ear. Usual etiologic agents are *Streptococcus, Staphylococcus,* and *Haemophilus,* although anaerobes also have been implicated. The infection extends to the lymph nodes located in the space between the posterior pharyngeal wall and prevertebral fascia. The infection occurs predominantly in early childhood; 75% of patients are younger than 5 years.[36] In older children and adults, factors leading to retropharyngeal cellulitis/abscess include regional trauma, foreign body ingestion, complication of prior surgical

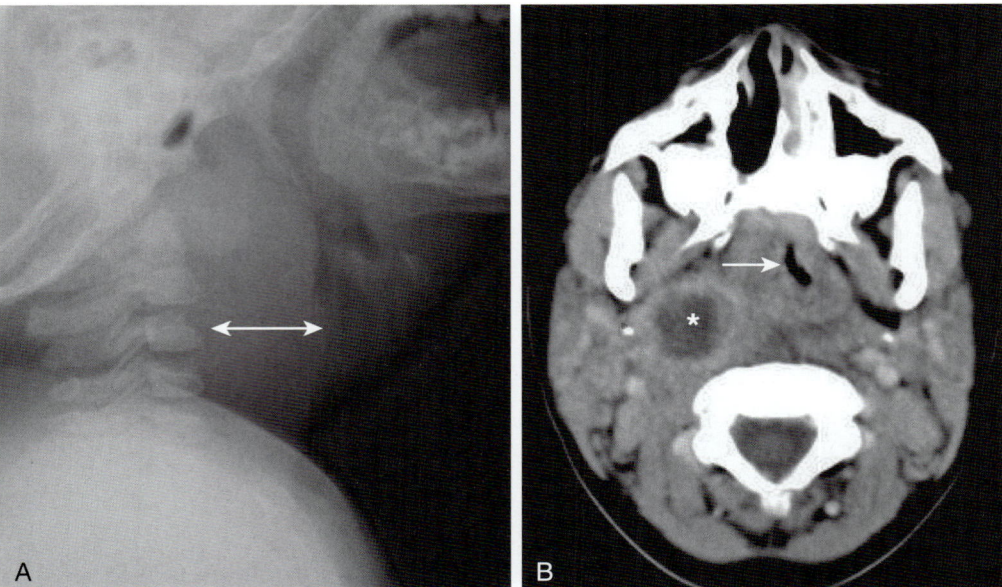

Figure 51-10 A retropharyngeal abscess in a 3-year-old girl. **A,** A lateral soft tissue neck radiograph shows markedly widened retropharyngeal soft tissue (*double arrow*). **B,** An axial computed tomography scan through the upper airway demonstrates a rounded area of hypoattenuation with enhancing border compatible with abscess (*asterisk*) and associated soft tissue swelling effacing the airway (*arrow*).

procedures, or immunocompromised states. Typical clinical symptoms are fever, neck stiffness, and dysphagia, but occasionally affected patients will present with signs of upper airway obstruction.[1,4] Diagnosis is based on clinical suspicion with supportive imaging studies.

Imaging   The retropharynx, a potential space between the pharynx and the cervical spine, is easily appreciated on the lateral radiograph of the airway. In infants and children, the prevertebral space is wider because the vertebrae are not fully ossified. As a general guide, the thickness of the prevertebral soft tissue space from C1 to C4 is equal to half of the vertebral body width. In the older child, the vertebral bodies become larger and the prevertebral space becomes smaller. Below C4, the thickness of the prevertebral space normally equals the adjacent vertebral body width. If the thickness of the prevertebral space is greater than the adjacent vertebral body width below C3, it usually is abnormal.[2] Attention to imaging technique is important when interpreting the lateral neck radiograph because a poorly obtained neck radiograph that is taken obliquely, on expiration, or with the neck flexed can accentuate the thickness of the retropharyngeal space and mimic pathology. Typical findings of retropharyngeal cellulitis/abscess on a lateral neck radiograph include a fixed soft tissue widening of the retropharyngeal soft tissue, anterior displacement of the airway, and often reversal of the cervical lordotic curvature.[1,4] A plain radiograph cannot distinguish between retropharyngeal cellulitis and an abscess, but if air is seen in the widened retropharyngeal space, an abscess can be diagnosed with confidence.[4] CT is now the preferred imaging modality to confirm the diagnosis and demonstrate the size, extent, and location of the pus collection from a retropharyngeal abscess.[1,37,38] Lesions with a low-density center surrounded by an enhancing thick rim are more characteristic of a retropharyngeal abscess rather than cellulitis (Fig. 51-10).

Treatment and Follow-up   Although retropharyngeal abscesses traditionally have been treated with surgical drainage of the pus collection, some cases may be managed with antibiotics alone. The role of operative drainage varies between studies[38,39] and also depends on the appearance and extent of disease. Nonoperative management is evolving, and a trial of antibiotics is considered in cases of retropharyngeal cellulitis and some small retropharyngeal abscesses with no evidence of airway compromise.[37]

Other Causes of Upper Airway Abnormalities

OBSTRUCTIVE SLEEP APNEA

Etiology   Obstructive sleep apnea syndrome (OSA) is a disorder of breathing during sleep that is characterized by prolonged partial or complete upper airway obstruction that disrupts normal ventilation and sleep patterns. Typical symptoms of OSA include snoring, disturbed sleep, and daytime neurobehavioral problems. Common complications from OSA are neurocognitive impairment, behavioral problems, failure to thrive, and cor pulmonale in severe cases. Risk factors for developing OSA include adenotonsillar hypertrophy, obesity, craniofacial anomalies, and neuromuscular disorders.[40] Nocturnal polysomnography (sleep study) is the only diagnostic technique shown to quantify the ventilatory and sleep abnormalities associated with sleep-disordered breathing.

Imaging   For imaging assessment of OSA, a lateral soft tissue neck radiograph can be obtained to evaluate adenoid size.[1] The adenoidal-nasopharyngeal ratio derived from the lateral soft tissue neck radiograph is a clinically useful index of pharyngeal patency.[41,42] Videofluoroscopic evaluation of the airway while the child is asleep also can be performed to

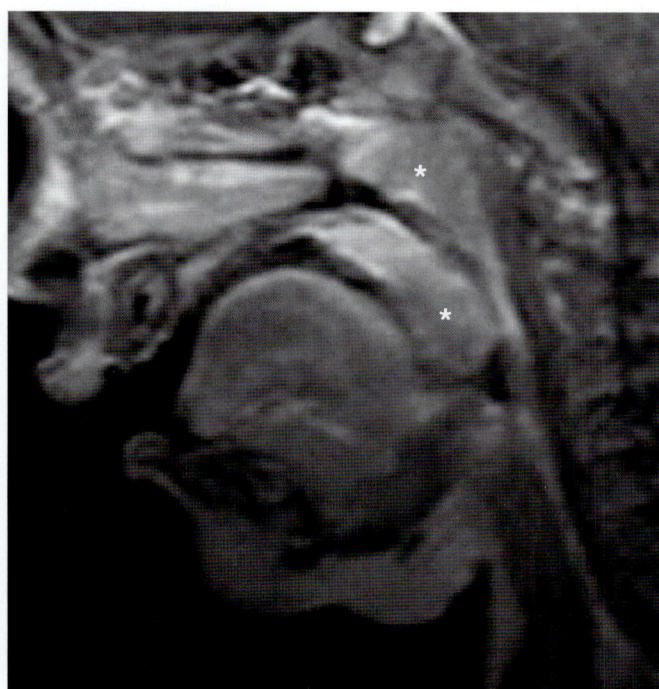

Figure 51-11 Obstructive sleep apnea in a 2-year-old girl with snoring. A sagittal magnetic resonance imaging sequence of the upper airway shows markedly enlarged adenoids (*upper asterisk*) and palatine tonsils (*lower asterisk*) causing narrowing of the nasopharyngeal airway.

investigate inspiratory collapse of the nasopharynx and oropharynx as a result of proximal airway obstruction acting in concert with sleep-related hypotonia of the pharyngeal musculature.[43] More recently, cine MRI has been advocated as the more accurate diagnostic imaging technique because it shows the volumetric dimension of the adenoids and palatine tonsils (Fig. 51-11). Furthermore, it also can demonstrate dynamic motion of the upper airway, thereby allowing evaluation of the relationship between the size of the adenoid and palatine tonsils and the degree of airway motion.[44]

Treatment and Follow-up Treatment of mild cases of OSA include lifestyle changes such as weight loss. For moderate to severe OSA, the two most commonly used treatments include a continuous positive airway pressure or automatic positive airway pressure device that can maintain the patency of the patient's airway during sleep by providing the pressurized air flow into the upper airway. Additionally, several surgical treatments currently are available in patients with anatomic causes of upper airway obstruction, including septoplasty, turbinate surgery, tonsillectomy, and uvulopalatopharyngoplasty.

FOREIGN BODY

Etiology Most patients who present with foreign bodies in the upper airway are children between 6 months to 3 years of age. In these patients, the most commonly aspirated foreign bodies are food, plastic toys, and small household items. A diagnosis of foreign body aspiration often is missed or delayed because the causative event is usually unobserved and the symptoms are nonspecific in children.[45] Nasal foreign bodies tend to be located on the floor of the nasal passage, just below the inferior turbinate, or in the upper nasal fossa anterior to the middle turbinate (Fig. 51-12).[46] Affected pediatric patients often present with unilateral, foul-smelling nasal discharge.

Imaging Radiography can be helpful in localizing radiopaque foreign bodies such as coins, buttons, and batteries, but because most foreign bodies are radiolucent, management should not be based solely on imaging.[47] Plain radiography is sufficient to demonstrate radiopaque upper airway and esophageal foreign bodies. On frontal radiographs, coins in the esophagus are seen en face, whereas coins in the trachea are seen in tangent because of a posterior gap in the tracheal cartilage rings. Food and other nonradiopaque foreign bodies in the upper airway often are identified only with an endoscopy.[4]

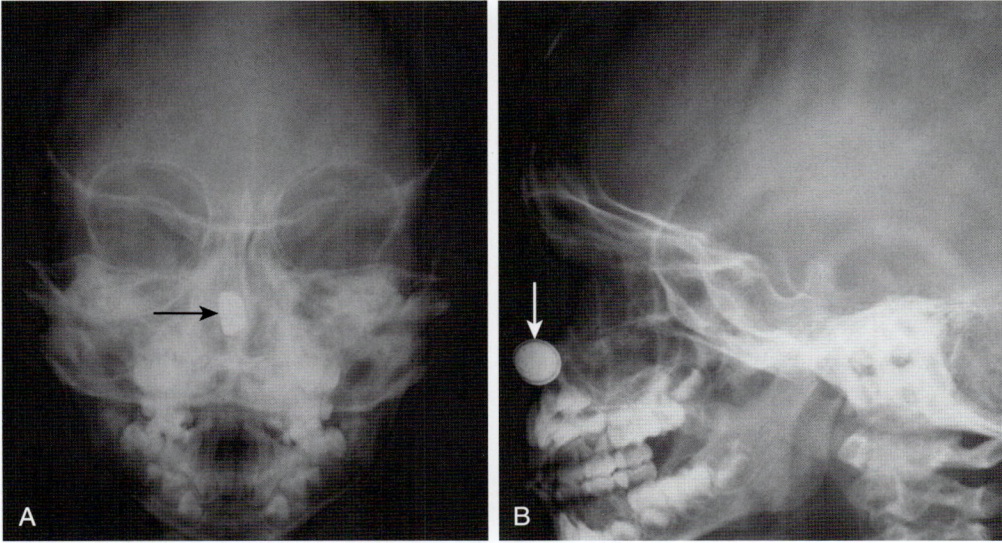

Figure 51-12 A nasal foreign body in a boy who presented with nasal congestion and foul-smelling discharge for 1 week. Frontal (**A**) and lateral (**B**) radiographs of the nasal airway show a metallic foreign body (battery; *arrow*) in the right nasal cavity.

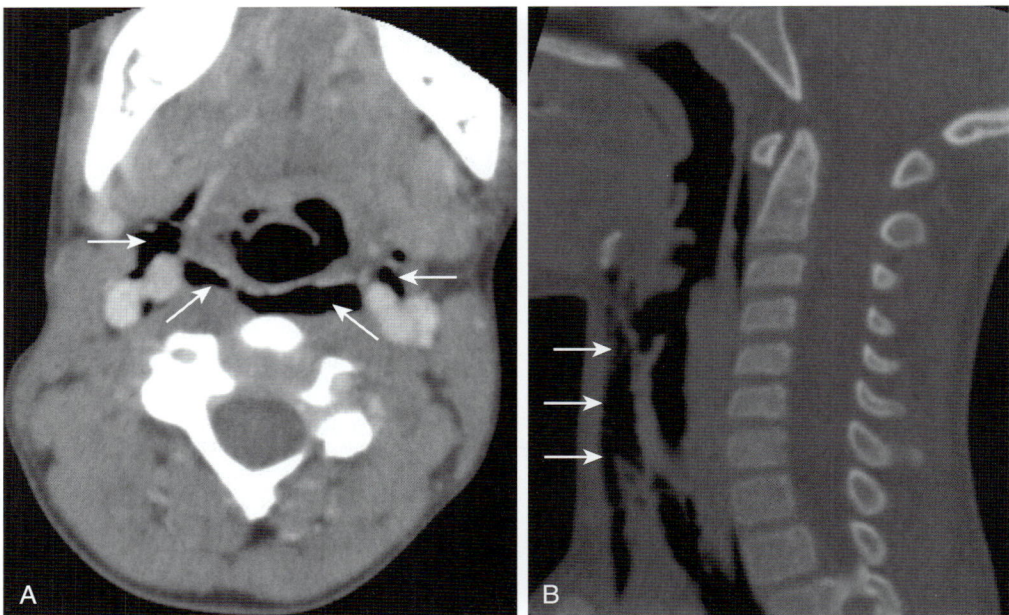

Figure 51-13 Laryngeal trauma in a 10-year-old boy who tripped and struck his anterior neck across a log. Axial (**A**) and sagittal reconstruction (**B**) computed tomography scans of the neck show air dissecting along the parapharyngeal region (*arrows*) compatible with laryngeal trauma. (Courtesy Elizabeth H. Ey, MD, Dayton, OH.)

Treatment and Follow-up Most nasal foreign bodies can be removed by a skilled physician, although attempts at removal may push the nasal foreign body into the pharynx, creating an airway hazard. Pharyngeal and laryngeal foreign bodies are medical emergencies because airway obstruction usually occurs at the time of aspiration and results in immediate respiratory distress. Flexible or rigid endoscopy usually is required to confirm the diagnosis, remove the foreign body, and avoid complications including airway obstruction, laryngeal edema, and pushing the foreign body into the subglottic space or trachea.[47]

TRAUMATIC INJURIES

Etiology Pediatric laryngotracheal injuries are infrequent because of the softer cartilages and the protection provided by the prominent mandible.[48,49] The degree and presentation of blunt and penetrating injuries are diverse. External evidence of trauma often associated with laryngotracheal injuries in children includes bruising, cuts, abrasions, and subcutaneous emphysema. Airway compromise is suggested if dysphonia, dysphagia, or dyspnea is present.[50] The most important clinical signs of laryngeal injury include hoarseness and subcutaneous emphysema.[49] Injuries may be subtle and present with minimal initial symptoms that, if undiagnosed, may rapidly progress to loss of the airway. Thus a high index of suspicion is needed to promptly and accurately diagnose and manage pediatric laryngotracheal injuries. Fiberoptic laryngoscopy is mandatory when injury to the larynx and trachea is suspected.[49,50]

Imaging In any pediatric patient with possible upper airway injury, plain radiographs of the neck and chest may aid in the diagnosis. Radiographs also can be useful to assess the cervical spine. Findings of laryngotracheal injuries in pediatric patients vary considerably according to the mechanism of injury, but radiographic evidence of soft tissue air and wounds opening into the airway are common findings. CT is also useful and can play a primary role in localizing the injury and determining its extent (Fig. 51-13).[49-52]

Treatment and Follow-up Most laryngotracheal injuries in children can be managed conservatively. However, extensive injuries, including displaced fractures of the cartilage, injuries to the recurrent nerves, and laryngotracheal separation, require surgical intervention.[51]

NEOPLASMS

Subglottic Hemangioma

Etiology Subglottic hemangioma, a congenital vascular tumor, is the most common primary neoplasm affecting the subglottic trachea. Although the tumor is present at birth, patients with subglottic hemangioma usually become symptomatic between 1 and 6 months of age because of the rapid growth of hemangiomas at this stage. Affected infants usually present with the sudden onset of acute respiratory difficulty that varies in severity and includes stridor and crouplike symptoms. The symptoms are intermittent at first, but they eventually become persistent, especially as the hemangioma grows. If the subglottic hemangioma extends superiorly to involve the true cords, hoarseness also may be present. The sudden enlargement of a hemangioma as a result of hemorrhage can cause varying degrees of acute upper airway narrowing, potentially resulting in life-threatening asphyxia. Fifty percent of patients also have concomitant cutaneous hemangiomas. During its initial proliferative phase, the mass grows rapidly during the first 18 months of life, followed by a gradual involution that may last until age 10 years. Generally, a subglottic hemangioma is a self-limiting condition, and

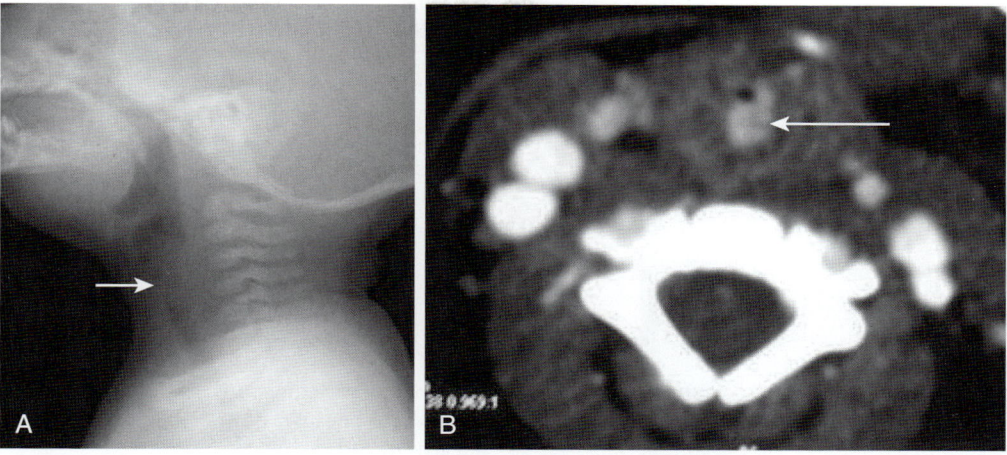

Figure 51-14 Subglottic hemangioma in a 6-month-old boy with stridor. **A,** A lateral neck radiograph demonstrates haziness and soft tissue densities in the subglottic tracheal region (*arrow*). **B,** An axial computed tomography scan at the subglottic region shows the hemangioma (*arrow*), an intensely enhancing soft tissue mass causing marked narrowing of the subglottic trachea.

the respiratory distress tends to diminish and may disappear. However, the behavior of the individual lesion is unpredictable, and the symptoms are variable in severity.[53]

Imaging Plain radiographs of infants and children with subglottic hemangiomas typically show an irregular, small, soft tissue mass below the true vocal cords (Fig. 51-14). These lesions have a characteristic radiographic appearance of a soft tissue shadow bulging into the airway lumen, often with asymmetric subglottic narrowing. However, symmetric narrowing of the trachea can be caused by a hemangioma if it is located central to the plane of projection. CT or MRI can show the mass at the subglottic region with intense enhancement following the administration of contrast material (see Fig. 51-14).[53]

Treatment and Follow-up The currently available treatment options for subglottic hemangioma include conservative monitoring in mildly symptomatic patients with a small subglottic hemangioma and laser therapy, laryngotracheoplasty, and direct surgical excision in patients with severe airway compromise. It has recently been recognized that propranolol may work for the treatment of hemangiomas.

Lymphoma

Etiology Lymphoma is a neoplasm in the lymphatic cells of the immune system. It is the most common malignancy involving the extracranial head and neck in children. Hodgkin and non-Hodgkin lymphoma together account for 10% to 15% of all childhood malignancies in developed countries.[54] Most children with head and neck lymphoma present with cervical lymph node involvement. They may present with nodal disease involving Waldeyer's ring (i.e., lymphatic tissue in the nasopharynx, base of the tongue, tonsils, and soft palate). Hodgkin lymphoma, characterized histologically by the presence of Reed-Sternberg cells, is more commonly seen in adolescents. Non-Hodgkin lymphoma is more common than Hodgkin lymphoma in children younger than 10 years. Lymphomas typically present with enlarged, painless cervical

lymph nodes, but other symptoms, including airway obstruction, are dependent on the extent and involvement of surrounding structures.

Imaging Plain radiographs typically show a masslike opacity in the region of neck (Fig. 51-15). Narrowing and displacement of the upper airway also may be seen on plain radiographs. Compared with plain radiographs, cross-sectional imaging such as CT or MRI can better demonstrate the location, degree, and extent of the upper airway compromise. Both CT and MRI with intravenous contrast can be used for diagnosis, staging, and follow-up.[55]

Treatment and Follow-up Pediatric patients with lymphoma compromising the upper airway usually respond well to chemotherapy and do not require emergent tracheostomy placement. With the reduction in size of lymph nodes after chemotherapy, the patency of the upper airway subsequently can be regained.

Rhabdomyosarcoma

Etiology Rhabdomyosarcoma is the most common soft tissue sarcoma arising from the connective tissues in children younger than 15 years. It accounts for 8% of all childhood malignancies.[56] Most rhabdomyosarcomas occur in the first decade of life, with a slight male predominance. The head and neck is the primary site of the disease in 40% of children with rhabdomyosarcoma.[57]

Imaging Plain radiographs usually show a large masslike opacity, and ultrasound often demonstrates a heterogeneous mass in patients with cervical rhabdomyosarcoma. However, a complete evaluation, particularly for any upper airway obstruction, requires a cross-sectional imaging study such as CT or MRI. MRI is the imaging modality of choice for rhabdomyosarcoma. Typically it is hyperintense on T2-weighted sequences and isointense or minimally hyperintense on T1-weighted sequences. Moderate to intense enhancement usually is seen after administration of

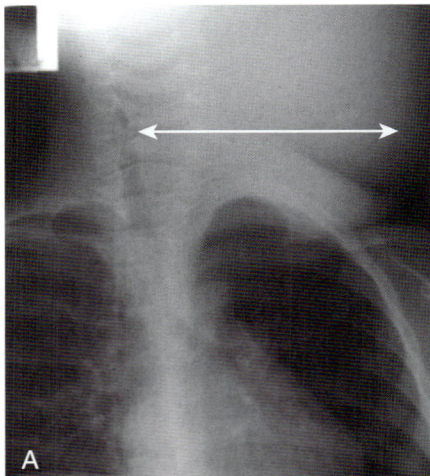

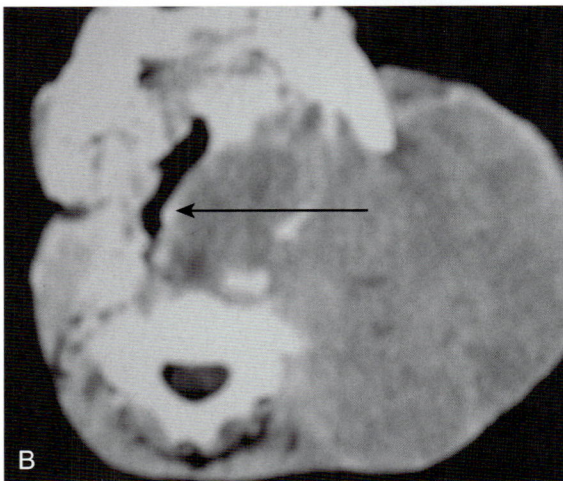

Figure 51-15 Lymphoma in a 9-year-old boy with difficulty breathing. **A,** A frontal neck radiograph shows a large left-sided neck mass (*double arrow*). **B,** An axial computed tomography scan of the upper neck demonstrates the large mass effacing and displacing the airway to the right (*arrow*).

Key Points

Upper airway disease is a common problem in infants and children because of the narrow diameter of the airway early in life.

Upper airway diseases in children can be categorized as acute or chronic, but the etiology is diverse and includes congenital, infectious/inflammatory, foreign body, post-traumatic, and neoplastic causes.

Radiographs maintain an integral role in the initial evaluation of a patient with upper airway disease, but attention to proper positioning and technique is important to avoid pitfalls.

Cross-sectional imaging (CT and MRI) is capable of multiplanar reconstruction, which allows a detailed evaluation of airway anatomy and disease on both static and dynamic states.

Endoscopy is still the gold standard in evaluating upper airway diseases, but CT with three-dimensional–virtual endoscopy has the ability to produce a realistic presentation of the inner walls of the airway, simulating a real endoscopic examination even if the lumen cannot be passed endoscopically because of stenosis.

contrast.[55] CT is less effective than MRI in determining the extent of the mass but is important in determining bone involvement.

Treatment and Follow-up   Treatment of rhabdomyosarcoma with upper airway obstruction includes chemotherapy, radiation therapy, and sometimes surgical resection. Urgent tracheostomy placement to secure the airway below the level of obstruction and provide sufficient air flow for respiration may be required in pediatric patients who do not respond to nonsurgical treatment.

Other malignant neoplasms involving the head and neck that have the potential to affect the airway include nasopharyngeal carcinoma, thyroid cancers, and salivary gland tumors, although these entities are uncommon in children.

Suggested Readings

Bradshaw K. Imaging the upper airways. *Paediatr Respir Rev.* 2001;2:46-56.
Goodman TR, McHugh K. The role of radiology in the evaluation of stridor. *Arch Dis Child.* 1999;81:456-459.
John SD, Swischuk LE. Stridor and upper airway obstruction in infants and children. *Radiographics.* 1992;12:625-643.
Laya BF, Lee EY. Congenital causes of upper airway obstruction in pediatric patients: updated techniques and review of imaging findings. *Semin Roentgenol.* 2012;47(2):147-158.
Lee EY, Restrepo R, Dillman JR, et al. Imaging evaluation of trachea and bronchi: systematic review and updates. *Semin Roentgenol.* 2012;47(2):182-196.
Lloyd C, Mchugh K. The role of radiology in head and neck tumors in children. *Cancer Imaging.* 2010;10:49-61.
Macpherson RI, Leithiser RE. Upper airway obstruction in children: an update. *Radiographics.* 1985;5(3):339-376.

References

Full references for this chapter can be found on www.expertconsult.com.

Chapter 52

Lower Large Airway Disease

EDWARD Y. LEE, RICARDO RESTREPO, and PHILLIP M. BOISELLE

Overview

Disorders of the lower large airways are common in the pediatric population and have the potential to be life threatening.[1-3] Because these disorders are associated with nonspecific clinical symptoms, the diagnosis frequently is missed or delayed, particularly in infants and young children. After careful investigation of the clinical history and physical examination, imaging evaluation is the next management step. Imaging plays an important role in the diagnosis of congenital and acquired lower large airway disorders. By becoming familiar with the characteristic imaging findings of lower large airway disorders, radiologists can play an important role in ensuring prompt diagnosis and guiding appropriate management of these often acute and complex conditions in pediatric patients.

This chapter reviews the etiology, imaging findings, and management of the most frequently encountered congenital and acquired lower large airway disorders in the pediatric population. Large airway disorders due to primary benign neoplasms and extrinsic compression due to mediastinal vascular anomalies are not included in this chapter because they are discussed in detail in other chapters (Chapters 51 and 77, respectively) in this book.

Spectrum of Lower Large Airway Disease

CONGENITAL ANOMALIES

Tracheobronchial Branching Anomalies

Tracheal Agenesis

Etiology Tracheal agenesis, which is a rare congenital anomaly of unknown etiology, is characterized by either partial or complete tracheal underdevelopment.[4-6] This condition frequently is associated with maternal polyhydramnios, and a tracheoesophageal or bronchoesophageal fistula often is present concomitantly.[4-7] Three main types of tracheal agenesis exist. Type 1 consists of absent upper trachea and connection of the lower trachea to the esophagus; type 2 consists of a common bronchus connecting bilateral main bronchi to the esophagus; and type 3 consists of independent bilateral main bronchi arising from the esophagus (Fig. 52-1, *A*). Of these three types, type 2 is the most common. Affected patients typically present with severe respiratory distress and absence of an audible cry, and the airway cannot be intubated

below the larynx immediately after birth.[4-7] The diagnosis of tracheal agenesis should be considered in any infant who demonstrates improved lung ventilation after placement of the endotracheal tube in the esophagus following an initial unsuccessful intubation attempt. Once tracheal agenesis is diagnosed, radiologists should look carefully for other congenital anomalies that frequently are associated with this condition, such as congenital heart disease, duodenal atresia, and radial ray anomalies.[4-7]

Imaging Chest radiographic imaging findings of tracheal agenesis often are nonspecific, such as absent or decreased lung volume. However, the diagnosis of tracheal agenesis should be considered when absence of the normal tracheal air lucency, abnormal carinal position, and placement of the endotracheal tube in the esophagus are seen on chest radiographs of infants with severe respiratory distress immediately after birth (Fig. 52-1, *B* and *C*). The diagnosis is confirmed by computed tomography (CT) and/or bronchoesophagoscopy.[4-8] These studies can show both the partial or complete tracheal underdevelopment and anomalous bronchi connected to the esophagus (Fig. 52-1, *D*).

Treatment and Follow-up Because of difficulties related to both early diagnosis and treatment, tracheal agenesis usually is a fatal condition.[4-7] The initial management of tracheal agenesis is aimed at early diagnosis at birth and immediate maintenance of airway patency, usually via the esophagus in the presence of a bronchoesophageal fistula. Although several surgical approaches have been proposed in the past, definitive treatment currently has not been established, and long-term survival of affected patients is rare. However, patients with short-segment tracheal agenesis may be amenable to direct tracheal anastomosis.[5,7]

Tracheal Bronchus

Etiology Tracheal bronchus is a congenital bronchial branching anomaly in which an ectopic (more frequently) or supernumerary bronchial branch arises from the lateral tracheal wall just above the carina.[9-15] This condition also is known as bronchus suis because it is a normal finding in pigs. The incidence of tracheal bronchus in the pediatric population is between 0.1% and 5%.[16] Although tracheal bronchus most frequently occurs on the right side, it also can present on the left side or bilaterally. Most patients with tracheal bronchus are asymptomatic, and it is usually an incidental finding detected on imaging studies obtained for the workup of other medical conditions. However, patients with tracheal

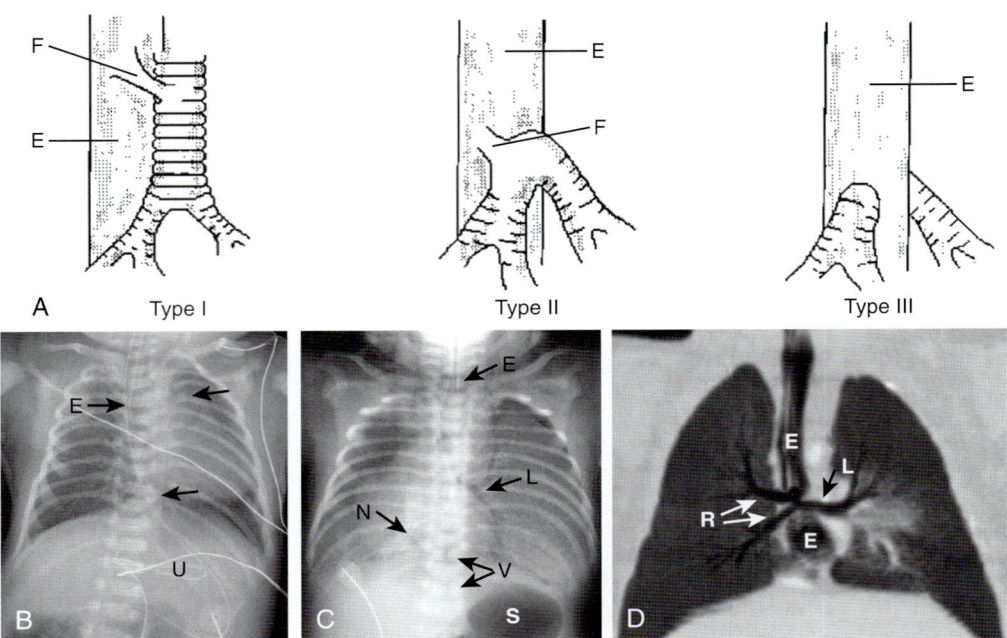

Figure 52-1   A, Three types of tracheal agenesis. In type I, part of the proximal trachea is absent with a short distal trachea communicating to the esophagus via a tracheoesophageal fistula. In type II, the most common type, the trachea is completely absent with a carina connecting the two main bronchi. A bronchoesophageal fistula is usually, but not always, present. In type III, the trachea and carina are absent with the bronchial orifices separately arising directly from the esophagus. **B,** A newborn with type II tracheal agenesis. The chest radiograph shows lungs that are relatively normal in aeration, although haziness is present, which may represent retained fetal fluid. The endotracheal tube (E) is slightly low but otherwise is unremarkable. The nasogastric tube also is present and is in the stomach. Segmentation abnormalities of the spine and upper left ribs are noted (arrows). The umbilical venous catheter (U) is malpositioned. **C,** A newborn with type III tracheal agenesis. A chest radiograph obtained during resuscitation shows poorly aerated lungs with pneumomediastinum and a left pneumothorax. The endotracheal tube (E) is at the thoracic inlet level. The nasogastric tube (N) is in the right bronchial tree, which appears to originate lower than normal. Note the low position of the left main bronchus (L). "Butterfly" vertebral (V) are seen. **D,** A newborn with type III trachea agenesis (the same condition as the patient in part **C**). A coronal maximum intensity projection reformatted image shows two right bronchi (R) and the left bronchus (L) arising near the midline from the esophagus (E). The trachea is absent with the possible exception of a small segment connecting the bronchi. The nasogastric tube is present in the esophagus (E). E, Esophagus; F, fistula; S, stomach. (**A,** From Effmann EI, Spackman TJ, Berdon WE, et al. Tracheal agenesis, *AJR Am J Roentgenol* 125:767, 1975. **B** to **D,** From Strouse PJ, Newman B, Hernandez RJ, et al. CT of tracheal agenesis, *Pediatr Radiol.* 36:920-926, 2006.)

bronchus also may present with symptoms such as persistent or recurrent upper lobe pneumonia, atelectasis, or air trapping.[11] Additionally, tracheal bronchus may unexpectedly be discovered after intubation as a result of upper lobe atelectasis related to inadvertent occlusion of the ectopic upper lobe bronchial orifice by a low-lying endotracheal tube.[14]

Imaging   On chest radiographs, secondary imaging findings of tracheal bronchus such as upper lobe atelectasis or pneumonia can be detected, but the anomalous upper lobe bronchus cannot be reliably visualized. In the past, tracheal bronchus was evaluated with tracheobronchography. However, CT with two-dimensional (2D) and three-dimensional (3D) reconstructions is now the imaging technique of choice for evaluating anomalous tracheal bronchus and associated lung abnormalities[17-19] (Fig. 52-2). Bronchoscopy can confirm the diagnosis of tracheal bronchus when necessary.

Treatment and Follow-up   Pediatric patients with incidentally detected tracheal bronchus generally do not require any treatment. However, symptomatic children with recurrent upper lobe infection due to tracheal bronchus may require surgical resection, especially if permanent lung damage has developed or they are considered at risk for the development of permanent lung damage.[1]

Esophageal Bronchus or Lung

Etiology   Esophageal bronchus or lung is a rare congenital anomaly.[11,20] The term "esophageal bronchus" refers to the condition in which a lobar bronchus, typically the medial basal segment of the right lower lobe, arises directly from the esophagus. The term "esophageal lung" is used when the main bronchus arises directly from the esophagus. This condition most commonly presents in infants but may be diagnosed at any age. It is associated with a wide spectrum of clinical presentations ranging from asymptomatic to recurrent severe pulmonary infections or even death depending on the size and location of the anomaly. In general, symptomatic pediatric patients with esophageal bronchus or lung typically present with feeding difficulties and recurrent respiratory tract infections. Other associated congenital anomalies include congenital heart disease, duodenal atresia, duodenal stenosis, distal tracheoesophageal fistula, and esophageal atresia.

Imaging   On chest radiographs, affected patients typically present as a result of aspiration during feeding, with air space opacification in the medial lower lobe in the case of esophageal bronchus and air space opacification that involves the entire lung in the case of esophageal lung.[1,11] An esophagogram can provide a definitive diagnosis by allowing

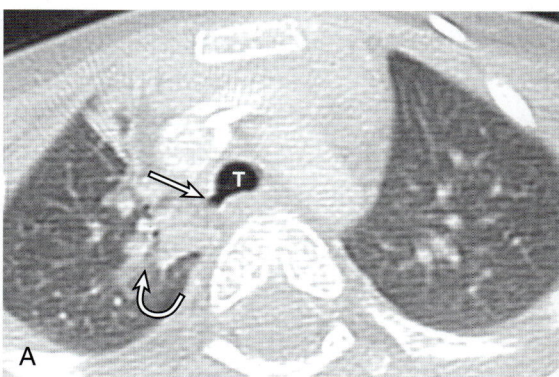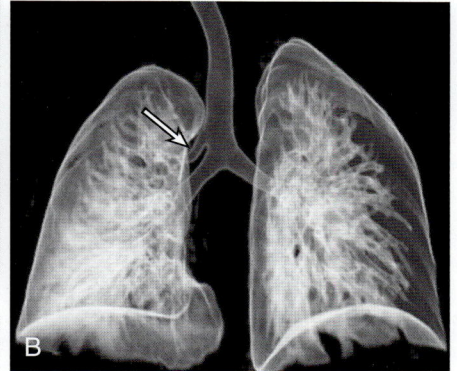

Figure 52-2 Tracheal bronchus in a 1-year-old boy with recurrent right upper lobe atelectasis. **A,** An axial lung window computed tomography (CT) image shows an anomalous right upper lobe bronchus (*straight arrow*) directly arising from the trachea (*T*). Atelectasis (*curved arrow*) is present in the medial right upper lobe. **B,** A frontal three-dimensional (3D) volume-rendered image of the central airways and lungs shows an anomalous right upper lobe bronchus (*arrow*) directly arising from the trachea. The location, size, and course of this anomalous right upper lobe bronchus (i.e., tracheal bronchus) are better demonstrated on a 3D volume-rendered image than on an axial CT image (A).

visualization of a direct communication between a bronchus and the esophagus (Fig. 52-3). CT may be helpful for evaluating associated lung parenchymal abnormalities and guiding surgery.

Treatment and Follow-up Surgical lobectomy or pneumonectomy is the current management of choice for symptomatic patients with esophageal bronchus or lung, respectively.[20]

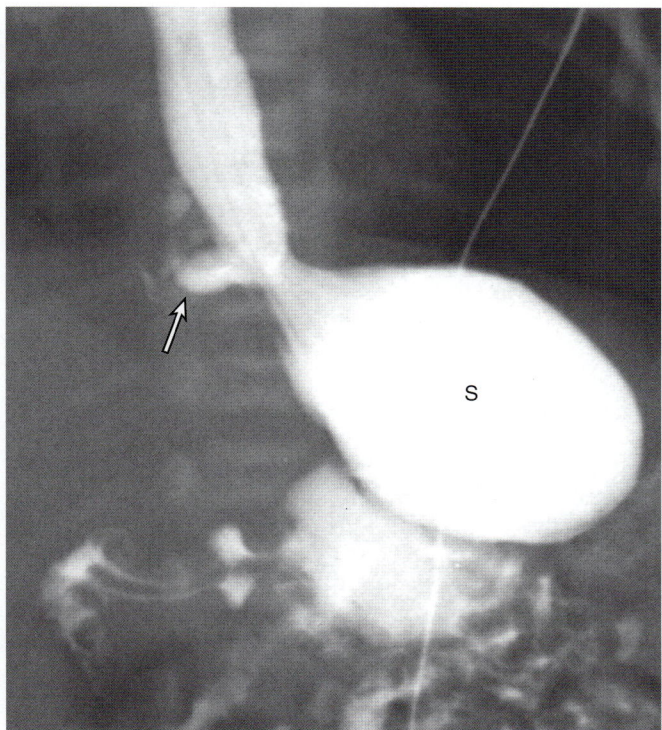

Figure 52-3 Esophageal bronchus in a 4-day-old infant girl who presented with acute respiratory distress during feeding. An esophagogram shows a barium-filled medial right lower lobe bronchus (*arrow*) directly arising from the distal esophagus. *S,* stomach.

Congenital Tracheal Stenosis

Etiology Congenital tracheal stenosis is a rare condition characterized by intrinsic narrowing of the tracheal lumen, usually as a result of underlying complete cartilaginous rings.[2,3,21,22] Such cartilaginous rings with an absent or deficient posterior membranous portion render the tracheal lumen smaller and less pliable. Affected patients present in the first year of life with expiratory stridor, wheezing, and respiratory distress.[2,3,21,22] Congenital tracheal stenosis traditionally is classified into three types, including (1) focal (50%), (2) generalized (30%), and (3) funnel shaped (20%).[23] Other congenital anomalies often associated with congenital tracheal stenosis are tracheoesophageal fistula, pulmonary agenesis or hypoplasia, pulmonary artery sling type 2, and bronchial stenosis.[2,3,11,24]

Imaging Although neck and chest radiographs or fluoroscopy may lead to the suspicion of congenital tracheal stenosis when a narrowed trachea is encountered in pediatric patients with respiratory symptoms, CT is the imaging modality of choice for diagnosis and characterizion.[2,4,24] With CT, the diagnosis of congenital tracheal stenosis is based on the identification of decreased caliber of the trachea without evidence of tracheal wall thickening. The size of the subglottic region (which does not contain tracheal cartilage) can serve as an internal reference standard. The use of 2D/3D reconstructed CT imaging is particularly helpful for increasing detection of subtle stenoses, improving measurement of craniocaudal extent of disease, and enhancing evaluation of its anatomic relationship with other mediastinal structures for preoperative assessment (Fig. 52-4).[2,4,24] Virtual bronchoscopic images can confirm the diagnosis of complete rings by showing concentric rings extending along the posterior wall of the trachea.[25] This appearance contrasts with the normal appearance in which the C-shaped rings do not extend to the posterior membranous wall.[25] In addition, virtual bronchoscopy has the capability of evaluating the airways distal to high-grade trachea stenoses, beyond which a conventional bronchoscope cannot pass.[2,4,24,25] CT also may aid in the detection of other associated anomalies that often have an abnormal lung component.

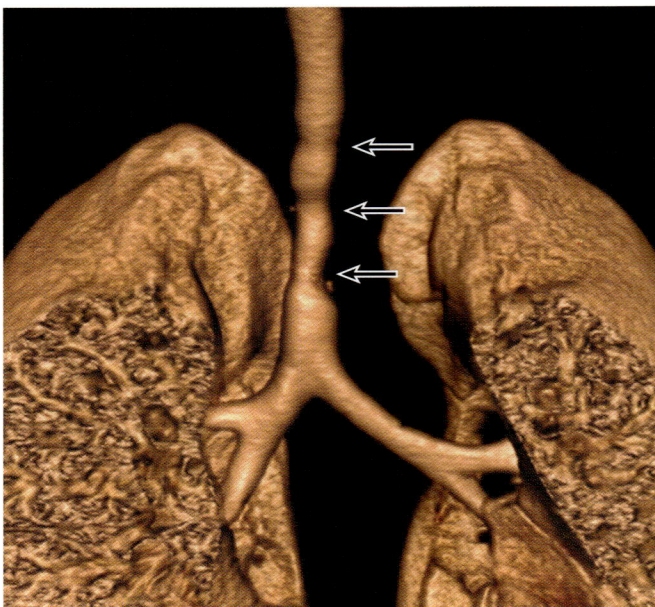

Figure 52-4 Congenital tracheal stenosis in a 3-month-old boy with expiratory stridor and respiratory distress. A frontal three-dimensional volume-rendered image of the large airways and lungs shows several areas of mild to moderate mid to distal tracheal narrowing (*arrows*).

Treatment and Follow-up Treatment of congenital tracheal stenosis mainly depends on the following three factors: (1) degree, (2) location, and (3) extent of the tracheal narrowing. A short tracheal stenosis may be treated by end-to-end anastomosis, whereas a longer lesion may require a patch or autograft repair.[22] Other available options for short-segment tracheal stenosis include stent placement or balloon dilatation, although these methods are used more commonly to treat acquired tracheal stenosis.

Tracheobronchomegaly

Etiology Tracheobronchomegaly, also known as Mounier-Kuhn syndrome, is a rare disorder characterized by dilatation of the trachea and main bronchi.[26-28] Although the exact etiology of this condition currently is unknown, a defect in the elastic and muscular tissues of the large airways is presumed to be a potential underlying cause. The increased compliance of the large airway walls as a result of the atrophy of longitudinal elastic fibers with thinning of the muscularis mucosa often results in the development of broad, diverticulum-like protrusions of redundant musculomembranous tissue between the cartilaginous rings. It may occur either as a familial condition or in association with a connective tissue disorder such as Ehlers-Danlos syndrome.[29] It typically occurs in pediatric patients who have received prolonged ventilatory support or who have a chronic pulmonary infection such as cystic fibrosis. Although the clinical manifestations of tracheobronchomegaly are nonspecific, affected patients may present with a harsh cough, copious purulent sputum, occasional hemoptysis, and progressive dyspnea.

Imaging Chest radiographs alone may be adequate to detect the enlargement of trachea and bronchi in severe cases (Fig. 52-5), but CT is the imaging modality of choice for diagnosing tracheobronchomegaly, potential tracheal diverticulum, and associated lung abnormalities (Fig. 52-6).[1] Because of the increased incidence of tracheobronchomalacia (TBM) in patients with tracheobronchomegaly, a dynamic CT study consisting of both inspiratory and expiratory phase imaging may be beneficial for detecting concomitant TBM.

Treatment and Follow-up Asymptomatic pediatric patients with tracheobronchomegaly require no specific treatment. For symptomatic patients, treatment usually is conservative, including chest physiotherapy for assistance with clearing of

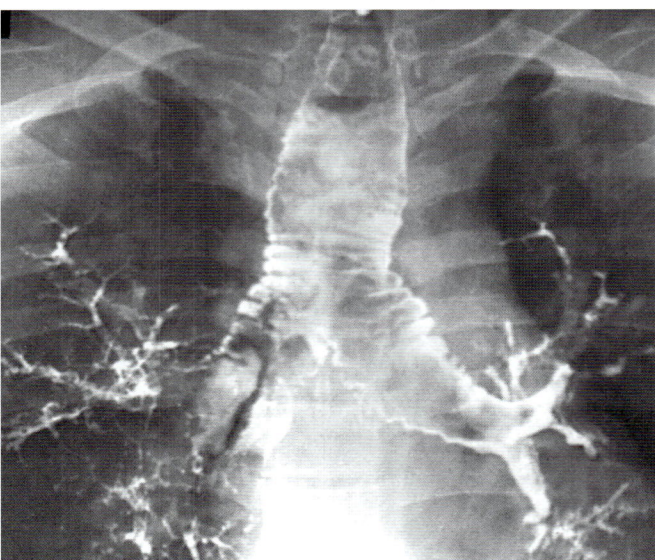

Figure 52-5 Tracheobronchomegaly. A tracheogram shows marked dilatation of the trachea and larger bronchi and indentations of the tracheal wall between the cartilaginous rings. (From Katz I, Levine M, Herman P. Tracheobronchomegaly: the Mounier-Kuhn syndrome, *AJR Am J Roentgenol* 88:1084, 1962.).

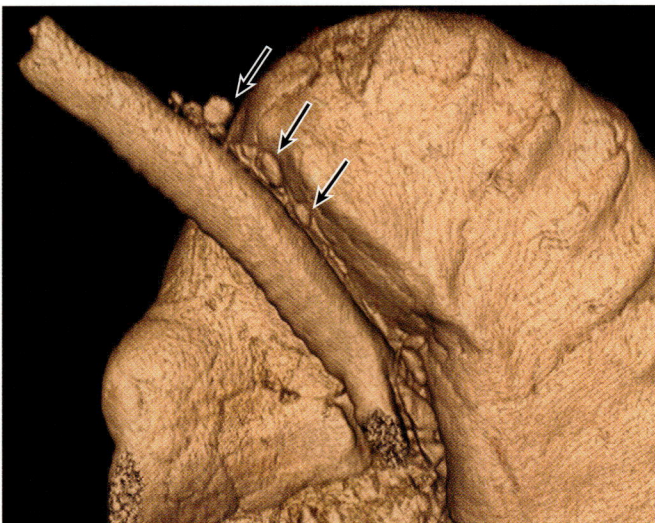

Figure 52-6 Tracheomegaly with tracheal diverticuli in an adolescent girl with cystic fibrosis. A three-dimensional volume-rendered lateral view of the large airway shows multiple diverticuli (*arrows*) arising from the posterior aspect of the enlarged trachea.

secretions and antibiotics for treatment of pulmonary infections.[30,31] Unfortunately, the generalized nature of this disorder limits possible benefits from surgical management.

ACQUIRED ABNORMALITIES

Foreign Body Aspiration

Etiology Foreign body aspiration into the tracheobronchial airway is a frequent cause of acute respiratory distress in pediatric patients, especially those between 6 months and 3 years of age.[1-3,32,33] Each year, aspirated foreign bodies are responsible for approximately 160 deaths in children aged 14 years or younger in the United States alone, along with substantial additional morbidity.[32,33] Although some pediatric patients may present with a clinical history of possible aspiration followed by cough, wheezing, respiratory distress, or decreased breath sounds, most affected pediatric patients present with a history that is either lacking or misleading.[1-3,32,33] Therefore a high clinical suspicion and thorough investigation are required for any infants and young children with respiratory symptoms suspicious for possible foreign body aspiration.

Only approximately 10% of aspirated foreign bodies within the tracheobronchial airway are radiopaque.[34] The remaining 90% of nonradiopaque foreign bodies are particularly difficult to diagnose early in pediatric patients. Nearly 70% of aspirated foreign bodies lodge in the bronchi, with the right side (52%) affected more frequently than the left side (18%).[32] The remaining 30% of aspirated foreign bodies lodge in the trachea (13%) and less common locations (17%).[32] In the early phase of foreign body aspiration, affected patients typically present with cough, wheezing, respiratory distress, or decreased breath sounds. During the late phase of missed foreign body aspiration, affected patients often present with episodic wheezing and/or recurrent pneumonias.

Imaging Radiographic findings of foreign body aspiration depend on the size, location, duration, and nature of the aspirated foreign body (Fig. 52-7). Radiopaque foreign bodies usually are detected easily with radiographic studies, which should include frontal and lateral films encompassing the upper airway from the nasopharynx to the upper abdomen. When the foreign body is not radiopaque, careful inspection of the tracheobronchial airway with high-kilovoltage films or fluoroscopy may show a faintly visible opacity interrupting the air column within the large airways. If the foreign object is located in the trachea, the chest radiograph may be normal or may show bilateral hypoinflation or hyperinflation depending on the degree of obstruction. Many intratracheal foreign bodies escape detection without the use of CT.

Rather than lodging in the trachea, most foreign bodies lodge in the main bronchi. In approximately 20% of cases, the foreign body migrates into a segmental bronchial branch.[32] The chest radiograph may show a variety of findings, the most common of which is a unilateral hyperlucent lung. If the bronchial obstruction becomes more complete, postobstructive atelectasis, pneumonia, or bronchiectasis may develop. A chest radiograph obtained at full inspiration can appear normal in approximately 20% to 30% of patients with bronchial foreign bodies; close inspection may show relatively increased volume on the normal side with a slight mediastinal shift toward the partially obstructed side. If a foreign body is suspected clinically, an expiratory chest radiograph always should be obtained, because it is critical for diagnosis. Lateral decubitus films may be diagnostic if satisfactory inspiration-expiration chest radiographs cannot be obtained. When air trapping is present in a dependent lung on the decubitus view, the affected lobe or segment tends to remain hyperlucent rather than deflating, as would normally occur (Fig. 52-8). Fluoroscopic examination of the chest also is valuable for detecting air trapping. It can show inspiratory mediastinal shift toward the affected side and restricted diaphragmatic excursion on the affected side.

The sensitivity and specificity of chest radiographs for foreign body detection were only 74% and 45%, respectively, in a series of 93 patients examined by Silva et al[35] and 68% and 67%, respectively, in a series of 83 patients examined by Svedstrom et al.[36] Because of this relatively poor accuracy, Silva and colleagues have suggested that chest radiographs should not be relied upon for diagnosis, but rather that all patients with suspected foreign body aspiration should undergo

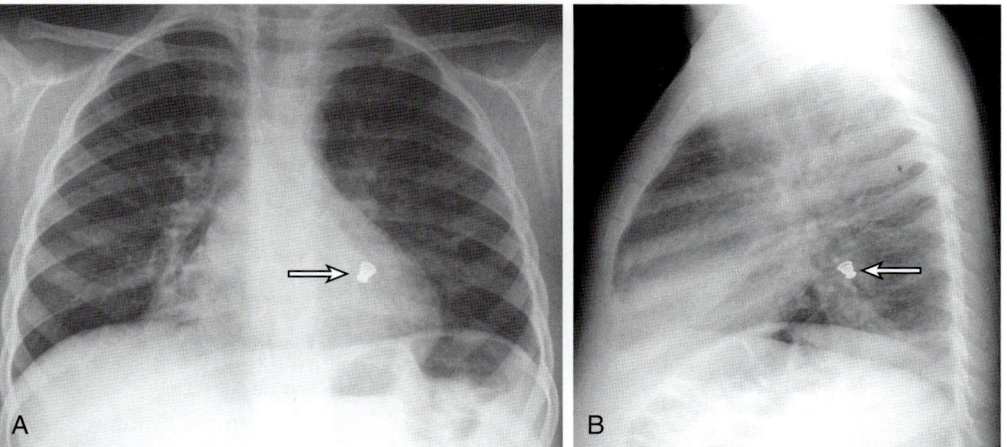

Figure 52-7 Radiopaque foreign body aspiration in a 4-year-old boy who presented with acute onset of coughing and respiratory distress. After a chest radiograph was performed, the patient underwent bronchoscopy, which showed a metallic bottle cap lodged in the left lower lobe bronchus. **A,** A frontal chest radiograph shows a radiopaque foreign body (*arrow*) located in the left lower lobe, retrocardiac region. **B,** A lateral chest radiograph confirms the location of the foreign body (*arrow*) in a left lower lobe bronchus. (From Lee EY, Restrepo R, Dillman JR, et al. Imaging evaluation of pediatric trachea and bronchi: systematic review and updates, *Semin Roentgenol.* 47(2):183, 2012.)

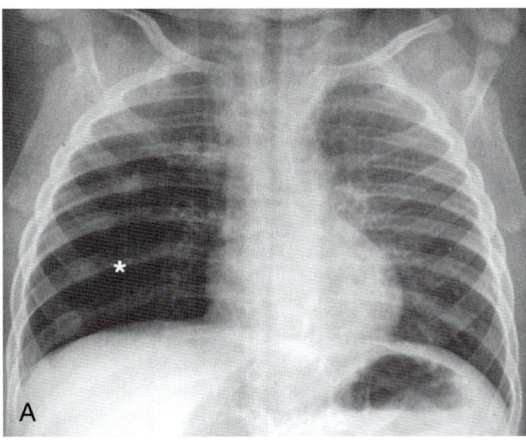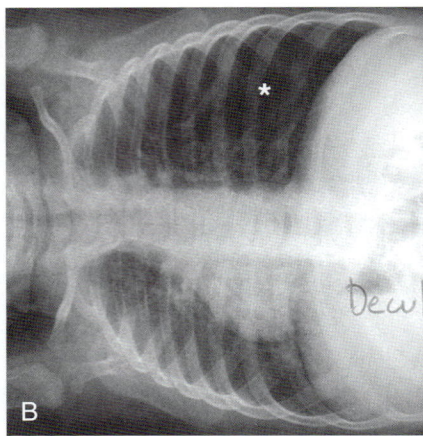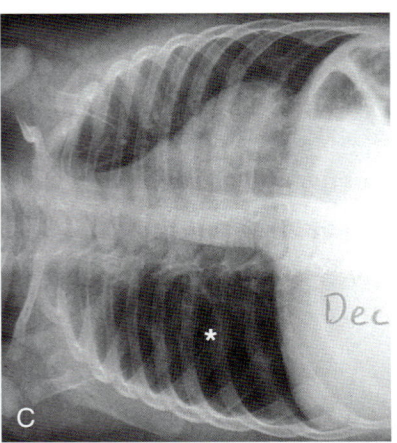

Figure 52-8   Nonradiopaque foreign body aspiration in a 5-year-old girl who presented with persistent coughing and respiratory distress while eating popcorn. **A,** A frontal chest radiograph obtained at end-inspiration shows mild hyperinflation (*asterisk*) of the right lower lobe. **B,** A frontal chest radiograph obtained at end-inspiration in the left lateral decubitus position demonstrates normal volume loss in the left lung and mild hyperinflation (*asterisk*) of the right lower lobe. **C,** A frontal chest radiograph obtained at end-inspiration in the right lateral decubitus position shows persistent hyperinflation (*asterisk*) of the right lower lobe.

bronchoscopy.[35] This approach results in a false-negative bronchoscopy rate of at least 20% in most series, however.[35]

CT is the most sensitive diagnostic imaging technique, but in general it should be reserved for patients for whom chest radiography is either normal or nonspecific. With use of CT, the diagnosis of a foreign body can be established with nearly 100% accuracy.[2] Either the foreign body is visualized or a focal pulmonary abnormality such as postobstructive air trapping, atelectasis, or consolidation is seen. If none of these findings is present, it is extremely unlikely that a foreign body is present. However, CT is less likely to visualize the foreign body directly if the lung is consolidated unless the foreign body is calcified or opaque.

Preliminary studies of low-dose multidetector computed tomography (MDCT) virtual bronchoscopy suggest that it may play a potential role in children with suspected foreign body aspiration by (1) identifying the precise location of a foreign body prior to bronchoscopy and (2) excluding a foreign body in children with a low level of suspicion and normal or nonspecific findings on chest radiography.[36-39] Because CT is less expensive and less invasive than bronchoscopy, it may be a viable alternative for selected patients.

Treatment and Follow-up   Once an aspirated foreign body is diagnosed on imaging studies, bronchoscopy and removal of the aspirated foreign body should be performed. Although imaging findings may be nonspecific or normal, symptomatic pediatric patients with high clinical suspicion and a convincing history of possible foreign body aspiration require bronchoscopy for a complete assessment. CT after bronchoscopy also is valuable because it provides additional diagnostic information regarding the presence and pattern of bronchial obstruction in symptomatic children with suspected residual foreign body.[34]

Infection/Inflammation

Tuberculosis

Etiology   Tuberculosis (TB) is caused by *Mycobacterium tuberculosis*. Although advances in diagnosis and treatment have

been made in the past two decades, TB continues to be a major cause of morbidity and mortality, particularly in infants, elderly persons, and immunocompromised patients.[40,41] In developed countries, TB most commonly is transmitted to infants and children by an adult family member infected with active TB. Although most pediatric patients who have primary TB are asymptomatic, some patients may present with nonspecific symptoms such as a mild cough, a low-grade fever, weight loss, fatigue, and malaise. Respiratory distress may be the primary symptom in pediatric patients with large airway involvement from TB infection. The diagnosis usually can be made by TB skin testing, whereas sputum and gastric aspirates are confirmatory in anergic patients.

Imaging   Large airway involvement of TB infection mainly results from either extrinsic compression of airways by enlarged mediastinal and/or hilar infectious lymph nodes or direct infection of the airway wall through peribronchial lymphatic pathways.[1-3,40-43] Although chest radiographs may show mediastinal and/or hilar lymphadenopathy with resultant large airway narrowing, the location, degree, and extent can be better evaluated with CT with 2D/3D reconstructions (Fig. 52-9).[1-3] Direct tracheobronchial infection from TB eventually may result in irreversible large airway stricture/stenosis.[1-3,40-43] Such narrowing of the large airway is best assessed with CT with 2D/3D reconstructions. Additionally, CT also can show lung abnormalities associated with TB infection such as "tree-in-bud" nodular opacities and airspace consolidation.

Treatment and Follow-up   Pediatric patients affected with TB currently are treated with 6 months of a combination of antibiotics containing rifampin along with isoniazid, pyrazinamide, and ethambutol for the first 2 months, followed by isoniazid alone for the following 4 months. Large airway narrowing due to extrinsic compression from the enlarged mediastinal lymph nodes often resolves after medical treatment, whereas irreversible stricture/stenosis from direct tracheobronchial TB infection may require surgical management, including primary end-to-end anastomosis after stricture resection.

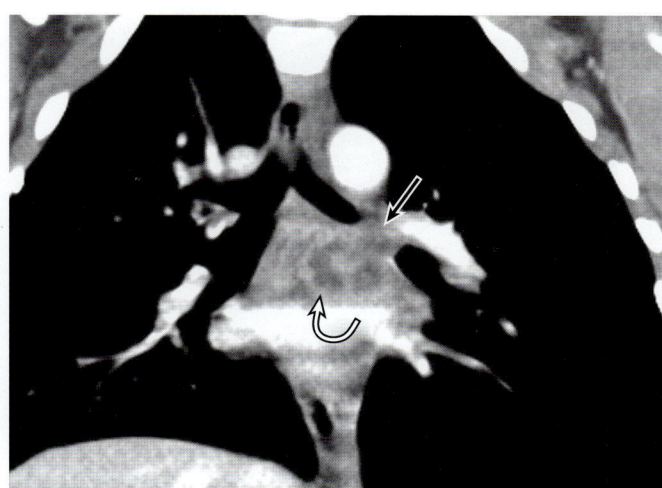

Figure 52-9 Left main bronchial obstruction due to subcarinal lymphadenopathy from tuberculosis infection in a 4-year-old girl. A coronal enhanced computed tomography image shows left main stem bronchial obstruction (*straight arrow*) as a result of the necrotic subcarinal lymphadenopathy (*curved arrow*).

Histoplasmosis

Etiology Histoplasmosis is caused by the dimorphic fungus *Histoplasma capsulatum*. Although *H. capsulatum* is found throughout the world, it is endemic in certain areas, including states bordering the Ohio River valley, the lower Mississippi River, and caves in southern and East Africa. Although acute histoplasmosis is attributed to airborne primary infection, chronic progressive histoplasmosis is the consequence of reactivation of a prior infection. Large airway involvement from histoplasmosis often results from fibrosing mediastinitis.[44-46] Affected patients may present with respiratory or esophageal symptoms related to complete or partial obstruction of large airways and the esophagus.[45,46] The definitive diagnosis of histoplasmosis is made by finding the fungus in samples taken from sputum, blood, or infected organs. It also can be diagnosed by identifying antigens in blood or urine samples by enzyme-linked immunosorbent assay polymerase chain reaction protocol.

Imaging On chest radiographs, typical imaging findings of pediatric patients with histoplasmosis infection include multiple, ill-defined pulmonary nodules (1 to 3 cm in diameter) and hilar and/or mediastinal lymphadenopathy, both of which often are calcified.[44] CT currently is the imaging modality of choice for evaluating large airway compromise, particularly related to underlying fibrosing mediastinitis.[1-3] These patients typically show heterogeneous and often calcified mediastinal soft tissue densities resulting in complete or partial obstruction of mediastinal structures such as the tracheobronchial airway, superior vena cava, and esophagus (Fig. 52-10).[1-3,45,46] CT also can demonstrate abnormal lung findings from histoplasmosis infection.

Treatment and Follow-up In severe cases, antifungal medications such as itraconazole and amphotericin B are used to treat acute, chronic, and disseminated histoplasmosis infection. Unfortunately, no pharmacologic treatment has been

shown to affect the outcome of fibrosing mediastinitis related to histoplasmosis infection. Large airway occlusion due to fibrosing mediastinitis is particularly difficult to treat because surgery often is ineffective and placement of metallic airway stents is avoided because of recurrent obstruction from ingrowth of granulation tissue.

Neoplasm

Tracheobronchial tumors are rare in children. Two of the most common primary benign large airway neoplasms, subglottic hemangioma and recurrent respiratory papillomatosis, were discussed in Chapter 51. The most common malignant lower large airway primary neoplasm, carcinoid tumor, is discussed in the next section.

Carcinoid Tumor

Etiology A carcinoid tumor is a neuroendocrine neoplasm that encompasses a spectrum of histology ranging from slow-growing, locally infiltrative lesions to a metastasizing neoplasm.[47-52] Carcinoid tumors traditionally have been classified into two types based on typical or atypical histologic findings. Affected patients typically present with a cough, wheezing, and recurrent pneumonia as a result of airway obstruction. Because of the underlying hypervascularity of carcinoid tumors, hemoptysis may be the presenting symptom. The carcinoid syndrome rarely occurs in pediatric patients with a large airway carcinoid tumor. The diagnosis is confirmed by bronchoscopy and biopsy.

Imaging Imaging findings of a carcinoid tumor within the large airway depend on the size and location of the tumor.[47-52] Most tracheobronchial carcinoid tumors are intrabronchial (Fig. 52-11). Centrally located carcinoid tumors

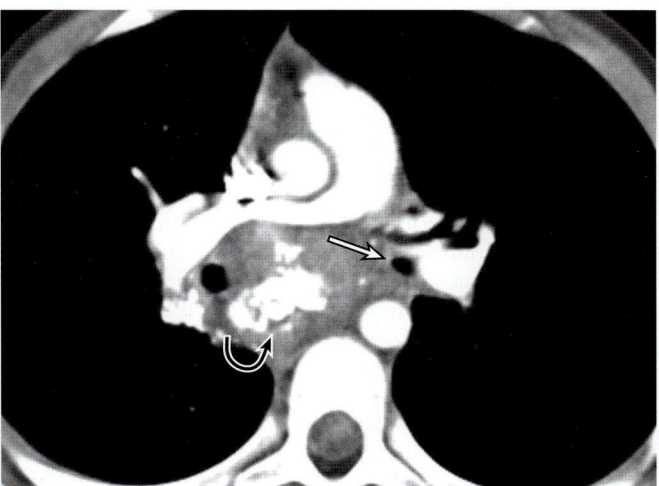

Figure 52-10 Fibrosing mediastinitis caused by histoplasmosis in a 9-year-old girl who presented with one month of cough and dyspnea. An axial contrast-enhanced computed tomography image shows narrowing of the left main stem bronchus (*straight arrow*) from a heterogeneously enhancing and partially calcified subcarinal soft tissue mass (*curved arrow*). (From Lee EY, Greenberg SB, Boiselle PM. Multidetector computed tomography of pediatric large airway diseases: state-of-the-art, *Radiol Clin North Am.* 49(5):886, 2011.)

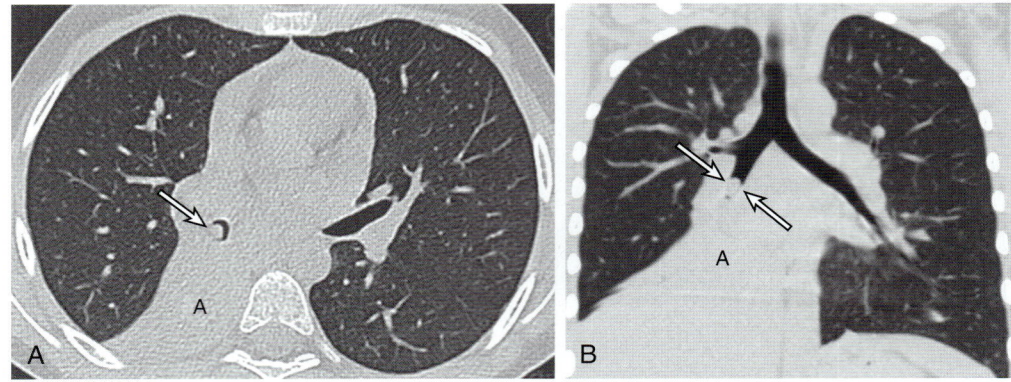

Figure 52-11 An endobronchial carcinoid tumor in a 17-year-old girl who presented with a cough and recurrent right lower lobe pneumonia for the past 18 months. Surgical pathology confirmed the diagnosis of an endobronchial carcinoid tumor. **A,** An axial bone window computed tomography (CT) image shows an endobronchial mass (*arrow*) located within the right bronchus intermedius with postobstructive atelectasis (*A*). **B,** A coronal lung window CT image demonstrates an endobronchial mass (*arrows*) in the right bronchus intermedius. The overall shape, size, and location of the mass is better visualized on this coronal multiplanar reformatted CT image than on the axial CT image (*A*). Again, postobstructive atelectasis is seen (*A*).

may mimic foreign bodies and may cause postobstructive air trapping, atelectasis, recurrent infection, abscess, or bronchiectasis.[51] Peripherally located carcinoid tumors usually are not associated with bronchial obstruction and have the appearance of a pulmonary nodule.[51] Chest radiographs may be normal in 10% of cases or may show either a well-defined hilar or perihilar opacity representing an underlying tumor or secondary signs such as focal air trapping or consolidation.[47-52] CT characteristically shows an enhancing spherical or ovoid mass with a well-defined lobulated contour.[51,52] Although calcification may not be clearly visible on chest radiographs, either punctate or diffuse calcifications may be detected in up to 30% of cases on CT.[52] The tumor may recur locally after resection, but distant metastases are rare.

Treatment and Follow-up The current treatment of choice for large airway carcinoid tumors is complete surgical resection with primary reanastomosis or sleeve resection. Prognosis is excellent.

Trauma

Acquired Tracheobronchial Stenosis

Etiology Acquired tracheobronchial stenosis in children usually is caused by previous instrumentation such as endotracheal intubation or use of a tracheostomy tube.[1-3] Granulation tissue and fibrosis can develop at the stoma, at the tip of the tube, or at the site of the cuff. Scott and Kramer[53] reported tracheostomy-related complications in 26% of intubated children. The duration of intubation is a major factor in determining the incidence and severity of complications. Microscopic lesions occur after approximately 48 hours of intubation. Epithelial metaplasia is seen in children intubated for longer than 7 days, although occasionally granuloma may develop after very brief periods of intubation. Bronchial stenosis, like tracheal stenosis, usually is acquired and occurs at the site of surgical anastomosis in pediatric patients after lung transplantation.[1-3]

Imaging The diagnosis of tracheobronchial stenosis may be suspected on chest radiographs when large airway narrowing is observed. However, CT, which can measure cross-sectional areas of the large airways accurately, is the current choice for evaluating tracheobronchial stenosis, especially preoperatively.[1-3] Such stenosis may be weblike or fusiform, or it may have an irregular shape (Fig. 52-12).[1-3,54] Newer techniques such as paired inspiratory and expiratory CT or real-time dynamic four-dimensional CT can help differentiate a fixed tracheobronchial stenosis from TBM.[54-59] In some patients, these conditions may coexist.

Treatment and Follow-up A short tracheobronchial stenosis may be treated by balloon dilatation, stent placement, or end-to-end anastomosis after surgical resection of the stenotic segment. A longer stenosis may require a patch or autograft repair.[58]

Tracheobronchial Injury

Etiology Tracheobronchial injury is a potentially life-threatening condition that may be caused by either penetrating or blunt chest trauma.[60-66] Although tracheobronchial injury is relatively rare with a reported incidence between 0.7% and 2.9%, it is associated with a substantial mortality of 30%.[60-71] Tracheobronchial injury typically occurs within 2.5 cm of the carina.[60-69] In the setting of trauma, abnormal endotracheal tube position, rib fractures (particularly involving the anterior ends of the first three ribs), and persistent pneumothoraces and/or pneumomediastinum despite the presence of a well-functioning chest tube and/or mediastinal tube should raise the possibility of underlying tracheobronchial injury.[70,71]

Imaging Radiographic imaging findings of a traumatic tracheobronchial injury depend on the location and degree of injury. In the setting of mild injury, a small amount of pneumothorax and/or pneumomediastinum may be the only findings. Such nonspecific and subtle radiographic findings often delay the accurate diagnosis of tracheobronchial injury, particularly in pediatric patients.[60,61,66] Extensive pneumothorax and/or pneumomediastinum, often extending into subcutaneous tissues of the neck and chest wall, typically are seen with severe injuries such as a displaced laceration or transection.[60-71] When the collapsed lung is observed in a

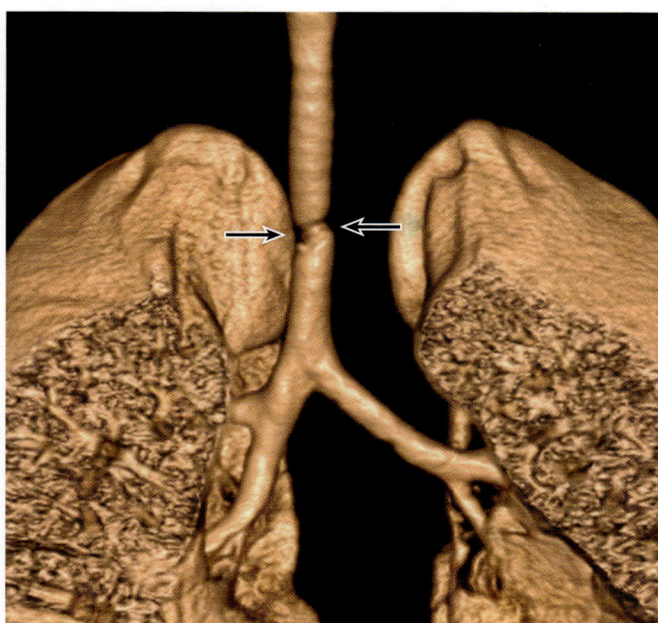

Figure 52-12 Acquired tracheobronchial stenosis in a 4-year-old girl with progressively worsening stridor after long-term endotracheal tube placement. A frontal three-dimensional volume-rendered image of the central airways and lungs shows a focal irregular narrowing (*arrows*) at the level of the previous endotracheal tube placement.

dependent position, hanging on the hilum only by its vascular attachments (the "fallen lung sign"), a complete transaction or rupture of the main stem bronchus should be considered.[1] MDCT with thin-section axial and 2D/3D reconstruction can provide accurate diagnosis and preoperative guidance in these patients (Fig. 52-13).[1,68,70,71]

Treatment and Follow-up Individualized surgical repairs depend on the location and severity of injury and are performed via primary anastomosis or reimplantation.

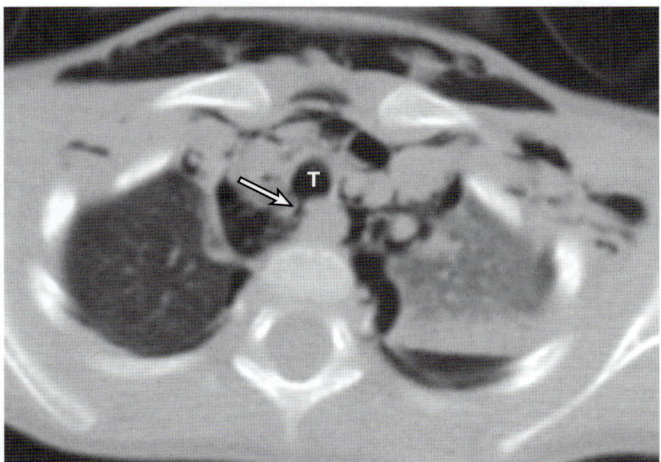

Figure 52-13 Traumatic tracheal injury in a 3-year-old boy as a result of a motor vehicle accident. An axial computed tomography image shows a focal disruption (*arrow*) of the posterior wall of the trachea at the 7 o'clock position, with an adjacent collection of air within the mediastinum, indicating tracheal rupture. Extensive pneumomediastinum and subcutaneous emphysema also are seen. *T*, Trachea.

DYNAMIC TRACHEOBRONCHIAL DISORDER

Tracheobronchomalacia

Etiology TBM is attributed to an abnormal weakness of the underlying airway walls and/or supporting cartilage.[57,58,72] Despite increasing recognition of this condition in recent years, diagnosing TBM continues to be challenging mainly because clinical symptoms of affected patients are nonspecific and overlap with those of other chronic respiratory disorders.[57,58,72] TBM can be divided into two types: primary and secondary.[58,72] Primary TBM often is seen in premature infants or children with a variety of syndromes and in persons with systemic disease affecting cartilage, such as Larsen syndrome and relapsing polychondritis.[58,72] Secondary TBM is seen in infants or children with tracheoesophageal fistula, extrinsic pressure by vessels, and mediastinal masses.[58,72] It also may arise as a result of tracheal injury, most commonly intubation. Affected patients typically present with expiratory stridor and a cough that often is described as barking or brassy. Undiagnosed TBM may result in chronic tracheobronchial and lung infections.

Imaging Chest radiographs and airway fluoroscopy have been used to evaluate TBM in pediatric patients in the past.[1] Fluoroscopy may show an exaggerated decrease (>50%) in the caliber of the trachea during expiration in patients with tracheomalacia[1,2] (Fig. 52-14); however, evaluation of the bronchi is markedly limited with this technique. MDCT has become the imaging modality of choice for a complete assessment of TBM and underlying causes in pediatric populations.[55-59] MDCT provides noninvasive evaluation of TBM with diagnostic accuracy that is similar to the historical reference standard of bronchoscopy, and 2D and 3D evaluation with MDCT in particular has become an important preoperative assessment of TBM because it offers information regarding the precise location, accurate degree and extent, and underlying predisposing conditions of TBM.[57,58,72] For the diagnosis of TBM with MDCT in children, tracheobronchial collapse >50% currently is used (Fig. 52-15).[57,58] The very large detector array CT scanners that have become available recently allow real-time evaluation of large airway collapsibility even in nonsedated infants and young children, which is a promising technique.[1,2]

Treatment and Follow-up Conservative therapies such as treatment of underlying respiratory infections, humidified oxygen therapy, and pulmonary physiotherapy are the mainstay of

> **✓ WHAT THE CLINICIAN NEEDS TO KNOW**
>
> - The spectrum of congenital and acquired lower large airway lesions
> - Underlying etiologies for congenital and acquired lower large airway lesions
> - Imaging modalities of choice for optimal evaluation of large airway lesions
> - The location, degree, and extent of the abnormality and associated airway obstruction
> - Current management of various lower large airway lesions in pediatric patients

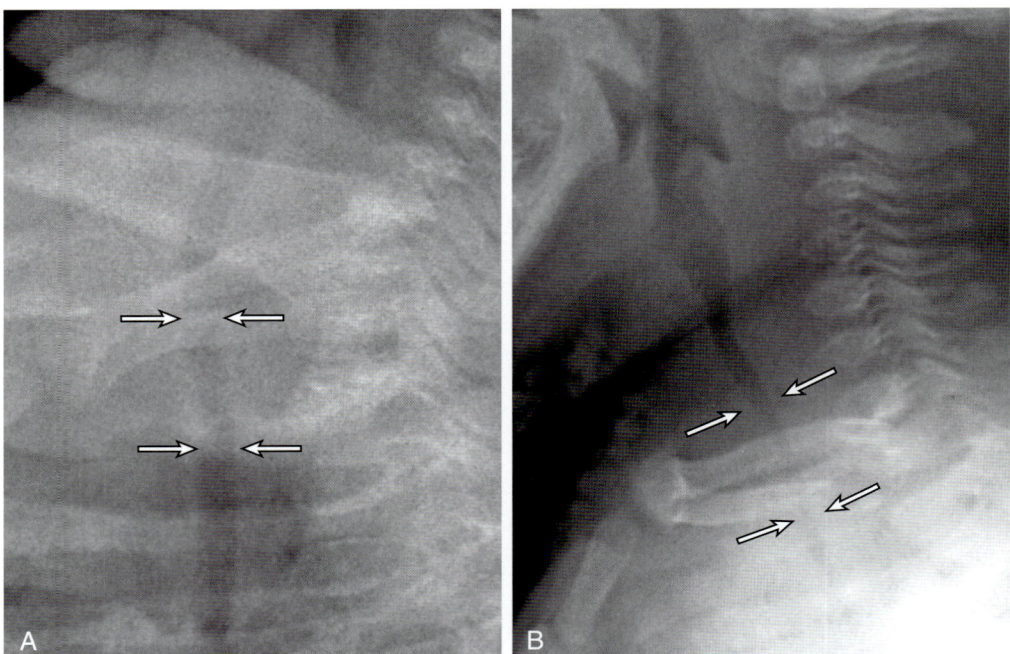

Figure 52-14 Tracheomalacia in a 2-year-old girl who presented with a chronic cough and recurrent pulmonary infections. **A,** A lateral radiograph obtained at end-inspiration during airway fluoroscopy study shows a patent trachea (*arrows*). **B,** A lateral radiograph obtained at end-expiration during airway fluoroscopy study demonstrates marked (>75%) collapse of the trachea (*arrows*), consistent with tracheomalacia.

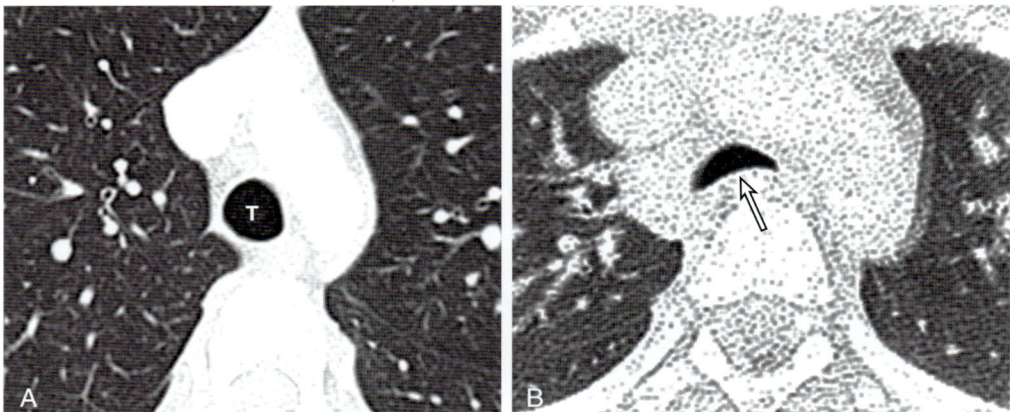

Figure 52-15 Tracheomalacia in a 15-year-old girl who presented with a chronic cough and recurrent pulmonary infections. Bronchoscopy showed marked tracheomalacia. **A,** An axial computed tomography (CT) image obtained at end inspiration shows a normal patent trachea (*T*). **B,** An axial CT image obtained at end expiration demonstrates a collapse of the trachea (*arrow*) >50%, which is consistent with tracheomalacia. Increased attenuation of the lungs is a result of decreased lung volume related to end expiration.

management in pediatric patients with a mild to moderate degree of TBM.[72-74] However, pediatric patients with severe and progressively worsening TBM may require more aggressive treatment including tracheostomy placement, stent placement, and surgical intervention such as a tracheoplasty.[75-86]

Key Points

Congenital and acquired lower large airway disorders are common and may be life threatening in the pediatric population.

The diagnosis of lower large airway disorders is frequently missed or delayed, particularly in infants and young children, mainly because of nonspecific clinical symptoms.

After careful investigation of the clinical history and physical examination, imaging evaluation is the next management step and plays an important role in the diagnosis of a variety of congenital and acquired lower large airway disorders.

Although conventional radiographs may be sufficient for making an accurate diagnosis of several lower large airway disorders, such as radiopaque foreign body aspiration, CT is usually necessary for a complete assessment, particularly for surgical lesions.

Bronchoscopy is still the reference standard in evaluating lower large airway diseases, but CT with 2D/3D reconstructed images may provide sufficient information to avoid this invasive procedure in many patients. In selected cases, CT may provide information to help guide diagnostic and therapeutic bronchoscopic procedures.

Suggested Readings

Carden KA, Boisell PM, Waltz DA, et al. Tracheomalacia and tracheobronchomalacia in children and adults: an in-depth review. *Chest.* 2005; 127:987-1005.

Lee EY, Restrepo R, Dillman JR, et al. Imaging evaluation of pediatric trachea and bronchi: systematic review and updates. *Semin Roentgenol.* 2012;47(2):182-196.

Lee EY, Greenberg SB, Boiselle PM. Multidetector computed tomography of pediatric large airway disease: state-of-the-art. *Radiol Clin North Am.* 2011;49:869-893.

Lee EY, Siegel MR. MDCT of tracheobronchial narrowing in pediatric patients. *J Thorac Imaging.* 2007;22:300-309.

Shin SM, Kim WS, Cheon JE, et al. CT in children with suspected residual foreign body in airway after bronchoscopy. *Am J Roentgenol.* 2009; 192:1744-1751.

References

Full references for this chapter can be found on www.expertconsult.com.

Chapter 53

Congenital Lung Anomalies

MONICA EPELMAN, PEDRO DALTRO, GLORIA SOTO,
CELIA M. FERRARI, and EDWARD Y. LEE

Congenital lung anomalies refer to a heterogeneous group of pulmonary developmental disorders that affect the lung parenchyma, the arterial supply, and the venous drainage to the lung, or a combination of these entities. The reported incidence of congenital lung anomalies ranges from 1.2 : 10,000 to 1 : 35,000 pregnancies; however, these reports may be an underestimate of their true incidence.[1-3] Although prenatal sonography (ultrasound), advances in postnatal imaging, and, more recently, fetal magnetic resonance imaging (MRI) have enhanced our understanding of congenital lung anomalies, substantial controversy continues regarding the nomenclature, classification, pathogenesis, description, and management of these lesions. In addition, considerable variability exists in their prenatal clinical presentation and outcome, ranging from in-utero involution to severe hydrops and fetal demise. Likewise, their postnatal clinical presentation also is variable, ranging from the completely asymptomatic newborn to the older child or young adult with recurrent pneumonias. In this chapter, the underlying etiology, clinical presentation, imaging findings, and management of various congenital lung anomalies encountered in the pediatric population are discussed.

Spectrum of Congenital Lung Anomalies

The classification of congenital lung anomalies is challenging and continuously controversial from embryologic, radiologic, pathologic, and clinical viewpoints. Several classifications and terminologies with their own advantages and disadvantages have been suggested.[4-6] Some investigators have used embryology as a basis and have classified congenital lung anomalies according to the stage of intrauterine development in which the insult resulting in the malformation developed.[4] Other investigators have categorized lesions based on their morphologic-radiologic features and divided them into two groups: whole lung malformations (e.g., lung hypoplasia) and focal malformations (e.g., bronchial atresia).[5,7] Recently the Langston[6] classification has become one of the most accepted classification systems for congenital lung anomalies, particularly from the pathological standpoint, although it is by no means the most widely used classification by all clinical

groups. Langston categorizes the wide spectrum of respiratory tract malformations primarily as bronchial atresia, congenital pulmonary airway malformation (CPAM), extralobar bronchopulmonary sequestration (BPS), congenital lobar hyperinflation (CLH), and bronchogenic cysts. These five congenital lung anomalies comprise approximately 90% of the anomalies seen in clinical practice. However, this classification system is limited because other congenital lung anomalies (e.g., pulmonary arteriovenous malformation [AVM]) are not included.

For the purpose of relatively clear classification, easy differentiation on imaging studies, and preoperative assessment of surgical lesions, congenital lung anomalies discussed in this chapter are categorized according to their morphologic-radiologic-pathologic features. Such a classification system views congenital lung anomalies as a continuum ranging from predominantly parenchymal abnormalities (i.e., abnormal lung parenchyma, relatively normal vasculature, airway, and foregut derivatives, e.g., CPAM), to predominantly vascular abnormalities (i.e., normal lung parenchyma, normal airway, and no foregut abnormality but abnormal vasculature; e.g., AVM), to combined parenchymal and vascular abnormalities (e.g., pulmonary sequestration and scimitar syndrome) in which influencing factors (foregut and airway components) play an important role and the major abnormalities are intertwined (Fig. 53-1).

Given that specific terminology for these lesions may be controversial and occasionally confusing, we and other authors[8-11] recommend that radiologists thoroughly describe all imaging findings of congenital lung anomalies rather than try to categorize the lesions by pathologic terminology. Specific imaging findings of congenital lung anomalies that need to be evaluated and described include (1) location of lesions, (2) associated anomalous vascular supply and drainage of the lesions, (3) internal components and the degree of aeration, (4) exclusion of communication with the gastrointestinal (GI) tract, (5) integrity of the diaphragm, and (6) an assessment of associated anomalies, such as vertebral anomalies.[8,10]

Predominantly Parenchymal Lesions

BRONCHIAL ATRESIA

Etiology Bronchial atresia refers to atresia of a lobar, segmental, or subsegmental bronchus at or near its origin

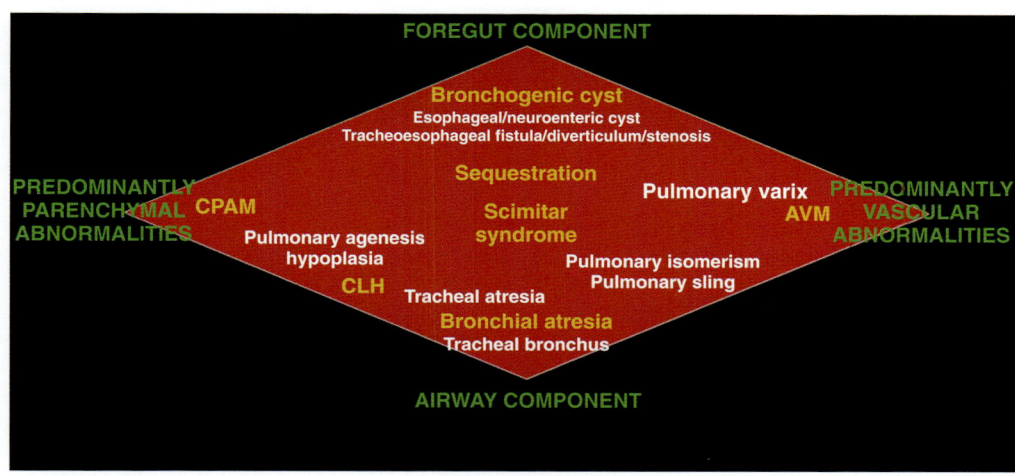

Figure 53-1   Diagram of the spectrum of congenital lung anomalies, including foregut and airway components. The lesions in yellow denote those most commonly encountered in this entity, whereas the lesions in white represent additional lesions that can be considered part of the spectrum. *AVM,* Arteriovenous malformation; *CPAM,* congenital pulmonary airway malformation; *CLH,* congenital lobar hyperinflation. (Adapted from Newman B. Congenital bronchopulmonary foregut malformations: concepts and controversies. *Pediatr Radiol.* 2006;36:773-791.)

resulting in a blind-ended atretic proximal bronchus. Bronchial atresia most frequently affects a segmental bronchus. The precise etiology of bronchial atresia remains unknown, but etiologies such as a vascular insult to the involved atretic or stenotic portion have been proposed.[6,8] Several authors who used modern dissecting techniques found that bronchial atresia is more common than originally thought.[6,12,13] Furthermore, bronchial atresia and BPSs coexist in nearly all cases,[6,12,13] whereas it is found in nearly 70% of CPAM lesions.[12] A malformation sequence resulting from airway obstruction during development has been proposed as the unifying element for such a wide spectrum of imaging appearances. Differences in degree, level, and timing of the bronchial obstruction are thought to be responsible for the association of bronchial atresia and other congenital lung anomalies.[6,8,12] Bronchial atresia usually is diagnosed as an incidental finding on chest radiographs later in life in asymptomatic older children or adults.[6,10] However, bronchial atresia increasingly is being diagnosed in utero, given the widespread use of prenatal imaging.[6,9,10,12,13]

Imaging   Prenatally, the involved portion of the lung appears hyperexpanded and shows increased homogenous echogenicity on ultrasound and high T2 signal on fetal MRI[14] (Fig. 53-2). On occasion, it is possible to identify the centrally located, mucus-filled bronchocele/mucocele on prenatal ultrasound or MRI[9,15] (e-Fig. 53-3).

Characteristically, the apicoposterior segmental bronchus of the left upper lobe is most commonly affected, followed by the segmental bronchi of the right upper, right middle, and lower lobes.[16] In children, radiographic and computed tomography (CT) imaging features of bronchial atresia are characterized by a tubular or glove-shaped opacity representing mucus plugging in the region distal to the atretic bronchus, surrounding segmental hyperlucency due to air trapping, and decreased underlying vascularity[15,17] (e-Fig. 53-4). However, in neonates, a portion of the lung distal to the atretic segment may remain atelectatic as a result of the in-utero mucostasis. Therefore some authors recommend avoiding immediate postnatal imaging evaluation because the under-aerated lung related to bronchial atresia may be

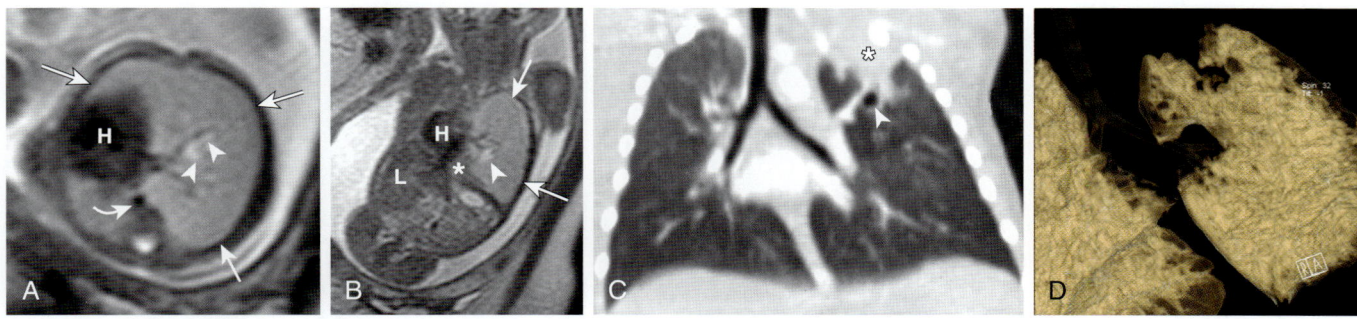

Figure 53-2   Bronchial atresia. Axial (**A**) and coronal (**B**) T2-weighted fetal magnetic resonance images in a 22-week gestational age fetus demonstrate a large homogeneous lesion in the left upper lobe (*arrows*). Central fluid-filled bronchi are noted (*arrowheads*). The left lower lobe (*asterisk*) is compressed inferiorly and displaced medially adjacent to the fetal heart (*H*). The *curved arrow* denotes the aorta, which is also displaced to the right. *L,* Liver. **C,** A coronal multiplanar reconstruction computed tomography (CT) image shows partial opacification (*asterisk*) of the left upper lobe, presumably due to mucostasis related to bronchial atresia. In addition, a small air bubble is seen (*arrowhead*), reflecting a bronchocele. **D,** A volume-rendered reconstructed CT image could not delineate the left upper lobe bronchus.

difficult to differentiate from the normal lung with expected fetal fluid retention in the newborn period.[10] Identification of the hallmark atretic bronchus and the "bronchocele/mucocele" by means of two-dimensional (2D) multiplanar or three-dimensional (3D) reconstructions either on prenatal or postnatal imaging may be helpful.[10,18]

Treatment and Follow-up   Management of bronchial atresia is somewhat varied. In general, surgical resection is primarily recommended in symptomatic pediatric patients because of recurrent infection.[17,18] Although opinions vary, some centers advocate elective surgical resection of bronchial atresia even in asymptomatic pediatric patients because of potential future lung infection and increased association with CPAM.[13,20]

BRONCHOGENIC CYSTS

Etiology   Bronchogenic cysts result from abnormal tracheobronchial branching and presumably originate from an aberrant bud of the developing foregut, similar to other foregut duplication cysts. Bronchogenic cysts typically are unilocular, fluid-filled, or mucus-filled cysts lined by respiratory epithelium and are attached to but do not communicate with the tracheobronchial tree.[5,17,19] Although most bronchogenic cysts are located within the mediastinum (predominantly near the carina), they may be encountered anywhere from the suprasternal area to the retroperitoneum. Bronchogenic cysts also may be found within the lung parenchyma, usually in the lower lobes.[17,19] Such intrapulmonary bronchogenic cysts do not communicate with the airway unless superimposed infection with wall necrosis occurs,[6] which may further predispose them to recurrent infections. The clinical symptomatology of affected pediatric patients primarily depends on the mass effect the lesion exerts on its neighboring structures including the airway, GI tract, and cardiovascular structures. Airway compression is usually mild, but it may be life threatening in some instances when large bronchogenic cysts are located near the carina regions.[21]

Imaging   A bronchogenic cyst typically presents as a round or oval-shaped cystic lesion located near the right paratracheal or subcarinal area within the middle mediastinum. Bronchogenic cysts are anechoic on prenatal ultrasound and show high signal intensity on T2-weighted prenatal MRI imaging[14,19] (e-Fig. 53-5). On chest radiographs, a bronchogenic cyst manifests as a well-delineated round or oval-shaped middle mediastinal mass. On CT, approximately 50% of bronchogenic cysts demonstrate fluid attenuation value (~0 Hounsfield unit) (Fig. 53-6). The remaining bronchogenic cysts may have CT attenuation higher than water because of thick mucoid, milk-of-calcium, proteinaceous, or hemorrhagic contents. MRI, which can confirm the cystic nature of the bronchogenic cysts on T2-weighted images, is helpful for differentiating bronchogenic cysts with high attenuation value from a mildly enhancing solid mass on CT. Typically, no internal contrast enhancement is seen within the uncomplicated bronchogenic cysts on CT or MRI. The presence

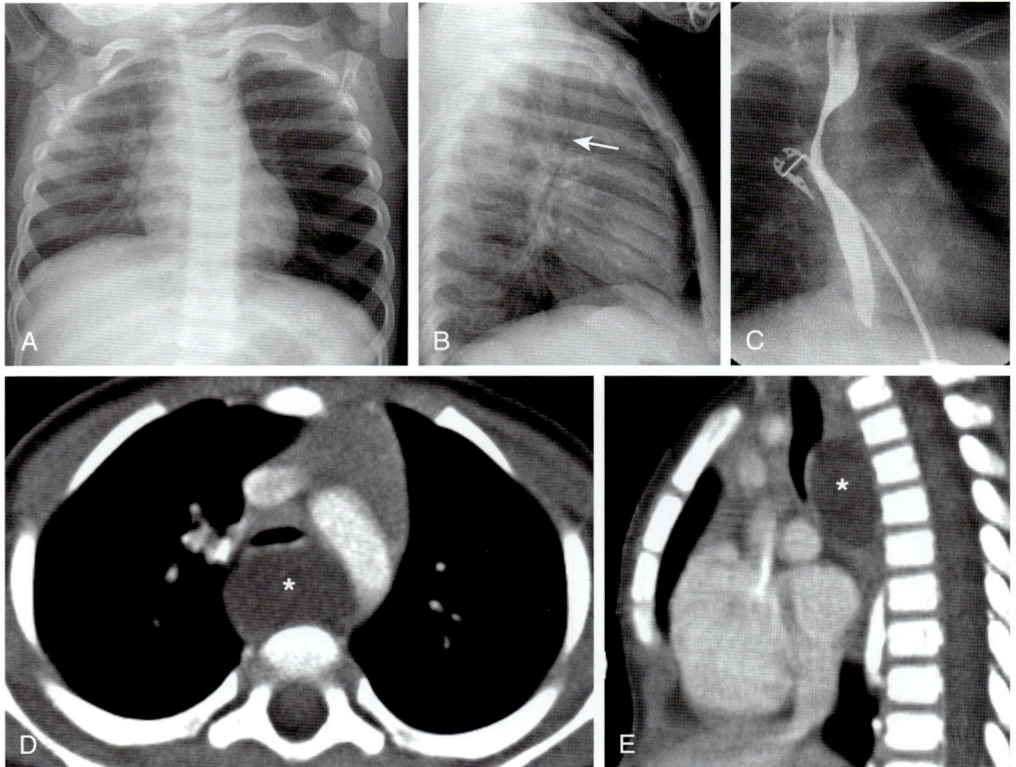

Figure 53-6   A bronchogenic cyst in a 15-month-old child with stridor. The frontal chest radiograph (**A**) shows hyperinflation of the left lung. The lateral radiograph (**B**) reveals the effect of the mass and posterior displacement of the airway (*arrow*). **C,** An upper gastrointestinal image shows an esophageal displacement by a soft tissue density mass. Enhanced axial (**D**) and sagittal (**E**) computed tomography images show a fluid density lesion (*asterisks*) posterior to the lower trachea consistent with a bronchogenic cyst.

of an air–fluid level, thick wall enhancement, or surrounding inflammatory changes often is associated with superimposed infection.[11,16,17]

Treatment and Follow-up   Complete surgical resection is the current management of choice for bronchogenic cysts, particularly in symptomatic pediatric patients.[22] Temporizing or palliative procedures such as transparietal, transbronchial, or mediastinal aspiration may be considered in symptomatic pediatric patients who are not surgical candidates.

CONGENITAL LOBAR HYPERINFLATION

Etiology   CLH, also referred to as infantile lobar emphysema or congenital lobar emphysema, presumably is caused by an intrinsic or extrinsic bronchial narrowing, resulting in subsequent air trapping. Intrinsic bronchial narrowing can be caused by weakness or absence of underlying bronchial cartilage, whereas extrinsic bronchial narrowing may be due to the compression from adjacent mediastinal masses or enlarged vessels. CLH clinically presents with respiratory distress in the newborn period[14,17,19] in nearly half of the cases and by the age of 6 months in 80% of cases.[23] There is a slight male predominance, and the upper lobes are affected more frequently than the lower lobes, with the left lung affected more often than the right.[23]

Imaging   On prenatal imaging, CLH manifests as a homogeneously hyperechogenic lesion on ultrasound or as a T2 hyperintense lesion on MRI without visible cysts.[9,24] On prenatal imaging, CLH often is indistinguishable from other congenital lung anomalies, particularly bronchial atresia.[9,24] CLH usually is diagnosed by its typical clinical presentation and characteristic radiographic features of progressive lobar hyperexpansion and hyperlucency, producing displacement or compression of adjacent structures. In the immediate postnatal period, CLH initially may appear as an area of increased opacity related to retained fetal lung fluid, which will clear on subsequent studies.[6,17,19,23] Similar imaging findings are noted on CT, and the attenuated pulmonary vasculature is a helpful clue to distinguish CLH from a pneumothorax or other entities in cases of inconclusive chest radiographic findings[17] (Fig. 53-7).

Treatment and Follow-up   Surgical lobectomy is the current management for symptomatic pediatric patients with CLH.[22] Some medical centers advocate expectant management for cases with minimal or no symptoms.[21,25]

CONGENITAL PULMONARY AIRWAY MALFORMATION

Etiology   CPAMs, formerly known as cystic adenomatoid malformations of the lung, were first described in the literature by Ch'In and Tang in 1949 as rare lung lesions occurring in premature or stillborn infants with significant hydrops.[26,27] CPAMs are characterized by a heterogeneous group of congenital cystic and noncystic lung masses that communicate with an abnormal bronchial tree lacking supporting cartilage.[8,17,28]

In 1977, Stocker et al.[28] classified these lesions based on their clinical and pathologic features, with subdivisions based on the size of the cysts (types I, II, and III) and according to the location of suspected development of the malformation along the airway. Type I CPAMs consist of cysts larger than 2 cm, with presumed bronchial/bronchiolar origin. Type II CPAMs consist of cysts smaller than 2 cm, with presumed bronchiolar origin. Type III CPAMs appear solid, with a presumed bronchiolar/alveolar origin. However, Stocker later expanded his CPAM classification into five types that included type 0 CPAMs, with presumed tracheobronchial origin, and type IV CPAMs, with presumed distal acinar origin. The term CPAM was now implemented instead of cystic adenomatoid malformations, because cystic changes were observed in only three of the aforementioned types (types, I, II, and IV), and adenomatoid change was observed only in type III.[9,17,29,30] Increasing evidence indicates that type IV CPAM lesions and type I pleuropulmonary blastomas may represent the same entity.[6,31] It is important to recognize that although Stocker's classification is widely used, it is by no means universally accepted. For an example, Langston[6] classifies CPAM lesions into two types and terms the Stocker type I CPAM as "large cyst type lesions" and the Stocker type II CPAMs as "small cyst type lesions" based on cyst size and pathologic criteria.[6] Langston proposed that the type III CPAM actually represents a form of pulmonary hyperplasia and should be excluded from the CPAM classification.

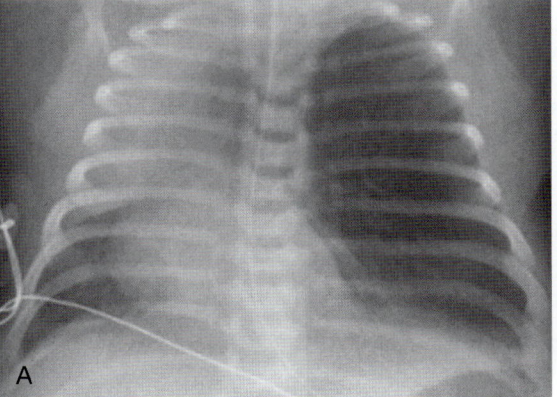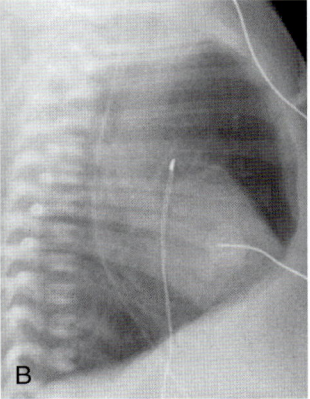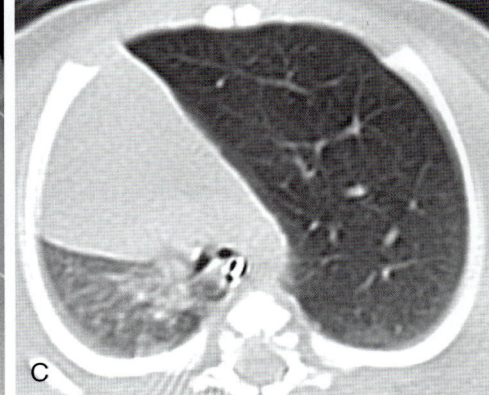

Figure 53-7   Congenital lobar hyperinflation in a 3-day-old with increasing tachypnea. Frontal (**A**) and lateral (**B**) chest radiographs and an axial computed tomography image (**C**) show hyperexpansion and hyperlucency of the left upper lobe consistent with congenital lobar emphysema.

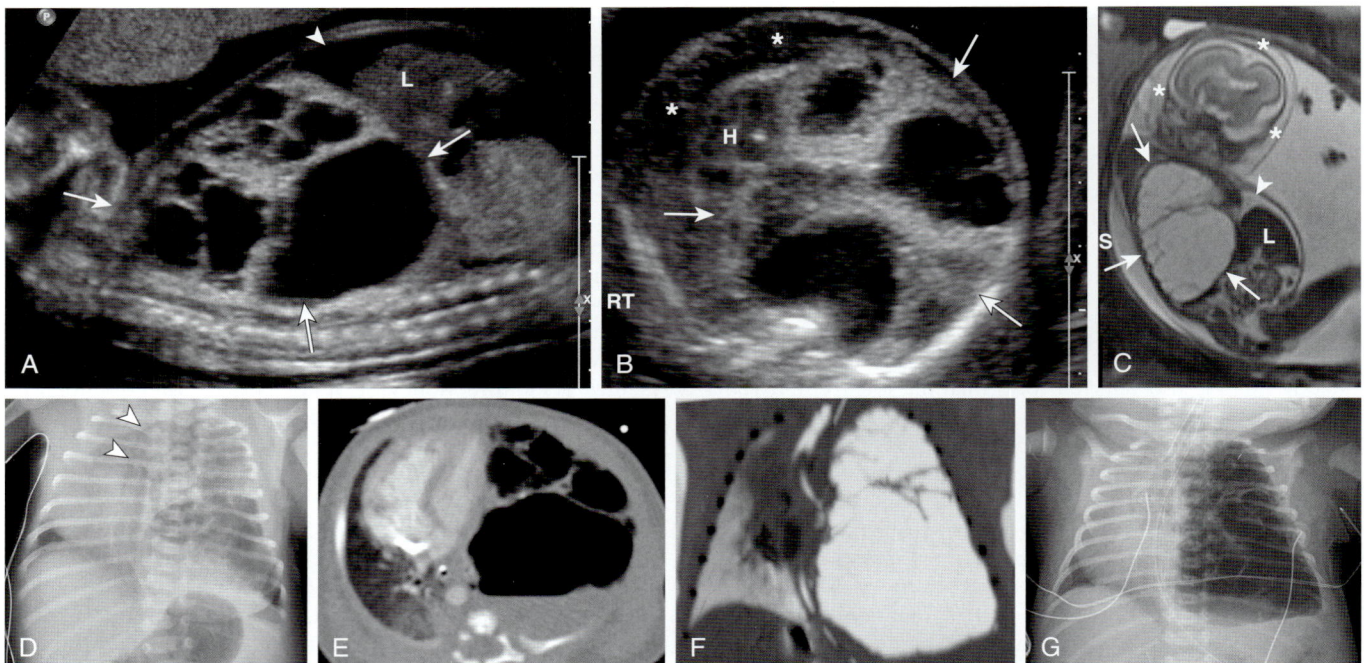

Figure 53-8 Congenital pulmonary airway malformation type I. Sagittal ultrasound (**A**), axial ultrasound (**B**), and fetal T2-weighted magnetic resonance sagittal (**C**) images in a 22-week gestational age fetus show a large, heterogeneous, multicystic lesion occupying the vast majority of the left hemithorax (*arrows*) and resulting in inversion of the left hemidiaphragm. Note the ascites in the abdomen (*arrowhead*) and the skin thickening and edema (*asterisks*), which are reflective of hydrops. *H,* Heart; *L,* liver. **D,** A radiograph immediately after delivery shows the complex, partially aerated lesion resulting in significant mediastinal shift. The arrowheads denote the severe tracheal deviation. Axial computed tomography angiography (**E**) and minimum intensity projection (**F**) images obtained the following day show the large, heterogenous lesion with multiple macrocysts of varying sizes. Fluid is identified in some of the cysts. **G,** As fetal fluid is cleared from the lungs, the lesion appears more aerated and further mediastinal shift occurs.

Imaging Prenatally, CPAMs are classified on the basis of cyst size as microcysts (<5 mm) and macrocysts (≥5 mm) on fetal ultrasound and MRI.[32] Type 1 CPAMs may contain one, several, or multiple macrocysts, some of which are ≥5 mm in diameter[9] (Fig. 53-8). Type II CPAMs have variable appearances, ranging from homogeneously hyperechoic or hyperintense lesions to microcystic lesions exhibiting multiple, uniform cysts that measure <5 mm[9,14,19] (e-Figs. 53-9 and 53-10).

Postnatal imaging findings of CPAMs usually correlate with underlying histopathologic features.[17] Large cyst type or type I CPAMs typically present with one or several larger air-filled cystic structures with intervening solid, unaerated lung parenchyma. The cysts of type I CPAMs are larger than 2 cm and may be accompanied by several microcysts, whereas small cyst type or type II CPAMs usually manifest as partially air-filled multicystic masses, with individual cysts smaller than 2 cm and with variable degrees of solid-appearing, unaerated lung tissue.[10,17] Type 3 CPAMs typically appear as solid lesions with mild contrast enhancement because of microscopic cysts that can be identified only at histologic evaluation. Type IV CPAMs usually present as large cysts arising from the peripheral portion of the lung and can be radiographically indistinguishable from a predominantly cystic type 1 pleuropulmonary blastoma (see Chapter 55) (e-Fig. 53-11).

In their pure forms, CPAM blood supply is from the pulmonary artery and venous drainage is into the pulmonary veins. Although unilobar involvement of CPAM is far more common, multilobar and even bilateral lung involvement may occur.[3,27,30] Although any lobe of the lung can be involved, predilection exists for the lower lobe.[3] CPAMs that are complicated as a result of superimposed infection may have an imaging appearance similar to pneumonia or a lung abscess (Fig. 53-12).

Treatment and Follow-up The generalized consensus is that symptomatic CPAMs should be resected, typically by lobectomy, regardless of the patient's age at presentation.[17,22,33] However, considerable controversy exists with regard to the management of prenatally diagnosed, asymptomatic, small CPAM lesions, and no consensus exists on the timing of[34] or need for resection.[35-39] Although some persons advocate a nonsurgical strategy with imaging follow-up, most medical centers advocate surgical resection before 1 year of age because of the potential risk of associated complications, such as infection, pneumothorax, and the small risk of malignant transformation, particularly in the case of CPAM type I lesions.[3,21,22,33,40]

Predominantly Vascular Lesions

ANOMALIES OF THE PULMONARY ARTERY

Pulmonary Agenesis, Aplasia, and Hypoplasia

Etiology Pulmonary underdevelopment may be classified into three main types: (1) lung agenesis, consisting of the absence of the lung, bronchus, and pulmonary artery; (2) lung

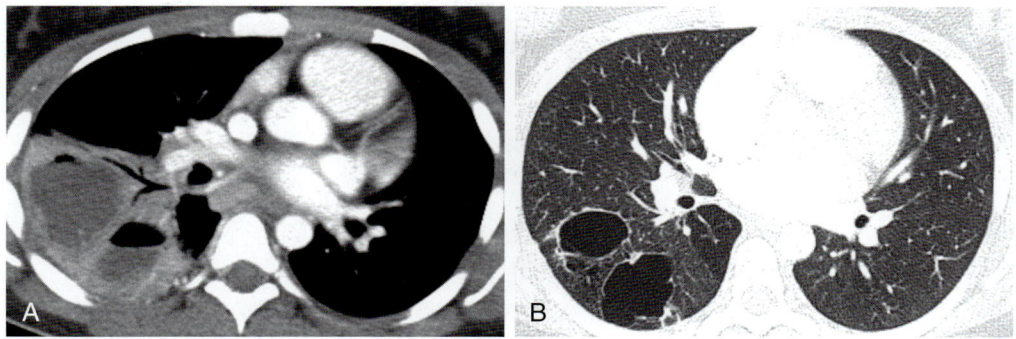

Figure 53-12 An infected congenital pulmonary airway malformation (CPAM) type I lesion in a 15-year-old girl. **A,** An initial computed tomography (CT) enhanced image shows consolidation, with areas of low attenuation representing superimposed infection of the cystic components. **B,** A follow-up CT image obtained 7 months later shows resolution of the infection and visualization of CPAM cystic components.

aplasia, that is, the presence of a rudimentary bronchus but the lack of lung tissue and pulmonary artery; and (3) lung hypoplasia, which consists of a hypoplastic bronchial tree and pulmonary artery with a variable amount of lung parenchyma.[17,41]

The etiology of lung agenesis or aplasia remains uncertain. Genetic, teratogenic, and mechanical factors may play a role.[17] Pulmonary agenesis associated with ipsilateral radial ray defects or hemifacial microsomia may be the result of an abnormal development of the first and second arch derivatives or abnormal blood flow at this level inciting the developmental event, given the common association.[42] On the other end of the spectrum, no identifiable cause has been found for lung hypoplasia.[17]

Persons with pulmonary agenesis, aplasia, and hypoplasia either are asymptomatic or present with variable degrees of respiratory distress, depending on the extent of lung underdevelopment. Associated congenital malformations may be seen in 50% to 80% of cases involving the heart, gastrointestinal tract, skeleton, and vascular and genitourinary systems.[17,42-44]

Imaging On chest radiographs, affected pediatric patients may or may not present with a small, radiopaque hemithorax, depending on the degree of the abnormality. Ipsilateral displacement of mediastinal structures and elevation of the hemidiaphragm usually are present. The normal contralateral lung shows compensatory hyperinflation and herniation across the anterior midline, which is best seen on the lateral projections as a band of increased retrosternal lucency[17] (Fig. 53-13). Left lung agenesis is more common than right lung agenesis. Multidetector CT with multiplanar 2D and 3D imaging

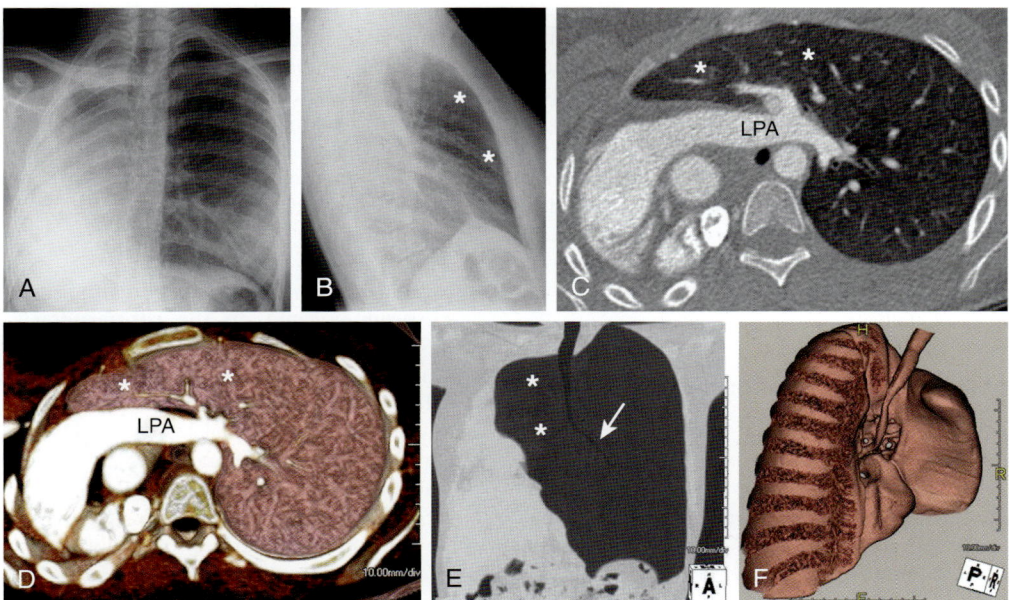

Figure 53-13 Pulmonary agenesis. Frontal (**A**) and lateral (**B**) radiographs in a 15-year-old with worsening asthma demonstrate marked hyperinflation of the left lung that extends across the midline anteriorly and herniates toward the right, as evidenced by a band of retrosternal lucency on the lateral projection (*asterisks*). Associated dextroposition of the heart into the right hemithorax is seen. Enhanced axial computed tomography (**C**), axial volume-rendered (**D**), minimum intensity projection (**E**) and three-dimensional volume-rendered (**F**) images of the central airway and lungs demonstrate complete agenesis of the right bronchus and lung. Associated dextroposition of the heart and compensatory hyperexpansion is present, particularly of the left upper lobe (*asterisks*), which herniates into the right hemithorax. A normal left mainstem bronchus (*arrow*) is seen. *LPA,* Left pulmonary artery.

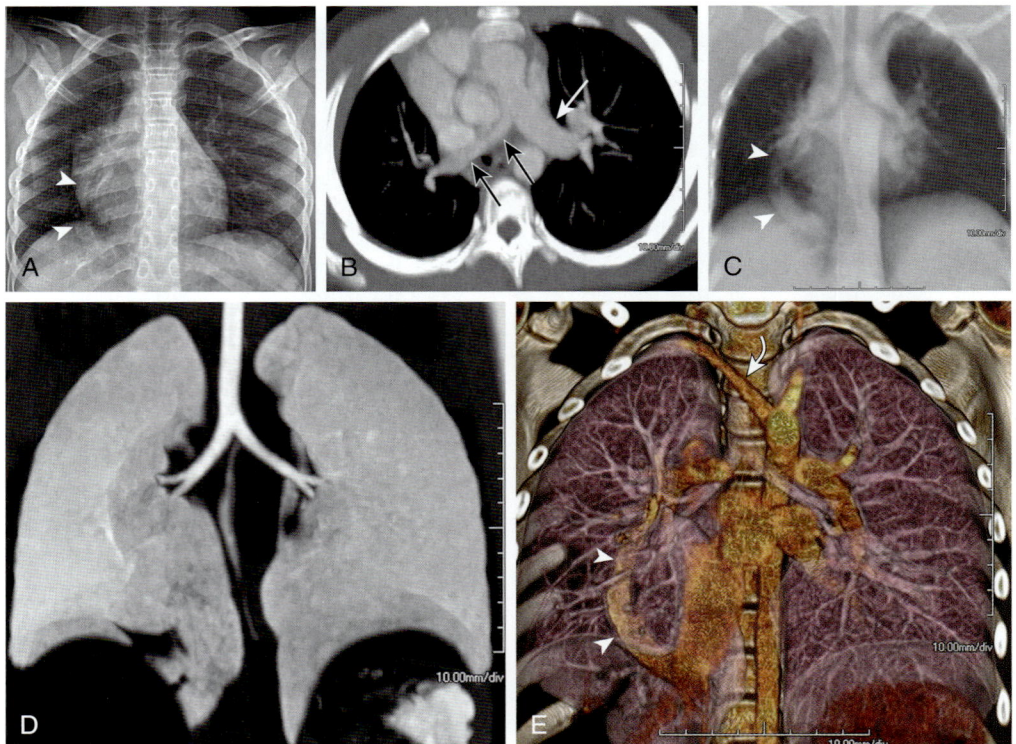

Figure 53-16 Hypoplastic right lung and scimitar syndrome in an 8-year-old. **A,** A frontal chest radiograph shows asymmetric lung volumes with dextroposition of the heart and a vertically oriented curvilinear opacity (*arrowheads*) projecting over the right lower hemithorax. An axial maximum intensity projection computed tomography image (**B**) confirms mild dextroposition of the heart and hypoplastic right pulmonary artery (PA) (*black arrows*) relative to the normal left pulmonary artery (*white arrow*). Coronal thick multiplanar reconstruction (**C**), inverted minimum intensity projection (**D**), and three-dimensional volume rendered (**E**) images show hypoplasia of the right lung with absence of the right upper lobe bronchus and partial anomalous pulmonary venous return of a vast portion of the right lung via a scimitar vein (*arrowheads*) into the inferior vena cava. Incidentally noted is a right aberrant subclavian artery (*curved arrow*).

capabilities can be used to distinguish among pulmonary agenesis, pulmonary aplasia, and pulmonary hypoplasia by clearly identifying the bronchial stump and/or the rudimentary bronchial tree[17,45] (e-Figs. 53-14 and 53-15, Fig. 53-16, and e-Fig. 53-17).

Treatment and Follow-up The prognosis of pediatric patients with pulmonary underdevelopment primarily depends on the extent of underdevelopment and the severity of other associated congenital malformations. Treatment usually is aimed at improving the respiratory status and symptoms related to concomitant congenital malformations.

Proximal Interruption of the Pulmonary Artery

Etiology Proximal interruption of the pulmonary artery results from the abnormal involution of the proximal sixth aortic arch. Such involution causes the "absence" of the proximal pulmonary artery and a persistent connection of the hilar pulmonary artery to the distal sixth aortic arch, which ultimately becomes the ductus arteriosus. The hilar pulmonary artery supplying the ipsilateral affected lung continues to develop via the blood supply received from the ductus arteriosus (which originates either from the base of the right innominate artery or occasionally from an aberrant right subclavian artery).[8,17] Progressive closure of the ductus arteriosus eventually results in loss of blood supply to the hilar

pulmonary artery and the lung. Perfusion of the affected lung subsequently becomes dependent on collateral systemic vessels, mainly aortopulmonary and bronchial arteries but also transpleural branches of the intercostal, internal mammary, subclavian, and innominate arteries.[17,46-48] Although asymptomatic pediatric patients with this anomaly may be detected incidentally, some children present with symptoms related to recurrent pulmonary infections, hemoptysis, and pulmonary hypertension.[8,11,17]

Imaging The interrupted proximal pulmonary artery is characteristically located on the contralateral side of the aortic arch. Proximal interruption of the pulmonary artery is more commonly seen on the right side. Interruption of the proximal left pulmonary artery is less common and frequently is associated with congenital heart disease, typically tetralogy of Fallot and ventricular septal defect.[8,17,45] On chest radiographs, the affected lung and hilum are smaller than those of the contralateral side (Fig. 53-18). Ipsilateral mediastinal shift, narrowed intercostal spaces, or rarely rib notching in the case of prominent intercostal collaterals also may be present.[11,17,49] CT or MRI can definitely confirm and characterize this condition (e-Fig. 53-19). On CT, the interrupted pulmonary artery terminates within 1 cm of its origin from the main pulmonary artery. However, the hilar portion of the pulmonary artery and the intrapulmonary vascular network remain patent. A serrated pleural thickening and subpleural

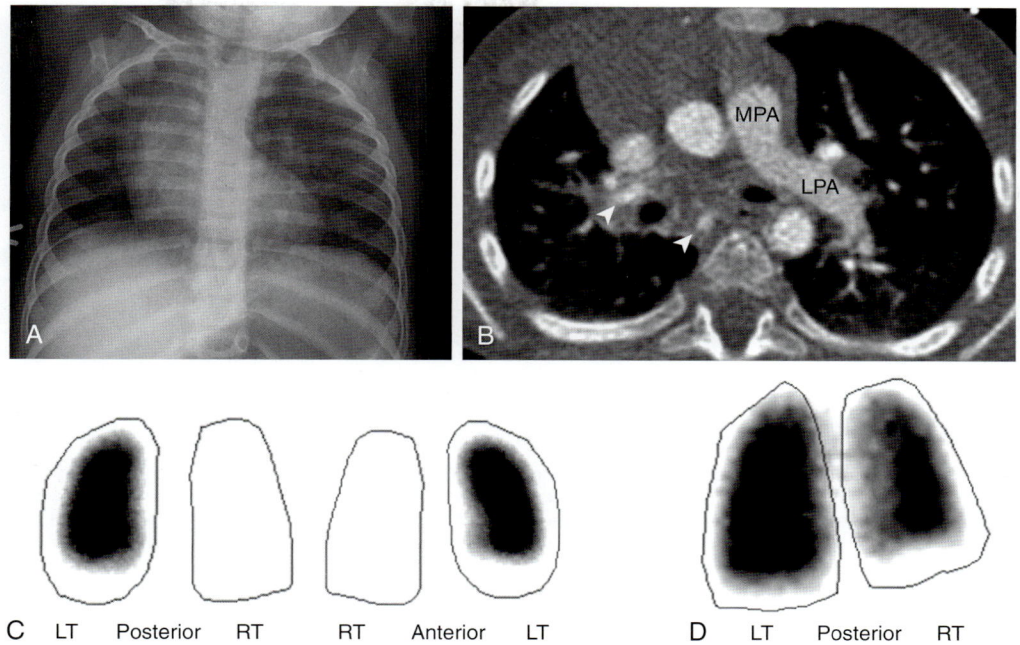

Figure 53-18 An interrupted proximal right pulmonary artery in a 16-month-old with a persistent abnormal chest radiograph following resolution of respiratory syncytial virus bronchiolitis. **A,** A frontal chest radiograph shows dextroposition of the cardiomediastinal silhouette and mild asymmetry on pulmonary vascularity, decreased on the right. **B,** An axial computed tomography image reveals absence of the right pulmonary artery. Several collaterals to the right lung are present (*arrowheads*). Pulmonary blood flow is from the main pulmonary artery (*MPA*) to the left pulmonary artery (*LPA*). The aortic arch is left sided, and overall findings are consistent with proximal interruption of the right pulmonary artery. **C,** Techtetium-99m macroaggregated albumin lung perfusion images show absent blood flow to the right lung. **D,** A xenon-133 posterior planar image of the lungs shows decreased airflow to the right lung. *LT*, Left; *RT*, right.

parenchymal bands also may be observed, which reflect the direct anastomosis of transpleural systemic collaterals with peripheral pulmonary arterial branches. Airway branching and pulmonary lobation anomalies are not uncommon. Additional imaging findings may include tiny peripheral cystic and possibly dysplastic lung changes, areas of mosaic attenuation, bronchiectasis, and an asymmetric thoracic cage.[8,11,17,45,47,48]

Treatment and Follow-up Treatment of this anomaly is aimed at prompt diagnosis and early surgical intervention, which may provide adequate blood supply to the affected lung, allowing improved pulmonary arterial and lung growth. Surveillance is indicated for patients with a late presentation who are considered unsuitable for intervention. Patients who present with recurrent hemoptysis or pulmonary hypertension may benefit from coil embolization of large systemic collaterals.[8,17,50]

Pulmonary Artery Sling

Etiology Pulmonary artery sling (PAS) is a rare congenital anomaly in which the left pulmonary artery arises from the posterior aspect of the right pulmonary artery and courses between the trachea and esophagus to reach the left hilum. The anomalous left pulmonary artery forms a sling around the distal trachea and/or the proximal right mainstem bronchus.[17,48,51,52] It is hypothesized that PAS develops as a result of proximal left sixth arch involution, and a secondary connection is acquired to the right sixth branchial arch via the embryonic peritracheal primitive mesenchymal vessels.[48,51,52] The concurrent presence of a left ligamentum arteriosum

connecting the main or right pulmonary artery and the left descending aorta results in a complete vascular ring that encircles the trachea but spares the esophagus.[17,51]

Two main types of PAS exist. In type I PAS, the position of the carina is normally situated at the T4-T5 level. In these instances, the airway is intrinsically normal or with an associated tracheal bronchus. The aberrant left pulmonary artery may compress the posterior wall of the distal trachea and/or the lateral aspect of the right mainstem bronchus, resulting in right lung air trapping.[8,17,52] Type II PAS is more common[52,53] and is associated with a more inferiorly located carina at the T6 level. Type II PAS often is associated with long-segment tracheal stenosis with complete cartilaginous rings and abnormal bronchial branching, including a T-shaped carina and a right-bridging bronchus. Other cardiovascular, GI, and right lung anomalies (e.g., lung hypoplasia, aplasia, agenesis, and scimitar syndrome) may coexist with PAS.[8,17,52] Patients usually present as infants with respiratory symptoms, such as stridor, apneic spells, and/or hypoxia. The timing and severity of the respiratory symptoms depend on the severity of the accompanying airway abnormalities.[8,11,52]

Imaging Imaging findings of PAS depend on its type and other coexisting congenital anomalies. On frontal chest radiographs, either hyperinflation or hypoinflation of the right lung as a result of partial or complete obstruction of the right mainstem bronchus may present in patients with type I PAS. In patients with type II PAS associated with long-segment tracheal stenosis, bilateral hyperinflation may be observed.[8,52] On occasion, a small, rounded soft tissue density representing the anomalous left pulmonary artery may be seen between

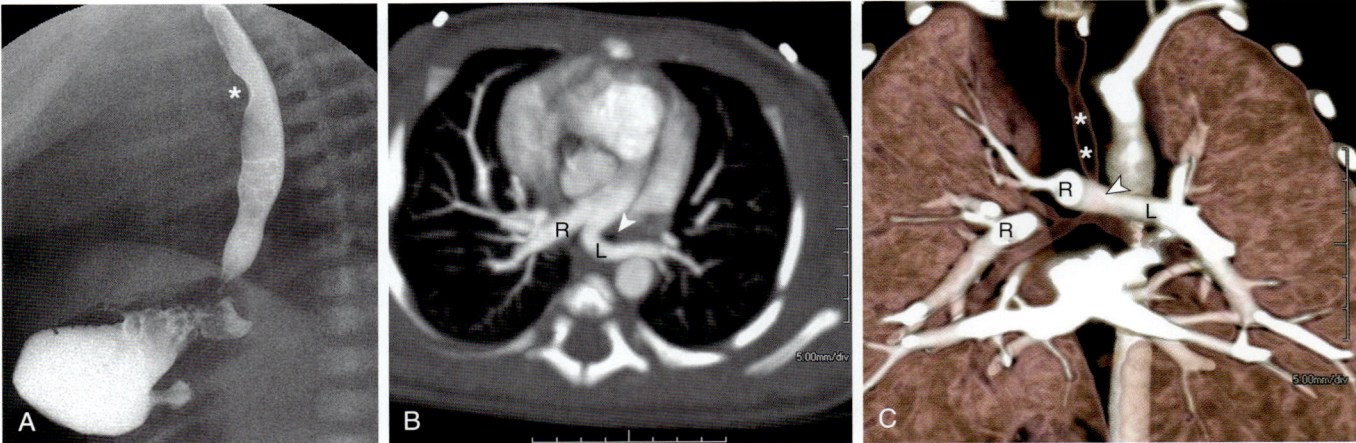

Figure 53-20 A neonate with respiratory distress and a left pulmonary artery (LPA) sling. **A,** An esophagogram shows soft tissue density (*asterisk*) between the trachea and the esophagus, suggesting an LPA sling. **B,** An axial maximum intensity projection computed tomography angiography (CTA) image shows that the left pulmonary artery (*L*) originates from the proximal right pulmonary (*R*) before crossing behind the trachea (*arrowhead*) to feed the left lung. **C,** A coronal volume-rendered CTA image shows severe distal trachea narrowing (*arrowhead*) at the level of the anomalous course of the LPA, which originates off the right pulmonary artery (*R*) consistent with an LPA (*L*) sling. The distal trachea shows long segment narrowing (*asterisks*) from complete tracheal rings. Note the low T-shaped carina.

the midtrachea and esophagus on lateral chest radiographs in patients with both types of PAS (Fig. 53-20, *A*). Multidetector CT or MRI with 2D and 3D reconstructions are useful for evaluating the origin, size, and entire course of the anomalous vasculature (Fig. 53-20, *A* and *B*). CT is advantageous over MRI for evaluating associated central airway and lung abnormalities (Fig. 53-20, *C*). Inspiratory and expiratory imaging is particularly useful for assessing for associated tracheobronchomalacia.[17,54]

Treatment and Follow-up Asymptomatic pediatric patients with PAS may be followed up clinically. Symptomatic pediatric patients with PAS require surgical reimplantation of the anomalous left pulmonary artery to the main pulmonary artery or anterior translocation in conjunction with excision of the coexisting patent ductus arteriosus or ductal ligament. In patients with type II PAS, reimplantation or anterior translocation of the anomalous left pulmonary artery by itself may not result in respiratory improvement if the coexisting long-segment tracheal stenosis is not repaired, usually by slide tracheoplasty.[52]

ANOMALIES OF THE PULMONARY VEINS

Partial Anomalous Pulmonary Venous Return

Etiology In partial anomalous pulmonary venous return (PAPVR), one or several, but not all, pulmonary veins return anomalously to the systemic circulation. Such anomalous veins typically drain into the superior or inferior vena cava, the azygos vein, or the left innominate vein. The right cardiac chambers and pulmonary vasculature frequently become enlarged because of volume overload. In the pure forms of PAPVR, pulmonary hypertension and right heart failure subsequently may develop. Unlike patients with total anomalous pulmonary venous return, most patients with PAPVR are either mildly symptomatic or asymptomatic.

PAPVR usually is an isolated finding and is more frequent on the right. The most common type of PAPVR is right

upper lobe pulmonary veins draining anomalously into the superior vena cava, with or without an associated sinus venosus defect. Other forms of PAPVR sometimes are associated with a secundum type of atrial septal defect or a patent foramen ovale. The second common type of PAPVR is an anomalous connection of the left upper pulmonary vein to the left innominate vein. This connection is followed by anomalous connections of pulmonary veins from the right lung to the inferior vena cava, which may be encountered in association with an intact atrial septum and bronchopulmonary sequestration. Unlike in total anomalous pulmonary venous return, obstruction of the anomalous venous drainage pathway is rare in PAPVR.[45,51,55,56]

Imaging Imaging findings of PAPVR vary depending on the site of anomalous venous connection and the presence or lack of obstruction. On chest radiographs, mild to moderate increase in pulmonary blood flow with a pattern of overcirculation may be seen (e-Fig. 53-21). If overcirculation of blood is substantial and sufficient time has elapsed, mild to moderate right-sided cardiomegaly may be observed. CT and MRI can accurately depict the anomalous venous connections (see e-Fig 53-21 and Fig. 53-22). MRI provides the additional physiologic information necessary to determine whether surgical repair is warranted. The pulmonary to systemic (Qp/Qs) flow ratio can be calculated from phase-contrast velocity mapping of the right and left pulmonary arteries and the ascending aorta, obviating the need for invasive cardiac catheterization in most cases.[55,57,58]

Treatment and Follow-up In asymptomatic pediatric patients with PAPVR, particularly those who have a single anomalous draining vein that does not produce right ventricular volume overload, surgical management is not necessary. Although indications for surgical repair currently are not clearly established, surgical repair is recommended in symptomatic patients with a substantial volume-loaded right ventricle. The surgery type is determined by the location of the anomalous venous connection and generally consists of reconnection of the

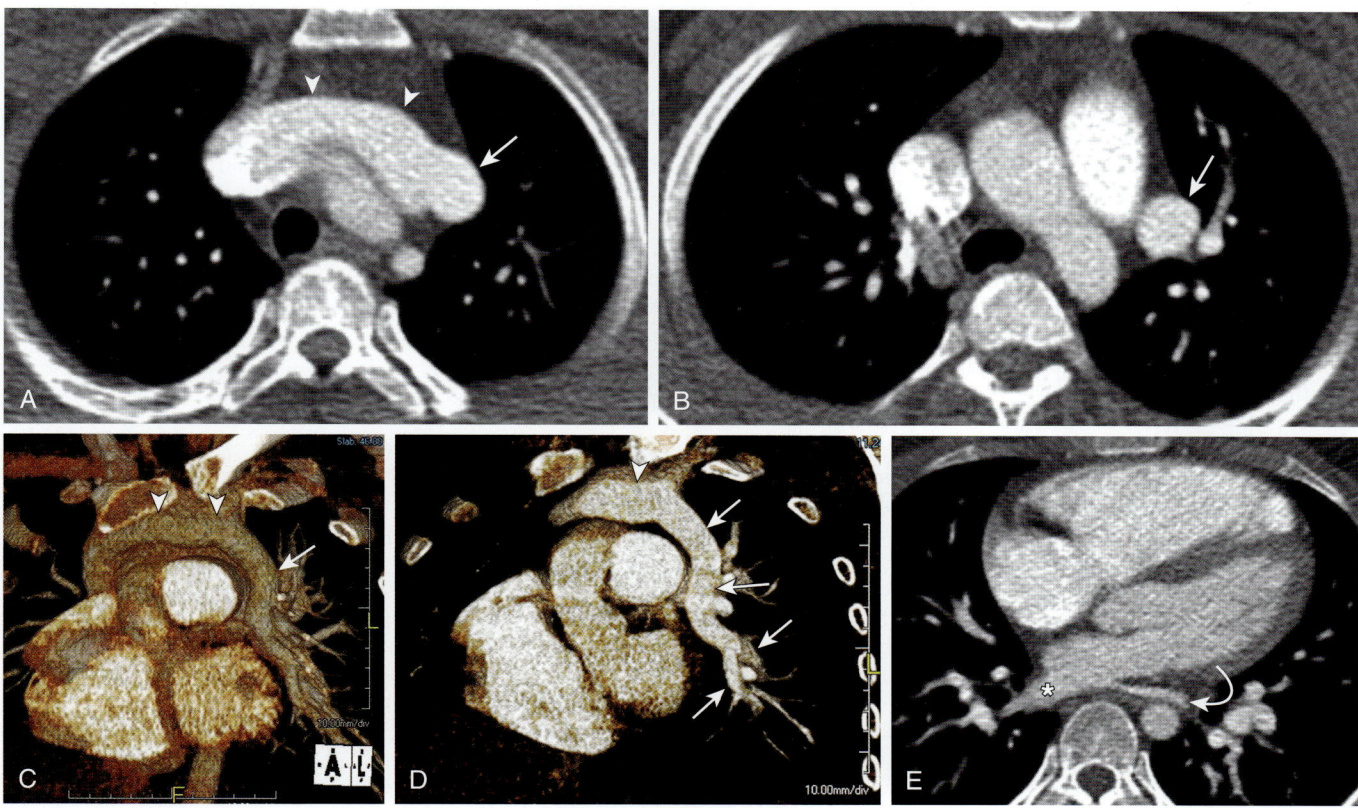

Figure 53-22 Partial anomalous pulmonary venous return to the left innominate vein. Enhanced axial computed tomography images (**A** and **B**) show an anomalous left pulmonary vein (*arrow*) draining into the left innominate vein (*arrowheads*). Volume-rendered images (**C** and **D**) depict a large anomalous vein (*arrows*) draining a vast portion of the left lung into a prominent left innominate vein (*arrowheads*). **E,** An enhanced axial image shows a relative small size of the left inferior pulmonary vein (*curved arrow*) when compared with the right (*asterisk*). Only a portion of the left lower lobe drained into the left inferior pulmonary vein (*curved arrow*).

anomalous veins to the left atrium, either by direct anastomosis or through a baffle in most instances.[59]

Pulmonary Vein Atresia/Hypoplasia

Etiology Pulmonary venous atresia is an uncommon anomaly associated with high morbidity and mortality. It is typically unilateral,[8] and if bilateral and surgical repair is not performed on an emergency basis, the condition typically is fatal.[57,60] The etiology is believed to represent the result of the unsuccessful incorporation of the common pulmonary vein into the left atrium, resulting in the lack of long segments of the central pulmonary veins.[8] If unilateral, the condition may be asymptomatic or may manifest in infancy or childhood with recurrent episodes of pneumonia, hemoptysis (as a result of the systemic collateral supply to the affected lung), exercise intolerance, and pulmonary hypertension.[8,61] Nearly half of the cases are associated with other forms of congenital heart disease.[8,61,62]

Imaging Chest radiographs typically show a small affected hemithorax and hilum with ipsilateral mediastinal shift. The affected lung demonstrates circumferential pleural thickening, diffuse reticular opacities, and septal lines reminiscent of pulmonary edema, which are most pronounced in the lower lung zones.[8,61] On enhanced CT examinations, the margins

of the left atrium at the expected level of the pulmonary vein ostia appear smooth, and some adjacent enhancing soft tissue density may be present, reflecting collateral pulmonary-to-systemic venous channels. Additional collaterals may be seen in other portions of the mediastinum. The ipsilateral pulmonary artery appears small. On lung windows, diffuse ground-glass attenuation and smooth thickening of the interlobular septa and bronchovascular bundles may be observed.[61] This constellation of findings is believed to represent prominent bronchial veins, dilated lymphatics, and patchy parenchymal fibrosis as a result of pulmonary infarcts[61] (e-Fig. 53-23).

Treatment and Follow-up In cases of unilateral pulmonary venous atresia, surgical repair usually is not possible, depending on the age at diagnosis. Most patients present late in life once irreversible changes have occurred. Pneumonectomy may be necessary to prevent repeated pulmonary infections, to relieve the left-to-right shunt, and to remove the dead space contributing to exercise intolerance.[62]

Pulmonary Vein Stenosis

Etiology Congenital pulmonary vein stenosis (PVS) is believed to be the result of an uninhibited myofibroblast-like proliferation causing endoluminal thickening and narrowing of the pulmonary veins.[11,63] However, the term "primary" pulmonary vein stenosis would be more accurate, because increasing evidence exists that the disease is progressive and may not even be present at the time of delivery. Association with other congenital heart defects is high, ranging from 30% to 80%.[11,64] Therefore echocardiographic evaluations of all forms of congenital heart defects should include assessment of the pulmonary veins.[65] A strong association between PVS and prematurity has been recently reported, with a preponderance in premature newborns with cardiac shunt lesions.[66] However, PVS also may occur in isolation, and in these cases, PVS usually progresses rapidly.[64]

Generally, the age at diagnosis and severity of symptoms are contingent on the number of pulmonary veins involved and the severity of pulmonary venous obstruction to individual pulmonary veins.[57,64] Patients with more than three stenotic pulmonary veins have a poorer prognosis; their mortality rate approaches 85%, versus 0% in patients with one or two stenosed pulmonary veins.[65] Most cases of PVS present in infancy with a history of worsening respiratory distress and recurrent pneumonias. With disease progression, pulmonary hypertension develops and becomes progressive. Therefore PVS always should be excluded in young patients with unexplained pulmonary hypertension. Hemoptysis may occur, particularly in older patients.[64] Secondary PVS in pediatric patients typically occurs after anomalous pulmonary vein surgery. In approximately 10% of these patients, substantial stenosis develops either at the anastomotic site or within the central portions of the pulmonary veins.[67,68]

Imaging Echocardiography usually can visualize all pulmonary veins in neonates and infants. Turbulent flow on color Doppler with flow velocities >1.6 m/s indicate hemodynamically significant pulmonary venous obstruction.[69] Findings on chest radiographs include patchy reticular opacities and thickened septa, reflecting the impaired venous drainage in the affected lung. On CT, pulmonary vein thickening and narrowing can be seen. Although it typically affects the pulmonary venous–left atrial junction, it may involve more central and peripheral segments, resulting in long-segment narrowing, particularly in cases of advanced disease[11,17] (Fig. 53-24). In advanced cases of PVS, lung and pleural findings may be indistinguishable from pulmonary venous atresia, with smooth septal thickening, reticular opacities, patchy ground-glass areas, and pleural thickening. MRI may show similar although lesser findings, because CT has better spatial resolution. However, MRI may provide additional physiologic information in patients.[57]

Treatment and Follow-up PVS may be amenable to balloon dilatation occasionally followed by stent placement, although restenosis seems universal. Care should be taken, because stent implantation before surgery may limit the surgical approaches. The restenosis rate after surgery approaches 10%, despite advanced techniques reducing trauma to the veins to avoid any stimulus for regrowth of obstructive tissue. In severe cases with multiple vein involvement, lung transplantation may be necessary.[64]

Pulmonary Varix

Etiology Congenital pulmonary varix is a rare congenital or acquired vascular anomaly resulting in focal aneurysmal dilatation of a pulmonary vein.[11] Acquired congenital pulmonary varix typically is seen in pediatric patients who have underlying cardiac conditions resulting in pulmonary venous hypertension, such as mitral valve disease, aortic coarctation, and pulmonary vein stenosis.[11] In most instances, pulmonary varices are incidental findings in otherwise asymptomatic patients. Rare complications such as rupture or thromboembolism may produce symptoms.[11,17]

Imaging On chest radiographs, pulmonary varices usually present as well-defined pulmonary or mediastinal lesions in close proximity to the cardiac silhouette. They should be differentiated from other masses such as congenital lung anomaly, a neoplasm, or an infectious process. CT is particularly helpful in showing the characteristic imaging features of pulmonary varix, including contiguity between the pulmonary vein and the varix, simultaneous contrast enhancement within both structures, and lack of a feeding artery.[11,17] Some authors advocate for the use of imaging modalities that can provide information regarding flow direction and pattern within the lesion, such as ultrasound, MRI, or conventional angiography to avoid confusion with a pulmonary AVM[70] (e-Fig. 53-25).

Treatment and Follow-up Surgical resection of pulmonary varix is indicated in symptomatic pediatric patients, particularly with complications such as rupture or thromboembolism.[17,70]

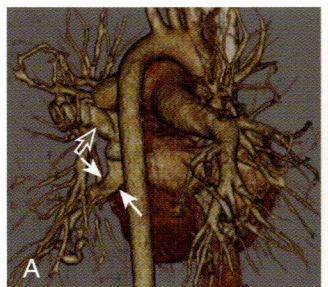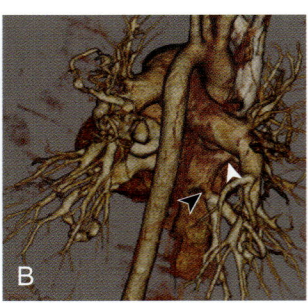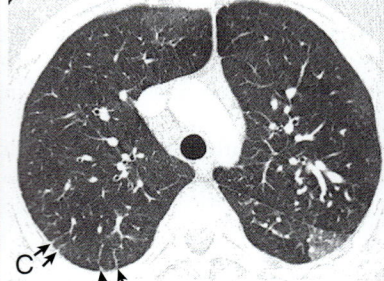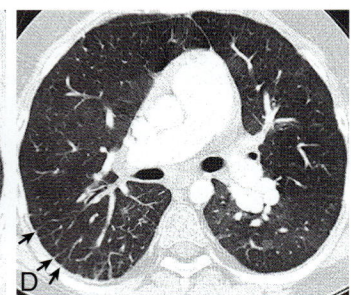

Figure 53-24 A 10-year-old boy with pulmonary venoocclusive disease. Posterior oblique volume-rendered three-dimensional images (**A** and **B**) show severe right inferior pulmonary vein narrowing in the anteroposterior dimension resulting in flattening of the vein (*solid arrows*). Compensatory varicous enlargement of the right superior pulmonary vein is present (*open arrow*), likely because of the redirection of flow. The left inferior pulmonary vein shows approximately 50% stenosis (*black arrowhead*), whereas the left superior pulmonary vein (*white arrowhead*) remains patent. Axial computed tomography images on lung windows (**C** and **D**) show smooth interlobular septal thickening (*arrows*) and mild patchy areas of ground-glass opacity.

COMBINED ANOMALIES OF THE PULMONARY ARTERY AND VEIN

Pulmonary Arteriovenous Malformation

Etiology Pulmonary AVM is a vascular malformation due to an underlying direct connection between the pulmonary arteries and veins without an intervening capillary network.[11] This bypass of the capillary network has two important physiologic consequences. First, the direct communication acts as a right-to-left shunt. Second, blood flowing through a pulmonary AVM circumvents the filter function of the normal pulmonary capillary bed, predisposing patients to paradoxical emboli.

Pulmonary AVMs can be congenital or acquired. The acquired form of pulmonary AVM usually is seen in patients with a prior history of congenital heart disease surgeries, chronic liver disease, or infections such as tuberculosis or actinomycosis.[11,17] Congenital pulmonary AVMs may occur sporadically, although characteristically they are seen in 30% to 40% of family members with hereditary hemorrhagic telangiectasia (HHT), also known as Rendu-Osler-Weber syndrome. HHT is an autosomal-dominant condition, which is diagnosed clinically on the basis of Curaçao criteria (cerebral, pulmonary, or hepatic AVMs, epistaxis, family history of HHT, and telangiectasias).[71] Given that each offspring of an affected person has a 50% chance of having inherited the condition, family members of patients with HHT should be screened for pulmonary AVMs.[17,72]

Pediatric patients with small pulmonary AVMs often are asymptomatic. Typical clinical symptoms of patients with larger or multiple pulmonary AVMs include dyspnea on exertion, cyanosis, chest pain, palpitations, and hemoptysis.[73] Direct right-to-left shunting through larger or multiple pulmonary AVMs bypassing the pulmonary capillary bed can result in paradoxical emboli to the brain. Such paradoxical emboli may cause a stroke or brain abscess.

Imaging On chest radiographs, pulmonary AVM may appear as a well-circumscribed serpiginous or lobulated opacity. Occasionally, curvilinear opacities directed toward the hilum representing the feeding artery or draining vein may be observed. Most pulmonary AVMs are located within the lower lobes. Small pulmonary AVMs or lesions in areas obscured by normal structures, such as the retrocardiac area or the pulmonary hila, may be overlooked easily.

In the past, pulmonary AVM traditionally was evaluated with conventional pulmonary angiography. Multidetector CT is now the preferred imaging modality for a complete assessment of pulmonary AVMs and can clearly show the often complex angioarchitecture of the pulmonary AVM with its feeding artery and draining vein. Reconstructed 2D and 3D images play an important role in the treatment of pulmonary AVMs by allowing preinterventional planning prior to embolization, which is of outmost importance when managing large or complex lesions[17,73] (Fig. 53-26). MRA technology has narrowed the gap for the assessment of pulmonary AVMs.[74]

Pulmonary AVMs may be simple or complex. Approximately 80% to 90% of the simple angioarchitecture of pulmonary AVMs, consisting of single or multiple feeding

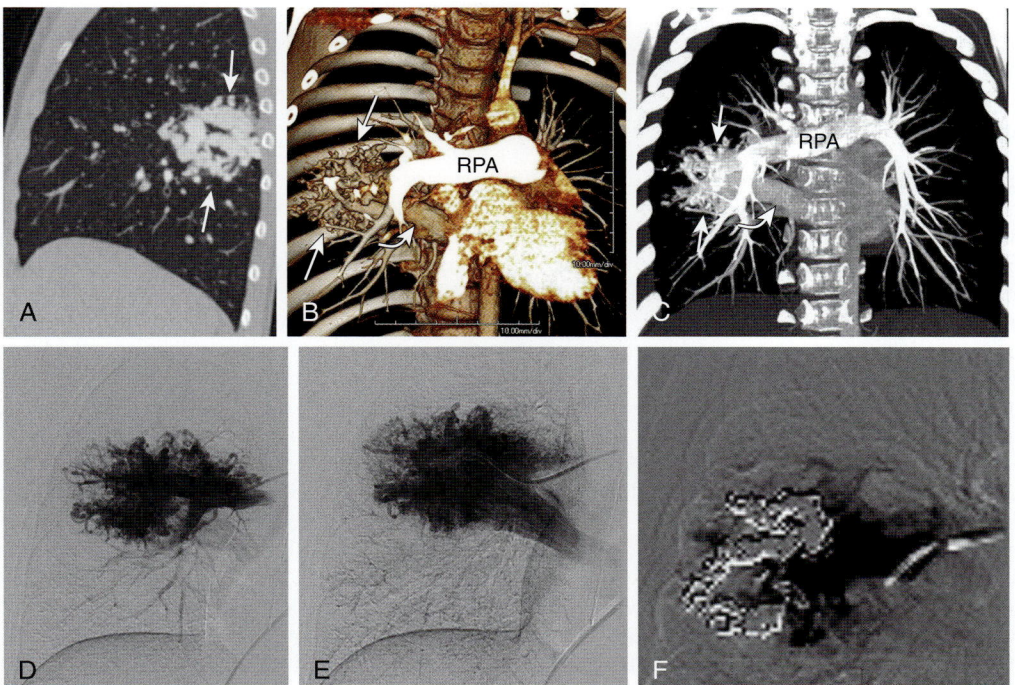

Figure 53-26 An 8-year-old with a family history of hereditary hemorrhagic telangiectasia and a positive echocardiogram for a pulmonary arteriovenous malformation (AVM). **A,** An enhanced sagittal reformatted computed tomography (CT) image shows a large AVM (*arrows*) in the superior segment of the right lower lobe. Coronal-oblique volume-rendered (**B**) and coronal maximum intensity projection (**C**) CT angiography images show a large AVM (*straight arrows*) with a feeding artery from the right main pulmonary artery (*RPA*) and a large draining vein into an enlarged right inferior pulmonary vein (*curved arrow*). Pulmonary angiogram images (**D** and **E**) demonstrate a large AVM that correlates well with the CT angiography findings. A postembolization image (**F**) with platinum coils shows partial obliteration of a large portion of the lesion.

arteries, all originate from one segmental artery and are connected directly to a single draining vein.[11] Typically, both the artery and vein are dilated and are connected by the aneurysmal sac. The remaining 10% to 20% of cases involve complex architecture lesions, with two or more feeding arteries arising from at least two different segmental arteries and connecting with at least two draining veins.[11] Nearly 5% of patients with HHT have multiple pulmonary AVMs.[75]

Treatment and Follow-up As a general rule, treatment is offered for pulmonary AVMs with feeding arteries larger than 3 mm. However, symptomatic paradoxical emboli have been reported in patients with sub–3-mm feeding arteries. Consequently, many HHT centers currently are treating pulmonary AVMs with feeding arteries of less than 3 mm.[76] The current management choice for pulmonary AVM is transvenous transcatheter embolotherapy, which can be performed using a variety of devices including coils, detachable balloons, and, most recently, with the Amplatzer vascular occluder (AGA Medical, Plymouth, MN). The latter, with the addition of at least one platinum coil, is believed to be the combination that most effectively prevents pulmonary AVM recanalization.[73]

Regarding pulmonary AVMs in pediatric patients, far less agreement exists with regard to who should be treated, particularly with children who are asymptomatic and younger than 12 years.[75,77] Developing lungs in this setting may be at increased risk for reperfusion via pulmonary collaterals, which are even more difficult to treat. Symptomatic pulmonary AVMs should be treated regardless of the age of patients.[73]

Combined Parenchymal and Vascular Lesions

HYPOGENETIC LUNG SYNDROME (SCIMITAR SYNDROME)

Etiology Hypogenetic lung syndrome, also known as scimitar syndrome, refers to an anomalous connection of the right pulmonary veins to the inferior vena cava, in which an anomalous pulmonary vein drains part of or the entire right lung. The anomalous vein may on occasion drain into the hepatic veins, portal veins, azygos vein, coronary sinus, or right atrium. The anomalous vein often resembles a scimitar, a curved Turkish sword, hence the name "scimitar syndrome." Hypogenetic lung syndrome frequently is associated with various degrees of right lung hypoplasia and abnormal lobation, along with heart dextroposition.[45,78] Additional reported anomalies associated with hypogenetic lung syndrome include bronchogenic cyst, horseshoe lung, accessory diaphragm, hernia, and arterial supply of parts of the right lung by collateral arterial blood vessels, usually from the descending aorta.[17,45] Affected infants may present with clinical signs and symptoms related to congestive heart failure from right-heart volume overload. Hypogenetic lung syndrome also may be seen as an incidental finding in older children or alternatively may manifest as recurrent right basilar pneumonia.[17,79]

Imaging The classic vertically oriented curvilinear opacity, representing the scimitar vein, which projects over the right lower hemithorax in conjunction with a hypoplastic right lung, is usually seen on frontal chest radiographs. On lateral chest radiographs, a dense retrosternal band of variable width typically is observed, which is a result of the decrease in anteroposterior diameter of the hypoplastic lung, resulting in a lung–soft tissue interface.[7,55] CT or MRI are the preferred imaging modalities for confirming and characterizing hypogenetic lung syndrome in pediatric patients (e-Figs. 53-27 and 53-28). Multidetector CT with 2D and 3D images have been reported as being particularly useful for displaying the entire course of the anomalous scimitar vein as a preprocedural or preoperative evaluation.[11,45] In addition, they also are helpful noninvasive imaging tools for evaluating postoperative complications, including thrombosis or stenosis of a reimplanted anomalous vein. Furthermore, abnormal lung parenchymal changes, abnormal lung lobation, and anomalous bronchial branching patterns often are seen in patients with hypogenetic lung syndrome and also can be well evaluated with multidetector CT.[11,45] The absence of an ipsilateral inferior pulmonary vein is a helpful finding that supports the diagnosis.

Treatment and Follow-up For symptomatic pediatric patients with scimitar syndrome, several surgical techniques currently are available that aim to reconnect the anomalous vein to the left atrium with or without the creation of an intracardiac baffle. However, complications related to either restenosis or baffle obstruction are not uncommon.[80] In addition, occlusion of the collateral arteries may be necessary in affected patients.[59]

PULMONARY SEQUESTRATION

Etiology BPSs are congenital lung malformations that consist of nonfunctioning lung tissue that does not connect with the tracheobronchial tree. A BPS has a systemic arterial supply, usually from the aorta, although occasionally it may arise from branches of the celiac, splenic, intercostal, or subclavian arteries.

Sequestrations traditionally are classified as either extralobar (25%) or intralobar (75%). Extralobar sequestration (ELS) is defined as an isolated mass of lung tissue with its own pleural investment and aberrant systemic vascular supply. An ELS is believed to develop from a supernumerary lung bud that separates from the tracheobronchial tree and parasitizes its own vascular supply from the systemic circulation.[6,81] Venous drainage is into the azygous or hemiazygous systems in most cases. However, an ELS may drain into the pulmonary veins or the systemic circulation, including the subclavian and intercostal veins, as well as the portal venous system.[6,10,81] Although most ELSs are identified in isolation, occasionally an ELS may be associated with congenital heart defects, abnormal communications with the GI tract, pulmonary hypoplasia, ectopic pancreas, vertebral anomalies, and congenital diaphragmatic hernia, which is the most commonly associated anomaly.[6,10,17,19,81] Associated microcystic maldevelopment or CPAM type 2 components have been described in many of these cases,[10,82] an anomaly referred to by many investigators as hybrid lesions.[83,84] Most patients with an ELS are asymptomatic.

Intralobar sequestration (ILS) lesions are defined as developmental malformations composed of isolated, nonfunctioning lung tissue without communication to the tracheobronchial tree and with an aberrant systemic vascular supply, typically embedded within a normal lobe.[6,19,85] Unlike ELS lesions, ILS lesions do not have their own pleural coat, and venous drainage primarily occurs into the pulmonary veins.[10,17,19,85] ILS has been considered an acquired lesion resulting from a chronic inflammatory process that recruited collateral flow from aortic branch arteries.[85] Increasing reports of antenatal ILS detection, confirmed by postnatal resection, has challenged this previous concept. Although still uncertain, the hypothesis that ILS represents a developmental malformation rather than an acquired entity is most accepted.[10] Pediatric patients with ILS often clinically present with a recurrent lung infection.

Imaging Imaging findings of BPS may vary primarily on the basis of association with superimposed infection (e-Fig. 53-29), CPAM lesions (Fig. 53-30), or GI tract communication.[10,17] In fetal imaging, BPS lesions present as echogenic lesions on ultrasound and as hyperintense lesions on T2-weighted images.[24] Similar to CPAM and bronchial atresia, sequestrations can be detected as early as in the twelfth week of gestation,[22] although most usually are diagnosed on routine ultrasound at 19 to 20 weeks. They exhibit a characteristic increase in volume from the twentieth to the twenty-sixth week and usually reach a plateau by the twenty-eighth week of gestation.[3,9,22,24,40] These lesions usually decrease in size during the third trimester and seem to vanish in nearly half of the cases. However, they do not truly

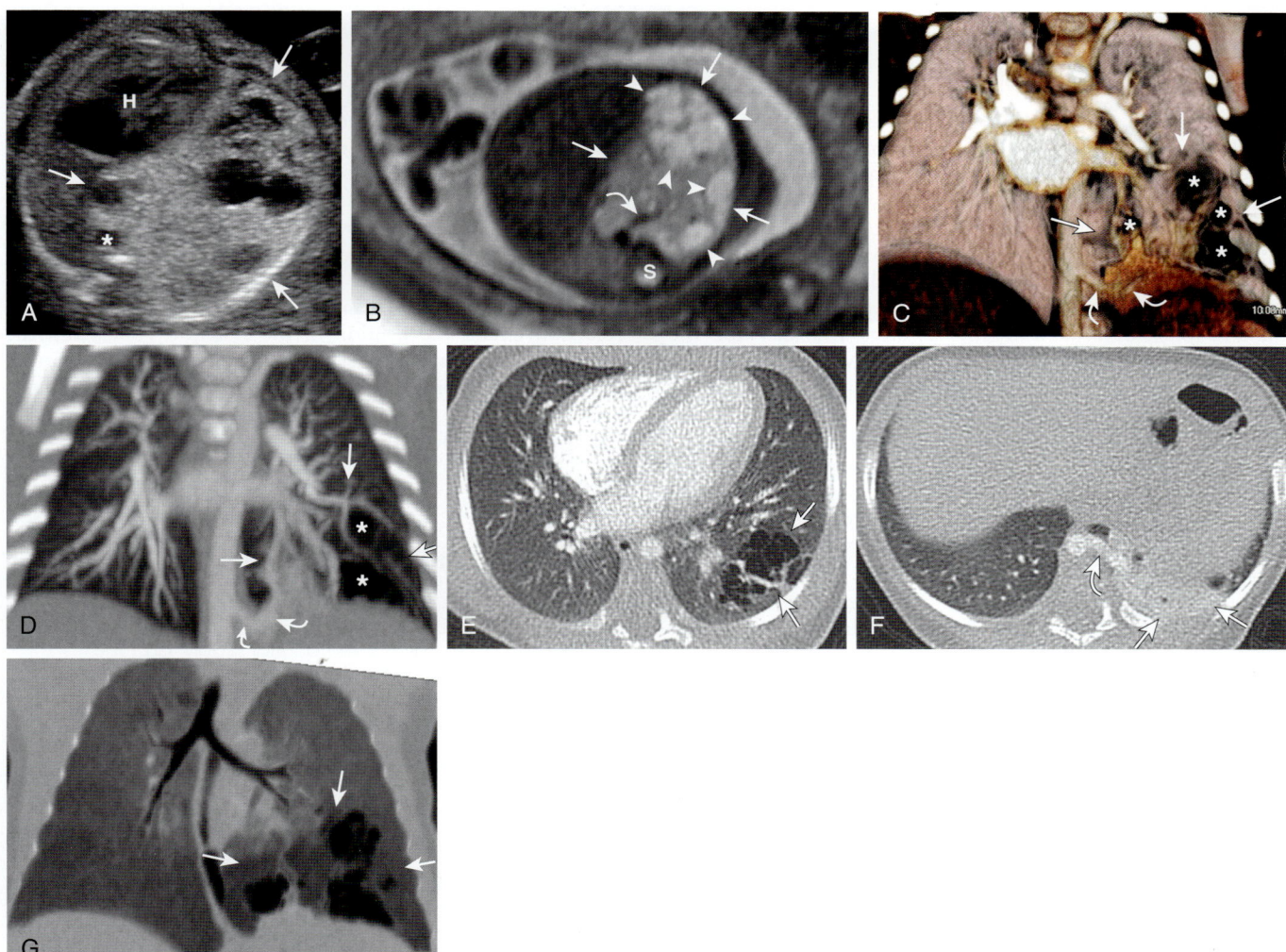

Figure 53-30 A hybrid lesion, intralobar sequestration, and microcystic maldevelopment (congenital pulmonary airway malformation (CPAM) type 2). **A,** A transverse fetal ultrasound image shows a large left lower lesion (*arrows*) resulting in significant cardiac heart (*H*) and aortic (*asterisk*) displacement. Internal cystic components are noted mainly at the periphery of the lesion. **B,** An axial T2-weighted fetal magnetic resonance image shows the extensive hyperintense lesion within the left lower lobe. Cystic peripheral components consistent with CPAM are noted (*arrowheads*). An aortic feeder (*curved arrow*) is seen supplying the lesion. *S,* Spine. **C-F,** Postnatal imaging shows a complex, partially aerated left lower lesion supplied by an aberrant aortic vessel (*curved arrows*) with aerated, mainly peripheral cysts (*asterisks*) and overall findings consistent with a hybrid lesion (*arrows*). The lesion appears relatively smaller when compared with the prenatal images. Volume-rendered (**C**), maximum intensity projection (**D**), and axial computed tomography angiography (**E** and **F**) images show a systemic, aortic feeder (*curved arrows*) to the lesion (*arrows*). Internal cystic components are noted predominantly at the periphery (*asterisks*) of the lesion. A portion of unaerated lung is seen at the base of the lesion. **G,** A coronal reformatted minimum intensity projection image shows the internal cystic components of the CPAM (*arrows*) to better advantage.

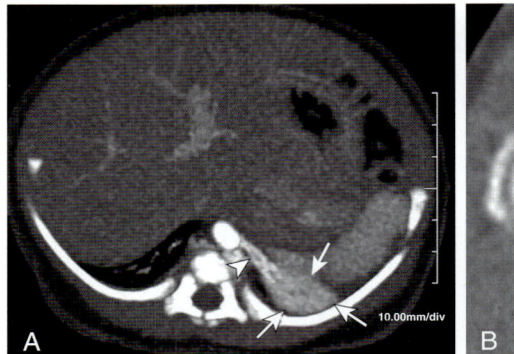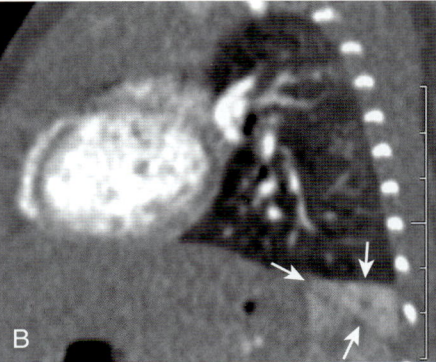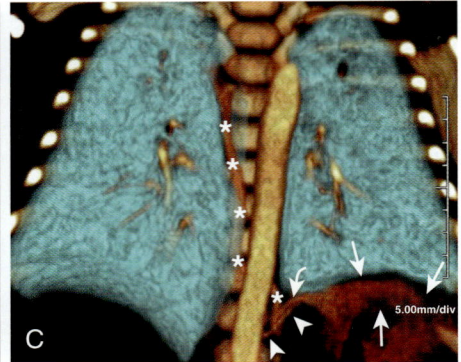

Figure 53-31   Extralobar bronchopulmonary sequestration in a 1-month-old infant. Axial maximum intensity projection (**A**) and a sagittal multiplanar reconstruction (**B**) computed tomography images show unaerated, enhancing lung tissue in the left costophrenic sulcus with a small aortic feeder (*arrowhead*), consistent with extralobar sequestration (ELS) (*arrows*). ELS in this location easily could be confused with atelectasis. A coronal volume-rendered three-dimensional image (**C**) demonstrates the relationship of the sequestration (*arrows*) to the left lung and depicts the course of the aortic feeder (*arrowheads*) and the draining vein (*curved arrow*) into the azygos system (*asterisks*).

disappear. This phenomenon probably is partially related to the decrease in the size of the lesion, but technically it also is related to the relative increase in echogenicity of the adjacent normal lung parenchyma, which makes recognition challenging.[24] Because complete regression is extremely unusual, follow-up cross-sectional postnatal imaging is recommended in all cases[3,9,24] because these lesions may be overlooked on chest radiographs.[86] In our experience, ultrasound duplex appears to be a highly sensitive modality for the depiction of the aberrant feeders. On fetal MRI, these feeders sometimes are difficult to identify and appear as low-signal linear structures extending from the aorta into the sequestration; they usually are best seen on coronal images.

On chest radiographs, ELS lesions typically present as a focal lung mass. ILS lesions often present as a focal lung mass and/or cyst but also may manifest as an area of consolidation or lung abscess, particularly in the setting of recurrent superimposed infection. Although ELSs may be encountered anywhere from the neck to below the diaphragm, they are found most commonly within the lower hemithorax, on the left side more often than the right side.[6,10,81]

On CT, ELS lesions characteristically appear as solid, unaerated lesions, although in nearly half of the cases, coexistent pathology with CPAM type 2 has been reported (Fig. 53-31). In these cases, internal cystic components may be identified.[6,10,82] Because ILS lesions do not have a pleural investment, they typically manifest as aerated lesions, presumably from collateral air drift, if enough time has elapsed to adequately clear any retained fetal lung fluid[10] (Fig. 53-32). Anomalous vascular components of BPS can be evaluated with either CT or MRI. When interpreting these studies, the real-time and interactive 2D and 3D imaging evaluation at the 2D/3D work stations can facilitate the accurate assessment of the anomalous vascular structures, which are better displayed in the z-plane.[10,17,45]

Treatment and Follow-up   Many authors support the elective surgical resection of ILSs because of the risk of complications, such as superimposed infection, pneumothorax, hemorrhage, sudden respiratory compromise, and the small risk of malignant transformation.[21,22,33] Lobectomy performed via

video-assisted thoracoscopic surgery is performed in many institutions, because segmentectomies may result in incomplete resection and air leaks.[21,22,33]

Management of ELSs is more controversial, because persons with an ELS appear to be at lower risk for the development of complications.[21] Nonoperative, expectant management frequently is applied to an extrathoracic ELS, whereas an intrathoracic ELS usually is resected surgically. Their resection entails the ligation of the systemic vessels and the removal of the lesion. Arterial embolization has been reported as a successful alternative management, particularly for infants presenting with congestive heart failure,[21] as evidenced by shrinkage of the lesion on follow-up imaging.[87,88]

✓ WHAT THE CLINICIAN NEEDS TO KNOW

- Congenital lung anomalies refer to a heterogeneous group of pulmonary developmental disorders that affect the lung parenchyma, the arterial supply, and the venous drainage to the lung, or a combination of these entities.

- Despite the advent of prenatal imaging and advancement in postnatal imaging evaluation that has substantially enhanced our understanding of congenital lung anomalies, substantial controversy continues to exist regarding the nomenclature, classification, pathogenesis, description, and management of congenital lung anomalies.

- It is important to recognize that specific terminology for these lesions may be controversial and occasionally confusing. Therefore, careful evaluation and thorough understanding of all imaging findings are more important for practical care than trying to categorize the lesions by pathological terminology.

- Specific imaging findings of congenital lung anomalies that need to be evaluated include (1) location of lesions, (2) associated anomalous vascular supply and drainage of the lesions, (3) internal components and the degree of aeration, (4) exclusion of communication with the gastrointestinal tract, (5) integrity of the diaphragm, and (6) an assessment of associated anomalies, such as vertebral anomalies.

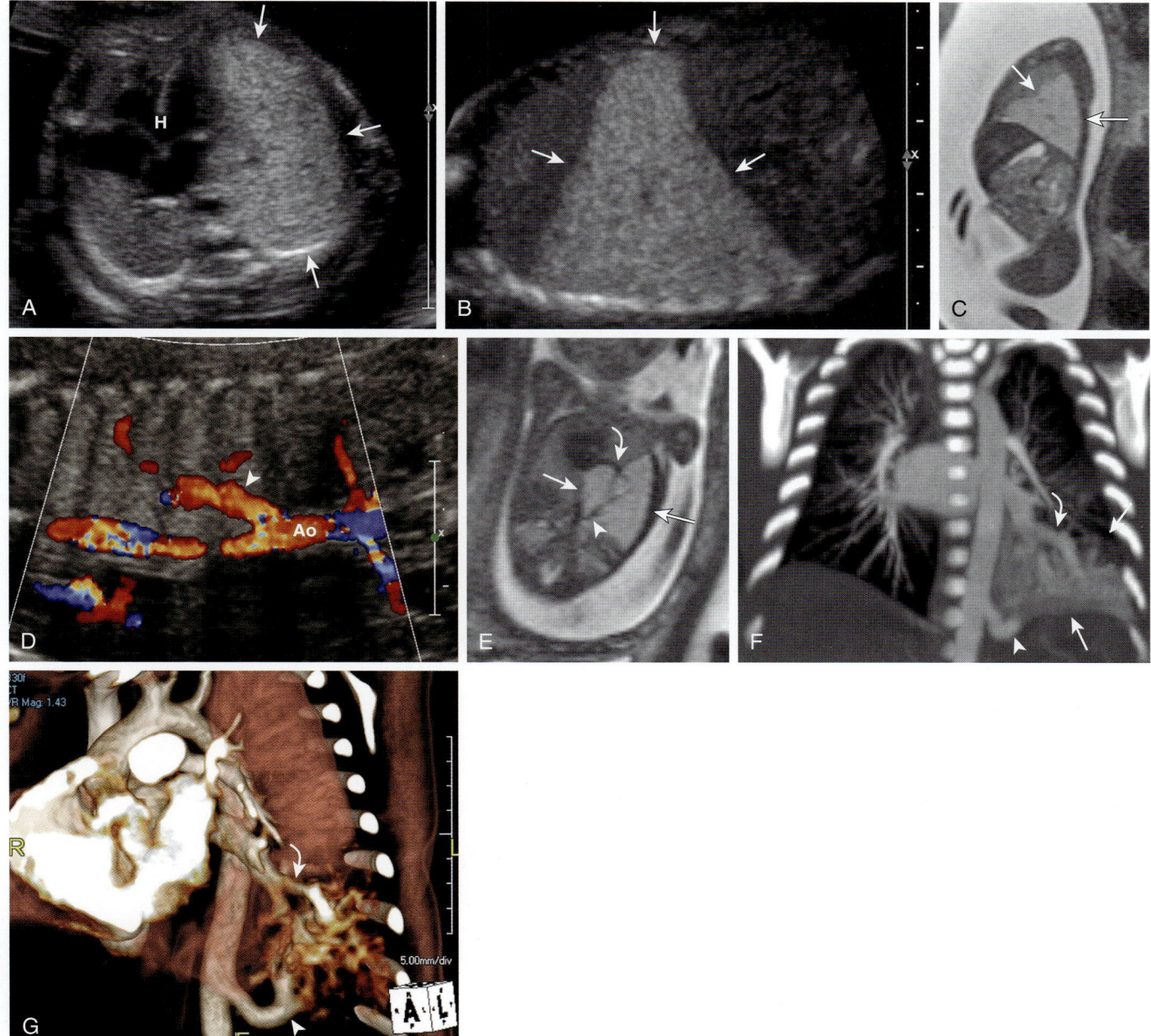

Figure 53-32 Intralobar sequestration. A transverse ultrasound scan (**A**) through the chest shows a large, homogeneously hyperechoic lesion (*arrows*) in the left lower chest resulting in mild mediastinal shift and cardiac heart (*H*) displacement. Sagittal ultrasound (**B**) and sagittal T2-weighted fetal magnetic resonance (MR) (**C**) images show a homogeneous large left lower lesion without visible cysts (*arrows*). **D,** A coronal fetal ultrasound image shows an aortic feeder (*arrowhead*). *Ao,* Aorta. **E,** A coronal oblique T2-weighted fetal MR image shows a prominent aortic feeder (*arrowhead*) and a slightly prominent pulmonary vein (*curved arrow*) draining the large hyperintense lesion (*arrows*) within the left lower lobe. Coronal maximum intensity projection (**F**) and volume-rendered (**G**) computed tomography angiography images show a prominent aortic feeder (*arrowhead*) in a 7-day-old neonate. The lesion (*straight arrows*) is only partially aerated and drains into a prominent pulmonary vein (*curved arrows*) consistent with an intralobar bronchopulmonary sequestration. Note the relative decrease in the size of the lesion compared with prenatal imaging.

Key Points

Congenital lung anomalies vary widely in their clinical manifestation and imaging appearance.

Congenital lung anomalies can be classified into three groups: predominantly parenchymal abnormalities, predominantly vascular abnormalities, and combined parenchymal and vascular abnormalities, based on morphologic-radiologic-pathologic classification.

Although radiographs play a role in the incidental detection and initial imaging evaluation in pediatric patients with clinically suspected congenital lung anomalies, cross-sectional imaging such as CT with 2D/3D imaging evaluation often is required for confirmation of diagnosis, further characterization, and preoperative evaluation in cases of surgical lesions.

Understanding proper imaging techniques and characteristic imaging appearances of congenital lung anomalies can enhance the accurate diagnosis and proper management of pediatric patients who have these often complex congenital lung malformations.

Suggested Readings

Epelman M, Kreiger PA, Servaes S, et al. Current imaging of prenatally diagnosed congenital lung lesions. *Semin Ultrasound CT MR.* 2010;31(2):141-157.

Hellinger JC, Daubert M, Lee EY, et al. Congenital thoracic vascular anomalies: evaluation with state-of-the-art MR imaging and MDCT. *Radiol Clin North Am.* 2011;49(5):969-996.

Langston C. New concepts in the pathology of congenital lung malformations. *Semin Pediatr Surg.* 2003;12:17-37.

Lee EY, Dorkin H, Vargas SO. Congenital pulmonary malformations in pediatric patients: review and update on etiology, classification, and imaging findings. *Radiol Clin North Am.* 2011;49(5):921-948.

Lee EY, Boiselle PM, Cleveland RH. Multidetector CT evaluation of congenital lung anomalies. *Radiology.* 2008;247(3):632-648.

Yikilmaz A, Lee EY. CT imaging of mass-like non-vascular pulmonary lesions in children. *Pediatr Radiol.* 2007;37(12):1253-1263.

References

Full references for this chapter can be found on www.expertconsult.com.

Chapter 54

Pulmonary Infection

SJIRK J. WESTRA, BRENT ADLER, ALI YIKILMAZ, and EDWARD Y. LEE

Pneumonia and other pulmonary infections, defined as those involving the lower respiratory tract below the glottis, continue to be the most common cause of illness in children, affecting over 150 million children under the age of 5 years per year worldwide, and are implicated in 20 million hospitalizations annually in the United States.[1-5] Since clinical signs and symptoms are poor predictors of pediatric pulmonary infections, and the value of microbial studies is limited, chest radiography with the use of standardized reporting criteria continues to be the best available diagnostic standard.[1,3,6,7] The value of lateral radiograph in diagnosis continues to be debated, but the hyperinflation that is a radiographic hallmark of pulmonary infections in young children is more reliably detected on the lateral radiograph than on the frontal radiograph.[1,8,9]

In the ambulatory care setting, performing routine chest radiography has not been shown to improve the outcomes of pulmonary infections in young children, and it is not indicated in first-time wheezing episodes presumed to be viral or reactive in etiology.[10-12] The yield of radiography is greater in the presence of a high temperature and in the absence of a family history of asthma.[13] Radiography is most helpful when an inconsistency exists among the data from history, physical examination, and observation.[14] Negative chest radiography provides justification to withhold antibiotics in symptomatic children.[1] Valid indications for chest radiography, therefore, are severe disease, confirmation or exclusion of diagnosis in the presence of an atypical presentation, assessment of complications, and exclusion of other causes of respiratory distress.[10]

Maternal antibodies protect newborns against viral pulmonary infections, and bacterial infections are most common in this age group, usually caused by pathogens acquired during labor and delivery. With dropping maternal antibodies, viral infections become more prevalent between ages 2 months and 2 years. After this, bacterial infections again become more common.[3] Tuberculosis, fungal infections, and parasitic infestations continue to add substantially to the disease burden of children who are immunocompromised or live in endemic areas.[2]

The spectrum of pulmonary infections in childhood is categorized in Table 54-1.[2,15] However, the distinctions between these categories are arbitrary, since considerable overlap exists both at presentation and during evolution of disease. In young children, the lungs can only respond to insult in a limited number of ways, and this response is more age specific than antigen dependent.[16-20] Viral and bacterial infections frequently coexist, and radiographic criteria alone do not reliably distinguish between them.[21-23] This is compounded by a reported high interobserver variability for interpretation of chest radiographs.[24-27] Use of inexact terminology may hamper communication between radiologists and referring physicians, who agree with radiologists' interpretations in only 78% of cases, and antibiotics are frequently prescribed even when no bacterial agent can be proven.[6,28,29]

Pulmonary Infections Caused by Viruses

Viral pulmonary infections usually occur after the inhalation of infected air droplets.[2] The clinical presentation depends on the infectious agent, patient age, and immune response (mainly cellular, T-cell–mediated immunity). In young children, degrees of mucosal swelling within the small-caliber terminal airways, which would not compromise air exchange in older individuals with relatively larger-caliber airways, lead to diffuse alveolar air trapping. This, in combination with lack of development of collateral pathways of ventilation via the pores of Kohn and canals of Lambert, leads to fixed hyperinflation of the lungs (Fig. 54-1). In addition, more hypersecretion occurs in the inflamed airways in young children, contributing to mucous plugging of the airways; this leads to (sub)segmental atelectasis mimicking alveolar consolidations, which are frequently misinterpreted to represent bacterial pneumonia.[1,29-31]

Etiology The most common viral agents causing pulmonary infections in childhood are listed in Table 54-2.

RNA Viruses Respiratory syncytial virus (RSV) consists of 10 genes encoding 11 proteins that are associated with inhibiting type 1 interferon activity. It is the most common cause of pulmonary infections in infants and young children. The disease can be virulent and is fatal in up to 1% of healthy infants, but those with chronic lung disease from prematurity and cardiovascular disease are at much higher risk.[32] Clinical signs range from mild coryza to severe respiratory distress with wheezing, tachypnea, cyanosis, dyspnea, and retractions. Hypoxemia, possibly caused by a ventilation–perfusion imbalance, may be profound and last for several weeks.[33] The diagnosis of RSV infection is made by examining the nasoepithelial cells by using direct fluorescent antibody detection.

Table 54-1

Classification of Pulmonary Infections in Childhood		
By Pathology, Clinical Presentation	**By Primary Location**	**By Radiographic Feature**
Acute focal	Trachea: tracheitis	Alveolar
Atypical	Large airways: bronchitis	Interstitial
Miliary or nodular	Small airways: bronchiolitis	Volume loss (atelectasis)
Progressive or fulminant	Small airways and parenchyma: bronchopneumonia	Pulmonary nodule(s) Necrosis, cavitation
Aspiration	Parenchyma	Lymphadenopathy
"Pulmonary infiltrates with eosinophilia"	Alveoli ("alveolitis")	Pleural effusion
Chronic or recurrent	Interstitium	

From Eslamy HK, Newman B. Pneumonia in normal and immunocompromised children: an overview and update. *Radiol Clin North Am.* 2011;49:895-920.

Human metapneumovirus (HMV) is a negative single-stranded ribonucleic acid (RNA) virus of the family *Paramyxoviridae*, and the second most common cause of viral pulmonary infections in young children after RSV.[34] It affects children who are slightly older than those infected by RSV, and the disease is less severe, except when seen as a coinfection. HMV has a worldwide distribution and causes a disease spectrum indistinguishable from influenza and RSV infection, with the same seasonal variation.

Parainfluenza virus is a common community-acquired virus with a seasonal pattern distinctly different from that of RSV. Parainfluenza virus types 1 and 2 fluctuate biannually,

typically in the fall, and parainfluenza virus type 3 is common in the late winter or early spring.

The various subtypes of the influenza virus are common causes of pneumonia requiring hospitalization in young and school-age children, ranking behind RSV and parainfluenza. Influenza attacks the ciliated respiratory epithelium, and lesions may extend to the distal airways, producing severe pneumonia. The onset is often more abrupt and intense than that of RSV or parainfluenza. The newly isolated avian influenza virus (H1N1), originating in Asia from infected poultry, has spread over many parts of the world from 2003 to 2007.[34-36] A novel H1N1 infection resulting from antigenic shift of the virus has been reported since 2009 and has been associated with a higher rate of shock, acute respiratory distress syndrome (ARDS), and neurologic complications in children compared with seasonal (non–H1N1) infections.[37]

Severe acute respiratory distress syndrome (SARS) is caused by a coronavirus, which was recognized in 2003, and in the following year, it was diagnosed in over 8000 patients, primarily in China, Taiwan, Hong Kong, Vietnam, and Toronto.[34,38] After 2004, the outbreak appeared to have been contained; since then, SARS has only been sporadically reported. Like most respiratory viral diseases, it is spread by face-to-face contact. SARS typically has a brief prodrome of fever, with or without constitutional symptoms. This quickly progresses to severe respiratory symptoms by day 6 of the fever.[39] Most patients require hospitalization. It has an overall mortality of 10%, but children have constituted only 5% of reported cases, and no pediatric deaths have been reported.[34] Children have a mild clinical course and recover with no sequelae.[38] Recently, newer coronaviruses (NL63 and HKU1), which cause milder forms of respiratory disease, have been discovered.[34]

Pneumonia as a complication of childhood measles is diminishing in frequency because of vaccination, but it is still

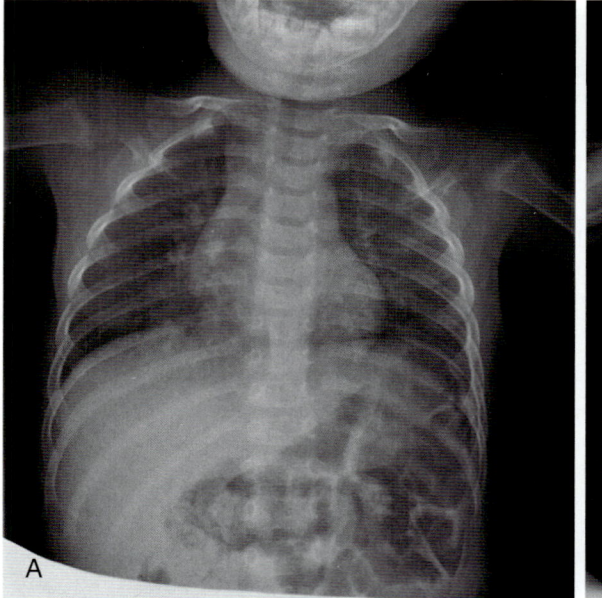
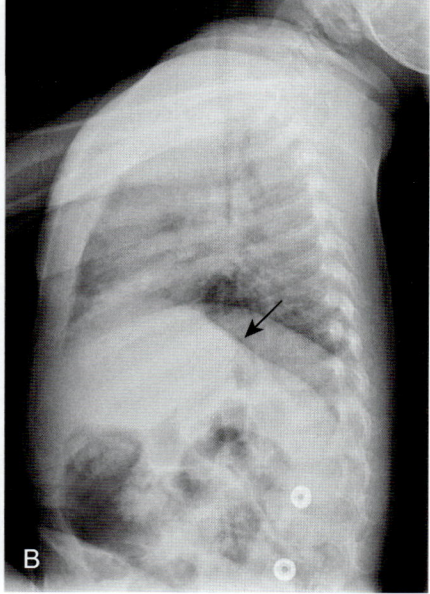

Figure 54-1   Respiratory syncytial virus pneumonia in a 1.5-year-old boy. **A,** The frontal chest radiograph shows perihilar streaky lung opacities and peribronchial thickening, typical of viral infections, with more focal opacity medially in the right lung base, from superimposed atelectasis. This was mistaken for alveolar consolidation indicative of bacterial pneumonia, and antibiotic treatment was given unnecessarily. **B,** The lateral chest radiograph better demonstrates air trapping in the right lung base, with flattening of the right hemidiaphragm (*arrow*).

Table 54-2

Most Common Organisms Causing Pulmonary Infections in Childhood

Organism	Characteristic Clinical Features	Typical Radiographic Findings and Sequelae
Viruses		
RNA Viruses		
RSV	Bronchiolitis (winter)	Interstitial pneumonia
HMV	Bronchiolitis (winter)	Interstitial pneumonia
Parainfluenza	Bronchiolitis (fall, spring)	Interstitial pneumonia
Influenza	"Bird flu," pandemic flu	Interstitial pneumonia
Corona	SARS	Interstitial pneumonia
Measles	Nonimmunized, opportunistic	Atypical pneumonia
DNA viruses		
Adenovirus	Necrotizing bronchopneumonia	Bronchiolitis obliterans
CMV	Congenital, opportunistic	Ground glass opacity
Varicella	Opportunistic	Pulmonary calcifications
EBV	Infectious mononucleosis, PTLD	Lymphadenopathy
Bacteria		
Aerobic/Facultative		
Streptococcus pneumoniae	De novo, postviral	Acute focal pneumonia
Streptococcus A	Pharyngitis	Bronchopneumonia
Streptococcus B	Prematurity, neonatal pneumonia	Diagnosis of hyaline membrane disease
Staphyloccocus aureus	Postviral, embolic	Bronchopneumonia
Haemophilus Influenzae B	Epiglottitis, vaccination	Atypical pneumonia
Bordetella pertussis	Whooping cough	Atypical pneumonia, "shaggy heart"
Pseudomonas	Opportunistic (CF)	Findings of CF, bronchiectasis
Legionella	Opportunistic	Atypical pneumonia
Anaerobic	Aspiration, debilitated	Lung necrosis, abscess
Bacteria-like		
Chlamydia trachomatis	Infancy, conjunctivitis	Interstitial pneumonia
Chlamydia pneumoniae	School age, bronchitis	Peribronchitis
Mycoplasma	School age, atypical pneumonia	Interstitial pneumonia, atypical
Mycobacterium tuberculosis	TB, opportunistic	Primary, miliary, postprimary
NTM	NTM disease, opportunistic	Mimics TB
Fungi		
Aspergillus	Aspergilloma, invasive disease	Halo, air crescent signs
Histoplasma	Histoplasmosis	Mimics TB, calcified granulomas
Coccidioides	Coccidioiodomycosis	Mimics TB
Pneumocystis	Opportunistic	Ground glass opacities, interstitial pneumonia
Candida	Opportunistic, debilitated	Nodules
Parasites		
Paragonimus	Ingestion of uncooked crustaceans	Nodules, ring shadows
Echinococcus	Contact with infestated dogs	Fluid-filled masses, with or without rupture
Others	Visceral larva migrans, Löffler syndrome	PIE

DNA, deoxyribonucleic acid; *CF,* cystic fibrosis; *CMV,* cytomegalovirus; *EBV,* Epstein-Barr virus; *HMV,* human metapneumovirus; *NTM,* nontuberculous mycobacteria; *PIE,* pulmonary infiltrates with eosinophilia; *PTLD,* posttransplantation lymphoproliferative disorder; *RNA,* ribonucleic acid; *RSV,* respiratory syncytial virus; *SARS,* severe acute respiratory syndrome; *TB,* tuberculosis.

occasionally seen in nonimmunized or immunosuppressed children. An atypical measles pneumonia was noted during the 1970s and 1980s in patients who were immunized with a killed measles vaccine that was in use from 1963 to 1967. Atypical measles pneumonia followed exposure to measles or vaccination with the live vaccine and was characterized by a prodromal period of rash and flulike illness.

DNA Viruses Adenovirus pneumonia is responsible for about 5% of respiratory tract disease in infants and children, with a peak age between 6 months and 5 years.[31] It is a common cause of viral pneumonia, along with RSV, parainfluenza virus, and influenza virus. Adenovirus has also been associated with a pertussis–like syndrome. Although often relatively benign, adenoviral infection may be severe and even fatal in young infants, particularly when caused by the recently identified serotype Ad14.[34]

Cytomegalovirus (CMV) is a cause of congenital infection of the lungs, the liver, and the central nervous system, and causes hematologic changes of petechiae, purpura, hemolytic anemia, and atypical lymphocytes. These same systems are involved in acquired disease, but the disease is less severe. Children with a compromised immune status are at lifelong risk for CMV infection, and it is frequently seen in patients with acquired immunodeficiency syndrome (AIDS) and in children treated with cyclosporine.

Varicella (chickenpox) pneumonia is relatively rare, but immunocompromised children are at risk for progressive varicella and more severe pulmonary involvement as well as for meningoencephalitis and hepatitis. These children are severely ill, with extensive rashes and high fever; chest pain and hemoptysis are frequent. Epstein-Barr virus (EBV) infects B-lymphocytes and pharyngeal and possibly pulmonary epithelial cells. It is associated with infectious mononucleosis, a common disease in older children and young adults, presenting with fever, pharyngitis, and adenopathy. The disease may be suspected if the tonsils and adenoid are markedly enlarged. EBV is frequently associated with posttransplantation lymphoproliferative disorder, lymphomas complicating immune deficiency disorders, and lymphocytic interstitial pneumonitis (with or without associated human immunodeficiency virus [HIV] infection).

Imaging Bilateral interstitial opacities with peribronchial thickening and hyperinflation (see Fig. 54-1), thought to represent viral bronchiolitis, are nonspecific and are, in fact, indicative of an acute pulmonary infection of any cause (viral or bacterial) in young children.[1,15] Pleural effusions are rare in purely viral lung infections. Radiologic abnormalities often clear slowly and lag behind clinical improvement. Complications are superimposed bacterial infection (often hospital-acquired), and postinfectious bronchiolitis obliterans, bronchiectasis, or both.[2] These latter conditions, which frequently follow an adenovirus infection, are characterized by features of chronic air trapping and atelectasis resulting from bronchial dysfunction; mosaic perfusion abnormalities, peribronchial thickening, chronic atelectasis and bronchiectasis, best seen on computed tomography (CT).[2] Swyer-James-MacLeod syndrome is characterized by a unilateral small hyperlucent lung, which exhibits hypoperfusion and chronic bronchiectasis (e-Fig. 54-2).

In RSV infection, the lungs are often quite clear, or focal areas of superimposed atelectasis may be noted (see Fig. 54-1); when present, these predict a need for more prolonged mechanical ventilation.[40]

In mild influenza infection, initial chest radiographs are normal or may demonstrate nonspecific prominence of peribronchial markings and hyperinflation. In children with a more severe clinical course, bilateral symmetric and multifocal areas of consolidation, often associated with ground-glass opacities, are seen (e-Fig. 54-3).[41]

The radiographic manifestations of SARS are typically mild, with interstitial thickening, which may progress to focal consolidation.[42,43] In children, unlike in adults, no lymphadenopathy, pleural effusion, or cavitation is reported.[44] However, abnormalities may persist on thin-section CT in older children for up to 12 months following infection.[45]

Measles virus is thought to be the cause of giant cell pneumonia, which produces a diffuse reticulonodular bronchopneumonia-like radiographic pattern (e-Fig. 54-4), with hilar node enlargement and superimposed bacterial infection, usually affecting the lower lobes. Atypical measles pneumonia following vaccination with, or exposure to, live virus was characterized by extensive nonsegmental parenchymal consolidation, with pulmonary nodules, hilar lymph node enlargement, and pleural effusion being common.

Adenovirus may cause necrotizing bronchopneumonia, bronchitis, or bronchiolitis. Radiographic features are nonspecific but usually include bronchial wall thickening, peribronchiolar densities, air trapping, and patchy or confluent consolidations.[30] Adenopathy is more common than in other viral pneumonias. Bronchiectasis or bronchiolitis obliterans may be a permanent sequel (see e-Fig. 54-2).[30,31,46]

In children infected with CMV, often, a progressive interstitial pneumonitis is seen (e-Fig. 54-5). Gallium-67 scintigraphy may show abnormal uptake in the lungs of patients who have a normal chest CT.[47]

Findings in varicella are similar to those of measles pneumonia. Multiple focal calcifications frequently develop after severe chickenpox pneumonia (e-Fig. 54-6).

In EBV infection, hilar and mediastinal lymph node enlargement may be seen (e-Fig. 54-7). Pulmonary involvement is uncommon but is characterized by bilateral reticular perihilar infiltrates.[48]

Treatment and Follow-up Effective antiviral therapies have not been established, and treatment of viral pulmonary infections is mainly supportive. Experimental treatments to correct the acquired surfactant deficiency and dysfunction that occurs in critically ill infants with viral pulmonary infections are actively being investigated.[37] With a few exceptions, the use of extracorporeal membrane oxygenation to treat severe respiratory failure from ARDS, which frequently complicates severe infections, has not lead to better outcomes than that of optimal less invasive supportive care.[37] Certain high-risk infants may qualify for prophylactic injection of monoclonal antibodies against the F-glycoprotein of RSV. Since the most important complication of viral pulmonary infection is a superimposed bacterial infection, this should be actively looked for and treated with antibiotics when confirmed.[2]

Pulmonary Infections Caused by Bacteria and Bacteria-Like Organisms

Bacterial pulmonary infections are acquired through inhalation, hematogenously, or rarely by direct extension of chest wall or extrathoracic sites. Their course is determined by the balance between the virulence of the organism and the host immune response (mainly humoral, B-cell–mediated immunity, and macrophageal activity). They are characterized by alveolar airspace consolidation, visible as one or more focal lung opacities that exhibit air bronchograms and obliterate normal air–soft tissue interfaces (the silhouette sign). Pleural effusions are common. The most common bacteria and bacteria-like agents causing pulmonary infections in children are listed in Table 54-2.

In young children, the classic segmental or lobar airspace consolidation is rarely present, and it is nearly absent in neonates. This is reflected by the reported low 30% positive predictive value of radiographic criteria for a bacterial cause of pneumonia, accounting for a widespread overprescription of antibiotics and development of antibiotic resistant bacteria.[1,21] On the other hand, the high 92% negative predictive value of radiographic criteria for bacterial pneumonia is helpful, allowing clinicians to withhold antibiotics in symptomatic children with a negative chest radiograph and to focus on other potential sources of the fever.[1,21] It is, therefore, important not to overcall pediatric chest radiographs for the presence of a pulmonary infection, which is the most common interpretation error made by radiologists unfamiliar with pediatric imaging.[49,50]

Clinically occult pneumonia may be diagnosed with radiography in up to 19% of children less than 5 years old with fever of unknown origin and leucocytosis, although a more recent study found a lower incidence (5.3%) and a low utility of radiography when cough was not one of the presenting symptoms in this setting.[51,52]

AEROBIC AND FACULTATIVE ORGANISMS

Streptococcus pneumoniae

Etiology   This organism is the most common cause of bacterial pneumonia in children less than 5 years of age. It is a gram-positive diplococcus, which infects healthy patients but also commonly attacks those with underlying illness, including the hospitalized and immunocompromised, and children with sickle cell anemia.[53] A strong association with a preceding viral infection, in particular influenza, is seen.[54] The virally activated respiratory epithelium has an increased expression of receptors for pneumococcal attachment.[55] In the usual case of an infected but otherwise healthy child, the onset is acute with fever, headache, and abdominal or chest pain. The pulse and respirations are rapid. By the second day, cough, expiratory grunts, rales, and pleural friction rub may be heard. Rapid clinical resolution usually occurs within 24 to 48 hours after treatment with antibiotics in patients with uncomplicated infections. However, a rapid increase has been seen in the incidence of partially or fully penicillin-resistant strains of *S. pneumoniae*.[56] Following the institution of conjugate pneumococcal vaccination, the proportion of children younger than 5 years with suspected occult pneumococcal pneumonia confirmed by radiography decreased from 15% to 9%.[57]

Imaging   Pneumococcal pneumonia is usually confined to one lobe, but only rarely is the entire lobe consolidated. A pattern of homogeneous airspace consolidation is usual but not invariable, especially in the presence of underlying lung disease. This pneumonia may initially have a strikingly round appearance in children younger than 8 years (Fig. 54-8), simulating an intrapulmonary mass or abscess, until it spreads

further to reach a normal anatomic boundary such as a fissure.[1,58,59] Pleural effusion, empyema (e-Fig. 54-9), and lung necrosis (e-Fig. 54-10) are infrequent complications, seen in less than 30% of patients. Resolution on radiographs is usually complete by 6 to 8 weeks.

Streptococcus Pyogenes (Group A Streptococci) and *Agalactiae* (Group B Streptococci)

Etiology   Group A streptococcus usually produces tonsillitis or pharyngitis. In the 1990s, *S. pyogenes* pneumonia, often associated with the toxic shock syndrome, was increasingly reported in childhood. It may occur de novo in a healthy child or follow a viral infection. In neonates, group B streptococcus is a leading cause of sepsis, including pneumonia and meningitis.

Imaging   Group A *Streptococcus* produces a bronchopneumonia in a segmental configuration with either homogeneous or patchy consolidation, which frequently affects a lower lobe. It may be bilateral. Pleural effusion and empyema are common in untreated cases. Lung abscess may be a complication. Clinically and on imaging studies, this pneumonia is very similar to staphylococcal pneumonia, although pneumatoceles are less commonly seen. Group B *Streptococcus* may accompany or mimic hyaline membrane disease in neonates, and is radiographically difficult to distinguish from it, although the presence of pleural effusion favors (concomitant) infection.

Staphylococcus aureus

Etiology   This gram-positive, catalase-positive coccus primarily affects infants under the age of 1 year (70%). In debilitated patients, it occurs as a superinfection, particularly in the hospital. The incidence of "primary" staphylococcal pneumonia has decreased markedly since the early 1950s. However, staphylococcal pneumonia secondary to septicemia rather than inhalation of organisms is increasing and occurs in older children. This form of "embolic" disease may present with multiple nodular masses or abscesses (e-Fig. 54-11). This evolving pulmonary pattern in a child with sepsis should

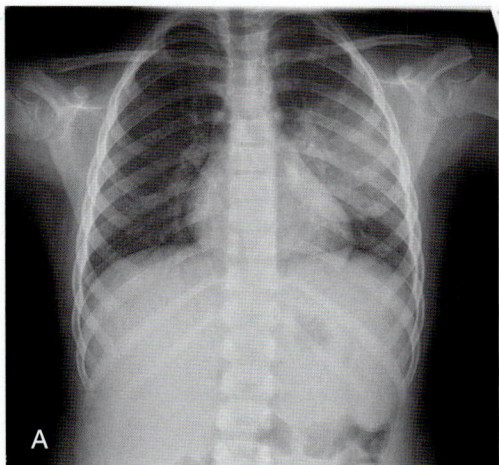
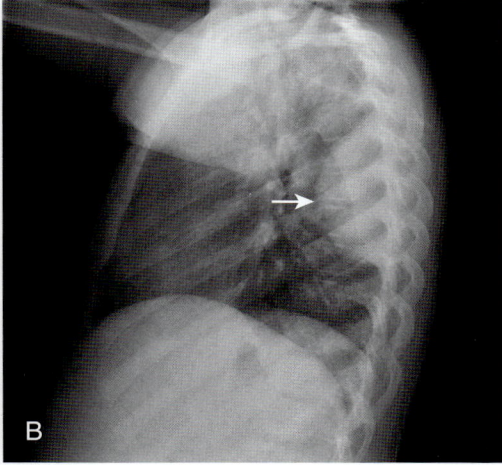

Figure 54-8   Streptococcal round pneumonia in a 5.5-year-old girl presenting with fever and left-sided back and rib pain. Frontal (**A**) and lateral (**B**) radiographs show alveolar consolidation in the superior segment of the left lower lobe with a rounded appearance (*arrow in B*). Note in *A* the visibility of the left hilar shadow, which is superimposed on the posteriorly located pulmonary pseudomass (hilar overlay sign).

initiate a search for a distant source of infection, often in bones, joints, or skin.[60] Despite extensive pulmonary disease, if recovery occurs it is usually without sequelae. In comparison with methicillin-sensitive strains, methicillin-resistant strains of community-acquired *S. aureus* cause more serious pneumonias in younger children.[61,62]

Imaging In contrast to pneumococcal pneumonia, staphylococcal pneumonia is a lobular or bronchopneumonia, which begins in the airways rather than in the alveoli. Consolidation of peribronchiolar acinar units occurs initially in a segmental distribution. This infectious agent is very virulent, and severe hemorrhagic pulmonary edema may develop rapidly. Pneumatoceles are more common than in any other type (also reported in *S. pneumoniae*, *H. influenzae*, and *Escherichia coli* pneumonia) and occur in 40% to 60% of patients.[61,63,64] They usually appear during the first week of the pneumonia and resolve within 3 months. Pneumatoceles often appear as the child is getting better, and their presence does not have prognostic significance. Ten percent of children with staphylococcal pneumonia have a pneumothorax, which may result from the rupture of a pneumatocele.[61,63,64] Pleural effusion and empyema are also very frequent, occurring in more than 90% of children (Fig. 54-12).[64]

Haemophilus Influenzae Type B

Etiology *Haemophilus influenzae* is a gram-negative, rod-shaped bacterium, which was first discovered in 1892 during an influenza pandemic. In infants and young children, it causes bacteremia, pneumonia, cellulitis, epiglottitis, and meningitis. Since 1990, vaccination has markedly reduced the incidence of this pneumonia (<95%).

Imaging The radiographic appearance is nonspecific: pulmonary opacities that often begin as a segmental, interstitial-appearing process progresses to airspace consolidation.[65] Approximately two thirds of cases have unilateral involvement, but more than one lobe is involved 25% of the time.[65] Empyema is a common complication, occurring in about 40%.[65]

Bordetella pertussis

Etiology *Bordetella pertussis* is a gram-negative, aerobic, capsulated coccobacillus. The incidence of pertussis (whooping cough) has decreased significantly with immunization, but it is still seen in young infants, particularly in the unimmunized. This agent is spread by airborne droplets. A characteristic

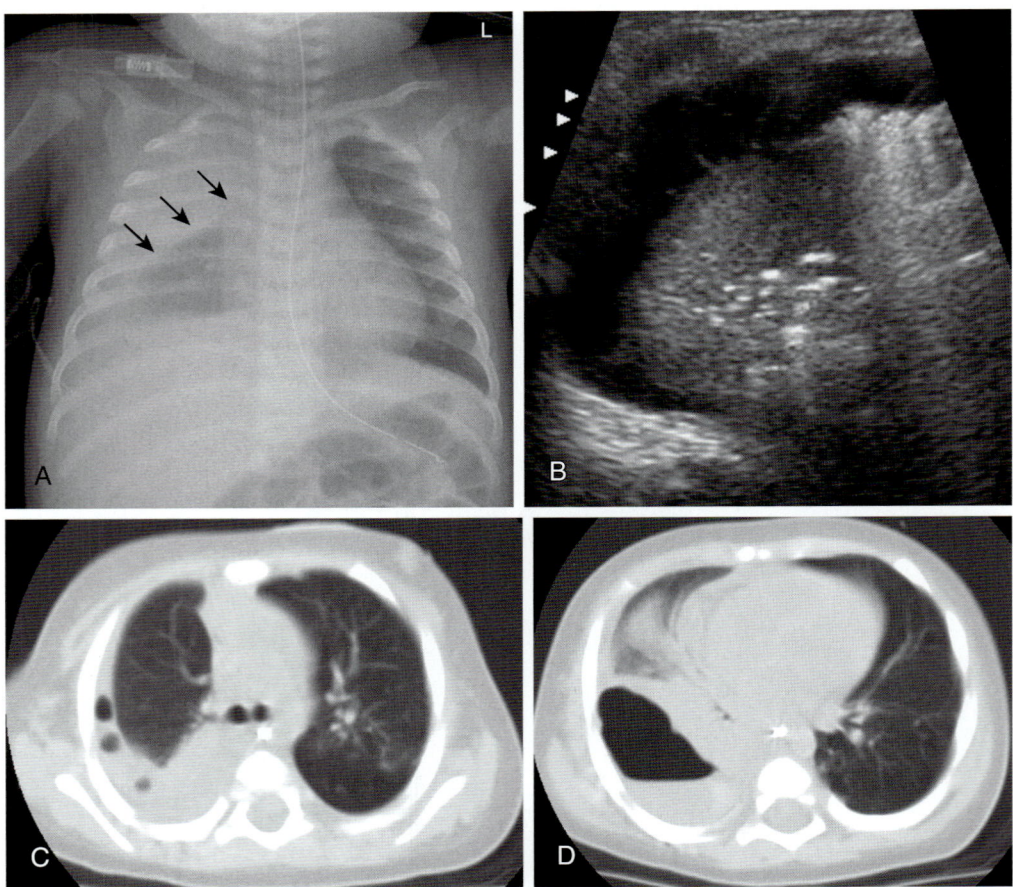

Figure 54-12 Role of cross-sectional imaging in a 7-month-old girl with staphylococcal pneumonia and empyema. **A,** The radiograph demonstrates right pleural thickening, which has a convex margin toward the lung (*arrows*). **B,** The transverse ultrasound image of the right chest shows a complex pleural effusion, containing thin septations. **C** and **D,** Computed tomography confirmed the presence of loculated pleural fluid collections, containing trapped gas bubbles (**C**) and, more inferiorly, an air-fluid level (**D**). (Reprinted with permission granted by Springer-Verlag of Westra SJ, Choy G. What imaging should be performed for the diagnosis and management of pulmonary infections?. *Pediatr Radiol.* 2009;39(suppl 2):S178-S183 (Figure 1, page S179)).

clinical sign is the paroxysmal cough (whoop). Even after convalescence, the patient's cough may persist for weeks or months. In China, the disease has been termed "the cough of 100 days."

Imaging Abnormal but nonspecific findings are present in most patients with pertussis. Because this is an airways-centered disease, it may mimic viral airways disease and pneumonia. The classic appearance is that of the "shaggy heart" (e-Fig. 54-13). However, nonspecific findings such as hyperaeration, atelectasis, segmental consolidations, and hilar lymphadenopathy are seen more commonly. Radiographic changes may persist for several weeks. Bronchiectasis may be a long-term complication.

Pseudomonas aeruginosa

Etiology *Pseudomonas aeruginosa* is a gram-negative, aerobic, rod-shaped bacterium, which is an opportunistic pathogen in humans. Lungs, urinary tract, and kidneys are the common sites of infection. *P. aeruginosa* usually occurs as a nosocomial infection and is a major problem for patients with cystic fibrosis, in which thick layers of lung mucus and alginate produced by the bacteria may limit the diffusion of oxygen. Diagnosis of this infection depends on the Gram stain of sputum or other bacteriologic specimens (e.g., lung tissue, bronchoscopic aspiration, and bronchoalveolar lavage fluid).

Imaging When the patient is infected by airway contamination, the process tends to involve both lung bases, with extensive bilateral parenchymal consolidation, patchy areas of disease with small abscess formation, or small regions of lobular emphysema. In the bacteremic form, widespread patchy or nodular shadows may be found throughout both lungs. Lung necrosis may also occur.

Legionella pneumophila

Etiology *Legionella pneumophila* is an aerobic, pleomorphic, flagellated, gram-negative bacterium. It is the cause legionnaires' disease, is mainly seen in immunocompromised patients and is rare in children.[66,67]

Imaging Typically, initial radiographs show poorly marginated opacities that progress to more widespread consolidation, often accompanied by pleural effusion. Presentation as multiple pulmonary nodules has been reported but is less common.[67] Cavitation and abscess formation are complications.

ANAEROBIC ORGANISMS

Etiology Anaerobic bacteria are uncommonly responsible for pneumonia and lung abscess.[68] Aspiration is the most common route of exposure, and *Fusobacterium* species, *Bacteroides* species, *Peptococcus*, and *Peptostreptococcus* may be cultured from the abscess or the pleural fluid.

Imaging Usually, consolidation occurs in the lower respiratory tract, and clinical course is slowly progressive (e-Fig. 54-14). Lung abscess (e-Fig. 54-15) and fulminant necrotizing pneumonia may eventually develop.

BACTERIA-LIKE ORGANISMS

Chlamydophila trachomatis and pneumoniae

Etiology *Chlamydia trachomatis* is an intracellular bacterium commonly found in the genital tract, where it causes urethritis in men and cervicitis in women. In neonates, it causes conjunctivitis, which is contracted during passage through an infected birth canal. Chlamydia is a common cause of pneumonia in infants between 2 and 14 weeks of age.[69] The infant is affected by a staccato-like cough and may have conjunctivitis and eosinophilia, although these are not invariable findings. Usually, the patient is afebrile, with a radiographic appearance suggesting an illness more severe than the clinical findings indicate. Recently, *C. pneumoniae* has been recognized as a common agent causing community-acquired bronchitis and mild atypical pneumonia in school-age children.[3] The clinical response to appropriate therapy is usually rapid.

Imaging The radiographic findings of *C. trachomatis* infections are nonspecific (e-Fig. 54-16), but when they are analyzed in conjunction with clinical findings, the disease may be suspected. Bilateral involvement is usual.[70] The lungs are usually hyperaerated with increased linear density and patchy areas of consolidation, probably representing subsegmental atelectasis. Lobar consolidation is rare.[70]

Mycoplasma pneumoniae

Etiology This organism is one of the most common causes of pulmonary infection in childhood, accounting for 10% to 30% of pediatric pneumonias.[71] It is most often seen in school-age children and is uncommon in children less than 3 years of age. It is acquired by droplet inhalation, and it is most commonly noted in families, in schools, and among military recruits. The disease is usually mild, with low-grade malaise, headache, fever, and cough. Stevens-Johnson syndrome (erythema multiforme) may complicate the disease. The diagnosis is established by culturing the organisms from sputum or by demonstration of rising specific *Mycoplasma* titers. A rise in the titer of cold agglutinins is seen in about 50% of cases but is nonspecific; of greater diagnostic value are immunofluorescent and complement fixation tests for specific antibodies and the recently developed molecular probes.[72]

Imaging This classic "atypical pneumonia" has a radiographic appearance that frequently mimics viral pulmonary infection (Fig. 54-17).[1] In early cases, a fine reticular pattern suggestive of interstitial inflammation may be seen.[73] This tends to be in a segmental distribution and in some cases progresses to airspace consolidation suggestive of bacterial pulmonary infection.[74,75] Small pleural effusions are seen in up to 20% of patients. Hilar adenopathy is common. Bilateral involvement occurs in approximately one third of cases. The radiographic changes are frequently more severe compared with the patient's clinical condition. Resolution is often slow and lags behind clinical improvement.

Treatment and Follow-up Treatment of bacterial pulmonary infections is with antibiotics and other chemotherapeutic agents, focused on the causative agent, either presumed

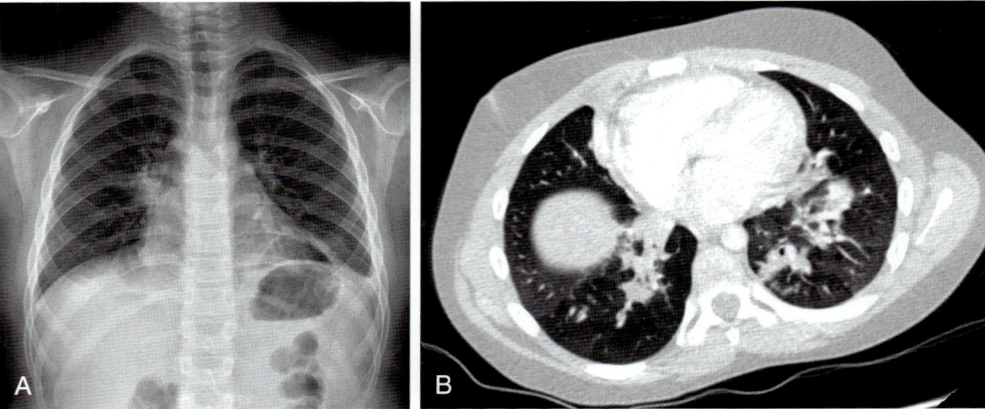

Figure 54-17 Mycoplasma atypical pneumonia in an 8-year-old girl who presented with fatigue, low-grade fever, and cough. **A,** The chest radiograph shows irregularity of the right hilum and bibasillar infiltration. **B,** Contrast-enhanced computed tomography demonstrates bilateral bronchopneumonia in the lower lobes. A direct fluorescent antibody test from nasopharyngeal aspirate confirmed the diagnosis.

(empirical treatment) or preferably directed by the results of culture or immunoassay. Complications of bacterial pulmonary infections are lung necrosis, abscess, empyema, and bronchopleural fistula.[2] Ultrasonography is the most effective initial cross-sectional modality when pleural complications are suspected, whereas CT is the preferred modality to diagnose parenchymal complications.[76-82] A review of the diagnostic performance of CT versus radiography confirms the expected higher sensitivity of CT.[78,83-90] CT is more sensitive than radiography to determine the cause of a delayed response to medical and percutaneous treatment of pediatric chest infections, but it is unclear whether this affects the eventual outcomes of treatment.[78,89] Cavitary lung necrosis is demonstrated well by CT.[90] However, most of the affected children recover without permanent sequelae on clinical and imaging follow-up.[1] For this reason, documentation of complete resolution of pneumonia in children who are otherwise healthy is not indicated.[1,22,91] CT and, potentially, magnetic resonance imaging (MRI) are helpful, however, to fully investigate any underlying focal anatomic cause such as anomalous bronchi, bronchogenic cysts, sequestrations, or bronchial atresia (Fig. 54-18), which may underlie recurrent or chronic pneumonia.[1,92-94] Conversely, the value of CT to monitor diffuse processes that predispose to repeated pulmonary infections such as chronic granulomatous disease of childhood and cystic fibrosis remains controversial.[95,96] Children with these chronic conditions will accumulate a substantial radiation burden from repeated examinations during their lifetime, and the theoretical risks of these procedures with regard to the induction of cancer will have to be balanced against the immediate clinical benefits, which remain unproven.[97] MRI has promise as a nonradiating cross-sectional imaging alternative for examination of these conditions.[92]

Mycobacterial Infection—Pulmonary Tuberculosis

Etiology TB is caused by *Mycobacterium tuberculosis*, an aerobic, nonmotile, non–spore-forming rod. Although the resurgence of TB noted in the United States in the 1980s and 1990s has declined, in 2003, 15,000 new cases were reported, and the rate of decline appears to be slowing.[98] The incidence continues to increase worldwide.[99-101] Of all new cases of TB, 5% to 6% are in children less than 15 years of age, and approximately 60% of new childhood infections occur in children less than 5 years of age.[99] A significant number of new cases occur in immunocompromised patients, particularly in those with HIV infection.[102-104] The incidence of TB has decreased in the general population but has increased in the foreign-born population, accounting for 50% of new cases in the United States.

Inhalation of the tubercle bacillus is the most common route of infection in children. Congenital infection is extremely rare and is most often secondary to hematogenous spread across the placenta during pregnancy or from contaminated amniotic fluid. Pulmonary TB infection may be categorized into three groups: (1) primary infection; (2) miliary infection; and (3) reactive or postprimary infection.

The length of the incubation period of TB depends on the size of the initial inhaled inoculum and varies from 2 to 10 weeks; it ends when the patient becomes sensitized (i.e., has a positive skin test). Annual skin testing in high-risk groups is recommended. In the low-risk child, skin testing at 12 to 15 months, at 4 to 6 years, and in adolescence is a reasonable approach.[105] In asymptomatic primary tuberculosis, the disease is detected because of a routine skin test, and chest radiography is most often normal. In endemic areas, radiographs may demonstrate hilar lymphadenopathy only.[106-108] Because children produce little sputum, they do not transmit the disease to one another, and a search for the infected adult must be undertaken. The index child is always treated with antibiotics. Following this treatment, no evidence suggests that the few children with a positive skin test and abnormal findings on chest radiography have a clinical course or prognosis different from that of the majority of children with a positive skin test and normal chest radiographs.

If radiographs are positive, usually, a single small primary focus is present (70%), located in the subpleural region. From there, the bacilli spread through the lymphatics to regional hilar and mediastinal lymph nodes (primary complex, e-Fig. 54-19). In postobstructive tuberculosis, large lymph nodes may cause extrinsic bronchial compression, and granuloma formation may cause endobronchial obstruction, leading to segmental air trapping, atelectasis (e-Fig. 54-20), or both. The presence of airway obstruction in a child who does not appear to be sick may spuriously suggest the possibility of an inhaled foreign body.[109] For a few patients, bronchoscopy is

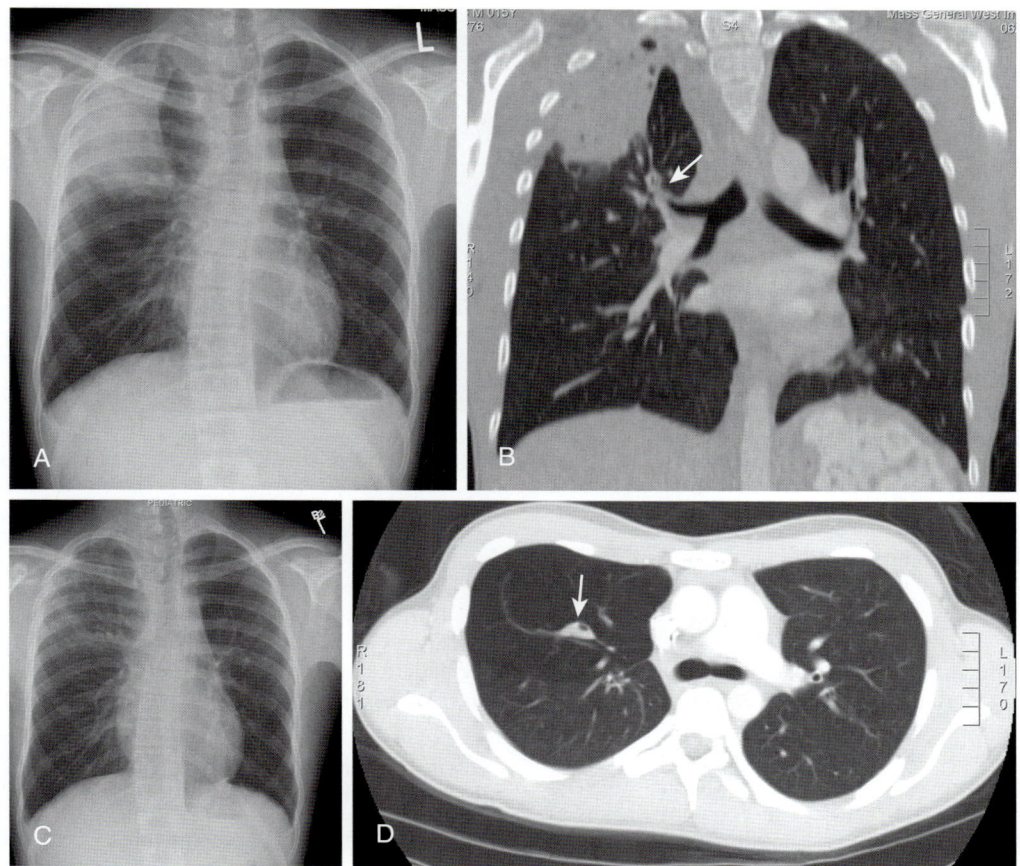

Figure 54-18   Role of computed tomography (CT) in recurrent pneumonia in a 15-year-old boy with bronchogenic cyst and bronchial atresia. **A,** The chest radiograph shows consolidation in the right upper lobe and right upper mediastinal widening. **B,** The CT scan shows atresia in the apical bronchus of the right upper lobe (*arrow*) and right mediastinal widening caused by a bronchogenic cyst. **C** and **D,** The follow-up chest radiograph (**C**) and CT scan (**D**) show near-complete resolution of the pneumonia, with persistent architectural distortion of the right upper lobe. The atretic bronchus contains inspissated mucus (*arrow in D*). Right upper lobectomy and resection of the bronchogenic cyst was performed.

required to diagnose the initial endobronchial lesion.[110] Chronic obstruction may lead to bronchiectasis. Calcification occurs after caseation of the primary lesion and is seen earlier in infants (6 months after infection, e-Fig. 54-21) than in older children (2 to 3 years after infection, e-Fig. 54-22).

Progressive primary pulmonary tuberculosis is a serious but rare complication.[111] Progressive enlargement of the primary complex occurs, with caseation of the lesion followed by liquefaction (Fig. 54-23). The lesion may rupture into a bronchus, establishing new foci of disease (Fig. 54-24). Affected children are usually quite ill, with weight loss, dyspnea, anorexia, and failure to thrive. Pleural involvement in TB (e-Fig. 54-25) is usually noted in children older than 2 years, who present with fever, chest pain, and symptoms of pneumonia.[112] The pleural fluid usually has few organisms, many white cells, a high protein content, and a low glucose content.

The host response to lymphohematogenous spread is varied, with immunosuppressed patients being at greatest risk. A few children present with high spiking fevers, hepatomegaly, and positive blood culture (chronic tuberculous bacteremia, e-Fig. 54-26). Miliary tuberculosis usually occurs within 6 months of the primary infection and results from lymphohematogenous dissemination of *M. tuberculosis* from the primary complex (e-Fig. 54-27).

Reactivation or postprimary TB infection is the classic adult or adolescent form of the disease. It is the result of growth of previously dormant bacilli in the apices of the lung. The reactivated lesions in the apical and posterior segments of the upper lobes are composed of foci of caseous necrosis with surrounding edema, hemorrhage, and mononuclear cells. These lesions may liquefy and rupture into a bronchus, spreading the bacilli (e-Fig. 54-28). Cavitation with scarring occurs (Fig. 54-29). Reactivation of tuberculosis is rare in children who were infected with primary tuberculosis before the age of 2 years. It is much more frequent in children whose primary infection occurred after the age of 7 years, particularly if they were initially infected near puberty.[98]

Imaging   Primary TB infection of the lung falls under the subcategory of subacute dense focal (atypical) pneumonia (see e-Fig. 54-19).[15,113-115] Chest radiography is insensitive to primary infection.[116,117] In children with a positive skin test, screening with only a frontal radiograph is sufficient in nonendemic areas, whereas in endemic areas the addition of the lateral radiograph is beneficial for improved detection of hilar lymphadenopathy.[106,118] Almost half (43%) of children diagnosed with tuberculous meningitis have normal chest radiographs.[119] CT typically shows a subtle parenchymal opacity

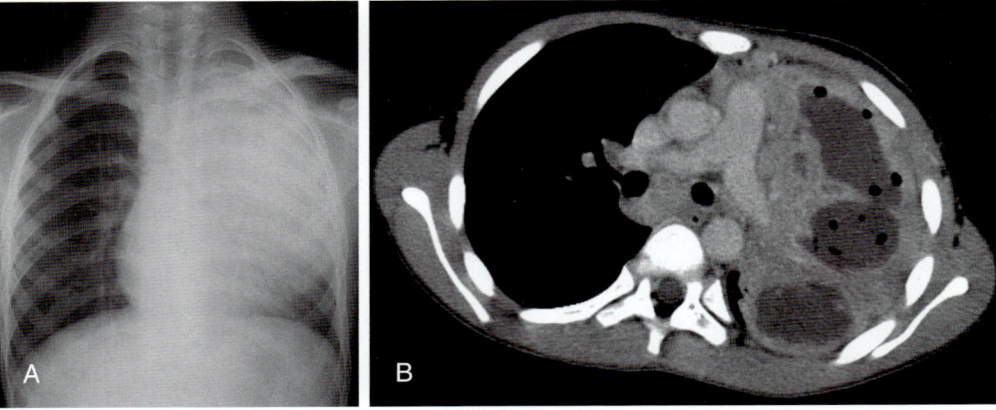

Figure 54-23   Progressive primary tuberculosis in an older child. **A,** The radiograph shows dense consolidation with expansion in the left upper lobe, which contains an air-filled cavity. **B,** Contrast-enhanced computed tomography demonstrates extensive liquefactive parenchymal disease (Courtesy of Bernard Laya, M.D.).

with associated lymph node enlargement. In a large study of children with TB, when initial chest radiography was positive, hilar and peritracheal lymphadenopathy was the most common finding, present in 92% of the cases.[102,104] Studies using CT confirm that infected patients frequently have abnormal lymph nodes (see e-Figs. 54-19 through 54-21), but 50% may not have nodes larger than 1 cm.[120] Affected nodes typically are large and of low density with rim enhancement and calcify later in the course of the disease. The adenopathy may be contralateral to the parenchymal disease in one third of patients. Chest radiography is most useful for following the course of disease in children with recent conversion to tuberculin sensitivity and for the early detection of miliary TB infection (see e-Fig. 54-27), which produces a "snowstorm" pattern in the lung, liver, and spleen.[121] Occasionally, this may be present before there is overt clinical manifestation of the disease; as expected, CT is more sensitive than chest radiography.[99,100] Regression of abnormalities is slow and may require from 6 months to 2 years to resolve on radiography and up to 15 months on CT evaluation (see e-Fig. 54-21 and Fig. 54-29).[104,122]

Treatment and Follow-up   TB is treated with a combination of antibiotics and chemotherapeutic agents to which the organism is sensitive.[123] Multidrug resistance to the regimens is an increasing problem worldwide, but strategies for

effective treatment and reinforcing patient adherence have proven successful, even in the developing world.[123] Because of the limited sensitivity of radiography, cross-sectional imaging with CT, when locally available, is frequently helpful for patient management (see e-Figs. 54-19 and 21, Figs 54-23, and 54-24; and e-Figs. 54-26 and 54-28).[100,103,110-112,121]

Nontuberculous Mycobacterial Pulmonary Infection

Etiology   Nontuberculous mycobacteria (NTM) are widely distributed in the environment and may produce infection in patients with normal immunity, although infection is significantly more frequent in patients with immunodeficiencies (particularly HIV infection) or with altered local defenses (e.g., in cystic fibrosis or ciliary dyskinesia). Although the signs and symptoms of NTM pulmonary infection are variable and nonspecific, affected pediatric patients usually present with chronic cough, fever, chills, night sweats, dyspnea on exertion, and weight loss. The diagnosis is based on clinical, radiographic, and bacteriologic criteria.

Imaging   Although the radiologic findings of pulmonary NTM disease are variable, depending on the presence or absence of underlying disease, typical findings include multiple nodules, consolidation, and cavitation. Mediastinal or

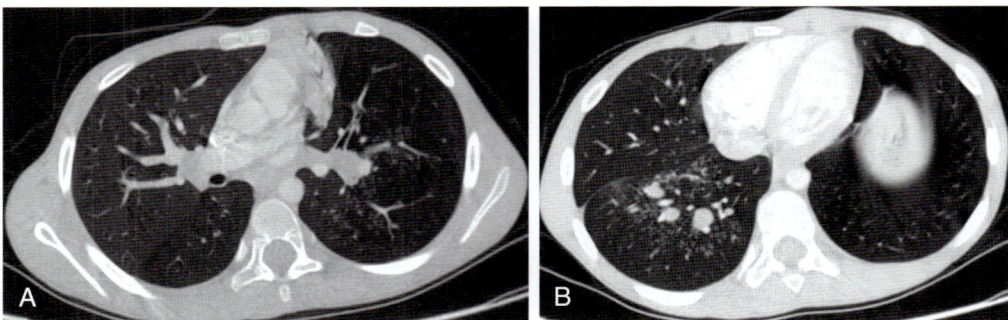

Figure 54-24   Active pulmonary tuberculosis in a 9-year-old boy who presented with cough and fever. **A** and **B,** Contrast-enhanced computed tomography demonstrates centrilobular nodules and branching linear opacities ("tree-in-bud" pattern) in both lower lobes. Dilated fluid-filled bronchi are adjacent to areas of parenchymal abnormality. Atelectasis is also present in the paramediastinal parenchyma of the left lung. Culture of bronchial lavage fluid confirmed the diagnosis.

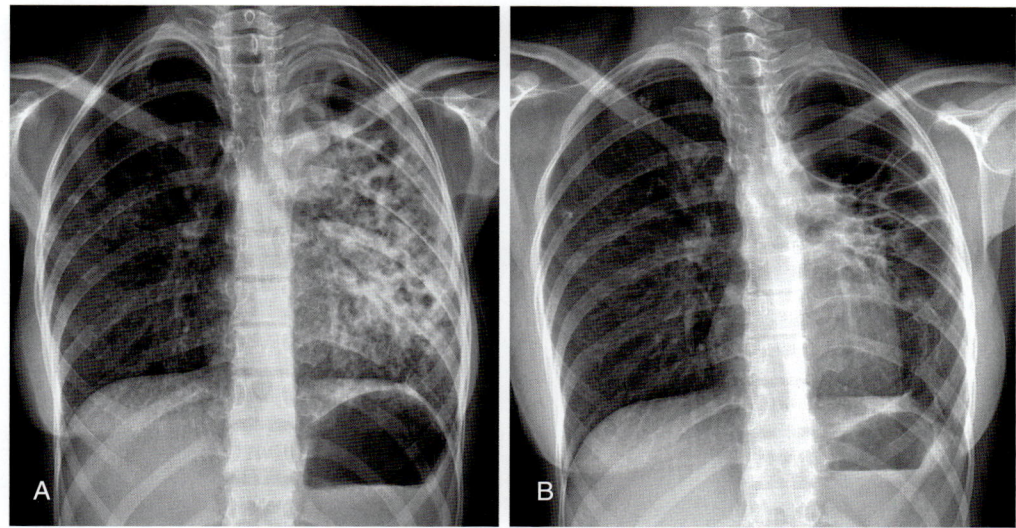

Figure 54-29 Postprimary tuberculosis (TB) with scarring and cavitation in a 13-year-old girl who presented with weight loss and productive cough, and whose mother had a history of TB. **A,** The initial radiograph shows diffuse opacities in the left lung associated with bronchiectasis. Sputum culture indicated *Mycobacterium tuberculosis* infection. **B,** After 1 year of appropriate anti-TB therapy, the abnormalities had markedly improved, with extensive scarring in the left lung. The disease was no longer clinically active.

hilar adenopathy similar to that of TB may be present (e-Fig. 54-30). NTM may also complicate or cause bronchiectasis.

Treatment and Follow-up Successful treatment depends on tailoring drug treatment to the type of NTM cultured. Because NTM pulmonary infection could be indolent, long-term clinical and radiological study follow-up (months to years) may be required at relatively short intervals.

Pulmonary Infections Caused by Fungi

Fungal infections of the lung predominantly affect children with a suppressed immune system, mainly those with defective T-cell immunity and granulocyte function, either congenital (DiGeorge syndrome, chronic granulomatous disease of childhood) or acquired (AIDS, those undergoing chemotherapy for malignancies). In immunocompromised children, CT may add both sensitivity and specificity to radiography and should be performed with a low threshold.[84,88] The imaging appearance of fungal infections is typically within the miliary or nodular pneumonia category.[15] The nodules may be surrounded in the acute phase by a ground-glass halo, indicating the angioinvasiveness of the organism, and may eventually calcify.[2,15] Hilar and mediastinal lymphadenopathy is frequently seen, and the lymph nodes often calcify, as in TB. The most common fungal agents causing pulmonary infections in children are listed in Table 54-2.

ASPERGILLOSIS

Etiology *Aspergillus* species are a group of ubiquitous molds within the environment that may be cultured from a wide variety of soils, water sources, and decaying organic matter. Pulmonary infection is most often caused by *Aspergillus*

fumigatus. Although pulmonary infection with *Aspergillus* species may take a variety of clinical courses and imaging appearances mainly depend on the affected patients' immune status, it can be grouped into three main categories: (1) fungal ball, (2) allergic bronchopulmonary aspergillosis (ABPA), and (3) invasive aspergillosis.[124] A fungal ball or mycetoma typically grows saprophytically in immunocompetent children with a preexisting cavity often related to cystic fibrosis or postprimary TB. ABPA, characterized by a hypersensitivity response to *Aspergillus* antigens, typically develops in children with cystic fibrosis or asthma.[125] Invasive aspergillosis almost exclusively occurs in immunocompromised children with underlying neutropenia related to bone marrow or solid organ transplantations and others receiving systemic chemotherapy.[124] The organism may produce a bronchocentric or angiocentric lesion and is associated with a high morbidity and mortality.[126] A semi-invasive, less aggressive form of *Aspergillus* infection may be seen in patients with underlying lung disease or in mildly immunocompromised patients.[127]

Imaging A fungal ball typically appears on chest radiographs as an intracavitary mass within a thick-walled cavity usually located in an upper lobe, especially the apical segment (e-Fig. 54-31). CT shows a round or oval-shaped cavity containing a freely mobile soft tissue mass surrounded by a crescent of air (Monad sign).[128] The most common features of ABPA are mucoid impaction within bronchiectasis and segmental and lobar atelectasis. Such dilated bronchi filled with inspissated mucus often cause a homogeneous branching opacity referred to as the *finger-in-glove sign.* Invasive aspergillosis characteristically appears as one or a few nodular opacities randomly distributed throughout the lungs. Distinctive but nonspecific characteristics include the halo sign and the air crescent sign. The *halo sign* refers to an irregular ground-glass opacity surrounding a nodule of infection (Fig. 54-32). The indistinct halo probably represents hemorrhage in lung adjacent to the nodule, resulting from vascular invasion. The *air crescent sign* is an air collection that partially outlines a masslike lesion that

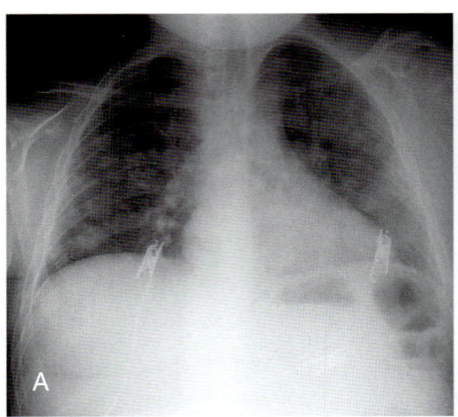
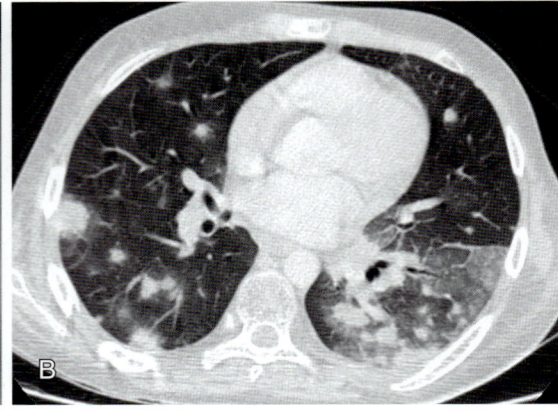

Figure 54-32 Invasive pulmonary aspergillosis in a 14-year-old boy with leukemia, who presented with neutropenia, fever, and a positive serum galactomannan enzyme-linked immunosorbent assay test. **A,** The radiograph shows bilateral ill-defined nodular opacities. **B,** Contrast-enhanced computed tomography demonstrates multiple nodules with, with ground-glass opacity around some of these nodules (the "halo" sign). The diagnosis of invasive pulmonary aspergillosis was made based on the clinical, laboratory, and radiologic findings.

represents a contracting nodule.[128] This sign is noted in well-established *Aspergillus* infections when the host's defense mechanisms have partially recovered.

Treatment and Follow-up   The main treatment goal in children with pulmonary aspergillosis is to correct any underlying immune deficiency and to control the infection with antifungal medications such as voriconazole and liposomal amphotericin B.

HISTOPLASMOSIS

Etiology   Histoplasmosis, caused by *Histoplasma capsulatum*, is common in many parts of the United States. Initial infection is similar to that of the primary tuberculous complex except that in histoplasmosis, large numbers of pulmonary foci are the rule. Histoplasmosis may be categorized into three phases: (1) acute infection, characterized by nonspecific respiratory symptoms that usually develop 12 to 14 days after initial exposure; (2) chronic infection, which may resemble TB; and (3) disseminated infection. The diagnosis of pulmonary histoplasmosis rests on the identification of antigen and the demonstration of *Histoplasma*-specific antibodies. Rapid diagnosis may be obtained from biopsy of the granulomas with special fungal stains. *Histoplasma* may be cultured from lavage or blood specimens, but cultures take a long time to grow and have a low sensitivity.

Imaging   Radiographic findings are similar to TB in all phases of these diseases, and in some cases, they resemble those in coccidioidomycosis (e-Fig. 54-33).[129] Approximately 95% of patients are asymptomatic during the initial infection, and thus the initial exudative phase of the disease is much less obvious radiographically compared with the sequelae of infection.[129] The first phase of the infection is characterized by single or multiple pulmonary nodules that are 1 to 3 cm in size, as well as mediastinal and hilar lymphadenopathy. Pulmonary nodules that have been present for more than a few months usually show central or dystrophic calcification. Calcified mediastinal and hilar lymph nodes are often seen in patients with calcified pulmonary nodules (e-Fig. 54-34). Sarcoidosis may exhibit similar adenopathy. Because

treatment of sarcoidosis involves immunosuppression, histoplasmosis must be excluded, particularly in endemic areas. In children with chronic histoplasmosis, upper lobe consolidations simulating TB infection, sometimes associated with cavitation, may be present. Disseminated histoplasmosis has been observed in infancy, and the imaging findings are similar to those in miliary tuberculosis. Massive hepatosplenomegaly is common in disseminated cases. Granulomatous or calcified foci in the spleen are a frequent incidental finding in endemic regions and are almost diagnostic of disease exposure in an otherwise healthy patient. A rare but devastating result of chronic pulmonary histoplasmosis is mediastinal fibrosis, which may lead to pulmonary artery compression (see e-Fig. 54-33) and terminal pulmonary artery hypertension. It may also result in compression of the superior vena cava, esophagus, trachea, and bronchi.

Treatment and Follow-up   Treatment is merely supportive in asymptomatic and mild cases, but when disseminated histoplasmosis is present, a combination therapy of antifungal agents is given (itraconazole, amphotericin B).

COCCIDIOIDOMYCOSIS

Etiology   Coccidioidomycosis, caused by *Coccidioides immitis* or *C. posadasi*, is acquired by inhalation. Endemic areas in the United States include the semi-arid regions of California, Arizona, New Mexico, and western Texas. The infection is usually self-limiting, and affected children present with mild flulike illness, with fever, cough, headaches, rash, and myalgia. However, severe pulmonary infection may develop in immunocompromised children (particularly those with HIV infection). The diagnosis may be made by positive reaction to the coccidioidin skin test or by positive culture of the sputum or gastric washings.

Imaging   Radiographic examination during the early stages of disease usually shows lobar or segmental airspace consolidation and enlargement of the regional lymph nodes.[130] The pulmonary opacity of primary coccidioidomycosis is similar to that in primary tuberculosis (e-Fig. 54-35). It usually clears after a few weeks—its duration is usually much shorter than in tuberculosis—and residual calcified foci appear later within both the lung and lymph nodes. Small localized or large free pleural effusions may be visualized early.[131] Although small, sharply defined, thin-walled pulmonary cavities are commonly noted in adults, they are uncommon in children.

Treatment and Follow-up Affected children with mild symptoms often do not require treatment. However, immunocompromised children with progressive or disseminated disease are treated with a combination of antifungal agents (amphotericin B, fluconazole, itraconazole, or ketoconazole).

PNEUMOCYSTIS JIROVECI

Etiology *Pneumocystis carinii*, a unicellular organism, that infects humans, was recently renamed *Pneumocystis jiroveci*. Originally considered a parasite, it is currently categorized as a fungus on the basis of molecular similarities to fungal RNA. This potentially life-threatening opportunistic infection most often affects immunodeficient children, particularly those who are infected with HIV and have CD4 counts of less than 100 cells/mm[3]. The clinical onset is variable but often abrupt, with tachypnea, cough, and cyanosis. A marked decrease in the arterial oxygen saturation is seen, with a normal carbon dioxide level.

Imaging The characteristic radiographic findings of *P. jiroveci* pneumonia are symmetric bilateral ground-glass opacities (Fig. 54-36). Such opacities may be diffuse but tend to involve predominately the perihilar regions or middle and lower lung zones.[132,133] Disease progression may result in more confluent, mainly perihilar or diffuse, bilateral airspace consolidation. The underlying pathophysiologic process is alveolar filling by a foamy exudate consisting of surfactant, fibrin, and cellular debris.[134-137] Associated interstitial edema or cellular infiltration may present on CT as septal thickening, intralobular thickening, or both.[138] The combination of such interstitial thickening and ground-glass opacities may produce a CT pattern known as "crazy paving".[139] Terminally, massive consolidation may occur, often complicated by pneumothorax and pneumomediastinum.[140] Pleural effusions are rare.[141]

In 10% to 30% of patient with AIDS who received prophylaxis with aerosolized pentamidine and trimethoprim-sulfamethoxazole, a cystic form of the disease may evolve, characterized by either unilateral or bilateral upper lobe predominant thin-walled cysts.[138] Such pulmonary cysts are associated with pneumothoraces.[142] In recent years, in spite of the advances in the prevention and treatment of *P. jiroveci* infection, several atypical presentations have emerged, including multiple pulmonary nodules, mass lesions, pleural effusion, and lymph node enlargement.[143-146]

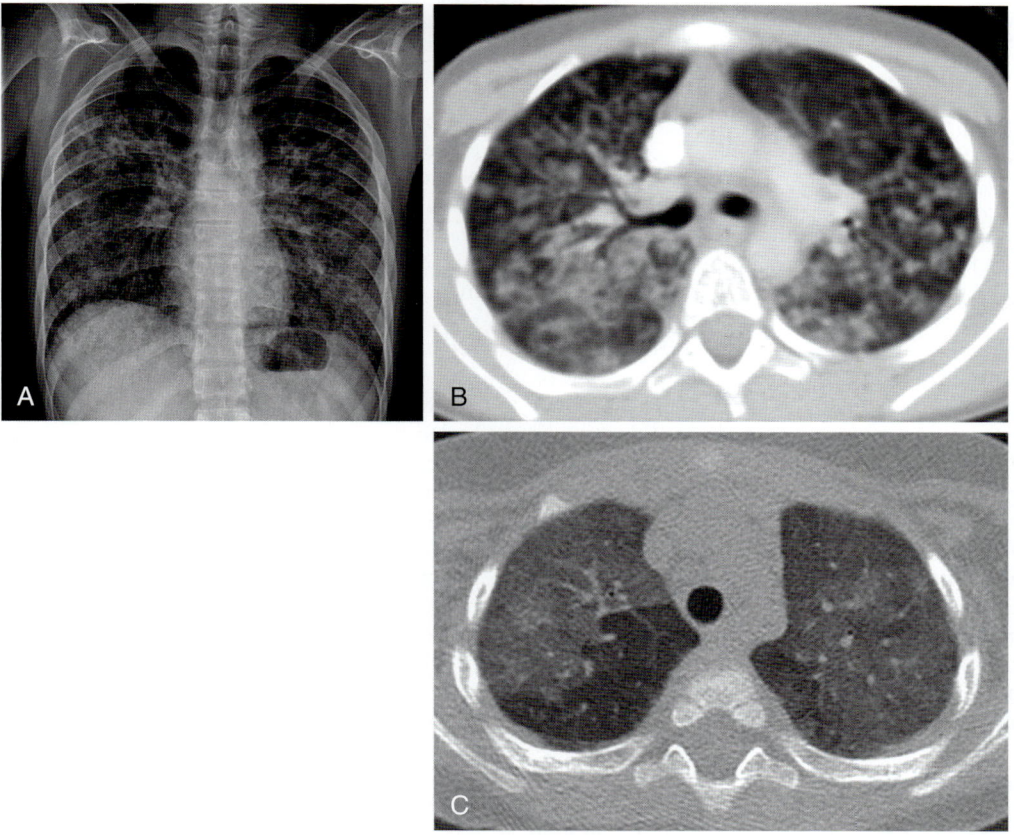

Figure 54-36 Pneumocystis jiroveci infection in a 17-year-old boy with acute lymphoblastic leukemia and immunodeficiency, who presented with dyspnea, fever, nonproductive cough, and decreased white blood cell counts. **A,** The radiograph shows diffuse bilateral interstitial opacity throughout the lungs. **B,** Contrast-enhanced computed tomography (CT) confirms the bilateral patchy and ground-glass opacities in both lungs. The diagnosis was confirmed by a positive polymerase chain reaction test from bronchial lavage fluid. **C,** CT in a different patient demonstrates a typical "crazy paving" pattern in both upper lobes.

Treatment and Follow-up   Although imaging findings are not specific for *P. jiroveci* infection, the presence of bilateral ground-glass opacities in immunocompromised children should lead to this diagnosis.[147] Tracheal washings or lung biopsy, when performed, may show the organisms on microscopic examination after silver methenamine staining.

CANDIDIASIS

Etiology   Pulmonary candidiasis is almost always encountered in immunocompromised children, those with indwelling catheters, those who are undergoing prolonged antibiotic therapy, or those who are on steroids. *Candida albicans* is the responsible organism in the majority of candidal infections.[148] The organism regularly colonizes the upper respiratory tract and then spreads to the lungs. Pulmonary candidiasis may be either a primary infection (limited to the lungs) or a secondary infection (caused by hematogenous dissemination from other sites of infection).

Imaging   Although radiographs are often normal in the earliest stages of infection, nonspecific features of bronchopneumonia and lung nodules may be noted (e-Fig. 54-37).[148,149] Those nodules may cavitate, and unilateral or bilateral lobar or segmental opacities may also be seen.

Treatment and Follow-up   Children who are severely ill with pulmonary candidiasis receive antifungal therapy with triazole compounds and echinocandins, which are known for their excellent lung penetration.

Pulmonary Manifestations of Parasitic Infestations

Pulmonary manifestations of parasitic infestations are predominantly encountered in the developing world, in those who have recently traveled to or from these regions, or in immunocompromised patients. A variety of imaging findings are seen, predominantly in the multinodular pneumonia category, as in paragonimiasis and echinococcus (hydatid) disease. However, several types of parasitic infestation may produce clinical and radiographic signs as a consequence of the passage of larval forms through the lung in the course of the parasite's life cycle. These include *Ascaris lumbricoides*, *Necator americanus*, *Ancylostoma duodenale* (hookworms), *Strongyloides stercoralis*, and *Toxocara cati* and *canis*.[150] *T. cati* and *T. canis* may produce a localized granulomatous reaction, termed *visceral larva migrans*, with resultant opacities in the lungs. The first four mentioned species as well as a number of rarer parasites may be associated with Löffler syndrome (acute allergic eosinophilic pneumonia).[2] The most common parasitic agents with pulmonary involvement are listed in Table 54-2.

PULMONARY PARAGONIMIASIS

Etiology   The lung fluke *Paragonimus westermani* is endemic in parts of Southeast Asia, South America, and Western Africa. In the United States, pulmonary paragonimiasis has affected refugee Indochinese children and Latin-American immigrants.[151,152] Children are usually infected after ingestion of undercooked crustaceans, including crabs or crayfish, or by drinking contaminated water. In Southeast Asia, infestation of the lungs by *P. westermani* is said to be a common cause of pediatric lung necrosis and calcification, but it is difficult to differentiate from TB and fungal diseases on the basis of radiographic criteria alone (e-Fig. 54-38). Affected children usually present with fever, pleuritic chest pain, and respiratory symptoms such as chronic cough or hemoptysis. The diagnosis depends on a combination of findings, including history, peripheral blood eosinophilia, identification of ova in the stool or the sputum, and a positive ELISA (enzyme-linked immunosorbent assay) test result.

Imaging   Imaging findings depend on the stage of the disease. The early stage is characterized by (1) linear opacities, which are 2 to 4 mm thick and 3 to 7 cm long, extending inward from the pleura representing the migration of juvenile worms; (2) focal airspace consolidation, representing exudative or hemorrhagic pneumonia caused by the migrating worm; (3) pneumothorax; or (4) hydropneumothorax. Features of the late stage of infection include nodules, thin-walled crescent-shaped worm cysts (the "signet ring" sign), dense masslike consolidation, or bronchiectasis. As the flukes move from the abdomen to the chest, they penetrate the diaphragm and pleural layers, and thus pleural effusions and thickening are commonly noted.

Treatment and Follow-up   Pulmonary paragonimiasis is treated with antiparasitics such as praziquatel and bithionol.

ECHINOCOCCUS DISEASE OF THE LUNG

Etiology   Echinococcosis or hydatid disease in humans is caused by infestation with *Echinococcus granulosus* (dog tapeworm). Humans are infected by direct contact with definite hosts (e.g., dogs) or by ingestion of eggs present in infected water, food, or soil. The eggs of *E. granulosus* hatch into larvae in the duodenum and are typically trapped within the liver (~75%) or lungs (~5% to 15%). They pass through the portal system in the liver or pulmonary alveolar capillaries, respectively. These larvae eventually develop into round or oval-shaped cysts within the liver or lungs (e-Fig. 54-39). Although most children with pulmonary involvement by hydatid disease are asymptomatic, they may present with fever, shortness of breath, cough, chest pain, which is usually a sign of cyst rupture. Diagnosis of hydatid disease depends on the combination of imaging and serology.

Imaging   The radiologic findings are characterized by single or multiple (~25%), round or oval-shaped, cystic nodules or masses (1-20 cm in diameter) with well-defined walls, surrounded by normal lung parenchyma (see e-Fig. 54-39). Other findings include an air-crescent sign, when a cyst communicates with a bronchus, or the water-lily sign (Fig. 54-40), when a cyst membrane floats in residual fluid after cyst rupture.[140,141] Pericystic emphysema may be a sign of impending rupture. After rupture of the cysts, cavitation or abscess formation and bronchiectasis may occur.

Treatment and Follow-up   Traditionally, surgical removal of the pulmonary cysts, often with supplemental medication such as benzimidazole, has been performed. Despite the risk

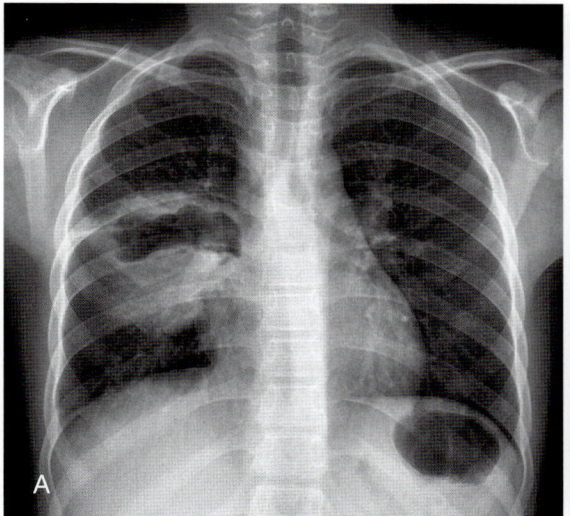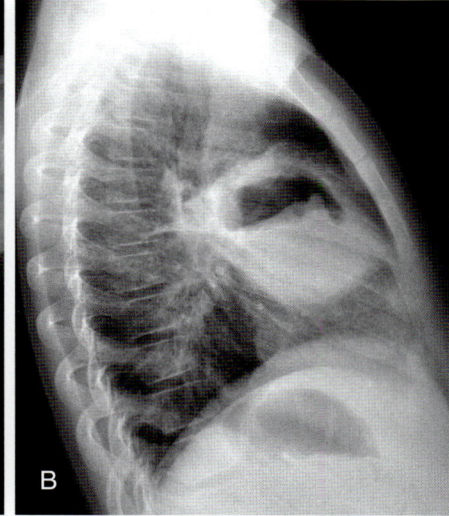

Figure 54-40   Hydatid disease in a 12-year-old boy, who presented with cough. **A** and **B,** Radiographs show a cavitary lesion with an irregular air-fluid level in the right middle lobe. The floating germinative membranes account for the classic "water lily" sign. Histopathologic diagnosis after surgical resection was consistent with hydatid infection.

of anaphylactic reactions following cyst aspiration, careful image-guided percutaneous techniques appear to be sufficiently safe.[153]

Key Points

Imaging studies have limited value in the differentiation between viral and bacterial pulmonary infections in young children, and these infectious agents frequently coexist.

Patient age, salient details of the clinical presentation, and pretest probability (knowledge of seasonal variations in disease) must be considered in an attempt to make a distinction between viral and bacterial infections of the lung.

Clear, well-defined and mutually understood terminology should be used in reports of chest radiographs obtained in children suspected to have pulmonary infections to optimally impact on treatment decisions.

Overcalling bacterial pneumonia is the most common interpretive error on pediatric chest radiographs.

Ultrasonography is used as the initial modality to detect and characterize complex effusions from pulmonary infection, and CT is used to identify underlying etiologies and complications.

MRI should be considered a potential alternative to CT when cross-sectional chest imaging is needed for diagnosing pulmonary infections with complications.

Generally, it is not necessary to monitor uncomplicated pediatric pulmonary infections with radiographs until resolution.

In the embolic form of staphylococcal lung infection, a search should be undertaken for the primary source in skin, joints, or bones.

Children who recently tested positive to tuberculin skin testing need to be evaluated with chest radiography for possible acute or chronic pulmonary TB infection.

CT may improve the diagnosis and management of symptomatic pulmonary tuberculosis, fungal infection, and parasite infestation, particularly if an associated immune deficiency exists.

The appearance of ground-glass opacities in combination with interstitial thickening seen on CT in children with AIDS is sufficiently specific to institute an empirical treatment for *Pneumocystis jiroveci*.

Infestations by parasites may be associated with the Löffler syndrome (acute allergic eosinophilic pneumonia).

Suggested Readings

Bradley JS, Byington CL, Shah SS, et al. The management of community-acquired pneumonia in infants and children older than 3 months of age: Clinical practice guidelines by the Pediatric Infectious Diseases Society and the Infectious Diseases Society of America. *Clin Infect Dis.* 2011; 53(7):e25-e76.

Daltro P, Santos EN, Gasparetto TD, et al. Pulmonary infections. *Pediatr Radiol.* 2011;41(Suppl 1):S69-S82.

Eslamy HK, Newman B. Pneumonia in normal and immunocompromised children: An overview and update. *Radiol Clin North Am.* 2011; 49(5):895-920.

McIntosh K. Community-acquired pneumonia in children. *N Engl J Med.* 2002;346:429-437.

Ventre KM, Wolf GK, Arnold JH. Pediatric respiratory diseases: 2011 update for the *Rogers' textbook of pediatric intensive care. Pediatr Crit Care Med.* 2011;12(3):325-338.

Westra SJ, Choy G. What imaging should we perform for the diagnosis and management of pulmonary infections? *Pediatr Radiol.* 2009;39(suppl 2):S178-S183.

References

Full references for this chapter can be found on www.expertconsult.com.

Chapter 55

Neoplasia

WINNIE C.W. CHU, MONICA EPELMAN, DAVID A. MONG, and EDWARD Y. LEE

Neoplasia

Pulmonary neoplasm is much less common in children than in adults. Affected children may present clinically with respiratory symptoms or pulmonary neoplasm may be detected incidentally on a chest radiograph in an asymptomatic child. In a recent series of 204 pediatric lung tumors, the ratio of primary benign to primary malignant to secondary malignant pulmonary neoplasms (i.e., metastases) is 1.4 : 1 : 11.6.[1] Primary lung tumors represent only 0.19% of all pediatric neoplasms. Metastatic lung tumors are approximately 12 times more common than primary lung tumors in children. A list of benign and malignant lung neoplasms is summarized in Table 55-1.

Primary Benign Pulmonary Neoplasms

Primary benign pulmonary neoplasms in children are far less common malignant pulmonary neoplasms, including both primary and secondary lesions. The imaging characteristics of benign lung neoplasms are summarized in Table 55-2.

HAMARTOMA

Etiology Pulmonary hamartoma, originally thought to represent a congenital lesion, is now considered a true benign mesenchymal neoplasm. It contains predominantly cartilage, fat, and fibrous tissue. Occasionally, pulmonary hamartoma may also have smooth muscle, bone, and entrapped respiratory epithelium, which grow slowly.[2] Pulmonary hamartoma is rare in children (the peak incidence is in the fourth to sixth decades); however, it is the most common primary benign pulmonary neoplasm accounting for 7% to 14% of all solitary pulmonary nodules in children.[3] Ninety percent of pulmonary hamartomas are parenchymal in location. They usually present as incidental findings, although a large pulmonary hamartoma could cause respiratory distress.

Imaging The typical radiographic appearance of pulmonary hamartoma is a smooth or slightly lobulated, solitary pulmonary nodule or mass, usually located in the peripheral portion of the lungs. Characteristic punctuate or popcorn-like

calcifications may be seen in approximately 10%. On computed tomography (CT), it is typically a well-circumscribed pulmonary nodule that is less than 2.5 cm in diameter. Pulmonary hamartoma often contains fat or calcification, which, in a solitary pulmonary nodule, is considered diagnostic (Fig. 55-1).[4]

Treatment and Follow-up Pediatric patients with pulmonary hamartoma require no further treatment unless it grows rapidly or the patient becomes symptomatic because of recurrent pneumonia or atelectasis caused by the mass effect from the tumor.[5] In such situations, surgical resection is usually curative.

CHONDROMA

Etiology Pulmonary chondroma is a benign tumor composed of a well-differentiated benign cartilage with lack of bronchial epithelium.[6] Pulmonary chondroma tends to occur before 30 years of age (82%), mainly in young women (85%). Affected persons are usually asymptomatic. Pulmonary chondroma is associated with the Carney triad.[7] This syndrome commonly affects three organs: (1) stomach (gastrointestinal stromal tumor, 75%) (Fig. 55-2, *B*), (2) lung (pulmonary chondroma, 15%), and (3) paraganglionic system (paraganglioma, 10%). However, tumors arising from the adrenal gland (adrenal adenoma or pheochromocytoma, 20%) and the esophagus (leiomyoma, 10%) have also been reported in association with the Carney triad. The majority of patients present with two of three neoplasms. Seventy-five percent of patients with the Carney triad have pulmonary chondroma(s).

Imaging Pulmonary chondroma may be single (40%), multiple unilateral (25%), or bilateral (15%) without predilection for specific lobe or side of lung.[7] Chest radiography usually shows well-demarcated, often multiple, lung masses with central or popcorn-like calcification (Fig. 55-2, *A*). When calcified (45%), the appearance of chondroma is indistinguishable from that of pulmonary hamartoma on imaging studies.

Treatment and Follow-up Although surgical resection is sometimes performed, pulmonary chondroma may be left in situ because it is benign and usually indolent. Periodic screening of patients is currently recommended for metachronous development of paragangliomas or gastrointestinal stromal tumors.

Table 55-1

List of Benign and Malignant Lung Neoplasms	
Benign lung neoplasm	Hamartoma
	Chondroma
	Papillomatosis
	Lymphangioma
	Lymphoproliferation
	Plasma cell granuloma or inflammatory myofibroblastic tumor
	Mucosa-associated lymphoid tissue
	Bronchus-associated lymphoid tissue
	Lymphomatoid granulomatosis
	Posttransplantation lymphoproliferative disorder
Malignant lung neoplasm	Primary
	Bronchial adenoma, carcinoid or salivary gland tumor
	Bronchogenic carcinoma
	Pleuropulmonary blastoma
	Epithelioid hemangioma
	Secondary malignant conditions
	Metastases
	Osteogenic sarcoma
	Wilms tumor
	Leukemia
	Lymphoma

RECURRENT RESPIRATORY PAPILLOMATOSIS

Etiology Recurrent respiratory papillomatosis (RRP) is characterized by mucosal papillomas, which are ingrowths of squamous cell–lined fibrovascular core in the lumen of central airways. It is the most common neoplasm that occurs in the larynx of children. RRP is caused by the human papilloma virus (HPV) types 6 and 11, which is typically acquired during vaginal birth. The primary lesions commonly affect the larynx but may spread to the lung parenchyma (1.8%) especially if surgical or laser therapy had been provided earlier.[8] The ultimate prognosis is poor when pulmonary involvement occurs. Malignant transformation into squamous cell carcinoma may occur.[9]

Table 55-2

Imaging Characteristics of Benign Lung Neoplasm (Nonlymphoproliferative)	
Neoplasm	**Imaging Characteristics**
Hamartoma	Smooth or slightly lobulated, sharply defined mass, occasionally calcified ("popcorn") Fat and calcification in solitary pulmonary mass on computed tomography is diagnostic
Chondroma	Solitary or multiple nodules; commonly (45%) calcified; associated with the Carney triad
Respiratory papillomatosis	Rarely (<1%) intrapulmonary; Bilateral, multiple subpleural solid or cystic nodules; may be associated with bronchiectasis or atelectasis
Lymphatic malformation	Rarely intrapulmonary; well-marginated, nonenhancing cystic mass; may simulate congenital pulmonary airway malformation or diaphragmatic hernia in neonates; or solid, low-attenuation mediastinal or pulmonary mass in older children

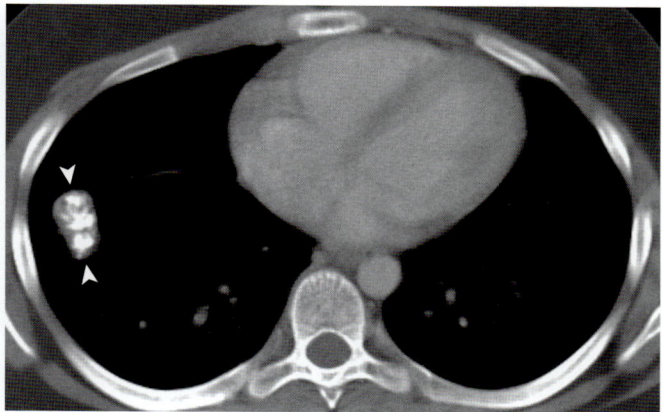

Figure 55-1 Pulmonary hamartoma. A 14-year-old boy with incidental calcified lesion noted on chest radiograph (*image not shown*). Axial enhanced computed tomography image shows a peripherally located, well-circumscribed, oval shaped smooth mass (*arrowheads*) with popcorn calcifications.

Imaging On chest radiography, RRP typically presents as bilateral, multiple nodular and cystic lesions of varying size containing air or debris. Postobstructive atelectasis, bronchiectasis, or secondary infection presenting as consolidation may be also seen.[10] On CT, usually, scattered nodules are seen in the lungs (Fig. 55-3), and these nodules may enlarge, become air-filled cysts, or form large cavities with thin or thick walls.[11] CT virtual bronchoscopy may be useful to evaluate mural nodules within the central airways.

Treatment and Follow-up The typical management of RRP in the central airway is by endoscopic surgery with cryotherapy, laser, or microdebrider treatment.[12] Intravenous cidofovir has been used recently for treating pulmonary involvement of RRP but with inconsistent results.[13]

LYMPHATIC MALFORMATION

Etiology Lymphatic malformation, previously referred to as *lymphangioma*, is characterized by a benign proliferation of nonfunctional lymphatic tissue that may involve nearly every organ of the body. Only 1% of lymphatic malformations remain confined to the chest. Primary pulmonary lymphatic malformation is even less common.[14] Affected persons are often asymptomatic. However, some may present with compressive symptoms such as cough, dyspnea, stridor, or even pneumothorax. Younger patients tend to have lesions that affect the lung.[15]

Imaging On chest radiography, lymphatic malformation typically presents as a masslike opacity. The most common CT finding is a smooth, well-marginated, nonenhancing, cystic mass. In neonates and infants, this may simulate congenital pulmonary airway malformation (CPAM) or diaphragmatic hernia. Older children may have a solid, low-attenuation, masslike lesion that may mimic pneumonia or tumors (e-Fig. 55-4).

Treatment and Follow-up Early surgical removal of lymphatic malformation is currently recommended to prevent local growth and the resultant compression of vital structures.[16]

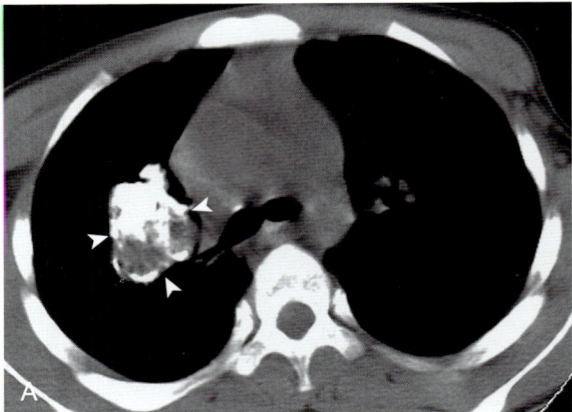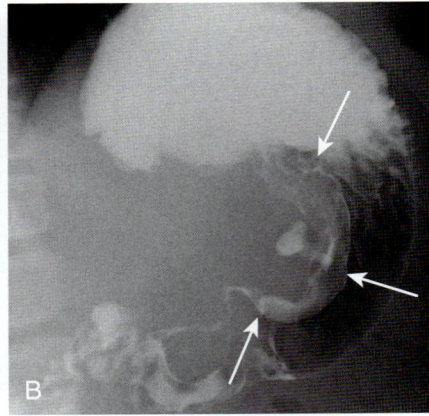

Figure 55-2 Pulmonary chondroma. **A,** A 14-year-old boy in the setting of the Carney triad. Axial unenhanced computed tomography image shows a large right parahilar mass (*arrowheads*) with extensive calcifications. **B,** Upper gastrointestinal study of the same patient demonstrates a large ulcerated exophytic soft tissue mass (*arrows*) in the stomach consistent with gastric leiomyosarcoma.

Lymphoproliferation

In recent years, the incidence of lymphoproliferative disorders has increased because of increase in pediatric organ transplantation, prevalence of human immunodeficiency virus (HIV) infection, and development of more potent immunosuppressive therapies. The most common lymphoproliferative disorders affecting lungs in children are plasma cell granuloma, mucosa-associated and bronchus-associated lymphoid tissue, lymphocytic interstitial pneumonitis, lymphomatoid granulomatosis, and posttransplantation lymphoproliferative disorder. The imaging characteristics of lymphoproliferative disorders involving lungs are listed in Table 55-3.

PLASMA CELL GRANULOMA OR INFLAMMATORY MYOFIBROBLASTIC TUMOR

Etiology Plasma cell granuloma is the most common tumor-like abnormality in the lungs of children. It arises in the lung parenchyma but may also involve the mediastinum or pleura.

Due to the complexity and variable histologic characteristics, it is known by several different terms, including *inflammatory or postinflammatory pseudotumor, fibroxanthoma, myofibroblastic tumor, fibrous histiocytoma, xanthogranuloma,* or *histiocytoma.*[17,18] Recently, it has been termed *inflammatory myofibroblastic tumor (IMT)* because myofibroblasts, fibroblasts, and histiocytes are the main constituents of this tumor (Fig. 55-5, *B*).[19] A substantial proportion of tumors have *ALK1* gene mutations.[20] The World Health Organization (WHO) currently recognizes IMT as a low-grade mesenchymal malignancy. The majority of children with IMT are older than 5 years, although it has been reported in younger children and even infants. Approximately 60% of affected children are symptomatic, typically presenting with fever, cough, chest pain, dyspnea, wheezing, or hemoptysis.

Imaging Radiographically, IMTs may be seen as solitary (95%) or multiple (5%). IMTs are usually sharply circumscribed, lobulated mass(es) of varying sizes, typically located in the peripheral portion of the lungs. IMT may occasionally

Table 55-3

Lymphoproliferative Disorders of the Lungs	
Disorder	**Imaging Characteristics**
Plasma cell granuloma or inflammatory myofibroblastic tumor	Solitary or multiple; sharply circumscribed mass; may be locally invasive; 15% to 25% have calcification; may be composed of both solid and cystic components
Mucosa-associated lymphoid tissue proliferation (pseudolymphoma)	2- to 5-cm discrete lesions with air bronchograms; may evolve into malignant lymphoma; pleural effusion common
Bronchus-associated lymphoid tissue proliferation	Diffuse reticulonodular pattern on chest radiography Small centrilobular nodules and ground glass opacity on computed tomography
Lymphoid interstitial pneumonia	Seen in patients with acquired or congenital immunodeficiency as reticular or reticulonodular opacities on chest radiography; diffuse centrilobular and subpleural nodules on high-resolution computed tomography; associated with ground-glass opacity; bronchovascular and interstitial thickening
Lymphomatoid granulomatosis	Seen in immunocompromised patients Multiple nodules or confluent masses that frequently cavitate; basal predominance
Posttransplantation lymphoproliferative disorder	Solitary or multiple lung masses or consolidation noted months to years after solid organ or bone marrow transplantation; may have associated mediastinal and extrathoracic adenopathy; large lesions may cavitate

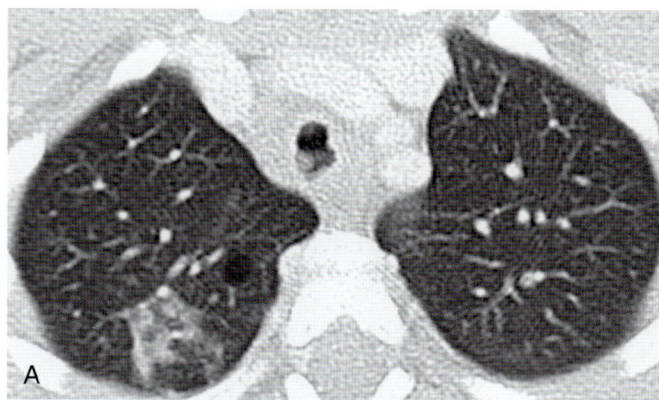
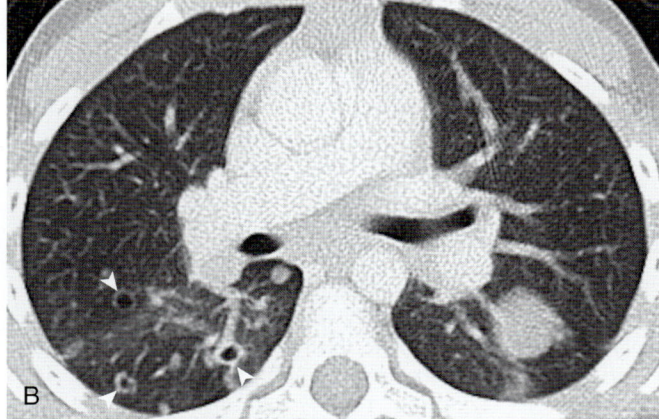
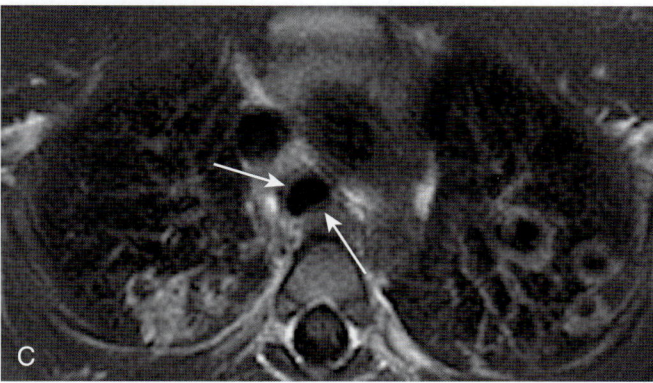

Figure 55-3 Recurrent respiratory papillomatosis. **A,** Axial lung window computed tomography image obtained in a 5-year-old girl with recurrent respiratory papillomatosis shows multiple intratracheal soft tissue nodules. **B,** Multiple parenchymal papillomas are also present, some of which show cavitation (*arrowheads*). **C,** An axial T1-weighted magnetic resonance image shows cavitating lesions in both lungs and mildly thickened tracheal walls (*arrows*).

be endobronchial. On CT, it usually presents as a soft tissue mass with either homogeneous or heterogeneous attenuation (see Fig. 55-5, *A*). Although IMT does not enhance substantially, a thick enhancing rim has been reported. Less commonly, it may present with both solid and cystic components. IMT may also have an infiltrative pattern simulating an aggressive malignancy.[21] If the mediastinum is involved or the mass contains calcifications (15% to 25%), IMT may mimic a germ cell tumor, neuroblastoma, or metastatic osteosarcoma in pediatric patients.

Treatment and Follow-up Complete surgical resection is the treatment for IMT typically leading to excellent results. Irradiation, chemotherapy, and antiinflammatory medications have been proposed as adjuvant therapies but have not been successful in most patients.

MUCOSA-ASSOCIATED LYMPHOID TISSUE AND BRONCHUS-ASSOCIATED LYMPHOID TISSUE

Etiology Mucosa-associated lymphoid tissue (MALT, or pseudolymphoma) is rare in children. Affected persons generally are not severely ill but may have nonspecific respiratory symptoms. Lymphoma has been reported to develop in some cases of MALT. It may be quite difficult to clearly differentiate pseudolymphoma from a true lymphoproliferative condition, even by using modern immunofluorescence techniques. Experts currently disagree about whether MALT should be considered a premalignant or a postinflammatory condition. Bronchus-associated lymphoid tissue (BALT) is a subcategory of the more widely distributed MALT. BALT is a lymphoid aggregate located in the submucosal area of bronchioles, which may become hyperplastic because of chronic antigen stimuli.[22] It has been suggested that BALT is related to a hypersensitivity response to unidentified antigens. BALT has two forms: (1) lymphoid interstitial pneumonia and (2) follicular bronchitis or bronchiolitis. Lymphoid interstitial pneumonia type BALT is commonly seen in pediatric patients with acquired immunodeficiency syndrome (AIDS) or other immune compromise. Follicular bronchitis or bronchiolitis type of BALT typically occurs in children with chronic infection, connective tissue disorders, or immunodeficiency disorders and as a hypersensitivity reaction.

Imaging On chest radiography, MALT typically presents as discrete, often multiple lesions, usually with air bronchograms ranging from 2 to 5 cm in diameter. A pleural effusion is commonly seen. A diffuse reticulonodular opacity, often associated with hyperinflation, is the common radiographic finding of BALT (e-Fig. 55-6, *A*). On CT, the usual imaging appearance of BALT consists of small centrilobular nodules (foci of lymphoid proliferation) and a ground-glass opacity predominantly involving the lower lobes (see e-Fig. 55-6, *B*). In patients with advanced BALT, bronchiectasis and peribronchovascular consolidation caused by recurrent infection and chronic airway obstruction may present.

Treatment and Follow-up Aggressive management (e.g., complete surgical excision, radiotherapy, chemotherapy, or a combination of all of these) is the current treatment of choice for MALT. Because of the wide extent of disease often associated with BALT, surgical excision may be considered only for a minority of patients. Chemotherapy is the treatment of choice for the majority of patients with BALT.

LYMPHOCYTIC INTERSTITIAL PNEUMONITIS

Etiology Lymphocytic interstitial pneumonitis (LIP) is characterized by diffuse proliferation of polyclonal lymphocytes and plasma cells in the pulmonary parenchymal interstitium, which expands to the alveolar septa. It is considered an AIDS-defining illness in children younger than 13 years

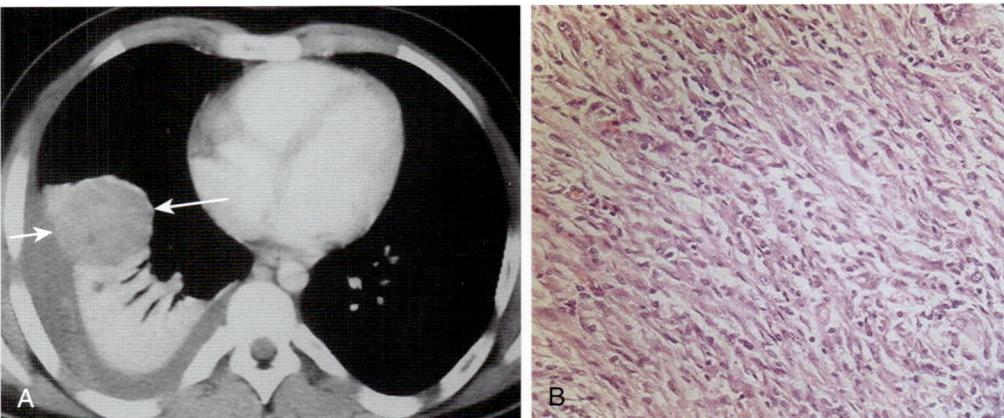

Figure 55-5   **Inflammatory myofibroblastic tumor.** An afebrile 13-year-old boy who presented with increasing dyspnea and right-sided pleuritic chest pain. **A,** An axial contrast-enhanced computed tomography of the chest shows a rounded heterogeneously enhancing lesion (*arrows*) located adjacent to an area of atelectatic lung. Pleural fluid at the same level demonstrates increased attenuation consistent with a hemothorax. **B,** A photomicrograph (hematoxylin-eosin stain) of the surgical specimen reveals the presence of both spindle-shaped myofibroblasts and inflammatory cells consistent with an inflammatory myofibroblastic tumor of the lung.

old who are infected with HIV because LIP is rarely idiopathic.

Imaging   On chest radiography, LIP typically presents with reticular or reticulonodular opacities predominantly in the bilateral lower lung zones.[23] On high-resolution CT, diffuse centrilobular and subpleural nodules (representing local proliferation of lymphoid germinal centers), areas of ground-glass opacity, and bronchovascular and interstitial thickening in both lungs are often seen (Fig. 55-7). Thin-walled cysts and bronchiectasis may be also present.[24]

Treatment and Follow-up   Steroid and other immunosuppressive agents are used for treating LIP with variable results. Prognosis of children with LIP depends on the associated underlying disease. Progressive honeycomb fibrosis or infectious complications may lead to increased mortality. Low grade B-cell lymphoma may develop in rare cases.[25]

LYMPHOMATOID GRANULOMATOSIS

Etiology   Lymphomatoid granulomatosis, also known as *pseudolymphoma, angiocentric lymphoma,* or *angiocentric immuno-proliferative lesion,* is characterized pathologically by an angiocentric and angiodestructive lymphocytic infiltration. It is considered an aggressive multisystem disease with a poor prognosis. The lung is often the primary site of involvement. This disease is associated with Epstein-Barr virus (EBV) infection in immunocompromised individuals. Progression of lymphomatoid granulomatosis to lymphoma occurs in 12% to 47% of patients, with the mortality rate over 50%.[26]

Imaging   On chest radiography, bilateral, poorly defined, nodular and confluent lesions with a basilar predominance are usually seen (e-Fig. 55-8). Characteristic CT findings of lymphomatoid granulomatosis include peribronchovascular distribution of nodules (which reflects the tendency of

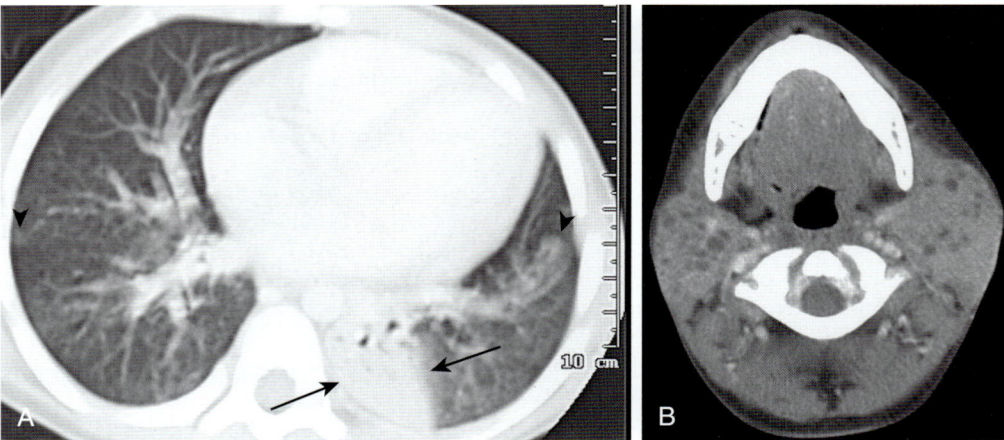

Figure 55-7   **Lymphocystic interstitial pneumonitis.** An 8-year-old girl with human immunodeficiency virus (HIV) infection with increasing shortness of breath. **A,** An axial computed tomography (CT) image shows bilateral patchy areas of ground-glass attenuation, right greater than left, poorly defined nodules (*arrowheads*) and an area of consolidation in the left lower lobe (*arrows*). **B,** An axial, enhanced CT image of neck demonstrates multiple, bilateral parotid lymphoepithelial cysts consistent with HIV parotitis.

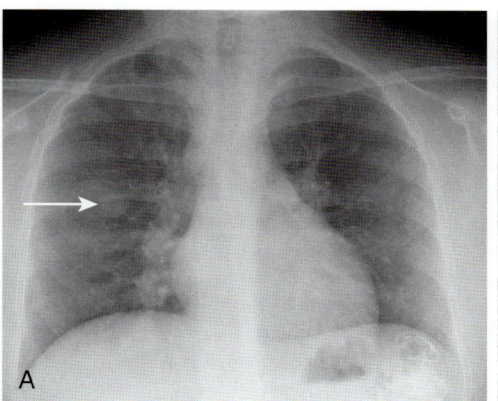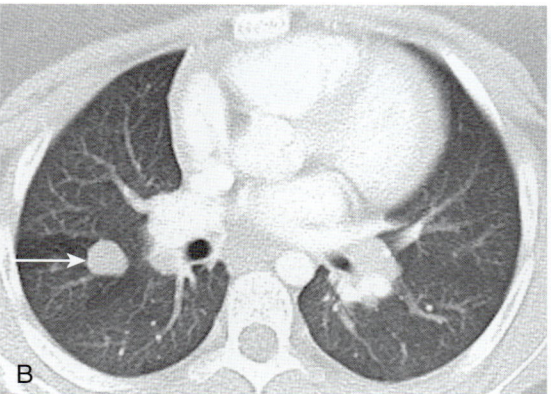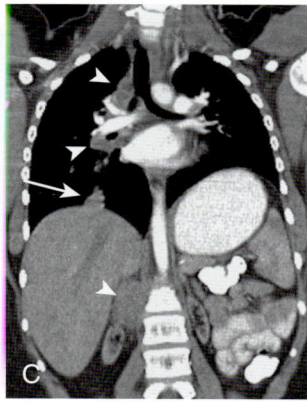

Figure 55-9 Posttransplantation lymphoproliferative disorder (PTLD). An 11-year-old girl who presented with PTLD following renal transplantation. **A,** A chest radiograph shows a nodular opacity (*arrow*) in the right upper lobe and bilateral hilar lymphadenopathy. **B,** An axial lung window computed tomography (CT) image demonstrates a right upper lobe lung nodule (*arrow*) corresponding to the opacity noted on chest radiograph. **C,** A coronal reformatted CT image shows mediastinal, hilar, and retroperitoneal lymphadenopathy (*arrowheads*) and an additional nodule at the right lung base (*arrow*). Note the atrophic native bilateral kidneys.

lymphomononuclear cells to infiltrate the subintimal region of medium-sized arteries and veins), small thin-walled cysts, and conglomerate small nodules.[24,27] Lesions may cavitate, mimicking Wegener granulomatosis.

Treatment and Follow-up Lymphomatoid granulomatosis may be resistant to ordinary chemotherapy. Retuximab, combined with other conventional chemotherapy, has been used with promising results.[28]

POSTTRANSPLANTATION LYMPHOPROLIFERATIVE DISORDER

Etiology Posttransplantation lymphoproliferative disorder (PTLD) is a consequence of chronic immunosuppression following solid organ transplantation or, less often, bone marrow transplantation.[29-32] It is believed to be induced by exposure to EBV. The lesions consist of uncontrolled proliferation of B lymphocytes ranging from benign lymphoid hyperplasia to invasive malignant lymphoma. The incidence of PTLD (1% to 18%) varies with the type of organ transplanted. It occurs most frequently in lung or heart-lung transplantation patients, likely because of the higher levels of immunosuppression required for these organ transplantations.[29,33-35] It is also more common in pediatric patients than in adult transplantation patients, possibly because of the lack of prior exposure to EBV. Improved surveillance, earlier diagnosis, and close monitoring of immunosuppression have led to a decreased incidence of PTLD in recent years, as well as a more favorable outcome. The most common sites for PTLD are the tonsils, cervical nodes, gastrointestinal tract, and the chest.[36,37] Intrathoracic PTLD tends to present earlier compared with extrathoracic PTLD. PTLD tends to occur within the allograft organ itself, as well as in adjacent anatomic regions.[38] Heart transplantation is the sole exception to this predilection.[39] Clinical symptoms of PTLD are often vague and include lethargy, fever, and weight loss. Biopsy is typically required to confirm the diagnosis.

Imaging The imaging appearance of PTLD is not specific and overlaps with that of many opportunistic infections. On chest radiography, the most common finding in PTLD is the presence of multiple well-defined pulmonary nodules with or without mediastinal adenopathy (Fig. 55-9).[39] These are best visualized on CT. Large pulmonary nodules and mediastinal adenopathy tend to show central low attenuation, likely representing necrosis. Other less frequent patterns of thoracic involvement include air space consolidation, pleural or chest wall masses, pleural or pericardial effusions, and thymic enlargement.[40-42] For a more confident diagnosis, it is helpful to search for extrathoracic PTLD such as thickening of bowel loops, enlarged abdominal lymph nodes, cervical adenopathy, or enlarged oropharyngeal lymphatic tissues.[39,43] Fludeoxyglucose positron emission tomography or CT may also increase sensitivity and specificity for the diagnosis.[44]

Treatment and Follow-up Reduction in immunosuppressive therapy remains a primary component of treatment for EBV-positive PTLD, which may lead to resolution of disease in the majority of cases.[45] Chemotherapy is used when reduced immunosuppression fails to control disease progression. Newer treatments of PTLD include B-lymphocyte–depleting antibodies, adoptive T-cell immunotherapy using allogeneic, or autologous EBV-specific cytotoxic T-lymphocytes.[46] EBV vaccination is advocated to be effective prophylaxis against PTLD.

Primary Malignant Pulmonary Neoplasms

Primary malignant pulmonary neoplasms are rare in children and are histologically diverse. The current WHO classification system of primary malignant pulmonary neoplasms differs substantially from the prior classification system, particularly with regard to new tumors (e.g., pleuropulmonary blastoma) and reclassification of benign and malignant tumors (e.g., IMT).[47] A series published in 2008 showed that the most common primary lung malignancies in children are pleuropulmonary blastoma and carcinoid tumor.[1] Because of the rarity of these malignant neoplasms and the nonspecific

Table 55-4

Imaging Characteristics of Primary Malignant Lung Tumors	
Neoplasm	**Imaging Characteristics**
Carcinoid or salivary gland tumor	Centrally located lesion: intraluminal soft tissue mass with distal atelectasis or obstructive pneumonitis Peripherally located lesion: oval or lobulated intraluminal or exophytic mass and occasionally calcify
Bronchogenic carcinoma	Central mass lesions with bronchial obstruction or, less commonly, small peripheral lesions
Pleuropulmonary blastoma	Cystic or mixed cystic and solid lesions adjacent to pleura; usually very large, with mediastinal displacement
Epithelioid hemangioendothelioma	Multiple well- or ill-defined nodular opacities up to 3 cm in diameter; very rare in childhood

clinical symptoms, they are often not considered in the differential diagnosis in children presenting with persistent pneumonitis, cough, and atelectasis. This often leads to delayed definitive treatment and generally a worse prognosis. The imaging characteristics of primary malignant lung tumors are listed in Table 55-4.

BRONCHIAL ADENOMA (CARCINOID TUMOR OR SALIVARY GLAND TUMOR)

Etiology   The term *bronchial adenoma*, which implies a benign disease process, was recently recategorized as either carcinoid or salivary gland tumors by the WHO.[47] Historically, bronchial adenomas encompassed bronchial carcinoid tumor, mucoepidermoid tumor, and adenoid cystic carcinoma. Carcinoid tumor accounts for approximately 80% of previously classified pediatric bronchial adenomas, which are low-grade neuroendocrine carcinoma arising in lobar bronchi (75%), main stem bronchi (10%), or the lung parenchyma (15%).[48-50]

Mucoepidermoid carcinoma (e-Fig. 55-10) and adenoid cystic carcinoma (cylindromas) (Fig. 55-11) arise from the salivary-type mucous cells of the submucosa along the tracheobronchial tree. Adenoid cystic carcinoma is extremely rare in children.[51] Patients with carcinoid tumor and mucoepidermoid carcinoma frequently present with wheezing, cough, hemoptysis, or pneumonia.[48,52,53] Association with the carcinoid syndrome in children with carcinoid tumor is exceedingly rare. The differential diagnosis of these rare tumors includes foreign body aspiration, granulomatous infection, and asthma with mucus plugging.

Imaging   The radiographic presentation depends on the size and location of tumor within the airway or lungs. A centrally located tumor is typically seen as an intraluminal soft tissue attenuation mass with associated distal atelectasis or obstructive pneumonitis. A peripherally located tumor is commonly seen as a sharply marginated, oval, or lobulated intraluminal or exophytic mass.[54-58] Associated stippled calcification is seen in up to 30% of carcinoid tumors. CT is particularly helpful for detecting and defining extrabronchial portion of the tumor and associated adenopathy.

Treatment and Follow-up   The current treatment of choice is surgical resection. Chemotherapy and radiotherapy are reserved for tumors with incomplete surgical resection. Overall survival rate for carcinoid and mucoepidermoid carcinoma is approximately 90%, whereas adenoid cystic carcinoma has a poorer survival rate of 55% because of higher likelihood of distant metastases.[59]

BRONCHOGENIC CARCINOMA

Etiology   Traditionally, the term *bronchogenic carcinoma* has been used to include both small cell and non–small cell lung cancers (including squamous cell carcinoma, large cell carcinoma, and adenocarcinoma). These tumors are very rare in childhood. In the most recent WHO classification guideline, the term *bronchogenic carcinoma* is not used and each tumor type is listed individually.[47] Among these tumors, adenocarcinoma is the most common in children.[51] Most children with adenocarcinoma present with advanced disease, which

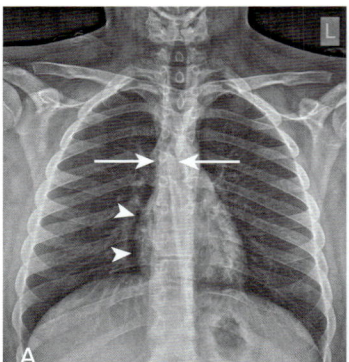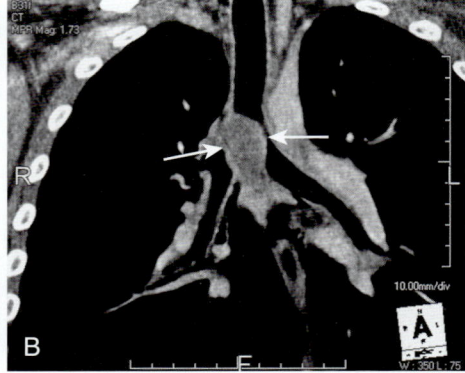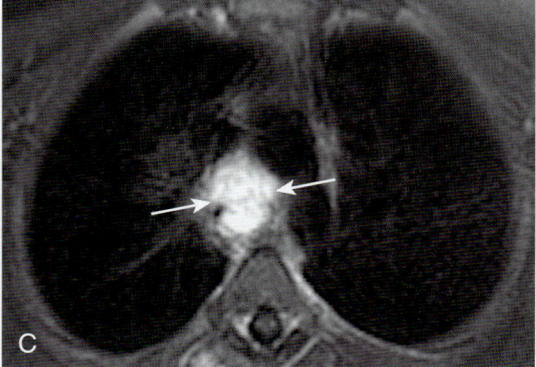

Figure 55-11   Adenoid cystic carcinoma. A 14-year-old boy with progressively worsening chronic cough and respiratory difficulty for 1 year who presented with hoarseness and crepitations over the neck. **A,** A chest radiograph shows pneumomediastinum (*arrowheads*) and an apparent soft tissue density projecting over the carina (*arrows*). **B,** A coronal enhanced computed tomography image shows a lobulated soft tissue mass (*arrows*) centered near the carina, which results in narrowing of the adjacent airway. **C,** An axial contrast-enhanced T1-weighted magnetic resonance image demonstrates avid enhancement of the mass (*arrows*).

results in high mortality. Small cell carcinoma, squamous cell carcinoma, and large cell carcinoma are very rare in children.[60,61]

Imaging On chest radiography, these tumors often present as a solitary pulmonary nodule or central mass, often associated with postobstructive atelectasis or consolidation (e-Fig. 55-12). On CT, the attenuation and enhancement of masses vary substantially among different types of tumors. Concomitant mediastinal or hilar adenopathy as well as malignant pleural effusion may also present. Aggressive tumors may also invade adjacent mediastinal or osseous structures.

Treatment and Follow-up Surgical resection often combined with subsequent chemotherapy and radiotherapy is the current management of choice. Unfortunately, bronchogenic carcinoma of childhood has been known for its unusually rapid disease course with early metastases.

PLEUROPULMONARY BLASTOMA

Etiology Pleuropulmonary blastoma (PPB) is an embryonal tumor of the lung, and it only occurs in young children. Over 90% of affected patients are below 6 years old at diagnosis. It recapitulates the morphogenesis of the fetal lung and may be regarded as a dysontogenetic analog to Wilms tumor, neuroblastoma, and hepatoblastoma. PPB contains primitive mesenchyma and varying degrees of more mature cartilage, skeletal and smooth muscle, and fibrous tissue. PPB is associated with hereditary tumor predisposition syndrome. Of the affected children, 25% to 30% have family members at risk of other dysplastic and neoplastic conditions.[62] The three PPB types are (1) type I (purely cystic with primitive mesenchymal cells beneath an intact epithelium), (2) type II (cystic and solid, mesenchymal cells overgrow the septa), and (3) type III (purely solid, complex sarcomatous neoplasm). Type I lesions occur earlier at a median age of 9 months and have a more favorable prognosis, with 85% to 90% overall survival rate.[63] Type II and III lesions occur at a median age of 36 and 42 months, with an overall survival of 60% and 45%, respectively.[64] It has been suggested that PPB is probably the same malignant tumor that has been reported in previous studies as mesenchymal sarcoma, malignant mesenchymoma, embryonal sarcoma, primary pulmonary rhabdomyosarcoma, embryonal sarcoma, primary pulmonary rhabdomyosarcoma arising in congenital lung cysts, or pulmonary blastoma in children.[65,66] Current data support the assertion that congenital lung cysts do not degenerate to become PPB but that cystic type I PPB may progress to more aggressive type II or type III PPB.[67-71] PPB may metastasize to the central nervous system, bone, and liver.

Imaging Imaging appearances of PPB depend on the type. PPBs present as solid, cystic, or mixed lesions. On chest radiography, the tumor may appear as a nodule or small mass that rapidly grows or as a large mass occupying the hemithorax. A large PPB may often result in mass effect on mediastinal structures. On CT, type 1 PPB is typically a cystic lesion often associated with multiple septations (Fig. 55-13), whereas type 3 PPB is a heterogeneously enhancing solid mass. Type 2 PPB has a combination of both cystic and solid components (Fig. 55-14). Type 1 PPB is often indistinguishable from CPAM on the basis of radiologic evaluation.[72] Approximately, 25% of patients with PPB have other embryonal tumors, most commonly renal cystic nephroma.[73,74] Other tumors less commonly seen in patients with PPB include medulloblastoma, thyroid dysplasia, germ cell neoplasms, and ovarian teratoma.[75]

Treatment and Follow-up The current treatment of choice for PPB is lobectomy or pneumonectomy.[76] Chemotherapy and local radiotherapy are adjuvant therapies if residual disease is present. Many congenital cystic lung lesions are removed surgically because of the risk of recurrent infection and the possibility of underlying neoplasm. Lesions that are not removed should be monitored closely. If the cystic lesion develops a solid component or if a family history of pediatric neoplasm exists, surgical resection is recommended.

EPITHELIOID HEMANGIOMA

Etiology Pulmonary epithelioid hemnagioendothelioma (PEH) is a rare tumor arising from endothelium with borderline malignant potential. PEH was first described by Dail

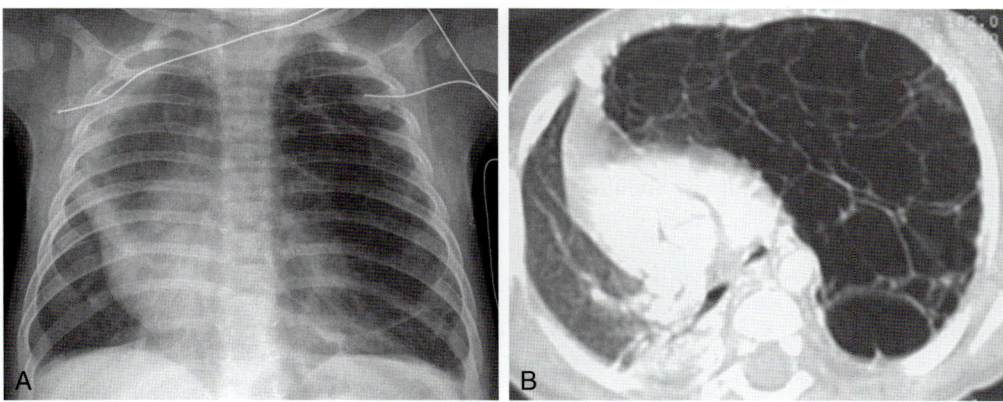

Figure 55-13 Cystic pleuropulmonary blastoma. A 4-month-old boy with worsening respiratory distress. **A,** A chest radiograph demonstrates a large radiolucent lesion with fine septations and multiple cysts within the left lung resulting in mediastinal shift. **B,** An axial lung window computed tomography image shows multiple cysts of varying sizes with mass effect on the mediastinum and contralateral right lung.

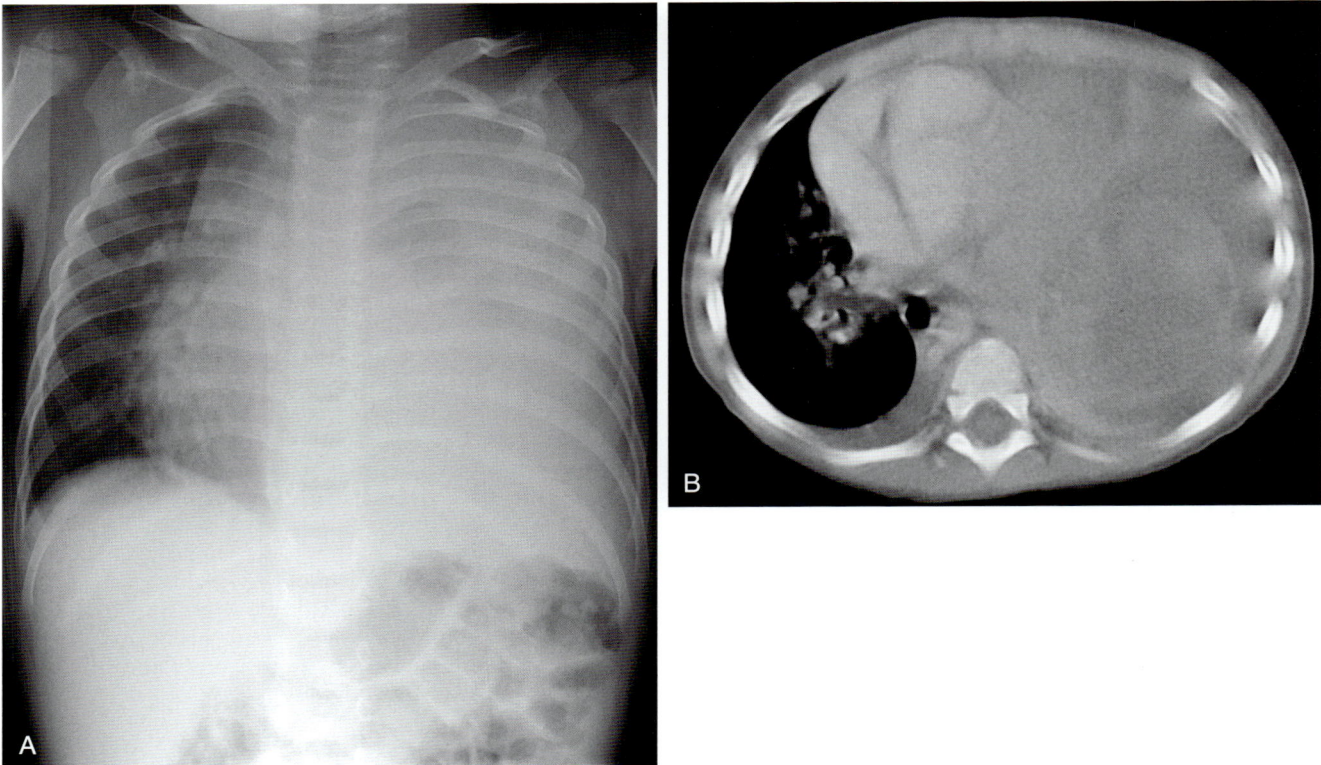

Figure 55-14 Mixed cystic and solid pleuropulmonary blastoma in a 2-year-old boy. **A,** A chest radiograph shows a completely opacified left hemithorax with mass effect producing a rightward cardiomediastinal shift. **B,** An axial enhanced computed tomography image demonstrates bilateral pleural effusion and a large, left-sided predominantly solid, pulmonary and mediastinal heterogeneously enhancing mass.

and Liebow in 1975 as an intravascular bronchoalveolar tumor that may affect bone, soft tissue, liver, and lung. Later studies revealed that intravascular bronchoalveolar tumor and PEH are different manifestations of the same disease.[77,78] Although most of the affected patients are adult women, it may also occur in children.[79] The majority of patients are asymptomatic, and lesions are typically detected incidentally.[80]

Imaging On chest radiography, PEH typically presents as bilateral multiple pulmonary nodules ranging from 5 mm to 2 cm in diameter (e-Fig. 55-15, *A*). Some patients may present with a solitary lesion. Concomitant hilar adenopathy and pleural effusion are seen in less than 10% of cases.[81] On CT, multiple well-defined or ill-defined perivascular nodules located near medium-sized vessels and bronchi are usually seen (see e-Fig. 55-15, *B*). Some pulmonary nodules may show calcification.[82,83]

Treatment and Follow-up Surgical resection is preferred in patients with solitary or a limited number of pulmonary lesions localized within the one lobe. Chemotherapy, radiotherapy, and interferon are other treatment choices that are associated with variable results.[84] Close follow-up with no active therapy is usually used for asymptomatic patients with multiple lesions.[80] Recently, vascular endothelium growth factor was proposed as a potential treatment for PEH.

Secondary Malignant Conditions

Secondary malignant conditions of the lungs may be caused by metastatic disease or from systemic diseases such as leukemia or lymphoma. Metastatic disease is, by far, the most common cause of pulmonary malignancy in childhood. Metastatic tumors accounts for approximately 80% of all lung tumors in children.[1] Osteogenic sarcoma and Wilms tumor are most common tumors with pulmonary metastasis in children. Secondary pulmonary involvement in systemic diseases such as leukemia or lymphoma is rare but could occur.

METASTASES

Etiology Pulmonary metastatic disease most often occurs hematogenously via the pulmonary arterial system. However, it may also occur via lymphatics, airways, or direct invasion. Pediatric tumors that have a propensity to metastasize to the lung are listed in the order of frequency by anatomic system in Table 55-5.

Imaging On imaging studies, most metastatic lesions are seen as round and sharply marginated and of homogeneous soft tissue attenuation. They tend to be located subpleurally in the outer two thirds of the lung. Metastatic lesions often appear to be directly contiguous with a pulmonary artery

Table 55-5

Pediatric Tumors that Metastasize to the Lung	
Primary site	**Tumor**
Bone	Osteosarcoma Ewing sarcoma Chondrosarcoma (rare) Ameloblastoma (very rare)
Musculoskeletal	Rhabdomyosarcoma Soft tissue sarcomas (e.g., synovial sarcoma, malignant fibrous histiocytoma)
Gastrointestinal	Hepatoblastoma, hepatocellular carcinoma Leiomyosarcoma (rare) Adenocarcinoma of colon (rare) Embryonal sarcoma of liver (very rare)
Genitourinary	Wilms tumor Gonadal germ cell tumor Malignant rhabdoid tumor of kidney (rare) Neuroblastoma (rare) Pheochromocytoma (rare) Trophoblastic choriocarcinoma (rare) Clear cell sarcoma of kidney (rare)
Thyroid	Thyroid carcinoma

branch, reflecting their hematogenous origin. A greater number of metastatic lesions are located at the lung bases rather than in the upper lobes, likely because of gravity-dependent increased basilar blood flow. Lymphangitic tumors usually present as reticular or reticulonodular opacities on chest radiography. Thickening of interlobular or interlobar septa and bronchovascular bundles are often seen on CT of children with lymphangitic tumor spread.

CT is sensitive but not specific in detecting pulmonary metastasis. No specific CT features (e.g., location, attenuation, size, margin characteristics) can reliably distinguish benign lesions from malignant pulmonary lesions. However, in general, solitary pulmonary lesion larger than 5 mm in diameter with sharp margins, especially when multiple, are usually malignant.[85] Pulmonary nodules that decrease in size during antineoplastic therapy are usually assumed to be malignant, whereas those that decrease in size without therapy or remain stable during 12 months of follow-up are likely benign.

Although the imaging appearances of the majority of metastatic pulmonary nodules are nonspecific, some primary tumors may have a characteristic appearance of pulmonary metastasis. Metastatic osteosarcoma may ossify (Fig. 55-16), cavitate, or present with acute pneumothorax. Lymphangitic spread is most commonly seen in children with rhabdomyosarcoma, neuroblastoma, and lymphoma.

Treatment and Follow-up Pulmonary metastases have been reported in 10% to 20% of patients with osteogenic sarcoma at initial diagnosis. Approximately 40% to 55% of patients with nonmetastatic osteosarcoma develop lung metastases in the later stages of the disease.[86-90] Number, distribution, and timing but not the size of lung metastases are of prognostic value for survival.[91,92] The best treatment for this group of patients is a combination of metastatectomy and adjuvant chemotherapy.[93,94]

The lung is the most common site of metastatic disease in children with Wilms tumor. Traditionally, treatment strategy for metastatic Wilms tumor has been based on lung lesions detectable with chest radiography. Currently, controversy exists over the optimal way for managing small pulmonary lesions that are detected only with CT and are not apparent on chest radiography because of the potential lung toxicity associated with aggressive therapy.[95] Previous studies[96,97] suggested that majority of these pulmonary lesions represent metastases and patients with these lesions probably require more potent chemotherapy than those children without metastatic disease.[98]

LEUKEMIA

Etiology Approximately 20% to 60% of patients with leukemia have histologic evidence of lung involvement at autopsy; but fewer than 5% of these patients present with lung abnormality suggesting leukemic infiltrates on chest radiography.[99] Pulmonary involvement of leukemia is most often seen in patients with acute monocytic and myelogenous leukemia.[100]

Imaging On chest radiography, leukemic infiltrates usually show a diffuse reticular pattern of opacities (Fig. 55-17). Pulmonary nodules and focal homogeneous opacities are also reported in patients with leukemic involvement of lungs. On CT, interstitial thickening in peribronchial distribution, small pulmonary nodules in centrilobular or peribronchovascular distribution, and focal areas of consolidation are common imaging findings.[101,102]

Treatment and Follow-up Lung biopsy is required for a definitive diagnosis of lung involvement from leukemia. Once the diagnosis is established, chemotherapy is currently the treatment of choice in pediatric patients with pulmonary leukemic involvement.[103]

LYMPHOMA

Etiology The lung is not commonly involved in lymphoma; involvement is 12% with Hodgkin disease (HD) and 10%

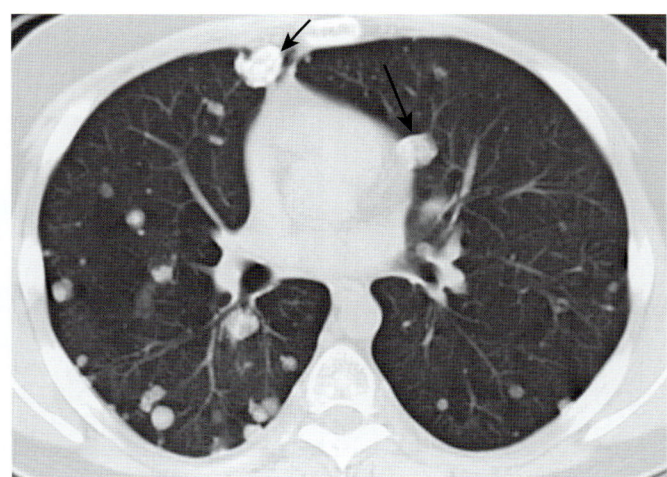

Figure 55-16 **Pulmonary metastases.** A 17-year-old boy with metastatic osteosarcoma. **A,** An axial computed tomography image demonstrates numerous, smooth lung nodules of varying sizes, some of which show internal calcification (*arrows*).

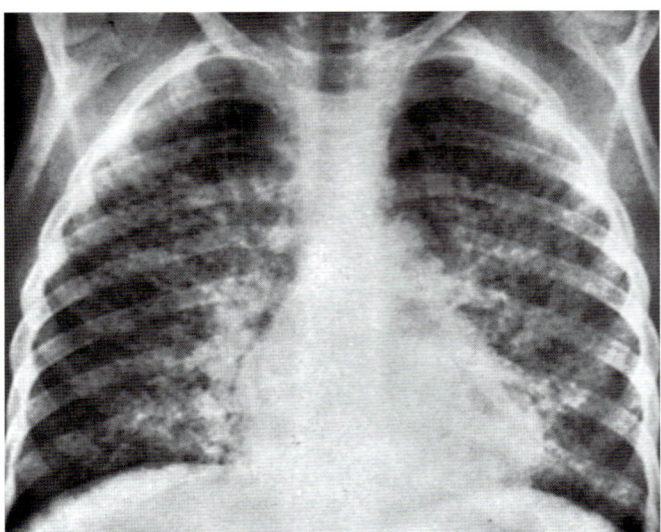

Figure 55-17 Pulmonary leukemia. A 7-year-old boy with biopsy-proven leukemia of the lungs. A chest radiograph shows a reticulonodular pattern opacity with central confluence. Relative sparing of the apices and the lateral segments of both lungs is evident. No radiographic evidence for adenopathy is present.

lymphatic obstruction caused by hilar or mediastinal adenoapthy, or from interstitial tumor deposition; and (3) lobar or segmental consolidation, which may mimic an infectious process.[105-108] Occasionally, multiple tiny pulmonary nodules in a miliary pattern in children with HD may simulate miliary tuberculosis.[109,110] Pleural effusion is found in less than 5% of children with lymphoma.

Although the imaging appearance of lung involvement in children with HD and NHL is similar on imaging studies, lung involvement is usually concomitantly present with mediastinal or hilar lymphadenopathy in children with HD, whereas lung involvement may occur without associated lymphadenopathy in NHL.[105,111]

Treatment and Follow-up Chemotherapy is the current treatment of choice. Although infection is more common in pediatric lymphoma patients, especially those undergoing treatment, development of new pulmonary lesions with a poor response to antibiotics may represent lymphoma lesions and therefore should promptly be biopsied for a definitive diagnosis. Pulmonary lesions from lymphoma usually decrease in size, disappear, or leave a parenchymal scar after chemotherapy treatment.[112]

with non–Hodgkin lymphoma (NHL) in pediatric patients. Lung involvement is almost always seen at initial presentation rather than at disease relapse.[104] In both HD and NHL, the underlying mechanisms of lung involvement from lymphoma are hematogenous spread, lymphangitic dissemination, and, less frequently, direct invasion.

Imaging Lung involvement of lymphoma in pediatric patients typically presents as one of three patterns: (1) presence of single or multiple pulmonary nodules with irregular borders and sometimes central cavitation, which is the most common radiographic pattern (Figs. 55-18 and 55-19); (2) reticular interstitial opacities, which result from venous or

---

✓ **WHAT THE CLINICIAN NEEDS TO KNOW**

1. Pulmonary mass: size, number, site (parenchymal, intraluminal, extraluminal)
2. Characteristics of mass: fat, calcification, cyst, cavitation, enhancement
3. Reticulonodular interstitial pattern: distribution (centrilobular, intralobular, peribronchial, perivascular, subpleural)
4. Associated parenchymal changes: consolidation, atelectasis, ground glass opacification
5. Associated features: mediastinal adenopathy, pleural effusion, extrathoracic manifestation, associated tumoral lesions (syndrome)

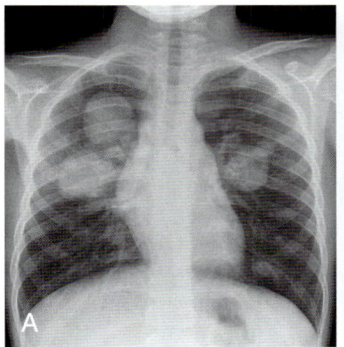
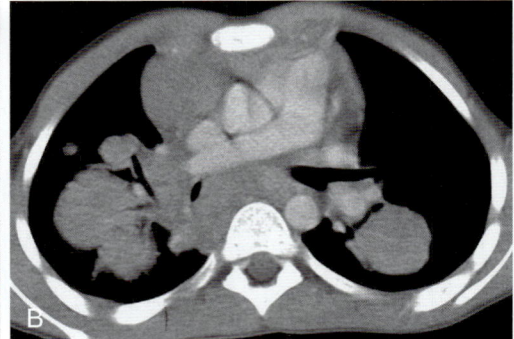
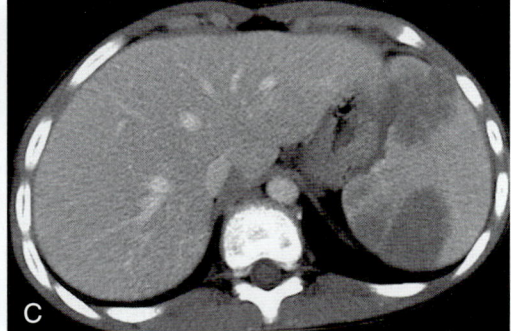

Figure 55-18 Hodgkin lymphoma. A 13-year-old boy who presented with a cough that had lasted for 6 months. **A,** A chest radiograph shows several pulmonary masses in both lungs of varying sizes predominantly in central location. **B,** An axial enhanced computed tomography (CT) image demonstrates several, bilateral pulmonary masses of soft tissue density and varying sizes in addition to anterior and posterior mediastinal lymphadenopathy. **C,** An axial enhanced CT image of the upper abdomen shows several hypodense lesions in the spleen likely representing splenic involvement of lymphoma.

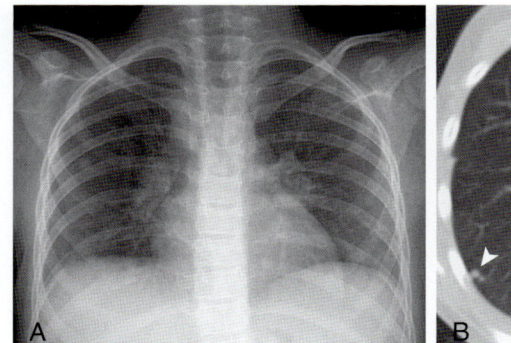 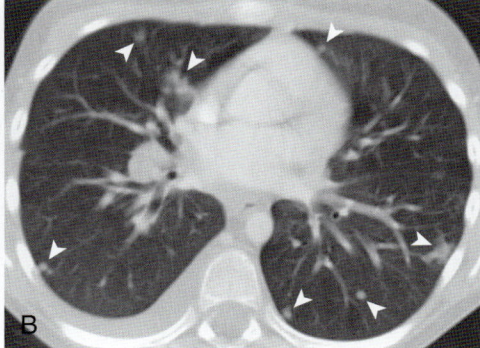 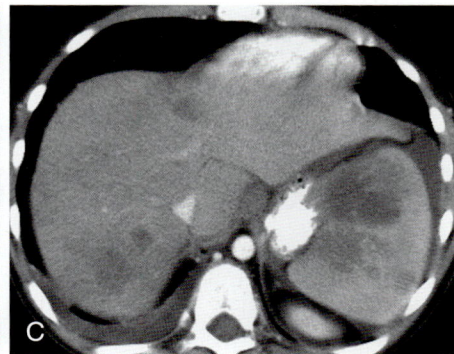

Figure 55-19 Hodgkin lymphoma. A 12-year-old boy with a history of ataxia telangiectasia, who presented with fevers and intermittent dry cough. He had daily fevers with a maximum temperature of 104°F, worse at night, and night sweats. **A,** A chest radiograph shows mediastinal and hilar lymphadenopathy, which prompted computed tomography (CT) evaluation. **B,** An axial lung window CT image demonstrates multiple, small, bilateral ill-defined pulmonary nodules (*arrowheads*), a small right pleural effusion in addition to lymphadenopathy. **C,** An axial enhanced CT image shows numerous low attenuation lesions in the liver and spleen. Biopsy samples from his liver and pleural fluid confirmed the diagnosis of Hodgkin lymphoma.

Key Points

Pulmonary parenchymal masses are more commonly congenital or inflammatory lesions rather than neoplasms in children.

Benign pulmonary neoplasms in children are far less common than malignant lesions. The ratio of primary benign to primary malignant to secondary malignant neoplasms is 1.4 : 1 : 11.6.

Lymphoproliferative disease is common in immunocompromised children, including those who have received transplantation. CT features range from pseudotumor, nodules, reticular interstitial pattern, to cysts. Definitive diagnosis relies on tissue biopsy.

Metastatic disease is, by far, the most common cause of pulmonary malignancy in childhood. The most frequent causes are osteogenic sarcoma and Wilms tumor.

Secondary pulmonary involvement in systemic diseases such as leukemia or lymphoma is uncommon in children. CT features are nonspecific and include nodules, reticular interstitial pattern, and consolidation, which mimic infectious lung changes. Lung biopsy is required for definitive diagnosis.

Suggested Readings

Dishop MK, Kuruvilla S. Primary and metastatic lung tumors in the pediatric population: a review and 25-year experience at a large children's hospital. *Arch Pathol Lab Med.* 2008;132(7):1079-1103.

Do KH, Lee JS, et al. Pulmonary parenchymal involvement of low-grade lymphoproliferative disorders. *J Comput Assist Tomogr.* 2005;29(6): 825-830.

McCahon E. Lung tumours in children. *Paediatr Respir Rev.* 2006; 7(3):191-196.

Pickhardt PJ, Siegel MJ, et al. Posttransplantation lymphoproliferative disorder in children: clinical, histopathologic, and imaging features. *Radiology.* 2000;217(1):16-25.

Yikilmaz A, Lee EY. CT imaging of mass-like nonvascular pulmonary lesions in children. *Pediatr Radiol.* 2007;37(12):1253-1263.

References

Full references for this chapter can be found on www.expertconsult.com.

Chapter 56

Diffuse Lung Disease

EVAN J. ZUCKER, R. PAUL GUILLERMAN, MARTHA P. FISHMAN,
ALICIA M. CASEY, CRAIG W. LILLEHEI, and EDWARD Y. LEE

Childhood interstitial lung diseases (ChILDs), which are associated with significant morbidity and mortality, represent a rare and heterogeneous group of chronic diffuse lung disorders characterized clinically by dyspnea, tachypnea, crackles, and hypoxemia. Although termed "interstitial," the diseases additionally may involve the alveoli, airways, blood vessels, lymphatic channels, and pleural spaces. With advances in imaging, improved thoracoscopic lung biopsy techniques, and in particular a revised ChILD classification scheme, substantial progress has been made in understanding these previously enigmatic disorders.[1-4] In this chapter, we provide an overview of pediatric chronic diffuse lung disease, first discussing the recognized disorders of infancy as defined by the revised ChILD criteria (Box 56-1). We then focus on selected, practically relevant examples of ILDs occurring in older children; even under the new classification system, these diseases remain too numerous to review in their entirety.

Disorders of Infancy

DIFFUSE DEVELOPMENTAL DISORDERS

Etiology Diffuse developmental disorders are characterized by marked alveolar gas exchange impairment and are thought to arise early in prenatal lung development. The three main entities within this category are acinar dysplasia, congenital alveolar dysplasia, and alveolar capillary dysplasia with misalignment of pulmonary veins (ACD/MPV). Acinar dysplasia is characterized by arrest of lung development in the pseudoglandular or early canalicular phase. Arrest in the late canalicular/early saccular phase is typical of congenital alveolar dysplasia. ACD/MPV results from an abnormal location of the pulmonary vein branches next to the pulmonary artery branches rather than within the interlobular septae; medial hypertrophy of the pulmonary arterioles, reduced alveolar capillary density, and maldevelopment of pulmonary lobules also occur. A proportion of ACD/MPV cases are caused by *FOXF1* gene mutations or 16q24.1 microdeletions.[1-3,5-9]

Imaging Generally, only portable chest radiographs are available because of the severity of disease. Initial chest radiographs may be unremarkable, but follow-up examinations typically demonstrate progressive hazy bilateral pulmonary opacities, similar to that seen in children with surfactant

deficiency of prematurity or inborn errors of surfactant metabolism. Typically, lung volumes initially are normal to decreased but may be increased with ventilator support. Air leaks such as pneumothorax and pneumomediastinum develop in about half of patients, likely because of barotrauma (Fig. 56-1). Radiographs may show enlargement of the main pulmonary artery in patients with concurrent pulmonary hypertension (PHT). Although imaging findings are nonspecific, this group of disorders should be considered in a full-term neonate with severe respiratory distress similar to PHT of the newborn in the absence of such risk factors as meconium aspiration, asphyxia, prematurity, or sepsis.[1-3,10-13]

Treatment and Follow-up Diffuse developmental disorders carry an extremely poor prognosis and are nearly universally fatal, with rapidly progressive respiratory failure typically developing in the first 2 months of life despite such measures as treatment for PHT, intensive ventilation, and extracorporeal membrane oxygenation. Serial chest radiographs can monitor the progression of the disease and help identify acute complications that may be seen with prolonged ventilatory support. Lung transplantation is the only viable treatment. However, patients generally do not survive long enough to receive a transplant, and many families elect to withdraw care upon diagnosis. More than 80% of patients with ACD/MPV have associated extrapulmonary anomalies (e.g., cardiac, gastrointestinal, or genitourinary) for which screening studies may be performed. Because 10% of reported ACD/MPV cases demonstrate a familial association, genetic counseling may be offered to family members.[1-3,5-14]

ALVEOLAR GROWTH DISORDERS

Etiology The most common form of neonatal ILD, alveolar growth disorders, are characterized by defects in alveolar formation with lobular simplification, lack of alveolar septation, and enlargement of airspaces. Unlike diffuse developmental disorders, in which lung development is preprogrammed to be abnormal, growth disorders are caused by a secondary condition or event affecting lung development. Entities in this category include: (1) pulmonary hypoplasia due to such conditions as oligohydramnios, space-occupying lesions, or neuromuscular disease; (2) postnatal conditions such as prematurity-related chronic lung disease (bronchopulmonary dysplasia [BPD]) and full-term chronic lung disease;

alveoli are just beginning to develop, a shift in the imaging features of BPD has occurred, termed "new" BPD. Findings on chest radiography and CT in infants with new BPD and other alveolar growth abnormalities range from near normal to markedly disordered, variably sized pulmonary lobules, thick perilobular reticular opacities, linear and triangular subpleural opacities, ground-glass opacities, and hyperlucent areas, some of which resemble cysts (Fig. 56-2). These features may be mistaken for "emphysematous changes." In infants with trisomy 21, small subpleural cysts are particularly common (Fig. 56-3). Chest imaging in patients with abnormal alveolar growth related to X-linked filamin A gene mutations is characterized by central pulmonary artery enlargement, atelectasis, progressive severe pulmonary hyperinflation, hyperlucency, and peripheral pulmonary vascular attenuation similar to congenital lobar or acquired emphysema (e-Fig. 56-4).[1-3,5,15-20]

Treatment and Follow-up Reduction in BPD severity and incidence may be achieved by decreasing respiratory support interventions causing lung injury. Additional treatment strategies including nasal respiratory support, low-dose corticosteroids, fluid restriction, vitamin A, and medical/surgical patent ductus arteriosus closure have shown only lackluster results. The linear and subpleural opacities seen on computed tomography (CT) correspond to interstitial fibroproliferation and are associated with low functional residual capacity, supplemental oxygen, and mechanical ventilation, but they do not correlate with the severity of symptoms. Because a significant proportion of patients with growth abnormalities also have patchy pulmonary interstitial glycogenosis (PIG) (detailed later), which is potentially responsive to steroids, a lung biopsy may be considered to help establish a concurrent diagnosis. Patients with filamin A mutations may experience especially severe respiratory decline requiring lung transplantation for survival.[1-3,5,14-22]

(3) structural pulmonary changes seen with such chromosomal abnormalities as trisomy 21; and (4) changes as a result of congenital heart disease in the absence of chromosomal abnormalities.[1-3,5,15-20]

Imaging Imaging findings are variable on both plain radiographs and high-resolution computed tomography (HRCT). Chest radiography in infants with classic BPD demonstrates coarse reticular opacities, cystic lucencies, and disordered lung aeration due to alveolar septal fibrosis and hyperinflation. With advances in perinatal medicine allowing delivery as early as 23 weeks' gestation, when the alveolar ducts and

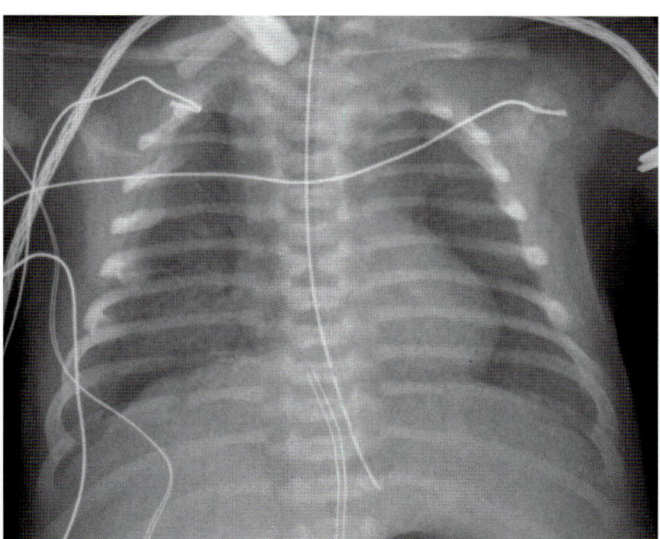

Figure 56-1 A chest radiograph of a full-term newborn with alveolar capillary dysplasia/malalignment of the pulmonary veins demonstrates hazy bilateral pulmonary opacities, pneumomediastinum, and a right pneumothorax.

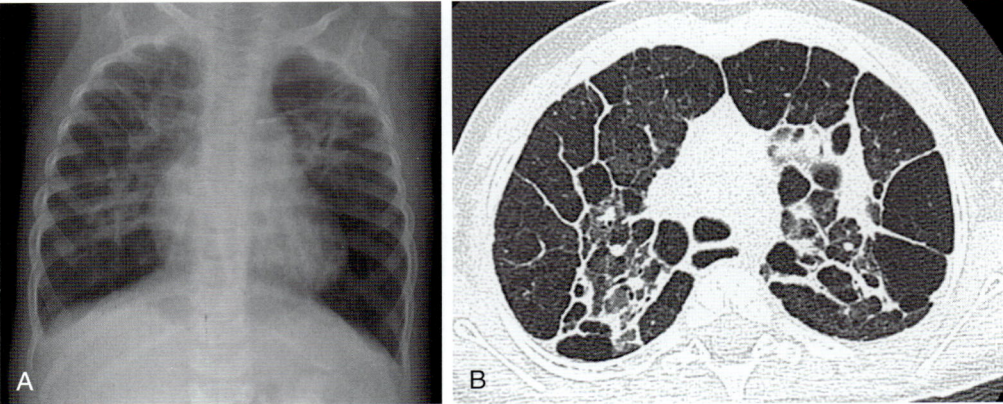

Figure 56-2 A chest radiograph at 21 months of age (**A**) and an axial computed tomography image at 2 years of age (**B**) in a child born prematurely at 25 weeks' gestation with alveolar growth disorder show pulmonary architectural distortion with pulmonary lobules of variable size and attenuation, perilobular reticular opacities, ground-glass opacities, and hyperlucent areas resembling cysts.

SURFACTANT DYSFUNCTION DISORDERS AND RELATED ABNORMALITIES

Etiology Diseases in surfactant dysfunction disorders and related abnormalities are caused by genetic mutations resulting in surfactant dysfunction. Mutations in surfactant proteins B (SpB) and C (SpC) and the adenosine triphosphate–binding cassette transporter protein A3 (ABCA3) directly impair surfactant metabolism. SpB and ABCA3 mutations demonstrate an autosomal-recessive inheritance pattern, whereas SpC defects are autosomal-dominant loss of function mutations. Other rare genetic disorders such as thyroid transcription factor-1 abnormalities ("brain-lung-thyroid syndrome"), lysinuric protein intolerance, and granulocyte-macrophage colony-stimulating factor–Rα mutations also affect surfactant metabolism and also are included in this category. Additional uncharacterized disorders of surfactant metabolism exist.[1-3,21-42]

Imaging Chest radiographs in infants presenting with a surfactant disorder demonstrate diffuse or patchy hazy granular pulmonary opacities. HRCT is characterized by diffuse ground-glass opacity, consolidation, interlobular septal thickening, or a crazy-paving pattern typical of pulmonary alveolar proteinosis (PAP) (detailed separately in a later section) (Fig. 56-5). With increasing age, the ground–glass opacities decrease in extent and thin–walled parenchymal cysts develop, becoming larger and more numerous over time (e-Fig. 56-6). Pectus excavatum is common in patients surviving past infancy, possibly because of the effects of chronic lung disease on the growing chest wall.[1-3,21-42]

Treatment and Follow-up Often the diagnosis of inherited surfactant disorder can be established through testing of blood or buccal swab–derived samples for surfactant gene mutations, obviating the need for lung biopsy. The mainstay of treatment is chronic ventilator support in children with respiratory failure. Anecdotal evidence suggests a possible role for pulse corticosteroids, hydroxychloroquine (Plaquenil), and azithromycin. Nutritional supplementation via a gastrostomy tube often is required for growth. Palivizumab (Synagis) may be considered to help prevent lung infections. Patients with rapidly progressive disease may be eligible for lung transplantation. Investigational efforts focus on targeted therapies for the specific genetic mutations involved.[1-3,14,21-42]

SPECIFIC CONDITIONS OF UNKNOWN OR POORLY UNDERSTOOD ETIOLOGY

Neuroendocrine Cell Hyperplasia of Infancy

Etiology The etiology of neuroendocrine cell hyperplasia of infancy (NEHI) is unknown. Histopathologically, the disease (previously referred to as persistent tachypnea of infancy) is characterized by increased numbers of pulmonary neuroendocrine cells (PNECs) and innervated clusters of PNECs called neuroepithelial bodies in the epithelium of peripheral airways. PNECs function in oxygen sensing and fetal lung development; they usually rapidly decrease in number after the neonatal period. Although increased numbers of PNECs are seen in persons with a variety of pulmonary disorders, the diseases are not likely to be confused with NEHI histopathologically. Some patients with NEHI demonstrate mild inflammation or fibrosis of the airways. Additionally, some cases are familial, suggesting a genetic component.[1-3,5,14,43-50]

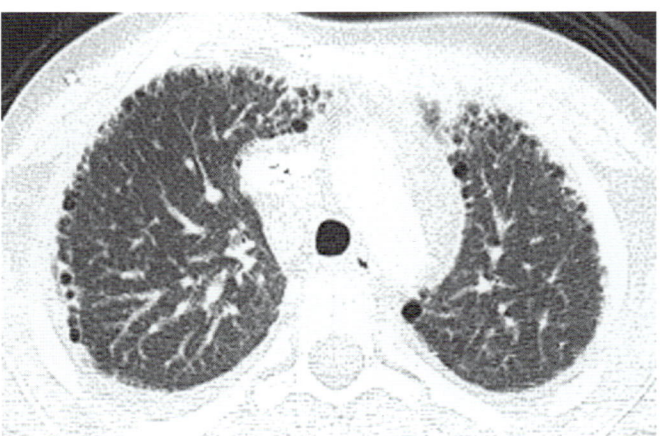

Figure 56-3 An axial computed tomography image from a 10-year-old with alveolar growth disorder related to trisomy 21 reveals numerous bilateral subpleural cysts.

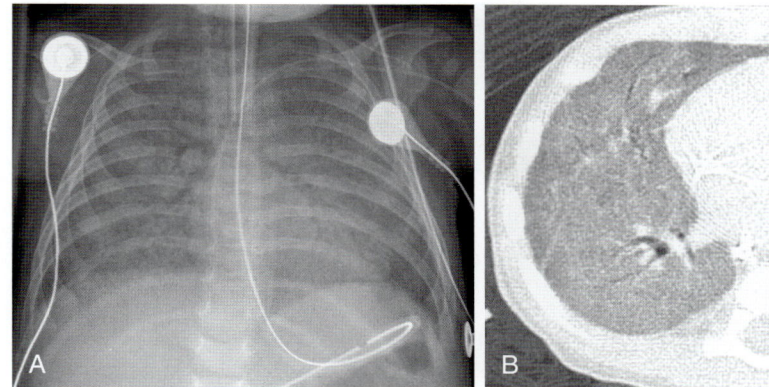

Figure 56-5 A chest radiograph (**A**) and an axial computed tomography image (**B**) from a 3-month-old full-term infant with surfactant dysfunction related to *ABCA3* gene mutations show diffuse hazy ground-glass pulmonary opacification.

Imaging Chest radiographs demonstrate hyperinflation and variable increased perihilar opacity resembling bronchiolitis or reactive airways disease (Fig. 56-7). HRCT findings are characteristic with air trapping and a mosaic attenuation pattern affecting at least four lobes and geographic ground-glass opacities most prominent in the right middle lobe, lingula, and paramediastinal lung regions (Fig. 56-8). The sensitivity and specificity of HRCT for the diagnosis is reported to be 78% to 83% and 100% when examinations are interpreted by experienced pediatric thoracic radiologists. Thus in the correct clinical setting, CT may obviate the need for a lung biopsy.[1-3,5,14,43-50]

Treatment and Follow-up Treatment of NEHI at present is supportive and is geared toward preventing hypoxemia and infection and maintaining nutritional support. Corticosteroids are not helpful and are not recommended, except for temporary glucocorticoid pulses if a patient has a concurrent viral

infection. Although patients with NEHI have persistent symptoms and require prolonged oxygen therapy, the prognosis is generally favorable with no reported deaths, progression to respiratory failure, or need for lung transplantation attributable to this disorder. However, it should be noted that patients in later life (i.e., adolescence) may experience symptoms such as exercise intolerance related to persistent air trapping and can relapse in the setting of respiratory infection.[1-3,5,14,43-50]

Pulmonary Interstitial Glycogenosis

Etiology The etiology of pulmonary interstitial glycogenosis (PIG), previously known as infantile cellular interstitial pneumonitis and histiocytoid pneumonia, remains unknown. PIG is characterized histopathologically by infiltration of the interstitium with immature mesenchymal cells containing copious cytoplasmic glycogen and staining positively for vimentin. Inflammation and fibrosis are not typical. Patchy PIG and alveolar growth abnormalities commonly coexist. The lack of PIG in lung biopsies from children older than 10 months suggests that the disorder may be related to lung growth and development.[1-3,5,14-15,51-56]

Imaging Chest radiographs have been reported to demonstrate progressive hyperinflation and evolution from a fine interstitial to a coarse interstitial or alveolar pattern. HRCT findings may include pulmonary architectural distortion, hyperinflated/hyperlucent areas, ground-glass opacities (diffuse, segmental, or subsegmental), interlobular septal thickening, and linear opacities (Fig. 56-9). Because patchy PIG often coexists with alveolar growth abnormalities, the specific imaging features of "pure" PIG are uncertain. In one reported case of PIG, the multiple, small, scattered, air-filled, cystic-appearing changes were most likely attributable to the concomitant alveolar growth abnormality.[1-3,5,14-15,51-56]

Treatment and Follow-up Most patients require supplemental oxygen. PIG may respond favorably to pulse glucocorticoids, which are recommended at many ChILD centers. Overall, the prognosis of pure PIG is favorable, with no reported deaths attributable to the disease. However, greater mortality and morbidity rates are expected with concomitant growth abnormalities and PHT. During the first several months of

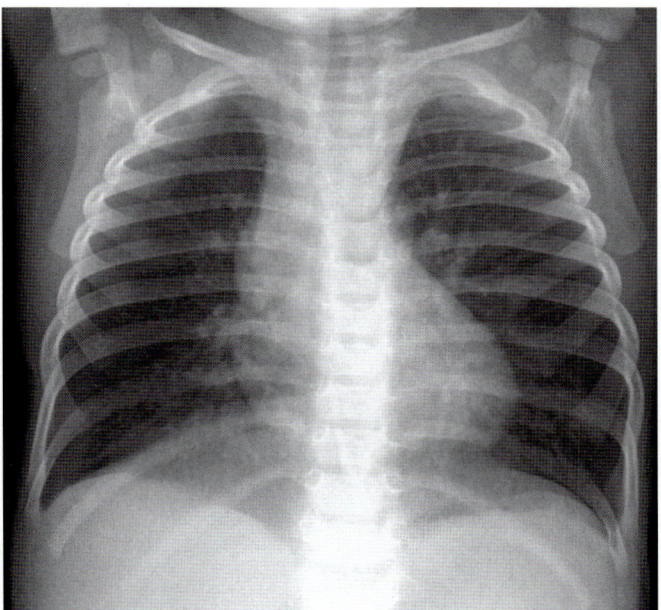

Figure 56-7 A chest radiograph of a 15-month-old with neuroendocrine cell hyperplasia of infancy demonstrates pulmonary hyperinflation and parahilar opacities resembling reactive airways disease or bronchiolitis.

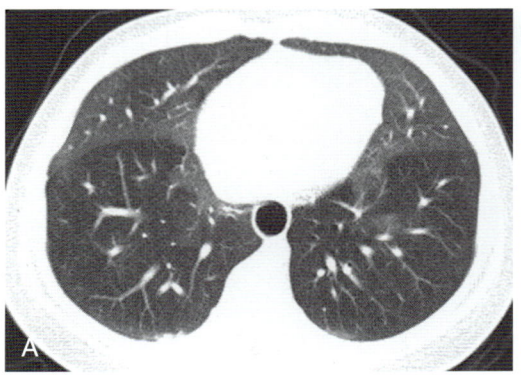 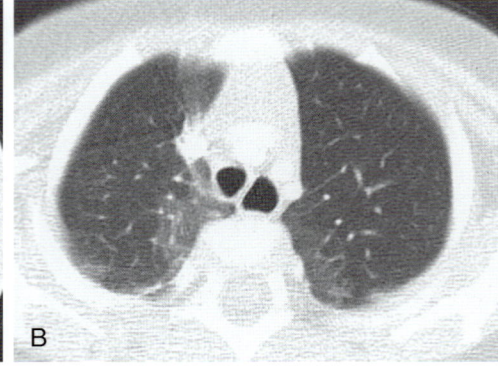

Figure 56-8 Axial computed tomography images of an 11-month-old with neuroendocrine cell hyperplasia of infancy depict characteristic geographic ground-glass opacities of the right middle lobe and lingula (**A**) and of the paramediastinal lung regions (**B**).

life, marked improvement often occurs clinically, radiologically, and histologically, although hyperinflation may persist for years.[1-3,5,14-15,51-56]

Disorders of Childhood

PULMONARY ALVEOLAR PROTEINOSIS

Etiology PAP is characterized by the abnormal accumulation of surfactant, a lipoproteinaceous material, within the alveoli that prevents normal gas exchange. As discussed previously, PAP may arise congenitally as the result of a genetic surfactant deficiency. The acquired form of PAP seen in older children and adults is most commonly an autoimmune process in which autoantibodies to granulocyte macrophage colony-stimulating factor (GM-CSF) are produced. Because GM-CSF normally participates in alveolar macrophage signaling, the disease results in impaired clearance of surfactant-derived intraalveolar lipoproteins. PAP also may be a result of a variety of processes including leukemia, chemotherapy, toxic exposure to fumes and dusts, and other entities that impair alveolar macrophage function.[1-3,5,57-63]

Imaging The various etiologies of PAP cannot be differentiated by imaging. Chest radiographs demonstrate symmetric perihilar opacities extending to the peripheral portions of the lungs. These opacities generally are not as consolidative and dense as would be expected for a bacterial pneumonia. HRCT shows bilateral ground-glass opacities with smooth intralobular and interlobular septal thickening in polygonal shapes, an appearance known as "crazy paving"[1-3,5,57-63] (Fig. 56-10).

Treatment and Follow-up After the diagnosis is confirmed, preferably by bronchoscopy with bronchoalveolar lavage and transbronchial biopsy but by a surgical lung biopsy if necessary, serologic testing for GM-CSF antibodies should be performed to distinguish between autoimmune and secondary PAP. For secondary PAP, treatment efforts should focus on identifying the underlying cause. For autoimmune PAP, repeated whole-lung lavage is the current treatment of choice. Aerosolized GM-CSF therapy has shown very promising results in observational studies, although randomized controlled trials are not yet available. Immunosuppression with

Figure 56-9 An axial computed tomography image from a 5-month-old former 25-week premature infant with concomitant alveolar growth disorder and pulmonary interstitial glycogenosis shows cystlike hyperlucent lobules, thick reticular perilobular opacities, and ground-glass opacities.

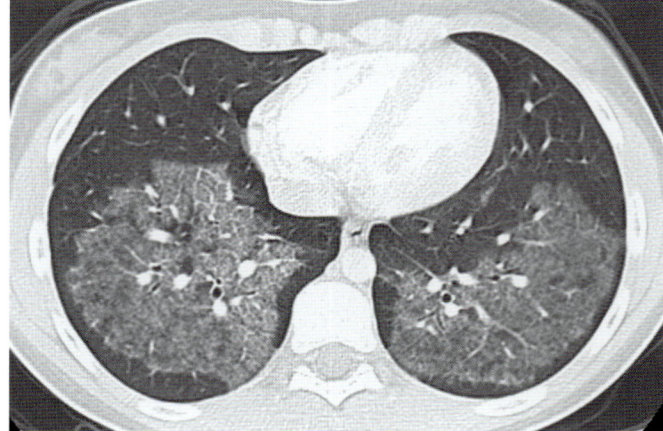

Figure 56-10 An axial computed tomography image of an 11-year-old with pulmonary alveolar proteinosis due to autoantibodies to anti-granulocyte macrophage colony-stimulating factor demonstrates a crazy-paving pattern of ground-glass opacities and septal thickening.

rituximab or mycophenolate mofetil also has been tried. CT can be used to monitor the response to therapy.[1-3,5,57-63]

PULMONARY LYMPHANGIECTASIA AND LYMPHANGIOMATOSIS

Etiology Lymphatic disorders are considered "masqueraders" of ILD according to the ChILD classification. However, primary pulmonary lymphangiectasia and lymphangiomatosis can be regarded as true ILDs because they involve the pulmonary interstitium. Pulmonary lymphangiectasia is characterized by dilatation of the lymphatics draining the pulmonary interstitial and subpleural spaces, either on a congenital basis (including some associated genetic syndromes) or an acquired basis (as a result of pulmonary lymphatic or venous obstruction). Pulmonary lymphangiomatosis is characterized by a proliferation of complex lymphatic channels with secondary lymphatic dilatation. In both disorders, the disease may be limited to the lung or may involve additional thoracic and/ or extrathoracic manifestations.[1-3,15,64-70]

Imaging Chest radiographs in patients who present with the classic sign of severe respiratory distress demonstrate diffuse hazy opacification of the lungs similar to the findings of surfactant deficiency of prematurity or genetic surfactant deficiency. A chest CT scan shows diffuse, smooth thickening of the interlobular septae and peribronchovascular interstitium, patchy ground-glass opacities, and pleural effusions (often chylous) (e-Fig. 56-11). Less diffuse opacity, less severe septal thickening, and greater hyperinflation are characteristic of surviving neonates or patients presenting later in infancy. Magnetic resonance imaging (MRI) demonstrates hyperintensity of the pulmonary interstitium on T2-weighted sequences and pleural effusions. Lung findings are very similar in pulmonary lymphangiectasia and lymphangiomatosis. Unlike lymphangiectasia, lymphangiomatosis usually presents in late childhood and often involves extrapulmonary sites, with lytic bone lesions and mediastinal soft tissue edema occurring frequently.[1-3,15,64-70]

Treatment and Follow-up Patients with congenital disease may be stillborn or present at birth with severe respiratory distress, which often results in death within the first few hours of life. Mechanical ventilation and pleural drainage invariably are required. Patients with long-term survival have variable degrees of respiratory compromise and are managed with supplemental oxygen at home, symptomatic therapy, fluid restriction, and dietary measures.[1-3,15,64-71]

BRONCHIOLITIS OBLITERANS

Etiology Bronchiolitis obliterans (BO) is characterized by a fibroblastic reparative response to injury of the small airways, resulting in occlusion of the lumen. The inciting injury is usually a respiratory viral infection (often adenovirus or influenza) with marked airway mucosal necrosis. Other preceding conditions include graft-versus-host disease, chronic allograft rejection in patients who have had a lung transplant, and Stevens-Johnson syndrome. Swyer-James-Macleod syndrome is a particular form of BO that predominantly affects one lung and presents several months or years after the initial infection. Terminology for BO in the literature is inconsistent, leading

to confusion. The clinical manifestation may be termed "bronchiolitis obliterans syndrome," whereas the histopathologic correlate is a spectrum termed "constrictive bronchiolitis" or "obliterative bronchiolitis," depending on the degree of airway lumen occlusion that is present.[1-3,5,72-77]

Imaging Findings of chest radiographs are nonspecific and may be normal. The most common abnormality is hyperinflation. A hyperlucent lung on the affected side that is relatively underperfused with normal or decreased volume is characteristic of Swyer-James-Macleod syndrome. CT findings consist of air trapping accentuated on expiration, parenchymal hyperlucency, mosaic attenuation, bronchial wall thickening, bronchiectasis, and pulmonary vascular attenuation. The presence of both hyperlucency and pulmonary vascular attenuation is highly specific for moderate/severe nontransplant BO (e-Fig. 56-12). With a correlating clinical history and a fixed obstructive pattern on pulmonary function testing, CT is diagnostic, bypassing the need for a lung biopsy. In the Swyer-James-Macleod variant, chest radiographs suggest a unilateral abnormality, but in fact, abnormal findings on CT are bilateral in 50% of cases.[1-3,5,72-77]

Treatment and Follow-up In the absence of bronchiectasis, BO can be difficult to distinguish from the more common acute viral bronchiolitis with CT. Follow-up imaging thus can be helpful. Imaging findings in persons with acute viral bronchiolitis will normalize on subsequent examinations after symptom resolution (with up to several months lag), whereas persistent or worsening abnormalities will be present in irreversible BO. CT provides valuable prognostic information in postinfectious BO; in children younger than 3 years of age with severe CT abnormalities, lung function is generally poor even after several years. In lung transplant recipients, CT is valuable in screening for posttransplant BO, which is an important contributor to mortality after the first postoperative year. For the BO variant associated with lung transplantation, corticosteroids and the antibiotic azithromycin have shown benefit.[1-3,5,72-79]

HYPERSENSITIVITY PNEUMONITIS

Etiology Also known as extrinsic allergic alveolitis, hypersensitivity pneumonitis is characterized by pulmonary inflammation related to inhalational exposure of organic antigens usually from birds, fungi, or dusts carried by family members from the workplace. Other inciting antigens include a variety of highly reactive low molecular weight compounds found in spray paints, glues, epoxy resins, insecticides, and drugs such as methotrexate. Histopathologically, lymphocytic infiltration of the bronchioles and interstitium is seen with giant cells and poorly developed granulomas situated around bronchioles. Three subtypes of hypersensitivity pneumonitis have been described: (1) acute, with symptoms occurring by 4 to 6 hours and lasting up to 22 hours; (2) subacute, characterized by repeated low-level antigen exposure over weeks to months; and (3) chronic, manifested by an insidious, progressive course over months to years, or, alternatively, recurrent acute episodes.[1-3,5,64,80-84]

Imaging The acute and subacute forms of hypersensitivity pneumonitis have similar imaging features. Common abnormal findings on chest radiographs are diffuse micronodular interstitial prominence and opacities in the mid to lower lungs, which may resemble pulmonary edema or pneumonia. However, many radiographs will appear normal, with 40% of cases having abnormalities visible only on CT. HRCT demonstrates small (1 to 3 mm) poorly defined centrilobular nodules (reflecting bronchiolitis), ground-glass opacities (reflecting alveolitis), and air trapping, with relative sparing of the upper lungs. On radiography and CT, the chronic form is characterized by volume loss and fibrotic changes predominantly with irregular linear/reticular opacities, architectural distortion, and honeycombing (e-Fig. 56-13).[1-3,5,64,80-84]

Treatment and Follow-up The most important aspect of treatment is identifying and eliminating exposure to the inciting antigen. The imaging findings associated with the acute and subacute forms of the disease regress with removal of the antigen. However, the chronic fibrotic changes persist and may even progress. Systemic corticosteroids are the only dependable drug therapy but do not affect the long-term outcome.[1-3,5,64,80-84]

DIFFUSE PULMONARY HEMORRHAGE DISORDERS

Etiology Diffuse pulmonary hemorrhage disorders can be subcategorized according to the presence or absence of capillaritis, which is characterized pathologically by inflammatory disruption of the interstitial capillary network. Disorders with capillaritis include idiopathic pulmonary capillaritis, Wegener granulomatosis (recently renamed granulomatosis with polyangiitis), microscopic polyangiitis, Goodpasture syndrome, idiopathic pulmonary-renal syndrome, systemic lupus erythematosus, and drug-induced capillaritis. Disorders without capillaritis include idiopathic pulmonary hemosiderosis, acute idiopathic pulmonary hemorrhage of infancy, Heiner syndrome (pulmonary disease caused by food sensitivity, usually to cow's milk), coagulation disorders, and cardiovascular disorders such as pulmonary venoocclusive disease and pulmonary arteriovenous malformation.[1-3,85-89]

Imaging The classic radiographic appearance of acute diffuse pulmonary hemorrhage consists of bilateral symmetric airspace opacities in a "butterfly" or "batwing" pattern. However, opacities may be asymmetric or unilateral. HRCT is more sensitive and shows patchy ground-glass opacities and consolidation acutely. With organizing or repetitive hemorrhage, findings evolve to interlobular septal thickening, nodular opacities, and potentially a crazy-paving pattern (Fig. 56-14).[1-3,85-89]

Treatment and Follow-up Distinguishing between pulmonary hemorrhage with capillaritis versus without capillaritis is critical, because pulmonary capillaritis often requires aggressive immunosuppressive therapy. Because imaging findings are similar in the many conditions causing pulmonary hemorrhage, a lung biopsy often is necessary for a definitive diagnosis. With treatment, CT findings typically improve.[1-3,85-89]

NONSPECIFIC INTERSTITIAL PNEUMONIA

Etiology Nonspecific interstitial pneumonia (NSIP) can be idiopathic, familial, or the final common pathway of several other disorders, including autoimmune connective tissue and collagen vascular diseases, genetic surfactant disorders, and hypersensitivity pneumonitis. Histopathologically, there is a characteristic appearance with temporally and spatially uniform interstitial lymphoplasmacytic inflammation and varying degrees of fibrosis. Cellular and fibrotic subtypes have been described.[1-3,5,90-93]

Imaging Best characterized by HRCT, the typical imaging findings are ground-glass and fine linear or reticular opacities, predominantly at the lung periphery (e-Fig. 56-15). Traction bronchiectasis, volume loss (predominantly in the lower lobe), and honeycombing may develop over time.[1-3,5,90-93]

Treatment and Follow-up HRCT findings of NSIP can resolve or persist, depending on the degree of fibrosis. Immunosuppressive therapy often is beneficial. However, patients with progressive disease may require lung transplantation.[1-3,5,90-93]

CONNECTIVE TISSUE AND COLLAGEN-VASCULAR DISEASES

Etiology Connective tissue and collagen-vascular diseases are a heterogeneous group of rheumatologic disorders characterized by chronic inflammation and generally thought to have an autoimmune basis. Included entities are systemic lupus

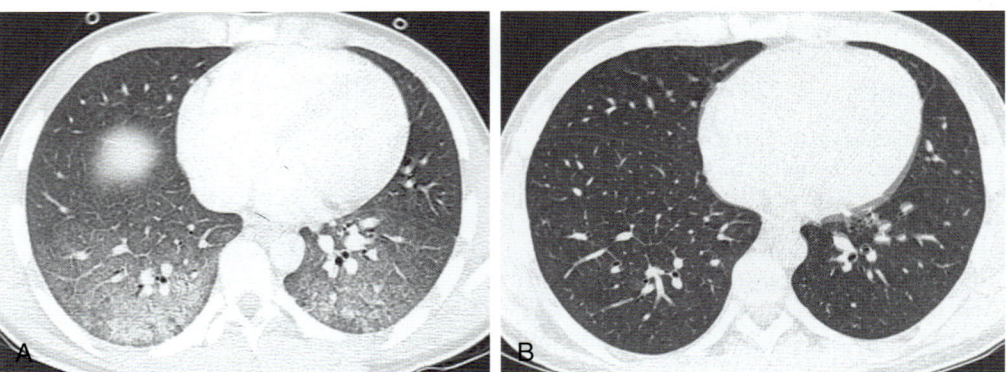

Figure 56-14 Axial computed tomography images of a 15-year-old with pulmonary capillaritis show posterior ground-glass opacities and consolidation at time of diagnosis (**A**) and normalization after 2 weeks of corticosteroid therapy (**B**).

erythematosus, rheumatoid arthritis, dermatomyositis, systemic sclerosis, Sjögren syndrome, and mixed connective tissue disease. Most commonly, an NSIP histopathologic pattern (previously detailed) is found. Pulmonary lymphoid hyperplasia, organizing pneumonia (detailed later), vasculopathy, and pleuritis also may occur.[1-3,5,90-96]

Imaging Because they share an NSIP pattern, the various entities usually cannot be differentiated by imaging. Occasionally, ancillary findings may suggest the diagnosis, such as a dilated esophagus in a person with systemic sclerosis (e-Fig. 56-16). Childhood-onset systemic lupus erythematosus presents with vasculitis and pulmonary hemorrhage much more commonly than it does with ILD, unlike its adult counterpart.[1-3,5,90-96]

Treatment and Follow-up Treatment generally involves immunosuppression. As with NSIP, imaging findings may abate with clinical improvement, but fibrotic changes persist. Newer investigational efforts focus on targeting specific genes involved in inciting inflammatory pathways.[1-3,5,90-96]

ORGANIZING PNEUMONIA

Etiology Organizing pneumonia is characterized histologically by intraluminal organizing fibrosis in the distal airways and airspaces (bronchioles, alveolar ducts, and alveoli). Organizing pneumonia may be idiopathic and termed "cryptogenic organizing pneumonia," or it can be a result of a variety of causes including asthma, drug reaction, aspiration pneumonia, autoimmune disease, chemotherapy, bone marrow transplantation, and other conditions stimulating a lung reparative response. The term "bronchiolitis obliterans organizing pneumonia" is no longer favored because of potential confusion with the distinct entity of BO.[1-3,97-99]

Imaging Imaging findings are variable, with CT most frequently showing peripheral patchy consolidation with or without surrounding ground-glass opacity. Commonly, air bronchograms and mild bronchial dilatation are found within areas of consolidation. Other recognized findings include the atoll or reverse halo sign (central ground-glass opacity surrounded by consolidation) (Fig. 56-17), small pulmonary nodules along bronchovascular bundles, linear and bandlike subpleural opacities, perilobular thickening, and progressive fibrosis.[1-3,97-99]

Treatment and Follow-up Although organizing pneumonia has many underlying causes, overall, corticosteroids are the best treatment option. The prognosis is generally favorable, with up to an 80% cure rate reported. Imaging findings related to inflammation will improve/resolve on follow-up, whereas irreversible fibrotic changes may persist or worsen.[1-3,78,97-99]

PULMONARY INFILTRATE WITH EOSINOPHILIA

Etiology The eosinophilic lung diseases are a diverse group of disorders characterized by peripheral or tissue eosinophilia, with interstitial and intraalveolar eosinophils typically present on pathology. Three subcategories are recognized: eosinophilic disease of unknown cause, eosinophilic disease of

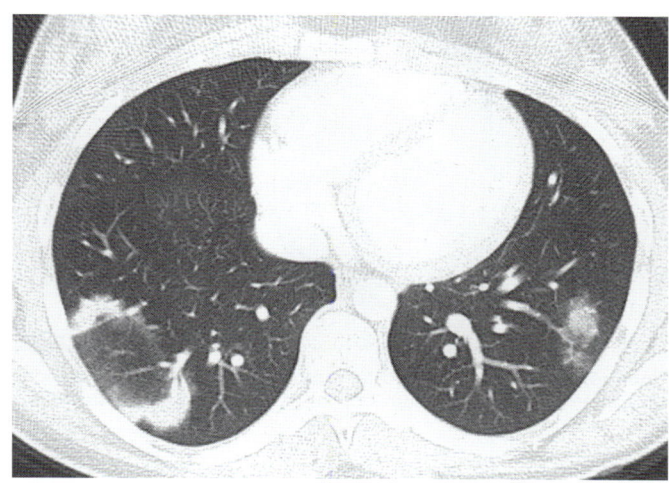

Figure 56-17 An axial computed tomography image from a 15-year-old with Sjögren syndrome depicts a patchy consolidation of the peripheral left lower lobe and a ground-glass opacity surrounded by consolidation ("atoll" or "reverse halo" sign) of the peripheral right lower lobe representing sites of organizing pneumonia.

known cause, and eosinophilic vasculitis. Diseases of unknown cause include simple pulmonary eosinophilia (or Löffler syndrome), acute eosinophilic pneumonia (AEP), chronic eosinophilic pneumonia (CEP), and idiopathic hypereosinophilic syndrome. Diseases of known cause include allergic bronchopulmonary aspergillosis (ABPA), bronchocentric granulomatosis, parasitic infections, and drug reactions. Eosinophilic vasculitis includes allergic angiitis and granulomatosis, also known as Churg-Strauss syndrome.[1-3,100-103]

Imaging Imaging findings of interstitial, alveolar, or mixed interstitial-alveolar opacities are in general nonspecific, but certain key features may suggest the underlying diagnosis. CEP and drug-induced pulmonary infiltrate with eosinophilia (PIE) demonstrate a characteristic pattern of peripheral consolidation with sparing of the central lung zones (a "photographic negative" or "reversed" pulmonary edema pattern), allowing a highly specific diagnosis in the setting of peripheral eosinophilia (Fig. 56-18). AEP presents radiographically with bilateral reticular opacities, possibly with consolidation and pleural effusion. On CT, bilateral patchy ground-glass opacity and often interlobular septal thickening, consolidation, or poorly defined nodules are seen. The imaging findings of AEP mimic those of more common entities such as pulmonary edema and acute respiratory distress syndrome, which may result in a delayed diagnosis. ABPA demonstrates central bronchiectasis with or without mucoid impaction; the presence of mucoid impaction of the large airways is referred to as the "finger-in-glove" sign. Simple pulmonary eosinophilia and idiopathic hypereosinophilic syndrome characteristically demonstrate pulmonary nodules with ground-glass halos. Bronchocentric granulomatosis demonstrates focal masses and nodules or lobar consolidation with atelectasis. Findings in persons with Churg-Strauss syndrome include subpleural consolidation, centrilobular nodules, bronchial wall thickening, and interlobular septal thickening.[1-3,100-103]

Treatment and Follow-up Imaging findings, even if nonspecific, can localize potential sites for lung biopsy.

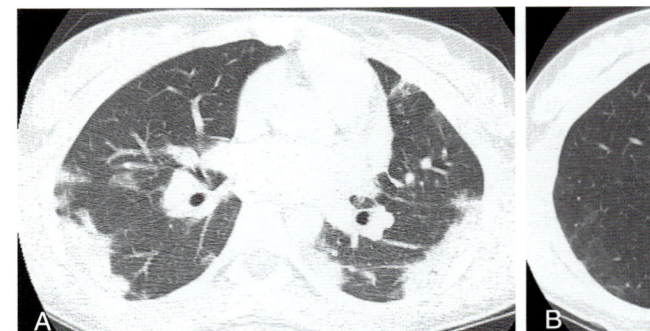

Figure 56-18 Axial computed tomography images of an 18-year-old with drug-induced (minocycline) pulmonary infiltrate with eosinophilia show characteristic peripheral consolidations at the time of diagnosis (**A**) and marked improvement after 2 weeks of corticosteroid therapy and cessation of the inciting drug (**B**).

Corticosteroids are the treatment of choice, resulting in prompt and complete response. In persons with AEP, relapses do not occur after cessation of corticosteroids, although they can occur in persons with CEP. Therapy may be tailored to the underlying cause; for example, antiparasitic medications may be used in a case of parasite-induced PIE.[1-3,100-103]

STORAGE DISEASES

Etiology The lysosomal storage diseases are a group of genetic metabolic disorders resulting in impaired lysosomal function. In the case of Gaucher disease and Niemann-Pick disease, lipid-laden "foamy" macrophages (Gaucher cells or Niemann-Pick cells, respectively) accumulate in tissues. These lipid-laden macrophages may infiltrate the lung, causing pulmonary symptoms. Gaucher disease is the most common lysosomal storage disorder.[2-3,104-107]

Imaging Pulmonary findings, if they appear at all, occur late in the course of Gaucher disease, most commonly in the neuronopathic type III form. Chest radiographs may show reticulonodular opacities. CT may reveal a variety of findings, including ground-glass opacities, consolidation, interstitial thickening, bronchial wall thickening, thymic enlargement, and lymphadenopathy. Diffuse interstitial thickening is characteristic of chest radiographs and CT in Niemann-Pick disease type B (Fig. 56-19). A crazy-paving pattern is typical of Niemann-Pick disease type C2[2-3,104-107] (e-Fig. 56-20).

Treatment and Follow-up Enzyme replacement therapy, approved by the U.S. Food and Drug Administration, is now available for several of the lysosomal storage disorders. In persons who have Gaucher disease with pulmonary involvement, the imaging findings gradually improve with treatment, although complete resolution typically is not achieved. Currently, chest radiographs are recommended every 2 years in persons with Gaucher disease to monitor the lungs.[2-3,104-107]

CHRONIC GRANULOMATOUS DISEASE

Etiology Chronic granulomatous disease (CGD) is a rare inherited immunodeficiency disorder that usually is caused by a mutation in one of the four genes encoding subunits of the phagocyte nicotinamide adenine dinucleotide phosphate. The mutation results in impaired phagocyte nicotinamide adenine

dinucleotide phosphate oxidase activity and therefore reduced superoxide production and an impaired oxidative burst. As a result, mechanisms for killing intracellular catalase-positive bacterial organisms and fungal organisms are impaired. The lungs are the most common location of infection. Histologically, granulomatous inflammation is present, often with necrosis, with surrounding chronic inflammation and fibrosis, hence the name chronic granulomatous disease.[1-2,108-110]

Imaging A variety of imaging findings may present in patients who have chronic, recurrent infections, including consolidation, ground-glass opacities, tree-in-bud opacities, and centrilobular or random (even miliary) nodules acutely, with bronchiectasis, septal thickening, air trapping, abscess formation, fibrosis, cysts, and honeycomb lung in persons with long-standing disease. Other common thoracic findings include mediastinal and/or hilar lymphadenopathy, pleural thickening, empyema, vertebral or rib osteomyelitis, and chest wall invasion[1-2,108-110] (Fig. 56-21).

Treatment and Follow-up CGD is treated with lipophilic antibiotics, antifungal agents, interferon-γ, abscess drainage,

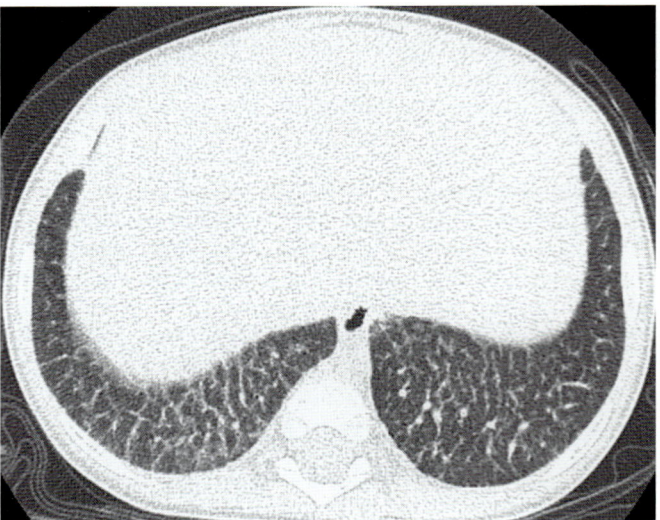

Figure 56-19 An axial computed tomography image from a 22-month-old with Niemann-Pick disease type B shows diffuse interstitial septal thickening.

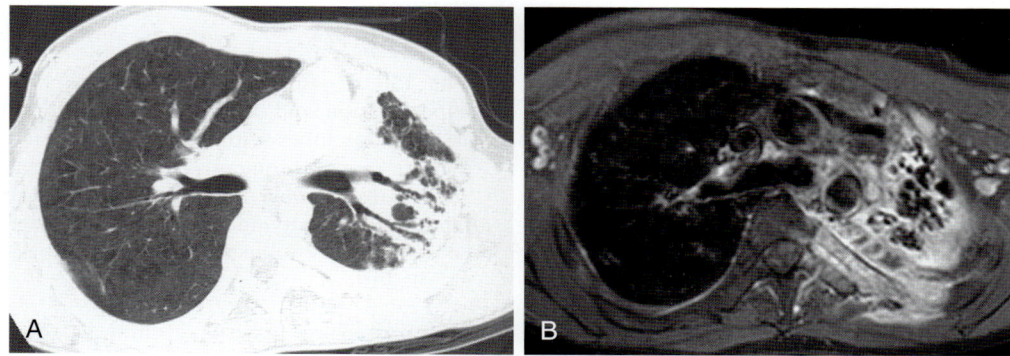

Figure 56-21 An axial computed tomography image from a 15-year-old with chronic granulomatous disease demonstrates left lung consolidation, bronchiectasis, and fibrotic volume loss (**A**). A gadolinium-enhanced T1-weighted fat-saturated axial magnetic resonance image from the same patient at 18 years of age reveals left pleural and chest wall involvement with empyema and costovertebral osteomyelitis (**B**).

surgical resection, and stem cell transplantation. Prophylactic antibiotics are beneficial. Fluorine-18 fluorodeoxyglucose positron emission tomography is more reliable than CT for distinguishing between active and dormant disease activity (e-Fig. 56-22). Improved ability to diagnose and treat CGD has allowed persons with this disease to survive into adulthood.[1-2,108-110]

CYSTIC FIBROSIS

Etiology The most common genetic disorder causing chronic pulmonary disease in children, cystic fibrosis (CF) is caused by mutations in the CF transmembrane regulator (CFTR) gene, which is inherited in an autosomal-recessive fashion. Chronic recurrent infections develop, in addition to numerous extrapulmonary manifestations such as meconium ileus in infancy. With progressive disease, chronic inflammatory changes occur that lead to alteration of airway walls with epithelial erosion, partial replacement of the mucosa by granulation tissue, progressive airway dilatation resulting in bronchiectasis, and fibrotic/obliterative changes involving the small airways.[1,102,111-113]

Imaging Chest imaging in persons with early CF may be normal or show mild to moderate air trapping and/or bronchiectasis (Fig. 56-23). In more advanced disease, bronchiectasis that is predominant in the upper lobe, bronchial wall

thickening, centrilobular nodular and tree-in-bud opacities, and mucus plugging with air trapping occur (Fig. 56-24). A finger-in-glove pattern of mucoid impaction similar to ABPA may be observed. Because of chronic/recurrent infections, mediastinal and hilar lymphadenopathy often is present. CT is much more sensitive than pulmonary functions tests for detecting mild or localized lung disease. Although they are not widely used and are of unclear benefit in individualized treatment, CT scoring systems to assess the extent and severity of CF are a valid surrogate endpoint for outcomes in clinical trials. There is a statistically significant correlation of the number of respiratory tract exacerbations and the CT score at baseline and change in score over a 2-year period.[111-113]

Treatment and Follow-up Treatment traditionally has focused on the managing/preventing the sequelae of the disease. The standard of care most recently has included oral azithromycin, inhaled tobramycin, hypertonic saline solution, and dornase alfa (Pulmozyme), which functions to break down thick secretions. Additional antibiotics are used depending on the type of infections present and the resistance pattern. Recently, the novel small molecule ivacaftor (Kalydeco) received and Drug Administration approval for CF in patients with at least one *G551D* mutation. By directly potentiating CFTR with significant improvements in lung function, the medication heralds a new era in drug development for CF, focusing on personalized medicine.[114]

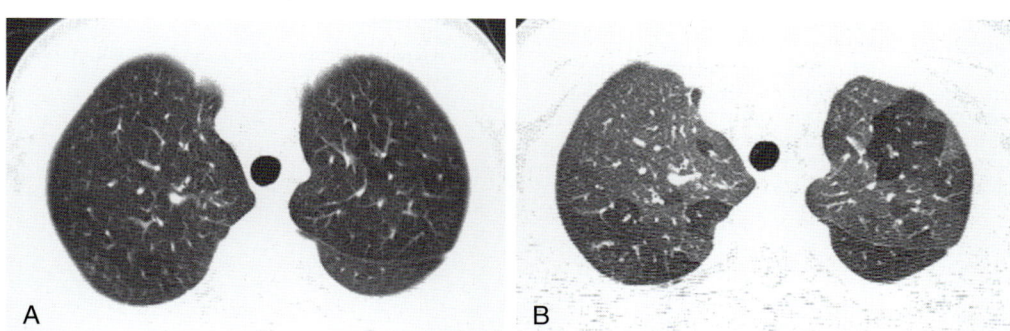

Figure 56-23 Paired inspiratory (**A**) and expiratory (**B**) phase axial computed tomography images from a 12-year-old with mild pulmonary cystic fibrosis show no bronchiectasis but demonstrate mosaic attenuation from air trapping that is accentuated on the expiratory phase.

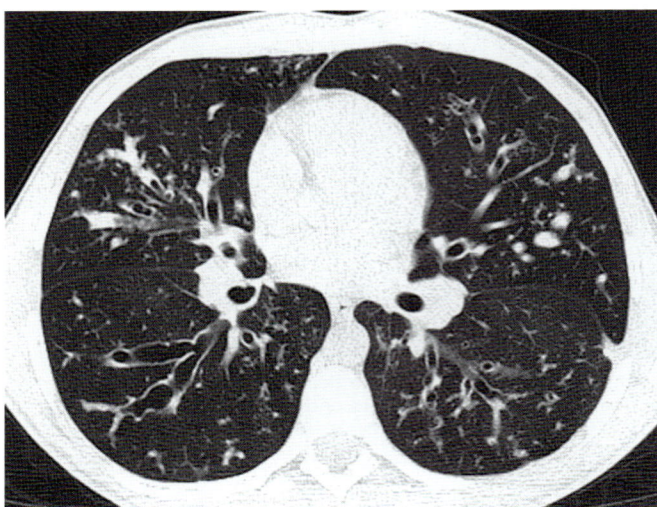

Figure 56-24 An axial computed tomography image from an 18-year-old with advanced cystic fibrosis shows saccular bronchiectasis, bronchial wall thickening, and airway plugging.

✓ WHAT THE CLINICIAN NEEDS TO KNOW

- The revised ChILD classification scheme has allowed substantial progress in our understanding of pediatric ILD.

- Many pediatric ILDs have a genetic basis with associated anomalies. If ILD is clinically suspected, screening for extrapulmonary abnormalities and a genetic basis should be considered. Additionally, genetic counseling should be offered to family members.

- Alveolar growth abnormalities commonly coexist with a patchy pattern of PIG; because glucocorticoids are recommended for the latter condition, a lung biopsy should be considered for definitive diagnosis. In contrast, the characteristic CT findings of NEHI are reported to have 100% specificity among experienced pediatric radiologists, thus potentially avoiding a lung biopsy.

- BO syndrome is the clinical correlate for the histopathologic entity of constrictive or obliterative bronchiolitis. In distinction, bronchiolitis obliterans organizing pneumonia falls under the category of organizing pneumonia and is termed cryptogenic organizing pneumonia if it is idiopathic.

- Lung transplantation may be the only curative treatment option for infants with respiratory failure from severe alveolar growth abnormalities or genetic surfactant disorders. Specific treatments exist for many etiologies of ILD in children presenting past infancy, including aerosolized GM-CSF therapy, in addition to whole-lung lavage for autoimmune PAP; inciting antigen cessation and corticosteroids for hypersensitivity pneumonitis; immunosuppression for pulmonary hemorrhage with capillaritis; corticosteroids for pulmonary infiltrates with eosinophilia; enzyme replacement therapy for lysosomal storage diseases; antibiotics, interferon-γ, and stem cell transplantation for CGD; and antibiotics, hypertonic saline solution, and dornase alfa for CF, along with the CFTR-potentiator ivacaftor for persons with the *G551D* mutation.

Key Points

The HRCT findings in NEHI are characteristic with hyperinflation and a mosaic attenuation pattern affecting at least four lobes with geographic ground-glass opacities that are most prominent in the right middle lobe, lingula, and paramediastinal lung regions. This pattern confers a reported sensitivity and specificity for diagnosis of 78% to 83% and 100%, respectively, among experienced pediatric radiologists.

A crazy-paving pattern (ground-glass opacity superimposed on interlobular septal thickening) is suggestive of but not specific for PAP and also can be observed with diffuse pulmonary hemorrhage, for example. PAP itself is a histopathologic entity with numerous underlying causes.

Chylous pleural effusions are typical of pulmonary lymphangiectasia and lymphangiomatosis.

On HRCT the connective tissue and collagen-vascular diseases most often demonstrate an NSIP pattern. This pattern is characterized by ground-glass and fine linear or reticular opacities predominantly at the lung periphery, with traction bronchiectasis, volume loss (predominantly lower lobe), and honeycombing developing over time.

Important radiologic patterns and signs in pediatric ILD include the photographic negative or reversed pulmonary edema pattern in CEP and drug-induced PIE; the atoll or reversed halo sign (central ground-glass opacity surrounded by consolidation) in organizing pneumonia; and the finger-in-glove sign (mucoid impaction of large airways) in ABPA and CF.

Suggested Readings

Deterding RR. Infants and young children with children's interstitial lung disease. *Pediatr Allergy Immunol Pulmonol.* 2010;23:25-31.
Guillerman RP, Brody AS. Contemporary perspectives on pediatric diffuse lung disease. *Radiol Clin North Am.* 2011;49:847-868.
Guillerman RP. Imaging of childhood interstitial lung disease. *Pediatr Allergy Immunol Pulmonol.* 2010;23:43-68.
Langston C, Dishop MK. Infant lung biopsy: clarifying the pathologic spectrum. *Pathol Int.* 2004;54:s419-s421.
Lee EY, Cleveland RH, Langston C. Interstitial lung disease in infants and children: new classification system with emphasis on clinical, imaging, and pathologic correlation. In: Cleveland RH, ed. *Imaging in pediatric pulmonology.* New York: Springer; 2011.

References

Full references for this chapter can be found on www.expertconsult.com.

Chapter 57

Systemic Conditions with Lung Involvement

JULIE CURRIE O'DONOVAN, EDWARD Y. LEE, and ERIC L. EFFMANN

Pulmonary involvement is a frequent component of systemic illness. Pediatric patients often present for chest imaging before the diagnosis of a specific systemic disorder has been made. Therefore, the radiologist plays an important role in directing the diagnostic workup by recognizing that the pulmonary findings reflect an underlying condition. The first imaging study in pediatric patients with respiratory symptoms is usually chest radiography. In some patients such as those with pulmonary edema or sickle cell disease, radiography shows the pulmonary findings adequately to continue appropriate clinical care. In many patients, however, chest radiography is nonspecific, provides initial clues to the diagnosis, or both, prompting further investigation with computed tomography (CT) of the chest. In recent years, the advent of multidetector CT and controlled ventilation techniques (see Chapter 49) has dramatically improved the detailed assessment of lungs in children with systemic disorders.

Specific Systemic Diseases

VASCULITIS AND COLLAGEN VASCULAR DISEASE

Although medium- and large-vessel vasculitides more commonly affect mediastinal vasculature structures and rarely the lung parenchyma, small-vessel vasculitides are the most likely to cause pulmonary parenchymal disease. Pediatric patients with pulmonary vasculitis typically present in their teen years. Of these disorders, Wegener polyangiitis (WP), previously known as granulomatosis, is the most common one in children. Microscopic polyangiitis (MPA) and Churg-Strauss syndrome (CSS) are rarely seen in children. Pulmonary nodules and airspace opacities are typically seen on imaging studies.[1-3]

Pulmonary involvement, most commonly interstitial changes, may be seen in children with collagen vascular diseases (CVD) such as juvenile arthritis, dermatomyositis, systemic sclerosis (scleroderma), systemic lupus erythematosus (SLE), and mixed connective tissue disease. Pulmonary involvement is less common in children than in adults. Pulmonary disease is seen more frequently in children with systemic sclerosis (59% to 91%) than in the other CVDs, and it is associated with significant morbidity and mortality.[4,5] A recent study found that abnormal pulmonary function tests (PFTs) were correlated with the severity of abnormalities on high-resolution CT (HRCT). Thus PFTs provide a monitoring tool to identify children who would benefit from further lung disease evaluation with HRCT.[5] Symptomatic lung disease is significantly less common in juvenile rheumatoid arthritis and SLE, reported in only 5% of patients.[6]

Both the vasculitides and CVDs may cause pulmonary renal syndrome, which is the association of both pulmonary hemorrhage and glomerulonephritis. It is often seen in WP and SLE.[1,2] Pulmonary hemorrhage may be seen in both the vasculitides and in CVDs (e-Fig. 57-1) and has a high morbidity and mortality (50% to 90%).[1,7]

Etiology WP is, by far, the most common of the pulmonary vasculitides seen in children and typically presents with a triad of necrotizing granulomatous lesions in both the upper and lower respiratory tract, as well as glomerulonephritis. MPA is a nongranulomatous necrotizing vasculitis almost always seen with glomerulonephritis. CSS (also known as *allergic granulomatosis* and *angiitis*) typically presents with asthma and blood eosinophilia but is rare in children.[1] Most of the pulmonary vasculitides are immunologically mediated. WP, MPA, and CSS are associated with antineutrophil cytoplasmic antibodies (ANCA) and are sometimes referred to as *ANCA-associated systemic vasculitides*.

Most of the CVDs also have an autoimmune mechanism, SLE being the classic autoimmune condition associated with antinuclear antibody. These disorders are associated with a variable degree of inflammation of multiple organ systems, including the lung. Depending on the specific disorder, patients may present with arthritis, serositis, vasculitis, other soft tissue inflammation, or all of these.

Imaging The common imaging findings of pulmonary vasculitis and CVDs are summarized in Table 57-1. The frequent imaging findings of WP are variable sized nodules, followed by ground-glass opacities and air space consolidation; 17% of the nodules show cavitation.[8] The nodules are frequently surrounded by a halo of ground-glass opacity, which represents hemorrhage (e-Fig. 57-2 and Fig. 57-3). Airway wall thickening may also be seen, but airway strictures are significantly less common in children (3%) compared with adults (up to 59%).[8] Diffuse alveolar hemorrhage (occurring in 44% of pediatric WP) is characterized by lobular or

Table 57-1

Pulmonary Imaging Findings in Systemic Diseases							
	Nodules (some cavitary)	Ground-Glass Opacities	Airspace Opacities	Diffuse Alveolar Hemorrhage*	Interstitial Disease	Pleural/Pericardial Disease	Lung Cysts
Wegener polyangiitis	++++ 90%	++ 52%	++ 45%	++ 44%	—	+	—
Microscopic polyangiitis	—	+	+	+++ 57%	+	+	—
Churg-Strauss syndrome	++ 38%	+++ 75%	+++ 75%	—	—	—	—
Juvenile arthritis	+†	++	—	—	++	+++ 60%	—
Systemic lupus erythematosus	—	++	++	++	+	+++	—
Systemic sclerosis (Scleroderma)	++ 64%‡	+++ 73%	—	—	++++ 91%	+	—
Mixed connective tissue disease	—	++	—	—	++	—	—
Dermatomyositis	—	++	—	—	+	—	—
Acute chest syndrome	—	—	++++	—	—	++	—
Langerhans cell histiocytosis	+++	—	—	—	—	++	++++
Gaucher/Neimann-Pick disease	+	+	—	—	+	—	—

*Specific imaging findings are a spectrum from ground-glass opacities to airspace consolidation.
†Nodules in juvenile arthritis seen in lipoid pneumonia.
‡Seen as subpleural micronodules and were not considered a dominant finding.
Data from references 1, 4, 6, 7, and 11; and Feng RE, Xu WB, Shi JH, et al. Pathological and high resolution CT findings in Churg-Strauss syndrome. *Chin Med Sci J.* 2011;26(1):1-8.

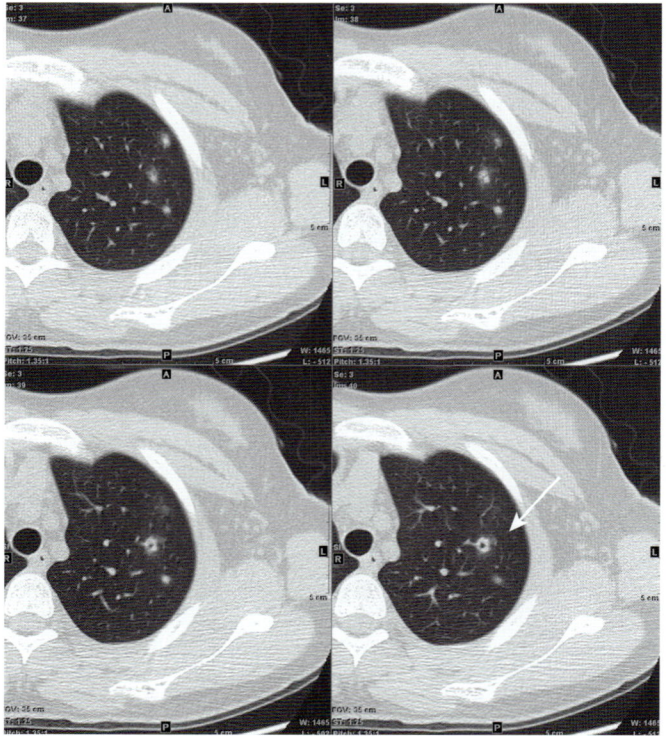

Figure 57-3 Wegener polyangiitis. This 16-year-old girl had a history of vasculitic skin lesions and headache. Computed tomography (CT) of the sinuses revealed inflammatory changes (*not shown*). Axial CT images of the chest show left upper lobe cavitary lesion (*arrow*) with surrounding ground-glass halo as well as several solid pulmonary nodules, also with surrounding halos of ground-glass opacity. Lung biopsy was positive for Wegener polyangiitis.

lobar regions of ground-glass opacity or airspace consolidation on CT.[9-11] It may also show the "crazy paving" pattern on CT, especially as it evolves.[12]

In the case of CVDs, pleural and pericardial effusions are the most common findings in the chest. Pulmonary findings are significantly less common but follow a similar pattern for most of these disorders and include ground-glass opacity and interstitial septal thickening, which may progress to pulmonary fibrosis. Despite normal chest radiographs or only minimal radiographic abnormalities in children with systemic sclerosis, HRCT demonstrates ground-glass opacities, peripheral areas of pulmonary fibrosis, and subpleural micronodules (Fig. 57-4).[4] Some authors have reported occurrence of lipoid pneumonia in children with juvenile idiopathic arthritis, not associated with mineral oil ingestion.[12] "Shrinking lung syndrome" has been described in SLE and represents decrease in lung volume that manifests radiographically by an elevated diaphragm.[7,12,13]

Treatment and Follow-up Treatment for vasculitides and CVDs is primarily aimed at suppressing the immune response, typically with corticosteroids and chemotherapeutic agents. In patients with vasculitis, CVDs, or both, who experience diffuse alveolar hemorrhage, evolving changes may be seen on CT at follow-up. A more linear and interstitial type of pattern may develop with interlobular septal thickening and the appearance of the "crazy paving" pattern. If episodes of hemorrhage recur, this may also progress to interstitial fibrosis.[9] Pulmonary involvement with CVD may progress to interstitial pulmonary fibrosis regardless of treatment, with advanced stages showing honeycombing. Pulmonary artery hypertension may also develop with advanced lung disease, especially in systemic sclerosis.

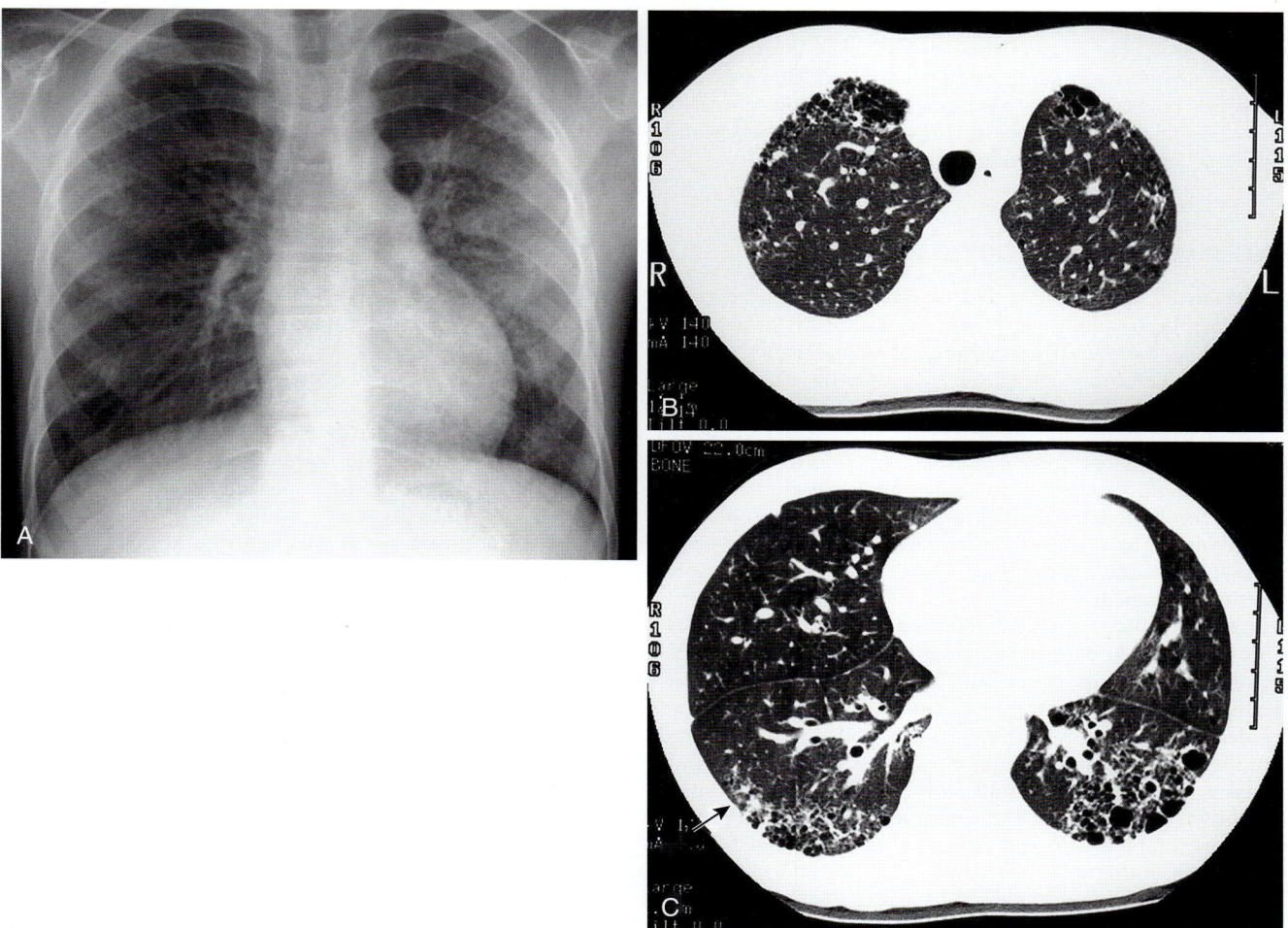

Figure 57-4 An 8-year-old girl with systemic sclerosis (scleroderma) diagnosed at age 5 years. **A,** The frontal chest radiograph shows mild increase in perihilar linear opacities. **B,** High-resolution computed tomography (HRCT) of upper lung zones shows thin-walled, small cystic areas anteriorly in both lungs and a few small scattered subpleural lucencies and opacities more posteriorly. **C,** HRCT through lower lung zones shows honeycomb pattern dependently in both lungs. More lateral area in right lung shows more ground-glass opacity (*arrow*) that may represent active disease.

Follow-up imaging is primarily determined by clinical needs, symptoms, or both but is best performed with HRCT, as radiographic findings may be too subtle to identify changes. Progression of abnormal PFTs in patients with juvenile systemic sclerosis over time (forced expiratory volume in 1 second and forced vital capacity) correlate with worsening of changes on HRCT, suggesting that PFTs could potentially be used as a marker to determine when follow-up imaging may be needed.

SICKLE CELL DISEASE

Acute chest syndrome (ACS), a pulmonary illness that occurs in up to 50% of children with sickle cell disease (SCD), is characterized by chest pain, leukocytosis, fever, and a new pulmonary opacity. It is the leading cause of death (25%) and hospitalization in all patients with SCD and usually occurs between 2 and 4 years of age.[14] ACS also occurs in patients with other sickle hemoglobinopathies.[15] When not fatal, it may lead to chronic lung disease (4%) and pulmonary hypertension.[16]

Etiology The etiology of ACS is complex and not always known. In a large multicenter study of 671 episodes, causes were found to be microvascular occlusion and infarction (16%), infection (29%), fat emboli from bone marrow infarcts (9%), and unknown in 46%. *Chlamydia, Mycoplasma,* and viral agents were the most common pathogens in cases caused by infection. One third of patients presented with symptoms of long bone pain caused by vasoocclusive crisis and developed ACS 2 to 3 days later.[17]

Imaging Radiographic findings of ACS are nonspecific but, by definition, include the presence of a pulmonary opacity (e-Fig. 57-5). Opacities were noted in the lower lobes in about 90%, and pleural effusion was noted in 55% of cases in a large multicenter study (see Table 57-1).[17]

Although CT is not generally used in the setting of ACS, chronic sickle cell lung disease has been studied by using HRCT. Abnormal findings most pronounced at the lung bases include parenchymal bands, interlobular septal thickening, architectural distortion, and traction bronchiectasis. Honeycombing is unusual, in contrast to other types of pulmonary fibrosis.[18]

Treatment and Follow-up   Therapy for ACS includes hydration, analgesia, respiratory support (including bronchodilators), broad-spectrum antibiotics, transfusion therapy, and sometimes corticosteroids.[19] Imaging follow-up is primarily dictated by clinical progression, improvement, or both and may be accomplished by using radiography.

LANGERHANS CELL HISTIOCYTOSIS

Langerhans cell histiocytosis (LCH) is now the preferred term describing the condition showing a proliferation of a group of histiocytes known as *Langerhans cells*. Langerhans cells are of myeloid dendritic cell origin and contain characteristic Birbeck bodies on histology.[20] The peak age at initial diagnosis is 1 to 3 years, and most patients present with osseous lesions.[20] LCH is currently classified according to the extent of involvement, whether it involves a single site (better prognosis) or multiple sites (higher risk of long-term problems). The involvement of "risk organs" (liver, spleen, lung, bone marrow) indicates a poorer prognosis and demands more aggressive treatment.[21]

Pulmonary involvement is reported to be present in 23% to 50% of children with multisystem LCH.[12,20] The mean age of patients with lung disease was 11.9 months in one study. Disease-free survival in these patients was 69%, with 3 out of 4 deaths occurring when "risk organs" other than the lung were involved.[22] Although lung disease was traditionally considered a poor prognostic indicator in LCH, recent studies have shown that it does not adversely affect outcome. Primary pulmonary LCH (single site) is rare in children and is typically seen in young adult smokers.[21,22]

Etiology   The etiology of LCH is not known. Most investigators believe it to be an immune-mediated condition, in which the Langerhans cells accumulate and cause an inflammatory reaction. In the lungs, destructive granulomatous lesions occur in the interstitial tissues, bronchial and bronchiolar epithelium, and subpleural septa that may eventually lead to cystic lesions.[20,21] Pulmonary fibrosis occurs later in 10% of children and may demonstrate multiple small cysts giving the lung a honeycomb appearance.[23]

Imaging   Radiologic findings of LCH vary widely with the extent of the disease and are summarized in Table 57-1. Initial chest radiography may be normal. Small nodules and cysts may be seen, with upper lobe involvement equal to or more extensive than lower lobe involvement (Fig. 57-6). The reticular appearance noted on chest radiography is often from multiple small cysts.[20,24] LCH is the most common cause of acquired extensive cystic lung disease in children (e-Fig. 57-7). Spontaneous pneumothorax occurs in about 11% of patients with pulmonary involvement and may be the first indicator of pulmonary disease.[25] However, it may be also a manifestation of more advanced disease, as in adolescents who more often have large coalescent cysts (see e-Fig. 57-7).[12]

CT is indicated for neonates with LCH and any patient with abnormalities on chest radiography.[21] HRCT findings in LCH are characterized by small nodules (with or without cavitation) with upper and middle lobe predominance (e-Fig. 57-8).[12,20,26] The pleura may be thickened and sometimes replaced by a thick layer of granulomatous tissue. However, pleural effusions are rare.[27] Mediastinal and hilar adenopathy is also rare in children with pulmonary LCH.[20,24]

Treatment and Follow-up   Treatment of pulmonary LCH depends on the extent of disease and whether "risk" organs are involved. Generally, the first line of treatment is corticosteroids, vinblastine, or both, with duration of therapy being determined by response. Radiation therapy has fallen out of favor except for treating unstable bone lesions.[21] Imaging follow-up for pulmonary LCH depends on clinical symptoms and is best performed with CT.

GAUCHER DISEASE AND NIEMANN-PICK DISEASE

Gaucher disease and Niemann-Pick disease are both autosomal-recessive inherited lysosomal storage disorders with a wide range of pathologic expression in different organ systems. Affected children are usually normal at birth and have variable age at onset, which is usually followed by progressive disease.

Etiology   Gaucher disease is caused by a deficiency of the enzyme glucocerebrosidase that results in an accumulation of

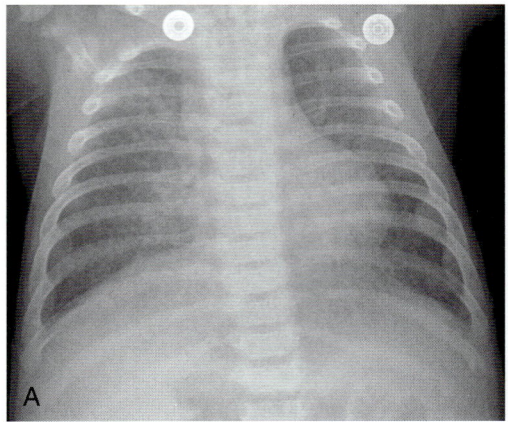
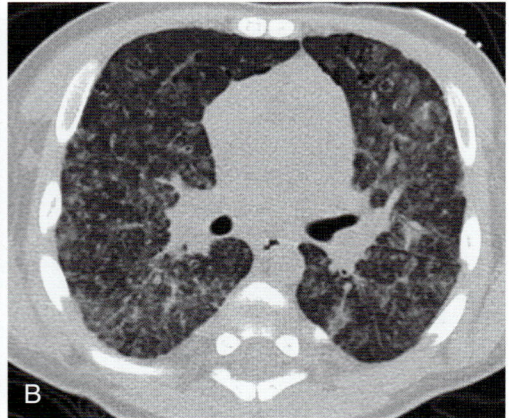

Figure 57-6   Langerhans cell histiocytosis of the lungs in a 2.5-month-old boy who initially presented with a skin rash. **A,** An anteroposterior chest radiograph shows a coarse reticulonodular interstitial pattern. **B,** An axial computed tomography image in a lung window shows the coarse reticulonodular interstitial pattern with some small thin-walled cysts seen in the anterior lung bilaterally.

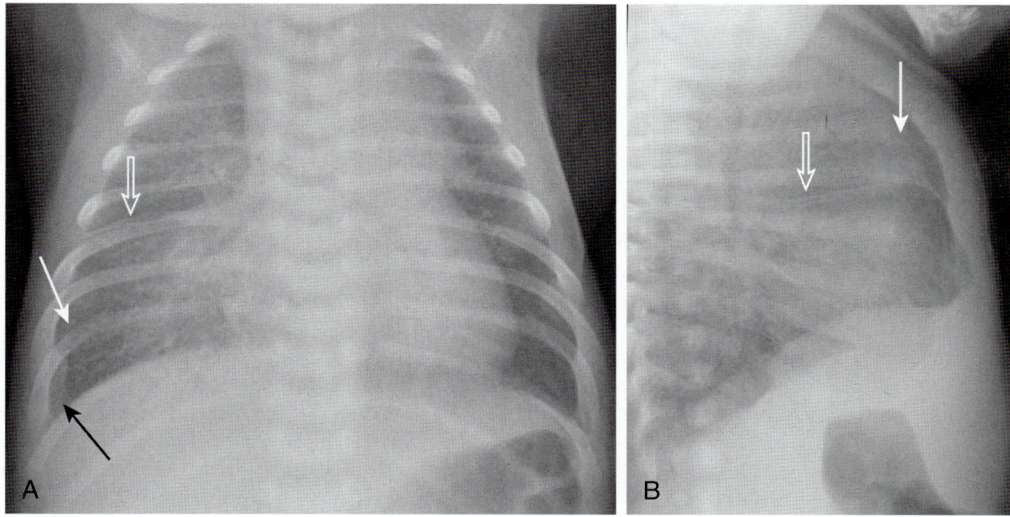

Figure 57-9 Pulmonary edema caused by obstructed pulmonary venous return. This 6-week-old infant presented to the emergency room with tachypnea and feeding difficulties. **A** and **B,** Anteroposterior and lateral chest radiographs show normal heart size and subtle interstitial edema characterized by hyperinflation, septal lines (*white arrows*), fissural thickening (*open arrows*), and tiny right pleural effusion (*black arrow*). Diagnosis of cor triatriatum was made with echocardiography.

glucocerebroside in phagocytic cells. Pulmonary involvement is most common in patients with neuronopathic types. Neimann-Pick disease is caused by a deficiency of sphingomyelinase, resulting in accumulation of sphingomyelin. Progressive pulmonary fibrosis has rarely been reported in Neimann-Pick disease.[28]

Imaging A diffuse reticular lung pattern may be seen on chest radiography with Gaucher disease.[29] Niemann-Pick disease may produce similar findings.[27] Lipoid pneumonia has been described in patients with Neimann-Pick disease.[30] Imaging findings are summarized in Table 57-1.

Treatment and Follow-up Visceral involvement may improve with enzyme replacement therapy in Gaucher disease, and this therapy may offer an alternative to lung transplantation. The current treatment for Neimann-Pick disease is whole lung lavage.[28,30] CT is more sensitive than plain radiography for imaging follow-up, when clinically warranted.

Pulmonary Conditions Occurring with Generalized Systemic Illness

PULMONARY EDEMA

Pulmonary edema is the excessive accumulation of water and solute in the lung tissues. Functionally, pulmonary edema is divided into two general categories: (1) those cases having elevated pulmonary venous pressure (cardiogenic or hydrostatic) and (2) those associated with increased capillary permeability with normal microvascular pressure (noncardiogenic). Pulmonary edema may also have mixed etiologies, and sometimes the actual mechanism is unknown.

In the pediatric population, cardiogenic edema usually presents in infants less than 6 months of age and is the result of congenital heart disease (CHD) (Figs. 57-9 and 57-10). In an older child, cardiomyopathy may be the cause of cardiogenic edema. Affected infants often present with nonspecific symptoms, including feeding difficulties, grunting, diaphoresis, wheezing, and retractions.[31] Rarely, pulmonary edema may be the presenting manifestation of CHD.

The frequent causes of noncardiogenic pulmonary edema in children include acute respiratory distress syndrome

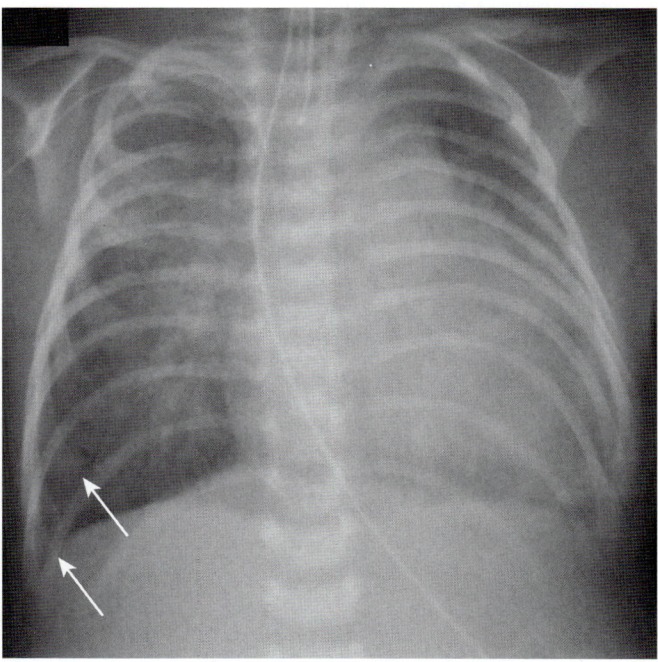

Figure 57-10 Cardiogenic edema. A 5-week-old male infant with known ventricular septal defect presenting with tachypnea and respiratory distress requiring intensive care unit admission. An anteroposterior chest radiograph shows cardiomegaly, hyperinflation, and pulmonary edema characterized by perihilar airspace opacity, indistinct hilar vessels, and septal lines (*arrows*).

(ARDS), near-drowning, neurogenic pulmonary edema, renal disease, and upper airway obstruction. Other less common causes of noncardiogenic pulmonary edema include aspiration pneumonia, hydrocarbon pneumonitis, smoke inhalation, and drug reactions.[32]

Cardiogenic Pulmonary Edema

Etiology Cardiogenic pulmonary edema occurs significantly less frequently in children than in adults. The common underlying causes for cardiogenic pulmonary edema include left-to-right shunting lesions, left ventricular outlet obstruction, obstruction of pulmonary venous return, or cardiomyopathy (e-Fig. 57–11).[31] Cardiogenic pulmonary edema progresses in severity as pulmonary capillary wedge pressure increases.

Imaging On chest radiography, cardiomegaly is usually found except in instances of pulmonary venous obstruction, in which interstitial edema is present in the absence of cardiac enlargement (see Fig. 57-9).

Early findings in interstitial edema in children with cardiogenic pulmonary edema are indistinct vascular margins and bronchial wall thickening. Interlobular septal thickening (septal lines or Kerley B lines) and interlobar fissural thickening are also often seen. In infants and young children, fissural thickening is often more easily recognized than Kerley lines and is therefore an important clue for diagnosing cardiogenic pulmonary edema in children (see Fig. 57-9). An indirect radiographic finding often seen in children with CHD is hyperinflation. This may be a pitfall for the imager if he or she attributes the findings of peribronchial thickening and hyperinflation to airways disease and does not recognize them as subtle findings of interstitial edema (see Fig. 57-9). Alveolar edema usually occurs after development of interstitial edema and is the most recognizable radiographic finding of pulmonary edema (see Fig. 57-10 and e-Fig. 57-11). The classic appearance of acute alveolar edema is a central or "butterfly" distribution of airspace disease, with central edema and sparing of the lung periphery. Pleural effusions are also usually present (see e-Fig. 57-11).

Although not commonly used to diagnose pulmonary edema, CT is sensitive for the detection of pulmonary edema of any etiology. CT shows peribronchial cuffing, septal lines, ground-glass opacities, and air space consolidation in order of increasing severity (e-Fig. 57-12).[33,34]

Occasionally, pulmonary edema is asymmetric or unilateral. This may be related to patient position (given the dependent nature of the edema) or to the presence of asymmetric pulmonary arterial supply or pulmonary venous drainage, particularly in patients with CHD.

Treatment and Follow-up Treatment for cardiogenic pulmonary edema is generally supportive and includes corrective or palliative treatment for CHD. Diuretics and inotropes may be used for cardiac dysfunction. Ventilator support is provided, if needed. Extracorporeal membrane oxygenation and other types of ventricular assist devices are now being used more frequently in the setting of pediatric cardiac failure.[35] Typically, imaging follow-up with chest radiography is adequate, although CT may be used to clarify the vascular anatomy.

Noncardiogenic Pulmonary Edema

Etiology Many episodes of noncardiogenic pulmonary edema progress to ARDS. ARDS accounts for 1% to 3% of pediatric intensive care admissions, and the mortality in various series ranges from 40% to 60%.[32] Sepsis, near-drowning, pneumonia, and smoke inhalation are the most frequent antecedents to pediatric ARDS. In most cases, ARDS progresses through stages of immediate lung injury, exudative alveolitis, fibroproliferative repair, and, in survivors, recovery. Ventilation–perfusion imbalance leads to varying degrees of hypoxemia.[32]

Neurogenic pulmonary edema may occur with increased intracranial pressure, which, in theory, causes a shift of blood from the systemic to the low-resistance pulmonary circulation. Pulmonary edema caused by renal disease (chronic renal failure, glomerulonephritis, nephrotic syndrome, or all of these) is felt to be multifactorial in mechanism, including factors such as fluid retention and hypoproteinemia (see e-Fig. 57-12). Although uncommon, postobstructive pulmonary edema may also occur in upper airway obstruction from conditions such as croup, epiglottitis, foreign body obstruction, and near-strangulation or when relief of upper airway obstruction occurs. The mechanism is thought to be an abrupt decrease in intrathoracic pressure caused by an attempt to inhale against a closed upper airway, also called *negative-pressure pulmonary edema*.[31]

Pulmonary edema may also develop after inhalation of a variety of noxious fumes or soluble aerosols. Aspiration of hypertonic water-soluble contrast agents may also produce pulmonary edema.

Imaging The radiographic pattern for ARDS is a multiple stage continuum (Fig. 57-13).[36,37] First, the radiograph is reflective of the initial insult, or it may be clear, or both. In 12 to 24 hours, bilateral pulmonary opacities develop, consistent with noncardiogenic pulmonary edema, and opacities become progressively more confluent.[37] Subsequent improvement or continued worsening may be seen in the next several days. For patients with progression, the course often is then complicated by air leak phenomenon (pneumothorax, pneumomediastinum, pulmonary interstitial emphysema), with or without ventilator-associated infections. Additionally, further progression to chronic changes of fibrosis may occur.[32,36,37]

The pulmonary findings of noncardiogenic pulmonary edema (e.g., ARDS) are similar to that of cardiogenic pulmonary edema, but the radiographs typically do not show cardiomegaly (see e-Fig. 57-12, Fig. 57-14, and e-Fig. 57-15).[37] Pleural effusions may not be a dominant finding, but they are frequently seen, particularly in patients requiring maximum clinical support as a manifestation of anasarca.

Glomerulonephritis and nephrotic syndrome are often sufficiently characteristic, aiding the radiologist to suggest the correct diagnosis. A child or teenager presents without a known cardiac history with a basilar predominant interstitial edema pattern, often with pleural effusions (see e-Fig. 57-12). Glomerulonephritis may be distinguished from nephrotic syndrome by its tendency to show mild cardiomegaly and increased pulmonary vascularity.[38]

Treatment and Follow-up Treatment of noncardiogenic pulmonary edema is directed toward the primary cause, is

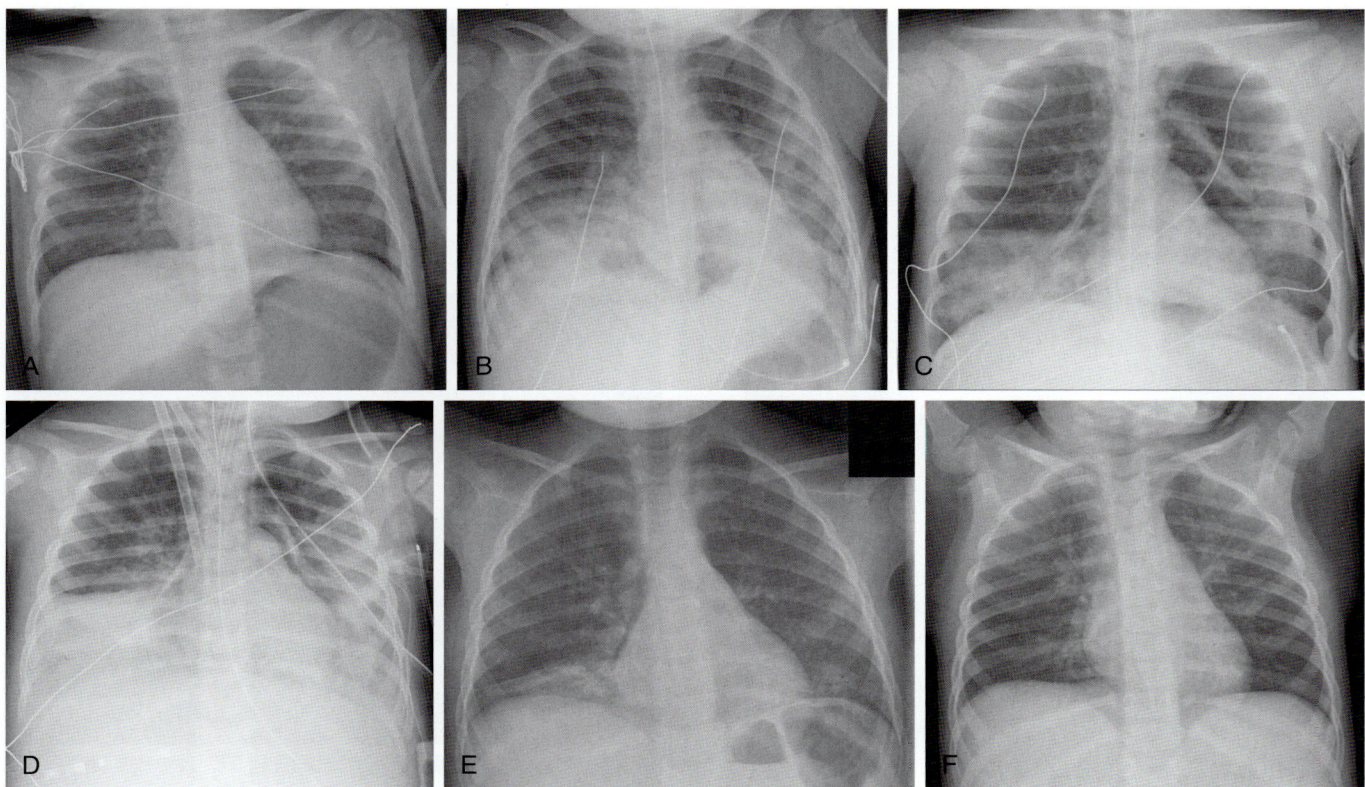

Figure 57-13 A 17-month-old girl who ingested citronella oil from a backyard lamp and developed acute respiratory distress syndrome. **A,** The chest radiograph at presentation is near-normal. **B,** At day 2, bibasilar airspace disease developed. She then deteriorated clinically, with increasing hypoxia that required intubation. **C,** Shortly thereafter, air leak developed, with pneumomediastinum and left pneumothorax at day 4. Further clinical deterioration occurred, and bacterial cultures from the endotracheal tube were positive consistent with ventilator associated pneumonia. **D,** She was then placed on arteriovenous extracorporeal membrane oxygenation with cannulas at day 7. Eventually, she clinically improved and was discharged from the hospital. **E** and **F,** Follow-up radiographs at 2 and 4 months show gradual clearing of interstitial type opacities in the bilateral lung bases.

generally supportive, or both. Ventilatory support is often needed. The use of positive end-expiratory pressure with mechanical ventilation has been shown by CT to improve ventilation of dependent regions of the lung in a setting of ARDS.[37,39] Extracorporeal membrane oxygenation is increasingly being used for children with severe respiratory failure. Pulmonary edema from neurogenic causes or upper airway obstruction usually resolves fairly rapidly, often within 12 to 48 hours (see Fig. 57-14).[31] Typically, imaging follow-up will be performed with chest radiography, as needed.

Survivors of ARDS may have long-term sequelae, often demonstrable by pulmonary function testing. Follow-up chest radiography most often show a return to normal (80%) but may demonstrate increased interstitial markings, hyperaeration, or both (see Fig. 57-13, E and F).[32,37,40]

PULMONARY THROMBOEMBOLIC DISEASE

Pulmonary thromboembolic disease was traditionally thought to be much less common in children than in adults but is being seen with increasing frequency in children. A 25-year pediatric autopsy series found an incidence of pulmonary embolism (PE) of 3.7% of 3600 autopsies.[41] More recent studies have reported a prevalence of 14% to 15% in a population of children undergoing computed tomography pulmonary angiography (CTPA) for clinical suspicion of PE.[42,43] Venous thromboembolism (including PE) is associated with

an underlying risk factor in 95% of children.[42-46] Surprisingly, however, a recent study of pediatric patients undergoing CTPA showed no significant difference in prevalence of risk factors between patients diagnosed with a PE compared with the control group without PE.[42] A bimodal age distribution exists for PE in children, which may present in the neonatal time frame or more commonly in late childhood or adolescence.[42,43,46]

Clinical diagnosis of PE remains a challenge. Many episodes of PE are probably asymptomatic in both children and adults. When signs and symptoms of PE do occur, they are often nonspecific. For example, patients may present with pleuritic chest pain, dyspnea, and tachypnea. Unlike the promising data in adults, D-dimer is not helpful for diagnosis of PE in children. Studies have shown that both pediatric patients at risk for PE as well as patients with a diagnosis of PE had elevated D-dimer.[43,46] In addition, no pediatric studies have been done to show that a negative D-dimer may be used to exclude PE in children.

Besides thrombotic emboli, septic embolization is a recognized cause of pulmonary embolic disease in children. Common sites of origin include osteomyelitis, soft tissue infections, infected central venous catheters, endocarditis, and tonsillitis or pharyngitis; the latter may lead to Lemierre syndrome.[47,48]

Pulmonary fat embolism is characterized clinically by a triad of progressive pulmonary insufficiency, cerebral

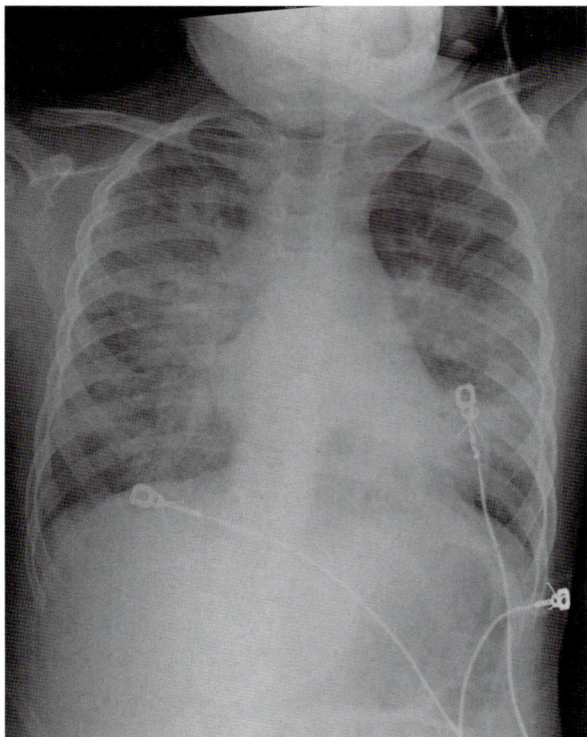

Figure 57-14 A 4-year-old girl was admitted to the intensive care unit for asthma with hypoxia and wheezing. She had an acute exacerbation one night and was noted to also have obstructive sleep apnea. The following morning this anteroposterior view of the chest showed pulmonary edema pattern caused by upper airway obstruction, which promptly resolved when her symptoms were addressed more aggressively.

dysfunction, and petechiae. Fat embolism is a cause of ACS following bone marrow infarcts in sickle cell patients.[17] Most other cases of pulmonary fat emboli occur after trauma, especially from fractures of the femora and tibiae. Autopsy studies have shown an incidence of 60% to 97%, but the risk for fat embolism from a single long bone fracture is reported to be 1% to 3%.[49] Symptoms usually do not develop until 24 to 48 hours after injury.

Thrombotic Emboli

Etiology   Deep venous thrombosis (DVT) is a common precursor to PE in children. In one study, 56% of PEs in children were found to be associated with thrombosis at another location.[46] However, even occurrence of a DVT in a child will usually have a predisposing cause such as the presence of a central venous catheter. Whereas lower extremity DVT is most common in adults, upper extremity DVT is more common in children (accounting for two thirds of DVTs) because of the association with central venous lines.[44,46,50] Other factors predisposing to thromboembolism include malignancy, hypercoagulable states (such as SCD, SLE, or coagulation disorders), CHD, trauma, infection, recent surgery, nephrotic syndrome, and use of birth control pills (see Fig. 57-16 and e-Fig. 57-17).[46] A recent study found a nearly 2% prevalence of unsuspected PE in pediatric oncology patients undergoing routine thoracic CT studies.[51]

Imaging   Radiographic findings of PE are unfortunately nonspecific. If the embolic episode occurs without infarction, the result of chest radiography is most often normal. If it is abnormal, it may show localized or generalized oligemia (Westermark sign), an enlarged pulmonary artery, or loss of lung volume. PE with associated infarct classically appears as a truncated cone of homogeneous opacity located at the lung

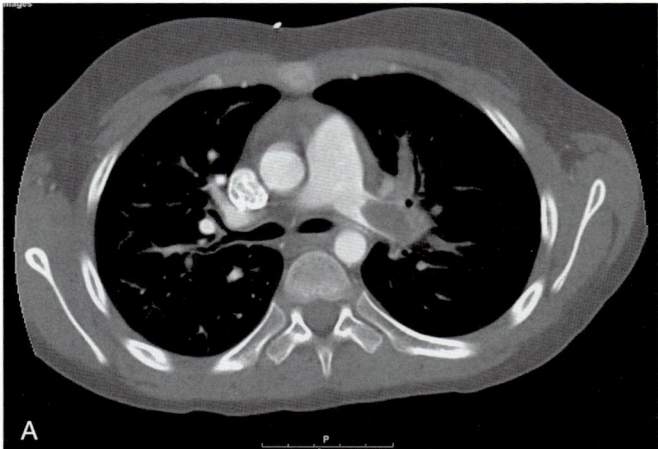

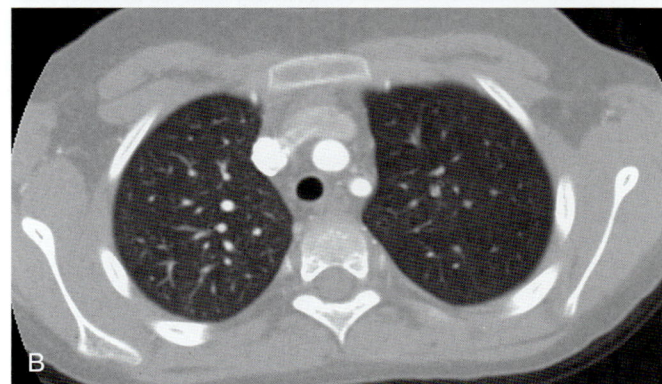

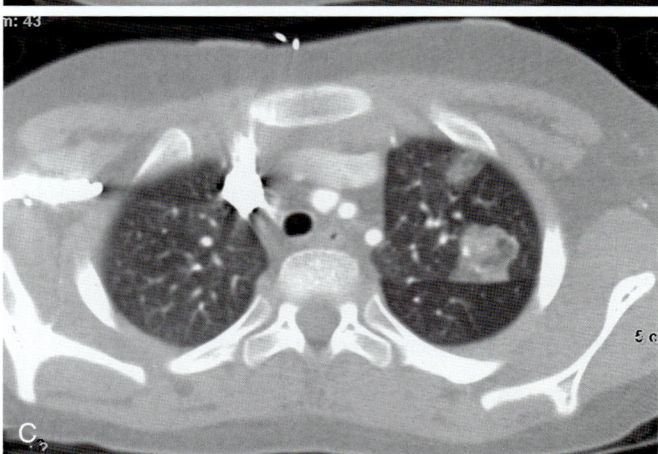

Figure 57-16 Pulmonary embolism found on computed tomography (CT) scan in a 9-year-old patient with a history of nephrotic syndrome and new hypoxia. **A,** An axial CT image clearly shows filling defects in the left proximal pulmonary artery and the branch to the left upper lobe. **B,** Lung window from the initial CT shows paucity of pulmonary vessels in the left upper lobe. **C,** Follow-up CT image obtained 36 hours later shows interval development of a focal pulmonary infarct in the left upper lobe.

periphery and abutting the pleural surface (Hampton hump), but in fact, this pattern is uncommon.

CTPA has a variable but high sensitivity (60% to 100%) and high specificity (81% to 100%) for the diagnosis of PE and provides direct visualization of emboli in central and in smaller, peripheral pulmonary arteries (Fig. 57-16 and e-Fig. 57-17).[44] Successful technique requires a multidetector helical scanner and the use of a well-timed contrast bolus, which allows detection of the pulmonary artery filling defects. The interpretation is more challenging if the contrast enhancement is suboptimal or if patient movement limits the image quality. Adjacent hilar lymph nodes may be a pitfall but reformatted images in multiple planes usually clarify their extrinsic location. In addition to the direct vascular findings, CT may also reveal a region of oligemia, peripheral pulmonary consolidation (infarct) with absent or poor enhancement, or both (see Fig. 57-16 and e-Fig. 57-17). Wedge-shaped peripheral consolidation was found to be significantly associated with presence of PE on a review of CTPA studies in children.[52]

Nuclear medicine assessment of pulmonary ventilation and perfusion (V/Q scan) remains an available imaging modality for evaluation of PE in children. A single segmental or larger perfusion defect, with mismatched normal ventilation, signals a high probability of PE. Although some are advocating continued use of V/Q scans in select populations with normal chest radiography results, CTPA is currently preferred in most centers, likely because of the many advantages of CT: it requires minimal patient cooperation, it is rapidly available, and it screens for alternate diagnoses.[45,46,53-56]

Many studies are underway to determine the utility of contrast-enhanced magnetic resonance angiography (CEMRA) for the diagnosis of PE. This technique would be particularly advantageous in children given the lack of radiation exposure and potential to screen upper extremity veins for thrombosis at the same time as the evaluation for PE.[44] PIOPED III (Prospective Investigation of Pulmonary Embolism Diagnosis III) results showed sensitivity of 78% and specificity of 99% in technically adequate CEMRA studies, but unfortunately 25% of studies were not considered technically adequate. Sensitivity was better for the central pulmonary arteries and decreased progressively in the more distal branches.[56] The advent and use of new blood pool magnetic resonance imaging contrast agents may improve the capabilities of CEMRA.

Conventional pulmonary angiography is still considered the gold standard for diagnosis of PE, but it is rarely necessary and is infrequently used.

Treatment and Follow-up Anticoagulation therapy is generally used to prevent extension of thrombus and the development of late complications such as recurrences and postthrombotic syndrome. Most children are treated primarily on the basis of recommendations for adults, since large clinical trials of antithrombotic therapy in children are lacking.[44,46] Traditionally, the first-line anticoagulant used was unfractionated heparin, but bleeding complications are 2% to 18%, depending on patient population, and it requires intravenous access for administration. The low-molecular-weight heparins being used more frequently have several advantages: lower bleeding complications (0% to 5%), subcutaneous administration, and reduced need for monitoring. These advantages make it ideal for outpatient treatment.[44,46]

Thrombolytic therapy causes faster resolution of the embolus, but data regarding efficacy and safety in children are lacking. The agent most commonly used is tissue plasminogen activator. A substantially higher risk of bleeding complications exists, with one study reporting bleeding in 68% of patients and transfusion required in 39% of treated children. Given that risk, most feel that thrombolytic therapy should only be considered in pediatric patients with unstable hemodynamic condition, massive PE, or both.[44,46]

Imaging follow-up for PE is based on clinical factors and is best performed with CTPA.

Septic Embolization

Etiology In septic emboli, hematogenous spread of infection from the original site occurs, as well as deposition of bacteria in end organs. Osteomyelitis is a common primary site of septic embolic disease (Fig. 57-18 and e-Fig. 57-19). In one study from Taiwan, 8 out of 10 pediatric patients with septic

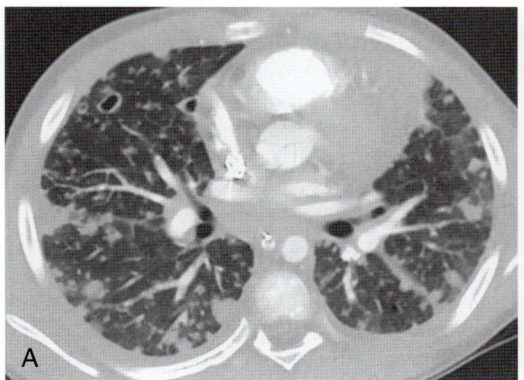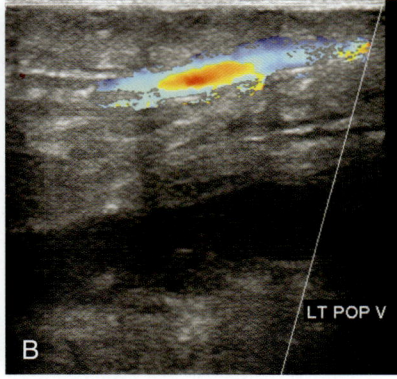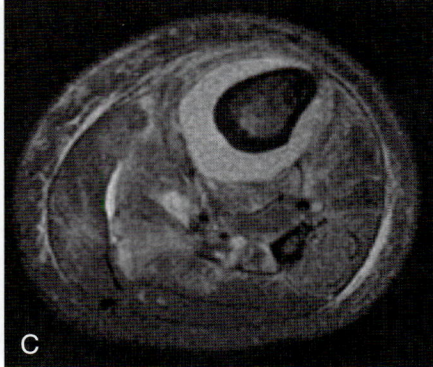

LT POP V

Figure 57-18 Septic emboli. A 12-year-old male who presented in septic shock with history of left leg swelling. Blood cultures were positive for methicillin-resistant *Staphylococcus aureus*. **A,** Initial study was the chest computed tomography showing multiple cavitary and noncavitary pulmonary nodules. **B,** Lower extremity ultrasonography showed a deep venous thrombosis in the popliteal vein, initially thought to be the source of sepsis. **C,** A lower leg axial magnetic resonance image (fat-saturated, T2-weighted) obtained 2 days later shows subperiosteal abscess around the tibia. This patient was subsequently found to have osteomyelitis in multiple sites, including right hip and iliac bone, thoracic spine, left sided ribs, left clavicle, and scapula.

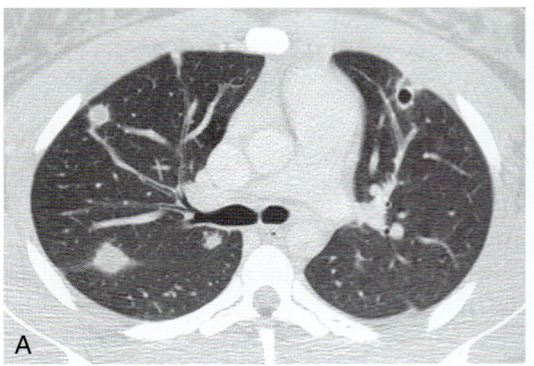 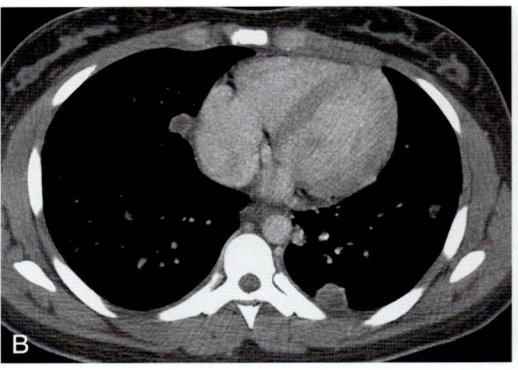 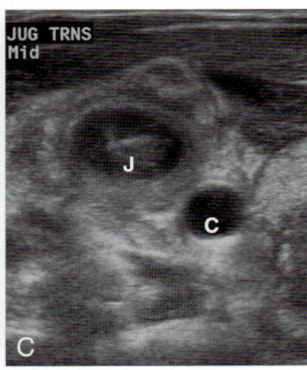

Figure 57-20   Lemierre's syndrome. A 16-year-old female seen initially in urgent care for pharyngitis. Ten days later, she presented to the emergency room with persistent fever, night sweats, and cervical lymphadenopathy. Pneumonia reported on radiographs (*not shown*). **A,** An axial chest computed tomography (CT) scan showing cavitary and noncavitary nodules. **B,** An axial chest CT image showing low-attenuation center in multiple nodules. **C,** A transverse ultrasonographic image through the neck shows thrombus in the right internal jugular vein (*J*) adjacent to the normal anechoic carotid artery (*C*).

emboli had methicillin-resistant *Staphylococcus aureus* as the responsible organism, and most patients had primary skin, soft tissue, or bone infections.[48] Lemierre syndrome is septic thrombophlebitis of the internal jugular vein secondary to bacterial pharyngitis or tonsillitis, usually from *Fusobacterium necrophorum*, with subsequent septicemia and systemic spread of infection and lung involvement in 97% of cases (Fig. 57-20).[47,57,58]

Imaging   The classic radiologic finding is one or more cavitary peripheral nodules, although radiographs more often show nonspecific airspace consolidation (see e-Fig. 57-19). CT is the most sensitive imaging test, more frequently demonstrating cavitation of the nodules (in 85% to 100%) and presence of a "feeding vessel" (in 50% to 71%). Hilar lymph node enlargement and pleural effusions may also be seen.[47,48]

Treatment and Follow-up   Antibiotics is the mainstay for treating the primary source of infection. If the source is unknown, echocardiography is indicated to look for endocarditis. Drainage of focal abscesses is indicated. Currently, no consensus exists on the use of anticoagulation in the setting of Lemierre syndrome.[47] Imaging follow-up may be performed with radiography or CT. Generally, if clinical improvement is prompt, radiography will be adequate. If fever or other symptoms persist, CT may be needed to better assess for persistent sources of infection.

Pulmonary Fat Embolism

Etiology   Fat droplets, typically from the marrow cavity, appear in blood and lodge in the capillaries of the lungs, brain, and other organs. Dyspnea, cyanosis, and tachycardia with cough and fever are the common clinical symptoms, and fat globules may usually be found in blood and urine on laboratory evaluation.

Imaging   Most often, the result of chest radiography is normal. Abnormalities, when present, are usually nonspecific and include airspace consolidation from alveolar hemorrhage and edema, more commonly peripheral and basilar in location. The time lapse between trauma and the development of radiographic findings is usually 1 to 2 days. Such delay

may be helpful in differentiating fat embolism from traumatic lung contusion; in the latter, the chest radiograph is abnormal initially.[59]

Treatment and Follow-up   Treatment of pulmonary fat embolism is generally supportive. Radiographic changes resulting from fat embolism usually disappear gradually within a week to 10 days.

Lung Injury Caused by Extrinsic Agents

DRUG-INDUCED PULMONARY DISEASE

Although a large number of pharmacologic agents may cause or exacerbate pulmonary disease in adults, the incidence and types of pulmonary effects in children are largely unknown.[60] Cause and effect are difficult to establish, and the time between drug administration and reaction is highly variable.

Etiology   Chemotherapeutic agents (such as cyclophosphamide, bleomycin, busulfan, cisplatin, nitrosureas, mitomycin-C, and methotrexate) are the most common drugs associated with pulmonary toxicity (occurring in up to 10% of patients).[61,62] These medications may cause interstitial pneumonitis or fibrosis, hypersensitivity reaction, ARDS, or bronchiolitis obliterans with organizing pneumonia. Amiodarone may cause interstitial thickening, bronchiolitis obliterans with organizing pneumonia, or both.[61]

Airway hyperreactivity has been associated with ingestion of aspirin and nonsteroidal antiinflammatory agents. Hypersensitivity reactions may be produced by reactions to methotrexate, sulfonamides, and nitrofurantoin.[61] Noncardiogenic pulmonary edema may result from overdoses of heroin, morphine, methadone, and cocaine.[61,63] Pulmonary hemorrhage may be seen after administration of anticoagulants, surfactants, and penicillamine.[52]

Imaging   Radiographic findings of drug-induced reactions are generally nonspecific, consisting of heterogeneous pulmonary opacities, homogeneous pulmonary opacities, or both.[60]

HRCT is most useful for early diagnosis of pulmonary toxicities. The findings depend on the histologic process and may include interstitial disease, alveolar disease, or both.[60,61] Interstitial pneumonitis and fibrosis, typical of bleomycin, produce ground-glass opacities, areas of consolidation, and irregular linear opacities that tend to predominate in the lower lung zones. Methotrexate hypersensitivity resembles hypersensitivity pneumonia, showing ground-glass opacities and poorly defined centrilobular nodules. ARDS results in predominantly dependent airspace consolidation. The least common reaction, a bronchiolitis obliterans with organizing pneumonia-like reaction, causes peribronchial or subpleural areas of consolidation.[61]

Airway reactivity is associated with air trapping on imaging. The appearance of noncardiogenic pulmonary edema and pulmonary hemorrhage has been previously discussed earlier in this chapter.

Treatment and Follow-up Removal of the causative agent is the ideal management for drug-induced pulmonary disease if the toxicity can be recognized and the removal is feasible. Unfortunately, some pulmonary toxicities are often irreversible. If symptoms persist, radiography and CT may help in follow-up management.

RADIATION DAMAGE TO THE THORAX

Lung damage may follow radiation therapy given primarily to the lungs, the mediastinum, the chest wall, or the total body. The incidence of radiation damage to the lung in adult patients treated for lung cancer, mediastinal lymphoma, and breast cancer ranges from 5% to 20%.[64] An even larger portion of patients may have changes in pulmonary function tests, although symptoms are present in only a few.[65]

In pediatric patients, whole-lung irradiation to 12 gray (Gy) was used in the third national Wilms tumor study, and 15 patients (approximately 10%) developed radiation pneumonitis.[65] Data from the Childhood Cancer Survivor Study showed a relative risk of lung fibrosis of 4.3 at 5 years or more after diagnosis among children who received chest radiation, total body irradiation, or both. The cumulative incidence of lung fibrosis at 20 years after diagnosis was 3.5%, and the incidence continued to increase from diagnosis up to 25 years. An increased risk for other pulmonary conditions such as supplemental oxygen use, recurrent pneumonia, chronic cough, and pleurisy was also seen in this population.[62]

Etiology Important factors in determining whether the lungs are damaged include the volume of tissue irradiated, the dosage and its fractionation, the relative biologic effectiveness of the therapy employed, and the use of concomitant chemotherapy. Radiation-induced lung injury is typically categorized as early pneumonitis (1-6 months) and late pulmonary fibrosis (>6 months).[66]

Imaging Radiographic changes, if present, usually appear a few months after the cessation of radiation therapy. The radiographic appearance initially is that of an ill-defined alveolar process. CT typically shows ground-glass opacity in a sharply defined zone not conforming to anatomic boundaries. As the process evolves, it becomes more interstitial in appearance until changes recognized as radiation fibrosis appear (e-Fig. 57-21). CT is more sensitive than chest radiography in showing these findings. If the mediastinum has been irradiated, a central perimediastinal, sharply delineated area of linear increased opacity corresponding to the radiation portal is typically seen (see e-Fig. 57-21).[64,66]

Treatment and Follow-up Corticosteroids are sometimes used for managing acute radiation-induced pneumonitis, and long-term treatment is aimed at control of symptoms.[66] Choice of follow-up imaging is largely determined by clinical factors. CT will be more sensitive to identify subtle findings of fibrosis.

INHALATION INJURIES

Children are rarely exposed to the industrial gases, chemicals, and particulates that adult workers may encounter. Pediatric inhalation injury is usually secondary to substances encountered in the home, the most common of which is smoke from house fires. Other causes, far less common, include chlorine gas (pool disinfectant), talcum powder, and household cleaning agents.[32]

Etiology Inhalation injuries are rare in pediatric fire victims but should be suspected in those with burns in the head-and-neck area, blackened sputum, and respiratory symptoms. Thermal injury is most likely to produce upper airway edema. More peripheral airway and airspace injuries are usually secondary to toxic chemical effects of the products of combustion. Typically, pulmonary burns progress through three distinct clinical stages: (1) bronchospasm (1 to 12 hours after the burn), (2) pulmonary edema (6 to 72 hours), and (3) bronchopneumonia (after 60 hours) (Fig. 57-22). Bacterial pneumonia is very frequent after the third or fourth day of injury and should be anticipated.[32]

Inhalation injury from chlorine gas inhalation has been reported in children. This irritant gas is found in swimming pool disinfectants and household cleaning agents. It reacts with the water in tissue to produce hydrochloric acid, which leads to mucosal necrosis. Irritation of the upper respiratory tract, cough, and wheezing are early findings.[32,67]

Another inhalation injury that may occur in infants is caused by inhalation of the small (approximately 5 micrometers) particles of hydrous magnesium silicate present in talcum powder. Inhaled talc produces airway obstruction and impairs ciliary action, which leads to inflammation. Symptoms of cough and respiratory distress are rapid after exposure.[68]

Passive smoking is associated with an increased rate of respiratory illness in infancy and childhood. The frequency of reactive airways disease is increased in exposed infants.[69,70]

Imaging The results of early radiographs are often normal in smoke inhalation, but diffuse or focal patchy opacities or pulmonary edema may be noted (see Fig. 57-22). More diffuse opacities, which usually appear after a latent period of 12 to 48 hours, may clear slowly. Rapid appearance of total or subtotal lung consolidation has been described in up to 10% of burned children and is associated with high early mortality. ARDS is a serious and common complication of inhalation injuries and burns.[32]

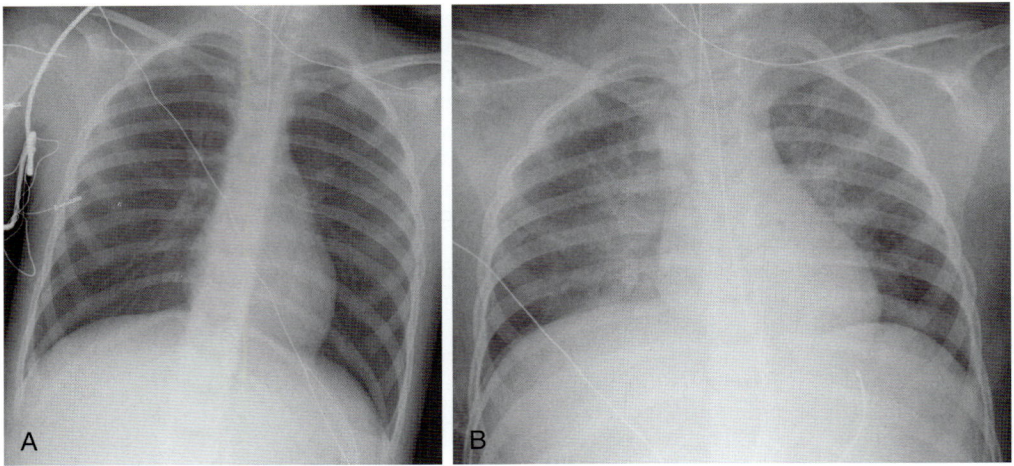

Figure 57-22 A 4-year-old girl rescued from a house fire. **A,** Portable anteroposterior chest radiograph at admission shows clear lungs and hyperinflation. **B,** One day later, bilateral pulmonary edema is developing and lung volumes are lower.

With chlorine gas inhalation, the onset of pulmonary edema is often rapid. The results of chest radiography may be normal or may show hyperinflation or pulmonary edema.[67,68] With talcum powder inhalation, chest radiography may show hyperinflation and patchy opacities.[68]

Treatment and Follow-up Treatment, as for noncardiogenic pulmonary edema, is primarily supportive. Late sequelae, including severe bronchiectasis, asthma, and bronchiolitis obliterans, may be noted after smoke inhalation.[32] Follow-up radiography is adequate if the patient shows clinical improvement. CT may be needed if clinical symptoms persist in a delayed setting.

HYDROCARBON PNEUMONITIS

Hydrocarbon pneumonitis occurs in 40% of children following ingestion of hydrocarbons such as lamp oil, lighter fluid, cleaning fluid, furniture and floor polishes, kerosene and gasoline.[71] These low-viscosity materials are aspirated when ingested. In the United States, such exposures continue to account for 12% to 25% of lethal poisonings in children less than 5 years old.[32]

Etiology Aspirated or inhaled material usually results in an intense chemical pneumonitis causing damage to the respiratory epithelium and development of cyanosis through displacement of alveolar gas by the hydrocarbon.[32]

Imaging Although changes may be evident on chest radiography as early as 30 minutes after aspiration, the findings may be delayed several hours; virtually all affected children with lung disease have abnormal chest radiographs by 12 hours (see Fig. 57-13 and e-Fig. 57-23).[32] The typical pattern of hydrocarbon pneumonitis is one of patchy airspace consolidation and alveolar edema involving predominantly the medial basilar portions of the lungs bilaterally. Pneumatoceles are a well-known complication of hydrocarbon aspiration but only develop in 10% of children.[71]

Treatment and Follow-up Treatment is supportive. Resolution of the radiographic changes usually lags behind clinical improvement and may take weeks or months. CT may be performed if improvement does not progress as expected.

LIPOID PNEUMONIA

Oral administration of mineral oil for constipation is the most common cause of exogenous lipoid pneumonia. In a study of affected children in Brazil, 79% of patients were less than 24 months of age.[72]

Etiology Lipids aspirated during oral administration of mineral oil may result in an insidious chronic process that produces an intense lung response and may result in severe lung injury. Histologic proof of exposure is gained by finding lipid-laden macrophages and lipid material in alveoli on biopsy. However, the current diagnostic method of choice for diagnosing lipoid pneumonia is by analysis of bronchoalveolar lavage fluid.[72]

Imaging The typical radiographic pattern of lipoid pneumonia is perihilar and basilar airspace opacities (Fig. 57-24 and e-Fig. 57-25). CT shows areas of ground-glass opacity or more confluent airspace disease (see Fig. 57-24 and e-Fig. 57-25). On CT, the presence of fat attenuation values of the airspace disease (occurring in 71% of children) should alert the radiologist to the diagnosis of lipoid pneumonia.[73] In adults and children with lipoid pneumonia, the crazy-paving pattern has also been noted on thin-section CT.[72-74]

Treatment and Follow-up Cessation of exposure and clearing of the oil by multiple bronchoalveolar lavages is usually followed by slow clearing of lung opacities and clinical improvement.[72] CT and chest radiography are usually used for follow-up.

NEAR-DROWNING

Drowning is the second most frequent, after motor vehicle accidents, cause of accidental death in children. The most common site for near-drowning is the backyard swimming pool. Accidental submersion injuries demonstrate a bimodal age peak of 6 months to 4 years and 18 to 24 years.[32]

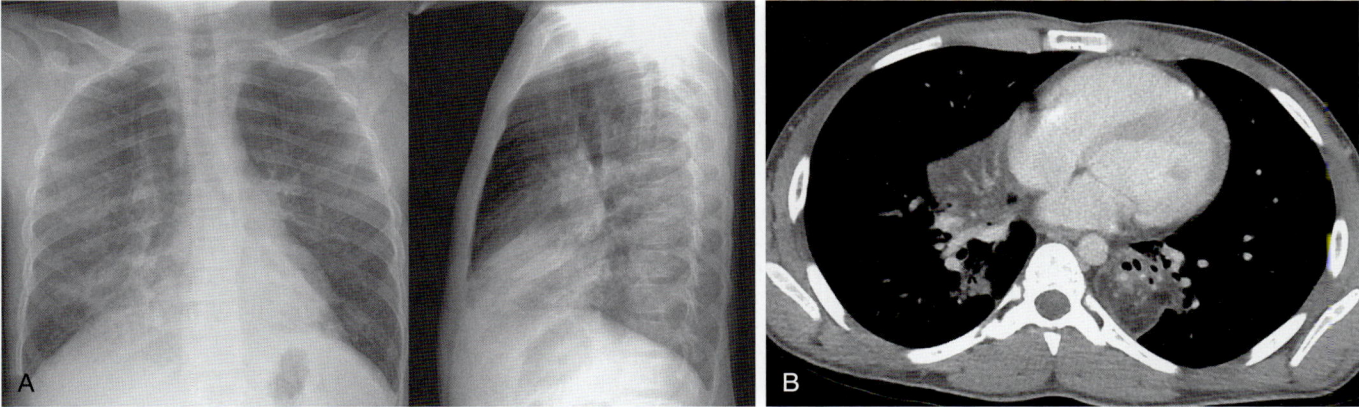

Figure 57-24 Lipoid pneumonia. This 11-year-old boy presented with chronic cough and drainage, with recent-onset difficulty breathing. He had a history of treatment with oral mineral oil for constipation. **A,** Bilateral airspace opacities are noted on the initial posteroanterior and lateral chest radiographs, predominantly in the lung bases. **B,** An axial chest computed tomography image shows fat attenuation and focal consolidation in the left lower lobe and right middle lobe.

Etiology Submersion time, volume of water aspirated, severity of acidosis, and length of delay in cardiopulmonary resuscitation all correlate directly with morbidity and mortality. Most submersion victims aspirate a small amount of water that may contain vomitus or a variety of contaminants. Laryngospasm occurs, which may prevent further aspiration. In about 15% of patients, laryngospasm persists and death is by anoxia (i.e., "dry drowning").[32]

Imaging The radiologic pattern of near-drowning is of pulmonary edema, and the severity depends predominantly on the amount of water aspirated. Opacities are usually bilateral and symmetric, and a significant delay, sometimes as long as 24 to 48 hours after near-drowning, may occur in the appearance of edema (Fig. 57-26).[32]

Treatment and Follow-up Treatment is primarily supportive with ventilatory support, if needed, in cases of severe respiratory distress. Radiography is usually adequate for imaging follow-up.

Conditions with Pulmonary Calcifications

PULMONARY ALVEOLAR MICROLITHIASIS

Pulmonary alveolar microlithiasis (PAM) is a rare disease characterized by the presence of innumerable calcium phosphate microliths in the alveoli. Many cases are familial and inherited as an autosomal-recessive trait.[75] In one review, 17% of affected patients presented at 12 years of age or younger.[76]

Etiology The etiology of PAM is currently unknown. However, the tiny stones in the alveoli consist of concentric calcium rings, which measure from 0.01 to 3 mm in size, are similar to bone histologically, radiographically, and metabolically. The number and size of the calculi and the amount of interstitial reaction increase with the age of the patient and the duration of the disease.[75,76]

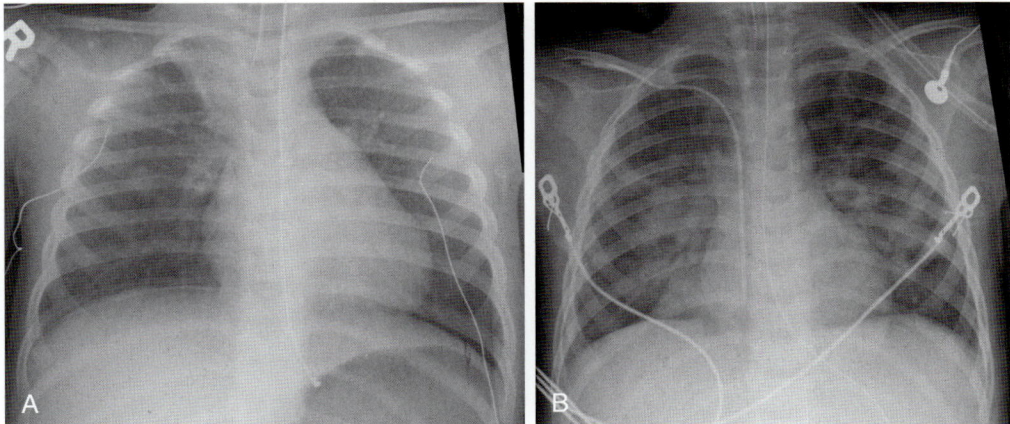

Figure 57-26 A 3-year-old male who suffered a near-drowning episode in a creek. **A,** The chest radiograph at presentation is near normal except for atelectasis at the medial right apex. **B,** The chest radiograph 2 days later shows development of perihilar airspace disease consistent with noncardiogenic edema.

Imaging On chest radiography, in children with PAM, diffuse ground-glass opacities were more common than nodular calcific densities. HRCT shows ground-glass opacities and calcific densities in the lung, pleura, and interlobar septae.[77] The calcified lung lesions demonstrate an avidity for bone scintigraphy agents.[76]

Treatment and Follow-up Virtually all types of treatment for PAM have been ineffective except lung transplantation.[76] CT or chest radiography may be used for follow-up, but CT shows the distribution and size of the calcifications more reliably.

MISCELLANEOUS PULMONARY CALCIFICATIONS

A wide variety of clinical conditions may be associated with pulmonary calcifications, which are not always readily apparent on chest radiography.

Etiology Focal pulmonary calcifications in childhood are usually the result of granulomatous infection, most commonly tuberculosis or histoplasmosis. Diffuse calcifications are probably dystrophic (calcification caused by tissue damage) and are most commonly seen after varicella infection. Metastatic calcification (calcification in normal tissue) is caused by abnormal calcium and phosphorous metabolism, usually in one of the following clinical situations: chronic renal failure and secondary hyperparathyroidism, acute renal failure, after renal transplantation, and after cardiac surgery.[78]

Imaging Initially, plain radiography shows airspace consolidation or nonspecific nodular opacities, which may demonstrate a progressive increase in opacity. These opacities may be mistaken for an infectious process such as pneumonia. CT is more sensitive than chest radiography for the definitive diagnosis of pulmonary calcification.

Treatment and Follow-up Besides treatment for a discovered active granulomatous process, no treatment or follow up is needed for the majority of pulmonary calcifications.

Key Points

The most common radiologic findings of vasculitis are best delineated by high-resolution CT and include nodules (often cavitary), ground-glass opacities, and airspace opacities.

Collagen vascular disease is rarely associated with interstitial lung opacities, best demonstrated by HRCT. Common thoracic findings of CVD are pleural and pericardial effusions.

Lung involvement with LCH is virtually always associated with multisystem disease and shows mostly cysts and nodules predominantly in the upper lobes and may progress to honeycombing.

Subtle radiographic findings of interstitial pulmonary edema in infants and children include peribronchial cuffing, perihilar vascular haziness, fissural thickening, septal lines, hyperinflation, and small pleural effusions.

Pulmonary embolus in children almost always occurs in the setting of a predisposing condition such as central venous catheter, DVT, malignancy, CHD, recent surgery, trauma, infection, renal disease (nephrotic syndrome), SCD, SLE, or clotting disorder.

Of pediatric patients with hydrocarbon pneumonitis, only 10% develop pneumatoceles despite the widely recognized association of this complication.

Exogenous lipoid pneumonia is usually caused by mineral oil ingestion for constipation and is associated with fat attenuation opacities on CT.

Suggested Readings

Dinwiddie R, Sonnappa S. Systemic diseases and the lung. *Paediatr Respir Rev.* 2005;6:181–189.

Garcia-Pena P, Boixadera H, Barber I, et al. Thoracic findings of systemic diseases at high-resolution CT in children. *RadioGraphics.* 2011; 31:465–482.

Patocka C, Nemeth J. Pulmonary embolism in pediatrics. *J Emerg Med.* 2012;42:(1):105–116.

Schmidt S, Eitch G, Geoffray A, et al. Extraosseous Langerhans cell histiocytosis in children. *RadioGraphics.* 2008;28:707–726.

Seely JM, Effmann EL. Acute lung injury and acute respiratory distress syndrome in children. *Semin Roentgenol.* 1998;33:163–173.

References

Full references for this chapter can be found on www.expertconsult.com.

Chapter 58

The Mediastinum

GERALD G. BEHR, RICARDO RESTREPO, and EDWARD Y. LEE

The intrathoracic compartment, which is situated between the sternum anteriorly and the vertebral column posteriorly and is bounded laterally by the parietal pleura, is considered the *mediastinum*. The thoracic inlet and the diaphragm form the superior and inferior boundaries, respectively. In humans, the mediastinum completely separates the left and right pleural spaces. The mediastinum contains several fundamental structural components including soft tissues, vessels, and nerves. A wide variety of congenital and developmental anomalies, inflammatory and infectious diseases, and benign and malignant neoplasms can affect these structural components in pediatric patients. An up-to-date knowledge of the practical diagnostic approach combined with a clear understanding of the characteristic imaging appearances of these conditions can lead to optimal patient management. This chapter reviews the etiology, imaging findings, and treatment and follow-up of various congenital and acquired anomalies and abnormalities that occur within the mediastinum in the pediatric population.

Spectrum of Mediastinal Anomalies and Abnormalities

PNEUMOMEDIASTINUM

Overview

Pneumomediastinum, also known as mediastinal emphysema, is a condition in which air is present within the mediastinum.[1] Pneumomediastinum occurs more frequently in infants than in older children.[2] Affected pediatric patients typically present with a sensation of retrosternal fullness, dysphagia, sore throat, chest pain, or dyspnea.

Etiology Pneumomediastinum may be spontaneous or iatrogenic. Spontaneous pneumomediastinum results from a sudden forceful increase in intraalveolar pressure such as forceful inhalation or the Valsalva maneuver. In this instance, an alveolus can rupture, allowing gas under pressure into the low-pressure pulmonary interstitial compartment. The air then travels via the peribronchovascular space medially toward the hilum, which opens into the mediastinum.[3,4] Occasionally, the air dissects along the lymphatics as well and extends to the visceral pleura, where a concomitant pneumothorax may occur. Iatrogenic pneumomediastinum may result from abdominal and cardiac surgery, endotracheal intubation, or cardiac catheterization. Additionally, pneumomediastinum also can occur after foreign body ingestion, trauma to the neck or chest, or any disruption of the tracheobronchial tree or esophagus (e.g., Boerhaave syndrome).[2]

It is not uncommon for pneumomediastinum and pneumothorax to coexist.[5] This phenomenon sometimes can be attributed to a common mechanism of injury, or the pneumothorax may arise as a result of a pneumomediastinum. In addition, potential communications between the mediastinum and the peritoneal cavity exist via anatomic diaphragmatic defects, such as the esophageal hiatus. As such, the pneumoperitoneum can dissect superiorly into the mediastinum and vice versa. Retroperitoneal extension of the pneumomediastinum also may be observed.[6] Rarely, air within the mediastinum can enter the spinal canal, which is termed *pneumorrhachis*.[7]

Imaging The air within the mediastinum typically displaces the pleura and lung laterally (Fig. 58-1). It may decompress into the superior mediastinum and dissect along fascial planes into the subcutaneous tissues of the neck and retropharynx (e-Fig. 58-2). In infants and younger children, air within the mediastinum may displace the thymus superiorly to produce the "spinnaker sail" sign (see Fig. 58-1).

With small pneumomediastinum, sometimes only a sliver of curvilinear radiolucency is seen adjacent to the cardiac border, most often on the left. This sliver may sharply outline the aortic arch and descending aorta. When air is adjacent to the pulmonary artery or a branch (typically on the right), the "ring around the artery" sign is seen on the lateral view.[6,8] The often-quoted "continuous diaphragm sign" results from air interposed between the pericardium and the diaphragm,[8] which effectively erases the normal "silhouetting" of the diaphragm that allows it to be visualized as the single structure that it is.

A large pneumomediastinum may be confused with a pneumothorax, especially when the patient undergoes imaging while in the supine position. In such an equivocal situation, a decubitus radiographic view may be helpful because the mediastinal air does not move, whereas the pneumothorax rises nondependently.[5]

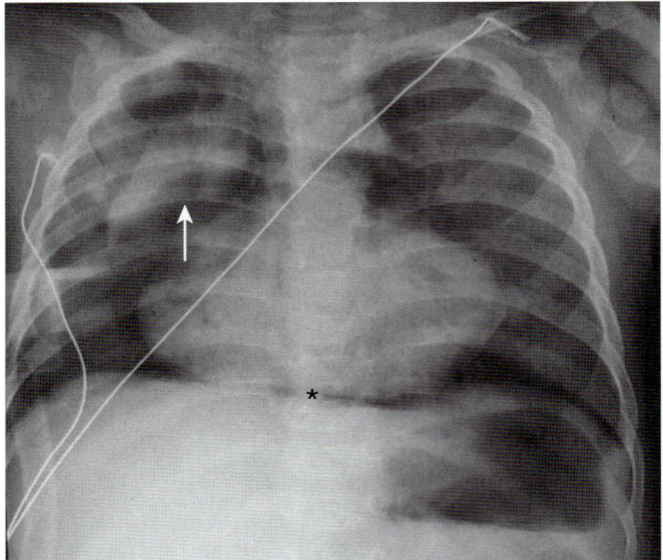

Figure 58-1   Pneumomediastinum in a 6-month-old boy. A frontal chest radiograph demonstrates a lifted thymic shadow (*arrow*), the so-called "spinnaker sail sign." Mediastinal air (*asterisk*) also is interposed between the central diaphragm and pericardium, and lucency is seen surrounding the heart.

At times, pneumomediastinum may be difficult to differentiate from pneumopericardium. In contrast to pneumomediastinum, pneumopericardium does *not* lift the thymus or outline the aortic arch. The air is contained by the pericardium, which can have a dome-shaped superior margin. Pneumopericardium is almost always seen in association with pneumomediastinum except after open-heart surgery.[5]

Treatment and Follow-up   Treatment of pneumomediastinum is aimed at the underlying cause. For most spontaneous cases of pneumomediastinum, treatment is supportive, including rest, pain control, and avoidance of Valsalva maneuvers.[2] If concern exists about the possibility of esophageal rupture, an esophagram using water-soluble contrast may be performed, and a timely surgical consultation should be obtained when

the possibility of rupture is present.[9,10] Very rarely, pseudotamponade, laryngeal compression, tension pneumomediastinum, tension pneumothorax, or mediastinitis occur and require surgical intervention.

MEDIASTINAL HEMORRHAGE

Etiology   Mediastinal hemorrhage in pediatric patients usually is due to venous bleeding from blunt trauma.[5] Large mediastinal hemorrhage as a result of mediastinal vessel rupture often is due to iatrogenic causes related to central catheter placement or cardiothoracic procedures in pediatric patients. However, mediastinal hemorrhage in children also can occur spontaneously in the context of hemophilia, in which case the hemorrhage may be retropharyngeal and dissect into the mediastinum.[5,11] Additionally, rare cases of neonatal thymic hemorrhage have been reported,[12] possibly related to vitamin K deficiency.[13,14]

Imaging   Although imaging findings of mediastinal hemorrhage may be nonspecific, the possibility of mediastinal hemorrhage should be considered when mediastinal widening, blurring of the aortic stripe margin, deviation of a nasoenteric tube, and/or left apical "capping" are present on chest radiographs (Fig. 58-3, *A*). When evaluating mediastinal widening on chest radiographs, attention must be paid to the technique (i.e., the portable anteroposterior vs. standard posterolateral view). A portable anteroposterior chest radiograph may exaggerate the size of the mediastinum. Therefore in equivocal cases, confirmation with a subsequent posterolateral view or a cross-sectional imaging study such as computed tomography (CT) may be necessary. On CT, mediastinal fluid with a Hounsfield unit greater than water (>20 HU) suggests mediastinal hemorrhage (Fig. 58-3, *B*).

Treatment and Follow-up   When mediastinal hemorrhage is considered on chest radiographs, further imaging studies such as echocardiography and/or contrast-enhanced CT using CT angiography protocol with subsequent multiplanar and three-dimensional reconstruction evaluation is warranted. With rapid clinical deterioration, urgent surgical exploration is an option to avoid delaying proper treatment.

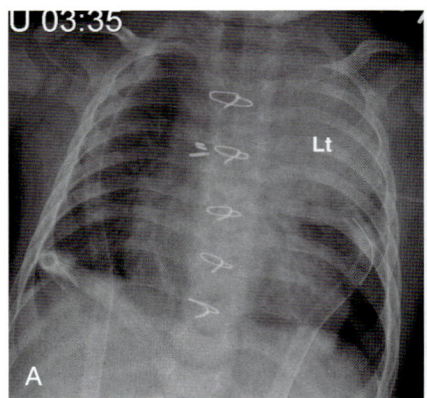
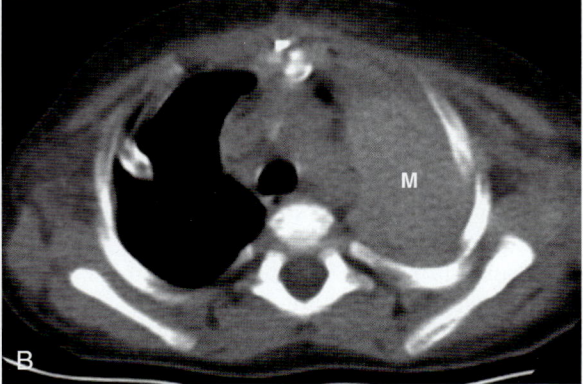

Figure 58-3   A mediastinal hematoma in a 2-year-old girl after open-heart surgery. **A,** A frontal chest radiograph shows large left upper lung zone opacity (*Lt*). No ipsilateral mediastinal shift or other evidence suggestive of atelectasis is present. Also noted are bilateral chest tubes, median sternotomy wires, and surgical clips within the mediastinum. **B,** An axial unenhanced computed tomography image at the level of the upper thorax reveals a large, left-sided, high-attenuation, masslike area (*M*) in the left extrapleural (mediastinal) space, indicative of a postprocedural mediastinal hematoma.

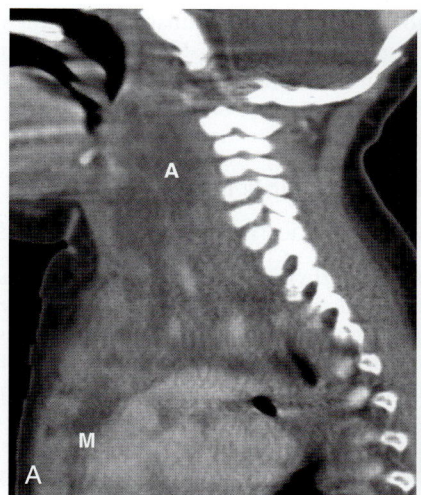
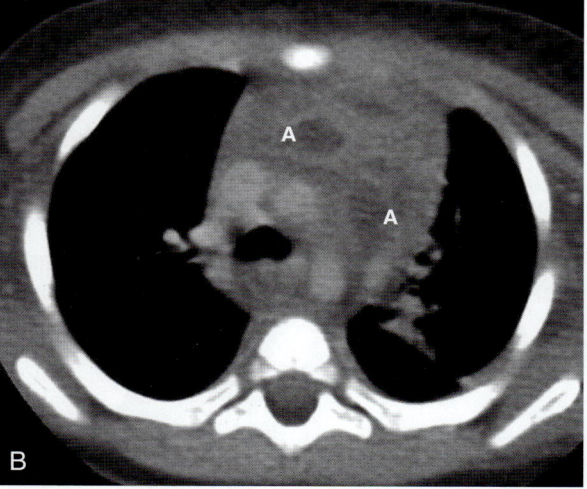

Figure 58-4 Acute mediastinitis resulting from a retropharyngeal abscess in a 1-year-old boy. **A,** A sagittal enhanced multiplanar computed tomography (CT) image through the neck shows a large, complex fluid collection (*A*) extending caudally into the mediastinum (*M*). **B,** An axial enhanced CT image obtained at the level of the aortic arch demonstrates two of the better defined abscesses (*A*) in the anterior mediastinal compartment embedded in an inflamed and heterogenous thymus.

MEDIASTINAL INFECTION

Overview

Infections arising de novo in the mediastinum are rare in the pediatric population. Mediastinal infections can be classified into two types: acute and chronic fibrosing mediastinitis. Whereas acute mediastinal infections usually are due to perforation of the esophagus and/or trachea with subsequent cellulitis or abscess formation,[15,16] chronic fibrosing mediastinitis typically results from tuberculosis or Histoplasmosis infections.[17-19]

Acute Mediastinitis

Etiology Acute superior mediastinal infections typically are due to cervical infection or sternoclavicular osteomyelitis.[20-22] The frequent underlying causes for acute anterior and middle mediastinal infections in pediatric patients include the incorrect passage of instruments (e.g., a nasogastric tube or endotracheal tube), impacted foreign bodies, child abuse, or leakage at the sites of surgical anastomoses.[23] Posterior acute mediastinal infections usually are due to the extension of osteomyelitis of the vertebrae. Affected pediatric patients typically present with pain, fever, and an elevated white blood cell count.

Imaging Plain radiographic findings of acute mediastinitis are nonspecific. However, mediastinal widening, obliteration of normal mediastinal contours, and displaced or narrowed trachea should suggest possible underlying acute mediastinitis in the appropriate clinical setting. The more specific radiological imaging finding of acute mediastinitis is the presence of gas within the mediastinum, which can be better evaluated with CT. CT also can show complications from acute mediastinitis such as mediastinal abscess formation or empyema (Fig. 58-4).

Treatment and Follow-up Acute mediastinitis is treated aggressively with a combination of antibiotics and surgical irrigation. More recently, a combination of continuous mediastinal irrigation and vacuum-assisted closure has been proposed.[24,25]

Chronic Fibrosing Mediastinitis

Etiology Chronic fibrosing mediastinitis, also known as sclerosing mediastinitis, is rare in the pediatric population. It is a condition characterized by abnormal proliferation of dense acellular collagen and fibrous tissue in the mediastinum.[26,27] Although it is most frequently attributed to the sequelae of granulomatous infection such as Mycobacterium tuberculosis or Histoplasmosis infection, it also can arise as an idiopathic condition or as the sequelae of autoimmune disease, radiotherapy, or drugs such as methysergide and metoprolol.[25,28] Additionally, chronic fibrosing mediastinitis also is associated with retroperitoneal fibrosis, sclerosing cholangitis, Riedel thyroiditis, and pulmonary granuloma.[29] Affected pediatric patients often present with respiratory distress related to airway narrowing, dysphagia due to esophageal compromise, and/or facial and neck swelling resulting from obstruction of the superior vena cava.

Imaging The widening of the mediastinum with a lobular paratracheal and/or subcarinal mass that may be calcified is a typical imaging finding on chest radiographs. CT imaging findings of chronic fibrosing mediastinitis can be categorized into two patterns: focal or diffuse.[26,30] Patients affected with focal-type chronic fibrosing mediastinitis typically present with a soft tissue mass, often associated with calcification (63%),[30] that is located in the right paratracheal, subcarinal, or hilar regions (Fig. 58-5). On the other hand, pediatric patients affected with diffuse-type chronic fibrosing mediastinitis present with a diffusely infiltrating mass without calcification that often affects entire mediastinal compartments.

Treatment and Follow-up Treatment of acute mediastinitis consists of the administration of antibiotics that target the offending organisms. Localized mediastinal abscess formation

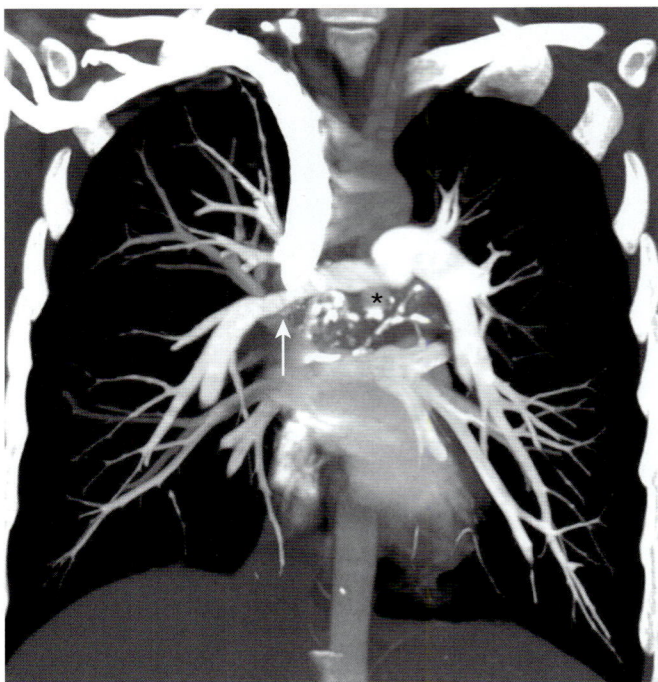

Figure 58-5 Chronic fibrosing mediastinitis in a 17-year-old girl. A coronal maximum intensity projection computed tomography image of the chest shows a middle mediastinal ill-defined mass that narrows the right pulmonary artery (*arrow*). Also note the calcifications (*asterisk*). (From Daltro PA, Santos EN, Gasparetto TD, et al. Pulmonary infections. *Pediatr Radiol.* 2011;41(Suppl 1):S69-S82.)

due to acute mediastinitis can be managed with either a surgical or percutaneous abscess drainage procedure. Although no consensus or widely accepted guidelines currently exist for the treatment of chronic fibrosing mediastinitis, systemic antifungal or corticosteroid treatment, surgical resection, and local therapy for complications are the management options currently available. Surgical resection may be necessary for symptomatic pediatric patients who have extensive and aggressive chronic fibrosing mediastinitis that results in either obstruction or compression of mediastinal structures such as central airways, the esophagus, or mediastinal large vessels.

MEDIASTINAL MASSES

Overview

The mediastinum is the most common location of chest masses in the pediatric population. Mediastinal masses in infants and children can be benign or malignant neoplasms, congenital anomalies, infections, vascular malformations, or pseudomasses. As with adult patients, it is useful to locate the mediastinal mass within one of the three mediastinal compartments (anterior, middle, or posterior) (Fig. 58-6). However, such a system of compartmentalizing the mediastinum may have shortcomings. For example, the borders of the anterior, middle, and posterior mediastinum, which are defined by anatomic landmarks as assessed on a lateral radiograph of the chest, do not have true and definite fascial planes. In addition, several disorders that may present as mediastinal masses cross boundaries or arise in multiple compartments. Nonetheless, the practice of assigning a mediastinal

mass to a specific mediastinal compartment is still useful because such a method enables one to formulate a manageable differential diagnosis and effectively direct further imaging workup, and it yields valuable information, particularly for surgical planning.

Anterior Mediastinal Masses

Congenital Abnormalities of the Thymus

Etiology The thymus is a bilobed organ that serves as the site of T-cell maturation. The thymus develops from the third pharyngeal pouch. It begins a process of caudal and ventromedial elongation during the seventh and eighth week of gestation whereby the two sides fuse at about the level of the aortic arch. Partial failure of descent may result in ectopic thymic tissue in the neck or superior mediastinum. Absence of the thymus is a component of DiGeorge syndrome,[31] with an incidence of 1 per 2000 to 4000.[32-34]

Imaging The appearance of the thymus on frontal chest radiographs is variable and largely dependent on the age of the patient (Fig. 58-7).[5,35,36] The thymus is prominent in size with a quadrilateral shape and convex margins during infancy (Fig. 58-8). After approximately the fifth year of life, the thymus becomes more triangular in shape with straight margins (e-Fig. 58-9). By the age of 15 years, the margins of the thymus are either straight or concave (Fig. 58-10). Absent thymic tissue in pediatric patients with DiGeorge syndrome is usually evident on chest radiographs in infants and young

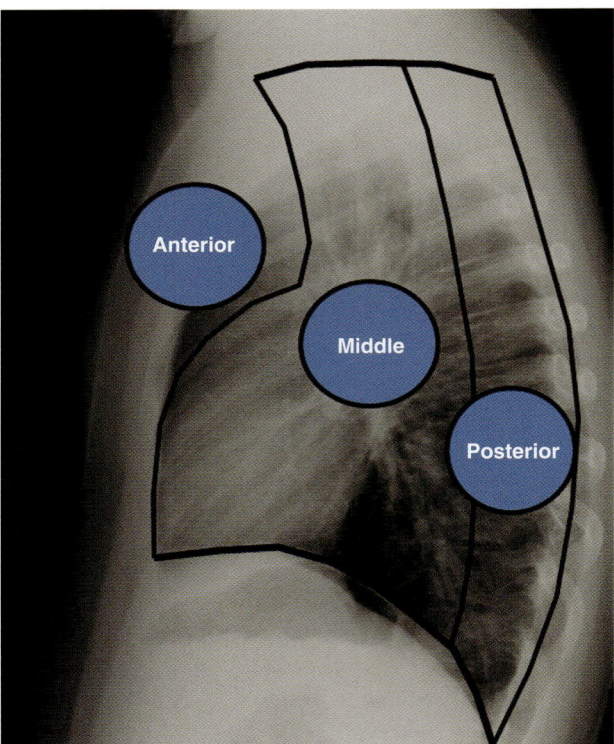

Figure 58-6 Anatomic landmarks demarcating the anterior, middle, and posterior compartments of the mediastinum labeled on a lateral chest radiograph. *Anterior* indicates the anterior mediastinal compartment, *Middle* indicates the middle mediastinal compartment, and *Posterior* indicates the posterior mediastinal compartment.

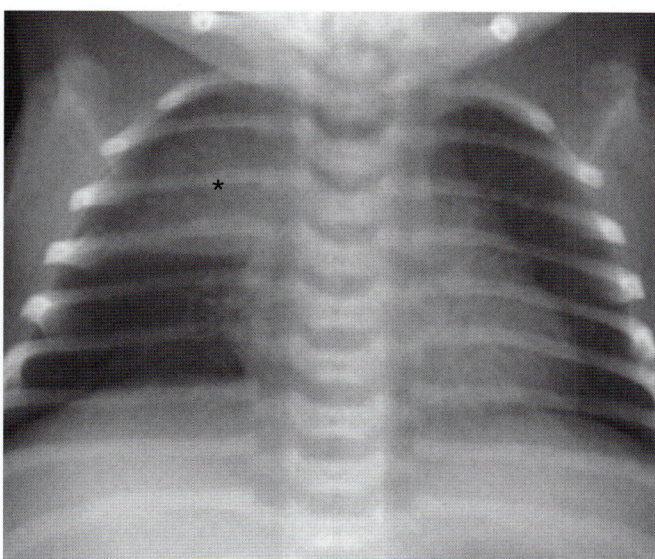

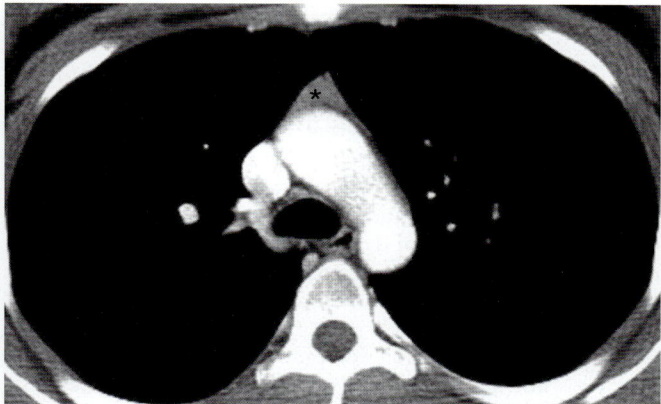

Figure 58-10 A normal thymus in an adolescent boy. An axial enhanced computed tomography image at the level of the aortic arch shows the expected appearance of the thymus (*asterisk*) in the anterior mediastinal compartment at this age. The thymus has a triangular shape with a straight margin.

Figure 58-7 A normal thymus in a female neonate. The frontal chest radiograph shows a thymic sail sign, which is created by the right lobe of the thymus (*asterisk*) abutting the minor fissure.

children. However, an atrophic thymus due to a stress response may appear similarly.[37,38] The clinical context is often helpful in distinguishing these two conditions without the need for cross-sectional studies.

Treatment and Follow-up Treatment of DiGeorge syndrome is targeted to the associated defects such as hypocalcemia, frequent infections, and conotruncal cardiac defects. Because DiGeorge syndrome is a component of the 22q11 deletion syndrome, many patients with this syndrome also have velo-cardiofacial syndrome.[39]

Normal Variants of the Thymus

Etiology The two most common anatomic variants of the thymus are either superior or posterior extension of the normal thymus (e-Fig. 58-11 and Fig. 58-12). These variants usually are seen before 2 years of age. The thymus may extent superiorly to the level of the lower neck[40,41] or posteriorly to the middle or posterior mediastinal compartment.[42,43] The posterior extension of the thymus typically is posterior to the superior vena cava on the right or the aortic arch on the left. After puberty, the thymus undergoes slow involution. During stress, a rapid transient decrease in the size of the gland occurs, and it regains its original size after the offending mechanism (e.g., intubation, surgery, or chemotherapy) is withdrawn—the so-called *thymic rebound*.[38,44]

Imaging An ectopic thymus rarely presents as a mass and is most commonly discovered incidentally as thymic tissue extension on cross-sectional imaging with similar signal characteristics and density as the orthotopic thymus on magnetic resonance imaging (MRI) and CT, respectively (see e-Fig. 58-11 and Fig. 58-12). Occasionally, however, retrocaval

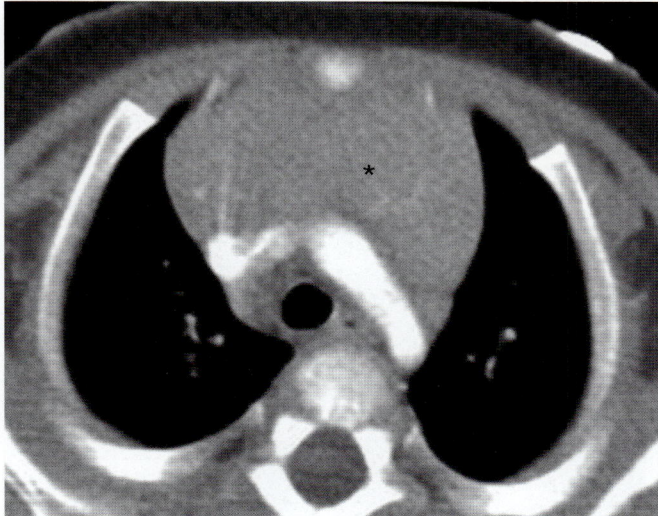

Figure 58-8 A normal thymus in a 5-month-old girl. An axial enhanced computed tomography image at the level of the aortic arch shows the expected appearance of the thymus (*asterisk*) in the anterior mediastinal compartment at this age. The thymus has a quadrilateral shape and a convex margin. It is homogeneous in attenuation without an associated cystic, calcific, or fat component.

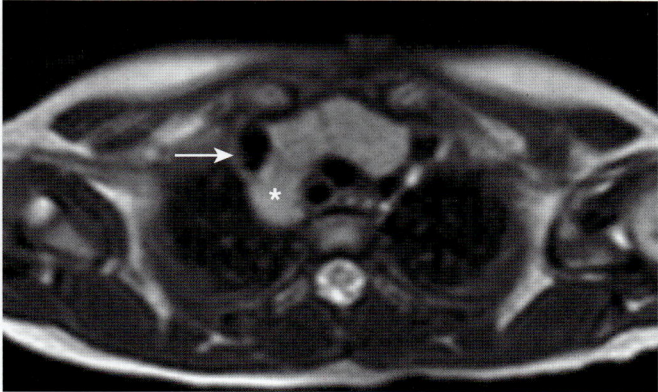

Figure 58-12 Posterior thymic extension as a normal variant in a 1-year-old boy. An axial T2-weighted magnetic resonance image at the level of the brachiocephalic vein shows posterior extension (*asterisk*) of the thymus behind the superior vena cava (*arrow*).

thymus may be mistaken for a mediastinal mass on radiographs. With superior mediastinal extension, the diagnosis may be made with ultrasound using a high-frequency linear array transducer. The ectopic thymus should exhibit homogenous echotexture with internal bright specular reflections, similar to the orthotopic thymus.[45] Further, contiguity with the orthotopic thymus may be demonstrated on ultrasound. The appearance of rebound thymus on chest radiographs may be impressive in terms of degree and rapidity of development. Any displacement or compression of adjacent airway or vessels by the thymus should raise suspicion for a neoplasm.

Treatment   Treatment for ectopic thymic tissue or rebound thymus is not necessary. However, its diagnosis is potentially important to avoid unnecessary procedures.

Thymic Cyst

Etiology   A thymic cyst is a rare, fluid-filled lesion typically representing a cystic remnant of the thymopharyngeal duct.[38,46] Although a thymic cyst can occur anywhere from the pyriform sinus to the anterior mediastinum, it is most commonly found in the lateral infrahyoid neck region.[47] A fibrous cord may connect the thymic cyst to the mediastinal thymus. When the cyst is large, affected pediatric patients present with a slowly enlarging neck mass that may be associated with respiratory compromise, dysphagia, or vocal cord paralysis. Although most thymic cysts are derived from a remnant of the thymopharyngeal duct, thymic cysts also have been described in patients infected with human immunodeficiency virus and in patients with Langerhans cell histiocytosis involving the thymus.[48,49] Cysts in the latter group may feature small calcifications.[50]

Imaging   Thymic cysts appear as a spherical, fluid-filled lesion or as multilocular cystic spaces with a thin wall. The thymic cyst is usually occult on chest radiographs. In infants and young children, ultrasound may confirm the fluid-filled nature of the mass. On CT and MRI, thymic cysts typically present as a nonenhancing cystic mass (e-Fig. 58-13). The MR signal of a thymic cyst is variable depending on whether the contents are proteinaceous and/or hemorrhagic. The differential diagnosis of a thymic cyst in pediatric patients includes branchial cleft cyst, lymphatic malformation, thyroglossal duct cyst, dermoid cyst, bronchogenic cyst, and teratoma.

Treatment   The current choice for managing a thymic cyst, particularly in symptomatic pediatric patients, is surgical resection, which is associated with an excellent prognosis.

Thymolipoma

Etiology   A thymolipoma is an uncommon benign thymic mass composed of both thymic and mature adipose tissue. Thymolipomas account for approximately 2% to 9% of all thymic neoplasms.[38,51] The presumed underlying etiologies include a variant of a thymoma, hyperplasia of mediastinal fat, and a neoplasm of mediastinal fat that encases thymic tissue.[51,52] Affected patients typically are asymptomatic because a thymolipoma is very soft and pliable, exerting little mass effect.

Imaging   On chest radiographs, a thymolipoma may present as a low-density lesion because of its underlying fatty component. On cross-sectional imaging studies, thymolipomas are characterized by an enlarged thymus with areas of low attenuation (on CT) and high signal intensity (on T2-weighted MRI) in a whorled pattern representing the underlying fatty component (Fig. 58-14).

Treatment and Follow-up   Although a thymolipoma is not a malignant lesion, surgical resection often is undertaken because the diagnosis may be uncertain solely on the basis of imaging findings.

Thymoma

Etiology   Thymomas arise from the thymic epithelial cells and account for approximately 1% to 2% of anterior mediastinal masses in the pediatric population.[47,53] Thymomas traditionally are classified into two types (i.e., noninvasive or invasive thymoma) depending on the presence of well-defined margins without extension through its fibrous capsule. Because thymomas may be locally invasive but typically do not metastasize, many authorities prefer the term "invasive thymoma"

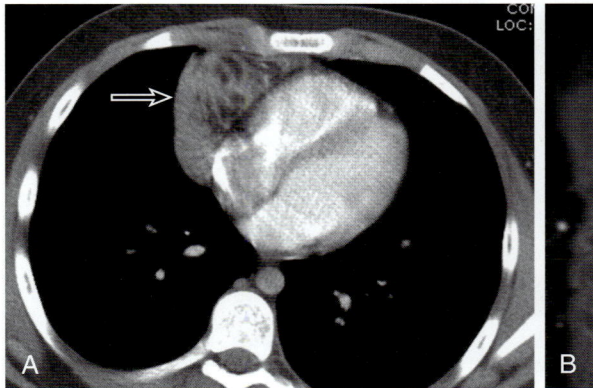
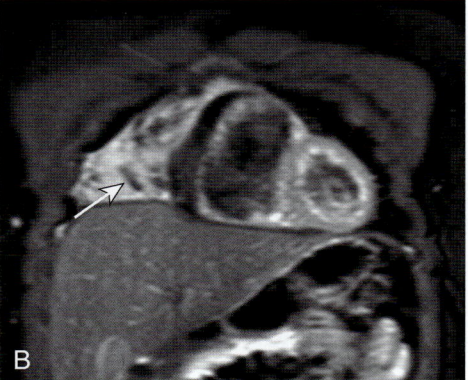

Figure 58-14   A thymolipoma in an 8-year-old girl. **A,** An axial enhanced computed tomography image at the level of the mid heart shows an anterior mediastinal mass (*arrow*) with whorls of low attenuating regions consistent with fat. **B,** A coronal fluid-sensitive magnetic resonance imaging sequence with fat saturation shows the linear low signal fatty striations (*arrow*) through the mass.

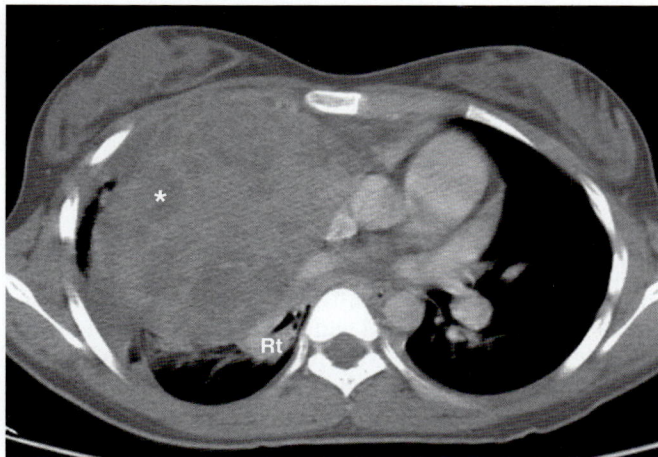

Figure 58-15 A thymoma in a 15-year-old girl. An axial enhanced computed tomography image at the level of the main pulmonary artery shows a large bulky thymus with irregular margins, heterogeneity, and areas of internal low attenuation (*asterisk*). Although the effect of the mass is seen, including posterior displacement of the bronchus intermedius and right sided atelectasis (*Rt*), no evidence is seen of vascular or soft tissue invasion.

rather than "malignant thymoma." Similar to adult patients with thymoma, about 15% to 30% of affected pediatric patients present with myasthenia gravis.[48,54,55] Other associated autoimmune conditions include pure red cell aplasia and hypogammaglobulinemia.[54,55]

Imaging On chest radiographs, a thymoma usually appears as an ovoid mass that occasionally is associated with thin peripheral capsular calcification located within the anterior mediastinum. Pleural nodules also may be seen in patients with an invasive thymoma. Cross-sectional imaging studies typically show an enlarged and homogeneous anterior mediastinal soft tissue mass sometimes associated with an area of low attenuation representing underlying cystic necrosis (Fig. 58-15)[47] Imaging findings suggestive of invasive-type thymoma include irregular margins, obliterated adjacent mediastinal fat planes, or extension to the pleura or chest wall. A search for these imaging features is particularly important, because the histology between invasive and noninvasive type thymoma is similar, apart from surgical evidence of capsular extension.

Treatment and Follow-up All thymomas that are deemed surgically resectable are removed. However, thymomas usually require radiation therapy and/or chemotherapy.

Thymic Carcinoma

Etiology A thymic carcinoma is an aggressive epithelial tumor of the thymus characterized by overt cellular atypia. Thymic carcinomas are rare in the pediatric population; they usually occur in adults during the fifth or sixth decade.[56] Affected pediatric patients most often present with chest pain and constitutional symptoms including fatigue, weight loss, and night sweats.[47] A paraneoplastic phenomenon such as myasthenia gravis is uncommon with a thymic carcinoma, in contradistinction to a thymoma.[57,58] Metastatic disease or

invasion is detected in most new diagnoses.[58,59] Prognosis is poor.

Imaging On imaging studies, a thymic carcinoma typically presents as a large anterior mediastinal mass with irregular margins, heterogeneous contrast enhancement, and local invasion of adjacent mediastinal structures (Fig. 58-16). Calcification and areas of necrosis are common.[60] Although differentiation from a thymoma is difficult, features such as local invasion of adjacent structures, lymphadenopathy, and metastasis favor the diagnosis of a thymic carcinoma over a thymoma.

Treatment The current treatment of a thymic carcinoma in pediatric patients includes neoadjuvant chemotherapy, surgery, and postoperative radiation therapy.[61]

Lymphoma

Etiology Lymphoma results from abnormal proliferation of lymphocytes, which are cells that are a component of the immune system. Lymphoma is the most common cause of mediastinal masses in the pediatric population. It also is the third most common group of malignancies after leukemia and central nervous system tumors in the pediatric population.[5] Lymphoma accounts for approximately 46% to 56% of all mediastinal masses.[5] Lymphoma is traditionally classified into two types: non-Hodgkin lymphoma and Hodgkin lymphoma. These two types of lymphoma have many similarities, including their appearance on imaging, but because of their many important differences, especially in clinical behavior, they are discussed separately in the following sections. Pulmonary involvement by lymphoma is discussed in Chapter 55.

Non-Hodgkin lymphoma typically occurs in pediatric patients who are younger than 5 years. It more frequently affects boys than girls by a ratio of 3:1.[5] The four main types of non-Hodgkin lymphoma include (1) lymphoblastic or T

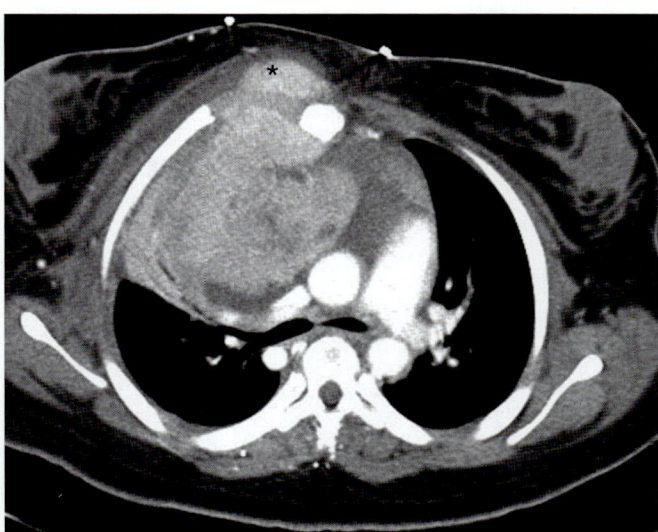

Figure 58-16 A thymic carcinoma in a 14-year-old girl. An axial enhanced computed tomography image at the level of the carina shows an anterior mediastinal mass with poorly defined areas of low attenuation. Note the anterior chest wall invasion by the mass (*asterisk*).

cell (the most common type); (2) Burkitt; (3) non-Burkitt; and (4) large cell or histiocytic. Pediatric patients with lymphoblastic or T-cell type non-Hodgkin lymphoma commonly present with a mediastinal mass. Although large cell or histiocytic types may involve either the thorax or the abdomen, Burkitt and non-Burkitt types nearly always present in the abdomen. In general, more than one third of patients with non-Hodgkin lymphoma present with a mediastinal mass.[62] Pediatric patients often present with clinical symptoms related to obstruction or compression related to adjacent mediastinal airways and vascular structures.

Hodgkin lymphoma is rare in younger children and occurs with increasing frequency in children older than 5 years.[5] It more frequently affects boys than girls by a ratio of 2:1.[5] Hodgkin lymphoma is divided into four main types based on the relative amounts of lymphocytes and Reed-Sternberg cells and the type of connective tissue proliferation: (1) nodular sclerosing; (2) mixed cellularity; (3) lymphocyte depletion; and (4) lymphocyte predominant. Among these four types of Hodgkin lymphoma, the nodular sclerosing type (the most common subtype) accounts for approximately 75%[5,63] of mediastinal masses in children. Although affected pediatric patients may present with asymptomatic cervical or axillary lymphadenopathy on physical examination, the majority of them present with chest pain and discomfort. Shortness of breath or wheezing should suggest underlying airway compression. More suggestive clinical symptoms of Hodgkin lymphoma include weight loss, night sweats, and unexplained fevers.

Imaging   Hodgkin lymphoma may present as bulky hilar nodes or an anterior mediastinal mass on chest radiographs (Fig. 58-17, *A* and *B*), although the chest radiographs may be entirely normal in the setting of minimal lymphadenopathy. When Hodgkin lymphoma is suspected, a contrast-enhanced CT scan of the chest should be performed to confirm the presence of a mass or enlarged nodes and to characterize its extent for disease staging (Fig. 58-17, *C*).[64,65] Common nodes involved in persons with Hodgkin lymphoma include the superior prevascular and pretracheal nodes. The appearance of affected nodes can range anywhere

between small lymph nodes to large, conglomerate nodular masses that fill in the mediastinum and displace adjacent structures. The presence of calcifications before treatment is rare.[47] On MRI, signal characteristics of Hodgkin lymphoma are variable but usually are intermediate on T1-weighted images and have an increased signal on T2-weighted images. However, MRI generally plays no additionally useful role in the diagnosis or workup of Hodgkin lymphoma. Positron emission tomography (PET) and/or PET/CT scans are now widely used and have been well validated in the literature for evaluating adult patients with lymphoma.[66-68] Although fewer studies have been conducted with pediatric patients, a growing body of evidence suggests very high accuracy of these modalities in children, especially when they are compared with CT used alone.[69-71]

Non-Hodgkin lymphoma is more variable than Hodgkin lymphoma with regard to its sites of disease predilection because it often may arise in the abdomen, thorax, or head/neck regions. When non-Hodgkin lymphoma occurs in the thorax (in about 50% of cases[47]), its most common appearance is that of a large anterior mediastinal mass on chest radiographs (Fig. 58-18, *A*). As with any anterior mediastinal mass, such imaging findings should prompt a CT scan, which typically shows discrete or conglomerate mediastinal lymph nodes (Fig. 58-18, *B*). After the administration of contrast, areas of heterogeneity and low-density necrosis are a frequent finding, particularly within the large masses. Because the lesion infiltrates or arises from the thymus, the mass can be confused with an enlarged, normal thymus in young children. Differentiating imaging features include unusually lobular, bulky borders, heterogeneity, and displacement of adjacent structures such as airway or vessels—features that a normal thymus should never have. Hilar, subcarinal, and posterior nodal chain involvement frequently is present. In contradistinction to Hodgkin lymphoma, pleural disease may be present, manifesting as pleural-based masses or effusion.[47] MRI may be useful in the evaluation of sites beyond the anterior mediastinum, including the chest wall. As with Hodgkin lymphoma, PET or combined PET/CT can assist in staging. PET is particularly helpful in discriminating between a viable tumor versus a scar, detecting active disease in "normal"-sized nodes

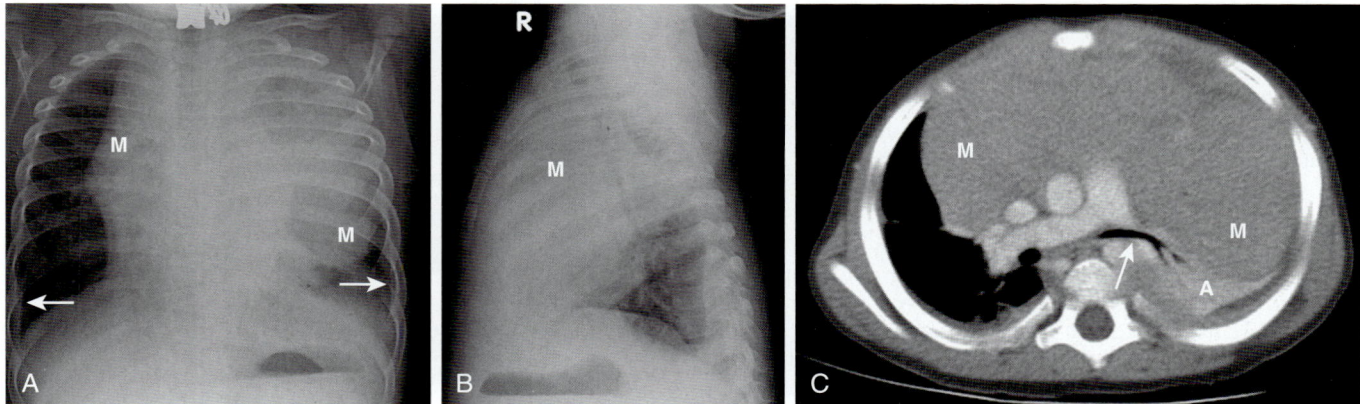

Figure 58-17   Hodgkin lymphoma in a 2-year-old girl. **A,** A frontal chest radiograph shows a large mediastinal mass (*M*) with lobulated and bulky margins. Small pleural effusions (*arrows*) also are present. **B,** A lateral chest radiograph confirms that the location of this mass (*M*) is within the anterior mediastinal compartment. **C,** An axial enhanced computed tomography image at the level of the right pulmonary artery shows a large anterior mediastinal mass (*M*) with effect of the mass showing on the left main stem bronchus (*arrow*). Left-sided atelectasis (*A*) is present.

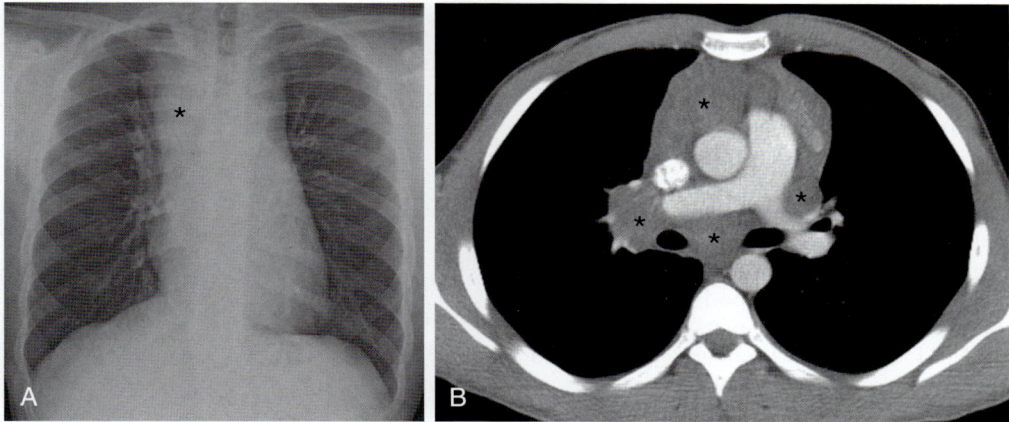

Figure 58-18 Non-Hodgkin lymphoma in an 8-year-old girl. **A,** A frontal chest radiograph shows a mediastinal mass (*asterisk*). **B,** An axial enhanced computed tomography image at the level of the pulmonary artery shows a mediastinal mass (*asterisks*) located within the mediastinum. Note both the anterior, subcarinal, and hilar components.

on CT, and searching for extranodal disease such as in the liver, spleen, and kidneys. Pitfalls of interpretation include the presence of increased metabolic activity in the thymus and brown fat.[72,73]

Treatment and Follow-up The prognosis of lymphoma in pediatric patients depends on the type and stage. The prognosis of Hodgkin lymphoma, which has a cure rate of approximately 90%,[47,74] is better than that of non–Hodgkin lymphoma, for which the cure rate among pediatric patients is 80%.[75] Currently, multiple chemotherapeutic treatment regimens are used in combination with radiation therapy to treat pediatric patients with lymphoma. In pediatric patients with non–Hodgkin lymphoma, a bone marrow transplant also is an option.

Lymphatic Malformation

Etiology Lymphatic malformation represents a congenital malformation of lymphatic channels, lined by single layer endothelium.[76] It typically occurs in the cervical region (often posterior to the sternocleidomastoid muscle) but may extend caudally into the superior and/or anterior mediastinum. Lymphatic malformation currently is classified into two types, macrocystic or microcystic, depending on the size of the cysts, although mixed lesions comprising both forms are common. Outdated terms include *cystic hygroma* and *lymphangioma* (for the macro and micro forms, respectively); use of these terms should be avoided. The term *lymphatic malformation* adheres to the currently recommended nomenclature of the International Society for the Study of Vascular Anomalies.[77] Lymphatic malformations may "grow" as more lymph fills the sacs. Lymphatic malformations typically present early in life as a palpable, pliable soft tissue mass and grow commensurate with the patient's growth. Sudden enlargement also may occur if they undergo hemorrhage (from the vascularized intervening septae) or become infected.

Imaging Plain radiographs have little role in the evaluation of lymphatic malformations. However, a lymphatic malformation may first be noted as a mediastinal opacity and enlargement (Fig. 58-19, *A*). CT can suggest the diagnosis,

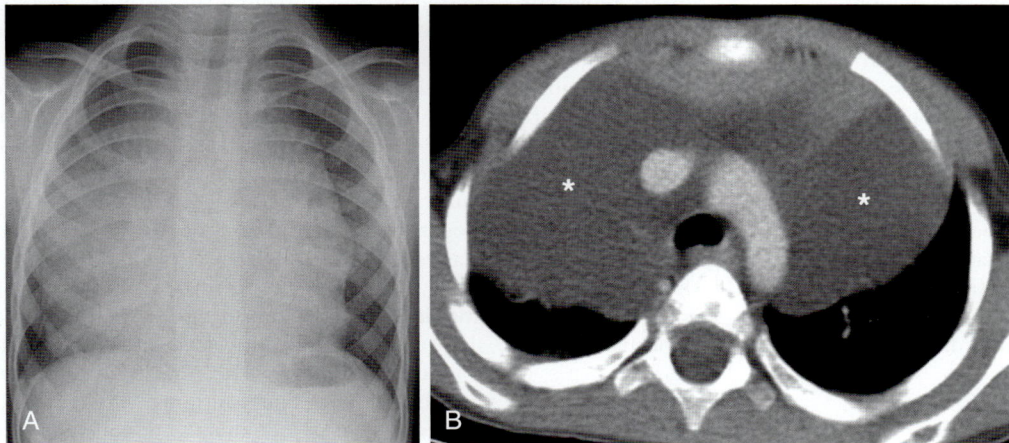

Figure 58-19 Mediastinal lymphatic malformation in a 1-year-old boy. **A,** A frontal chest radiograph shows a large mediastinal mass. **B,** An axial enhanced computed tomography image at the level of the aortic arch shows a large, predominantly anterior mediastinal mass (*asterisks*) of fluid attenuation that crosses midline and extends laterally, consistent with a macrocystic lymphatic malformation.

but because of proteinaceous debris and/or internal hemorrhage, the density may be higher than would be expected for simple fluid (Fig. 58-19, *B*). Because associated calcification is rare, the presence of calcification on CT should suggest an alternate diagnosis. MRI is superb for the evaluation of the lymphatic malformations because of its excellent capability for soft tissue characterization and multiplanar imaging assessment. The septa with the lymphatic malformation are particularly well visualized on MRI and may enhance as they are vascularized. The cystic components should not enhance. Because of proteinaceous debris and/or blood products within the lymphatic malformation, variability exists in T1 and T2 signal intensities on MRI. Fluid/fluid levels are common and strongly support the diagnosis of lymphatic malformation.

Treatment and Follow-up Because there is no known risk of malignant transformation of lymphatic malformation, some controversy exists with regard to treating smaller asymptomatic lesions. If treatment is elected, both surgery and/or percutaneous sclerotherapy currently are used in management. The macrocystic-type lymphatic malformation is particularly well suited for sclerotherapy. Laser therapy is another option for more superficially accessible lesions (typically of the microcystic-type lymphatic malformation).[78]

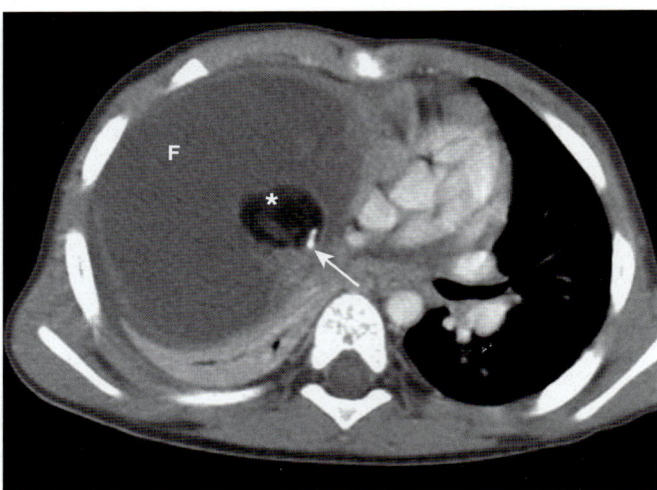

Figure 58-20 A teratoma in a 2-year-old girl. An axial enhanced computed tomography image at the level of the heart shows a large, right-sided, anterior and middle mediastinal mass, largely of fluid attenuation (*F*) with a well-defined plug of fat density (*asterisk*) and internal calcification (*arrow*). The surgical pathology confirmed the diagnosis of a mediastinal mature and benign teratoma.

Germ Cell Tumor

Etiology Germ cell tumors usually arise from the testes or ovaries. However, primitive germ cell rests may reside in the mediastinum and give rise to neoplasms.[79,80] Primary mediastinal germ cell tumors account for 6% to 18% of anterior mediastinal tumors in children,[65] and 60% of these tumors are teratomas.[47] The teratomas usually are further divided into mature and immature types, with the latter being malignant. Of all mediastinal germ cell tumors, 14% are malignant.[81] Infants with teratomas tend to present with airway compression, whereas older children often are asymptomatic.[5] Other symptoms include sudden onset of pain, dyspnea, or cough. The tumor can even rupture into the tracheobronchial tree or pleural space with expectoration or deposition of its contents.[5]

Imaging On chest radiographs, germ cell tumors typically appear as round, sharply demarcated anterior mediastinal masses. Calcifications occur in approximately 25% to 53% of teratomas[5,46,47,82] and may be seen on radiographs. As for most anterior mediastinal masses, CT can better characterize their extent and may allow definitive diagnosis. Typically, teratomas (both mature and immature) demonstrate fat, fluid, and calcifications, which, when seen, allow a confident diagnosis (Fig. 58-20). However, approximately 15% of mature teratomas display no fat or calcium on imaging.[5] Although calcifications may be difficult to detect on MRI, the intralesional fat and fluid are seen readily. Invasion of adjacent structures (as opposed to mere displacement) is suggestive of malignant, immature tumors.

Treatment and Follow-up The prognosis of mature, benign teratomas is excellent after complete excision. However, immature teratomas generally require chemotherapy and radiation in addition to surgical excision.

Middle Mediastinal Masses

Masses arising from the middle mediastinum may be classified into vascular and nonvascular lesions. Most nonvascular middle mediastinal masses in the pediatric population are developmental malformations of the embryonic foregut or adenopathy resulting from underlying infection, primary neoplasm, or metastatic disease.

Foregut Duplication Cysts

Etiology Foregut duplication cysts arise from developmental malformations of the embryonic foregut and are of three main types: bronchogenic, esophageal, and neurenteric cysts. Bronchogenic cysts develop from errors in lung budding during development of the ventral foregut during the first trimester. Errors in development of the posterior division of the embryonic foregut may result in an esophageal duplication cyst. Neurenteric cysts arise from a failure of complete separation between the gastrointestinal tract and the primitive neural crest during early embryonic life and represent one form of the split notochord syndrome. The distinction among these three types of foregut duplication cysts can be made histologically by demonstrating either respiratory, gastrointestinal, or mixed neural/gastrointestinal lining, respectively. Together, these three account for 11% of all mediastinal masses in children.[65]

Imaging Chest radiographs often show an oval or round-shaped middle mediastinal mass (e-Fig. 58-21, *A*). In cases of a neurenteric cyst, an accompanying vertebral anomaly also may be present. The position of the cyst in the mediastinum suggests its type. Bronchial duplication cysts typically are located within the middle mediastinum. Esophageal duplication cysts are in the middle or posterior mediastinum. Neurenteric cysts most often are in the posterior mediastinum but

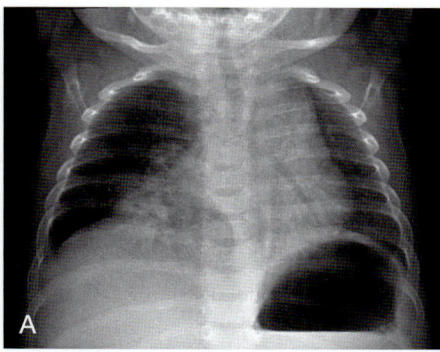 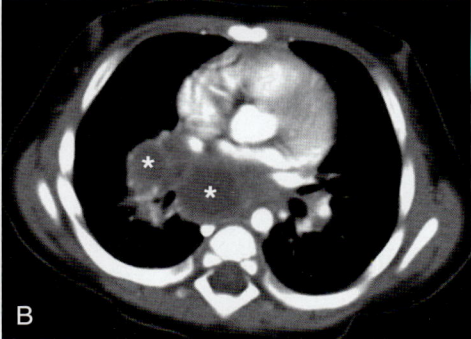 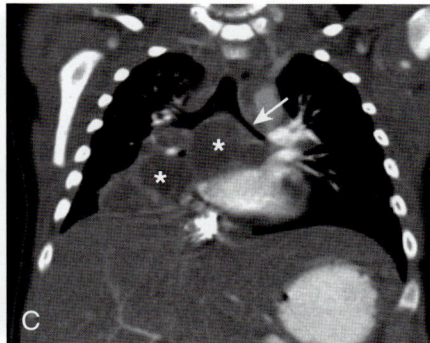

Figure 58-22 Primary *Mycobacterium tuberculosis* in a 2-year-old boy. The sputum culture confirmed the diagnosis of *Mycobacterium tuberculosis* infection. **A,** A frontal chest radiograph shows right hilar and infrahilar opacity. In addition, the distal trachea has a slight leftward deviation, suggesting an effect of the mass. **B,** An axial enhanced computed tomography (CT) image demonstrates low attenuation hilar, infrahilar, and subcarinal lymphadenopathy (*asterisks*). **C,** A coronal enhanced CT image shows a narrowing of the left main stem bronchus (*arrow*) as a result of a large mediastinal lymphadenopathy (*asterisks*).

are discussed here because they fall into the same differential. Cross-sectional imaging studies typically demonstrate a non-enhancing, fluid-filled cystic mass with well-marginated borders (e-Fig. 58-21, *B*). Internal proteinaceous material can increase the Hounsfield units on CT and signal intensity on T1-weighted MRI. The high water content usually results in adequate T2 prolongation to reveal its cystic nature on T2-weighted MRI when CT density is equivocal. On both CT and MRI, foregut duplication cysts should lack internal enhancement and appear homogeneous unless superimposed infection is present.

Treatment and Follow-up The current management choice of foregut duplication cyst is complete surgical resection, particularly in symptomatic pediatric patients. In some institutions, endoscopic ultrasound-guided fine-needle aspiration is used to preoperatively confirm the imaging diagnosis.[83] This procedure is generally considered safe, although reports have been made of complications such as infection.[84]

Lymphadenopathy

Etiology Lymphadenopathy may occur in any mediastinal compartment but is most prevalent in the middle mediastinum. Most enlarged mediastinal lymph nodes in children are reactive. Children with cystic fibrosis frequently demonstrate prominent mediastinal nodes. Particularly prominent hilar lymph nodes may be seen in the setting of granulomatous diseases such as Mycobacterium tuberculosis, Mycobacterium avium-intracellulare, Histoplasmosis, or sarcoidosis.

As discussed elsewhere in this chapter, lymphoma is the most common cause of a primary mediastinal neoplastic mass that presents as a conglomeration of lymph nodes. Although nodes commonly are found in the anterior mediastinum, they may extend or arise in the middle mediastinum as well, particularly in the setting of non-Hodgkin lymphoma. Although it is less common, mediastinal lymphadenopathy also may be seen as a result of metastatic disease from tumors such as Wilms tumors, Ewing tumors, and osteosarcoma.

Imaging Lymphadenopathy often is first detected on chest radiographs. The presence of hilar involvement, bilaterality,

and calcification should be investigated carefully. Most commonly, except when acute infection is the suspected cause, a CT scan is subsequently obtained for further evaluation after chest radiographs. Intravenous contrast always should be administered except when it is medically contraindicated, because lymph nodes on CT may be confused with vessels. MRI may be helpful in selected cases but is seldom needed. On T1-weighted MRI sequences, nodes are isointense to muscle and are hyperintense on T2-weighted sequences and are easily distinguished from adjacent vessels.

Calcified lymph nodes suggest a history of treated lymphoma or the presence of granulomatous disease such as Mycobacterium tuberculosis, *Histoplasmosis capsulatum*, or sarcoidosis. Low-density or centrally necrotic nodes should suggest Mycobacterium tuberculosis (Fig. 58-22)[85] or Mycobacterium avium-intracellulare.[86,87] Sarcoidosis may occur in children but is rare. Large hilar lymphadenopathy also has been described in persons with lymphoma, infectious mononucleosis, and Castleman disease (angiofollicular lymphoid hyperplasia) (e-Fig. 58-23).

Posterior Mediastinal Masses

Neurogenic Tumors

Etiology The vast majority (88%) of masses arising in the posterior mediastinum are of neurogenic origin and together account for about 34% of all mediastinal masses in children.[65] Ganglion cells in the paravertebral sympathetic chain and peripheral nerve sheaths within the posterior mediastinum are responsible for most of posterior mediastinal neurogenic masses. Sympathetic chain tumors are more common than nerve sheath tumors in the pediatric mediastinum.

Tumors arising from the sympathetic chain include neuroblastomas, ganglioneuroblastomas, and ganglioneuromas, in order of increasing cellular differentiation and increasing age of presentation. These tumors are related by their structure of origin but are distinguished by their underlying histologic cellular differentiation. The least differentiated (and hence most malignant) and most common of these tumors is the neuroblastoma, which usually arises in children younger than 5 years. About 10% to 16% of all neuroblastomas arise in the mediastinum. Clinical manifestations of neuroblastoma

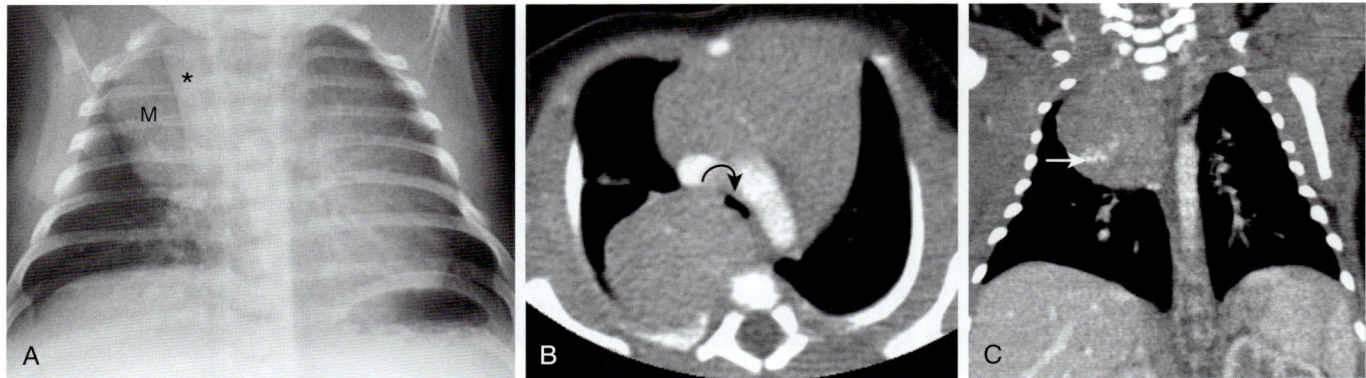

Figure 58-24 A neuroblastoma in a 1-year-old boy. The surgical pathology confirmed the diagnosis of neuroblastoma. **A,** A frontal chest radiograph shows a right upper mediastinal mass (*M*) that does not silhouette the anterior vascular structures such as the superior vena cava (*asterisk*). No bony changes are evident. **B,** An axial enhanced computed tomography (CT) image at the level of the aortic arch shows a large, right posterior, mediastinal, paravertebral mass with effect of the mass against the carina (*curved arrow*). **C,** A coronal enhanced CT image shows a large right upper paravertebral mass extending into the right apex with calcifications (*arrow*).

include constitutional symptoms and several paraneoplastic syndromes. However, presentations that are unique to the mediastinal location of neuroblastoma include Horner syndrome if the mass involves the superior mediastinum. Still, many children with thoracic neuroblastoma present with incidentally discovered masses on chest or abdominal radiographs. Seventy-six percent of thoracic neuroblastomas are positive for urinary catecholamines.[88]

The two most common nerve sheath masses are neurofibromas and schwannomas, both of which are benign tumors composed of spindle cells and myxoid stroma. Plexiform neurofibromas commonly are seen in children with neurofibromatosis type 1. These tumors tend to arise in the superior/posterior mediastinum and are usually bilateral. Posterior mediastinal schwannomas are more often seen in adults.

Imaging Most posterior mediastinal neurogenic tumors are first detected on chest radiographs as a soft tissue opacity (Figs. 58-24 and 58-25). Associated adjacent bone destruction or scalloping in addition to silhouetting of posterior

mediastinal structures such as the descending aorta also may be seen. Assessment of calcification is of paramount importance because its presence suggests a sympathetic chain tumor such as a neuroblastoma as opposed to a nerve sheath tumor.

On CT, posterior mediastinal neurogenic tumors typically present as soft tissue masses with a varying degree of contrast enhancement (see Figs. 58-24 and 58-25). Approximately 40% of neuroblastomas in the posterior mediastinum show speckled or curvilinear calcification.[5] Twenty percent of ganglioneuroblastomas have calcification.[5] Nerve sheath tumors typically do not calcify. Further characterization and differentiation among different types of posterior mediastinal neurogenic tumors with CT is limited.

In contradistinction to anterior and middle mediastinal masses, MRI is currently the best imaging modality for evaluating posterior mediastinal tumors in pediatric patients because of its high sensitivity for detecting the intraspinal (extradural) extension that often is found with these tumors without ionizing radiation exposure.[65] Moreover, MRI offers exquisite soft tissue contrast, which is an advantage when assessing a

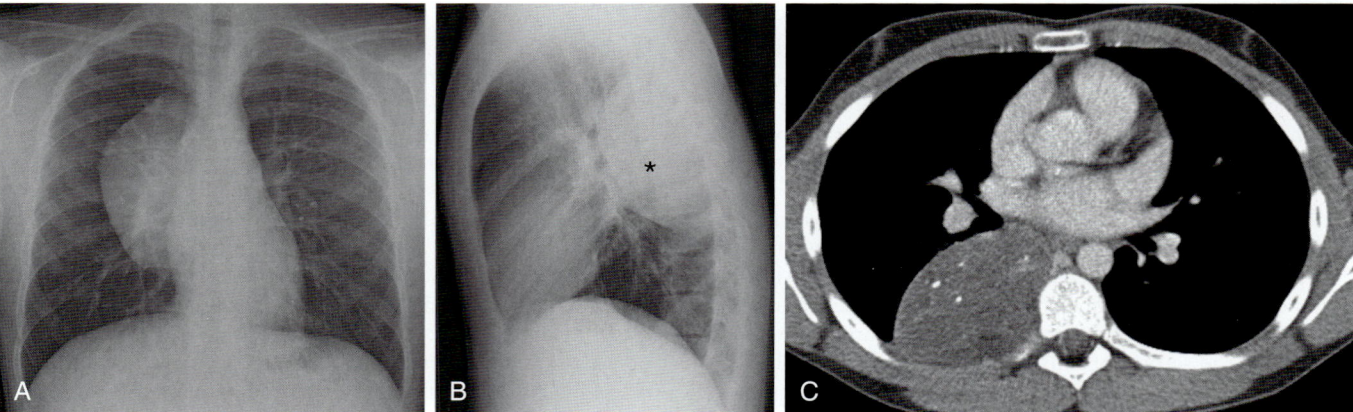

Figure 58-25 A ganglioneuroma in a 13-year-old boy. The surgical pathology confirmed the diagnosis of ganglioneuroma. **A,** A frontal chest radiograph shows a mediastinal mass without silhouetting of either the cardiac border or the right hilus, which is seen through the mass. **B,** A lateral chest radiograph confirms that the mass (*asterisk*) is centered posteriorly within the posterior mediastinal compartment. **C,** An axial enhanced computed tomography image at the level of the left atrium/pulmonary veins shows the right paravertebral posterior mediastinal mass with punctate internal calcification.

region such as the posterior mediastinum with similar soft tissue densities and minimal fat. Finally, MRI is sensitive for assessing bone marrow involvement.

The sympathetic chain tumors have a similar appearance on all imaging studies. These masses appear as T2-hyperintense, well-circumscribed, sausage-shaped structures in a paraspinal distribution along the expected region of the sympathetic chain. Intraspinal extension is common with widening of the neural foramina. After intravenous administration of contrast material, variable, heterogeneous enhancement occurs. A metaiodobenzylguanidine scan can confirm the diagnosis of a neuroblastoma and assess for distant sites of disease.

Nerve sheath tumors appear as sharply demarcated, rounded, or elliptic paravertebral masses in the posterior mediastinum. Whereas neuroblastomas course along several vertebral bodies, nerve sheath tumors usually are localized to one or two intervertebral spaces. However, plexiform neurofibromas can involve multiple levels and extend into the middle mediastinum. On T2-weighted imaging, plexiform neurofibromas have a distinct high signal periphery with an intermediate signal centrally—the so-called "target" appearance (Fig. 58-26). Associated findings include thoracic dural ectasia and scalloping of the posterior vertebral bodies.

Treatment and Follow-up Sympathetic chain neurogenic tumors are treated entirely differently from nerve sheath tumors because the sympathetic chain tumors are considered malignant (although to a varying degree depending on their cellular differentiation). Chemotherapy usually is initiated after a histologic diagnosis is rendered and surgical resection is performed for sympathetic chain neurogenic tumors. Radiation therapy generally has no role in treating sympathetic chain neurogenic tumors.[5] The prognosis depends on the patient's age. Younger patients (particularly infants) have a far better prognosis than older children. Overall, patients with a thoracic neuroblastoma have a better prognosis than patients

with retroperitoneal disease.[47] Patients with benign nerve sheath tumors such as neurofibromatosis type 1 do not undergo routine resection of their masses. However, imaging surveillance may be used because of risks of malignant transformation and other tumors arising de novo.

Other Posterior Mediastinal Lesions and Lesions Simulating Posterior Mediastinal Masses

Etiology Benign masses and even lung parenchymal processes may mimic one of the more sinister posterior mediastinal masses. For example, in a patient with severe, long-standing anemia, extramedullary sites of hematopoiesis include the posterior mediastinal paravertebral space.[89] Rarely, the posterior mediastinum may be the site of ectopic structures such as diaphragmatic hernias, both congenital and acquired. These structures may contain not only bowel loops but retroperitoneal structures such as kidneys (e-Fig. 58-27). Ectopic thymic extension into the posterior mediastinal compartment was discussed previously in the section on normal variants of thymus in this chapter. Cystic structures in the posterior mediastinum may be from neuroenteric cysts, esophageal duplication cysts (both of which are discussed in the section on middle mediastinal masses in this chapter), or from meningoceles, which usually are associated with neurofibromatosis type 1. Finally, pulmonary airspace disease, which is seen through the mediastinal structures on chest radiographs, may mimic a mediastinal mass or vice versa.

Imaging A focus of hematopoietic tissue is most often seen in a paravertebral position as abnormal smooth or lobulated soft tissue. Other clues such as bone marrow reconversion or evidence of sickle cell disease may suggest the diagnosis. An airspace consolidation such as that seen with pneumonia may mimic a posterior mediastinal mass, particularly when it is seen in the lower lobes medially and obscures posterior

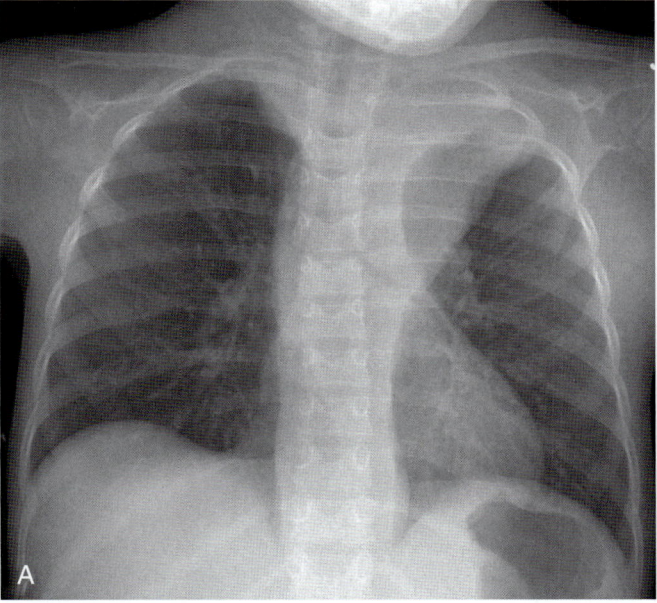
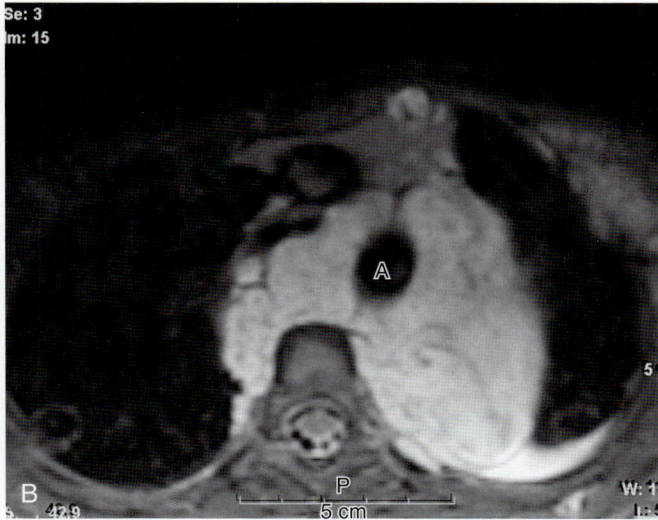

Figure 58-26 Neurofibromatosis type 1 in a 6-year-old boy who presented with cough. **A,** A frontal chest radiograph shows a large left apical and paraspinal mass that cascades down each side of the spine. **B,** An axial T2-weighted image demonstrates the "target sign" and the lobulated shape of the plexiform neurofibromas. The multilayered lobules of the neurofibromas appear as targets. *A,* Aorta; *P,* paraspinal muscle.

mediastinal structures such as the descending aorta and/or azygoesophageal fissure on a frontal chest radiograph. Conversely, a posterior mediastinal mass such as a neuroblastoma may be confused with lung consolidation, particularly when it occurs in the upper lobes. Ectopic intraabdominal structures such as the bowel, kidney, pancreas, and spleen may be seen in the posterior mediastinum with a large diaphragmatic hernia. The hernia is usually obvious, particularly if air-filled loops of bowel are present. In confusing cases, reconstructed thin-section CT in the coronal plane is useful.

Treatment and Follow-up Treatment and follow-up of posterior mediastinal structures mimicking posterior mediastinal masses are dictated entirely by the nature of the underlying lesion. As such, determination of the etiology is essential.

Key Points

Pneumomediastinum is most often attributed to alveolar rupture. Elevation of the thymus is a very helpful imaging clue for pneumomediastinum in neonates and infants on chest radiographs.

The mediastinum is the most common location of chest masses in the pediatric population.

The thymus is variable in size and shape, particularly among pediatric patients, and it changes dramatically over time for each patient, depending on disease/stress burden, recovery, and age.

Most nonvascular middle mediastinal masses in the pediatric population are developmental malformations of the embryonic foregut or adenopathy as a result of underlying infection, a primary neoplasm, or metastatic disease.

Most masses arising in the posterior mediastinum are of neurogenic origin and together account for about 34% of all mediastinal masses in children.

WHAT THE CLINICIAN NEEDS TO KNOW

- The imaging characteristics of pneumothorax and pneumomediastinum, because the management is different
- How to locate the mediastinal mass into one of the three mediastinal compartments (i.e., anterior, middle, and posterior) on a lateral chest radiograph, which is helpful for formulating a manageable differential diagnosis, narrowing the differential diagnosis, and determining the next step in imaging evaluation
- The differential diagnosis for anterior mediastinal masses in the pediatric population
- The differential diagnosis for middle mediastinal masses in the pediatric population
- The differential diagnosis for posterior mediastinal masses in the pediatric population

Suggested Readings

Lee EY. Evaluation of non-vascular mediastinal masses in infants and children: an evidence-based practical approach. *Pediatr Radiol.* 2009;39(suppl 2):S184-S190.

Lee EY. Imaging evaluation of mediastinal masses in infants and children. In: Medina LS, Applegate KE, Blackmore CC, eds. *Evidence-based imaging in pediatrics: optimizing imaging in pediatric patient care.* New York: Springer-Verlag; 2010.

Nasseri F, Effekhari F. Clinical and radiologic review of the normal and abnormal thymus: pearls and pitfalls. *Radiographics.* 2010;30(2):413-428.

Toma P, Granata C, Rossi A, et al. Multimodality imaging of Hodgkin disease and non-Hodgkin lymphomas in children. *Radiographics.* 2007;27(5):1335-1354.

Zylak CM, Standen JR, Barnes GR, et al. Pneumomediastinum revisited. *Radiographics.* 2000;20(4):1043-1057.

References

Full references for this chapter can be found on www.expertconsult.com.

Chapter 59

The Chest Wall

RICARDO RESTREPO, DONALD A. TRACY, and EDWARD Y. LEE

The chest wall provides support and protection to the various thoracic vascular and nonvascular structures. In addition, it allows the important physiologic motion of the lungs and airways. The chest wall is less rigid and more cartilaginous in children than in adults and consists of several fundamental structural components, including bones (ribs, sternum, and vertebrae), nerves, muscles, vessels, and subcutaneous soft tissues.[1] Within these structural components, a wide variety of localized or systemic processes (e.g., congenital and developmental anomalies, inflammatory and infectious diseases, benign and malignant neoplasms, and traumatic lesions) can occur in pediatric patients.[1-3]

Congenital and Developmental Anomalies

OVERVIEW

During childhood, congenital and developmental anomalies of the thorax typically manifest as deformities or anterior chest wall defects that can be isolated or part of a syndrome. Most of these lesions do not have serious physiologic consequences but rather cause cosmetic problems. However, pediatric patients with severe degrees of congenital or developmental anomalies of the chest wall may present with pain, respiratory distress, or cardiovascular compromise. Reconstructive surgery can be offered to correct the chest wall deformities or defects in both asymptomatic and symptomatic pediatric patients. Imaging can provide a road map for the surgeon in evaluating the anatomy and associated anomalies that can affect the reconstructive options, as well as the timing of surgery. Furthermore, accurate recognition of the radiologic manifestation of congenital and developmental conditions that affect the chest wall often provides important clues that point to the correct diagnosis.[4]

DEFORMITIES OF THE ANTERIOR CHEST WALL

Etiology Most asymptomatic palpable anterior chest wall lesions in pediatric patients are normal anatomic osseous or cartilaginous variants of the shape of the costal cartilage, ribs, and sternum.[5,6] These normal anatomic variations occur in approximately one third of children.[5] The most common cause of an asymptomatic, palpable anterior chest wall mass on physical examination is prominent anterior convexity of a solitary rib, costal cartilage, or sternal tilt (Fig. 59-1).[6] Symptoms that may raise concern and require further evaluation are focal pain and rapid growth of the mass.[3,5]

Imaging In the case of a palpable but otherwise asymptomatic anterior chest wall lesion in children, a chest radiograph with a BB marker is usually adequate to exclude a potentially aggressive or malignant underlying condition. When chest radiographic findings are equivocal, ultrasound can be performed.[7] To minimize ionizing radiation exposure, computed tomography (CT) should be reserved for situations in which further characterization is still necessary after radiographic and ultrasound evaluation.[3,6] Although it often is less available than CT, magnetic resonance imaging (MRI), which is not associated with ionizing radiation exposure, is a particularly helpful imaging modality for confirming and characterizing congenital and developmental chest wall lesions.

Treatment and Follow-up If the diagnosis of an anterior chest wall developmental variant can be made confidently by imaging studies in asymptomatic infants and children, no further treatment or follow-up is necessary.[5]

PECTUS DEFORMITY

Etiology Two of the most common abnormalities of the chest wall are pectus excavatum and pectus carinatum, with the former being the most common congenital deformity of the sternum and the most common sternal deformity requiring surgery. The current leading theory for the development of pectus excavatum is a misdirected, rapid growth of the lower costal cartilages. Such abnormal growth of the lower costal cartilages, which often intensifies during growth spurts, displaces the sternum either inward or outward, resulting in pectus deformity.[8] Pectus excavatum occurs in between 1 in 400 and 1 in 1000 live births.[9] In persons with pectus excavatum, the inferior aspect of the sternum is depressed inward, resulting in varying degrees of anterior chest wall concavity and anterior protrusion of the costochondral junctions. Although most cases of pectus excavatum are isolated, approximately 45% of cases are familial.[10,11]

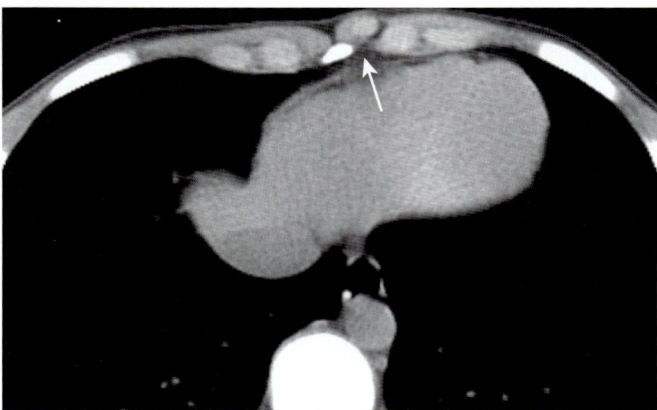

Figure 59-1 A chondral nodule in an adolescent boy who presented with a focal, palpable, painless lump in the anterior chest wall. An axial computed tomography soft tissue window image shows a small, round, well-defined structure (*arrow*) protruding anteriorly in the chest wall to the left of the sternum with the same density as the adjacent costochondral junctions.

Pectus carinatum is a less common chest wall deformity that occurs in approximately 1 in 1500 live births and has a familial occurrence of approximately 25%.[9] In persons with pectus carinatum, outward displacement of the sternum occurs, with secondary abnormal protrusion of the ribs.

Pectus deformities may occur in association with scoliosis (more frequently with pectus excavatum), Marfan syndrome, Ehlers-Danlos syndrome, Poland syndrome, and congenital heart disease. In addition to cosmetic issues, severe pectus deformities also can cause chest pain, dyspnea, palpitations, and restrictive lung disease.[3]

Imaging On frontal chest radiographs, the sternal depression of pectus excavatum may cause a pseudo-infiltrate over the right side of the heart and various degrees of leftward cardiac shift. On the lateral chest radiograph, the sternal depression causes narrowing of thoracic anteroposterior (AP) diameter (Fig. 59-2). Pectus carinatum usually is diagnosed on a lateral chest radiograph, which shows an increased AP diameter of the thoracic cavity and an extended retrosternal space (Fig. 59-3).[3,8]

The Haller or pectus index is used to estimate the severity of pectus excavatum. It is calculated from an axial CT image by dividing the maximum transverse dimension of the thorax from the inner aspect of the ribs by the AP dimension of the thoracic cavity at its narrowest point (Fig. 59-4). A pectus index greater than 3.25 in symptomatic pediatric patients typically initiates corrective surgery, whereas an index less than 2.56 is considered normal.[12] Recent studies have advocated the use of chest radiographs instead of CT to preoperatively evaluate the severity of the deformity.[13] In more severe cases, the use of a limited, low-dose CT scan with selective 5-7 axial CT images through the deformity can be obtained to generate the pectus index.[14] When the primary purpose of imaging is to assess the Haller index, axial MRI can be used to avoid ionizing radiation.[15]

Treatment and Follow-up Severe pectus deformity requires surgical correction, particularly in symptomatic pediatric patients. The Ravitch procedure for pectus excavatum

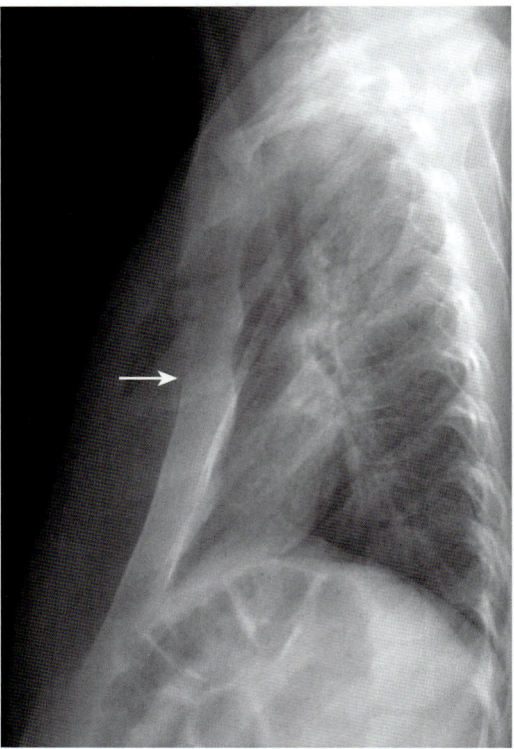

Figure 59-2 Pectus excavatum in an 8-year-old girl. A lateral chest radiograph shows the sternal depression (*arrow*) causing narrowing of the anteroposterior diameter of the thorax.

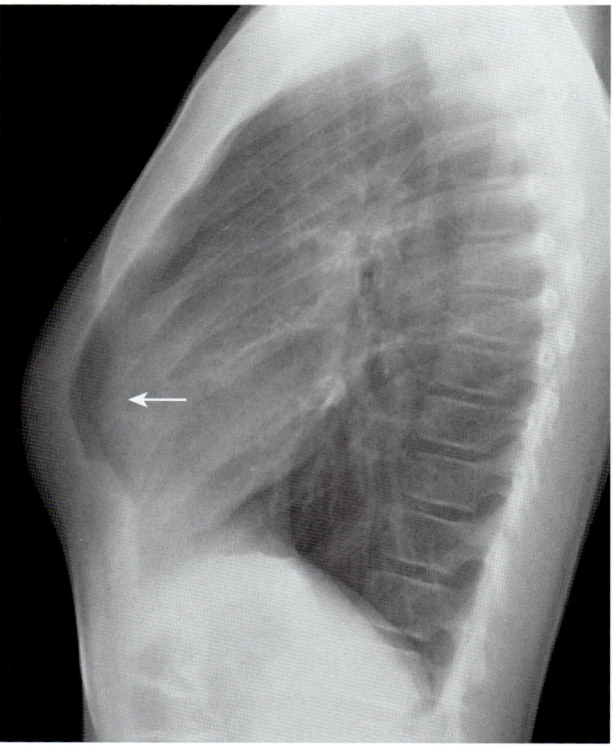

Figure 59-3 Pectus carinatum in an adolescent boy. A lateral chest radiograph demonstrates an increased anteroposterior diameter of the thoracic cavity and extended retrosternal space (*arrow*).

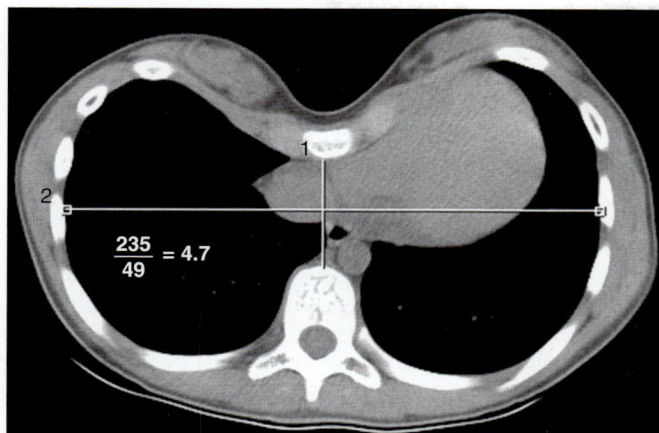

Figure 59-4 Pectus index. An axial computed tomography soft tissue window image shows severe anterior depression of the sternum that is compressing and displacing the heart. The pectus index is 4.7.

includes resection of deformed cartilages and correction of the sternum by a wedge osteotomy in the upper sternal cortex. In the Nuss procedure, a convex metal bar is placed behind the sternum, pulling the sternum anteriorly. Corrective surgery for pectus carinatum also requires costochondral resection and a wedge osteotomy, but the sternum is pushed inward. The Nuss procedure has a 4% to 11% complication rate,[16] and thus follow-up imaging is necessary to monitor the implanted bar and its complications. Infection and dislocation of the metallic bar are the two most common complications following the Nuss procedure.[16-18]

CLEIDOCRANIAL DYSOSTOSIS

Etiology Cleidocranial dysostosis is a rare syndrome usually caused by an autosomal dominant gene with high degree of penetrance and variable expression. In this condition, a mutation is present in the *CBFA1* gene located in the chromosome 6p21, which encodes a protein necessary to activate osteoblast differentiation. The triad of partial or complete absence of the clavicles, supernumerary or impacted teeth, and delayed fontanel closure is highly suggestive of this syndrome. Other features of the syndrome include midface hypoplasia, short stature, and pelvic and distal phalangeal hypoplasia that causes brachydactyly.[19-21]

Imaging Typical chest radiographic findings include a bell-shaped thorax, short ribs, and either complete or partial absence of the clavicles (e-Fig. 59-5). When the clavicle is partially absent, the distal portion of the clavicle usually is involved. Scoliosis may be present. Because many of the characteristic manifestations only become evident during adolescence, early clinical diagnosis may be difficult and often requires a skeletal survey. Other features of the syndrome can support the diagnosis.[19-21]

Treatment and Follow-up Multidisciplinary management by a team of specialists including pediatricians, geneticists, and orthodontists is the optimal approach for patients with cleidocranial dysostosis. Genetic counseling is recommended. No imaging follow-up is required once the diagnosis has been made.[19]

POLAND SYNDROME

Etiology Poland syndrome is a form of chest wall and breast hypoplasia that occurs in 1 in every 20,000 to 30,000 live births.[22] The syndrome includes absence of the pectoralis muscles and ipsilateral syndactyly. Other associations include rib aplasia, amastia/athelia, and absence of axillary hair. Poland syndrome typically is unilateral and (more often) sporadic and occurs more frequently in boys than in girls, with a ratio of 2-3:1.[23] The tendency toward unilaterality (with the right side affected more frequently than the left side) has raised the hypothesis that this anomaly is perhaps a result of interrupted or insufficient blood supply during limb bud development in the sixth week of gestation.[23] Poland syndrome is diagnosed clinically by the apparent asymmetry of the chest wall (e-Fig. 59-6) and syndactyly. Cardiopulmonary impairment and functional deficiency of the shoulder, although rare, also can be present.[3,22,23]

Imaging On chest radiographs, hyperlucency of the affected hemithorax is usually apparent in unilateral cases because of the absent pectoralis muscle and breast (Fig. 59-7). Because the extent of involvement is difficult to assess with clinical examination or chest radiographs, cross-sectional imaging with CT or MRI is useful (Fig. 59-8). Furthermore, it is imperative to preoperatively assess the presence of all of the chest wall and anterior abdominal wall muscles (e.g., the latissimus dorsi and rectus abdominis muscles), because muscle flaps are used in surgical reconstruction.[2,22]

Treatment and Follow-up Corrective surgery often is performed for cosmetic reasons, particularly in girls. Such surgery includes (1) restoration of the structural integrity of the

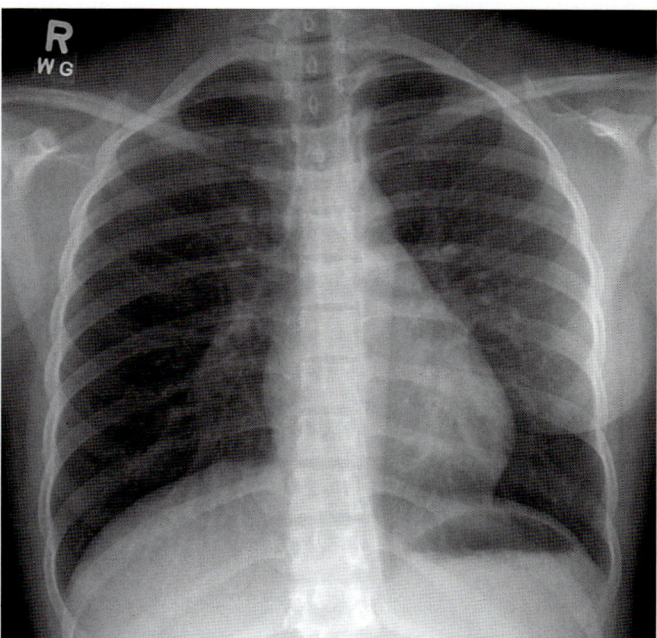

Figure 59-7 Poland syndrome in an adolescent girl. A frontal chest radiograph shows a hyperlucent right lung as a result of the absence of right chest wall soft tissues, including the breast.

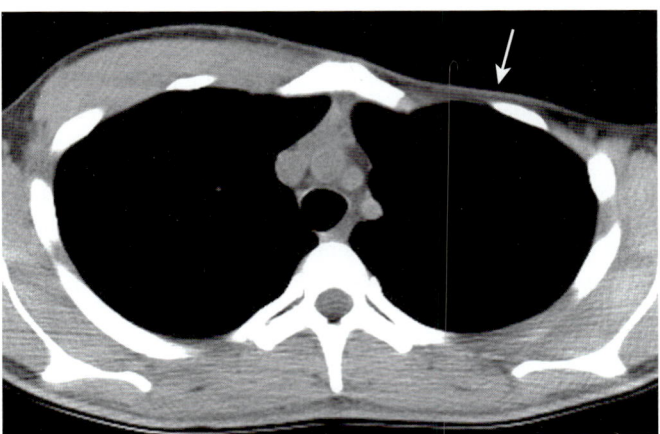

Figure 59-8 Poland syndrome in an adolescent boy. An axial computed tomography soft tissue window demonstrates complete absence of the left pectoralis muscles (*arrow*), causing asymmetry of the anterior chest wall.

rib cage and (2) improvement in the appearance of the chest by performing transposition of musculocutaneous flaps (most commonly with latissimus dorsi and rectus abdominis muscles), as well as concomitant breast implants in female patients.[8,22,23]

Infectious Diseases

OVERVIEW

Chest wall infections are relatively rare in children. Chest wall infections occur either by direct extension or, less frequently, by hematogenous spread. Such infectious processes can involve the soft tissues, cartilage, and osseous structures. Chest wall infections can be the result of bacterial, mycobacterial, or fungal infections. They range from superficial cellulitis to deeper infections, which include myositis, abscess, necrotizing fasciitis, and osteomyelitis.[24,25]

BACTERIAL INFECTION

Etiology Bacterial infections of the chest wall are rare in children. The common organisms that cause bacterial infections of the chest wall are *Staphylococcus aureus* and Salmonella species in persons with sickle cell disease. Sternal osteomyelitis may occur in patients with an underlying disease, such as immunodeficiency and hemoglobinopathies.[11] Rib osteomyelitis is most commonly acquired by direct spread from an adjacent pleuropulmonary infection, such as severe pneumonia or empyema. Empyema necessitatis is a rare complication of empyema characterized by the extension of the infection from the pleural space into the chest wall. Pediatric patients with a bacterial chest wall infection often present with focal soft tissue erythema, edema, and pain. Additionally, other signs of infection, such as leukocytosis and elevated erythrocyte sedimentation rate, often are present.[3,11,26,27]

Imaging Chest radiographs may reveal localized soft tissue edema in cases of cellulitis or fasciitis. Bone changes such as periosteal reaction or lytic or sclerotic lesions can be present, particularly in the late stage of disease. Concomitant pulmonary consolidation, empyema, and subcutaneous emphysema also may be present. Ultrasound, CT, and MRI are more sensitive than chest radiographs in detecting and characterizing chest wall infections. Ultrasound should be reserved for superficial and more localized chest wall infections because of the limited field of view (Fig. 59-9, *A*). The extent of the chest wall infection is best demonstrated on CT or MRI. For evaluation of chest wall abscess and bone marrow edema in the earlier stage of osteomyelitis, MRI is the most sensitive imaging modality (Fig. 59-9, *B*). CT is the imaging modality of choice for evaluating concomitant pulmonary parenchymal infection.[2,11,26-28]

Treatment and Follow-up Antibiotics are administered to treat bacterial chest wall infections. In cases of abscesses localized to the chest wall or empyema, drainage may be necessary to relieve the focus of infection and avoid further spread. Prolonged antibiotic therapy is necessary for cases of

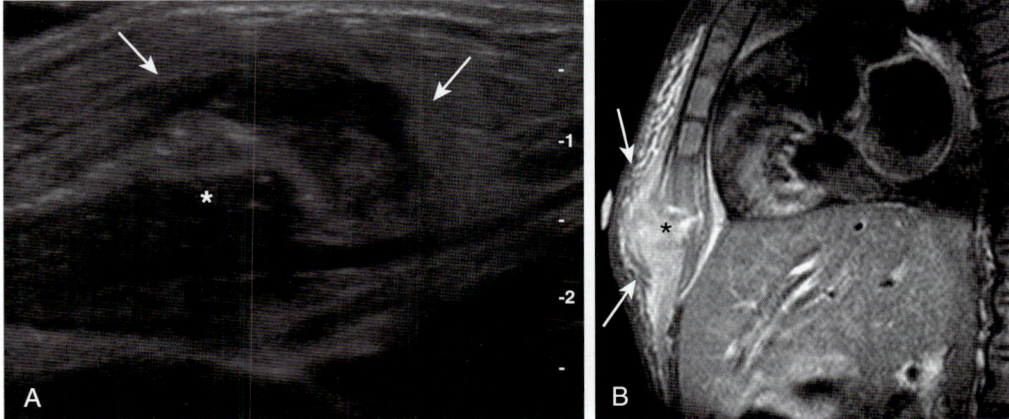

Figure 59-9 Sternal osteomyelitis in a 6-year-old girl who presented with prolonged fever and a painful, palpable, and erythematous sternal lump.
A, A longitudinal ultrasound view of the inferior aspect of the sternum (*asterisk*) shows marked surrounding soft tissue edema and swelling (*arrows*).
B, A sagittal contrast T1-weighted image of the chest with fat saturation demonstrates focal destruction of the distal ossification center of the sternum (*asterisk*) with contrast enhancement and edema of the adjacent soft tissues (*arrows*).

osteomyelitis.[27,29] Evaluation of response to treatment by monitoring C-reactive protein in pediatric patients with osteomyelitis has dramatically decreased both the average duration of therapy (now 3 to 4 weeks) and the need for follow-up imaging.[30]

TUBERCULOSIS

Etiology Tuberculosis (TB) is a potentially deadly infectious disease caused by various strains of mycobacteria, usually Mycobacterium tuberculosis in humans. Tuberculosis infection of the chest wall often is a result of the hematogenous spread of pulmonary TB infection.[31] However, tuberculosis of the chest wall also can occur as an isolated primary infection with no evidence of pulmonary disease, although this presentation is rare.[32] Skeletal TB infection accounts for 10% to 20% of extrapulmonary cases and 1% to 2% of all TB infection cases.[33] Affected patients present with a slow-growing soft tissue chest wall mass, often without associated pain or fever. Respiratory symptoms may be present in cases of lung involvement.[32,34]

Imaging TB infection can involve any bone of the chest wall; however, the ribs are most commonly affected. On radiographs, osseous TB infections are usually lytic and sharply marginated. Associated periosteal reaction is a relatively rare finding.[35] On CT or MRI, TB chest wall infections usually present as a rim-enhancing chest wall mass. CT and MRI can play an important role in demonstrating bone involvement from a chest wall TB infection that may not be seen on radiographs.[32] Expansion and destruction of the bone with an adjacent soft tissue mass from a TB infection of the chest wall may mimic an underlying malignancy. Rim-enhancing masses with central necrosis and sequestrum indicating abscess formation, regional hypodense adenopathy, and vertebral body involvement also may occur in affected patients.[31,33,34]

Treatment and Follow-up Treatment of chest wall TB infection currently is not well established. Some persons advocate the use of an antituberculous medication regimen alone for at least 6 months. Others suggest more aggressive management consisting of surgical excision of affected bones and soft tissues, in addition to preoperative and postoperative antituberculous medication regimens.[32,36]

ACTINOMYCOSIS

Etiology In humans, actinomycosis is most commonly caused by Actinomyces israelii, a branching gram-positive, facultative anaerobe. Actinomycosis infection typically affects the cervicofacial region in patients with dental caries. Pulmonary and chest wall involvement of actinomycosis in children is less frequent without underlying predisposing pulmonary conditions. Actinomycosis infection initially involves the lungs and then usually spreads to the adjacent soft tissues. Clinically, affected patients present with cough, intermittent fever, and weight loss. Pain develops once the microorganism invades the pleura and chest wall.[37,38]

Imaging On a chest radiograph, the classic radiologic appearance of actinomycosis infection is a chronic lung consolidation that crosses the fissures with a pleural effusion. Because actinomycosis infection does not respect tissue boundaries, it tends to invade the surrounding tissues with fistulous tracts and abscess formation that are best seen on CT or MRI. Rib periostitis, pulmonary cavitation, and diaphragmatic invasion also may occur in more advanced cases and are very suggestive of actinomycosis infection.[38,39] Advanced actinomycosis infection of the chest wall may mimic TB or a malignancy of the Ewing sarcoma family of tumors (ESFT).[37]

Treatment and Follow-up A definite diagnosis of actinomycosis of the chest wall requires either microscopic visualization of the typical sulfur granules representing the colonies of the microorganism or recovery of the Actinomyces organisms in an anaerobic culture. The standard treatment of actinomycosis is long-term, high-dose penicillin. In cases with an abscess, image-guided percutaneous drainage may help expedite recovery and isolate the organism. Rarely, surgical resection of the area involved is required in cases that are unresponsive to medical treatments.[37,38]

Tumors of the Chest Wall

OVERVIEW

Because the chest wall is composed of several different types of tissues, a wide variety of both benign and malignant tumors may occur, including vascular, cartilaginous, osseous, muscular, or adipose tumors. Imaging evaluation plays a pivotal role in (1) initial detection, (2) assessment of the extent of disease, (3) guidance for tissue sampling, (4) evaluation of the response to treatment, and (5) surveillance for recurrence.[7,25]

BENIGN TUMORS

Soft Tissue Tumors

Infantile Hemangioma

Etiology Infantile hemangiomas are benign vascular tumors of abnormally proliferating endothelial cells that follow a predictable course. Infantile hemangiomas are the most common tumor of childhood, with a reported incidence of approximately 10% in the general population.[40,41] The etiology of hemangiomas currently is unknown. Several proposed theories include placental emboli, somatic mutation, and clonal expansion of progenitor stem cells.[42,43] Infantile hemangiomas are more common in premature white children, with female predominance ratios ranging from 1.4:1 to 3:1.[41] Hemangiomas can involve any part of the body, including the chest wall and breast bud. At birth, these lesions frequently are underdeveloped, with only a macule or discoloration representing a "precursor" lesion. Soon after birth, infantile hemangiomas grow during the so-called proliferative phase and become raised and red in color. Around the first year of life, they involute, leaving a fibro-fatty scar. Multiple lesions are found in 15% to 30% of patients.[41,43]

Imaging Ultrasound is usually the first imaging modality of choice, especially for evaluating localized, superficial hemangiomas. For large and extensive lesions with a deep soft tissue component, MRI often is necessary for a complete evaluation. Although CT can be used when MRI is not available, it is less preferable because of the associated radiation and inferior soft tissue characterization. The imaging appearance of infantile hemangiomas may change according to the stage of disease. On ultrasound, hemangiomas are well-defined, lobulated, hyperechoic masses that become more heterogeneous during the involuting phase. Increased vascularity, containing arteries, veins, and even evidence of shunting, often is seen on color Doppler, especially during the proliferative phase (e-Fig. 59-10). On MRI, infantile hemangiomas are isointense or slightly hyperintense compared with muscle on T1-weighted images, and they are hyperintense on T2-weighted images, containing flow voids that represent arteries or rapid venous flow. Hyperintense fatty elements may be seen on T1-weighted images. The pattern of contrast enhancement also varies according to the stage of disease. Marked contrast enhancement usually is seen during the proliferative phase, whereas heterogeneous contrast enhancement reflecting areas of necrosis often is observed during the involuting phase. On CT, hemangiomas present as well-defined soft tissue masses that are isodense to muscle with marked postcontrast enhancement.[43,44]

Treatment and Follow-up Most infantile hemangiomas require no treatment because they typically involute. A pulsed dye laser can be used for the cosmetic management of superficial lesions. In the past, corticosteroids were the cornerstone of management of hemangiomas; however, secondary effects, such as cushingoid features, were commonly seen.[30] Propranolol has been used recently in the treatment of hemangiomas with promising results and minor complications, such as hypoglycemia and hypotension.[45,46]

Lymphatic Malformation

Etiology Lymphatic malformations are a subtype of slow-flow vascular malformations. These lesions are fully developed at birth and grow commensurate to the patient's growth. Lymphatic malformations consist of dilated lymphatic channels and spaces, with walls lined by mature endothelium that have normal rates of endothelial cell turnover. These lesions occur anywhere in the body, but the cervicofacial, axillary, and chest regions are the most common locations. Lymphatic malformations have no sex predilection. Except for very small lesions, these lesions present as a mass that usually is discovered at birth. The lesions have normal overlying skin and often display positive transillumination. With superimposed hemorrhage or infection, a sudden increase in the lesion size is typical.[3,47]

Imaging Plain radiography plays no role in the evaluation of lymphatic malformations in the chest wall of pediatric patients. The imaging workup of lymphatic malformations includes ultrasound and MRI, with the former more commonly used for localized and superficial lesions. More extensive lesions are better evaluated with contrast-enhanced MRI, with CT as an alternative imaging modality. On ultrasound, lymphatic malformations appear as multiloculated cystic lesions that are macrocystic or microcystic, depending on the size of the locules. No internal blood flow is seen on color Doppler imaging. With associated bleeding or superimposed infection, echogenic material, low-level echoes, or fluid-fluid levels can be observed (Fig. 59-11, A). On MRI, the cystic lesions are hyperintense on T2-weighted images (Fig. 59-11, B) and hypointense on T1-weighted images. Lymphatic malformations display no solid components and have minimal, if any, peripheral and septal enhancement, unless superimposed infection is present. Hyperintense elements on T1-weighted images suggest proteinaceous material, bleeding, or infection. Because of their pliable nature, lymphatic malformations typically insinuate and displace, rather than invade, adjacent structures.[3,44,48]

Treatment and Follow-up The treatment for lymphatic malformation is percutaneous sclerosis, surgical resection, or frequently a combination of both. Sclerotherapy is the preferred method for macrocystic lymphatic malformations. The treatment of microcystic lesions is more difficult and can include observation, sclerotherapy, and/or surgical resection. Multiple agents, including doxycycline, sodium tetradecyl sulfate, and alcohol currently are used for sclerotherapy. Sclerotherapy usually requires several interventions.[44,47,48]

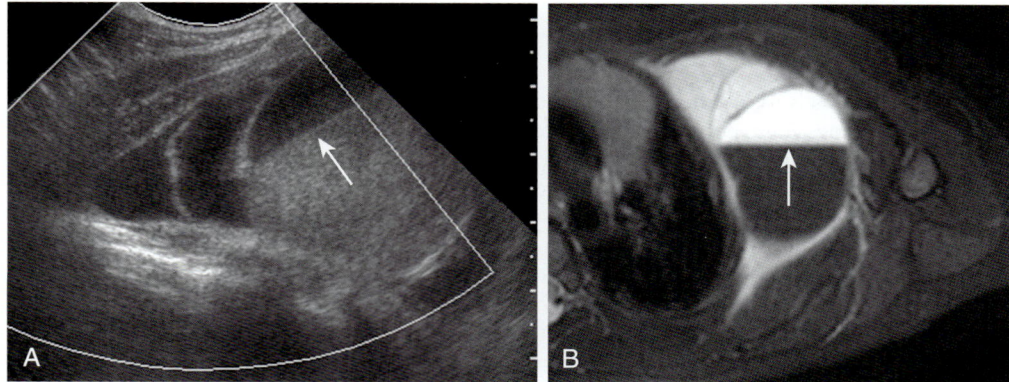

Figure 59-11 Lymphatic malformation in a 2-year-old boy who presented with an enlarging chest wall lump after a fall. **A,** A longitudinal view of color Doppler ultrasound shows a multiloculated avascular cystic mass in the anterolateral chest wall. Some of the locules are anechoic, but a fluid-fluid level (*arrow*) is present in the most dominant one, likely indicating recent bleeding. **B,** An axial T2-weighted image of the chest demonstrates the multiseptated mass with hyperintense elements representing lymphatic fluid and hypodense elements with a fluid-fluid level (*arrow*) indicating recent bleeding. The patient has minimal, if any, adjacent soft tissue edema, and no soft tissue component is seen in the lesion.

Infantile Fibrous Hamartoma

Etiology An infantile fibrous hamartoma is a tumor of neonates, infants, and young children, with approximately 90% occurring in the first year of life.[49] They are more common in boys than in girls. The most common location is around the shoulder girdle. The tumor usually presents as a painless, mobile soft tissue mass. Histologically, an infantile fibrous hamartoma contains fibrocollagenous tissue, primitive mesenchyma, and mature fat.[49-51]

Imaging An infantile fibrous hamartoma is a well-defined lesion with a heterogeneous echotexture on ultrasound, attenuation on CT, and signal intensity on MRI because of different underlying tissue components. Hyperechoic elements seen on ultrasound and T1 hyperintensities seen on MRI represent the fatty elements, which is an important clue in the diagnosis. On MRI, the fibrous component of infantile fibrous hamartoma is seen as hypointense areas on T1- and T2-weighted images.[49]

Treatment and Follow-up Local surgical resection of infantile fibrous hamartoma is usually curative, with a low risk of recurrence. No metastatic disease from infantile fibrous hamartoma has been reported.[51,52]

Osseous Tumors

Fibrous Dysplasia

Etiology Fibrous dysplasia is a benign, intramedullary, fibro-osseous lesion thought to occur as a result of a developmental failure in the remodeling of primitive bone to mature lamellar bone and failure of the bone to realign in response to mechanical stress. The etiology of fibrous dysplasia has been linked to an activating mutation in the gene that encodes the alpha subunit of stimulatory G-protein located at 20q133.2-13.3.[53] The true incidence of fibrous dysplasia is difficult to estimate, but the lesions are not rare and typically are discovered before the age of 30 years. Fibrous dysplasia has been reported to represent 20% to 30% of chest wall masses, with the rib being the most commonly affected bone.[3,54] Fibrous dysplasia can be monostotic or polyostotic; however, monostotic disease does not progress to polyostotic disease. Although a focal mass or chest wall deformity can be seen with fibrous dysplasia, most cases of monostotic fibrous dysplasia are discovered incidentally when radiographs of the area are obtained for different reasons. Localized pain may be the presenting symptom in cases with pathologic fractures or effects of the mass upon adjacent thoracic structures.[53,54]

Imaging The diagnosis of fibrous dysplasia usually is made with plain radiographs. Radiographic characteristics of fibrous dysplasia include a focal, well-defined, expansile, intramedullary lytic lesion with a lucent, ground glass, or sclerotic matrix, causing cortical thinning and loss of trabecular definition (e-Fig. 59-12). Rarely, fibrous dysplasia can produce adjacent soft tissue proliferation, or it can be cystic with fluid-fluid levels. Fibrous dysplasia is usually a radiographic diagnosis that requires no further imaging.[3,55] When seen on CT, amorphous calcification inside the lesion with bone expansion is usually present. Pathologic fractures also can be confirmed on CT if they are not detected on radiographs. MRI is helpful in assessing the extent of the disease. Despite its name, fibrous dysplasia does not follow the same signal characteristics of pure fibrous tissue. The lesions are isointense to muscle on T1-weighted images. On fluid-sensitive sequences, the lesions are predominantly hyperintense, with focal hypointense, isointense, or markedly hyperintense foci. The heterogeneous signal of fibrous dysplasia on MRI is due to the presence of calcifications, fat, cystic changes, or septations. Fibrous dysplasia displays various contrast enhancement patterns that can be patchy, peripheral, or homogeneous.[55,56]

Treatment and Follow-up Fibrous dysplasia of the chest wall usually requires no treatment unless symptoms such as nerve or vascular compression develop. In such cases, resection of the affected bone, usually a rib, can alleviate the symptoms. Impending bone collapse also is an indication for preventive surgical excision and bone grafting.[57,58] In symptomatic polyostotic cases, bisphosphonates can be used because of their inhibitory effect on bone resorption. When the lesions are discovered incidentally and the radiographic features are characteristic, no biopsy is indicated; a follow-up study every 6 months to ensure stability currently is advised.[53]

Osteochondroma

Etiology An osteochondroma is a benign cartilage-capped developmental lesion rather than a true neoplasm. It affects bones with epiphyses and apophyses. These lesions result from the separation of a fragment of epiphyseal growth plate cartilage, which subsequently herniates through the periosteal bone cuff normally surrounding the physis. An osteochondroma usually is diagnosed in the first three decades of life and may be inherited as a multifocal, familial, autosomal-dominant disease. Solitary lesions have a male predilection; they occur in approximately 1% to 2% of persons undergoing radiographic evaluations and constitute 10% to 15% of all bone tumors.[59] Osteochondromas are the most common benign osseous neoplasm involving the chest wall.[3] Most solitary osteochondromas are asymptomatic. Symptomatic lesions tend to occur in younger patients, with 75% to 80% of those cases discovered before the age of 20 years.[59] Lesions in the chest wall usually present with a palpable, painless mass or focal deformity. Pain may occur as a result of mechanical irritation, fracture, and nerve or vascular compression.[3,55,60]

Imaging Osteochondromas usually can be diagnosed on the basis of plain radiographs. In patients with multiple osteochondromatosis, a skeletal survey usually is obtained to assess the overall extent of disease. In the chest wall, the lesions arise most frequently from the ribs or scapula (Fig. 59-13). They can be sessile or pedunculated, depending on whether a narrow or broad pedicle is located at the base. Corticomedullary continuity is the characteristic imaging finding of an osteochondroma, but this finding may be difficult to completely assess on radiographs. Although both CT and MRI demonstrate the corticomedullary continuity, MRI has an advantage over CT in evaluating the thickness of the cartilaginous cap that should be thin, uniform, and hyperintense on fluid-sensitive sequences. Additionally, MRI can be helpful in assessing the adjacent soft tissue edema and bursa formation that are indicative of the irritation often resulting from osteochondromas. It has been reported that CT with

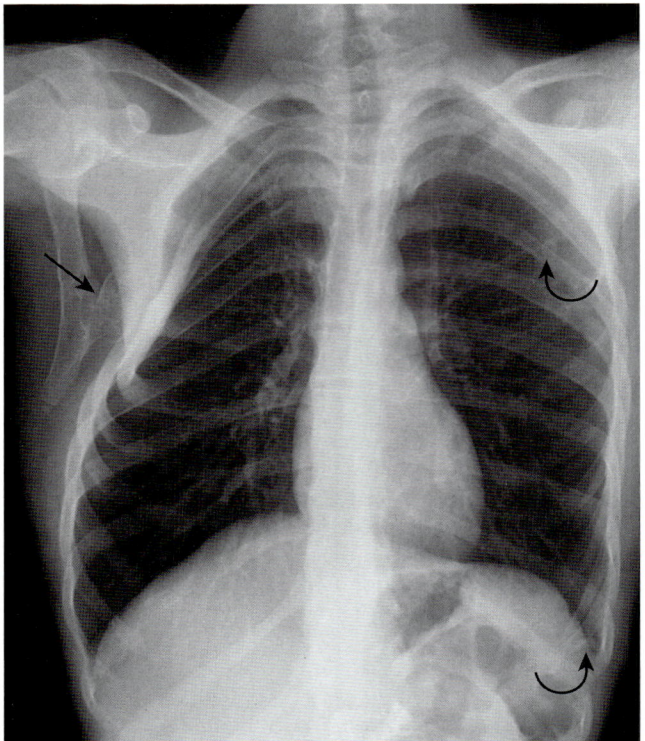

Figure 59-13 Multiple osteochondromas in an adolescent boy with hereditary exostosis. A frontal chest radiograph shows a large pedunculated osteochondroma (*straight arrow*) arising from the undersurface of the scapula that is causing remodeling of the underlying right ribs and chest wall deformity. Smaller lesions (*curved arrows*) are seen in the left scapula and the tenth left rib at the mid axillary line, producing focal rib deformity.

three-dimensional reconstructions can be valuable for the surgeon in preoperative planning.[27,55,59,60]

Treatment and Follow-up Indications for surgical resection of solitary osteochondromas include pain, cosmetic deformity, and nerve impingement. The treatment choice for multiple hereditary exostoses is more complicated and often is directed to correct bone deformity.[59,60] Malignant transformation of the cartilaginous cap into a chondrosarcoma occurs in fewer than 1% of solitary cases and in up to 25% of multiple hereditary exostoses.[59] The risk of malignant transformation is proportional to the size and number of lesions and is only found in adulthood. Solitary osteochondromas in children do not require routine follow-up unless symptoms or rapid growth occur.[60] In cases of multiple lesions, close clinical and radiographic monitoring is required to evaluate the progression of deformities and the development of complications.[59]

Mesenchymal Hamartoma

Etiology A mesenchymal hamartoma of the chest wall is a rare, benign lesion. It typically presents at birth as a large, extrapleural mass arising from a rib that causes chest wall deformity or respiratory distress because of mass effect. Mesenchymal hamartomas, which are not considered true neoplasms, are composed of maturing, proliferating normal skeletal elements with a prominent cartilaginous component and hemorrhagic cavities as a result of aneurysmal bone cyst (ABC) formation. To date, no instances of malignant degeneration of mesenchymal hamartoma of the chest wall have been reported.[61-63]

Imaging A mesenchymal hamartoma may have an ominous imaging appearance, despite its benign nature. On chest radiographs, it usually presents as a partially calcified extrapleural mass causing erosion of one or more ribs. A mass effect on the adjacent lungs and mediastinum often is present.[64] CT or MRI scans show that a mesenchymal hamartoma is a well-circumscribed lesion with solid and cystic components, the latter representing ABC, a feature specific to this lesion (Fig. 59-14). Cortical bone partially surrounding the lesion and mineralization also can be seen. In one series, mineralization was present in 100% of cases and hemorrhagic cystic areas of aneurysmal bone cyst were present in more than half of patients with a mesenchymal hamartoma.[61] On MRI, the signal intensity of mesenchymal hamartoma is variable. Hyperintense areas on fluid-sensitive sequences represent ABC formation and chondroid elements, whereas areas of low signal on T1 and fluid-sensitive sequences represent areas of mineralization.[61,65] Multifocal cases of mesenchymal hamartoma also have been reported.[61,65]

Treatment and Follow-up Surgical excision of a mesenchymal hamartoma with rib resection and chest wall reconstruction is recommended if cardiorespiratory symptoms from mass effect or chest wall deformity are present. Mesenchymal hamartomas, which are benign lesions, generally are cured with en bloc resection. Smaller lesions can be monitored with chest radiographs and ultrasound because spontaneous regression of the lesion has been reported, and the lesions typically stop growing after age 1 year.[61,62,66]

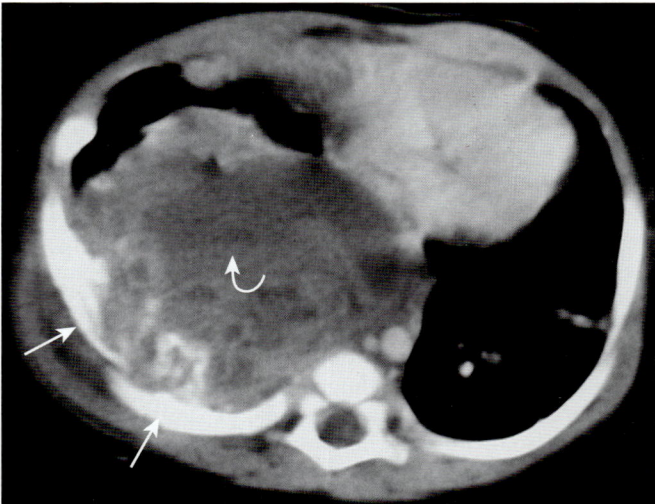

Figure 59-14 A mesenchymal hamartoma in a newborn girl with respiratory distress and a palpable mass in the right chest wall. A postcontrast axial computed tomography soft tissue window image shows a very large, round mass in the posterior right hemithorax with erosion of two consecutive ribs (*straight arrows*). The lesion has a heterogeneous parenchyma with a fluid-fluid level (*curved arrow*) corresponding to the aneurysmal bone cyst component.

Other Osseous Tumors (Langerhans Cell Histiocytosis, Enchondroma, and Aneurysmal Bone Cyst)

Etiology   Several other benign tumors can involve the chest wall in the pediatric population, including eosinophilic granuloma (EG), enchondroma, and ABC. These tumors can arise from any bone in the chest wall, including the ribs, scapula, and (less frequently) the sternum.

An EG that is localized to bone is the most common form of Langerhans cell histiocytosis. An EG is characterized by a proliferation of Langerhans cells, which is a type of histiocyte that originates from the bone marrow and plays a role in the immune system. In the chest wall, an EG most commonly affects the thoracic vertebral bodies, causing vertebrae plana, but it can involve any bone. Bone destruction, pain, localized swelling, and a palpable mass often are present in pediatric patients with EG involving the chest wall.[67,68]

Enchondromas occur less frequently in children than osteochondromas and represent benign, mainly hyaline cartilage tumors arising from the medullary canal of a bone. Most enchondromas are solitary and usually are found incidentally; they also may be multiple, such as in patients with Ollier or Maffucci syndromes.[3,26,55,69]

ABCs are benign, expansile, osteolytic lesions that contain multiple blood-filled spaces of different sizes and are lined by fibroblasts and giant cells of the osteoclast type. An ABC is a hyperplastic lesion reactive to a subperiosteal or intraosseous hemorrhage. The pathogenesis of the hemorrhage of an ABC currently is unclear. Although they are benign, these lesions can grow rapidly, causing bone destruction and pathologic fractures that produce pain and a palpable mass. ABCs may be found either as primary osteolytic lesions or as a reactive process as part of another lesion. The primary ABC is found mostly in the second decade of life and more frequently in females, with a ratio of 2:1.[55,70] In the chest wall, the most common sites of involvement from ABCs are the posterior elements of the spine and the ribs.[55]

Imaging   The classic imaging finding of an EG when it involves the thoracic spine is vertebrae plana, characterized by flattening of vertebral bodies. When it involves other bones of the chest wall, the radiographic appearance of EG varies. In the acute phase of the disease, the lesion develops rapidly and has a more aggressive appearance. In this phase, the lesions typically are lytic with poorly defined borders (Fig. 59-15). Periosteal reaction occurs when the lesion involves the cortex. A soft tissue component of an EG often is present and is best seen on CT or MRI. In the later phase of disease, the lesions can be lytic and sclerotic, and they may adopt a bubbly appearance and have sharp, sclerotic borders.[3,67,68]

Enchondromas are osseous lesions arising from the medullary portion of bone with well-defined, lobulated borders and endosteal scalloping. Localized bone expansion and a chondroid matrix frequently are present in enchondromas (Fig. 59-16).[3,55,69] ABCs are well-defined, lytic, expansile, intramedullary lesions. In the short and flat bones, such as the ribs, the cyst usually appears as an eccentric osteolytic area extending into the cancellous bone with overlying cortical thinning. Because of the rapid growth, a more aggressive appearance with cortical disruption also can be seen (Fig. 59-17, *A*). On CT or MRI, ABCs are typically cystic, with

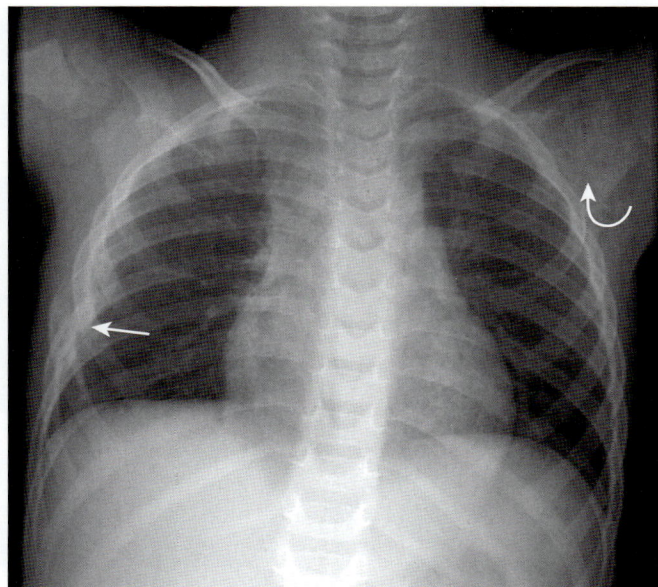

Figure 59-15   Eosinophilic granuloma of a rib and left scapula in a young boy who presented with chest pain. A frontal chest radiograph shows a lytic, slightly expansile lesion involving a segment of the right sixth rib (*straight arrow*) with cortical disruption. A second lytic lesion (*curved arrow*) with rather defined borders involves the left scapular neck.

multiple locules and fluid–fluid levels representing the underlying hemorrhagic nature of the lesion (Fig. 59-17, *B*). Fluid–fluid levels, which frequently are seen within the lesions, are not pathognomonic of ABCs. ABCs do not have an associated soft tissue component.[55,70]

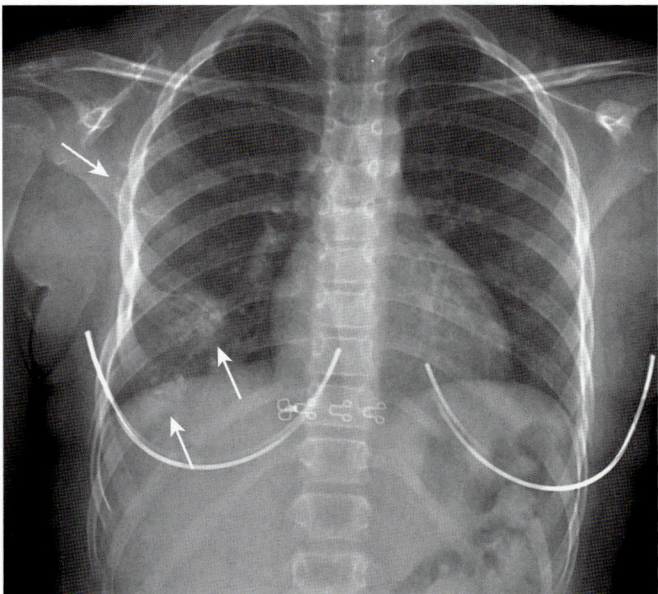

Figure 59-16   Chest wall enchondromas in an adolescent girl with Ollier disease. A frontal chest radiograph shows several well-defined lytic lesions involving the costochondral junction of the right sixth and seventh ribs and the mid aspect and superior border of the right scapular wing (*arrows*). Chondroid matrix is better identified in the rib lesions.

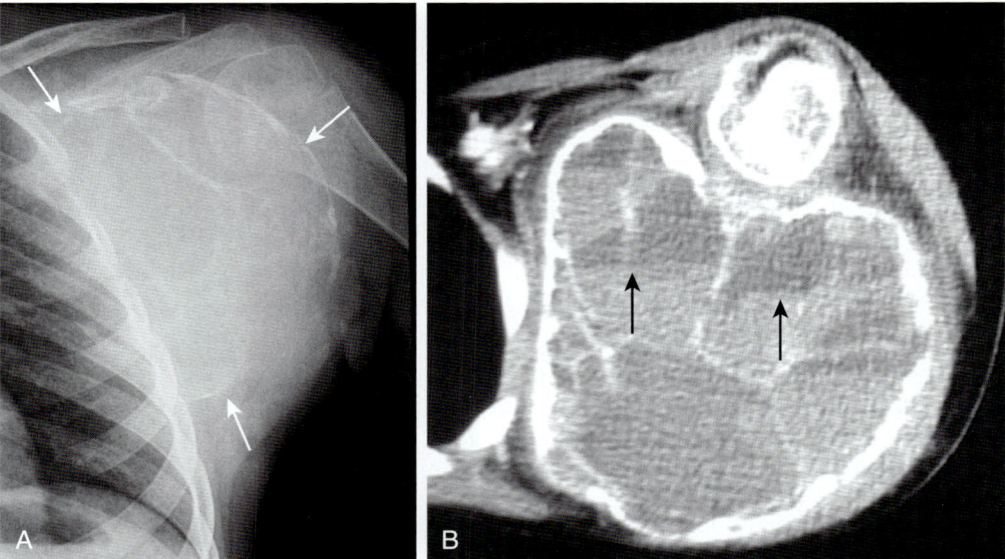

Figure 59-17   A large aneurysmal bone cyst in a patient with a slowly growing left shoulder mass. **A,** A frontal view of the left shoulder demonstrates a very large expansile lytic lesion (*arrows*) arising from the left scapular wing. Thin bony septations are seen inside the lesion. The inferior margin of the lesion is indistinct. **B,** An axial contrast computed tomography soft tissue image clearly shows the expansile lytic lesion containing multiple bony septae arising from the left scapular wing and its relationship with the rib cage and humerus. Several slightly hyperintense fluid-fluid levels are seen in some of the internal locules (*arrows*).

Treatment and Follow-up   The treatment for an EG currently is not standardized. Solitary EG lesions initially can be managed conservatively with close radiographic follow-up, because some of these lesions may heal spontaneously with bone remodeling. Alternatively, the lesion can be treated with curettage and bone graft implantation. More disseminated disease may require systemic chemotherapy.[67,68] Enchondromas, especially the solitary ones, can be incidental findings and, as such, require no treatment. For symptomatic lesions that often are associated with pathologic fractures, curettage and bone grafting usually are curative.[71] The progression of ABCs is variable. Some of the lesions display an aggressive growth pattern, whereas other lesions grow slowly, mature, and may regress spontaneously. ABCs can be treated with selective arterial embolization, percutaneous sclerotherapy, or intralesional excision with bone grafting.[72,73] En bloc resection of ABC is recommended for small lesions located in the ribs. For large lesions, excision with bone grafting may be necessary.[70]

MALIGNANT TUMORS

Soft Tissue Tumors

Rhabdomyosarcoma

Etiology   Rhabdomyosarcoma (RMS) tumors are the second most common primary malignancy that occurs in the chest wall in children.[74] An RMS arises from primitive mesenchymal cells committed to develop into striated muscles. It can arise from any tissue anywhere in the body, except from cortical bone.[74] In children, the age-standardized annual incidence rate for RMS is 4 to 7 per million. Tumors of the trunk account for 7% of all RMS tumors.[75] In a study of 15 chest wall tumors out of 303 RMS tumors, the mean age of diagnosis was 16 years.[76] Affected children typically present with a painful and rapidly enlarging chest wall mass. Respiratory distress can be the presenting symptom in children with large RMS tumors because of mass effect on the adjacent lung or when an associated pleural effusion is present.[76,77]

Imaging   On ultrasound, an RMS presents as a heterogeneous soft tissue mass with increased internal vascularity. The outer margin of the tumor may be either well defined or ill defined. For a complete assessment of tumor extension, CT or MRI is necessary. Although CT is more sensitive than MRI for the evaluation of osseous abnormality and pulmonary metastatic disease in pediatric patients with an RMS mass, MRI is better than CT for assessment of the local extension of the tumor because of its higher soft tissue characterization capability. On CT and MRI, chest wall RMS usually presents as a large, heterogeneous, soft tissue mass with intrathoracic extension. The tumor tends to show a heterogeneously increased signal on T1 and fluid-sensitive sequences on MRI. After administration of intravenous contrast material, an RMS mass typically displays enhancement that is heterogeneous in cases of underlying tumor necrosis.[5,78-80] In comparison with ESFT, bone involvement is much less frequent in children with an RMS, and if present, it tends to occur later in the course of the disease (Fig. 59-18).[78]

Treatment and Follow-up   The current treatment of RMS tumors of the chest wall is chemotherapy to control local disease and reduce the size of the mas before surgical resection. Radiotherapy also often is used if surgical resection margins are positive.[74,77] Because of its higher sensitivity in detecting residual, recurrent, or metastatic disease, CT positron emission tomography (PET) in conjunction with MRI currently is recommended as the follow-up imaging modality of choice.[81-83]

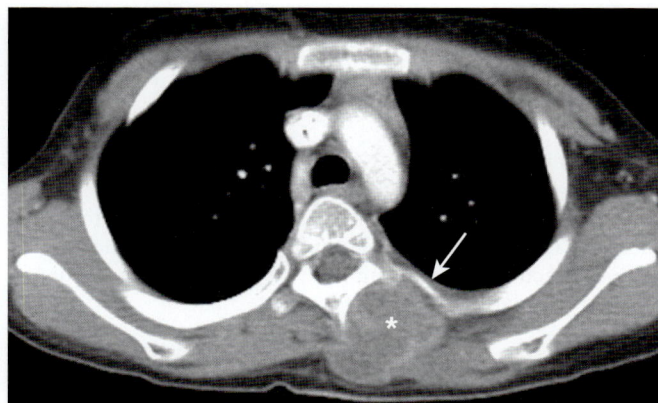

Figure 59-18 A rhabdomyosarcoma of the left paraspinal musculature in a 14-year-old girl who presented with a painful, palpable, soft tissue lump. A postcontrast axial computed tomography soft tissue window image shows a well-defined, slightly hypodense mass in the left paraspinal region (*asterisk*). The mass causes mild remodeling of the underlying bone but no destruction (*arrow*).

Osseous Tumors

Ewing Sarcoma Family of Tumors

Etiology The ESFT represents the most common primary chest wall malignancies in children and young adults.[84] They comprise the classic Ewing sarcoma, atypical Ewing sarcoma, primitive neuroectodermal tumor, and Askin tumor. These tumors belong to the small, round, blue cell tumors that originate from unique mesenchymal cells capable of multilineage differentiation. Based on their varied but similar underlying neural differentiation, their immunohistochemical, cytogenetic, and molecular uniformity, and their identical response to Ewing-based chemotherapy regimens, tumors such as ESFT are regarded as being related to sarcomas. A common chromosomal translocation (t11; 22) (q24; q12) has been implicated in 80% to 95% of cases. ESFT lesions have been reported in all age groups, but most cases are diagnosed in the second decade of life, with a median age of 15 years.[85,86] The occurrence of an ESFT lesion is more common in males, with a ratio of 1.3 to 1.5 : 1; in addition, a predilection for white persons has been noted.[85] Affected children usually present with a rapidly growing palpable chest wall mass that often is painful. In cases with pleural effusions and substantial mass effect on the lung, dyspnea can be the predominant symptom. Pediatric patients with an ESFT lesion in a paraspinal location may present with symptoms related to neurologic impairment. Systemic symptoms, such as fever, and laboratory test abnormalities, including leukocytosis and an elevated erythrocyte sedimentation rate, may simulate infectious processes such as osteomyelitis.[77,85]

Imaging On chest radiographs, an ESFT lesion usually presents as an extraparenchymal and lytic osseous mass with associated bone destruction and aggressive periosteal reaction. An associated soft tissue component can be suggested on plain radiographs but is best seen on CT or MRI (Fig. 59-19).[85,87,88] Calcifications within the mass may be present in approximately 10% of cases.[88] Because of its higher intrinsic contrast resolution and soft tissue characterization, MRI can better depict soft tissue and marrow involvement; local spread,

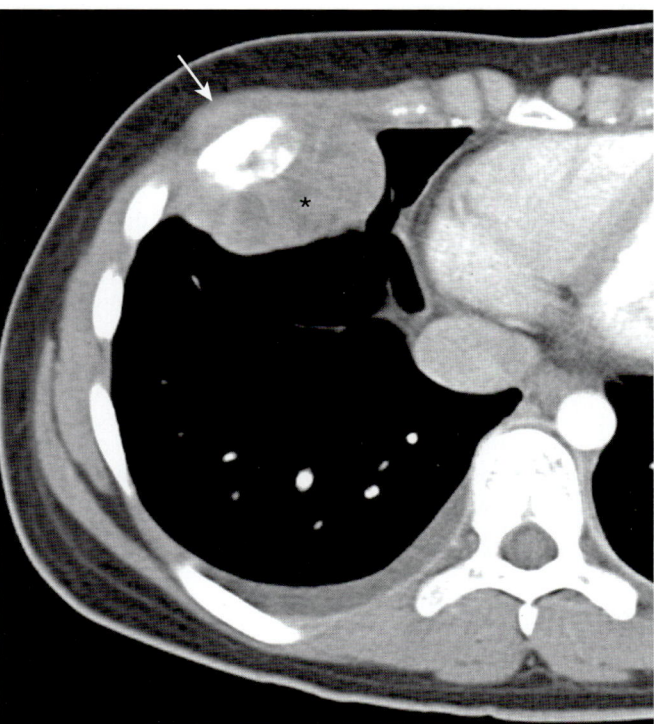

Figure 59-19 A Ewing sarcoma of a rib in an 11-year-old boy who presented with a painful, palpable lump in the anterior chest wall. A postcontrast axial computed tomography soft tissue window image shows focal thickening of the anterior aspect of a right rib (*arrow*) surrounded by a soft tissue mass (*asterisk*).

especially into the spinal canal when the lesion has a paraspinal location; and the relationship with adjacent organs or neurovascular structures. On CT and MRI, an ESFT mass typically presents as a lytic and destructive osseous lesion associated with aggressive periosteal reaction and heterogeneous soft tissue components (Fig. 59-20). On MRI, the soft tissue component of an ESFT lesion is isointense or

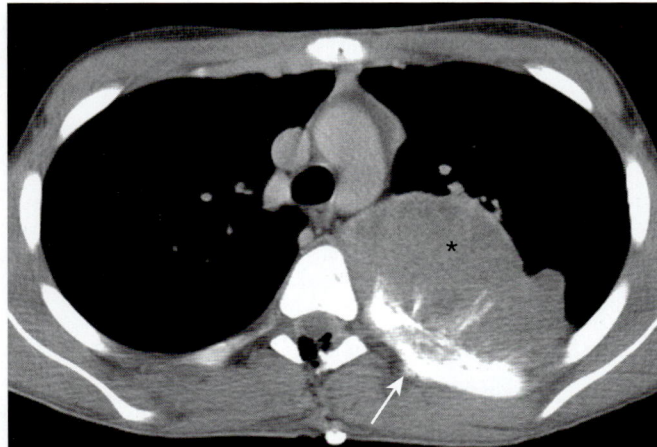

Figure 59-20 A primitive neuroectodermal tumor of a rib in a 10-year-old boy with back pain. A contrast axial computed tomography soft tissue window image shows a large, extrapleural, soft tissue mass arising from the medial aspect of a left rib (*asterisk*). The patient has aggressive associated periosteal reaction, sclerosis, and thickening of the rib (*arrow*).

slightly hyperintense to muscle and hyperintense on fluid-sensitive sequences. Heterogeneous contrast enhancement is seen frequently, except in areas of necrosis. Pleural effusions that obscure the soft tissue mass can be present. Regional lymphadenopathy in patients with an ESFT lesion is unusual.[85,87,88]

Treatment and Follow-up　An ESFT lesion of the chest wall currently is treated with chemotherapy to reduce the size of the tumor and achieve optimal local control and control of distant microscopic metastatic lesions, followed by surgical resection.[74,77,84,85] Currently, CT-PET is used to stage the tumor and monitor patients with an ESFT mass. CT in the follow-up of these patients plays an important role in detecting pulmonary metastasis, because surgical resection of the pulmonary metastasis and radiotherapy may be curative. Fluorine deoxyglucose PET has a limited sensitivity in the detection of small pulmonary metastasis.[81,89]

Osteosarcoma

Etiology　A chest wall osteosarcoma is rare. Osteosarcomas that do present in this location occur more frequently in younger children. A chest wall osteosarcoma can arise from a rib, scapula, or clavicle or can be a focus of metastatic disease.[77] The incidence of osteosarcomas is 4.8 per 1 million children, with about 1% located in the chest wall and spine.[77] The peak incidence of osteosarcoma lesions occurs in the second decade of life.[90] Much like the other malignant chest wall tumors, osteosarcomas typically present as rapidly growing and usually painful chest wall masses.[2]

Imaging　An osteosarcoma typically demonstrates prominent new bone formation on all imaging modalities. Chest radiographs show a lytic or blastic osseous lesion with a soft tissue mass containing calcifications. On CT, areas of bone formation characteristically are seen at the center, rather than the periphery, of the lesion (Fig. 59-21). On MRI, the areas of bone formation are seen as hypointense relative to muscle

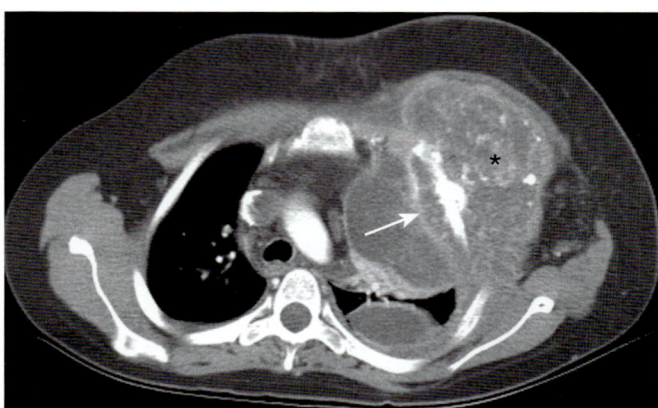

Figure 59-21　An osteosarcoma lesion in an adolescent boy who presented with a painful asymmetry of the anterior chest wall. A postcontrast axial computed tomography soft tissue image shows destruction of a left rib with aggressive periosteal reaction (*arrow*) and a large, partially calcified soft tissue mass (*asterisk*) that is causing deformity of the anterior left chest wall.

on T1-weighted images. A mixed but predominantly hyperintense mass is seen on fluid-sensitive sequences. Heterogeneous contrast enhancement of the soft tissue component of an osteosarcoma indicates necrosis.[80]

Treatment and Follow-up　Chemotherapy and surgical resection constitute the current treatment of choice for a chest wall osteosarcoma; this lesion is relative insensitivity to radiotherapy. The possibility of complete surgical resection is the primary factor in determining the ultimate outcome of affected patients.[74]

Trauma of the Chest Wall

OVERVIEW

The chest wall in children is more elastic and flexible than in adults because of its larger cartilaginous component, and thus less force is absorbed by the chest wall with impact and proportionally more force is transmitted to intrathoracic organs. Thus intrathoracic injury may occur without visible damage to the chest wall. Trauma is the leading cause of mortality in children. Although death from a chest injury is uncommon, after head injury, chest trauma is the second most common cause of death in pediatric patients. In children younger than 12 years, 60% to 80% of chest injuries are the result of blunt trauma, and more than half are accounted for by impact with motor vehicles.[91-93] However, among infants and young children, it is important to recognize that rib fractures occur most commonly as the result of nonaccidental trauma.[94-97]

Etiology　Rib fractures constitute the majority of chest wall injuries in children. In a prospective study of 80 children after thoracic trauma, 28 (35%) had rib fractures, and one (1%) had a sternal fracture.[94] Rib fractures occur as a result of blunt trauma, such as falls or motor vehicle accidents. In pediatric trauma, the location of rib fractures is more a function of the mechanism of injury than the magnitude of the force that is transferred, although the number of fractured ribs is proportional to the severity of the trauma and the likelihood of associated multisystemic injury. This situation occurs because a greater force is necessary to deform and fracture multiple ribs in pediatric patients.[97]

In infants or young children (<3 years) without underlying metabolic bone disease, rib fractures are very unusual and highly suggest nonaccidental trauma as a result of abuse.[98] Although fractures related to abuse can occur along any part of the ribs, when they are posterior in location, they are highly specific for nonaccidental trauma. This specificity occurs because of the substantial posterior levering force that the transverse processes exert over the posterior aspect of the ribs, resulting in fracture during a tight squeeze by the perpetrator.[26,98] In addition to abuse, birth trauma and diseases associated with underlying bone fragility, such as rickets and osteogenesis imperfecta, are other rare causes of rib fractures in infants and young children.[99]

Imaging　In the acute setting, the initial assessment of possible chest wall injury in pediatric patients with trauma usually

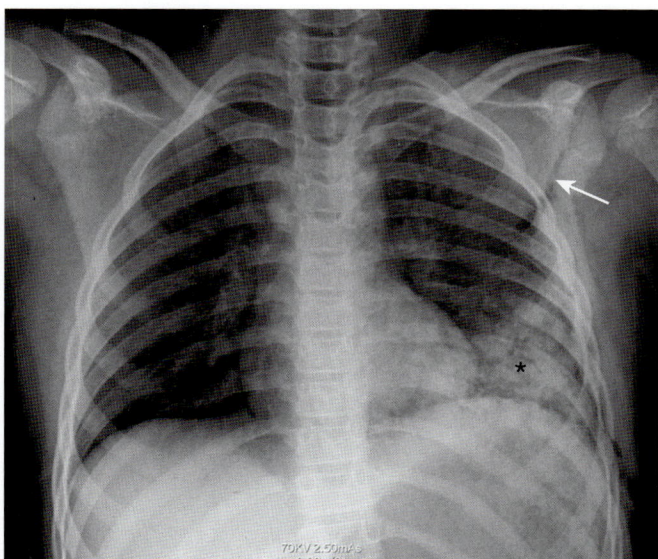

Figure 59-22 Multiple fractures of the left ribs and a left scapular fracture in a young boy involved in a high-speed jet ski accident. A frontal chest radiograph shows fractures of the seventh through ninth left ribs posterolaterally and more subtle fractures of the left tenth and eleventh ribs. A minimally diastatic fracture (*arrow*) is seen through the neck and body of the left scapula. Subcutaneous emphysema is seen along the lateral side of the left chest wall, as well as a fluffy consolidation (*asterisk*) in the left lower lobe consistent with a pulmonary contusion.

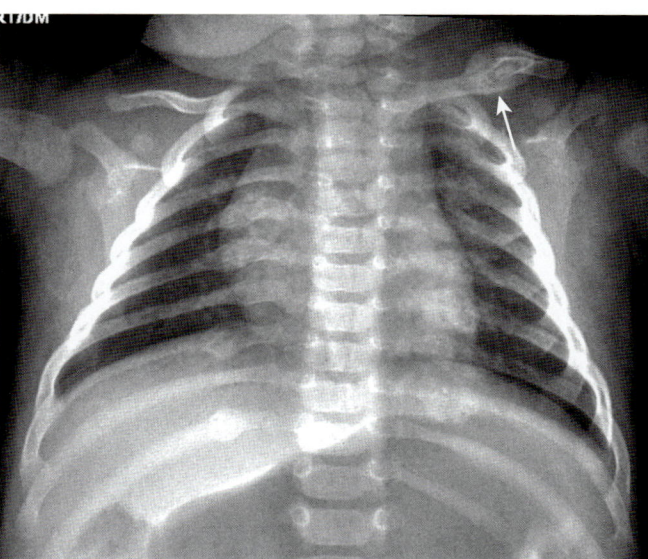

Figure 59-23 Multiple bilateral rib fractures in a young girl who has sustained nonaccidental trauma. A frontal chest radiograph shows multiple, consecutive, bilateral, posterior rib fractures in the stage of healing. A healing fracture of the left clavicle is also present (*arrow*).

requires chest radiographs. Radiographs can be obtained portably and rapidly, and they provide not only an overview of the severity of the trauma and evaluation of the bones but also the location of the support tubes and lines. Once the diagnosis of rib fractures is established, careful attention to exclude associated intrathoracic injury must be provided. The most commonly associated nonosseous abnormality with chest wall injury is pulmonary contusion (Fig. 59-22), followed by pneumothorax. However, other injuries such as hemothorax and fractures of other bones also may be present and can be detected on chest radiographs. In the case of unconscious and hemodynamically unstable pediatric patients, a CT of the chest with contrast using the CT angiography technique can be performed to evaluate the intrathoracic vascular and nonvascular structures.[94,93] First rib fractures are uncommon but suggest severe trauma and increased risk of intrathoracic vascular injury.[100] Likewise, flail chest is rare in the pediatric population compared with adults. Flail chest occurs when a segment of the rib cage fractures and becomes detached from the rest of the chest wall.[101] Lower rib fractures can be associated with traumatic injury to the upper abdominal organs, such as the liver, spleen, and kidneys.[102]

In cases of suspected child abuse, a skeletal survey must be obtained. Acute nondisplaced rib fractures can be difficult to detect on radiographs in infants and young children. These fractures become more apparent during healing, when callus is present (Fig. 59-23). Fractures involving the anterior and posterior ends of a rib can be seen better on oblique radiographic views. The presence of acute and healing rib fractures is highly suggestive of abuse.[26,98,99] First rib fractures can be seen in the setting of child abuse.[103] Because not all chest wall

fractures are detected on radiographs, a bone scintigraphy or follow-up radiographs may be necessary.[26,98] Assessment of the chest wall musculature and tendon injury can be performed with ultrasound or MRI. Ultrasound also allows dynamic evaluation of the muscle function.[104]

Treatment and Follow-up   The treatment of rib fractures is supportive with pain medications and aggressive respiratory therapy to prevent atelectasis and pneumonia. In cases of flail chest, ventilatory support during the healing phase may be necessary.[93,96] Because nondisplaced acute rib fractures can be difficult to identify on plain radiographs, follow-up chest radiographs or bone scintigraphy can be obtained approximately 1 week later to increase the detection of fractures in cases of suspected child abuse.[26,98] Nonoperative, conservative treatment currently is advocated for the low-grade muscular and musculotendinous injury of the chest wall. Early surgical intervention is recommended for patients who have complete tears or avulsion of tendon from the bone.[104]

✔ WHAT THE CLINICIAN NEEDS TO KNOW

- The common congenital and developmental anomalies of the chest wall in children, including their workup and treatment
- Infections that can involve the chest wall, including bacterial, mycobacterial, and fungal infections
- Benign and malignant chest wall tumors in children, along with their clinical presentation, workup, and follow-up
- Traumatic injury to the thorax, its mechanisms, and possible etiologies, including child abuse

Key Points

Palpable but otherwise asymptomatic chest wall masses in children usually are congenital or developmental osseous or cartilaginous normal anatomic variants.

Congenital malformations of the chest wall can be isolated or part of a syndrome. These malformations usually cause cosmetic rather than physiologic problems. The two most common chest wall deformities are pectus excavatum and pectus carinatum.

Chest wall infections in children are rare and usually occur as a result of hematogenous dissemination or local spread. Unusual organisms causing chest wall infections in children include actinomycosis and tuberculosis, and the imaging manifestations may be confused with malignancies.

Malignant chest wall tumors in children are uncommon and usually present with a rapidly growing, painful mass. Malignant chest wall tumors include RMSs, which usually involves the soft tissues, the ESFT, and osteosarcomas, which most commonly involve a rib.

The chest wall in children is more elastic and flexible than in adults; therefore the chest wall absorbs less impact force, and more force is transmitted to intrathoracic organs. This mechanism allows intrathoracic injury to occur without visible chest wall injury. The presence of rib fractures in pediatric patients indicates a significant traumatic force, and associated internal injuries must be suspected and investigated.

Suggested Readings

Donnelly LF, Taylor CN, Emery K, et al. Asymptomatic, palpable, anterior chest wall lesions in children: is cross-sectional imaging necessary? *Radiology*. 1997;202:829-831.

Fefferman NR, Pinkney LP. Evaluation of chest wall disorders in children. *Radiol Clin North Am*. 2005;43:355-370.

Glass RB, Norton KI, Mitre SA, et al. Pediatric ribs: a spectrum of abnormalities. *Radiographics*. 2002;22:87-104.

Groom KR, Murphey MD, Lonergan GJ, et al. Mesenchymal hamartoma of the chest wall: radiologic manifestations with emphasis on cross-sectional imaging and histopathologic comparison. *Radiology*. 2002;222:205-211.

La Quaglia MP. Chest wall tumors in childhood and adolescence. *Semin Pediatr Surg*. 2008;17:173-180.

Laffan EE, Ngan BY, Navarro OM. Pediatric soft tissue tumors and pseudotumors: MR imaging features with pathologic correlation. Part 2. Tumors of fibroblastic/myofibroblastic, so called fibrohistiocytic, muscular, lymphomatous, neurogenic, hair matrix and uncertain origin. *Radiographics*. 2009;29(4):e36.

References

Full references for this chapter can be found on www.expertconsult.com.

Chapter 60

The Pleura

RICARDO RESTREPO and EDWARD Y. LEE

The pleura is a serous membrane consisting of two layers the visceral and the parietal pleura. The parietal pleura covers the inner aspect of the chest wall and the diaphragm. The visceral pleura is strongly adherent to the surface of the lungs and interlobar fissures. In healthy persons, the space between the visceral and parietal pleura is nothing more than two apposed pleural surfaces separated by a trace of glycoprotein-rich fluid. In normal conditions, no imaging study can visualize the pleural space because pleural membranes are only 0.2 to 0.4 mm thick, and the physiologic volume of pleural fluid forms a thin 5- to 10-micron layer. However, in children, various pathologic processes can occur within this space that require imaging evaluation. In this chapter, etiologies, imaging characteristics, treatment, and follow-up of pathologic processes involving the pleura are discussed.[1-4]

Pleural Effusion

Etiology The lymphatic system, which is part of the immune system and comprises a network of lymphatic vessels, plays an important role in the homeostasis of pleural fluid. Excess production or decreased absorption of lymphatic fluid can result in an increased volume of pleural fluid.[1,5] Pleural effusions may be caused by systemic diseases or local infectious/inflammatory processes.

Pleural effusions traditionally are classified into two types: transudates and exudates. Transudates usually result from underlying systemic diseases that alter the normal balance of formation and absorption of pleural fluid. Transudative pleural effusions commonly are seen in patients with nephrotic syndrome, heart failure, and cirrhosis. Exudates typically are caused by local infectious or inflammatory processes that result in the increased formation of pleural fluid. Exudative pleural effusions usually are seen in patients with pulmonary infections, neoplasms, hemothorax, and collagen vascular diseases.[3-5]

Causes of pleural effusion in pediatric patients differ substantially from those in adults. Whereas the most frequent cause of effusions in adults is congestive heart failure, pleural effusions in children are most commonly a result of underlying pleuropulmonary infection (Table 60-1).[3] Although pediatric patients with small pleural effusions are usually asymptomatic, large pleural effusions can result in symptomatic respiratory distress or inspiratory pleuric chest pain as a result of stretching of the parietal pleura.[3] When infection is the underlying cause, the predominant symptoms are cough, dyspnea, fever, and elevated white blood cell counts.[1,3]

Imaging The first-line imaging modality, chest radiography, plays an important role in the initial diagnosis of pleural effusions in children. The radiographic appearance of pleural effusions depends on the volume and consistency of the pleural fluid, the patient's position, and the presence of septations and/or loculations. On chest radiographs, a free-flowing effusion forms an internally concave meniscus paralleling the chest wall that changes in position on lateral decubitus radiographs. On supine radiographs, a mobile fluid may layer over the hemithorax, resulting in a diffuse opacity. The presence of a lentiform-shaped effusion with internal convex margins is suggestive of a loculated pleural effusion.[2,6]

The most common indication of chest ultrasound in children is to characterize an opaque hemithorax seen on a chest radiograph (Fig. 60-1).[6,7] Ultrasound is the best imaging modality in diagnosing and characterizing pleural fluid.[7] Ultrasound is more sensitive than radiographs in detecting pleural fluid, particularly when the amount is small (~5 mL).[2,8]

The internal echogenicity of pleural effusions on ultrasound can be categorized into four types (Table 60-2): (1) homogeneously anechoic (see Fig. 60-1, B); (2) nonseptated with internal low-level echoes (Fig. 60-2); (3) septated (Fig. 60-3, A); and (4) homogeneously echogenic (Fig. 60-4, A).[7,9] Anechoic and free-flowing effusions are called simple pleural effusions, whereas the remainder are classified as complex pleural effusions.

Computed tomography (CT) also is more sensitive than chest radiographs in detecting small pleural effusions. The advantage of CT is that it provides an unobstructed view of the entire underlying lung parenchyma, mediastinum, and chest wall; however, it is associated with ionizing radiation exposure. Intravenous administration of contrast material is necessary to optimally visualize and assess the pleura and lung parenchyma (Fig. 60-4, B). In comparison to ultrasound, CT is limited in characterizing pleural effusions and demonstrating internal septations (see Fig. 60-3).[2]

Treatment and Follow-up The main treatment of choice for pleural effusions is thoracentesis, which can be helpful in evaluating the underlying cause of the pleural effusion and also in relieving symptoms. Indications for thoracentesis in children with pleural effusions are persistent fever, respiratory compromise, mediastinal shift, pleuritic pain, and underlying

Table 60-1

Phases of Pleural Infection	
Phase	**Description**
Exudative	Pleural inflammation leads to accumulation of free-flowing clear liquid
Fibrinopurulent	Deposition of fibrin in the pleural space results in septation/loculations limiting the flow of fluid; pus accumulates in the pleural cavity
Organizing phase	Fibroblasts infiltrate the pleura, forming a rigid pleura and preventing lung expansion

Table 60-2

Pleural Effusions on Ultrasound Based on Internal Echogenicity	
Type of Effusion	**Description**
Simple	Homogeneously anechoic
Complex	Nonseptated with internal low-level echoes Multiseptated Homogenously echogenic

lung disease.[3] The management of parapneumonic effusion is discussed in the following section.

Parapneumonic Effusion and Empyema

Etiology   A parapneumonic pleural effusion refers to a pleural fluid collection in association with an underlying pneumonia, whereas empyema is the presence of pus in the pleural space.[1,10] *Streptococcus pneumoniae* is still the main etiological agent in parapneumonic effusions in children, although the number of cases caused by *Staphylococcus aureus* has increased.[1,10] More recently, the *Streptococcus milleri* group, typically found in the oropharynx and upper respiratory and gastrointestinal tracts, has been recognized as an important pathogen causing purulent pleuropulmonary infections, especially in immuno-compromised patients.[11]

Pleural infection can be classified into three phases based on the progression of infection: exudative, fibrinopurulent, and organizing (Box 60-1). During the exudative phase, the inflammatory process associated with the underlying pneumonia leads to the accumulation of free-flowing clear fluid within the pleural cavity. During the fibrinopurulent phase, deposition of fibrin in the pleural space results in septations and loculations, limiting the flow of pleural fluid. The

fibrinopurulent phase may be divided into two stages: (1) early fibrinopurulent stage A and (2) late fibrinopurulent stage B. The early fibrinopurulent stage A is characterized by an increase in white blood cell accumulation, which causes thickening of the pleural fluid consistency. The late fibrino-purulent stage B is defined as the accumulation of pus in the pleural space. The organizing phase begins when fibroblasts infiltrate the pleural cavity, forming a thick rigid pleural rind. This pleural rind prevents lung reexpansion, impairs lung function, and creates a persistent pleural space with ongoing potential for infection. At this stage, spontaneous healing eventually may occur, or a chronic empyema may develop.[1,6,12]

Imaging   A chest radiograph is the initial imaging modality for assessing the presence of parapneumonic effusions. Ultrasound subsequently can be obtained for characterization of the parapneumonic effusion. In most cases, parapneumonic effusions are exudates and therefore are complex in appearance on ultrasound, although they may be simple in appearance during the early stage.[9,13] As the underlying infection progresses, parapneumonic effusions may develop low–level internal echoes and floating debris (see Fig. 60-2) followed by septations and loculations (see Fig. 60-3, *A*), preventing free motion of the fluid. The internal echoes indicate increased underlying cellularity of fluid; these pleural effusions are usually exudates but not necessarily empyemas.[1,6,7,9,13] The parapneumonic effusion eventually may become semi–solid in appearance on ultrasound (see Fig. 60-4, *A*). The development of pleural thickening indicates the presence of a fibrous capsule.

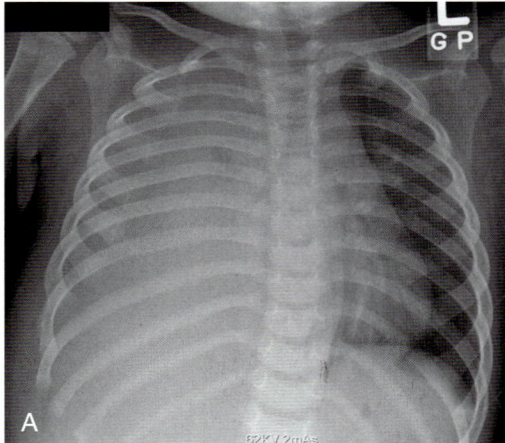
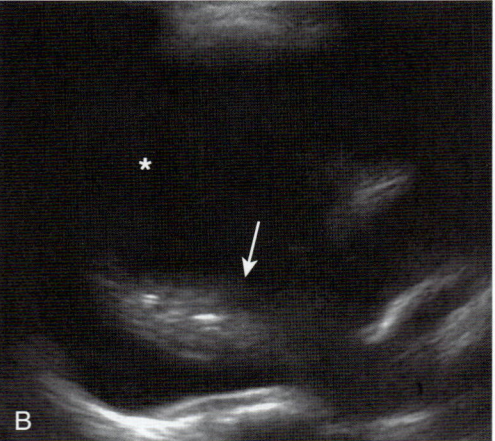

Figure 60-1   Simple effusion in a 2-year-old boy. **A,** Complete opacification of the right hemithorax with obliteration of the right side of the mediastinum and hemidiaphragm. The cardiac and tracheal deviations to the left are imaging findings suggestive of a pleural effusion. **B,** Ultrasound of the right hemithorax confirms the presence of a large simple pleural effusion (*asterisk*). Consolidation (*arrow*) of the underlying lung also is seen.

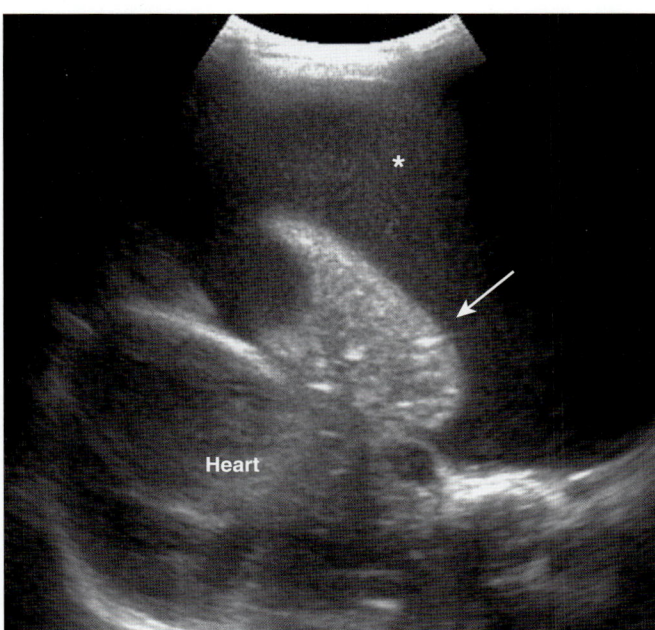

Figure 60-2 Complex effusion with low-level echoes in a 9-year-old girl with bacterial pneumonia. An ultrasound image of the left hemithorax reveals a large pleural effusion with floating low-level echoes indicating debris (*asterisk*) and the consolidated underlying lung (*arrow*).

smooth indentations due to fibrin strands that produce intrapleural adhesions, or in the presence of a lentiform-shaped pleural fluid collection.[2] The presence of air or gas in the dependant portion of the effusion also is an imaging finding that suggests loculation (see Fig. 60-4, *B*). In the absence of a previous thoracentesis or thoracostomy tube placement, the presence of air/gas or an air-fluid level in the pleural cavity in a patient with pneumonia is diagnostic of a bronchopleural fistula (see Fig. 60-5).[1,2,6,16,17] If a bronchopleural fistula is peripheral in location, the direct communication between the lung and the pleural space occasionally can be visualized on CT.[16,17]

The routine use of CT is not necessary to evaluate parapneumonic pleural effusions, particularly in pediatric patients, because it entails exposure to ionizing radiation.[1,6,14] However, CT with intravenous contrast may aid in the evaluation of the lung parenchyma when a complication such as a bronchopleural fistula is suspected (Fig. 60-5) or in the differentiation of a parapneumonic effusion from a lung abscess.[2] An imaging finding suggestive of empyema on CT is a lentiform-shaped fluid collection with pleural thickening and/or enhancement.[15] In contrast, lung abscesses tend to be round and are embedded within the lung parenchyma rather than displacing it.[2] Loculations in parapneumonic effusions, which are best visualized by ultrasound, can be suggested on CT indirectly when the surface of the underlying lung shows

Treatment and Follow-up Anechoic simple pleural effusions can be managed by thoracentesis or percutaneous placement of a chest tube. Because 50% of parapneumonic effusions recur after aspiration in children, the routine placement of a drainage catheter currently is recommended after aspiration.[7] Distinction between parapneumonic pleural effusions and empyema in children is less important than in adults because diagnostic thoracentesis is rarely performed before definitive treatment in children with clinically suspected pleuropulmonary infection.[1,6] However, the optimal management of parapneumonic effusions and empyemas in children currently is not clearly established.

The management choice for complex pleural effusions in children, particularly in the presence of septations, is currently

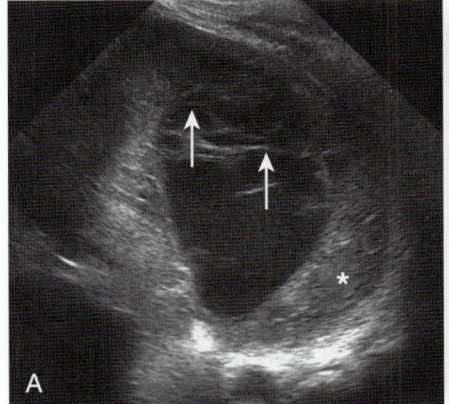
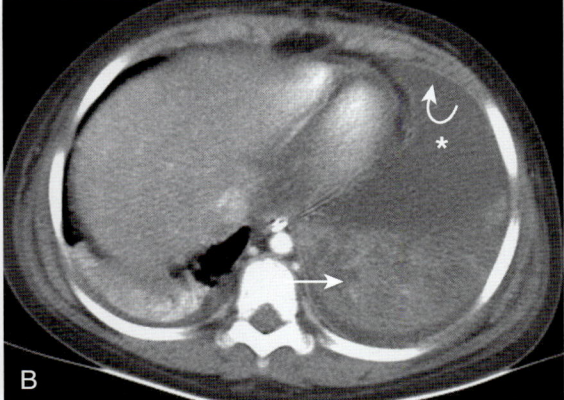

Figure 60-3 Complex septated effusion in a 6-year-old patient with bacterial pneumonia. **A,** An ultrasound image of the left hemithorax shows a large parapneumonic effusion with multiple septations (*arrows*). Consolidation of the adjacent lung also is present (*asterisk*). **B,** An axial postcontrast computed tomography (CT) image shows the pleural effusion (*asterisk*) in the anterior aspect of the left base. The septations seen on the ultrasound are not clearly visualized on CT; however, pleural enhancement is present (*curved arrow*). The adjacent consolidated lung also is noted (*straight arrow*).

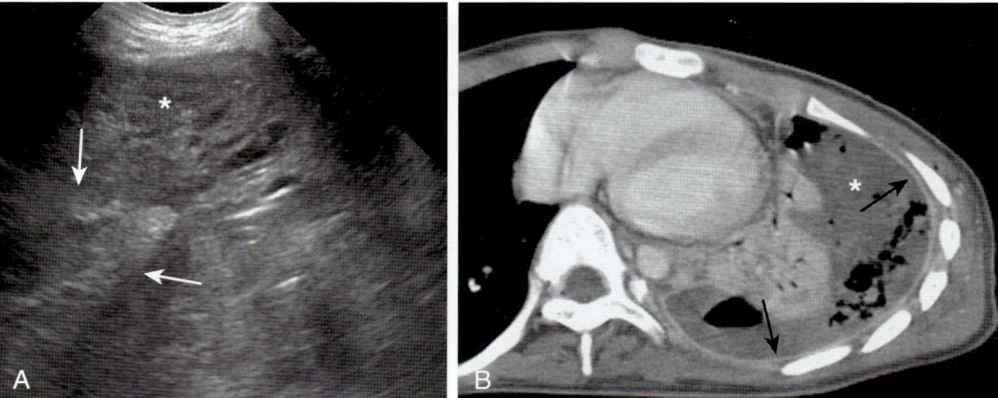

Figure 60-4   Complex effusion in a 6-year-old patient with bacterial pneumonia. **A,** An ultrasound image shows a mostly solid-appearing parapneumonic effusion (*arrows*). The consolidated underlying lung (*asterisk*) also is seen. **B,** An axial contrast-enhanced computed tomography image shows the large pleural effusion (*asterisk*) with pleural enhancement (*arrows*).

somewhat controversial. Some investigators advocate the use of percutaneous insertion of a chest tube combined with instillation of a fibrinolytic agent, whereas others support the use of video-assisted thoracoscopy (VATS).[1,18-22] The presence of septations or complex effusions is not necessarily a contraindication for percutaneous drainage. However, concomitant fibrinolytic therapy typically is required and should be started promptly to maximize the benefit of the procedure.[23,24] In a retrospective study consisting of 54 pediatric patients with parapneumonic effusions, chest tube insertion with intrapleural instillation of a fibrinolytic agent was successful, safe, and less costly as the first therapeutic option compared with VATS.[25] A recent cost-effective analysis study of the management of empyema in children that was conducted with a Bayesian tree approach showed that chest tube insertion with instillation of a fibrinolytic agent was the most cost-effective strategy for treating pediatric empyema based on the length of hospital stay.[26] The management of bronchopleural fistulas is initially medical, including pleural space decompression with a thoracotomy tube and nutritional support. When conservative management is ineffective, closure of the fistula must be considered through VATS for peripheral fistulas and through an open thoracotomy for central fistulas.[16,27]

In children with parapneumonic effusions or empyema that is successfully treated, most chest radiographs return to the baseline between 3 and 6 months. The British Thoracic Society currently recommends follow-up chest radiographs in 4 to 6 weeks after treatment of parapneumonic effusion or empyema.[1] In cases of no improvement on follow-up chest radiographs, either a subsequent ultrasound or a CT scan may be beneficial to exclude underlying complications.[1,6,28]

Pneumothorax

Etiology   Pneumothorax is the presence of air in the potential space between the parietal and visceral pleura. Pneumothorax can be classified into two categories based on the underlying etiology: spontaneous and traumatic. Spontaneous pneumothorax can be further subdivided into primary and secondary. Primary spontaneous pneumothorax occurs in an otherwise healthy child and often is attributed to a ruptured preexisting apical bleb or bulla. Secondary spontaneous pneumothorax occurs as a complication of an underlying pulmonary disease, most commonly asthma and cystic fibrosis in children.[29,30] In the United States, the incidence of spontaneous pneumothorax is approximately 1.8 to 7.4 per 100,000 in boys and 1.2

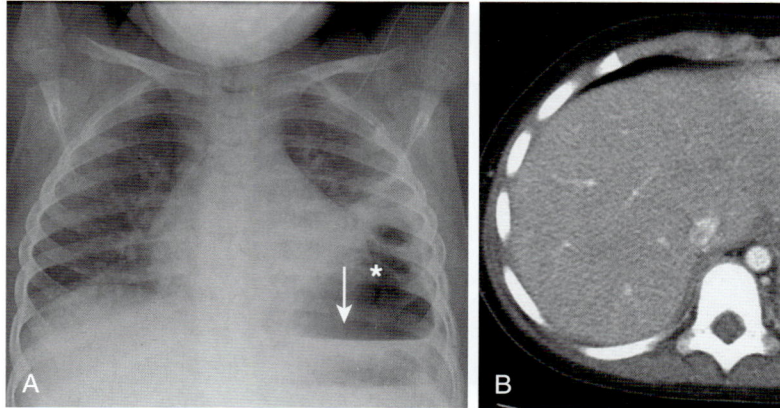

Figure 60-5   A bronchopleural fistula in a 4-year-old boy with necrotizing pneumonia. **A,** A frontal chest radiograph shows a collection of air in the left pleural space superior to the gastric bubble (*asterisk*), with an air-fluid level (*arrow*) indicating a hydropneumothorax. **B,** An axial contrast-enhanced computed tomography image of the same patient confirms the presence of air in the pleural space (*asterisk*) and the air-fluid level (*arrow*).

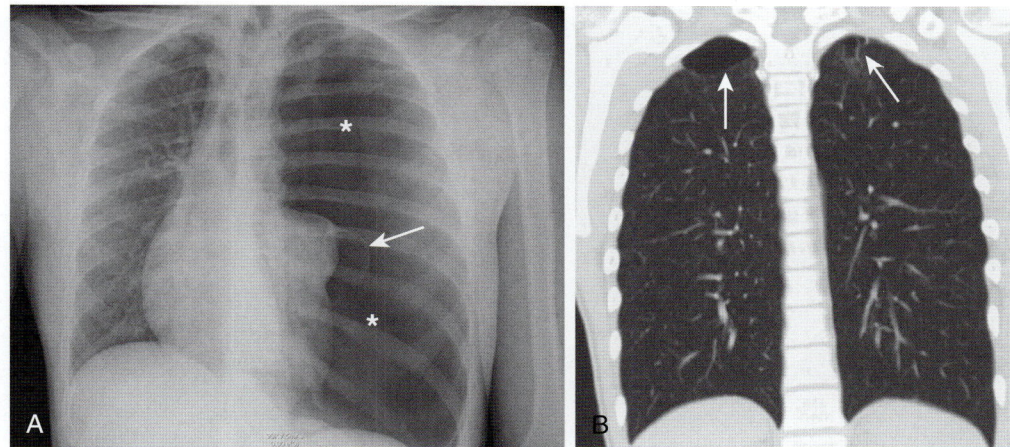

Figure 60-6   Spontaneous pneumothorax in a tall, thin teenager presenting with tachypnea and tachycardia but a normal blood pressure reading. **A,** A frontal chest radiograph shows a large pneumothorax occupying the entire left hemithorax (*asterisks*), with a mild cardiomediastinal shift to the right. A bleb is noted along the surface of the collapsed left lung (*arrow*). **B,** A coronal computed tomography image using a lung window obtained 1 month after thoracotomy tube removal shows biapical blebs (*arrows*), which are larger on the right. The right apical bleb was not seen on the chest radiographs.

to 6 per 100,000 in girls. The mean age at presentation is 14 to 15.9 years.[29,31] The classic phenotype is a thin, tall male with a low body mass index. Children with primary spontaneous pneumothorax typically present with a sudden onset of unilateral chest pain and dyspnea at rest. Patients with secondary spontaneous pneumothorax often present with cardiopulmonary distress.[29,31] Traumatic pneumothorax occurs as a result of blunt or penetrating mechanisms, with iatrogenic pneumothorax being a subset resulting from medical procedures. The outcome of traumatic pneumothorax that causes the most concern is progression to tension pneumothorax. Tension phenomenon occurs when the lung or airway defect acts as a check-valve mechanism, allowing flow of air into, but not out from, the pleural cavity. The diagnosis of tension pneumothorax is based on both radiologic and clinical findings. Hemodynamic and ventilatory compromise may be present with rapid cardiorespiratory collapse. On physical examination, signs of tension include neck vein distension, tracheal deviation away from the affected side, and cyanosis.[29] Tension pneumothorax in the absence of trauma is rare in pediatric patients, occurring in 1% to 3% of cases.[32]

Imaging   Chest radiography is the initial test in the diagnosis of a pneumothorax by visualizing the visceral pleural with absence of pulmonary markings beyond the pleural margin (Fig. 60-6, *A*). For evaluation of pneumothorax, an upright chest radiograph is the procedure of choice, with a lateral decubitus as an alternative.[29,31] Inspiratory and expiratory views are reported to be equally sensitive in the detection of pneumothorax, and thus the expiratory view does not need to be obtained routinely.[33] On chest radiographs, a tension pneumothorax is characterized by a large pneumothorax, resulting in collapse of the ipsilateral lung and shifting of the mediastinum, including the trachea, to the contralateral side.[29] Widened ipsilateral rib spaces and flattening of the diaphragm are also often seen in patients with a tension pneumothorax.

Although ultrasound is rarely used for evaluating pneumothorax, it is important to recognize the sonographic finding of a pneumothorax, because it may be encountered during ultrasound evaluation of the pediatric chest performed for other reasons. Without a pneumothorax, the strong acoustic interface between the pleura and aerated lung produces posterior reverberations. The normal sliding motion of the lung during respiration also is visualized. When air is introduced into the pleural space, the normal tension between the pleural layers is lost and a gap is created between the parietal and visceral pleura, disrupting the normal acoustic interface. The sliding of the underlying lung no longer can be seen, and the normal reverberation is replaced by a static homogeneous acoustic shadowing.[7,29] A recent literature review reported a sensitivity between 86% and 98% and a specificity between 97% and 100% for ultrasound compared with a sensitivity between 28% and 75% for supine chest radiographs in detecting pneumothorax.[34]

In cases of primary spontaneous pneumothorax, a CT scan may play a role in identifying pre-existing subpleural blebs and bullae (Fig. 60-6, *B*). The exact relationship between blebs and primary spontaneous pneumothorax is not clear. However, with CT, there is an increased recognition of subpleural blebs in patients with primary spontaneous pneumothorax and, in particular, in patients presenting with recurrent pneumothoraces.[35-40]

Treatment and Follow-up   No pediatric-specific management guidelines for primary spontaneous pneumothorax have been developed to date. Pediatric patients have not been addressed separately in the available international guidelines.[30,31] In the setting of primary spontaneous pneumothorax, observation should be the initial management of choice for small closed pneumothoraces separated less than 2 cm from the chest wall in asymptomatic patients. Administration of oxygen should be considered because it may increase the rate of reabsorption of the pneumothorax. Symptomatic pneumothoraces, whether primary or secondary, require active intervention with a simple aspiration or placement of a thoracostomy tube in cases of a large pneumothorax.[29,30] When a tension pneumothorax is present, a large-bore needle or angiocatheter should be inserted in the affected side at the second intercostal space to decompress the tension pneumothorax in a timely fashion.[29]

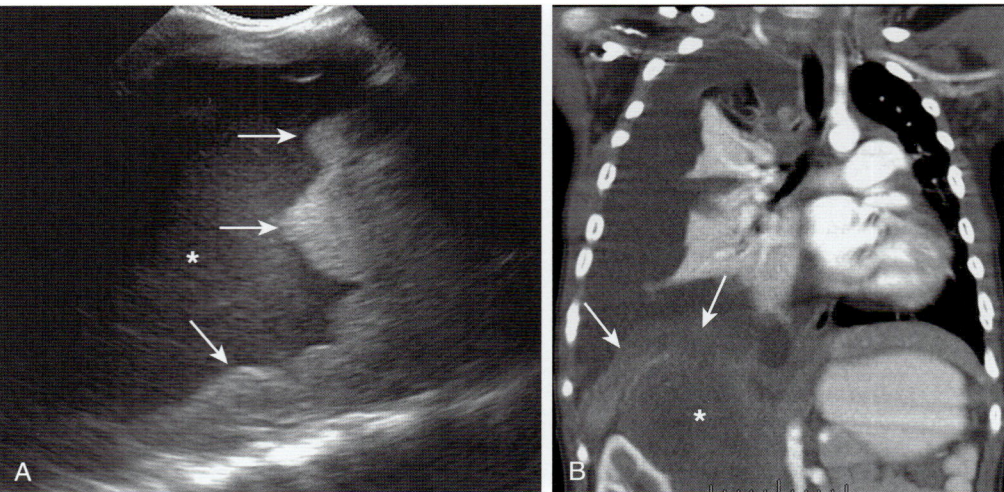

Figure 60-7 A primary retroperitoneal rhabdomyosarcoma with metastasis to the pleura in a 3-year-old girl. **A,** Ultrasound of the right hemithorax shows a large complex effusion with low-level echoes (*asterisk*) and nodularity of the pleura (*arrows*). **B,** A coronal contrast-enhanced computed tomography image shows the large right suprarenal rhabdomyosarcoma (*asterisk*). The soft tissue along the right diaphragm and pleura indicate metastasis (*arrows*). A secondary large right pleural effusion causing collapse of the right lung also is seen.

The risk of recurrence after a single episode of spontaneous pneumothorax with conservative treatment ranges from 16% to 52%.[40] Patients with a primary spontaneous pneumothorax that is treated successfully by a simple aspiration should be observed before discharge. Patients with a spontaneous pneumothorax who are discharged without intervention should have a follow-up chest radiograph after 2 weeks. Patients who have a secondary pneumothorax that is treated with simple aspiration should be admitted for 24 hours for a repeat chest radiograph to ensure no recurrence.[30] The exact indications for CT in the pediatric population in the setting of spontaneous pneumothorax currently are not well established. It has been advocated that a limited CT scan of the lung apices with coronal reconstruction may suffice in children because most blebs and bullae occur in this location, thus allowing a decrease in radiation exposure.[31,38]

Pleural Neoplasms

Etiology Pleural tumors in children are rare and much less common than in adults. Secondary neoplasms (i.e., metastasis or direct invasion) are more common than are primary tumors.[7] Metastatic neoplasms involving the pleura include lymphoma, neuroblastoma, Wilms tumors, rhabdomyosarcoma, and other sarcomas.[7] A metastatic Wilms tumor may involve the peritoneal, pleural, and pericardial cavities and is one of the most common causes of malignant effusions in children.[41]

Primary malignant tumors of the pleura include desmoplastic small round cell tumors and mesotheliomas. The former more commonly occur in the peritoneal cavity but may arise primarily from the pleura.[42,43] Mesotheliomas are regarded as an adult-type neoplasm that rarely occur in children in the second decade. Clinicopathologic features of mesothelioma are similar to those in adults, with a predilection for the pleura, a male predominance, and a poor prognosis.[44] Malignant pleural tumors typically present with chest pain and respiratory distress, especially in the presence of a large pleural effusion.

The most common benign lesions of the pleura include a calcifying fibrous tumor, myofibromatosis, and lipomas.[42] Calcifying fibrous tumors usually are found in subcutaneous and deep soft tissues, but on rare occasions have been reported in the pleura.[42]

Imaging Malignant pleural neoplasms, whether primary or secondary, usually manifest with pleural effusions that initially are identified on chest radiographs. Ultrasound subsequently can be used for the confirmation and characterization of pleural neoplasms. Pleural metastases tend to produce large effusions with hemorrhage presenting as increased cellularity and low-level echoes on ultrasound. The presence of pleural fluid aids in the detection of nodules or masses adherent to the parietal or visceral pleura on ultrasound (Fig. 60-7).[7] CT and magnetic resonance imaging are helpful imaging modalities for evaluating the tumor, its extent, and its relationship with adjacent organs. Because of the markedly overlapping imaging findings among different types of primary and secondary pleural neoplasms, definitive diagnosis is based on histopathologic analysis. If the neoplasm is visible on ultrasound, biopsy under ultrasound guidance can be performed for the diagnosis.[7]

Treatment and Follow-up The current treatment of primary malignant pleural neoplasms is surgical resection, often combined with chemotherapy. When pleural metastasis is discovered, it usually indicates advanced disease, and the treatment is aimed at treating the primary tumor. In cases of recurrent intractable pleural effusions, pleurodesis as a palliative treatment can be performed.[45]

WHAT THE CLINICIAN NEEDS TO KNOW

- Chest radiography is an initial imaging modality for evaluating pleural effusion in children.
- Ultrasound is the best imaging modality for diagnosing and characterizing pleural fluid.
- The routine use of CT is not necessary to evaluate parapneumonic pleural effusions, particularly in pediatric patients, because of exposure to ionizing radiation.
- A bronchopleural fistula may be present as a complication of a parapneumonic effusion.
- Types of pneumothorax and their etiology are required knowledge.

Key Points

Pleural effusions are best characterized on ultrasound as simple and complex. Simple effusions are anechoic, whereas complex effusions contain floating low-level echoes, septations, and/or semi-solid components.

Parapneumonic effusions and empyema are part of a spectrum of pleural infection.

The three phases of pleural infection include exudative, fibrinopurulent, and organizing.

The diagnosis of a tension pneumothorax is both clinical and radiologic, based on cardiorespiratory deterioration in the presence of a large pneumothorax.

Primary spontaneous pneumothorax occurs in an otherwise healthy child and often is attributed to ruptured pre-existing apical blebs or bullae.

Suggested Readings

Balfour-Lynn IM, Abrahamson E, Cohen G, et al. BTS guidelines for the management of pleural infection in children. *Thorax.* 2005;60:i1–i21.
Calder A, Owens CM. Imaging of parapneumonic effusions and empyema in children. *Pediatr Radiol.* 2009;39:527-537.
Chen HJ, Tu CY, Ling SJ, et al. Sonographic appearances in transudative pleural effusions: not always an anechoic pattern. *Ultrasound Med Biol.* 2008;34:362-369.
Coley BD. Chest sonography in children: current indications, techniques, and imaging findings. *Radiol Clin N Am.* 2011;49(5):825-849.
Johnson NN, Toledo A, Endon EE. Pneumothorax, pneumomediastinum and pulmonary embolism. *Pediatr Clin N Am.* 2010;57:1357-1383.

References

Full references for this chapter can be found on www.expertconsult.com.

Chapter 61

The Diaphragm

RICARDO RESTREPO, KARUNAMOY DAS, and EDWARD Y. LEE

Overview

The diaphragm is a dome-shaped musculofibrous membrane that separates the thoracic from the abdominal cavity. It also performs an important function in respiration. The diaphragm has a fibrous portion centrally (i.e., a central tendon) surrounded by a peripheral muscular portion. The diaphragm has three major musculofibrous groups, based on their origins: sternal, lumbar, and costal. Major structures pass through three openings: the caval opening (for the inferior vena cava and some branches of the right phrenic nerve), the esophageal hiatus (for the esophagus, anterior and posterior vagal trunks, and some small esophageal arteries), and the aortic hiatus (for the aorta, azygous vein, and thoracic duct). The diaphragm is innervated by the phrenic nerve, which is formed from the central nerves of C3, C4, and C5.[1,2] Diaphragmatic lesions can arise from a variety of congenital, traumatic, infectious, and neoplastic conditions, as discussed in the following sections.

Congenital Anomalies

DUPLICATION OF THE DIAPHRAGM (ACCESSORY DIAPHRAGM)

Etiology Duplication of the diaphragm, also known as an accessory diaphragm, is a rare congenital anomaly. It is almost always located on the right side and frequently is associated with lobar agenesis-aplasia complex.[3,4] Although the precise pathogenesis of duplication of the diaphragm is currently unknown, it is suggested that this anomaly is the result of a defect of synchronization between the caudal migration of the septum transversum and the development of the bronchial system.[3,5] Instead of developing independently, these two structures mutually interfere in each other's growth. In gross pathology, the accessory diaphragm is a fine fibromuscular membrane with a serosal lining that is united to the anterior part of the diaphragm.[3] It follows a posterosuperior direction to join the posterior chest wall, separating the right hemithorax into two parts.[3,4] It is crescentic in form and usually has an opening (i.e., central hiatus) medially, through which vessels and bronchial structures pass. Affected patients may be asymptomatic, but most present with respiratory difficulties of varying degrees.[5]

Imaging On chest radiographs or computed tomography (CT), the accessory diaphragm may have two different appearances.[3] When the central hiatus is markedly narrowed and the trapped lung is not aerated, it appears like a mass. However, when the trapped lung is aerated, the accessory diaphragm is seen as a fissurelike structure in the right base extending from the anterior aspect of the hemidiaphragm cephalad toward the posterior chest wall. On CT, it is seen as a bandlike structure with crowding of pulmonary structures as the bronchi and vessels traverse the central hiatus (Fig. 61-1).[4,5]

Treatment and Follow-up Most duplicated diaphragms require no surgical intervention. Surgical repair should be performed only when dyspnea or recurrent respiratory infections occur. In asymptomatic patients, treatment is not necessary.[3,5]

CONGENITAL DIAPHRAGMATIC HERNIA

Overview

Traditionally, congenital diaphragmatic hernias (CDHs) have been classified according to their anatomic location. Almost 90% of CDHs are reported to involve the posterolateral aspect of the diaphragm and are referred as to Bochdalek hernias.[6] Nonposterolateral CDHs occur most often in the anterior portion of the diaphragm and are known as Morgagni hernias. However, diaphragmatic defects do not exclusively localize to these two areas, and thus some defects do not follow this classification. To further complicate the classification, some diaphragmatic hernias have a sac, which is thought to represent focal thinning of the diaphragmatic musculature. Thus the terms *sac hernia* and *eventration* currently are poorly defined. Despite its limitations, an anatomic-based classification system continues to be used (Box 61-1).[6]

Congenital Diaphragmatic Hernia: Bochdalek

Etiology CDH of the Bochdalek type is a birth defect that is associated with significant morbidity and mortality.[7] The average prevalence of CDH, derived from a meta-analysis of 16 population-based studies, is 1 in 4000 births.[7] The Bochdalek hernia is the most common subtype, accounting for approximately 90% to 95% of all CDHs.[6] Approximately 85% of these hernias occur on the left side, whereas right-sided and bilateral hernias represent only 13% and 2% of cases, respectively.[8] Bochdalek hernias can be divided into two main categories—isolated and complex—based on the presence of additional associated malformations.[6]

The underlying pathogenesis of CDH is poorly understood. However, much more is currently known about the cellular events and molecular cues that control early

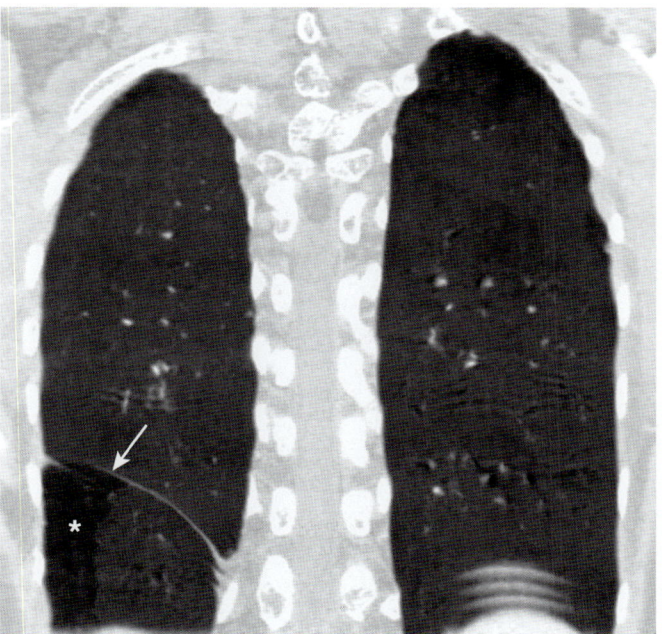

Figure 61-1 A duplicated diaphragm in a 12-year-old girl who initially presented with a cough. A coronal lung window computed tomography image shows a bandlike structure (*arrow*) in the right base with the hyperlucent (*asterisk*) lateral aspect of the right lower lobe, indicating air trapping.

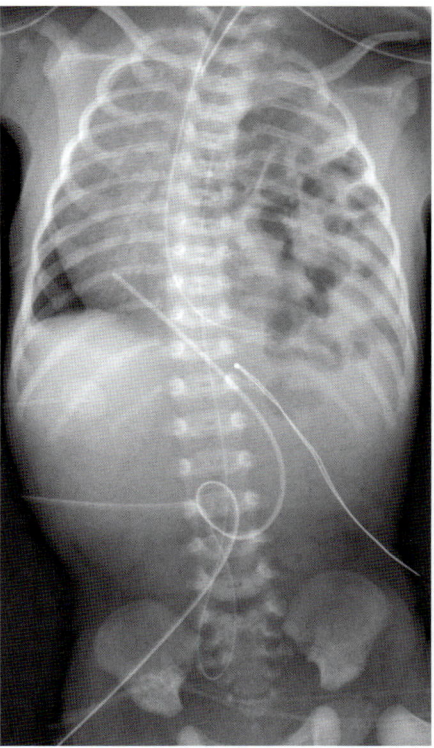

Figure 61-2 A Bochdalek hernia in a newborn. A chest and abdomen radiograph shows multiple air-filled bowel loops in the left hemithorax with cardiomediastinal shift to the right and a paucity of bowel gas in the abdomen.

differentiation of the diaphragm. The diaphragm initially develops as a septum between the heart and the liver, progresses posterolaterally, and closes at the Bochdalek foramen at approximately 8 to 10 weeks of gestation.[8,9] Studies have suggested that the primary abnormality resulting in a Bochdalek hernia is failure or delay of the pleuroperitoneal fold and transverse septum to properly fuse with the intercostal muscles around the eighth week of gestation.[9] More recent evidence suggests that a diaphragmatic hernia and lung hypoplasia are associated, but they may not be causally related.[8]

Imaging A Bochdalek hernia may appear at birth as an opacified hemithorax with contralateral cardiomediastinal shift. As the infant swallows air, the air-filled gut located within the hemithorax may become apparent (Fig. 61-2). In the case of intraabdominal solid organ herniation such as the liver and spleen, the hemithorax can remain homogeneously opacified. When large and with herniation of the bowel, a paucity of air in the abdomen causing the so-called "scaphoid abdomen" can be seen on abdominal radiographs.[9] The position of catheters and tubes is helpful in confirming the presence of a Bochdalek hernia. The nasogastric (NG) tube deviates to the side opposite to the hernia in the chest. If the stomach is herniated within the hemithorax, the tip of the

NG tube can project in the chest. The position of umbilical venous catheters also is affected according to the location of the liver, which is shifted either in the abdomen or chest. In contrast, the position of umbilical arterial catheters is rarely affected because of their retroperitoneal location.[10] In the postoperative period, an ipsilateral pneumothorax is a common finding and should not be rapidly evacuated. A rapid evacuation of a pneumothorax in this situation may cause mediastinal rotation and subsequent venae cavae obstruction because of the increased mobility of the neonatal mediastinum.[9] The pleural air subsequently reabsorbs by itself and sometimes is replaced by fluid. Ultrasound with color Doppler may help delineate the venae cavae and the hepatic vasculature, and it may identify the presence of herniated solid organs before surgery. CT and magnetic resonance imaging (MRI) may play an occasional role in excluding a congenital lung anomaly such as congenital pulmonary airway malformation or pulmonary sequestration.[9]

Treatment and Follow-up Treatment of all types of CDH, including the Bochdalek hernia, can be classified into medical or surgical management. The medical management of CDH focuses on addressing the underlying major causes of neonatal death as a result of CDH, such as pulmonary hypoplasia and pulmonary hypertension. It includes the use of extracorporeal membrane oxygenation, high-frequency ventilation, and inhaled nitric oxide.[11–13] Surgical repair of CDH is performed with a transabdominal or transthoracic approach, and more recently, surgery is performed laparoscopically or thoracoscopically. The herniated abdominal viscera are removed

---

Box 61-1 Anatomic Classification of Congenital Diaphragmatic Hernias

Posterolateral (Bochdalek)
Parasternal (Morgagni)
Central
Posteromedial
Anterolateral

from the chest and repositioned in the abdomen. The posterolateral diaphragmatic defect is usually closed with nonabsorbable sutures if the defect is small or with a prosthetic patch if the defect is larger than 5 cm.[14] Currently no specific guideline exists for following up on children with a repaired CDH. However, chest radiographs often are obtained routinely for confirmation of an intact diaphragm and early detection of a possible CDH recurrence. On follow-up chest radiographs, abnormalities including persistent lung hypoplasia, decreased pulmonary vascularity, and mediastinal shift may be observed.

Congenital Diaphragmatic Hernia: Morgagni

Etiology The foramen of Morgagni is an anterior opening in the diaphragm that extends between the sternum medially and the eighth rib laterally. In Morgagni hernias, also known as retrosternal hernias, the underlying congenital defect results from developmental failure of the fibrotendinous elements of the sternal part of the diaphragm to fuse with the costal part.[15-17] They account for 9% to 12% of the diaphragmatic defects in infancy. These hernias usually are unilateral and are right sided in 90% of cases.[9] A Morgagni hernia may occur as one of the components of the pentalogy of Cantrell, which is characterized by omphalocele, anterior diaphragmatic hernia, sternal cleft, ectopia cordis, and intracardiac defect such as a ventricular septal defect or a diverticulum of the left ventricle.[9,17] A Morgagni hernia can be seen in association with congenital heart disease, intestinal malrotation, and chromosomal abnormalities, most frequently Down syndrome.[9,17]

Imaging Most cases of Morgagni hernias are discovered incidentally on chest radiographs that are obtained for evaluation of other conditions in older children and adults. On chest radiographs, the diagnosis is made when anterior herniation of bowel loops is identified on the lateral chest radiograph (Fig. 61-3). When solid organs such as the liver or spleen are involved, the appearance may not be specific and can resemble focal diaphragmatic eventration, lymphadenopathy, or a foregut duplication cyst. Ultrasound, CT, or MRI can be helpful in the diagnosis when solid organs are herniated.[9,16,17]

Treatment and Follow-up The current treatment of choice for a Morgagni hernia is surgical repair at the initial diagnosis, even in the absence of symptoms, because of the increased risk of developing bowel obstruction and subsequent incarceration. Most Morgagni hernias can be repaired laparoscopically.[1,9,16]

Delayed Presentation of Congenital Diaphragmatic Hernia

Etiology Approximately 5% to 20% of pediatric patients may present with a delayed CDH.[18] Although currently it is not clear whether the diaphragmatic defect in these patients is congenital or acquired, it has been assumed that the defect may have been present prenatally but was either small or temporarily occluded by solid organs such as the liver or spleen.[18,19] In a recent multicenter retrospective study by the Congenital Diaphragmatic Hernia Study Group,[19] the location, male/female ratio, birth weight, and gestational age all

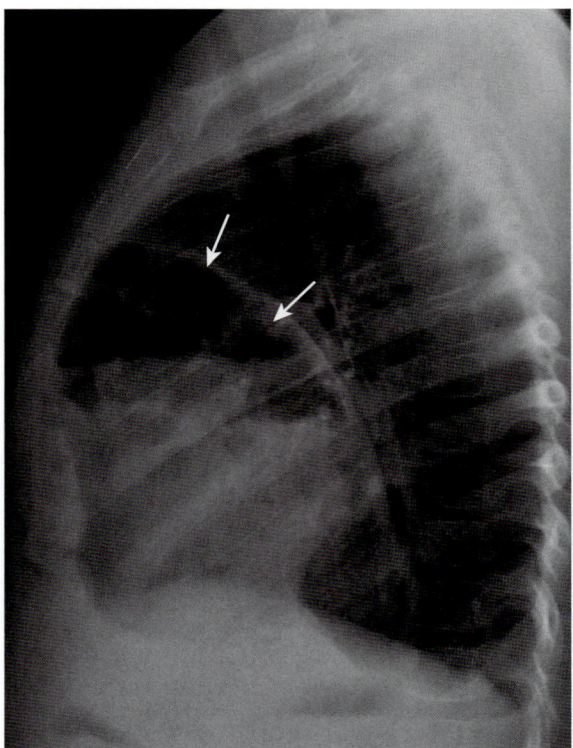

Figure 61-3 A Morgagni hernia in an 8-year-old boy who presented with cough and fever. A lateral chest radiograph shows multiple bowel loops (*arrows*) projecting in the anterior aspect of the chest.

were similar between children with neonatal CDH and infants or children with delayed presentation of CDH. These findings support the assumption that the defect of late-presenting CDH is most likely congenital in nature. Because of the widely varied presenting symptoms and the rarity of this entity, the diagnosis of late-presenting CDH may be delayed or missed.[20,21]

Delayed presentation of a diaphragmatic hernia can be categorized into two groups: (1) infants who present with respiratory symptoms and (2) older children who present with gastrointestinal symptoms. Infants with delayed presentation of CDH usually present in the first few months of life. It often is associated with right-sided pneumonia caused by group B streptococcal infection and initially may be obscured by the consolidative changes. In contrast, the larger group of older children often present with a history of abdominal pain or recurrent vomiting later in life. Approximately two thirds of this delayed presentation of CDH occurs on the posterolateral right side (i.e., Bochdalek). Asymptomatic cases discovered incidentally also occur.[18-21]

Imaging Several studies have shown that delayed presentation of a CDH often can be missed on initial chest radiographs.[18,20] The chest radiograph of a neonate with this type of hernia may be normal in the neonatal period. When only solid organs are herniated, a homogeneous opacity may be seen. Unfortunately, such opacity can be confused with pneumonia or a pleural effusion (Fig. 61-4). In the case of a herniated bowel, tubular air-filled, radiolucent structures projecting into the chest may mimic pneumatoceles or a pneumothorax. Such situations may cause mismanagement such as

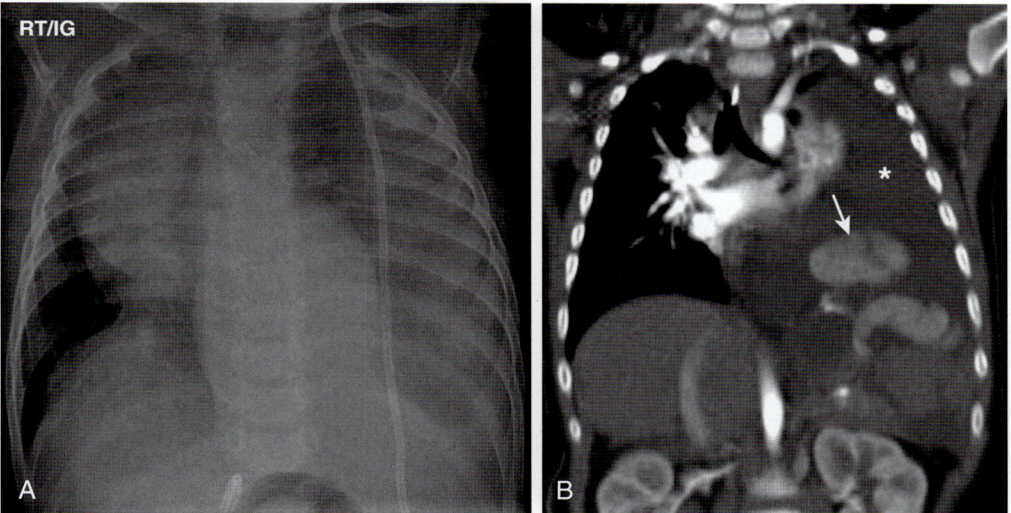

Figure 61-4 A late-presenting congenital diaphragmatic hernia in a 16-month-old boy with shunted hydrocephalus and vomiting. **A,** A frontal chest radiograph shows an opacity in the left hemithorax without clear visualization of the left hemidiaphragm. Cardiomediastinal shift to the right side is also present. Note a left shunt catheter. **B,** A coronal soft tissue window computed tomography image shows a left pleural effusion (*asterisk*) and herniated spleen (*arrow*) into the left hemithorax and poor visualization of the left hemidiaphragm. The left pleural effusion was attributed to a malfunctioning shunt catheter.

insertion of a chest tube, which is associated with a potential risk of gastrointestinal perforation or bleeding. A gas-filled herniated stomach may mimic a pneumothorax or a lung abscess. A delayed presentation of an anteriorly located Morgagni hernia, if it is not gas filled, may simulate cardiomegaly or a mediastinal mass.[18-21] A chest radiograph after insertion of an NG tube has been shown to be the most useful imaging study in confirming a late-presenting hernia.[22] Not infrequently, chest radiography is supplemented by other diagnostic modalities aimed at confirming the hernia. An upper gastrointestinal study can be useful if it demonstrates the presence of bowel in the chest; however, it may yield false negative results in cases of exclusive solid organ herniation. To correctly diagnose a hernia containing only large bowel, it is important to obtain a delayed image during an upper gastrointestinal study. Ultrasound is particularly useful for patients with intrathoracic herniation of only solid organs, or when the hernia mimics a pleural effusion. CT or MRI has the advantage of demonstrating the diaphragmatic defect and herniating mesentery and bowel.[18,21]

Treatment and Follow-up The treatment of delayed diaphragmatic hernia is surgical, with repositioning of the herniated organs in the abdomen and primary closure of the defect or placement of mesh to patch the defect when it is large. The outcome is generally favorable, but misdiagnosis may result in significant morbidity or death. Gastrointestinal obstruction with visceral incarceration is a possible presentation beyond the neonatal period. The role of routine follow-up chest radiographs after surgical repair currently is unclear; however, it may be beneficial for assessing possible recurrence rather than evaluating underlying pulmonary hypoplasia.[20,23]

EVENTRATION

Etiology Diaphragmatic eventration is defined as an abnormal elevation of all or a portion of an attenuated but otherwise intact diaphragmatic leaf. It may be congenital or may develop as a result of paralysis, with the former situation being more common. Congenital diaphragmatic eventration occurs when the fetal diaphragm fails to muscularize, leaving a layer of pleura and peritoneum in that region.[1,24] Among cases that develop as a result of paralysis, diaphragmatic eventration has been described in association with poliomyelitis, herpes zoster, diphtheria, lead poisoning, various infections, and infantile cortical hyperostosis. It can be focal or diffuse, with the former presentation being more common. The focal type of diaphragmatic eventration frequently occurs anteromedially on the right side, and the diffuse type occurs on the left side.[16] Pediatric patients with focal diaphragmatic eventration usually are asymptomatic. With diffuse eventration, symptoms of respiratory insufficiency are seen more frequently in newborns and infants because of a mobile mediastinum causing pulmonary and venous compression by the elevated viscera.[16,17,25]

Imaging Focal diaphragmatic eventration, which is a common incidental finding on a chest radiograph, appears as a focal diaphragmatic bulge in the anteromedial side of the right hemithorax (Fig. 61-5).[16,17] Radiographs may show the elevated diaphragm, allowing distinction in some cases from CDH, in which the diaphragm is in a normal position but the intestinal contents have herniated through an opening in the diaphragm.[16,20] After chest radiographs are obtained, ultrasound can be used to exclude a possible underlying mass and also to evaluate the diaphragmatic mobility using M-mode.[17] Total eventration of the diaphragm in older children and adults often is indistinguishable from diaphragmatic paralysis on chest radiographs. A helpful differentiating sign is that an eventration typically will not have adjacent areas of atelectasis, whereas paralysis of the diaphragm will have such areas. During fluoroscopy, an eventrated diaphragm typically displays an inspiratory lag followed by delayed downward motion. However, slight paradoxic movement, little movement, or no movement

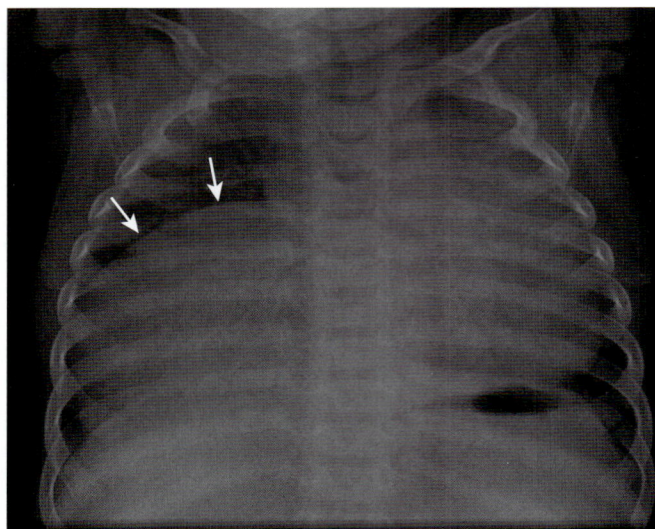

Figure 61-5 Diaphragmatic eventration in a 2-year-old boy who presented with a cough and fever. A frontal chest radiograph shows an elevation of the right hemidiaphragm (*arrows*).

may occur in cases of an eventrated diaphragm, which sometimes makes the distinction from paralysis challenging.[16,17]

Treatment and Follow-up A focal diaphragmatic eventration usually requires no treatment or follow-up because it is usually of no clinical significance. In pediatric patients with a focal diaphragmatic eventration that causes respiratory distress, eventration is plicated. Plication involves a folding and subsequent suturing of the eventrated diaphragm to reduce the excess diaphragmatic tissue. Although surgical techniques of diaphragmatic plication technically are relatively simple, the indication and the timing of surgery are still somewhat controversial.[1,25]

Diaphragmatic Injuries

DIAPHRAGMATIC PARALYSIS

Etiology Injury or abnormality of the phrenic nerve leading to diaphragmatic motion abnormalities may occur unilaterally

or bilaterally as a result of birth trauma or after surgical interventions, most commonly cardiac surgery.[2] The prevalence of diaphragmatic paralysis is 0.03% to 0.5%.[2] The prevalence following thoracic surgery in children has been reported to range between 0.5% and 10%.[2,26–28] In infants, diaphragmatic paralysis may result in life-threatening respiratory insufficiency and ventilatory failure. Unexplained difficulty in weaning a patient from mechanical ventilation or an increasing oxygen requirement should raise the suspicion of diaphragmatic paralysis.[17,27]

Imaging Several imaging modalities have been used to diagnose diaphragmatic paralysis. Diaphragmatic paralysis usually is suggested on chest radiographs when they show persistent elevation of the affected hemidiaphragm. However, the position of the diaphragm may not be reliable in the newborn period. Fluoroscopic assessment of diaphragmatic motion, which previously was the gold standard, largely has been replaced by ultrasound. Ultrasound with the use of M-mode is superior to fluoroscopy in the evaluation of the diaphragm because of its portability, lack of ionizing radiation, and ability to visualize the entire diaphragm (Fig. 61-6).[27] Diaphragmatic movement is considered normal if the diaphragm moves toward the transducer during inspiration, with excursion of greater than 4 mm and a difference in excursion between the domes of less than 50%.[16,17,26–28]

Treatment and Follow-up The initial treatment of patients with diaphragmatic paralysis is supportive, which includes positioning the affected patients ipsilateral to the affected side and providing oxygen and mechanical ventilation in cases of respiratory failure.[2,29] After 30 days of unsuccessful noninvasive treatment, plication usually is needed, especially in patients younger than 1 year and those with iatrogenic injuries of the phrenic nerve.[1,2,17,30]

DIAPHRAGMATIC RUPTURE

Etiology Diaphragmatic rupture, which is rare in children, typically occurs after a blunt or penetrating trauma. In a large study of 20,500 pediatric trauma patients, the incidence of traumatic diaphragmatic rupture was found to be 0.07%, with a mean age of 7.5 years.[31] It was slightly more frequent in boys and occurred more commonly as a result of blunt, rather than penetrating, trauma.[31] Associated injuries such as a head

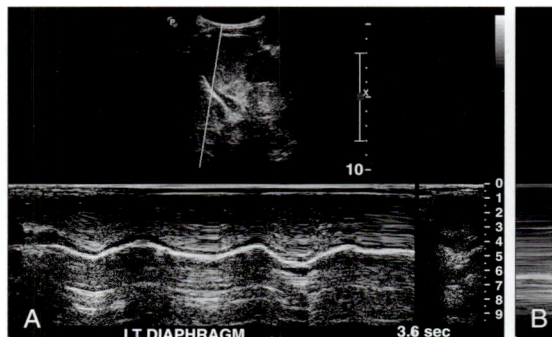
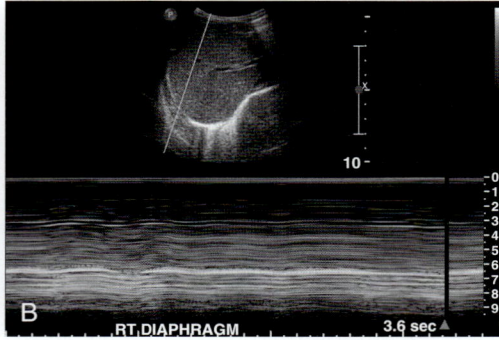

Figure 61-6 Diaphragmatic paralysis in a 10-month old boy after tetralogy of Fallot repair who was unable to be weaned from the ventilator. **A,** An ultrasound image using M-mode of the left hemidiaphragm reveals a normal diaphragmatic waveform. **B,** An ultrasound image using M-mode of the right hemidiaphragm reveals a flat waveform, indicating paralysis.

injury, pelvic fractures, and splenic and renal injuries are common. However, isolated diaphragmatic injuries have been reported more often in children than in adults. Diaphragmatic rupture is more common on the left than on the right. The left-sided predominance probably is the result of a protective effect by the liver on the right diaphragm.[32] Because of its rarity, the correct diagnosis of diaphragmatic rupture often is delayed or missed, often leading to intestinal obstruction and subsequent bowel ischemia.[31]

Imaging Diaphragmatic rupture in children is difficult to detect clinically and on imaging, and it requires a high index of suspicion.[31-33] Several studies show that chest radiographs have suggestive findings in 64% to 77% of cases; however, they are diagnostic in only 25% to 50% of cases.[33] Nonspecific but suggestive imaging findings of diaphragmatic rupture on chest radiographs include (1) an archlike soft tissue opacity in the lower chest; (2) unusual densities or gas bubbles resulting from bowel herniation; and (3) atelectasis, pleural effusions, and a mediastinal shift to the nonaffected side.[33] Imaging findings considered diagnostic of a diaphragmatic rupture after trauma are the presence of herniated abdominal organs (e.g., bowel loops or solid organs) and an NG tube in the chest (Fig. 61-7).[33] CT, especially coronal reformations, may confirm the diagnosis of diaphragmatic rupture by showing irregularity and thickening of the diaphragmatic leaflet and herniated abdominal organs.[32,33] Fluoroscopy and contrast studies have limited use in the acute setting.[34]

Treatment and Follow-up The treatment of diaphragmatic rupture is surgical, whether the patient presents in the acute or delayed setting. Repair of the acute traumatic diaphragmatic rupture is directed by other injuries that may be present. Small defects are repaired by direct suturing, whereas larger defects are patched with mesh.[1,32] Although fluoroscopy plays little role in the preoperative diagnosis of diaphragmatic rupture, it can be useful in assessing the diaphragm after repair to evaluate diaphragmatic motion and hernia recurrence.

Diaphragmatic Neoplasms

Etiology Primary diaphragmatic tumors are very rare.[17] In a study by Cada et al,[34] 41 cases were found in patients younger than 18 years with equal gender frequency and a mean age at diagnosis of 10 years. Most diaphragmatic tumors are malignant, with rhabdomyosarcoma being the most common tumor found in the diaphragm.[17,35] Other primary diaphragmatic malignant tumors in children are undifferentiated sarcomas, germ cell tumors, and the Ewing sarcoma family of tumors.[17,35-37] Secondary involvement of the diaphragm by adjacent malignant tumors also can occur.[17,35] Benign tumors include neurofibromas, lipomas, myofibroblastic tumors, and hemangiomas.[17] Cystic lesions (not necessarily neoplasms) involving the diaphragm include mesothelial cysts, bronchogenic cysts, cystic teratomas, and hydatid cysts.[17,38]

Affected patients—especially those with benign lesions—usually are asymptomatic, and the diagnosis of diaphragmatic neoplasm is made incidentally as part of unrelated imaging, at surgery, or even at autopsy. Patients with a large or malignant diaphragmatic tumor usually present with symptoms such as chest pain, cough, dyspnea, nausea, vomiting, and dysphagia.[17,35,37] An exophytic, large diaphragmatic tumor also may be palpable on physical examination.

Imaging The greatest challenge in assessing a diaphragmatic tumor is determining its exact site of origin. Especially on right-sided lesions, the site of origin frequently has been mistakenly assigned to the liver. No single imaging modality has demonstrated superiority in diagnosing diaphragmatic tumors, and frequently a combination of ultrasound, CT, and MRI is necessary for a correct diagnosis.[17,35] The majority of malignant tumors present as large masses with advanced local disease or metastasis to the pleura and lung.[36] The claw sign, the pattern of organ displacement, and the presence of an obtuse angle between the tumor and the diaphragm may help determine diaphragmatic origin (Fig. 61-8).[35] Not infrequently, the diaphragmatic origin of the tumor becomes more evident after size reduction following chemotherapy. In cases of a palpable mass or a mass seen on chest or abdominal radiographs, ultrasound may be the initial study of choice to begin the investigation. Ultrasound can confirm the presence of a mass and excludes the presence of a pleural effusion, which is one of main differential diagnostic considerations. To further evaluate the precise extent of the mass, including invasion to adjacent organs, cross-sectional imaging studies such as CT or MRI with two-dimensional and three-dimensional reconstructions can be of great value.[35]

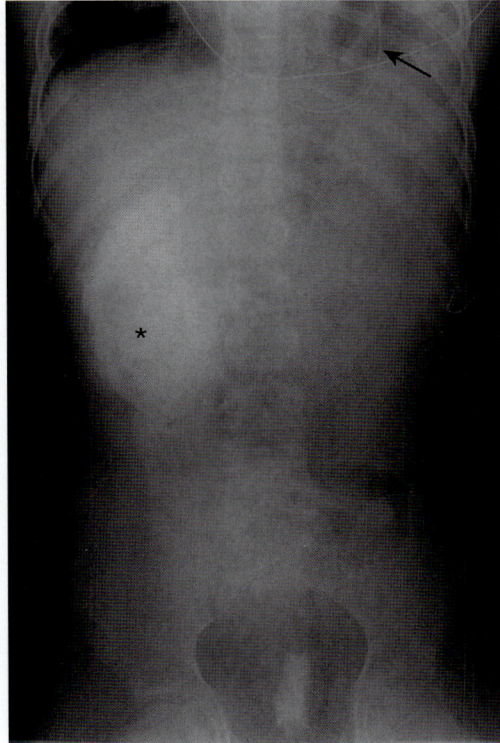

Figure 61-7 Diaphragmatic rupture in a 5-year-old boy who fell from playground equipment. An abdominal radiograph shows obliteration of the left hemidiaphragm with soft tissue and lucencies projecting in the left base. The tip (*arrow*) of a nasogastric tube projects in the chest, confirming a left diaphragmatic rupture. The hyperdensity in the right flank is due to perinephric intravenous contrast extravasation as a result of a shattered kidney (*asterisk*).

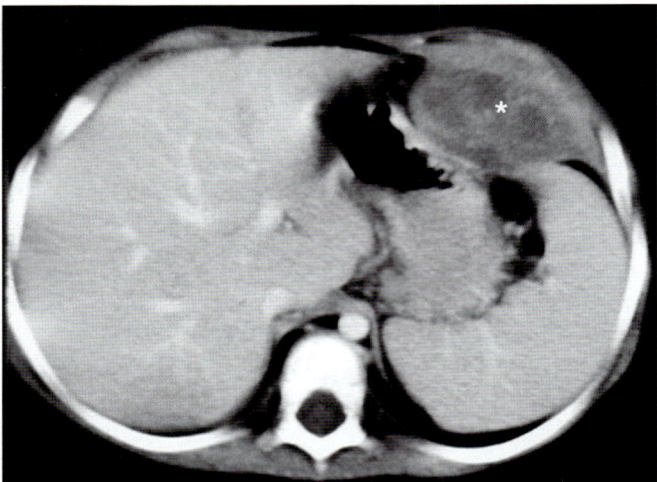

Figure 61-8 A germ cell tumor of the diaphragm in a 7-year-old boy with a palpable mass. An axial computed tomography image at the thoracoabdominal junction shows a heterogeneous anteriorly located mass (*asterisk*) with obtuse angles in relation to the diaphragm.

Treatment and Follow-up After imaging studies, a definitive diagnosis of diaphragmatic tumors can be made on the basis of histopathological evaluation of a biopsy specimen. Once a histopathological diagnosis is made, chemotherapy usually is instituted to reduce the size before surgical resection. Adjuvant preoperative radiation therapy may help in cases of infiltrative tumors. Germ cell tumors may go into remission after chemotherapy because of their high chemosensitivity.[17,35,36]

WHAT THE CLINICIAN NEEDS TO KNOW

- Types of CDHs, imaging appearances, and workup
- Clinical presentation and radiographic findings of late-onset CDH, diaphragmatic paralysis, and diaphragmatic rupture
- Potential complications of late-onset CDH and diaphragmatic rupture
- Types of tumors involving the diaphragm and their workup

Key Points

The Bochdalek hernia, which involves the posterolateral aspect of the diaphragm, is the most common subtype, accounting for approximately 90% to 95% of all CDHs.

The clinical presentation of late-onset CDH is varied and may require multiple imaging modalities to reach a diagnosis.

Ultrasound with M-mode is the imaging modality of choice to evaluate diaphragmatic paralysis.

The diagnosis of diaphragmatic rupture is usually delayed because of its rarity and multiple associated injuries, and it requires a high index of suspicion.

Primary diaphragmatic tumors are very rare in children. Most diaphragmatic tumors are malignant, with rhabdomyosarcoma being the most common diaphragmatic tumor.

Suggested Readings

Baglaj M, Dorobisz U. Late presenting congenital diaphragmatic hernia in children: a literature review. *Pediatr Radiol.* 2005;35:478-488.

Chavhan GB, Babyn PS, Chohen RA, et al. Multimodality imaging of the pediatric diaphragm: anatomy and pathologic conditions. *Radiographics.* 2010;30:1797-1817.

Mata JM, Caceres J. The dysmorphic lung: imaging findings. *Eur Radiol.* 1996;6:403-414.

Ramos CT, Koplewitz BZ, Babyn PS, et al. What have we learned about traumatic diaphragmatic hernias in children? *J Pediatr Surg.* 2000;35:601-604.

Schumpelick V, Steinau G, Schluper I, et al. Surgical embryology and anatomy of the diaphragm with surgical applications. *Surg Clin North Am* 2999;80:213-239.

References

Full references for this chapter can be found on www.expertconsult.com.

SECTION 5

Heart and Great Vessels

Chapter 62

Introductory Embryology

JAMES RENÉ HERLONG

Cardiac Development

The major task in cardiac development is to form a four-chambered heart that functions in a coordinated fashion from a straight tube that functions merely by peristalsis. Cardiac development can be thought of as proceeding along various phases: fusion of myocardium and endocardium in the ventral midline to form a simple tube, onset of function, looping to the right side, specification and formation of chambers, development of specialized conduction tissue, formation of the coronary circulation, innervation of the heart, and formation of mature valves. The approximate times at which these various events occur in human development are shown in Table 62-1.

Three main groups of cells contribute to the morphogenesis of the heart. These main groups are the mesoderm of the primary heart fields (located in the splanchnic layer of lateral plate mesoderm bilaterally), the secondary heart fields (located in the pharyngeal mesenchyme), and the cardiac neural crest (a subdivision of the cranial portion of the neural crest). These tissues and their roles in the developing heart are illustrated in e-Figure 62-1, along with the two important extracardiac populations of cells described later in this chapter.

The first stage in the development of the heart is the formation of a single midline heart tube from the bilateral cardiogenic fields. This process is illustrated in e-Figure 62-2. The heart begins to beat even at this single tubular stage. Cells are then added to each end of the heart tube, and the tube begins to loop to the right. During looping, the tube is further lengthened by the addition of cells from the secondary heart field to the outflow pole. Looping and convergence bring the inflow and outflow poles of the heart into proximity (Fig. 62-3), setting the stage for septation and definitive chamber formation. The traditional names of the various segments of the recently looped heart are illustrated in Figure 62-4. Note that the heart in this configuration is set up to become a double-inlet left ventricle and a double-outlet right ventricle; if septation proceeds properly, these forms of congenital heart disease are avoided. Formation of a four-chamber heart requires the right ventricle to obtain an inlet and the left ventricle to obtain an outlet.

The atrioventricular canal of the heart is divided into right and left sides by endocardial cushions that develop at the atrioventricular junction and ultimately form the septum of the atrioventricular canal and the atrioventricular valves (Fig. 62-5). The right atrioventricular canal and right ventricle expand to the right, and the atria are septated from one another. Septum primum, the primary atrial septum, is led by the spina vestibuli (vestibular spine) and ultimately fuses with the endocardial cushions to close the first interatrial communication, or ostium primum. As the septum primum is growing, fenestrations begin to develop within it. These fenestrations coalesce to form the secondary interatrial communication, or ostium secundum (see Fig. 62-5). A second septum, or septum secundum, forms to the right of the septum primum much later, and postnatal fusion of the two septa obliterates any interatrial communication. Note that septum primum is ultimately a left atrial structure and that septum secundum is considered a right atrial structure, even though it expresses left-sided molecular markers. Note further that, in the common parlance of naming atrial septal defects, the defect is named for the embryonic ostium that persists, not for the embryonic tissue in which the defect exists. Thus, for example, a secundum atrial septal defect is persistence of the embryonic ostium secundum, even though the defect itself is most often in the septum primum. This naming practice is one of the more confusing points in the nomenclature of congenital heart disease.

Just as the atria and the atrioventricular canal portions of the heart are septated, so are the ventricles. The muscular ventricular septum arises from the deepest convexity of the cardiac loop and grows toward the atrioventricular septum. The membranous septum ultimately will bridge the gap between these two portions of the septum. The outlet, conal, or infundibular septum (i.e., the portion of the septum that ultimately will lie just below the semilunar valves and between the outflow tracts) forms from the conal cushions. Initially it is mesenchymal and only later muscularizes. Ventricular septal defects tend to occur at the locations where these various primordia of the ventricular septum fuse.

The aorticopulmonary septum is derived from the cardiac neural crest and functions to separate the aortic sac into the aorta and pulmonary artery and to separate the truncus into the aortic and pulmonic valve orifices. This septum is contiguous proximally with the conal septum. The aorticopulmonary septation complex segregates the ventricular outflows from one another just as the septation of the atrioventricular canal segregates the ventricular inflows.

Table 62-1

Timing of the Onset of Various Events in Human Cardiovascular Development	
Event	**Gestational Age (wk)**
Formation of a heart tube	3
Aortic arches form	3
Onset of function	4
Looping	4
Onset of chamber septation	5
Development of specialized conduction tissue	5
Formation of the coronary circulation	5-6
Onset of innervation of the heart	7-8
Formation of mature valves	10
Definitive venous system established	12

The cardiac electrical system, which is composed of pacemaking cells and a specialized conduction system, develops from regions of specialized myocardial cells that are set aside from working myocardium for this purpose. One of the most important processes involved in the electrical coordination of cardiac function is the electrical isolation of the atria from the ventricles by the fibrous skeleton of the heart. Only the penetrating bundle of His normally electrically connects (via muscle to muscle) the atria and the ventricles. This atrioventricular discontinuity is established by the incorporation of nonmyocardial tissue into the atrioventricular junction.

The epicardium of the heart is derived from an extracardiac population of cells known as the proepicardium. These cells come from the mesenchyme of the septum transversum or liver and literally jump across the coelomic cavity to reach the heart (see e-Fig. 62-1). The proepicardium not only forms the definitive epicardium of the heart but also the endothelium and smooth muscles of the coronary arteries, as

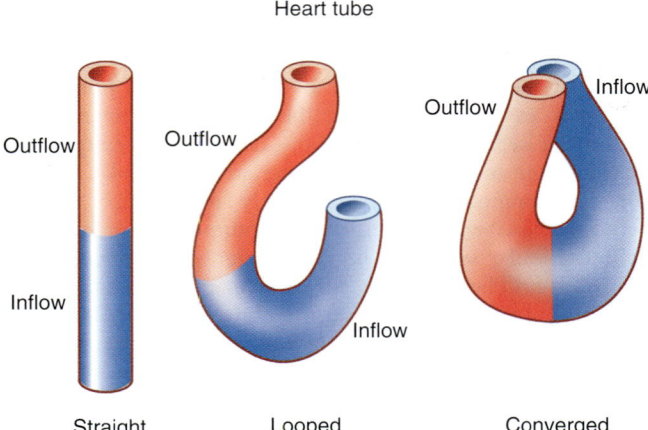

Heart tube

Figure 62-3   The heart tube begins as a straight midline tube with blood entering caudally via the inflow tract and exiting cranially via the outflow tract. Under normal circumstances, the tube loops to the right, creating an inflow limb (*blue*) and an outflow limb (*red*). The distal extremities of the inflow and outflow limbs grow toward each other in a process called *convergence*. Convergence is necessary before septation can create a four-chambered heart. (From Kirby ML. *Cardiac development.* New York: Oxford University Press; 2006.)

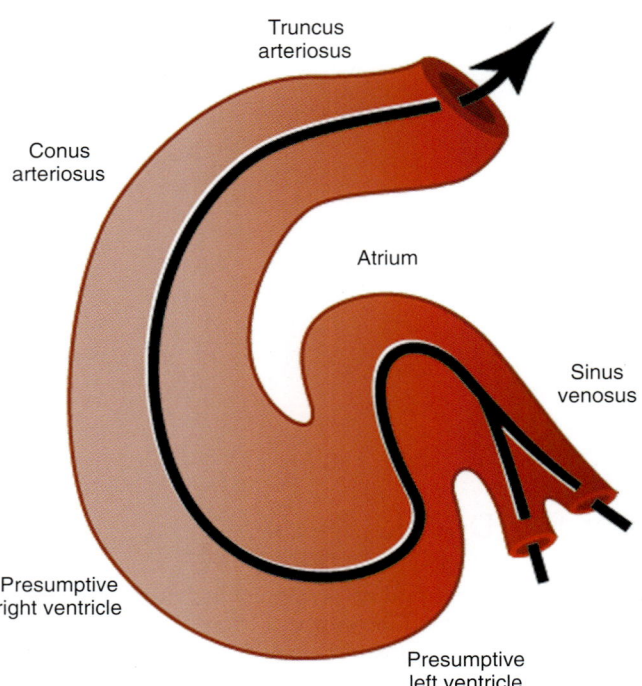

Figure 62-4   Traditional names of the various parts of the tubular heart. (From Kirby ML. *Cardiac development.* New York: Oxford University Press; 2006.)

well as the connective tissue of the heart. The formation of the coronary arteries and the connective tissue of the heart is made possible by a process known as epithelial to mesenchymal transformation. The epicardium of the outflow tract is distinct from that of the remainder of the heart and is derived from the splanchnic mesoderm of the ventral pharynx. Because of the diversity of cells that the proepicardium provides, many investigators consider the proepicardium to be an important potential source of cardiac stem cells.

Before the development of the coronary arteries, the loosely packed myocardium of the embryonic heart is nourished from the cavities by sinusoids. As the myocardium becomes more compact, arteries and veins develop within the epicardial layer, with the intramyocardial circulation developing within the myocardium itself. The arterial channels then grow into the developing aortic valvar sinuses to form true coronary arteries arising from the aorta.

Innervation of the heart is a late development and is not complete until well after birth. Parasympathetic ganglia are intrinsic to the heart and develop from the cardiac neural crest. Sympathetic ganglia are paravertebral and develop from the truncal neural crest. All postganglionic neurons develop from the cardiac neural crest.

The final step in cardiac development is sculpting of the endocardial cushions at the ventricular inflow and outflow to form functional valves. This process occurs at the atrioventricular junction by undermining of the cell layers just underneath the luminal cells to free the leaflets from the myocardium and to create the support apparatus (papillary muscles and chordae tendineae) of the valves. At the ventriculoarterial junction, the sculpting occurs distal to the cushions themselves, and no such support apparatus is formed.

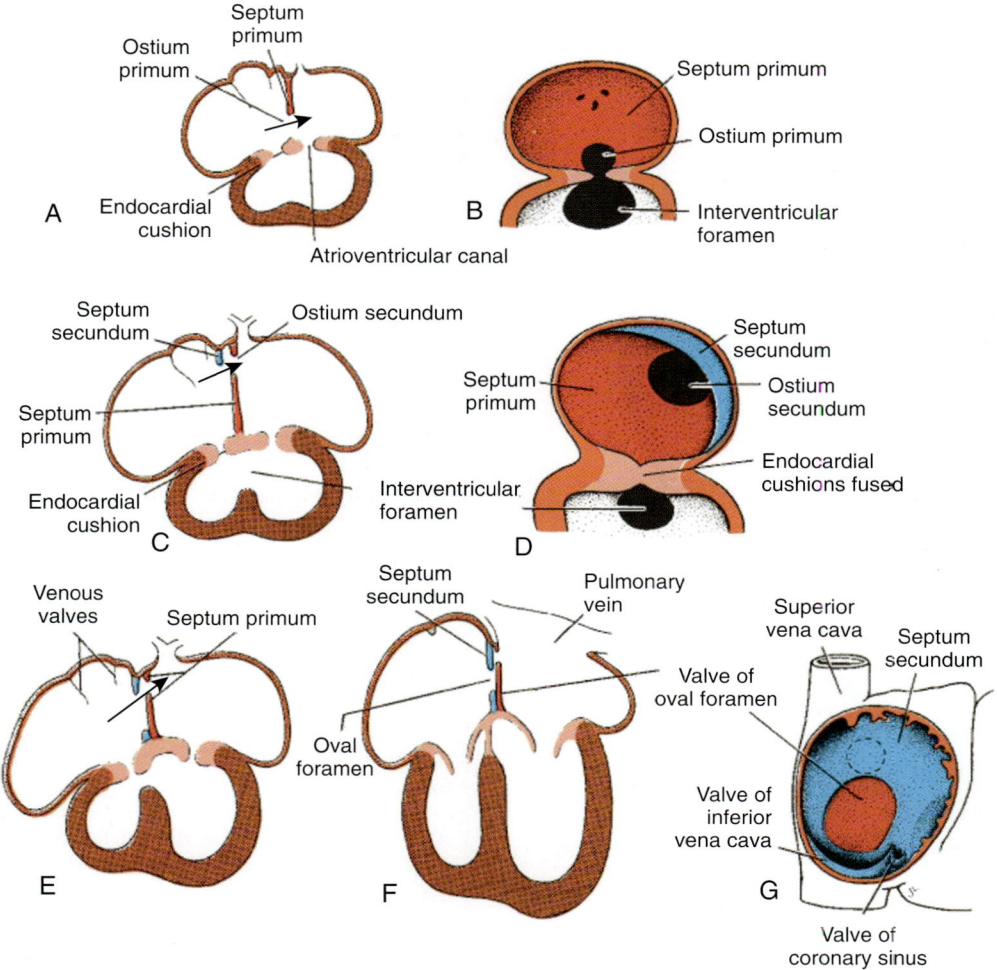

Figure 62-5 **A-G,** Development of the atrial septum. **A** (cross sectional) and **B** (en face from the right atrium) show the atrial septum at 30 days of gestation. **C** (cross sectional) and **D** (en face from the right atrium) show the atrial septum at 33 days of gestation. **E** shows the atrial septum at 37 days of gestation. **F** (cross sectional) and **G** (en face from the right atrium) show the atrial septum immediately after birth. (From Sadler T. *Langman's medical embryology.* 10th ed. Philadelphia: Lippincott Williams & Wilkins; 2004.)

Vascular Development

The arteries and veins are developed by a combination of vasculogenesis and angiogenesis. Vasculogenesis occurs first to form the major arteries and veins, and vessels sprout from these larger vessels by angiogenesis. The vasculature of the embryo begins as a bilaterally symmetric system of arteries and veins. This symmetry is maintained in the head and limbs as well as in the derivatives of the somites and spinal cord.

The central vessels, however, lose their symmetry and are extensively remodeled. The great arteries begin as bilaterally symmetric, paired arch arteries that connect the ventral aortic sac to the bilateral dorsal aortae. These symmetrical arch arteries undergo involution and remodeling to form the aortic arch, arch vessels, main and branch pulmonary arteries, and the ductus arteriosus (e-Fig. 62-6). This patterning is supported by cells from the cardiac neural crest. Abnormal arterial remodeling leads to aberrant origins of arch arteries and to vascular rings. To understand the embryonic origin of various arch anomalies, it is useful to consider a "totipotential arch" that includes all the relevant arch arteries and

imagine how this arch may be "cut" to produce each anomaly. The "totipotential arch" is a theoretic construct. Such an arch never exists in fetal life; because of involution and remodeling, all of the represented components never exist simultaneously. However, the concept (illustrated in Fig. 62-7) is quite useful in understanding how various arch anomalies occur and which of them produce vascular rings.

The embryonic venous system is also extensively remodeled. Originally there are bilaterally symmetric vitelline, umbilical, and cardinal systems. The original systems drain to ipsilateral horns of the sinus venosus portion of the developing heart. Because the left sinus horn regresses and systemic venous return is directed solely to the right atrium, the left system of veins must involute or form anastomotic connections with the right system. The inferior vena cava is composed of elements of four separate systems (e-Fig. 62-8). When the inferior vena cava is interrupted, as in cases of the polysplenic form of heterotaxy, bilateral symmetry of all but the intrahepatic portion is largely maintained. The inferior venous drainage then proceeds to one or both superior venae cavae via azygous or hemiazygous veins.

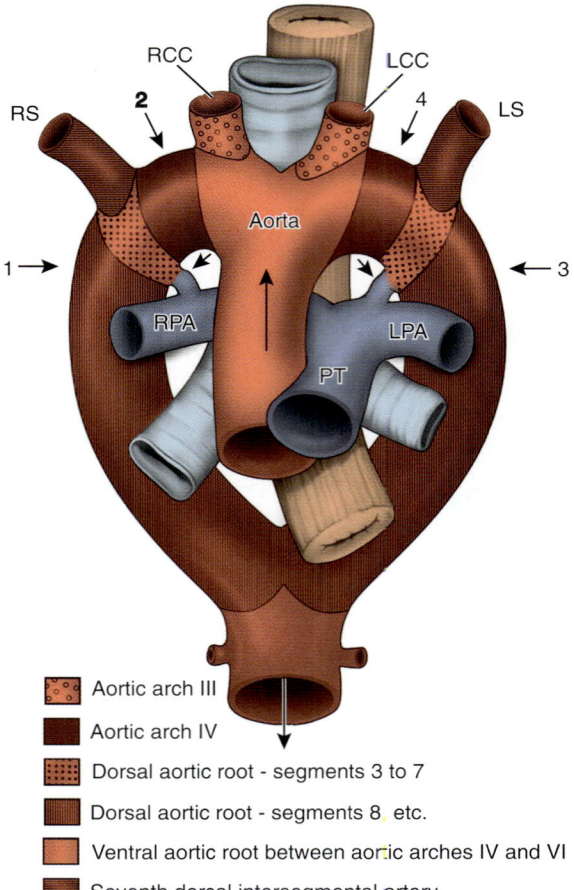

▦	Aortic arch III
▦	Aortic arch IV
▦	Dorsal aortic root - segments 3 to 7
▦	Dorsal aortic root - segments 8 etc.
▦	Ventral aortic root between aortic arches IV and VI
▦	Seventh dorsal intersegmental artery

Figure 62-7 Ventral view of Dr. Jesse Edward's "totipotential arch" or hypothetic double aortic arch and bilateral ductus arteriosi. The numbered arrows point to the four key locations where regression occurs in various anomalies. Arrow 1 indicates the eighth segment of the right dorsal aortic root; arrow 2, the right fourth arch; and arrows 3 and 4, the corresponding two positions on the left. The small black arrows point to the ductus arteriosi bilaterally, and the larger black arrows indicate the direction of blood flow. *LCC,* Left subclavian artery; *LPA,* left pulmonary artery; *LS,* left subclavian artery; *PT,* pulmonary trunk; *RCC,* right common carotid artery; *RPA,* right pulmonary artery; *RS,* right subclavian artery. (From Stewart JR, Kincaid OW, Edwards JE. *An atlas of vascular rings and related malformations of the aortic arch system.* Springfield, IL: Charles C. Thomas; 1964.)

The head and neck veins derive from the anterior cardinal veins. The left anterior cardinal vein involutes, and anastomotic channels drain the left head, neck, and arm to the remnants of the right anterior cardinal system and ultimately to the heart by the right superior vena cava. A persistent left superior vena cava is a common variant of normal. This vein drains into the coronary sinus, which is a remnant of the left horn of the sinus venosus.

The pulmonary veins form from fusion of the veins developing in the mesoderm surrounding the bronchial buds with the common pulmonary vein that develops as an evagination of the developing left atrium. Prior to this fusion, connections of the developing pulmonary veins to the systemic venous system are formed. These connections persist as "vertical veins" when atresia of the common pulmonary vein occurs, a condition known more commonly as totally anomalous pulmonary venous connection.

To understand common associations in congenital malformations, it is important to realize that the heart develops in close juxtaposition to the forebrain, face, and anterior neck as part of what has been called the cardiocraniofacial field. The simultaneous occurrence of defects in these other organ systems with congenital heart defects therefore is not surprising.

Acknowledgement

I thank Dr. Margaret L. Kirby for her lucid teaching, her patience with this clinician, her sharing of figures, her review of this manuscript, and her enormous contributions to the field of cardiovascular development.

Key Points

Looping and convergence of the primitive heart tube set the stage for cardiac septation and definitive chamber formation.

Atrial septal defects are named for the embryonic ostium that persists, not for the embryonic tissue in which the defect exists.

The proepicardium gives rise to a very diverse population of cells and is an important potential source of cardiac stem cells.

The vasculature of the head, limbs, and derivatives of the somites maintains its embryonic symmetry, whereas the central vessels are remodeled extensively.

Suggested Readings

Bogers AJJC, Gittenberger-de Groot AC, Poelmann RE, et al. Development of the origin of the coronary arteries, a matter of ingrowth or outgrowth. *Anat Embryol (Berl).* 1989;180:437-441.

Harvey RP, Rosenthal N, eds. *Heart development.* San Diego, CA: Academic Press; 1998.

Horsthuis T, Christoffels VM, Anderson RH, et al. Can recent insights into cardiac development improve our understanding of congenitally malformed hearts? *Clin Anat.* 2009;22:4-20.

Hutson MR, Kirby ML. Neural crest and cardiovascular development: a 20-year perspective, *Birth Defects Res.* 2003;69:2-13.

Kirby ML. *Cardiac development.* New York: Oxford University Press; 2007.

Moorman AFM, Christoffels VM. Cardiac chamber formation: development, genes and evolution. *Physiol Rev.* 2003;83:1223-1267.

Wessels A, Pérez-Pomares JM. The epicardium and epicardially derived cells (EPDCs) as cardiac stem cells. *Anat Rec A Discov Mol Cell Evol Biol.* 2004;276(1):43-57.

Chapter 63

Cardiovascular Anatomy and Segmental Approach to Imaging of Congenital Heart Disease

RAJESH KRISHNAMURTHY

Because of the large variety of human hearts in nature, a standardized approach and nomenclature are needed to understand and describe cardiac anatomy and physiology in the setting of congenital heart disease (CHD). The most widely used approach is the segmental approach to heart disease, which was first proposed by Richard Van Praagh in 1972 and later modified by others. It is strongly rooted in embryologic principles and follows a logical sequence from evaluation of cardiac morphology and physiology to treatment decision making.

Embryologic Basis for the Segmental Approach to Heart Disease

Embryology of the heart is covered in Chapter 62. In this chapter, some embryologic events that are fundamental to understanding the segmental approach to heart disease are reiterated.

The heart develops from two simple epithelial tubes that fuse to form a single tube (Fig. 63-1) with the following components:

Sinus venosus consists of right and left horns. Each horn receives blood from three important veins: the umbilical vein, the common cardinal vein, and the vitelline vein.

Paired primitive atria will later fuse to form a common atrium.

The atrioventricular (AV) sulcus divides the common atrium and the primitive ventricle.

The primitive ventricle becomes the left ventricle (LV).

The interventricular sulcus divides the primitive ventricle and the bulbus cordis.

The bulbus cordis may be divided as follows: the proximal third gives rise to the body of the right ventricle (RV). The distal-most section is the truncus arteriosus, which develops into the aortic root and part of the pulmonary artery (PA). The remaining mid portion is the conus cordis, which connects the primitive RV to the truncus arteriosus. The conus cordis partitions to form the outflow tracts of the RV and LV.

Although the two ends of the heart tube remain relatively fixed, rapid growth of the middle section results in the development of a large S-shaped curve called the *bulboventricular loop* (see Fig. 63-1). As the heart tube grows and becomes longer, it usually bends to the right, termed *D-looping* by Van Praagh. D-looping is responsible for the proximal bulbus cordis (RV) lying anterior and to the right of the primitive ventricle (LV). If the heart tube loops to the left, termed *L-looping,* the RV will lie anterior and to the left of the LV.

In the heart tube stage, the primitive LV and the proximal bulbus cordis (primitive RV) are separated from the truncus arteriosus (which gives rise to both great arteries) by the conus or infundibulum. The conus consists of the subpulmonary and subaortic conus cushions. Normally, expansile growth of the subpulmonary conus occurs, causing it to protrude anteriorly on the left, carrying the pulmonary valve anteriorly, superiorly, and to the left of the aortic valve. Resorption of the subaortic conus occurs. Hence the aortic valve lies posterior, inferior, and right-sided, in direct fibrous contiguity with the mitral valve (Fig. 63-2). The anterior pulmonary artery rises above the anterior ventricle (RV) and leads to the posterior sixth arterial arch, which forms the branch pulmonary arteries. The posterior aorta originates above the posterior LV and leads to the anterior fourth arterial arch (which forms the aortic arch).

The segmental approach involves the analysis of the three major cardiac segments: atria, ventricles, and great arteries, along with the two connecting segments: the AV canal and the conotruncus. These segments of the heart can be distinguished in the very early embryo. Some important embryologic concepts underlie the segmental approach to heart disease:

1. The development of the suprahepatic portion of the inferior vena cava (IVC) is closely linked to the growth of the liver, and thus the anatomic right atrium (RA) and the liver almost invariably develop on the same side of the body. This concept of visceroatrial situs is fundamental to the segmental approach.
2. Ventricular looping is independent of the visceroatrial situs. This phenomenon gives rise to the concept of concordance (RA-RV and left atrium [LA]-LV) and discordance (RA-LV and LA-RV).

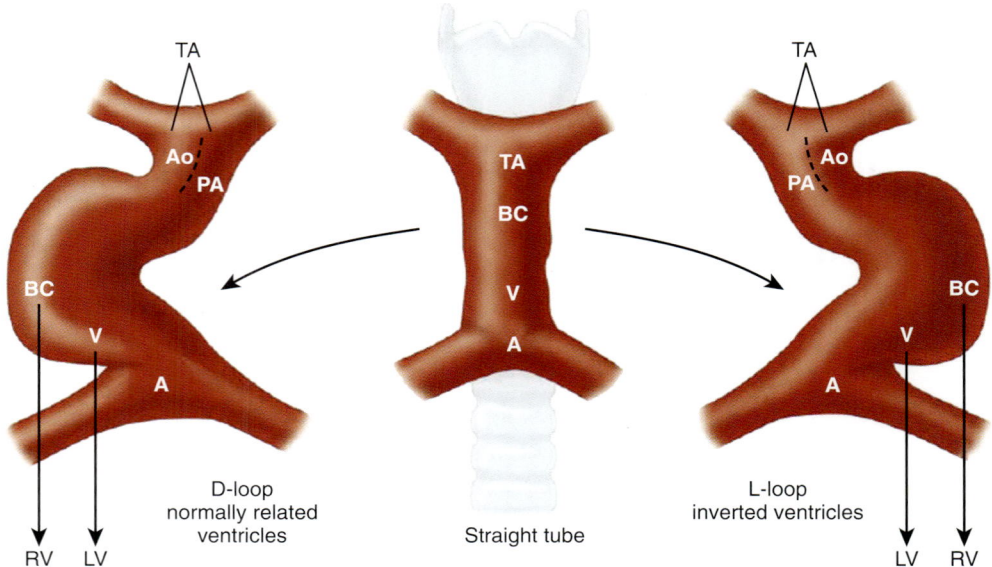

Figure 63-1 Bulboventricular looping of the primitive heart tube may occur to the right (D-looping) or to the left (L-looping). *Ao,* aorta; *BC,* bulbus cordis; *LV,* left ventricle; *PA,* pulmonary artery; *RV,* right ventricle. (Modified from Van Praagh R, Weinberg PM, Matsuoka R, et al. Malposition of the heart and the segmental approach to diagnosis. In: Adams FH, Emmanouilides GC, eds. *Moss' heart diseases in infants, children and adolescents.* 3rd ed. Baltimore: Williams & Wilkins, 1983.)

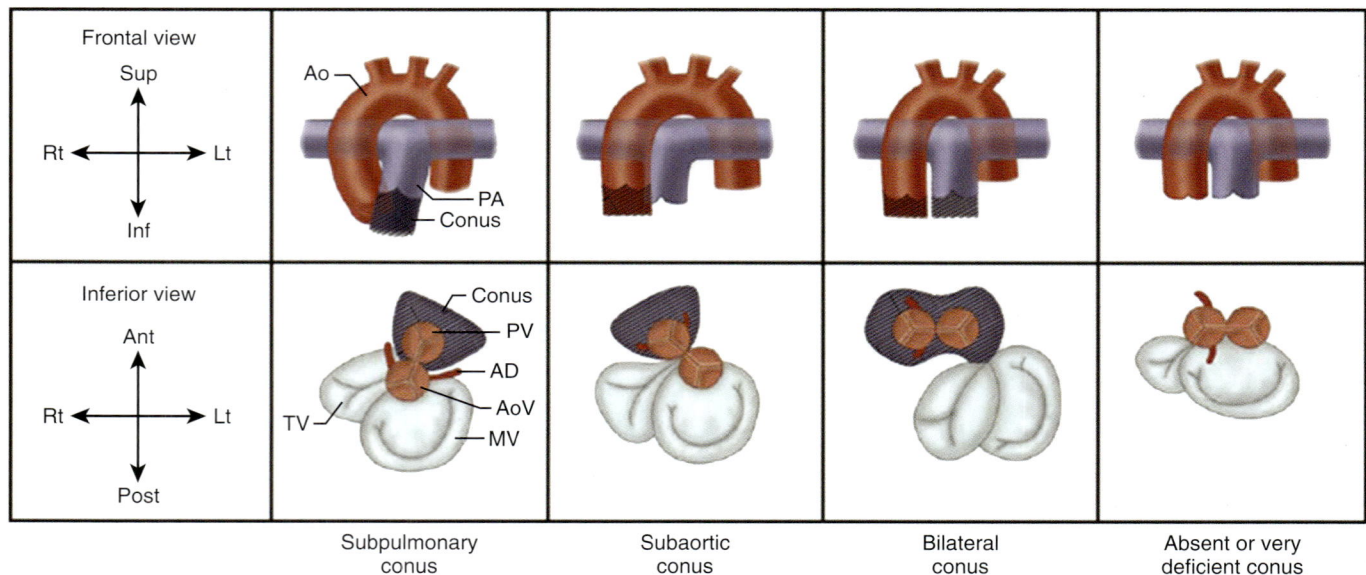

Figure 63-2 Normal and abnormal conal development. **A,** Subpulmonary conus seen in normally related great arteries. **B,** Subaortic conus in typical transposition of the great arteries. **C,** Bilateral conus, as in double-outlet right ventricle. **D,** Absent or deficient conus, as in double-outlet left ventricle. On the side of the conus, the semilunar valve sits atop the muscular infundibulum, and no direct fibrous contiguity exists between the semilunar valve and the atrioventricular (AV) valve. On the side of the deficient conus, direct fibrous contiguity usually exists between the AV valve and the semilunar valve. *Ant,* anterior; *Ao,* aorta; *AoV,* aortic valve; *Inf,* inferior; *Lt,* left; *MV,* mitral valve; *PA,* pulmonary artery; *Post,* posterior; *PV,* pulmonary valve; *Rt,* right; *Sup,* superior; *TV,* tricuspid valve. (Modified from Van Praagh R, Weinberg PM, Matsuoka R, et al. Malposition of the heart and the segmental approach to diagnosis. In: Adams FH, Emmanouilides GC, editors: *Moss' heart diseases in infants, children and adolescents.* 3rd ed. Baltimore: Williams & Wilkins; 1983.)

3. Ventricular looping and the great arterial relationship are independent entities. The direction of bulboventricular looping and the development of the conotruncus are responsible for the ultimate relationship of the great arteries to each other and to the underlying ventricles and AV valves.

Segmental Approach to Diagnosis of Congenital Heart Disease

Any imaginable combination of visceral, atrial, ventricular, and great vessel morphology can and does occur in CHD. A simple, logical, step-by-step approach to diagnosis and

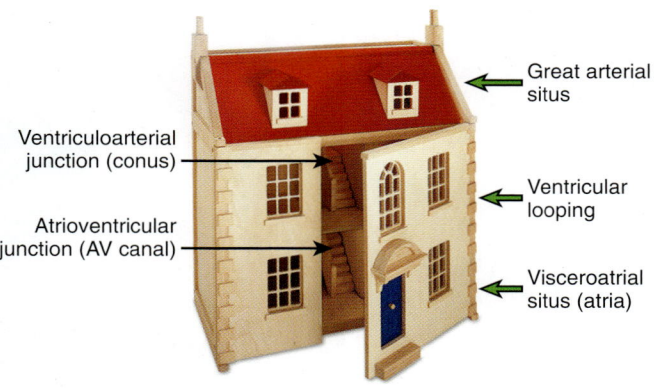

Great arterial
situs

Ventriculoarterial
junction (conus)

Ventricular
looping

Atrioventricular
junction (AV canal)

Visceroatrial
situs (atria)

Figure 63-3 The "house" model of the heart. The three levels (major cardiac segments) are the atria, ventricles, and great arteries. The house has two connecting walls with doors (connecting segments): the atrio-ventricular junction and the ventriculoarterial junction. The house has two entrances: the systemic veins and the pulmonary veins.

decision making and a standardized nomenclature go a long way in advancing patient care by ensuring that different caregivers have similar understanding of the disease and are speaking the same language.

One can think of the heart as a three-level house (Fig. 63-3). The first level is the visceroatrial situs, the middle level is the ventricular loop, and the third level is the conotruncus. To describe it simply, the three levels are the atria, ventricles, and great arteries. The heart has two staircases: the AV ventricular junction and the ventriculoarterial junction. The levels represent the major cardiac segments. The staircases represent the connecting segments.

The segmental approach to heart disease comprises the following steps:
1. What is the anatomic type of each of the three major cardiac segments: the atria, the ventricles, and the great arteries?
2. How is each segment connected to the adjacent segment?
3. What are the associated anomalies involving the valves, atrial and ventricular septum, the great vessels, and the systemic and pulmonary veins?
4. How do the segmental combinations and connections, with or without the associated malformations, *function*?

The first three steps in the segmental approach are concerned with morphology, whereas the last step concerns physiology.

Van Praagh used a segmental set to provide a shorthand description of the floor plan of the heart. The first letter stands for the visceroatrial situs, the second for the ventricular loop, and the third for the great arterial relationship. In a person with situs solitus of the viscera and atria, D-looping of the ventricles, and solitus relationship of the great arteries, the segmental set is {S,D,S}.

Identification of the Major Cardiac Segments

Reliable identification of the cardiac chambers based on specific morphologic features is the first step in the segmental

approach to heart disease. It is important to remember that right and left do not refer to the side of the body on which the chamber lies but to specific morphologic criteria that identify each component of the heart. For instance, "right atrium" does not refer to the atrium that is on the right side of the body but to the atrium that receives the insertion of the IVC and the coronary sinus and has a triangular append-age with a broad base. Hence the morphologic RA will be on the right side of the body in persons with situs solitus and on the left side in persons with situs inversus.

ATRIAL IDENTIFICATION

The defining features of the morphologic RA (systemic venous atrium) and LA (pulmonary venous atrium) are based on their venous connections, as well as their appendage and pectinate muscle morphology. Using venoatrial connections for atrial identification is based on the fact that the sinus venosus, which carries the systemic venous return, is an integral part of the morphologic RA. Hence the morphologic RA receives the IVC and the superior vena cava (SVC) and the orifice of the coronary sinus. However, the SVC and coronary sinus have a high incidence of variation, which can be a source of diagnostic confusion. These variations include left SVC to an unroofed coronary sinus and bilateral SVC with the left SVC draining to an unroofed coronary sinus. In these cases, the SVC would appear to drain into the LA. In rare instances, even the IVC may drain into the coronary sinus, which may be unroofed, or the coronary sinus septum may be absent. In spite of this rare exception, the most reliable means of identifying the morphologic RA by cross-sectional imaging is by recognizing its connection to the IVC (Fig. 63-4). Even in the setting of an interrupted IVC, a suprahepatic segment of the IVC is present entering the RA, allowing accurate identification.

The morphologic LA is defined as the atrium that receives all or half of the pulmonary veins and none of the systemic veins (except an SVC to an unroofed coronary sinus). The LA is also the chamber that may receive no veins at all (in the setting of total anomalous pulmonary venous return). When all systemic veins and part or all of the pulmonary veins drain into one atrium, this atrium represents the morphologic RA.

Anderson has described the morphologic RA (systemic atrium) as being characterized by the presence of a triangular appendage with a broad junction and by the recognition of pectinate muscles extending to the AV junction. The morphologic LA is characterized by a tubular narrow-based appendage and lack of pectinate muscle extension. Because determination of pectinate muscle morphology is beyond the resolution of magnetic resonance imaging (MRI) or computed tomography (CT), atrial identification is performed by recognition of venoatrial connections and morphology of the appendages. If this analysis fails to yield a confident identification of the RA and LA, then a diagnosis of atrial situs ambiguous is made. Even in the setting of visceral situs ambiguous, reliable identification of atrial situs may be made in more than 80% of cases.

VENTRICULAR IDENTIFICATION

Ventricles are defined by their morphologic features, not by their spatial relationships. The morphologic RV is defined by the following features:

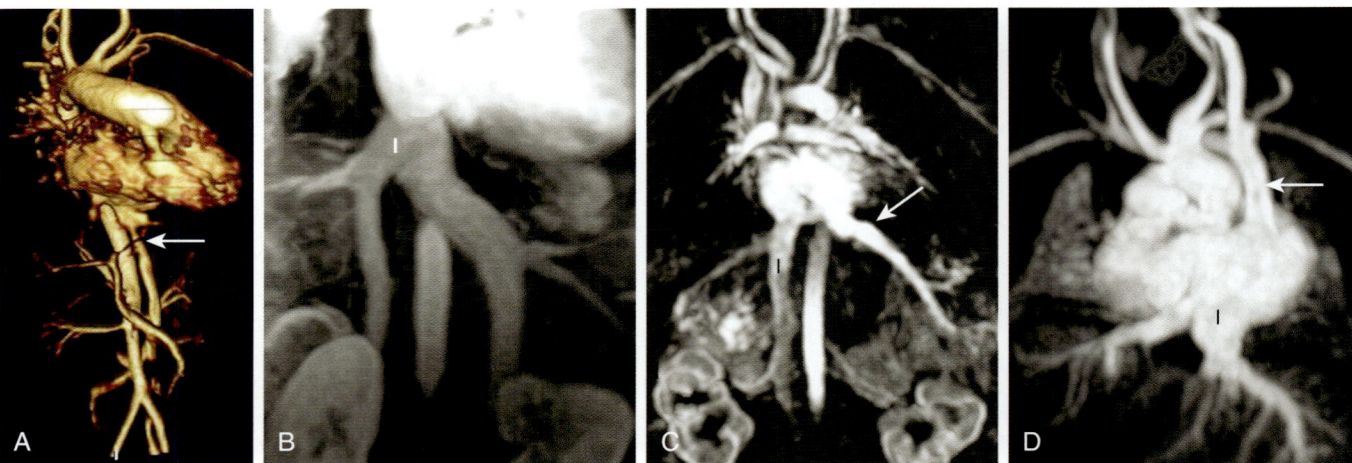

Figure 63-4   The inferior vena cava (IVC) as a marker of the morphologic right atrium (RA). **A,** The IVC (*arrow*) and aorta are on the left and the IVC enters the left-sided atrium, which represents the morphologic RA. **B,** Bilateral IVC that fuse (*I*) prior to entering the right atrium. **C,** The right hepatic vein enters the IVC (*I*), which drains into the RA, while the remaining hepatic veins (*arrow*) drain separately into the left atrium. **D,** Left sided-interrupted IVC with azygos continuation. A suprahepatic segment of the IVC (*I*) drains into the left-sided right atrium in this patient with atrial situs inversus. A left superior vena cava also is present (*arrow*).

1. Muscular connection between the free wall and the interventricular septum (moderator band) (Fig. 63-5, *A*)
2. The septal attachment of the AV valve of the RV (tricuspid valve) is more apically placed relative to the LV (Fig. 63-5, *B*)

3. Presence of a conus/infundibulum; the infundibulum is identified as a muscular cone of tissue that separates the AV valve from the semilunar valve on the same side, resulting in a lack of fibrous contiguity between the two valves (Fig. 63-5, *C*)

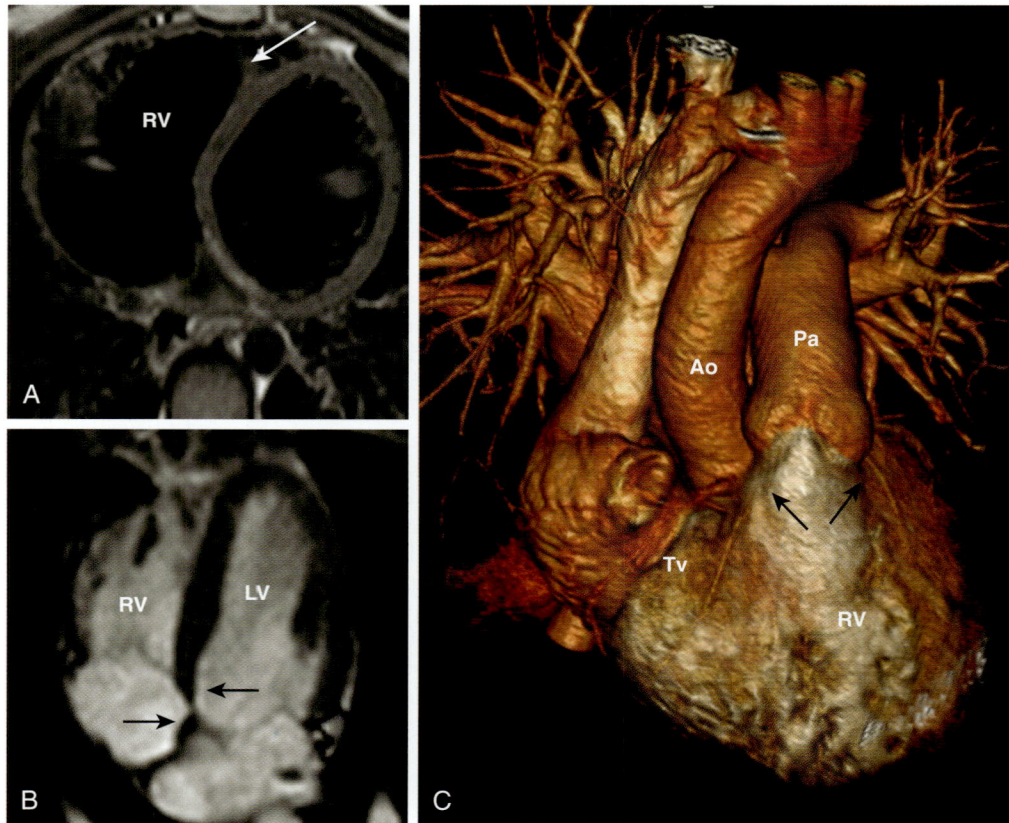

Figure 63-5   Right ventricular identification. **A,** Moderator band of the right ventricle (*RV*) (*arrow*). **B,** The atrioventricular (AV) valve of the RV (tricuspid valve) is more apically displaced (*arrow*) than the AV valve of the left ventricle (*LV*) (mitral valve) (*arrow*). **C,** The conus (*arrows*) is a marker of the RV. It is a muscular cone of tissue that separates the AV valve (*Tv*) from the semilunar (pulmonary) valve on the same side. *Ao,* Aorta; *Pa,* pulmonary artery.

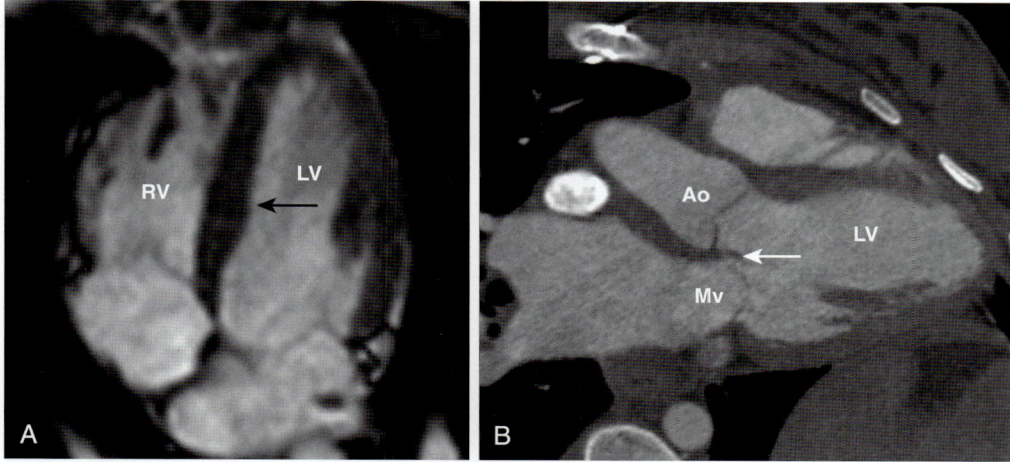

Figure 63-6 **Left ventricular identification. A,** Smooth septal surface of the left ventricle (*LV*) (*arrow*). **B,** The LV does not have a conus, resulting in mitral (*Mv*) to aortic (*Ao*) fibrous contiguity (*arrow*). *RV,* Right ventricle.

The morphologic LV is identified by the following features:

1. Smooth surface of the interventricular septum without any muscular attachments to the free wall (Fig. 63-6)
2. The septal attachment of the AV valve of the LV (mitral valve) is more cranially located relative to the RV (see Fig. 63-6, *B*)
3. Absence of a conus/infundibulum, resulting in fibrous contiguity between the AV valve and the semilunar valve on that side (see Fig. 63-6)

The AV valves follow the ventricle rather than the atrium. Thus the tricuspid valve is related to the morphologic RV and the mitral valve is related to the morphologic LV. The tricuspid valve typically has papillary muscle attachments to the right ventricular septal surface (septophilic valve), whereas the mitral valve is septophobic and only attaches to the free wall of the LV.

Neither the shape of the ventricle nor the degree of trabeculation or hypertrophy is considered a reliable marker for ventricular identification, because they frequently are affected by pressure or volume changes.

GREAT ARTERIAL IDENTIFICATION

The pulmonary artery gives rise to branches to the lungs and no branches to the body. The aorta gives rise to branches to the body as well as the coronary arteries. A common vessel arising from the ventricles that gives rise to the coronaries and branches to the body as well the lungs is termed a *common arterial trunk* or *truncus,* and a segmental relationship is not assigned (labeled "X" for undetermined). On transverse cross-sectional imaging at the level of the outflow tract, the coronary artery origin is used to identify the aortic annulus. The intercoronary commissure of the aortic valve is pointed toward the right-left commissure of the pulmonary valve and is an important landmark for determining great arterial relationship (Fig. 63-7). In a solitus relationship of the great arteries, the aortic valve annulus lies posterior and to the right of the pulmonary valve annulus.

Analysis of the Three Major Cardiac Segments

FIRST MAJOR SEGMENT: VISCEROATRIAL SITUS

Situs refers to the position of the atria and viscera relative to the midline. Three types of situs exist: solitus (S), inversus (I), and ambiguous (A) (Fig. 63-8). Heterotaxy is synonymous with situs ambiguous.

Visceral situs solitus is characterized by the presence of a right-sided liver, a single or dominant left-sided spleen, a three-lobed right lung with an eparterial bronchus, and a two-lobed left lung with a hyparterial bronchus. Atrial situs solitus is characterized by the presence of the systemic venous atrium on the right and the pulmonary venous atrium on the left. Situs inversus is defined as the "mirror image" of situs solitus. Hence visceral situs inversus is characterized by a left-sided liver, a single or dominant right-sided spleen, a three-lobed left lung with an eparterial bronchus, and a two-lobed right lung with a hyparterial bronchus. Atrial situs inversus is characterized by the presence of the systemic venous atrium on the left and the pulmonary venous atrium on the right. Although the location of the cardiac apex and the stomach is usually on the left in persons with situs solitus and on the right in persons with situs inversus, they are not considered reliable markers of visceral situs because of the high incidence of variation in the setting of normal situs.

Because heterotaxy is defined as "situs other than solitus or inversus," it is not a specific disease but a constellation of cardiac, vascular, and visceral abnormalities, including situs ambiguous of the viscera, lung symmetry, atrial appendage symmetry, anomalous systemic venous return, anomalous pulmonary venous return, and associated intracardiac defects. No single finding is pathognomonic. A tendency exists to cluster defects into two syndromes based on the predominance of right-sided or left-sided structures:

1. Asplenia complex—Manifestations include bilateral three-lobed lungs with eparterial bronchi, a transverse or symmetric liver, a bilateral SVC, and bilateral triangular broad-based atrial appendages. The spleen is absent.

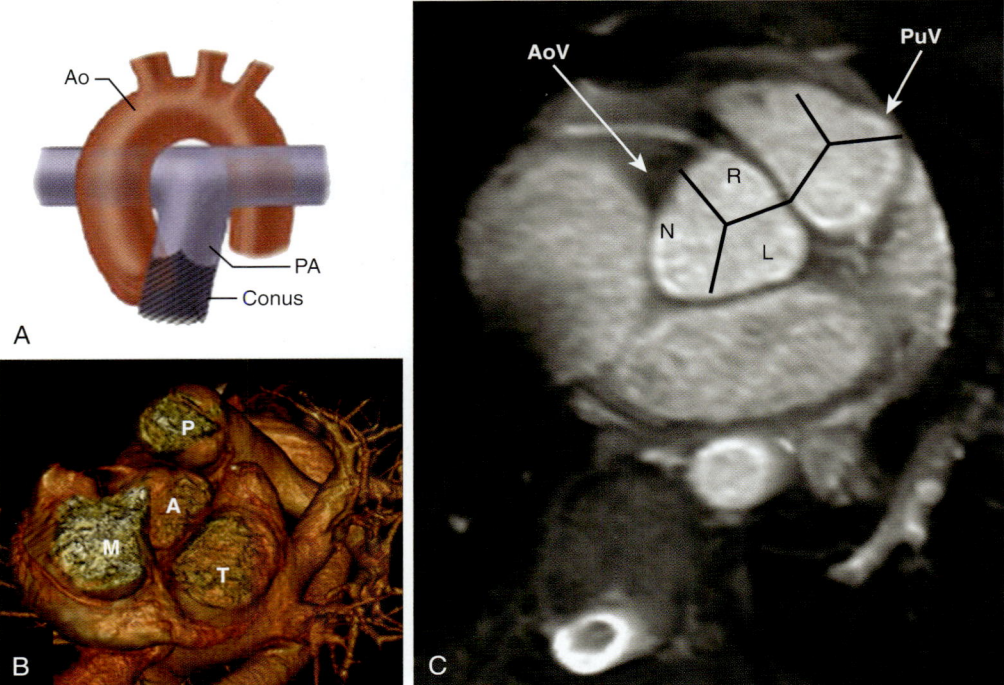

Figure 63-7   **A,** Solitus (normal) relationship of the great arteries. **B,** Three-dimensional view of the heart from above. The aortic valve (A) has direct fibrous contiguity with the mitral (M) and tricuspid (T) valves, whereas the pulmonary valve (P) lies ventrally, and is separated from the atrioventricular valves by the conus. **C,** The aortic valve annulus (AoV) lies posterior and to the right of the pulmonary valve annulus (PuV). The intercoronary commissure of the aortic valve is pointed toward the right-left commissure of the pulmonary valve. Ao, Aorta; L, left sinus of Valsalva; N, noncoronary sinus of Valsalva; PA, pulmonary artery; R, right sinus of Valsalva.

2. Polysplenia complex—Manifestations include bilateral two-lobed lungs with hyparterial bronchi, a transverse liver, multiple splenic fragments, and bilateral tubular atrial appendages. The renal to hepatic segment of the IVC is frequently absent, with associated azygos continuation.
3. Van Praagh has added a third syndrome of heterotaxy manifested by levocardia with a single right-sided spleen. Features of this syndrome are similar to that of right isomerism.

The use of the terms *atrial isomerism, bilateral right-sidedness,* or *bilateral left-sidedness* as substitutes for the syndromes of situs ambiguous is discouraged because they are semantically inaccurate representations of the anatomy found in these patients.

SECOND MAJOR SEGMENT: VENTRICULAR LOOP

Depending on the direction of ventricular looping during development, the RV may be located spatially on the right or left side of the heart (Fig. 63-9). If the bulboventricular loop occurs to the right, it is termed a *D-loop,* and the morphologic RV lies anterior and to the right of the morphologic LV. If the bulboventricular loop occurs to the left, it is termed an *L-loop,* and the morphologic RV lies anterior and to the left of the morphologic LV.

THIRD MAJOR SEGMENT: GREAT ARTERIAL RELATIONSHIP

Normally the aortic annulus lies posterior, inferior, and to the right of the pulmonary valve annulus. This position is called *solitus* (S) (Fig. 63-10, *A*). In situs inversus, the aorta lies posterior and to the left of the pulmonary valve, termed *inversus* (I) (Fig. 63-10, *B*). Any other position of the aorta and pulmonary artery other than solitus or inversus is termed *malposition.* If the aorta lies to the right of the PA, it is called *D-malposition* (Fig. 63-10, *C*). If the aorta lies to the left of the PA, it is termed *L-malposition* (Fig. 63-10, *D*).

Different Types of Human Hearts

The segmental possibilities at each level are as follows:
   Atria: Solitus (S), inversus (I), and ambiguous (A)
   Ventricles: D and L
   Great arteries: Solitus (S), inversus (I), D-malposition, and L-malposition

Based on the various permutations and combinations of atrial, ventricular, and great arterial relationships, as well as on the anatomy of the conus, Van Praagh provided an overview of the diversity that exists in human hearts (Fig. 63-11). It becomes immediately apparent that a pattern-based approach or an approach based on connections or the direction of flow of blood will not do justice to the complexity of the disease process. The segmental approach not only takes into account the morphologic variations at each level but also provides structural landmarks to distinguish the variations from each other and determine their impact on physiology, thereby allowing informed decision making regarding management.

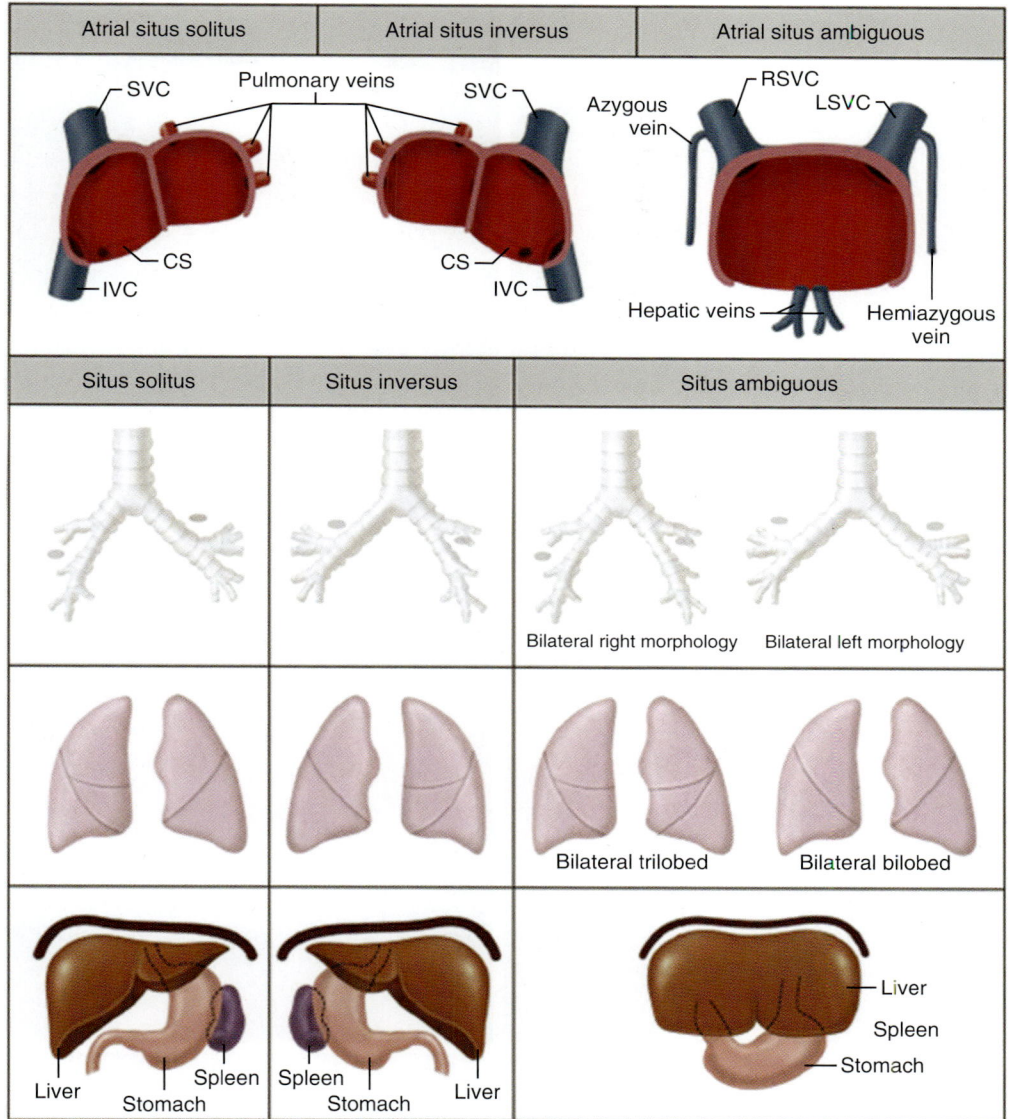

Figure 63-8 First major cardiac segment: visceroatrial situs. The three types of visceroatrial situs: situs solitus, situs inversus, and situs ambiguous. *CS,* coronary sinus; *IVC,* inferior vena cava; *LSVC,* left-sided vena cava; *RSCV,* right-sided vena cava; *SVC,* superior vena cava. (Modified from Van Praagh R, Weinberg PM, Matsuoka R et al. Malposition of the heart and the segmental approach to diagnosis. In Adams FH, Emmanouilides GC, editors: *Moss' heart diseases in infants, children and adolescents,* ed 3. Baltimore: Williams & Wilkins; 1983.)

Analysis of the Connecting Segments

FIRST CONNECTING SEGMENT: ATRIOVENTRICULAR JUNCTION

The anatomic possibilities at the AV junction level may be classified on the basis of the number of ventricles as follows:
1. Biventricular AV connections
2. Univentricular AV connections

The types of biventricular AV connections (Fig. 63-12) include:
1. Concordant AV connections (RA-RV and LA-LV)
2. Discordant AV connections (RA-LV and LA-RV)
3. Straddling AV valve, in which attachment of the tensor apparatus of the valve to the opposite ventricle is abnormal
4. Overriding AV valve, in which the AV valve annulus crosses the interventricular septum and partly overlies the opposite ventricle
5. Overriding and straddling AV valve
6. Balanced common AV canal with two symmetric-sized ventricles

The types of univentricular AV connections (Fig. 63-13) include:
1. Unilateral left AV valve atresia (mitral atresia)
2. Unilateral right AV valve atresia (tricuspid atresia)
3. Double inlet LV

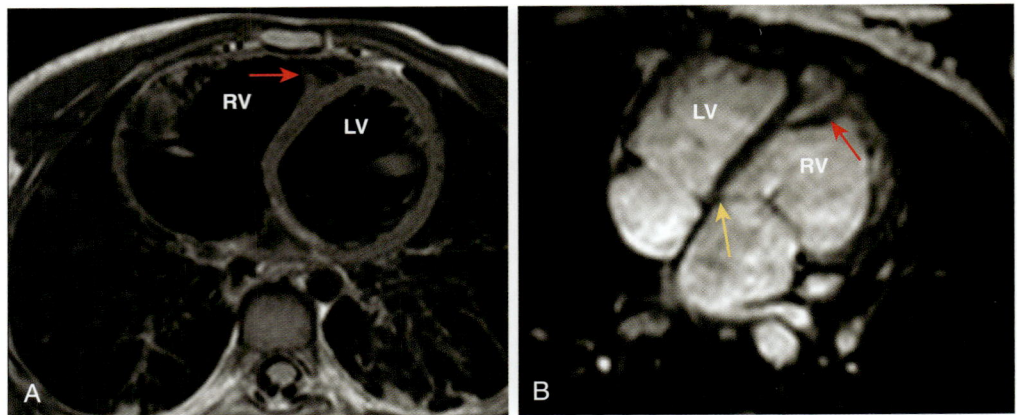

Figure 63-9 The second major cardiac segment: ventricular looping. **A,** D-looping with the right ventricle (*RV*) lying anterior and to the right of the left ventricle (*LV*). **B,** L-looping, with the RV lying anterior and to the left of the LV. The RV is identified by the moderator band (*red arrow*), apical displacement of the AV valve (*yellow arrow*), and the conus (not shown).

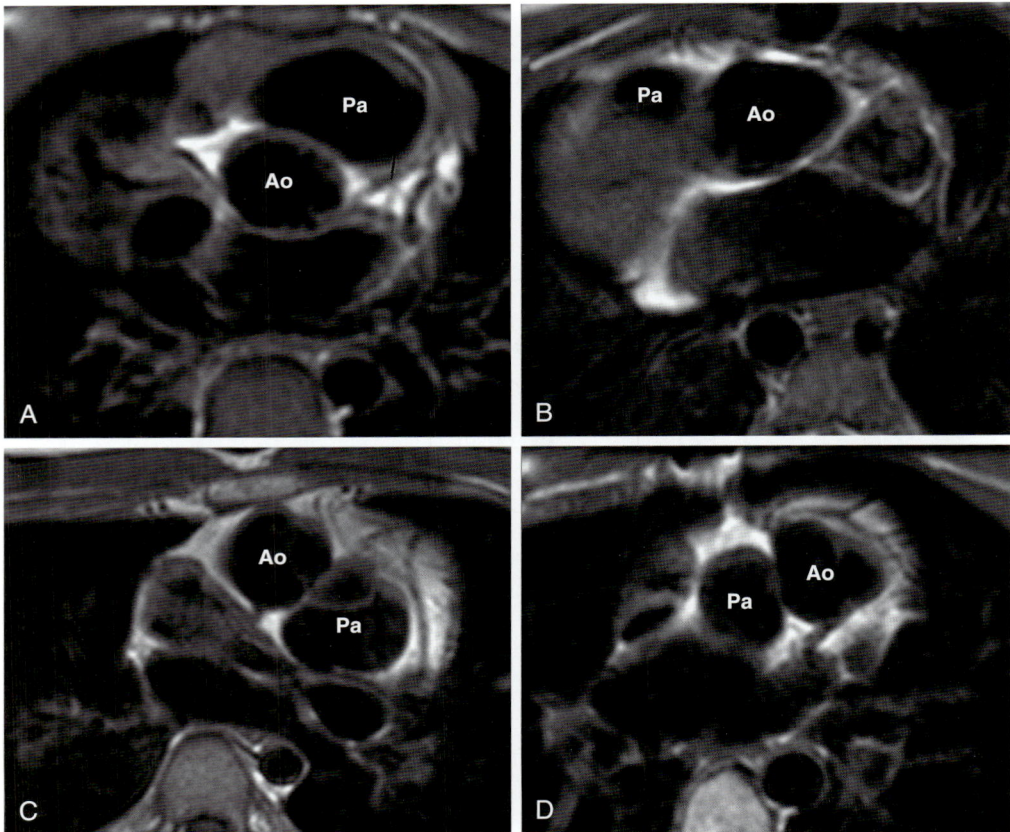

Figure 63-10 The third major cardiac segment: arterial relationship. **A,** Solitus: the aortic annulus (*Ao*) lies posterior, inferior, and to the right of the pulmonary valve annulus (*Pa*). **B,** Inversus: the aorta lies posterior and to the left of the pulmonary valve. **C,** D-malposition: the aorta lies anterior and to the right of the pulmonary artery. **D,** L-malposition: the aorta lies anterior and to the left of the pulmonary artery.

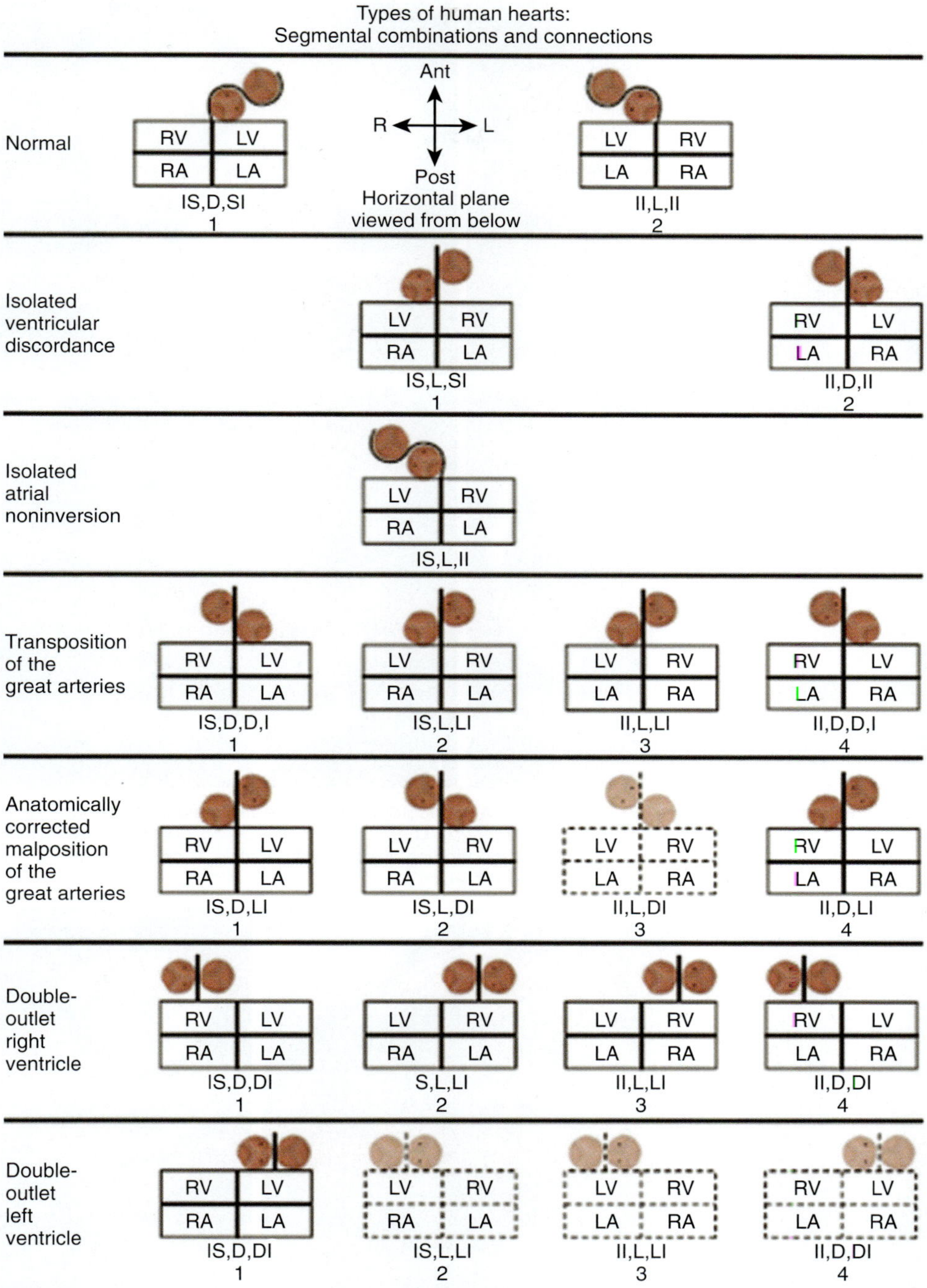

Types of human hearts:
Segmental combinations and connections

Figure 63-11 Van Praagh's types of human hearts, based on segmental combinations of visceroatrial situs, ventricular looping, and great arterial situs. The segmental combination is expressed as a set, within braces. For instance, a normal heart would be expressed as {S,D,S} for visceroatrial situs solitus, D-looping of the ventricles, and solitus relationship of the great arteries. The segmental connections and associated anomalies are expressed outside the braces. For instance, physiologically corrected transposition would be expressed as {S,L,L} transposition of the great arteries for solitus atria, L-looped ventricles, and L-malposition of the great arteries. If this patient also had straddling atrioventricular valve and an inlet ventricular septal defect (VSD), it would be expressed as {S,L,L} transposition of great arteries, straddling tricuspid valve, and inlet VSD. *Ant,* Anterior; *LA,* left atrium; *LV,* left ventricle; *Post,* posterior; *R,* right; *RA,* right atrium; *RV,* right ventricle. (Modified from Van Praagh R, Weinberg PM, Matsuoka R, et al. Malposition of the heart and the segmental approach to diagnosis. In: Adams FH, Emmanouilides GC, editors: *Moss' heart diseases in infants, children and adolescents.* 3rd ed. Baltimore: Williams & Wilkins; 1983.)

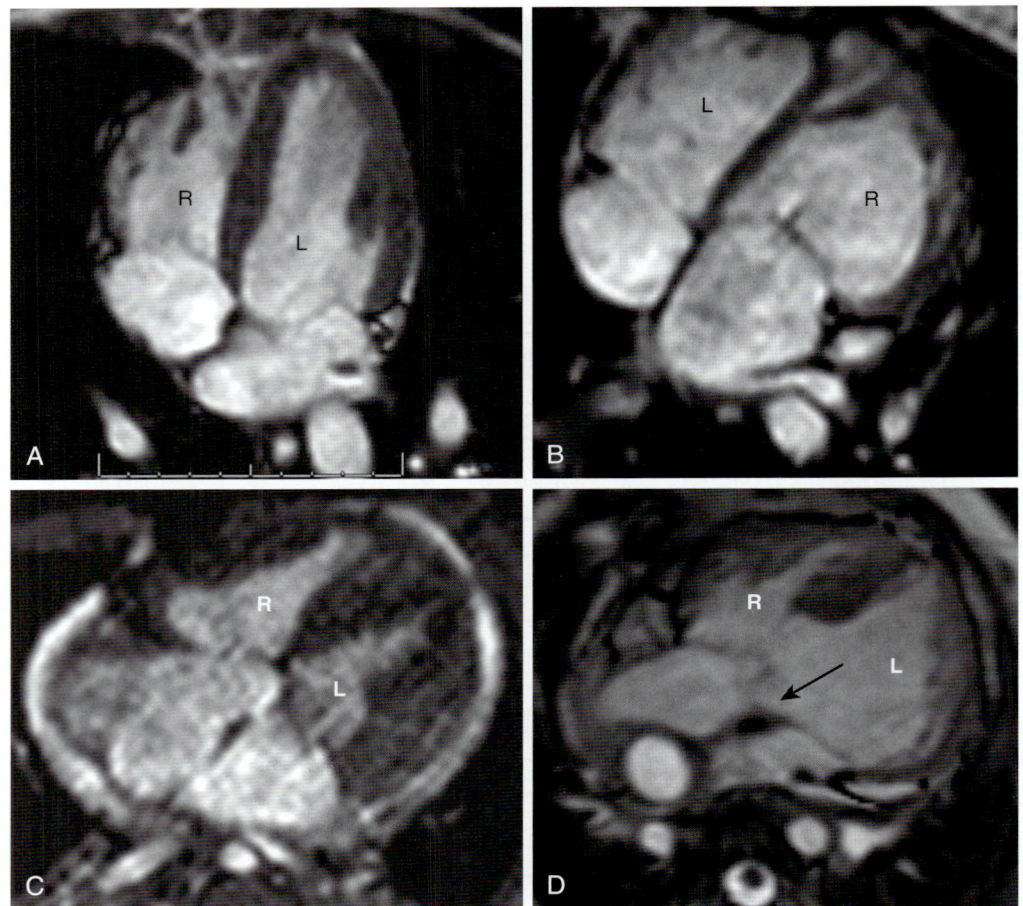

Figure 63-12 Types of biventricular atrioventricular (AV) connections. **A,** Concordant AV connections (right atrium-right ventricle (RA-RV) and left atrium-left ventricle (LA-LV)) **B,** Discordant AV connections (RA-LV and LA-RV). **C,** Balanced common AV canal with two symmetric sized ventricles. **D,** Straddling and overriding tricuspid valve (*arrow*) in a patient with D-looped ventricles. *L,* Left ventricle; *R,* right ventricle.

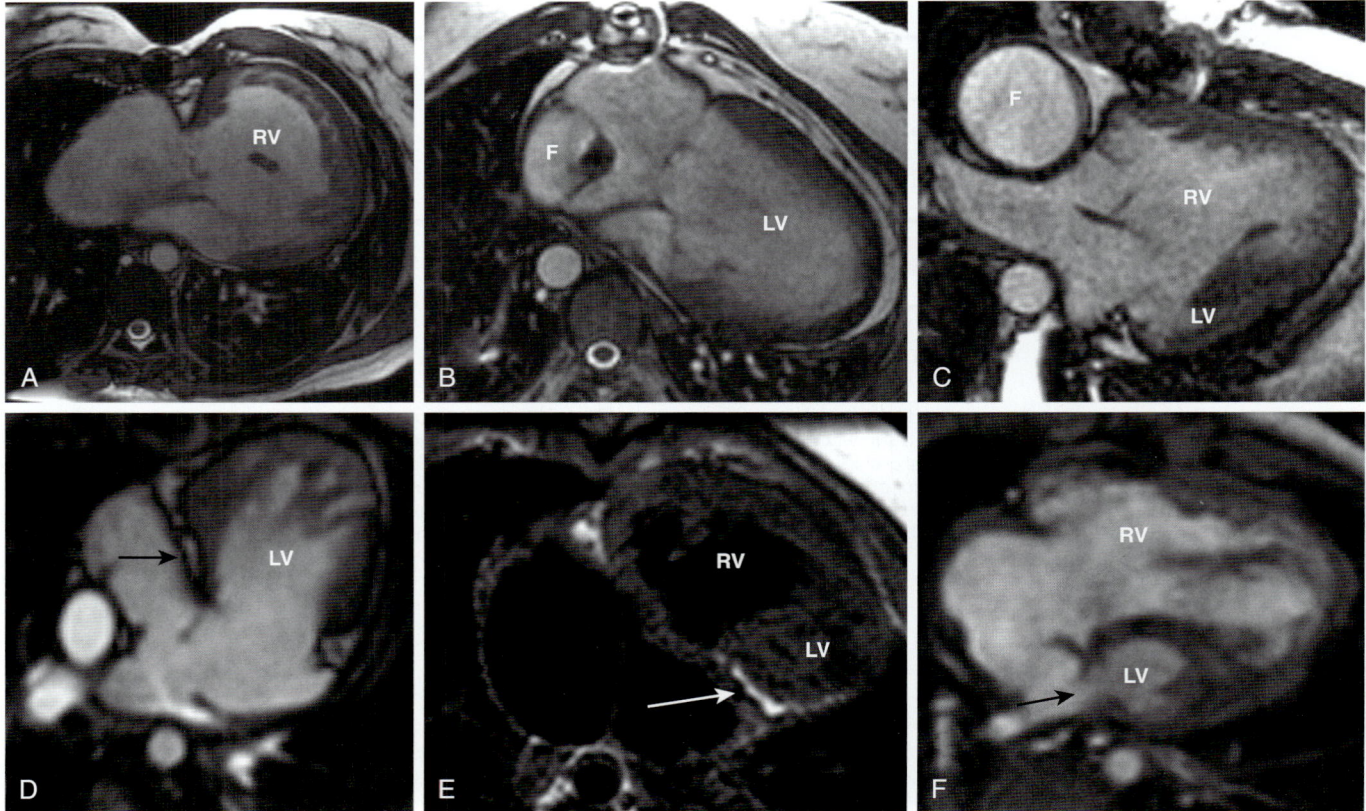

Figure 63-13 Types of univentricular atrioventricular (AV) connections. **A,** Double inlet right ventricle (*RV*). **B,** Double inlet left ventricle (*LV*). **C,** Right dominant unbalanced common AV canal. **D,** Tricuspid atresia (*arrow* shows atretic tricuspid valve plane). **E,** Mitral atresia (*arrow* shows atretic fatty mitral valve plane). **F,** Severe mitral stenosis (*arrow*) in hypoplastic left heart syndrome. *F,* Fontan.

4. Double inlet RV
5. Left dominant unbalanced common AV canal
6. Right dominant unbalanced common AV canal

In the setting of univentricular AV connections, one of the AV valves is atretic, or both AV valves open partly or wholly into the same ventricle. The second ventricular chamber subsequently is very small or is just an outflow chamber and is of little functional use, apart from serving as a conduit for one of the great arteries. Single ventricles may be of an LV, RV, or indeterminate morphology. The functional single LV is characterized by the presence of a bulbo-ventricular foramen, which connects the LV chamber to the small anteriorly located infundibular outlet chamber of the RV. The RV sinus (inflow portion) is typically absent. A functional single RV is characterized by the presence of a septal band, and in most cases, by a rudimentary posterolaterally located LV chamber.

SECOND CONNECTING SEGMENT: CONOTRUNCUS OR VENTRICULOARTERIAL JUNCTION

The development of the conotruncus is the most important variable in the genesis of outflow tract anomalies. The differential growth of the subpulmonary and subaortic conus cushions largely determines the relationship between the semilunar valves, between the semilunar valves and the ventricles, and between the semilunar valves and the atrioventricular valves. It also determines the presence of distal infundibular stenosis and the location of the ventricular septal defect in outflow tract anomalies. Based on conal development, the following anatomic types of conus (Fig. 63-14) may be recognized:

1. Development of subpulmonary conus and resorption of the subaortic conus results in ventriculoarterial concordance and normal relationship of great arteries. The aorta lies posterior and to the right in a D-loop heart (solitus), and posterior and to the left in an L-looped heart (inversus).

2. Development of the subaortic conus and resorption of the subpulmonary conus results in ventriculoarterial discordance and transposition of the great arteries. Transposition means that the LV is connected to the main pulmonary artery and the RV is connected to the aorta. The aorta lies anterior and to the right in a D-looped heart (D-malposition) (Fig. 63-15) and anterior and to the left in an L-looped heart (L-malposition).

3. Persistence and development of both the subaortic and subpulmonary conus leads to a double-outlet RV, meaning that both great vessels arise predominantly from the RV (Fig. 63-16). Variable development of the pulmonary and aortic conus may occur, resulting in variable location of the ventricular septal defect in relation to the great arteries.

4. Resorption of both the subpulmonary and subaortic conus results in double-outlet LV, meaning that both vessels arise predominantly from the LV.

A rare form of conal maldevelopment is anatomically corrected malposition of the great arteries, in which the malposed aorta originates above the LV and the malposed pulmonary artery originates above the RV. Malalignment of the conal septum also is the cause of infundibular obstruction

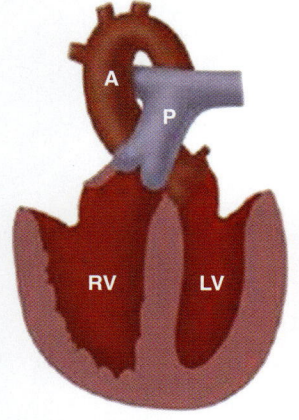
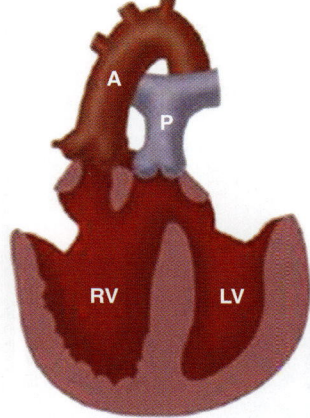

A   Concordant connection   B   Double-outlet right ventricle

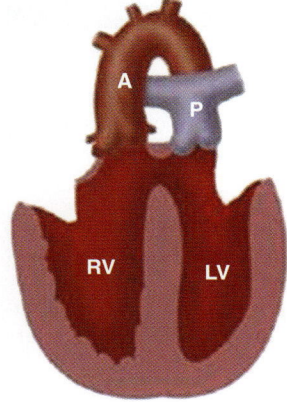
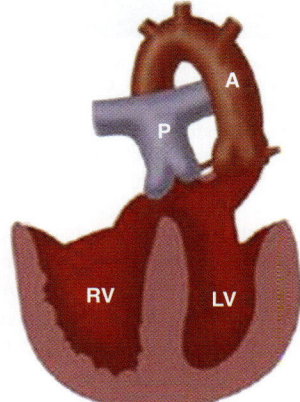

C   Discordant connection   D   Double-outlet left ventricle

Figure 63-14 Types of ventriculoarterial connections based on conal development. **A,** Concordant ventriculoarterial connection: solitus great arteries with subpulmonary conus. **B,** Double-outlet right ventricle (*RV*) with bilateral conus. **C,** Discordant ventriculoarterial connection: dextraposed transposition of the great arteries with subaortic conus. **D,** Double-outlet left ventricle (*LV*) with absent conus. *A,* Aorta; *P,* pulmonary artery. (From Krishnamurthy R. Embryologic basis and segmental approach to imaging of congenital heart disease. In: Ho V, Reddy GP, eds. *Cardiovascular imaging.* 1st ed. Philadelphia: Saunders Elsevier; 2010.)

in tetralogy of Fallot (anterior malalignment) and subaortic stenosis with interrupted aortic arch (posterior malalignment).

Evaluation of Associated Anomalies

The presence of associated anomalies involving the atrial and ventricular septum, AV and semilunar valves, aorta, pulmonary arteries, pulmonary veins, and systemic veins plays an important part in the functional outcome of the patient, and screening for these conditions is an integral part of the segmental approach to heart disease.

Evaluation of Function

The final step in the segmental approach to heart disease is to determine how the segmental combinations and

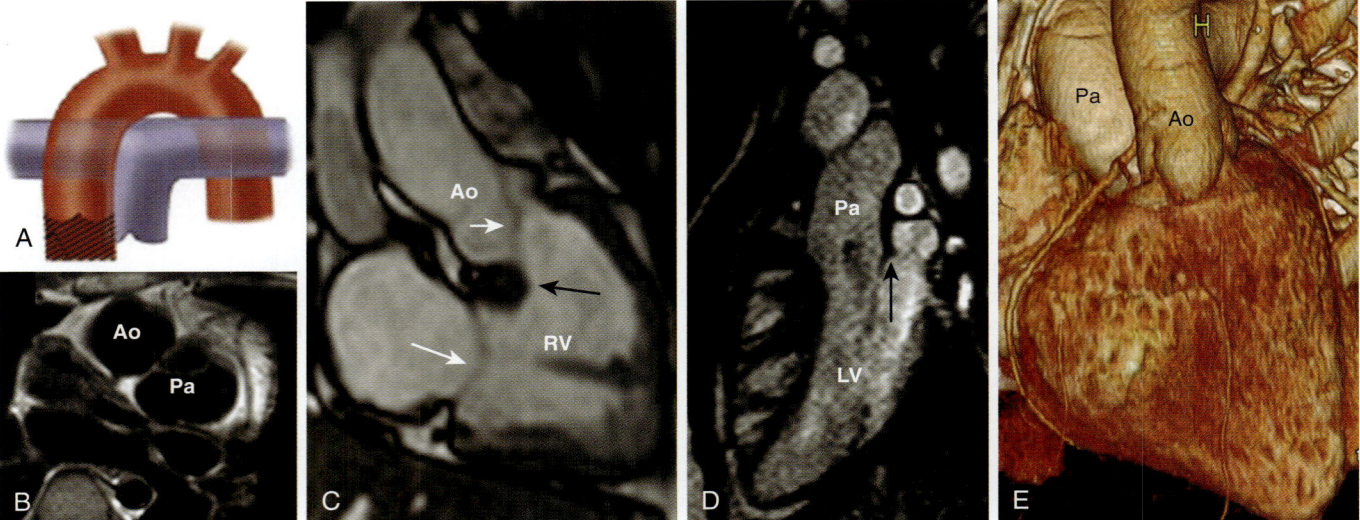

Figure 63-15 Conus in dextroposed transposition of the great arteries (D-TGA). **A** and **B,** The aorta (*Ao*) lies anterior and to the right of the pulmonary artery (D-malposition). **C,** The right ventricle (*RV*) is connected to the aorta by a muscular infundibulum (*black arrow*), resulting in lack of fibrous contiguity between the tricuspid valve (*long white arrow*) and the aortic valve (*short white arrow*). **D,** The left ventricle (*LV*) is connected to the main pulmonary artery (*Pa*) with absence of an intervening conus, resulting in direct fibrous contiguity between the aortic and pulmonary valves (*arrow*). **E,** Three-dimensional volume rendering of a patient with D-TGA. *H,* heart.

connections, with the associated anomalies, function. Broadly, abnormal function of the congenitally malformed heart may be classified into the following subgroups:

1. Pressure overload related to phenomena such as valvular stenosis, coarctation, and branch pulmonary artery stenosis
2. Volume overload related to phenomena such as valvular regurgitation and left to right shunts
3. Intermixing, in which there is mixing of oxygenated blood with deoxygenated blood before entering the systemic circulation; this phenomenon typically occurs in the setting of a common chamber, vessel, or valve or in a right–left shunt
4. Poor contractility of the myocardium related to conditions such as cardiomyopathy or ischemia

When all relevant information regarding morphology and function has been collected, decisions regarding management may be made, which may be in the form of medical therapy, surgical therapy, or both.

Illustrated Case Discussion

A case study of a segmental approach to imaging of CHD is illustrated in Figure 63-17.

- Situs solitus of the atria (S): The coronary sinus and IVC enter the right-sided atrium, which therefore represents the morphologic RA. The pulmonary veins enter the morphologic LA. The RA connects to the right pulmonary artery via an atriopulmonary anastomosis. The SVC also connects to the right pulmonary artery.
- AV connection: The right AV valve (tricuspid valve) is atretic and fatty replaced. The left AV valve (mitral valve) is normal.

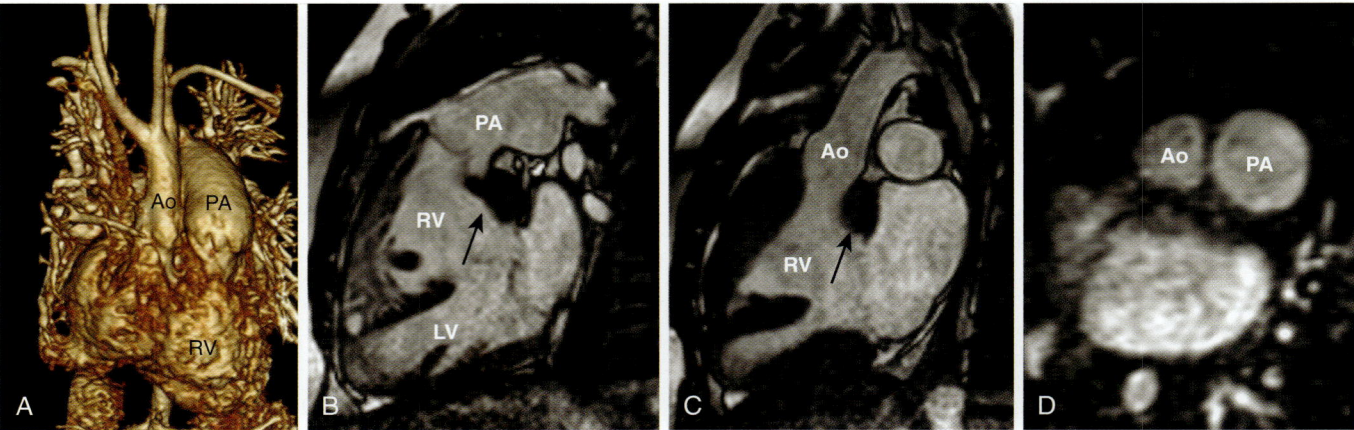

Figure 63-16 Double outlet right ventricle (*RV*) with bilateral conus and side-by-side great arteries. **A,** Three-dimensional volume rendering of double outlet RV showing both great arteries arising from the RV. **B** and **C,** Presence of a subpulmonary and subaortic conus (*arrows*). **D,** Side-by-side great arteries. *Ao,* Aorta; *LV,* left ventricle; *PA,* pulmonary artery.

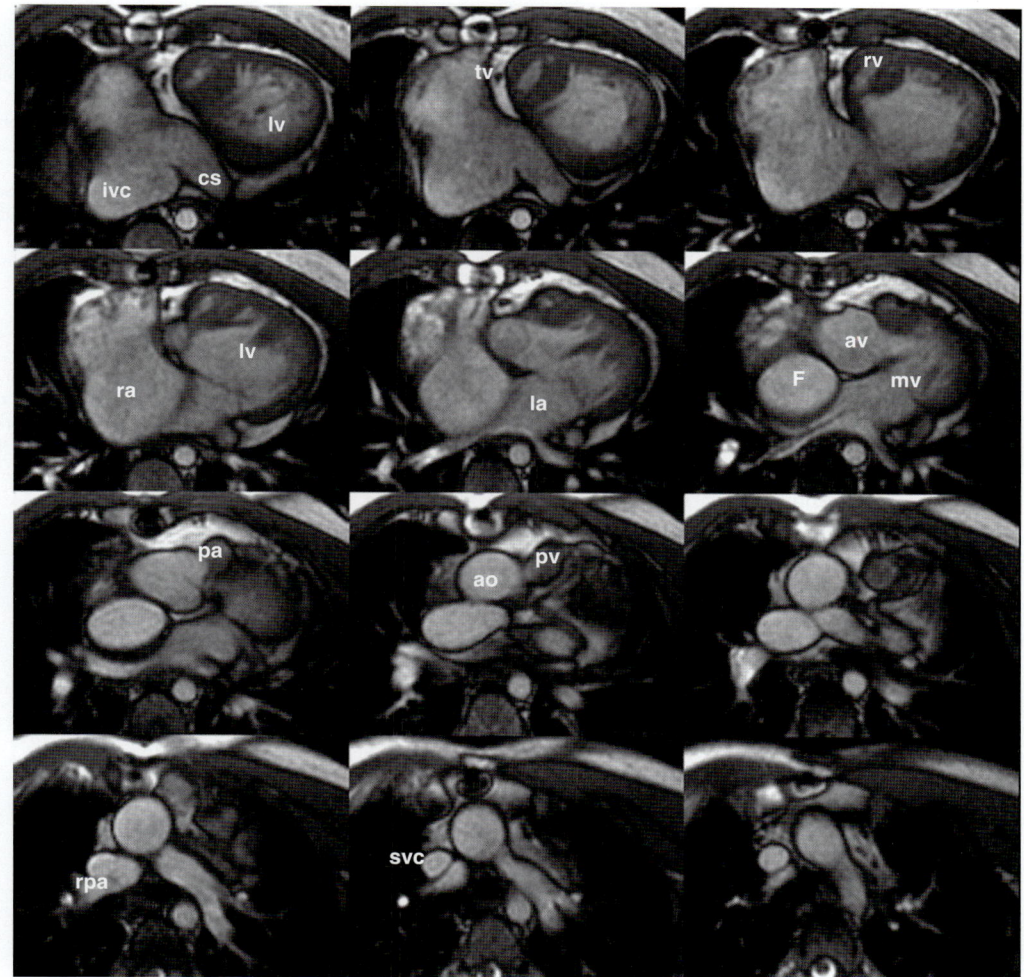

Figure 63-17 Illustrative case study of segmental approach to imaging of congenital heart disease. *ao,* Aortic outflow; *av,* aortic valve; *cs,* coronary sinus; *F,* Fontan; *ivc,* inferior vena cava; *la,* left ctrium; *lv,* left ventricle; *mv,* mitral valve; *pa,* pulmonary artery; *pv,* pulmonary veins; *ra,* right atrium; *rpa,* right pulmonary artery; *svc,* superior vena cava; *tv,* tricuspid valve.

- D-looping of the ventricles: The large left-sided ventricle has a smooth septal surface consistent with a morphologic LV. The small blind-ending chamber to the right is the infundibular outlet chamber of the RV, which fills via a bulboventricular foramen.
- Ventriculoarterial connection: RV-PA outflow is atretic. Aortic outflow from the LV is normal.
- Solitus relationship of the great arteries (S): The aortic valve lies posterior and to the right of the atretic pulmonary valve.

The final diagnosis is {S,D,S} tricuspid atresia, pulmonary atresia, status postoperative Fontan completion.

Conclusion

In summary, the segmental approach to heart disease provides an elegantly simple method to break down the complexity of CHD on cross-sectional imaging. It creates a template for standardizing nomenclature in CHD, thereby ensuring that caregivers from different specialties understand each other. It is firmly rooted in embryologic principles and is therefore fairly intuitive to the beginner in the field. MRI and CT almost rival pathologic evaluation of specimens in the detail that they provide on cardiovascular morphology. Additionally, MRI provides unique information regarding function, flow, and tissue characterization that decreases the need for more invasive means of diagnosis. Thus MRI and CT are ideal vehicles for the segmental approach to heart disease.

Key Points

The segmental approach is a simple, logical, step-by-step approach to diagnosis and decision making in CHD and is rooted in sound embryologic concepts.

The segmental approach involves the analysis of the three major cardiac segments (atria, ventricles, and great arteries), the two connecting segments (the AV canal and the conotruncus), and associated anomalies involving the atrial and ventricular septum, great arteries, and systemic and pulmonary veins. The final step is evaluation of physiology and function, which paves the way for decision making regarding management.

Continued

Reliable identification of the cardiac chambers based on specific morphologic features is the first step in the segmental approach to heart disease. These features may be appreciated easily on cross-sectional imaging.

Characterizing the specific type of visceroatrial situs, ventricular looping, and great arterial situs is the next step. Based on the various permutations and combinations of atrial, ventricular, and great arterial relationships, Van Praagh created a chart that outlines the diversity that exists in human hearts.

Analysis of connecting segments—the AV junction and the ventriculoarterial junction—leads to an understanding of the pathogenesis of single ventricle and outflow tract anomalies, respectively.

The final step in the segmental approach to heart disease is to determine how the segmental combinations and connections, with the associated anomalies, function. This determination paves the way for appropriate decision making regarding management, which may be medical, surgical, or both.

Suggested Readings

Colvin EV. Single ventricle. In: Garson Jr A, Bricker JT, McNamara DG, eds. *The science and practice of pediatric cardiology*. Philadelphia: Lea and Febiger; 1990.

Krishnamurthy R. Embryologic basis and segmental approach to imaging of congenital heart disease. In: Ho V, Reddy GP, eds. *Cardiovascular imaging*. 1st ed. Philadelphia: Saunders/Elsevier; 2010.

Shinebourne EA, Macartney FJ, Anderson RH. Sequential chamber localization-logical approach to diagnosis in congenital heart disease. *Br Heart J*. 1976;38:327-340.

Van Praagh R. Diagnosis of complex congenital heart disease: morphologic-anatomic method and terminology. *Cardiovasc Intervent Radiol*. 1984;7:115-120.

Van Praagh R. The segmental approach to diagnosis in congenital heart disease *Birth Defects*. 1972;8:4-23.

Van Praagh S, Kreutzer J, Alday L, et al. Systemic and pulmonary venous connections in visceral heterotaxy, with emphasis on the diagnosis of the atrial situs: a study of 109 postmortem cases. In: Clark E, Takao A, eds. *Developmental cardiology, morphogenesis and function*. Mt. Kisco, NY: Futura; 1990.

Chapter 64

Pediatric Echocardiography

JAMES RENÉ HERLONG

Echocardiography is the primary imaging modality used to assess the heart and the vasculature proximal to the heart in pediatrics. Vascular ultrasound typically is used to assess the remainder of the vasculature. Echocardiography is sufficiently robust to be used as the sole imaging modality in assessing cardiac anatomy before surgical repair in most pediatric patients with congenital heart disease. Thus familiarity with echocardiography is important for anyone involved in diagnostic imaging in pediatric patients.

Technique

Transthoracic echocardiography is an ultrasound technique that is optimized for imaging the moving heart. Standard imaging windows that are free of interference from the lungs are illustrated in Figure 64-1. These windows allow imaging of the heart in multiple planes. These planes are based on the axes of the heart and not on the axes of the body (Fig. 64-2).

In each acoustic window, the heart is imaged in orthogonal planes. Because the heart is a three-dimensional structure and because ultrasonography is a tomographic imaging technique, slow sweeps in each view are necessary to understand the complex relationships between various segments of the heart. Three- and four-dimensional echocardiography are becoming ever more robust, but they are not yet capable of high-resolution imaging of the entire heart. Currently, the utility of these techniques is largely in the assessment of the cardiac valves, particularly the atrioventricular valves.

Assessment of ventricular systolic function is performed in every echocardiographic examination. Among the various techniques of quantifying left ventricular systolic function, the left ventricular shortening fraction is the most easily accomplished and universally used. Figure 64-3 illustrates this technique. Standards for left ventricular dimensions and shortening fraction according to body surface area are available in standard references. Assessment of left ventricular diastolic function is less exact, and techniques continue to be developed to evaluate this rather elusive entity. The method with the most promise is tissue Doppler imaging, which uses the Doppler principle to measure the high amplitude but low velocity signals derived from myocardial motion.

Doppler echocardiography uses color and spectral Doppler in the same manner as in vascular ultrasound imaging. One important difference is that when using color Doppler, the color map is always set so that flow toward the transducer is red, whereas flow away from the transducer is blue. Color Doppler imaging is useful for screening for valvar stenosis or regurgitation, septal defects, and arterial and venous stenoses. Color Doppler should be used to complement two-dimensional imaging, not to replace it, because color Doppler obscures anatomy.

In a typical echocardiographic examination, all cardiac valves are assessed by spectral Doppler, as are the aortic arch at the isthmus and any identified septal defects. As with all Doppler applications, the most accurate assessment is obtained by aligning the angle of interrogation exactly along the direction of flow. The simplified Bernoulli equation states that the pressure gradient across an area is approximately equal to four times the measured Doppler velocity squared ($4v^2$). By using this equation, gradients are estimated in each of the locations that are assessed by spectral Doppler. In general, peak instantaneous pressure gradients across semilunar valves and in the arterial system should be less than 15 mm Hg, and mean gradients in veins and across atrioventricular valves should be less than 3 mm Hg.

Other differences from noncardiac ultrasound involve sedation and image archiving. Because accurate assessment of anatomy and function requires images free of patient movement and because accurate assessment of pressure gradients requires the patient to be in a resting state, sedation often is necessary in patients younger than about 3 years. Because assessment of function and complex anatomy requires viewing moving images, echocardiograms are archived as video clips rather than as still-frame images.

Transesophageal echocardiography in the pediatric population is used primarily in the operating room during surgery for congenital heart disease and in the interventional cardiac catheterization laboratory. Techniques are similar to those previously described.

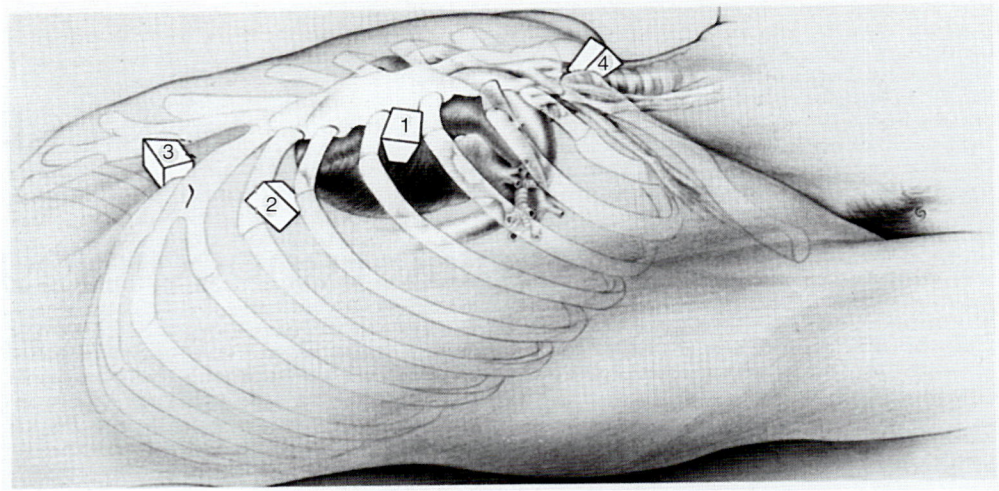

Figure 64-1   Probe positions for the four standard windows used in transthoracic echocardiography. Position 1, parasternal; position 2, apical; position 3, subcostal; position 4, suprasternal. (From Snicer AR, Serwer GA, Ritter SB: *Echocardiography in pediatric heart disease.* 2nd ed. St Louis: Mosby–Year Book; 1997.)

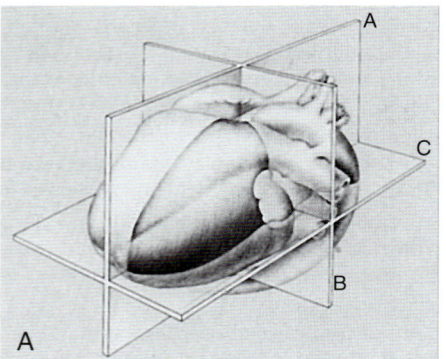

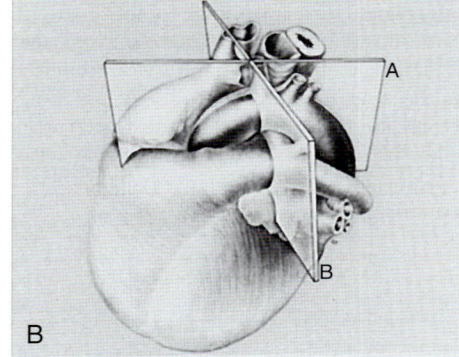

Figure 64-2   **A,** Three standard cardiac imaging planes. Plane A is a long-axis plane parallel to the major axis of the left ventricle. Plane B is a short-axis plane perpendicular to the major axis of the left ventricle. Plane C is a coronal plane of the heart through the cardiac apex that produces a standard four-chamber view. **B,** Two standard suprasternal notch imaging planes. Plane A is a long-axis plane parallel to the major axis of the aortic arch. Plane B is a short-axis plane perpendicular to the major axis of the aortic arch. (From Snider AR, Serwer GA, Ritter SB: *Echocardiography in pediatric heart disease.* 2nd ed. St Louis: Mosby–Year Book; 1997.)

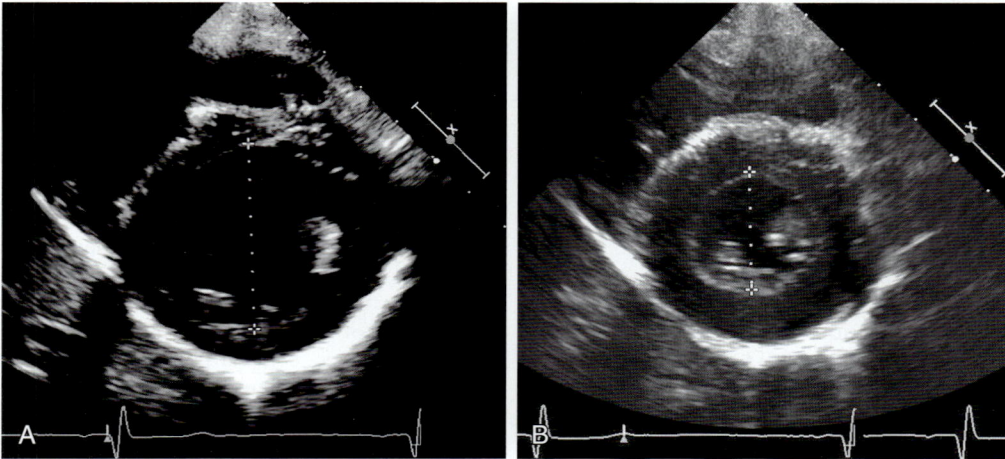

Figure 64-3   Parasternal short-axis views of the left ventricle at the midventricular level. **A,** End-diastolic frame. **B,** End-systolic frame. Measurements of left ventricular end-diastolic dimension (LVEDD) (**A**) and left ventricular end-systolic dimension (LVESD) (**B**) are depicted. The cursor is placed perpendicular to the ventricular septum and the left ventricular free wall. Left ventricular shortening fraction is defined as (LVEDD – LVESD)/LVEDD × 100.

Box 64-1 Format for Organizing the Report of an Echocardiogram

Cardiac position
Description of venoatrial segment
Description of atrioventricular canal, including atrioventricular valves
Description of ventricles
Description of conotruncus
Description of semilunar valves
Description of coronary arteries
Description of aorta, including arch sidedness and branching as well as presence or absence of coarctation
Description of main and branch pulmonary arteries
Description of ductus arteriosus
Description of ventricular function
Description of pericardium and pericardial effusion
Description of any masses, vegetations, or thrombi
Presence or absence of pleural effusions
Comment upon diaphragm motion

Formulating a Diagnosis

Once the images have been obtained, a comprehensive diagnosis must be constructed, which is accomplished by using the segmental approach to cardiac anatomy (see Chapter 63). A common template for reporting the findings of an echocardiogram is presented in Box 64-1. Note that the scheme is logical and largely follows the blood flow through the various segments of the heart.

Key Points

Most pediatric patients with congenital heart disease are taken to the operating room on the basis of an echocardiographic diagnosis alone.

Standard imaging planes for echocardiography relate to the axes of the heart, not to the axes of the body.

The heart is best understood by considering its anatomy segmentally.

Suggested Readings

Ayers NA, Miller-Hance W, Fyfe DA, et al. Indications and guidelines for performance of transesophageal echocardiography in the patient with pediatric acquired or congenital heart disease: a report from the Task Force of the Pediatric Council of the American Society of Echocardiography. *J Am Soc Echocardiogr.* 2005;18:91-98.

Eidem BW, Cetta F, O'Leary PW, eds. *Echocardiography in pediatric and adult congenital heart disease.* Philadelphia: Lippincott Williams & Wilkins; 2010.

Lai WW, Geva T, Shirali GS. Guidelines and standards for the performance of a pediatric echocardiogram: a report from the Task Force of the Pediatric Council of the American Society of Echocardiography. *J Am Soc Echocardiogr.* 2006;19:1413-1430.

Lai WW, Mertens L, Cohen MS, et al, eds. *Echocardiography in pediatric and congenital heart disease: from fetus to adult.* Hoboken, NJ: Wiley-Blackwell; 2009.

Lopez L, Colan SD, Frommelt PC, et al. Recommendations for quantification methods during the performance of a pediatric echocardiogram: a report from the Pediatric Measurements Writing Group of the American Society of Echocardiography Pediatric and Congenital Heart Disease Council. *J Am Soc Echocardiogr.* 2010;23:465-495.

Chapter 65

Chest Radiography in Pediatric Cardiovascular Disease

J. A. GORDON CULHAM and JOHN B. MAWSON

The role of chest radiography in the diagnosis and evaluation of congenital cardiovascular disease continues to evolve. At one time a major tool in the assessment of heart disease, radiography now occupies an ancillary role, with echocardiography serving as the major primary investigation after physical examination, especially in the neonatal period. However, the chest radiograph still may provide the first indication of unsuspected cardiovascular disease, and in infants and children with known cardiac disease, radiography offers an important overview of the heart and pulmonary circulation. Moreover, chest radiography is a vital tool in the early postoperative period and is useful in the follow-up of heart disease. These latter topics are beyond the scope of this chapter.

The major chest radiographic findings in patients with cardiac disease are cardiomegaly, pulmonary vascular changes (predominantly overcirculation or undercirculation), and signs of pulmonary venous hypertension and edema. However, several caveats need to be emphasized. First, children with relatively mild structural defects and even some children with severe or complex disease may have normal chest films. This situation is particularly true in newborns. In addition, the chest radiograph usually does not provide useful information about specific chamber size, hypertrophy, or intracardiac connections or malformations. Echocardiography, magnetic resonance imaging, computed tomography, or angiography are needed for precise evaluation of intracardiac structure and function. Furthermore, findings such as a boot-shaped or egg-shaped heart are nonspecific for tetralogy of Fallot or transposition of the great arteries. On the other hand, plain film findings may be specific for some extracardiac lesions, such as supracardiac total anomalous pulmonary venous return, aortic arch anomalies, pulmonary stenosis, and coarctation of the aorta.

A systematic approach to evaluation of the chest film consists of an assessment of heart size, shape, and position; pulmonary vasculature; the airway and mediastinum; visceral situs; and skeletal abnormalities. Applying such an approach often results in a diagnosis of a cardiovascular disease category such as a shunt or a right- or left-sided obstructive lesion, which in turn leads to a differential diagnosis and the identification of the likely etiology of nonspecific clinical findings, such as congestive heart failure or cyanosis (Box 65-1).

Technique

As in all medical imaging, attention to detail is necessary to optimize the examination and its interpretation. Proper exposure, centering, collimation, patient positioning, and inspiration are necessary (e-Fig. 65-1).

Many films of infants are obtained using the anteroposterior projection and supine position. Because of the small size of the chest, this technique results in little magnification of the heart, as can be seen in larger children. Beam angulation also may affect the appearance of the heart and great vessels. With lordotic positioning, the heart may appear more globular, with an uplifted apex and accentuation of the pulmonary outflow tract; with reverse lordosis, much of the heart may be obscured by the hemidiaphragms. Oblique views are not useful for cardiac evaluation, and barium should be used only if a vascular ring or sling is suspected (and when such findings are likely, cross-sectional imaging should be considered for complete evaluation). Chest fluoroscopy is rarely used except to evaluate prosthetic valve function, the diaphragm, or airway dynamics.

Systematic Interpretation

NORMAL ANATOMY AND PHYSIOLOGY

One of the challenges in evaluating the chest radiograph of younger children is their variable anatomy and physiology. For example, the thymus is variable in size and position and may mimic cardiomegaly, abnormally positioned vessels, pericardial fluid, or a mediastinal mass (e-Fig. 65-2).

It is rare for the thymus to extend posteriorly. The thymus usually causes few problems in the interpretation of chest radiographs in children older than 6 years.

Newborn infants have physiologic pulmonary hypertension, and as a result, large shunt lesions do not appear until the pulmonary vascular resistance falls, which usually occurs by 4 to 6 weeks (Fig. 65-3). Similarly, newborn infants may not show the expected changes of severe pulmonary stenosis or atresia if the ductus arteriosus is patent.

The physiology of small airways in infants and young children (up to approximately 2 years of age) results in unique

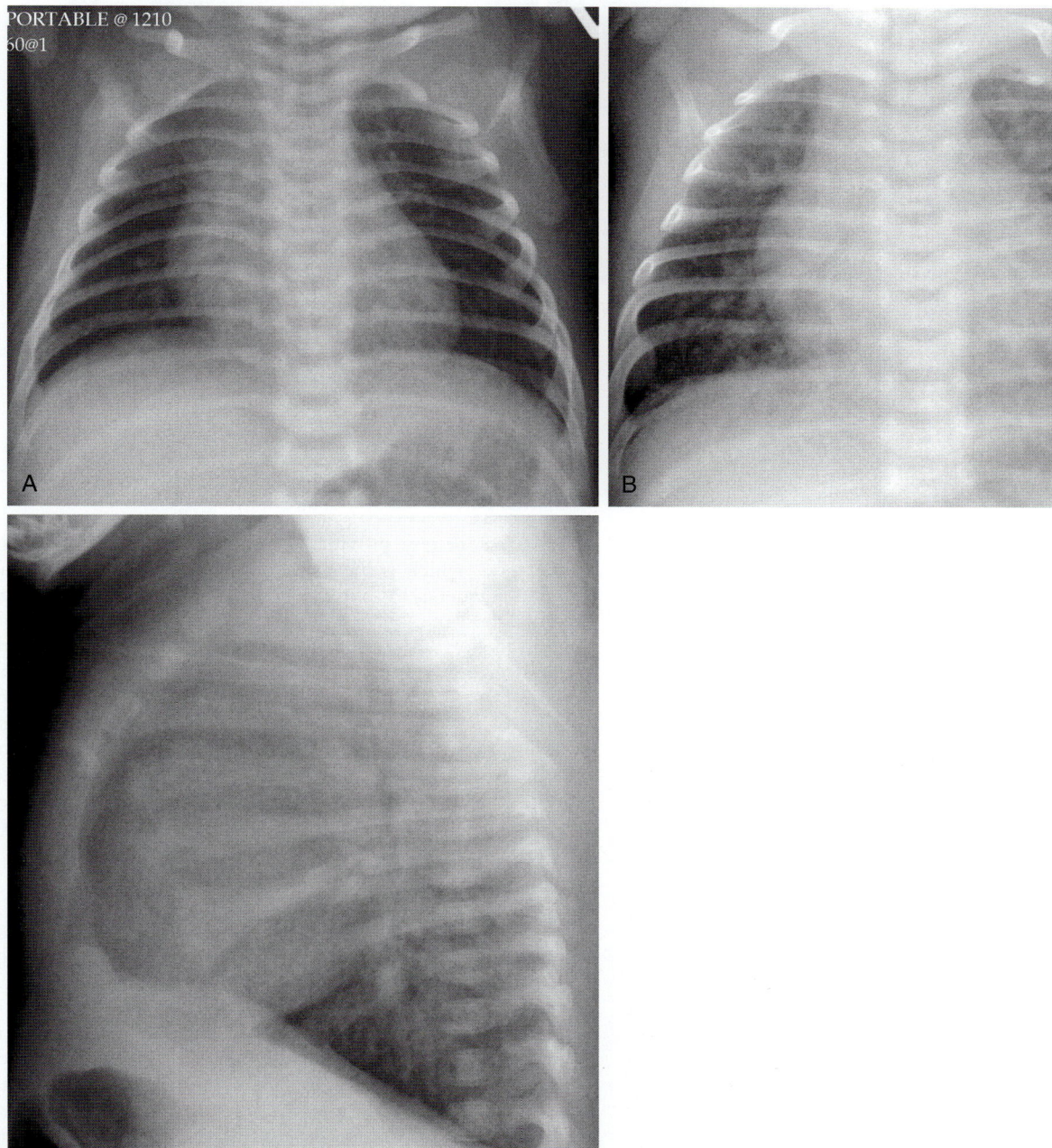

Figure 65-3 **Complete transposition of the great arteries in a neonate.** A frontal radiograph (**A**) on day 1 of life shows a heart that is within normal limits in size and shows normal pulmonary vascularity. The same child at 7 weeks of age (**B** and **C**) has an enlarged heart and increased pulmonary vascularity. Volume loading of the heart and pulmonary circulation has occurred as pulmonary vascular resistance has dropped.

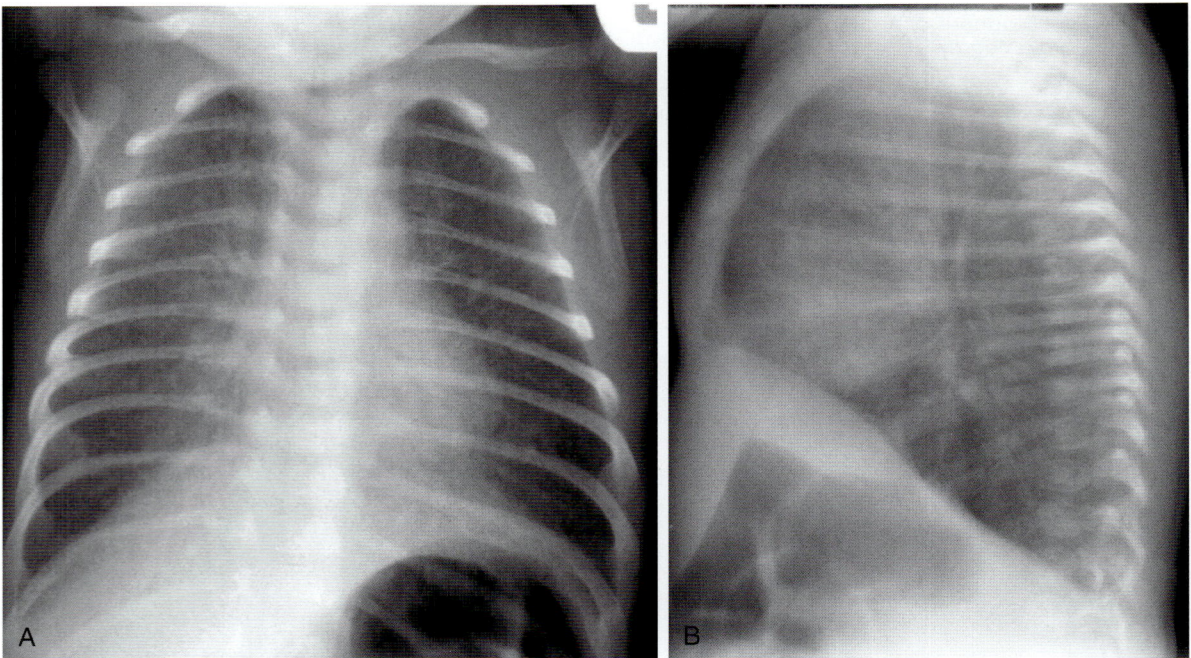

Figure 65-4 Total anomalous pulmonary venous return with obstruction in an infant. Frontal (**A**) and lateral (**B**) radiographs show normal heart size, hyperinflation, and interstitial thickening consistent with pulmonary edema.

manifestations of pulmonary edema. Specifically, infants show hyperinflation as a response to interstitial edema, as would happen in the presence of airway inflammation with bronchiolitis (Figs. 65-3 and 65-4).

The hyperinflation occurs as an adaptive response to the interstitial edema to prevent small airway closure. In the absence of clinical signs of a respiratory infection, hyperinflation is an important sign of early pulmonary edema.

HEART SIZE

The size of the heart can be difficult to assess in the frontal projection of infants and young children because of the presence of the relatively large thymus and poor inspiration (see e-Figs. 65-1 and 65-2). Measurement of the cardiothoracic ratio is of little use. The lateral view provides a more reliable indication of true heart size by permitting an assessment of the anteroposterior dimension without interference from the thymus. However, the thymus does fill in the retrosternal space, obscuring the right ventricular outflow tract. In older children, the frontal radiograph is more useful, and the radiologist should evaluate both views to assess the three-dimensional volume of the heart. In a child with pectus excavatum, the heart may appear large in the frontal view but compressed in the lateral film. Marked cardiomegaly is seen in children with severe valve regurgitation, especially tricuspid valve disease (Ebstein anomaly), pericardial effusion, and cardiomyopathy, and it is rarely seen in children with cardiac tumors. Mediastinal masses may mimic cardiomegaly (e-Fig. 65-5).

PULMONARY VASCULATURE

Chest radiography provides a window into the pulmonary circulation, which is the main area in which chest radiography supplements the information gained from echocardiography. The pulmonary vasculature may show evidence of increased flow, decreased flow, normal flow, or pulmonary venous hypertension. The pulmonary flow may be asymmetrical in the setting of tetralogy of Fallot, pulmonary atresia, or other rare lesions. The assessment of the pulmonary vasculature is both important and difficult. Poor-quality films that are rotated or obtained during expiration are difficult to interpret (see e-Fig. 65-1). Many radiographs in younger children are obtained in the supine position, and therefore flow is symmetrical from base to apex.

Increased Pulmonary Vascularity

The size of the pulmonary vessels is noticeably larger only when the amount of flow doubles (thus when the pulmonary/systemic ratio is 2 : 1) (e-Figs. 65-6 and 65-7).

Because of this phenomenon, smaller shunts are not detectable. Detecting moderate increases in flow requires considerable experience. One useful sign is to compare the end-on pulmonary artery to the adjacent bronchus. An arterial dimension greater than that of the bronchus is suggestive of increased flow. However, a slightly larger dimension can be seen normally. The larger vessels extend more peripherally into the lung. Increases in pulmonary blood flow should be accompanied by a proportional increase in heart size because of volume loading.

Decreased Pulmonary Vascularity

Identifying decreased vascularity is even more difficult than identifying increased flow (e-Fig. 65-8).

A cyanotic child beyond the newborn period whose flow appears to be within normal limits very likely has a right-to-left shunt Box 65-2.

Normal Pulmonary Vascularity

The pulmonary vascularity is normal in the presence of valve lesions without shunting or congestive heart failure, in small to moderate shunts, and even in certain cases of balanced complex congenital heart disease. For example, in a patient with a single ventricle and moderate pulmonary stenosis, the flow to the lungs is neither increased nor decreased.

Pulmonary Venous Hypertension and Pulmonary Edema

Early pulmonary venous hypertension often manifests as hyperinflation in infants younger than 2 years (see Fig. 65-4 and e-Fig. 65-6). As interstitial fluid accumulates, the perihilar bronchi and vessels become poorly defined. Septal (i.e., Kerley) lines are uncommon in children. Eventually, frank alveolar pulmonary edema is seen. In the presence of severe heart failure, it can be difficult to determine whether the failure is caused by pulmonary venous hypertension alone or is associated with an underlying large left-to-right shunt (e-Fig. 65-9) (Box 65-3). Pulmonary edema can obscure vessel detail, and left heart failure can distend the vessels. The detection of heart disease can be difficult in the child who presents with an acute viral respiratory illness because the

inflammation can produce ill-defined vascular markings and hyperinflation similar to the findings in congestive heart failure. In a supine patient, pleural fluid will layer posteriorly. Unlike in children with large shunts, with left-sided obstruction or pump failure, the heart often is disproportionate to the vascularity (e-Fig. 65-9, *A*)

Centralized Pulmonary Vascularity

Prominence of the perihilar vessels with rapid tapering as a sign of pulmonary arterial hypertension is rarely seen in children. In a rare variation of tetralogy of Fallot with absent pulmonary valve (not to be confused with pulmonary atresia), large hilar vessels may be seen even during the newborn period, but they are not caused by pulmonary arterial hypertension (e-Fig. 65-10).

Asymmetrical Pulmonary Flow

The chest film must be carefully evaluated for asymmetrical flow, which can occur as a result of pulmonary arterial stenosis or hypoplasia, pulmonary venous obstruction, or disturbances in ventilation with secondary vasoconstriction, as well as postoperatively. Care must be taken to avoid misinterpretation of the rotated radiograph (see e-Fig. 65-1). In children with decreased pulmonary blood flow as a result of tetralogy of Fallot or pulmonary atresia, stenosis of the pulmonary artery (usually the left at the site of ductal insertion) is a common problem (e-Fig. 65-11).

The left pulmonary artery can even become isolated, and the lung will fail to grow. Early recognition of this complication can allow repair and lead to normal lung growth.

AIRWAY AND MEDIASTINUM

The chest film is evaluated for the presence of the thymus, a mediastinal mass, the side of the aortic arch, and the presence of a vascular ring. The size and position of the trachea is an important indicator of arch abnormalities. A careful search should be made on both frontal and lateral films for displacement or narrowing of the trachea (e-Fig. 65-12).

Mechanical displacement or obstruction of large airways occurs in anomalies of the aortic arch, pulmonary arteries, and more severe forms of cardiomegaly (see e-Figs. 65-5, 65-6, 65-7, 65-9, 65-10, and 65-12). The position and contour of the descending aorta should be carefully examined. In coarctation of the aorta, the only sign in younger children may be a leftward convexity to the descending aorta (e-Fig. 65-13). Such a contour is seen often in older adults as a result of age-related ectasia, but it is abnormal in children.

SITUS

The chest film assessment is incomplete unless abnormalities of abdominal and thoracic situs (the anatomic location of organs that are asymmetrically positioned in the body) are sought and the cardiac position relative to visceral situs is determined. Dextrocardia in situs solitus is strongly associated with complex cardiac abnormalities. Abnormal situs can be subtle, with a normal-appearing liver and stomach. Airway anatomy and lung morphology are valuable indicators of visceral situs. Symmetrical bronchi are seen in almost all patients with right isomerism (asplenia) (e-Fig. 65-14) and in 68% of patients with left isomerism (polysplenia). Splenic dysfunction and intestinal malrotation occur in these children.

BONY ABNORMALITIES

A complete evaluation of the chest radiograph must include the bony thorax. Few skeletal abnormalities are strongly associated with congenital heart disease, but abnormalities of the spine (e.g., scoliosis, segmentation anomalies, and rib anomalies) and sternum (e.g., an abnormal number of ossification centers and caudal deficiency) occur. Rib notching is rarely seen in younger children with aortic coarctation, but it may be present in adolescents and teenagers in whom intercostal artery collaterals have developed (e-Fig. 65-15). Bony changes are common after a thoracotomy.

Conclusion

The role of chest radiography has changed with the development of echocardiography. Previous texts and articles have either overstated or understated the utility of the chest film. The carefully performed and thoughtfully interpreted chest radiograph continues to play a useful role in the care of children with congenital cardiovascular disease.

Key Points
Changes in pulmonary vascular resistance influence the manifestations of cardiovascular disease in the newborn.
Hyperinflation is a sign of congestive heart failure in infants.
Chest films may appear normal even in children with serious heart disease

Suggested Readings

Donnelly LF, Gelfand KJ, Schwartz DC, et al. The "wall to wall" heart: Massive cardiothymic silhouette in newborns. *Appl Radiol.* 1997;26: 23-28.

Kellenberger CJ. Aortic arch malformations. *Pediatr Radiol.* 2010;40: 876-884.

Laya BF, Goske MJ, Morrison S, et al. The accuracy of chest radiographs in the detection of congenital heart disease and in the diagnosis of specific congenital cardiac lesions. *Pediatr Radiol.* 2006;36:677-681.

Markowitz RI, Fellows KE. The effects of congenital heart disease on the lungs. *Semin Roentgenol.* 1998;33:126-135.

Strife JL, Sze RW. Radiographic evaluation of the neonate with congenital heart disease. *Radiol Clin North Am.* 1999;37:1093-1107.

Chapter 66

Pediatric Cardiothoracic Computed Tomographic Angiography

DONALD P. FRUSH

Remarkable advances have occurred in noninvasive imaging evaluation of pediatric cardiothoracic vascular disorders. One such technologic advancement is multidetector array computed tomography (MDCT). MDCT, using the computed tomography angiographic (CTA) technique, has become a primary imaging consideration for structural cardiovascular evaluation beginning as early as the newborn period.[1-5] Attention to technique is fundamental for pediatric CTA.[6-8] Without optimal or at least sufficient technical performance, diagnostic capabilities may be limited. This technical aspect (in addition to the diagnostic interpretation and communication of results) is the responsibility of the imaging expert. Therefore the objective of this chapter is to provide technical guidelines for performing pediatric thoracic CTA. The clinical examples provided illustrate these technical considerations.

Costs and Benefits

Pediatric CTA offers several advantages over other contemporary imaging modalities, including echocardiography, magnetic resonance imaging (MRI), and conventional cardiac catheterization and angiography. First, computed tomography (CT) provides the best global assessment of the lungs and airways, as well as other regional structures, in both congenital[9] and acquired vascular disorders (e-Figs. 66-1 and 66-2).

Congenital cardiovascular disorders may affect the respiratory system by causing tracheal compression or deviation (e.g., from vascular rings or pulmonary slings) with resulting obstructive effects on the lungs, or by causing air trapping at the parenchymal level, such as diffuse hypoinflation or mosaicism as a result of cardiogenic pulmonary edema. In addition, CT can suggest or demonstrate associated primary abnormalities of the respiratory system, such as pulmonary hypoplasia or tracheomalacia. Although conventional angiography could supply information on the lungs and airway, it is focused primarily on the evaluation of the vascular intraluminal anatomy. In addition, sedation is needed less frequently in younger children for CT than for magnetic resonance (MR) vascular imaging, echocardiography, or conventional angiography.

With newer technology, such as volume MDCT (e.g., 320 detector array single rotation acquisition)[10] or dual-source MDCT (Fig. 66-3),[11] a complete examination of the entire chest of an infant can be completed in less than 1 second. With echocardiography, MR vascular imaging, or angiography, imaging times typically exceed 20 minutes and may occur over hours. A reduced examination time means that CT is better tolerated by infants, children, and patients in the intensive care unit who may have a limited ability to hold still or require the examination to be performed quickly for other reasons. The technical quality, including display, also is more consistent with CT compared with echocardiography, which is a more operator-dependent examination, and compared with MR evaluation, where operators select parameters and sequences that may give a different study quality from one examination to the next. CT also allows better patient monitoring than does MRI. In addition, many of the contraindications of MRI (e.g., pacemakers, internal support apparatus, and some surgical devices) are not contraindications with CTA and produce less image artifact than with MR angiography. Unlike with conventional angiography, the multiplanar and three-dimensional capabilities of CTA provide for off-line review of information in virtually any plane. For conventional angiography, this feature is limited to the planes selected during a particular sequence, and for echocardiography, the examination planes or views recorded are the only information available for off-line evaluation. The cost of CT is comparable with that of Doppler echocardiography, in general is less than that of MR, and is much less than conventional angiography.

CTA has some disadvantages. CTA involves the use of radiation, which is an issue with angiocardiography but not with MRI or echocardiography. CT radiation dosages depend on the technique used. In general, CTA can be performed with a dosage similar to or lower than that of a routine chest CT. CTA dose estimates in young children can be less than 1.0 mSv.[12,13] With gated technology, employing prospective gating and newer volume scanning, doses also can be substantially lower than with older CT technology and retrospective gating.[13-16] With rare exceptions, properly performed pediatric CTA results in a lower radiation dose than conventional diagnostic angiographic evaluation. Electrocardiographic-gated CTA usually involves a greater radiation dosage than

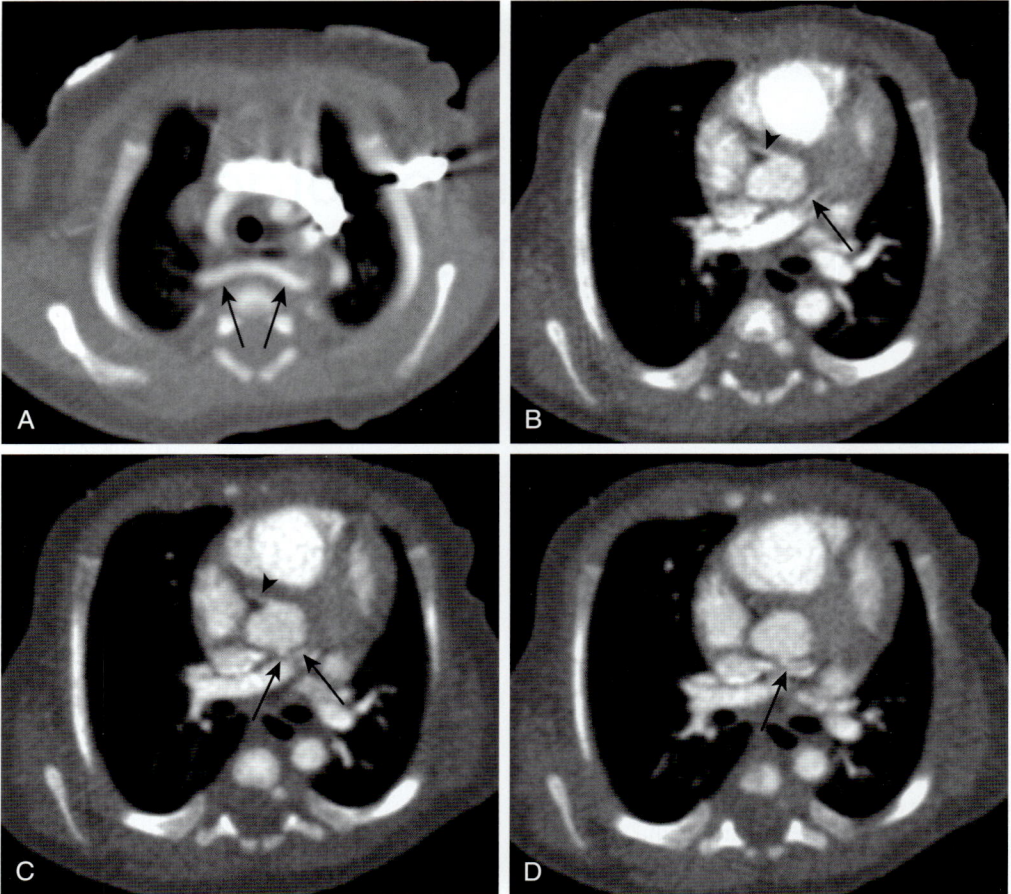

Figure 66-3 A newborn boy with labored stridor. Aortic arch anatomy was incompletely assessed on echocardiography. Nongated dual-source cardiac computed tomographic angiography was performed using high-pitch 3.2, 80 kVp, 60 effective mA, and 6.0 mL of 300 mg/mL iodine yielding an estimated radiation dose of approximately 1.4 mSv. The scan was performed over about 0.6 seconds. **A,** An aberrant right subclavian artery (*arrows*) is seen to pass behind a normal caliber trachea. No cause for respiratory difficulty was identified. **B** to **D,** Note excellent depiction of small structures as a result of high-pitch scanning, demonstrating the normal origin of the right coronary artery (**B** and **C**) (*arrowheads*) and the relatively posterior origin and course of the left main coronary artery, probably still from the left coronary cusp in **B** to **D** (*arrows*).

limited diagnostic conventional angiography or a nongated CTA. Intravenous (IV) contrast material is required for CTA but also is required for conventional angiography and for MR angiography. The risk of major adverse effects (e.g., airway spasm and cardiovascular collapse) from iodinated IV contrast material is extremely small in children.[17,18] Unlike with echocardiography, MRI, and conventional angiography, pediatric thoracic CTA typically is used for morphologic assessment, although cardiac function and other hemodynamic information can be obtained.[19] CT for cardiovascular evaluation also is not portable.

Various factors must be taken into consideration in choosing an appropriate imaging algorithm. Individual expertise is a strong consideration, as is the availability of the modality desired. Personnel must be able to perform these examinations, and imaging experts, such as radiologists, may have preferences. Performing CTA on an MDCT device that offers less than 16 slice (e.g., a 4- and 8-slice MDCT device) is problematic, and image quality (both contrast enhancement and multiplanar reformations) is more limited. A CT scan that can be performed within the same day or relative quickly may be preferred compared with waiting several days for an

MR evaluation. In general, echocardiography should be the first examination considered, with MR being second, unless contraindications are present.

Technique

Box 66-1 shows the steps taken in performing a pediatric CTA (see e-Fig. 66-2).[6-8]

Pediatric cardiovascular CT evaluation is less protocol driven than is cardiovascular CT evaluation for adults. The examination should be constructed to obtain the appropriate diagnostic information while minimizing radiation dosage. Patient preparation includes understanding the clinical indications for the examination and understanding the anatomy in question. Optimal vascular opacification and minimization of streak artifacts depend in part on familiarity with abnormal congenital anatomy, and an understanding of palliative and corrective cardiovascular anatomy is critical.

Patient motion needs to be controlled (e-Fig. 66-4), which may require sedation of younger children. Breath holding is preferred during CTA but is not a requisite, especially with

---

Box 66-1 Steps in Performing Pediatric Computed Tomography Angiography

The subject is an otherwise healthy, 4-week-old, 4.0-kg male infant with congenital stridor. Findings of an echocardiogram suggest the presence of a vascular ring (see Fig. 66-6).

Planning the Computed Tomography Angiogram

1. **Determine that computed tomographic angiography (CTA) is the appropriate examination.** Echocardiography was inconclusive. Magnetic resonance would require sedation and a 2- to 3-week wait for a sedation slot. CTA had a 1-day turnaround.

2. **Define the question to be answered.** Aortic arch and airway. A high-detail examination (e.g., for small vessels) is not necessary. It is not necessary to image below the mid to lower thoracic aorta (thus the radiation dose can be lower).

3. **Understand the anatomy.** Aortic rings, including innominate compression; a pulmonary sling is not exhibited with true stridor.

4. **Patient limitations.** Essentially none. The patient will be fed immediately before the CTA but after the intravenous line is in place.

Performing the Computed Tomography Angiogram

1. **Intravenous contrast material**
   Type: Low osmolar, nonionic iodine, 300 mg/mL
   Dose: Total volume of 6.0 mL (4.0 kg at 1.5 mL/kg)
   Rate and route: 24-gauge angiocatheter in hand vein; manual administration as quickly as possible

   Onset of scanning: Determined with a test bolus of 0.6 mL contrast in a tuberculin syringe. Short extension tubing. Start monitoring images at 2-second intervals and begin push of the test bolus when the first monitoring image appears. Contrast reaches the right ventricle in 5 seconds and the left ventricle in 6 to 7 seconds. Add 2 seconds, so the scan onset will be 8 to 10 seconds after starting administration of contrast for the diagnostic study.

2. **Select scan parameters:** 16-detector row
   Scan field of view: small
   Detector thickness: 16 × 0.625 mm, anticipating multiplanar and three-dimensional reconstruction, especially for airway depiction
   Slice thickness and interval for axial review: 2.5 mm at 2.5-mm reconstruction interval
   Tube current: 60 mA
   Peak kilovoltage: 80 kVp
   Gantry cycle time: 0.5 sec (yields 30-mA examination)
   Pitch: 1.375

3. **Scan interpretation**
   Reconstruct an axial data set at 0.625-mm thickness; 0.5-mm interval; soft algorithm
   Coronal and sagittal reformations at 2.5-mm thickness and 2.5-mm interval; axial data set can also be used for volume-rendered three-dimensional reconstruction

From Frush DP. Technique of pediatric thoracic CT angiography. *Radiol Clin North Am.* 2005;43:419-433.

---

volume scanning and other fast (e.g., dual-source, high-pitch) scanning technology. If the child is intubated, an inspiratory hold during the CTA evaluation is recommended. Metal (e.g., pacemakers, intracardiac leads, sternal wires, stents, clips, and valves) and arms (Fig. 66-5) may cause streak artifact. Monitors and associated leads should be positioned outside the scan field if possible to minimize streak artifact across the chest. Knowing the location and caliber of angiocatheters used for IV contrast administration will help determine the rate of administration and the time it takes contrast material to reach the heart.[20] Finally, because cardiac CT evaluation may involve patients with left-to-right shunts or admixture lesions, extreme care must be taken to avoid injection of air or a thrombus through the line when contrast is administered. This situation is rarely, if ever, a problem with adult cardiac evaluation.

Technical considerations regarding the IV contrast material include type and concentration, dosage, rate of administration, and timing of scan onset after administration.[21] In general, low osmolar, nonionic contrast media are recommended for contrast–enhanced CT scanning in the pediatric population. The iodine concentration varies but usually is around 300 mg/mL. For newborns and small children, higher concentrations such as 370 mg/mL will afford better enhancement of their smaller vessels. A dosage of 1.5 mL/kg is usually adequate, with a maximum total volume of 125 mL. With gated cardiac evaluation, the contrast dose can be smaller (e.g., <100 mL). If a second CT scan must be performed while the patient remains on the scanner, then 1 to 1.5 mL/kg of additional contrast can be administered. In this case, the maximal dosage would be 3.0 mL/kg, which is still reasonable for a single examination.

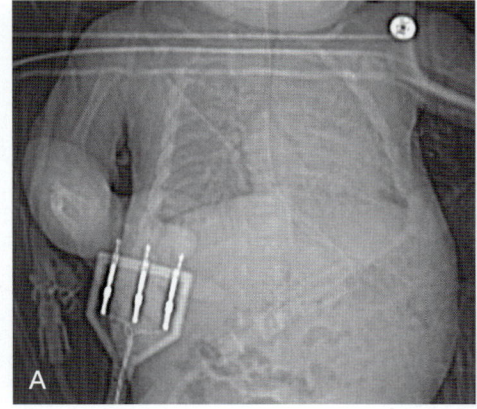
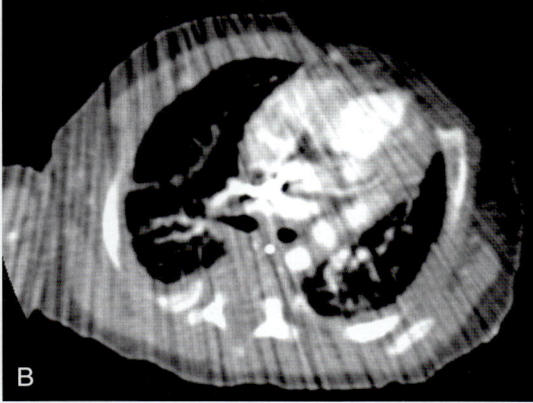

Figure 66-5 Artifact from leads. **A,** A topogram demonstrates the leads that were in the scan range. **B,** Note substantial streak artifact. (From Frush DP: Thoracic cardiovascular CT: technique and applications, *Pediatr Radiol.* 2009;39(3):464-70. Reprinted with permission.)

The rate of administration depends on whether a manual injection or a power injector is used and also on the size of the angiocatheter. Most peripherally inserted central catheters are not amenable to contrast administration for CTA. Suggested rates of administration are 1.5 mL/sec for a 24-gauge angiocatheter, 2.0 to 2.5 mL/sec for a 22-gauge angiocatheter, and 3.0 to 4.0 mL/sec for a 20-gauge angiocatheter. When possible, contrast should be administered through a power injector, which gives a more predictable and consistent enhancement curve. However, performing manual administration as quickly as possible can provide adequate enhancement when power injection is not appropriate. Use of central venous catheters for power administration varies based on individual practice and preferences.

The timing of contrast administration with respect to scanning initiation is a critical factor in CTA. In general, scanning is started either during administration of the contrast or immediately after administration is completed. Timing depends on the structures that need to be opacified. Later scan initiation is used for opacification of the thoracic aorta and major branches or systemic venous structures, whereas earlier scan initiation is appropriate for right-sided structures, especially pulmonary arteries. An empiric delay can be used, but because of the wide range of sizes that may be encountered in pediatric CTA (i.e., 1.0 to 100 kg), a single recommendation is impossible. A range of delays could be determined depending on the rate of administration. In general, most cardiac CTA, even in the smallest child, does not begin before 5 seconds after the onset of contrast administration. For large children, the empiric delay may be as long as 50 seconds. Bolus tracking technology, which obviates the need for this estimation, can be used to start the CTA. Alternatively, a test bolus can be administered and the arrival of contrast to the desired location (for cardiac CT, the right side versus the left side of the heart) can be used (Fig. 66-6).

This test bolus technique works even in neonates. A test bolus of 10% of the total expected volume is used, which requires a tuberculin syringe and minimization of catheter and tubing dead space for a child receiving a test bolus of less than 1.0 mL. The arrival of the test bolus at the appropriate side of the heart is timed, and this time is used to set the delay for the start of scanning. In neonates, usually about 2 to 3 seconds is added to this arrival of the test bolus for optimal enhancement. Tracking without a test bolus is simple to perform, and a test bolus rarely is used for nongated CTA in children. Fontan circuits may require special contrast administration techniques.[22]

Scan techniques include adjustment of technical parameters such as the number of detector rows, the thickness of detectors, the gantry cycle time, tube current (milliamperes [mA]), and peak kilovoltage (kVp). Parameters such as scan thickness and interval are adjustable after the scan volume is obtained (these parameters usually are in protocols). Suggestions for a CTA technique are provided in Table 66-1.[21]

The isotropic images obtained with 16-slice and higher MDCT scanners provide excellent multiplanar reformations and three-dimensional evaluation, which show complicated anatomy in a way to which clinical care providers (e.g., cardiac surgeons) are accustomed (e-Figs. 66-7 to 66-9). The thinnest detector option should be chosen for pediatric CTA, because thinner slices improve the quality of reformations. The fastest gantry cycle time is recommended to minimize motion artifact and to obtain the fastest scanning time possible, which is important in children who may be anxious or otherwise fidgety. Pitch, essentially representing table speed (mm/second) divided by effective collimation (mm), generally is in the range of 1 to 1.5 for nongated CTA. Tube current, including tube current modulation technology,[23] varies depending on patient size; recommendations can be found in Table 66-1.

Because contrast is relatively high in cardiothoracic CTA, consideration should be given to lowering the peak kilovoltage.[8,24] This step will improve image contrast and, although some increased noise occurs, the increase in contrast is greater than the increase in noise in small children, which produces an improved contrast-to-noise ratio and better image quality.

Table 66-1

Technical Guidelines for Pediatric Cardiovascular Multidetector Array Computed Tomography Angiography									
				Pitch‡			Thickness of Detector (mm)		
Weight (lb)	kVp	mA*	Slice Thickness (mm)†	4-	8-	16-, 64-	4-, 8-	16-, 64-	Increment (mm)
10-19	80-100	60	1.25-2.5	1.5	1.35	1.375	1.25	0.625	1.0-2.5
20-39	80-100	70							
40-59	100	80							
60-79	100	100							
80-99	120	120							
100-149	120	140-160							
>150	120	≥170							

The technique shown is based on General Electric computed tomography (CT) equipment options. Similar parameters can be used as a guideline for other CT equipment.

*Slightly higher than body CT protocols. Use fastest gantry rotation time.

†Displayed thickness. For coronal and sagittal reformats and three-dimensional reconstructions, reconstruct an axial data set at thickness of the detector (e.g., 0.625 for a 16-slice scanner) at 0.5- to 1.0-mm intervals, soft algorithm. Multiplanar thickness and interval should be similar to axial. For evaluation of larger structures (e.g., the aorta), especially in larger children, the larger detector configuration (2.5 for an 8-slice scanner and 1.25 for a 16-slice scanner) and a larger reconstructed thickness and interval can be used.

‡For larger children and larger vessels, the highest pitch can be used for multidetector array computed tomography.

Modified from Frush DP. Evidence-based principles and protocols for pediatric body multislice computed tomography. In Knollman F, Coakley FV, editors: *Multislice CT: principles and protocols*, Philadelphia: Elsevier; 2005.

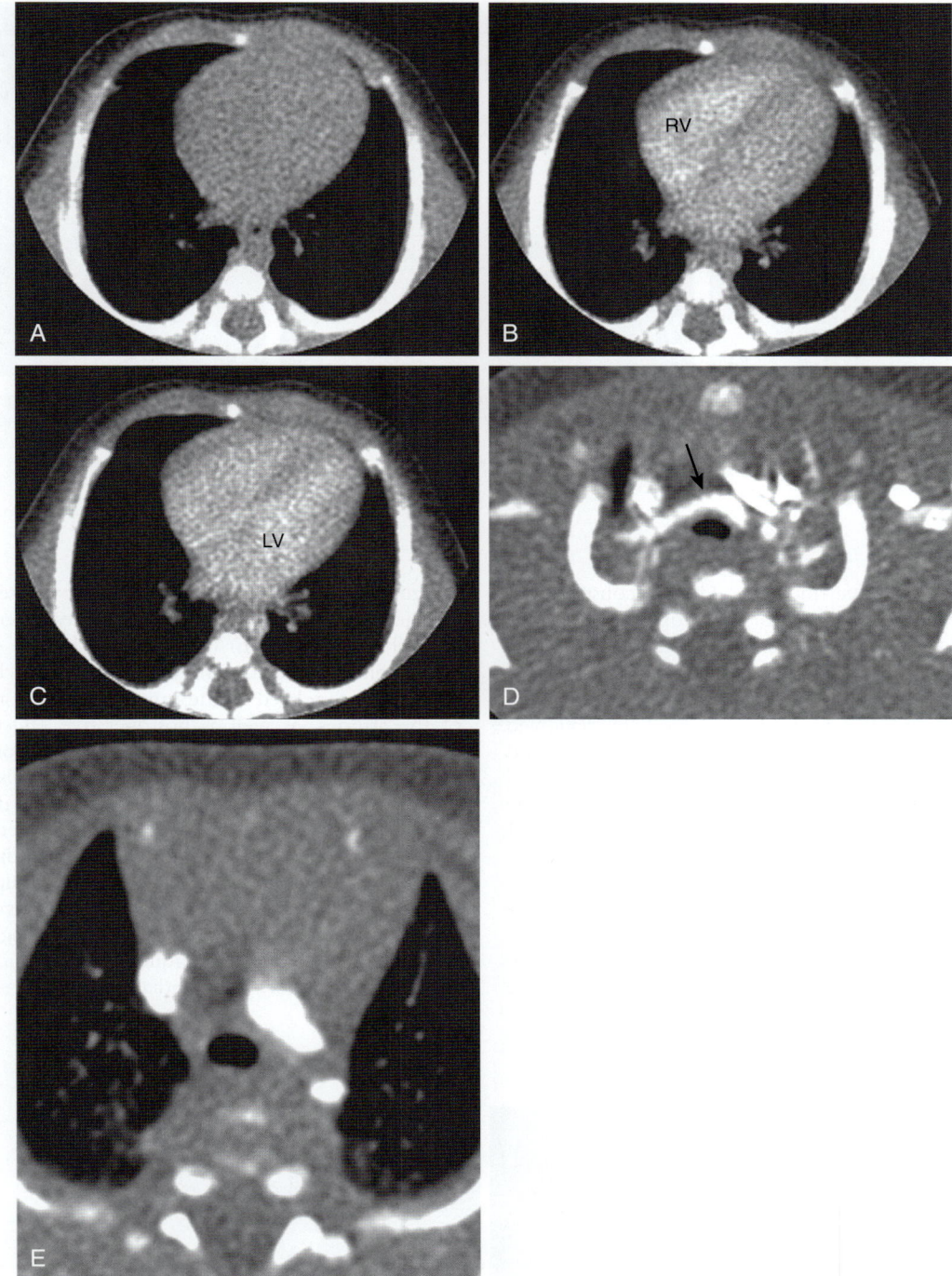

Figure 66-6 **A 4-week-old infant boy with congenital stridor.** An echocardiogram was not able to fully assess for a suspected vascular ring. Axial serial isolevel monitoring images during bolus tracking at the midventricular level show precontrast appearance (**A**) and the arrival of a 0.6-mL test bolus in the right ventricle (*RV*) at 5 seconds (**B**) and the left ventricle (*LV*) and descending thoracic aorta at approximately 7 seconds (**C**). **D,** After the diagnostic computed tomography angiogram, the trachea is narrowed at the level of the thoracic inlet to about 50% of normal anteroposterior diameter brachiocephalic artery (*arrow*), but no distal tracheal or aortic branching abnormality was present (**E**). (From Frush DP. Technique of pediatric thoracic CT angiography, *Radiol Clin North Am.* 2005;43:419-433. Reprinted with permission.)

Therefore 80 kVp (Fig. 66-10) for newborn through young school-age children and 100 kVp for older but still young school-age children (up to about 10 years assuming normal body habitus) is acceptable. A value of 120 kVp can be used for older children.

With advances in image processing time and storage and the availability of off-line workstations, evaluation of the pediatric heart and great vessels in multiple perspectives is now performed rapidly. Images should be reconstructed at the narrowest slice thickness possible (submillimeter) and at

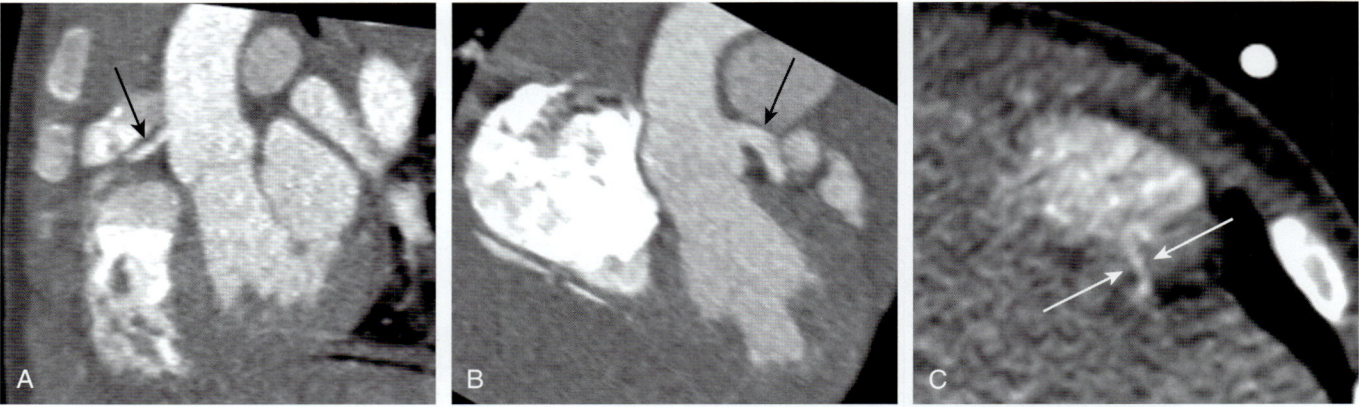

Figure 66-10   A coronary cameral fistula in a 10-month-old boy. Oblique reformatted maximum intensity projection images through the origins of the left (**A**) (*arrow*) and right (**B**) (*arrow*) coronary arteries demonstrate a larger left coronary artery. **C,** A coned down axial image demonstrates the distal portion of the left sided coronary-cameral fistula (*arrow*) coursing through the myocardium to the right ventricular chamber. (From Lerner C, Frush DP, Boll DT. Evaluation of a coronary-cameral fistula: benefits of coronary dual source MDCT angiography in children, *Pediatr Radiol.* 2008;38:874-878. Reprinted with permission.)

intervals just under the slice thickness. These reconstructions generally are performed with use of low noise kernels.

Cardiac gated CTA became more practical after the availability of 16-detector row technology with improved spatial resolution. As previously noted, prospective gating reduces radiation dose. Technical considerations have been reviewed recently[13]; a detailed description of gated techniques is beyond the intent of this chapter. Even more than with the nongated angiographic technique, presence at the scanner by the imaging expert usually is necessary to determine contrast details, particularly with the timing bolus, and scan parameters (e.g., scan range, tube current, and peak kilovoltage), as well as performance of postacquisition processing. Applications include improved depiction of the great vessels (e.g., for aortic dissection). However, evaluation in children usually is focused on coronary artery anatomy. Recently, dual-source design (i.e., two x-ray tubes) has improved temporal resolution (obviating β-blockage of heart rates, even to heart rates around 120 beats/min) (see Figs. 66-10 and 66-11).[25] Pediatric applications of coronary artery CTA include congenital abnormalities related to the number, site of origin, or course of the arteries, as well as postoperative effects on coronary arteries (e.g., after correction of transposition of the great vessels). In addition, the effect of systemic disorders, such as Kawasaki disease, on coronary arteries (and development of stenosis or aneurysm) increasingly is reported using cardiac gated techniques. As with adults, intracardiac anatomy is better displayed with use of gating, although dual-source high-pitch technology can provide improved intracardiac detail compared with non–high pitch and single-source scanners. Applying adult techniques to pediatric scanning can result in excessively high radiation dosages—as high as 30

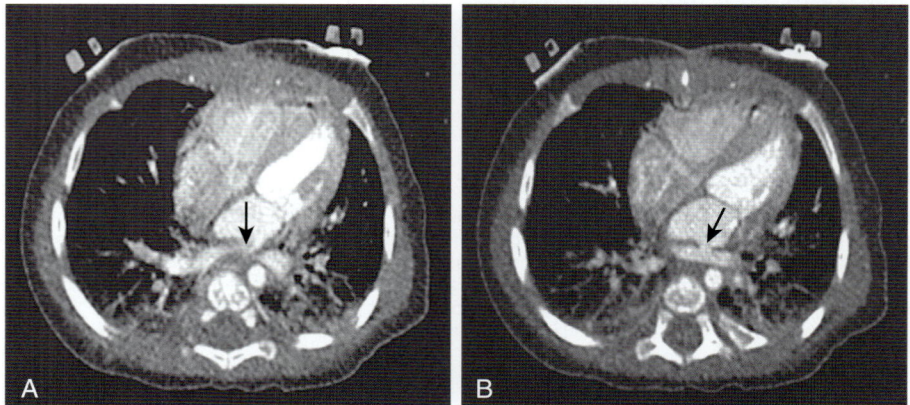

Figure 66-11   Postoperative evaluation of total anomalous pulmonary venous return in an infant. Pulmonary vein stenosis was suspected after echocardiography was performed. A gated cardiac computed tomography examination, without β-blockade (heart rate, approximately 120 beats/min) was performed using 110 mA (approximately half of the adult tube current). Stenoses are present at insertion of the right upper pulmonary vein at the left atrium (*arrow*) (**A**) and the confluence of the remainder of the pulmonary veins (*arrow*) (**B**). A twisting of the confluence of all pulmonary veins was encountered in the operating room and corrected. (From Frush DP, Yoshizuma T. Conventional and CT angiography in children: dosimetry and dose comparisons, *Pediatr Radiol.* 2006;36:154-158.)

millisieverts (mSv)—which is approximately 10 to 20 times the dosage of a normal chest CT examination in a child. Dosages and image quality for gated cardiac evaluation should reflect reduced-dosage techniques for other body applications in infants and children, with consideration of lower tube current and kilovoltage (see Fig. 66-6).

The use of bismuth breast shields to reduce breast dose has lowered radiation dose and maintained image quality for pediatric chest CT,[26] although the benefit of shielding is debated given the availability of other techniques for dose reduction.[27] The use of organ–based dose modulation, where the tube current is reduced over an arc to reduce surface dose such as for the breasts, has yet to be systematically studied in pediatric chest CT. In addition, iterative reconstruction technology[28] likely will provide new opportunities to reduce dose or improve image quality for pediatric thoracic cardiovascular CTA.

Conclusion

CT evaluation of intrathoracic cardiovascular anatomy has increased dramatically in both adults and children during the past decade. In certain pediatric populations, including very young children, technical challenges need to be considered before and during performance of cardiac CT angiography. Considerations include proper patient preparation and individualization of scanning techniques to address the specific clinical questions, as well as considerations unique to that child (such as size). These considerations also will minimize radiation exposure. Despite these challenges, excellent cardiac angiographic evaluation can be obtained even in the most challenging cases.

Key Points

Technique is critical for optimizing pediatric cardiovascular CT angiography in children.
Pediatric CT angiography is less protocol driven than with adults.
If performed properly, nongated and even gated CT angiography in children can result in dose estimates at or below 1.0 mSv in certain circumstances.
Familiarity with clinical questions and anatomy with congenital disorders will afford the greatest potential for safe and high-quality pediatric examinations.
Lower peak kilovoltage (e.g., 80 and 100 kVp) can be used in CT angiography compared with other body imaging because of high contrast vascular enhancement.

Suggested Readings

Frush DP. Thoracic cardiovascular CT: technique and applications. *Pediatr Radiol.* 2009;39(3):464-470.

Frush DP. Evidence-based principles and protocols for pediatric body multislice computed tomography. In: Knollman F, Coakley FV, eds. *Multislice CT: principles and protocols.* Philadelphia: Elsevier; 2005.

Siegel MJ. Computed tomography of pediatric cardiovascular disease. *J Thorac Imaging.* 2010;25:256-266.

Young C, Taylor A, Owens C. Paediatric cardiac computed tomography: a review of imaging techniques and radiation dose consideration. *Eur Radiol.* 2011;21:518-529.

References

Full references for this chapter can be found on www.expertconsult.com.

Chapter 67

Magnetic Resonance Imaging for Congenital Heart Disease

SADAF T. BHUTTA and S. BRUCE GREENBERG

Electrocardiographic-gated spin echo and gradient echo pulse sequences are staples for anatomic and functional assessment of congenital heart disease. Technologic innovations in the magnetic resonance imaging (MRI) hardware and software continue to refine cardiovascular imaging techniques. Steady-state free precession (SSFP) cine sequences of the heart in multiple planes have become a mainstay for both anatomic and functional evaluation in congenital heart diseases. Parallel imaging protocols reduce scan times and thus decrease the need for prolonged sedation in children. New sequences for magnetic resonance angiography (MRA) permit time-resolved imaging or nonintravenous contrast acquisitions. Perfusion imaging is becoming more commonplace.

Pulse Sequences

Spin echo and gradient echo sequences are used for cardiac evaluation. Spin echo, or "black blood," imaging gives excellent contrast resolution between the endocardium or vessel wall and the blood-filled lumen. Double inversion recovery imaging adds additional nonselective and selective 180-degree pulses to further null the blood signal. The double inversion recovery pulse sequence is the current backbone of spin echo morphologic cardiac imaging in teenagers and adults, but it requires that the patient hold his or her breath (Fig. 67-1). More traditional T1-weighted sequences are used in uncooperative or sedated children. T1-weighted sequences are longer but do not require that patients hold their breath.

Blood has a high signal in gradient echo sequences and is the basis for "white blood" or "bright blood" imaging. Balanced SSFP (b-SSFP) is the state-of-the-art gradient echo sequence for bright blood imaging. b-SSFP sequences are faster than earlier gradient echo sequences and have better contrast between myocardium and blood. As with double inversion recovery imaging, b-SSFP is ideally performed with the patient holding his or her breath. Respiratory motion artifacts are minimized in the sedated or uncooperative patient by increasing the number of excitations. This technique is the preferred sequence for evaluating cardiac motion and quantifying cardiac function. Stenosis and turbulent flow appear as a black jet in the white blood on gradient imaging (Fig. 67-2).

Functional Evaluation

MRI is the gold standard for cardiac function assessment and is markedly superior to echocardiography in assessing right ventricular function. A stack of short-axis cine images through the ventricles in end-systole and end-diastole is used to measure ventricular volumes.[1] The product of the endocardial cross-section tracing and the section thickness is the section volume. The section volumes are summated to determine end-diastolic and end-systolic volumes for the right and left ventricles. The same images are used to measure the left ventricle mass by performing epicardial and endocardial tracings. The difference in the volumes circumscribed by the epicardium and endocardium is the left ventricle myocardium volume, from which mass is determined.

Cardiac measurements need to be indexed by dividing by the patient body surface area because children vary greatly in size. Ejection fractions and stroke volumes are calculated from the ventricle end-diastolic and end-systolic measurements. The cardiac output is the product of stroke volume and heart rate. The cardiac index is the cardiac output divided by the body surface area. The left ventricle mass divided by the body surface area is the myocardial index. The myocardial index is particularly helpful in evaluating the deconditioned left ventricle in the older infant or child before performing an arterial switch procedure.

The stroke volumes of the right and left ventricles are the same in the structurally normal heart. Differences in stroke volumes are caused by shunts and valve regurgitation. Using MR, both shunt size and regurgitant fraction can be calculated from the stroke volumes. Shunt size, or the pulmonary to systemic flow ratio (Qp:Qs), is determined by dividing the larger stroke volume by the smaller. The valvular regurgitant fraction is determined by dividing the regurgitant volume, which is the difference of ventricle stroke volumes, by the larger ventricle stroke volume (Fig. 67-3). The regurgitant volume may result from atrioventricular valve or semilunar valve or a combination of both.

$$Qp{:}Qs = \text{Ventricle stroke volume}_1 / \text{Ventricle stroke volume}_2$$

$$\text{Valvular regurgitant fraction} = (\text{ventricle stroke volume}_1 - \text{ventricle stroke volume}_2)/\text{ventricle stroke volume}_1$$

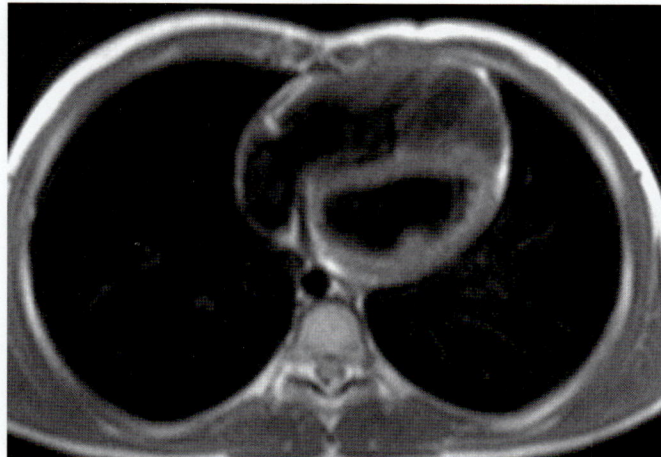

Figure 67-1 An axial double inversion recovery spin echo image shows both ventricles and the right atrium. The nulled blood signal provides excellent visualization of the static myocardial tissue.

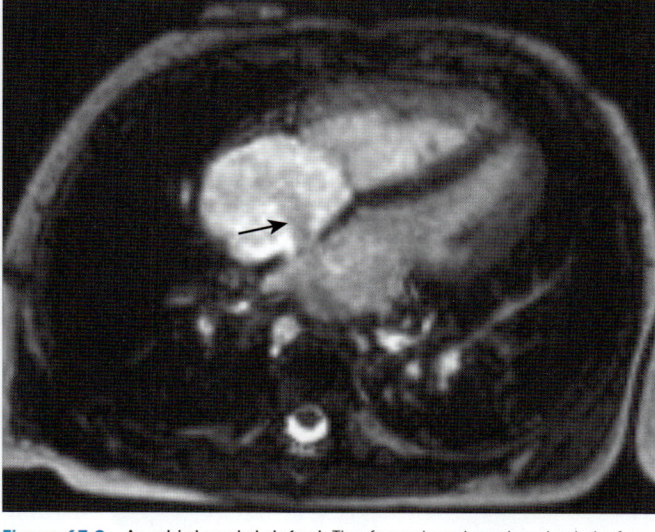

Figure 67-2 **An atrial septal defect.** The four-chamber steady-state free-precession view shows mild right atrial and right ventricular enlargement. A small atrial septal defect is seen with a jet of blood passing from the left atrium to the right atrium, indicating a left-to-right shunt (*arrow*).

where *volume*₁ is the larger of the two ventricular stroke volumes.

Quantitative phase-contrast imaging uses gradient echo sequences to measure phase shift. Flow quantification using a plane of imaging perpendicular to the vessel or valve of interest allows quantification of blood flow and velocity. Flow quantification gives both magnitude and directional information (Fig. 67-4). Shunt volumes and regurgitant fractions are quantified. Regurgitation is quantified by:

Vessel regurgitant fraction = Regurgitant volume/

Antegrade volume

The pressure gradient across a stenosis is calculated using the modified Bernoulli equation:

$$\Delta P = 4v^2$$

where ΔP is the peak instantaneous pressure gradient across the stenosis and v is the velocity across the stenosis measured by flow analysis.

Magnetic Resonance Angiography

Contrast-enhanced magnetic resonance angiography (CE-MRA) is performed after injection of a gadolinium chelate bolus. The technique relies on T1 shortening of blood and requires rapid imaging. A time-of-flight spoiled gradient sequence with a short echo time is used. Conventionally, CE-MRA is not an electrocardiographic–gated technique but ideally is performed as the breath is held. Recently the free-breathing time-resolved CE-MRA technique has proved to

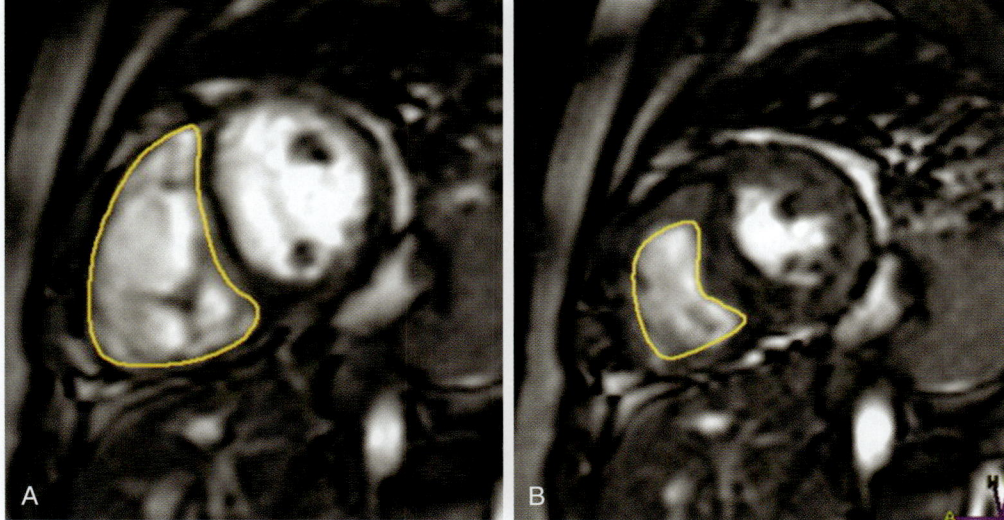

Figure 67-3 **Pulmonary regurgitation.** Endocardial contours are drawn on a short-axis steady-state free precession image of the right ventricle from base to apex in end-diastole (**A**) and end-systole (**B**) in a patient with a history of pulmonary stenosis after a pulmonary valvectomy and now with pulmonary regurgitation. The pulmonary regurgitant fraction was calculated to be 37% by right and left ventricular stroke volume differences.

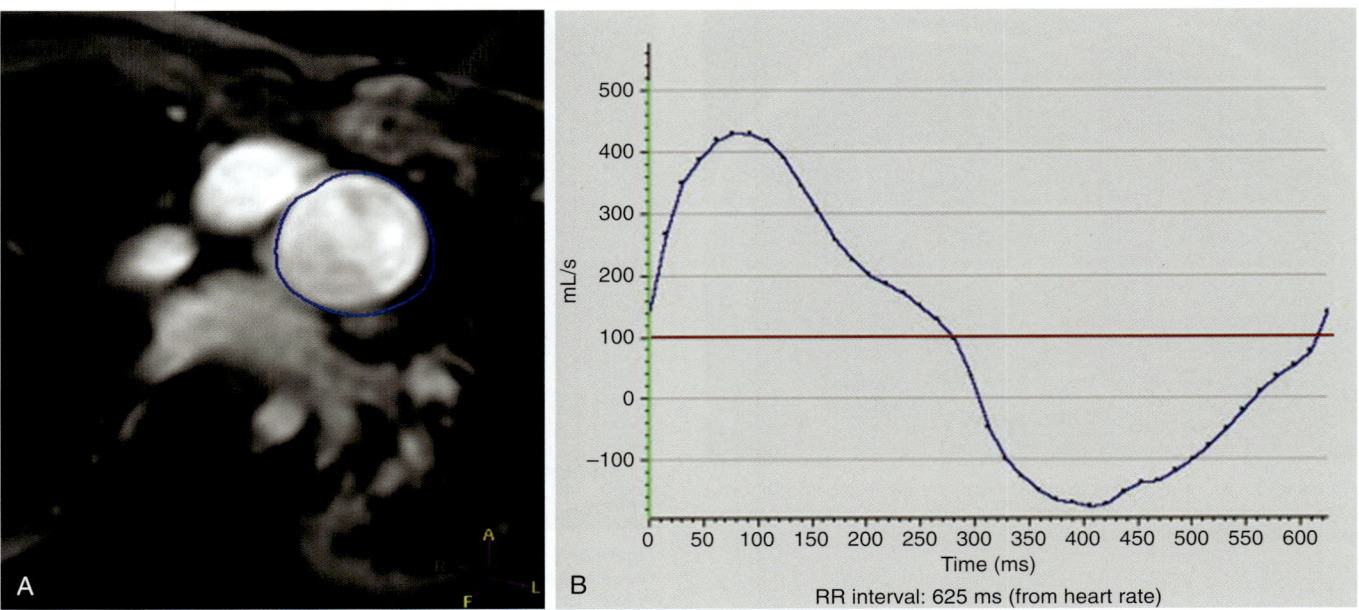

Figure 67-4 Tetralogy of Fallot. Phase contrast velocity mapping of the pulmonary artery in a 15-year-old with a history of tetralogy of Fallot after patch augmentation of the subpulmonary outflow tract obstruction. The blue region of interest is around the pulmonary outflow tract (**A**). The flow curve demonstrates moderate pulmonary regurgitation of 34% (**B**).

be feasible in children with a higher heart rate with use of a keyhole approach with parallel imaging.[1]

CE-MRA can be performed on sedated children and younger children who cannot hold their breath. Some image degradation is present because of the breathing motion, but it can be minimized by shortening the acquisition time with use of parallel imaging techniques or by decreasing the time of the MRA acquisition by decreasing the number of excitations to less than 1.

CE-MRA creates a volume data set with high contrast resolution (Fig. 67-5). Three-dimensional volume renderings and multiplanar reformations are created in any plane or view.

Overlapping structures are eliminated. Simultaneous imaging of multiple vessels with a single injection is another advantage.

Time-resolved CE-MRA has been performed successfully when acquiring angiographic data in various body parts in the pediatric population.[2] In contrast to conventional CE-MRA, time-resolved MRA achieves greater temporal resolution.[3,4] By oversampling the center of k-space compared with the periphery, portions of k-space are shared to create higher temporal resolution than with spiral k-space ordering. Before contrast material is injected, a mask volume is obtained. The contrast material is then injected and the scan is initiated. The precontrast mask is subtracted from each

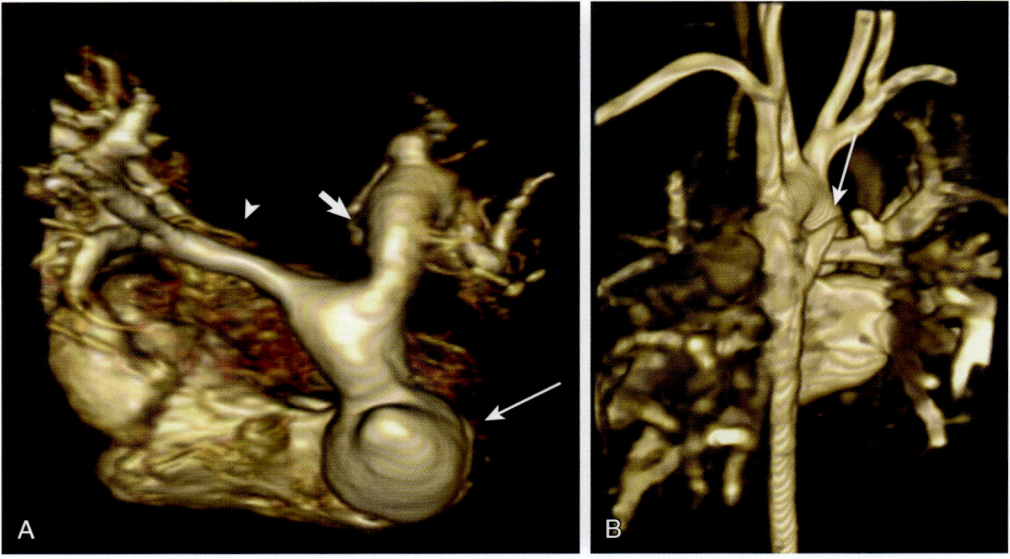

Figure 67-5 Tetralogy of Fallot after patch augmentation for right ventricular outflow tract obstruction. A three-dimensional volume-rendered image of the pulmonary artery and branches (**A**) from a superior to inferior view. A pseudoaneurysm of the right ventricular outflow tract is seen (*arrow*). Hypoplasia of the right branch pulmonary artery is present (*arrowhead*), along with ectasia of the left branch pulmonary artery (*short bold arrow*). A posterior image of the chest (**B**) in the same patient shows a major aortopulmonary collateral artery to the upper lobe segment of the right lung (*arrow*).

subsequent volume to obtain a series of maximum intensity projection images obtained over time (Video 67-1).

A respiratory- and cardiac-gated, fat-suppressed, three-dimensional MRA technique (b-SSFP sequence) has been developed for whole-heart imaging that provides high resolution for the evaluation of intracardiac anatomy and coronary arteries (Fig. 67-6 and Video 67-2).[5,6] This technique can be used either without or with contrast and is very is helpful in evaluating patients with severe renal dysfunction who cannot undergo testing with gadolinium-chelate contrast agents because of the risk of developing nephrogenic systemic fibrosis.[7]

Perfusion and Delayed Enhancement

First-pass contrast-enhanced perfusion images, with or without vasodilators, provide assessment of myocardial perfusion reserve. Perfusion imaging has limited application in children. Delayed enhanced images provide information about abnormal myocardium in both ischemic and nonischemic cardiomyopathies and can be used frequently in pediatric protocols for cardiac MR.[8] Stress imaging to detect decreased coronary flow is assessed by cine spoiled gradient echo sequences or SSFP sequences. The ventricular function at rest is compared with the regional function during pharmacologic stress. Infarction is always seen in the subendocardium, and delayed hyperenhancement is seen in ischemia (Fig. 67-7 and Video 67-3). Myocardial perfusion is acquired by rapid imaging during multiple cardiac cycles, which allows visualization of a contrast bolus through the heart. Perfusion is delayed with the decreased appearance of contrast in a myocardial territory

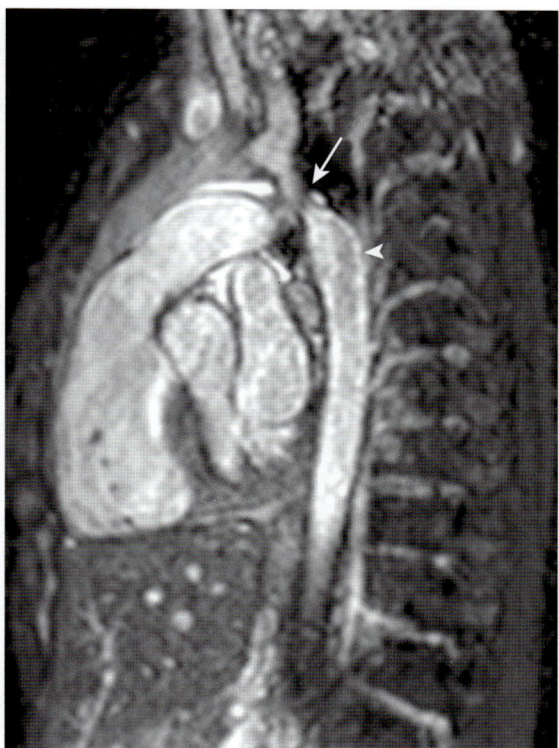

Figure 67-6 **Aortic coarctation.** A 3-year-old patient with a recently diagnosed coarctation of the aorta had a preoperative magnetic resonance imaging scan. Per protocol, a nonenhanced three-dimensional magnetic resonance angiogram of the chest was performed. The arrow points to a focal area of high-grade stenosis in the postductal aorta, whereas the arrowhead shows the turbulent flow distal to the coarctation consistent with a hemodynamically significant obstruction (see Video 67-2).

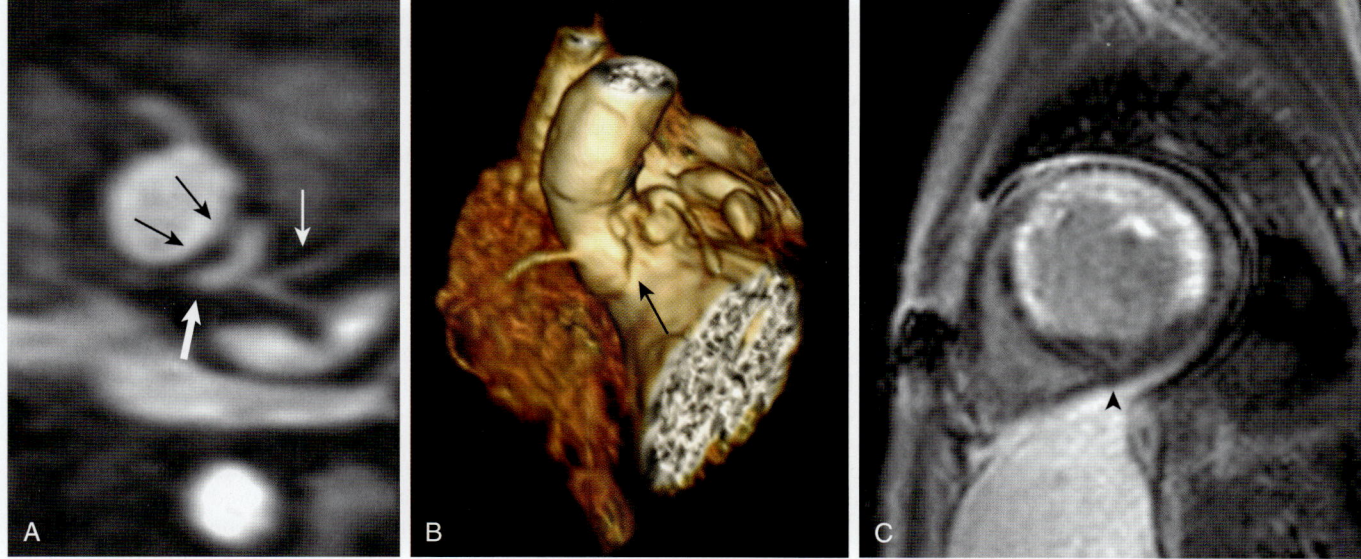

Figure 67-7 A multiplanar reformatted image (**A**) of the nonenhanced three-dimensional (3D) magnetic resonance angiogram shows the hypointense pericardial tissue (*thin black arrows*) causing partial isolation of the left coronary cusp (*thick white arrow*). The left main coronary artery and the left descending and the left circumflex branches are well visualized (*thin white arrow*). A 3D volume-rendered image of the aorta (**B**) shows the defect in the aortic root (*arrow*) consistent with the pericardial tissue seen on the multiplanar reformatted image. A 10-minute delayed gadolinium enhancement image (**C**) shows late enhancement of the left ventricular free wall, the anterior wall, and the interventricular septum. There is sparing of the right coronary artery distribution (*arrowhead*) (See Video 67-3).

distributed by a stenosed artery. Delayed enhancement is assessed 10 minutes after the injection of gadolinium. Depending on the extent of delayed enhancement and specific patterns of distribution, a distinction can be made between different nonischemic causes of cardiomyopathies. For example, hypertrophic cardiomyopathy shows predominantly patchy rather than confluent late enhancement and is localized predominantly to the interventricular septum. Nonischemic dilated cardiomyopathy occurs as a result of several causes and shows a variable pattern of late enhancement. This late enhancement is shown to have two distinct patterns: patchy with mid wall late enhancement or transmural or subendocardial late enhancement that cannot be distinguished from the ischemic heart disease. Arrhythmogenic right ventricular cardiomyopathy may show late enhancement in regions of fibrofatty infiltration of the right ventricular wall (see Chapter 80).[9,10]

Protocols

PREOPERATIVE IMAGING

Protocols should be individualized on the basis of patient needs. MRI is performed to complement echocardiography for evaluation of cardiovascular anomalies and function. For example, echocardiography may provide adequate cardiac imaging in a child with tetralogy of Fallot, but it may not adequately visualize the branch pulmonary arteries. CE-MRA of the pulmonary arteries would complement the echocardiogram and is less invasive than digital angiography.

Because MRI examinations contain a large number of images, an organized segmental approach is necessary for image interpretation. The morphologic assessment includes determining atrial, bronchial, and abdominal situs. The cardiac situs and segments, including the atrioventricular and ventriculoarterial connections, are evaluated (see Chapter 63). The number and connections of the pulmonary veins are noted. Septal defects, pulmonary artery anomalies, aortic anomalies, shunts, and valvular and vascular stenoses or regurgitations are assessed.

Most intrinsic cardiac anomalies do not require MRI for initial diagnosis or treatment, although a rare anomaly or complex anomaly may benefit from this modality. Axial spin echo imaging usually is adequate for morphology, but coronal and sagittal imaging may be helpful. Long- and short-axis gradient echo cine imaging is useful for function and to detect flow disturbances associated with septal defects or regurgitant valves. Short-axis cine images are used to measure shunts and regurgitant fractions but seldom are necessary before an initial surgery. Children suspected of having arrhythmogenic right ventricular cardiomyopathy need high-quality T1-weighted imaging of the myocardium to evaluate for fat deposition, focal myocardial thinning, or microaneurysm formation. Cine imaging in the long and short axis is necessary for observing abnormal right ventricle segmental wall motion and right ventricular volume.

Extracardiac abnormalities of the aorta and pulmonary artery are evaluated with a combination of spin echo imaging and CE-MRA. Like other forms of angiography, CE-MRA provides intraluminal structural information, or lumenograms. A spin echo imaging sequence complements CE-MRA by

allowing visualization of the vessel wall. Aortic and pulmonary valve stenosis can result in poststenotic dilation that is well imaged by CE-MRA. Progressive dilation of the ascending aorta associated with Marfan syndrome or aortic valve stenosis can be difficult to measure by echocardiography, but it is easily imaged with CE-MRA. Vascular rings are well delineated by CE-MRA but require additional spin echo imaging to identify the degree of associated airway compression. Sagittal spin echo imaging of the trachea may be helpful. Coarctation of the aorta and associated collateral arteries are identified by CE-MRA, but flow analysis is helpful in determining the associated pressure gradient. Collateral flow in the descending aorta can be quantified by measuring flow in the aorta proximal to the coarctation and at the diaphragm.[11,12]

POSTOPERATIVE IMAGING

MRI of the heart is performed more commonly in children after surgery than before surgery for preoperative diagnosis. Palliative procedures such as Blalock-Taussig shunts, central shunts, cavopulmonary shunts, and Fontan procedures for treatment of complex congenital heart disease with single ventricle physiology are well evaluated by a combination of SSFP cardiac imaging and a CE-MRA of the great vessels. Stenoses, aneurysms, and collateral flow can be evaluated, but care must be taken in planning CE-MRA because streaming is associated with possible imaging pitfalls.[13] The shunts can be studied for patency or stenosis by CE-MRA. Shunt flow is quantified by flow analysis. Flow patterns in the superior vena cava and inferior vena cava can be analyzed to determine the flow (e.g., whether the target of continuous flow is present versus reduced or even physically reversed through the circuit) of Fontan conduits.

Cardiac evaluation in the child with right ventricle dilation resulting from pulmonary regurgitation is among the most common indications for cardiac MRI following tetralogy of Fallot repair or pulmonary stenosis that has been treated by disruption of the pulmonary valve (see Chapter 76). Cardiac MRI can provide essential quantitative data and prognostic information to cardiothoracic surgeons that echocardiography and cardiac computed tomography or catheterization cannot provide.[14,15]

Postoperative MR evaluation also is useful in assessment after repair of transposition of the great arteries. Transposition of the great arteries was palliated by atrial switch procedures in the past, but currently, the arterial switch procedure is preferred. Persons with atrial baffles can experience baffle stenosis or leaks that can be evaluated with spin echo and white blood techniques. The morphologic right ventricle functions as the systemic ventricle and is prone to failure. Patients undergoing the arterial switch procedure are prone to pulmonary artery and branch pulmonary artery stenosis, which are well evaluated by CE-MRA.

MR can be helpful in evaluating complications that can occur after other congenital heart anomalies have been corrected. The protocols need to be tailored to the individual's clinical needs. In general, vascular stenoses and aneurysms require some form of MRA evaluation. Valvular regurgitation requires at least one method to determine flow properties. Cardiomyopathies that develop after surgery require ventricular function measurements and may benefit from perfusion and delayed enhancement sequences.

Key Points

Time-resolved MRA produces better temporal resolution than conventional contrast-enhanced MRA. The shorter acquisition time with parallel imaging makes it an ideal choice for pediatric cardiovascular imaging.

The b-SSFP noncontrast three-dimensional MRA technique gives excellent intracardiac and coronary artery detail and is especially suited for patients with renal failure, for whom administration of gadolinium chelate contrast agents is contraindicated.

Delayed enhanced images can be used to assess ischemic and nonischemic cardiomyopathies and can be used frequently in pediatric cardiac imaging.

Suggested Readings

Chung T. Magnetic resonance angiography of the body in pediatric patients: experience with a contrast-enhanced time-resolved technique. *Pediatr Radiol.* 2005;35:3-10.

Krishnamurthy R, Slesnick T, Taylor M, et al. Free breathing high temporal resolution time resolved contrast enhanced MRA (4D MRA) at high heart rates using keyhole SENSE CENTRA in congenital heart disease. *J Cardiovasc Magn Reson.* 2011;i12(suppl 1):O31.

Lim R, Srichai M, Lee V. Non-ischemic causes of delayed myocardial hyper-enhancement on MRI. *AJR Am J Roentgenol.* 2007;188:1675-1681.

Varaprasathan GA, Araoz PA, Higgins CB, et al. Quantification of flow dynamics in congenital heart disease: applications of velocity-encoded cine MR imaging. *Radiographics.* 2002;22(4):895-905.

Vasanawala SS, Chan FP, Newman B, et al. Combined respiratory and cardiac triggering improves blood pool contrast-enhanced pediatric cardiovascular MRI. *Pediatr Radiol.* 2011;41(12):1536-1544.

References

Full references for this chapter can be found on www.expertconsult.com.

Chapter 68

Nuclear Cardiology

S. TED TREVES and JAN STAUSS

Nuclear cardiovascular examinations complement anatomic imaging modalities by providing noninvasive methods to assess myocardial perfusion, myocardial viability, myocardial function (including ejection fraction and wall motion), cardiac shunts, and regional pulmonary blood flow in children with congenital and acquired anomalies of the heart and great vessels. Among the different nuclear cardiology techniques, myocardial and pulmonary perfusion imaging are the most commonly used in children.

Myocardial Perfusion

Myocardial perfusion images are obtained by using single photon emission tomography (SPECT) after administration of an intravenous tracer during a time of peak stress and while the patient is at rest. A time of peak stress can be achieved by having the patient exercise in the form of walking on a treadmill or riding a stationary bicycle. For children who are too young to cooperate with exercise testing (usually, children younger than 4 or 5 years), pharmacologic stress testing with use of vasodilators such as dipyridamole and adenosine or inotropic drugs such as dobutamine can be performed safely. Different radiotracers are available for myocardial SPECT in children, including technetium-99m hexakis-2-methoxyisobutylisonitrile (^{99m}Tc-MIBI), technetium-99m (^{99m}Tc) tetrofosmin, and thallium-201 (^{201}Tl). ^{99m}Tc-MIBI and ^{99m}Tc-tetrofosmin are both rapidly taken up by the myocardium, reflecting regional perfusion at the time of injection, and show only negligible redistribution compared with ^{201}Tl. The use of technetium-labeled compounds in pediatric nuclear cardiology is favorable compared with ^{201}Tl because of the lower radiation dose, the potentially higher tracer activities for better counting statistics, the advantageous photon energy, and the longer retention in the myocardium, which facilitates acquisition of gated SPECT to assess ventricular wall motion. The ^{99m}Tc-labeled compounds (MIBI and tetrofosmin) have largely replaced ^{201}Tl for the evaluation of myocardial perfusion in children.

Myocardial perfusion SPECT is useful for identification of fixed or stress-induced myocardial perfusion abnormalities in patients with a history of Kawasaki disease, transposition of the great arteries after an arterial switch operation, cardiac transplants, cardiomyopathy, chest pain, chest trauma, an anomalous left coronary artery from the right sinus of Valsalva, an anomalous right coronary artery from the left sinus of Valsalva, and a left coronary artery from the pulmonary artery. Other less frequent indications include hyperlipidemia, supravalvular aortic stenosis, syncope, coarctation of the aorta, and pulmonary atresia with an intact ventricular septum. In children with Kawasaki disease and coronary aneurysms (which has surpassed acute rheumatic fever as the leading cause of acquired heart disease in children in the United States), cardiac stress testing for reversible ischemia is indicated to assess the existence and functional consequences of coronary artery abnormalities (Figs. 68-1 and 68-2). It has been shown that myocardial perfusion SPECT is a safe and sensitive diagnostic method for identifying coronary stenosis in these children.

Because ^{99m}Tc-MIBI does not show significant redistribution, two injections of the radiopharmaceutical agent are necessary to obtain resting and peak exercise myocardial perfusion images. For a single study (rest or exercise), a dose of 0.25 mCi (9.25 MBq)/kg can be used with a minimum total dose of 2 mCi (74 MBq) and a maximum dose of 10 mCi (370 MBq). If rest and exercise studies are done on separate days (i.e., a 2-day protocol), the same dose of ^{99m}Tc-MIBI can be used for both studies. For rest and exercise studies performed on the same day (i.e., a 1-day protocol), 0.15 mCi (5.55 MBq)/kg, with a minimum dose of 2.0 mCi (74 MBq) and a maximum dose of 10 mCi (370 MBq), should be used for the study while the patient is at rest. At 2 to 4 hours after the rest study is completed, the exercise study is performed, using a dose of 0.35 mCi (12.95 MBq)/kg, with a minimum dose of 4 mCi (148 MBq) and a maximum dose of 20 mCi (740 MBq), administered at the time of peak exercise. Imaging is performed 0.5 to 1.0 hour after administration of the tracer. The acquisition protocols should be adapted to individual SPECT systems. SPECT is usually acquired using 120 total projections with a 128 × 128 matrix for a total acquisition of 30 minutes. Appropriate magnification should be used, which depends on the patient's heart size.

Myocardial perfusion also can be assessed using positron emission tomography (PET) with a variety of tracers such as rubidium-82, nitrogen-13 (^{13}N) ammonia, and oxygen-15. Cardiac PET remains underused in the pediatric patient population. Observed agreement between perfusion abnormalities on ^{13}N-ammonia PET and coronary angiography suggests a potential for ^{13}N-ammonia PET to serve as a valid noninvasive screening tool and an important adjunct to invasive angiography in selected populations. However, PET imaging with short-lived radiotracers such as ^{13}N-ammonia requires access to an on-site cyclotron and therefore is not yet widely available.

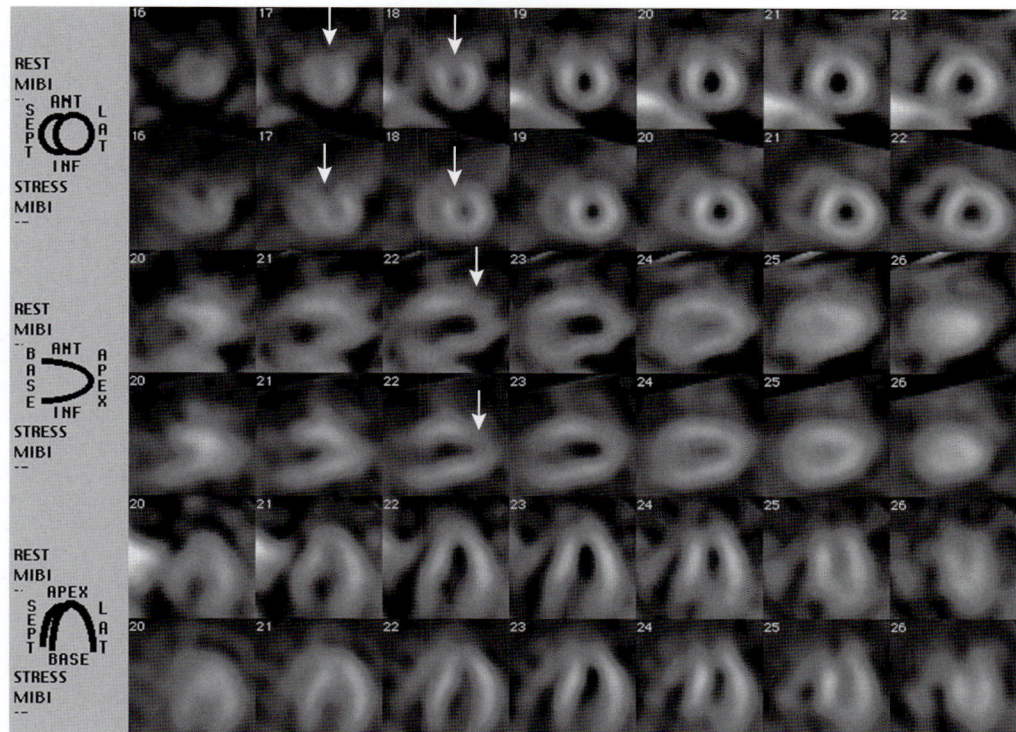

Figure 68-1 Single photon emission tomography images of a patient with Kawasaki disease. An exercise stress test with technetium-99m MIBI was ordered for a 20-year-old man with a history of Kawasaki disease who had giant coronary artery aneurysms. Single photon emission tomography images were acquired after injection of the tracer material at rest, and the procedure was repeated during a period of stress on the same day. A small fixed perfusion defect on rest, along with stress images involving the distal anterior wall of the left ventricle and the apex (*arrows*), most likely represent an area of prior infarction. No evidence was found of additional stress-induced ischemia. *Ant*, Anterior; *Inf*, inferior; *Lat*, lateral; *MIBI*, hexakis-2-methoxy-isobutylisonitrile; *Sept*, septal.

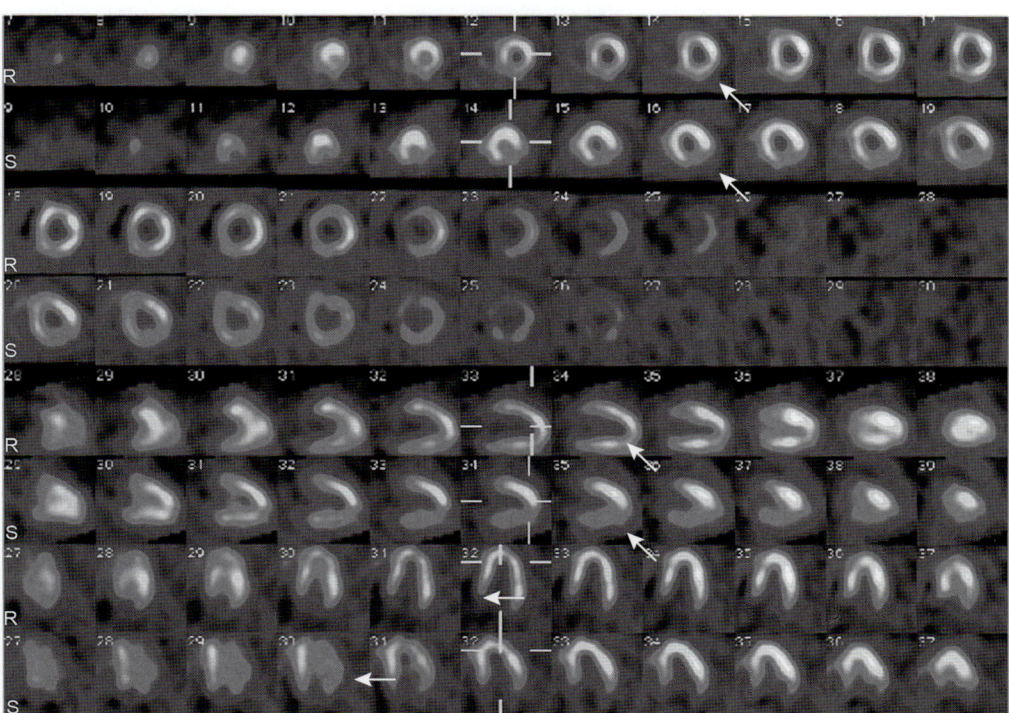

Figure 68-2 Single photon emission tomography images of a patient with Kawasaki disease. A 4-year-old boy with a history of Kawasaki disease underwent exercise stress testing with technetium-99m MIBI. Short-axis images, as well as vertical and horizontal long-axis stress images (S rows of images), show a perfusion defect (*arrows*) in the inferolateral wall that is reversible on rest images (R rows of images), consistent with stress-induced ischemia. *MIBI*, hexakis-2-methoxyisobutylisonitrile.

Myocardial Viability

Fixed defects on 4-hour ^{201}Tl or ^{99m}Tc-MIBI images could represent either scarred or viable chronic ischemic (hibernating) myocardium. To differentiate between these two possibilities, delayed images after 12 to 24 hours or reinjection techniques with ^{201}Tl traditionally have been used to allow a maximum of redistribution in viable myocardial cells. Alternatively, cardiac PET imaging with fluorine-18-2-fluorodeoxyglucose (^{18}F-FDG) can be used for viability testing.

^{18}F-FDG is a glucose analog that is phosphorylated and trapped in the myocardial cell without further metabolism. ^{18}F-FDG PET images reflect regional myocardial glucose metabolism, which is preserved in viable myocardium but not in scarred tissue. Compared with ^{18}F-FDG PET, imaging with ^{201}Tl may underestimate the extent of viable myocardium. In adult nuclear cardiology, ^{18}F-FDG PET has become the gold standard for viability evaluation. Only limited data on the role of ^{18}F-FDG PET in pediatric cardiology has been available until now. In children, the usefulness of ^{18}F-FDG PET has been evaluated for myocardial viability after arterial switch operation and suspected infarction. In these children, ^{18}F-FDG PET may provide pertinent information to guide further therapy by identifying patients with viable myocardium who will more likely benefit from revascularization.

Myocardial Function

Nuclear medicine techniques available for the assessment of ventricular function include electrocardiography-gated myocardial perfusion SPECT, gated metabolic PET, gated blood pool scintigraphy, and first-pass radionuclide angiography. The main purpose of these methods is to assess ventricular function such as right and left ventricular ejection fractions and to detect wall motion abnormalities.

Gated scintigraphy is based on synchronization of data recording with the patient's electrocardiogram, which allows repetitive sampling of the cardiac cycle until an appropriate count density is acquired. The data acquisition during each R-R interval is subdivided into a number of frames. At least 16 frames per cardiac cycle are required to calculate an accurate ejection fraction. In gated blood pool scintigraphy, autologous red blood cells are labeled in vivo or in vitro with ^{99m}Tc, and imaging should be performed using SPECT. Because of its excellent interobserver and intraobserver reliability, SPECT is used clinically to track serial changes in quantitative measurements of left ventricular ejection fraction. In pediatrics, it has been used to monitor the left ventricular ejection fraction in patients undergoing chemotherapy regimens involving drugs with high cardiotoxicity such as Adriamycin to reduce chemotherapy-related morbidity and mortality through early detection of a decline in cardiac function.

Shunts

LEFT-TO-RIGHT SHUNTS

First-pass radionuclide angiocardiography is a rapid, accurate, and noninvasive method for diagnosis and quantitation of left-to-right shunts. A bolus of ^{99m}Tc-pertechnetate is injected intravenously and imaged at two or four frames per second for 25 seconds on a 128 × 128 matrix. In a normal radionuclide angiocardiogram, tracer material is seen as it circulates sequentially through the superior vena cava, right atrium, right ventricle, pulmonary artery, lungs, left atrium, left ventricle, and aorta. The left ventricle and the aorta are clearly visualized with only minimal pulmonary activity. With left-to-right shunting, the radionuclide angiocardiogram shows persistent tracer activity in the lungs caused by early pulmonary recirculation of the tracer due to the intracardiac shunt. The left side of the heart and the aorta therefore are not well visualized on the angiogram of these children. The amount

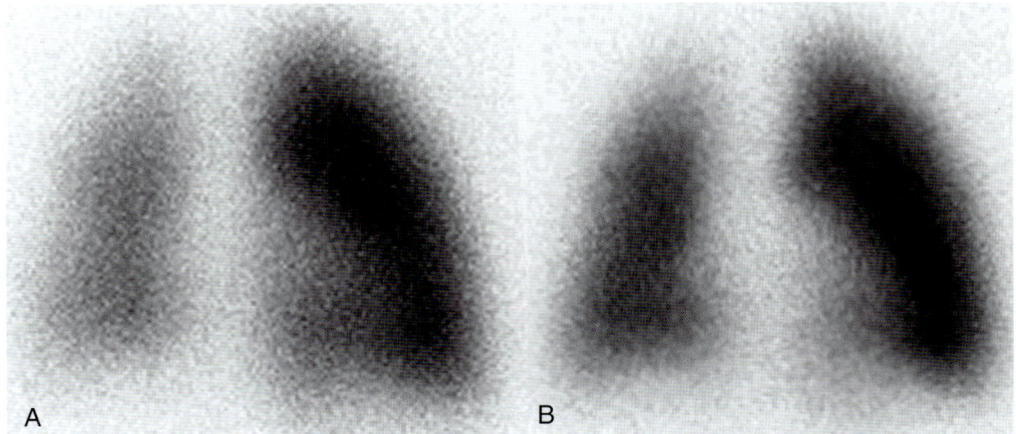

Figure 68-3 Lung perfusion scan images of a patient with tetralogy of Fallot. After surgical repair, a 4-year-old girl with a history of tetralogy of Fallot underwent a lung perfusion scan to evaluate the distribution of regional pulmonary perfusion. A recent echocardiogram had revealed a slight size discrepancy between her branch pulmonary arteries. **A,** Her first lung scan showed an asymmetric perfusion of 80% to the left lung and 20% to the right lung. Because of this perfusion asymmetry, she was admitted for a hemodynamic cardiac catheterization study and balloon dilation of her right pulmonary artery branch. **B,** After intervention, the second lung scan demonstrates increased relative perfusion of the right lung, quantified as 34% to the right lung and 66% to the left lung.

of tracer activity in the lungs relates to the magnitude of shunt flow. Regions of interest are drawn over the lung fields, and a pulmonary time activity curve can be used to calculate the pulmonary-to-systemic flow ratio (Qp/Qs). The radionuclide method allows precise detection and quantitation of left to right shunts with Qp/Qs ratios of 1.2 to 3.0.

RIGHT-TO-LEFT SHUNTS

Two nuclear medicine techniques are used for detection and quantitation of right-to-left shunts. The angiocardiographic technique is based on the principle described earlier for left-to-right shunting. Alternatively, large-molecular-weight radioactive particles such as ^{99m}Tc-macroaggregated albumin (MAA) can be used. This technique is based on the assumption that the particles are completely extracted from the circulation in one pass through either the pulmonary or the systemic capillary beds. After intravenous administration of ^{99m}Tc-MAA in a patient with suspected right-to-left shunt, the ratio of particles that enter the pulmonary and systemic circulations equals the ratio of pulmonary blood flow to systemic blood flow and can be quantified scintigraphically. Although no adverse reactions have been reported from the intravenous administration of particles in patients with right-to-left shunting, a relatively small number of particles (<10,000) should be used to reduce microembolization in the systemic vascular bed.

Regional Pulmonary Blood Flow

A more frequent indication for pulmonary scintigraphy with ^{99m}Tc-MAA in pediatric nuclear cardiology is to assess regional pulmonary blood flow in children with congenital or acquired anomalies of the heart and great vessels. This rapid and safe technique often is used to quantify the percent distribution of total pulmonary blood flow in the left and right lungs before and after interventional procedures to relieve obstruction to pulmonary blood flow (Fig. 68-3). This technique is used, for example, before and after catheter or surgical arterioplasty in patients with tetralogy of Fallot and peripheral pulmonary artery stenosis, in patients with pulmonary vein stenosis, and to assess the effect of intravascular stent placement or coil occlusion of vascular communications.

Suggested Readings

Agarwala S, Kumar R, Bhatnagar V, et al. High incidence of Adriamycin cardiotoxicity in children even at low cumulative doses: role of radionuclide cardiac angiography. *J Pediatr Surg.* 2000;35:1786-1789.

Askenazi J, Ahnberg DS, Korngold E, et al. Quantitative radionuclide angiocardiography: detection and quantitation of left to right shunts. *Am J Cardiol.* 1976;37:382-387.

Hernandez-Pampaloni M, Allada V, Fishbein MC, et al. Myocardial perfusion and viability by positron emission tomography in infants and children with coronary abnormalities: correlation with echocardiography, coronary angiography, and histopathology. *J Am Coll Cardiol.* 2003;41: 618-626.

Hurwitz RA, Treves S, Kuruc A. Right ventricular and left ventricular ejection fraction in pediatric patients with normal hearts: first-pass radionuclide angiocardiography. *Am Heart J.* 1984;107:726-773.

Jan SL, Hwang B, Fu YC, et al. Usefulness of pharmacologic stress 201Tl myocardial tomography: comparison of 201Tl SPECT and treadmill exercise testing in patients with Kawasaki disease. *Nucl Med Commun.* 2000;21:431-435.

Kondo C, Hiroe M, Nakanishi T, et al. Detection of coronary artery stenosis in children with Kawasaki disease. *Circulation.* 1989;80:615-624.

Maltz DL, Treves S. Quantitative radionuclide angiocardiography: determination of Qp:Qs in children. *Circulation.* 1973;47:1049-1056.

Miyagawa M, Mochizuki T, Murase K, et al. Prognostic value of dipyridamole-thallium myocardial scintigraphy in patients with Kawasaki disease. *Circulation.* 1998;98:990-996.

Newburger JW, Takahashi M, Gerber MA, et al. Diagnosis, treatment, and long-term management of Kawasaki disease: a statement for health professionals from the Committee on Rheumatic Fever, Endocarditis and Kawasaki Disease; Council on Cardiovascular Disease in the Young; American Heart Association; American Academy of Pediatrics. *Circulation.* 2004; 110:2747-2771.

Quinlivan RM, Robinson RO, Maisey MN. Positron emission tomography in paediatric cardiology. *Arch Dis Child.* 1998;79:520-522.

Rickers C, Sasse K, Buchert R, et al. Myocardial viability assessed by positron emission tomography in infants and children after the arterial switch operation and suspected infarction. *J Am Coll Cardiol.* 2000;36: 1676-1683.

Treves ST, Blume ED, Armsby L, et al. Cardiovascular system. In: Treves ST, ed. *Pediatric nuclear medicine.* 3rd ed. New York: Springer-Verlag; 2007.

Chapter 69

Pediatric Cardiac Catheterization and Electrophysiology

JOHN F. RHODES and RONALD J. KANTER

Pediatric Cardiac Catheterization

INTRODUCTION

During the past few decades, noninvasive imaging techniques including echocardiography, magnetic resonance angiography, and computed tomography angiography have evolved significantly in the assessment of complex congenital cardiovascular anatomy. Consequently, use of the catheterization laboratory has evolved to include both diagnostic procedures to assess complex congenital abnormalities before surgery and interventional procedures that permit therapeutic options and often preclude surgery.[1]

PROCEDURAL TECHNIQUES

Catheterizations are performed with use of the standard Seldinger technique in the femoral artery and/or vein. Alternative venous access includes the internal jugular, subclavian, or transhepatic approaches. Arterial access also may be obtained via the arteries of the upper extremities or the carotid artery, but these approaches typically are restricted to larger patients or emergent conditions. Anticoagulation is managed with heparin, 80 to 100 U/kg or 5000 U in patients who weigh more than 50 kg, for an activated clotting time goal of 200 to 250 seconds, depending on the procedure to be performed. Antibiotics are administered to patients who receive an implanted device. Baseline hemodynamics (including pressures and oxygen saturations) and angiography are obtained in room air, whenever possible. Subsequently, relative blood flows and vascular resistances are calculated. The ratio of pulmonary blood flow (Qp) to systemic blood flow (Qs) is calculated according to the following formula: $Qp/Qs = [(A_{O_2} - Mv_{O_2})/(Pv_{O_2} - Pa_{O_2})]$, where A_{O_2} is the aortic oxygen saturation, Mv_{O_2} is the mixed venous oxygen saturation, Pa_{O_2} is the pulmonary arterial saturation, and Pv_{O_2} is the pulmonary venous saturation. These data then determine whether additional information or interventions are necessary.

SEMILUNAR VALVE STENOSIS AND BALLOON VALVULOPLASTY

Since transcatheter balloon pulmonary valvuloplasty for valvar pulmonary stenosis in infants was first reported in the early 1980s, it has become the first line of therapy. The recommended balloon/annulus diameter ratio is 120%.[2] The reported success rate is greater than 90%, with major adverse events occurring in fewer than 1% of the procedures.[3] Hemodynamic measurements include the right ventricular pressure compared with systemic arterial pressure and the peak-to-peak systolic pressure gradient across the pulmonary valve. The indication for balloon pulmonary valvuloplasty is the presence of at least moderate pulmonary valve stenosis. We use as a guideline the "rule of 50," which is defined as a peak right ventricular systolic pressure of more than 50 mm Hg, a peak right ventricular systolic pressure more than 50% of the systemic systolic pressure, or a peak-to-peak systolic gradient across the pulmonary valve of more than 50 mm Hg.

Valvar aortic stenosis can be classified into two groups: disease that is severe enough that it presents at birth or within 1 year of age (10% to 15%), and disease that is not diagnosed until after age 2 years and will progress much more slowly, if at all.[4,5] Mortality and the need for intervention are significantly skewed toward the infantile group. As with pulmonary stenosis, noninvasive imaging techniques have advanced to the point that nearly all anatomic and functional information about the valve may be obtained without catheterization. Catheterization is performed for valves that clearly merit intervention or when symptoms and imaging findings are incomplete or confounding.

Aortic valve stenosis is classified into the following categories: trivial, mild, moderate, severe, and critical. Critical aortic stenosis is not defined by a specific pressure gradient or valve orifice size but on the basis of physiologic manifestations. If the stenosis is such that the patient is unable to produce and maintain an adequate cardiac output, the stenosis is critical. Patients in this group may have a low valve gradient, as measured by echocardiography, because of decreased cardiac function and low cardiac output. Although some controversy still exists with regard to the most beneficial treatment method for this population (i.e., surgical valvotomy vs. percutaneous balloon valvuloplasty), most centers have adopted balloon valvuloplasty as the initial treatment of choice. Patients in this category do not tolerate the stress of any procedure well, and catheterization has immediate results comparable with those of surgery (i.e., a reduction in gradient and resultant valve regurgitation) with a shorter course in the intensive care unit after the procedure and a shorter overall hospital stay.

Balloon valvuloplasty has been associated with an increased rate of reintervention compared with surgical valvotomy as a result of recurrent stenosis or worsening regurgitation. Given that residual aortic valve disease, especially regurgitation, may progress over time, the recommendation for the valvuloplasty technique is more conservative, with a smaller maximal balloon diameter (80% to 100% of the annulus) than that recommended for the pulmonary valve (100% to 120%). The valve may be approached retrograde from the aorta, using a soft-tipped J-wire to cross the narrowed valve orifice and obtaining arterial access in the femoral artery (more commonly) or the carotid artery. The valve also may be approached prograde by crossing an existing atrial communication or by performing a transseptal puncture to access the left side of the heart. Once in the left ventricle, angiography is performed to measure the annulus of the valve and obtain landmarks for valvuloplasty. The diameter of the balloon should not exceed 80% to 90% of the valve annulus. The smaller balloon diameter, compared with a similar sized pulmonary valve annulus, is recommended to decrease the amount of valve tearing and resultant acute regurgitation.

Many centers have adopted rapid right ventricular pacing at the time of balloon inflation. This rapid pacing transiently reduces cardiac output and the shearing force transmitted to the balloon as it is inflated across the valve annulus. The goal is to reduce the motion on the fragile valve leaflets and prevent excessive damage and regurgitation. Repeat angiography and echocardiography after inflation are essential to evaluate the success of the valvuloplasty and monitor for regurgitation or other complications.

The differentiation between noncritical stenosis categories is made by noninvasive echocardiographic measurements of valve area and Doppler gradient. A normal valve area is $2 \text{ cm}^2/\text{m}^2$. Mild obstruction is consistent with valve areas less than $2 \text{ cm}^2/\text{m}^2$ but greater than $0.7 \text{ cm}^2/\text{m}^2$, and severe obstruction is consistent with valve areas less than $0.5 \text{ cm}^2/\text{m}^2$. Mean echocardiographic Doppler gradients are good predictors of the peak-to-peak pressure gradient measured at catheterization. Gradients less than 25 mm Hg are considered trivial, those 25 to 50 mm Hg are mild, those 50 to 75 mm Hg are moderate, and those >75 mm Hg are severe. These measurements are made with the understanding that the cardiac function and cardiac output are normal.

Catheterization is not recommended for trivial or mild stenosis. Moderate and severe stenoses are approached with primary balloon valvuloplasty using the techniques previously described.

BALLOON OR STENT ANGIOPLASTY

Since the late 1980s, when balloon angioplasty was performed with low-pressure balloons (<5 atmospheres), balloons capable of dilations at higher pressure have been introduced. Since the introduction of high-pressure balloons, standard balloon angioplasty has resulted in a successful result of more than 70% for pulmonary artery angioplasty. As for coarctation or recoarctation, balloon angioplasty also has been used with some success. Patients who have severely hypoplastic pulmonary arteries with multiple stenoses that are refractory to high-pressure angioplasty may not be treatable using currently available medical, surgical, or catheter-based tools. In such cases, a "waist" persists during angioplasty at the maximum recommended inflation pressure, or even at pressures exceeding the recommended maximum, because of inadequate stretching or tearing of the vessel wall. For this patient population, cutting balloon angioplasty has become a therapeutic option with use of balloons up to 8 mm in diameter. Cutting balloon angioplasty often is followed by standard angioplasty for the best final result. Balloon-expandable stents have improved results in proximal vessels, eliminating the need for surgery in most patients, but they are of limited value in distal pulmonary vessels. Furthermore, stents are contraindicated in noncompliant vessels that cannot be expanded using high-pressure balloons. Stent angioplasty also has been utilized for coarctation of the aorta in postoperative and native lesions.

Pulmonary artery stenosis is a form of congenital heart disease that can occur in isolation or as part of more complex malformations such as tetralogy of Fallot. Although obstructions confined to the main or proximal branches can be repaired surgically, many patients can receive adequate palliation with transcatheter balloon angioplasty techniques. In addition, more distal obstructions that cannot be repaired operatively require angioplasty with balloons delivered to the distal stenotic segments as previously described. The inflation of a balloon whose maximum diameter is two to three times the diameter of the lesion will tear the vessel wall within the stenotic segment, resulting in an increase in lumen diameter. Although balloon catheters have not specifically been approved by the Food and Drug Administration as a treatment for pulmonary artery stenoses, transcatheter techniques have become the mainstay of treatment for distal vessel obstruction.

Often, aortic obstruction after an end-to-end surgical repair at the isthmus is a result of aortic narrowing within the transverse arch. These obstructive lesions are further defined as either the proximal transverse arch between the innominate artery and left carotid artery or the distal transverse arch, defined as the region between the left carotid artery and the left subclavian artery. Although few data exist regarding stent angioplasty within the distal transverse aortic arch, general experience has been that this procedure is safe and effective. An arterial monitoring catheter is placed in the right upper extremity and a 4 Fr sheath is used to advance a 4 Fr pigtail to the aorta from the right radial artery. This catheter is used to monitor pressures during stent angioplasty of the distal transverse arch and to perform cine angiograms to determine appropriate stent placement distal to the takeoff of the left carotid artery.

Transcatheter stent angioplasty for postoperative recoarctation of the aorta at the isthmus has been demonstrated to be safe and effective.[5] The technique usually involves a femoral arterial approach. An exchange length wire is placed in the ascending aorta or right subclavian artery. An angioplasty balloon is used with a maximum diameter that is equal to or less than the diameter of the normal aortic segments adjacent to the stenotic region and/or the diameter of the descending thoracic aorta at the diaphragm. The stent is mounted on the angioplasty balloon and passed through a sheath at least 1 to 2 Fr larger than that required by the balloon. The stent length is dependent on the lesion length but usually is at least 36 mm in adults. The stent is fully dilated in most cases, but at times it is deemed safer to serially dilate the lesion over two procedures.

SEPTAL AND VASCULAR OCCLUSION DEVICES

Although diagnosing the presence of an atrial septal defect (ASD) rarely requires cardiac catheterization, today many patients are undergoing cardiac catheterization for therapeutic device closure.[6] These patients require assessment of associated anomalies such as abnormalities of pulmonary venous connections. A step-up in oxygen saturations in the right atrium and pulmonary arteries is characteristic for an ASD, and the degree of left-to-right shunting or the pulmonary to systemic blood flow ratio (Qp : Qs) can be determined. The ideal age or timing for elective ASD closure is 2 to 5 years of age or within 6 to 12 months of diagnosis. Rarely, a child with an ASD presents with severe congestive heart failure and requires intervention in the first year of life.

Percutaneous ASD closure has been established as a safe and effective alternative to operative repair. The technique involves transcatheter delivery of a device in its retracted state via the femoral vein under fluoroscopic and echocardiographic guidance. Echocardiographic guidance can be transthoracic in young children and transesophageal, intracardiac, or even three-dimensional (3D) in older children. The most commonly available devices today consist of a double disc design made of nickel and titanium (Nitinol) with deployment of the first disc on the left atrial aspect of the septum followed by deployment of the second opposing disc on the right atrial wall. The expanded discs are tightly approximated, thus closing the defect. The device becomes endothelialized during the next 3 to 12 months while the patient is treated with antiplatelet medications. Contraindications include some very large defects, the absence of adequate septal tissue

margins, close proximity to vital cardiac structures, and very small children. ASD devices require an adequate tissue margin (minimum 7 to 8 mm) for deployment. The ASD must be small enough that the device can be deployed and held in the atrial septum (an adequate margin must be present on all sides other than the anterior superior rim by the aorta, where some splay of the device around the aorta will compensate for deficient rim) without impingement on adjacent structures or significant pressure on the walls of the atrium. Venous inflow to both the right and left atria must not be impeded, and the tricuspid and mitral valves should not come into contact with the device.

The world experience of transcatheter ASD closure using the Food and Drug Administration–approved Amplatzer Septal Occluder (AGA Medical Corporation, Golden Valley, MN) has been reported with a greater than 97% immediate success rate.[7] The occlusion rate reached 100% by 3 years. An overall 2.8% adverse event rate was found, and no procedural deaths occurred. Several studies regarding comparisons of device occlusion versus surgical closure have been performed prospectively. These reports include the Amplatzer and Helex (W.L. Gore & Associates, Flagstaff, AZ) devices for ASD closure. Findings include shorter hospital stays, less discomfort, and shorter durations for convalescence in patients undergoing successful closure with use of a device. Hospital costs are similar. Regression of right ventricular dilatation was similar for both groups of patients; however, it was dependent on the patient's age at the time of closure, with greater regression following earlier intervention.

Procedural adverse events are uncommon but include embolization into the right or left atrium, pulmonary artery, left ventricle, and aorta; stroke as a result of a clot or air embolization; and bleeding complications.[8] Both acute and late embolization have been reported, and thus it is critical for the radiologist to be familiar with the location of the interatrial septum on radiography to ascertain correct device position in the anteroposterior and lateral chest radiograph. Figure 69-1, *A*, demonstrates a septal occluder device in the appropriate position within the interatrial septum, and Figure 69-1, *B*, demonstrates the device positioned incorrectly in the left pulmonary artery.

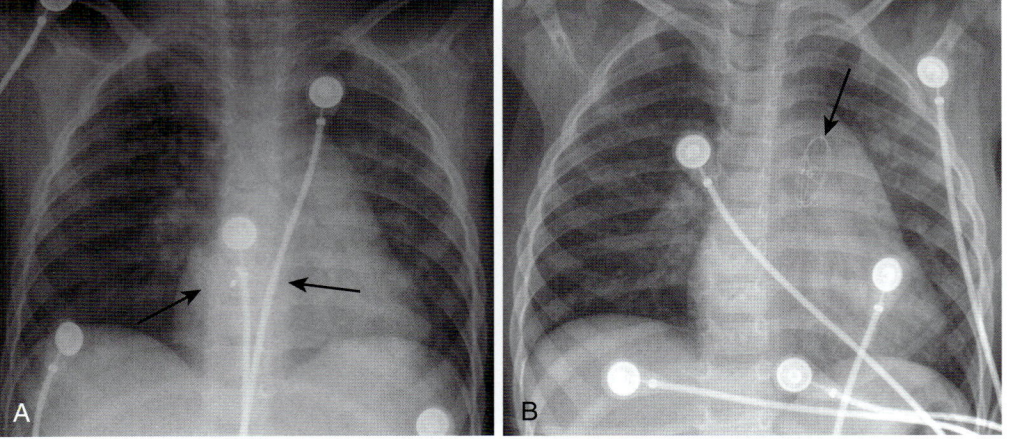

Figure 69-1   A, An atrial septal device (*arrows*) in the correct position within the atrial septum on anteroposterior fluoroscopy. **B,** An atrial septal device (*arrow*) in the incorrect position in the proximal left pulmonary artery.

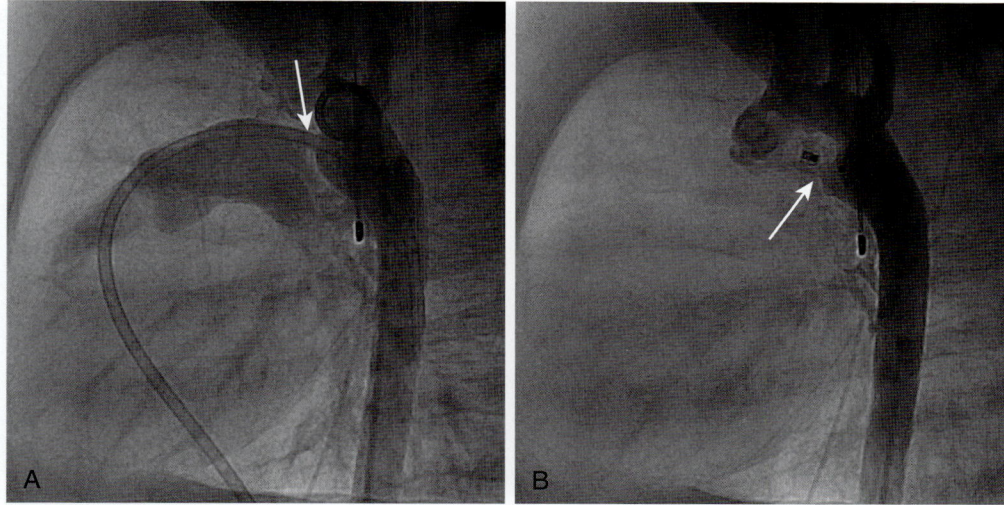

Figure 69-2 **A,** Lateral projection of patent ductus arteriosus (PDA) before placement of the device. A pigtail catheter is located in the aorta at the level of the distal arch. A venous catheter extends out the pulmonary outflow tract and across the PDA (*arrow*) to enter the descending thoracic aorta. **B,** Lateral projection with the Amplatzer Duct Occluder (*arrow*) deployed in the ductus arteriosus.

The first transcatheter interventional procedure was closure of a persistently patent ductus arteriosus (PDA), which was performed by Portsmann in 1967. Since that time a number of different PDA closure devices have been studied, some of which are no longer available. The goal of the procedure has always been to achieve 100% closure of the PDA without obstruction of either adjoining blood vessel (i.e., the aorta and the left pulmonary artery) with minimal risk of complications. The difficulty is that the PDA exhibits extreme variability in size and shape. Krichenko et al.[9] classified the PDA into five anatomic types based on the lateral aortic angiogram. The most common ("type A") ductus is conical with a narrowed pulmonary arterial end and large aortic ampulla. Other types include those with a narrowed aortic end, narrowing at both ends, and a tubular configuration. Early device closure procedures were complicated by a lack of choices for vessels of different sizes and shapes. The early devices had unsatisfactory rates of complications and residual leaks and were abandoned. In 1992, the first report was published using the Gianturco embolization coil (Cook Medical, Bloomington, IN) for closure of small PDAs. The Gianturco coil, which is available in multiple lengths and diameters, has now been in use for more than 20 years for blood vessel occlusion, including unwanted collateral vessels, fistulae, and arteriovenous malformations. The successful use of the coil in PDA closure, combined with sharing of ingenious techniques to deploy multiple coils and secure the coils before deployment by individual operators, provided the needed variety of approaches for successful PDA closure. At present, tens of thousands of patients around the world have had PDAs closed with embolization coils.

As expected, the recommended technique for coil embolization is variable, depending on the size and shape of the PDA. The vessel can be approached from the venous or arterial side, and the coils may be deployed "free hand" or secured with a bioptome or modified catheter. Smaller coils, such as the Flipper coil (Cook Medical), also are available; these coils are attached to a delivery system and are released once they are verified to be in the proper position.

A more recent addition to the interventional cardiologist's armamentarium for PDA closure is the Amplatzer Duct Occluder.[10] The PDA occluder is a self-expanding wire mesh device that is attached to a delivery cable and deployed through a long sheath from the venous system. Figure 69-2, A, demonstrates a lateral projection angiogram of the descending thoracic aorta and a left-to-right shunting PDA. Figure 69-2, B, demonstrates device occlusion of the PDA. The device has a retention skirt to occupy the aortic ampulla and tapers slightly to the pulmonary artery end. The device is filled with a polyester mesh that stimulates thrombus formation within the lumen of the PDA. The shape of the device and self-expanding properties exert radial force on the walls of the PDA, holding the device in place until endothelialization occurs. The device has excellent closure rates approaching 100% at 1 month after the procedure. The main limitation is the size and bulky nature of the device. The PDA must have an aortic ampulla adequate to accommodate the retention skirt without creating aortic obstruction. Furthermore, the device can create left pulmonary artery stenosis by compressing adjoining structures once it is released.

Accessory blood vessels are a common area of concern for the interventional radiologist and interventional cardiologist. These accessory blood vessels may include aortopulmonary or venovenous collaterals, arteriovenous fistulae and malformations, surgically placed shunts, and transhepatic access tracts. Techniques for closure are similar to those described for the PDA, predominately involving Gianturco and similar coils, the Amplatzer Duct Occluder, or the Amplatzer Vascular Plug. The vascular plug is similar to the duct occluder in that it is a self-expanding wire mesh design. It differs in that it is cylindrical in shape with no retention skirt, no tapering through its length, and no polyester mesh interior fabric. The device has excellent occlusion results but has been unsuccessful in short arterial vessels, such as aortopulmonary collaterals and the PDA. It is thought that the lack of occlusive material through the center of the device does not provide enough restriction to arterial blood flow to stimulate thrombosis and occlude the vessel.

Pediatric Electrophysiology

INTRODUCTION

With regard to imaging, the clinical practices of the pediatric radiologist and pediatric electrophysiologist intersect in two regards: Both subspecialists are interested in detailed internal anatomy and both subspecialties have evolved toward performing therapeutic procedures. In particular, advances in imaging have helped improve outcomes of catheter ablation for nearly every tachyarrhythmia.

This section is divided into two parts: (1) items of interest to the radiologist pertaining to activities in the electrophysiology laboratory, especially newer imaging technologies to guide catheter ablation and radiation exposure risks during catheter ablation, and (2) cardiac rhythm device therapy and special concerns in the radiology department.

CATHETER ABLATION IN CHILDREN

History and Indications

The surgical elimination of an accessory atrioventricular pathway in 1968 heralded the era of curative therapy of tachycardia substrates.[11] Transvascular catheter delivery of direct current to create atrioventricular block in adults with troublesome atrial fibrillation was first reported in 1983.[12] However, the modern era of catheter ablation began in 1987 with the use of alternating current in the radiofrequency range (about 550 kHz) to ablate an accessory pathway.[13] Unlike direct current, radiofrequency current causes resistive heating, thus creating a fairly well-circumscribed lesion and minimizing collateral damage. This technology rapidly expanded to include children[14] and patients with congenital heart disease.[15] Almost no tachyarrhythmia substrate is now considered exempt from catheter ablation therapy thanks to newer catheter designs, new electroanatomic mapping technologies, and additional energy sources, especially cryoenergy. Indications to perform catheter ablation in children remain somewhat limited by the benign natural history of some tachyarrhythmia substrates,[16] continued concern of damage to nearby structures, and concern for scar expansion with somatic growth.[17] The arrhythmia substrates that commonly undergo ablation in children appear in e-Table 69-1, and published indications for performing ablation appear in e-Box 69-1.[18]

Technical Considerations

The guiding principle of electrophysiologic testing and catheter ablation involves coupling of anatomic structures to electrical phenomena. Most cases can be accomplished with standard fluoroscopy and multiple multielectrode catheters positioned in the right ventricle, right atrium, coronary sinus, and His bundle region of the tricuspid valve annulus, with one for mapping and ablation (Fig. 69-3). In a normal heart, these anatomic sites can be easily accessed from a combination of femoral, internal jugular, and subclavian venous approaches. However, in some patients with complex congenital cardiovascular anomalies (e.g., interrupted inferior vena cava in some patients with heterotaxy) and in others having undergone certain congenital heart operations (e.g., cavopulmonary connection or extracardiac conduit in

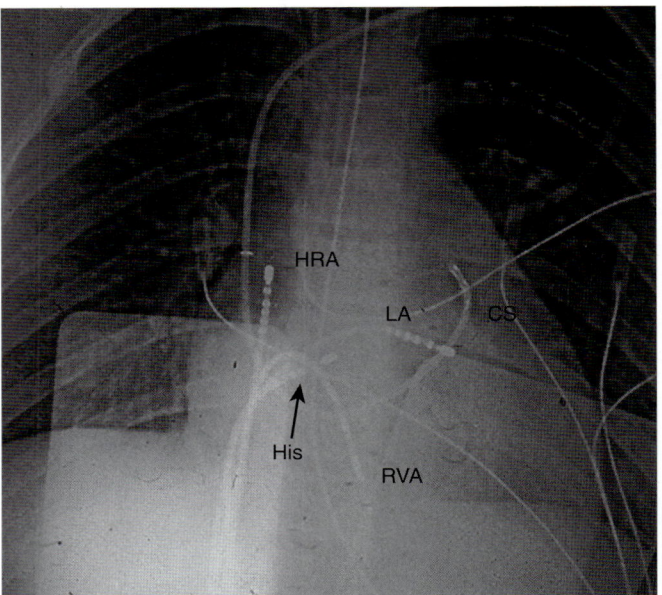

Figure 69-3   Anterior-posterior projection of a chest fluorograph during a radiofrequency catheter ablation procedure in a teenager with Wolff-Parkinson-White syndrome and a left lateral accessory pathway. Standard multipole electrode catheters are positioned in the high right atrium (*HRA*), across the tricuspid valve in the His bundle region (*His*), in the right ventricular apex (*RVA*), in the coronary sinus (*CS*), and at the mapped location of the accessory pathway along the mitral valve annulus (accessed from the left atrium (*LA*) via transseptal puncture).

patients having single ventricle physiology), some or all of these venous sites will not allow access to the heart. Moreover, patients who have undergone multiple prior procedures may have permanent venous occlusion of some of these access pathways. In these instances, alternate approaches may include transhepatic venous,[19] arterial/retroaortic, and transthoracic access.[20] Furthermore, occasional arrhythmia substrates are primarily epicardial, requiring transpericardial access. Transthoracic or intracardiac echocardiography[21] may aid in understanding anatomic details and in the positioning of catheters.

Even high-resolution fluoroscopy in multiple projections is insufficient to display the internal cardiac topography after complex congenital heart surgery. Therefore technologies using mathematically derived reconstructions have been developed for real-time creation of 3D cardiac chambers and associated structures.

The CARTO system (Biosense Webster, Diamond Bar, CA) allows an endocardial map to be created using a low-energy, triple-source transmitter located on a position pad mounted beneath the patient, a receiver in the tip of the specialized mapping/ablation catheter, and global positioning system technology. A second electrode catheter in a fixed intracardiac position serves as a temporal reference, thus permitting electroanatomic coupling by the mapping catheter as it is manipulated to create an anatomic rendition of the chamber(s) of interest. Isochronal activation, isopotential, and animated activation maps may be produced (e-Fig. 69-4).

The Ensite system (St. Jude Medical, St. Paul, MN) uses a noncontact multielectrode array that is mounted on a balloon catheter and centrally positioned in the chamber of interest (intracavitary). Ring electrodes on this catheter, proximal and distal to the array, serve as receivers from a low-current "locator" signal delivered from any second standard electrode catheter. As this second catheter is rapidly swept along all endocardial surfaces of the chamber of interest, a 3D computer model of the endocardium is generated. Far-field electrical activity recorded from each electrode on the array is enhanced and resolved based on an inverse solution to Laplace's equation. The inverse solution considers how a signal detected at a remote point (the array) will appear at its source (endocardial surface), thus superimposing a real-time isopotential map on the geometry matrix, even from a single heartbeat (e-Fig. 69-5).[22]

Both of these systems now have the capacity to merge previously obtained digital imaging and communication in medicine–formatted computerized tomographic or magnetic resonance images (MRI) of the patient's heart chambers with the real-time anatomic renderings previously described (e-Fig. 69-6).

This technology has been of greatest value in the mapping and ablation of atrial or ventricular muscle tachycardias whose substrates are within the wall of a chamber and are defined by areas of slow or absent conduction and not only by structural conduction boundaries, such as venous ostia or valve annuli. Each system has its own idiosyncrasies and limitations and requires extra equipment with attendant costs.

Radiation Exposure

Fluoroscopy remains the workhorse for cardiac catheter ablation procedures in most institutions. Under the direction of John Kugler, the Pediatric Electrophysiology Society began a pediatric radiofrequency registry in 1990, which has demonstrated a progressive reduction in procedural fluoroscopy duration from 61.5 minutes in 1994[14] to 38.3 minutes in 2004,[23] at least among patients with supraventricular tachycardia. Most operators limit x-ray exposure by reducing frame rates to 15 and even 7.5 frames/sec and by minimizing the use of magnification. That said, clever use of electroanatomic mapping systems may markedly reduce the duration of fluoroscopy.[22,24] St. Jude Medical's Ensite NavX system permits continuous, real-time, 3D rendering of all electrode catheters, anatomic features, and tagged structures (including locations of previously delivered ablation lesions) with use of a global positioning system–like technology, which is facilitated by three pairs of skin surface patches, serving as x-y-z axis low-energy transmitters. Using continuous impedance measurements, the electrode catheters are the receivers. Virtual elimination of ionizing radiation for simple catheter ablation procedures has been reported with use of this system.[25]

Data on actual x-ray exposure during catheter ablation procedures comes largely from adult series, in which thermoluminescent dosimeters and/or anthropomorphic radiologic phantoms were used.[26-30] Considering fluoroscopy times ranging from 41 to 60 minutes, a single procedure has been estimated to carry a risk of fatal malignancy in 0.03% to 0.13% of individuals and to result in birth defects in 0.00012%.[27,28,30] These figures are approximately equivalent to 1% and 0.1% of the spontaneous incidences, respectively. Geise and colleagues[31] reported that radiation doses to exposed skin were 6.2 to 49 mGy/min in nine children,

which calculated to total doses of 0.09 to 2.35 Gy. In our laboratory, our median fluoroscopy time is 32 minutes per case, and we limit fluoroscopy times to 120 minutes, even for complicated cases.

DEVICE THERAPY IN CHILDREN

Fundamentals of Pacing Hardware

Bradycardia devices (i.e., pacemakers) and antitachycardia devices (i.e., implantable cardioverter defibrillators [ICDs]) require two basic hardware components, the pulse generator and conductors (primarily, "leads"). The pulse generator consists of an energy source (battery), microcircuitry, titanium alloy housing, and a plastic connector block for conductor attachment. In addition, the ICD contains capacitors to store deliverable energy. The lead consists of one (unipolar) or two (bipolar) wires, silicon or polyurethane insulation, a connector pin (or pins) that insert(s) into the pulse generator connector block, and a fixation end that attaches to myocardium (via a tiny screw, fish hook, plaque, or other device). Transvenous bipolar leads generally have a radiodense distal electrode and a slightly more proximal "ring" electrode, whereas the unipolar lead has only a distal electrode. Epicardial leads are mostly unipolar, but bifurcated plaque electrodes and in-line bipolar leads also exist. In addition, the ventricular lead for an ICD may have one or two additional insulated conductors that are exposed on the outer surface of the lead (so-called coils) and participate in the shock field. Arrays and patches may be necessary to optimize cardioversion or defibrillation and are inserted in subcutaneous or intrapericardial sites. Figures 69-7 and 69-8 illustrate the radiographic appearance of this hardware. An entirely subcutaneous cardioverter-defibrillator (which can sense and shock only) is currently in clinical trials.

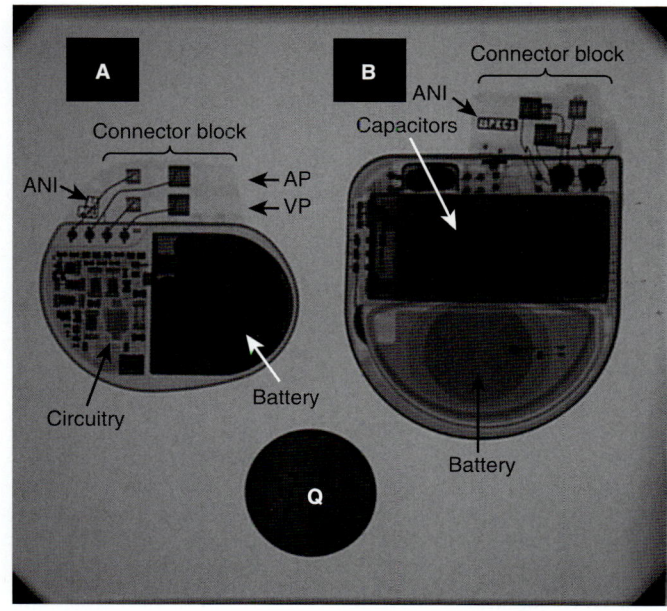

Figure 69-7 Fluoroscopic image of a modern dual-chamber pacemaker (**A**) and implantable cardioverter-defibrillator (**B**). *ANI,* Alphanumeric identifier; *AP,* atrial port (the portion of the connector block that accepts the connector pin of the atrial lead); *Q,* quarter (for size comparison); *VP,* ventricular port (the portion of the connector block that accepts the connector pin of the ventricular lead).

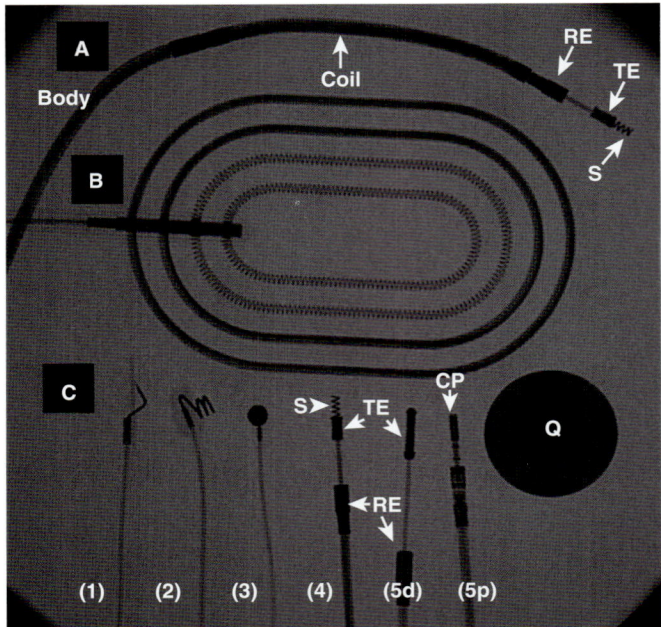

Figure 69-8   A fluoroscopic image of several types of conductors used for cardiac device therapy in children and teenagers. **A,** A transvenous, active fixation, bipolar, ventricular lead used with implantable cardioverter-defibrillators (ICDs) and containing a coil for participation in shock delivery. **B,** A patch, which is placed in either pericardial or subcutaneous locations, and is used with ICDs for participation in shock delivery. **C,** A variety of leads used with either pacemakers or ICDs. *1,* The distal (cardiac) end of a unipolar, epicardial active fixation (stab-on or fish hook) lead. *2,* The distal end of a unipolar, epicardial active fixation (screw-in) lead. *3,* The distal end of a unipolar, epicardial passive fixation (plaque, suture-on) lead. *4,* The distal end of a bipolar, transvenous active fixation lead (with a retractable screw). *5d* and *5p* illustrate the distal (cardiac) and proximal (connector block of pacemaker) ends of a bipolar, passive fixation lead, respectively. *CP,* Connector pin; *Q,* quarter (for size comparison); *RE,* ring electrode; *S,* screw; *TE,* tip electrode.

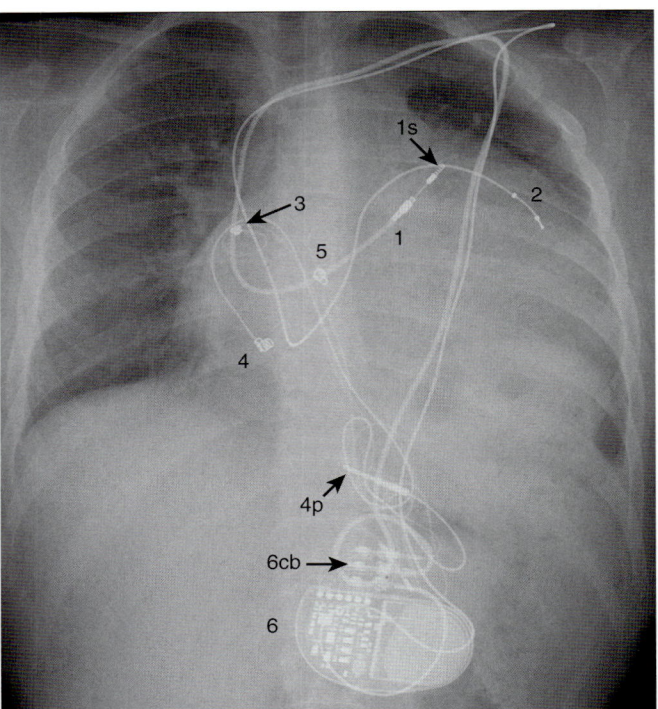

Figure 69-9   Posterior-anterior chest radiograph from an 11-year-old girl who underwent repair of an atrioventricular septal defect and who has postoperative heart block, severe mitral regurgitation, and left ventricular dysfunction. 1, A transvenous, bipolar, active fixation (1s, screw) lead positioned in the right ventricular outflow tract. 2, A transvenous, bipolar, passive fixation lead positioned in the posterolateral cardiac vein via the coronary sinus for the purpose of synchronizing ventricular activation. 3, An epicardial, unipolar, passive fixation (plaque electrode) lead positioned on the right atrium. 4, An epicardial, unipolar, active fixation (screw-in) lead positioned on the right atrium, abandoned, with the proximal end (4p, connector pin) in the abdominal pacemaker pocket. 5, An epicardial, unipolar screw fragment positioned on the right ventricle. 6, Pacemaker (6cb, pacemaker connector block).

Radiography of Pacing Systems

The radiologist will be called upon to interpret radiographs from children with devices immediately after device implantation, during routine follow-up, and when component failure is suspected.

A systematic approach will enable the radiologist to interpret the appearance of the hardware. The first step is to identify the location of the pulse generator. When the device is infraclavicular, the conductors usually are transvenous. Epicardial leads are generally tunneled to a subcutaneous abdominal device, but subcostal and flank locations (especially in premature infants) also may be used. Hybrid systems imply use of a combination of transvenous, epicardial, and/or subcutaneous conductors, configured to accommodate restricted venous access, and/or a preexisting lead that is considered valuable, and/or an optimized shock vector in the case of ICDs. The pulse generator will be positioned in a location optimal to the complex configuration of the conductors. The second step is to describe each conductor, including the type (e.g., lead, lead with coils, array, or patch), its course from the pulse generator to the heart or other thoracic site, its form of attachment to the heart in the case of leads, and whether the lead is unipolar or bipolar. Magnification of the lead tip

may be required. In young children with epicardial lead(s), redundant lead body is coiled anterior to the heart. Lead may be partially looped within the right atrium in the case of transvenous leads (the so-called *growth loop*). The third step is to correlate the congenital and surgical anatomy with lead locations and courses. Understanding the appropriateness of the course of each lead often requires some knowledge of the surgical anatomy. Figures 69-9 and 69-10, and e-Figure 69-11 illustrate the radiographic appearance of patients who have complex cardiac device therapy. Finally, leads attached to both right and left ventricles suggest an attempt at ventricular resynchronization as a result of ventricular dysfunction. The left ventricular lead may be transvenous to the coronary sinus or epicardial surface of the heart.

In children undergoing chronic device therapy, symptoms suggestive of device malfunction may develop, such as syncope, skeletal muscle twitching, hiccoughs, new onset of fatigue, palpitations, and, in the case of ICDs, inappropriate shocks. Radiographic abnormalities that may suggest the etiology include lead conduction fracture, lead dislodgement (especially if symptoms occur soon after implantation), lead stretch as a result of somatic growth, and connector pin separation from pulse generator. Transvenous leads usually fracture

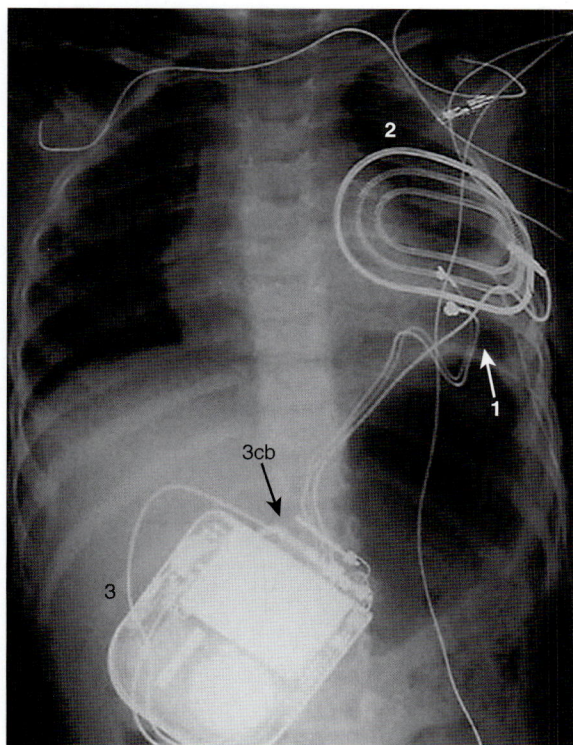

Figure 69-10 A posterior-anterior chest radiograph from a 3-month-old male infant with ventricular tachycardia associated with Brugada syndrome. *1*, An epicardial, bifurcated (hence, bipolar), passive fixation (plaque electrodes) lead positioned on the left ventricle for purposes of ventricular pacing and sensing. *2*, A patch placed posteriorly and in a subcutaneous location for participation in possible shock delivery. *3*, An implantable cardioverter-defibrillator (ICD) in a subcutaneous pocket over the left abdomen (*3cb*, ICD connector block).

beneath the clavicle, and epicardial leads tend to fracture at the level of the diaphragm or within the active fixation component (especially when it is a screw). A caveat: The Medtronic model 4968 (Medtronic, Minneapolis, MN) bifurcated, epicardial, double-plaque lead always has the appearance of near-fracture at the union of the two conductors (Fig. 69-12). Finally, the radiologist may be called upon to identify the type of implanted device (i.e., the manufacturer and model number) that is in a patient. Each pulse generator has a radiodense alphanumeric identifier (often its model number) that can be referenced in any of the major companies' device encyclopedias (see Fig. 69-7). Unfortunately, if the face of the device is facing posteriorly or if sufficient obliquity is present, it may not be readable.

Caring for Children with Devices While in the Radiology Department

Cardiac devices became interactive with the first inclusion of demand circuitry, which was developed in 1965 to allow sensing of intrinsic electrical activity. We now communicate with these devices for purposes of reprogramming, functional testing, and telemetry using a computerized programmer and radiofrequency signals. Hence, despite various forms of protective shielding and electronic filters, all devices may be affected by certain sources of electromagnetic interference (EMI) that may be present in the radiology department. It should be emphasized that ionizing radiation used for diagnostic procedures usually is not a source of EMI. High-dose x-rays during computerized tomography, only when applied directly to the device, can rarely result in oversensing.[32] This effect theoretically can inhibit a device, resulting in loss of output. However, the effect is transient and reverses as the beam moves away from the device.

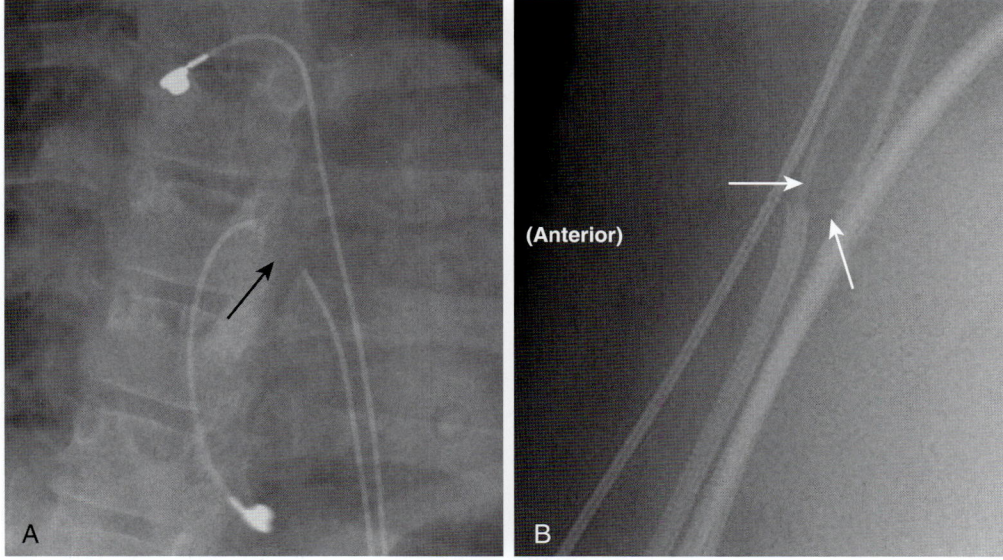

Figure 69-12 **A,** Posterior-anterior projection of the chest showing an epicardial lead fracture (*arrow*). **B,** Lateral projection of the upper abdomen in a different child showing a pseudofracture in the Medtronic 4968 epicardial lead. The proximal conductors are identified by white arrows just superior to their union at the bifurcation. The lower arrow identifies the smallest caliber component of the conductor. This image shows the normal appearance of this lead.

Repeated high-dose radiation therapy may damage the silicone and silicone oxide insulation necessary for the complementary metal oxide semiconductor chip technology of cardiac devices. Device manufacturers have provided guidelines to minimize risk of damage to ICDs resulting from radiotherapy.[33] EMI-device interactions may result from MRI, defibrillation, electrocautery, peripheral nerve stimulation, transcutaneous electrical nerve stimulation, diathermy, radiofrequency ablation, and lithotripsy. Untoward responses by the device may include oversensing, noise reversion, power-on reset, permanent circuit failure, and damage to the lead-tissue interface, causing a permanent rise in the stimulation threshold. A glossary of these terms appear in e-Box 69-2. Some of these potentially harmful medical procedures, specific responses to EMI, and ways to prevent these responses appear in e-Table 69-2.[34] MRI theoretically may cause device malfunction as a result of static magnetic, gradient, and radiofrequency fields and may cause tissue heating at the conductor-cardiac interface. Nevertheless, the performance of a nonthoracic MRI (at 1.5 T) in a patient with a pacemaker[35] or ICD[36] has been upgraded to a relative, not absolute, contraindication. An MRI-compatible pacemaker (but not ICD) manufactured by Medtronic also recently has become available.

Summary

Cardiac catheterization for congenital heart disease has evolved from its early days when it was exclusively a diagnostic tool to a dynamic and continuously growing field of therapeutic interventional procedures for children and adults with cardiac abnormalities. Clinicians and industry have a history of working together to push the field forward and find novel solutions to difficult problems while making the products to accomplish these goals smaller and safer. The interventional cardiologist and cardiothoracic surgeon have truly become an organized team in the treatment of once uniformly fatal conditions to offer longer and better quality of life to a diverse group of medically complex and rewarding patients.

Suggested Reading

Burney K, Burchard F, Papouchado M, et al. Cardiac pacing systems and implantable cardiac defibrillators (ICDs): a radiological perspective of equipment, anatomy and complications. *Clin Radiol.* 2004;59:1145.

References

Full references for this chapter can be found on www.expertconsult.com.

Chapter 70

Surgical Considerations for Congenital Heart Disease

ASVIN M. GANAPATHI and ANDREW J. LODGE

Congenital cardiac defects may be categorized in a variety of ways. One approach is to separate them based on the presence or absence of cyanosis in the patient presenting to the pediatric cardiologist or cardiac surgeon. Cyanotic lesions are associated with shunting of deoxygenated blood into the systemic arterial circulation or with severely reduced pulmonary blood flow. These lesions include transposition of the great arteries, tetralogy of Fallot (TOF), truncus arteriosus, total anomalous pulmonary venous connection, and hypoplastic left heart syndrome (HLHS). Acyanotic lesions include (1) obstructions to left ventricular outflow, such as aortic stenosis or coarctation of the aorta, and (2) defects with shunting of blood from the systemic circulation to the pulmonary circulation, including atrial, ventricular, and atrioventricular septal defects and patent ductus arteriosus (PDA). Often a combination of lesions exists, and associated anomalies must be thoroughly identified by preoperative imaging studies. This chapter will review the pathophysiology and clinical and imaging evaluation of patients with congenital heart disease as they relate to surgical planning. Discussion will reference treatments, particularly with regard to choice of surgical approach, along with intraoperative and postoperative considerations pertinent for radiologists.

General Considerations

Many congenital heart defects are fatal if they are not corrected surgically. Other defects can lead to long-term complications or a shortened life expectancy if timely surgical treatment is not undertaken. Surgery for congenital heart disease has advanced quite rapidly in the past several decades, with progress in surgical techniques and instrumentation and substantial improvements in anesthesia, critical care, and diagnostic imaging. As a result, many congenital heart defects can be treated effectively, with consistently improving results.

Surgical Approaches

Surgery for congenital heart disease is most commonly performed via a median sternotomy incision. Such an incision involves an anterior midline thoracic incision with dissection through the subcutaneous tissues down to the sternum. Once the sternum has been exposed, a sternal saw is used to split the sternum and a retractor is placed to define the operative field within which the pericardial sac is contained (Fig. 70-1). Because this incision offers excellent access to all of the structures contained within the mediastinum, including all chambers of the heart, ventricular outflow tracts, and venous returns, it is useful when multiple lesions are present or if a complicated repair must be performed.

Less invasive options for repair of congenital heart lesions also exist, such as a partial median sternotomy or a thoracotomy. In the case of a partial median sternotomy, the skin incision is kept small and only the upper or lower sternum is divided (e-Fig. 70-2). Depending on the necessary exposure, thoracotomy incisions can be anterior, lateral, or posterior (e-Fig. 70-3). Historically, thoracotomy incisions involved the sectioning of a rib; in general these incisions now are made simply by dividing the intercostal muscles and leaving the ribs intact.

The type of lesion being repaired determines the choice of surgical incision. Straightforward repair of extracardiac lesions such as aortic coarctation, vascular rings, or PDA generally can be performed through a left thoracotomy (e-Fig. 70-4). In addition, in the case of simple intracardiac repairs such as an atrial septal defect (ASD), a minimally invasive approach can be used even though the operation requires the use of cardiopulmonary bypass (CPB). As techniques have been refined in recent years, interest has increased in operating on simple defects, as well as the mitral, tricuspid, and aortic valves, through minimally invasive incisions. In addition, interest has developed in performing relatively straightforward operations, including some heart valve surgery, using thoracoscopic or robotic techniques. In these cases, several very small incisions are made through which specially designed instruments can be placed and used to perform the procedure (e-Fig. 70-5). Advantages touted include an improved cosmetic result and potentially shorter recovery times inside and outside the hospital.

For most complex congenital heart defects, such as repair of an atrioventricular (AV) septal defect lesion, a median sternotomy is used. In this case the repair includes a right

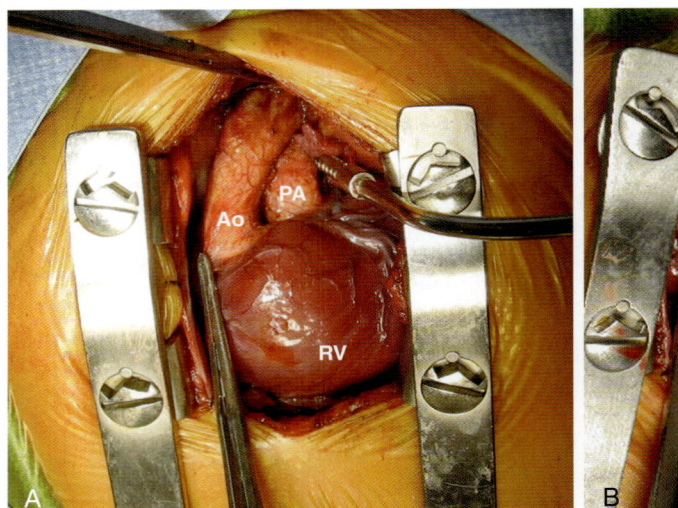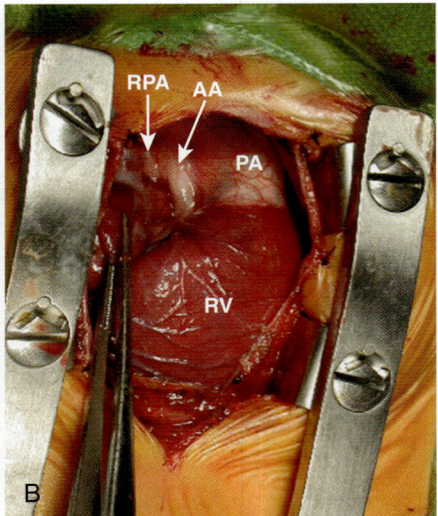

Figure 70-1   Median sternotomy. **A,** A sternal retractor is in place in a patient with transposition of the great arteries. The pericardium has been opened and sutured to the margins of the incision to expose the heart. The aorta (*Ao*) arises from the right ventricle (*RV*) and the pulmonary artery (*PA*) from the left ventricle. The left coronary artery and some of its branches also are seen. Note that the left ventricle, which is a posterior structure, is not well exposed. **B,** Similar exposure in a patient with hypoplastic left heart syndrome. The main *PA* is large and the ascending aorta (*AA*) is diminutive. The right pulmonary artery (*RPA*) is visible emerging from behind the aorta. The right atrial appendage is being grasped with a forceps. The right ventricle (*RV*) is also exposed. The cut pericardial edge, which is sutured to the skin edge, is more easily seen in this picture.

atriotomy, closure of a ventricular septal defect (VSD), repair of the ASD, and partitioning of the common AV valve into right and left components, with closure of the "cleft" in the left-sided AV valve (e-Fig. 70-6). Additionally, repair of cyanotic lesions typically requires the use of a median sternotomy incision. The reasoning is that these lesions often require greater exposure of both intracardiac and extracardiac structures that need to be repaired. One example of the need for a median sternotomy incision is a repair in a patient with TOF where an approach through the right atrium and the pulmonary artery is needed to close the VSD and relieve the right ventricular outflow obstruction. In some cases in which a very small pulmonary annulus or significant infundibular stenosis is present, the incision might even need to be extended to the right ventricular cavity (e-Fig. 70-7).

The choice of surgical approach also is important in the case of staged operations. A patient with HLHS generally will undergo three operations for complete palliation, and the need for a repeat sternotomy carries both operative and radiographic implications. Radiographically, imaging of the chest can help with operative planning because repeating median sternotomy incisions carries a greater risk of damage to the thoracic contents as a result of the formation of postoperative adhesions. For example, the aorta or other structures can be found very close to the sternum (e-Fig. 70-8) and might be damaged upon entry to the chest during the sternotomy, requiring the emergent institution of CPB. Careful review of chest imaging and the potential use of alternative, peripheral cannulation (discussed later) can help make the redo operation safer. Lesions that commonly require multiple operations include HLHS, TOF, and truncus arteriosus.

Other scenarios influencing operative planning and the choice of incision include the presence of multiple lesions or when a complete repair is not indicated and a palliative procedure is indicated instead. Many congenital heart defects can occur together, such as coarctation of the aorta and VSD. In

this case, a surgical procedure that might have been accomplished through a thoracotomy incision for isolated coarctation (e-Fig. 70-9) would necessitate a median sternotomy to address both lesions. As a result, preoperative imaging to determine all the lesions that are present is essential. Alternatively, for some patients a palliative procedure rather than a complete repair is indicated. This situation affects the necessary surgical exposure. One example of such a defect is complicated TOF, where placement of a Blalock-Taussig shunt initially may be performed, with later definitive repair.

The incision used for surgery has a variety of clinical and radiographic consequences. Patients who have had median sternotomy incisions often will have steel wires reapproximating the sternum, although in children, sutures that are not radio-opaque often are used. Occasionally chest wall deformities may develop in children who have sternotomy incisions as the children grow. Children who have had surgery for congenital heart disease also are at higher risk for developing scoliosis than the general population (e-Fig. 70-10). Thoracotomy incisions can produce distortion of the ribs on the side that has been operated upon and also can lead to scoliosis in children.[1] In the current era, ribs usually are not cut or sectioned during thoracotomy procedures, but sometimes inadvertent rib fractures can occur, which would be noted on the postoperative chest radiograph.

Cardiopulmonary Bypass and Extracorporeal Membrane Oxygenation

Most congenital heart operations are performed using CPB to support the circulation. The principal components of the system are a blood pump, commonly a roller or centrifugal pump, and an artificial lung (Fig. 70-11). The artificial lung

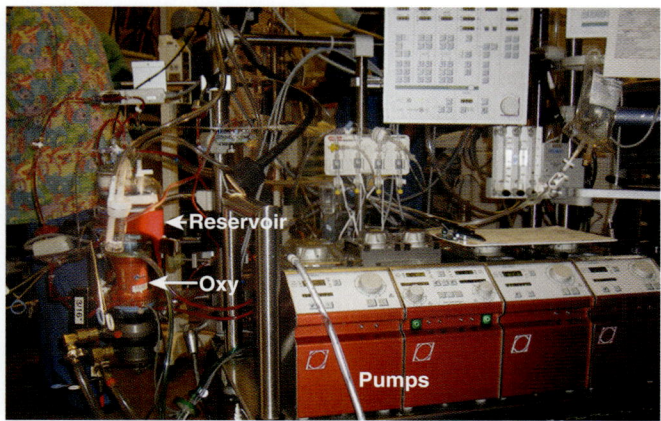

Figure 70-11 Pediatric cardiopulmonary bypass (heart-lung) machine. The blood reservoir, oxygenator (*oxy*), and pumps are labeled. The blood tubing connecting the components can be seen. Below the oxygenator is a temperature coil to which water lines are attached, allowing control of the patient's body temperature. Some of the monitoring equipment for the apparatus can be seen in the upper right.

and lungs by emptying the heart of blood, stopping ventilation, and, if necessary, arresting the heart. This apparatus has become progressively sophisticated and includes many built-in safety features, such as continuous online blood gas monitoring, bubble detectors, biocompatible surfaces, and filters that have contributed to a decrease in CPB–related complications. The evolution of this technology has reduced CPB–related morbidity such as the systemic inflammatory response, catastrophic air embolism, myocardial injury, and pulmonary dysfunction.[2-4]

When required for the repair of intracardiac defects, diastolic cardiac arrest is accomplished through the use of cardioplegia, a potassium-rich solution that is circulated through the coronary vasculature after clamping the aorta between the coronary arteries and the CPB arterial inflow. This solution may be crystalloid or blood based. In the case of severe left ventricular dysfunction, it has been suggested that blood cardioplegia offers potentially better outcomes.[5,6] This strategy is effective because arrest of the heart eliminates approximately 90% of the energy requirements of the heart. In addition, cooling of the myocardium leads to a reduction of approximately 10% of myocardial energy demands.[7]

Some surgery on extracardiac structures, such as modified Blalock–Taussig shunts and pulmonary artery banding, can be performed without CPB if the patient remains hemodynamically stable. In these cases, CPB generally is readily available should circumstances change. Intracardiac defects require the use of CPB. Sometimes extracorporeal circulatory support is necessary after surgery to allow for recovery of the heart over an extended period, or as a bridge to transplant in the case of an unsuccessful repair. In these cases, a modified CPB circuit is used for extracorporeal membrane oxygenation (ECMO) (Fig. 70-13). ECMO can be continued for days to

(called an *oxygenator*) in modern CPB contains a network of microporous membranes through which oxygen and carbon dioxide can be added to or removed from the blood. CPB is established by the placement of arterial and venous cannulae (e-Fig. 70-12), usually in the ascending aorta and right atrium, respectively, to deliver blood to the heart-lung machine and return it to the patient. However, the femoral, iliac, or axillary arteries can serve as alternatives for arterial cannulation, and in surgeries necessitating opening of the heart, venous cannulation is accomplished by separate superior and inferior vena cavae cannulae. CPB replaces the heart

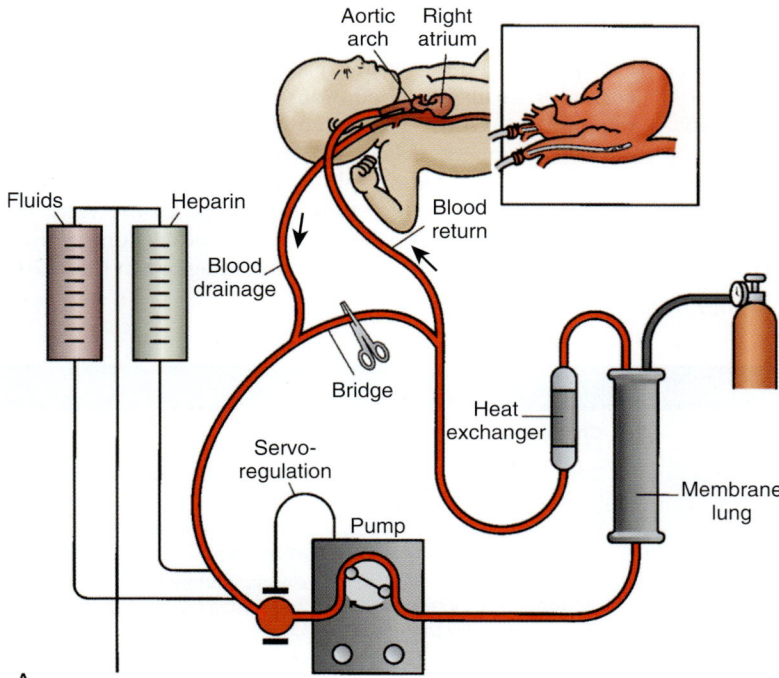

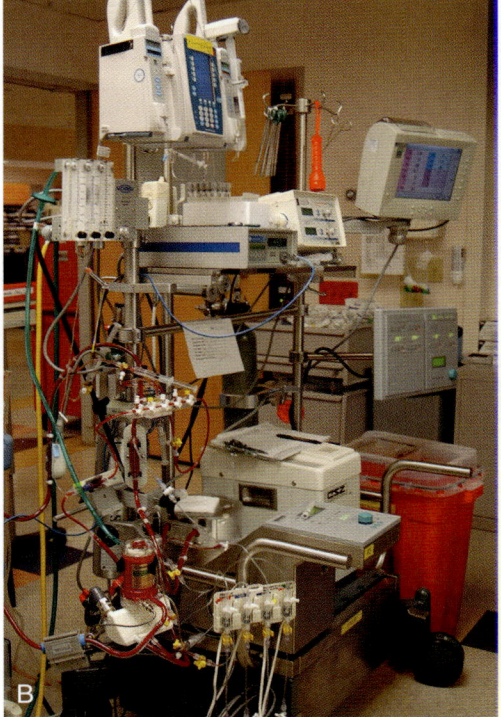

Figure 70-13 Extracorporeal membrane oxygenation (ECMO). **A,** A schematic diagram of an ECMO circuit. **B,** An actual ECMO circuit in clinical use. (**A,** From http://www.nichd.nih.gov/publications/pubs/images/Efig1p26.gif. Accessed April 2, 2012.)

weeks if necessary. Survival rates in patients who require ECMO after surgery range from 38% to 53%.[8]

Circulatory Arrest and Regional Cerebral Perfusion

In very complex cases such as those involving small neonates or complex aortic arch reconstruction, it occasionally is desirable to temporarily stop the entire circulation for a period. This technique, termed "deep hypothermic circulatory arrest" (DHCA), uses total body cooling to approximately 18° C, thus allowing the circulation to be safely suspended for up to 30 to 45 minutes. The safety of circulatory arrest and its effect on long-term neurologic outcome are controversial. A landmark study known as the Boston Circulatory Arrest Study suggested that neurodevelopmental abnormalities became significantly more prevalent after 41 minutes of DHCA.[9] However, it should be noted that data from other studies suggest that DHCA has little or no effect.[10-12] One limitation of all of these studies is the relatively small sample size.

Examples of operations in which patients possibly may be subjected to DHCA include the Norwood procedure for HLHS or repair of total anomalous pulmonary venous connection. As techniques have evolved, the use of DHCA has decreased, and many surgeons prefer to use regional cerebral perfusion, a technique that uses selective arterial inflow at a lower rate to the innominate or carotid artery and thereby limits periods of total ischemia. One advantage of this technique is blood flow not only to the brain but also to subdiaphragmatic organs.[13] For some operations, a combination of all of the aforementioned perfusion techniques may be used.

Chest Radiography

Chest radiographs are critical both before and after cardiac surgery. From a preoperative standpoint, the chest radiograph can be used for diagnostic purposes, because many lesions have characteristic findings, as well as a means to determine the severity of disease. With regard to disease severity, a chest radiograph also is very useful because often it will reveal evidence of congestive heart failure, pulmonary edema, or atrial/generalized cardiac enlargement. These findings may influence medical management before surgery or help to predict the postoperative course. In addition, a chest radiograph provides an important baseline to which to compare postoperative films.

Chest radiographs are the most common radiographic study obtained after heart surgery. A chest radiograph is obtained immediately upon arrival at the recovery room or intensive care unit (e-Fig. 70-14). These images are used to verify the positioning of central venous lines, chest tubes, the endotracheal tube, sternal wires, and prostheses, as well as to assess the degree of lung expansion and to rule out unsuspected pleural effusions or pneumothoraces. In small children with limited percutaneous vascular access, pressure monitoring lines sometimes are inserted directly into the cardiac chamber (and later removed at the bedside). The most common points of insertion, in decreasing order of frequency, are the right atrium, left atrium (usually via the right superior pulmonary vein, but it also can be through the left atrial appendage), and pulmonary artery.

Obtaining and interpreting the immediate postoperative film in a timely fashion is critical because delays can be life threatening. For instance, mediastinal widening—a new or enlarging opacity in the vicinity of the aorta after the repair of coarctation of the aorta—may represent postoperative bleeding. An unsuspected pneumothorax can be life threatening if it is not detected early. A pneumothorax may arise in the case of a patient who undergoes PDA ligation via a left thoracotomy but does not have a pleural drain left in at the end of the operation (a common scenario). Additionally, if a patient has undergone a procedure requiring a left thoracotomy, one might observe asymmetry of the lung fields because of congestion or atelectasis of the right lung paired with hyperinflation of the left lung (e-Fig. 70-15). This asymmetry occurs because the patient is positioned with the right side down for an extended period and the left lung is partially or completely collapsed during the procedure for surgical exposure purposes. Many patients have mild pulmonary edema or small pleural effusions related to the inflammatory response to CPB. These findings generally resolve with diuretic treatment. Many current valve prostheses also are visible on a chest radiograph because of the presence of radiopaque material in the sewing ring, stent, or the valve itself. However, some bioprosthetic valves, including homografts and autografts, will not be apparent on radiographs (Table 70-1).

Table 70-1

Cardiac Valve Prostheses			
Prosthesis Type	Synonym	Definition	Characteristics
Bioprosthetic	Xenograft, heterograft	Manufactured valve; uses tissue from other species such as pig or cow	Does not require long-term anticoagulation; subject to structural deterioration
Mechanical	—	Manufactured valve, generally composed of metal and pyrolytic carbon	Requires long-term anticoagulation; the most durable prosthesis; magnetic resonance imaging compatible
Homograft	Allograft	Cryopreserved human valve or valved conduit	Included segment of aorta or pulmonary artery offers greater reconstructive potential; subject to structural deterioration; aortic valve particularly prone to calcification
Autograft	—	Patient's own tissue	Pulmonary autograft used to replace aortic valve in Ross procedure
Stentless	—	Bioprosthetic valve that does not have a rigid plastic or metal stent built in	Technically more difficult to implant; may have greater effective orifice area

Daily chest radiographs frequently are obtained for patients after cardiac surgery. Posterior-anterior and lateral films generally are preferred for patients who are stable enough to travel to the radiology department, including patients with indwelling appliances such as chest tubes. However, it is common practice to obtain daily portable films while the patient requires intensive care unit monitoring. Neonates and infants who remain intubated with small bore endotracheal tubes are at risk for the development of atelectasis, which can be a major impediment to clinical care. The presence, extent, and distribution of atelectasis and the position of the endotracheal tube are critically important elements of the chest radiograph that may require daily assessment. Follow-up films generally are obtained immediately after the removal of pleural chest tubes, but they are not routinely necessary after the removal of intracardiac lines, pacing wires, and pericardial (mediastinal) drains. Although these films primarily are used to observe if a pneumothorax is present after removal of the chest tube, they also can help identify other conditions such as pleural or pericardial effusions.

Other Considerations

Imaging studies performed or interpreted by radiologists are important in many other situations in the evaluation and surgical management of congenital heart disease. Many patients with complex congenital heart disease, particularly patients requiring intervention as neonates or infants, may have associated syndromes or anomalies. In these cases it is common practice to obtain imaging studies such as ultrasound of the brain and/or kidneys before surgery to establish baseline diagnoses. It has been increasingly recognized that neonates with complex congenital heart disease have brain pathology that exists even before neonatal surgical correction, and at some centers, preoperative magnetic resonance imaging (MRI) studies of the brain have become routine in such patients (e-Fig. 70-16). Such imaging of the brain also becomes important when considering ECMO or during the use of ECMO because findings of a severe neurologic insult may affect decision making.

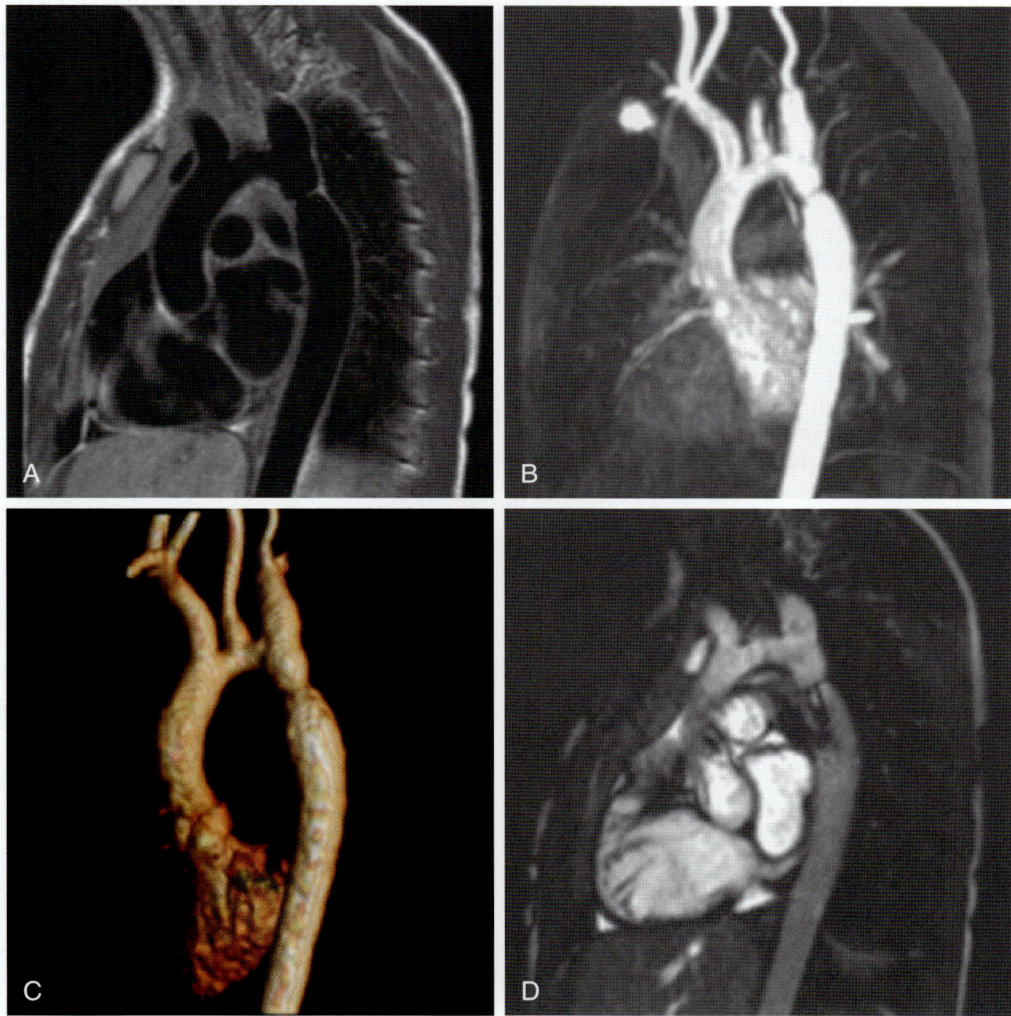

Figure 70-17 Aortic coarctation magnetic resonance images showing the relationship of the coarctation to the brachiocephalic vessels and aortic arch. Images such as these are helpful for planning the surgical approach or stenting. (From Atilli AK, Parish V, Valverde I, et al. Cardiovascular MRI in childhood, *Arch Dis Child* 2011;96:1147-1155.)

Feeding problems in patients who undergo congenital heart surgery as infants also are common and involve the use of radiology services. In certain subsets of patients, such as those with HLHS, gastroesophageal reflux is particularly common. These patients may require diagnostic tests such as upper gastrointestinal series and gastric emptying studies to help establish a diagnosis or to plan for antireflux surgery. They also may require placement or repositioning of feeding tubes with fluoroscopic guidance.

Other studies may be required to aid in the assessment of postoperative complications. Renal insufficiency is relatively common in the postoperative period. Renal ultrasound with Doppler assessment of renal artery and vein flow may be helpful in these patients. Many patients who require prolonged ventilation have a confusing combination of lung and pleural space disease, and chest ultrasound imaging can be very helpful in differentiating pathologic processes in the chest. Occasionally, image-guided drainage using either ultrasound or computed tomography (CT) can be helpful in treating more complicated effusions. Infants who require ECMO and are at risk for ongoing coagulopathy require serial cranial ultrasound imaging procedures to assess for bleeding.

Imaging studies also have become increasingly useful for preoperative planning in complicated cases. CT and MRI play an increasingly important role in these situations. In patients who have had previous cardiac surgery and are at risk for injury to the heart with a repeat sternotomy, CT scans can be very helpful in risk assessment or surgical planning by showing the relationship of the heart and great vessels to the sternum. CT angiography also can be helpful in patients with aortic coarctation who have complex anatomy or late diagnosis, both for operative planning and assessing candidacy for stent placement. CT or CT angiography also are useful in the diagnoses or characterization of complicated pulmonary artery or vein anatomy, such as in patients who have had repair of anomalous pulmonary venous connections, TOF, or transposition of the great arteries. Cardiac MRI is being used more commonly for many of these same indications, such as aortic coarctation (Fig. 70-17). In addition, cardiac MRI can be used to evaluate intracardiac shunts and plan therapy, such as in the case of transcatheter device closure of ASD. MRI also has become quite useful for evaluating right ventricular function and pulmonary insufficiency in patients who have had repair of TOF (Videos 70-1 and 70-2). CT and MRI are the best imaging modalities for most vascular rings (e-Fig. 70-18). Some patients require cannulation of peripheral vessels for the institution of CPB but also may have had multiple heart catheterizations or cutdowns. In these cases, ultrasound imaging with Doppler can help establish the patency of peripheral vessels such as the femoral artery and vein.

Summary

Congenital heart disease can present with a variety of symptoms in patients at any age. Surgical and catheter-based techniques, as well as pediatric cardiac anesthesiology, have evolved during the past 30 years, and interventions are being performed at an earlier age and through smaller incisions, with improving short- and long-term survival. Diagnosis is established by echocardiography in most circumstances, although MRI and CT may be useful in a number of preoperative and postoperative circumstances. Management decisions are based on the overall clinical picture, which takes into consideration patient symptoms, physical findings, and results of imaging studies. Imaging studies performed and interpreted by radiologists during the preoperative and postoperative phases are critical for the successful treatment of these patients.

Key Points

Incisions for pediatric cardiac surgery range from minimally invasive options such as small incisions for robotic procedures and thoracotomies to large midline, sternal incisions requiring splitting of the sternum.

Radiographic studies are extremely important for both the diagnosis and operative planning of congenital heart disease. These studies consist primarily of chest radiographs, CT scans, and MRI. Echocardiography also plays a significant role in diagnosis.

Chest radiographs are perhaps the most important study utilized in patients undergoing congenital heart surgery. They provide important diagnostic, preoperative, and postoperative information. Additionally, they serve to verify correct positioning of intraoperatively placed lines, chest tubes, and endotracheal tubes.

Because many children with congenital heart disease have other comorbidities involving other organ systems, radiographic studies for diagnosis and management of these processes are essential, such as renal and vascular ultrasound, brain imaging, and a variety of gastrointestinal studies.

Suggested Readings

Castaneda AR, Jonas RA, Mayer JE, et al. *Cardiac surgery of the neonate and infant*. Philadelphia: W. B. Saunders; 1994.

Jonas RA. *Comprehensive surgical management of congenital heart disease*. London: Hodder Arnold; 2004.

Mavroudis C, Backer C. *Pediatric cardiac surgery*. 3rd ed. St Louis: Mosby; 2003.

Selke F, del Nido P, Swanson S. *Sabiston and Spencer surgery of the chest*. 7th ed. Philadelphia: Saunders; 2004.

Stark JF, de Laval MR, Tsang VT, eds. *Surgery for congenital heart defects*. 3rd ed. Hoboken, NJ: John Wiley & Sons; 2006.

References

Full references for this chapter can be found on www.expertconsult.com.

Chapter 71

Prenatal Imaging and Therapy of Congenital Heart Disease

ANITA KRISHNAN and MARY T. DONOFRIO

Congenital heart disease, the most common birth defect, occurs in 3 to 8 per 1000 newborns.[1-3] The incidence is higher prenatally, affecting 5.8% to 16.9% of fetuses undergoing screening echocardiograms.[4-6] Despite advances in imaging techniques, routine obstetric ultrasound is only 30% to 50% sensitive for detection of congenital heart defects.[7-12] With the addition of careful delineation of outflow tracts, sensitivity improves significantly.[13] The most difficult lesions to diagnose prenatally are transposition of the great arteries and outflow tract abnormalities. A complete fetal echocardiogram includes two-dimensional, M-mode, and color Doppler imaging to assess fetal cardiac structure, rhythm, and function. Novel techniques include tissue Doppler and strain analysis.

Fetal Physiology and Flow

The fetal cardiac circulation has been studied in human and animal models (Fig. 71-1). Fetal and postnatal cardiovascular physiology differs markedly. Key differences include the following:

1. Right ventricular output is greater than left ventricular output.
2. Oxygen saturation of blood to the brain is higher than of blood to the body because maternal blood is directed from the umbilical vein to the ductus venosus and across the foramen ovale by the eustachian valve.
3. A ductus arteriosus is present. Deoxygenated blood from the superior vena cava travels to the right ventricle to the ductus arteriosus and then to the placenta.
4. Pulmonary vascular resistance is increased, resulting in decreased flow to the lungs. This changes after birth to allow an increase in pulmonary blood flow.
5. In utero, afterload for the left ventricle decreases but increases dramatically with umbilical cord clamping.

Fetuses with congenital heart disease have additional alterations of fetal physiology. They can have restricted intrauterine growth, neurologic abnormalities, and poor neurodevelopmental outcome. Circulatory alterations that accompany specific cardiac defects may cause blood flow disturbances that affect normal development. Doppler ultrasound of the middle cerebral artery, umbilical artery, umbilical vein, and ductus venosus can provide clinically useful information when combined with an understanding of fetal physiology.

CEREBRAL RESISTANCE

Fetal cerebral vessels can vasodilate during stress, which decreases resistance and increases diastolic flow in the middle cerebral artery. Peripheral vessels vasoconstrict to direct blood to the brain; this causes increased resistance and decreased diastolic flow in the descending aorta. This represents an autoregulatory mechanism (Fig. 71-2). This phenomenon of increasing cerebral blood flow has been described in growth-restricted fetuses as a predictor of poor perinatal outcome (Fig. 71-3). This phenomenon also occurs in fetuses with congenital heart disease (Table 71-1), although the clinical significance of this finding as a predictor of outcome is still in question.[14]

UMBILICAL ARTERY FLOW PATTERNS

Umbilical artery flow is used to assess fetal and placental well-being. It can be altered in high-risk pregnancies, hydrops fetalis, and certain forms of congenital heart disease. Absent diastolic flow in the umbilical artery is a poor prognostic marker.

VENOUS FLOW PATTERNS

Flow patterns in the umbilical vein and ductus venosus can be used to assess right ventricular filling. Impaired relaxation, associated with placental insufficiency or cardiac dysfunction, can cause decreased or reversed diastolic venous flow, particularly in atrial systole (Fig. 71-4). Absent or reversed flow in the ductus venosus and pulsatility of the umbilical vein flow associated with elevated atrial pressure have been recognized as markers of poor outcome in hydropic fetuses.

Fetal Anatomy

A complete fetal echocardiogram includes imaging of the atria, ventricles, atrioventricular (AV) and semilunar valves, foramen ovale, pulmonary veins (at least two), ductal and aortic arches, branch pulmonary arteries, and cardiac rhythm

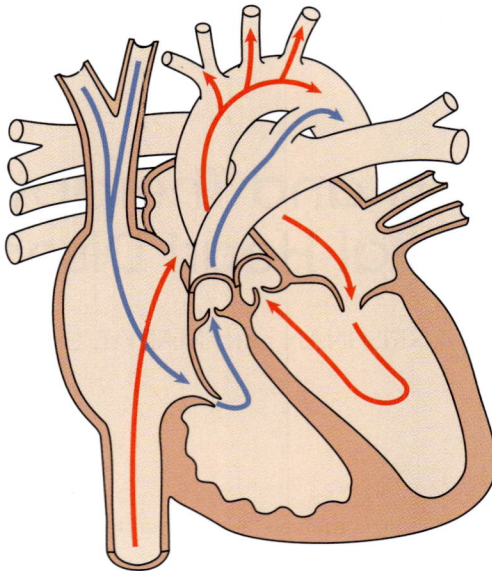

Figure 71-1 Diagram of the normal fetal cardiac circulation. Oxygenated umbilical venous blood enters the right atrium from the inferior vena cava and is directed across a patent foramen ovale, into the left atrium, from which it enters the fetal systemic circulation. Unoxygenated fetal systemic venous blood enters the right atrium via the superior vena cava. This blood is directed into the right ventricle and then out into the main pulmonary artery. High pulmonary vascular resistance and a patent ductus arteriosus causes preferential flow into the descending aorta.

and function. Measurements vary by gestational age and should be compared with normative data. Doppler and color interrogation of each structure should be performed.

SITUS

Situs of heart and abdominal viscera should be assessed, and delineation of normal drainage of systemic veins should be performed. The vena cavae normally enter the morphologic right atrium, and at least two pulmonary veins are seen entering the morphologic left atrium. The flap valve of septum

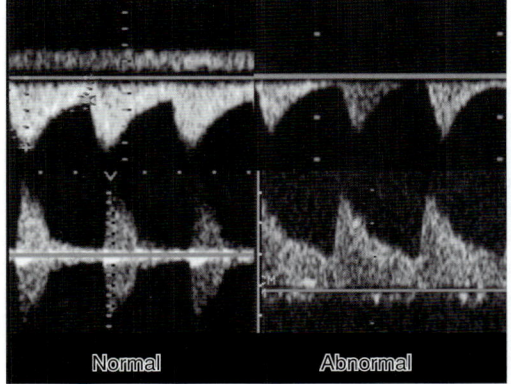

Figure 71-2 Normal and abnormal arterial spectral Doppler signals from the umbilical and middle cerebral arteries. Fetal compromise results in increased peripheral and placental resistance (decreased diastolic flow in umbilical artery) and decreased cerebral resistance (increased diastolic flow in middle cerebral artery); this is known as the *brain-sparing effect.*

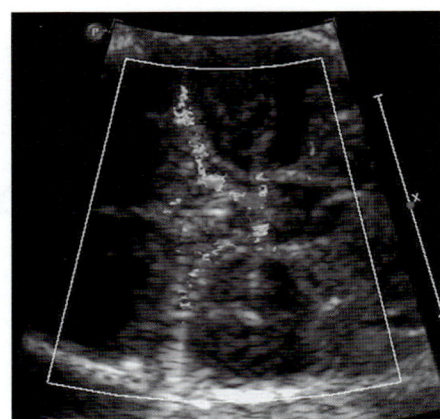

Figure 71-3 Color Doppler image of normal fetal cerebral blood flow in the circle of Willis.

primum, associated with the morphologic left atrium, can help identify it in situs abnormalities. Morphology of the atrial appendages (broad-based right-sided appendage vs. finger-like left atrial appendage) can help identify each atrium.

ATRIOVENTRICULAR AND SEMILUNAR VALVES

Tricuspid and pulmonary valve annuli measure slightly larger compared with mitral and aortic valves, respectively. Size discrepancy (ratio >1.5) between right-sided and left-sided structures suggests disease. The tricuspid valve annulus is positioned more apically compared with the mitral valve annulus. Two left ventricular papillary muscles should be identified. Biphasic flow patterns should be seen on Doppler evaluation of both the tricuspid valve and the mitral valve.

AORTIC AND DUCTAL ARCHES

The relationship of the aorta and pulmonary outflow to the ventricles should be determined, and peak velocities in aortic and ductal arches should be obtained. Arch sidedness can be determined from the three-vessel view. The aorta, main pulmonary artery, and the SVC are seen relative to the trachea (Fig. 71-5) An aorta positioned right of the trachea suggests

Table 71-1

Hypothesized Alterations in Circulatory Dynamics for Specific Congenital Heart Defects Compared with Normal			
Defect	Resistance to Cerebral Flow	Oxygen Content of Cerebral Blood	No. Ventricles
HLHS	↑↑	↓	1
LVOTO	↑	Normal	2
TGA	Normal	↓↓	2
TOF	Normal	↓	2
HRH	Normal	↓	1

HLHS, hypoplastic left heart syndrome; *HRH,* hypoplastic right heart; *LVOTO,* left ventricular outflow tract obstruction; *TGA,* transposition of the great arteries; *TOF,* tetralogy of Fallot.

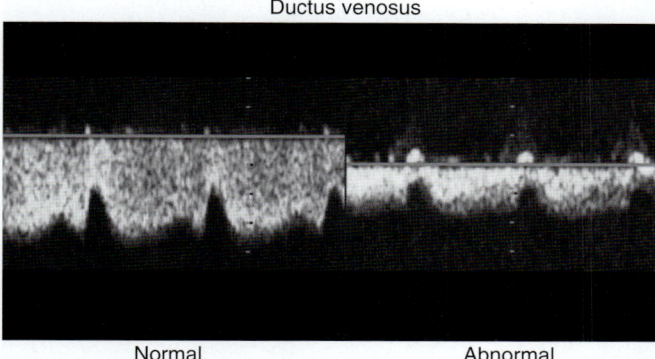

Figure 71-4 Normal and abnormal arterial spectral Doppler signal from the ductus venosus. Late fetal compromise or impaired cardiac filling or both result in decreased forward and some reversal of late diastolic flow in the ductus venosus.

a right aortic arch and calls for careful evaluation for vascular rings and congenital heart disease.

RIGHT AND LEFT VENTRICLES

Key morphologic features for the right ventricle are moderator band, attachments of tricuspid valve to ventricular septum, plane of tricuspid valve annulus lower than mitral valve annulus, and coarse trabeculations. The left ventricle, in contrast, has smooth trabeculations, and the mitral valve attachments are located away from the septum.

Prenatal Imaging: Timing and Indications

Fetal echocardiography has been in use since the late 1980s. The optimal time for transabdominal imaging of the fetal heart is between 20 and 28 weeks of gestation. Transvaginal imaging can be performed as early as 8 weeks, with successful diagnosis of heart defects possible as early as 11 weeks.[15-16] Third-trimester imaging, although possible, is limited by paucity of the amniotic fluid and limited variability in fetal

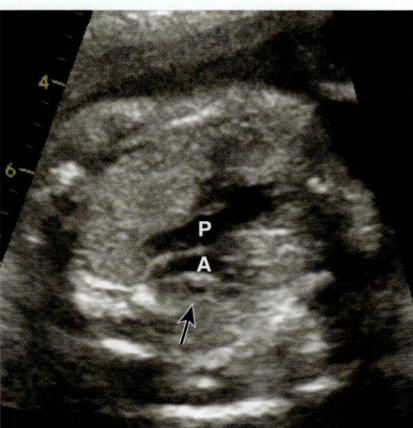

Figure 71-5 The three-vessel view, showing pulmonary artery, aorta, and superior vena cava relative to the spine. Note the position of the trachea (*arrow*) relative to the aorta (*A*) and pulmonary artery (*P*).

position. Indications for fetal echocardiography include maternal and fetal risk factors (Box 71-1). The most common reasons are family history of congenital heart disease, fetal dysrhythmia, maternal diabetes, and extracardiac defects. Indications that are most predictive of cardiac disease are an abnormal four-chamber view on routine ultrasound (30% to 50%), fetal dysrhythmia (30%), hydrops (30%), and polyhydramnios (25%).

Cardiac Defects

SEPTATION DEFECTS

Atrial Septal Defects

The most common atrial septal defects (ASDs) are ostium secundum defects. Sinus venosus defects (superior or inferior type) are often associated with anomalous drainage of the right pulmonary veins. Ostium primum defects are an endocardial cushion defect, and often associated with Down syndrome. A patent foramen ovale is a normal structure of the fetus and newborn (Figs. 71-6 and 71-7); it may be difficult to distinguish a normal foramen ovale from a secundum ASD prenatally. Secundum defects are amenable to catheter closure; other defects require surgical correction.

Ventricular Septal Defects

Ventricular septal defects (VSDs) are the most common type of congenital heart defect. They can occur in the membranous, AV canal, muscular, or conal (outlet) septum. Perimembranous (around the membranous septum) defects are the most common. Moderate to large defects require surgical intervention in infants with congestive heart failure; small defects often close on their own. Muscular defects are the second most common; small defects usually close on their own, but multiple defects can cause congestive heart failure (Fig. 71-8).

Box 71-1   Indications for Fetal Echocardiography

Maternal Factors
- Maternal congenital heart disease
- Congenital heart disease in older siblings
- Maternal systemic disease (diabetes mellitus, systemic lupus erythematosus)
- Maternal teratogenic exposure (drug, environmental)

Fetal Factors
- Fetal chromosomal abnormality
- Fetal genetic syndrome
- Fetal extracardiac anomaly
- Fetal distress or hydrops
- Abnormal heart on routine ultrasound scan
- Fetal dysrhythmia
- Multiple gestation with discordant twin syndrome
- In vitro fertilization
- Monochorionic twins
- Unexplained polyhydramnios
- Increased nuchal translucency

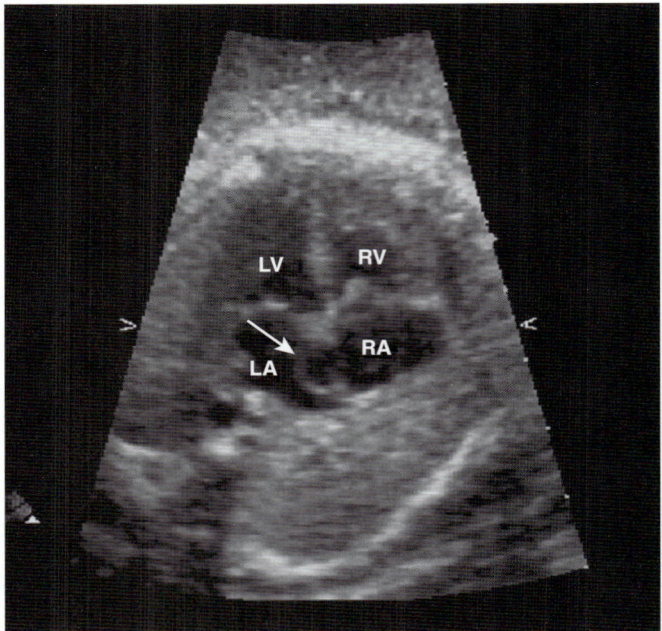

Figure 71-6 Fetal four-chamber image of normal patent foramen ovale and bulging of atrial septum (*arrow*) into the left atrium (*LA*). *RA*, right atrium; *LV*, left ventricle; *RV*, right ventricle.

Atrioventricular Canal defects

AV canal (endocardial cushion) defects are easily diagnosed prenatally (Fig. 71-9) and can be associated with Down syndrome. They include a primum ASD, inlet VSD, and common AV valve. VSDs can be isolated. The cross-sectional anatomy of the common valve is best determined from short-axis imaging. Partial AV septal defects have a primum ASD with a cleft mitral valve. Transitional AV septal defects have an atrial defect, common AV valve, and restrictive VSD.

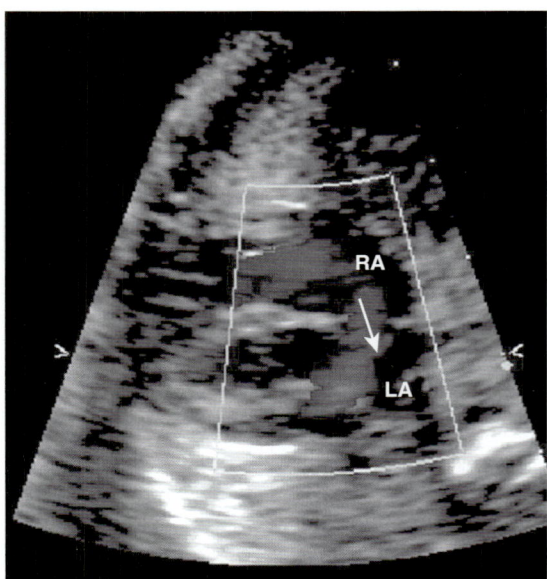

Figure 71-7 Fetal color Doppler four-chamber image of normal right-to-left atrial shunting (*arrow*). *LA*, left atrium; *RA*, right atrium.

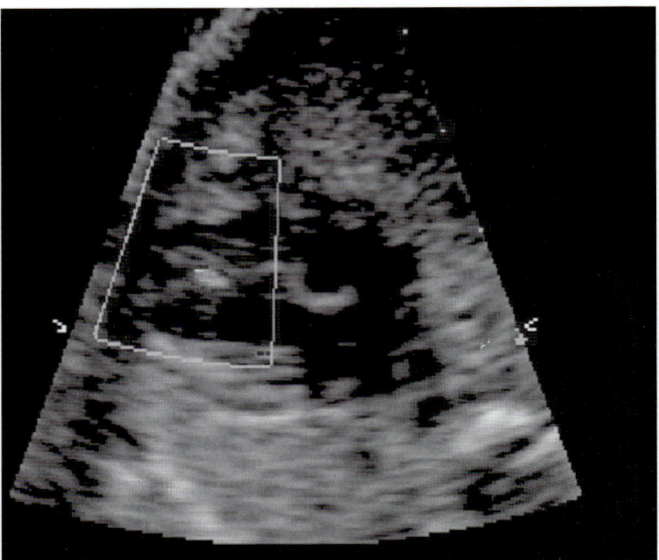

Figure 71-8 Fetal color Doppler four-chamber image of small midmuscular ventricular septal defect with small left-to-right shunt.

INFLOW/OUTFLOW

Right-Sided Inflow Lesions

Right ventricular inflow lesions include Ebstein anomaly, tricuspid valve dysplasia, and tricuspid stenosis or atresia. The tricuspid valve orifice is displaced apically in Ebstein anomaly, with abnormal delamination of the septal leaflet and tricuspid valve regurgitation. (Fig. 71-10) Milder disease may not present until the first decade of life with arrhythmias and tricuspid regurgitation; severe forms can cause fetal hydrops, death, or neonatal cyanosis. Ebstein anomaly can be associated with pulmonary stenosis or atresia, causing cyanosis and requiring initiation of prostaglandin therapy to maintain

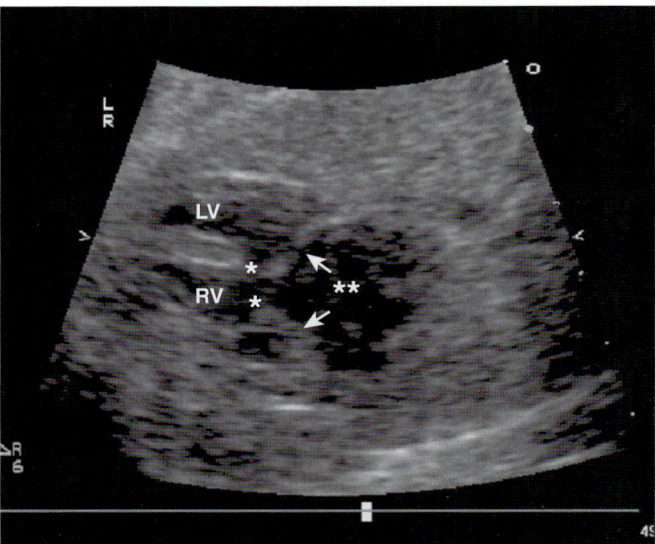

Figure 71-9 Fetal four-chamber image of complete atrioventricular septal defect with large atrial (*double asterisk*) and ventricular (*asterisk*) septal defects. *Arrows* show common atrioventricular valve. *LV*, left ventricle; *RV*, right ventricle.

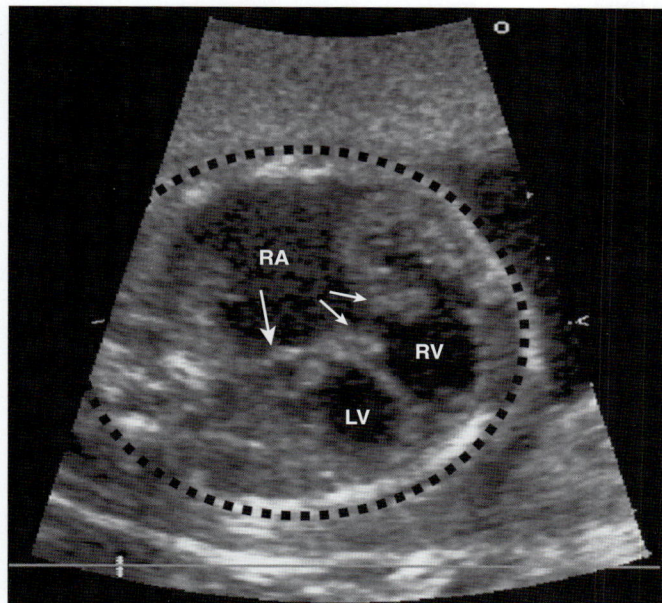

Figure 71-10 Fetal four-chamber image of highly thickened and api-cally displaced (Ebstein anomaly) tricuspid valve (*thin arrows*). Cardio-megaly from tricuspid valve regurgitation is severe, with the cardiac mass taking up most of the cardiothoracic space (*dotted black circle*). Nor-mally, the cardiothoracic area ratio is less than 33%. The right atrium (*RA*) is severely dilated, compressing the atrial septum (*single thick arrow*) and left atrium. *LV*, left ventricle; *RV*, right ventricle.

Figure 71-11 Fetal image of tetralogy of Fallot with large malaligned ventricular septal defect with overriding aorta (*asterisk*). *Ao*, aorta; *LV*, left ventricle; *RV*, right ventricle.

ductus arteriosus patency. Tricuspid valve dysplasia has similar features but without apical displacement of the valve annulus. Tricuspid atresia or stenosis can be associated with hypoplasia of the right ventricle and pulmonary outflow obstruction; without a VSD, this lesion requires postnatal prostaglandin to maintain ductal patency prior to neonatal single-ventricle palliation surgery.

Right-Sided Outflow Lesions

Pulmonary outflow obstruction can be subvalvular, valvular, or supravalvular. The disease spectrum ranges from severe cyanosis and pulmonary atresia in newborns to normal oxygen saturation and a near normal pulmonary outflow tract in infants. Fetal echocardiography can predict the degree of subvalvular and valvular stenosis.

Isolated pulmonary valve stenosis is diagnosed by identify-ing domed and thickened pulmonary valve leaflets. The annulus may be hypoplastic. Fetal Doppler echocardiography may not accurately predict the postnatal pulmonary valve gradient. This lack of agreement between prenatal and post-natal gradients is attributed to in utero physiology, elevated pulmonary vascular resistance, and right-to-left shunting at the atrial level. Supravalvular pulmonic stenosis is associated with Williams syndrome. Subvalvular obstruction is usually seen in combination with other defects such as tetralogy of Fallot (Fig. 71-11).

Left-Sided Inflow Lesions

Left ventricular inflow abnormalities include cor triatriatum, congenital mitral stenosis, and congenital mitral insufficiency.

In cor triatriatum, a membrane within the left atrium causes obstruction to pulmonary venous return and is usually associ-ated with an ASD. Congenital mitral valve anomalies may occur in isolation or in combination with aortic valve anoma-lies and arch anomalies. Shone's complex is a combination of these defects and includes supravalvular mitral ring, parachute mitral valve, subaortic stenosis, and aortic coarctation.

Left-Sided Outflow Lesions

Left-sided outflow tract obstruction can occur at the subval-vular, valvular, or supravalvular levels. Infants of mothers with diabetes, especially of mothers with poor glucose control, are at risk for hypertrophic cardiomyopathy (with or without obstruction).[17] Even in severe cases, the hypertrophy usually regresses by 3 months of age. Valvular aortic stenosis seen in utero can be associated with left ventricular dysfunc-tion and progressive hydrops. Supravalvular stenosis is associ-ated with Williams syndrome and can occur in combination with right-sided outflow tract obstruction. Left-sided obstruc-tive lesions can be associated with Turner syndrome.[18]

CONOTRUNCAL DEFECTS

Conotruncal defects include abnormalities of the connection between the ventricles and the great vessels, including tetral-ogy of Fallot, transposition of the great arteries, truncus arteriosus, and double-outlet right ventricle. The lesions can be associated with deletions in chromosome locus 22q11 (DiGeorge sequence, velocardiofacial syndrome, CATCH 22 [cardiac defects, abnormal facies, thymic hypoplasia, cleft palate, hypocalcemia]).[19]

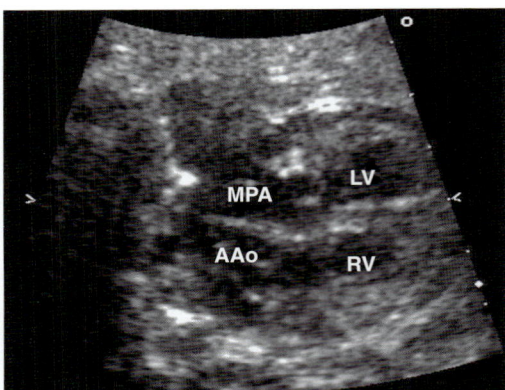

Figure 71-12   Fetal image of transposition of great arteries with the aorta arising from the right ventricle (*RV*) and the pulmonary artery arising from the left ventricle (*LV*). *AAo*, ascending aorta; *MPA*, main pulmonary artery.

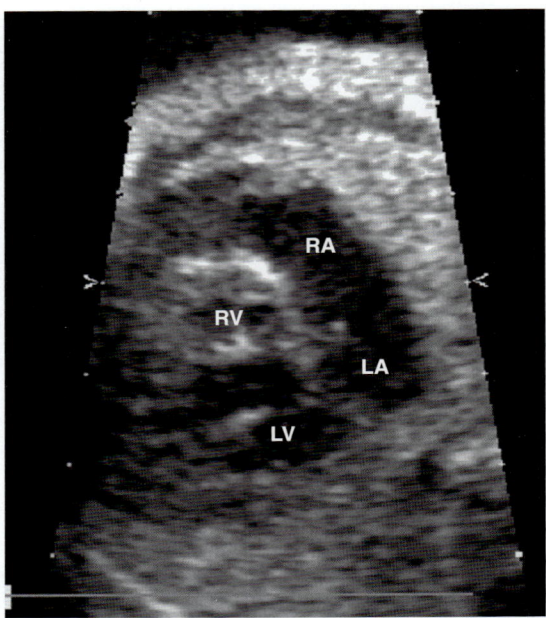

Figure 71-13   Fetal four-chamber image of pulmonary atresia with intact ventricular septum and very hypoplastic and hypertrophied right ventricle (*RV*). *LA*, left atrium; *LV*, left ventricle; *RA*, right atrium.

Tetralogy of Fallot (right ventricular outflow obstruction, right ventricular hypertrophy, overriding aorta, and large anterior malaligned VSD) is the most common form of cyanotic congenital heart disease, with transposition of the great vessels being the second most common. In transposition, the aorta originates from the right ventricle, and the pulmonary artery arises from the left ventricle. Echocardiography shows parallel great vessels with aorta located anterior and rightward of the pulmonary artery (Fig. 71-12). A laterally branching vessel (left pulmonary artery) from the great artery is seen related to the left ventricle. Additional abnormalities such as VSDs (one third of cases) also are identified. The four-chamber view is normal, making diagnosis quite difficult.

In the double-outlet right ventricle, the presence of sub-aortic conus causes anterior displacement of the aorta. A VSD is present. The disease can encompass a spectrum of physiology from single ventricle lesions, to tetralogy of Fallot or transposition of the great arteries. In truncus arteriosus, a single outflow tract originates from the heart, with a malalignment-type VSD. Pulmonary arteries vary in size, and originate from the truncal outflow. The truncal valve can range from unicuspid to quadricuspid and often is stenotic or insufficient.

VENTRICULAR HYPOPLASIA

Underdevelopment of either ventricle can result in a univentricular heart. After birth, patients require staged surgical palliation and possible heart transplantation later. Hypoplastic right heart syndrome can result from tricuspid atresia or pulmonary atresia with an intact interventricular septum (Fig. 71-13). Hypoplastic left heart syndrome may have severe aortic and mitral stenosis or atresia (Fig. 71-14) and requires intervention or surgery in the neonatal period. Double-inlet left ventricle with a right ventricular outlet chamber is another, more complex form of a single ventricle heart (see Fig. 71-14) and can be associated with a normal or hypoplastic outflow tract.

FIBROELASTOSIS

Endocardial fibroelastosis is an abnormality of the endocardial surface. Prenatally, thickening and fibrosis of the endocardium due to inflammation or hypoxia result in an echobright appearance. These areas can be either focal or diffuse. It has been described in fetuses with maternal Sjogren's antibody exposure; structural anomalies such as hypoplastic left heart syndrome; anomalous coronaries; aortic stenosis; fetal infections such as parvovirus infection; metabolic diseases; and cardiomyopathy (Fig. 71-15).[20] Once diagnosed, serial assessment of ventricular function, venous flow patterns, and valve regurgitation is warranted to evaluate for development of fetal hydrops fetalis.

VENOUS AND AORTIC ARCH ANOMALIES

Systemic venous abnormalities often have no clinical consequences. A common abnormality, existing in 3% of the normal population, is bilateral superior vena cavae with the left superior vena cava draining into the coronary sinus. It may be suspected when an enlarged coronary sinus is seen and is more prevalent in patients with congenital heart disease.

Some or all of the pulmonary veins can drain anomalously to the systemic (right) circulation, entering supracardiac (through a vertical vein into the innominate vein), intracardiac (directly into the right atrium or coronary sinus), or infracardiac (through the liver or inferior vena cava). In obstructed total anomalous pulmonary venous drainage, neonates may be critically ill and require immediate surgery. This lesion is suspected when a small left atrium is seen in combination with dilated right heart. It is difficult to diagnose prenatally because of the decreased pulmonary venous return.

Aortic arch abnormalities include vascular rings, coarctation of the aorta, and interrupted aortic arch. Vascular rings can be associated with a right-sided aortic arch, aberrant left subclavian artery, and Kommerell's diverticulum or ligamentum arteriosus. Depending on the type of ring, infants may

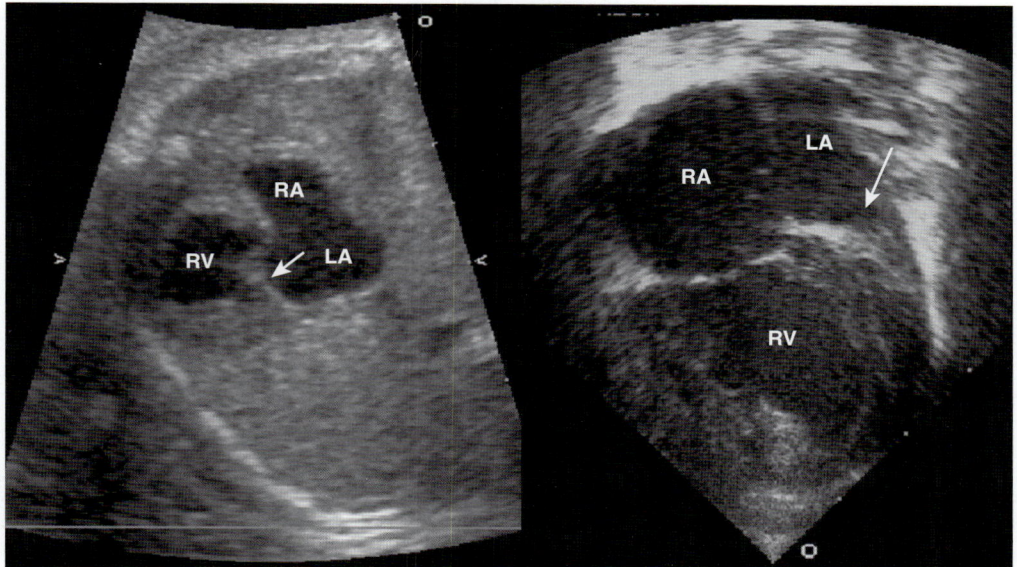

Figure 71-14   Fetal (*left*) and postnatal apical (*right*) four-chamber images of the same patient with hypoplastic left heart syndrome. The mitral valve (*arrow*) is atretic. *LA*, left atrium; *RA*, right atrium; *RV*, right ventricle.

be asymptomatic, have airway narrowing, or have feeding difficulties. Finding a right aortic arch warrants further evaluation for associated anomalies. Coarctation of the aorta may present in early infancy with cardiogenic shock after ductal closure or in later life with hypertension. Coarctation may be difficult to diagnose in the fetal period when the ductus arteriosus is still open. Interrupted aortic arch is a severe type of coarctation, in which the ascending and descending aorta are discontinuous, with the descending aorta supplied by the ductus arteriosus. When associated with a VSD, this form is considered a conotruncal abnormality. Patent ductus arteriosus is a normal fetal structure; its premature closure can lead to right-sided heart failure in utero (Fig. 71-16). Indomethacin and other nonsteroidal antiinflammatory drugs predispose to this condition. The heart normalizes at delivery.[21]

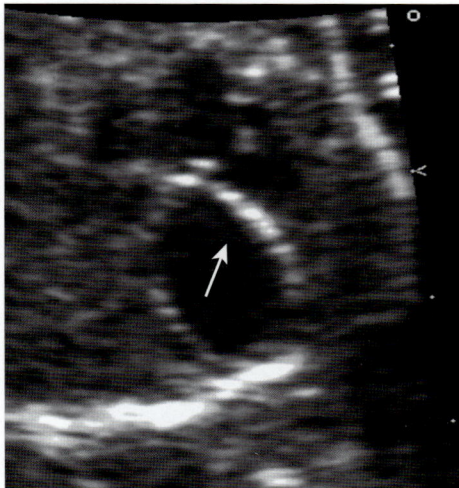

Figure 71-15   Endocardial fibroelastosis of a fetus with aortic stenosis. Scarring and fibrosis of the endocardium result from ischemic insult to the left ventricle. The *arrow* indicates endocardial fibroelastosis.

HETEROTAXY SYNDROMES: SITUS/CARDIAC MASSES/ARRHYTHMIAS

Situs abnormalities and complex congenital heart disease can be diagnosed by carefully evaluating abdominal and cardiac situs and intracardiac relationships (Fig. 71-17).[22] Correct determination of abdominal and cardiac situs depends on the delineation of fetal position and right or left orientation. Double-outlet right ventricle, atrioventricular septal defects, and venous anomalies are frequently associated with abnormalities of abdominal situs resulting in asplenia (bilateral "right-sidedness") or polysplenia (bilateral "left-sidedness"). Abnormal looping of the fetal heart may result in ventricular inversion (right-sided morphologic left ventricle and left-sided morphologic right ventricle) in these patients.

CARDIAC MASSES

Tiny echogenic objects in the left ventricular papillary muscles are frequently noted on fetal echocardiography (Fig. 71-18) and are considered normal variants.[23] Larger, more numerous masses suggest the presence of cardiac tumors. The most common prenatal cardiac tumors are rhabdomyomas (Fig. 71-19). They usually are associated with tuberous sclerosis. Although benign and usually regressive after birth, these tumors can cause obstruction or arrhythmias.[24]

Fetal Arrhythmias

Echocardiography provides accurate diagnosis of fetal arrhythmias.[25,26] Premature atrial contractions (Fig. 71-20) are common and usually benign. Supraventricular tachycardia and atrial flutter can be diagnosed with M-mode and Doppler ultrasound (Figs. 71-21 and 71-22). Bradycardia may be benign and is often caused by blocked premature atrial contractions. Complete heart block, a rare complication of maternal Sjögren antibody exposure, can be diagnosed by

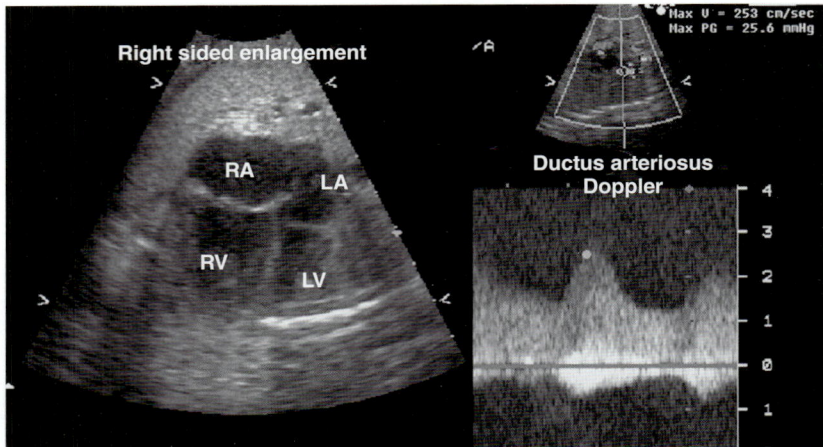

Figure 71-16   Fetal four-chamber (*left*) and spectral Doppler (*right*) images of a fetus with a restrictive ductus arteriosus causing significant right-sided enlargement. The increased Doppler velocity and diastolic "drag" is consistent with a restrictive flow pattern. *LA*, left atrium; *LV*, left ventricle; *RA*, right atrium; *RV*, right ventricle.

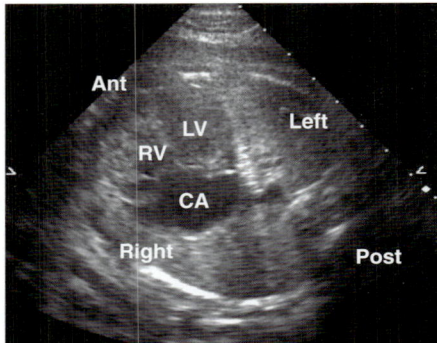

Figure 71-17   Fetal image of dextrocardia with abdominal situs inversus and a partial atrioventricular septal defect. The heart is in the right chest, and the ventricles are inverted. There is a common atrium. *Ant*, anterior; *CA*, common atrium; *LV*, left ventricle; *Post*, posterior; *RV*, right ventricle.

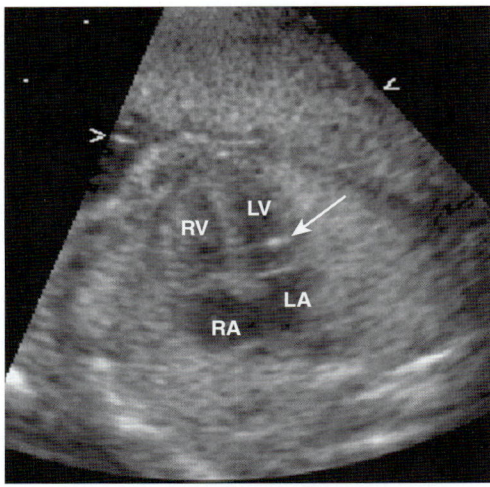

Figure 71-18   Fetal four-chamber image of benign calcification (*arrow*) on papillary muscle of the left ventricle (*LV*). *LA*, left atrium; *RA*, right atrium; *RV*, right ventricle.

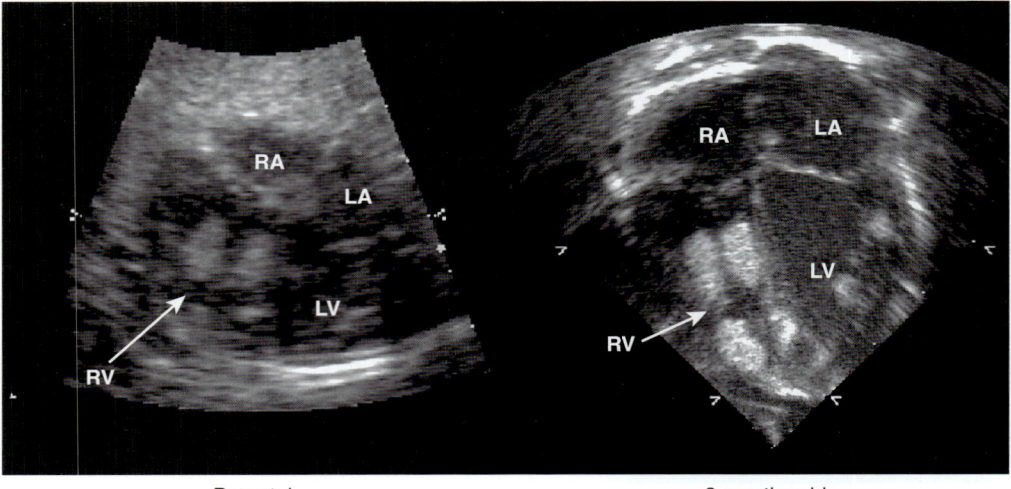

Prenatal   2 months old

Figure 71-19   Fetal (*left*) and postnatal apical (*right*) four-chamber image of the same patient with large rhabdomyomas in the right ventricle (*RV*) and smaller lesions in the left ventricle (*LV*). *LA*, left atrium; *RA*, right atrium.

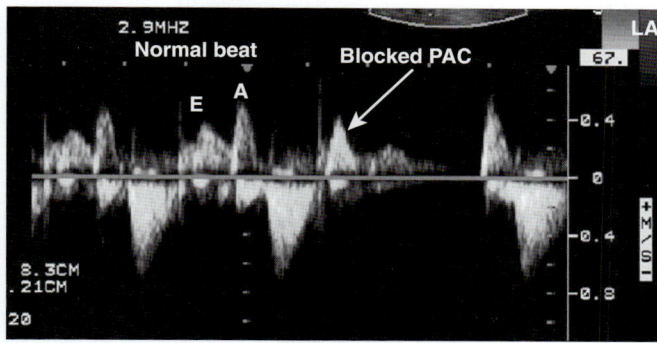

Figure 71-20 Fetal spectral Doppler image of mitral inflow and aortic outflow showing a blocked premature atrial contraction (*arrow*; PAC). *A*, mitral valve A wave; *E*, mitral valve E wave; *V*, ventricular outflow.

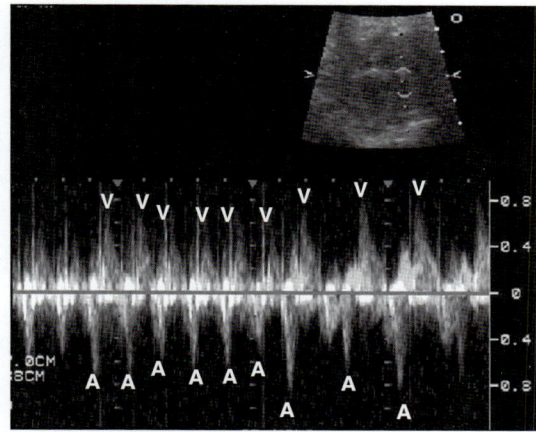

Figure 71-21 Fetal spectral Doppler image of mitral inflow and aortic outflow showing a short run of supraventricular tachycardia with 1:1 conduction. *A*, mitral valve A wave; *V*, ventricular outflow.

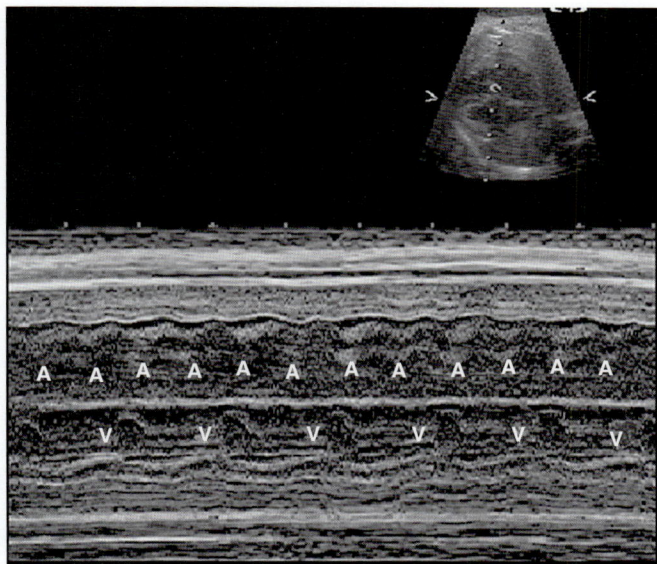

Figure 71-22 Fetal M-mode image of atrial and ventricular contraction showing atrial flutter with 2:1 conduction. The atrial rate is approximately 400 beats per minute, and the ventricular rate is approximately 200 beats per minute. *A*, atrial wall contraction; *V*, ventricular wall contraction.

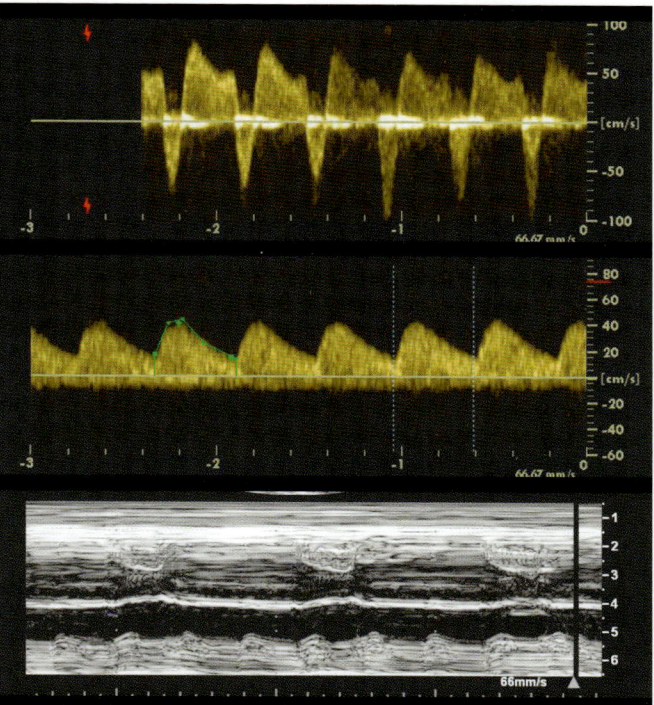

Figure 71-23 Fetal M-mode image of atrial and ventricular contractions showing complete heart block with atrioventricular dissociation. The atrial rate is approximately 150 beats per minute, and the ventricular rate is approximately 55 beats per minute.

M-mode or Doppler ultrasound (Fig. 71-23).[27] Serial Doppler assessment of the time between atrial and ventricular contractions is used in maternal Sjögren antibody carriers to follow the fetal conduction system (Fig. 71-24).

Fetal Management

Fetal echocardiography can provide crucial information that improves the outcomes of newborns with certain types of

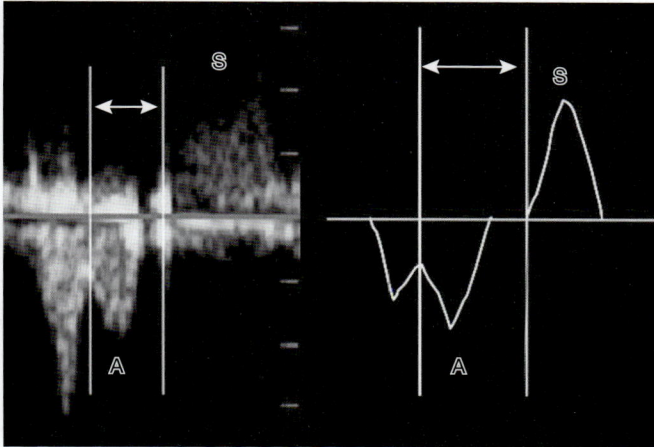

Figure 71-24 Fetal spectral Doppler image and drawing of diastolic atrial contraction (*A*) and systolic ventricular contraction (*S*). The mechanical atrioventricular interval (analogous to the P–R interval on an electrocardiogram) is measured from the beginning of the A wave to the beginning of the S wave (*lines and arrows*).

22 weeks
dilated left ventricle

33 weeks
small left ventricle

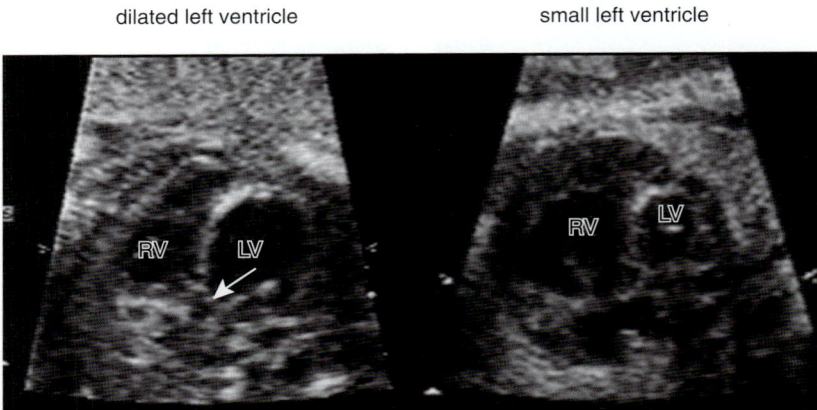

Figure 71-25 Side-by-side four-chamber images of the same fetus with critical aortic valve stenosis at 22 and 33 weeks' gestational age. At 22 weeks, the left ventricle (*LV*) is dilated, and the apex is forming; at 33 weeks, the LV is hypoplastic. Arrow indicates aortic valve. *RV*, right ventricle. (Courtesy Wayne Tworetzky, MD, Division of Cardiology, Children's Hospital Boston, Boston, MA.)

congenital heart disease. It is invaluable in counseling families and guiding prenatal and delivery room treatments of structural heart disease and arrhythmias.

The most common rhythm disturbances in the fetus do not require treatment. Persistent supraventricular tachycardia or atrial flutter can result in cardiac dysfunction and hydrops if left untreated. Administration of digoxin to the mother is often successful as first-line therapy for fetuses with supraventricular tachycardia, but it is less effective in fetuses with atrial flutter or those who are hydropic. Higher dosages of digoxin are required during pregnancy because of increased maternal volume of distribution. Sotalol can be considered as a first-line drug for atrial flutter. Second-line drugs for supraventricular tachycardia (other than atrial flutter) include sotalol, flecainide, or amiodarone. Close monitoring of the mother and fetus is required, and initiation of drug therapy may necessitate hospitalization. Administration of adenosine via the umbilical cord may be considered in severely compromised fetuses with supraventricular tachycardia. Complete heart block is difficult to manage. Maternal steroid and β-agonist treatment has been used with variable success in these patients. Early delivery may be required if hydrops and fetal compromise are present.

Fetuses with ductal-dependent systemic or pulmonary blood flow require prostaglandin treatment immediately after birth. If the diagnosis is unknown and the ductus closes, severe cyanosis, acidosis, and compromised cardiac output are likely to occur, resulting in potential multisystemic organ damage. Patients with hypoplastic left heart syndrome and transposition of the great arteries with intact atrial septum are at highest risk for compromise at birth. They may require immediate interventional cardiac catheterization to open the atrial communication for survival. Considerable planning is required to deliver these infants in a setting where a pediatric cardiac catheterization laboratory and intervention are available immediately or soon after delivery.

Although the heart develops by 8 weeks' gestation, fetal flow patterns can affect development of the heart throughout gestation. Disproportionate flow to one side of the circulation may lead to underdevelopment of either side of the heart. Fetuses with aortic or pulmonary valve stenosis at 18 to 20 weeks' gestation can progress to hypoplastic left or right heart by 30 weeks' gestation (Fig. 71-25). Fetal catheter-based intervention to relieve aortic stenosis, pulmonary stenosis, or a restrictive atrial septum has been performed.[28-31] Technically successful fetal balloon aortic valvuloplasty in fetuses with critical aortic valve stenosis with likely evolving hypoplastic left heart syndrome was reported in 2004. Improved left heart growth and postnatal two-ventricular circulation was seen in some of the successful cases (Figs. 71-26 through 71-28).

Conclusion

Fetal echocardiography is an important adjunct to other prenatal evaluations, including ultrasound and genetic screening. Radiologists, cardiologists, perinatologists, neonataologists,

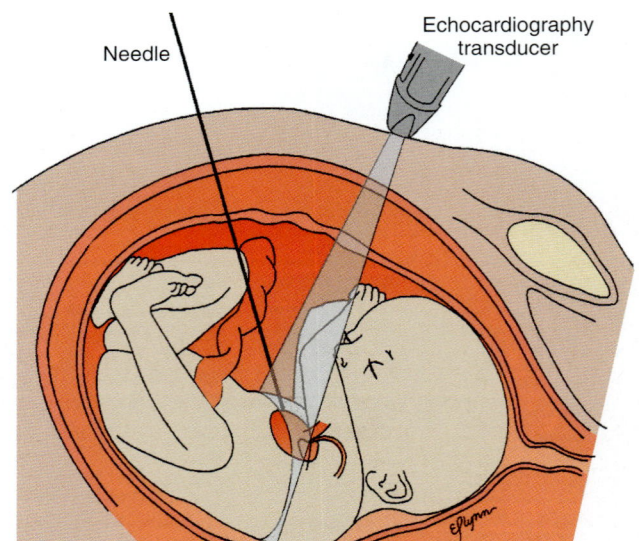

Needle

Echocardiography transducer

Figure 71-26 Needle insertion through maternal abdomen, uterine wall, fetal chest, and fetal heart under ultrasound guidance. (Courtesy Wayne Tworetzky, MD, Division of Cardiology, Children's Hospital Boston, Boston, MA.)

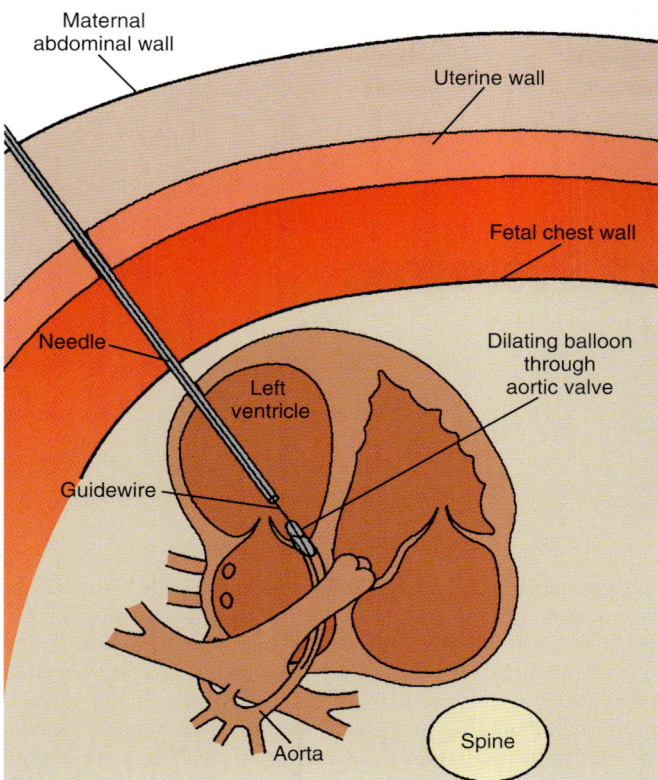

Figure 71-27 Needle, wire, and balloon catheter insertion through fetal left ventricle and across the aortic valve under ultrasound guidance. (Courtesy Wayne Tworetzky, MD, Division of Cardiology, Children's Hospital Boston, Boston, MA.)

and other pediatric subspecialists must work together to provide a multidisciplinary treatment and counseling approach to patients with complex diagnoses (Fig. 71-29). Newer imaging modalities of the fetal heart, including three-dimensional echocardiography and magnetic resonance imaging,

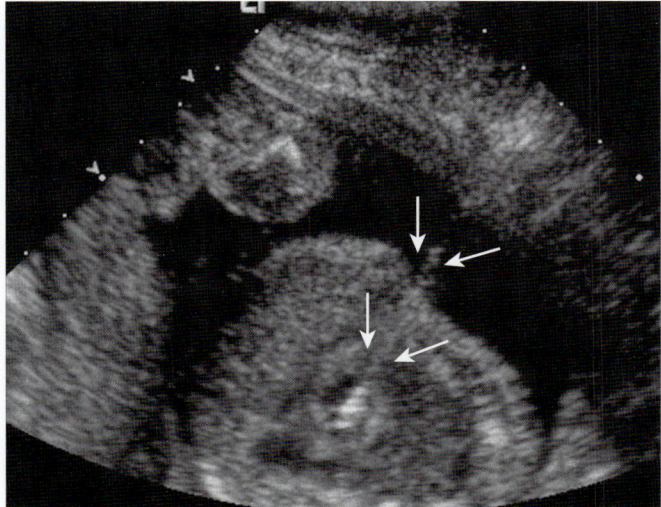

Figure 71-28 Fetal ultrasound image of needle (*arrows*) being inserted through the uterine wall, fetal chest, and fetal heart. (Courtesy Wayne Tworetzky, MD, Division of Cardiology, Children's Hospital Boston, Boston, MA.)

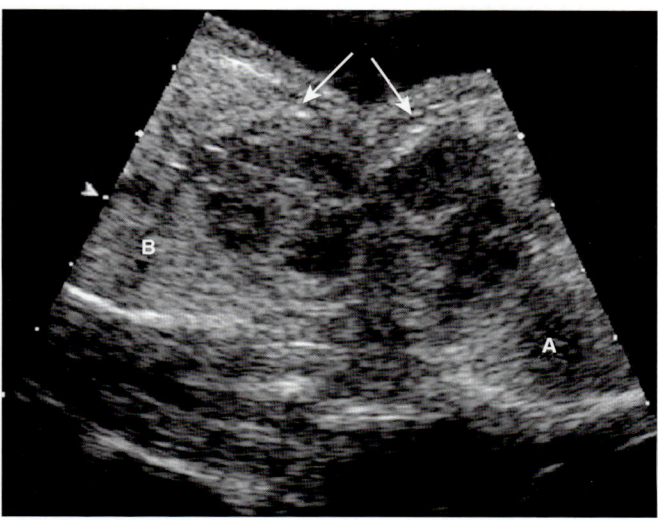

Figure 71-29 Fetal image of conjoined twins with a shared heart (*arrows*). **A,** twin A. **B,** twin B.

will further contribute to fetal cardiac management. As technology and treatments evolve, fetal cardiology represents an area of tremendous potential for early diagnosis and in utero treatment of abnormalities. In the future, intervention during the fetal period may allow physicians to actually alter the evolution of structural cardiac disease, thus helping improve long-term outcome.

Key Points

- Congenital heart disease is the most common birth defect in 0.3% to 0.8% of newborns.

- Fetal cardiovascular physiology is unique with right-to-left shunting to provide high oxygen saturation of blood to the fetal brain.

- Optimal timing for imaging of the fetal heart is 20 to 28 weeks' gestation.

- Indications for fetal echocardiography include family history, dysrhythmia, maternal diabetes, the presence of fetal extracardiac defects, or all of these factors.

Suggested Readings

Allan LD. Fetal cardiology. *Ultrasound Obstet Gynecol.* 1994;4:441-444.
Ferencz C, Neill CA. Cardiovascular malformations: prevalence at live birth. In: Freedom RM, Benson LN, Smallhorn JF, eds. *Neonatal heart disease.* London: Springer-Verlag; 1992:19-29.
Rychik J, Ayres N, Cuneo B. American Society of Echocardiography guidelines and standards for performance of a fetal echocardiogram. *J Am Soc Echocardiogr.* 2004;17:803-810.
Simpson LL. Fetal supraventricular tachycardias: diagnosis and management. *Semin Perinatol.* 2000;24:360-372.

References

Full references for this chapter can be found on www.expertconsult.com.

Chapter 72

Abnormal Pulmonary and Systemic Venous Connections

CYNTHIA K. RIGSBY, ANGIRA PATEL, BRIAN REILLY, and GRACE R. CHOI

Partial Anomalous Pulmonary Venous Connection and Scimitar Syndrome

Overview Partial anomalous pulmonary venous connection (PAPVC) is present when one or more pulmonary veins drain into a systemic vein. Because a single anomalous connection may be unrecognized, the incidence is difficult to establish, but it has been reported to be present in one in 200 postmortem examinations.[1,2]

Etiology, Pathophysiology, and Clinical Presentation All pulmonary veins from one lung may have anomalous drainage, or parts of the lung may have anomalous drainage to the same or different systemic veins. Anomalous drainage of the left pulmonary veins is most often to the brachiocephalic vein or coronary sinus.[3] On the right, anomalous drainage is most often to the superior vena cava (SVC), right atrium, and inferior vena cava (IVC).[4] When there is anomalous pulmonary venous drainage of all the right pulmonary veins, or just the middle and lower lobe veins to the IVC, scimitar syndrome is present. Other anomalies associated with scimitar syndrome include hypoplasia of the right lung and bronchial system, hypoplasia of the right pulmonary artery, systemic arterial supply to the right lower lung, and pulmonary sequestration.[5-8]

Approximately 67% of patients with partial anomalous pulmonary venous return also have atrial-level defects, most commonly a sinus venosus defect (see Chapter 73).[9] Sinus venosus defects are not true atrial septal defects (ASDs) but occur as a result of deficiency of the wall between the SVC and the right upper pulmonary veins or of the wall between the right atrium and the right upper and lower pulmonary veins. Thus although a sinus venosus defect does not represent an abnormal pulmonary venous connection with a systemic vein, a superior sinus venosus defect often is associated with anomalous drainage of the right pulmonary veins to the SVC or to the right atrium.

With an intact atrial septum, the amount of blood draining through anomalous veins depends on the number of anomalous draining veins, the compliance of the atria, and the resistance of the pulmonary vascular beds. Anomalous connection of one pulmonary vein usually is not clinically apparent in childhood, but these patients may present in the third and fourth decades with cyanosis resulting from increased pulmonary vascular resistance.[10] If all but one of the pulmonary veins drains anomalously, the clinical manifestations may be similar to total anomalous pulmonary venous connection. If they are associated with a sinus venosus septal defect, signs and symptoms usually are related to the amount of shunting through the defect. Patients with scimitar syndrome may present in infancy with pulmonary hypertension from the arterial supply to the right lower lung, stenosis of the anomalous pulmonary veins, or pulmonary infections. Otherwise, this syndrome may be detected in adulthood in persons who do not have significant symptoms.[11]

Imaging With anomalous drainage of multiple veins, cardiomegaly with right heart enlargement and increased pulmonary flow are seen on chest radiography. Findings with scimitar syndrome include a crescent-shaped anomalous pulmonary vein (resembling a Turkish sword or scimitar) paralleling the lower right heart border (Fig. 72-1). Patients generally have associated hypoplasia of the right lung, a small right pulmonary artery, and varying degrees of cardiac dextroposition.

Cross-sectional imaging goals include identifying the anomalous pulmonary to systemic venous connection, locating each pulmonary vein and its drainage relative to the left atrium, and determining the location of venous obstruction, if present (e-Fig. 72-2). Evaluation for the presence and size of either an ASD or sinus venosus defect, is necessary (e-Figs. 72-3 and 72-4). The heart and great vessels are evaluated for other abnormalities, and when scimitar syndrome is present, the upper abdomen should be assessed for anomalous venous drainage and systemic supply to the lung (Fig. 72-5). Both computed tomography (CT) and magnetic resonance imaging (MRI) are highly sensitive and specific for evaluation of anomalous pulmonary venous drainage, and three-dimensional CT or magnetic resonance angiography is very useful for identifying the relationship between the anomalous pulmonary veins and the left atrium.[12,13] MRI also is useful for ASD evaluation and for quantification of systemic to pulmonary

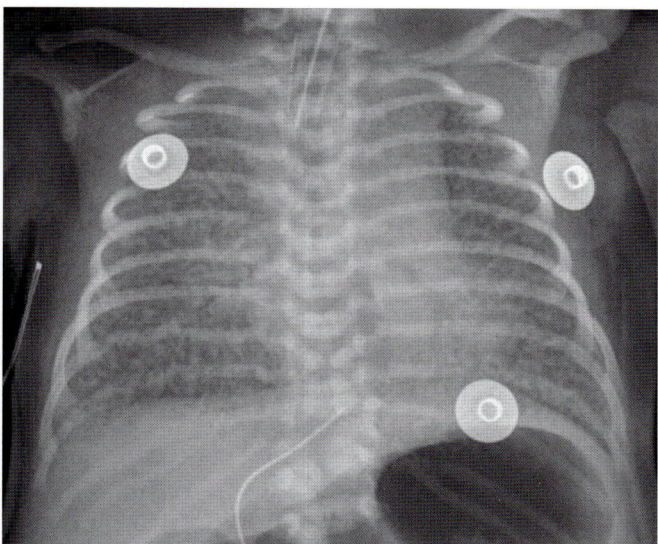

Figure 72-10 Obstructed total anomalous pulmonary venous connection (TAPVC). A chest radiograph in a newborn with obstructed TAPVC shows a normal heart size and pulmonary edema pattern as a result of venous obstruction.

Cor Triatriatum and Other Anomalies of the Pulmonary Veins

Overview Cor triatriatum sinister or "divided left atrium" is rare, representing only 0.1% to 0.4% of congenital heart disease cases.[22,23] It is associated with other cardiac anomalies in 12% to 50% of cases.[24]

Etiology, Pathophysiology, and Clinical Presentation In cor triatriatum, the pulmonary veins connect to an accessory left atrial chamber, which is separated from the true left atrium by a fibromuscular membrane with a typically small, obstructed opening (e-Fig. 72-11).[23] An ASD may be present. The embryology is thought to result from incomplete incorporation of the common pulmonary vein into the left atrium, and the accessory chamber represents the embryologic common pulmonary vein.[25] Localized stenosis, hypoplasia, or atresia of individual or all pulmonary veins also can occur, with abnormal absorption of the common pulmonary vein into the left atrium.[26] With these variants, an accessory left atrial chamber does not exist, but there is either focal stenosis of pulmonary veins near the left atrial junction, diffuse long-segment hypoplasia or narrowing of individual pulmonary veins, or unilateral or bilateral atresia of the common pulmonary vein or of individual pulmonary veins in extreme cases.[27]

Because of the typically obstructed opening between the accessory left atrium and the true left atrium, the predominant physiology is that of pulmonary venous obstruction. With very small openings and more severe obstruction, patients tend to present in the neonatal period with low cardiac output and right heart failure.[28] With larger, less obstructed openings, patients may not present with symptoms until older childhood or even adulthood. The pathophysiology of individual or total pulmonary vein hypoplasia, stenosis, or atresia is similar to that of cor triatriatum. Complete atresia of all the individual pulmonary veins is not compatible with life unless significant bronchopulmonary venous collaterals are present (e-Fig. 72-12).[29]

Imaging The chest radiograph may show evidence of right ventricular enlargement and pulmonary edema related to the pulmonary venous obstruction. Enlargement of the left atrial region, representing both left atrial chambers, also may be present.

Cross-sectional imaging goals include evaluation of the two left atrial chambers and the intervening membrane and complete evaluation of the pulmonary vein and the relationship of the veins to the membrane (Fig. 72-13). CT is ideal for evaluation of pulmonary vein stenosis and for evaluation of the lung.[30,31]

Treatment Surgery for cor triatriatum is generally performed as soon as the diagnosis is made. The intervening septum of

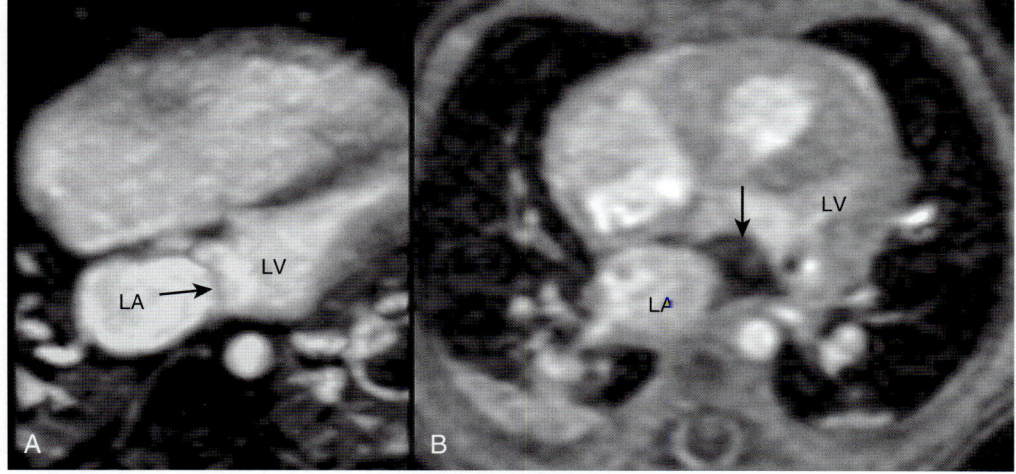

Figure 72-13 Magnetic resonance imaging of cor triatriatum. **A,** Four-chamber steady-state free-precession image showing a linear membrane in the left atrium (*arrow*) proximal to the mitral valve. **B,** Cine gradient echo showing dephasing (*arrow*) distal to the membrane indicating obstruction of pulmonary venous blood flow. *LA,* Left atrium; *LV,* left ventricle. (Courtesy Rajesh Krishnamurthy, Texas Children's Hospital, Baylor College of Medicine, Houston, Texas.)

the left atrium is resected and if an ASD is present, it is closed. The prognosis is good for patients who survive the perioperative period and who have no associated cardiac anomalies.[28] Operative management of individual pulmonary vein hypoplasia, stenosis, or atresia is variable. The prognosis is not as favorable, and balloon angioplasty has led to disappointing results.[32,33] Atresia of the common pulmonary vein with a sizable pulmonary venous confluence may be repaired, similar to TAPVC.[34,35]

Anomalies of Systemic Venous Connections

Abnormal systemic venous connections represent a heterogeneous group of malformations with clinical manifestations that can range from none to severe desaturation. The anomalies can involve the venous return from the head and neck and from the lower body.

ANOMALIES OF THE SUPERIOR VENA CAVA

Persistence of the left SVC results from failure of the left anterior and left common cardinal veins to involute.[36] In patients with congenital heart disease, the incidence varies from 11% to 34%.[37,38] Bilateral SVCs usually have normal drainage, with the right SVC into the right atrium and the left SVC to the coronary sinus and the right atrium (92%); however, abnormal drainage to the left atrium via an unroofed coronary sinus occurs in 8% of cases (e-Fig. 72-14).[39] Although bilateral SVCs with normal drainage have no hemodynamic consequences, technical implications can be present during cardiac catheterization or surgery. Abnormal SVC drainage into the left atrium can result in cyanosis. A left SVC may be suspected based on a shadow in the left upper border of the mediastinum on a chest radiograph. Imaging will show an associated dilated coronary sinus, and the caliber of the brachiocephalic vein is inversely proportional to the size of the left SVC (Fig. 72-15).

ANOMALIES OF THE INFERIOR VENA CAVA AND HEPATIC VEINS

IVC anomalies include interrupted IVC, which is defined by the absence of the hepatic or infrahepatic segment of the IVC with azygous or hemiazygous continuation into the right or left SVC (e-Fig. 72-16)[40] and is seen in up to 86% of patients with visceral heterotaxy and polysplenia.[41] Patients with asplenia usually have normal IVC but can have a prominent azygous vein and separate drainage of the hepatic veins into the right atrium (e-Fig. 72-17).[42,43]

ANOMALIES OF THE BRACHIOCEPHALIC VEINS

The normal course of the left brachiocephalic vein is obliquely downward to the right, passing anterior to the aortic arch. A retroaortic brachiocephalic vein is characterized by an abnormal position behind the ascending aorta (e-Fig. 72-18).[44] An anomalous retroesophageal brachiocephalic vein is characterized by an abnormal course posterior to the trachea and esophagus and joining the azygous vein before draining to the SVC (e-Fig. 72-19).[45]

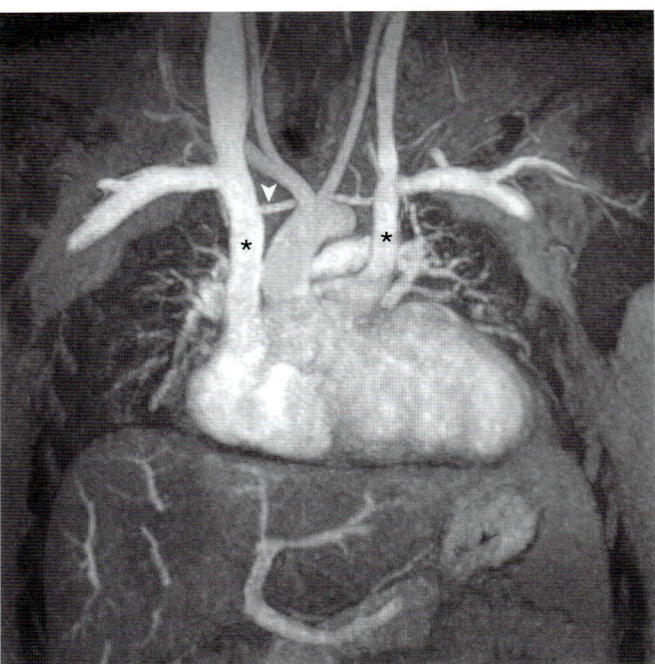

Figure 72-15 Magnetic resonance angiogram (MRA) of left superior vena cava (SVC). A coronal thick maximum intensity projection MRA showing bilateral SVCs (*asterisks*). A small bridging vein is present (*arrowhead*).

Key Points

PAPVC and partial anomalous pulmonary venous return present with right side volume overload similar to an ASD. Assessment of the degree of left-to-right shunting and associated cardiovascular defects is important.

TAPVC presents in early infancy with variable cyanosis and pulmonary edema on a chest radiograph. The ascending or descending vein course needs to be accurately described, with assessment for any obstruction to the pulmonary venous drainage.

Anomalous systemic venous connections can present with no clinical manifestations or cyanosis depending on the route of drainage. Diagnosis can be important for surgical planning such as placement of central lines and/or cannulation for cardiopulmonary bypass.

Suggested Readings

Dillman JR, Yarram SG, Hernandez RJ. Imaging of pulmonary venous developmental anomalies. *AJR Am J Roentgenol.* 2009;192(5):1272-1285.

Kafka H, Mohiaddin RH. Cardiac MRI and pulmonary MR angiography of sinus venosus defect and partial anomalous pulmonary venous connection in cause of right undiagnosed ventricular enlargement. *AJR Am J Roentgenol.* 2009;192(1):259-266.

Martinez-Jimenez S, Heyneman LE, McAdams HP, et al. Nonsurgical extracardiac vascular shunts in the thorax: clinical and imaging characteristics. *Radiographics.* 2010;30(5):e41.

References

Full references for this chapter can be found on www.expertconsult.com.

Chapter 73

Septal Defects

JOSHUA D. ROBINSON, CYNTHIA K. RIGSBY, and DARSHIT THAKRAR

Atrial Septal Defect

Overview An atrial septal defect (ASD) is a defect in the atrial septum that allows communication between the right and left atria. Isolated ASDs account for 6% to 10% of all cases of congenital heart disease.

Etiology Two primary types of ASDs occur and are classified by their relationship to the fossa ovalis (e-Fig. 73-1). Secundum defects (which comprise 80% to 90% of all ASDs) occur in the region of the fossa ovalis. Although a patent foramen ovale is in a similar location, it usually is not considered a septal defect but is the remnant of the normal interatrial communication present during fetal life and is present in 27% to 34% of the general population (Fig. 73-2).[1,2] Ostium primum defects occur caudal to the fossa ovalis at the base of the atrial septum, are usually large defects, and almost always are associated with other types of structural heart disease. Additionally, two defects—a sinus venosus septal defect and an unroofed coronary sinus—do not involve the atrial septum but are physiologically equivalent to an ASD because they allow blood to shunt from the left atrium to the right atrium.[3,4] Sinus venosus septal defects are located posterior to the fossa ovalis and occur as a result of a deficiency in the sinus venosus septum, which separates the right pulmonary veins from the superior vena cava and from the posterior aspect of the right atrium. This defect is usually located in the wall between the posterior and inferior border of the superior vena cava and the right atrium, and it is commonly associated with anomalous drainage of the right upper, middle, or lower pulmonary veins draining to either the right atrium or superior vena cava (see Chapter 72).[5] An unroofed coronary sinus is rare and occurs as a result of a partial or complete absence of the wall between the inferior left atrium and the roof of the coronary sinus. An unroofed coronary sinus generally is associated with drainage of a left superior vena cava to the coronary sinus or left atrium.[6]

Pathophysiology and Clinical Presentation Small secundum ASDs may close spontaneously[7]; however, primum ASDs, sinus venosus septal defects, and coronary sinus defects generally do not decrease in size. Shunt volume is related to the size of the defect, right and left heart compliance, and pulmonary vascular resistance. With larger shunt volumes, right atrial, right ventricular, and pulmonary artery sizes increase. Over time, pulmonary hypertension may develop.

Most infants and young children with ASDs are asymptomatic. ASDs usually are detected at about 6 months of age,[8] often during evaluation for a murmur or as an incidental finding on a chest radiograph. Older children with moderate to large ASDs may have symptoms of fatigue and dyspnea. In addition to pulmonary hypertension, older children with ASDs may have atrial tachyarrhythmias or paradoxical strokes, a risk that increases with age.[9-12]

Imaging Chest radiography in the neonate usually shows that the heart is normal in size and pulmonary flow is normal. Findings in infancy and childhood include mild cardiomegaly related to right atrial and right ventricular enlargement (Fig. 73-3). The left atrium is not enlarged, which distinguishes an ASD from other left-to-right shunt lesions. Usually main pulmonary artery enlargement and increased pulmonary vascularity is found if the pulmonary to systemic flow ratio is greater than two to one. If the patient has significant pulmonary hypertension, enlarged central pulmonary arteries and peripheral pulmonary arterial vessel tapering may be seen (e-Fig. 73-4).

Echocardiography is the imaging modality of choice to determine the location and direction of flow across the defect, to evaluate atrial and ventricular chamber size and ventricular function, and to assess for associated cardiovascular abnormalities. Magnetic resonance imaging (MRI) or computed tomography (CT) also may be used for evaluation of the atrial septum in cases of poor acoustic windows[13] or to evaluate the pulmonary veins in patients with suspected sinus venosus defects (Videos 73-1 to 73-3). Left and right ventricular size and quantitative systolic function can be assessed, and right ventricular volume overload is detected as diastolic septal flattening or diastolic bowing of the septum from right to left with severe volume overload. Comparison of right and left ventricular stroke volumes can be used to calculate the ratio of pulmonary to systemic arterial flow (Qp:Qs). Right ventricular pressure is assessed by evaluating the degree of tricuspid regurgitation and septal systolic position. Systolic septal flattening is indicative of elevated right ventricular pressure. Phase contrast MRI can be used to estimate the size of the ASD and to determine the direction

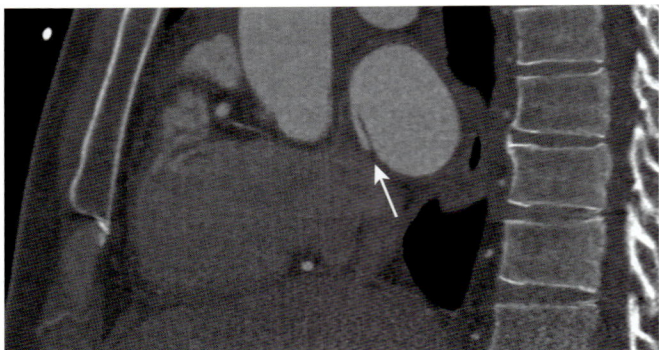

Figure 73-2 Short axis angiography image of the heart at the level of the atria shows the flap valve of a patent foramen ovale (*arrow*). (Courtesy B. Kelly Han, Minneapolis Heart Institute/Children's Hospitals and Clinics of Minnesota.)

and amount of shunting at the atrial level by calculation of Qp:Qs (e-Fig. 73-5).[14]

Treatment Closure should be performed in childhood to avoid complications of arrhythmia, right ventricular dysfunction, pulmonary hypertension, and paradoxical embolus.[15] ASD closure can be performed surgically or via transcatheter closure; the latter procedure largely has become primary therapy for anatomically favorable secundum defects. After closure, children with ASDs have an excellent prognosis.

Atrioventricular Septal Defect

Overview Atrioventricular septal defects (AVSDs) account for 4% of all cases of congenital heart disease.[16] Most patients with complete AVSD have Down syndrome.[17] AVSD also is associated with the visceral heterotaxy syndromes.[18,19]

Etiology AVSD results from abnormal development of the embryologic endocardial cushions and produces a spectrum of disease (Fig. 73-6). In its mild form or in partial AVSD, a crescent-shaped defect is found in the inferior portion of the atrial septum immediately adjacent to the atrioventricular (AV) valve, along with an associated "cleft" mitral valve with separate mitral and tricuspid valve orifices. Persons with the complete form have an ostium primum, a large inlet ventricular septal defect (VSD) beneath the plane of the AV valves, and a single or common AV valve, with variable leaflet size, location, and morphology. Most importantly, the common valve has two components that "bridge" the ventricular septum and may form attachments to the septal surface and/or both the right and left sides of the heart.[20] In most cases, the common AV valve is shared equally between the right and left ventricles, but the valve orifice may be unequally shared and may favor either the right or left ventricle.[19]

Pathophysiology and Clinical Presentation With complete AVSD, the amount of left-to-right shunting is generally large but is related to the size of the ASD and VSD, right and left heart compliance, and pulmonary vascular resistance. The shunting may be interatrial or interventricular. The cleft mitral valve can lead to significant mitral insufficiency and can exacerbate congestive heart failure.

Infants with complete AVSD present with tachypnea, tachycardia, and signs of congestive heart failure as pulmonary resistance falls during the newborn period. Patients with partial AVSD may be asymptomatic as infants and young children, although they may have symptoms earlier in life if significant associated mitral valve regurgitation is present.[21]

Imaging The amount of left-to-right shunting is reflected on the chest radiograph and may reflect the physiology of either the ASD or VSD or both. With complete AVSD, findings include moderate to marked cardiomegaly with right atrial and right ventricular enlargement and increased pulmonary vascularity (Fig. 73-7). Left atrial enlargement may be seen if associated mitral insufficiency is present. Children with large left-to-right shunts commonly have lung hyperinflation, which may be related to an increase in airway resistance from enlarged pulmonary arteries and veins or to an increase in lung volume related to the increase in blood volume.

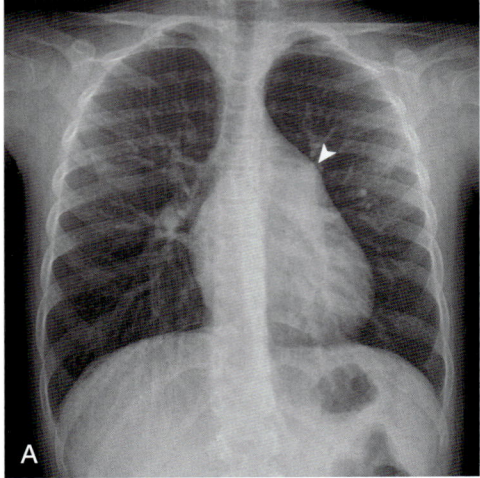
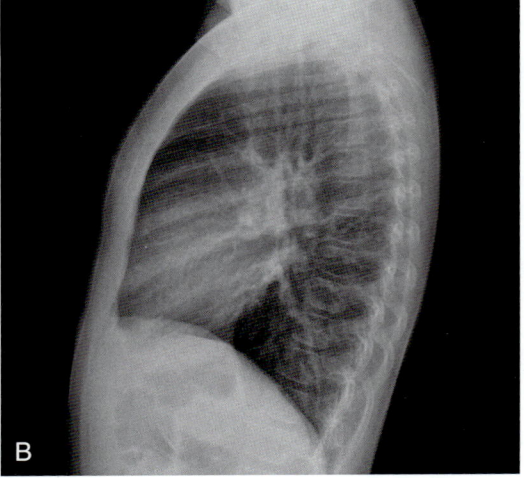

Figure 73-3 Atrial septal defect, secundum type, in a 7-year-old. Frontal (**A**) and lateral (**B**) views of the chest show mild cardiomegaly, a prominent pulmonary artery (*arrowhead*), and increased pulmonary vascularity without left atrial dilation.

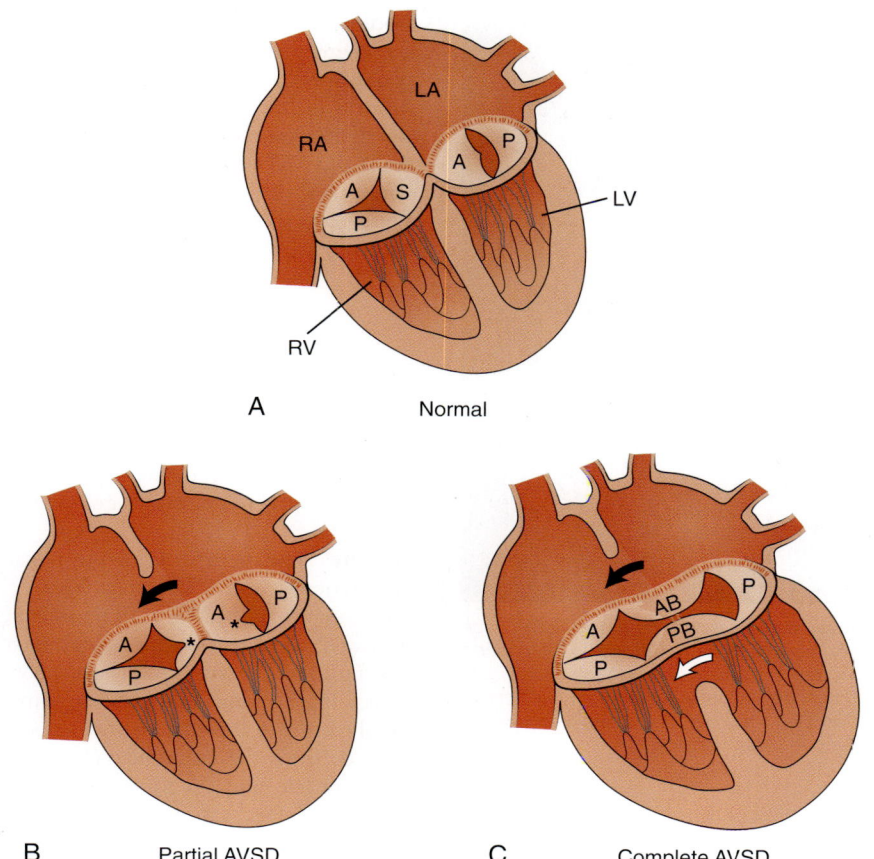

Figure 73-6 Diagrams illustrating the spectrum of atrioventricular septal defect (AVSD). **A,** The normal tricuspid valve has three leaflets, anterior (*A*), posterior (*P*), and septal (*S*), and the normal mitral valve has two leaflets, anterior (*A*) and posterior (*P*). **B,** Partial AVSD showing the clefts (*asterisks*) in the septal leaflet of the tricuspid valve, the anterior leaflet of the mitral valve, and the ostium primum atrial septal defect (ASD) (*arrow*). **C,** Complete AVSD showing the common atrioventricular valve with the anterior bridging (*AB*) and posterior bridging (*PB*) leaflets, the ostium primum ASD (*black arrow*), and the inlet ventricular septal defect (*white arrow*). *LA,* Left atrium; *LV,* left ventricle; *RA,* right atrium; *RV,* right ventricle. (Modified from Park MK. Left-to-right shunt lesions. In Park MK, editor: *Pediatric cardiology for practitioners,* St. Louis: Mosby Elsevier; 2002.)

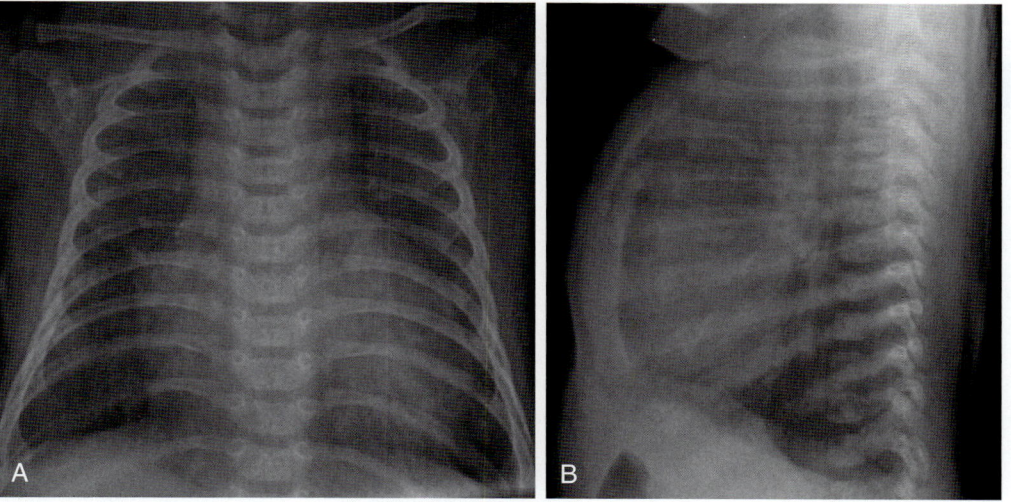

Figure 73-7 Atrioventricular septal defect in a 6-week-old. Frontal (**A**) and lateral (**B**) views of the chest show moderate cardiomegaly with enlargement of the right atrium and ventricle, increased pulmonary vascularity, and lung hyperinflation.

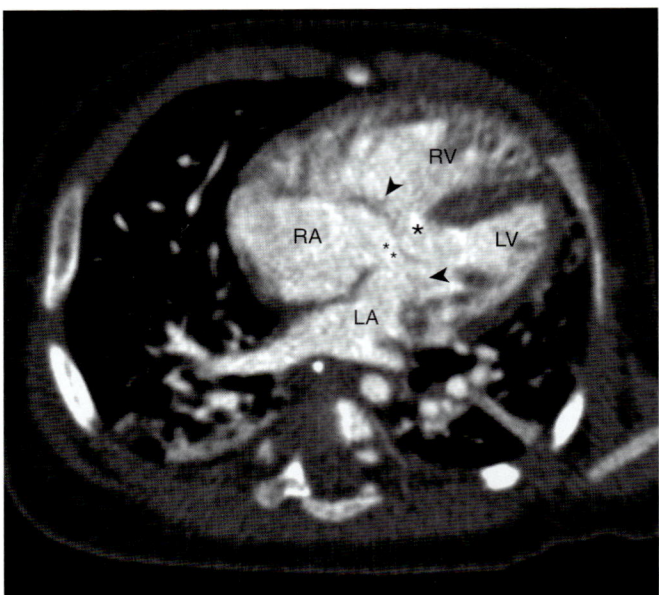

Figure 73-8 Complete atrioventricular septal defect (AVSD). Four-chamber computed tomography view in an infant with a balanced AVSD shows the ostium primum defect (*double asterisks*), inlet ventricular septal defect (*single asterisk*), and common atrioventricular valve (*arrowheads*) that bridges the right and left sides of the heart. *LA,* Left atrium; *LV,* left ventricle; *RA,* right atrium; *RV,* right ventricle.

Echocardiography is the primary modality for evaluation of AVSD, but MRI can be used as an adjunct in complex cases, especially when an accurate assessment of right and left ventricular size is needed. Components to evaluate include the ostium primum portion of the atrial septum and the inlet portion of the ventricular septum, the AV valve leaflet morphology and attachments, the papillary muscle architecture, the level and direction of shunting, ventricle size and systolic function, and the presence of outflow tract obstruction or other cardiovascular anomalies (Fig. 73-8).

Treatment Patients with partial AVSD generally undergo complete surgical repair between 1 and 4 years of age. For patients with complete AVSD, early repair between 2 and 4 months of life is recommended to avoid the development of significant pulmonary hypertension.[19] Surgical goals include ASD and VSD closure with creation of two patent and competent AV valves and preservation of the conduction system. Long-term survival after repair for partial and complete AVSD survival is excellent.[17,22-24]

Ventricular Septal Defect

Overview Isolated VSD accounts for approximately 20% of all cases of congenital heart disease, with an incidence of approximately two per 1000 live births.[25] Isolated VSDs are slightly more common in girls than in boys.[26,27] VSD may be isolated or part of a complex congenital heart malformation.[28-30]

Etiology The ventricular septum can be divided into four components, and VSDs may involve one or more of these components (Table 73-1). The inlet septum extends from the tricuspid annulus to the septal attachments of the tensor apparatus of the tricuspid valve. AVSD is associated with a defect in this portion of the septum. The muscular septum involves the trabeculated portion of the right ventricle and extends from the tricuspid valve attachments to the apex of the ventricle and up to the septal band. Single or multiple muscular defects can be present in this portion of the septum. The outlet or conal portion of the ventricular septum separates the ventricular outflow tracts and, when viewed from the right ventricle, extends from the septal band to the pulmonary valve. The thin, membranous septum lies adjacent to the anteroseptal commissure of the tricuspid valve on the right side of the heart and to the right and noncoronary cusps of the aortic valve on the left side. Approximately 80% of VSDs involve the area around the membranous septum (e-Fig. 73-9).[31,32]

Table 73-1

Classification of Ventricular Septal Defects			
Type	**Synonym**	**Frequency**	**Associated Features**
Membranous	Perimembranous	80%	Adherence of tricuspid valve tissue to defect with left ventricle–right atrial shunt
	Paramembranous		
	Conoventricular		Extension to muscular, inlet, or outlet septum
	Infracristal		Anterior malalignment of the infundibular septum causing aortic override
			Posterior malalignment of the ventricular septum causing subaortic stenosis
			Small defects may spontaneously close
Inlet	Atrioventricular septal defect	5%-8%	—
	Atrioventricular canal type		
Outlet	Conal	5%-7%	Right coronary leaflet prolapse through defect
	Subpulmonary		Aortic regurgitation
	Doubly committed juxtaarterial		Dilation of the right sinus of Valsalva
	Supracristal		
	Infundibular		
Muscular	Trabecular	5%-20%	Small defects may spontaneously close
	Marginal		Defects may be multiple

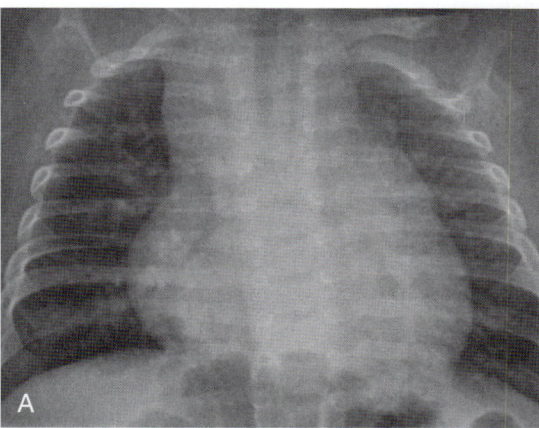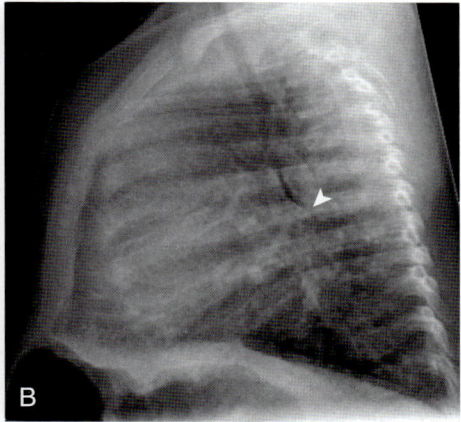

Figure 73-10   Ventricular septal defect in a 3-month-old. Frontal (**A**) and lateral (**B**) views of the chest show right atrial, right ventricular, and left atrial enlargement with posterior displacement of the left main stem bronchus (*arrowhead* in **B**) and increased pulmonary vascularity.

Pathophysiology and Clinical Presentation   The physiologic effect of a VSD is determined by its size, right and left heart compliance, and pulmonary vascular resistance. Small defects offer high resistance to flow, and large defects offer low resistance to flow. Large defects subject the pulmonary vasculature to high flow and high pressure, which frequently results in pulmonary hypertension.

Symptoms vary depending on the size of the VSD and the degree of left-to-right shunting. At birth, pulmonary resistance is high, limiting left-to-right shunting. As pulmonary resistance falls during early infancy, left-to-right shunting increases. When shunting becomes significant, failure to thrive, dyspnea, and congestive heart failure may be seen. Irreversible pulmonary hypertension can develop within 2 to 3 years and frequently is seen in young adults.[29]

Imaging   Chest radiograph findings vary depending on the size of the VSD. A chest radiograph appears normal in a person with a small VSD. Common findings with moderate to large VSDs include cardiomegaly with enlargement of the left atrium, left ventricle, and pulmonary arteries and increased pulmonary blood flow (Fig. 73-10). Congestive heart failure occurs frequently in infants with a moderate or large defect. Pulmonary hypertension may be evident in older children or young adults.

Echocardiography is the imaging method of choice for evaluation of VSDs. Imaging goals include addressing the size, number, and location of VSDs and the degree of left-to-right or right-to-left shunting. Estimates of right ventricular and pulmonary artery pressures and right and left heart volumes are obtained. The tricuspid and aortic valves are evaluated for possible tethering of valve tissue into the borders of the defect. MRI and CT are useful for noninvasive evaluation of VSDs and hemodynamic consequences, with a reported 90% accuracy in detection (Fig. 73-11).[33,34] Phase contrast MRI measurements in the aorta and pulmonary artery or a comparison of right and left ventricular stroke volumes can be used to evaluate Qp:Qs, and qualitative assessment of the septal position can be used as a measure of ventricular volume and/or pressure overload.

Treatment   During the first year of life, 80% to 90% of small (<0.5 cm) VSDs become smaller or completely close.[27] Operative correction is preferable before 6 months of age in patients with large VSDs to decrease the chance of having irreversible pulmonary hypertension develop. Consideration for early closure of outlet defects is recommended to prevent development of aortic sinus prolapse and progressive valve regurgitation. The results of operative closure are excellent, with a very low risk of morbidity or mortality. VSDs are closed most frequently via a right atrial approach, but transpulmonary artery and transaortic approaches also are used. Transcatheter device closure is an alternative to surgery for selected single or multiple VSDs, usually in the muscular septum, and also has been used intraoperatively (e-Fig. 73-12).

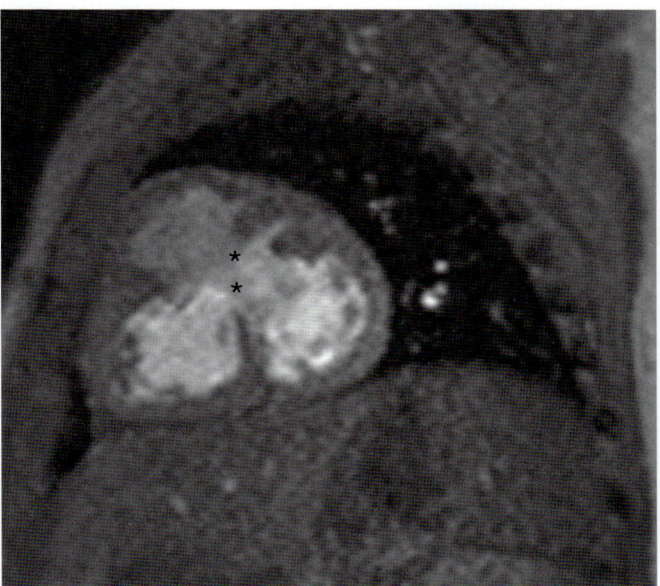

Figure 73-11   A ventricular septal defect in a 2-year-old. A short-axis steady-state free-precession magnetic resonance image shows a large muscular ventricular septal defect (*asterisks*).

Patent Ductus Arteriosus

Overview Patent ductus arteriosus (PDA) accounts for approximately 10% of all cases of congenital heart disease.[35] Approximately 20% to 30% of premature infants have a PDA, and the incidence increases with increased prematurity.[36] Complex congenital heart disease may include PDA with ductal dependent pulmonary or systemic blood flow.

Etiology and Pathophysiology PDA represents the persistence of the embryologic sixth aortic arch, which most commonly connects the left pulmonary artery with the descending aorta just beyond the origin of the left subclavian artery (see Chapter 62). With a right arch, the ductus arteriosus may be on the right. Prostaglandins maintain ductal patency during fetal life. At birth, increased blood oxygen concentration causes functional constriction of the duct, usually within hours after birth. Ductal closure is delayed in premature infants with respiratory distress and hypoxia, because the immature ductal tissue is less sensitive to oxygen-mediated constriction. In a majority of cases of PDA in term infants, the etiology is unknown.[37-39]

Clinical Presentation The amount of left-to-right shunting depends on the length and diameter of the duct and the degree of pulmonary hypertension. Pulmonary hypertension may develop if a large PDA is left untreated. In premature infants without significant lung disease, a PDA may become clinically apparent 24 to 72 hours after birth. Congestive heart failure occurs if the shunt is large. In premature infants with significant lung disease, the prevalence of PDA is greater than 80%. Screening echocardiography may detect a PDA in these infants before clinical manifestations occur. A term infant with a small PDA is generally asymptomatic, and the PDA often is detected because of the presence of a murmur. Term infants with moderate to large PDAs may display poor feeding, irritability, and failure to thrive and may have congestive heart failure.[40]

Imaging Pulmonary edema and cardiomegaly may be seen as signs of a PDA on a chest radiograph. In premature infants who exhibit lung infiltrates after the first few days of life, particularly with an increase in heart size, PDA should be considered. Chest radiographs of term infants with significant shunting show increased pulmonary blood flow and cardiomegaly (e-Fig. 73-13).

Echocardiography is the standard imaging technique for evaluating PDA. Goals of imaging are to measure the PDA size and diameter, assess the amount of left-to-right or right-to-left shunting and the degree of pulmonary hypertension, and identify possible complicating factors such as a ductal aneurysm. CT or MRI may be used in conjunction with echocardiography to define anatomy in complicated cases and to determine Qp:Qs (Fig. 73-14).[41,42]

Treatment Indomethacin and/or ibuprofen therapy often is successful in achieving PDA closure in premature infants, followed by surgical ligation if medical therapy fails. Nonsurgical transcatheter closure is the method of choice for small to moderate PDAs in most term infants.[43,44] Larger PDAs in term infants generally are managed surgically. Patient

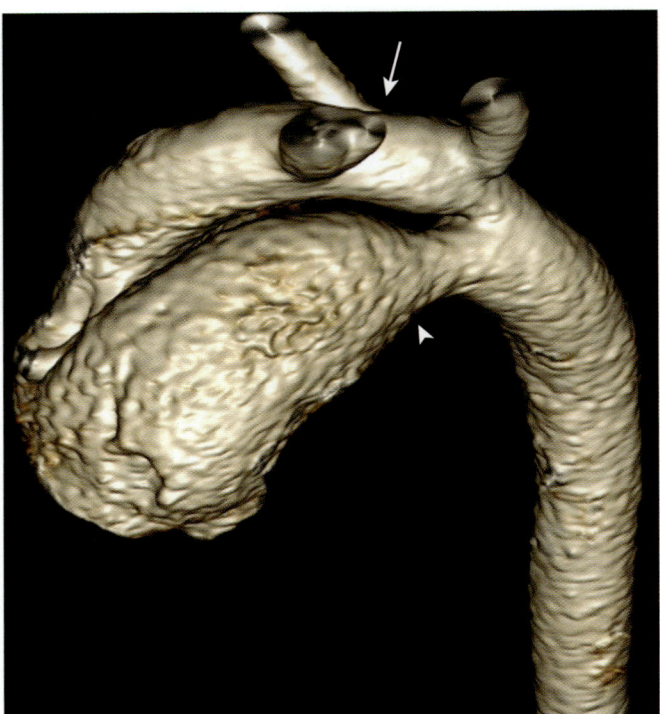

Figure 73-14 Patent ductus arteriosus (PDA). An anterior oblique volume-rendered computed tomography angiogram shows near-parallel configuration between the aortic arch (*arrow*) and the PDA (*arrowhead*).

prognosis is excellent if ductal closure is performed between 6 and 24 months of age.[45]

Aortopulmonary Window

Aortopulmonary window is rare and accounts for 0.2% cases of congenital heart disease.[46-49] Aortopulmonary window is the result of incomplete aortopulmonary septation, and as a result, communication occurs between the ascending aorta and pulmonary artery. This defect creates a large, high-pressure, left-to-right shunt that usually is apparent clinically in the first weeks of life and is similar to a large PDA in pathophysiology.

Imaging Chest radiograph findings include cardiomegaly with left atrial and left ventricular enlargement, increased pulmonary blood flow, and prominence of the ascending aorta and pulmonary artery related to the left-to-right shunt at the level of the great vessels. Imaging is performed to evaluate the anatomy of the aortopulmonary window and its relationship to the aortic and pulmonary valves, to define the coronary anatomy, to estimate pulmonary pressure and ventricular function, to assess Qp:Qs, and to evaluate for other cardiovascular defects. Differentiation from truncus arteriosus is critical and is accomplished by the identification of two separate semilunar valves (Fig. 73-15).

Treatment Early surgical patch repair for large defects or suture repair for small defects to separate the great vessels should be performed before the development of pulmonary vascular hypertension. The outcome following surgery generally is excellent.

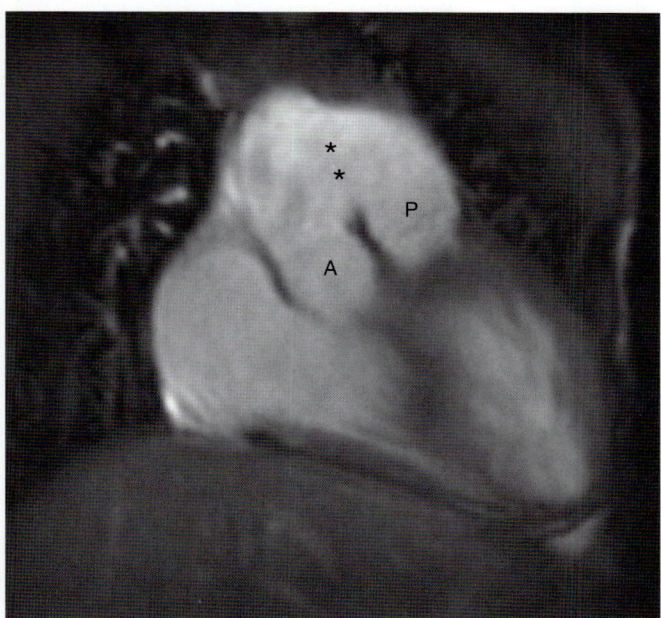

Figure 73-15 **Aortopulmonary window.** A coronal steady-state free-precession magnetic resonance image shows separate origins of the aortic root (*A*) and pulmonary trunk (*P*) with a large communication (*asterisks*) between the ascending aorta and the pulmonary trunk. (Courtesy Deborah L. Thompson, MD. Dalhousie University.)

Key Points

The most common cause of cardiomegaly in an acyanotic patient with increased pulmonary vascularity is VSD. Differential diagnosis includes ASD, AVSD, PDA, and aortopulmonary window.

ASD does not cause left atrial enlargement, which distinguishes ASD from other left-to-right shunts.

Phase contrast MRI can be used to assess the direction of flow and to determine the amount of shunting by calculation of the ratio of pulmonary to systemic flow (Qp : Qs).

Suggested Readings

Rojas CA, El-Sherief A, Medina HM, et al. Embryology and developmental defects of the interatrial septum. *AJR Am J Roentgenol.* 2010;195(5):1100-1104.

Van Praagh R, Geva T, Kreutzer J. Ventricular septal defects: how shall we describe, name and classify them? *J Am Coll Cardiol.* 1989;14(5):1298-1299.

Wang ZJ, Reddy GP, Gotway MB, et al. Cardiovascular shunts: MR imaging evaluation. *Radiographics.* 2003;23(Spec No):S181-S194.

References

Full references for this chapter can be found on www.expertconsult.com.

Chapter 74

Right Heart Lesions

ANDRADA R. POPESCU, DARSHIT THAKRAR, STANLEY T. KIM, EMMA E. BOYLAN, R. ANDREW DEFREITAS, and CYNTHIA K. RIGSBY

Ebstein Anomaly

Overview Ebstein anomaly accounts for fewer than 1% of all cases of congenital heart disease.[1] Associated malformations include ventricular septal defect (VSD), pulmonary stenosis and atresia, tetralogy of Fallot, congenitally corrected transposition of the great arteries, and patent ductus arteriosus (PDA) or atrial septal defect (ASD).[1] Conduction system abnormalities and arrhythmias, including Wolff-Parkinson-White syndrome and right bundle branch block, have been seen in 22% to 42% of patients.[2]

Etiology, Pathophysiology, and Clinical Presentation The Ebstein anomaly is named for Wilhelm Ebstein, who described the abnormality in 1866.[3] The anomaly is characterized by abnormal development and positioning of the tricuspid valve leaflets, with apical displacement of the septal and posterior valve leaflets into the right ventricle (RV). This phenomenon leads to partitioning of the RV into an atrialized basal segment and an apical outflow chamber. The displaced valve leaflets may be either adherent or nonadherent to the right ventricular wall. The anterior valve leaflet tends to be normally positioned, is frequently large and redundant, and sometimes is adherent to the right ventricular free wall with a "sail-like" appearance.[4]

The pathophysiology of this lesion varies, depending on the degree of tricuspid valve dysplasia and displacement of the tricuspid valve leaflets and the presence and severity of associated defects. With greater degrees of dysplasia and displacement, severe tricuspid insufficiency is increasingly present, resulting in elevated right atrial pressures and thus right-to-left shunting through either the ASD or the patent foramen ovale (PFO). Patients with mild forms of Ebstein anomaly may be asymptomatic in childhood and present with symptoms of cyanosis, right heart failure, or arrhythmia in adulthood. Patients with severe forms present in early neonatal life with severe combined cyanosis and acidosis and a duct-dependent circulation.[5]

Imaging The chest radiographic appearance depends on the degree of tricuspid valve dysplasia and displacement. Classically, the chest radiographic appearance includes a globular or box-shaped heart as a result of right atrial enlargement associated with normal to diminished pulmonary vascularity (Fig. 74-1).[6] Patients with significant valvular dysplasia and severe tricuspid insufficiency have marked enlargement of the right heart and decreased pulmonary blood flow. With less marked valve displacement and tricuspid insufficiency, only mild right heart enlargement may be present (e-Fig. 74-2).

Ebstein anomaly can be readily diagnosed by both prenatal and postnatal echocardiography.[5] Cardiac magnetic resonance imaging (MRI) has emerged as a more complete method to evaluate the RV both anatomically and functionally.[7,8] The characteristic features include displacement and tethering of the septal and posterior leaflets of the tricuspid valve and enlargement of the right atrium, including the atrialized RV (Fig. 74-3). Imaging goals include evaluation of the appearance of the tricuspid valve and the severity of tricuspid regurgitation; determination of the degree of right-to-left shunting through the ASD or PFO, which typically is present; evaluation of the volume of the atrialized and functional portions of the RV and RV systolic function; imaging for areas of fibrosis in the thin atrialized ventricular wall and septum on delayed gadolinium enhancement imaging[9]; assessment of the pulmonary valve and branch pulmonary arteries for stenosis; evaluation of left ventricle size and systolic function; and assessment of the heart and great vessels for other congenital abnormalities.[2,7-9]

Treatment Patients with mild forms of Ebstein anomaly may not require surgical treatment, or the need for surgery may not arise until later in life if right heart dysfunction develops. Indications for surgical intervention/reintervention and/or medical therapy include limited exercise capacity (greater than New York Heart Association class II), increasing heart size (cardiothoracic ratio >65%), cyanosis (resting oxygen saturations of <90%), severe tricuspid regurgitation with symptoms, transient ischemic attack, or stroke.[10]

If surgery is required, valvuloplasty with either the Carpentier or cone procedures may be performed. The Carpentier procedure uses reimplantation of the anterior and posterior tricuspid valve leaflets at the level of the neotricuspid annulus, resulting in a monocuspid or bicuspid valve configuration.[11] In the more recently developed cone procedure, the tricuspid valve leaflets and subvalvar apparatus are mobilized and reanastomosed to form a cone-shaped valve with improved inflow and valve competence.[4] Other possible treatments include tricuspid valve replacement or, rarely, oversewing of

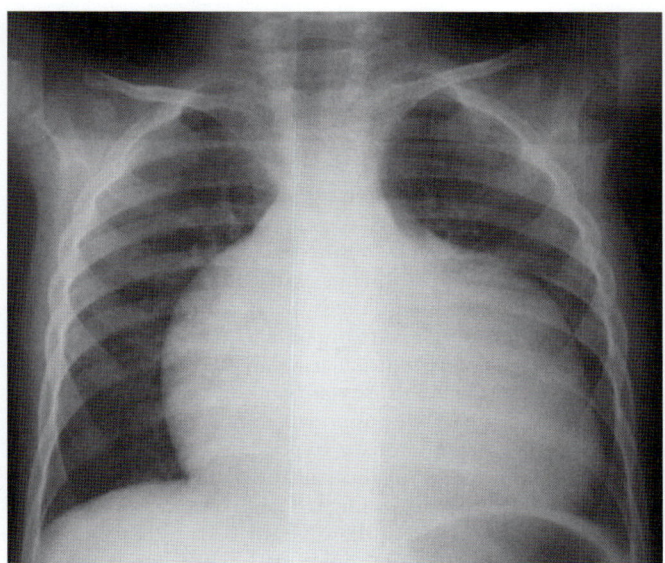

Figure 74-1 The classic radiographic appearance of Ebstein anomaly. A frontal view of the chest shows globular box-shaped heart enlargement and diminished pulmonary vascularity.

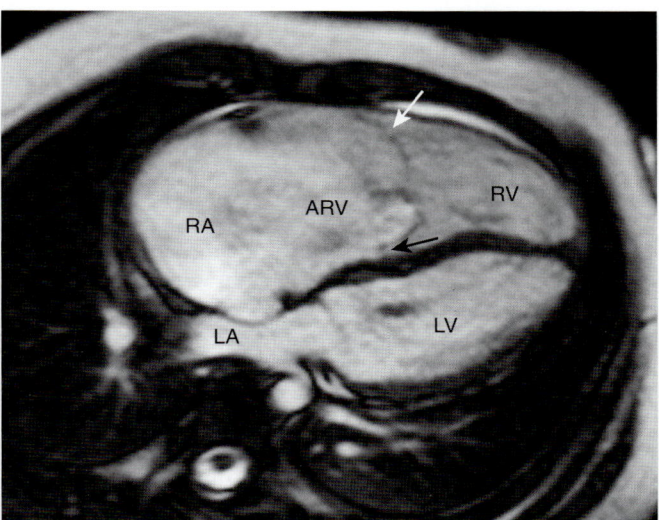

Figure 74-3 Ebstein anomaly magnetic resonance image (MRI). Axial steady-state free-precession MRI demonstrates right heart enlargement with redundancy of the anterior tricuspid valve leaflet (*white arrow*) and displacement of the septal tricuspid valve leaflet (*black arrow*) into the right ventricle (*RV*). As a result, a large atrialized portion of the right ventricle (*ARV*) is present. *LA,* Left atrium; *LV,* left ventricle; *RA,* right atrium.

the tricuspid valve and creation of a central shunt in infancy. Transcatheter closure of the ASD may be considered if severe cyanosis is present without tricuspid insufficiency necessitating valve repair.[12] In rare situations, cardiac transplantation may be indicated.[5] Clinically significant arrhythmias develop in some patients and require transcatheter or surgical ablation procedures.[2]

Tricuspid Atresia

Overview Tricuspid atresia features an absence of the tricuspid valve with a resultant lack of a direct connection between the right atrium and RV. Tricuspid atresia accounts for approximately 3% to 4% of congenital heart disease.[13] Most cases of tricuspid atresia are sporadic, but familial cases and association with 22q11 microdeletions have been reported.[14]

Pathophysiology and Clinical Presentation The tricuspid valve is usually absent; instead, muscular tissue or, less commonly, fibrous tissue is present in the floor of the right atrium. Because of the absence of a communication between the right atrium and the RV, an obligatory ASD or PFO is present to allow blood returning to the right side of the heart to reach the left side of the heart. This phenomenon results in mixing of systemic venous and pulmonary venous return

and a variable degree of cyanosis. A VSD also may be present, with the degree of RV development related to the size of the VSD.[13] In 70% of cases, the ventriculoarterial connections are concordant, and usually severe pulmonary or subpulmonary stenosis is present. In 30% of cases, the ventriculoarterial connections are discordant (transposition of the great arteries), and associated mild pulmonary stenosis and obstruction to aortic outflow is present. The most commonly used classification system was developed by Tandon and Edwards in 1974; they describe tricuspid atresia as types I, II, and III (Table 74-1).[15]

The clinical presentation is variable. The severity of cyanosis is related to the degree of RV outflow obstruction, the size of the VSD, the origins of the great arteries, the presence or absence of a PDA, and the pulmonary vascular resistance. All these factors will determine the relative blood flow to the pulmonary versus the systemic vasculature. If an infant has a large VSD and no obstruction to pulmonary outflow or a large PDA, the relative flow to the pulmonary circulation is much greater than that to the systemic circulation. This phenomenon may result in mild cyanosis with overcirculated, congested lungs. In contrast, restricted pulmonary blood flow results in more severe cyanosis.[13]

Table 74-1

Anatomic Classification of Tricuspid Atresia			
Type	**A**	**B**	**C**
I, with normally positioned great arteries (70%)	Pulmonary atresia	Small ventricular septal defect, pulmonary artery hypoplasia	Large ventricular septal defect, normal pulmonary artery
II, with dextrotransposition of the great vessels (25%)	With pulmonary atresia/stenosis	Pulmonary or subpulmonary stenosis	Large pulmonary artery
III, with levotransposition of the great vessels (5%)	Pulmonary or subpulmonary stenosis	Subaortic stenosis	

Imaging The appearance of the heart on a chest radiograph depends on the specific anatomic type of tricuspid atresia; the heart usually appears normal or may be mildly enlarged. When pulmonary outflow obstruction is present, the chest radiograph shows normal to decreased pulmonary vascularity. When no pulmonary outflow obstruction is present, cardiomegaly and increased pulmonary vascularity usually are present (e-Fig. 74-4).

The characteristic imaging feature of tricuspid atresia is replacement of the tricuspid valve with a ridge of muscular and fatty tissue positioned between the enlarged right atrium and the hypoplastic RV (Fig. 74-5). The size of the coexistent VSD and the relationship of the pulmonary artery and aorta can be characterized to determine the specific type of tricuspid atresia present. Echocardiography generally is the imaging study of choice in infancy, but MRI or computed tomography (CT) can be used to determine cardiac or great vessel anatomy in complex cases. Although cardiac catheterization traditionally has been performed before the second and third stages of univentricular repair, MRI is playing an increasing role in preoperative evaluation and may obviate the need for catheterization in carefully selected patients (see Treatment section).[16] Important components of cross-sectional imaging before Glenn or Fontan procedures include assessment of anatomy and flow through the cavopulmonary pathway, atrioventricular valve function, and quantification of ventricular size and systolic function. MRI also allows detailed anatomic and functional assessment of the full Fontan pathway unless it is limited by artifact from implanted ferromagnetic material or pacemakers. MRI therefore is a valuable tool in the assessment of a "failing Fontan."

Treatment Ultimately, patients with tricuspid atresia require univentricular palliative repair because the hypoplastic RV is not capable of providing the cardiac output necessary to support a two-ventricle heart. Neonates with tricuspid atresia and associated pulmonary atresia or stenosis may require a prostaglandin infusion to keep the PDA open until surgical repair is performed. In an infant with a large VSD and no pulmonary stenosis, diuretics may be needed to decrease pulmonary overcirculation.

The goal of univentricular repair is to eliminate cyanosis.[17] This is accomplished by having the single left ventricle support the systemic circulation and by directing the systemic venous return to the pulmonary arteries, thus bypassing the nonfunctional RV. The first stage of single ventricle palliation performed in early infancy ensures adequate but not excessive pulmonary blood flow. Infants with pulmonary stenosis or atresia may require a modified Blalock-Taussig systemic to pulmonary artery shunt to maintain adequate pulmonary flow as the first stage of univentricular repair (see also Chapter 75). Alternatively, pulmonary arterial banding may be performed in infants with excessive pulmonary blood flow because of a large VSD and no pulmonary hypoplasia or stenosis.

At the second stage of the palliation, generally performed between 3 and 9 months of age, a bidirectional Glenn shunt is created by anastomosing the superior vena cava to the right pulmonary artery. The modified Blalock-Taussig shunt, if present, is taken down. Completion of the total cavopulmonary anastomosis with the modified Fontan procedure, which is performed between 1 and 5 years of age, involves anastomosing the inferior vena cava to the pulmonary arteries via an extracardiac conduit or an intracardiac "lateral tunnel," which usually is created in the lateral aspect of the atrium using a patch (Fig. 74-6).[18] This procedure completes the separation of the systemic and pulmonary circulations and eliminates cyanosis. Other approaches to creating a cavopulmonary connection, including direct anastomosis of the right atrium to the pulmonary artery, have been used in the past (Fig. 74-7).[17]

Surgical mortality rates for the modified Fontan procedure range between 1.1% and 2.7%.[18] Acute complications after the Fontan procedure include pleural effusions and ascites that may be slow to resolve.[19] Long-term complications of Fontan palliation include thrombosis within the cavopulmonary pathway, especially in a dilated right atrium in the original "classic" Fontan procedure, which incorporated the right atrium into the Fontan pathway; stenoses within the cavopulmonary pathway; cyanosis due to the development of pulmonary arteriovenous malformations or systemic venous to pulmonary venous collateral shunts; arrhythmias; congestive hepatopathy or cirrhosis; and protein-losing enteropathy (Fig. 74-8).[19] Cardiac transplantation remains the only definitive treatment for patients with failing Fontan procedure circulation.[19]

Pulmonary Atresia with Intact Ventricular Septum

Overview Pulmonary atresia with intact ventricular septum (PA/IVS), a rare cardiac disorder that is highly variable in its appearance and presentation, represents approximately 1% to 3% of all cases of congenital heart disease.[20] RV outflow tract obstruction is present because of atresia of the pulmonary valve or the pulmonary infundibulum and an intact ventricular septum. Obstruction of the outflow from the right heart in persons with PA/IVS necessitates an interatrial communication or PDA to allow for pulmonary blood flow.[21]

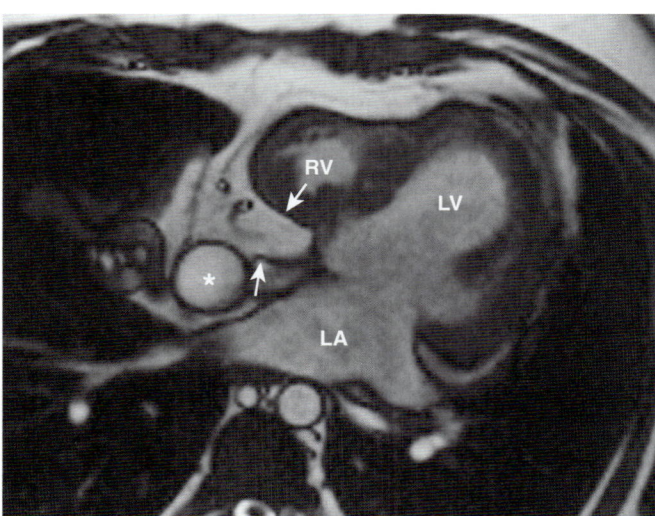

Figure 74-5 A 27-year-old with tricuspid atresia after extracardiac Fontan palliation (*asterisk*). An axial magnetic resonance image of the heart shows a ridge of fatty tissue (*arrows*) in the floor of the right atrium at the site of the atretic tricuspid valve. A small caliber right ventricle (*RV*) also is present. *LA,* Left atrium; *LV,* left ventricle.

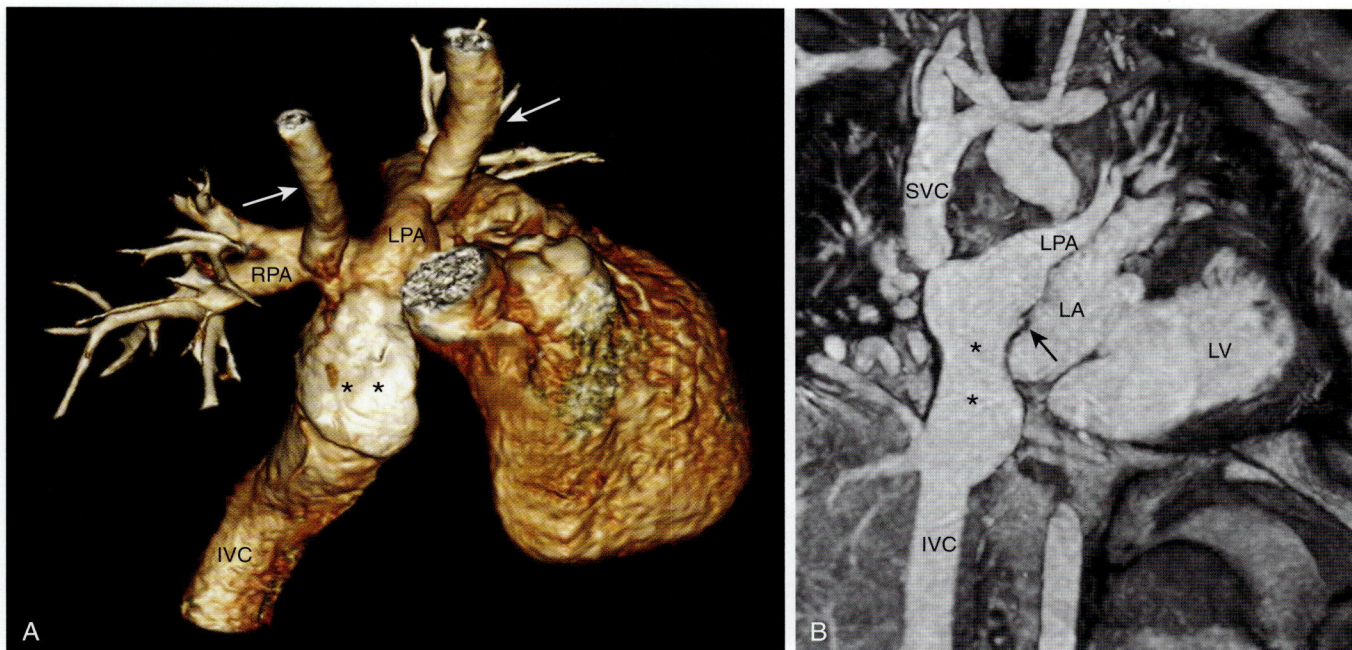

Figure 74-6 Fontan palliation. **A,** Extracardiac Fontan baffle (*asterisks*) extending from the inferior vena cava (*IVC*) to the right pulmonary artery (*RPA*), associated with bilateral Glenn anastomoses (*white arrows*). The right and left atria have been removed to show the anatomy. **B,** Lateral tunnel Fontan (*asterisks*) extending from the IVC to the left pulmonary artery (*LPA*) and classic Glenn anastomosis between the superior vena cava (*SVC*) and right pulmonary artery. *LA,* Left atrium; *LV,* left ventricle; *arrow,* patch.

Etiology, Pathophysiology, and Clinical Presentation In contrast to patients with pulmonary atresia with VSD, patients with PA/IVS generally have well-developed, confluent central pulmonary arteries.[22] The development of the tricuspid valve in these patients is highly variable, with both severe stenosis and marked insufficiency detected. The degree of RV development also is variable, with varying degrees of

hypoplasia (hypoplastic right heart syndrome). The RV is less hypoplastic in the setting of severe tricuspid regurgitation. Significant RV hypertrophy is common. Associated coronary artery anomalies may include RV to coronary connections. Some persons exhibit an RV-dependent coronary physiology.[23] In this condition, blood from the hypertensive RV perfuses the coronary arteries. Loss of elevated RV pressure (e.g., if a pulmonary valvotomy is performed) may result in myocardial ischemia and hemodynamic collapse. RV-dependent coronary circulation typically is seen in patients with small RVs and no significant tricuspid regurgitation (which lowers RV systolic pressure).[24] The major clinical manifestation of this entity is cyanosis, which typically is seen shortly after birth when the PDA begins to close. If significant tricuspid regurgitation or a small restrictive ASD is present, associated hepatic venous congestion may be detected.

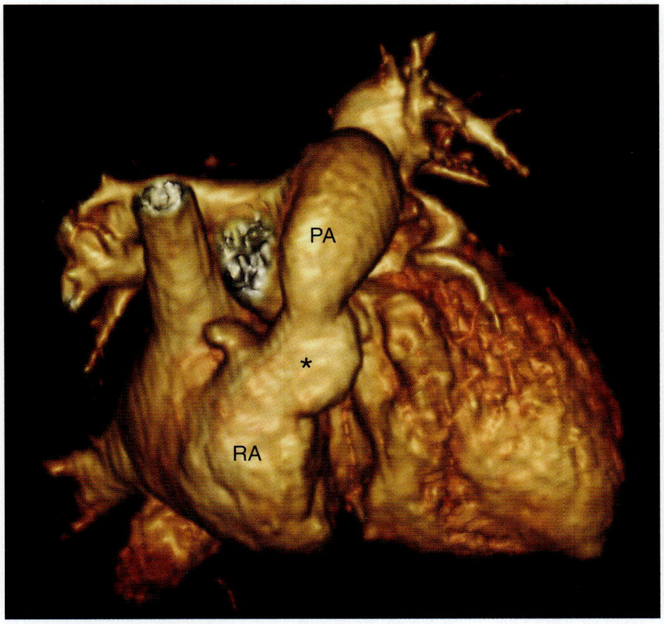

Imaging In infancy, the size of the heart on a chest radiograph correlates with the degree of tricuspid insufficiency, with larger cardiac size correlating with increasing tricuspid regurgitation. Severe cardiomegaly producing the "wall-to-wall" heart may be present with severe tricuspid regurgitation (Fig. 74-9).[25]

Echocardiography yields diagnostic imaging in infancy, and cardiac MRI may be used in complex cases.[26] Imaging features of PA/IVS include atresia of the pulmonary valve or infundibulum, intact ventricular septum, hypoplastic RV and tricuspid valve, an interatrial communication, and a PDA. Preoperative imaging goals include a comprehensive evaluation of the right heart structures. Attention to the anatomy and function of the hypoplastic tricuspid valve and RV is necessary, and MRI offers precise quantitation of RV morphology, volume, and systolic function (Fig. 74-10).

Figure 74-7 Right atrial (*RA*) to pulmonary artery (*PA*) Fontan anastomosis. *Asterisk* indicates the area of anastomosis.

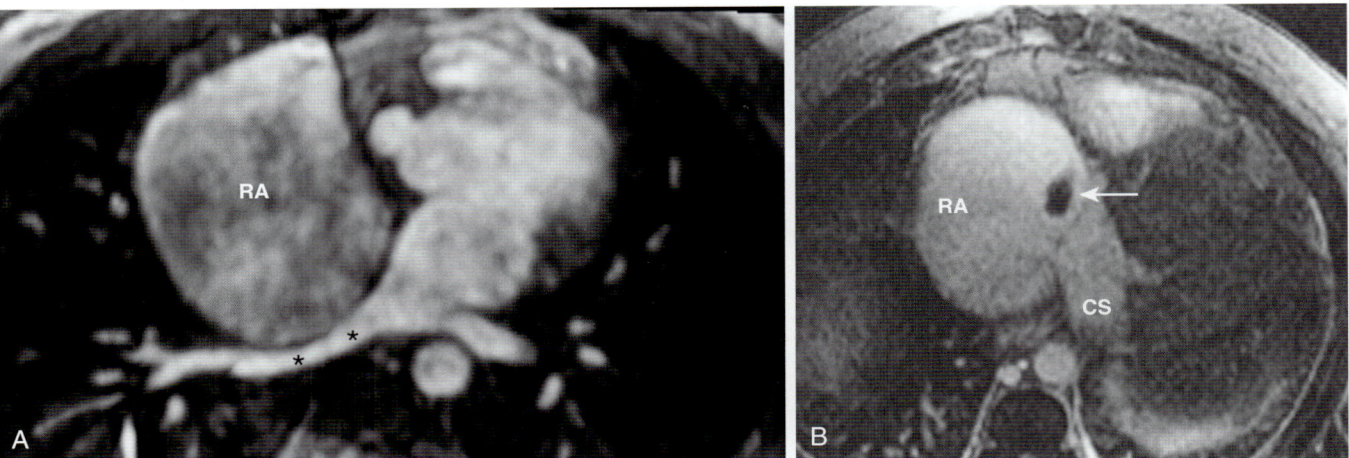

Figure 74-8 Fontan complications. **A,** A 25-year-old with tricuspid atresia after right atrial to pulmonary artery Fontan palliation. A four-chamber magnetic resonance steady-state free-precession view shows a markedly dilated right atrium (*RA*) compressing the right inferior pulmonary vein (*asterisks*). **B,** A 27-year-old with tricuspid atresia after RA to right ventricle Fontan palliation. A four-chamber magnetic resonance late gadolinium enhancement image shows a markedly dilated RA and coronary sinus (*CS*) with a thrombus (*arrow*) in the RA.

Coronary artery anatomy and ventriculocoronary communications may not be well visualized on echocardiography, and thus additional evaluation with angiocardiography, cardiac CT, or cardiac magnetic resonance angiography (MRA) may be necessary. Both computed tomographic angiography (CTA) and MRA studies offer a noninvasive assessment of pulmonary artery anatomy and the relationship of the right ventricular outflow tract to the pulmonary artery. Postoperatively, the type of imaging that is used will depend on the type of repair that has been performed. MRI may be important in these postoperative patients because RV evaluation is limited with echocardiography.

Treatment   Initial management of a neonate with PA/IVS includes the administration of prostaglandins to prevent closure of the PDA to maintain the pulmonary blood flow. Interventions in children with this disorder depend on the degree of RV and pulmonary arterial development and the coronary circulation pattern that is present. A pulmonary valvotomy is contraindicated in the presence of an RV–dependent coronary circulation.[23] A transcatheter pulmonary valvotomy and balloon dilation may be possible if the morphology of the imperforate pulmonary valve is favorable and if minimal separation of the RV outflow tract from the main pulmonary artery is present.[27] When the pulmonary anatomy is not favorable for a transcatheter intervention, a surgical valvotomy may be performed.[28] In the setting of significant RV hypoplasia, a one-and-one-half ventricular repair may be considered.[29] This repair used a bidirectional Glenn shunt to direct superior caval return to the pulmonary arteries. As a result, the hypoplastic tricuspid valve and RV receive venous return only from the inferior vena cava. Univentricular repair or cardiac transplantation may be considered with severe coronary anomalies.[30]

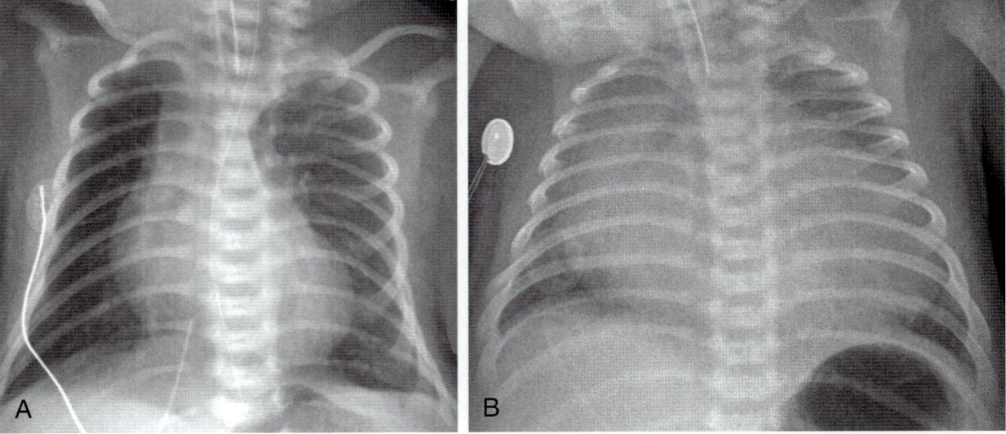

Figure 74-9 Pulmonary atresia with intact ventricular septum (PA/IVS). **A,** A frontal chest radiograph demonstrates mild cardiac enlargement in a cyanotic newborn boy. Additionally, asymmetric pulmonary vascularity is present with decreased pulmonary blood flow on the right compared with the left related to stenosis of the right pulmonary artery just proximal to the insertion of the patent ductus arteriosus. **B,** A frontal chest radiograph in a cyanotic newborn boy showing severe cardiomegaly as a result of significant tricuspid regurgitation producing severe cardiomegaly with a "wall-to-wall" appearance of the heart.

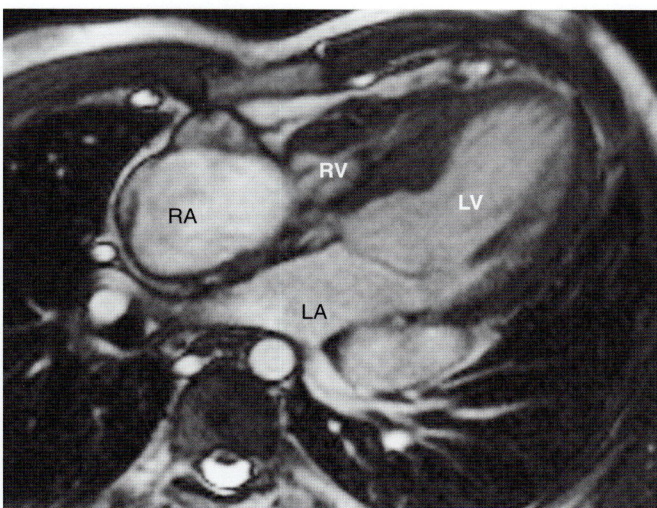

Figure 74-10 A 21-year-old with pulmonary atresia with intact ventricular septum after undergoing right classic Glenn and right atrium (*RA*) to pulmonary artery Fontan procedures. A four-chamber steady-state free-precession image shows the hypoplastic right ventricle (*RV*). The RA is mildly dilated. *LA*, Left atrium; *LV*, left ventricle.

Pulmonary Valve Stenosis

Overview Pulmonary valve stenosis (PVS) accounts for approximately 8% to 10% of all cases of congenital heart disease[31] and 80% to 90% of cases of RV outflow obstruction.[32] Less commonly, pulmonary stenosis occurs at the subvalvular, supravalvular, or peripheral pulmonary arterial levels. Peripheral pulmonary stenosis can be seen after maternal rubella infection and in Noonan, Alagille, and Williams syndromes (see Chapter 79).[33-35]

Etiology, Pathophysiology, and Clinical Presentation In most cases of PVS the valve leaflets are thickened, and fusion of the leaflets produces a domelike pulmonary valve with a small central or eccentric opening. The stenotic valve may be trileaflet, bicuspid, unicuspid, or dysplastic. In severe forms (10% to 20% of cases) and when associated with syndromes, the pulmonary valve is dysplastic, with markedly thickened, nonfused cusps and a hypoplastic annulus.[36] The peripheral pulmonary stenoses seen in persons with Williams and Alagille syndromes may be single or multiple.[33,34]

When severe or critical PVS manifests in infancy, the stenosis leads to decreased right ventricular output.[37] The RV and tricuspid valve may be hypoplastic because limited forward flow through these structures decreases the stimulus for their development. Right atrial pressures are increased, resulting in cyanosis caused by right-to-left shunting through an atrial level shunt. Pulmonary blood flow may depend on the patency of the ductus arteriosus (PDA). Closure of the PDA can lead to decreased pulmonary blood flow, cyanosis, hypoxemia, and death.[37]

Clinical presentation in childhood depends on the degree of RV outflow obstruction. Most children with mild to moderate PVS are asymptomatic and have only a systolic murmur. In cases of severely stenotic and dysplastic valves, symptoms include dyspnea, fatigue, and chest pain with right heart failure.[38]

Imaging Significant cardiomegaly due to right atrial and left heart enlargement may be seen in infants with critical PVS. In cases of moderate to severe PVS, poststenotic dilation of the main and left pulmonary arteries may be seen (Fig. 74-11). The chest radiograph of patients with mild PVS may appear normal. Enlargement of the main and left pulmonary arteries may be seen as a result of the extension of the flow jet from the pulmonary trunk directly posterior into the left pulmonary artery.[39] The pulmonary vascularity is normal if adequate RV output is present. RV hypertrophy with elevation and uplifting of the cardiac apex and associated filling in of the upper retrosternal space can be seen. Right atrial enlargement associated with tricuspid insufficiency may be present.

Echocardiography is the initial imaging method of choice in patients with PVS, but the role of cardiac MRI has increased during the past decade and is particularly important in adult patients, in whom echocardiographic views often are limited.[40] Imaging findings with valvar stenosis include systolic valve thickening and doming with poststenotic enlargement of the main and left pulmonary arteries (Fig. 74-12). With a dysplastic valve, a small pulmonary annulus is seen. Imaging goals include assessment of the level of the pulmonary outflow obstruction, evaluation of pulmonary valve anatomy, and determination of the peak systolic velocity across the pulmonary valve, which allows calculation of the maximal instantaneous gradient. The transvalvar gradient may be estimated from the flow velocity through the valve obtained from phase contrast imaging using the modified Bernoulli equation, $\Delta P = 4V^2$ (where ΔP is the pressure gradient and V is the peak velocity across the pulmonary valve in m/sec). This estimation allows assessment of the severity of the stenosis.[41] Lower peak velocities may be obtained with MRI phase contrast imaging relative to echocardiography.[42] Morphologic assessment of the right side of the heart with

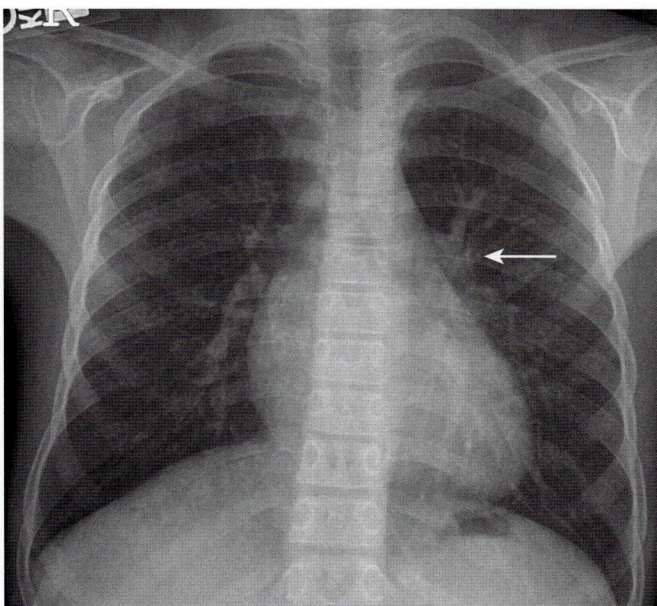

Figure 74-11 Pulmonary valve stenosis. Frontal view of the chest in a 10-year-old shows a normal heart size and pulmonary vascularity. Mild enlargement of the pulmonary trunk and left pulmonary artery is present (*arrow*).

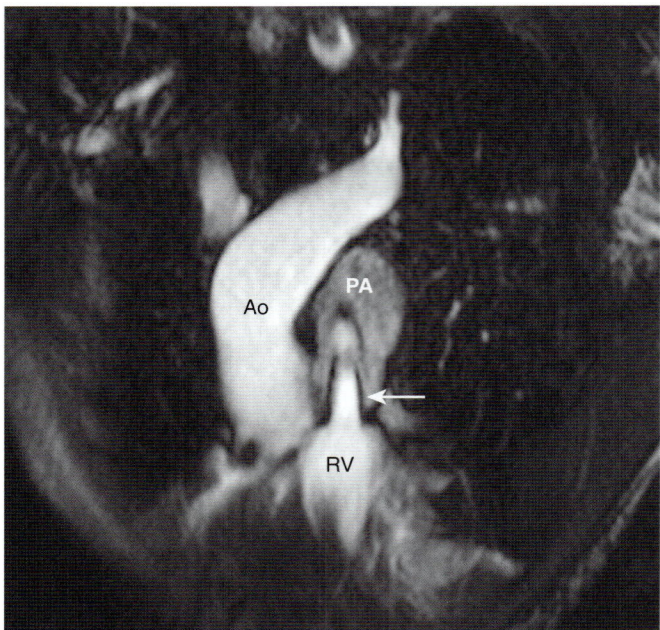

Figure 74-12 Pulmonary valve stenosis. A steady-state free-precession magnetic resonance image coronal to the right ventricular outflow tract (*RV*) shows a poststenotic jet of turbulent flow (*arrow*) across the pulmonary valve. *Ao*, Aorta; *PA*, pulmonary artery.

quantitative assessment of the RV size and systolic function is necessary, as is assessment of the left side of the heart.[36] MRA or CTA allows determination of peripheral pulmonary arterial stenosis. After intervention, imaging is used to determine the degree of residual pulmonary stenosis and the severity of pulmonary regurgitation and to evaluate RV size and systolic function.

Treatment Infants with critical PVS are treated medically with inotropic support and intubation. Prostaglandin E_1 infusion is initiated to maintain ductal patency.[37,38] Balloon valvuloplasty is the treatment of choice for isolated PVS in a nondysplastic valve, with excellent outcomes.[37,43-45] A systemic-to-pulmonary artery shunt is rarely indicated for continued cyanosis.[46] Balloon valvuloplasty often is used as the initial treatment for dysplastic pulmonary valves, but surgery may be necessary because of the lower response rate to this intervention.[31,47] Peripheral pulmonary stenoses often require repeat angioplasty procedures and/or stent placement because of lower angioplasty success rates.[48,49]

Indications for reintervention or surgery include residual RV outflow obstruction from severe infundibular hypertrophy, residual PVS, or peripheral arterial stenosis. Pulmonary valve replacement is indicated for symptomatic severe pulmonary insufficiency, RV dysfunction or dilation, or significant ventricular arrhythmia.[50-53]

Key Points

Enlargement of the main and left pulmonary arteries without increased pulmonary vascularity should represent pulmonary valve stenosis. However, it may be normal for the main pulmonary artery to be prominent in adolescence, and thus correlation with imaging and the clinical examination should differentiate these entities.

Using the peak velocity obtained by either echocardiography or phase contrast MRI and the modified Bernoulli equation, $4V^2$ (V = peak velocity beyond the pulmonary valve in m/s), the peak pulmonary valve pressure gradient in mm Hg can be calculated.

Suggested Readings

Attenhofer Jost CH, Connolly HM, Dearani JA, et al. Ebstein's anomaly. *Circulation*. 2007;115(2):277-285.

Fredenburg TB, Johnson TR, Cohen MD. The Fontan procedure: anatomy, complications, and manifestations of failure. *Radiographics*. 2011;31(2): 453-463.

Kawel N, Valsangiacomo-Buechel E, Hoop R, et al. Preoperative evaluation of pulmonary artery morphology and pulmonary circulation in neonates with pulmonary atresia—usefulness of MR angiography in clinical routine. *J Cardiovasc Magn Reson*. 2010;12:52.

References

Full references for this chapter can be found on www.expertconsult.com.

Chapter 75

Left Heart Lesions

CYNTHIA K. RIGSBY, JOSHUA D. ROBINSON, and DARSHIT THAKRAR

Hypoplastic Left Heart Syndrome

Overview Hypoplastic left heart syndrome (HLHS) is a spectrum of disease characterized by underdevelopment of the left ventricle with obstruction or atresia of ventricular inflow and outflow. HLHS accounts for approximately 2% to 3% of all cases of congenital heart disease, with a slight male predominance.[1,2] Chromosomal abnormalities associated with HLHS include Turner syndrome, trisomy 13 and 18, and terminal 11q deletion.[1-3]

Etiology and Pathophysiology The structural defects of HLHS include varying degrees of hypoplasia of left heart structures including a hypoplastic ascending aorta and arch, aortic valve atresia or stenosis, hypoplastic left ventricle, mitral atresia or stenosis, and patent ductus arteriosus (PDA) and patent foramen ovale or atrial septal defect (ASD) (Fig. 75-1). In a majority of cases, the ventricular septum is intact, and in severe cases, thickening of the left ventricular endocardium or endocardial fibroelastosis is present.[4] Coarctation of the aorta coexists in approximately 80% of patients.[5] The right heart structures often are enlarged.[5]

Both the pulmonary and systemic circulations depend on the right ventricle. Oxygenated pulmonary venous blood returns to the left atrium, and because of the significant left ventricular inflow obstruction and decreased compliance, an obligatory left-to-right shunt is present at the atrial level, most often through a patent foramen ovale or ASD. In the right atrium, the oxygenated pulmonary venous blood mixes with deoxygenated systemic venous blood and flows into the right ventricle. Blood is pumped to the pulmonary artery, with systemic blood then flowing from right to left through the PDA. The brachiocephalic vessels and coronary arteries are perfused through retrograde flow from the PDA into the arch and ascending aorta. The descending aorta is perfused from antegrade flow through the PDA.

Clinical Presentation Cyanosis and tachypnea generally are apparent within hours to 2 days after birth. Poor arteriovenous mixing as a result of inadequate interatrial communication can lead to early elevation of left atrial and pulmonary venous pressure, pulmonary edema, and right heart failure. Serious hemodynamic changes occur after the birth of an infant with HLHS when pulmonary vascular resistance begins to drop and the PDA begins to spontaneously close.[6] When pulmonary vascular resistance drops, an increase in pulmonary blood flow and a decrease in systemic blood flow occur, leading to a decrease in systemic perfusion. When the PDA constricts, a further decrease in the ductal-dependent systemic and coronary circulations occurs, leading to a decrease in systemic perfusion, myocardial ischemia, shock, and death.

Imaging HLHS is readily identified in utero. The condition is now discovered in approximately 60% of patients with use of prenatal echocardiography.[7,8] Chest radiographic findings are variable. The heart may be normal in size or may be enlarged with a globular configuration, suggesting multichamber enlargement (e-Fig. 75-2). Pulmonary vascularity may be normal in the first hours of life, with a subsequent progressive increase in vascularity if no restriction to blood flow exists at the atrial level. Indistinctness of the pulmonary vessels or pulmonary venous congestion with interstitial lines or pleural fluid may be seen with a restrictive atrial septum.

Echocardiography is the imaging method of choice and generally delineates all relevant presurgical anatomy. Cross-sectional imaging can be performed as an adjunct to echocardiography in complex cases.[9] Magnetic resonance imaging (MRI) may be especially useful when a marginally hypoplastic left ventricle is present and the possibility exists of a two-ventricle surgical repair (Fig. 75-3 and Video 75-1).[4] In these cases, MRI can be used to assess the size of the left atrium, atrial septum, mitral valve orifice, left ventricle, and aortic root to help plan the most appropriate surgical repair. MRI increasingly is being used after the first stage of the palliative single ventricle surgery to reliably quantify the systemic right ventricle systolic function, tricuspid regurgitation, and residual or recurrent coarctation and for pulmonary artery stenosis or hypoplasia before the second-stage bidirectional cavopulmonary anastomosis.[10-12]

Treatment Initial medical management includes intravenous prostaglandin E_1 (PGE_1) to maintain ductal patency. Medical therapy, including ventilator adjustments, inhaled agents, and medications, is used to optimize the ratio of pulmonary to systemic blood flow and to minimize the volume load on the single functional ventricle to maintain adequate systemic perfusion.[13]

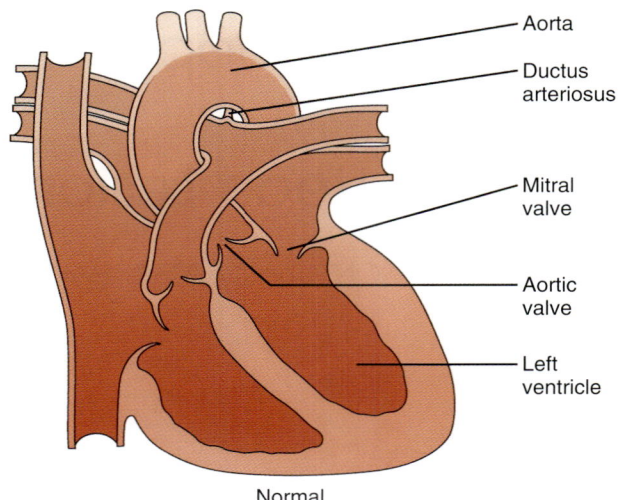

Normal

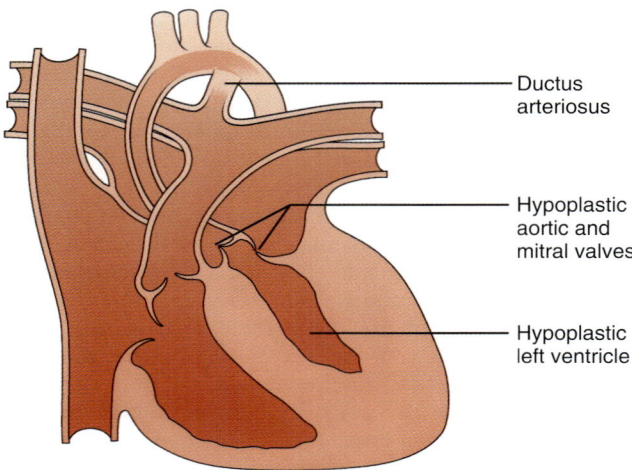

Hypoplastic left heart syndrome

Figure 75-1 Diagram of hypoplastic left heart syndrome. Compared with the normal heart, the mitral and aortic valves are severely hypoplastic or atretic, the left ventricular cavity and aorta are hypoplastic, and systemic blood flow is supplied by the patent ductus arteriosus. (From American Heart Association. Hypoplastic left heart syndrome. www.americanheart.org. © 2006, American Heart Association, Inc.)

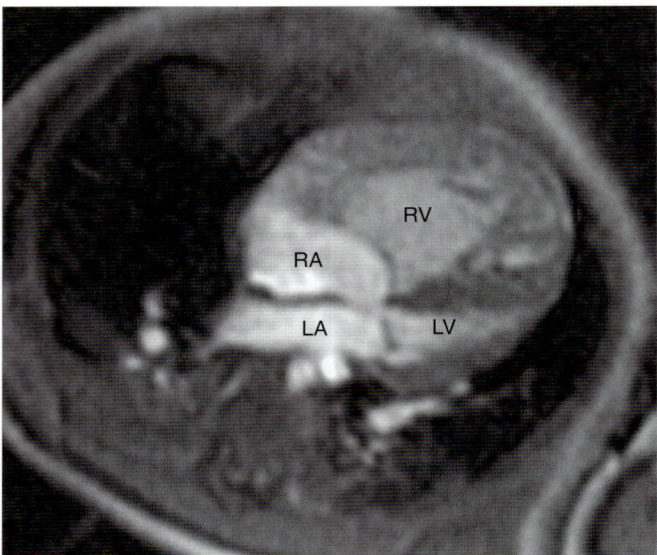

Figure 75-3 Hypoplastic left heart syndrome. Four-chamber steady-state free-precession (SSFP) magnetic resonance image (MRI) of a 12-week-old with a marginally hypoplastic left ventricle to evaluate for a two-ventricle versus single-ventricle repair. The left atrium (*LA*) and left ventricle (*LV*) are small, with the left ventricular volume calculated at 24.2 mL/m². The study also showed adequate mitral and aortic valve dimensions. Based on the MRI measurements, the patient underwent a successful two-ventricle repair. See Video 75-1 for a four-chamber cine SSFP MRI of the same patient. *RA*, Right atrium; *RV*, right ventricle.

brachiocephalic artery to the pulmonary artery. (Fig. 75-5). Alternatively, a right ventricle to pulmonary artery (RV-PA) conduit may be placed.[15] The potential benefit of the RV-PA conduit is elimination of the diastolic runoff that occurs with a BT shunt. Diastolic runoff can lead to coronary and systemic artery blood flow steal or an increase in the ratio of pulmonary blood flow to systemic blood flow. The potential disadvantages of the RV-PA conduit include right ventricular dysfunction due to the ventriculotomy, the potential for aneurysm formation at the site of the conduit insertion, and right ventricular volume overload from pulmonary regurgitation because there is no valve in the conduit.[1,15]

By approximately 3 to 6 months of age, pulmonary vascular resistance has physiologically dropped, and the second stage of the reconstruction—the bidirectional cavopulmonary (Glenn) anastomosis or hemi–Fontan procedure—is performed to redirect the upper body systemic venous return directly to the lungs. The bidirectional Glenn procedure involves anastomosing the superior vena cava (SVC) to the right pulmonary artery. The hemi–Fontan procedure involves anastomosing the pulmonary arteries to the superior caval-atrial junction and placing a patch into the superior aspect of the right atrium to isolate SVC return into the pulmonary arteries. At this time, the BT shunt is divided or the RV-PA conduit is obliterated and tricuspid valve repair and pulmonary artery angioplasty are performed, if necessary.

A "hybrid" approach, which combines surgical branch pulmonary artery banding to limit pulmonary blood flow with transcatheter ductal stenting to provide systemic flow, has more recently been advocated to achieve similar physiology to the stage I procedure without requiring cardiopulmonary bypass in the fragile neonate with HLHS (Fig. 75-6).[1,16]

Surgical treatment consists of a staged reconstruction procedure (Fig. 75-4). The staged reconstruction involves three surgical procedures with the goal of creating separate pulmonary and systemic circulations supported by the right ventricle and accounts for the high neonatal pulmonary vascular resistance and the subsequent decrease in pulmonary vascular resistance. The first stage of the reconstruction—the Norwood procedure—often is performed in the first week of life.[14] This procedure involves transection of the pulmonary trunk proximal to the pulmonary bifurcation and anastomosis of the pulmonary trunk to the aorta. A triangular patch of homograft material is used to augment the hypoplastic ascending aorta, aortic arch, and distal arch. The coronary arteries are then perfused retrograde through the small ascending aorta. The PDA is ligated. A complete atrial septectomy is performed. Blood flow to the lungs is reestablished via a modified Blalock–Taussig shunt (BT shunt) from the subclavian or

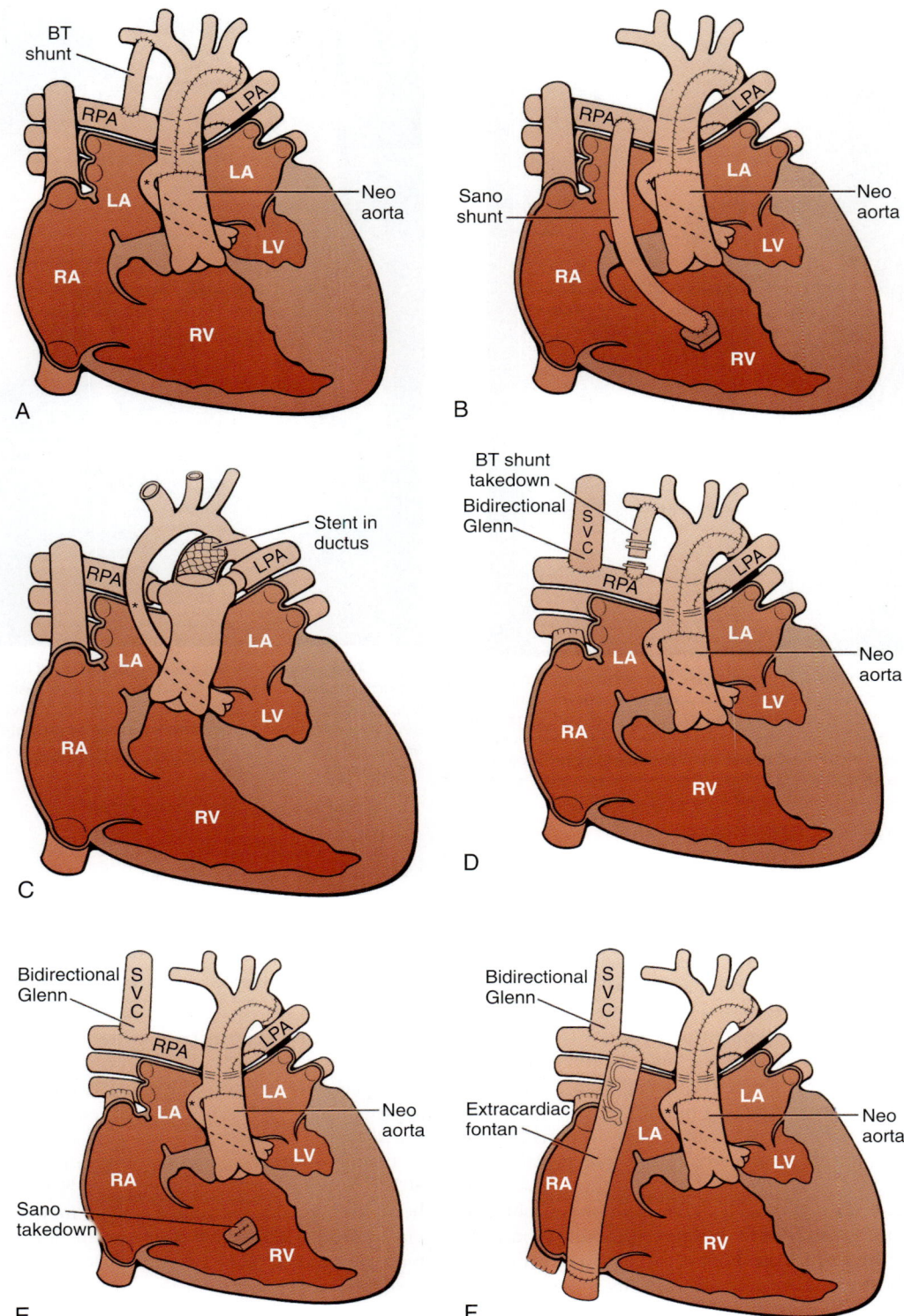

Figure 75-4 Staged reconstruction for hypoplastic left heart syndrome. **A,** Stage I of the Norwood reconstruction using a modified Blalock-Taussig (*BT*) shunt. **B,** Stage I of the Norwood reconstruction using the Sano modification. **C,** Hybrid procedure. **D,** Stage II of the Norwood reconstruction. **E,** Stage II of the Norwood reconstruction using the Sano modification. **F,** Fontan procedure. *Asterisk,* Native ascending aorta; *LA,* left atrium; *LPA,* left pulmonary artery; *LV,* left ventricle; *RA,* right atrium; *RPA,* right pulmonary artery; *RV,* right ventricle; *SVC,* superior vena cava.

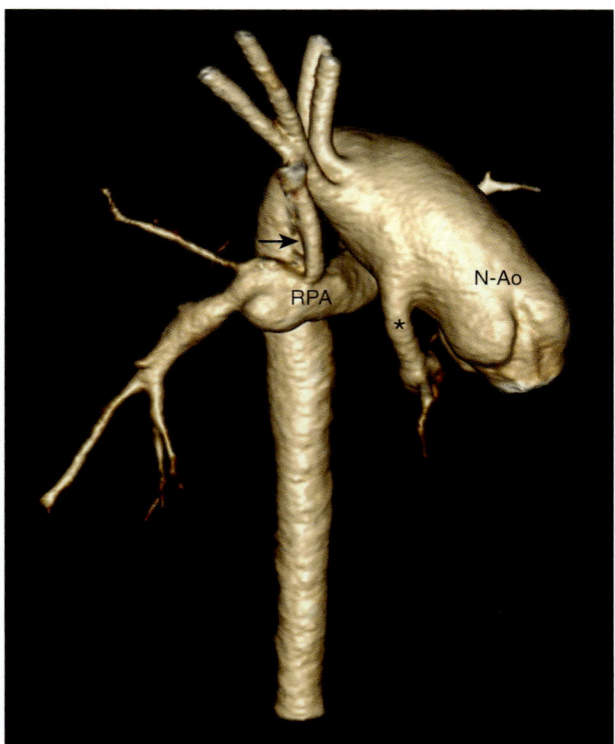

Figure 75-5 A 6-month-old with hypoplastic left heart syndrome after the Norwood I procedure. *Posterior oblique volume-rendered computed tomographic angiography shows the hypoplastic native aorta (*asterisk*) anastomosed with the native pulmonary artery (now neoaorta) and a Blalock-Taussig shunt (*arrow*) extending from the right brachiocephalic artery to the right pulmonary artery. N-Ao, Neo-aorta; RPA, right pulmonary artery.*

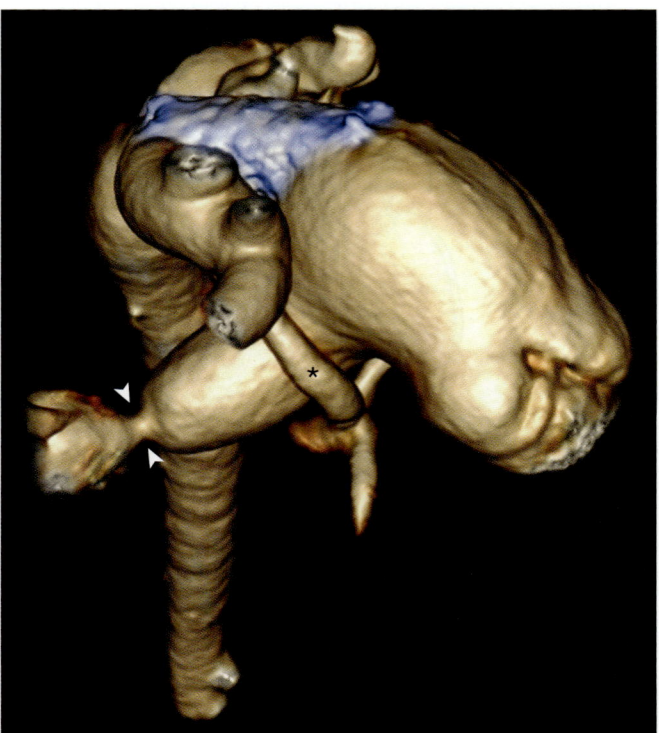

Figure 75-6 A 5-month-old with hypoplastic left heart syndrome after a hybrid procedure. *Posterior oblique volume-rendered computed tomographic angiography shows the hypoplastic native aorta (*asterisk*). A stent (*blue*) has been placed to keep the large patent ductus arteriosus open and a pulmonary artery band (*arrowheads*) has been placed to limit pulmonary blood flow.*

The comprehensive second-stage procedure then involves cardiopulmonary bypass, removal of the PDA stent and pulmonary artery bands, repair of the aortic arch and pulmonary arteries, division of the diminutive ascending aorta with reimplantation into the pulmonary root, main pulmonary artery to reconstructed aortic anastomosis, atrial septectomy, and a bidirectional Glenn or hemi-Fontan procedure.[1,16]

The third stage of the reconstruction—the Fontan completion procedure—is generally performed at 18 to 36 months of age. This stage involves directing inferior vena cava blood flow to the pulmonary arteries either via an extracardiac conduit or an intracardiac right atrial baffle (lateral tunnel). If a patch was placed in the right atrium during the second stage of the repair, it is removed. This third stage achieves separation of the systemic and pulmonary circulations. A fenestration may be left in the Fontan circuit so if pressures become high, there can be a pop-off from the Fontan circuit into the heart, which may lead to a more stable postoperative course.[17,18] Many fenestrations close spontaneously but also can be closed during a cardiac catheterization procedure.

Survival after the three-stage palliative procedure has improved steadily and now approaches 70%.[8] The stage I Norwood procedure carries the highest mortality, ranging from 7% to 19%.[15] Cardiac transplantation had been considered an alternative to staged Norwood palliation in the past, but because of limited donor availability and the recent improvement in survival following Norwood palliation,

transplantation now generally is reserved for patients for whom staged palliation has failed.[1,19]

Aortic Stenosis

Overview   Left ventricular outflow tract (LVOT) obstruction can occur at the level of the aortic valve or in the subvalvar or supravalvar regions. This spectrum of disease represents approximately 10% of cases of congenital heart disease.[20] Valvar aortic stenosis (AS) is by far the most common form of LVOT obstruction and has a male predominance of nearly 80%.[21] Supravalvar AS accounts for 1% to 2% of AS in childhood and occurs spontaneously or may be familial, usually via autosomal dominant transmission. Up to 50% of patients with supravalvar AS have Williams syndrome. Subvalvar AS is slightly more common than supravalvar AS[22]; it also has a male predominance and may be associated with more complex disease such as double-outlet right ventricle and transposition of the great arteries.

Etiology and Pathophysiology   Congenital aortic valve stenosis results from abnormal valve development rather than the degenerative disease commonly seen in adults. The stenotic valve has variable anatomy, with annular hypoplasia, thickened or tethered leaflets, and/or incompletely developed commissures. Valve morphology may predict clinical severity or associated disease.[23,24] Whereas neonatal critical AS often is associated with a unicuspid valve and a small eccentric orifice, bicuspid morphology accounts for up to 95% of cases of congenital valvar AS and is present in up to 30% to 60% of patients with coarctation.[25,26] In addition to the abnormality of the bicuspid valve, the aortic root tissue is abnormal in these patients and can lead to significant aortic dilation above a stenotic bicuspid valve. The aortic dilation has been thought to be due to poststenotic dilation, but histologic abnormalities of the ascending aorta can occur without significant valvar stenosis or regurgitation. The histology is similar to the medial disease seen in persons with Marfan syndrome in addition to abnormalities of the smooth muscle, extracellular matrix, elastin, and collagen.[27,28]

The narrowing in supravalvar AS most commonly is hourglass in shape, occurs immediately above the sinuses of Valsalva at the sinotubular junction, and may be associated with poststenotic dilatation of the aorta, diffuse aortic arch hypoplasia, aortic valve abnormalities, coronary artery ostial stenosis, or left ventricular hypertrophy.[29,30] Supravalvar AS often is part of a widespread arteriopathy.

Subvalvar AS can be discrete or diffuse. The discrete form, which represents the majority of cases, is a thin fibromuscular diaphragm encircling the LVOT. In the more severe diffuse form, a fibromuscular subaortic band is present along the length of the LVOT, producing a tunnel-like narrowing. The fibrous process often extends to involve the aortic valve cusps or the anterior mitral valve leaflet. The more diffuse form usually is associated with other left heart lesions, including mitral stenosis, supramitral ring, parachute mitral valve, valvar AS, or coarctation of the aorta.[31]

Clinical Presentation Severe or critical AS may be diagnosed prenatally or present early in infancy with severe left heart obstruction, congestive heart failure, dyspnea, and poor peripheral circulation. Systemic flow is ductal dependent in cases of critical AS. The clinical manifestations of AS in infancy depend on the degree of valvar obstruction, mitral insufficiency, left atrial hypertension, and left ventricular dysfunction, as well as the amount of shunted atrial and ductal flow and other associated left-sided obstructive lesions. In cases of severe obstruction, the left ventricle may be severely hypoplastic, dilated, or dysfunctional.

AS in children usually is the result of a bicuspid aortic valve, and the obstruction generally is not severe. The degree of ventricular obstruction progresses gradually with age. Children with mild to moderate AS generally are asymptomatic and usually present with a characteristic systolic ejection murmur. With more severe obstruction, symptoms include chest pain, dyspnea, decreased exercise tolerance, and syncope.

Hemodynamically, supravalvar AS mimics valvar AS. In the absence of Williams syndrome, cardiovascular symptoms are rare, but patients with supravalvar AS may experience left heart failure, dyspnea, angina, and syncope related to the degree of LVOT obstruction. Patients with peripheral systemic or pulmonary arterial stenoses may have associated left or right ventricular hypertension, respectively.

Subvalvar AS is generally progressive. The turbulent subaortic jet can cause shear stress on the aortic valve, leading to valve deformation and progressive insufficiency. Subvalvar AS is rarely detected in infancy but may be detected in childhood. Children may have an asymptomatic systolic ejection

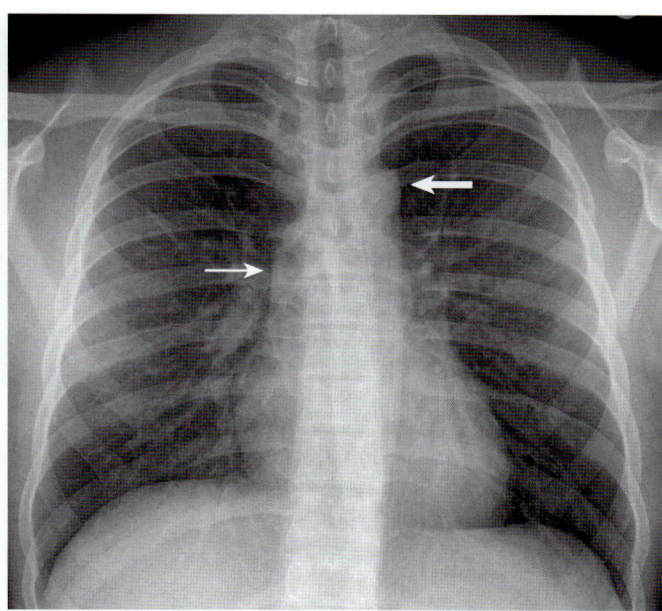

Figure 75-7 Aortic valve stenosis. A frontal view of the chest in an 18-year-old shows poststenotic dilation of the ascending aorta (*thin arrow*) and aortic arch (*thick arrow*).

murmur. A diastolic murmur of aortic insufficiency may be found in older children as regurgitation increases with age. In older patients with moderate to severe obstruction, signs of left ventricular failure with dyspnea, chest pain, syncope, and tachypnea may occur.

Imaging The chest radiograph in infants with critical AS shows cardiomegaly and pulmonary venous congestion. In older children with mild stenosis, the radiograph generally is normal. When moderate to severe stenosis and left ventricular hypertrophy are present, the cardiac apex is depressed toward the diaphragm and posteriorly to the inferior vena cava. Left atrial enlargement can be seen with severe stenosis. Poststenotic dilation of the ascending aorta is rare in young children (Fig. 75-7).

Echocardiography is the imaging procedure of choice for the evaluation of valvar AS. Cardiac MRI can be used to complement echocardiography in cases of poor acoustic windows or if larger field of view imaging is indicated. Goals of imaging include demonstration of the degree and location of obstruction, valve morphology, leaflet mobility and effective valve orifice area. Systolic valve area calculated by MRI planimetry correlates well with transesophageal echocardiography and cardiac catheterization measurements (Fig. 75-8 and Video 75-2).[32] The valve typically appears thickened and doming, with asymmetric or restricted leaflet excursion. The gradient across the aortic valve in millimeters of mercury is calculated using the modified Bernoulli equation ($4V^2$, where V is peak Doppler velocity beyond the aortic valve in meters per second). Aortic valvular regurgitant fraction is calculated with phase-contrast MRI (e-Fig. 75-9). Evaluation of left ventricular size, systolic performance, and diastolic dysfunction is necessary. Assessment of aortic root, ascending aorta, and arch size is crucial in infants with critical AS. These patients may have abnormal endocardium, which can indicate the presence of endocardial fibroelastosis (e-Fig. 75-10).

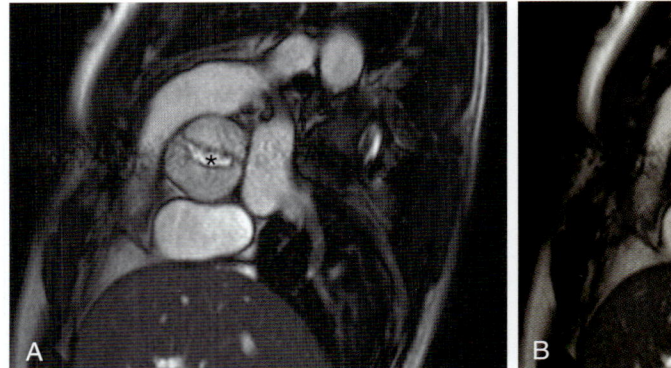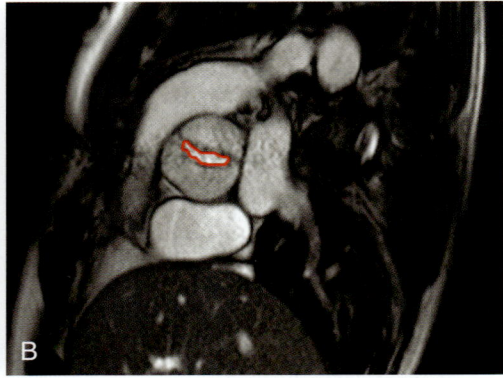

Figure 75-8   Bicuspid aortic valve in a 25-year-old with history of aortic coarctation. **A,** A cross-sectional steady-state free-precession (SSFP) systolic image of a severely stenotic bicuspid aortic valve (*asterisk*) with fusion of the right and noncoronary commissures, giving a "fish-mouth" appearance. See Video 75-2 for a cine SSFP image of the same. **B,** The aortic valve area (outlined in red) as measured by planimetry is 1.18 cm².

Surveillance of the thoracic aorta is indicated to evaluate for the development of aortic root dilation and aortic dissection associated with aortic valve disease (e-Fig. 75-11 and Video 75-3).[28]

In supravalvar AS, imaging is tailored to evaluate for the presence of discrete or diffuse supravalvar narrowing of the ascending aorta, the coronary ostia, the degree of left ventricular hypertrophy, ventricular function, supravalvar pulmonary stenosis, and other sites of vasculopathy as clinically indicated (Fig. 75-12). In patients with subvalvar AS, evaluation for the discrete subaortic membrane or ridge and

definition of the long subaortic area of the tunnel-type subaortic lesion is necessary (Fig. 75-13).

Treatment   Infants with severe or critical AS need urgent treatment. Patients are supported with a PGE_1 infusion to maintain ductal patency, mechanical ventilation, and inotropic medications. Urgent percutaneous balloon valvuloplasty is the treatment of choice. A neonatal Ross procedure (i.e., replacement of the aortic valve with a pulmonary valve annulus and trunk autograft, coronary reimplantation, and replacement of the pulmonary valve with a homograft conduit) has been advocated by some persons as the treatment of choice in patients with dysplastic valves or small aortic annuli[33,34]; however, increased mortality and higher rates of autograft deterioration in children compared with adults has resulted in less enthusiasm by others.[35,36] During the era of aggressive transcatheter intervention, early mortality for infants with severe or critical AS has fallen from as high as 43% to 4% to 13%.[37,38]

Balloon valvotomy is considered in older children with a peak systolic ejection gradient of 50 mm Hg or greater at

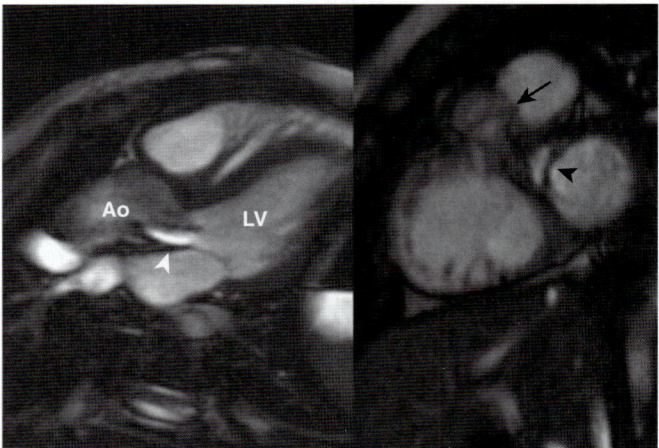

Figure 75-13   Subaortic stenosis. Steady-state free-precession magnetic resonance imaging long-axis (*left*) and short-axis (*right*) images of the left ventricular outflow tract (LVOT) show a subaortic membrane (*black arrowhead*) causing a jet of flow acceleration across the LVOT (*white arrowhead*) beginning just below the aortic valve plane (*arrow*). *Ao,* Aorta; *LV,* left ventricle.

Figure 75-12   Supravalvar aortic stenosis (AS). An oblique volume-rendered three-dimensional computed tomography angiographic image shows supravalvar AS with an abrupt caliber change in the proximal ascending aorta (*arrows*).

catheterization, for patients with angina, syncope, or congestive heart failure, and for persons who want to play competitive sports or become pregnant.[39,40] Routine follow-up is necessary to evaluate for aortic insufficiency and recurrent stenosis. Late surgical valve repair or replacement is necessary in approximately 25% to 35% of patients.[38,41] For patients who require valve replacement, a bioprosthetic or mechanical valve may be placed or a Ross procedure may be performed.

Patients with AS are at increased risk for sudden death and endocarditis. The risk of sudden death is thought to significantly increase with symptoms[40] but probably has decreased in the era of aggressive and effective transcatheter treatment.[42] The incidence of subacute bacterial endocarditis is rare but is approximately 35 times greater than in the general population and also increases with AS severity.[43,44]

Indications for interventions related to supravalvar AS are less clear, but surgery is performed in symptomatic cases. The high likelihood of progression influences consideration for aortoplasty or LVOT reconstruction. Balloon angioplasty and stenting of associated pulmonary stenoses may be necessary. Complications include aortic aneurysms and infective endocarditis, and surgical mortality is low.[45] Given the recurrent and progressive nature of diffuse arteriopathy, long-term follow-up is warranted.

In asymptomatic patients, the timing of surgical intervention for subvalvar AS is controversial and is related to the degree and progression of LVOT obstruction and other associated heart disease.[46-48] For persons with discrete subvalvar obstruction, fibromuscular resection with or without septal myectomy is performed, and operative mortality is low. Treatment for the tunnel-like narrowing form of obstruction varies, depending on the size and function of the aortic valve. The Konno procedure (i.e., aortoventriculoplasty, including replacement of the aortic valve) and modifications including valve repair or the Ross procedure (described earlier) may be performed (e-Fig. 75-14). A wide rage in the rates of recurrence and complications such as aortic regurgitation are reported; however, operative mortality, recurrence, and progressive AS are more common after repair of the diffuse type of subvalvar AS.

Coarctation of the Aorta

Overview Coarctation of the aorta accounts for approximately 7% of cases of congenital heart disease,[49] with a male to female ratio of approximately 1.5 : 1.[28] Coarctation of the aorta is isolated or present with a PDA in 82% of cases.[50] A bicuspid aortic valve is seen in up to 30% to 60% of patients,[25,26,51] and ventricular septal defect (VSD) is seen in 11% of patients.[50] Other associated lesions include ASD, left-sided obstructive lesions, transposition of the great vessels, double-outlet right ventricle, and atrioventricular septal defect in 7% of patients.[50] Eleven percent to 15% of patients with Turner syndrome have aortic coarctation.[52,53] Berry aneurysms are seen in up to 10% of patients.[54] Coarctation of the aorta is seen in 15% of patients with PHACES syndrome (posterior fossa defects, hemangiomas, arterial anomalies, cardiac defects and coarctation, eye anomalies, and sternal defects or supraumbilical raphe).[55]

Etiology and Pathophysiology Coarctation of the aorta is a narrowing of the thoracic aorta that generally occurs adjacent to the insertion site of the ductus arteriosus just distal to the left subclavian artery. The coarctation is almost always juxtaductal and discrete, but varying degrees of tubular hypoplasia of the transverse arch and isthmus may be present and are more commonly seen in infancy.[56] The embryology of aortic coarctation is not known, but two theories have been proposed. One theory, called the ductal sling theory, suggests that an abnormal extension of contractile ductal tissue occurs circumferentially around the aortic lumen. Contraction of this tissue with ductal closure leads to a shelflike aortic narrowing in the juxtaductal region.[56] The second theory, called the flow theory, postulates that aortic coarctation develops as a result of decreased blood flow through the aortic isthmus as a result of left-sided obstructive lesions. In fetal life the aortic isthmus normally receives a relatively low volume of blood flow. Most of the flow to the descending aorta arises from the right ventricle through the PDA. The left ventricle supplies highly oxygenated blood to the ascending aorta and brachiocephalic vessels, with a small amount of flow going through the aortic valve. With left-sided obstructive lesions, decreased isthmic flow occurs, promoting abnormal isthmic development and leading to aortic coarctation.[56,57]

The pathophysiology of coarctation of the aorta is related to the severity of the arch obstruction, the presence of collateral vessels, and associated cardiac lesions.[50] Initially, the neonate with coarctation will have a PDA, allowing blood flow to bypass the obstruction. With severe obstruction, left ventricular afterload is increased acutely following closure of the PDA, and patients then may present with congestive heart failure and shock. With less severe obstruction, collateral blood vessels develop to bypass the obstruction. The development of adequate collateral vessels may mask the presence of the coarctation until later in childhood or adulthood. Upper extremity hypertension is present in 90% of children and is thought to be secondary to three proposed mechanisms, including mechanical aortic obstruction, abnormal body baroreceptor settings proximal to the obstruction, and hyperactivation of the renin-angiotensin system caused by the underperfused kidneys.[50,58,59] Left-sided obstructive lesions may further increase left ventricular afterload, and the presence of a VSD may further increase left ventricular volume load, leading to pulmonary venous and arterial hypertension and heart failure.

Clinical Presentation Infants with critical coarctation of the aorta, especially when it is associated with other cardiac defects, typically present by 7 to 14 days of life as the PDA begins to close and they have dramatic signs of congestive heart failure and poor systemic perfusion. Clinical symptoms include dyspnea, poor feeding, tachycardia, and signs of shock, including oliguria, anuria, and severe acidemia. Femoral pulses are weak or absent, and differential blood pressures generally show a gradient between the upper and lower limbs.[50]

Coarctation of the aorta also may be diagnosed from infancy to adulthood in asymptomatic or mildly symptomatic patients, with a reported median age of 10 years (range, 1 to 36 years).[60] These patients present later because the coarctation is not significant or because adequate collateral circulation has developed. The diagnosis usually is made on the basis

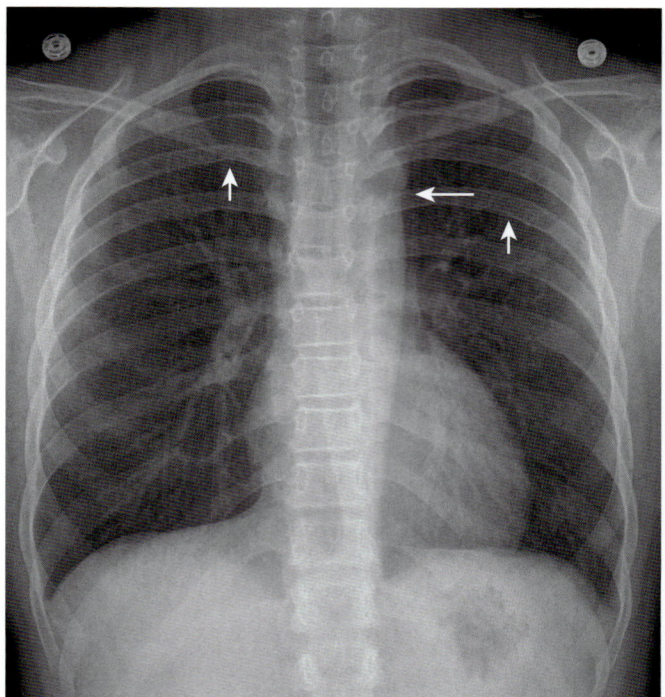

Figure 75-16 Coarctation of the aorta in a 10-year-old. A frontal view of the chest shows the "figure three" sign (*long arrow*), which is indicative of aortic coarctation, and bilateral posterior rib notching (*short arrows*), which is indicative of collateral vessels.

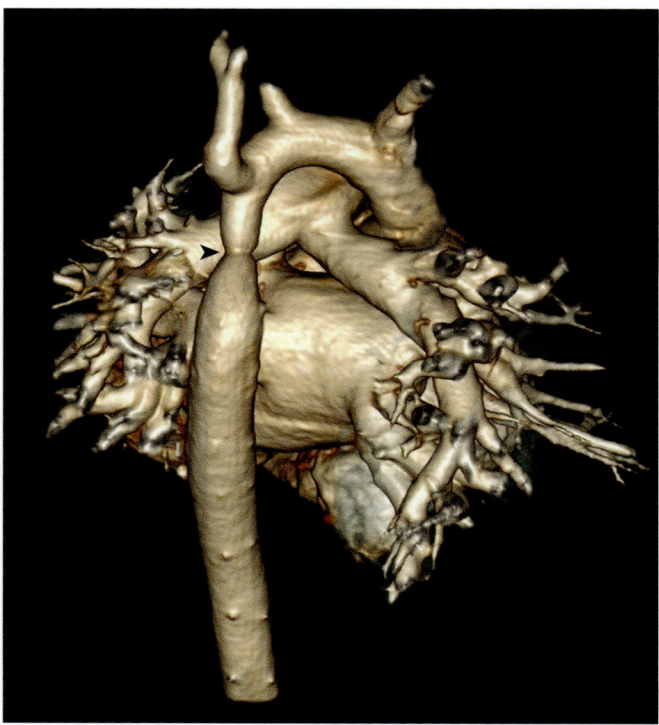

Figure 75-17 Aortic coarctation in a 3-year-old. Posterior projection from a volume-rendered magnetic resonance angiography image shows a discrete aortic coarctation (*arrowhead*) distal to the left subclavian artery. No significant collateral vessels are seen.

of routine physical examination findings such as an incidental murmur, hypertension, or absent or diminished lower extremity pulses.[60]

Imaging Infants with severe coarctation present with moderate to marked cardiomegaly and increased pulmonary vascular markings due to venous congestion from obstruction or overcirculation with an associated VSD (e-Fig. 75-15). Congestive heart failure presenting between the first and fourth weeks of life strongly suggests coarctation. Chest radiographs in children older than 1 year and younger than 5 years usually show a normal heart size, but cardiomegaly due to left ventricular hypertrophy can be seen. Rib notching as a result of dilated intercostal collateral arteries forming grooves on the rib undersurfaces is the hallmark of this condition and usually is seen after 5 years of age. The lower borders of the fourth through eighth ribs usually are involved posteriorly.[61] The rib notching is bilateral unless an aberrant subclavian artery arising distal to the coarctation is present. Poststenotic dilation of the aorta below the coarctation usually occurs. A "figure three" sign frequently is seen along the left upper mediastinal border, related to the prominent aortic knob and left subclavian artery proximal to the coarctation, the indentation from the coarctation, and the poststenotic aortic segment below the coarctation (Fig. 75-16). The imprint of the aorta on the adjacent barium–filled esophagus, which is known as the "E" sign or "reversed three" sign, is caused by indentation of the esophagus by the dilated aorta proximal and distal to the coarctation.

Echocardiography is the method of choice for imaging coarctation in infancy. Computed tomography and MRI can provide detailed anatomic imaging of the coarctation in older children or adults with limited acoustic windows (Figs. 75-17 and 75-18). MRI also can be used to assess the hemodynamic significance of the coarctation. A complete imaging examination involves imaging for ventricular systolic function, volume and mass; atrioventricular and semilunar valve assessment with particular attention to the aortic valve; and imaging of the aortic root, ascending aorta, arch, coarctation, and descending aorta to the renal arteries. Maximum blood flow velocity, blood flow volume, and flow pattern in the aorta just distal to the coarctation can be assessed using phase-contrast MRI sequences (e-Fig. 75-19 and Video 75-4). The maximal flow velocity obtained across the coarctation can be used in the Bernoulli equation (see the previous aortic stenosis imaging section) to estimate the gradient across the coarctation.[62] Aortic flow volume at the diaphragm also can be assessed using phase-contrast sequences. In patients with significant coarctation, the flow volume at the diaphragm may be increased relative to the volume just distal to the coarctation as a result of recruitment of collateral flow through the intercostal arteries and can be an indicator of the significance of the coarctation.[63-65]

Treatment Coarctation of the aorta that presents with congestive heart failure in the neonatal period is managed medically with inotropic drugs and PGE_1 to maintain ductal patency and improve blood flow to the descending aorta.

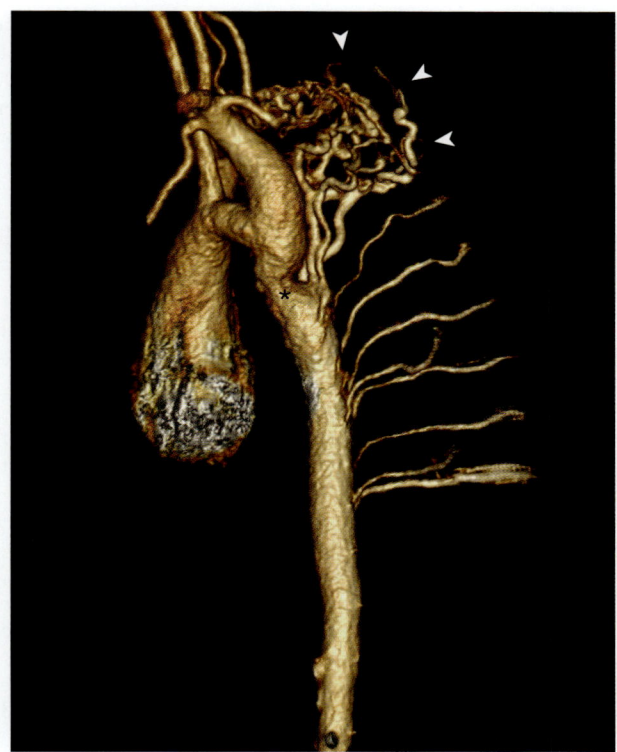

Figure 75-18   Aortic coarctation in a 14-year-old. Sagittal oblique three-dimensional magnetic resonance angiography reconstruction shows a discrete aortic coarctation distal to the left subclavian artery (*asterisk*) with multiple dilated tortuous collateral vessels arising proximal to the coarctation (*arrowheads*) and feeding the descending aorta distal to the coarctation.

After stabilization with medical therapy, urgent surgical repair is the treatment of choice.[66,67] Balloon angioplasty can be considered as an initial procedure for neonates at high surgical risk.[66]

Repair is performed on a more elective basis in patients who present in infancy or childhood with a murmur or upper extremity hypertension compared with critically ill neonates. Conventional therapy for aortic coarctation is surgical. Currently, the surgical procedure used most commonly in infants and children is resection of the coarctation with end-to-end or extended end-to-end anastomosis.[50,66,67] Other surgical procedures, including patch aortoplasty and subclavian flap repair, are less commonly performed as the procedure of choice in children because of the risk of aneurysm formation at the patch site with patch aortoplasty and left arm complications and remnant residual ductal tissue with the subclavian flap repair.[50,66] The efficacy of balloon angioplasty for native aortic coarctation in infants and children has been a topic of controversy because aneurysm formation and iliofemoral artery injury are reported as being higher[68] and the reintervention rate for recurrent stenosis may be higher than for conventional surgical therapy.[66] Stent placement can be considered for primary coarctation repair in children who weigh more than 10 to 15 kg.[69] The transcatheter approach is accepted therapy for treatment of recoarctation in all age groups.[66] Late complications after surgical or endovascular treatment include recurrent coarctation, aneurysm or pseudoaneurysm formation, aortic dissection, and hypertension.[50,66,70]

Interrupted Aortic Arch

Overview   Interrupted aortic arch (IAA) is rare and accounts for approximately 1.5% of congenital heart anomalies.[71] IAA consists of discontinuity between the ascending and descending aorta and is classified according to the location of the arch interruption.[72] Type A interruption is the second most common type (seen in 42% of cases), occurs at the isthmus just beyond the origin of the left subclavian artery, and is seen in association with aortopulmonary window with an intact ventricular septum and with transposition of the great arteries and VSD.[73] Type B interruption is most common (seen in 58% of cases), occurs between the left common carotid and left subclavian arteries, and usually is associated with conotruncal abnormalities, large posterior malalignment VSDs, and subaortic stenosis.[73] Type B interruption is associated with aberrant origin of the right subclavian artery from the descending aorta.[74] DiGeorge syndrome is relatively common in patients with type B IAA and often is associated with a right aortic arch.[75] Type C interruption is least common (appearing in 4% of cases) and occurs between the right and left common carotid arteries. A PDA is seen in nearly all persons with IAA. Other lesions reported in association with IAA include isolated VSD (73%),[71] ASD, bicommissural aortic valve, aortic stenosis, and more complex lesions including truncus arteriosus and the Taussig-Bing type of double-outlet right ventricle (see Chapter 76).[76]

Etiology, Pathophysiology, and Clinical Presentation   The embryology of IAA depends on the type of interruption. Type A is formed as a result of abnormal distal fourth arch regression during late development, after the ascent of the left subclavian artery. Type B results from an early regression of the fourth arch before migration of the left subclavian artery. Type C likely results from abnormal regression of portions of the left third and fourth arches.

The pathophysiology of IAA is similar to other obstructive left heart lesions such as aortic coarctation. Patients are dependent on blood flow through the PDA. Once ductal closure begins, patients may present with profound systemic acidosis, anuria, and ischemic injury to the abdominal organs and lower extremities. If adequate collateral vasculature develops, the clinical presentation can be delayed.

Imaging   IAA may be diagnosed prenatally. Postnatal imaging is directed at defining the arch sidedness and branching pattern, the site of arch interruption, the size of the proximal and distal portions of the arch, the distance of interruption, the size of the aortic annulus, and the presence of a PDA (Fig. 75-20).[71] Screening for other cardiovascular abnormalities also is performed. Echocardiography generally is sufficient for preoperative assessment. Cross-sectional imaging is obtained to better define arch branching or other cardiovascular anatomy as needed.

Treatment   PGE$_1$ infusion is begun upon patient presentation to keep the ductus arteriosus patent. Metabolic abnormalities are treated medically, and surgical repair is undertaken as soon as the infant is clinically stable.[71]

Complete surgical repair is performed in the neonatal period with generally good outcomes that depend on

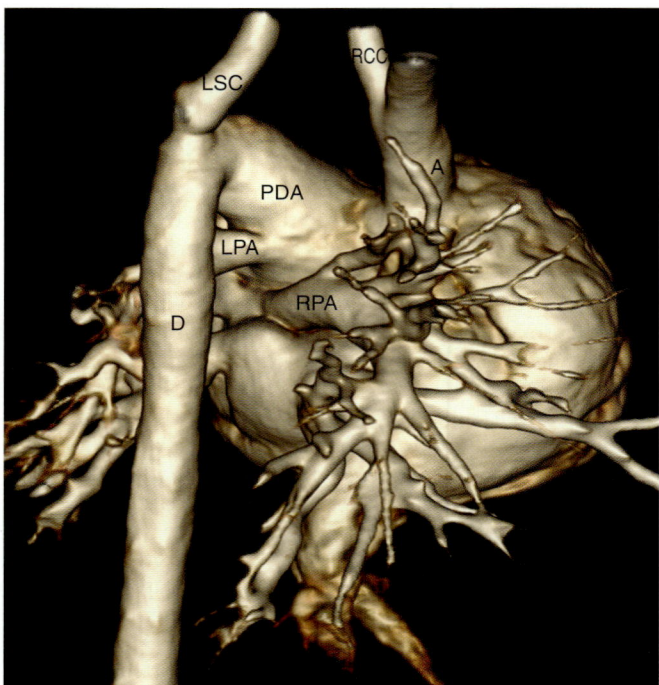

Figure 75-20 Newborn with type B interrupted aortic arch and truncus arteriosus. A three-dimensional computed tomography reconstruction right posterior view shows interruption of the aortic arch between the right common carotid (*RCC*) and left subclavian (*LSC*) arteries. The right (*RPA*) and left (*LPA*) pulmonary arteries arise from the pulmonary trunk. A large patent ductus arteriosus (*PDA*) supplies the descending aorta (*D*) from which the left subclavian artery arises. The common origin of the aorta and pulmonary artery from a single truncal valve is not shown. *A,* Ascending aorta.

associated cardiovascular lesions.[76] Direct arch anastomosis between the ascending and descending aorta with ductal ligation is the preferred technique. Homograft, pericardial patch, or autologous carotid artery augmentation may be needed if the arch is hypoplastic.[76] An intervening conduit generally is not placed unless associated anomalies are present. Surgical technique modifications performed as a result of associated anomalies are based on individual patient anatomy.[71]

Postoperatively, monitoring for arch obstruction or dilation at the site of anastomosis is necessary. The incidence of postoperative arch obstruction is low, with a reported 74%

actuarial freedom from arch obstruction necessitating reintervention at 15 years.[76] Assessment for complications related to other cardiovascular anomalies such as recurrent LVOT obstruction also is undertaken. Postoperative imaging generally is performed with echocardiography, with supplementary cross-sectional imaging as needed.

Key Points

Surgical palliation of HLHS is a staged reconstruction that involves three surgical procedures with the ultimate goal of creating separate pulmonary and systemic circulations supported by the right ventricle.

A bicuspid aortic valve is the most common cause of congenital aortic stenosis and is associated with aortic root dilation and aortic wall abnormalities.

The Ross procedure involves replacement of the aortic valve with a pulmonary valve annulus and trunk autograft, coronary reimplantation, and replacement of the pulmonary valve with an allograft conduit. It has the advantage of using the patient's own pulmonary valve.

Congestive heart failure presenting between the first and fourth weeks of life strongly suggests coarctation.

Suggested Readings

Abbruzzese PA, Aidala E. Aortic coarctation: an overview. *J Cardiovasc Med (Hagerstown).* 2007;8(2):123-128.

Egan M, Holzer RJ. Comparing balloon angioplasty, stenting and surgery in the treatment of aortic coarctation. *Expert Rev Cardiovasc Ther.* 2009;7(11):1401-1412.

Fernandes SM, Sanders SP, Khairy P, et al. Morphology of bicuspid aortic valve in children and adolescents. *J Am Coll Cardiol.* 2004;44(8):1648-1651.

Konen E, Merchant N, Provost Y, et al. Coarctation of the aorta before and after correction: the role of cardiovascular MRI. *AJR Am J Roentgenol.* 2004;182(5):1333-1339.

Ohye RG, Sleeper LA, Mahony L, et al. Comparison of shunt types in the Norwood procedure for single-ventricle lesions. *N Engl J Med.* 2010;362(21):1980-1992.

References

Full references for this chapter can be found on www.expertconsult.com.

Chapter 76

Conotruncal Anomalies

MARYAM GHADIMI MAHANI, PRACHI P. AGARWAL,
JIMMY C. LU, and ADAM L. DORFMAN

Conotruncal anomalies are a group of congenital heart defects involving the outflow tract of the heart and great vessels. The conotruncal anomalies include tetralogy of Fallot (TOF), transposition of the great arteries (TGA), double-outlet ventricles, and truncus arteriosus. Interrupted aortic arch type B also is a conotruncal anomaly that will be discussed with other aortic arch anomalies (see Chapter 75).

Conotruncal abnormalities are the result of abnormal division or rotation of the primitive truncus during embryologic development.[1,2] The common outlet of the embryonic univentricular heart normally undergoes a complex sequence of events to separate into the right ventricular outflow tract (RVOT) and left ventricular outflow tract (LVOT), the aorta, and the main pulmonary artery.[3] Control by numerous genes and migration of the mesenchymal cells from the embryonic neural crest are required for this development.[1] Mutations in a number of genes have been associated with conotruncal anomalies in humans and animal models.[4]

Echocardiography is the mainstay of clinical diagnosis. Conventional angiography is used primarily to evaluate coronary artery anatomy and aortopulmonary collaterals. Magnetic resonance imaging (MRI) and computed tomography (CT) occasionally are used to clarify anatomic details that are not fully delineated by echocardiography in the preoperative patient; these details often are related to the aortic arch, pulmonary arteries and their supply, and pulmonary veins. MRI and CT more often are requested for routine follow-up of patients with conotruncal anomalies, particularly as they reach their teenaged and adult years.

Tetralogy of Fallot

Overview TOF is the most common cyanotic congenital heart defect. The median described incidence of TOF is 356 per 1 million live births in the United States.[5] The classic manifestations include RVOT obstruction, ventricular septal defect (VSD), overriding of the aortic root above the VSD, and right ventricular (RV) hypertrophy (Fig. 76-1, *A*). These findings are a result of underdevelopment of the subpulmonary infundibulum,[6] which is associated with anterior deviation of the conal septum. Rather than sitting between the anterior and posterior limbs of the trabecula septomarginalis

(a Y-shaped bundle of muscle along the right side of the ventricular septum), the conal septum in TOF typically is fused with the anterior limb, bringing the aorta over the ventricular septum and leading to the malalignment VSD.[7,8] The septal malalignment and hypertrophy of the trabeculations of the infundibular free wall result in RVOT obstruction (Fig. 76-1, *B*). The VSD in TOF is located between the malaligned conal septum superiorly and the muscular septum inferiorly (i.e., a conoventricular septal defect),[9] and it typically is large, nonrestrictive, and subaortic. For further discussion of the trabecula septomarginalis, see the section of this chapter on double-outlet RV.

The anatomic appearance of TOF varies, including TOF with pulmonary atresia and TOF with dysplastic (absent) pulmonary valve syndrome. The extent of RVOT obstruction is variable, ranging from minimal obstruction to pulmonary atresia.[10] The pulmonary valve often is thickened or fused with doming leaflets and a variably hypoplastic annulus causing valvular stenosis. The size of the main and branch pulmonary arteries also varies. Patients with pulmonary valve atresia have no antegrade flow supplying the pulmonary arteries; instead, pulmonary blood flow is supplied by a patent ductus arteriosus, aortopulmonary collateral arteries, or both (e-Fig. 76-2). The central pulmonary arteries can be absent, discontinuous, or diminutive. In persons with TOF and a dysplastic pulmonary valve, congenital severe pulmonary regurgitation occurs, which often is associated with severe dilatation of the central pulmonary arteries and resultant airway compression (e-Fig. 76-3, *A* and *B*).[11]

Etiology, Pathophysiology, and Clinical Presentation Genetic abnormalities such as chromosome 22q11 deletion, which also leads to DiGeorge or velocardiofacial syndrome, may play an important role in some patients with this disease.[12] Many cases are sporadic, without any specific genetic abnormality identified.

Clinical manifestations are variable. Most patients have adequate pulmonary blood flow at birth, and increasing cyanosis develops early in life.[13] If RVOT obstruction is severe, right-to-left shunting occurs, resulting in cyanosis. When the obstruction is less severe, the shunting is predominantly left-to-right (so-called pink TOF); patients with this condition can present with congestive heart failure as a result of the

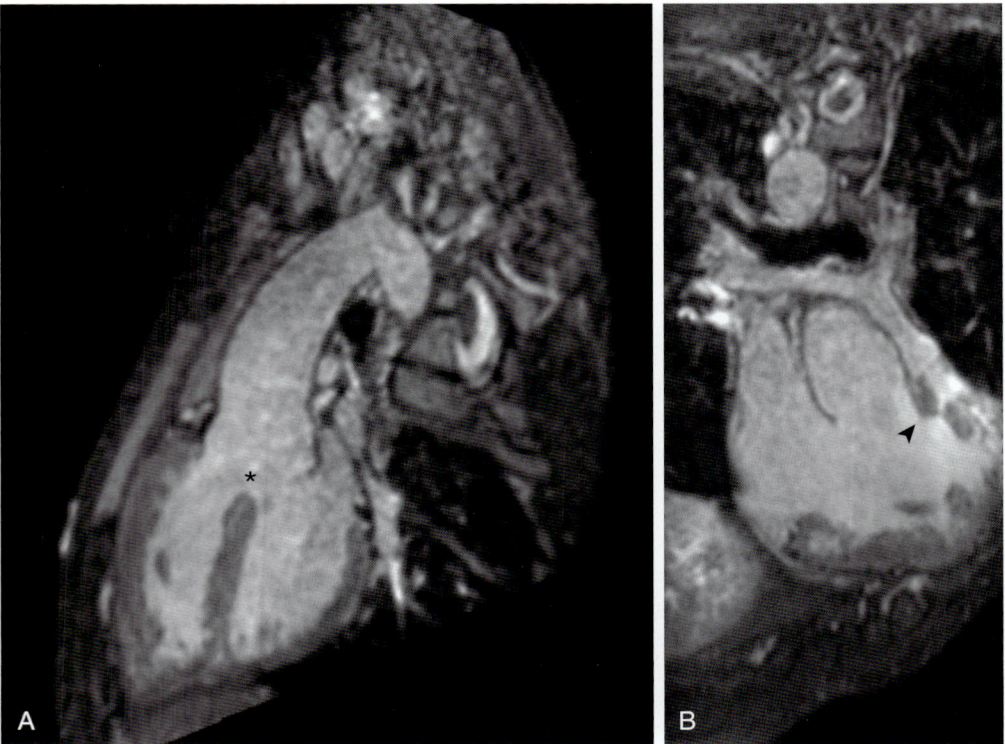

Figure 76-1   Three-dimensional steady-state free-precession imaging in an 18-year-old man with unrepaired tetralogy of Fallot. **A,** Sagittal oblique projection demonstrates the aorta overriding an anterior malalignment ventricular septal defect (*asterisk*). **B,** Coronal oblique projection demonstrates the deviation of the conal septum (*arrowhead*), leading to subvalvar and valvar pulmonary stenosis.

large VSD. Patients who have TOF with pulmonary atresia are dependent on the patent ductus arteriosus or aortopulmonary collaterals for pulmonary artery blood flow. If they are dependent on the patent ductus arteriosus, an infusion of prostaglandin E_1 is necessary to maintain ductal patency until a more stable supply of pulmonary blood flow can be established. In patients who have TOF with dysplastic pulmonary valve syndrome, presentation primarily may be with tracheo-bronchomalacia and air trapping, as well as cyanosis.

Other congenital heart anomalies can accompany TOF. These anomalies include right aortic arch (25%) and coronary artery anomalies such as abnormal origin of the left anterior descending (LAD) artery arising from the right coronary artery (5% to 6%) or dual LAD coronary arteries.[14] When the LAD artery arises from the right, it passes over the RVOT before supplying its usual territory (e-Fig. 76-4).

Imaging   RV hypertrophy causes uplifting of the cardiac apex. Concavity is present at the location of the main pulmonary artery because of underdevelopment, causing a "wooden shoe "or "boot shape" appearance of the heart (in French, *Coeur en sabot)* on frontal chest radiographs, a classic sign for TOF (Fig. 76-5). The shadow of the main pulmonary artery is absent, and pulmonary vascularity is decreased.[15] Rarely, dilatation of the pulmonary artery occurs as a result of an aneurysm or asymmetric pulmonary vascularity is present as a result of differential pulmonary artery stenosis and collateralization. In the absence of a thymus, the possibility

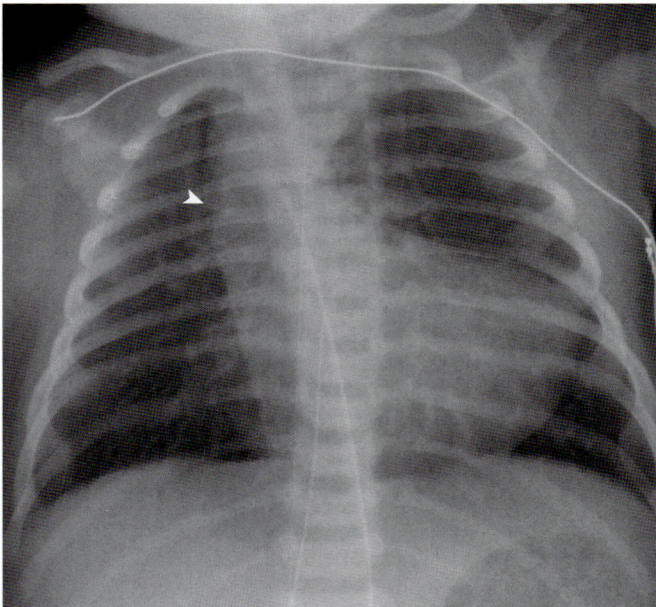

Figure 76-5   A 1-day-old girl who has tetralogy of Fallot with pulmonary atresia. Anteroposterior chest radiograph demonstrates the upturned apex and concavity in the region of the pulmonary artery (a boot-shaped heart). Note the shadow to the right of the trachea (*arrowhead*), which is indicative of a right aortic arch.

of DiGeorge syndrome should be considered. A right-sided aortic arch also can be seen on the frontal chest radiograph (see Fig. 76-5).

Complete anatomic diagnosis in a neonate with TOF usually is made by echocardiography, with an infrequent need for cross-sectional imaging. CT or MRI typically is requested to determine pulmonary artery anatomy and sources of pulmonary blood flow, including the central pulmonary arteries, patent ductus arteriosus, and aortopulmonary collaterals. CT angiography is an effective modality for delineating pulmonary artery and collateral anatomy in these patients, but it has the disadvantage of using ionizing radiation.[16] MRI also can accurately describe these anatomic details but without the risks of ionizing radiation. Turbo spin echo techniques can display vessels clearly, with the added advantage of demonstrating airway anatomy. The mainstay of MRI for these anatomic questions is three-dimensional, gadolinium contrast-enhanced magnetic resonance (MR) angiography, which is highly accurate compared with diagnostic catheterization.[17]

Treatment and Follow-up   Current management of TOF in most large centers is early single-stage reconstructive surgery, typically performed at 3 to 6 months of age.[18] Staged reconstruction can be required if significant hypoplasia of the central pulmonary arteries is present; a palliative shunt is placed from the systemic to the pulmonary circulation to provide stable pulmonary blood flow. When pulmonary supply is from multiple aortopulmonary collaterals, a staged approach of unifocalization of collaterals to either a shunt or the central pulmonary arteries is utilized, eventually bringing the major vessels into continuity with the RV. VSD closure often is not tolerated until later in life in this subgroup of patients.[18]

The goal of surgical repair of TOF is to close the VSD and relieve the RVOT obstruction, thus providing unobstructed flow to the pulmonary vessels from the RV. The approach depends on the anatomy, including the degree of

pulmonary valve annulus hypoplasia and anatomy of the pulmonary arteries. The entire repair can be performed transatrially, including VSD closure and division of muscle bundles within the RVOT to relieve obstruction, with no right ventriculotomy. If the pulmonary valve annulus is hypoplastic, a limited transannular patch may be needed to relieve the obstruction.[18] This procedure inevitably results in severe pulmonary regurgitation. In the past this operation was performed with a large right ventriculotomy, which now usually is avoided. In patients who have TOF with pulmonary atresia, a limited transannular patch may be sufficient to relieve RVOT obstruction. With a longer segment atresia, an RV to pulmonary artery conduit may be required. In patients with an LAD coronary artery arising from the right coronary artery and crossing the RVOT, an RV to pulmonary artery conduit occasionally is necessary to avoid damaging the vessel (see e-Fig. 76-4).[11]

In patients with a transannular patch, a pulmonary valve replacement may be indicated later in life to remove the volume load of pulmonary regurgitation from the RV (Video 76-1). The appropriate timing of this valve replacement is the subject of intense interest.[19] In patients who require an RV to pulmonary artery conduit, a conduit replacement will be needed in time because of the somatic growth of the patient. More recently, a percutaneous pulmonary valve has become available for placement within a conduit to relieve both stenosis and regurgitation (Video 76-2).

Repaired TOF is a frequent referral diagnosis for cardiac MRI. Chronic, severe pulmonary regurgitation can lead to RV pathology. Cardiac MRI is widely considered the gold standard for assessment of RV size and function, making it particularly useful in this patient population (Video 76-3). Other questions in this patient population include anatomy of the RVOT (Video 76-4), quantification of pulmonary regurgitation (Video 76-5 and Fig. 76-6, *A*), assessment of branch and segmental pulmonary artery anatomy, measurement of branch pulmonary artery flow, anatomy of

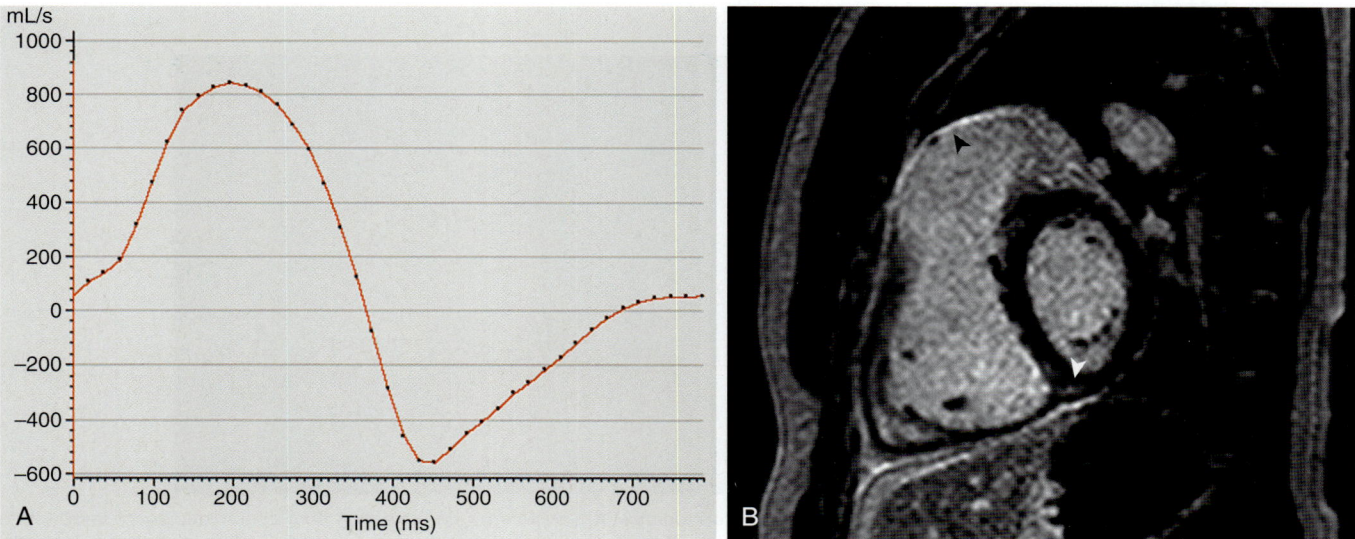

Figure 76-6   Cardiovascular magnetic resonance evaluation of a 31-year-old man with tetralogy of Fallot after he underwent repair of the lesion. **A,** Graphical representation (flux vs. time) of antegrade and regurgitant flow in the main pulmonary artery. This patient had severe pulmonary insufficiency, with a regurgitant fraction of 57%. **B,** Late gadolinium enhancement imaging in the short axis of the ventricles demonstrates enhancement (*arrowheads*) along the right ventricular outflow tract and at the inferior insertion point of the interventricular septum. See Videos 76-3, 76-4, and 76-5.

aortopulmonary collaterals, assessment of the left ventricle (LV), and aortic valve and root pathology.

These studies typically are performed with steady-state free-precession imaging in the vertical and horizontal long-axis planes and short axis of the ventricles, as well as parallel to the RVOT. Gadolinium-enhanced three-dimensional MR angiography offers high-resolution assessment of the distal pulmonary arteries and can evaluate for aortopulmonary collaterals. Velocity-encoded phase-contrast imaging assesses the ratio of pulmonary to systemic flow, differential pulmonary blood flow, and valve regurgitation. Delayed enhancement imaging reveals scarring or fibrosis in the heart (Fig. 76-6, *B*).[1,11]

Use of CT for patients with repaired TOF generally is restricted to evaluation of pulmonary artery anatomy and aortic size, particularly in patients in whom MRI is contraindicated (e.g., patients with an internal defibrillator). Electrocardiographic-gated multidetector array computed tomography can provide RV size and systolic function, although with less temporal resolution than MRI.

Transposition of the Great Arteries

Overview TGA is defined by discordant ventriculoarterial relations; the aorta is connected to the RV and the pulmonary artery is connected to the LV. The most common type of TGA, defined by the segmental anatomy of the heart, is {S, D, D} transposition—that is, visceral and atrial situs solitus (S), ventricular D loop (D), and dextroposition of the aortic valve (D) (see Chapter 63). The aortic valve is side by side or anterior and rightward of the pulmonary valve (Fig. 76-7, *A*) and usually is separated from the tricuspid valve by conal tissue. "D-looped TGA" also is acceptable terminology.[1]

{S, D, D} TGA is the second most common cyanotic congenital heart disease.[11] The median described incidence of {S, D, D} TGA is 303 per 1 million live births.[5]

Etiology, Pathophysiology, and Clinical Presentation TGA usually is not associated with extracardiac anomalies or syndromes.[15] It is associated with VSD in approximately 40% to 45% of cases. Other anomalies that can be seen in patients with TGA are LVOT obstruction, aortic coarctation or interrupted aortic arch, tricuspid valve abnormalities, or, less commonly, mitral valve abnormalities, leftward juxtaposition of the atrial appendages, and RV hypoplasia.[20]

Patients present with cyanosis as a result of parallel systemic and pulmonary circulations. Deoxygenated blood returns to the right atrium via systemic veins, then passes through the RV to the aorta. Pulmonary venous blood returns to the left atrium and LV, then back to the pulmonary artery. Survival depends on communications between the systemic and pulmonary circulations, typically via an atrial septal defect, patent ductus arteriosus, and/or VSD.

Imaging The radiographic appearance is variable. The classic finding of TGA by chest radiography is the "egg on a string" sign (Fig. 76-7, *B*), which is caused by a narrow mediastinum and the cardiac shadow. The narrow mediastinum is a result of stress-related thymic atrophy and the parallel position of the great vessels, with the pulmonary artery obscured by the aorta. The heart size varies from normal to enlarged.[15]

Cross-sectional imaging is seldom used for preoperative evaluation of TGA, but it can be helpful for specific questions that are unanswered by echocardiography, typically complex associated abnormalities of the aorta or pulmonary arteries. MRI often is preferred instead of CT to avoid the risks of ionizing radiation. In some centers, CT may be preferred because it offers greater accessibility and decreases the need for anesthesia or sedation as a result of shorter scanning times. CT scans should be performed with parameters optimized to minimize exposure of the patient to ionizing radiation.

Treatment and Follow-up In newborn infants with {S, D, D} TGA, adequacy of the communications between the pulmonary and systemic circulations is critical. Infusion of

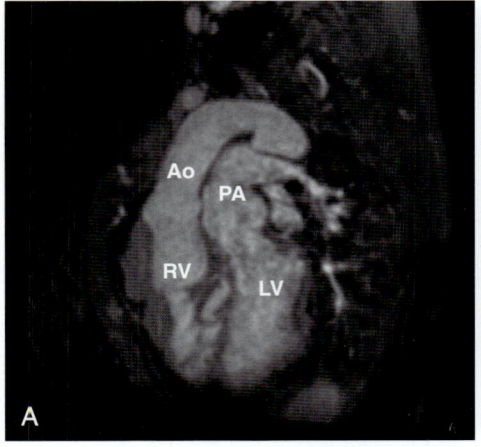
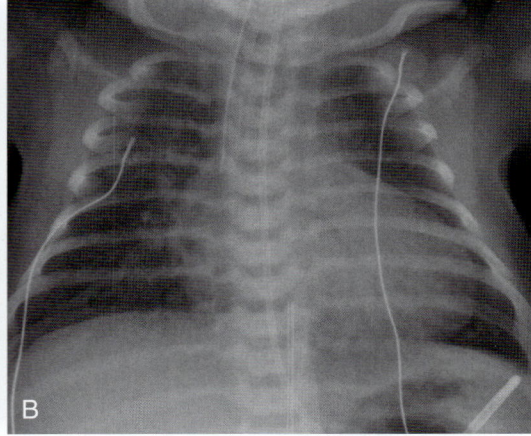

Figure 76-7 Imaging appearance of {S,D,D} transposition of the great arteries. **A,** Sagittal oblique projection from three-dimensional steady-state free-precession imaging in a 29-year-old woman with {S,D,D} transposition of the great arteries, after an atrial switch procedure, demonstrates parallel outflow tracts, with the aorta (*Ao*) arising from the right ventricle (*RV*) and the pulmonary artery (*PA*) arising from the left ventricle (*LV*). **B,** A chest radiograph of a neonate with {S,D,D} TGA prior to repair. As a result of the parallel, anterior-posterior relationship of the great arteries, patients with {S,D,D} transposition of the great arteries have a narrow mediastinum, which, combined with cardiomegaly and increased vascular flow, produces the classic "egg on a string" appearance.

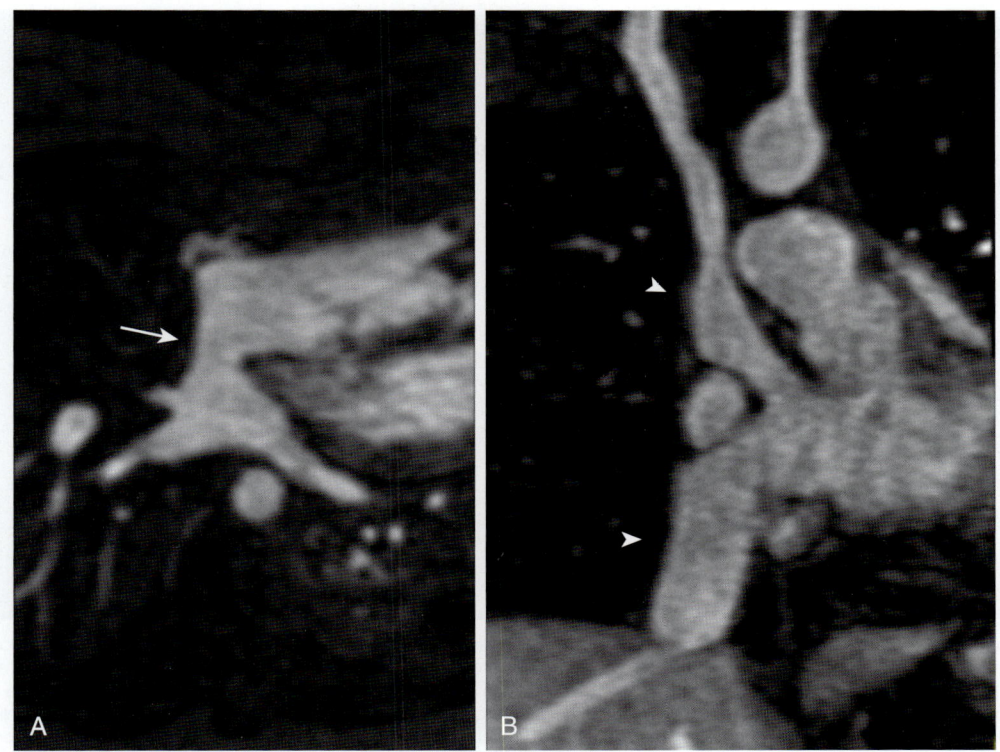

Figure 76-8 A contrast-enhanced magnetic resonance angiogram in a 29-year-old woman with {S,D,D} transposition of the great arteries, after an atrial switch procedure. **A,** Transverse oblique projection demonstrating an unobstructed pulmonary venous baffle (*arrow*) to the tricuspid valve. **B,** A coronal oblique projection demonstrating unobstructed pathways from the superior and inferior vena cavae (*arrowheads*) to the mitral valve. See Video 76-6.

prostaglandin E_1 maintains ductal patency. If the atrial septum is restrictive, urgent cardiac catheterization for balloon atrial septostomy often is required.[21] In this procedure, a balloon septostomy catheter is passed across the atrial septum into the left atrium. The balloon is inflated and the catheter is sharply pulled back, fracturing the septum and enlarging the opening, allowing for greater mixing of oxygenated and deoxygenated blood.

In the early days of surgical repair of TGA, the atrial switch was used (i.e., "Mustard" or "Senning" procedures). With the atrial switch procedure, an intraatrial baffle is created with use of pericardium or native atrial tissue, which directs systemic venous return to the morphologic LV and pulmonary artery, and pulmonary venous return to the morphologic RV and aorta (Fig. 76-8, *A* and *B*).

The atrial switch has been replaced by the arterial switch operation, which has been used widely in the United States since the mid to late 1980s. In this operation the ascending aorta and pulmonary artery are transected at the sinotubular junction and anastomosed to the concordant ventricle, the aorta to the left and the pulmonary artery to the right, after the pulmonary artery is relocated anterior to the aorta (the "Lecompte maneuver") (Fig. 76-9, *A*). The coronary arteries are relocated from the native aorta to the neoaorta (Fig. 76-9, *B*).[22]

In the presence of a VSD and LVOT obstruction, a Rastelli repair can be performed,[23] with baffling of the LV through the VSD to the native aortic valve, along with placement of an RV to the pulmonary artery conduit (e-Fig. 76-10).

Each of these procedures can be associated with early and late complications. Attention to these specific complications is essential on follow-up imaging.

For the atrial switch procedure, the following early and mid-term complications may occur:
1. Systemic baffle obstruction, most commonly affecting the superior limb of the baffle at the junction of the right atrium with the superior vena cava[24]
2. Baffle leaks (in approximately 20% of patients) (e-Fig. 76-11)[25]
3. Pulmonary venous obstruction (less common) (e-Fig. 76-12)

The most important complication after the atrial switch procedure, early or late, is failure of the systemic RV and tricuspid regurgitation. Less common complications include conduction and rhythm disturbances, which might require mechanical pacing or even cause sudden death.[11]

MRI is frequently used for assessment after the atrial switch procedure is performed. The MRI protocol is tailored for assessment of the aforementioned complications.[1,11] Specifically, MRI is useful for the following assessments:
1. Evaluation of the size and function of the ventricles (Video 76-6)
2. Evaluation of the systemic and pulmonary venous pathways for obstruction and/or baffle leak(s) (e-Fig. 76-13)
3. Assessment of tricuspid valve regurgitation
4. Evaluation of the LVOT and RVOT for obstruction
5. Late gadolinium enhancement for evaluation of fibrosis in the RV[26]

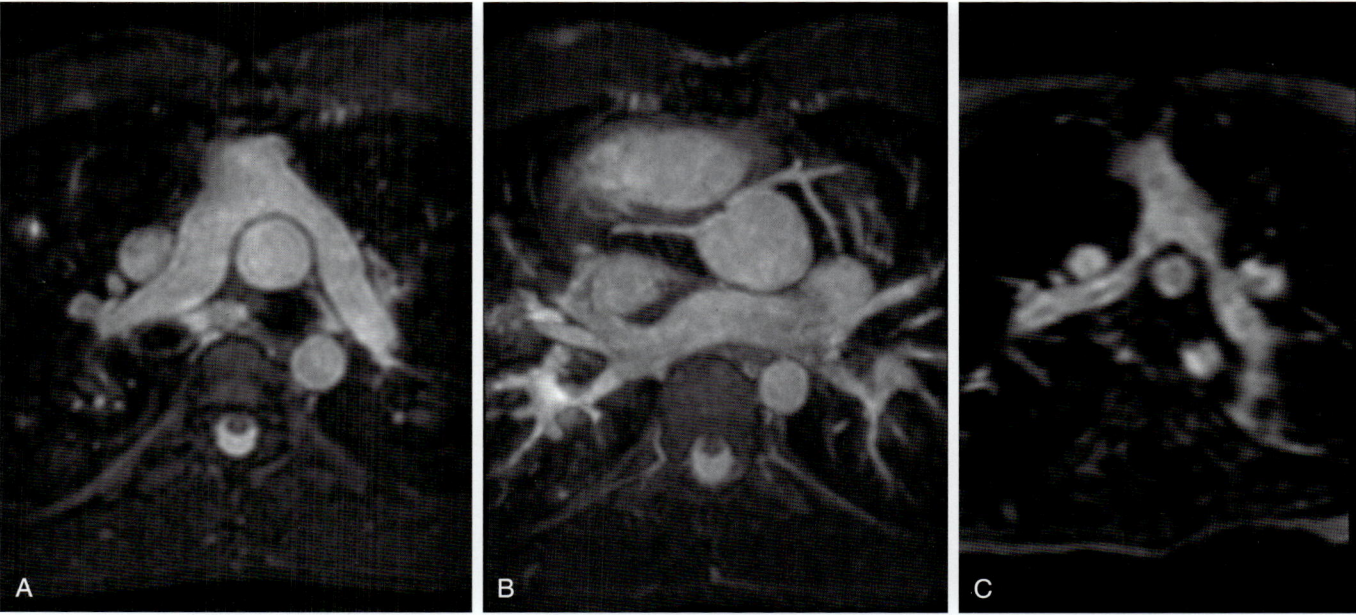

Figure 76-9 Cardiovascular magnetic resonance evaluation after arterial switch operation. **A,** Transverse projection demonstrating the pulmonary artery bifurcation anterior to the ascending aorta, with no narrowing of the proximal branch pulmonary arteries. **B,** Maximum intensity projection in the transverse oblique plane from three-dimensional steady-state free precession in a 16-year-old boy with {S,D,D} transposition of the great arteries, after an arterial switch operation, demonstrates unobstructed proximal coronary arteries that have been translocated to the facing sinuses of the native pulmonary (neoaortic) root. **C,** Transverse oblique projection of a contrast-enhanced magnetic resonance angiogram in a 19-month boy with {S,D,D} transposition of the great arteries, after an arterial switch operation, demonstrates proximal narrowing of both left and right branch pulmonary arteries.

The arterial switch procedure uses the LV as the systemic ventricle and therefore is favored. The following potential complications may occur after the arterial switch procedure is performed:

1. RVOT obstruction
2. Stenosis at the arterial anastomotic sites, most commonly pulmonary stenosis
3. Branch pulmonary artery obstruction (see Fig. 76-9, C)
4. Aortic root dilatation
5. Neoaortic valve regurgitation
6. Coronary artery ostial stenosis[27]

MRI also is used frequently for assessment of patients who have undergone an arterial switch procedure, with clinical questions dictated by the aforementioned potential complications[1,11]:

1. RV and LV size and function
2. Evaluation of the RVOT and LVOT for obstruction and for valvular regurgitation
3. Evaluation of the great arteries
4. Evaluation of the coronary arteries

The Rastelli repair includes a conduit that does not grow with the patient and can become stenotic and/or regurgitant. In addition, the baffle from the LV to the aorta can become obstructed, often at the level of the VSD, resulting in subaortic stenosis. After a Rastelli-type repair, answers to the following primary questions may be sought with MRI:

1. LV and RV size and systolic function
2. Anatomy and potential obstruction of the LV to aorta pathway
3. Stenosis and regurgitation of the RV to pulmonary artery conduit

MRI protocols are similar to those previously described for TOF, although additional sequences often are needed. For example, an axial steady-state free-precession stack can help define post-Lecompte pulmonary artery anatomy and the venous baffles of the atrial switch. Oblique steady-state free-precession imaging along the LVOT is performed to rule out obstruction of the Rastelli pathway.

CT is used postoperatively in selected cases to answer anatomic questions, particularly when MRI is contraindicated. CT is particularly useful for assessment of extracardiac anatomy such as repaired aortic coarctation, arterial anastomotic sites, and branch pulmonary arteries after an arterial switch procedure is performed (e-Fig. 76-14) and venous baffles after an atrial switch procedure is performed. Functional evaluation of the heart is limited compared with MRI.

Physiologically Corrected Transposition of the Great Arteries

Overview Physiologically corrected or {S,L,L} TGA is rare, with an estimated incidence of 30 per 1 million live births.[28] The segmental anatomy of this lesion is visceral and atrial situs solitus (S), L-ventricular loop (L), and levo-malposition of the aortic valve (L) (see Chapter 63). In L-looped TGA, atrioventricular and ventriculoarterial discordance occurs. The morphologic RV receives the pulmonary venous blood via the left atrium and connects to the aorta (Fig. 76-15, A, and Video 76-7). The LV receives systemic venous blood via

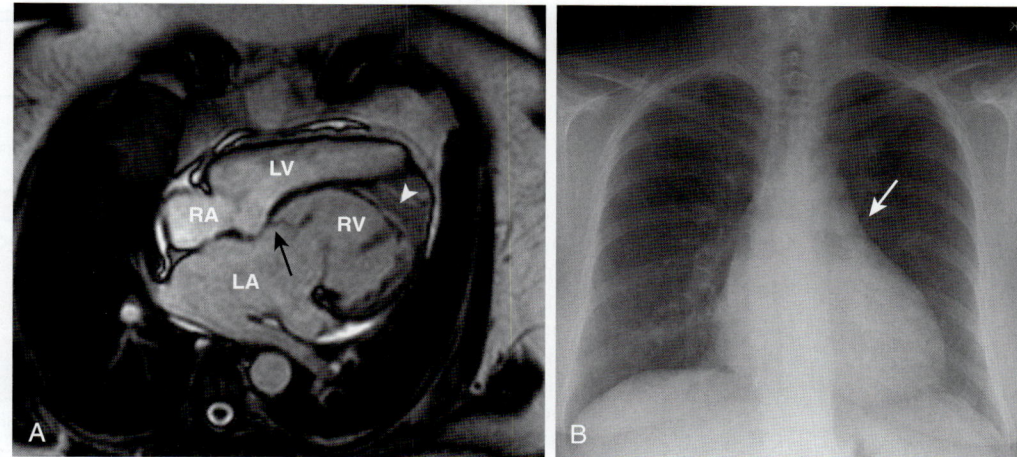

Figure 76-15 Imaging characteristics of {S,L,L} congenitally corrected transposition of the great arteries in a 56-year-old woman with no previous intervention. **A,** Steady-state free-precession imaging in the four-chamber view demonstrates apical displacement of the septal insertion of the left-sided atrioventricular valve (*black arrow*) and a moderator band (*white arrowhead*) and coarse trabeculation of the left-sided ventricle, consistent with a left-sided morphologic right ventricle (*RV*). Note the bowing of the septum into the right-sided, morphologic left (subpulmonary) ventricle (*LV*). **B,** A posterior-anterior chest radiograph demonstrates a straightened upper left heart border (*arrow*) as a result of leftward malposition of the aorta. *LA,* Left atrium; *RA,* right atrium. See Video 76-7.

the right atrium and connects to the pulmonary artery. The outflow tracts are parallel and the aorta is leftward and anterior to the pulmonary artery.

Etiology, Pathophysiology, and Clinical Presentation Physiologically corrected TGA is attributed to abnormal cardiac looping during embryologic development. It can be characterized as ventricular inversion, with the systemic and pulmonary circulations in series. Most patients have associated heart lesions, but if no associated lesions are present, the patient is not cyanotic and typically is asymptomatic in early life. Patients with this lesion can present for the first time in adulthood, although this presentation is not typical.

More than 90% of patients with physiologically corrected TGA have additional anatomic abnormalities. Associated anomalies include dextrocardia, tricuspid valve abnormalities such as Ebstein anomaly, VSD (e-Fig. 76-16), RV hypoplasia, subvalvar and valvar pulmonary stenosis (Video 76-8), and conduction abnormalities, including complete heart block.[1]

Imaging The ascending aorta is not visible on the right and the descending aorta and pulmonary artery may not be visible on the left. The vascular pedicle looks narrow, and straightening of the left heart border occurs as a result of the anterior and leftward position of the aorta. The cardiac silhouette has a "humped" appearance and is more vertical than usual (see Fig. 76-15, *B*).[29] In the presence of systemic atrioventricular valve regurgitation and ventricular dysfunction, the heart may be enlarged. Dextrocardia or mesocardia also occurs with {S,L,L} TGA; if the chest radiograph reveals the gastric bubble on the left (abdominal situs solitus) and the apex of the heart on the right, this lesion should be suspected. Findings seen with associated cardiac lesions such as VSD and pulmonary atresia also can be detected.

MRI is useful in patients with {S,L,L} TGA who have not undergone surgery mainly for the assessment of systemic RV function and tricuspid regurgitation. In preoperative patients, MRI can evaluate RV size and assess the morphology of the cardiac chambers, particularly in relationship to a VSD and the great arteries if a complex intraventricular baffle repair is planned.

CT can evaluate coronary artery and extracardiac anatomy. In patients who undergo pacing because of a complete heart block, electrocardiographic–gated multidetector array computed tomography can be used to assess RV size and systolic function.

Treatment and Follow-up The early management of patients with physiologically corrected TGA who have no associated structural anomalies is controversial. Because this lesion is noncyanotic and usually asymptomatic, it can be managed medically.[11,30] However, some physicians believe that earlier surgery should be performed, particularly in the presence of tricuspid valve (systemic) regurgitation.[31]

Until the early to mid 1990s, repair of physiologically corrected TGA was intended only to repair the pertinent associated anomalies, including VSD, pulmonary stenosis or atresia, and tricuspid valve abnormalities,[22] leaving the RV as the systemic ventricle. However, in many patients with physiologically corrected transposition, systemic (RV) ventricular failure develops over time.[32] Tricuspid (systemic atrioventricular) valve regurgitation also is associated with RV dysfunction and heart failure. In addition to RV failure and tricuspid regurgitation, complete heart block develops in many patients. These complications become more prevalent with increasing patient age and have led to greater interest in performing early surgery for an anatomic correction with a systemic LV. Depending on the individual anatomy, this correction can be accomplished with a combination of an atrial switch with an arterial switch (a "double switch"), or, in the presence of LVOT obstruction and a VSD, with a Rastelli procedure.[22] In the absence of significant LVOT obstruction, the LV is not prepared to function at systemic pressure. A pulmonary artery band is first placed to "train" the LV to pump at higher pressures. After approximately 6 months, the complete repair is undertaken.

The complications associated with these operations are the same as those associated with the individual procedures, previously described in detail. MRI and CT can assess the atrial switch and arterial switch or intraventricular baffle (Rastelli repair), as previously delineated.

Double-Outlet Right Ventricle

Overview According to the Congenital Heart Surgery Nomenclature and Database Project, double-outlet right ventricle (DORV) is "a type of ventriculoarterial connection in which both great vessels arise entirely or predominantly from the right ventricle."[33] DORV has been defined by some investigators as the degree of aortic override, with diagnosis if the aorta is more than 50% over the RV.[34] However, this definition can be difficult to apply practically, because the degree of override may appear different from various anatomic planes, which can lead to lack of clarity, for example, in differentiating DORV from TOF. The absence of fibrous continuity between the aortic and mitral valve also has been referred to as a criterion for diagnosis of DORV; however, according to the Congenital Heart Surgery Nomenclature and Database Project, this finding should not be used as an absolute prerequisite for the diagnosis of DORV.[33,35] Although the definition may be problematic, the median described incidence of DORV is 127 per 1 million live births.[5]

The anatomy and consequent physiology of a person with DORV is differentiated by the position of the VSD, the conal morphology, and the relationship of the great vessels. An understanding of these anatomic-physiologic variants is important to the surgical approach and management of the patients.[1] The VSD usually is found between the limbs of the trabecula septomarginalis (Fig. 76-17). The aorta can be located rightward and posterior, directly rightward, anterior and rightward, directly anterior, or anterior and leftward of the pulmonary artery (Fig. 76-18, *A*). Because both vessels arise from one ventricle, abnormal positioning of the great arteries is termed "malposition" rather than "transposition."[36]

The relationship of the VSD to the conal septum and great arteries has been used as the basis for one of the most widely used clinical classifications, in which DORV is classified into four anatomic subtypes (see Fig. 76-17). This clinical classification was first described by Lev et al. in 1972[35,37]:

1. DORV with subaortic VSD (most common): the conal septum (outlet septum) is attached to the anterior limbus of the trabecula septomarginalis
2. DORV with subpulmonary VSD: the conal septum is attached to the posterior limbus of the trabecula septomarginalis
3. DORV with doubly committed VSD: the conal septum is hypoplastic or absent
4. DORV with noncommitted VSD: the defect is located at the inlet or at the trabecular zone of the interventricular septum, usually as an atrioventricular canal–type or apical muscular defect

Etiology, Pathophysiology, and Clinical Presentation In one review, chromosomal abnormalities, including trisomies 13 and 18 and deletion of chromosome 22q11, were the most commonly associated cytogenetic lesions.[35]

DORV also can be classified by physiologic subtypes, which dictate clinical presentation[1]:

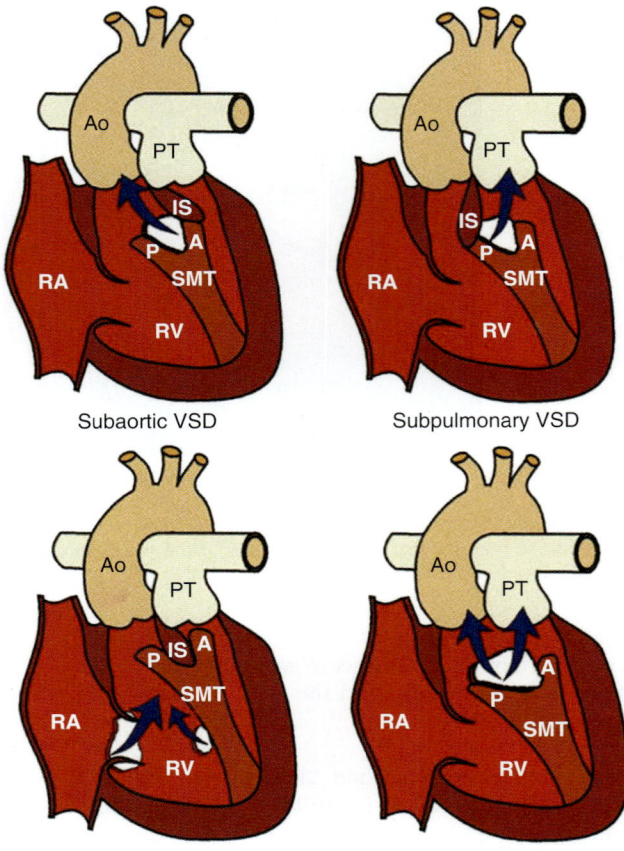

Subaortic VSD

Subpulmonary VSD

Noncommitted VSD

Doubly-committed VSD

Figure 76-17 Types of double-outlet right ventricle, classified by relationship of the ventricular septal defect and great arteries. *A,* anterior limb; *Ao,* aorta; *IS,* infundibular septum; *P,* posterior limb; *PT,* pulmonary trunk; *RA,* right atrium; *RV,* right ventricle; *SMT,* trabecula septomarginalis; *VSD,* ventricular septal defect. (From Peixoto LB, Leal SMB, Silva CES et al. Double outlet right ventricle with anterior and left-sided aorta and subpulmonary ventricular septal defect, *Arq Bras Cardiol.* 1999;73:446-450.)

1. VSD physiology: Subaortic VSD and no pulmonary stenosis
2. TOF physiology: Subaortic VSD and pulmonary stenosis
3. TGA physiology: Subpulmonary VSD, with or without systemic outflow obstruction
4. Single-ventricle physiology: DORV with mitral atresia, unbalanced atrioventricular canal, or severe hypoplasia of one of the ventricular sinuses (often in association with heterotaxy syndrome)

DORV is associated with several cardiac anomalies. VSD is almost ubiquitous. Obstruction to either pulmonary or systemic outflow is common. Coarctation of the aorta is common in patients with a subpulmonary VSD, particularly when aortic outflow is obstructed. Coronary artery anomalies often follow the physiology. For example, in DORV with subaortic VSD and pulmonary stenosis (TOF-type), supply of the LAD coronary artery from the right coronary artery can occur, crossing the subpulmonary outflow tract. In DORV with subpulmonary VSD (TGA-type), anomalies can vary, such as the circumflex coronary artery supplied from the right coronary artery.[11]

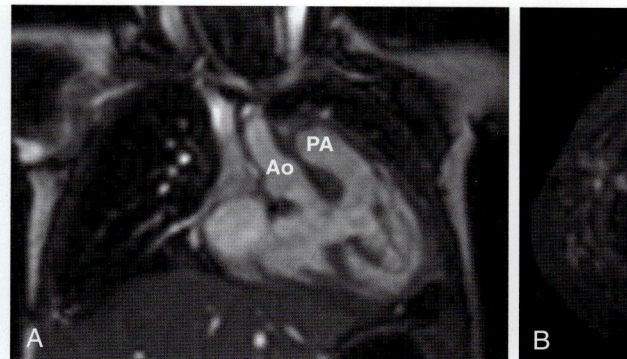
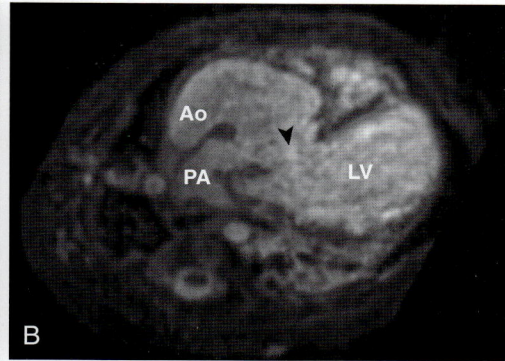

Figure 76-18 Examples of variations of double-outlet right ventricle (DORV). **A,** A coronal oblique steady-state free-precession image in a 5-month old girl with DORV, side-by-side great arteries (aorta to the right), with no subaortic or subpulmonary stenosis, requiring previous pulmonary artery banding. **B,** Transverse oblique projection from three-dimensional steady-state free-precession imaging in a 4-month-old boy with DORV, anterior-posterior great arteries (aorta anterior to the pulmonary artery), subpulmonary ventricular septal defect (VSD) (*arrowhead*), and subvalvar and valvar pulmonary stenosis. This patient subsequently underwent a Rastelli procedure, with complicated baffle of the VSD to the anterior aortic valve and a right ventricle to the pulmonary artery conduit. *Ao,* aorta; *PA,* pulmonary artery; *LV,* left ventricle.

Imaging Given the many anatomic and physiologic variants of DORV, no specific pattern is described in the chest radiograph of patients with DORV. Chest radiograph findings follow the anatomic-physiologic type of DORV, such as an enlarged heart and increased pulmonary vascular markings in persons with a VSD, decreased pulmonary vascularity, a concave main pulmonary artery shadow and upward lifted heart apex in persons with TOF, or varied findings in persons with TGA, sometimes including cardiomegaly and increased pulmonary vascularity.

Echocardiography is adequate for diagnosis and surgical planning in most newborns or infants with DORV. Cardiac MRI or CT is helpful in the evaluation of complex anomalies of the aortic arch, pulmonary arteries, aortopulmonary collaterals, and systemic or pulmonary venous anomalies that are not completely delineated by echocardiography. Considerations for CT versus MRI have been discussed previously. Assessment of the relationship between the VSD and the position of the great vessels in relation to the conal septum also can be answered by cardiac MRI (Fig. 76-18, *B*)[1] and can be helpful in planning complex surgical baffling of the LV to the aorta. In addition, MRI can accurately assess the size of the RV when its adequacy for a two-ventricle repair is in question.

Treatment and Follow-up The goal of surgical treatment of DORV is the connection of the LV to the systemic circulation and the RV to the pulmonary circulation. The preferred approach is to use an intraventricular tunnel repair, but such a repair may not be possible because of anatomic barriers, which may preclude a two-ventricle circulation. Alternative surgical procedures have been applied in these situations.[33]

In patients with a subaortic VSD, an intraventricular patch directing LV outflow to the aorta is the usual approach. Resection of RVOT obstruction, with or without an outflow patch, may be necessary, analogous to TOF repair. In persons with subpulmonary VSD, an intraventricular patch can be used to direct LV outflow to the pulmonary artery, which is accompanied by an arterial switch operation. Alternatively, the pulmonary artery can be closed proximally, the LV baffled through the VSD to the aorta, and a valved conduit placed between the RV and distal pulmonary artery (Rastelli

procedure).[36] More complex forms of DORV with heterotaxy syndrome, severe hypoplasia or absence of one of the ventricular sinuses, major straddling of an AV valve, or mitral atresia are palliated as a single ventricle.[1]

MRI is an important modality in the assessment of patients with repaired DORV. Questions for MRI depend on the anatomic-physiologic subtype of DORV and follow the descriptions in the previous sections for MRI of TOF and {S,D,D} TGA. In addition, assessment of the LV to aortic pathway for potential obstruction is crucial, similar to the aforementioned description for a Rastelli repair. Imaging for patients with single ventricle physiology can be found under the section regarding Fontan imaging in Chapter 74.

Similarly, CT is useful in assessing patients with repaired DORV, with questions analogous to those previously described for TOF and {S,D,D} TGA.

Truncus Arteriosus

Overview Truncus arteriosus is defined as a single vessel arising from the heart that has a single semilunar valve, giving rise to the coronary arteries, aorta, and at least one branch of the pulmonary artery. Truncus arteriosus is uncommon, with a reported incidence of 94 per 1 million live births.[5]

The classification of truncus arteriosus is based on the branching pattern of the pulmonary arteries. Van Praagh and Van Praagh modified the original classification of Collett and Edwards[1,38]:

- Type I: The branch pulmonary arteries arise from a short main pulmonary artery
- Type II: The branch pulmonary arteries arise directly from the arterial trunk through separate orifices (Fig. 76-19, *A* and *B*)
- Type III: One branch pulmonary artery arises from the ascending segment of the trunk; collateral vessels usually supply the contralateral lung
- Type IV: Truncus arteriosus with aortic arch hypoplasia, coarctation, or interruption (usually type B, between the common carotid and subclavian arteries) (see Chapter 75).

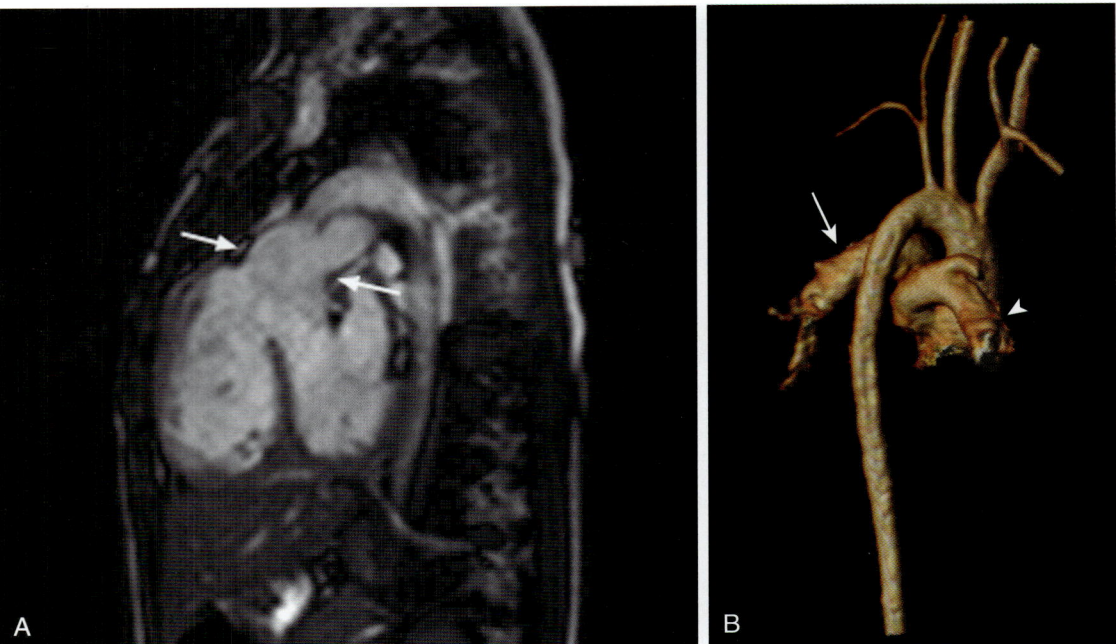

Figure 76-19 Cardiac magnetic resonance imaging of a 3-year-old girl with unrepaired truncus arteriosus, type II. **A,** A sagittal oblique steady-state free-precession image demonstrates a truncal root (*arrows*) overriding a conoventricular ventricular septal defect, with the origin of the pulmonary arteries from the truncal root. **B,** A three-dimensional reconstruction (viewed posteriorly) from a contrast-enhanced magnetic resonance angiogram demonstrates the origin of the left (*arrow*) and right (*arrowhead*) branch pulmonary arteries from the truncal root.

Etiology, Pathophysiology, and Clinical Presentation Truncus arteriosus results from failure of septation of the conotruncus into a separate aorta and pulmonary artery. It is associated with DiGeorge syndrome and chromosome 22q11 deletion.[39]

The semilunar valve of the truncus, that is, the truncal valve, is most often tricommissural. A bicommissural or quadricommissural valve occurs less frequently. The truncal valve often is thickened with deformed leaflets, causing stenosis or insufficiency. The conal septum is usually absent, and a malalignment VSD is present in almost all patients (>80%). An interrupted aortic arch is a common associated lesion (occurring in 11% to 14% of patients). Abnormalities of the mitral valve, coronary arteries, and pulmonary venous connections also are among the associated cardiac abnormalities.[11,38]

Neonates with truncus arteriosus generally are asymptomatic, while pulmonary vascular resistance remains elevated. As pulmonary vascular resistance decreases in early life, excessive pulmonary blood flow and symptoms of congestive heart failure develop. These children are at high risk for pulmonary vascular disease if they are not treated in the first 3 to 6 months of life.[18]

Imaging Cardiomegaly, increased pulmonary vascularity, and right-sided aortic arch (in 30% of cases) are consistent with truncus arteriosus (e-Fig. 76-20). A depressed diaphragm and thymic atrophy also are noted.

In most neonates with this diagnosis, echocardiography is sufficient for anatomic diagnosis and surgical planning. Evaluation with MRI or CT is helpful for extracardiac anatomy that is difficult to fully delineate by echocardiography, such as complex aortic arch or pulmonary arterial anomalies.

Treatment and Follow-up Surgical repair is undertaken within the first few weeks of life. In 1968, McGoon et al.[40] described the first surgical repair of truncus arteriosus. In this description, the pulmonary arteries were separated from the aorta, and a valved homograft was placed from the RV to the pulmonary arteries. The VSD was closed with a patch to align the truncal valve with the LV. This technique, which is similar to the Rastelli procedure, remains the predominant method of repair of truncus arteriosus.[18] Aortic arch interruption or coarctation is repaired at the same time. A severe valve abnormality can be addressed at the time of repair as well.[41]

In the absence of associated lesions, repair can be accomplished with very good survival rates in the neonatal and early infancy period.[42] Newborns with truncus arteriosus and associated interrupted aortic arch have a poorer prognosis.[43]

Important complications after truncal repair are RV–pulmonary artery conduit stenosis or regurgitation, branch pulmonary artery stenosis, neoaortic valve (truncal) insufficiency or stenosis, residual VSD, and aortic arch obstruction. Conduits require replacement over time because of somatic growth.[18,43] More recently, a percutaneous pulmonary valve is available for placement via cardiac catheterization for relief of conduit obstruction and regurgitation.

MRI and CT are useful for postoperative imaging of repaired truncus arteriosus. The anatomic and functional issues in patients who have undergone this repair are similar to those in patients with repaired TOF, specifically those with an RV to pulmonary artery conduit. Neoaortic valve dysfunction and aortic arch obstruction may require additional investigation. The postoperative MRI should address the following questions (e-Fig. 76-21)[1]:

1. Quantitative assessment of LV and RV volumes, function, and mass
2. Measurements of pulmonary (conduit) and neoaortic valve regurgitation
3. Imaging of the RVOT, conduit, and pulmonary arteries
4. Assessment of residual shunts
5. Imaging of the aortic arch and isthmus

WHAT THE CLINICIAN NEEDS TO KNOW

- Ventricular size and systolic function
- Status of the RVOT and LVOT, including anatomic or functional obstruction, and valve regurgitation
- Presence of obstruction of surgical baffles, such as the venous baffles in an atrial switch procedure or the intraventricular baffle in a Rastelli procedure
- Anatomy of pulmonary arteries and the aorta
- Interval change since the previous MRI or CT

Key Points

In neonates with conotruncal defects, echocardiography is the principal imaging modality for preoperative diagnosis. Cross-sectional imaging is used to clarify anatomy that is not adequately imaged by echocardiography, usually extra-cardiac vascular structures.

Cardiac MRI plays a crucial role in the routine follow-up of postoperative patients with conotruncal defects, particularly as they reach their teens and adulthood.

Assessment of the RV is an important part of follow-up imaging, whether there is a systemic RV (e.g., {S,D,D} TGA after an atrial switch procedure or uncorrected {S,L,L} TGA) or a pulmonary RV with abnormal pressure and/or volume loading conditions (e.g., free pulmonary regurgitation, conduit stenosis and regurgitation, and residual outflow tract obstruction).

Suggested Readings

Lai WW, Mertens LL, Cohen MS, et al. eds. *Echocardiography in pediatric and congenital heart disease: from fetus to adult.* Chichester, UK: Wiley-Blackwell; 2009.

Lewin MB, Salerno JC. Truncus arteriosus. In: *Echocardiography in pediatric and congenital heart disease: from fetus to adult.* Chichester, UK: Wiley-Blackwell; 2009.

Lopez L. Double outlet ventricle. In: *Echocardiography in pediatric and congenital heart disease: from fetus to adult,* Chichester, UK: Wiley-Blackwell; 2009.

Jonas RA. *Comprehensive surgical management of congenital heart disease.* London: Arnold; 2004.

Mertens LL, Otto Vogt M, Marek J, et al. Transposition of the great arteries. In: *Echocardiography in pediatric and congenital heart disease: from fetus to adult.* Chichester, UK: Wiley-Blackwell; 2009.

Oechslin E. Physiologically "corrected" transposition of the great arteries. In: *Echocardiography in pediatric and congenital heart disease: from fetus to adult.* Chichester, UK: Wiley-Blackwell; 2009.

Srivastava S, Parness IA. Tetralogy of Fallot. In: *Echocardiography in pediatric and congenital heart disease: from fetus to adult.* Chichester, UK: Wiley-Blackwell; 2009.

References

Full references for this chapter can be found on www.expertconsult.com.

Chapter 77

Congenital Anomalies of the Thoracic Great Arteries

FRANDICS P. CHAN

This chapter covers congenital anomalies of the aorta and the pulmonary arteries, with an emphasis on anomalies that produce clinical symptoms of airway and esophageal obstructions. Anomalies of the thoracic great arteries can be broadly classified into anomalous origins, anomalous connections, obstructions, and structural anomalies of the aortic arch. Important clinical entities under each category are listed in Box 77-1. This chapter will focus on structural anomalies of the aortic arch and pulmonary sling.

Vascular Rings

Overview Anomalies of the aortic arch and the cervical vessels are relatively common, with a prevalence estimated at 0.5% to 3%, depending on the inclusion criteria. Most variations, such as a left aortic arch with an aberrant right subclavian artery, common origin of the left common carotid and right innominate arteries (bovine arch), and ectopic origin of the left vertebral artery from the aortic arch, are of little or no clinical consequence.

"Vascular ring" is a term that refers to encirclement of the trachea and esophagus caused by the abnormal embryologic development of the aortic arch. The principal structural components responsible for this encirclement are derived from the aortic arch or arches, subclavian artery, circumflex aortic segment, ductus arteriosus, or ligamentum arteriosum. Structural anomalies of the aortic arch can be understood as the abnormal divisions in the totipotential arch, a theoretical construct proposed by Jesse Edwards (Fig. 77-1).[1] Only a small subset of aortic arch developmental anomalies leads to vascular rings, accounting for less than 1% of all congenital cardiovascular defects. Although about a dozen different types of vascular rings exist, double aortic arches and right aortic arch with left ligamentum arteriosum account for 90% of cases.[2]

Chromosome 22q11 deletion has been reported in 24% of patients with isolated arch anomalies.[3,4] This deletion was first identified in persons with DiGeorge syndrome, which consists of various degrees of immunodeficiency, thymic hypoplasia or aplasia, hypoparathyroidism, outflow tract cardiac defects, and dysmorphic appearance. Chromosome 22q11 deletion is now recognized as a major factor in many congenital heart defects. For example, it is detected in up to 50% of patients born with interrupted aortic arch or truncus arteriosus. Testing for this chromosomal abnormality can be performed using fluorescence in situ hybridization.

Clinical Manifestations The severity of symptoms and the age of onset depend on the extent of the compression about the esophagus and trachea.[5] Because different ring arrangements have different constrictive effects, not all vascular rings produce the same degree of symptoms; in fact, some rings produce no symptoms. Conversely, symptomatic vascular compression of the trachea and esophagus does not require a complete ring, as can be seen in an anomalously placed or aneurysmal innominate artery or a retroesophageal subclavian artery. Most cases of vascular ring, if they are symptomatic, present during infancy or early childhood.

Clinical symptoms related to constriction of the trachea include stridor, exertional dyspnea, cyanosis, respiratory distress, reflex apnea, and chronic cough. In cases of severe obstruction, intercostal retractions and lung hyperinflation can occur. Some patients have a history of recurrent respiratory infections. The pathophysiology involves external vascular compression, which leads directly to a reduced luminal cross-sectional area, as well as cartilage breakdown, tracheomalacia, and stenosis as a result of chronic, pulsatile mechanical compression. Clinical symptoms related to constriction of the esophagus are dysphagia, recurrent vomiting, difficulty feeding, and failure to thrive. Because the trachea and esophagus share the same space within the ring, respiratory symptoms can worsen during feedings. Of the different types of rings, double aortic arches produce the most severe symptoms. It is not uncommon for infants and children with vascular rings to be misdiagnosed with reactive airway disease.

Imaging Chest radiography may show tracheal compression by a vascular ring, but by itself a chest radiograph cannot confirm or exclude a vascular ring. Because a vascular ring is more likely in the presence of a right aortic arch, symptoms of tracheal compression in the presence of a right aortic arch should raise the possibility of a vascular ring.

In patients presenting with nonspecific symptoms, barium esophagography is a useful first test.[6] A normal barium esophagram usually excludes a clinically significant vascular ring. Classic S-shaped indentations in the frontal projection of an

Anomalous Origins

Aorta

Transposition of the great arteries

Pulmonary Artery

Transposition of the great arteries
Truncus arteriosus
Hemitruncus
Pulmonary sling
Accessory branch pulmonary artery
Pulmonary atresia with major aortopulmonary collateral arteries

Anomalous Connections Between Aorta and Pulmonary Artery

Truncus arteriosus
Aortopulmonary window
Patent ductus arteriosus

Structural Anomalies of the Aortic Arch

Double aortic arch
Right aortic arch, aberrant left subclavian artery, left ductus
    arteriosus
Right aortic arch, mirror-image branching, left ductus arteriosus
Right aortic arch, circumflex aorta, left ductus arteriosus
Right cervical aortic arch
Left aortic arch, aberrant right subclavian artery, right ductus
    arteriosus
Left aortic arch, circumflex aorta, right ductus arteriosus
Left cervical aortic arch

Obstructive Anomalies

Aorta

Aortic atresia
Interrupted aortic arch
Coarctation

Pulmonary Artery

Pulmonary stenosis
Pulmonary atresia
Absent branch pulmonary artery

---

esophagram are highly suggestive of double aortic arches. A posterior vascular indentation may or may not be a vascular ring but is more likely in the presence of a right aortic arch. An esophagram may reveal other causes of a patient's symptoms, such as gastroesophageal reflux, aspiration, or tracheoesophageal fistula.

Mediastinal ultrasonography or echocardiography with gray scale and color Doppler imaging may visualize the vascular ring directly in neonates and infants because these patients have excellent sonographic windows.[7] Echocardiography generally is not useful in older children or adolescents. Moreover, because ultrasound is primarily a two-dimensional imaging method, connecting tortuous vascular structures can be difficult, especially when ligamentous or interrupted vascular segments are present. The presence of a vascular ring has been diagnosed successfully in utero with fetal ultrasonography.[8]

Patients with severe symptoms or an abnormal results of an esophagram, chest radiograph, or mediastinal ultrasonography should undergo angiography to confirm the vascular abnormalities and to gather information for surgical planning. Conventional catheter angiography has been replaced by first-pass, contrast-enhanced computed tomographic angiography (CTA) or magnetic resonance angiography (MRA). Both modalities can visualize the aortic arch and the cervical

arteries well. MRA is usually preferred because it does not subject the patient to ionizing radiation.[9,10] However, in cases in which the airways and the lungs must be evaluated together with the vascular anomaly, CTA can accomplish both in a single scan and may be a better choice.

Treatment The definitive treatment is surgical relief of the obstruction.[11] A double aortic arch is repaired by dividing the nondominant arch between its last cervical artery and the point where the nondominant arch joins the descending aorta. If the ductus arteriosus or the ligamentum arteriosum forms a border of the ring, it is ligated to relieve the constriction. A thoracotomy is performed at the side of the planned ligation. Persistent stenosis or tracheomalacia may develop in the constricted trachea, requiring additional repair.

Anatomic, clinical, and imaging considerations for specific aortic arch anomalies are discussed in the following section.

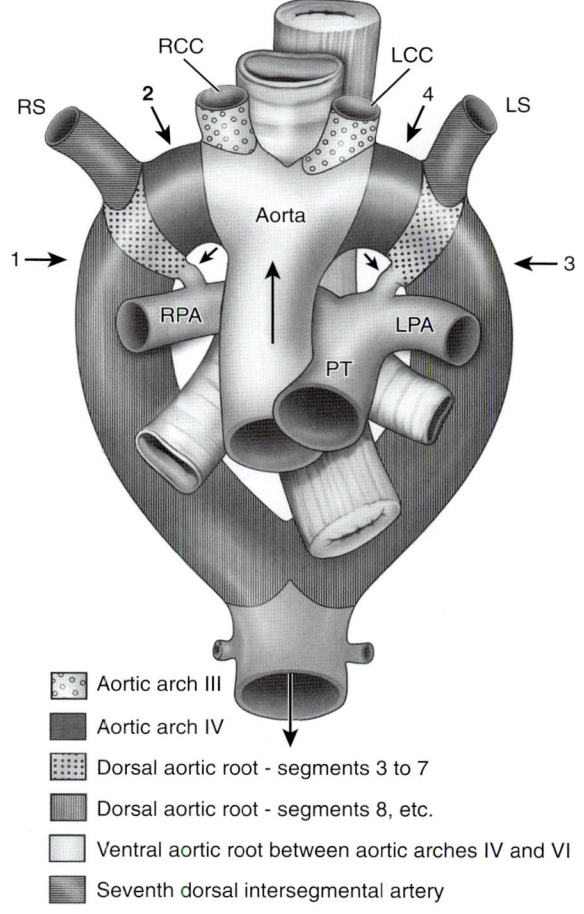

Aortic arch III

Aortic arch IV

Dorsal aortic root - segments 3 to 7

Dorsal aortic root - segments 8, etc.

Ventral aortic root between aortic arches IV and VI

Seventh dorsal intersegmental artery

Figure 77-1 Ventral view of Dr. Jesse Edward's "totipotential arch" or hypothetic double aortic arch and bilateral ducti arteriosi. The numbered arrows point to the four key locations where regression occurs in various anomalies. *Arrow 1* indicates the eighth segment of the right dorsal aortic root; *arrow 2*, the right fourth arch; and *arrows 3 and 4*, the corresponding two positions on the left. The *shortest black arrows* point to the ducti arteriosi bilaterally, and the *longest black arrow* indicates the direction of blood flow. *LCC*, Left subclavian artery; *LPA*, left pulmonary artery; *LS*, left subclavian artery; *PT*, pulmonary trunk; *RCC*, right common carotid artery; *RPA*, right pulmonary artery; *RS*, right subclavian artery. (From Stewart JR, Kincaid OW, Edwards JE: *An atlas of vascular rings and related malformations of the aortic arch system*, Springfield, IL, 1964, Charles C Thomas.)

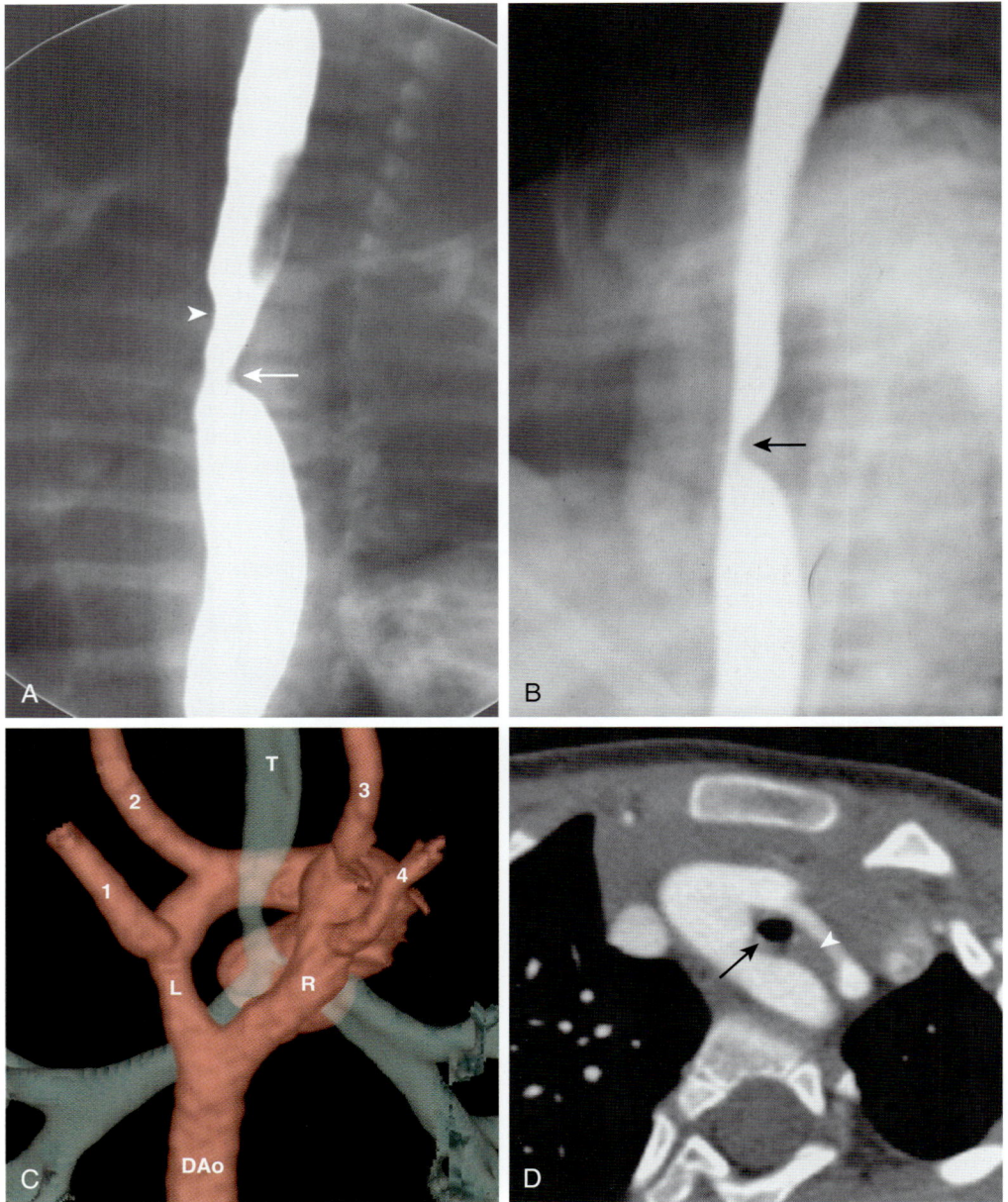

Figure 77-2   Bilaterally patent double aortic arches in a 7-year-old boy. **A,** The frontal view of a barium esophagram shows bilateral indentations of the barium column. The right arch indention (*arrowhead*) is higher than the left (*arrow*). **B,** The lateral view of a barium esophagram shows a posterior indentation (*arrow*) corresponding to the posterior right arch. **C,** A volume-rendered image from a computed tomography (CT) angiogram shows the aorta as seen from the back. A dominant right arch (*R*) and a nondominant left arch (*L*) are present, both draining into the descending aorta (*DAo*). Four cervical arteries arise from the arch: left subclavian artery (*1*), left common carotid artery (*2*), right common carotid artery (*3*), and right subclavian artery (*4*). The ring encloses the trachea (*T*), causing tracheal narrowing just above the carina. **D,** An axial CT scan shows a complete double aortic arch constricting the trachea (*black arrow*) and the esophagus (*white arrowhead*).

Special Considerations

DOUBLE AORTIC ARCHES

Double aortic arches can be categorized as bilaterally patent or as atretic in a portion of one of the two arches, usually the left. Bilaterally patent or complete double aortic arches represent persistence of both the right and the left embryologic fourth aortic arches. Two vessels arise from the ascending aorta and course dorsally, one on each side of the trachea and esophagus, to join posteriorly in a left descending aorta in 80% of cases. In this arrangement, the left arch is usually anterior and the right arch is posterior. In 20% of cases, the descending aorta lies on the right and the posterior-anterior relationship of the double aortic arches is reversed. The larger aortic arch is the dominant arch, and in 73% of cases, the right arch is dominant. The right arch normally is situated higher than the left arch, as can be seen in a typical esophagram, where the right arch indents the esophagus higher than does the left arch (Fig. 77-2). Double aortic arches usually are found without associated cardiac anomalies.

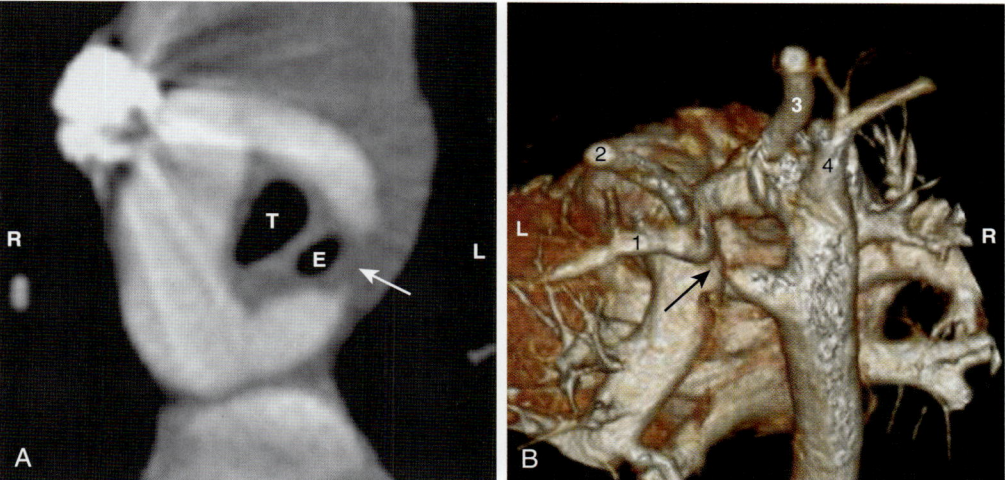

Figure 77-3 A double aortic arch with an atretic left arch in a 2-year-old girl. **A,** The axial view from a computed tomography (CT) angiogram shows a patent right arch and an incomplete left arch. A ligamentous connection (*arrow*) can be inferred from the tapered contour of the left arch, forming the left border of the vascular ring and constricting the trachea (*T*) and esophagus (*E*). **B,** A volume-rendered view from a CT angiogram shows the atretic segment in the left arch (*arrow*). The left subclavian artery (*1*) and the left common carotid artery (*2*) are supplied by the proximal portion of the left arch. The right arch gives off the right common carotid artery (*3*) and the right subclavian artery (*4*). The patient's right (*R*) and left (*L*) are labeled for reference.

Double aortic arches with left arch atresia develop from regression of varying segments of the left aortic arch, with fibrous continuity of the segments completing the vascular ring.[12] The atretic segment may lie between the left subclavian artery and the descending aorta (Fig. 77-3) or between the left common carotid artery and the left subclavian artery. The former configuration is similar to a right aortic arch with a mirror-image branching pattern, and the latter configuration is similar to a right aortic arch with an aberrant left subclavian artery. An aortic diverticulum may be present posterior to the esophagus, which is part of the distal left aortic arch, before connecting to the aberrant left subclavian artery. Double aortic arches with right arch atresia are theoretically possible but extremely rare, with very few reported cases. The clinical presentation, imaging approach, and surgical treatment are no different from those for other types of double aortic arches.

It may not be possible to distinguish double aortic arches with or without left arch atresia with an esophagram or chest radiograph. With ultrasonography, no Doppler flow is present in the atretic arch. CTA and MRA can readily visualize the atretic segment that appears to tether adjacent vascular structures and identify an aortic diverticulum.

RIGHT AORTIC ARCH WITH ABERRANT LEFT SUBCLAVIAN ARTERY

A right aortic arch with an aberrant left subclavian artery is a common cause of a vascular ring. The distal portion of the rudimentary left arch may persist as a diverticulum of Kommerell, giving origin to the left subclavian artery. Unlike double aortic arches with left arch atresia, no fibrous connection is present between the left common carotid artery and the left subclavian artery. Instead, the left border of the ring is completed by the left ligamentum arteriosum, which extends from the left subclavian artery to the pulmonary artery (Fig. 77-4). In 10% of cases, the ligamentum

arteriosum is on the right side, and thus there would be no vascular ring. Unlike double aortic arches, this vascular ring typically is loose, and many patients are asymptomatic or present with mild symptoms later in life.

RIGHT AORTIC ARCH WITH MIRROR-IMAGE BRANCHING

The right aortic arch with mirror-image branching pattern is associated with congenital heart disease in 90% of cases, typically tetralogy of Fallot and truncus arteriosus. In most instances, the aorta descends on the right. If the ductus is left sided, it usually connects between the anteriorly located innominate artery and the pulmonary artery, which does not form a vascular ring and does not result in posterior indentation on the esophagram. In rare cases, a true ring forms when a ligamentum arteriosum extends from the left pulmonary artery to an aortic diverticulum, resulting in a large posterior indentation on the esophagram.[13]

RIGHT AORTIC ARCH WITH CIRCUMFLEX AORTA

Unlike the typical right aortic arch, in which the descending aorta is right sided, a circumflex aorta descends on the left. To do so, the distal aortic arch travels from right to left, posterior to the esophagus, before turning downward (Fig. 77-5). A left ligamentum arteriosum connects the pulmonary artery to the descending aorta, completing the ring. The cervical branching can have a mirror-image pattern or an aberrant left subclavian artery. Neither type affects the formation of the ring. An aberrant left subclavian artery frequently arises from an aortic diverticulum with stenosis at its origin.

RIGHT CERVICAL AORTIC ARCH

A right cervical aortic arch occurs when abnormal cephalic migration of the aortic arch into the supraclavicular and neck

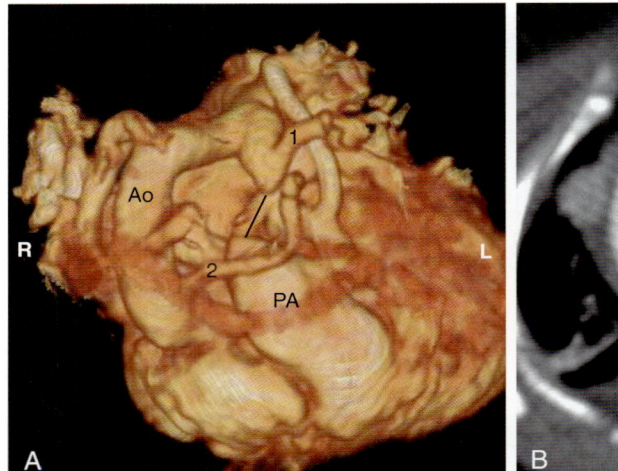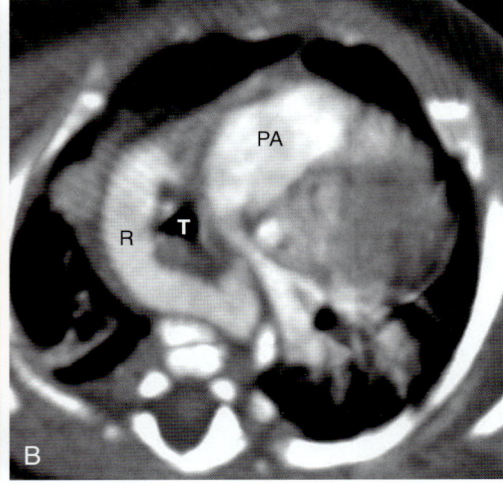

Figure 77-4 A right aortic arch with an aberrant left subclavian artery in a 1-year-old girl. **A,** A volume-rendered anterior and superior view reconstructed from a computed tomography (CT) angiogram. The right aortic arch (*Ao*) gives off the left common carotid artery (*2*) as the first branch and the left subclavian artery (*1*) as the last branch. A kink is seen between the diverticulum of Kommerell and the left subclavian artery, suggesting the attachment of a tight ligamentum arteriosum. The probable connection of the ligamentum arteriosum is drawn as a black line, which forms the left border of the vascular ring. The patient's right (*R*) and left (*L*) are labeled for reference. **B,** An axial CT angiogram of the same patient. The right aortic arch (*R*) forms the right and posterior border of the vascular ring; the ligamentum arteriosum forms the left border, enclosing the trachea (*T*). *PA,* Pulmonary artery.

region occurs. Embryologically, the cervical aortic arch forms from the third arch rather than the normal fourth arch. A cervical arch is more common on the right than on the left. The cervical branching pattern varies, and separate origins of the internal and external carotid arteries may arise from the cervical aortic arch. Disturbance of the carotid arteries can be anticipated, because they also are derived from the third arch. The right cervical aortic arch can give rise to a vascular ring in a manner similar to the other types of right aortic arch. Clinically, a pulsatile mass may be present in the supraclavicular region. Radiographic findings include right superior mediastinal widening, tracheal displacement to the left and anteriorly, a large oblique impression on the esophagram from cephalic right to caudal left, and a left descending aorta (Fig. 77-6).

LEFT AORTIC ARCH WITH ABERRANT RIGHT SUBCLAVIAN ARTERY

Compared with a right aortic arch, vascular ring formation in a left aortic arch is rare (Fig. 77-7) because the ductus arteriosus and ligamentum arteriosum usually are left-sided. To complete a ring with a left aortic arch would require a right ductus arteriosus. In the specific case of a left aortic arch with an aberrant right subclavian artery, very few proven cases of vascular ring have been reported. Although it is not part of a vascular ring, a large diverticulum of Kommerell at the retroesophageal right subclavian artery could cause difficulty swallowing; this association has been termed "dysphagia lusoria." This association is hard to prove, however, because although aberrant right subclavian artery is common, occurring in about 0.5% of the population, few persons experience symptoms.

LEFT AORTIC ARCH WITH CIRCUMFLEX AORTA

A left aortic arch with a circumflex aorta is analogous to a right aortic arch with a circumflex aorta, in that the distal

arch travels from left to right behind the esophagus before turning downward to become a right descending aorta. To complete a vascular ring, a right ligamentum arteriosum must connect the pulmonary artery to the descending aorta.[14]

LEFT CERVICAL AORTIC ARCH

Although a left cervical aortic arch is less common than the right-sided version, it similarly extends abnormally high in the upper mediastinal–low cervical region on the left side of the trachea. Symptoms depend on the cervical branching pattern and the presence of a vascular ring. Patients may present with a pulsatile left supraclavicular mass. The esophagram and angiographic findings are similar to those of right cervical aortic arch, except on the opposite side.

INNOMINATE ARTERY COMPRESSION SYNDROME

Anterior tracheal compression by the innominate artery may rarely cause symptoms of respiratory obstruction. Although such compression is not a form of vascular ring, it could mimic the symptoms. Infants may present with frequent respiratory infection, stridor, and respiratory arrest, and they frequently are misdiagnosed as having tracheomalacia. Bronchoscopy is diagnostic when a pulsatile impression is found on the anterior tracheal wall 1 to 2 cm above the carina. CTA or MRA can confirm the diagnosis.

Pulmonary Artery Sling

Overview A pulmonary artery sling (PAS) is a rare congenital anomaly of the pulmonary artery that produces obstructive symptoms of the upper airway. In a person with normal anatomy, the left main pulmonary artery branches off the pulmonary trunk in a shallow turn toward the left at a level slightly above the right main pulmonary artery. It then

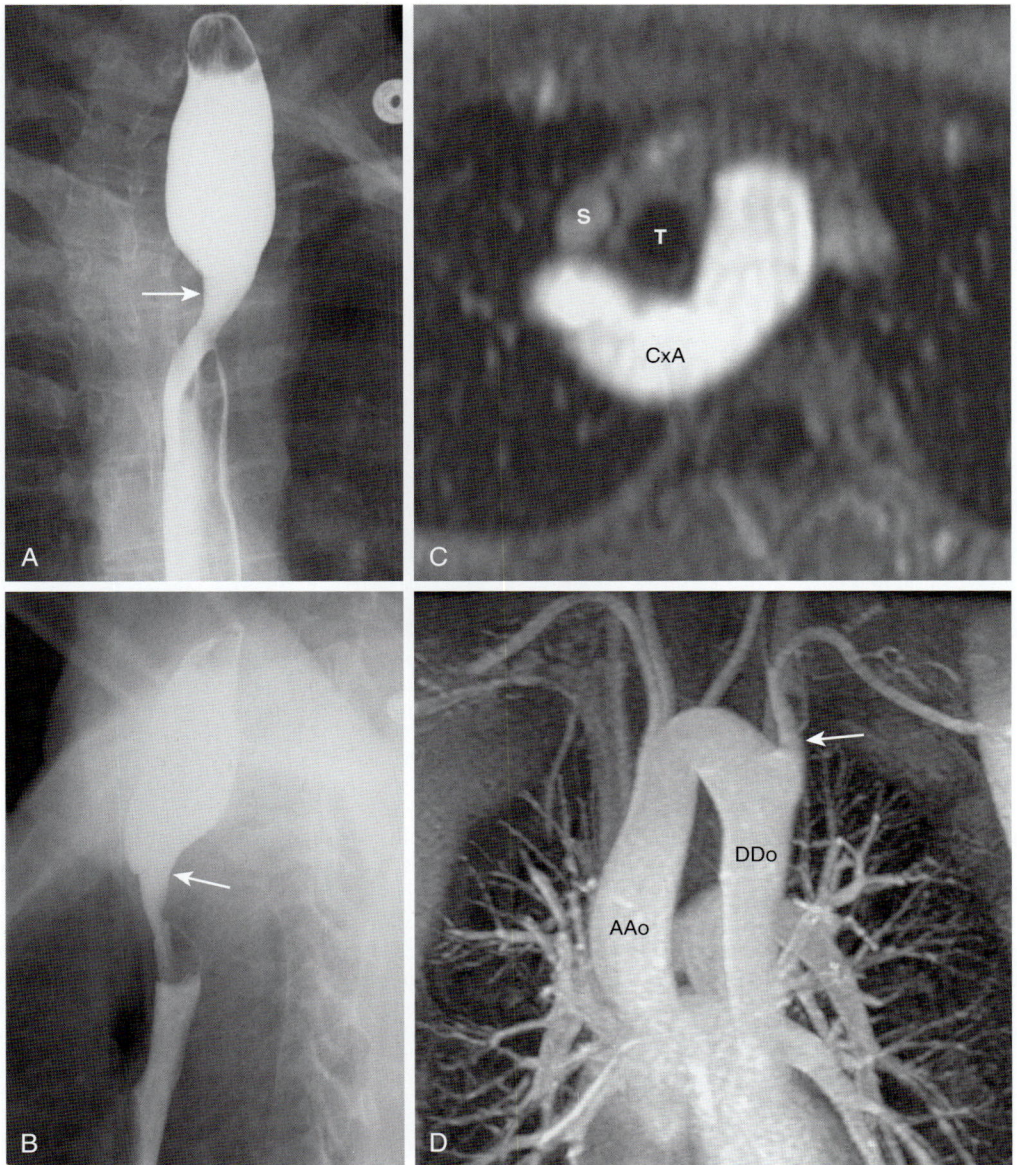

Figure 77-5 Circumflex aortic arch. **A,** The frontal esophagram of an 18-year-old woman shows a large right indentation (*arrow*) corresponding to a right aortic arch. **B,** The lateral esophagram shows a posterior indentation (*arrow*) larger than expected for an aberrant left subclavian artery. **C,** Axial reconstruction of a magnetic resonance (MR) angiogram shows that the aorta (*CxA*) passes behind the trachea (*T*) and the esophagus. The superior vena cava (*S*) is labeled for reference. **D,** Maximal intensity projection of an MR angiogram shows a right ascending aorta (*AAo*) and a left descending aorta (*DAo*). There is an aberrant left subclavian artery (*arrow*) as the last branch off the arch.

courses above the left main bronchus. In a person with a PAS, the left main pulmonary artery originates from the posterior aspect of the right pulmonary artery. It turns left behind the trachea at or near the level of the carina toward the left pulmonary hilum. The trachea is compressed between the left and right main pulmonary arteries (Fig. 77-8). The esophagus courses posterior to both pulmonary arteries and is not obstructed, unlike the situation in a person with a vascular ring.

The incidence of PAS is not known. In a large-scale screening study of more than 180,000 school-aged children with ultrasonography, 11 cases were found,[15] representing an in incidence of 1 in 17,000. A slight male predilection was noted. Patients present with clinical symptoms in childhood,

and 90% of patients present with symptoms before the first year of life.[16] Nonspecific respiratory symptoms include an asthmatic cough and acute and recurrent bronchopulmonary infections. Some patients are misdiagnosed with asthma for many years before PAS is discovered. Symptom severity depends on the degree of airway compression and coexisting airway abnormalities. Long-standing compression of the airways also may cause tracheobronchomalacia. Unlike with a vascular ring, the obstructive symptoms of the esophagus tend to be mild or absent in persons with a PAS.

Coexisting airway abnormalities are present in more than 50% of patients, including abnormal branching of the airways, complete tracheal rings, and tracheal stenosis.[17] The vertical position of the left pulmonary artery origin, along with the

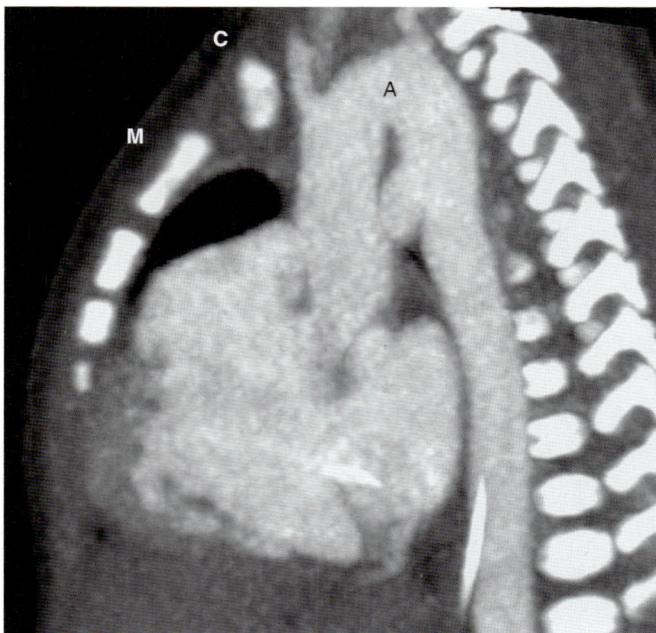

Figure 77-6 A cervical aortic arch in a 1-month-old boy. Sagittal reformation of a chest computed tomography angiogram shows a high aortic arch (*A*) with its apex above the level of the manubrium (*M*) at vertebral level T3-T4. *C*, Clavicle.

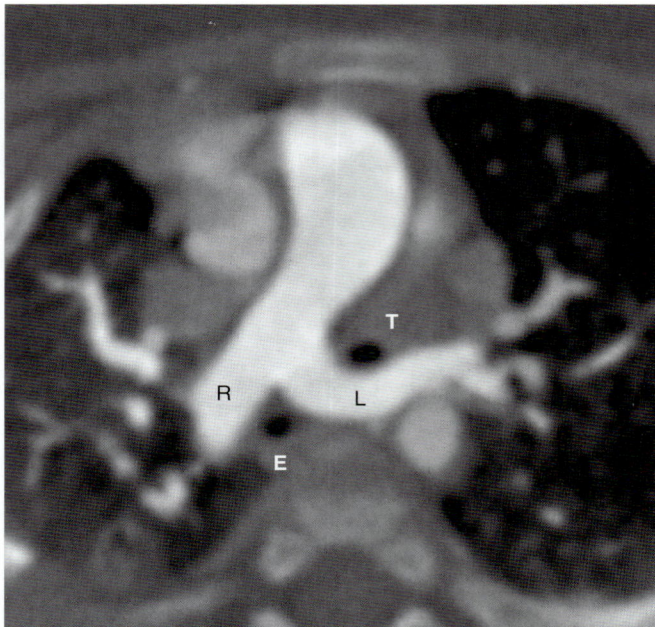

Figure 77-8 A pulmonary artery sling in a 6-month-old girl. An axial image from a computed tomography angiogram shows an anomalous left pulmonary artery (*L*) arising from the right pulmonary artery (*R*). It courses between the trachea (*T*) and the esophagus (*E*). The trachea is entrapped between the left and right pulmonary arteries.

branching pattern of the airways, has been used to classify PAS.[18] In type 1 PAS, the left pulmonary artery originates at T4–T5 vertebral levels, just above the normal level of the carina. Subtype 1A has normal branching pattern of the airways; subtype 1B has a tracheal bronchus. In type 2 PAS, the left pulmonary artery originates below the T5 vertebral level, below the normal carina. Subtype 2A has a right main bronchus connecting to the right upper lobe only. A separate "bridging" airway arises from the left main

bronchus, below the aberrant left pulmonary artery, that supplies the right middle and right lower lobes (Fig. 77–9, *A*). In subtype 2B, the right main bronchus is absent and the bridging airway defined in 2A supplies the entire right lung. Except for the level of the left pulmonary artery, the right main bronchus in type 2A superficially resembles the tracheal bronchus in type 1B. Regardless of the type, complete tracheal rings and stenosis frequently are present (Fig. 77–9, *B*).

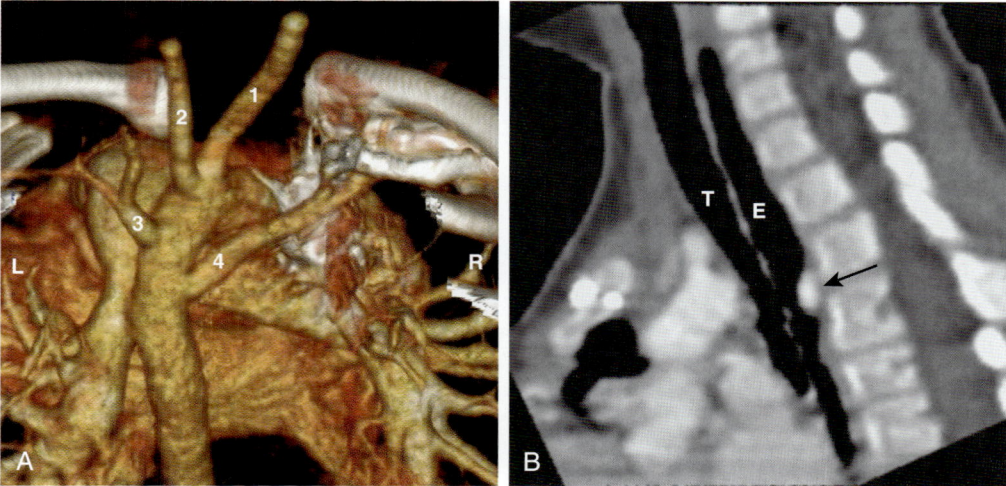

Figure 77-7 A left aortic arch with an aberrant right subclavian artery in a 4-year-old boy. **A,** A volume-rendered image from a computed tomography angiogram seen from the back shows the cervical arteries: right common carotid artery (*1*), left common carotid artery (*2*), left subclavian artery (*3*), and aberrant right subclavian artery (*4*). The patient's right (*R*) and left (*L*) are labeled for reference. **B,** A sagittal reformat view shows the air-filled trachea (*T*) and the esophagus (*E*). The esophagus is indented posteriorly by the aberrant subclavian artery (*arrow*).

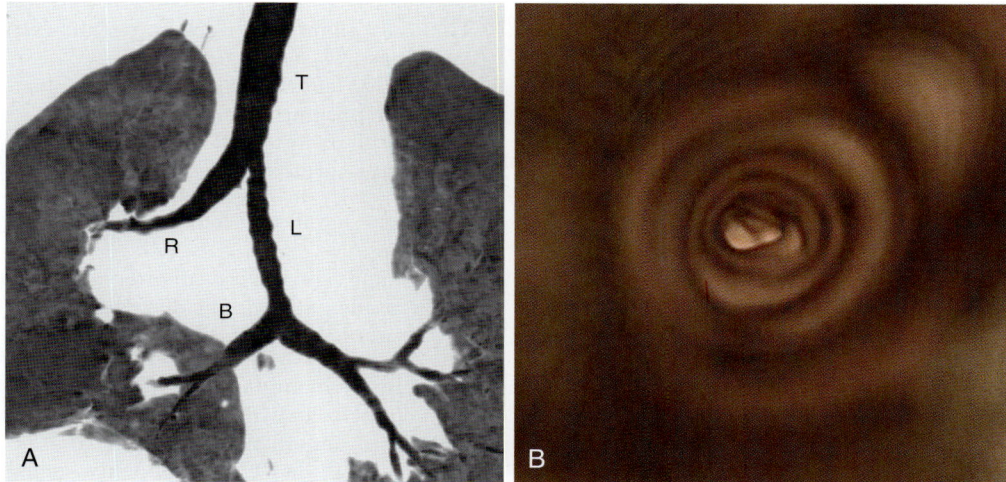

Figure 77-9 Abnormal central airways of a 40-year-old woman with a pulmonary artery sling. **A,** Coronal reformation with minimum intensity projection shows type 2A configuration where the trachea (*T*) bifurcates into a right main bronchus (*R*) and a left main bronchus (*L*). The right main bronchus supplies the right upper lobe airways only. A bridging artery (*B*) supplies the rest of the right lung. Superficially, the right main bronchus resembles a tracheal bronchus, except that it arises at the expected location of the carina, instead of high up from the trachea. **B,** The endoscopic view in the trachea shows complete tracheal rings.

About a third of PAS cases are associated with other cardiovascular anomalies, including ventricular septal defect, atrial septal defect, patent ductus arteriosus, tetralogy of Fallot, common ventricle, and coarctation.[16] Genetic associations include trisomies 18 and 21.[19]

Imaging As the left pulmonary artery wraps around the right side of the trachea, the right main bronchus or the bridging airway can be obstructed. In the newborn, this phenomenon may manifest as retained fluid in the right lung. In older children, this phenomenon may present as a hyperinflated right lung from air trapping. The most specific finding is the abnormal architecture of the central airways, often described as a low carina and an inverted T shape of the central airways (see Fig. 77-9, *A*). This finding is a result of the abnormal

airway structure found in type 2 PAS. The apparent low carina is the result of the low origin of the bridging bronchus. The horizontal course of the bridging bronchus gives the carina a flattened look, hence the inverted T shape.

Barium esophagography is a useful screening tool for PAS. The esophagus is indented anteriorly at the level of the carina (Fig. 77-10), unlike the posterior indentation seen with a vascular ring. In addition, on the lateral projection, the trachea is separated from the esophagus by the left main pulmonary artery.

Direct visualization of the anomalous left pulmonary artery can be performed with CTA or MRA.[20] Because assessment of the airways and the lungs is important for PAS, CTA is the preferred imaging modality. CTA images can be postprocessed to provide virtual endoscopic views to evaluate

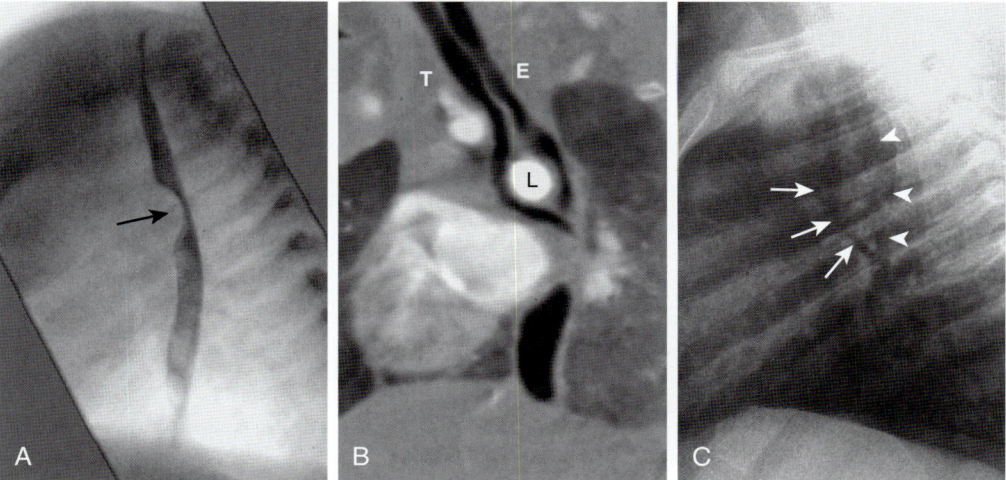

Figure 77-10 A pulmonary artery sling in a 6-month-old girl. **A,** An esophagram in the lateral projection shows an anterior indentation (*arrow*). **B,** A computed tomography angiogram reformatted in the same plane shows the left pulmonary artery (*L*) separating the trachea (*T*) from the esophagus (*E*) at the carina level. The anterior indentation seen in the esophagram is caused by compression by the left pulmonary artery. **C,** A lateral chest radiograph shows the same separation of the trachea (*arrows*) and the air-filled esophagus (*arrowheads*).

for focal stenosis, extrinsic vascular compression, and a tracheal ring (see Fig. 77-9, *B*). Endoscopic bronchoscopy is recommended to evaluate dynamic airway obstruction from tracheobronchomalacia and to confirm the extent of complete tracheal rings or stenosis for surgical planning.

Treatment The definite treatment is surgical reimplantation or relocation of the left pulmonary artery and release of the entrapped trachea. In many of these patients, stenosis of the trachea requires a sliding tracheoplasty or pericardial patch to augment the narrowed segment. A diameter of the trachea that is less than 3 mm is associated with the need for tracheoplasty or a poor outcome.[21] Airway narrowing that involves the carina or the bronchi is particularly difficult to repair.[22]

Key Points

Gene deletion at location 11 of the long arm of chromosome 22 is associated with a number of developmental abnormalities of the great arteries. In decreasing order of association, they are interrupted aortic arch, truncus arteriosus, tetralogy of Fallot, and other aortic arch anomalies.

A normal esophagram free of any abnormal vascular indentations excludes a clinically important vascular ring. Definitive diagnosis requires contrast-enhanced CTA and MRA.

On an esophagram, a posterior indentation is associated with a double aortic arch, a retroesophageal subclavian artery, or a circumflex aorta, whereas an anterior indentation is associated with a pulmonary artery sling.

Clinically significant right aortic arches may have these variations:
- Aberrant left subclavian artery, left ductus arteriosus
- Mirror-imaging branching, left ductus arteriosus
- Circumflex aorta, left ductus arteriosus
- Cervical aortic arch

Clinically significant left aortic arches may have these variations:
- Aberrant right subclavian artery, right ductus arteriosus
- Circumflex aorta, right ductus arteriosus
- Cervical aortic arch

Imaging evaluation of a pulmonary artery sling must include the central airways because of the frequent associations with abnormal branching of the airways, complete tracheal rings, and tracheobronchial stenosis.

Suggested Readings

Hellinger JC, Daubert M, Lee EY, et al. Congenital thoracic vascular anomalies: evaluation with state-of-the-art MR imaging and MDCT. *Radiol Clin North Am.* 2011;49:969-996.

Hernanz-Schulman M. Vascular rings: a practical approach to imaging diagnosis. *Pediatr Radiol.* 2005;35:961-979.

Momma K, Matsuoka R, Takao A. Aortic arch anomalies associated with chromosome 22q11 deletion (CATCH 22). *Pediatr Cardiol.* 1999;20:97-102.

Newman B, Cho Y. Left pulmonary artery sling-anatomy and imaging. *Semin Ultrasound CT MR.* 2010;31:158-170.

Oddone M, Granata C, Vercellino N, et al. Multi-modality evaluation of the abnormalities of the aortic arches in children: techniques and imaging spectrum with emphasis on MRI. *Pediatr Radiol.* 2005;35:947-960.

References

Full references for this chapter can be found on www.expertconsult.com.

Chapter 78

Coronary Artery Disease in Children

FRANDICS P. CHAN

Most coronary artery diseases in children are congenital.[1,2] A large number of anomalous arrangements of the coronary arteries exist, but only a few have clinical significance. Among acquired diseases of the coronary arteries in children, Kawasaki disease (KD) is the most common. Other diseases include sequelae from trauma, vasculitides (see Chapter 82), radiation injury after oncologic treatment, and rare cases of familial hyperlipidemia and idiopathic infantile arterial calcification. Box 78-1 outlines the two principal manifestations of coronary artery diseases, together with the diseases in which they are commonly seen in children. In clinical practice, patients presenting with syncope, arrhythmia, or near sudden death usually are referred for coronary computed tomography (CT) or magnetic resonance imaging (MRI) to diagnose a coronary anomaly, to confirm and clarify echocardiographic findings of coronary anomalies, to map out the coronary arteries for surgical planning, and to evaluate the coronary tree for aneurysms and stenosis.

Imaging Considerations

Catheter angiography is the gold standard for the determination of luminal coronary abnormalities, such as coronary stenosis.[3] During catheterization, the arterial wall can be characterized with intravascular ultrasound,[4] and the hemodynamic significance of a stenotic coronary lesion on myocardial perfusion can be measured using the fractional flow reserve technique.[5] In infants, transthoracic echocardiography is the first-line imaging tool for the evaluation of structural anomalies of the proximal coronary arteries. Echocardiography is usually adequate to exclude the major types of lethal anomalous coronary arteries. Echocardiography is less useful in older children, and it cannot visualize the entire coronary vasculature.

Cardiac-gated multidetector row CT angiography (CCTA) and cardiac magnetic resonance angiography (CMRA) are important noninvasive alternatives to catheter coronary angiography.[6] Both techniques record three-dimensional images of the heart, with the coronary vessels shown in the context of adjacent cardiac structures. Visualization is facilitated by three-dimensional postprocessing. These capabilities have made CCTA and CMRA the preferred method for the diagnosis and characterization of anomalous coronary arteries.

CCTA requires intravenous injection of an iodinated contrast agent. Cardiac synchronized images can be acquired in one of two modes: prospective or retrospective electrocardiographic (ECG) gating. Prospective ECG gating obtains a snapshot of the heart at a predetermined cardiac phase, whereas retrospective ECG gating scans throughout the cardiac cycle and can produce cine images of the heart. However, retrospective gating incurs a four to five times higher radiation dose compared with prospective gating. With 64-slice scanners, the typical scan time in either mode is less than 20 seconds. For young children who cannot hold their breath voluntarily, apnea is induced for a short interval with anesthesia. With an increasing number of detector rows, increasing gantry rotation speed, and multiple x-ray sources, it is conceivable that scan time will be shortened to a point where breath holding and anesthesia may not be necessary.

The greatest concern regarding CCTA is that it uses ionizing radiation (see Chapter 66). Every measure must be taken to reduce the dose of ionizing radiation delivered to a patient. First, CCTA should be undertaken only if the diagnostic goals are achievable and the results affect management of the patient's condition. As much as possible, scanning should be limited to a single pass over the heart only. Tube voltage and tube current should be kept to a minimum for the patient's size and acceptable image quality. If possible, the pitch factor should be adjusted to the heart rate. Prospective ECG gating and ECG dose modulation should be used when appropriate. With these measures, dose-equivalent radiation is less than 10 mSv for retrospectively gated CCTA and 3 mSv for prospective gated or nongated CCTA.[7] Noise reduction with iterative reconstruction currently is being investigated as a method to achieve diagnostic images at a very low radiation dose.[8] A dose equivalent to less than 1 mSv for prospectively gated or nongated CCTA likely is achievable.

The lack of ionizing radiation makes CMRA an attractive imaging choice. On most clinically available magnetic resonance (MR) scanners, whole heart CMRA is built on a three-dimensional, cardiac-gated, navigated echo, T2-prepared, steady-state, free-precession sequence.[9] Depending on coverage, spatial resolution, heart rate, and breathing pattern, imaging time typically is 10 to 20 minutes. For this amount of time, breath holding is impractical. Respiratory motion is managed by restricting data acquisition at a predetermined range of diaphragm position monitored in real time with the navigator echo technique. Contrast for the coronary vessels is based on the intrinsic long-T2 value of blood, and no gadolinium contrast administration is required, which is an important advantage in patients who have renal failure and the risk of gadolinium contrast–related nephrogenic systemic fibrosis.[10] However, the T2-contrast mechanism is not selective, and all vascular channels are equally bright. Furthermore, other materials with a high T2 value, such as pericardial effusion and pleural effusion, are as bright as blood. This lack of differentiation sometimes can confound diagnostic interpretation.

Compared with CCTA, CMRA lags in spatial resolution. In addition, CMRA is sensitive to metal artifacts from surgical clips and sutures, especially those made from ferromagnetic materials. Because CMRA has a long scan time, anesthesia is required for patients who cannot cooperate. The complexity of CMRA requires greater expertise to perform the procedure compared with other modalities, and high-quality results may not be achieved as consistently as with CCTA. Nonetheless, because it does not utilize ionizing radiation and intravenous contrast material, CMRA is a safer procedure compared with other procedures for patients who do not require anesthesia. For adolescents and young adults who are cooperative and have larger coronary arteries, trying CMRA first is a reasonable strategy. If CMRA fails to answer the clinical question, then CCTA or catheter angiography may be used as a backup. For infants and small children who must be anesthetized while they are studied, CCTA may be a more reliable option.

Normal Coronary Artery Anatomy

Many anatomic variations of the coronary arteries exist, and the separation of normal variants from anomalous coronary arteries is arbitrary (Fig. 78-1). In persons with conventional coronary anatomy, two main coronary arteries originate from two of the three aortic sinuses of Valsalva closest to the pulmonary trunk. The three aortic sinuses are labeled according to their attached coronary arteries: the right coronary sinus giving rise to the right coronary artery (RCA), the left coronary sinus giving rise to the left main coronary artery (LMCA), and the noncoronary sinus giving rise to no coronary branch.

After its takeoff from the right coronary sinus, the RCA courses anteriorly into the right atrioventricular groove. It gives rise to a right conal artery as the first branch 50% of the time. Otherwise, the right conal artery arises directly from the right coronary sinus. This conal artery supplies the myocardium of the right ventricular outflow tract (RVOT). In the majority of cases, a sinoatrial nodal artery branches from the proximal RCA (Fig. 78-2, *A*). Otherwise, it arises from the proximal left circumflex (LCx) artery. The middle portion of the RCA gives rise to one or more right ventricular branches (Fig. 78-2, *B*). These branches are called acute marginal branches, analogous to the obtuse marginal branches from the LCx artery. The distal portion of the RCA wraps around the inferior surface of the heart. In most people, the RCA gives rise to a posterior descending artery (PDA) (Fig. 78-2, *C*). The RCA then enters the "crux," the intersection between the interventricular septum and the atrioventricular groove. At the crux, the RCA bends and forms an inverted U and then continues into the left atrioventricular groove at the bottom of the heart, where it gives off multiple posterior left ventricular arteries that supply the basilar inferior wall of the left ventricle. This pattern of the distal RCA is called a right-dominant coronary system and occurs in 85% of the population. An atrioventricular nodal branch often arises from the RCA near the apex of the inverted U (Fig. 78-2, *D*). The PDA gives rise to many inferior septal perforator branches that supply the inferior septum, analogous to the anterior septal perforator branches that originate from the left anterior descending (LAD) artery.

The LMCA originates from the left coronary sinus and courses to the left for a short distance. In most people, it bifurcates into an LAD artery and an LCx artery. In other people, the LMCA trifurcates into an LAD artery, an LCx artery, and, in between, a ramus medianus branch (Fig. 78-3, *A*). This branch supplies the anterior left ventricular wall. The LAD artery gives rise to two sets of vessels: an epicardial set called the diagonal branches and an intramuscular set called the anterior septal perforator branches. The diagonal branches are responsible for perfusing the anterior left ventricular wall, whereas the septal perforator branches are responsible for the anterior septum. The distal LAD artery typically wraps around the cardiac apex and terminates at the inferior wall of the apex (Fig. 78-3, *B*). In a minority of cases, the LCx artery gives off a sinoatrial nodal branch (Fig. 78-3, *C*) before it enters the left atrioventricular groove. The LCx artery then gives rise to a number of obtuse marginal branches, which supply the lateral left ventricular wall (see Fig. 78-3, *B*). In 10% of the population, the LCx artery supplies the posterior left ventricular branches and the PDA instead of the RCA. This system is called a left-dominant coronary system. In 5% of the population, the RCA supplies the PDA while the LCx artery supplies the posterior left ventricular branches. This system is called a co-dominant coronary system.

Nomenclature of the coronary arteries can be confusing in the presence of ventricular malformations. In general, the coronary arteries are named relative to the morphology, not the position, of the underlying ventricles. For example, in l-looped ventricles where the morphologic left ventricle lies to the right, the coronary artery in the right-sided

CORONARY ARTERY DISTRIBUTION

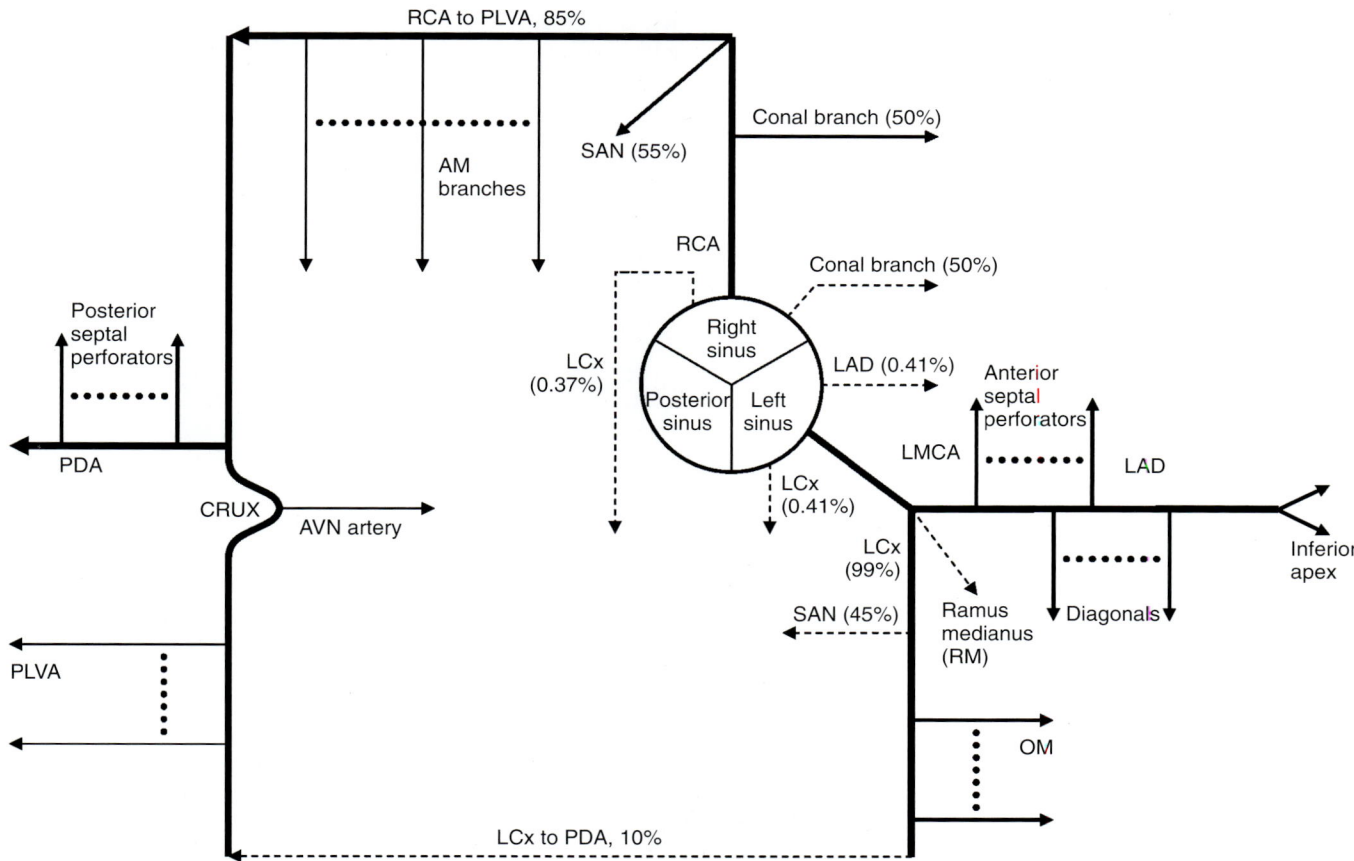

Figure 78-1 Coronary artery distribution diagram. *Solid lines* represent the most common coronary artery pattern. *Dashed lines* represent common variants (prevalences in percentages). *AM*, Acute marginal; *AVN*, atrioventricular nodal; *LAD*, left anterior descending; *LCx*, left circumflex; *LMCA*, left main coronary artery; *OM*, obtuse marginal; *PDA*, posterior descending artery; *PLVA*, posterior left ventricular artery; *RCA*, right coronary artery; *RM*, ramus medianus; *SAN*, sinoatrial nodal.

atrioventricular groove is named the left circumflex artery. When derangement of the ventricles is so severe that the ventricular morphology cannot be clearly identified, then the coronary arteries should be described relative to physical landmarks—for example, left-sided atrioventricular branch instead of LCx, right-sided atrioventricular branch instead of RCA, anterior interventricular septal branch instead of LAD, and posterior interventricular septal branch instead of PDA.

Congenital Coronary Artery Anomalies

EPIDEMIOLOGY

The true prevalence of congenital coronary artery anomalies is unknown. According to adult catheter angiographic data, 0.6% to 1.5% of patients were found to have coronary artery anomalies.[11,12] The largest study of this type reviewed more than 126,000 coronary studies and revealed a prevalence of 1.3%.[13] Of these anomalous cases, 80% were judged to have no clinical significance.[14] Ectopic coronary origin and aberrant course is estimated to affect 1% of the population. The

most common type is separate origins of the LAD and LCx arteries arising from the left sinus of Valsalva (0.41%) (Fig. 78-4, *A*). The next most common variation is an ectopic LCx artery arising from the right sinus or the RCA and then coursing posterior to the aorta (0.37%) (Fig. 78-4, *B*). Both configurations are clinically benign. Other examples of benign anomalies are an absent LCx artery with a superdominant RCA that reaches the anterior atrioventricular groove, an ectopic right or left coronary artery from the posterior sinus, and an ectopic left or right coronary origin from the ascending aorta. Clinically significant coronary artery anomalies are listed in Box 78-2.

CORONARY ARTERY WITH INTERARTERIAL COURSE

Overview An anomalous LMCA may originate from the right coronary sinus or from the RCA. Before bifurcating into the LAD and LCx arteries, the LMCA must travel toward the left by one of three routes: anterior to the RVOT, between the aorta and the pulmonary artery, or posterior to the aorta. Similarly, an anomalous RCA may originate from the left coronary sinus or from the LMCA. It must travel toward the right atrioventricular groove by one of these three

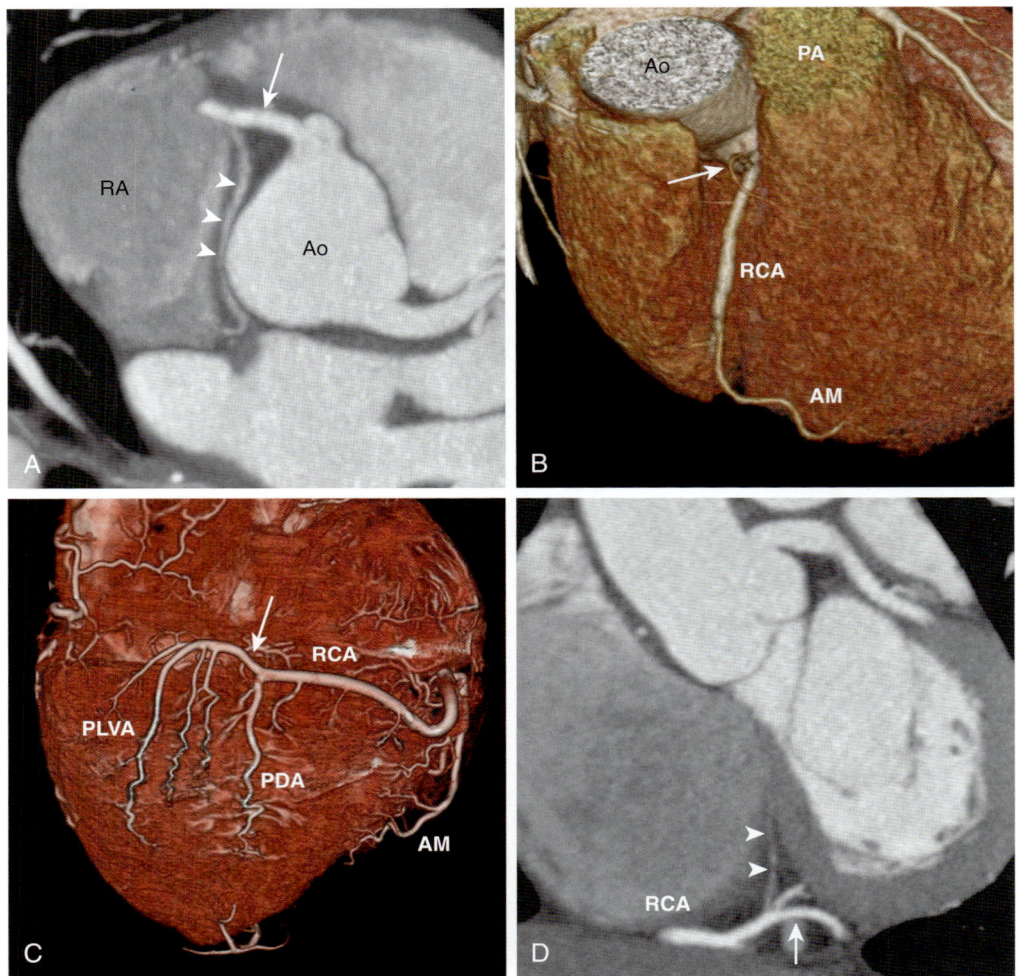

Figure 78-2 Major branches of the normal right coronary artery (*RCA*). **A,** Axial cardiac-gated multidetector row computed tomography angiography image shows the RCA (*arrow*) originating from the aorta (*Ao*) and extending toward the right atrioventricular groove. It gives off a sinoatrial nodal branch (*arrowheads*) that terminates at the right atrium (*RA*) near the atrial septum. **B,** A volume-rendered image shows an acute marginal (*AM*) branch arising from the RCA at the right ventricular free wall. The conal branch (*arrow*) is the first branch of the RCA. *PA,* pulmonary artery. **C,** A volume-rendered image shows the inferior surface of a heart. The RCA gives off in succession the AM branch, the posterior descending artery (*PDA*), and the posterior left ventricular arteries (*PLVA*), which lie on the left side of the crux (*arrow*). **D,** A short-axis view shows the RCA at the crux (*arrow*) giving off an atrioventricular nodal branch (*arrowheads*).

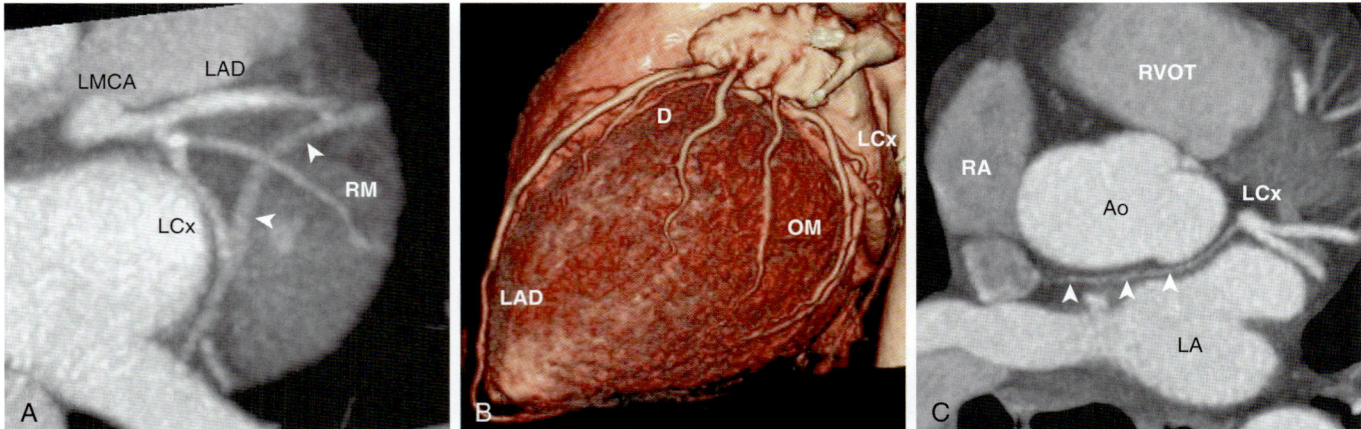

Figure 78-3 Major branches of the normal left main coronary artery (*LMCA*). **A,** Oblique axial cardiac-gated multidetector row computed tomography angiography image shows the trifurcation of the LMCA into a left anterior descending (*LAD*) artery, a ramus medianus (*RM*) branch, and a left circumflex (*LCx*) artery. The crossing vessel (*arrowheads*) is the greater cardiac vein. **B,** A volume-rendered image shows the LAD and several diagonal (*D*) branches. The LAD wraps around the apex to reach the apical inferior surface. The LCx artery gives off several obtuse marginal (*OM*) branches. **C,** An axial image shows the LCx giving off a sinoatrial nodal branch (*arrowheads*) that travels behind the aorta (*Ao*) and terminates at the right atrium (*RA*) near the atrial septum. *LA,* left atrium; *RVOT,* right ventricular outflow tract.

Box 78-2 Clinically Significant Coronary Artery Anomalies and Their Routes

Coronary Artery with Interarterial Course
- LMCA from RCA or right coronary sinus
- RCA from LMCA or left coronary sinus

Coronary Artery from Pulmonary Artery (PA)
- LMCA from PA (ALCAPA)
- RCA from PA (ARCAPA)
- LAD artery from PA
- LCx artery from PA

Large Coronary Artery Fistula
- From RCA > LAD > both
- To RV > RA > PA > LV > SVC

Coronary Artery-Associated Cardiac Anomalies
- Truncus arteriosus
- Tetralogy of Fallot
- Transposition of the great arteries
- Pulmonary atresia with intact ventricular septum
- Coronary artery hypoplasia

ALCAPA, Anomalous left coronary artery from the pulmonary artery; *ARCAPA,* anomalous right coronary artery from the pulmonary artery; *LAD,* left anterior descending; *LCx,* left circumflex; *LMCA,* left main coronary artery; *LV,* left ventricle; *PA,* pulmonary artery; *RA,* right atrium; *RCA,* right coronary artery; *RV,* right ventricle; *SVC,* superior vena cava.

routes. For both coronary arteries, the anterior and posterior courses are clinically benign, whereas the interarterial course—that is, between the aorta and the pulmonary artery (Fig. 78-5)—is associated with sudden death.[15] An aberrant LMCA with an interarterial course is estimated to affect 0.03% to 0.05% of the population. An anomalous RCA with an interarterial course is more common, with a prevalence estimated at 0.1%. The interarterial segment of the coronary artery may be intramural within the aortic wall, intramuscular within the myocardium, or free between the aorta and the pulmonary artery.

The association between an anomalous coronary artery with an interarterial course and sudden death in young athletes was discovered in autopsy series.[16-18] Sudden death in this otherwise healthy population is rare, with an incidence estimated to be 5 in 1 million people per year,[19] with anomalous coronary arteries found in up to 20% of these cases. Most autopsy series report a greater number of anomalous LMCAs than anomalous RCAs, some by a ratio of 3:1. Given that the anomalous RCA is three times more common, the autopsy results suggest that anomalous LMCA is a more lethal lesion. The mortality rate of these lesions is unknown, because most patients have not been diagnosed and followed up prospectively.

In patients with lethal types of coronary anomalies, sudden death almost always occurs during exertion. Most of these patients who died had no known premonitory symptoms.[20] In about 30% of the cases, syncope or chest pain occurred within 2 years of death, but resting ECG and stress ECG have been reported as normal. The pathophysiology of sudden death has not been conclusively determined. A lethal arrhythmia may be triggered by transient ischemia caused by inadequate coronary flow through either the slitlike opening of the anomalous coronary artery or the narrowed lumen compressed by the aorta and pulmonary artery.

In addition to interarterial coronary arteries, sudden death has been associated with an aberrant LMCA arising from the noncoronary sinus without an interarterial course.[21] In this configuration, the alignment of the LMCA origin and the anterior interventricular groove is such that the LMCA must have a more acute takeoff angle from the noncoronary sinus (Fig. 78-6). This acute takeoff angle creates a narrowing at the ostium that is thought to be a factor leading to ischemia and sudden death.

Imaging In neonates and young children, echocardiography sometimes provides sufficient visualization of the proximal coronary arteries to suggest the lethal anomalous coronary types previously discussed. These patients are referred for CMRA or CCTA to confirm the diagnosis and to map out the coronary vessels for surgical planning. In adolescents and young adults, the coronary arteries may not be adequately assessed with echocardiography. Anomalous coronary arteries are suspected on the basis of clinical symptoms, which often are nonspecific. The pretest probability of disease usually is low. To avoid exposing a large number of normal patients to radiation, CMRA should be the first test of choice. If the CMRA is not diagnostic, then CCTA can be used as a backup test. Diagnostic catheter angiography does not have much of a role for this indication.

Treatment Because most deaths occur in patients between 10 and 30 years of age, teenagers and young adults who are diagnosed with an anomalous coronary artery with an interarterial course or rare types of anomalous LMCA from the noncoronary sinus should consider surgery with the goal of preventing sudden death. Preventive surgery in patients outside this age group is controversial, because their risk of sudden death is not known. The surgical approach depends on whether the interarterial segment is intramural or free. If it is intramural, then the ostium can be surgically enlarged by unroofing the common wall between the aorta and the coronary segment. Otherwise, the coronary artery must be reimplanted or bypassed. Determination of the intramural course can be difficult with CCTA and CMRA. Correlation with surgical pathology suggests that CCTA findings of a slitlike orifice, an acute angle at vessel takeoff, and an elliptical cross section are related to an intramural coronary segment (Fig. 78-7).[22]

CORONARY ARTERY FROM PULMONARY ARTERY

Overview Origination of a coronary artery from a pulmonary artery includes anomalous origin of the LMCA, LAD artery, LCx artery, or RCA from the pulmonary trunk or the main branch pulmonary arteries. The most common and clinically most important type is the anomalous left coronary artery from the pulmonary artery (ALCAPA) (Fig. 78-8). The incidence is approximately 1 in 300,000 live births, accounting for 0.24% to 0.5% of congenital cardiac anomalies.[23] Origination of the anomalous right coronary artery from the pulmonary artery is four times less common than is ALCAPA.[24] The clinical presentation depends on how much of the coronary flow to the left ventricle is compromised.

In fetal circulation, the pulmonary artery pressure is higher than the aortic pressure because the pulmonary resistance is high. Furthermore, both the pulmonary artery and the aorta

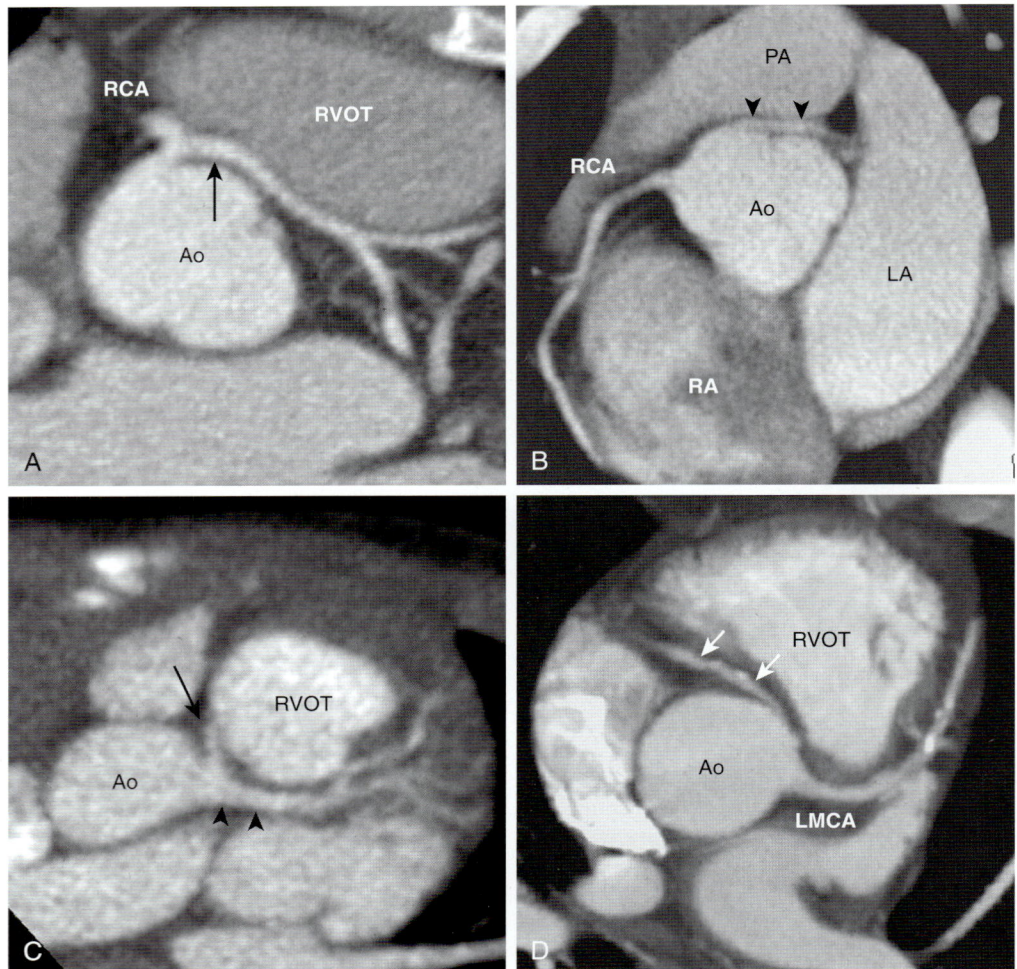

Figure 78-5 An anomalous coronary artery with an interarterial course. **A,** The axial view from a cardiac computed tomography angiogram of a 10-year-old boy shows a common origin of the right coronary artery (*RCA*) and the left main coronary artery (LMCA) (*arrow*) arising from the right sinus of the aorta (*Ao*). The LMCA has a long interarterial course as it travels between the aorta and the right ventricular outflow tract (*RVOT*). **B,** In this 20-year-old man, an LMCA (*arrowheads*) originates from the right sinus separate from the RCA, then travels between the Ao and the pulmonary artery (*PA*). **C,** In this 2-year-old boy, the RCA (*arrow*) arises from the LMCA (*arrowheads*). **D,** In this adult with calcific coronary plaques, an RCA (*arrows*) originates from the left sinus separate from the LMCA. A tapered narrowing is evident at the proximal, interarterial portion of the RCA. *LA*, Left atrium; *RA*, right atrium.

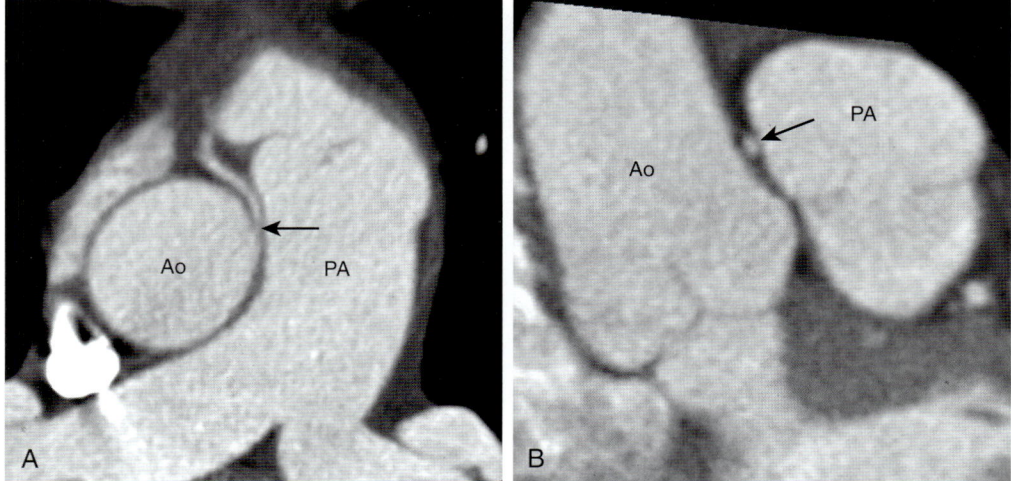

Figure 78-7 Coronary computed tomography angiogram of a surgically proven case of intramural right coronary artery (RCA) arising from the left coronary sinus in an 8-year-old girl. **A,** The short-axis view shows an interarterial RCA (*arrow*) arising from the aorta (*Ao*) in an acute angle. The proximal RCA tapers to a slitlike opening at the ostium. **B,** A longitudinal view shows the RCA compressed (*arrow*) by the Ao and the pulmonary artery (*PA*). The cross section of the RCA is elliptical in shape.

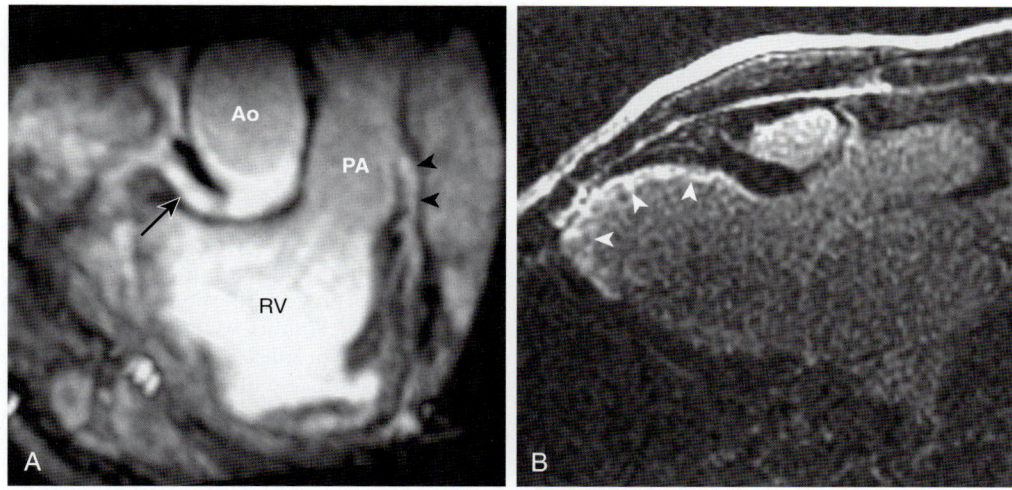

Figure 78-8 Magnetic resonance imaging of a 12-year-old boy with an anomalous left coronary artery from the pulmonary artery (PA). **A,** An oblique image reformatted from a noncontrast coronary magnetic resonance angiogram shows the right coronary artery (*arrow*) arising from the aorta (*Ao*) at the normal location and the left main coronary artery (LMCA) (*arrowheads*) originating from the PA. **B,** Three-chamber view from a delayed-enhancement study shows endocardial infarction at the left ventricular anteroseptal wall and the apex (*arrowheads*) caused by inadequate myocardial perfusion from the LMCA. *RV,* Right ventricle.

conduct oxygenated blood. Consequently, the coronary flow through the anomalous LMCA is essentially normal, and fetal development is unaffected. After birth, the pulmonary resistance decreases and the ductus arteriosus closes, and the pulmonary pressure and the LMCA pressure drop together. Flow through the LMCA slows and myocardial perfusion decreases. Eventually, the pressure difference between the high-pressure RCA and the low-pressure LMCA favors collateral flow from the RCA to the LMCA. Blood in the LMCA flows retrograde into the pulmonary artery. Coronary "steal" deprives myocardium in the LMCA territory of adequate perfusion, ensuring ischemia.

In 90% of patients with this condition, the RCA-to-LMCA collateral flow is not enough to sustain myocardial viability. Myocardial ischemia, infarction, congestive heart failure, ventricular dilation, mitral regurgitation, and pulmonary edema develop early during the sixth to eighth week of life, representing the infantile form of ALCAPA; the associated clinical syndrome is called the Bland-White-Garland syndrome. Without intervention, mortality can be as high as 90%. In 10% of patients with ALCAPA, collateral flow from RCA to LMCA was large enough to sustain myocardial viability. As a result of the high shunt flow, the coronary arteries can be abnormally large. These patients have few or no symptoms and survive into adulthood; this presentation is the adult form of ALCAPA. ALCAPA usually is an isolated lesion, but it can be associated with ventricular septal defect (VSD), atrioventricular canal, tetralogy of Fallot (TOF), truncus arteriosus, and aortic stenosis. Origination of the anomalous right coronary artery from the pulmonary artery, in contrast, usually is asymptomatic in the first 2 years of life and presents with exertional chest pain later in adolescence or adulthood.

Imaging Chest radiographs for patients with the infantile form of ALCAPA usually show an enlarged cardiac silhouette and signs of pulmonary venous congestion or pulmonary edema. ECG and other laboratory tests suggest myocardial

ischemia and infarction. When selective coronary angiography is performed, the catheter fails to engage the LMCA ostium. An aortogram fills a single right coronary artery in the early phase, with late opacification of the LMCA and retrograde flow of contrast material into the pulmonary artery. Echocardiography usually can detect the connection between the anomalous coronary artery and the pulmonary artery and can visualize the reversed coronary flow by color Doppler imaging. In difficult cases, the connection between the anomalous coronary artery and the pulmonary artery can be seen readily with CCTA or CMRA.[25]

Management The definitive treatment is surgery. The most straightforward approach is to reimplant the anomalous coronary artery from the pulmonary artery to the aorta.[26] With ALCAPA, reimplantation of the LMCA can be difficult because the LMCA may be too short to reach the centrally located aorta. This problem can be solved with the Takeuchi operation,[27] in which an aortopulmonary window is created first. Then a baffled tunnel is created inside the pulmonary trunk to connect the aortopulmonary window to the ostium of the anomalous LMCA. Blood flows from the aorta, through the aortopulmonary window, into the baffled tunnel, and then into the anomalous LMCA ostium.

CORONARY ARTERY FISTULA

Overview A coronary artery fistula is a common coronary abnormality seen in 0.3% to 0.8% of patients referred for cardiac catheterization.[28] It is an abnormal communication between a normal coronary artery and another cardiovascular structure. Although it usually is congenital, it can form after trauma or after a surgical procedure such as a myomectomy. Anatomically, a coronary fistula most frequently originates from the RCA (55%), followed in frequency by the LAD artery (35%), both arteries (5%), and others (5%). A coronary fistula terminates in the right side of the heart far more often than in the left side of the heart. The most common site of

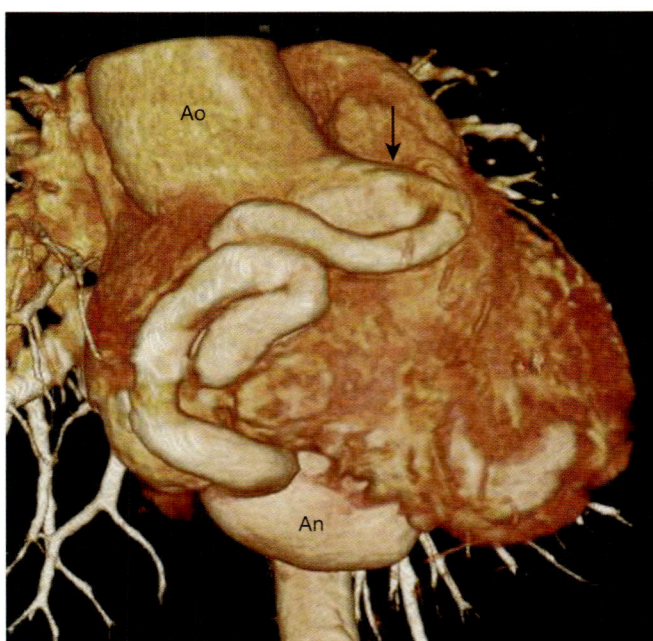

Figure 78-9 Coronary fistula to the right ventricle. A volume-rendered image from a coronary computed tomography angiogram of a 22-year-old woman shows a large and extremely tortuous right coronary artery arising (*arrow*) from the aorta (*Ao*). At the inferior surface of the heart, this coronary fistula connects to a giant aneurysm (*An*), which empties into the right ventricle (not shown).

termination is the right ventricle (41%) (Fig. 78-9), followed by the right atrium (26%), pulmonary trunk (17%) (Fig. 78-10), left ventricle (3%), and superior vena cava (1%).[29]

Coronary artery fistulae usually are isolated without associated cardiac anomalies. However, in pulmonary atresia with intact ventricular septum (PAIVS), coronary fistulae to the right ventricle are an integral part of the disease, with important consequences for treatment options. Coronary fistulae in PAIVS are discussed later in the context of complex congenital heart disease.

The clinical significance of a coronary artery fistula depends on the size of the fistulous communication, as well as its termination site. Most fistulae are small and conduct too little flow to be clinically significant. Patients with small fistulae usually are asymptomatic and may have a continuous murmur. A large fistula communicating to the right side of the heart is effectively a left-to-right shunt. It behaves clinically like a VSD and has complications normally associated with VSD, such as endocarditis and pulmonary hypertension. In contrast, a large fistula to the left side of the heart forms a left-to-left shunt. Clinically it behaves like aortic regurgitation, with signs and symptoms relating to volume overload of the left ventricle. Over time, the left ventricle enlarges and fails, leading to symptoms of heart failure, that is, fatigue, dyspnea, and orthopnea. In addition, a large coronary artery fistula can divert coronary flow from perfusing the myocardium to a great enough degree to cause myocardial ischemia and infarction. Finally, a large coronary fistula can expand like an arterial aneurysm and can thrombose or rupture.

Imaging A small coronary artery fistula may be detected incidentally when a screening echocardiography is ordered

for an unexplained murmur or for unrelated symptoms. If the fistula is large, the course and connections of the fistula, as well as aneurysmal or stenotic segments, should be defined with catheter angiography, CCTA, or CMRA. In addition, MRI can quantify the shunt flow and shunt ratio with use of phase–contrast techniques.

Management Patients with fistulae of any size should be given antibiotic prophylaxis to prevent endocarditis.[30] For patients with a shunt ratio greater than 1.5, the fistula should be closed to prevent the development of pulmonary hypertension. Some authors advocate elective closure of all fistulae to prevent myocardial ischemia, endocarditis, and aneurysm formation. Fistulae with favorable connections and shapes can be closed with catheter embolization. Otherwise, they can be closed with surgical ligation.[31,32] Aneurysmal segments should be surgically reduced to prevent rupture.

ANOMALOUS CORONARY ARTERY IN STRUCTURAL HEART DISEASE

The prevalence of anomalous coronary arteries is much greater in the presence of underlying cardiac malformations, especially conotruncal anomalies, such as truncus arteriosus, transposition of the great arteries (TGA), and TOF. The origins and courses of the anomalous coronary arteries can affect important surgical decisions, especially in the repair of TOF, TGA, and PAIVS. The role of the imager is to map out the coronary pattern in relationship to other cardiovascular structures to help a surgeon plan the surgical approach. Instead of describing all the possible coronary variations associated with cardiac malformations, the importance of certain coronary anomalies in the surgical repair of TOF, TGA, and PAIVS will be explained.

Tetralogy of Fallot

Overview TOF is the most common cyanotic congenital heart disease, accounting for 10% of all congenital heart defects (see Chapter 76). The standard treatment today is early total correction between 3 and 12 months of age. The surgical repair has two components: a patch closure of the VSD and a transannular patch augmentation of the RVOT and the pulmonary trunk. In 4% of patients with TOF, an anomalous LAD artery arises from the RCA and crosses anterior to the RVOT before entering the anterior interventricular septal groove (Fig. 78-11).[33] This LAD artery lies in the path of the transannular incision and can be accidentally transected. If it cannot be adequately mobilized, it may prevent sufficient augmentation of the RVOT.[34]

Imaging TOF usually can be detected with echocardiography, but some institutions advocate use of screening catheter angiography. Today, TOF can be evaluated reliably with CCTA.

Transposition of the Great Arteries

Overview TGA accounts for 5% of all congenital heart defects (see Chapter 76). Most patients with TGA have normal ventricular positioning (D-looping), atrioventricular concordance, and ventriculoarterial discordance with the

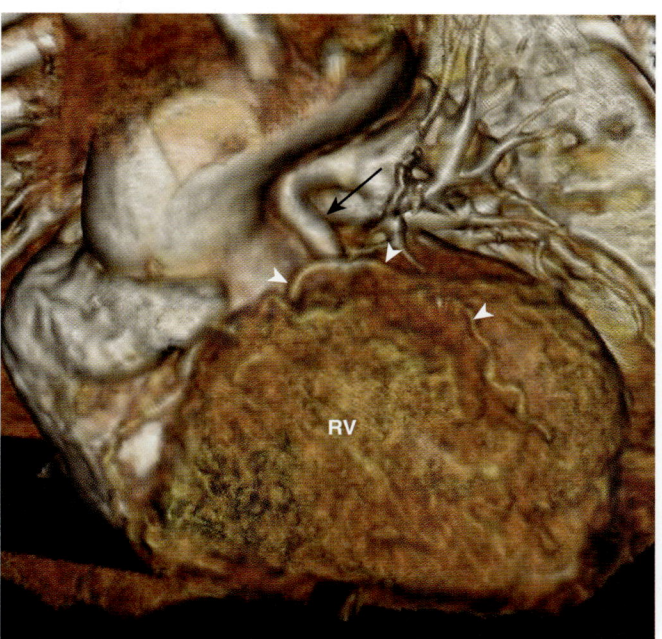

Figure 78-11 Aberrant left anterior descending (LAD) artery in a child with tetralogy of Fallot. A volume-rendered image from a 1-year-old boy viewed from the front shows an LAD artery (*arrowheads*) that travels in front of the stenotic pulmonary trunk (*black arrow*). The position of this LAD artery may complicate the surgical repair. *RV,* Right ventricle.

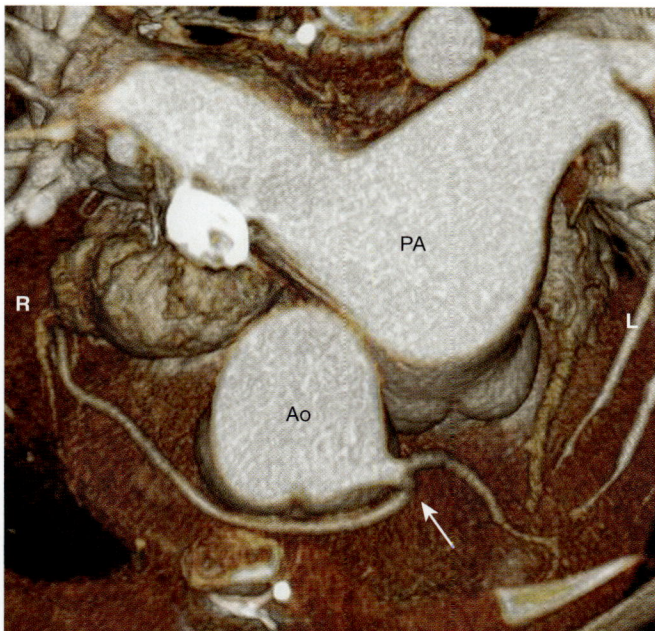

Figure 78-12 Coronary artery arrangement in d-transposition of the great arteries (d-TGA). A volume-rendered image from a coronary computed tomography angiogram of a 12-year-old girl shows an aorta (*Ao*) that is situated in front and to the right of the pulmonary artery (*PA*), consistent with a d-TGA. A single coronary ostium is present (*arrow*), and the right coronary artery courses in front of the Ao. This coronary pattern is not favorable for the arterial switch operation.

aorta anterior and to the right of the pulmonary trunk (Fig. 78-12).

Imaging and Treatment The preferred surgical treatment for complete TGA is the arterial switch, or Jatene operation. This surgery is a definitive operation in which the aorta and the pulmonary trunk are surgically transposed, thereby returning the circulatory anatomy to a "normal" state. In this operation, the coronary arteries also must be reimplanted from the aortic sinuses to the pulmonary sinuses. In normal truncal anatomy, the left and right coronary arteries arise from the aortic sinuses closest to the pulmonary trunk. This relationship usually is preserved even when the aorta and the pulmonary trunk are congenitally transposed. The close proximity of the coronary origins from both great arteries makes surgical translocation of the coronary arteries feasible. However, frequent variations of coronary origins and course occur that make this operation difficult or even impossible.[35] By mapping out the coronary anatomy, CCTA or CMRA can be very useful for surgical planning.[36]

After the arterial switch operation, the surgically manipulated coronary arteries are at risk for stenosis or even occlusion. In the past, patients who had this operation underwent regular catheter coronary angiography to assess this complication. Today, CCTA and CMRA are useful noninvasive alternatives, and catheter angiography is reserved for patients in whom signs and symptoms of myocardial ischemia develop.

Pulmonary Atresia with Intact Ventricular Septum

Overview PAIVS is believed to be caused by the in-utero obstruction of the pulmonary valve after the formation of the pulmonary infundibulum and the central pulmonary arteries (see Chapter 74). The reduced right ventricular flow prevents the normal growth of the right ventricle and the tricuspid valve, causing hypoplasia of both structures. Without an outlet, the right ventricular systolic pressure can rise above the left ventricular systolic pressure and the coronary arterial pressure. This mechanism, in turn, disrupts the normal regression of embryologic communications between epicardial coronary arteries and the right ventricle, resulting in coronary fistulae between the two in 75% of the patients at birth.

After birth, the right ventricular pressure remains high and blood flows from the right ventricle into the coronary system. If the right ventricle is decompressed by surgically relieving the pulmonary obstruction, blood flow in the coronary fistulae abruptly reverses, shunting blood away from the myocardium into the right ventricle and leading to myocardial ischemia and infarction. Normal coronary circulation, then, depends on a pressurized right ventricle. A pressurized right ventricle, in turn, precludes surgery that restores the right ventricle to a functioning pump for the pulmonary circulation. This physiology is called a "right ventricle–dependent coronary circulation."[37]

Imaging and Management Catheter coronary angiography is the standard imaging study to detect PAIVS-related coronary fistulae. Classic findings on coronary angiography include systolic retrograde filling of the RCA and the LAD artery during right ventriculography (Fig. 78-13) and end-diastolic filling of the right ventricle during coronary angiography. This type of coronary fistula can be seen readily with CCTA, although its role in the surgical decision of PAIVS is not defined.

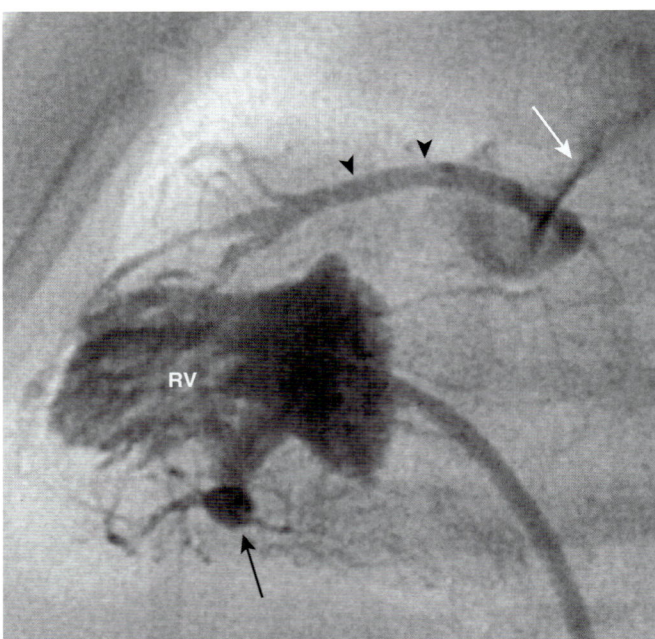

Figure 78-13   Catheter angiography of the right ventricle of a 1-year-old boy with pulmonary atresia and an intact ventricular septum. Contrast material injected into the right ventricle (*RV*) flows through the sinusoids (*black arrow*) into the coronary arterial system (*arrowheads*) and then flows retrograde out of the pulmonary artery (*white arrow*). This coronary circulation is judged right-ventricular dependent.

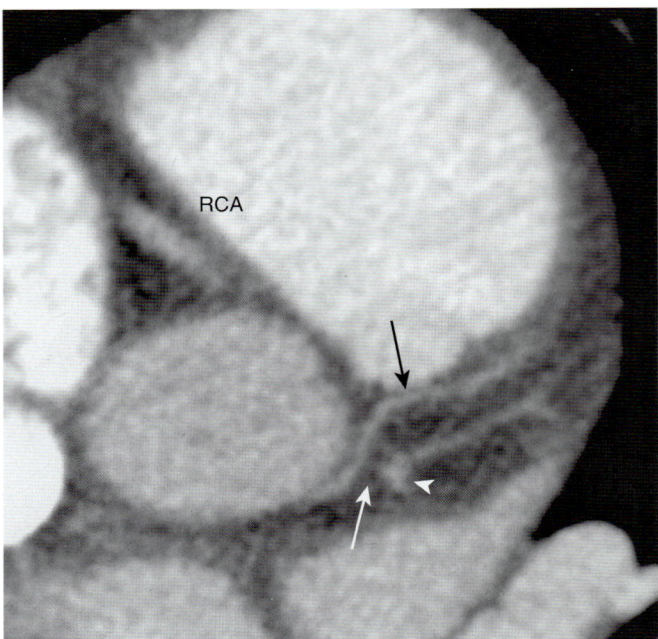

Figure 78-14   Coronary artery hypoplasia in a 15-year-old girl with exertional angina. An axial view from a coronary computed tomography angiogram shows diffusely small left coronary arteries compared with the right coronary artery (*RCA*). The left circumflex artery (*arrowhead*) is occluded (*white arrow*) from the left main coronary artery (*black arrow*).

CORONARY ARTERY HYPOPLASIA

Overview   Coronary artery hypoplasia (CAH) is a rare condition characterized by a diffusely narrowed, underdeveloped major coronary segment or branch.[38] The prevalence of CAH is estimated to be 0.03% based on adult coronary angiography, and it represents 6% of all coronary anomalies. Most reported cases involve the left coronary system (Fig. 78-14). The pathogenesis of this lesion is unknown, but an in-utero embolic event affecting a coronary artery may be a cause. The clinical significance of CAH also is unknown. In a few cases it was related to sudden death, but other persons with this anomaly led normal lives, with the diagnosis being made at autopsy after they died from unrelated causes.

Imaging and Management   CCTA can be used to visualize the threadlike epicardial coronary artery. However, catheter angiography is required to delineate all collateral vessels. The optimal treatment has not been determined, but in patients who have CAH along with documented arrhythmia or syncope, implantation of a defibrillator would be a prudent choice.

Acquired Coronary Artery Diseases

KAWASAKI DISEASE

KD, or mucocutaneous lymph node syndrome, was first described by Tomisaku Kawasaki in 1967. It is an acute, febrile, multisystem vasculitis of unknown etiology that affects primarily children younger than 5 years of age, with a slight male predominance. It is most common in Japan, although the number of cases in the United States is increasing. The number of children hospitalized for KD is estimated to be 3000 per year in the United States. KD is the most common acquired coronary artery disease in children. Diagnosis is made by clinical characteristics of prolonged high fever, conjunctivitis, red, cracked lips, a red oral mucous membrane, a strawberry tongue, a multiform rash, cervical lymphadenopathy, erythema of the palms and the soles, swollen hands and feet, and desquamation around fingers and toes 1 to 2 weeks after the onset of symptoms.[39] The disease usually is self-limiting, although recurrence has been seen in 3% of patients.

Imaging   The most important complication of KD is the development of coronary artery aneurysms. Coronary artery aneurysms develop in 15% to 30% of patients who do not receive gamma globulin therapy, usually 1 to 4 weeks after disease onset. Thromboembolism of coronary artery aneurysms (Fig. 78-15) and coronary artery stenosis are the causes of myocardial ischemia, infarction, heart failure, and sudden death in these patients. Expanding aneurysms may rupture. Echocardiography is the primary imaging tool in persons with KD. In young children, echocardiography is quite effective in detecting coronary aneurysms. Giant aneurysms (>8 mm in diameter) are associated with increased risk of myocardial infarction and sudden death. Echocardiography is less effective in older children and young adults, and serial angiography is needed to monitor progression of aneurysms and the development of stenosis. Both CCTA and CMRA are useful, noninvasive alternatives for this purpose.[40,41] In addition, MRI is useful in the assessment of myocardial ischemia, infarction, and ventricular function.

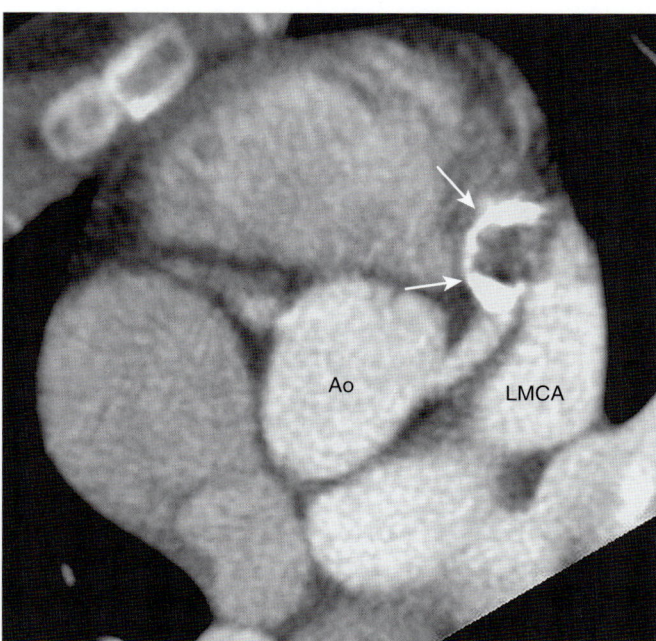

Figure 78-15 **Kawasaki disease.** An axial image from a coronary computed tomography angiogram shows chronic changes of Kawasaki disease, which include a calcified, thrombosed aneurysm (*arrows*) in the left main coronary artery (*LMCA*). *Ao,* Aorta.

Treatment In multiple studies, it has been shown that administration of intravenous gamma globulin therapy lowers the risk of aneurysm formation from more than 15% to 5%. High-dose aspirin is used as adjunctive therapy during the acute phase to lower coagulation activation. In 1970 the mortality rate of KD was 2%, mostly as a result of cardiac complications, but with improvements in treatment, it has dropped to 0.1%.

TRAUMA

Overview Trauma to the chest is relatively common in children; however, few reported injuries are specific to the coronary arteries. The most common cause of pediatric trauma is blunt trauma from motor vehicle accidents, although in urban areas, penetrating injuries from assaults and other violence occur not infrequently. Blunt injury to the coronary artery can cause an intimal tear, dissection, and acute thrombosis, leading to myocardial infarction and arrhythmia.[42,43] Both blunt and penetrating injury can cause rupture of the coronary arteries, resulting in hemorrhage, tamponade, and myocardial infarction. Commotio cordis, or concussion of the heart, has led to dramatic sudden death during play in otherwise healthy children.[44] The pathophysiology is not known, but postulated mechanisms include ventricular fibrillation brought on by mechanical shock to the myocardium during its vulnerable repolarization period, or by myocardial ischemia resulting from coronary vasospasm or dissection. Over time, the weakened or ruptured coronary vessel wall can form a pseudoaneurysm. Traumatic coronary artery fistulae to the ventricles have been reported. The infarcted or contused myocardium can become aneurysmal (Fig. 78-16), and if the injury to myocardium is extensive, heart failure can result.

Imaging and Management The initial management of chest trauma focuses on more common lethal injuries such as airway compromise, pneumothorax, aortic rupture, and tamponade. Conventional computed tomographic angiography is routinely performed to evaluate for these findings. If signs of cardiac injury such as an abnormal ECG, hemodynamic instability, and elevated myocardial enzymes are found, echocardiography is performed to evaluate wall motion abnormality, abnormal valvular function, myocardial hematoma, and pericardial effusion or blood. To assess for acute coronary injury, catheter angiography is the imaging modality of choice. Less acutely, CCTA can be used to assess structural damages in the heart, such as traumatic VSD and myocardial aneurysm. MRI is useful for the evaluation of myocardial infarction and ventricular functions.

Management of traumatic coronary artery injuries depends on the type of injury and the degree and extent of myocardial compromise. Initial management should focus on the preservation of viable myocardium. Acutely, dissection, intimal flap, and stenosis of the coronary artery can be treated with a stent to maintain coronary patency. Coronary aneurysms, traumatic coronary fistulae, and secondary cardiac abnormalities such as ventricular aneurysm, VSD, and injured valves require surgical repair.

Treatment Complications Involving Coronary Arteries

Surgical manipulation of the coronary arteries always carries the risk of postsurgical stenosis or occlusion of the arteries. Indeed, this risk was a concern during the early surgical experience with the arterial switch operation. Other pediatric cardiac operations that affect the coronary arteries are reimplantation of an anomalous coronary artery, the Takeuchi operation for ALCAPA, surgical augmentation for supravalvular aortic stenosis, composite valve-graft repair (the Bentall procedure) for a Marfan aortic aneurysm, and aortic valve replacement with an autologous pulmonary valve (the Ross procedure). Aneurysms of the coronary ostia after aortic root replacement can be seen in patients with connective tissue diseases, such as Marfan syndrome. Finally, radiation therapy that includes the aortic root in the radiation mantle causes accelerated atherosclerosis and stenoses of the proximal coronary arteries and the coronary ostia. Symptoms typically occur a decade or more after treatment.

Metabolic Diseases Affecting the Coronary Artery

FAMILIAL HYPERCHOLESTEROLEMIA

Familial hypercholesterolemia (FH) is an autosomal dominant disorder that causes a severe elevation in total cholesterol and low-density lipoprotein (LDL) levels. It is caused by mutations in the LDL receptor gene in chromosome 19. The prevalence of the heterozygous form of FH is 1 in 500 people, and the prevalence of homozygous FH is 1 in 1 million people.[45] Children with the heterozygous form usually are asymptomatic. Children with the rare but clinically much more severe homozygous form present with early atherosclerosis of the coronary arteries, leading to acute myocardial infarction and sudden death at as young as 1 to 2 years of age. These patients also experience peripheral vascular disease, cerebrovascular disease, aortic stenosis, cutaneous xanthomas, corneal arcus, and an LDL level of greater than 600 mg/dL. The role of imaging, except for echocardiography screening

Key Points

Patients usually are referred for CT or MR coronary imaging for diagnosis of a coronary anomaly; confirmation and clarification of echocardiographic findings of coronary anomalies; mapping out the coronary arteries for surgical planning; and evaluation for a coronary aneurysm or stenosis.

The following measures can minimize the CCTA radiation dose: the study must be indicated; a single pass scan should be used with no precontrast scan; the lowest tube voltage possible should be used; the tube current should be minimized for body size; the pitch factor should be maximized; nongated or a prospectively gated mode should be used; and ECG dose modulation should be used.

The following anomalous coronary arteries can be lethal: interarterial LMCA from the right coronary sinus; interarterial LMCA from the RCA; interarterial RCA from the left coronary sinus; interarterial RCA from the LMCA; and LMCA from the noncoronary sinus.

Evaluation of the following congenital heart diseases should include the coronary arteries: tetralogy of Fallot, preoperative; transposition of the great arteries; arterial switch procedure, postoperative; pulmonary atresia with intact ventricular septum; and Williams syndrome.

The following criteria are diagnostic for KD: fever that persists for 5 or more days, along with four of the following findings: changes in the hands and feet: erythema, edema, desquamation; bilateral conjunctivitis; multiform rash; cervical lymphadenopathy; and oral changes (e.g., cracked lips, a red mucous membrane, and a strawberry tongue).

for aortic stenosis, has not been defined for this rare disease. The mainstay of treatment is aggressive cholesterol-lowering medical therapy and treatments of atherosclerosis–related complications. Because FH is a disease of a defective LDL receptor in the liver, liver transplantation has been attempted as a curative procedure.

CORONARY CALCINOSIS

Although coronary calcification is rare in children, it can occur in children with chronic vasculitis, which is seen with KD, radiation, end-stage renal disease, and type I diabetes mellitus. Coronary calcification can be seen as part of idiopathic infantile arterial calcification, a very rare disease characterized by extensive depositions of hydroxyapatite in the elastic layer of the large and medium-size muscular arteries, including the coronary arteries.[46] Coronary stenosis is caused by intimal proliferation, and patients with idiopathic infantile arterial calcification experience myocardial infarction in infancy. Similarly, renal artery stenosis causes hypertension, and carotid stenosis causes cerebral infarction. Patients rarely survive beyond infancy, and many die prenatally. Diagnosis is made by radiologic demonstration of diffuse arterial calcification, arterial biopsy, or prenatal ultrasound demonstrating dilated cardiac ventricles, hydrops fetalis, and hyperechogenic large vessels. Patients are treated with etidronate, which inhibits calcific mineralization in addition to inhibiting bone resorption. Regression of arterial calcification has been shown after treatment, but vascular stenoses may not resolve.

Suggested Readings

Basso C, Maron BJ, Corrado D, et al. Clinical profile of congenital coronary artery anomalies with origin from the wrong aortic sinus leading to sudden death in young competitive athletes. *J Am Coll Cardiol*. 2000;35:1493-1501.

Frommelt PC, Frommelt MA. Congenital coronary artery anomalies. *Pediatr Clin North Am*. 2004;51:1273-1288.

Hellinger JC, Pena A, Poon M, et al. Pediatric computed tomographic angiography: imaging the cardiovascular system gently. *Radiol Clin North Am*. 2010;48:439-467.

Stuber M, Weiss RG. Coronary magnetic resonance angiography. *J Magn Reson Imaging*. 2007;26:219-234.

Tacke CE, Kuipers IM, Groenink M, et al. Cardiac magnetic resonance imaging for noninvasive assessment of cardiovascular disease during the follow-up of patients with Kawasaki disease. *Circ Cardiovasc Imaging*. 2011;4:712-720.

References

Full references for this chapter can be found on www.expertconsult.com.

Chapter 79

Syndromes and Chromosomal Anomalies

BEVERLEY NEWMAN, ALEXANDER J. TOWBIN, and FRANDICS P. CHAN

A large number of syndromes, dysplasias, and chromosomal anomalies are associated with congenital or acquired cardiac and vascular disease. This chapter discusses the cardiovascular features of some commonly encountered lesions. A more extensive list is provided in Tables 79-1 to 79-3.

Syndromes

SITUS AND CARDIOSPLENIC (HETEROTAXY) SYNDROMES

Overview The heterotaxy syndromes, that is, right and left isomerism, feature abnormalities of the visceral situs. These syndromes have an estimated incidence of 1 in 6000 to 1 in 20,000 live births and account for 1% of all congenital heart defects. Although heterotaxy usually occurs sporadically, familial cases have been described.

Although visceral and atrial situs do not always correspond, body situs (from the Latin word meaning location) generally is divided into three types: solitus, inversus, and ambiguus. Situs solitus is the normal arrangement of the viscera in the body (see Chapter 63). Situs inversus is the mirror image of normal; it is seen in 0.01% of the population and is associated with a slightly higher incidence of congenital heart disease (3% to 5%) compared with the solitus population (0.6% to 0.8%). The most common cardiac abnormalities seen in patients with situs inversus are a right-sided aortic arch, atrioventricular discordance, and transposition of the great vessels. Situs ambiguus, or heterotaxy, encompasses all other visceroatrial arrangements. By definition, in situs ambiguus, visceral malposition and dysmorphism associated with an indeterminate atrial arrangement are present.[1]

Heterotaxy syndrome with right isomerism or bilateral right-sidedness is usually, but not invariably, accompanied by asplenia.[1] The condition is more common in males and is characterized by bilateral systemic atria with broad trabeculated appendages (Fig. 79-1), bilateral trilobed lungs with bilateral minor fissures and short eparterial bronchi, a central horizontal liver, bowel malrotation, and the stomach in an indeterminate position (see Fig. 79-1). The abdominal aorta and inferior vena cava often are located on the same side of the spine, frequently in a posterior-anterior orientation. Other occasional anomalies include tracheoesophageal fistula, imperforate anus, absent gallbladder, pancreatic anomalies,

fused adrenal glands, and genitourinary abnormalities.[2] The prognosis for right isomerism is poor because of an abnormal immune status (asplenia) and the typically complex cardiac anomalies.

Cardiac anomalies are almost invariable and cause the most common presenting symptoms: cyanosis and severe respiratory distress. The "right isomerism heart" often consists of a common atrioventricular canal, a single ventricle, a large ventricular septal defect (VSD), and a double-outlet right ventricle and/or transposition of the great vessels, along with pulmonary outflow obstruction or atresia and total anomalous pulmonary venous drainage (frequently obstructed) (see Fig. 79-1). The spectrum of cardiovascular anomalies also can include cardiac malposition (dextrocardia or mesocardia), tricuspid atresia, truncus arteriosus, right aortic arch, anomalous systemic venous return, and bilateral superior vena cavae.[2,3]

Heterotaxy syndrome with left isomerism or bilateral left-sidedness most often accompanies polysplenia. It is characterized by bilateral pulmonary atria with narrow fingerlike appendages, bilateral bilobed lungs, bilateral long hyparterial bronchi, a centrally located liver, the stomach in an indeterminate position, bowel malrotation, and multiclefted or multiple spleens (either right sided or left sided) (Fig. 79-2). An interrupted inferior vena cava with azygos continuation is the most consistent abdominal finding in left isomerism (see Fig. 79-2). Left isomerism is slightly more common in females and generally has a better prognosis than right isomerism with less complex cardiovascular disease. Other associated anomalies include ciliary dyskinesia, biliary atresia, and other gastrointestinal abnormalities including bowel malrotation and pancreatic anomalies, as well as congenital portosystemic shunts (see Fig. 79-2).[2,4]

Cardiac anomalies are seen in more than 50% of patients who have heterotaxy syndrome with left isomerism. The common cardiovascular anomalies include abnormalities of the inferior and superior vena cavae, cardiac malposition, atrial septal defect (ASD), VSD, common atrioventricular canal, double-outlet right ventricle, and anomalous pulmonary venous return (usually partial).[2,3]

Imaging Eight major structures are appraised to evaluate situs in heterotaxy syndromes[1]:

- Atrial morphology
- Cardiac apex

Table 79-1

Syndromes, Dysplasias, and Their Associated Cardiovascular Anomalies

Syndrome	Cardiovascular Anomalies
Achondrogenesis	PDA, ASD, VSD, COA
Alagille syndrome (arteriohepatic dysplasia) (see e-Fig. 79-13)	PS, PPS, ASD, VSD, TOF, PDA, PAT, PAPVR, dysplastic AV valves, COA
Apert syndrome (acrocephalosyndactyly)	ASD, PDA, VSD, PS, TOF, EFE, DEXTRO, COA
Arthrogryposis	CMY
Beckwith-Wiedemann syndrome (EMG syndrome)	CM, CMY, ASD, PDA, TOF, HPLH, subvalvular AS, cardiac fibromas
Cardioauditory syndromes	LVH, RVH
Cantrell syndrome (pentalogy of Cantrell) (see e-Fig. 79-14)	Combined sternal, pericardial, intracardiac, diaphragmatic, and anterior abdominal wall defects Radiographic findings: sternal defect, ectopia cordis, CHD, ASD, VSD, PS, TOF, APVR, DEXTRO, ventricular diverticulum, intrapericardial herniation of abdominal organs; associated with Turner, trisomy 18, sirenomelia, and amniotic band syndromes
Cardiosplenic (heterotaxy) syndromes (see Figs. 79-1 and 79-2)	
Right isomerism (see Fig. 79-1)	TAPVR, AVSD, pulmonary outflow obstruction or PAT, DORV, TGA, single atrium (R), single common ventricle, DEXTRO, TAT, TRU (rare), AO-IVC juxtaposition, bilateral right PAs, bilateral SVC, interrupted IVC
Left isomerism (see Fig. 79-2)	Cardiac malposition, single atrium (L), single ventricle, VSD, AVSD, DORV, APVR, interrupted IVC, bilateral left PAs, bilateral SVC
Cayler syndrome (cardiofacial syndrome)	ASD, PDA, VSD, AVSD, TOF, RAA, COA
CHARGE association	ASD, VSD, conotruncal malformations, PDA, TOF, parachute mitral valve
Degos syndrome (malignant atrophic papulosis)	MI, pericarditis, constrictive pericarditis, myocardial fibrosis, and renal, cerebral, coronary, visceral, and peripheral arteriopathy
Diamond-Blackfan syndrome (congenital red cell aplasia)	VSD, ASD, mitral valve dysplasia
Ehlers-Danlos syndrome (see Fig. 79-3)	MVP, dilated AO root, coronary and aortic aneurysms, dissection or rupture, AS, AR, TR, PS, ASD, VSD, TOF, DEXTRO, LV rupture, arteriovenous fistula
Ellis–van Creveld syndrome (chondroectodermal dysplasia)	Common atrium, ASD, AVSD
Fryns syndrome	Septal defects, arch anomalies, TOF, cystic hygroma
Hallermann-Streiff syndrome (oculomandibulofacial syndrome)	PS, TOF, ASD, VSD
Holt-Oram syndrome (heart-hand syndrome) (see e-Fig. 79-10)	ASD, VSD, MVP, PDA, HPLH, TAPVR, TRU, conduction disorder, hypoplastic peripheral vessels
Jeune syndrome (asphyxiating thoracic dystrophy)	CHF
Kartagener syndrome (primary ciliary dyskinesia) (see e-Fig. 79-11)	DEXTRO, CHD
Klippel-Trénaunay-Weber syndrome (angioosteohypertrophy syndrome)	CHF, pericardial effusion, superficial varices, telangiectatic nevi, organ hemangiomas, lymphatic obstruction
LEOPARD syndrome (cardiomyopathic lentiginosis) (see e-Fig 79-8)	CMY, conduction defect, PS, sub-AS
Loeys-Dietz syndrome (see Fig. 79-5)	Congenital heart defects include patent ductus arteriosus, bicuspid aortic valve, bicuspid pulmonary valve, mitral valve prolapse, and atrial septal defect; arterial tortuosity, stenoses, aneurysms, dissection, diffuse arterial involvement; spontaneous rupture of viscera
Marfan syndrome (see Fig. 79-4)	MVP, MR, dilation of AO root, AR, CHF, aneurysms (AO, pulmonary, ductus), AO dissection, MI, arrhythmia, TR, ASD, TOF
MELAS syndrome	CMY, CHF, conduction abnormalities
Mucolipidosis III	AR
Mucopolysaccharidoses	
IH (Hurler syndrome)	Acute CMY associated with EFE, AR, MR, MS, arteriopathy (coronary, renal, AO, mesenteric)
IS (Scheie syndrome)	AS, MS
II (Hunter syndrome)	AR, CHF, valve thickening, CMY
III (Sanfilippo syndrome)	CMY, MR, AR
IV (Morquio syndrome)	AR, CMY, AS, MR, CAD
VI (Maroteaux-Lamy syndrome)	AS, MS, CMY
Neurofibromatosis type 1 (see Fig. 79-6)	PS, COA, ASD, VSD, CMY, MVP, AS, TOF, PDA, vasculopathy (coronary, pulmonary, renal, systemic), cardiac neurofibroma, arteriovenous fistula, lymphatic abnormality
Noonan syndrome (Turner phenotype with normal karyotype)	PS, dysplastic pulmonic valve, hypertrophic CMY, lymphatic abnormalities, PDA, ASD, COA, mitral valve abnormalities, AS, pericarditis, APVR, coronary anomalies

Continued

Table 79-1

Syndromes, Dysplasias, and Their Associated Cardiovascular Anomalies—cont'd	
Syndrome	**Cardiovascular Anomalies**
Oculoauriculovertebral dysplasia (Goldenhar syndrome)	TOF, VSD, DORV, PAT, TAPVR, RAA, COA, asplenia
PHACES	Arch atresia, aberrant subclavian origins, hypoplasia of the descending thoracic aorta, double aortic arch, COA, stenosis and aneurysm formation of the aorta and the cervical arteries, stroke
Progeria (Hutchinson-Gilford syndrome)	Accelerated atherosclerosis, CM, MI, CHF, stroke
Proteus syndrome	CHD, CMY, myocardial mass, conduction abnormality, venous dilation, hemangioma, lymphangioma
Ravitch syndrome (thoracoabdominal wall defect)	Ectopia cordis, pentalogy of Cantrell, TGA, PDA, ASD, VSD, PS, TOF
Robinow syndrome (fetal face syndrome)	CHD (right heart lesions)
Rubinstein-Taybi syndrome	ASD, VSD, PDA, COA, PS, bicuspid AO valve
Silver-Russell syndrome	CHD
Smith-Lemli-Opitz syndrome	ASD, complex cardiac anomalies
Thrombocytopenia–absent radius (TAR) syndrome	COA, ASD, VSD, PDA, AVSD, TOF
Tuberous sclerosis (Bourneville-Pringle syndrome) (see Fig. 79-7)	Rhabdomyoma, hamartoma, CHF, CMY, COA, arrhythmia, arterial aneurysm and stenosis (AO, cerebral, renal, peripheral)
VATER/VACTERL association (see Fig. 79-9)	VSD, ASD, PDA, TOF, TGA, single ventricle
Velocardiofacial syndrome (Shprintzen syndrome)	TOF, TRU, PA, VSD, absent pulmonary valve, TGA, AS, interrupted AO arch, RAA
Williams syndrome (e-Fig. 79-12)	Supravalvular AS, PPS, MR, ASD, VSD, TOF, MI, COA, interrupted arch, hypoplastic AO, aneurysm or stenosis (AO, systemic, renal, cerebral arteries)
Zellweger syndrome (cerebrohepatorenal syndrome)	CHD, PDA, VSD, DiGeorge

AO, Aorta or aortic; *APVR,* anomalous pulmonary venous return; *AR,* aortic regurgitation; *AS,* aortic stenosis; *ASD,* atrial septal defect; *AV,* atrioventricular; *AVSD,* atrioventricular septal defect; *CAD,* coronary artery disease; *CHARGE,* coloboma, heart defects, atresia choanae, retardation of growth and development, genitourinary problems, ear abnormalities; *CHD,* congenital heart disease; *CHF,* congestive heart failure; *CM,* cardiomegaly; *CMY,* cardiomyopathy; *COA,* coarctation of the aorta; *DEXTRO,* dextrocardia; *DORV,* double-outlet right ventricle; *EFE,* endocardial fibroelastosis; *EMG,* exomphalos, macroglossia, gigantism; *HPLH,* hypoplastic left heart; *IVC,* inferior vena cava; *L,* left; *LEOPARD,* lentigines, electrocardiographic conduction abnormalities, ocular hypertelorism, pulmonary stenosis, abnormal genitalia, retardation of growth, deafness; *LV,* left ventricle; *LVH,* left ventricular hypertrophy; *MELAS,* mitochondrial myopathy, encephalopathy, lactic acidosis, stroke; *MI,* myocardial infarction; *MR,* mitral regurgitation; *MS,* mitral stenosis; *MVP,* mitral valve prolapse; *PA,* pulmonary artery; *PAPVR,* partial anomalous pulmonary venous return; *PAT,* pulmonary atresia; *PDA,* patent ductus arteriosus; *PHACES,* posterior fossa brain malformations, hemangiomas of the face, arterial anomalies, cardiac anomalies, eye abnormalities, sternal clefting or supraumbilical raphe; *PPS,* peripheral pulmonary stenosis; *PS,* pulmonary stenosis; *R,* right; *RAA,* right aortic arch; *RVH,* right ventricular hypertrophy; *SVC,* superior vena cava; *TAPVR,* total anomalous pulmonary venous return; *TAT,* tricuspid atresia; *TGA,* transposition of the great arteries; *TOF,* tetralogy of Fallot; *TR,* tricuspid regurgitation; *TRU,* truncus arteriosus; *VACTERL,* vertebral, anal atresia, cardiac, tracheal, esophageal, renal, limb; *VATER,* vertebral defects, VSD, imperforate anus, tracheoesophageal fistula, radial and renal dysplasia; *VSD,* ventricular septal defect.

Table 79-2

Syndromes that Predominantly Affect the Cardiovascular System	
Syndrome	**Cardiovascular Defects**
Absent pulmonary valve leaflet syndrome (see e-Fig. 79-15)	Maldeveloped nodular myxoid pulmonary valve cusps with aneurysmal dilation of central PAs associated with TOF, airway compression, lobar emphysema and abnormal PA branching, CM, RAA, ASD, VSD, PDA, DORV, AVSD, Marfan syndrome, 18q deletion
Berry syndrome	Distal AP window with AO origin of the right PA and arch interruption
Bland-White-Garland syndrome	Anomalous origin of left coronary artery from PA
Congenital cardiomyopathy: hypertrophic cardiomyopathy	Asymmetric septal hypertrophy, systolic anterior motion of mitral valve, LVOT obstruction, myocardial scar arrhythmias
Arrhythmogenic right ventricular dysplasia	Fibrofatty infiltration of right ventricular myocardium, RV dyskinesia/aneurysms, arrhythmias
Eisenmenger syndrome	Pulmonary hypertension with bidirectional or reversed shunt at atrial, ventricular, or AP level; cyanosis; dyspnea; sudden death; peripartum CMY radiographic findings: dilated central PAs with tapering, PA calcification
Floppy valve syndrome	MVP, prolapse of other valves, CAD, congestive or hypertrophic CMY, ASD, MR, AR, papillary muscle or chordae tendineae rupture
Hypoplastic left heart syndrome	Combined mitral and AO obstruction (stenosis or atresia), underdeveloped LA and LV, hypoplastic ascending AO ± COA or AO interruption; may be associated with right diaphragmatic hernia, omphalocele, brain anomalies; radiographic findings: CM and pulmonary edema

Continued

Table 79-2

Syndromes that Predominantly Affect the Cardiovascular System—cont'd	
Syndrome	**Cardiovascular Defects**
Lutembacher syndrome	ASD associated with MS
Postmyocardial infarction syndrome (Dressler syndrome)	Chest pain, fever, polyserositis—several weeks postinfarction; radiographic findings: pericardial or pleural effusion, noncardiogenic edema
Postpericardiotomy syndrome	Chest pain, fever, joint pain—weeks or months after closed or open heart surgery; radiographic findings: pericardial or pleural effusion, noncardiogenic pulmonary edema, constrictive pericarditis
Romano-Ward syndrome	Familial Q-T prolongation, arrhythmias, syncope
Shone syndrome (or complex) (see e-Fig. 79-16)	Complex of multiple left-sided obstructions, parachute mitral valve, supravalvular ring of LA, sub-AS, COA
Sick sinus syndrome	Arrhythmias
Tetralogy of Fallot (see Fig. 79-9 and e-Fig. 79-15)	Combination of VSD, overriding AO, RVH, RV outflow obstruction; may be PS and PPS
Trilogy of Fallot	PS, ASD (or PFO), right-to-left shunting
Uhl syndrome (anomaly)	Congenital aplasia of RV myocardium, RV CMY
Wolff-Parkinson-White syndrome	Aberrant intracardiac ECG pathway producing arrhythmias; associated with Ebstein anomaly, IHSS, levo-TGA, giant RA diverticulum

AO, Aorta or aortic; *AP*, aorticopulmonary; *AR*, aortic regurgitation; *AS*, aortic stenosis; *ASD*, atrial septal defect; *AVSD*, atrioventricular septal defect; *CAD*, coronary artery disease; *CM*, cardiomegaly; *CMY*, cardiomyopathy; *COA*, coarctation of the aorta; *DORV*, double-outlet right ventricle; *ECG*, electrocardiogram; *IHSS*, idiopathic hypertrophic subaortic stenosis; *LA*, left atrium; *LV*, left ventricle; *LVOT*, left ventricular outflow tract; *MR*, mitral regurgitation; *MS*, mitral stenosis; *MVP*, mitral valve prolapse; *PA*, pulmonary artery; *PDA*, patent ductus arteriosus; *PFO*, patent foramen ovale; *PPS*, peripheral pulmonary stenosis; *PS*, pulmonary stenosis; *RA*, right atrium; *RAA*, right aortic arch; *RV*, right ventricle; *RVH*, right ventricular hypertrophy; *TGA*, transposition of the great arteries; *TOF*, tetralogy of Fallot; *VSD*, ventricular septal defect.

Table 79-3

Chromosomal Anomalies and Their Associated Cardiovascular Defects	
Chromosomal Anomaly	**Cardiovascular Defects**
Fragile X	MVP, MR, AR, TR, dilated AO root, COA
Trisomy 13 (Patau syndrome)	PDA, VSD, ASD, DEXTRO, capillary hemangioma, cervical cystic hygroma
Trisomy 18 (Edwards syndrome)	VSD, polyvalvular heart disease (pulmonary and AO valves), ASD, PDA, COA, TOF, TGA, HPLH, VACTERL, pentalogy of Cantrell
Trisomy 21 (Down syndrome) (see Fig. 79-18)	AVSD, VSD, ASD, TOF, PDA, PS, MVP, aberrant right SCA, intimal arterial fibrodysplasia, lymphatic abnormality, upper airway obstruction and CHF
Cat-eye syndrome (trisomy or tetrasomy 22)	TAPVR, TOF
Monosomy X, XO (Turner syndrome) (see Fig. 79-19)	COA, bicuspid AO valve, AO dissection, septal defects, abnormal mitral valve, sub-AS, PS, APVR, pentalogy of Cantrell, DEXTRO, RAA, hemangioma, lymphangiectasia, venous anomalies
XXY (Klinefelter syndrome)	MVP, Takayasu arteritis, cerebral aneurysms, varicose veins
Deletion Syndromes	
Monosomy 1p36 syndrome	Dilated CMY, PDA
22q11 (predominantly DiGeorge syndrome (CATCH 22), also velocardiofacial syndrome) (see Fig. 79-17)	Type B interrupted arch, RAA, VSD, TOF, TRU, COA, aberrant right SCA, isolated SCA
5p: Cri du chat syndrome	CHD
4p: Wolf-Hirschhorn syndrome	ASD, VSD, valve anomalies, complex CHD, persistent left SVC
17p: Miller-Dieker syndrome (lissencephaly type 1)	ASD, CHD, conduction abnormalities
18q syndrome	Absent pulmonary valve, PDA, AS, dilated ascending AO

AO, Aorta or aortic; *APVR*, anomalous pulmonary venous return; *AR*, aortic regurgitation; *AS*, aortic stenosis; *ASD*, atrial septal defect; *AVSD*, atrioventricular septal defect; *CATCH 22*, cardiac defects, abnormal facies, thymic hypoplasia, cleft palate, hypocalcemia, 22q11 deletions; *CHD*, congenital heart disease; *CHF*, congestive heart failure; *CMY*, cardiomyopathy; *COA*, coarctation of the aorta; *DEXTRO*, dextrocardia; *HPLH*, hypoplastic left heart; *L*, left; *MR*, mitral regurgitation; *MVP*, mitral valve prolapse; *PDA*, patent ductus arteriosus; *PS*, pulmonary stenosis; *RAA*, right aortic arch; *SCA*, subclavian artery; *SVC*, superior vena cava; *TAPVR*, total anomalous pulmonary venous return; *TGA*, transposition of the great arteries; *TOF*, tetralogy of Fallot; *TR*, tricuspid regurgitation; *TRU*, truncus arteriosus, *VACTERL*, vertebral, anal atresia, cardiac, tracheal fistula, esophageal atresia, renal, limb; *VSD*, ventricular septal defect.

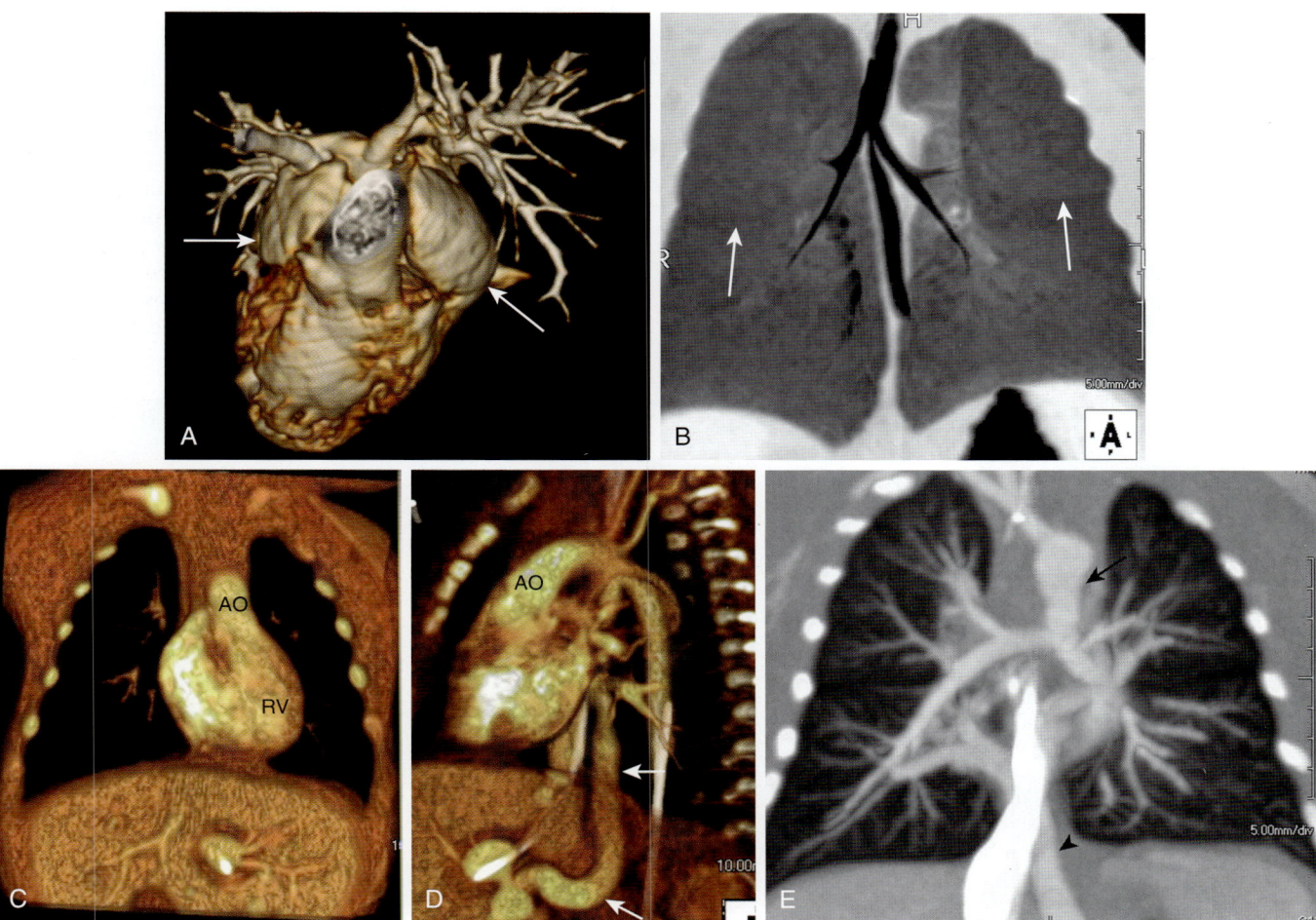

Figure 79-1 **A,** Right isomerism in a 3-year-old girl. Volumetric left anterior oblique, three-dimensional, computed tomographic angiography reconstruction demonstrates bilateral symmetric broad atrial appendages (*arrows*) consistent with right atrial morphology. Note also the anteriorly transposed ascending aorta. **B-E,** A newborn infant with complex congenital heart disease and heterotaxy with right isomerism. **B,** This coronal minimum intensity projection reconstruction demonstrates symmetric short mainstem bronchi consistent with bilateral right-sided bronchial branching. Bilateral minor fissures also are visible (*arrows*). **C,** A coronal volumetric reconstruction demonstrates a horizontal liver with no spleen. The patient has complex congenital heart disease consisting of a common atrioventricular canal (not shown), L-transposition and pulmonary atresia, and total anomalous pulmonary venous return. On this image the left-sided ascending aorta (*AO*) is seen arising from the left-sided morphologic right ventricle (*RV*). **D,** Sagittal volumetric reconstruction demonstrates the anteriorly positioned transposed ascending aorta (*AO*), absent pulmonary artery, and an anomalously draining confluence of pulmonary veins (*arrows*) extending below the diaphragm to the portal vein. **E,** Thin maximum intensity projection demonstrates a large patent ductus arteriosus (*arrow*) as the sole source of flow to the branch pulmonary arteries (the main pulmonary artery is absent). The anomalous inferiorly draining pulmonary veins (*arrowhead*) also are seen, partially obscured by dense contrast in the inferior vena cava.

- Aortic position
- Stomach and bowel position
- Liver and gallbladder position
- Spleen location and morphology
- Abdominal venous drainage
- Bronchial and pulmonary anatomy

Decreased pulmonary vascularity related to pulmonary outflow obstruction or pulmonary edema as a result of pulmonary venous obstruction is the most typical pattern seen on chest radiographs in persons with right isomerism. Cardiomegaly and increased vascularity on chest radiographs as a result of left–to-right shunting are the most common appearance in persons with left isomerism (see Fig. 79-2). Other chest radiographic features of the heterotaxy syndromes are related to duplicated structures, such as fissures and bronchi, as well as abnormal cardiac and visceral situs.

Echocardiography is the main imaging modality used to evaluate disordered intracardiac anatomy associated with heterotaxy. Both magnetic resonance imaging (MRI) and computed tomography (CT) have a role in fully defining this often complex anatomy. MRI, magnetic resonance angiography (MRA), and functional magnetic resonance (MR) assessment have partially replaced catheter–based angiography in evaluating these anomalies, especially the extracardiac vascular, airway, and visceral abnormalities (see Figs. 79-1 and 79-2).[1]

Ultrasound often is the first step in evaluating the abdominal anatomy because of its lack of ionizing radiation and ease of use. An upper gastrointestinal study should be performed to evaluate for malrotation. A small bowel follow through in conjunction with the upper gastrointestinal study is useful to determine the relative locations of the small and large bowel and to separate nonrotation from malrotation. Ultrasound, CT, MRI, or liver-spleen scans using technetium-99m sulfur colloid or p-isopropylacetanilidoimidodiacetic acid are used to evaluate the presence and location of splenic tissue, to assess other organs/anomalies, and to help diagnose biliary atresia (associated with polysplenia). Multimodality imaging may be needed to elucidate other less common anomalies associated with heterotaxy such as a congenital portosystemic shunt and a hypoplastic or absent portal vein (Abernethy malformation) with consequent hyperammonemic encephalopathy or hepatopulmonary syndrome (associated with left isomerism; see Fig. 79-2).[4]

EHLERS-DANLOS SYNDROME

Overview   Ehlers–Danlos syndrome (EDS) is an inherited group of disorders of connective tissue affecting the skin, ligaments, joints, vasculature, and visceral organs. It is characterized by joint and skin hyperextensibility, excessive bruisability, blood vessel fragility, and poor wound healing.[5] It occurs in as many as 1 in 5000 individuals. Although EDS is incompletely understood, six distinct varieties of EDS have been recognized based on genetics, biochemical structure, and clinical presentation.[5,6] Mitral valve prolapse (MVP) is the most common anomaly. Other cardiovascular anomalies

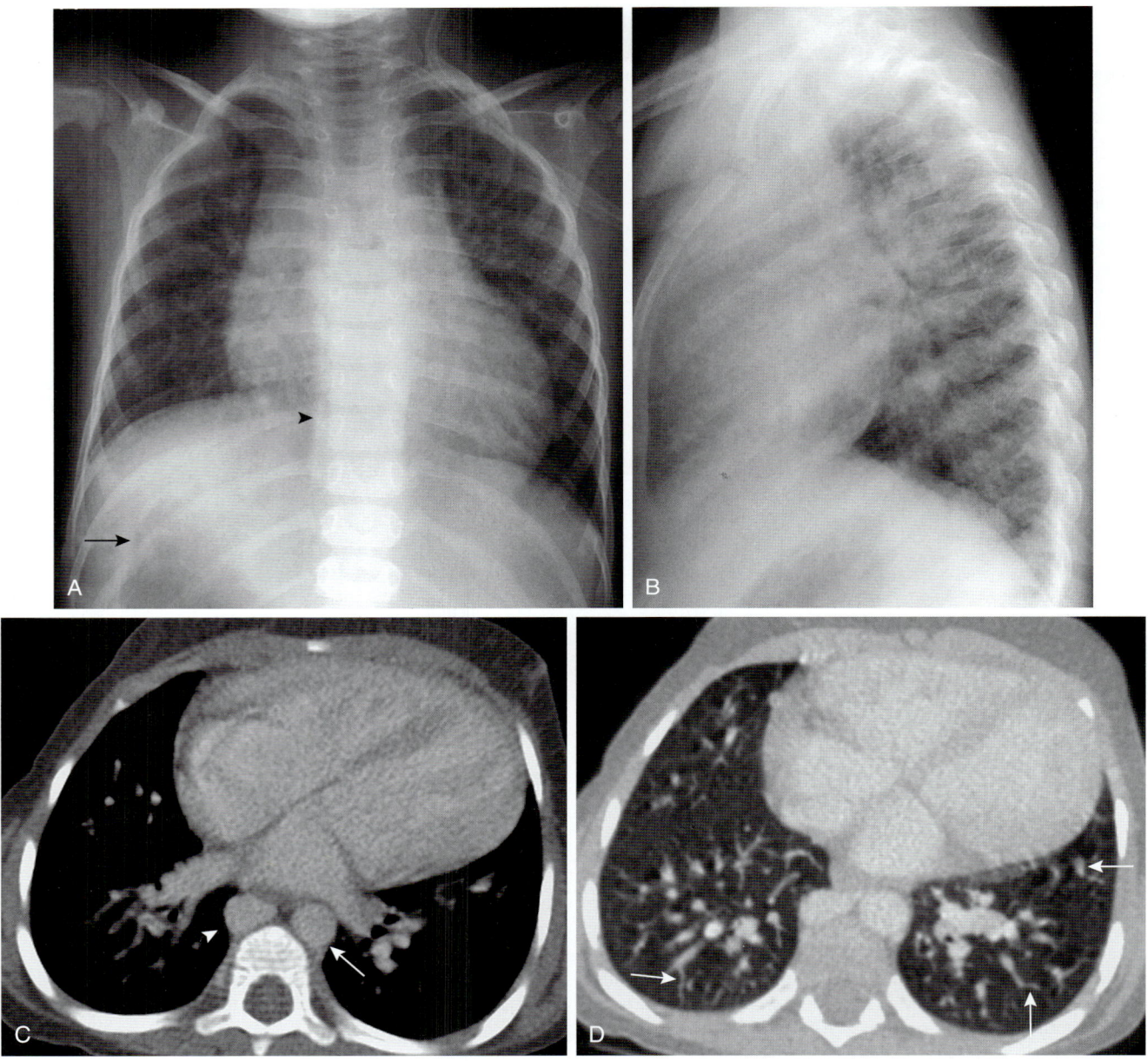

Figure 79-2   This 3-year-old girl, whose mother was diabetic, has polysplenia and Abernethy malformation with hepatopulmonary syndrome. **A,** A posteroanterior view of the chest shows heterotaxy with a left-sided cardiac apex, right-sided stomach (*arrow*), and left-sided liver. Cardiomegaly and increased pulmonary vascularity (a small atrial septal defect and pulmonary arteriovenous shunting) are present. It is difficult to see the bilateral left-sided bronchi. A prominent right paraspinal line is present as a result of an enlarged azygos vein (*arrowhead*). **B,** The lateral view of the chest is notable for the absence of the inferior vena cava shadow. **C,** Contrast-enhanced computed tomography (CT) scan of the chest shows cardiomegaly, a left-sided aorta (*arrow*), prominent pulmonary veins, and an enlarged azygos vein (*arrowhead*). **D,** A contrast-enhanced CT scan of the chest displayed in the lung window shows the presence of multiple dilated peripheral pulmonary vessels (*arrows*).

Continued

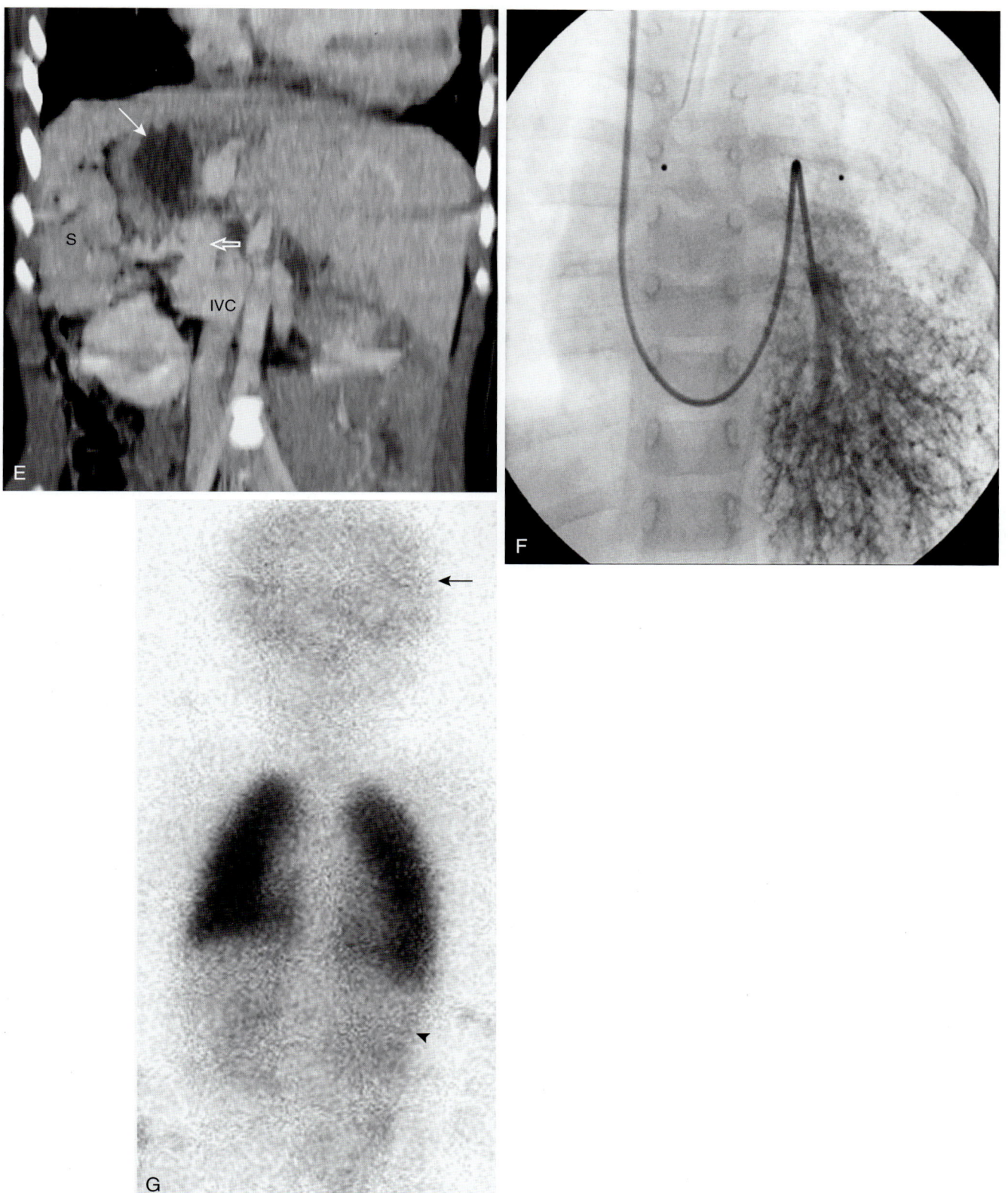

Figure 79-2, cont'd. **E,** Coronal reconstruction from a contrast-enhanced CT scan of the upper abdomen shows right-sided polysplenia (*S*), a right-sided stomach (*white arrow*), and a left-sided liver. A large right-sided portosystemic shunt (splenic vein to renal vein) is present (*open arrow*). Superiorly, there is interruption of the inferior vena cava (*IVC*) with azygos continuation (not shown). **F,** A left pulmonary artery angiogram from a right jugular approach shows dilated peripheral pulmonary arteries and micro arteriovenous connections, consistent with hepatopulmonary syndrome as a result of the congenital portosystemic shunt. This child does not have liver disease, and the intrahepatic portal veins are present but small (Abernethy malformation type II). **G,** Perfusion portion of a ventilation-perfusion scan using technetium-99m macroaggregated albumin performed after closure of the patient's atrial septal defect shows normal perfusion of the lungs. There is abnormal radiotracer uptake within the brain (*arrow*) and kidneys (*arrowhead*). The percentage of systemic tracer uptake was calculated at 44.7%. These findings are typical of a right-to-left arteriovenous shunt and confirm the presence of hepatopulmonary syndrome.

include a dilated aortic root, aneurysm, and aortic dissection or rupture (Fig. 79-3).[7] Papillary muscle dysfunction and left ventricular rupture also can occur.[6]

The vascular or arterial ecchymotic type of EDS is the most clinically severe form. It is an autosomal dominant disorder of the *COL3A1* gene on chromosome 2, which codes for type III procollagen. Patients are subject to spontaneous rupture of the bowel and other viscera. Vascular complications occur either spontaneously or after minor trauma and include arteriovenous fistulas and aneurysms of the aorta and medium-sized arteries, with degeneration and subsequent rupture or dissection (see Fig. 79-3). The thoracic and abdominal arteries are involved in half of the cases, with extremity and head and neck vessels each contributing 25%. Common neurovascular complications include carotid-cavernous fistula formation, carotid dissection, aneurysm formation, and rupture.[5-8]

Imaging, Treatment, and Follow-up Echocardiography is the mainstay for evaluation of the heart and valvular function. Ultrasound, CT, or MR vascular imaging is geared toward defining areas of aneurysm, dissection, and rupture. The size and the rate of growth of each aneurysm should be quantified. Because the neurovascular system may be involved, imaging of the cerebral circulation and the carotid arteries may be necessary.

The pattern of aneurysm distribution in persons with EDS differs from that in persons with Marfan syndrome. Whereas Marfan syndrome typically results in dilation of the aortic root and the sinuses of Valsalva, EDS produces discrete, fusiform aneurysms at different locations of the aorta, the iliac arteries, the cervical arteries, and their branches. Dissection in persons with EDS often has a complex morphology (see Fig. 79-3). The abnormal vessels usually are well characterized by noninvasive computed tomographic angiography (CTA) and MRA.[8] Catheter-based angiography carries significant hazards in these patients with a reported complication rate of 67%.[8]

Because of the rarity of the vascular form of EDS, data are lacking about the proper management of these patients. The substrate of the vascular wall is abnormal, and thus surgical repair often is complicated by the formation of new aneurysm, rupture, or dissection. As a result, surgery is a last resort.[8]

MARFAN SYNDROME

Overview Marfan syndrome is an autosomal dominant disorder of connective tissue caused by mutations in the gene that codes for the extracellular matrix protein fibrillin 1.[9,10] Marfan syndrome is present in 1 in 3000 to 1 in 5000 persons and is associated with skeletal, ocular, and cardiovascular manifestations.[10] The diagnosis of Marfan syndrome is based on clinical criteria—the 2011 revised Ghent nosology.[11]

Common cardiovascular features of Marfan syndrome include MVP, mitral regurgitation, aortic regurgitation, aortic root dilation, and ascending aortic aneurysm (Fig. 79-4). Aortic dissection and aortic rupture are the most life-threatening complications of Marfan syndrome.

MVP affects 35% to 100% of patients with Marfan syndrome and is more common in women and children.[12] More than 80% of children with Marfan syndrome have aortic root dilation, MVP, or both before age 18 years; aneurysms can

be present even in young children.[12,13] Symptoms of heart failure, usually related to valvular insufficiency, can develop in childhood or young adulthood.

Imaging On chest radiographs, a pectus deformity, kyphoscoliosis, and occasionally cystic lung disease may be present in addition to cardiomegaly and a dilated ascending aorta (see Fig. 79-4). Both MRI and transthoracic echocardiography are used for initial evaluation of the heart and aorta. Both have the advantage of being relatively noninvasive without exposing the patient to ionizing radiation. In Marfan syndrome, the dilated aorta/aneurysm typically is pear shaped because the most marked area of dilatation is at the level of the sinuses of Valsalva (see Fig. 79-4).

Long-term surveillance of the aortic root is performed via MRA or CTA, which have the advantage of providing a global view of the entire aorta. Reformatted and three-dimensional techniques provide excellent visualization of the anatomy in any plane and provide accurate long-term measurements (see Fig. 79-4).[14]

Treatment and Follow-up Measurement of the aortic root and assessment of aortic regurgitation are diagnostic criteria for Marfan syndrome. Affected individuals require long-term follow-up to identify progressive aortic root dilation and the appropriate timing for surgical intervention. In older children and adolescents, the incidence of complications such as dissection or rupture increases once the aortic root is larger than 5 cm in diameter.[12,15] Cystic medial necrosis is the underlying pathologic abnormality of the aortic wall. Currently, the Bentall procedure, or composite aortic valve graft replacement, is the standard surgical treatment with demonstrated marked improvement in survival. In some centers, the Bentall procedure has been superseded by the Tirone David procedure, which uses an aortic graft with a surgically resuspended native aortic valve, thus avoiding the need for anticoagulation.

It is now recognized that altered regulation of transforming growth factor-β (TGF-β), cytokines that affect cell performance, causes many of the manifestations of Marfan syndrome. Therapy using TGF-β antagonists appears to offer great promise.[9,15]

LOEYS-DIETZ SYNDROME

Overview Loeys-Dietz syndrome (LDS) is a rare condition associated with the dysregulation of TGF-β caused by mutations in the TGF-β receptor gene.[16] LDS is divided into two types; patients with type 1 LDS have both craniofacial anomalies (e.g., bifid uvula, cleft palate, hypertelorism, craniosynostosis, and cervical spine instability) and widespread vascular anomalies (Fig. 79-5 and Videos 79-1 and 79-2). Patients with type 2 LDS generally have less severe manifestations. They may have a bifid uvula but usually do not have other craniofacial anomalies.[16,17]

Vascular manifestations of LDS include elongated and tortuous large arteries, aneurysm formation, and stenoses (see Fig. 79-5 and Videos 79-1 and 79-2).[18] Abnormalities may be manifested in infancy. Dissection and aneurysm rupture occur commonly in persons with LDS at an earlier age and are associated with smaller sized aneurysms than are typical for persons with Marfan syndrome.[16,17] Although spontaneous

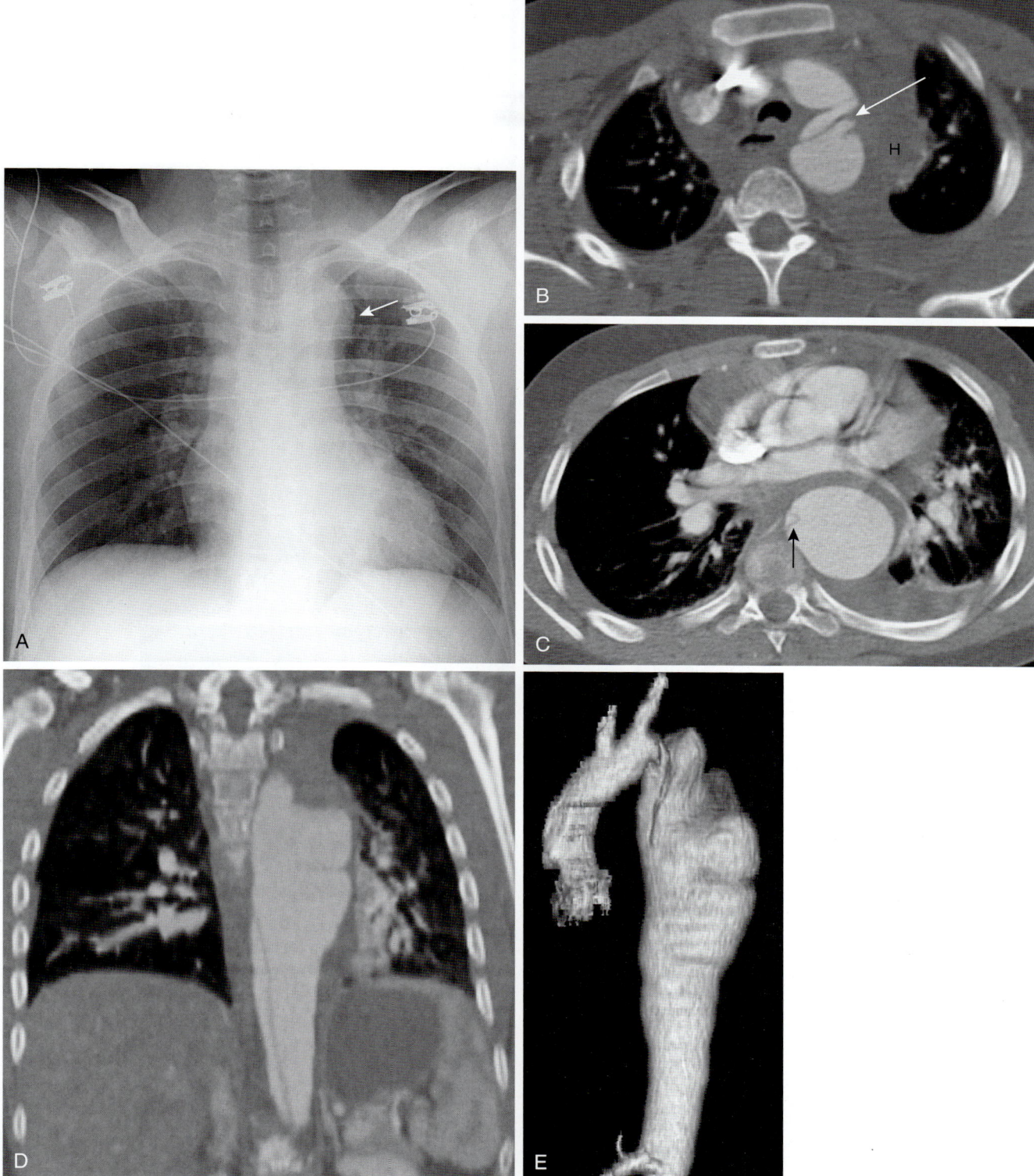

Figure 79-3   Ehlers-Danlos syndrome. This 14-year-old boy presented to the emergency department with chest pain and a family history of dissecting aortic aneurysm. **A,** Posteroanterior view of the chest shows a widened mediastinum and prominent aortic knob (*arrow*). **B,** Computed tomographic angiography (CTA) of the upper chest shows an intimal flap within the aortic arch (*arrow*), representing a dissection. Other findings include a mediastinal hematoma (*H*) and a left-sided pleural effusion. **C,** CTA of the chest at the level of the descending aorta shows a dilated descending aorta with a small intimal flap (*arrow*), a moderate amount of periaortic hematoma, and a small left pleural effusion. Coronal reconstruction (**D**) and three-dimensional reconstruction from the CTA (**E**) show a dissecting aortic aneurysm and irregular dilated aorta.

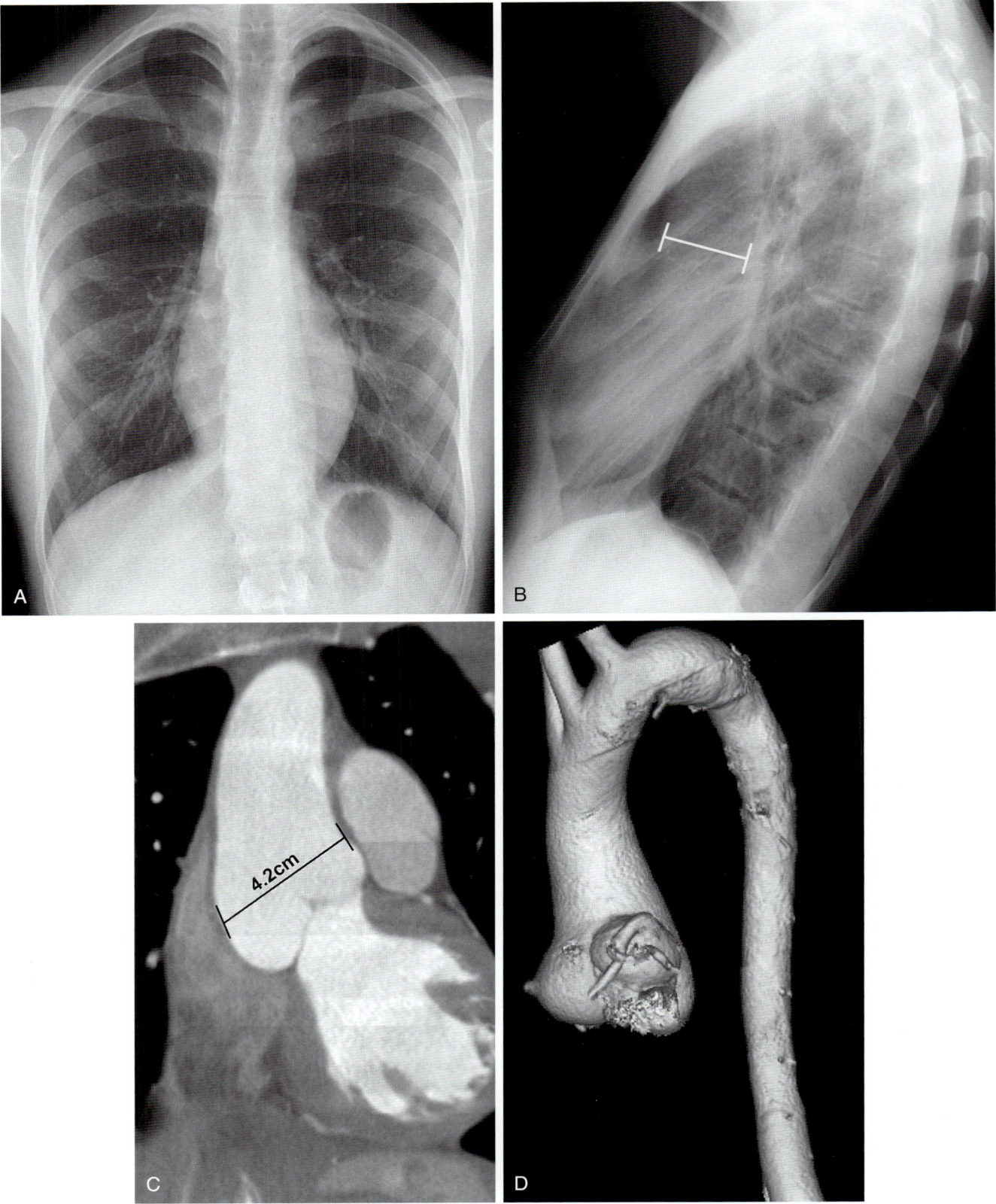

Figure 79-4   An 18-year-old man with a history of Marfan syndrome. **A,** A posteroanterior chest radiograph demonstrates a marfanoid appearance, with an elongated chest and little subcutaneous tissue. The anterior ribs are vertically oriented, suggesting a pectus deformity. **B,** A lateral view of the chest confirms the pectus excavatum and shows a dilated ascending aorta (*line*). Coronal reconstruction (**C**) and oblique sagittal three-dimensional reconstruction (**D**) from computed tomographic angiography of the chest demonstrates the dilated aortic root, which is largest at the level of the sinuses of Valsalva (measurement in **C**).

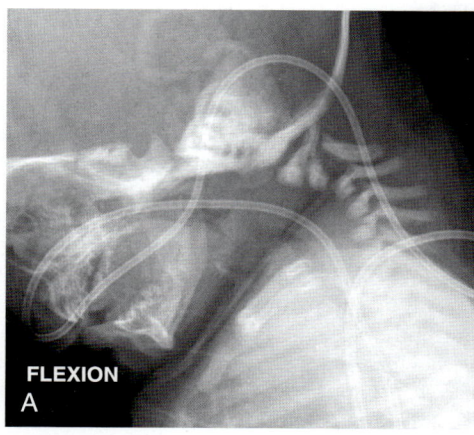 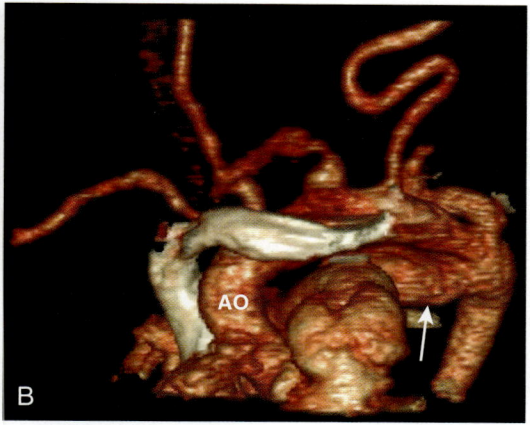

Figure 79-5   An infant with Loeys-Dietz syndrome. **A,** A flexion lateral view of the cervical spine demonstrates instability with marked subluxation, posterior hypoplasia, and kyphosis at C2-C3. **B,** Oblique coronal volumetric reconstruction of computed tomographic angiography. Note a very tortuous aortic (*AO*) arch and all cervical branches as well as an aneurysmal patent ductus arteriosus (*arrow*). See Video 79-1 for markedly tortuous aorta and iliac arteries with multiple stenoses and Video 79-2 for diffuse arterial tortuosity and multiple stenoses. (Courtesy Ron Cohen, Oakland Children's Hospital.)

visceral perforation may occur in patients with LDS (similar to patients with the vascular form of EDS), both the vascular and visceral lesions tend to do quite well with surgical intervention (unlike in patients with EDS).[17]

NEUROCUTANEOUS SYNDROMES

Neurocutaneous diseases affecting the cardiovascular system in children include neurofibromatosis type I, tuberous sclerosis complex, and the more recently described PHACES syndrome (see below).

Neurofibromatosis Type 1

Overview   Neurofibromatosis type 1 (NF1) is an autosomal-dominant disorder with multisystem involvement. It is seen in 1 in 3500 newborns. The classic clinical presentation includes café au lait spots, axillary freckling, dermal and plexiform neurofibromas, and learning disabilities.

Congenital heart defects are present in 2% to 4.3% of persons with NF1. The most common defect is pulmonary stenosis.[19] Other anomalies include tetralogy of Fallot (TOF), aortic stenosis, aortic coarctation, ASD, VSD, patent ductus arteriosus (PDA), and MVP.[2,19,20] Hypertrophic cardiomyopathy has been reported in a small number of patients with NF1. Neurofibromas occasionally can develop within the heart, obstruct cardiovascular blood flow by compression or invasion, or erode a vessel and cause hemorrhage.

Vascular manifestations include stenosis, aneurysms, fistulas, arteriovenous malformations, and spontaneous rupture of systemic arteries and veins (Fig. 79-6). Renovascular stenosis and hypertension are particularly common. Another vascular manifestation known as middle aortic syndrome is caused by the narrowing of the distal thoracic or abdominal aorta, leading to renal vascular hypertension and ischemia of the visceral organs and lower extremities (see Fig. 79-6).[21]

Imaging and Treatment   In addition to cardiovascular findings, chest imaging in persons with NF1 can show rib deformities ("penciling" and "twisted ribbon"), enlargement of the

neural foramen; intercostal, mediastinal, pleural, and soft tissue neurofibromas; and fibrosing alveolitis.

Typically, patients with NF1 are screened with frequent blood pressure measurements and undergo arterial imaging (i.e., CTA or MRA) if hypertension develops.[21] Vascular lesions may be treated with drug therapy, angioplasty, or surgery. Development of an aneurysm has been reported after stent or stent graft placement, consistent with an underlying disorder of the vascular wall.

Tuberous Sclerosis

Overview   Tuberous sclerosis is a disease characterized by hamartomas of multiple organs, cortical tubers, subependymal

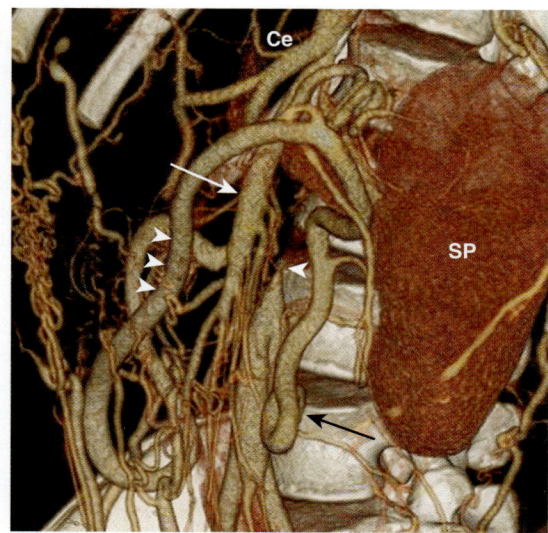

Figure 79-6   Aortic obstruction from neurofibromatosis type 1 in a 14-year-old boy. Volume rendering of an abdominal computed tomography angiogram shows a complete obstruction of the aorta beyond the origins of the celiac trunk (*Ce*) and the superior mesenteric artery (*white arrow*). The distal aorta (*single arrowhead*) is reconstituted through the superior mesenteric artery, the marginal artery of Drummond (*three arrowheads*), and the inferior mesenteric artery (*black arrow*). *SP,* Spleen.

giant cell astrocytomas, and renal angiomyolipomas.[22] It is inherited in an autosomal-dominant pattern and occurs in 1 in 6000 live births. The classic clinical triad is seizures, mental retardation, and skin lesions. The presentation and manifestations of tuberous sclerosis are quite varied, and the diagnosis can be missed for a prolonged period.[22]

Cardiac rhabdomyomas are the most common pediatric cardiac tumors, and 51% to 86% of all cardiac rhabdomyomas are associated with tuberous sclerosis (Fig. 79-7) (see Chapter 81).[23]

Other cardiovascular manifestations of tuberous sclerosis can include central and peripheral arterial aneurysms, aortic coarctation, and vascular stenotic–occlusive disease, including renal artery stenosis.[24] Aneurysms in the abdomen appear at an earlier age than do those in the thorax[25]; the pathologic process is medial atrophy and disruption.

Imaging, Treatment, and Follow-up   Rhabdomyoma is the earliest clinical sign of tuberous sclerosis in utero and can be diagnosed with prenatal or neonatal ultrasound. The presence of multiple cardiac tumors in utero is sufficient to establish a diagnosis of tuberous sclerosis.[26] On ultrasound, rhabdomyomas appear as rounded, homogeneous, hyperechoic areas within the myocardium (see Fig. 79-7).

Cardiomegaly with normal or decreased pulmonary vascular markings is the most common finding on chest radiographs after birth. The signal characteristics of rhabdomyomas on MRI are variable. They often are isointense to minimally hyperintense to the myocardium on T1-weighted images (see Fig. 79-7) and hyperintense on T2-weighted images. Rhabdomyomas may be hypointense to the myocardium after administration of gadolinium. They usually appear as low-density masses on contrast-enhanced CT (see Fig. 79-7).

Rhabdomyomas can cause obstruction of ventricular blood flow, arrhythmias, and loss of functional myocardium, which can lead to low cardiac output, congestive heart failure, and even myocardial infarction. Rhabdomyomas can arise anywhere in the myocardium and are more likely than any other cardiac tumor to arise from a valve. They often are multiple and can invade the pericardium. Areas of central necrosis may be present.

Rhabdomyomas are not considered true neoplasms. They tend to increase in size until 32 weeks of gestation and then progressively regress, especially during the first year of life.[20,23] Children can be monitored with serial echocardiograms; complete regression is observed in most patients by age 6 years.

Screening for aortic aneurysms (via ultrasound, MRA, or CTA) is recommended both at the time of diagnosis of the underlying disease and at frequent regular intervals thereafter.[25] Open elective repair of an identified aneurysm is important because one third of patients with tuberous sclerosis complex and aneurysms present with rupture.[25]

PHACES SYNDROME

Overview   PHACES syndrome, consisting of posterior fossa malformations, hemangiomas, arterial anomalies, cardiac defects, eye abnormalities, and sternal clefting or a supraumbilical raphe, is a recently described neurocutaneous complex with a strong female predominance.[27-30] Features overlap with Sturge-Weber syndrome, leading to confusion

as to the nature of the disease and associated vascular lesions.[29,30]

More than 30% of patients with PHACES syndrome have coarctation of the aorta or other congenital aortic abnormalities such as arch atresia, aberrant subclavian origins, hypoplasia of the descending thoracic aorta, and double aortic arch.[28,29] Progressive abnormalities such as stenosis of and aneurysm formation in the aorta and the cervical arteries are of particular concern. Patients with PHACES syndrome are at an unusually high risk of stroke (as a result of a progressive arterial vasculopathy) and cerebrovascular abnormalities.[27,29] Currently the imaging strategy is geared toward identification of vascular lesions, treatment planning, and monitoring of disease progression.

NOONAN SYNDROME

Overview   Noonan syndrome is an autosomal-dominant disorder that occurs in both male and female infants with an incidence of 1 in 1000 to 1 in 2000. It also is known as pseudo–Turner syndrome because it shares several phenotypic similarities with Turner syndrome. Noonan syndrome is typified by characteristic facies and a webbed neck, short stature, cardiac anomalies, deafness, motor delays, and mental retardation. According to Marino and colleagues,[31] Noonan syndrome is the second most frequent genetic anomaly associated with congenital heart disease after Down syndrome.

The most commonly reported heart defects in Noonan syndrome are pulmonary stenosis with or without a dysplastic pulmonary valve and hypertrophic cardiomyopathy with or without left ventricular outflow tract obstruction[32]; these defects are seen in 38.9% and 9.5% of individuals, respectively. Other abnormalities include ASD, VSD, PDA, TOF, anomalous pulmonary venous return, aortic coarctation, partial atrioventricular septal defect, mitral valve abnormalities, and coronary anomalies.[31] Lymphatic system abnormalities are particularly common and include lymphedema, lymphangiectasia, cystic hygroma, and chylothorax.[32]

The term "neurofibromatosis–Noonan syndrome" has been used for cases of NF1 with Noonan features such as pectus, broad neck, and congenital heart disease.[2] Noonan syndrome is allelic to, and may be associated with, LEOPARD syndrome (lentigines, electrocardiogram abnormalities, ocular hypertelorism, pulmonary stenosis, abnormalities of genitalia, retardation of growth, and deafness) (e-Fig. 79-8 and Video 79-3).[2]

VATER/VACTERL ASSOCIATION

Overview   The VATER (vertebral defects, VSD, imperforate anus, tracheo-esophageal fistula, radial and renal dysplasia) sequence or VACTERL (vertebral anomaly, anorectal atresia, cardiac lesion, tracheoesophageal fistula, renal anomaly, limb defect) association are nonrandom co-occurrences of birth defects. The VATER/VACTERL association occurs in between 2 and 13 per 10,000 births and is more frequent in infants of diabetic mothers and in persons with trisomy 18.[33] A child is diagnosed with the association when he or she has at least two of the characteristics.[34]

Large, population-based studies have examined the association of defects within this complex and suggested that the association of cardiac defects with other VATER components

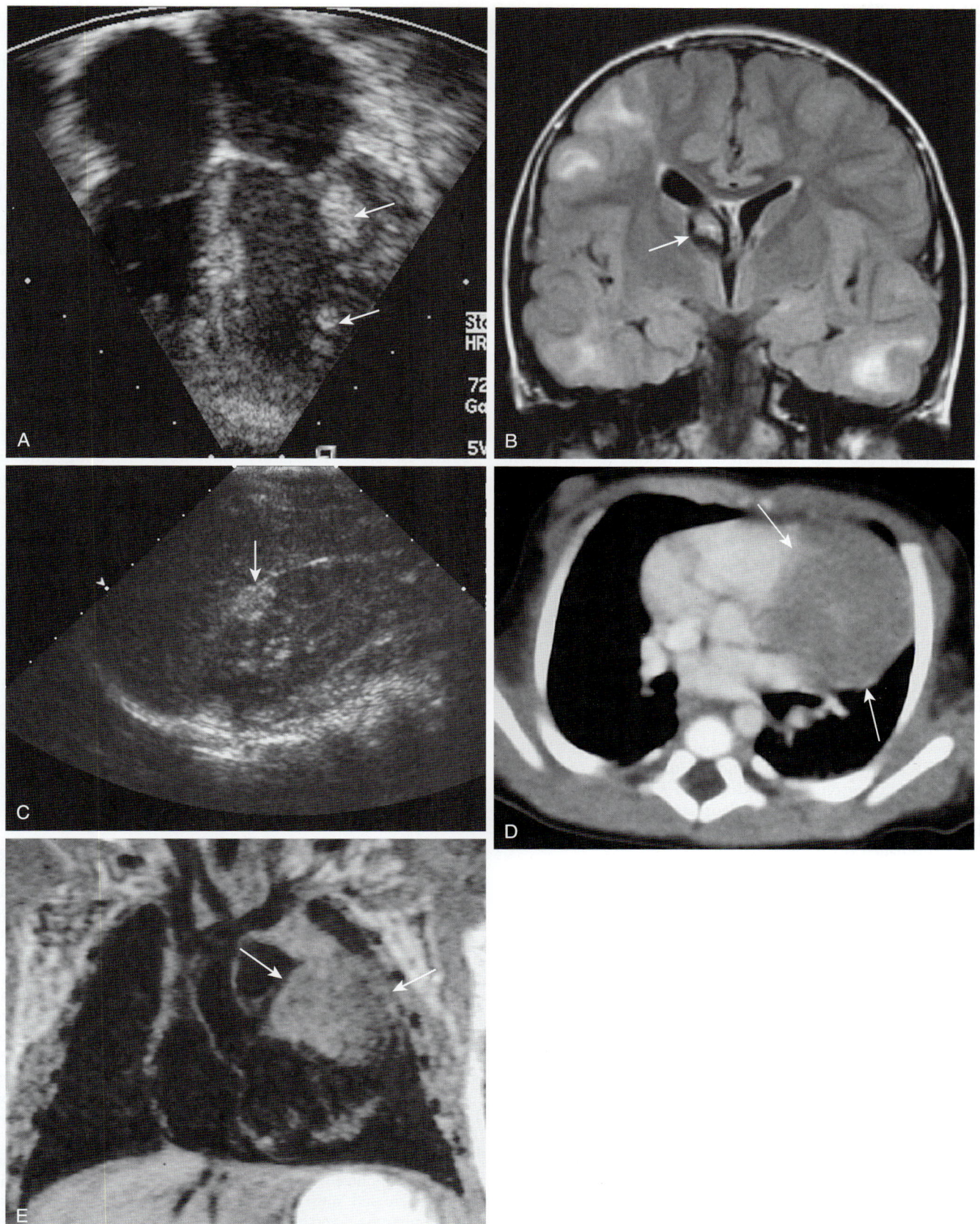

Figure 79-7 Tuberous sclerosis. **A,** Four-chamber view from an echocardiogram shows multiple echogenic masses within the free wall of the left ventricle (*arrows*). The cardiac tumors, representing rhabdomyomas, resolved spontaneously. **B,** Coronal fluid-attenuated inversion recovery magnetic resonance imaging of the brain from the same child 2 years later shows multiple hyperintense subcortical tubers and a mixed-signal giant cell astrocytoma (*arrow*) at the foramen of Monro. **C,** Sagittal ultrasonography of the right kidney shows a hyperechoic lesion in the anterior mid kidney (*arrow*) that is consistent with an angiomyolipoma. **D,** Contrast-enhanced computed tomography of a different 3-day-old boy with an abnormal chest radiograph demonstrates a large, hypodense, soft-tissue density mass of the left ventricular wall (*arrows*). **E,** A coronal T1-weighted magnetic resonance image demonstrates the large, isointense-to-muscle rhabdomyoma in the left ventricular free wall (*arrows*). (**A,** Courtesy Lizabeth Lanford, MD, Children's Hospital, Pittsburgh, PA.)

is no more frequent than with any other birth defect.[34] The cardiac anomalies described with the VACTERL association include VSD, ASD, PDA, dextrocardia, TOF, aortic coarctation, a single ventricle, and transposition of the great arteries (see Chapters 74, 75, and 76).

Bronchopulmonary foregut malformations other than the tracheoesophageal fistula complex also can be associated with a spectrum of anomalies similar to VACTERL. These malformations include tracheal agenesis, pulmonary hypoplasia and agenesis, pulmonary sling, scimitar syndrome, congenital lobar hyperinflation, congenital pulmonary airway malformation, bronchial atresia, and pulmonary sequestration. The exact incidence and frequency of anomalies vary somewhat. For example, children with tracheal agenesis tend to have more complex cardiac anomalies than do those who have a tracheoesophageal fistula.[35] Imperforate anus occurs much more frequently with a tracheoesophageal fistula than with tracheal agenesis.[35]

Imaging and Follow-up Prenatal diagnosis can be made with ultrasound. Prenatal findings include radial atresia or abnormality, vertebral anomalies, polyhydramnios, a single umbilical artery, intrauterine growth restriction, and renal and cardiac anomalies.[36] After delivery, echocardiography, plain films, fluoroscopy, CT, and MRI can supplement the clinical findings and confirm the diagnosis (Fig. 79-9). Part of the importance of recognizing this association of anomalies is that when one or more anomalies occur, others should be sought. Therefore infants with esophageal atresia, imperforate anus, or vertebral anomalies should undergo renal and cardiac ultrasound screening. Spinal ultrasound should be performed in the case of imperforate anus to look for occult dysraphism and cord tethering.

The prognosis of an infant diagnosed with VATER/VACTERL is variable and depends on the severity of disease. A study by Tongsong et al[36] described a neonatal mortality of 28% in infants with three or more anomalies.[36] Because of the variable prognosis, early diagnosis and clear identification of all anomalies are important.

OTHER SYNDROMES

Other less common syndromes and their associated cardiovascular components are listed in Table 79-1 (see e-Fig. 79-8, e-Figs. 79-10 through 79-14, and Video 79-4). The most common associated cardiac lesions are listed first. Many other rare syndromes have associated cardiac malformations; however, these syndromes are too numerous to mention specifically. Table 79-2 outlines syndromes that have cardiovascular manifestations almost exclusively (e-Figs. 79-15 and 79-16). This list is not exhaustive but includes the more common, important, and interesting entities.

Chromosomal Anomalies

22Q11 DELETION—DIGEORGE SYNDROME

Overview The 22q11 deletion is the most common chromosome deletion in DiGeorge syndrome and the velocardiofacial syndrome.[4] DiGeorge syndrome often is remembered by the acronym CATCH 22, which refers to the major

manifestations: Cardiac defects, Abnormal facies, Thymic hypoplasia, Cleft palate, Hypocalcemia (absent parathyroid) and 22q11 deletions. The defects seen in the DiGeorge syndrome are field defects of the third and fourth pharyngeal pouches. The most commonly associated cardiac anomalies are truncus arteriosus (Fig. 79-17) and interruption of the aortic arch (usually type B) (see Fig. 79-17), as well as TOF and aberrant or isolated subclavian artery.[37]

DiGeorge syndrome is associated with other syndromes including fetal alcohol syndrome, Noonan syndrome, and Zellweger syndrome. It also is associated with infants of diabetic mothers.[2]

The absence of the thymic shadow on radiographs in the first week of life in association with heart disease should raise strong consideration of DiGeorge syndrome. However, the thymus is not necessarily entirely absent and may just be hypoplastic.

Imaging and management depends on the severity of cardiac and other anomalies. Increased susceptibility to infections, especially respiratory infections, including unusual organisms seen in immunocompromised hosts (such as acid fast bacilli and pneumocystis), are a significant management concern.[2]

FRAGILE X SYNDROME

Overview Fragile X syndrome is the most common inherited form of mental retardation. Approximately 1 in 850 people carry the gene for this X-linked disorder; however, about 20% of males with the gene are unaffected. Affected individuals may have large heads and facial abnormalities along with learning disabilities and behavioral problems. Associated cardiac abnormalities include MVP, mitral regurgitation, aortic regurgitation, tricuspid regurgitation, a dilated aortic root, and coarctation.[2]

TRISOMY 21 (DOWN SYNDROME)

Overview Down syndrome, the most common chromosomal anomaly, is seen in 1 in 600 to 1 in 700 live births. Down syndrome is the most frequent genetic anomaly associated with congenital heart disease. Approximately 40% to 70% of patients with Down syndrome have congenital cardiac malformations, which represent the leading cause of death in the first 2 years of life.[38]

The most characteristic abnormality in Down syndrome is an ASD with a common atrioventricular junction, also known as a common atrioventricular canal, atrioventricular septal defect, or endocardial cushion defect (Fig. 79-18) (see Chapter 73). Almost 70% of endocardial cushion defects are associated with Down syndrome. Other common cardiac defects include VSD, PDA, TOF, and pulmonary stenosis.[2,38]

Arterial and lymphatic abnormalities also occur, the latter especially in utero.[2] Because persons with Down syndrome have decreased muscular tone, a relatively large tongue, a small pharynx, and laryngotracheomalacia, chronic upper airway obstruction may be a significant clinical problem and can result in congestive heart failure.

Imaging A combination of plain chest radiographs, echocardiography and ultrasound, and CT or MRI are used most

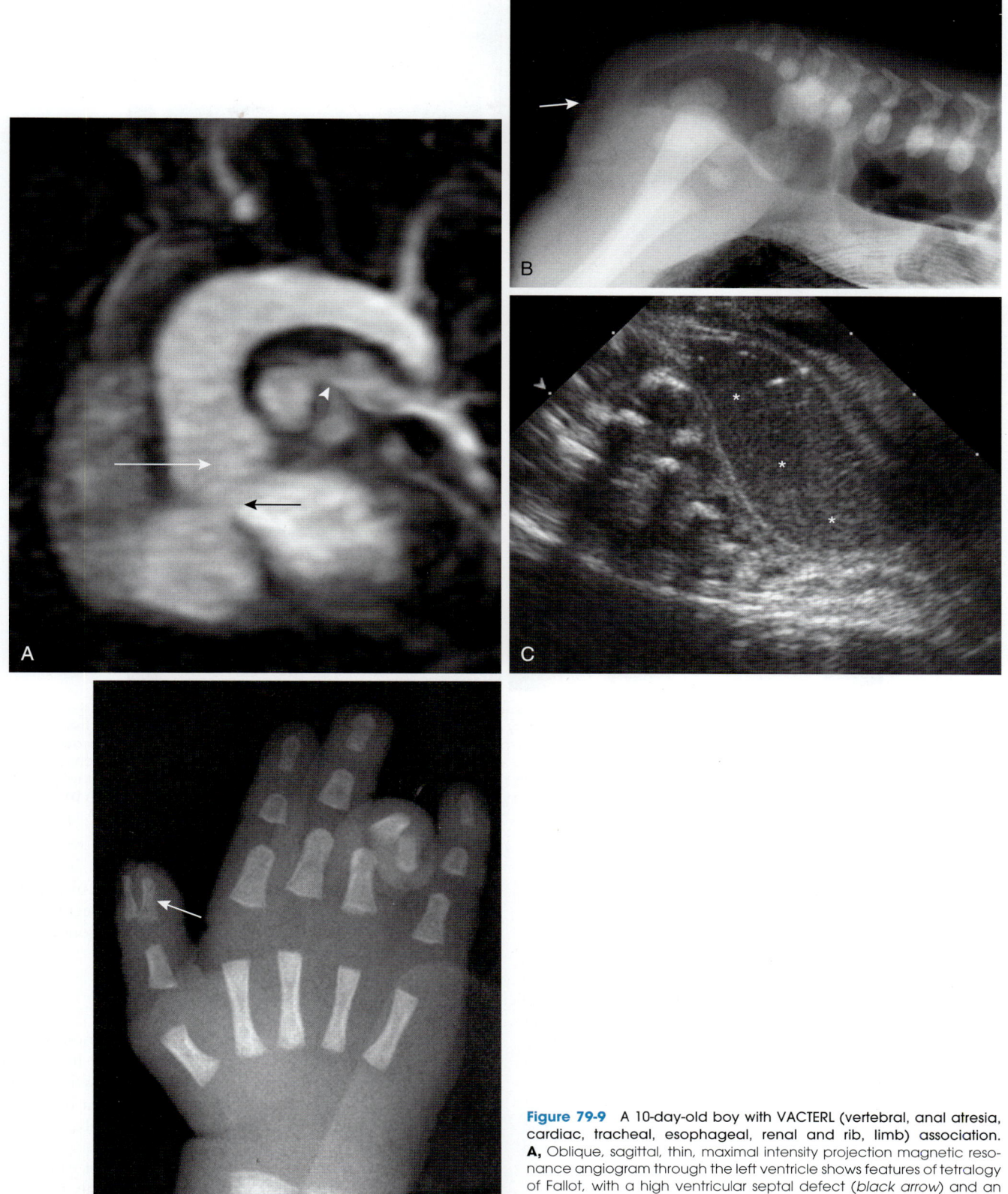

Figure 79-9 A 10-day-old boy with VACTERL (vertebral, anal atresia, cardiac, tracheal, esophageal, renal and rib, limb) association. **A,** Oblique, sagittal, thin, maximal intensity projection magnetic resonance angiogram through the left ventricle shows features of tetralogy of Fallot, with a high ventricular septal defect (*black arrow*) and an overriding aorta (*white arrow*). Stenosis of the proximal left pulmonary artery is present (*arrowhead*). A prone, cross-table lateral radiograph (**B**; *arrow* on anal dimple) and sagittal transabdominal ultrasonography (**C**) show an imperforate anus with a dilated, meconium-filled, distal sigmoid colon and rectum. **D,** A frontal radiograph of the left hand shows a duplicated distal first phalanx of the thumb (*arrow*). The child's ring finger is flexed.

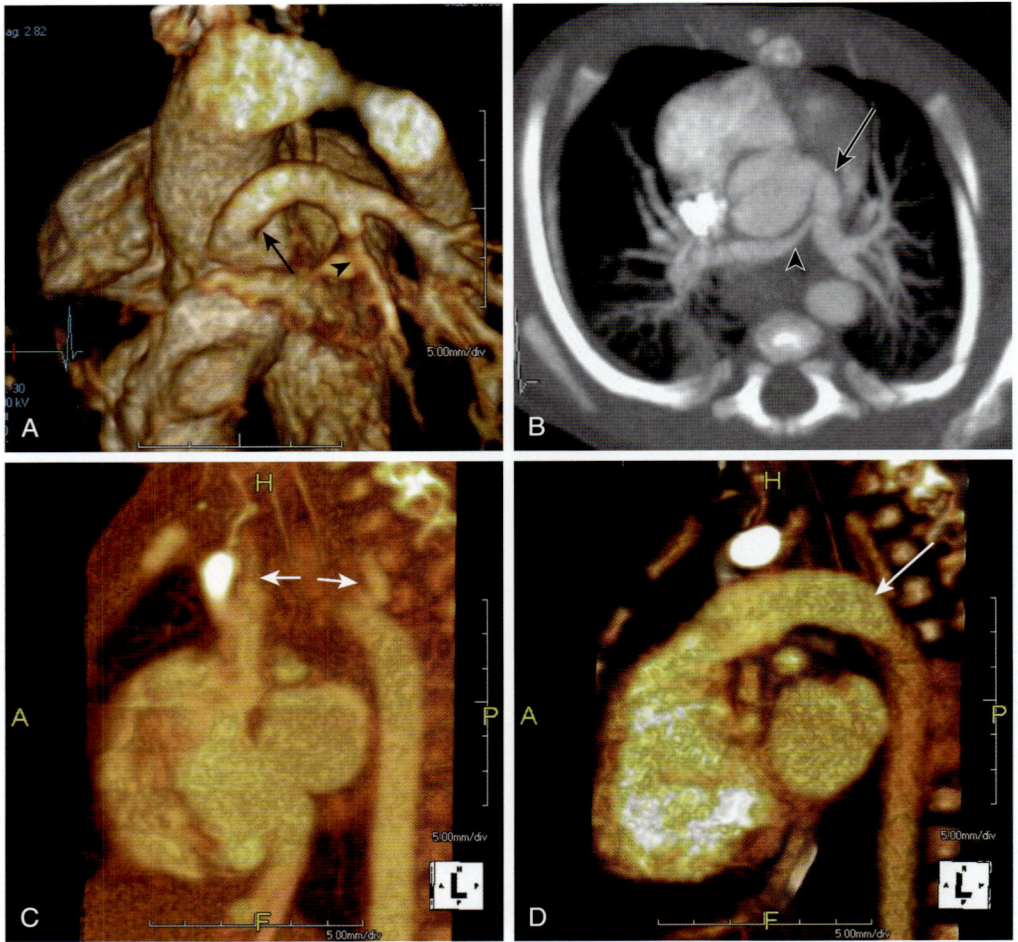

Figure 79-17   Two newborn infants with 22q11 deletion (DiGeorge syndrome). **A** and **B,** Truncus arteriosus type 1. A volume rendered, three-dimensional reconstruction, posterior oblique view (**A**) and axial thin maximum intensity projection (**B**) demonstrate a single great artery arising from the heart. The main pulmonary artery (*arrow*) arises from this vessel, which continues as the ascending aorta. Note branch pulmonary arteries with narrowing of the right pulmonary artery (*arrowhead*). **C** and **D,** Sagittal three-dimensional volumetric reconstructions show interruption of the aortic arch (type B). A marked gap exists between the ascending and descending aorta, with interruption between the left common carotid and left subclavian arteries (*arrows* in **C**). A large patent ductus arteriosus extends from the pulmonary artery centrally and supplies the descending aorta (*arrow* in **D**).

often to evaluate and manage cardiovascular lesions in persons with Down syndrome, supplemented by catheter angiography as needed (see Fig. 79-18).

Noncardiac chest imaging findings include the presence of 11 ribs and hypersegmentation of the manubrium, as well as multiple small peripheral and parafissural cysts thought to represent hypoplastic/dysplastic lung changes. Recurrent infection, follicular bronchiolitis, and increased tumor propensity, especially leukemia and lymphoma, are additional features related to immune dysfunction in persons with Down syndrome. Abdominal findings include a characteristic configuration of the pelvis (flattened acetabula and flared iliac wings), duodenal stenosis or atresia, annular pancreas, and Hirschsprung disease.

TRISOMY 13 (PATAU SYNDROME)

Overview   Patau syndrome is the least common and the most severe of the viable trisomies. It occurs in 1 in 29,000 live births. Eighty-two percent of patients die within the first

month of life. Congenital heart defects are seen in approximately 80% of patients. The most common defects include ASD, VSD, PDA, dextrocardia, and a double-outlet right ventricle.[2]

TRISOMY 18 (EDWARDS SYNDROME)

Overview   Trisomy 18 is the second most common autosomal trisomy, with prevalence at birth of about 1 in 7000. It is characterized by severe psychomotor and growth retardation, microcephaly, microphthalmia, micrognathia or retrognathia, microstomia, malformed ears, distinctively clenched fingers, and other congenital malformations.

Cardiac anomalies are seen in 90% to 100% of cases. The most common cardiac anomalies are VSD and valvular heart disease.[2] The pulmonary and aortic valves usually are affected. Other cardiac anomalies include ASD, PDA, aortic coarctation, TOF, transposition of the great arteries, and a hypoplastic left heart. Anomalies of the VACTERL spectrum also are associated with trisomy 18.

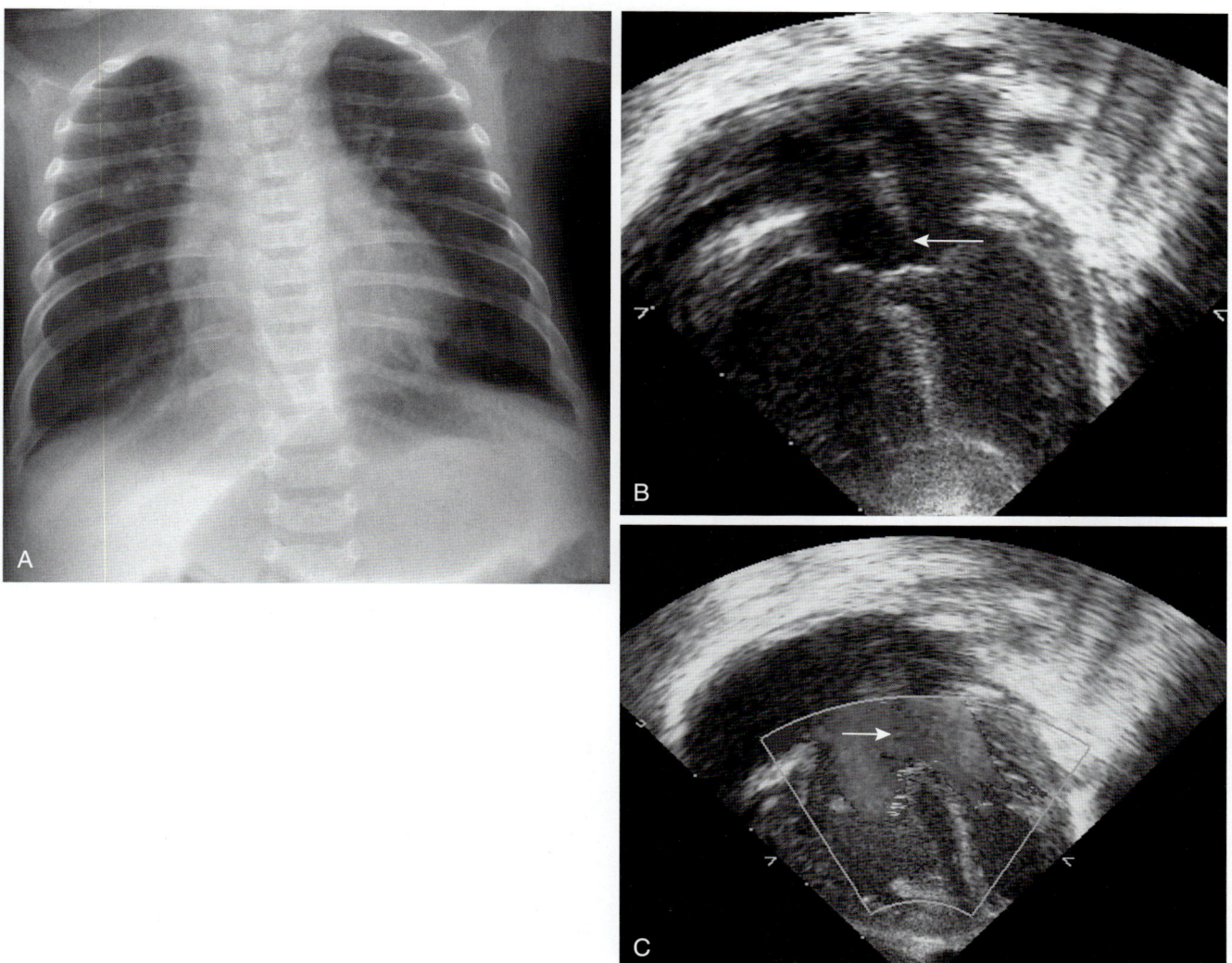

Figure 79-18 A 3-month-old girl with Down syndrome and a known atrioventricular septal defect. **A,** A chest radiograph shows increased vascularity, mild congestion, and accompanying hyperinflation of the lungs. Eleven ribs are present bilaterally. **B,** A four-chamber view from an echocardiogram shows a large atrioventricular septal defect (*arrow*). **C,** Left-to-right color Doppler flow is shown across the atrial defect (*arrow*). (**B** and **C,** Courtesy Liza-beth Lanford, MD, Children's Hospital, Pittsburgh, PA.)

TURNER SYNDROME (XO, MONOSOMY X)

Overview Turner syndrome is one of the most frequent chromosomal aberrations in females. It affects approximately 1 in 2000 live female births, but it has been estimated that only 1% of fetuses survive to term and that as many as 10% of spontaneous miscarriages have the 45,XO karyotype.[39] The characteristic clinical findings include a webbed neck, a shield chest with widely spaced nipples, short stature, gonadal insufficiency, and infertility.[40]

A congenital heart defect occurs in 20% to 40% of patients with Turner syndrome. The most common cardiac anomalies include coarctation of the aorta (30%) (Fig. 79-19) and bicuspid aortic valve (30% to 50%). Dilation of the aortic root is not as common (3% to 8%) but can have devastating consequences such as dissection and rupture.[39] Other less common malformations include MVP, aortic stenosis, aortic regurgitation, partial anomalous pulmonary venous drainage, and hypoplastic left heart syndrome. Lymphangiectasia, lymphedema, hemangiomas, and systemic venous anomalies also can occur.[40]

Imaging The approach to imaging of the cardiovascular system in both Turner and Noonan syndrome varies with the clinical scenario and is similar to other diseases with widespread cardiovascular manifestations such as Marfan syndrome and other collagen disorders.

KLINEFELTER SYNDROME (XXY)

Overview Klinefelter syndrome is present in 1 in 500 to 1 in 1000 live male births.[41] The clinical findings of Klinefelter syndrome include infertility, gynecomastia, hypogonadotropic hypogonadism, cognitive impairment, and predisposition to malignancy.[41]

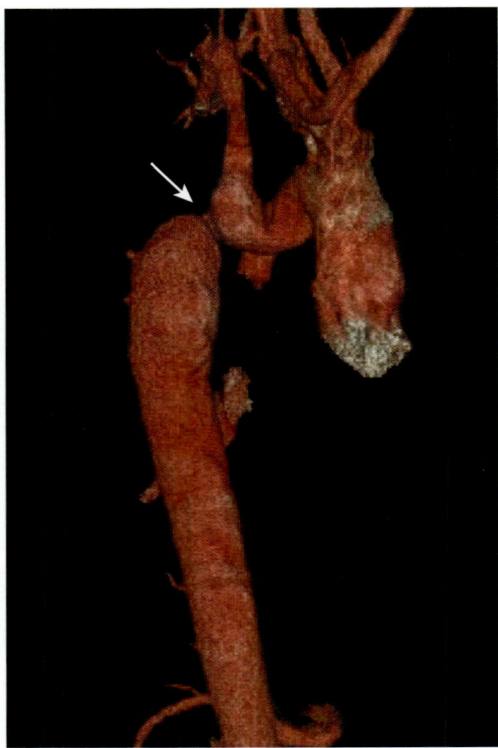

Figure 79-19 A 10-year-old girl with Turner syndrome. This sagittal oblique three-dimensional volumetric reconstruction of the aortic arch demonstrates marked tortuosity of the transverse arch along with focal coarctation immediately distal to the left subclavian artery (*arrow*).

MVP, the most common cardiac anomaly, occurs in 55% of patients. Other uncommon defects include TOF, ASD, VSD, tricuspid atresia, and aortic coarctation. Vascular abnormalities include cerebral aneurysms, varicose veins, venous thromboemboli, and arteritis.[42]

OTHER CHROMOSOMAL ANOMALIES

Less common chromosomal anomalies and their associated cardiovascular lesions are listed in Table 79-3. The most commonly associated defects are listed first, and cardiac lesions generally are listed before vascular malformations.

Suggested Readings

Syndromes

Araoz PA, Eklund HE, Welch TJ, et al. CT and MR imaging of primary cardiac malignancies. *Radiographics.* 1999;19:1421-1434.

Berdon WE, Willi U. Situs inversus, bronchiectasis, and sinusitis and its relation to immotile cilia: history of the diseases and their discoverers—Manes Kartagener and Bjorn Afzelius. *Pediatr Radiol.* 2004;34:3842.

Cyran SE, Martinez R, Daniels S, et al. Spectrum of congenital heart disease in CHARGE association. *J Pediatr.* 1987;110:576-578.

Elliott M, Bayly R, Cole T, et al. Clinical features and natural history of Beckwith-Wiedemann syndrome: presentation of 74 new cases. *Clin Genet.* 1994;46:168-174.

Greenhalgh KL, Howell RT, Bottani A, et al. Thrombocytopenia–absent radius syndrome: a clinical genetic study. *J Med Genet.* 2002;39:876-881.

Morrison PJ, Mulholland HC, Craig BG, et al. Cardiovascular abnormalities in the oculo-auriculo-vertebral spectrum (Goldenhar syndrome). *Am J Med Genet.* 1992;44:425-428.

Sletten LJ, Pierpont ME. Variation in severity of cardiac disease in Holt-Oram syndrome. *Am J Med Genet.* 1996;65:128-132.

Stevens CA, Bhakta MG. Cardiac abnormalities in the Rubinstein-Taybi syndrome. *Am J Med Genet.* 1995;59:346-348.

Wippermann CF, Beck M, Schranz D, et al. Mitral and aortic regurgitation in 84 patients with mucopolysaccharidoses. *Eur J Pediatr.* 1995;154:98-101.

Chromosomal Anomalies

Duarte AC, Menezes AIC, Devens ES, et al. Patau syndrome with a long survival: a case report. *Genet Mol Res.* 2004;3:288-292.

Versacci P, Digilio MC, Sauer U, et al. Absent pulmonary valve with intact ventricular septum and patent ductus arteriosus: a specific cardiac phenotype associated with deletion 18q syndrome. *Am J Med Genet A.* 2005;138:185-186.

References

Full references for this chapter can be found on www.expertconsult.com.

Myocardial, Endocardial, and Pericardial Diseases

ANA MARIA GACA, CHARLES M. MAXFIELD, and BEVERLEY NEWMAN

Myocardial Diseases

Cardiomyopathy is a chronic and often progressive disease of the myocardium with associated cardiac dysfunction. It is a rare but serious disorder; only 25% of children survive more than 5 years after the onset of symptoms. Although our understanding of the causes of pediatric cardiomyopathy has advanced, the prognosis has not changed considerably in the past 30 years and is the same in developing and industrialized nations.[1,2]

Cardiomyopathy can be classified according to the dominant pathophysiology and etiology (e-Box 80-1). Four major physiologic forms of cardiomyopathy exist: dilated, hypertrophic, restrictive, and arrhythmogenic. Hypertrophic and dilated cardiomyopathies are the most common forms in children.[2] Patients may be classified as having more than one physiologic form of cardiomyopathy.

Cardiomyopathy also may be classified according to etiology. Cardiomyopathies associated with particular cardiac or systemic diseases are referred to as specific cardiomyopathies. Inflammatory and isolated familial cardiomyopathies account for the majority of pediatric cases with a known cause.[3] Other specific cardiomyopathies that are less common in the pediatric population include those associated with metabolic disorders, general systemic diseases, muscular dystrophies, neuromuscular disorders, and sensitivity or toxic reactions (e.g., radiation and chemotherapy). In two thirds of children with cardiomyopathy, no etiology is found.[2,3]

Because of its availability, lack of radiation use, and portability, echocardiography is the most common method used to classify cardiomyopathy and evaluate cardiac function. With improvements in technology, cardiovascular magnetic resonance imaging (MRI) has become an accepted tool for assessing cardiomyopathy.[4,5] With the multiple techniques available, cardiac MRI can be used to assess myocardial morphology and function (cine sequences), myocardial perfusion reserve (first-pass contrast-enhanced perfusion), and myocardial viability and scar formation (delayed enhancement sequence).[4]

Treatment of cardiomyopathy typically involves medical therapy aimed at optimizing cardiac function through the use of medications, including antiarrhythmic agents, β-blockers, and diuretics. Pacemakers and defibrillation devices may be necessary, depending on the form of cardiomyopathy. Any known underlying cause also must be treated.

HYPERTROPHIC CARDIOMYOPATHY

Hypertrophic cardiomyopathy is commonly familial and is inherited in an autosomal-dominant fashion with variable penetrance and expression.[6] Although some children are asymptomatic, hypertrophic cardiomyopathy can present with arrhythmias and sudden cardiac death at any age.[4] Hypertrophic cardiomyopathy generally is characterized by left ventricular hypertrophy without a demonstrable cause. Although any region of the left ventricle can be involved, hypertrophy of the interventricular septum often is present, which may cause left ventricular outflow tract obstruction (Fig. 80-1 and Video 80-1). The right ventricle also may be affected.

Echocardiography is the standard method of diagnosing hypertrophic cardiomyopathy, but cardiac MRI can be used to assess the location and degree of hypertrophy, including areas difficult to visualize with echocardiography, such as the cardiac apex and portions of the right ventricle.[7] Cine gradient echo sequences can be used to evaluate the flow dynamics of the left ventricular outflow tract both before and after surgery. Contrast-enhanced MRI also may demonstrate delayed enhancement within scarred or fibrotic areas of myocardial hypertrophy—areas thought to play a role in the arrhythmias associated with hypertrophic cardiomyopathy.[8,9]

DILATED CARDIOMYOPATHY

Dilated cardiomyopathy is characterized by dilation and impaired contraction of the left ventricle or both ventricles, and patients typically present with progressive heart failure.[6] Most pediatric cases are idiopathic, but causes include infectious myocarditis, familial disease, and neuromuscular disorders (Duchenne and Becker muscular dystrophies).[10] Coronary

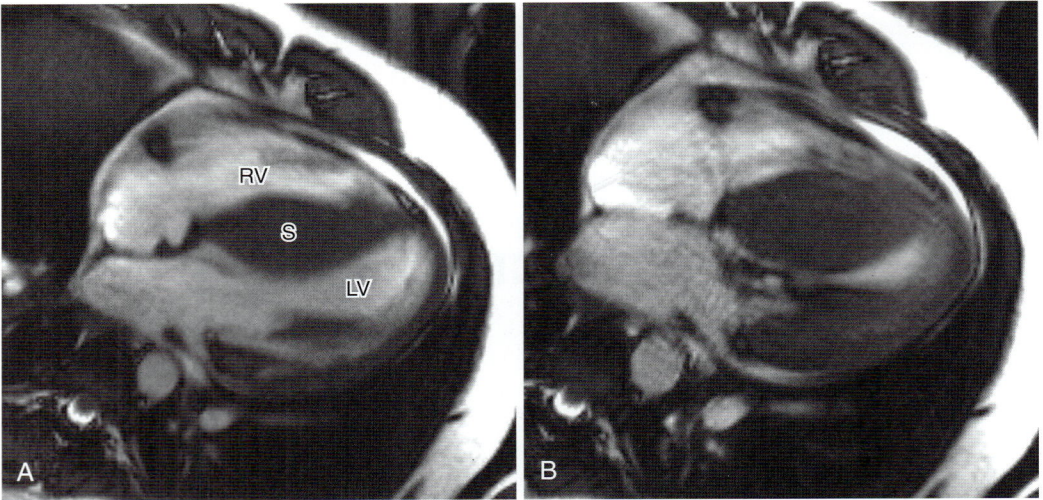

Figure 80-1 Hypertrophic cardiomyopathy. **A,** Four-chamber cine magnetic resonance view at end-diastole shows marked septal (*S*) thickening. **B,** During systole, near-complete obliteration of the left ventricular chamber occurs. *LV,* Left ventricle; *RV,* right ventricle. (Courtesy Laura Heyneman, Duke Medical Center.)

artery disease, a common cause of dilated cardiomyopathy in adults, is uncommon in childhood, although in children with sickle cell disease, ischemic cardiomyopathy related to micro-infarctions may develop.[1,11] Most children with dilated cardiomyopathy are diagnosed in the first year of life.[10]

The functional and anatomic changes associated with dilated cardiomyopathy can be well evaluated with cardiac MRI, including acute and chronic changes of myocarditis and changes in left ventricular mass, stroke volume, ejection fraction, and myocardial late enhancement.[5]

ARRHYTHMOGENIC RIGHT VENTRICULAR CARDIOMYOPATHY

Arrhythmogenic right ventricular cardiomyopathy (ARVC) is characterized by progressive fibrofatty replacement of right ventricular myocardium. This tissue replacement starts focally in the right ventricle but may progress to involve the entire right ventricle; it may involve the left ventricle as well. Areas of spared myocardium may act as foci of instability, resulting in ventricular arrhythmias and sudden death, which become more common in adolescents and young adults.[12] The fatty or fibrofatty myocardial infiltration and wall thinning of ARVC can be visualized on T1-weighted spin echo magnetic resonance (MR) sequences (Fig. 80-2). The most reliable MR findings include abnormal right ventricular regional and global wall motion, aneurysms, and dilation. Late gadolinium enhancement can also be seen.[5,13,14]

RESTRICTIVE CARDIOMYOPATHY

Restrictive cardiomyopathy, the least common type, is characterized by restricted filling and decreased diastolic volume of one or both ventricles, without ventricular dilation or hypertrophy.[6] Restrictive cardiomyopathy is usually idiopathic and may be associated with diseases that cause infiltration or fibrosis of the myocardium or endocardium, such as hemochromatosis, glycogen storage diseases, and Gaucher, Hurler, and Fabry diseases.[12] Although amyloidosis and sarcoidosis are rare in children, they also may cause restrictive

cardiomyopathy. Because both ventricles may be involved, patients may present with signs and symptoms of right or left ventricular failure or arrhythmias.[4] Restrictive cardiomyopathy should be considered in patients presenting with heart failure but without cardiomegaly or systolic dysfunction. It is important to distinguish restrictive cardiomyopathy from constrictive pericarditis, which has a similar clinical appearance but can be cured surgically.[15]

Radiographs of the chest in patients with restrictive cardiomyopathy may demonstrate a normal heart size. Pulmonary congestion, interstitial edema, and pleural effusions may be seen.[15] Cardiac MRI may demonstrate ventricles that are

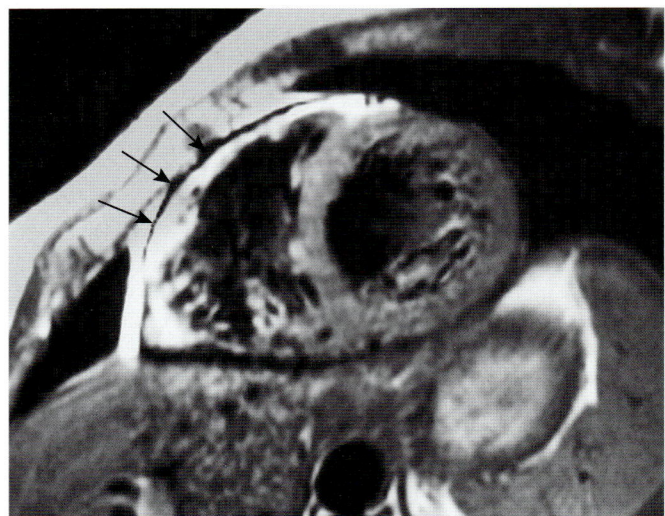

Figure 80-2 Arrhythmogenic right ventricular cardiomyopathy in an 18-year-old with recurrent supraventricular tachycardia. A T1-weighted short-axis image through the heart shows an abnormal high signal involving the anterior wall of the right ventricle (*arrows*) adjacent to the normally high T1 signal of pericardial fat. This appearance is consistent with the fibrofatty myocardial replacement and wall thinning seen with arrhythmogenic right ventricular cardiomyopathy.

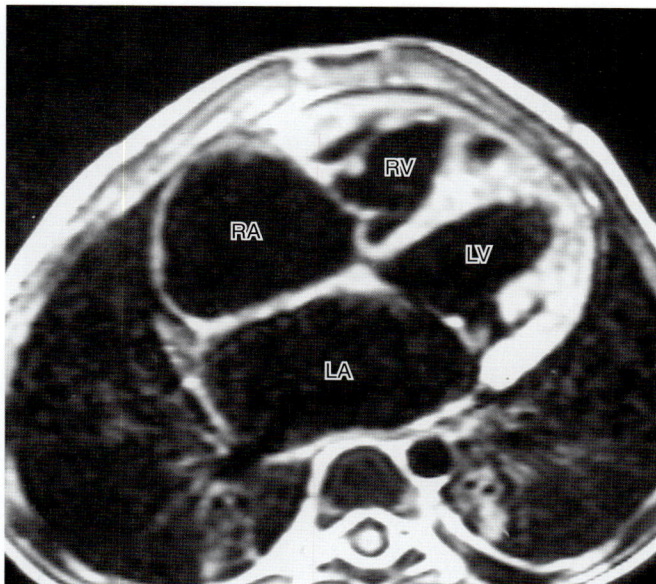

Figure 80-3 Restrictive cardiomyopathy. A T1-weighted four-chamber view in a 3-year-old boy with idiopathic restrictive cardiomyopathy demonstrates the relatively small size of the right (*RV*) and left (*LV*) ventricles, with dilation of the right atrium (*RA*) and left atrium (*LA*). There is no evidence of pericardial thickening to suggest restrictive pericarditis.

small to normal in size (Fig. 80-3); signs of poor ventricular filling may be present, including dilation of the atria, superior and inferior venae cavae, and hepatic veins.[4] These findings are similar to those of constrictive pericarditis, but the pericardial thickening (>4 mm) typical of constrictive pericarditis is absent.[16]

SPECIFIC CARDIOMYOPATHIES

Aside from inflammatory and neuromuscular cardiomyopathies, the other specific cardiomyopathies account for only a small fraction of cases in children. Of these, only cardiomyopathies associated with toxins and metabolic abnormalities are addressed here.

Inflammatory Cardiomyopathy

The inflammatory cardiomyopathies include both infectious and familial forms. Among cases with a known cause, nearly 30% are attributed to infection.[3] Although infectious cardiomyopathy, also known as myocarditis, can be caused by bacterial, fungal, or parasitic infection, viral myocarditis is most common. Enteroviruses, particularly Coxsackie virus B, are associated with 25% to 40% of cases of pediatric acute myocarditis and dilated cardiomyopathy.[17] The acute clinical presentation of myocarditis is characterized by dyspnea and tachypnea due to congestive heart failure. Myocardial involvement by tuberculosis is extremely rare and typically occurs in the setting of disseminated disease.[18] Eosinophilic myocarditis may be seen in the setting of eosinophilic syndromes or allergic reactions.[19]

Acute rheumatic fever, discussed later in more detail, is an autoimmune response that follows a small percentage of infections with group A β-hemolytic streptococcus. The sequela, rheumatic heart disease, is significant because of the associated morbidity that may include valvular disease (more common) and carditis (pericarditis, myocarditis, or endocarditis) in the acute setting.[20]

Isolated familial cardiomyopathy typically is defined as cardiomyopathy with no systemic features occurring in a patient with an identified genetic defect or in multiple family members. Familial cardiomyopathy accounts for approximately 20% to 25% of nonidiopathic cases of cardiomyopathy.[3,21]

Sarcoidosis

Sarcoidosis is a multiorgan disease characterized by noncaseating granulomas. It occurs most often in adolescents but has been reported in children as young as 2 years. Clinical manifestations vary according to age. In children younger than 5 years, the disease involves mainly the skin, eyes, and joints, whereas in older children, involvement of the lymph nodes, lungs, or eyes is more common.[22]

Cardiac disease is uncommon but has a wide spectrum of manifestations, including conduction abnormalities (usually ventricular arrhythmias) and heart block. Infiltration of the ventricular walls can compromise ventricular contraction and compliance, resulting in systolic and diastolic failure, respectively. Other cardiovascular manifestations include pericardial effusion, papillary muscle dysfunction, and valvular disease.[22] MRI has been used to make the diagnosis of cardiac involvement with infiltration of the myocardium.

Neuromuscular Cardiomyopathy

Neuromuscular cardiomyopathies include a variety of genetic and acquired disorders. Duchenne muscular dystrophy, the most common of the muscular dystrophies, is an X-linked recessive neurodegenerative disorder characterized by progressive skeletal muscle weakness. In children with Duchenne muscular dystrophy, dilated cardiomyopathy develops with alternating areas of hypertrophy, atrophy, and myocardial fibrosis.[23] Interestingly, dilated cardiomyopathy may be the only clinical manifestation of genetic carriers of Duchenne muscular dystrophy.[24]

Friedreich ataxia is a rare, autosomal recessive neurologic disorder characterized by progressive ataxia and musculoskeletal abnormalities (scoliosis and foot deformities). The cardiac disease of Friedreich ataxia includes hypertrophic cardiomyopathy that progresses to dilated cardiomyopathy, along with arrhythmias. Although patients typically present with neurologic symptoms, a small minority may present with symptoms of systolic dysfunction.[25]

Noonan syndrome is a relatively common genetic syndrome characterized by typical facies and short stature. Cardiac abnormalities associated with Noonan syndrome include pulmonary valve stenosis and hypertrophic cardiomyopathy, with or without obstruction.[26]

Metabolic Cardiomyopathy

The glycogen storage diseases (GSDs) constitute a group of rare diseases characterized by abnormal glycogen breakdown, with resultant storage in various tissues. Cardiac involvement is most common in types II (Pompe disease), III, and IV.[27]

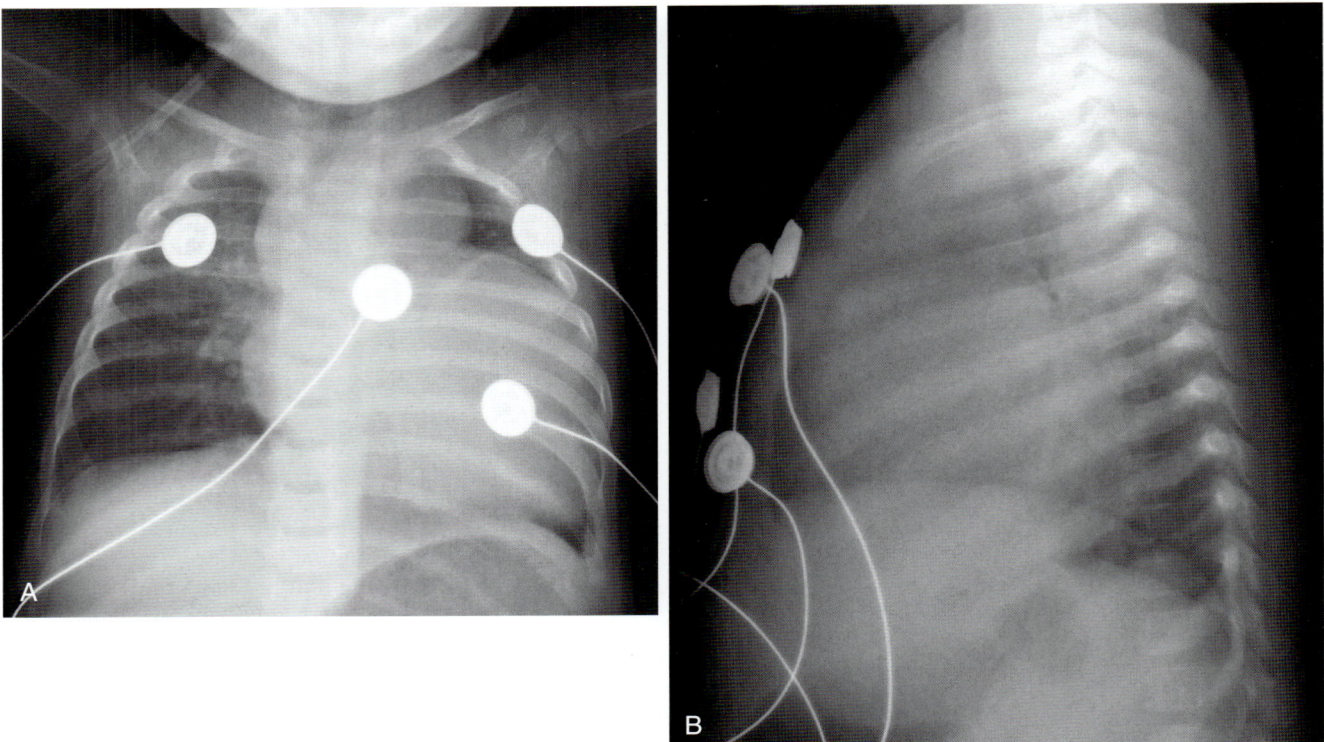

Figure 80-4   Glycogen storage disease of the heart (Pompe disease) in a 5-month-old girl. Marked cardiomegaly is seen on frontal (**A**) and lateral (**B**) radiographs. The prominent lobular shape of the superior mediastinum is due to the thymus.

Pompe disease (GSD type II), which is associated with a deficiency of acid α-glucosidase, has three major forms. A complete deficiency of acid α-glucosidase leads to the most severe infantile form, with progressive lethal cardiac and muscle disorder. Symptoms include failure to thrive, hypotonia, respiratory difficulties, and cardiac problems. The cardiac features include congestive heart failure, arrhythmias, cardiomegaly, biventricular hypertrophy, and outflow tract obstruction.[28] Marked cardiomegaly, with or without congestion, in an infant beyond the immediate newborn period should raise the possibility of this entity as a differential diagnosis (Fig. 80-4).[27] Partial deficiencies of acid α-glucosidase lead to milder, late-onset juvenile and adult forms of Pompe disease.

Nearly all patients with GSD type III have clinically silent heart disease. Patients with GSD type IV typically die of liver disease before their cardiomyopathy becomes clinically obvious. Echocardiography demonstrates cardiac hypertrophy, which may result in left ventricular outflow tract obstruction, but no cardiac dilation.[27]

The mucopolysaccharidoses are a group of rare inherited disorders characterized by a deficiency of lysosomal enzymes resulting in the abnormal storage of glycosaminoglycans. Of the mucopolysaccharidoses, Hurler, Hunter, Sanfilippo, Scheie, and Hurler-Scheie syndromes may have severe cardiac involvement. The myocardial cells become distended with storage material. Patients with these disorders also may have valvular thickening and short, thick chordae tendineae, resulting in valvular insufficiency.[27,29]

Fabry disease is an X-linked recessive storage disorder characterized by the accumulation of glycosphingolipid in different tissues. Patients with classic Fabry disease have diffuse organ involvement, with left ventricular hypertrophy and dilation, conduction abnormalities, valvular dysfunction, and myocardial infarcts. Some patients may have a cardiac variant of the disease that is limited to myocardial hypertrophy. Cardiac Fabry disease may be difficult to differentiate from hypertrophic cardiomyopathy; however, different patterns of enhancement can be seen on enhanced cardiac MRI.[30]

Hemochromatosis is a disorder of abnormal absorption and organ deposition of iron. Two types of primary hemochromatosis affect the young: juvenile hemochromatosis and neonatal hemochromatosis. Juvenile hemochromatosis is a severe form of hereditary hemochromatosis. Liver involvement is always present. Other manifestations, including cardiomyopathy, arrhythmias, and heart failure, are more common in the juvenile form than in the adult form. Systemic manifestations of the disease are present by the second or third decade. Death, often from intractable heart failure or arrhythmias, often occurs before the age of 30 years. A restrictive cardiomyopathy can be present because of myocardial iron deposition.[31,32]

Neonatal hemochromatosis is a disease of uncertain and complex etiology. Affected infants are small for gestational age and often are premature. The fetal period is complicated by oligohydramnios, placental edema, and intrauterine growth restriction. By the first several weeks of life, neonates usually have been diagnosed with the disorder after presenting with liver failure, hypoalbuminemia with secondary edema, hypoglycemia, coagulopathy, anemia, and hyperbilirubinemia. Although the liver is the most

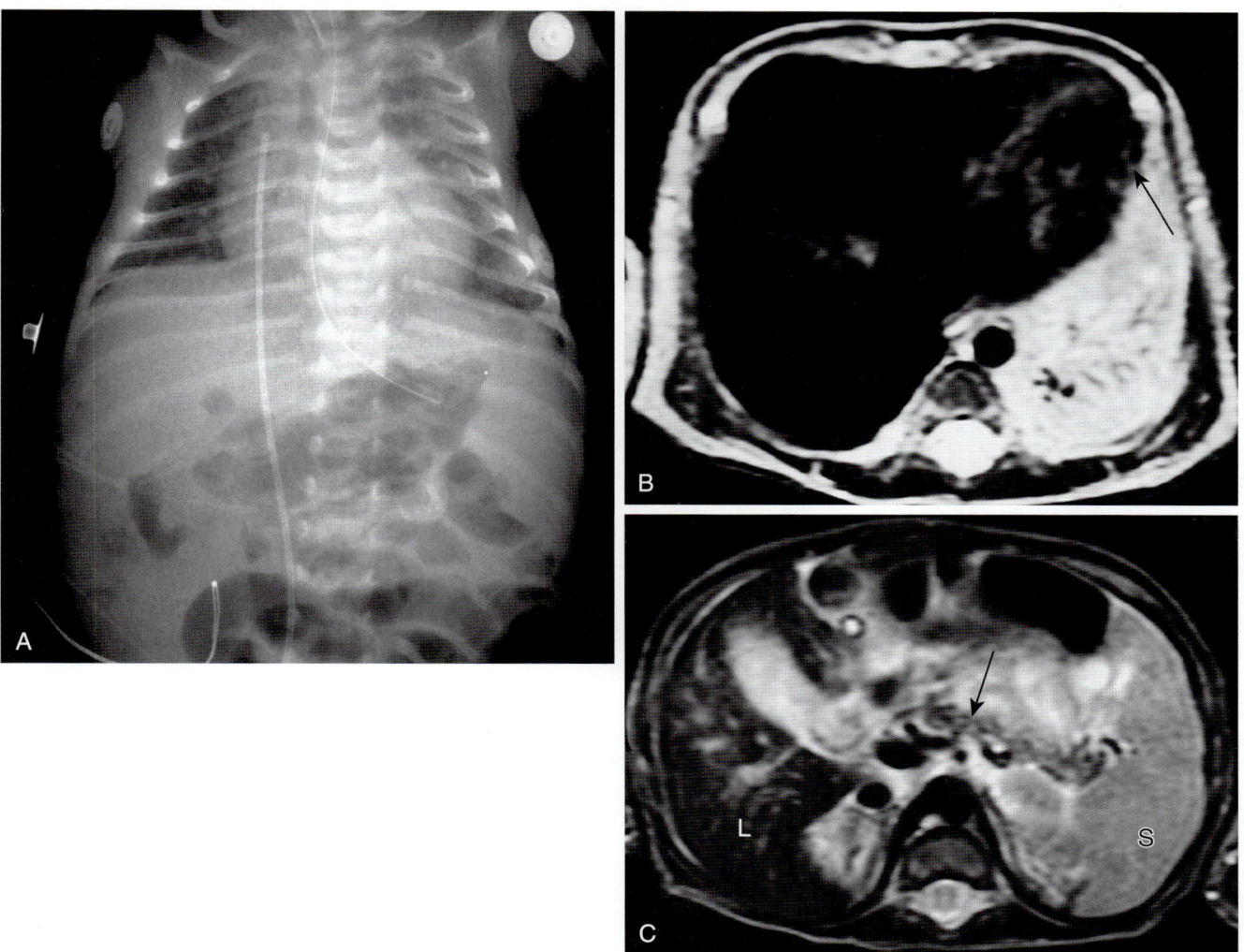

Figure 80-5 Neonatal hemochromatosis. This 2-week-old boy presented with liver failure and a distended abdomen and was later diagnosed with neonatal hemochromatosis. **A,** A radiograph of the chest and abdomen shows mild cardiomegaly and mild splenomegaly. The liver is small and the flanks are bulging with ascites. Multiple dilated loops of small bowel are present and represent an ileus. **B,** A T2-weighted axial magnetic resonance (MR) image of the chest shows the "disappearing heart" sign, a feature of hemochromatosis. The near-complete signal dropout of the myocardium (*arrow*) is caused by iron deposition. High signal intensity in the left hemithorax is the result of atelectasis of the left lower lobe. **C,** A T2-weighted axial MR image of the upper abdomen shows marked low signal intensity of the liver (*L*) and pancreas (*arrow*) compared with the relatively normal signal in the spleen (*S*). These findings are typical of primary hemochromatosis.

common site of iron deposition, other sites include the heart, pancreas, exocrine and endocrine organs, intestines, stomach, and salivary glands. Neonatal hemochromatosis is one of the more common reasons for neonatal liver transplantation.[31]

Both juvenile and neonatal hemochromatosis have similar MRI findings because of the paramagnetic effects of iron. Any tissue that contains iron will have low signal intensity on T1-weighted and especially T2-weighted and T2*-weighted sequences.[33] MRI can be used in the third trimester of high-risk pregnancies and after birth to evaluate the infant and help plan treatment options. In primary hemochromatosis, iron deposition is present in the liver, myocardium, and pancreas but not in the spleen (Fig. 80-5). In the secondary form—which often is the result of repeated blood transfusions, excess iron intake, or cirrhosis—splenic iron deposition is present.[34]

Toxins

Doxorubicin (Adriamycin) is a drug used to treat a variety of pediatric malignancies, including childhood leukemias and lymphomas, Wilms tumor, and neuroblastoma. Among its well-known cardiotoxic effects are cardiomyopathy and congestive heart failure (Fig. 80-6).[35] The elapsed time from treatment to heart failure is variable and may occur months to years after termination of therapy. The probability of developing heart failure increases with the cumulative dosage.[35] Female patients and those who have had prior mediastinal radiation that included the left ventricle are at increased risk for the development of heart failure.[36]

Unspecified Cardiomyopathy

Left ventricular noncompaction, also known as persistence of the spongy myocardium and left ventricular

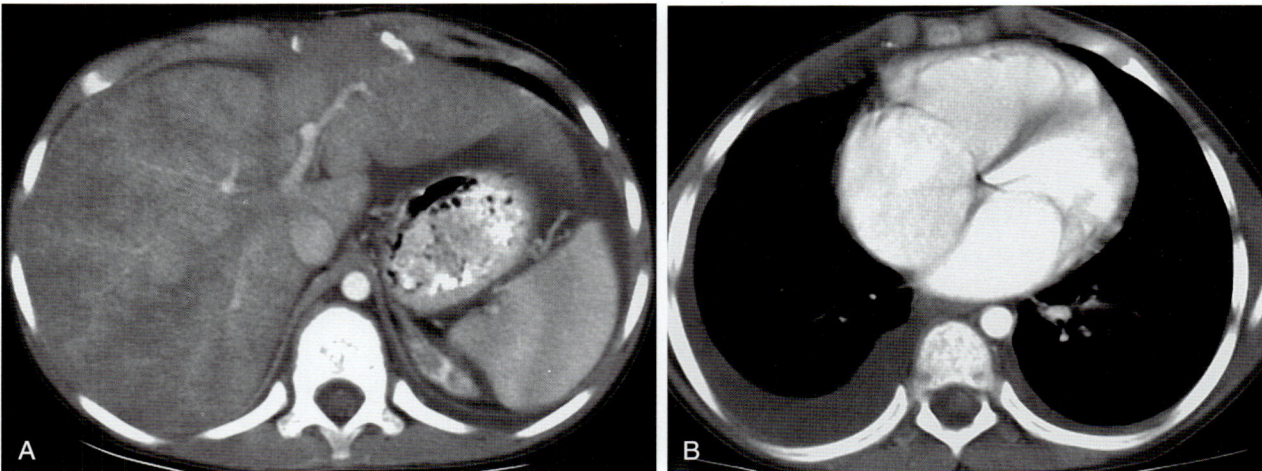

Figure 80-6 Doxorubicin cardiac toxicity in a 10-year-old boy with a history of rhabdomyosarcoma of the orbit. His chemotherapy regimen included doxorubicin, and he presented with abdominal pain and hepatomegaly. A computed tomography (CT) scan was obtained to evaluate for metastatic disease. **A,** Contrast-enhanced CT (CECT) of the abdomen shows hepatomegaly and a mottled appearance of the liver caused by passive conges-tion as well as dilation of the hepatic veins and inferior vena cava. **B,** CECT of the chest shows cardiomegaly, a dilated right atrium and ventricle, and bilateral pleural effusions consistent with right heart failure. These findings were attributed to doxorubicin toxicity.

hypertrabeculation, is a rare congenital cardiomyopathy that causes heart failure. It is characterized by excessively promi-nent ventricular trabeculations and deep intertrabecular recesses. Patients with this condition demonstrate systolic and diastolic dysfunction, arrhythmias, and embolic events. MRI can be useful in making the diagnosis by demonstrating thick trabeculae in the left ventricle and deep recesses within the myocardial wall.[37] The areas of left ventricular non-compaction may be focal or diffuse, and the diagnosis is suggested on computed tomography (CT) or MRI by a noncompacted to compacted wall ratio of greater than 2.3 in diastole (Fig. 80-7).[38]

Valves

INFECTIOUS ENDOCARDITIS

Pediatric valvular disease includes both congenital and acquired lesions with a predominance of congenital lesions. Infectious or rheumatic endocarditis is an inflammatory con-dition that involves the cardiac valves. In the past, rheumatic heart disease was the chief underlying cause of infectious endocarditis. However, given the decrease in rheumatic heart disease in developed countries and the improved survival of children with congenital heart disease, congenital heart disease is now a major predisposing factor for infectious endocardi-tis.[39] Although patients with prosthetic patches, grafts, or valves are at increased risk, all children who have undergone surgery for congenital heart disease are at a higher risk of endocarditis compared with children without congenital heart disease.[40] In patients without a history of congenital heart disease, infectious endocarditis often is associated with indwelling venous catheters.[39] In up to 10% of cases of child-hood infectious endocarditis, no identifiable risk factor or structural heart disease is present. These cases are believed to be a result of valve infection as a result of Staphylococcus bacteremia.[39]

Although children with infectious endocarditis may present acutely, with high spiking fevers, the presentation typically is more indolent, with prolonged low-grade fever and non-specific complaints including lethargy, weakness, arthralgia, myalgia, and weight loss.[39] In neonates, the symptoms may be more difficult to recognize and may include feeding dif-ficulties and neurologic signs and symptoms, including sei-zures, hemiparesis, and apnea. Gram-positive cocci, usually *Streptococcus,* are the most common causative agent, followed by *Staphylococcus.*[39]

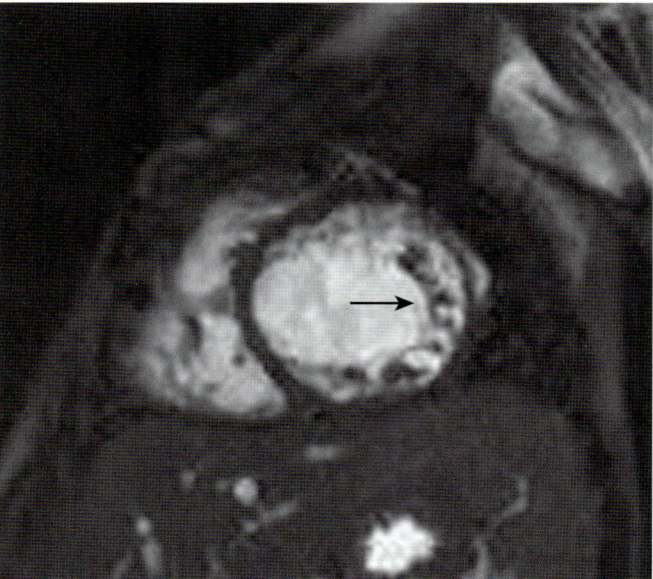

Figure 80-7 Left ventricular noncompaction. A short-axis diastolic steady-state free-precession magnetic resonance image of a 10-year-old with left ventricular noncompaction shows multiple deep intratra-becular recesses (*arrow*) communicating with the left ventricular cavity and a ratio of noncompacted to compacted myocardium of >2.3. (Case courtesy Cynthia Rigsby, MD, Chicago, IL.)

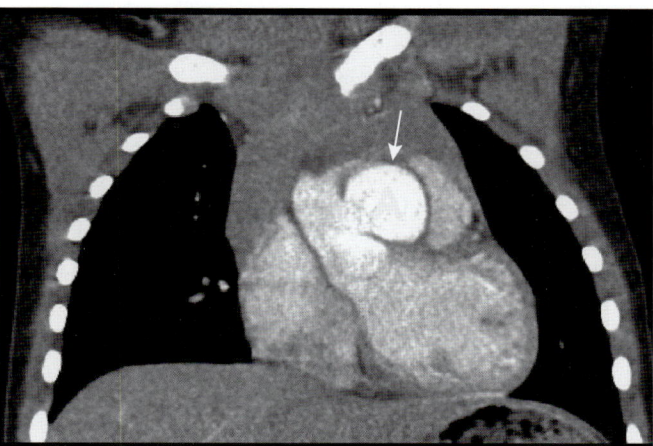

Figure 80-9 Mycotic aneurysm. Coronal reformation of a computed tomography angiogram shows a wide-necked saccular aneurysm (*arrow*) arising from the ascending aorta.

The diagnosis of infectious endocarditis is based on the modified Duke criteria.[41] These criteria involve a combination of major criteria, including positive blood cultures or evidence of endocardial or valve involvement by echocardiography (e.g., vegetations and valve dysfunction), and minor criteria, including fever, predisposing factors (e.g., a heart condition or intravenous drug use), and evidence of embolic disease (e.g., septic pulmonary emboli, intracranial hemorrhage, conjunctival hemorrhage, and Janeway lesions).[41]

Radiographic findings of infectious endocarditis may include cardiomegaly and congestive heart failure (e-Fig. 80-8). In the setting of right heart involvement, pulmonary parenchymal opacities may be related to septic emboli. Diagnostic imaging also is beneficial in assessing for sequelae of endocarditis. Mycotic aneurysms may develop when infections involve the great arteries or a patent ductus arteriosus. Prompt diagnosis of these life-threatening aneurysms by echocardiography, CT, MRI, or angiography is critical (Fig. 80-9). The valves themselves are best assessed with echocardiography from both a morphologic and a functional standpoint.

Surgery is indicated in patients with congestive heart failure, recurrent systemic embolization, acute valvular insufficiency, conduction abnormalities such as complete heart block, or persistent sepsis despite adequate antibiotic therapy. Surgery also may be indicated in patients who experience abscesses, mycotic aneurysms, or fistulous tracts (into the pericardium, between the cardiac chambers or vascular structures).[42]

RHEUMATIC FEVER

Rheumatic heart disease was once the leading cause of childhood-acquired heart disease in the United States and remains preeminent in many parts of the world. Rheumatic heart disease is the most serious manifestation of rheumatic fever, an autoimmune disease seen following pharyngitis with group A beta-hemolytic Streptococcus. The incidence of rheumatic fever and rheumatic heart disease has decreased dramatically with improved living conditions and the prompt use of antibiotics.[20]

Diagnosis of rheumatic fever is based on the Jones criteria. Rheumatic fever is diagnosed if the child has two major criteria or one major and two minor criteria, *plus* evidence of recent streptococcal infection. Major criteria include migratory arthritis of the large joints, carditis, Sydenham chorea, erythema marginatum, and subcutaneous nodules. Minor criteria for diagnosis include arthralgia, fever, elevated erythrocyte sedimentation rate, presence of C-reactive protein, prolonged PR interval on the electrocardiogram, and leukocytosis.[43,44]

Although all four cardiac valves may be affected by rheumatic heart disease, it is predominantly the mitral valve that is affected.[20] Acute valvular insufficiency develops, which, if severe, can result in congestive heart failure and death.[20] Noninfectious vegetations can be present on the valve leaflets. Other abnormalities that can be seen in persons with rheumatic heart disease include pericardial effusion and left atrial enlargement, characteristically involving the atrial appendage. In persons with chronic disease, affected valves may become stenotic in addition to the regurgitation that develops acutely (Fig. 80-10).

Pericardium

NORMAL PERICARDIUM

The pericardium is a conical structure that contains the heart and juxtacardiac origins of the great vessels. It consists of a tough, outer fibrous layer and an inner serosal layer; the serosa consists of an outer parietal layer and an inner visceral layer (the epicardium), separated by a potential space, the pericardial cavity, which normally contains as much as 30 mL of serous fluid in an adult.[45]

A complex three-dimensional arrangement of pericardial reflections extends between vessels off the principal cavity, forming recesses that contain a small amount of fluid. Familiarity with these normal recesses can help avoid mistaking the superior pericardial recess for precarinal adenopathy or the oblique pericardial recess, which is located dorsal to the left atrium, for a bronchogenic cyst.[46] The thickness of the normal pericardium is less than 2 mm, and it is best seen radiographically between the epicardial and anterior mediastinal fat, anterior to the right ventricle just above the diaphragm (Fig. 80-11).[47]

The pericardium and pericardial cavity are most often imaged using echocardiography,[48] but CT and MRI offer distinct advantages in certain clinical settings. Both modalities provide a larger field of view, superior tissue characterization, and excellent anatomic delineation. MR is superior to CT and CT is superior to echocardiography in characterizing pericardial effusions and pericardial masses. CT is most sensitive for pericardial calcifications.[49,50]

CONGENITAL ABSENCE OF THE PERICARDIUM

Congenital pericardial defects are rare. The defect may be partial, predominantly involving the left pericardium, or complete, which is less common and is of limited clinical significance. In approximately 30% of cases, associated cardiac and pulmonary anomalies are present.[51] Pericardial defects often are discovered incidentally at surgery, autopsy, or on chest radiograph, but they may present with periodic stabbing

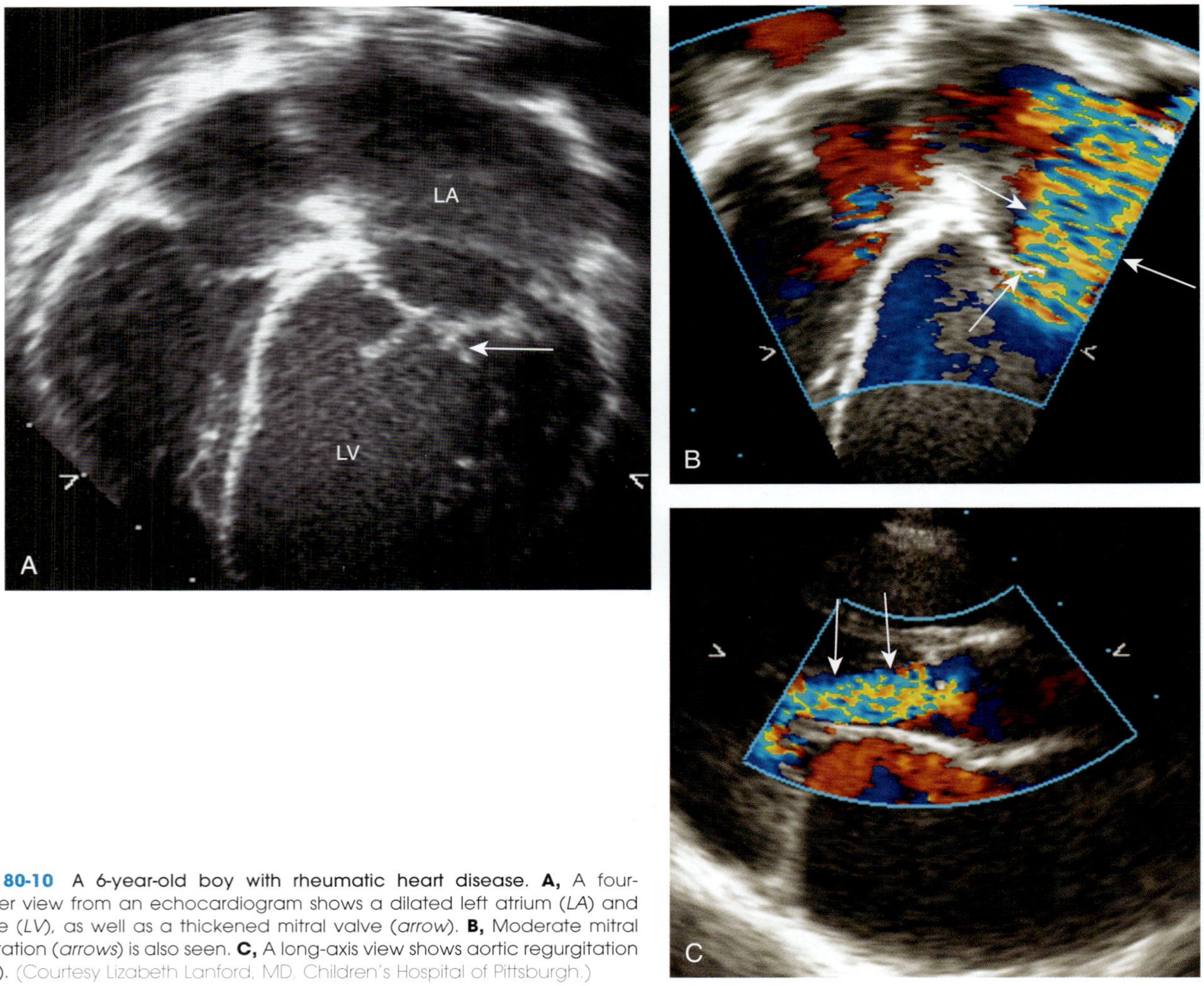

Figure 80-10 A 6-year-old boy with rheumatic heart disease. **A,** A four-chamber view from an echocardiogram shows a dilated left atrium (*LA*) and ventricle (*LV*), as well as a thickened mitral valve (*arrow*). **B,** Moderate mitral regurgitation (*arrows*) is also seen. **C,** A long-axis view shows aortic regurgitation (*arrows*). (Courtesy Lizabeth Lanford, MD. Children's Hospital of Pittsburgh.)

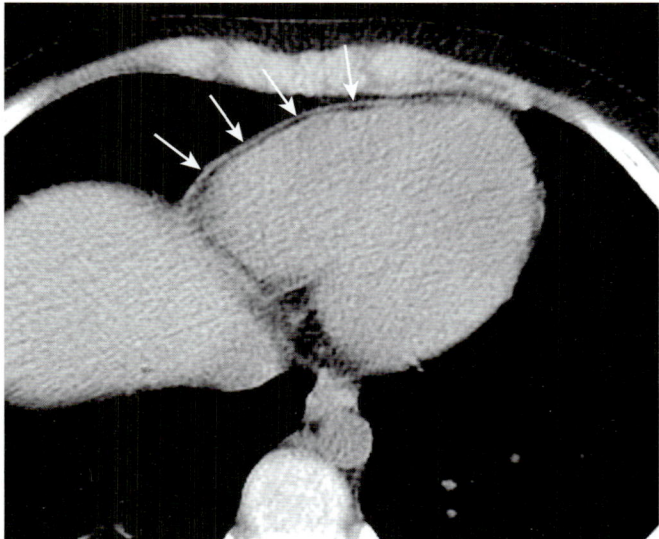

Figure 80-11 An axial non–contrast-enhanced computed tomography image shows the normal pericardium (*arrows*) outlined between anterior mediastinal and epicardial fat.

chest pains. Herniation of the left atrial appendage through a partial defect can be life threatening.[29] Partial defects may be suspected when there is focal prominence of the left atrial appendage along the upper left heart border. MRI can confirm this congenital anomaly by showing a defect in the thin, low signal intensity pericardium, as well as herniation of the left atrial appendage through the defect (Fig. 80-12).[51,52]

In complete absence of the pericardium, the chest radiograph typically demonstrates levocardia with varying degrees of prominence of the main pulmonary artery. Cross-sectional imaging best shows the characteristic findings of a thin tongue of lung tissue extending medially between the aorta and pulmonary trunk and between the inferior border of the heart and the left hemidiaphragm (Fig. 80-13). Surgical reconstruction of the pericardium can be performed to reduce the risk of death from strangulation of cardiac structures and to manage symptoms.[51]

PNEUMOPERICARDIUM

Pneumopericardium can be iatrogenic or posttraumatic but most often is seen in premature infants who undergo positive pressure ventilation.[53] Radiographs show a lucent halo of air

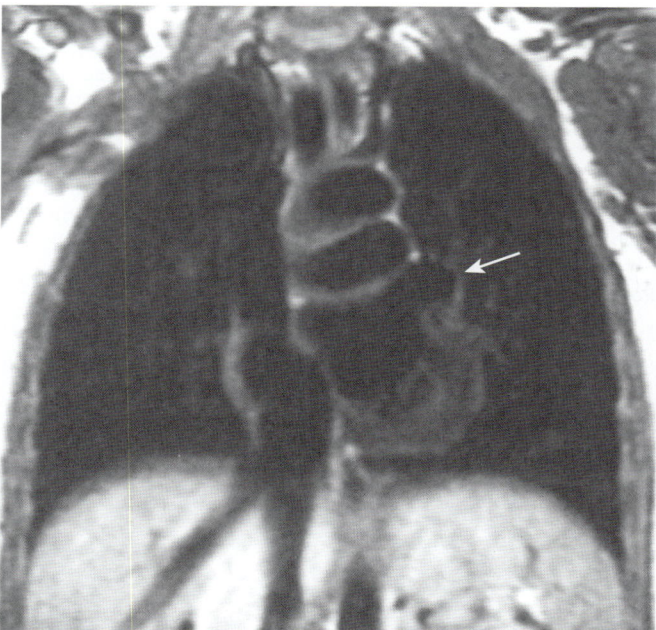

Figure 80-12 A 9-year-old girl with partial absence of the pericardium. A coronal T1-weighted image shows herniation of the left atrial appendage (*arrow*) through the partial pericardial defect.

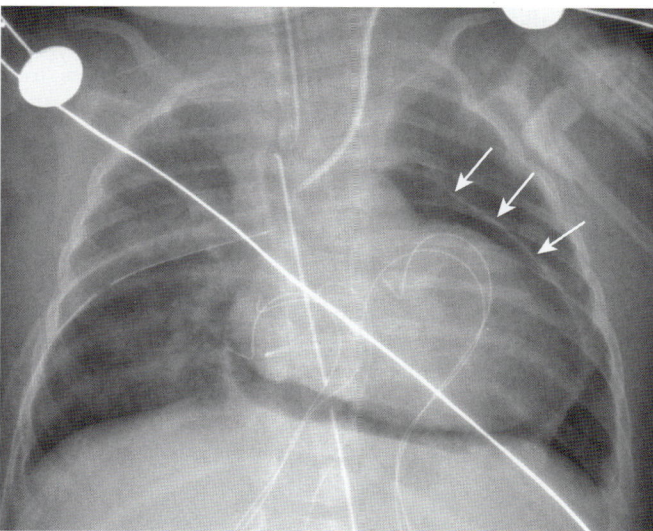

Figure 80-14 Pneumopericardium in a 16-day-old girl following surgery for atrioventricular septal defect repair, presumably due to positive pressure ventilation. Note the air encircling the heart but not extending above the origins of the great vessels. The pericardium is visible as a thin white stripe (*arrows*) encircling the heart.

encircling the heart, extending between the heart and diaphragm inferiorly and the origin of the great vessels superiorly (Fig. 80-14).[54] The parietal and fibrous pericardium sometimes can be seen as a thin white stripe contrasted between lung and pericardial air in the pericardial cavity. Pneumopericardium must be distinguished from pneumomediastinum, in which air also can outline the inferior aspect of the heart. In pneumomediastinum, however, air often extends above the origins of the great vessels, surrounding the thymus and occasionally extending into the neck.

The clinical significance of pneumopericardium depends on the amount of air in the pericardium. Large pericardial air collections can cause tamponade and must be evacuated.[54]

PERICARDIAL EFFUSION

The most common identifiable causes of pericardial effusion in children are infectious and iatrogenic. Neoplastic and connective tissue causes are less common. Infectious pericarditis is most often viral, but cases associated with significant pericardial fluid are more often of bacterial origin. Pericarditis from tuberculosis or fungal infection is unusual.[55] Large pericardial effusions often are due to bacterial pericarditis, malignancy, and immune disorders, but in some cases the cause is never determined.[56] Hemopericardium often is caused by trauma, either accidental or iatrogenic (Fig. 80-15). Special note should be made of pericardial effusions related to central

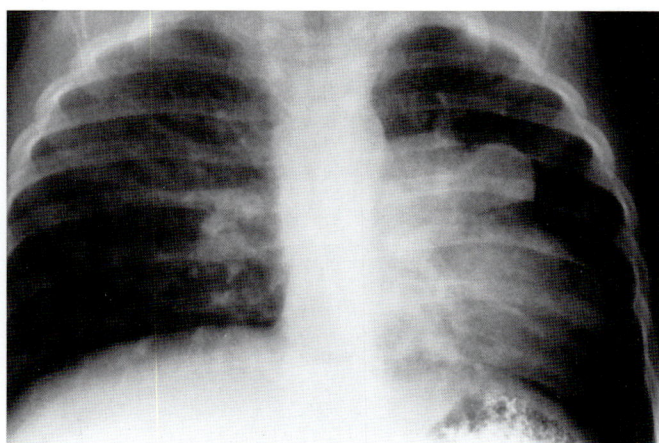

Figure 80-13 Complete absence of the left pericardium in a 9-year-old boy. The heart appears to be in the "oblique" position. The caudad surface is separated from the diaphragm (i.e., air is present between the heart and diaphragm). The heart is displaced to the left.

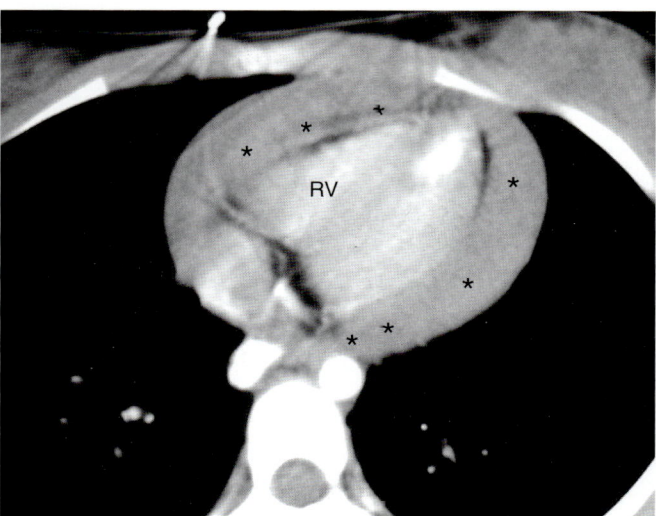

Figure 80-15 Traumatic hemopericardium in a juvenile involved in a motor vehicle crash. High-density fluid (*asterisks*) surrounds the heart, distending the pericardial space. Note compression of the right ventricle (*RV*).

venous catheter placement in children. Cardiac tamponade can result from vessel perforation, leading to hemopericardium or to intrapericardial infusion of fluid, such as total parenteral nutrition.[57]

Key Points

Cardiomyopathy may be categorized according to etiology and pathophysiology (dilated, hypertrophic, restrictive, and arrhythmogenic).

Idiopathic dilated cardiomyopathy is the most common cause of congestive heart failure in children.

Nearly two thirds of pediatric cases of cardiomyopathy are idiopathic. Of the cases of cardiomyopathy with an identified cause, 30% are infectious and 20% to 25% are familial.

Major factors predisposing to infectious endocarditis include congenital heart disease and indwelling venous catheters.

Cardiotoxicity and cardiomyopathy are well-known adverse effects of doxorubicin treatment related to cumulative dose, female sex, and cardiac radiation.

CT and MRI provide distinct advantages over echocardiography in the characterization of pericardial effusions and masses.

Suggested Readings

Breen JF. Imaging of the pericardium. *J Thorac Imaging*. 2001;16:47-54.

Durani Y, Giordano K, Goudie BW. Myocarditis and pericarditis in children. *Pediatr Clin North Am*. 2010;57(6):1281-1303.

Levine MC, Klugman D, Teach SJ. Update on myocarditis in children. *Curr Opin Pediatr*. 2010;22(3):278-283.

Schulz-Menger J, Friedrich MG. Magnetic resonance imaging in patients with cardiomyopathies: when and why. *Herz*. 2000;25(4):384-389.

Wang ZJ, Reddy GP, Gotway MB, et al. CT and MR imaging of pericardial disease. *Radiographics*. 2003;23:S167-S180.

References

Full references for this chapter can be found on www.expertconsult.com.

Chapter 81

Cardiac and Pericardial Tumors

S. BRUCE GREENBERG and CATHY MACDONALD

Primary cardiac tumors are rare in infants and children, with a reported prevalence of up to 0.32%.[1] Use of echocardiography has resulted in more frequent detection of cardiac tumors in the fetus and neonate.[2] More than 90% of cardiac tumors in infants and children are benign.[1] Symptoms are variable and usually depend on tumor location and size. Intracavitary cardiac tumors can cause cardiac valve obstruction or result in spread of tumor emboli into either the pulmonary or systemic vascular beds. Children with intracavitary cardiac tumors present with heart failure, dyspnea, or neurologic symptoms. Myocardial tumors compress the cardiac lumen, leading to obstruction or heart failure, and can be associated with arrhythmias. Pericardial tumors are associated with pericardial effusions. Conventional radiographs may show cardiomegaly, an abnormal cardiac shape, or pulmonary edema from congestive heart failure (e-Fig. 81-1). Cardiac tumors in children can be associated with several syndromes, as shown in Table 81-1. Computed tomography (CT) and magnetic resonance imaging (MRI) findings can help differentiate tumor types (Table 81-2).

Rhabdomyoma

Pathophysiology and Clinical Presentation Rhabdomyoma is the most common primary cardiac tumor of childhood and accounts for 60% to 79% of all cardiac tumors during the first year of life.[1,3] Rhabdomyomas are hamartomas that regress and have no potential for malignancy. More than half of fetuses with rhabdomyomas are asymptomatic. Patients with rhabdomyomas can present with nonimmune fetal hydrops, outflow tract obstruction, or arrhythmia. At least 50% of patients with rhabdomyomas have tuberous sclerosis, and rhabdomyomas can be the first detectable manifestation of tuberous sclerosis.[3]

Imaging Rhabdomyomas are round, hyperechoic, solid masses on echocardiography (e-Fig. 81-2). They usually are multiple and occur most commonly in the ventricular tissue but also can arise from atrial walls.[4,5] The rhabdomyoma signal characteristics on T1- and T2-weighted MRI are similar to those of myocardium, making MRI less sensitive than echocardiography.[6] Signal is increased on contrast-enhanced T1-weighted and proton-weighted imaging.[7] Rhabdomyomas are easier to detect when they extend into the cardiac lumen (Fig. 81-3). They have increased attenuation compared with myocardium on noncontrast-enhanced CT scans, and they have mild delayed enhancement with contrast (e-Fig. 81-4).[8] Small fat globules may be detected in rhabdomyomas.

Fibroma

Pathophysiology and Clinical Presentation Cardiac fibroma is the second most common and the most commonly resected primary cardiac tumor of childhood.[9,10] The tumors frequently are detected in the first year of life but can present throughout childhood. Fibromas are solitary tumors located in the myocardium. They are composed of fibroblasts and collagen. Calcifications are frequent and a differentiating finding compared with rhabdomyomas.[1,10] The tumor can be associated with Gorlin (basal cell nevus) syndrome.[7,9,10] Children can present with heart failure and arrhythmia.

Imaging Echocardiography reveals a heterogeneous, echogenic, solitary mass.[10] Cardiac fibroma signal intensity is isointense to slightly hypointense on T1-weighted imaging and low on T2-weighted imaging.[9,11] Classically, contrast-enhanced MRI of fibromas initially shows rim enhancement but decreased central enhancement compared with myocardium.[12] Enhancement on delayed imaging is characteristic (Video 81-1 and Fig. 81-5 and e-Figs. 81-6 and 81-7).[7,13] Calcifications may be detected by CT (e-Fig. 81-8).[14]

Myxoma

Pathophysiology and Clinical Presentation Myxomas are the most common cardiac tumor in adults, but they are rare in children.[1,3,9,10] A myxoma is an exophytic mass extending into a cardiac chamber. Most myxomas are pedunculated, irregular masses attached to the atrial septum, but myxomas can originate from other locations on the endocardium. Calcifications are common. Myxomas occurring in children frequently are associated with Carney syndrome.[15] Carney syndrome is an

Table 81-1

Cardiac Tumors Associated with Syndromes	
Tumor	**Association**
Rhabdomyoma	Tuberous sclerosis
Fibroma	Gorlin (basal cell nevus) syndrome
Myxoma	Carney syndrome

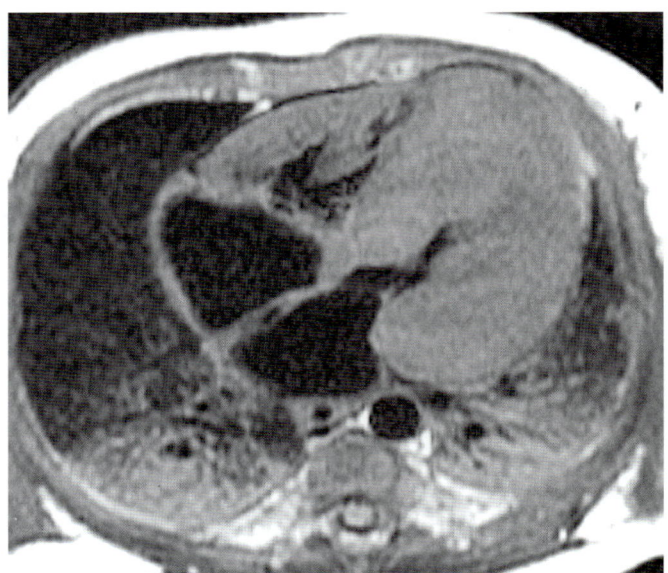

Figure 81-3 Rhabdomyomatosis in an infant shows multiple bulging tumors with isointense signal to the left ventricular myocardium on axial T1-weighted imaging.

autosomal–dominant condition that includes cardiac myxomas, skin myxomas, hyperpigmentation, and overactivity of the endocrine system. Myxomas in children are more likely to be multiple and to recur than in adults. Clinical symptoms include obstructive cardiac symptoms, embolic phenomena, and constitutional symptoms.

Imaging Echocardiography identifies a heterogeneous, spherical mass attached to the endocardial surface.[6,10] The pedunculated mass can be seen to prolapse across the mitral or tricuspid valve during the cardiac cycle. Myxomas have a heterogenous signal and myxoid regions; they have a low signal on T1-weighted imaging and a high signal on T2-weighted imaging[6,7,9,11]; and they enhance with administration of gadolinium (Fig. 81-9). Prolapse of the pedunculated mass can be identified with cine imaging.[14] Tumor attenuation is lower than nonopacified blood on CT sections. Calcifications may be visualized.[14] The mass is well outlined on contrast-enhanced CT scans.[9]

Teratoma

Pathophysiology and Clinical Presentation Cardiac teratomas overall are rare, but they are the most common pericardial tumors in infants, and most are identified during infancy.[3,10,16,17] Teratomas typically are attached to the pulmonary artery and aortic root and extend into the pericardium[3,16]; rarely, they originate from the myocardium.[18] Pericardial effusions usually are present. Fetal hydrops from caval obstruction can lead to spontaneous abortion.

Imaging Echocardiography, CT, and MRI show a mixed, solid, and multicystic tumor in the pericardium with a pericardial effusion[3] (e-Fig. 81-10). Calcification may be present. Echocardiography shows a heterogeneous, multilocular, cystic mass that may be associated with cardiac chamber compression.[10] MRI with both T1- and T2-weighted sequences can show high signal within a well-defined pericardial mass.[19] Calcifications and lipids within these tumors are well defined by CT.[16]

Other Cardiac Tumors

Other benign tumors, such as fibroelastomas, hemangiomas, and lipomas, are extremely rare in children. A fibroelastoma is an intracavitary tumor rarely found in children.[20,21] Unlike myxomas, fibroelastomas usually are attached to cardiac

Table 81-2

Cardiac Tumors: Computed Tomographic and Magnetic Resonance Imaging Findings				
Tumor	**Location**	**Number**	**CT**	**MRI Signal Intensity**
Rhabdomyoma	Myocardium	Multiple	– Calcification ↑ Attenuation* Mild contrast enhancement	Isointense T1- and T2-weighted images ↑ Contrast enhancement
Fibroma	Myocardium	Solitary	+ Calcification Heterogeneous enhancement	↓ T2-weighted images Early rim enhancement ↑ Delayed enhancement
Myxoma	Intracavitary	Solitary†	+ Calcification ↓ Attenuation, outlined by intracavitary contrast	↑ T2-weighted images Heterogeneous contrast enhancement
Teratoma	Pericardium	Solitary	+ Calcification + Fat Heterogeneous attenuation	↑ T2-weighted images ↑ T1-weighted images

*Relative to myocardium.
†Multiple and recurrent tumors associated with familial forms.
CT, computed tomography; MRI, magnetic resonance imaging.

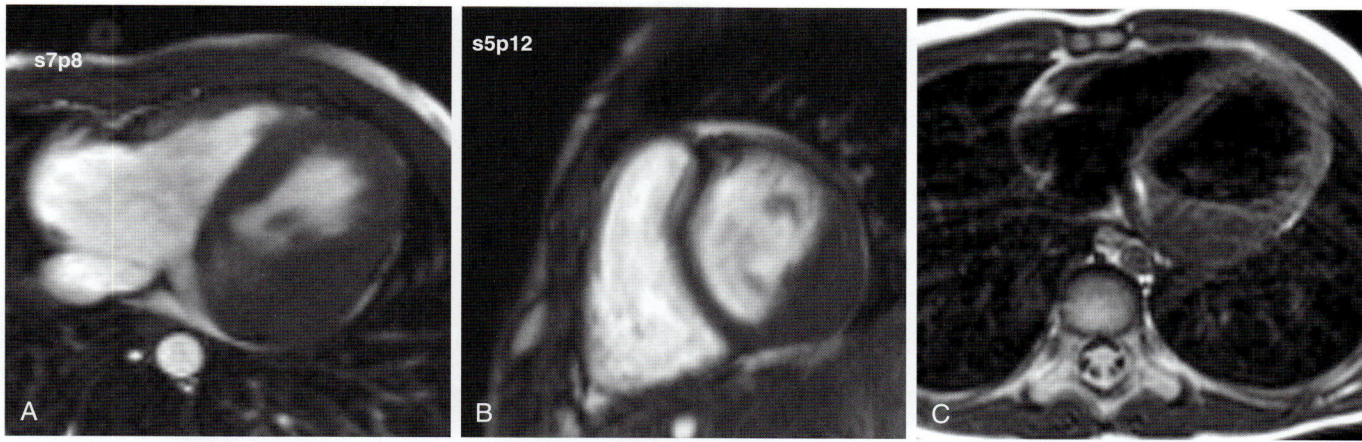

Figure 81-5   A cardiac fibroma in a 7-year-old boy with ventricular tachycardia shows a mass arising from the basal-mid posterolateral wall isointense with normal myocardium on steady-state free-precession imaging (A, B) and heterogeneous hypointensity due to the fibrous tissue on T2-weighting imaging (C).

valves.[20] Hemangiomas can occur in the heart and pericardium and also are associated with pericardial effusion.[3] Hemangiomas enhance intensely on CT (Fig. 81-11) and have a high signal on T2-weighted sequences and postgadolinium T1-weighted sequences (Fig. 81-12).[10,22] Lipomas can occur at any age but are rare in children.[23] CT and MRI demonstration of fat allows for the specific diagnosis.[19] (Fig. 81-13).

Malignant Tumors

Primary malignant tumors are so rare that frequently they are absent from series of cardiac tumors in children, appearing only in case reports.[1,2,24] Only four malignant primary cardiac tumors were confirmed in Great Britain during a 21-year period.[25] Sarcomas (Fig. 81-14),[26] primary lymphoma,[27] and kaposiform hemangioendothelioma[28] of the heart have been reported in children. Primary cardiac lymphoma is defined as lymphoma restricted to the heart and pericardium (Fig. 81-15). Kaposiform hemangioendothelioma can occur antenatally and is associated with pericardial effusion. CT shows a soft tissue mass without fat and MRI shows a high signal on T2-weighted images. Contrast uptake is similar to hemangiomas (Fig. 81-16). Metastatic tumors are more common than primary cardiac malignancies[19] and may be the result of leukemia, lymphoma, Wilms tumor, hepatoblastoma, neuroblastoma, Ewing sarcoma, and osteosarcoma. Spread may be from direct extension, by tumor extension through the inferior vena cava (Fig. 81-17), or via hematogenous metastases.

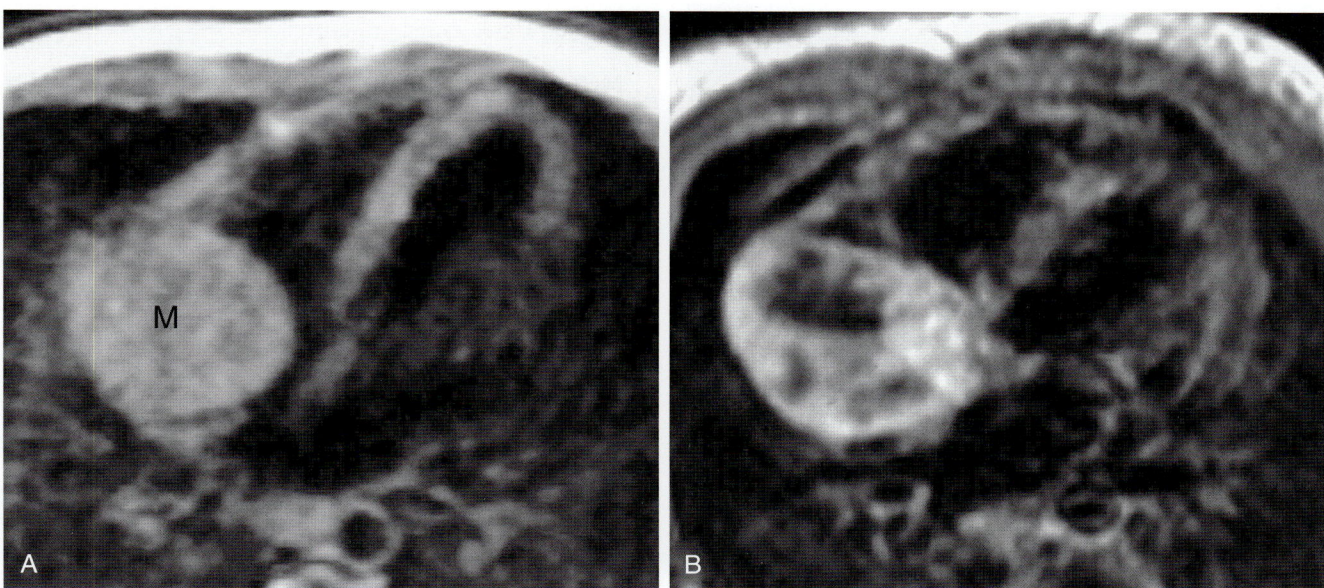

Figure 81-9   A right atrial myxoma in a child. **A,** Axial T1 magnetic resonance image shows an intraluminal right atrial mass (*M*). **B,** The mass enhances heterogeneously with gadolinium.

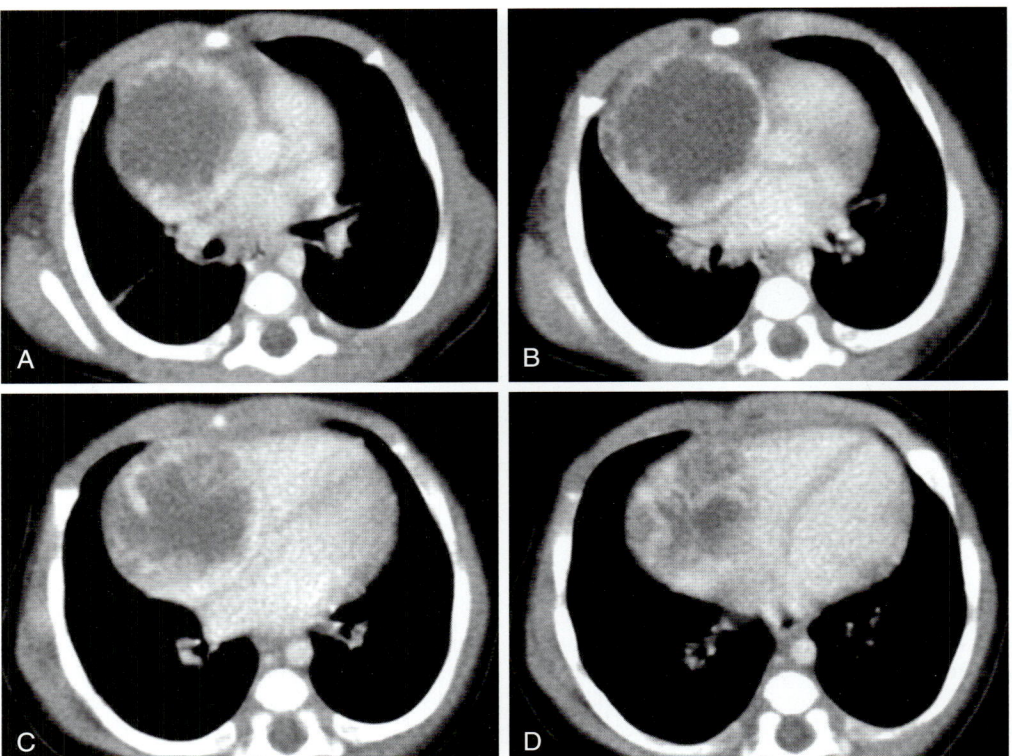

Figure 81-11   A pericardial hemangioma in a newborn. Computed tomography shows a hypodense pericardial mass arising from the right atrial wall that compresses the right atrium. Dense peripheral contrast enhancement is present.

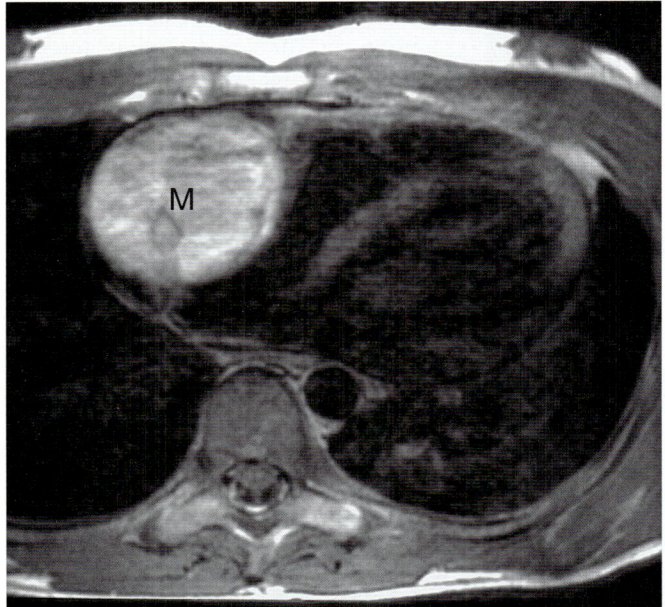

Figure 81-12   A pericardial hemangioma in an 8-year-old child. Magnetic resonance shows a high-signal mass (*M*) on T1-weighted imaging. The mass impinges on the right ventricle.

Key Points

Cardiac tumors are rare in infants and children.

Rhabdomyomas are the most common tumor in children and frequently are associated with tuberous sclerosis.

Fibromas demonstrate a lower T2-weighted imaging signal than do other cardiac tumors.

Metastatic tumors are more common than primary cardiac malignancies.

Suggested Readings

Beroukhim RS, Prakash A, Valsangiacomo Buechel ER, et al. Characterization of cardiac tumors in children by cardiovascular magnetic resonance imaging. *J Am Coll Cardiol.* 2011;58:1044-1054.

Bruce CJ. Cardiac tumours: diagnosis and management. *Heart.* 2011;97:151-160.

Isaacs H. Fetal and neonatal cardiac tumors. *Pediatr Cardiol.* 2004;25:252-273.

Salanitri J, Lisle D, Rigsby C, et al. Benign cardiac tumours: cardiac CT and MRI imaging appearances. *J Med Imaging Radiat Oncol.* 2008;52(6):550-558.

Van Beek EJR, Stolpen AH, Khanna G, et al. CT and MRI of pericardial and cardiac neoplastic disease. *Cancer Imaging.* 2007;7:19-26.

References

Full references for this chapter can be found on www.expertconsult.com.

Chapter 82

Cardiovascular Involvement by Systemic Diseases

BEVERLEY NEWMAN, ALEXANDER J. TOWBIN, and FRANDICS P. CHAN

Numerous systemic diseases can affect the heart and great vessels and are important causes of cardiac dysfunction. These systemic diseases include both prenatal and postnatal toxic and infectious exposures, adverse effects of therapeutic agents, and various nutritional, metabolic, inflammatory, granulomatous, infectious, and autoimmune entities. Endocrine, circulatory, and blood disorders frequently have secondary cardiac effects. Primary cardiac tumors can occur in association with underlying systemic disorders; although rare, neoplasms elsewhere can metastasize to the heart or locally invade the great vessels or pericardium. Both congenital and secondary lung and chest wall abnormalities are associated with structural and functional cardiac abnormalities.

These entities and the spectrum of their cardiac effects are outlined in Table 82-1. We have included both common diseases that have cardiovascular features and uncommon lesions in which cardiovascular manifestations are prominent. A small number of selected entities are discussed in the following sections. Many of the lesions outlined in Table 82-1 overlap with other chapters and thus are not specifically discussed here. Some well-known syndromes, such as Marfan syndrome, have both cardiac and other organ manifestations, but because they are covered in other chapters, further discussion is omitted here (see Chapter 79).

Toxins/Drugs

FETAL ALCOHOL EXPOSURE

Fetal alcohol syndrome is a common disorder affecting 0.5 to 2.0 per 1000 live births. Affected infants have moderate to severe growth retardation both in the prenatal and postnatal period, along with a characteristic facies. Most children with fetal alcohol syndrome have associated neurologic problems including mental retardation and learning disabilities, as well as altered behavior.[1,2]

Cardiac malformations are common with fetal alcohol exposure; the most frequent is ventricular septal defect. Other cardiac anomalies include pulmonary artery hypoplasia, coarctation or interruption of the aortic arch, atrial septal defect, patent ductus arteriosus, and tetralogy of Fallot (Fig. 82-1).[3]

Infectious, Inflammatory, and Autoimmune Disorders

INFECTIOUS AORTITIS

Overview Acute infectious aortitis in children often is caused by bacterial septicemia originating from infected lines and intravascular devices and from valvular endocarditis or occasionally by direct spread from an adjacent infection or abscess (Fig. 82-2).[4] Staphylococci and streptococci are the organisms most frequently responsible for acute infectious aortitis.[4,5] Predisposing conditions include congenital heart disease and an immunocompromised state. Once they are in the bloodstream, virulent organisms may adhere to and invade the aortic wall. The resulting inflammation leads to suppurative necrosis that weakens the aortic wall and forms an aneurysm (see Fig. 82-2, A). A contained leak may lead to pseudoaneurysm formation (see Fig. 82-2, B). Staphylococcal aortitis is particularly prone to overt rupture of the aneurysm or pseudoaneurysm and is the most serious complication of infectious aortitis. Fungal agents, especially Aspergillus or Candida, also may be the causative agent of infectious aortitis, especially in immune-compromised individuals.[6] Syphilitic and tuberculous aortic aneurysms are rare complications of chronic infection by those organisms and are very uncommon in children.

Diagnosis of infectious aortitis is difficult because many children with infected aneurysms are asymptomatic or they present with nonspecific complaints, such as fever and abdominal or back pain. Commonly used laboratory markers of infection can be normal. One adult study showed that blood cultures were negative in 28% of cases and white blood cell counts were normal in 42% of cases; however, an elevated erythrocyte sedimentation rate, a nonspecific finding of inflammation, was found in 92% of patients.[5]

Imaging Few clinical studies have evaluated the imaging appearance and distribution of infected aortic aneurysms in children. Experience from adult patients suggests that these aneurysms are more often saccular (93%) than fusiform (7%) and can be distributed throughout the course of the aorta:

Table 82-1

Cardiovascular Manifestations of Systemic Diseases or Disorders

Disease or Disorder Category	Cardiovascular Manifestations
Toxins/Drugs	
Carbon monoxide	Tachycardia, noncardiogenic pulmonary edema
Doxorubicin (Adriamycin)	Cardiomyopathy, CHF
Fetal alcohol exposure (see Fig. 82-1)	ASD, VSD, PDA, COA, arch interruption, PA hypoplasia, DORV, DEXTRO, TOF
Fenfluramine and phentermine (Fen-phen)	Valvular regurgitant heart disease, primary pulmonary hypertension
HAART (used to treat HIV)	Cardiomyopathy, CHF
Lead	Myocarditis, atherosclerosis
Radiation	Cardiomyopathy, MI, pericarditis, valvular disease, especially aortic
Steroids (chronic)	Cardiomyopathy, CHF, cardiomegaly
Theophylline	Arrhythmias
Metabolic	
Alkaptonuria	CAD, aortic and mitral valvulitis
Amyloidosis	Cardiomyopathy, CHF, arrhythmias
Carnitine deficiency	Dilated cardiomyopathy, CHF, endocardial fibroelastosis
Fabry disease	Cardiomyopathy, mitral valve disease, thromboembolism, arrhythmias, coronary aneurysm
Glycogen storage disease	
Type II (Pompe disease)	Cardiomyopathy, CHF, outflow tract obstruction
Type III	Hypertrophic cardiomyopathy
Type IV	Dilated cardiomyopathy
Danon disease (lysosomal glycogen-storage disease)	Hypertrophic cardiomyopathy
Hemochromatosis	Cardiomyopathy, arrhythmia, CHF
Gaucher disease (cerebroside lipidosis)	Cardiomyopathy, MR, MS, AS, coagulopathy
GM1 gangliosidosis	Infantile cardiomyopathy
Homocystinuria	Vascular stenoses and occlusions, aneurysms, thromboembolic episodes
Long-chain acetyl CoA dehydrogenase deficiency	Cardiomyopathy
Mucolipidosis III	AR, cardiomyopathy
Mucopolysaccharidosis	
IH (Hurler syndrome)	Acute cardiomyopathy associated with endocardial fibroelastosis, AR, MR, coronary narrowing
IS (Scheie)	AS, MS
II (Hunter syndrome)	AR
III (Sanfilippo syndrome)	Functional and morphologic mitral valve deterioration
IV (Morquio syndrome)	AR, MR, CAD
VI (Maroteaux-Lamy syndrome)	AS, MS
Oncocytic (histiocytoid) cardiomyopathy (infantile histiocytic cardiomyopathy, Purkinje cell tumor, focal lipid cardiomyopathy, idiopathic infantile cardiomyopathy)	Cardiomyopathy, ASD, VSD, nodular deposits on the ventricular endocardium or valves
Pseudoxanthoma elasticum	Premature atherosclerosis, MI, restrictive cardiomyopathy, mitral valve disease, AO dilation, vascular, coronary occlusions
Refsum disease (phytanic acid α-oxidase deficiency)	CHF, cardiomyopathy, conduction abnormality
Sitosterolemia (inherited plant sterol storage disease)	CAD, MI, CHF
Uremia	Pericardial effusion, constrictive pericarditis, CHF, cardiomyopathy
Granulomatous	
Histoplasmosis	Pericardial effusion, tamponade, AR, endocarditis, fibrosing mediastinitis
Sarcoid	Infiltrative cardiomyopathy, pericardial effusion, papillary muscle dysfunction, valvular disease, fibrosing mediastinitis, large vessel vasculitis
Tuberculosis	Myocarditis, ventricular aneurysms, calcific/constrictive pericarditis, fibrosing mediastinitis, vasculitis
Wegener granulomatosis	Pulmonary vasculitis, pericarditis, coronary arteritis, MI
Infectious/Inflammatory/Autoimmune/Connective Tissue Disorders	
Aortitis (infectious) (see Fig. 82-2)	Abscess, aneurysm, leak, pseudoaneurysm, rupture
Behçet syndrome	Aortic, pulmonary and coronary vasculitis and aneurysms, cardiac valvular vegetations

Table 82-1

Cardiovascular Manifestations of Systemic Diseases or Disorders—cont'd

Disease or Disorder Category	Cardiovascular Manifestations
Chagas disease (*Trypanosoma cruzi*)	Myocarditis, CHF, apical aneurysm
Dermatomyositis	Cardiomyopathy
Diphtheria	Cardiomyopathy, myocarditis
Enterovirus (Coxsackie B)	Myocarditis
Fetal rubella infection	PDA, pulmonary artery stenosis, COA, ASD, VSD, myocarditis, cardiomyopathy
HIV	Cardiomyopathy, CHF
Juvenile rheumatoid arthritis	Pericarditis, myocarditis, CHF
Kawasaki disease	Coronary artery aneurysm, coronary thrombosis, MR, papillary muscle dysfunction, MI, myocarditis, CHF, pericarditis, AR, systemic vasculitis
Polyarteritis nodosa	Cardiomyopathy, pericarditis, coronary artery aneurysms, MI, systemic vasculitis
Relapsing polychondritis	CM, AO dilation/aneurysm, AR, TR, MR
Rheumatic fever	Pancarditis, valve insufficiency, CHF, valvular stenosis (MS, AS, TS), atrial dilation, left atrial thrombus, constrictive pericarditis
Scleroderma	CM, pericarditis, myocarditis, conduction abnormality, cor pulmonale
Systemic lupus erythematosus	Pericarditis, cardiomyopathy, Libman-Sacks endocarditis, heart block, endocardial fibroelastosis, systemic/coronary vasculitis
Takayasu arteritis (see Fig. 82-3, e-Fig. 82-4, Fig. 82-5).	Widened mediastinum, AR, CHF, myocarditis, aortitis, pulmonary/coronary vasculitis, aneurysms, stenoses
Toxoplasmosis	Myocarditis
Malnutrition	
Anorexia	Decreased ventricular mass, MVP
Bulimia	Arrest, cardiac rupture, pneumomediastinum
Marasmus	Thinning of cardiac muscle, CHF, CHD
Obesity	CM, pulmonary hypertension, early atherosclerotic disease
Selenium deficiency (Keshan disease)	Congestive cardiomyopathy, cardiogenic shock, CHF
Vitamin B_1 (thiamine) deficiency (beriberi)	Cardiomyopathy, CHF
Cardiac Tumors Associated With Systemic Disease	
Fibromas (in Beckwith-Wiedemann syndrome, nevoid basal cell carcinoma syndrome, or Gorlin syndrome)	Cardiomyopathy, CHF, mass most commonly originates at the intraventricular septum, occasional calcification in the tumor
Myxomas (in Carney complex, LAMB/NAME syndrome) (see e-Fig. 82-9)	Attached to atrial septum and mitral apparatus in LA, can prolapse or embolize, multiple, can occur in any cardiac chamber, can recur at distant intracardiac and extracardiac sites, intracardiac valvular obstruction leading to CHF
Rhabdomyomas (in tuberous sclerosis)	Multiple intramural hamartomas, present in utero, abnormal valve function, outflow obstruction, cardiomyopathy, spontaneously regress
Metastases	
Lymphoma	Great vessel obstruction, SVC syndrome, CHF, pericardial infiltration
Wilms tumor (hepatoblastoma less commonly) (see Fig. 82-10)	IVC extension, CHF, cardiomyopathy
Endocrine	
Cushing disease	Cardiomyopathy, blood vessel fragility
Diabetes (acquired)	Early CAD
Diabetes gestational (Infant of a diabetic mother) (see Fig. 82-6)	Cardiomyopathy, cardiovisceral or atrioventricular discordance, outflow tract anomalies, TGA, AVSD, DiGeorge complex
Gigantism/acromegaly	Cardiac hypertrophy, LVH
Hyperthyroidism	CHF, cardiomyopathy
Hypothyroidism	Pericardial effusion, CHF
Circulatory/Blood Disorders	
Arteriovenous fistula (especially vein of Galen malformation, HHT and infantile hepatic hemangioma) (see e-Fig. 82-11)	CHF, high output; HHT: skin, visceral, single or multiple pulmonary AVM, angiodysplasia, coronary ectasia, Kasabach-Merritt syndrome (platelet trapping and consumptive coagulopathy)
Fanconi anemia	PDA, VSD, peripheral PS, cardiomyopathy, ASD, TOF, AS, COA, AO atheromas, hypoplastic AO, double AO arch

Continued

Table 82-1

Cardiovascular Manifestations of Systemic Diseases or Disorders—cont'd

Disease or Disorder Category	Cardiovascular Manifestations
Hepatopulmonary syndrome (chronic liver disease, hypoxemia, clubbing)	Pulmonary capillary microshunts, vasodilation, CHF—high output
Portopulmonary syndrome (Abernethy malformation): hepatopulmonary syndrome with no liver disease, portosystemic shunting (see Chapter 79)	Type I abnormal portal–systemic connection; absent intrahepatic portal vein; associated with VSD, AO arch anomalies
	Type II abnormal portal–systemic connection; intrahepatic portal vein present
Leukemia	SVC syndrome, cardiomyopathy, CHF, pericardial effusion
Polycythemia vera	MI, arterial and venous clots, CHF
Sickle cell disease (see Fig. 82-7)	Cardiomyopathy, MI, acute chest syndrome, CHF, vascular thromboses
Thalassemia (see Fig. 82-8)	CHF, cardiomyopathy, iron overload
Twin-to-twin transfusion	Shared placental circulation leads to unbalanced flow; CM and CHF may develop in both the anemic and the polycythemic twin
Musculoskeletal/Neurologic	
Abetalipoproteinemia	Arrhythmia, cardiomyopathy, CHF
Duchenne muscular dystrophy	Cardiomegaly, progressive cardiomyopathy, conduction abnormalities, CHF, MVP
Friedreich ataxia (spinocerebellar degeneration)	CM, cardiomyopathy, CHF, cardiac thrombus
Kyphoscoliosis	Cardiac, vascular, and airway displacement and compression
Osteogenesis imperfecta	MVP, AR, enlarged AO root
Pectus excavatum	Cardiac displacement, MVP, anterior compression of right ventricle

AO, Aorta/aortic; *AR,* aortic regurgitation; *AS,* aortic stenosis; *ASD,* atrial septal defect; *AVM,* arteriovenous malformations; *AVSD,* atrioventricular septal defect; *CAD,* coronary artery disease; *CHD,* congenital heart disease; *CHF,* congestive heart failure; *CM,* cardiomegaly; *CoA,* coenzyme A; *COA,* aorta coarctation; *DEXTRO,* dextrocardia; *DORV,* double outlet right ventricle; *HAART,* highly active anti-retroviral therapy; *HHT,* hereditary hemorrhagic telangiectasia; *HIV,* human immunodeficiency virus; *IVC,* inferior vena cava; *LA,* left atrium; *LAMB,* lentigines, atrial myxoma, mucocutaneous myxomas, blue nevi; *LVH,* left ventricular hypertrophy; *MI,* myocardial infarction; *MR,* mitral regurgitation; *MS,* mitral stenosis; *MVP,* mitral valve prolapse; *NAME,* nevi, atrial myxoma, myxoid neurofibromas, ephelides; *PA,* pulmonary artery; *PDA,* patent ductus arteriosus; *PS,* pulmonary stenosis; *SVC,* superior vena cava; *TGA,* transposition of great arteries; *TOF,* tetralogy of Fallot; *TR,* tricuspid regurgitation; *TS,* tricuspid stenosis; *VSD,* ventricular septal defect.

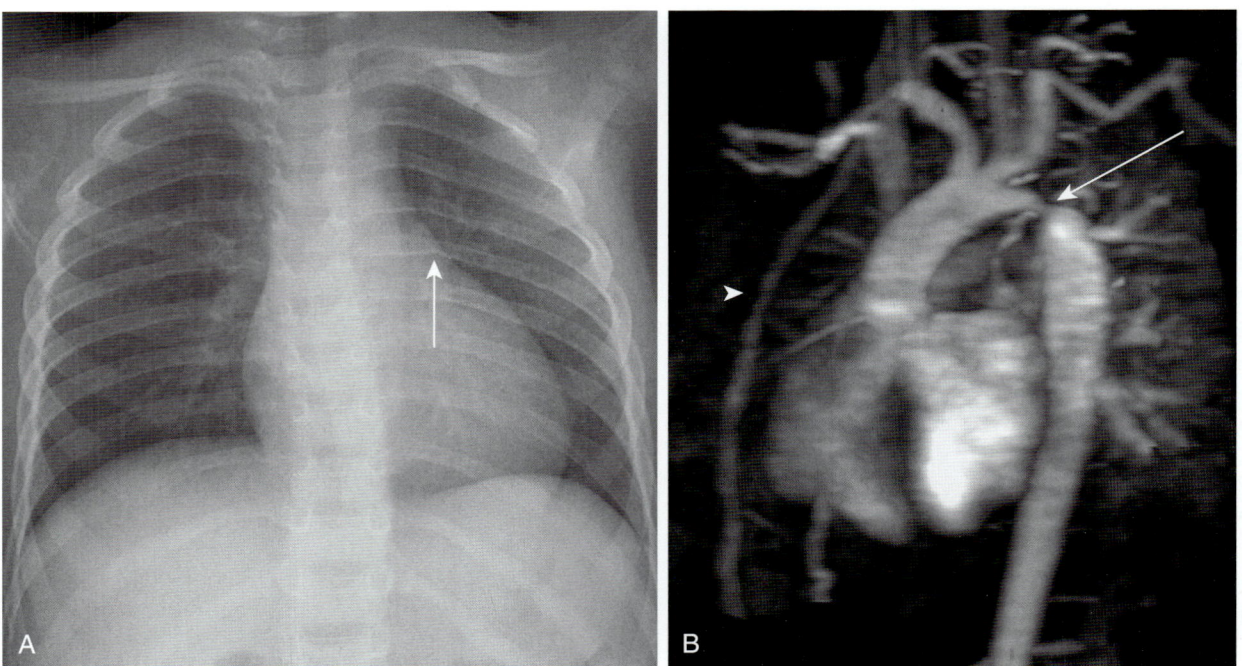

Figure 82-1   Fetal alcohol syndrome and aortic coarctation in a 4-year-old boy. **A,** A chest radiograph shows a prominent aortic arch and descending aorta. Notching of the posterior left sixth rib (*arrow*) from an intercostal aortic collateral vessel is present. **B,** Oblique sagittal three-dimensional magnetic resonance angiography image demonstrates marked coarctation of the aorta (*arrow*) distal to the left subclavian artery. Multiple large intercostal collateral vessels are present, as well as enlarged internal mammary collaterals (*arrowhead*).

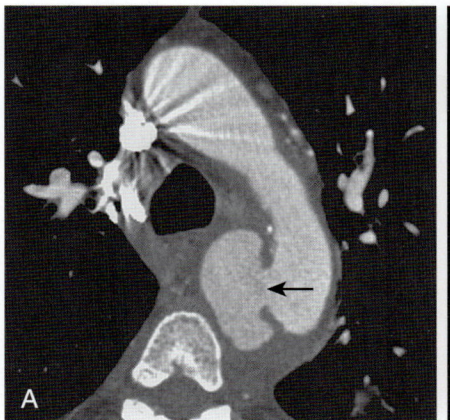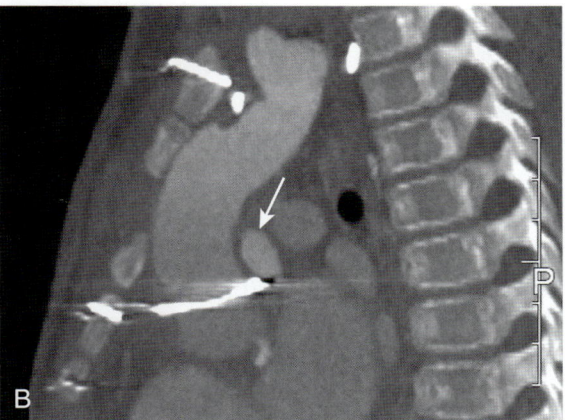

Figure 82-2 Infectious aortitis. **A,** Axial image from a computed tomography angiogram (CTA) shows a thick-walled saccular aneurysm communicating with the aortic arch through a narrow opening (*arrow*). **B,** An 8-year-old child after repair of aortic coarctation and aortic stenosis with prosthetic aortic valve replacement whose postoperative course was complicated by *Staphylococcus aureus* mediastinitis. A sagittal maximal intensity projection image from a gated CTA demonstrates a small posterior aortic pseudoneurysm (*arrow*) adjacent to the aortic valve. Note diffuse anterior soft tissue edema/inflammation.

6% in the ascending aorta, 23% in the descending thoracic, 19% in the thoracoabdominal aorta, 10% in the juxtarenal aorta, and 32% in the infrarenal aorta.[7] Periaortic fluid, stranding, or a soft tissue mass was present in 48% of patients with infectious aortitis. Periaortic gas, a specific sign, was present in only 7%. Rapid progression of aneurysm size was found in infected aneurysms in both adults and children.[7] Computed tomographic angiography (CTA) and magnetic resonance angiography (MRA) imaging have largely supplanted conventional angiography in the diagnosis of aortic aneurysms and their complications (see Fig. 82-2). Ultrasound may be an initial screening examination but usually is not definitive enough to support management decisions.

Treatment Antibiotic treatment with the goal of eradicating the offending organism is the first step in the treatment of infectious aortitis.[5] At the same time, imaging to document stability of the aortic lumen is necessary. If an aneurysm has formed, it should be surgically repaired after an adequate period of antibiotic treatment.[4,5] Deployment of endovascular stent grafts in infected aortic aneurysms has been attempted.[8] Although this deployment is not considered a treatment of choice, it may be useful to act as a bridge to open surgical repair, especially in the presence of low-virulence organisms or rapidly expanding aneurysms.

TAKAYASU ARTERITIS

Overview Takayasu arteritis, also known as pulseless arteritis, is a chronic inflammatory arteritis of large vessels.[9] The aorta is the artery that is most commonly involved, with the abdominal aorta involved in 59% to 75% of cases and the thoracic aorta involved in 40% to 56% of cases. Takayasu arteritis involvement is more common in the systemic arteries than in the pulmonary arteries.[10] Takayasu arteritis is a rare disease, occurring in 2.6 per 1 million people in North America.[11] It is more common in patients of Asian descent, and females make up 80% to 90% of patients.

Diagnosis of Takayasu arteritis is based on patient symptoms, physical findings, clinical laboratory values, serologic markers, and vascular findings.[9] The American College of Rheumatology criteria include arm or leg claudication, age younger than 40 years, a blood pressure difference between extremities of greater than 10 mm Hg, subclavian or aortic bruit, decreased brachial artery pulse, and aortic or branch narrowing.[12] Three of these criteria provide a diagnosis of Takayasu arteritis with a sensitivity of 90.5% and a specificity of 97.8%.[11] Other clinical manifestations of Takayasu arteritis that are not involved in diagnosis include fever, headache, neurologic symptoms including stroke, postural dizziness, arthralgias, weight loss, myalgias, and systemic or pulmonary hypertension.[11,13]

Takayasu arteritis has a triphasic pattern: a systemic non-vascular phase, a vascular inflammatory phase, and a quiescent "burnt out" phase, although the inflammatory and fibrotic changes often overlap.[10,11] In children, a long delay often occurs before Takayasu arteritis is diagnosed, especially when systemic symptoms predominate.[11,13,14]

The lesions of Takayasu arteritis are segmental with a patchy distribution. The vasculitis can lead to stenosis, occlusion, and aneurysm formation.[10] Severe stenosis or occlusive thrombosis of the pulmonary vasculature may lead to pulmonary infarction and pulmonary hypertension.[15] Cardiac symptoms include aortic regurgitation, dilated cardiomyopathy, myocarditis, pericarditis, congestive heart failure, and myocardial ischemia.

Etiology and Classification The specific cause of Takayasu arteritis is unknown, but it is probably a T-cell–mediated autoimmune process. Infection, particularly tuberculosis, has been linked to the development of Takayasu arteritis, especially in children.[13] The diseased vessel wall is thickened and shows granulomatous changes from the adventitia to the media. Giant cell (or temporal arteritis) has an identical pathologic appearance to Takayasu arteritis but affects an older population and typically involves the temporal artery.[16]

Takayasu arteritis currently is divided into six types depending on the location of aortic involvement. Coronary (C+) or pulmonary (P+) involvement may occur in all types (Fig. 82-3).[10]

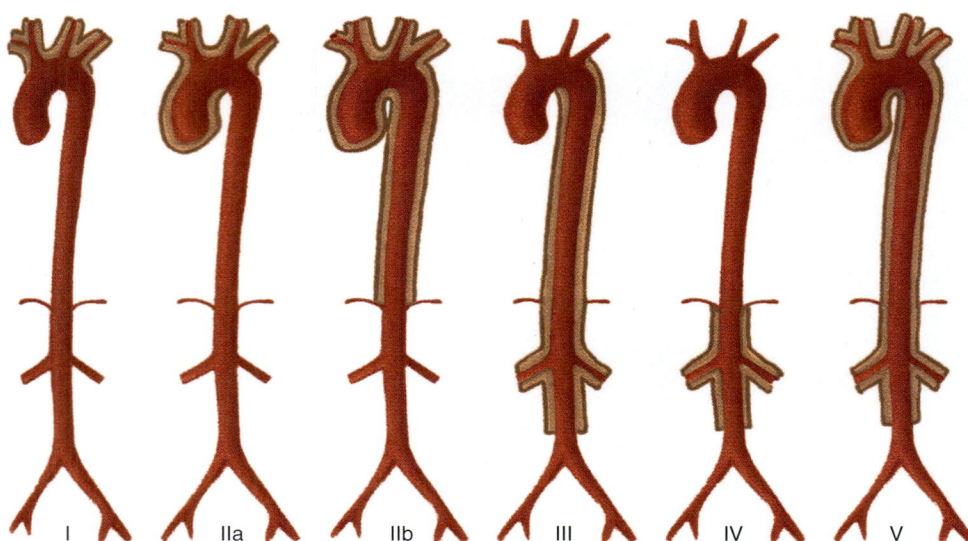

Figure 82-3   The classification schema of Takayasu arteritis. Coronary (C+) and/or pulmonary (P+) involvement can occur in all types. Type I involves aortic arch branches only; type IIa involves the ascending aorta, arch, and branches; type IIb involves the descending thoracic aorta, with or without involvement of the ascending aorta, arch, and branches; type III involves the descending thoracic aorta, abdominal aorta, and the renal arteries; type IV involves the abdominal vessels only; and type V is generalized. (From Nastri MV, Baptista LPS, Baroni RH, et al. Gadolinium-enhanced three-dimensional MR angiography of Takayasu arteritis. *Radiographics.* 2004;24:773-786.)

Imaging   Vascular stenosis and aneurysm are the primary causes of mortality and morbidity and therefore should be evaluated with angiographic techniques. Conventional angiography has been the gold standard for diagnosis, but it is being supplanted by MRA (e-Fig. 82-4 and Fig. 82-5).[10,11] MRA has several advantages, including its lack of ionizing radiation, its noninvasive nature, and its ability to show abnormal vascular wall signal and thickening before luminal narrowing becomes apparent.[9] It also does not require iodinated contrast agents. Active inflammation is suggested when a high T2 signal is noted within the vessel wall (see Fig. 82-5). Vessel wall enhancement can be seen with the administration of gadolinium and also is used to gauge the activity of the inflammatory process (see e-Fig. 82-4).[10,11,14] Inversion recovery delayed enhancement of the vessel wall also may be seen; the significance of this phenomenon is uncertain.[11]

Other imaging studies can be used to show the abnormalities of Takayasu arteritis. Ultrasound can show vessel wall thickening and CTA may demonstrate mural thickening and wall enhancement, as well as luminal dilation, narrowing, or occlusion (see Fig. 82-5).[9] Fluorodeoxyglucose positron emission tomography uptake also may be useful in evaluating active inflammation.[9,11]

Treatment and Follow-up   Medical therapy of Takayasu arteritis initially focuses on the suppression of the immunologic responses with corticosteroids, methotrexate, azathioprine, and cyclophosphamide. In refractory Takayasu arteritis, the anti–tumor necrosis factor-α agents Etanercept and Infliximab have been used to achieve sustained remission.[17] Follow-up with MRA or CTA helps document stability or progression of the vascular abnormalities and their complications.[9,14]

Patients with renovascular hypertension, severe coarctation of the aorta, claudication, progressive aneurysm enlargement, coronary artery disease, or cervicocranial vessel stenosis may benefit from surgical revascularization.[13] Bypass grafts, either synthetic or autologous, can be used, but restenosis has occurred in up to one third of cases in which synthetic grafts were used and in approximately 10% of procedures in which an autologous vessel was used. Other postoperative complications include heart failure, intractable hypertension, and graft deterioration with pseudoaneurysm formation. Postsurgical aneurysm formation at the anastomosis is a complication seen in up to 34% of patients. Angioplasty has been used with success in patients with Takayasu arteritis who have vascular stenosis, with an initial success rate of 92% and a restenosis rate of 22%. Surgical options preferably are performed during disease remission.[13]

OTHER VASCULITIDES

Aneurysmal disease of the aorta, which generally afflicts older patients, is a rare complication of systemic lupus erythematosus. The exact pathophysiology of the aortic aneurysm is unknown. It may be caused directly by the systemic lupus erythematosus–related inflammation of the vessel wall or as a result of chronic steroid treatment and the resultant accelerated aortic atherosclerosis.[18] Sarcoidosis has been reported as a rare cause of large-vessel vascular stenosis, and it has been recommended that children with early-onset sarcoidosis be evaluated for occlusive arterial disease.[19]

Other rare causes of vasculitis, especially in the pulmonary artery, include Behçet syndrome and Wegener granulomatosis.[12,20] Behçet syndrome is a multisystem inflammatory disease of unknown cause. Classically, Behçet syndrome describes a

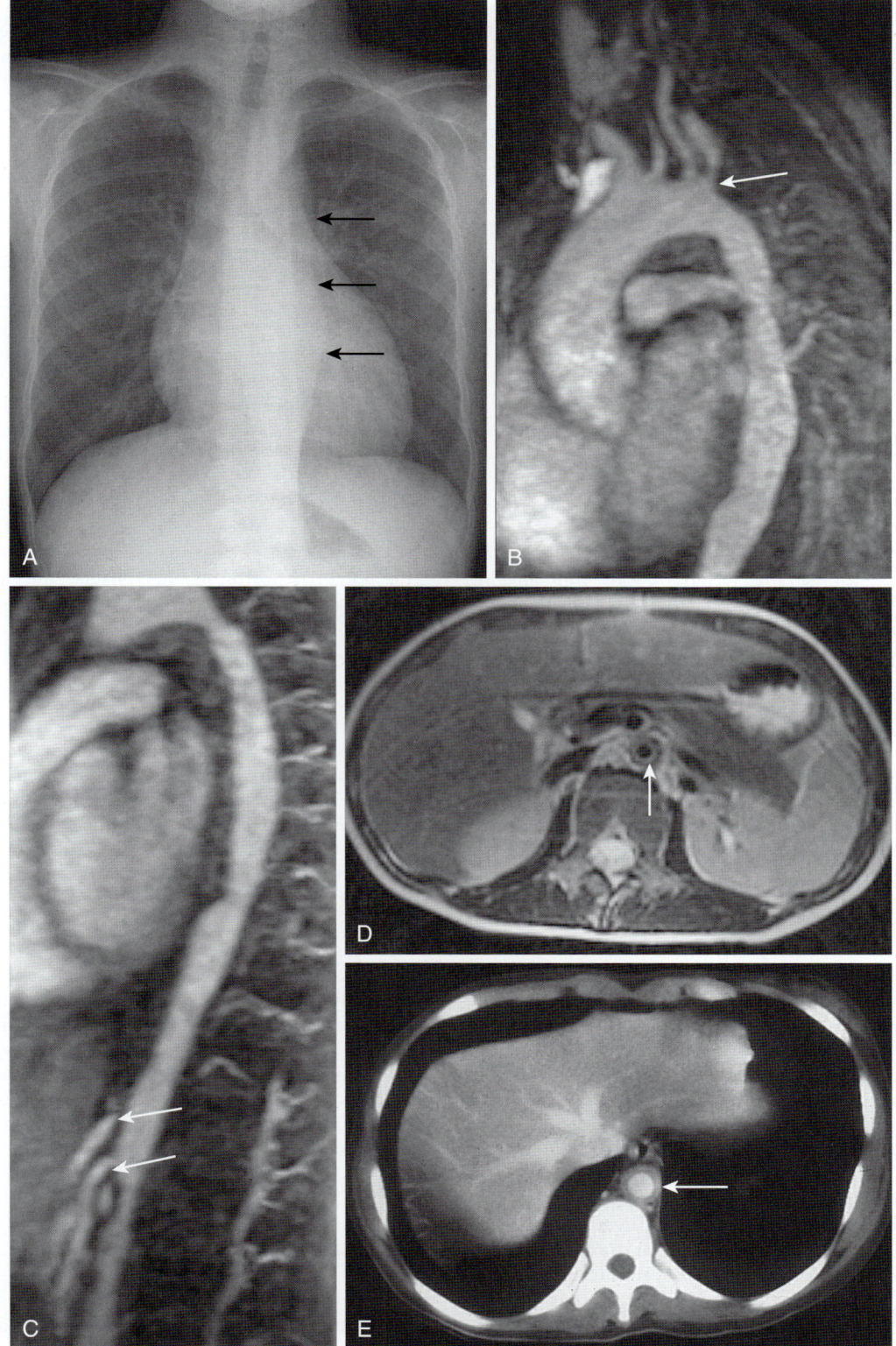

Figure 82-5 An 11-year-old girl with type V Takayasu arteritis. **A,** A chest radiograph shows a heart that is top-normal in size and has an abnormal wavy contour to the descending thoracic aorta (*arrows*). **B,** An oblique sagittal thin maximal intensity projection (MIP) from a magnetic resonance angiogram (MRA) image shows four vessels arising from the aortic arch: the right brachiocephalic artery, left common carotid artery, left vertebral artery, and left subclavian artery. Stenosis is present at the origin of the left subclavian artery (*arrow*) along with areas of stenosis and aneurysmal dilation of the visible portions of the descending aorta. **C,** Thin sagittal MIP image reconstruction of the MRA shows an irregular contour and narrowing of the descending aorta, as well as at the origins of the celiac and the superior mesenteric arteries (*arrows*). **D,** A T2-weighted axial magnetic resonance image shows increased signal and thickening of the wall with a narrowed lumen (*arrow*) of the inframesenteric abdominal aorta. **E,** A contrast-enhanced computed tomography image of a different patient shows wall thickening and enhancement (*arrow*) of the abdominal aorta.

combination of recurrent aphthous ulcers, genital ulceration, and uveitis. It also involves the central nervous system in 10% to 30% of cases and the vascular system, including systemic, pulmonary, and coronary vessels, in 10% to 40% of cases. Its prevalence in the United States is probably less than 5 cases per 100,000 people, but it is much more common in Turkey, with an estimated prevalence of 100 cases per 100,000 people. Although Behçet syndrome typically is an adult disease, onset in childhood is well recognized. When the pulmonary artery is affected by Behçet syndrome, the most common lesion is pulmonary artery aneurysm. Other findings include pulmonary artery stenosis and thrombosis, pulmonary infarct, and hemorrhage.[21] These lesions are readily evaluated with computed tomography (CT) pulmonary angiography.[20] Treatment, as for Takayasu arteritis, is focused on immunosuppression.[21] Resolution of aneurysms has been observed after remission of Behçet syndrome.

Malnutrition

ANOREXIA

Anorexia is a common eating disorder. It is characterized by an intense fear of gaining weight, undue influence of body shape or weight on self-image, the refusal to maintain a body weight of greater than 85% of that predicted, and the absence of at least three consecutive menstrual periods. It is 10 times more common in girls and occurs mostly during adolescence.

Cardiovascular complications occur in up to 80% of patients and are the cause of approximately one third of deaths in this disorder. The most common cardiac abnormality is decreased ventricular wall thickness caused by a loss of cardiac muscle. Other cardiac manifestations include sinus bradycardia, hypotension, arrhythmias, QT interval prolongation, and even sudden death.[22] These abnormalities are reversible in the early stages of disease.[22,23]

OBESITY

A worldwide epidemic of obesity is occurring among people of all ages.[24] The Obesity Consensus Working Group reported that the prevalence of overweight status has doubled among children 6 to 11 years of age and tripled in those 12 to 17 years of age from 1980 to 2000. Approximately 15% of all 15-year-olds can be classified as obese (defined as a body mass index greater than the 95th percentile) in the United States.

Obesity in children has led to an increase in type 2 diabetes mellitus, hypertension, fatty-related liver disease, and possibly asthma. Heart disease is a significant cause of morbidity in obese persons.[24] Excessive adipose accumulation induces increased blood volume and cardiac output, leading to cardiomegaly. Decreased alveolar ventilation and sleep apnea may contribute to both cardiomegaly and pulmonary hypertension (Pickwickian syndrome). Obesity and type 2 diabetes lead to the development of early atherosclerotic disease. It is uncertain whether childhood obesity increases the risk of myocardial infarction or stroke in adulthood.

The high incidence of obesity has led to a corresponding increase in the number of bariatric procedures used to treat patients, including children. Rapid loss of a large amount of weight and decreased absorption of nutrients postoperatively puts individuals at risk for nutritional deficiencies. Beriberi, a disorder of thiamine deficiency, has been reported after gastric bypass surgery.[25] The wet form of beriberi is associated with cardiac failure and edema.

Endocrine Disorders

TYPE 1 DIABETES MELLITUS

Overview   Type 1 insulin-dependent diabetes mellitus occurs relatively frequently in the United States; it develops in an estimated 3 of 1000 children by age 20 years. Cardiovascular complications are the most common causes of morbidity and mortality in persons with diabetes in childhood and are mainly the result of atherosclerotic disease.[26] Persons with diabetes are more likely than nondiabetic individuals to have severe narrowing of the coronary arteries, stenosis in all three major coronary vessels, and disease in more distal segments.

Etiology   The precise etiology of diabetes is unknown, but it is thought to be an autoimmune disorder of islet cells, possibly related to a prior viral infection. Most children present with polyuria, polydipsia, polyphagia, and weight loss with hyperglycemia, glycosuria, ketonemia, and ketonuria.

GESTATIONAL DIABETES

Gestational diabetes is associated with congenital abnormalities in infants born to affected mothers. The Baltimore-Washington Infant Study found that maternal diabetes was strongly associated with early cardiovascular malformations and with cardiomyopathy.[27] Early cardiovascular malformations refer to defects in early cardiac development such as laterality and cardiac looping defects, outflow tract anomalies with or without transposed great vessels, and atrioventricular septal defects. The data from this study also showed that maternal diabetes was not associated with obstructive and simple shunt defects.

Visceromegaly, hypoglycemia, and cardiomegaly occur commonly in neonates born to diabetic mothers (Fig. 82-6). The severity of these findings and of congenital heart defects may be related to how well the maternal blood sugar was controlled during pregnancy.[28] Left ventricular septal wall thickening and hypertrophic subaortic stenosis are characteristic and often transient features in affected neonates (see Fig. 82-6).

Blood Disorders

SICKLE CELL ANEMIA

Overview   Sickle cell anemia, which is the most common single gene disorder of African Americans, affects 1 in 375 African Americans. Almost 1 in 12 African Americans are heterozygous for the trait. Children with sickle cell anemia constitute the largest subgroup of patients with chronic anemia in the United States. Cardiac enlargement is the most common cardiac feature related to the chronic anemia.[29] Cardiomyopathy also may develop from coronary sickling and ischemia, along with cardiac dysfunction resulting from chronic transfusion and myocardial iron deposition.[29,30]

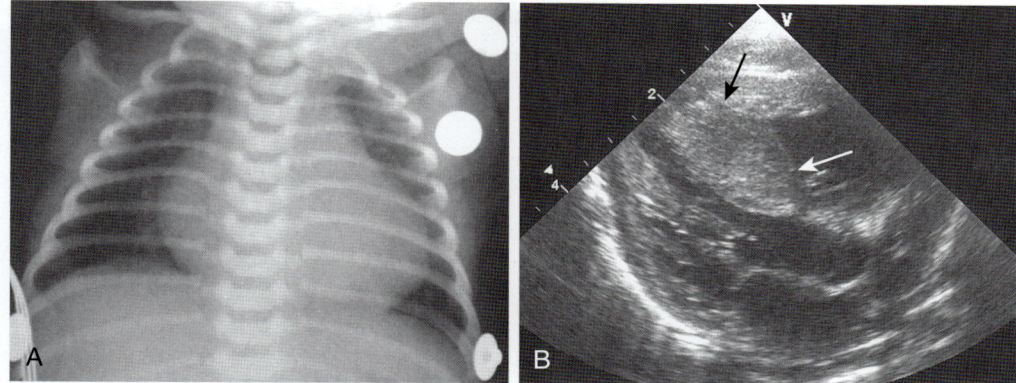

Figure 82-6 A newborn boy with a diabetic mother. **A,** A chest radiograph shows an enlarged heart and mild congestive heart failure. A hypoplastic left heart malformation was diagnosed on echocardiography. **B,** A Long-axis echocardiogram from another patient with neonatal diabetic cardiomyopathy shows septal hypertrophy (*arrows*), which partially impinges on the left ventricular outflow tract. (**B,** Courtesy Fred Sherman, MD, Children's Hospital of Pittsburgh.)

Imaging Acute chest syndrome is a common cause of hospitalization, morbidity, and mortality in children with sickle cell disease (Fig. 82-7). Clinical presentation includes chest pain, leukocytosis, and fever. Typical chest radiographic manifestations include cardiomegaly, venous congestion, new radiographic opacity (atelectasis or consolidation), and pleural effusion. The inciting etiology is not always apparent, but possibilities include infection, pulmonary sickling and infarction, and fat emboli from marrow infarction. Infection appears to be a more common underlying factor in younger children, whereas infarction is more common in older persons.

Imaging of the chest in children with sickle cell anemia depends on the clinical scenario. Plain chest radiographs are the mainstay but can be supplemented with echocardiography, CT, MRI, or a nuclear scan for such concerns as bone infarcts or osteomyelitis, pulmonary emboli, complicated pulmonary infection, myocardial ischemia or dysfunction, and liver/myocardial iron overload related to repeated transfusion.[30]

Children with sickle cell disease and specific risk factors have been shown by de Montalembert and coworkers[31] to be at risk for myocardial ischemia. Consequences of ischemia include include chest pain, heart failure, or a ventricular arrhythmia. Thallium-201 single–photon emission CT scans show that almost one third of symptomatic children have a fixed perfusion defect. These perfusion defects may not have a specific vascular pattern, suggesting involvement of the cardiac microcirculation.[31]

THALASSEMIA

Cardiac manifestations of thalassemia are primarily due to chronic anemia and vary with the severity of the disease.[32] Thalassemia major (homozygous) has more marked

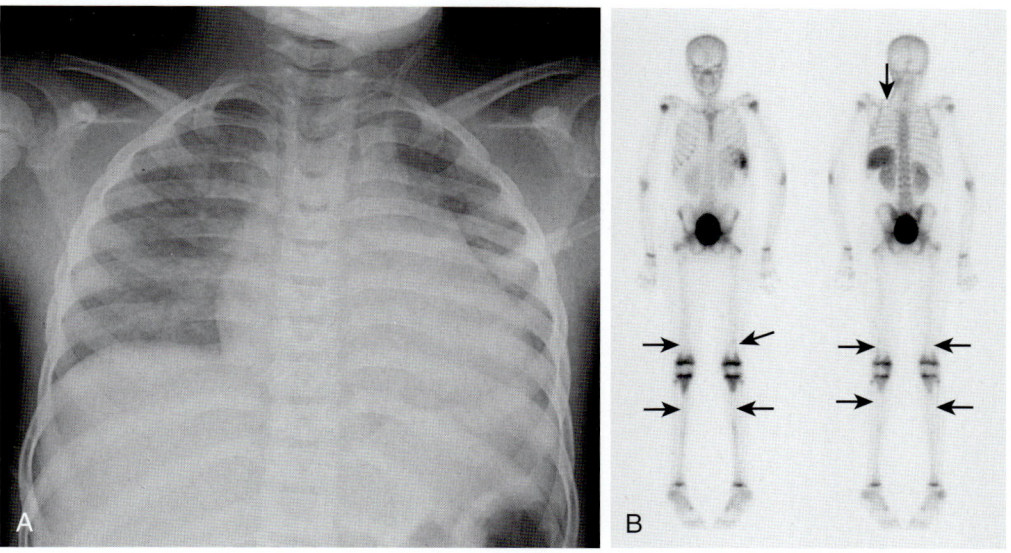

Figure 82-7 Acute chest syndrome in a patient with sickle cell disease. **A,** The frontal view of the chest in a patient with sickle cell disease shows a new opacity in the left lower lobe and a mildly enlarged heart. **B,** Anterior and posterior projection from a technetium-99m methylene-diphosponate bone scan in a different patient shows multiple areas of decreased uptake due to infarcts (*arrows*) in the distal femurs, proximal tibias, and left posterior third rib.

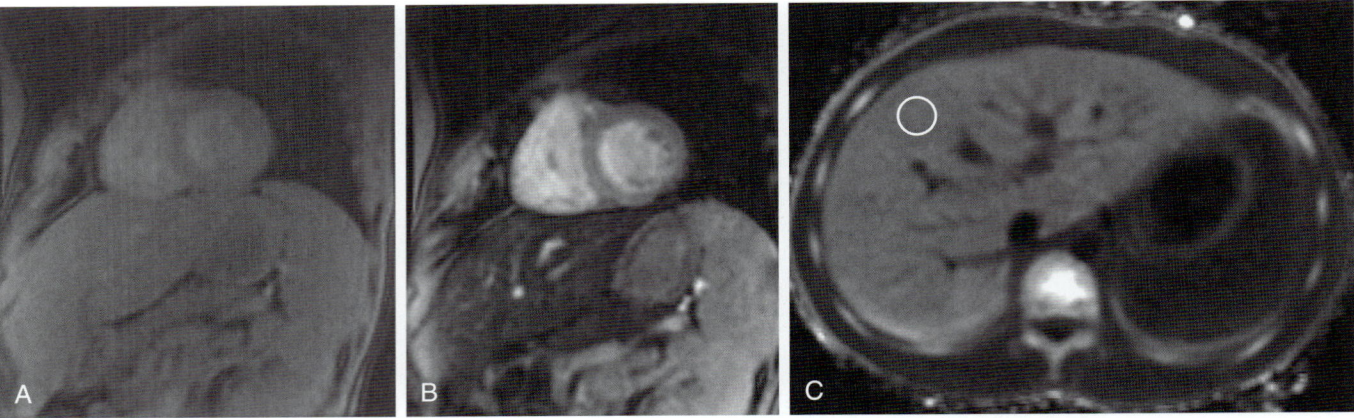

Figure 82-8 A 14-year-old boy with β-thalassemia who has received multiple transfusions. Magnetic resonance images were obtained of the liver and heart to evaluate iron deposition. **A** and **B,** Short axis gated, multiecho gradient echo sequence with increasing echo time shows progressive darkening of the liver but not the myocardium. **A,** Echo time (TE) 2.2. **B,** TE 13.4. **C,** An axial R2* map of the liver that was reconstructed from multiple gradient echo images. A region of interest in the liver as shown gave an R2* reading in the liver parenchyma of 124 Hertz. T2* can be calculated as the inverse of R2*, 8.1 msec. This T2* number reflects moderate iron deposition within the liver. Note the absence of iron in the spleen (dark on this image). T2* in the myocardium was similarly calculated (not shown) to be 30 msec (within normal limits).

hematologic, cardiac, and bone changes than thalassemia minor (heterozygous) and intermedia (the homozygous, milder form). A hyperdynamic circulation and congestive heart failure are the most common clinical cardiac findings.

Cardiomyopathy may develop as a result of ischemia or myocardial iron overload related to chronic transfusion. Widened and coarsely trabeculated rib changes are common in association with red marrow conversion. Extramedullary hematopoiesis occurs commonly in the liver and spleen as well as paraspinal soft tissues, most often in the lower thoracic region, with resultant visceromegaly and paraspinal soft tissue masses. MR imaging is useful for serial follow-up of children who undergo chronic transfusion to assess their visceral and myocardial iron burden and cardiac function (Fig. 82-8).

Other Systemic Disorders

Many other systemic disorders affect the cardiovascular system. These disorders are listed in Table 82-1 (also see e-Figs. 82-9 to 82-11).

References

Full references for this chapter can be found on www.expertconsult.com.

Chapter 83

Acquired Diseases of the Thoracic Great Vessels

FRANDICS P. CHAN

This chapter reviews acquired pediatric diseases of the thoracic aorta, venae cavae, pulmonary arteries, and pulmonary veins. Acquired pediatric aortic disease is uncommon, but radiologists and imagers play an important role in the care of patients who have sustained traumatic aortic injury. Pulmonary embolism is the most common acquired disease of the pulmonary artery. The most common acquired abnormalities of the pulmonary veins and venae cavae are obstruction or stenosis caused by luminal occlusion or extrinsic compression from mediastinal pathologies. Hemodynamically significant obstruction of the superior vena cava (SVC) leads to SVC syndrome, whereas obstruction of the pulmonary veins leads to pulmonary venous hypertension.

Acquired Diseases of the Thoracic Aorta

Pathology of the aorta can be categorized into aortic aneurysm, aortic dissection, and aortic stenosis.[1] Although each aortic disease may present one or more of these manifestations, it is the clinical consequences of aneurysm, dissection, or stenosis that determine mortality and morbidity (Table 83-1).

Normally, the caliber of the aorta gradually decreases in size from the sinotubular junction to the aortic hiatus. An aortic aneurysm is defined as an abnormal dilation of the aorta, which may undergo progressive expansion. An aortic aneurysm may form if wall stress increases, as in the case of systemic hypertension, or if the aortic wall weakens, as in the case of Marfan syndrome (see Chapter 79). The expansion rate of an aneurysm is determined by the wall stress, which increases with diameter. Thus a large aneurysm is more likely to expand than a small aneurysm, and the expansion is an accelerating process until rupture occurs.

Aortic dissection can occur in children as a complication of trauma or connective tissue diseases. A dissection is created when blood forces through a tear in the aortic intima and progressively separates the intimal layer from the aortic media, creating a true lumen that originally was connected to the aortic root and a false lumen that was not connected to the aortic root. Dissection can cause end-organ ischemia if the branch arteries supplying the organ are obstructed by the dissection flap. Dissection can weaken the aortic wall sufficiently to cause catastrophic rupture.

Aortic stenosis is defined as a narrowing that limits perfusion to organs supplied by the aorta distal to the stenosis. It may cause systemic hypertension, left ventricular pressure overload, and end-organ ischemia.

TRAUMA

Overview Trauma is a major cause of death in children and results primarily from motor vehicle accidents, although firearm injury (Fig. 83-1) and child abuse are other important causes of traumatic death. Survival of a child with a traumatic aortic injury until arrival at the emergency department is rare, accounting for one to two cases per year at large metropolitan level I pediatric trauma centers. Operative treatment involves fewer than 0.14% of all trauma patients, and only 6% of all traumatic ruptures of the aorta occur in patients younger than 16 years.[2,3] The outcome of traumatic aortic injury in the pediatric population is directly related to timely diagnosis, proper treatment, and hemodynamic status at the time of presentation.

Imaging Chest radiographic findings such as pleural capping at the left lung apex, obscuration of the aortic arch, mediastinal widening, pleural effusion, pneumothorax, pulmonary contusion, tracheal and nasogastric tube deviation, and upper rib and clavicle fracture in the setting of blunt trauma should raise clinical suspicion for an aortic injury (Fig. 83-2). Historically, the definitive diagnosis of traumatic aortic injury was made by conventional catheter angiography. Today, computed tomographic angiography (CTA) has supplanted catheter angiography as the diagnostic method of choice.[4,5] CTA allows speedy and precise visualization of the traumatic aortic injury. Care should be taken to identify the location of aortic rupture, active extravasation of arterial contrast, a dissection flap extending to major aortic branches, hemothorax and hemopericardium, and other organ and musculoskeletal injuries.

Table 83-1

Principal Etiologies of Acquired Aortic Diseases

Manifestation	Causes
Aortic aneurysm	Infectious aortitis
	Inflammatory aortitis
	Takayasu syndrome (acute, chronic)
	Systemic lupus erythematosus
	Sarcoid
	Connective tissue disease
	Marfan syndrome
	Ehlers-Danlos syndrome (vascular type)
	Loeys-Dietz syndrome
	Arterial tortuosity syndrome
	Neurocutaneous disease
	Tuberous sclerosis
	Trauma or postsurgical (pseudoaneurysm)
Aortic dissection	Connective tissue disease
	Marfan syndrome
	Ehlers-Danlos syndrome (vascular type)
	Trauma
Aortic stenosis	Inflammatory aortitis
	Takayasu syndrome (chronic)
	Congenital rubella syndrome
	Radiation
	Neurocutaneous disease
	Neurofibromatosis (type I)
	PHACES syndrome
	Postsurgical
	Coarctation repair
	Aortopulmonary shunts

PHACES, Posterior fossa malformations, hemangiomas, arterial anomalies, cardiac defects, eye abnormalities, sternal cleft and supraumbilical raphe.

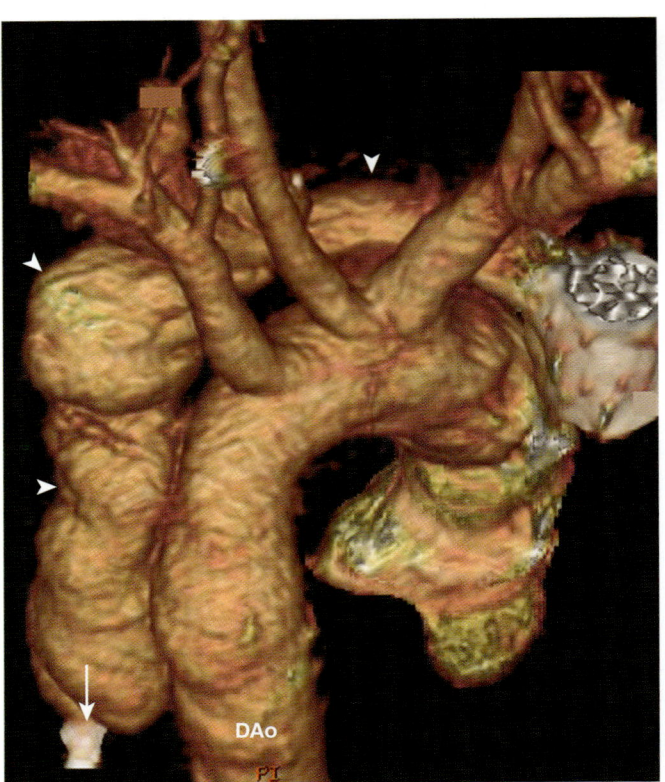

Figure 83-1   An aortic false aneurysm from a gunshot wound in an 18-year-old man. Volume rendering of a computed tomography angiogram shows a false aneurysm (*arrowheads*) that follows the track of a bullet. The bullet first entered the chest horizontally, parallel to the aortic arch, rupturing the aorta. Then it was deflected downward and came to rest (*arrow*) adjacent to the descending aorta (*DAo*).

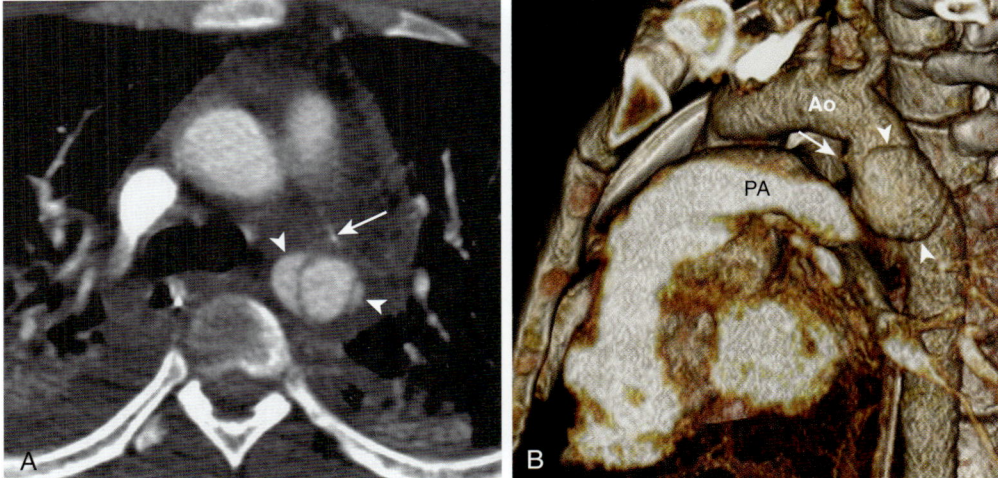

Figure 83-2   Aortic rupture in a 16-year-old boy as a result of a motor vehicle accident. **A**, An axial image from a computed tomography (CT) angiogram shows a ruptured descending aorta at the level of the ligamentum arteriosum (*arrow*) and two pseudoaneurysms (*arrowheads*) extending beyond the aortic wall. **B**, A volume-rendered image of the CT angiogram shows the relationship between one of the pseudoaneurysms (*arrowheads*) and the ligamentum arteriosum (*arrow*) between the aorta (*Ao*) and the pulmonary trunk (*PA*).

Treatment and Imaging Follow-up The goals of treatment of pediatric traumatic aortic rupture are identical to those in adults. The mainstay of treatment is operative repair of the aorta.[6] Patients for whom surgery poses a high risk have been treated successfully with endovascular stent grafts, with deployment during adenosine-induced cardiac arrest. CTA should be performed immediately after stent placement, with a follow-up study in 48 hours to document the stability of the repair. Rarely, observational management for an intimal tear has been utilized in patients with comorbidities too severe to allow intervention.

Acquired Diseases of the Pulmonary Artery

PULMONARY EMBOLISM

Overview Pulmonary embolism (PE) is an uncommon but potentially fatal disease in children.[7] In pediatric patients with deep venous thrombosis and PE, the mortality rate from all causes has been reported to be as high as 16%, whereas the mortality rate directly attributable to deep venous thrombosis or PE was 2.2%.[8] The most common risk factor for PE in children is catheter thrombosis, which develops in as many as 50% of patients with central venous catheters.[9] Other risk factors are peripartum asphyxia, dehydration, septicemia, trauma and burns, surgery, hemolysis, malignancy, and renal disease such as nephrotic syndrome. Rarely, PE can be seen in the setting of intracranial venous sinus thrombosis and Klippel–Trénaunay syndrome. Abnormal coagulation factors associated with adult PE that also have been reported in children are antiphospholipid antibodies, factor V Leiden mutation, and deficiencies in protein S, protein C, and antithrombin III.[10]

Clinical diagnosis of PE often is difficult because most cases of venous thrombosis in children are silent. Symptoms of PE may be masked by intrinsic lung disease or other underlying illness. In one series, 40% of proven cases of PE were negative in the D-dimer assay. Therefore a negative D-dimer assay in pediatric patients cannot exclude PE. A high level of clinical suspicion in the presence of risk factors is imperative.

Imaging Traditionally, catheter pulmonary angiography was considered the diagnostic gold standard.[11] In current clinical practice, catheter pulmonary angiography has been replaced by noninvasive CT pulmonary angiography (CTPA) performed with high-speed multidetector CT. The accuracy of the detection of PE by CTPA in an adult population has been studied in the Prospective Investigation of Pulmonary Embolism Diagnosis II trial.[12] With use of CT technology available before 2003, the sensitivity and specificity in this trial were reported as 83% and 96%, respectively. With advances in CT technology in the past decade that have improved spatial resolution, increased scan speed, and reduced contrast dose and radiation exposure, the diagnostic accuracy for PE likely is improved. Other imaging methods include nuclear ventilation-perfusion scanning and magnetic resonance pulmonary angiography.

As in adult patients, CTPA increasingly is being used to diagnose PE in children (Fig. 83-3), although its accuracy in

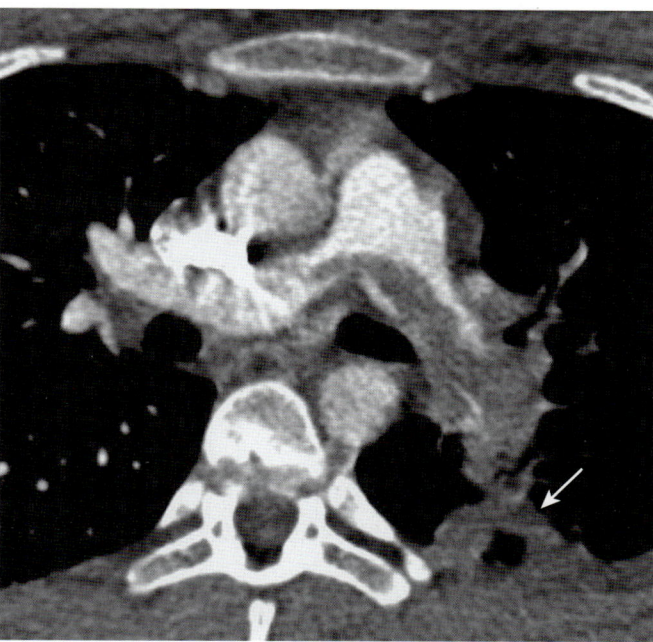

Figure 83-3 A saddle pulmonary embolus in a 15-year-old girl who recently started taking oral contraceptive pills. A filling defect spanning the left and right main pulmonary arteries is a large pulmonary embolism. A peripheral consolidation (*arrow*) that developed 2 days after her acute symptom is a pulmonary infarction.

children has not been studied by rigorous clinical trials. CTPA in children is technically challenging because of the small size of their pulmonary arteries, their inability to cooperate in holding their breath, and concerns about radiation exposure. The principal strategy for reducing radiation dose is to lower exposure factors such as x-ray tube voltage and tube current. Both maneuvers increase image noise and confound visual detection of PE. As a result, the CTPA protocol for children requires meticulous attention to optimize spatial resolution, scan speed, and exposure factors.

Treatment and Follow-up Anticoagulation is the mainstay of medical therapy for persons with a PE. Thrombolytic therapy is reserved for persons with hemodynamic instability. Surgical pulmonary thrombectomy has been successfully performed in persons with central or saddle emboli.

PE can be caused by materials other than bland thrombus. Septic emboli can be the result of endocarditis and of thrombophlebitis. Lemierre syndrome describes jugular vein thrombosis associated with anaerobic infection of the head and neck (classically by *Fusobacterium necrophorum*), and more than 50% of these cases are complicated by septic emboli to the lungs.[13] Tumor emboli may come from Wilms tumor, neuroblastoma, and hepatocellular carcinoma, because occasionally these tumors invade the inferior vena cava. Rarely, tumor emboli originate from primary cardiac tumors, such as atrial myxomas. Foreign bodies that embolize to the lungs include broken catheter tips and guide wires, misplaced embolization coils, and other endovascular devices. Finally, fat emboli may occur after major orthopedic trauma or surgery. In these situations, CT and magnetic resonance imaging (MRI) may help locate the source of emboli.

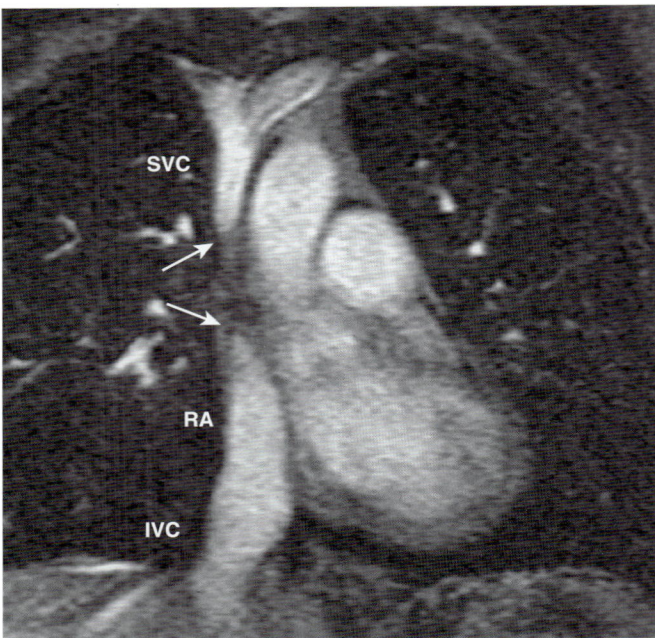

Figure 83-4 Superior vena cava (*SVC*) occlusion in a 14-year-old girl who had a long-term central venous catheter placed in the SVC. Coronal reconstruction of a magnetic resonance angiogram shows a complete obstruction (*arrows*) between the SVC and the right atrium (*RA*), whereas the inferior vena cava (*IVC*) drains freely into the RA.

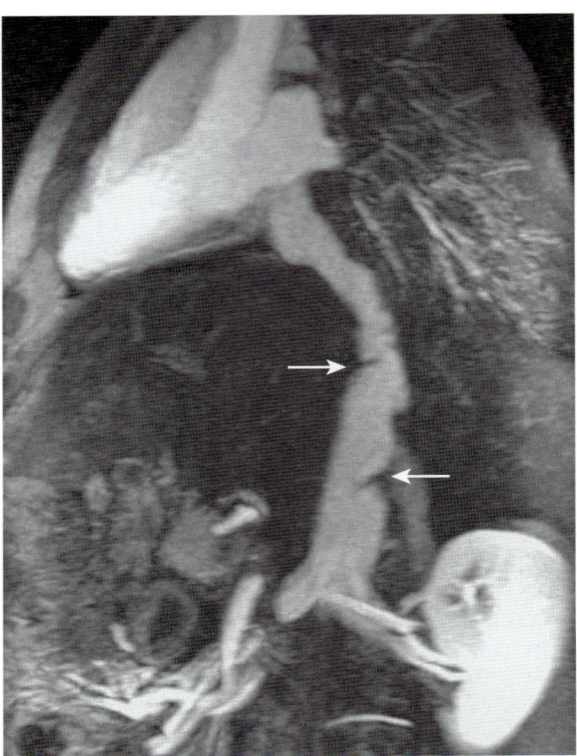

Figure 83-5 Inferior vena cava (IVC) stenosis in a 13-year-old boy who developed Budd-Chiari syndrome after trauma. Sagittal reconstruction of a magnetic resonance angiogram shows a narrowed IVC with multiple webs (*arrows*) protruding into the caval lumen.

Acquired Diseases of the Venae Cavae

SUPERIOR VENA CAVA SYNDROME

Overview SVC syndrome (SVCS) is a clinical manifestation of gradual obstruction of SVC flow, leading to elevated central venous pressure of the upper extremities and the head, interstitial edema and swelling of the upper body, and development of venous collaterals to the inferior vena cava (IVC). In children, SVCS is a medical emergency because swelling of the neck can compress and obstruct their small airway more easily than in adults. The most common pediatric cause of SVCS is extrinsic compression of the SVC by non-Hodgkin lymphoma.[14] The SVC can be compressed by other mediastinal masses, including germ cell tumor, infectious lymphadenopathy, aortic aneurysm, and mediastinal fibrosis.[15] Luminal occlusion (Fig. 83-4) can be the result of a thrombus forming around a central venous catheter or pacemaker wires, or of venous thrombosis secondary to Behçet syndrome (see Chapter 82). Intrinsic stenosis of the SVC can be caused by scarring from a chronic indwelling catheter and by infusion of caustic agents. Finally, SVC flow may be obstructed within the atrial baffle after the atrial switch procedure or the Mustard-Senning procedure[16] (see Chapter 76). Obstruction of the SVC above the azygos return precludes decompression by retrograde flow into the azygos vein and leads to more severe symptoms.

Imaging and Treatment The gold standard for the diagnosis of SVCS is catheter venography, with which the level of SVC obstruction, the presence of venous collaterals, and the central venous pressure can be assessed. Noninvasive tomographic techniques such as CT and MR venography can define the SVC stenosis and are helpful in evaluating any extrinsic mass.[17] An advantage of MRI is that venography can be done without use of a contrast agent through use of phase-contrast or time-of-flight inflow enhancement techniques. Treatment of SVCS depends on the underlying cause. Radiation or chemotherapy that reduces the tumor size may relieve the SVC obstruction. Thrombosed central venous catheters should be removed. Residual thrombosis may be treated with selective thrombolysis, and residual stenosis may be stented.

INFERIOR VENA CAVA OBSTRUCTION

Overview Reasons for acquired obstruction of the IVC are similar to those of the SVC. Thrombosis of the IVC can be the result of catheter access, placement of a caval filter, severe illness including sepsis and dehydration, and other hypercoagulopathy. The IVC can be obstructed at its entrance to the right atrium by abdominal tumors, such as Wilms tumor, neuroblastoma, hepatoblastoma, and hepatocellular carcinoma. The Budd-Chiari syndrome classically is attributed to hepatic venous obstruction, but the intrahepatic portion of the IVC can be involved, resulting in symptoms of hepatomegaly, ascites, and abdominal pain (Fig. 83-5).[18] Obstruction is caused by thrombus or an IVC web.

Imaging and Treatment Imaging evaluation can be performed with abdominal ultrasound, CT, and MRI, with the investigation focused on the location and severity of the obstruction and on the presence of a thrombus or extrinsic mass. Treatment is directed to correcting the underlying conditions. In the short term, patency of the IVC can be maintained with an endovascular stent.

SUPERIOR VENA CAVA ANEURYSM

Overview   Although a true SVC aneurysm is very rare, dilation of the SVC is more commonly seen in persons with elevated central venous pressure as a result of right heart failure or severe tricuspid valve regurgitation.[19] Dilation of the SVC also is associated with mediastinal lymphatic malformation, although the pathophysiology is not known.[20] Patients with saccular SVC aneurysms may be at risk for SVC thrombosis and PE.

Imaging and Treatment   Surgical resection of an SVC aneurysm has been performed successfully. CT and MRI can help aid surgical planning by defining the extent of the aneurysm and detecting involvement of other draining veins.

Acquired Disease of the Pulmonary Veins

PULMONARY VEIN STENOSIS

Overview   Acquired pulmonary vein stenosis in children is uncommon but can be seen in children with complications of surgical repair of congenital pulmonary vein anomalies. Children who undergo repairs for total anomalous pulmonary venous connection (Fig. 83-6) and scimitar syndrome are at

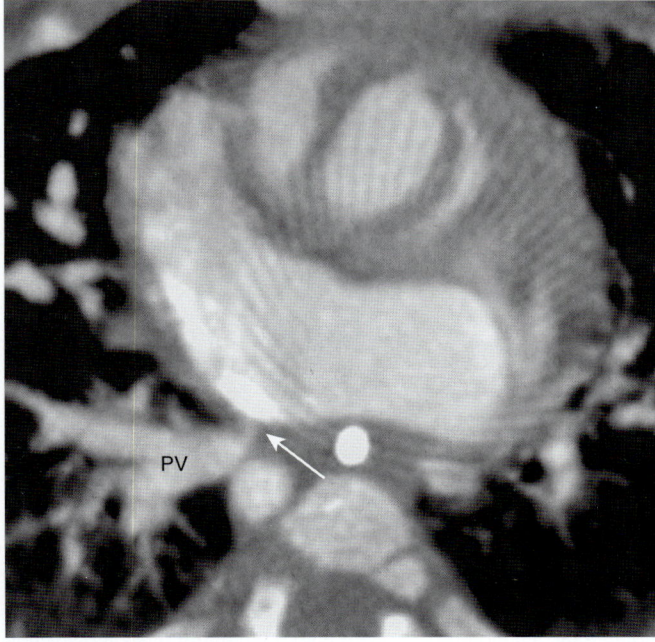

Figure 83-6   Pulmonary venous stenosis after surgical repair for total anomalous pulmonary venous connection in a 6-month-old girl. An axial computed tomographic angiography image shows a tight stenosis (*arrow*) at the origin of a right pulmonary vein (*PV*).

increased risk for acquired pulmonary vein stenosis. Pulmonary vein stenosis develops in up to 10% of infants who undergo repair of total anomalous pulmonary venous connection[21]; these patients often are very ill from pulmonary edema and poor oxygen saturation, with a mortality rate as high as 50%. The prognosis is worse for patients who have coexisting complex cardiac anomalies, often as part of the heterotaxy syndrome. Other acquired causes of pulmonary vein stenosis include mediastinal fibrosis and extrinsic compression by mediastinal tumors.

Imaging and Treatment   Catheter angiography is used to define the location of the pulmonary venous obstruction, and the severity of the stenosis can be evaluated by measuring the pressure gradient across the stenosis. With three-dimensional imaging capability, CTA and magnetic resonance angiography (MRA) often can identify the obstruction better than catheter angiography. CTA has the added advantage of evaluating the pulmonary parenchyma and airways for additional complications.

Pulmonary vein stenosis has been treated with angioplasty, endovascular stent placement, and surgical repair.[21,22] Despite immediate postoperative success, restenosis often occurs, and mortality is not substantially improved. The pathophysiology of pulmonary vein restenosis is not well understood. Medial fibrosis of the injured pulmonary veins, endothelial ingrowth into the stent, and abnormal reactivity of the pulmonary vascular bed have been proposed as possible mechanisms of restenosis.

PULMONARY VEIN VARIX

Overview   Pulmonary varices are rare aneurysmal dilations of the pulmonary veins[23] and may be congenital or acquired. Acquired pulmonary varices usually are the result of pulmonary venous hypertension, caused by central pulmonary vein stenosis, mitral regurgitation, mitral stenosis, and coarctation. Pulmonary varices generally are benign and require no specific treatment. They usually regress with correction of the underlying abnormality. However, it is important to distinguish pulmonary varices from pulmonary arteriovenous malformations, which can have a similar appearance. Pulmonary arteriovenous malformations carry the risk of stroke and other embolic events and require surgical removal or catheter embolization.

Imaging   Both CTA and MRA can detect pulmonary varices. In difficult cases, catheter angiography may be needed to differentiate varices from arteriovenous malformations.

NEOPLASMS OF THE GREAT VESSELS

Overview   Primary neoplasms of the great vessels are very rare; fewer than 400 cases have been reported in adults. Most of these malignant tumors are sarcomas. Of primary neoplasms that involve the aorta, fewer than 140 cases have been reported; most are undifferentiated sarcomas, with angiosarcoma being the next most common type of neoplasm.[24] These primary tumors have not been described in children. Secondary involvement of the great vessels by invasion or compression from a nearby, nonvascular tumor or by radiation vasculitis from radiation treatment can occur. Examples

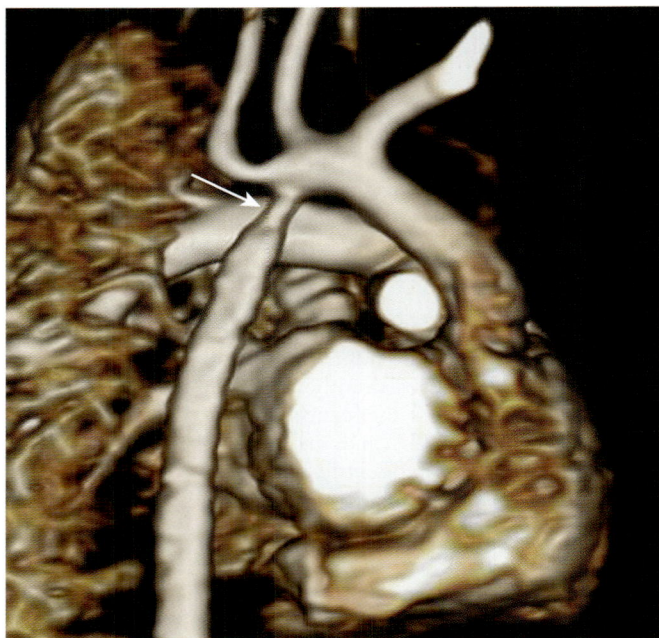

Figure 83-7 Restenosis 5 months after a surgical repair for coarctation in a 6-month-old boy. Volume rendering shows a segmental, circumferential narrowing (*arrow*) at the surgical site.

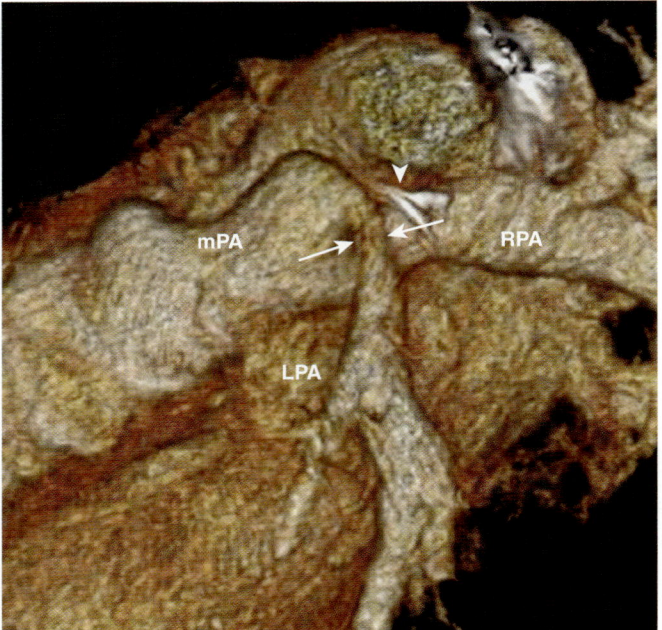

Figure 83-8 Postsurgical pulmonary artery stenosis in a 10-year-old boy. Volume rendering of a computed tomographic angiogram shows evidence of an arteriopulmonary shunt, now closed, identified by a surgical clip (*arrowhead*). Adjacent to this clip is a kink and a focal narrowing (*arrows*) of the left pulmonary artery (*LPA*). *mPA*, Main pulmonary artery; *RPA*, right pulmonary artery.

of secondary tumors include mediastinal lymphoma, germ cell tumor, teratoma, rare types of sarcomas, and mediastinal metastasis.[25,26]

Imaging and Treatment Because most great vessel tumors occur as a result of other disease processes, the tumor cell types and origins usually are known (see Chapter 81). The primary roles of imaging are to determine favorable sites for biopsy, evaluate the extent and the degree of vascular obstruction in preparation for vascular intervention, and monitor changes in vascular involvement after treatment. In most cases, CT or MRI is used for these purposes.[27] Treatment and imaging follow-up depend on the cell type and tumor staging.

POSTOPERATIVE COMPLICATIONS

Overview Pseudoaneurysm and stenosis can develop as complications of surgical repair or interventional treatment of pediatric thoracic great vessels, of which coarctation is the best studied. The average restenosis rates are 15% and 2% for balloon angioplasty and surgical repair of coarctation, respectively (Fig. 83-7).[28] Other surgical procedures that can be complicated by aneurysm or stenosis are surgical aortopulmonary and central shunts.[29] The Blalock-Taussig shunt, which classically connects the right subclavian artery to the right pulmonary artery, can lead to stenosis or obstruction of the right pulmonary artery (Fig. 83-8). The Potts shunt, which connects the descending aorta to the left pulmonary artery, often results in left pulmonary artery stenosis. The Waterston shunt connects the ascending aorta to the pulmonary trunk. Control of shunt flow is difficult, and excessive flow can create a massive aneurysm of the pulmonary artery (Fig. 83-9).

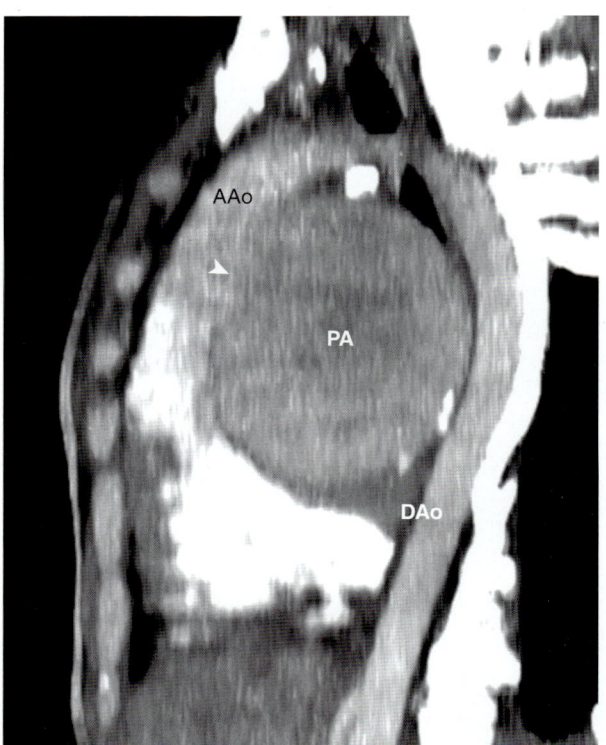

Figure 83-9 Pulmonary aneurysm from a Waterston shunt in a 20-year-old man. Sagittal reconstruction of a routine contrast-enhanced computed tomography scan shows the anastomosis (*arrowhead*) between the ascending aorta (*AAo*) and the massively dilated main pulmonary artery (*PA*). *DAo*, Descending aorta.

For these reasons, both Potts and Waterston shunts are rarely used today.

Imaging and Treatment Noninvasive imaging by CTA or MRA has largely supplanted catheter angiography for the purpose of detecting and characterizing these thoracic vascular lesions before surgical or interventional treatment. Catheterization is reserved for angioplasty and stenting of stenotic lesions and for stent graft deployment to exclude an aneurysm.

Key Points

Aortic pathology can be categorized as aortic aneurysm, aortic dissection, or aortic stenosis, and the clinical consequences of these three diagnostic entities directly determine mortality and morbidity.

The most common risk factor for pulmonary embolism in children is catheter thrombosis, which develops in as many as half of patients with central venous catheters.

A negative D-dimer assay in pediatric patients does not exclude PE.

SVCS is a medical emergency in children because swelling of the neck can cause compression and obstruction of the airway.

Restenosis of the pulmonary vein in children is common after surgical or interventional treatment and can be diagnosed with CTA or MRA.

Suggested Readings

Babyn PS, Gahunia HK, Massicotte P. Pulmonary thromboembolism in children. *Pediatr Radiol.* 2005;35:258-274.

Bendel EC, Maleszewski JJ, Araoz PA. Imaging sarcomas of the great vessels and heart. *Semin Ultrasound CT MR.* 2011;32:377-404.

Lowe LH, Bulas DI, Eichelberger MD, et al. Traumatic aortic injuries in children: radiologic evaluation. *AJR Am J Roentgenol.* 1998;170:39-42.

Stein PD, Fowler SE, Goodman LR, et al. Multidetector computed tomography for acute pulmonary embolism. *N Engl J Med.* 2006;354: 2317-2327.

Williams BJ, Mulvihill DM, Pettus BJ, et al. Pediatric superior vena cava syndrome: assessment at low radiation dose 64-slice CT angiography. *J Thorac Imaging.* 2006;21:71-72.

References

Full references for this chapter can be found on www.expertconsult.com.

Index

Page numbers followed by "f" indicate figures, "t" indicate tables, "b" indicate boxes, and "e" indicate online-only content.